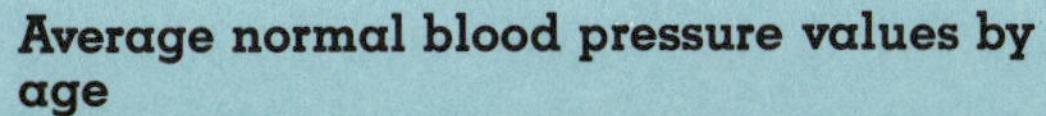

Average normal blood pressure values by age

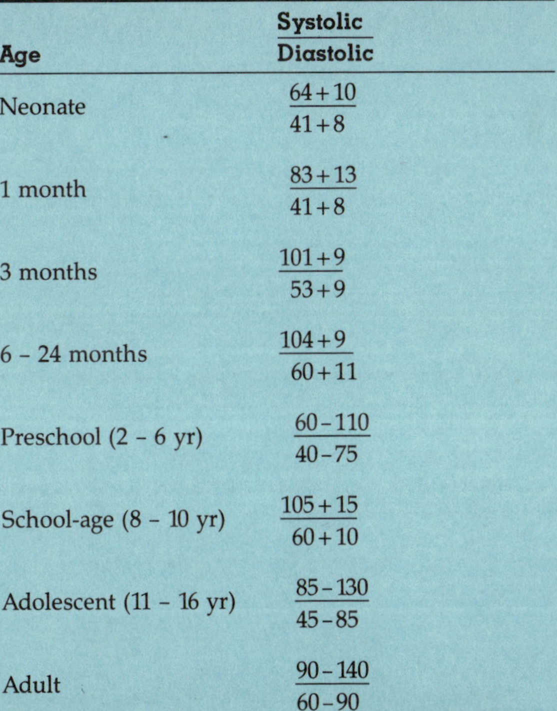

Age	Systolic / Diastolic
Neonate	64+10 / 41+8
1 month	83+13 / 41+8
3 months	101+9 / 53+9
6 - 24 months	104+9 / 60+11
Preschool (2 - 6 yr)	60-110 / 40-75
School-age (8 - 10 yr)	105+15 / 60+10
Adolescent (11 - 16 yr)	85-130 / 45-85
Adult	90-140 / 60-90

Average normal temperatures for children

	Celsius	Fahrenheit
Rectal	37.6°C (37.2–37.8)	99.6°F (99–100)
Oral	37°C (36.7–37.2)	98.6°F (98–99)
Axillary	36.3°C (36.1–36.7)	97.4°F (97–98)

Normal pulse and respiratory rates for specific ages

Age	Pulse	Respirations
Newborn	110-160	30-60
2 years	100-140	28-32
4 years	90-96	24-28
6 years	80-90	24-26
8 years	80-84	22-24
10 years	80-84	22-24
12 years	78-80	18-20

Caloric expenditures of children

Body weight in kilograms*	Caloric expenditure per day
3–10 kg	100 kcal/kg
11–20 kg	1000 kcal plus 50 kcal/kg for each kg over 10
Above 20 kg	1500 kcal plus 20 kcal/kg for each kg over 20

* 1 kg=2.2 lb.

Child and Family: Concepts of Nursing Practice

Second Edition

Child and Family: Concepts of Nursing Practice

Marjorie J. Smith

Associate Professor, College of Nursing and Health Sciences
Director, Masters Program in Nursing
Winona State University

Julie A. Goodman

Director of Continuing Education, School of Nursing
Rochester Community College

Nancy Lockwood Ramsey

Professor, Department of Nursing
Los Angeles City College

McGRAW-HILL BOOK COMPANY
New York St. Louis San Francisco Auckland Bogotá Hamburg Johannesburg London Madrid Mexico Milan Montreal New Delhi Panama Paris São Paulo Singapore Sydney Tokyo Toronto

NOTICE

As new medical and nursing research and clinical experience broaden our knowledge, changes in treatment and drug therapy are required. The editors and publisher of this work have made every effort to ensure that the drug dosage schedules herein are accurate and in accord with the standards accepted at the time of publication. Readers are advised, however, to check the product information sheet included in the package of each drug they plan to administer to be certain that changes have not been made in the recommended dose or in the contraindications for administration. This recommendation is of particular importance in regard to new or infrequently used drugs.

CHILD AND FAMILY: CONCEPTS OF NURSING PRACTICE

1 2 3 4 5 6 7 8 9 0 RMTRMT 8 9 2 1 0 9 8 7

ISBN 0-07-048726-X

This book was set in Primer by Waldman Graphics, Inc. (ECU). The editors were Sally J. Barhydt and Steven Tenney; the design was done by Caliber Design Planning; the production supervisor was Phil Galea. The drawings were done by J&R Services, Inc. Rand McNally & Company was printer and binder.

Library of Congress Cataloging-in-Publication Data

Child and family.

Includes bibliographies and index.
1. Pediatric nursing. 2. Family—Health and hygiene.
I. Smith, Marjorie J., R.N. II. Goodman, Julie A.
III. Ramsey, Nancy Lockwood. [DNLM: 1. Family—nurses' instruction. 2. Pediatric Nursing. WY 159 C533]
RJ245.C465 1987 610.73'62 86-20059
ISBN 0-07-048726-X

About the Authors

Marjorie J. Smith is an associate professor at Winona State University, Rochester Campus, Rochester, Minnesota. She is Director of the Master's Program. Her major teaching responsibilities include maternal-child nursing and nursing research. She received her Bachelor's degree in nursing with a major in management and teaching from the University of Wisconsin, and her Master's degree in childbearing-childrearing nursing and Ph.D. in adult education from the University of Minnesota. She has taught medical-surgical nursing, pediatric nursing, and maternity nursing at diploma, associate degree, and baccalaureate schools of nursing since 1963. A member of Sigma Theta Tau, she also served as Director of Continuing Education at Rochester Community College for six years. She has authored a computer simulation on oral contraceptives. She is a Certified Nurse Midwife, practices in a family planning clinic, and has served on the Family Planning Advisory Board for the Olmsted County Health Department. For the past several years she has also served as a site visit team member for the Central Regional Accrediting Committee of the American Nurses Association.

Julie A. Goodman is a member of the faculty of Rochester Community College, Rochester, Minnesota. Her Bachelor of Science degree with a major in nursing was earned at the College of Saint Catherine, St. Paul, Minnesota. After an interruption in her education of 13 years, she received a Master's in Science degree with a childbearing-childrearing focus and a clinical specialty of nurse midwifery from the University of Minnesota. She is licensed as a Certified Nurse Midwife. Currently she is a doctoral candidate in adult education at the University of Minnesota. Her job responsibilities at the University of South Dakota, St. Mary's School of Nursing, and Rochester Community College, over a 22-year period, have included many areas of nursing, but for the past 15 years maternal-child nursing has been her specialty. She has functioned as interim director of the Rochester Community College ADN Program and presently is the Director of Continuing Education in Nursing. As chairperson of the Minnesota League for Nursing Educator's Council, member of the Minnesota Nurses' Association Education Commission, chairperson of the continuing education approval committee, and member of Sigma Theta Tau, she participates fully in professional nursing activities. She is also proud to be a wife of 25 years and the mother of three nearly adult children. Her oldest daughter, Julia, has graduated from Julie's alma mater and is employed as a staff nurse and continues to provide feedback regarding "current nursing practice."

Nancy Lockwood Ramsey is a professor and the assistant chairperson at Los Angeles City College, Los Angeles, California. She received a Bachelor of Science degree in Nursing from Loma Linda University in Redlands, California. She then earned a Master of Science degree in nursing from Duke University in Durham, North Carolina. She has worked as a staff nurse primarily with pediatric and postsurgical patients. She has been Director of Nursing Education at Children's Hospital of Los Angeles and was also a nurse educator on the infant unit of that hospital. She has taught pediatric nursing at the University of North Carolina at Chapel Hill, North Carolina; California State University at Los Angeles; Azusa-Pacific University; and Los Angeles City College. She has also taught medical-surgical nursing at Los Angeles City College. At Loma Linda University she received several scholarships and is a member of the Honor Society at Azusa-Pacific University and is in *Who's Who in Professional Nursing*. She is a member of the Association for Children's Health and the Southern California Nursing Diagnosis Association. She is deeply committed to her husband of 13 years and to her children aged 3 and 12 and stepchildren of 19 and 21 years. They keep her constantly refining and learning new parenting methods and applying the theoretical principles of growth and development!

To those who said it was possible,
and to all those who made it possible.

Contents

List of Contributors

Pauline C. Beecroft, R.N., M.S.N.
Doctoral Student, University of Texas, Austin
Associate Professor and Pediatric Clinical Specialist
California State University Los Angeles and Children's Hospital of Los Angeles
Los Angeles, CA

Cindy S. Boehr, R.N., B.S.N., CCRN
Children's Hospital of Los Angeles
Los Angeles, CA

Margaret A. Brady, R.N., M.S.
Assistant Professor
California State University, Long Beach
Long Beach, CA

Shari Brumm, R.N., B.S.W.
Clinical Educator
Rochester Methodist Hospital
Rochester, MN

Marsha H. Cohen, R.N., M.S.
Doctoral Candidate, Department of Family Health Care Nursing
University of California
San Francisco, CA

Nancy A. Coulter, R.N., M.S.N.
Assistant Professor, Clinical Nursing
University of Southern California
Los Angeles, CA

Patricia Crisham, R.N., Ph.D.
Associate Professor
School of Nursing
University of Minnesota
Minneapolis, MN

Phyllis J. D'Ambra, R.N., B.S.N.
Nurse Coordinator
Orthopedics
Children's Hospital of Los Angeles
Los Angeles, CA

Maureen DeMaio-Esteves, R.N., M.A.
Ph.D. Candidate, New York University and Assistant Professor
College of Nursing, Rutgers, The State University of New Jersey
Newark, NJ

Dorothy J. DeMaio, Ed.D., R.N., F.A.A.N.
Dean and Professor
College of Nursing, Rutgers, The State University of New Jersey
Newark, NJ

Nancy Anne Eppich
Associate Director, Nursing Care of Children
Rainbow Babies and Children's Hospital
University Hospitals
Cleveland, OH

Phyllis Nie Esslinger, R.N., M.S.
Associate Professor
Azusa Pacific University
Azusa, CA

Mona Clare Lotz Finnila, R.N., P.H.N., P.N.P., M.S.
Formerly Family Health Coordinator
Family Development Project
Children's Hospital of Los Angeles
Los Angeles, CA

Marlene Singer Garvis, R.N., M.S.N., J.D.
Associate (Attorney)
Jardine, Logan, and O'Brien Law Firm
St. Paul, MN

Barbara Goergen, R.N., M.S., F.N.P., C.P.N.P.
Pediatric Nurse Practitioner
Community Pediatrics
Mayo Clinic
Rochester, MN

Julie A. Goodman, R.N., M.S.N., C.N.M.
Doctoral Candidate, University of Minnesota
Director, Continuing Education in Nursing
Rochester Community College
Rochester, MN

Cynthia Smith Greenberg, R.N., M.S., C.P.N.P.
Assistant Professor
Maternal-Child Nursing
California State University Long Beach
Long Beach, CA

Sandra Sonnessa Griffiths, R.N., M.N., M.B.A.
Formerly Instructor in Pediatric Nursing
Case Western Reserve University
Cleveland, OH

Marcia K. Henry, M.A.
Teaching Fellow and Doctoral Candidate
Stanford University
Stanford, CA

Carol J. Hill, R.N., M.S.N.
Associate Professor
College of Nursing
University of North Dakota
Grand Forks, ND

Kathleen W. Hinoki, R.N., M.S.
Nursing Unit Coordinator, NICU/Pediatrics
Glendale Adventist Medical Center
Glendale, CA

Diane M. Huse, R.D., M.S.
Pediatric Dietitian and Assistant Professor in Nutrition
Mayo Medical School
Mayo Clinic
Rochester, MN

Joanette Pete James, R.N., M.N., N.S.N., M.Ed.
Chairperson
Department of Nursing
University of West Florida
Pensacola, FL

Linda L. Jarvis, R.N., M.S.N., Ed.D.
Assistant Professor
School of Nursing
Curry College
Milton, MA

LiAnne M. Kitchen, R.N., M.S.
Director of Nursing
Lourdes Hospital
Paducah, KY
Formerly Clinical Educator
NICU, Saint Mary's Hospital, Rochester, MN

Nancy Kosiba Koster, R.N., M.S
Clinical Specialist
Pediatric Cardiovascular Surgery
Children's Memorial Hospital
Chicago, IL

Sheila Kramer, R.N., B.S.N.
Formerly Critical Care Coordinator
Saint Marys Hospital
Rochester, MN

Gay J. Lindquist, R.N., M.S.
Assistant Professor
University of Wisconsin-Eau Claire
Eau Claire, WI

Lois L. Lux, R.N., B.S.N.
Formerly Urology Nurse Clinician
Children's Hospital of Philadelphia
Philadelphia, PA

Madeleine Lynch Martin, R.N., M.S.N., Ed.D.
Professor and Department Chair
Medical-Surgical Nursing
University of Cincinnati
Cincinnati, OH

Ida M. Martinson, R.N., Ph.D., F.A.A.N.
Professor and Department Chair
Department of Family Health Nursing
University of California, San Francisco
San Francisco, CA

Mary Jo McCracken, R.N., B.S.N., P.N.P.
Pediatric Pulmonary Nurse Specialist
University of Minnesota Hospital and Clinics
Minneapolis, MN

Jean R. Miller, R.N., Ph.D.
Professor and Associate Dean of Research
College of Nursing
University of Utah
Salt Lake City, UT

Katherine Miller, R.N., M.S.N.
Nurse Educator
Children's Hospital of Los Angeles
Los Angeles, CA

Susan Steiner Nash, R.N., M.S.
Formerly Education Coordinator
Saint Marys Hospital
Rochester, MN

Sally Winn Nicholson, R.N., Ph.D.
Professor of Nursing
University of North Carolina at Charlotte
Charlotte, NC

Linda Waldrop Olivet, R.N., M.S.N., D.N.S.
Assistant Professor of Nursing
Capstone College of Nursing
University of Alabama
Tuscaloosa, AL

Kathy Orth, R.N., M.S.
Assistant Professor
Winona State University, Rochester Center
Rochester, MN

Roslyn Podratz, R.N., M.A.
Coordinator
Nursing Research Project
Rochester Methodist Hospital
Rochester, MN

Elizabeth C. Poster, R.N., Ph.D.
Assistant Director, Nursing Services
Neuropsychiatric Institute, UCLA
Los Angeles, CA

Susan J. Rabinovitz, R.N., B.A.
Nurse Coordinator, Teenage Health Center
Children's Hospital of Los Angeles
Los Angeles, CA

Nancy Lockwood Ramsey, R.N., M.S.N.
Professor
Los Angeles City College
Los Angeles, CA

Karen E. Roper, R.N., M.S.N.
Assistant Director of Nursing Education
Childrens Hospital of Philadelphia
Philadelphia, PA

Patricia J. Salisbury, R.N., M.S.N., P.N.P.
Assistant Professor
Department of Pediatrics and Human Development, College of Human Medicine
Michigan State University
East Lansing, MI

Gladys M. Scipien, R.N., M.S., F.A.A.N.
Associate Professor
School of Nursing
Boston University
Boston, MA

Elizabeth L'Estrange Simone
Formerly Clinical Nurse Specialist, Infants
Rainbow Babies and Children's Hospital
University Hospitals
Cleveland, OH

Ann R. Sloat, R.N., M.S.
Doctoral Candidate, University of Hawaii Associate Professor
School of Nursing
University of Hawaii
Honolulu, HI

Marjorie J. Smith, R.N., Ph.D., C.N.M.
Associate Professor
Director, Master's Program in Nursing
Winona State University
Rochester, MN

Susan M. Smith, R.N., M.S.
Associate Professor
School of Nursing
Azusa Pacific University
Azusa, CA

Connie L. Tooley, R.N., M.S.
Employee Assistance Counselor
Rochester Methodist Hospital
Rochester, MN

Sally Valentine, R.N., M.S.
Clinical Specialist, Infectious Disease
Children's Hospital of Los Angeles
Los Angeles, CA

Bonnie L. Westra, R.N., M.S.
Assistant Professor
Luther College
Decorah, IA
Former Head Nurse
Emergency Department
Rochester Methodist Hospital
Rochester, MN

Janet Louise Wilde, R.N., M.S.N.
School Nurse, Consultant
Sulphur Springs Union School District
Canyon Country, CA

Stephanie Wright, R.N., M.S.N.
Instructor
Nursing Program
Montgomery College
Takoma Park, MD

Preface

The second edition of *Child and Family* has been extensively revised to incorporate current research and pediatric nursing practice. We, the editors, have based the revision on feedback from students, educators, practitioners, and reviewers. Our goal was to keep all that was valuable from the first edition and incorporate the changing parameters of nursing of children and their families. The major organization is essentially the same. The writing style, tables, charts, and visual aids that students found so helpful in the first edition were retained and enhanced in the second. Most organizational changes were made to increase the internal consistency of the chapters and reduce repetition without sacrificing the book's manageable size.

Updated nursing care plans, using the nursing process framework, are included with most chapters on alterations in health. They are designed to illustrate the use of the nursing process in the actual care of children of different ages with illnesses characteristic of the various body systems.

In Part I the conceptual basis of the book is explained. The content on family has been integrated into one chapter and completely revised. New information has been included on the impact of culture on health care. The final chapter of Part I, which is entirely new, provides a method for use in examining moral dilemmas that occur in child health nursing.

Part II contains the basic growth and development content that helped make the first edition so valuable. Divided by age group, the chapter includes a description of physical and psychosocial maturation, developmental tasks, cognitive and moral development, nutritional assessment and needs, and common problems. The chapters on genetics and prenatal development remain essentially the same with new sections added on genetic engineering and prenatal therapy. Chapter 14, written by a pediatric nurse practitioner, provides the basic guide for the nurse's role in health assessment and maintenance and promotion of health. Developmental screening tests are reviewed and the components of routine health maintenance care described. The detailed sequence of the physical exam of each body system is described in the appropriate health alteration chapter in Part III.

Part III emphasizes the biophysical alterations in children and begins with the chapters that describe the basic nursing care of the hospitalized child. It is our intention to blend up-to-date theoretical content with practical applications to pediatric nursing practice to help overcome the student's inexperience when the nursing of children becomes a reality.

Chapters begin, where appropriate, with a brief review of embryology, anatomy, and physiology. Discussions of overall nursing assessment, diagnostic tests, etiology, manifestations, treatment, nursing management and prevention follow. All chapters in this section have been updated and revised and emphasize changes specific to children and those spanning all age groups. The chapters are sequenced to enhance continuity of learning concepts between chapters. Nursing care and treatment measures are included that represent a variety of geographic areas of the U.S.

Part IV emphasizes the psychosocial aspects of health alterations in children. While acute illness is the primary focus of Part III, chronic illness with care in the community and home or long-term care facility is stressed in Part IV. The chapters on chronic illness, behavioral problems, and substance abuse have been completely revised.

We again urge readers to regard this book as a companion through their nursing career. The book is generously furnished with information of reference value. In addition to the nursing procedures and guidelines summarized in tables, there are appendix sections devoted to metric conversion, growth charts, nutritional guidelines, poison treatment, and samples of personal information forms.

The editors and contributors appreciate the encouragement and positive feedback received from the many instructors and students using the first edition. We have endeavored to maintain the format that they all found so helpful while making the improvements that advances in knowledge and research demanded.

LEARNING AIDS

A totally new *instructor's manual* has been prepared by Sue Nash with the assistance of the editors and contributors. Its chapter-by-chapter format is keyed to each of the book's 39 chapters. It provides brief descriptions of how to use the text depending on curriculum plan, time allotment, and clinical or classroom grouping. For each chapter the instructor is given an overview, a brief outline, key concepts, classroom and clinical teaching strategies, a bibliography, and resources. The appendices include a growth and development assessment guide, a clinical experience checklist, options for organizing a pediatric nursing course using selected chapters from this book, suggestions for coordinating clinical assignments, and transparency masters.

Also available to the instructors who use this text is a *computerized test bank* and hard copy of over 800 multiple-choice questions keyed to each chapter and described according to difficulty level (easy, medium, difficult), cognitive type (knowledge, comprehension, application, analysis, decision making), and steps in the nursing process (assessment, nursing diagnosis, goals, interventions, evaluation, theory).

ACKNOWLEDGMENTS

We gratefully thank our contributors who have done an excellent job reviewing and writing chapters. They are the important nurses who have made this book what it is.

It would be impossible to acknowledge all the people—colleagues, students, and friends—who have contributed to this book, both its first and second editions. Nevertheless we do want to recognize some of those who have made a special contribution. The following have helped us with manuscript assistance and review: Marcia Anderson, R.N. and Mary Lou Stewart, R.N., Los Angeles City College Department of Nursing; Randy Adams and the staff at Los Angeles Children's Hospital Medical Library; Norma Blankenfeld, R.N., Winona State University, College of Nursing and Health Sciences; Allison Smith Cabalka, M.D., University of Wisconsin; Janet Cardle, photographer; Bradford Currier, M.D., Mayo Clinic; Phyllis D'Ambra, R.N., Los Angeles Children's Hospital; Phyllis Esslinger, R.N., Azusa-Pacific University School of Nursing; Robert W. Feldt, M.D., Mayo Clinic; Burton W. Fine, M.D., University of Southern California School of Medicine; Gail Jimenez, Rochester Community College; LiAnne Kitchen, R.N., Lourdes Hospital, Paducah, Ky; Andrea Piens Kuich, R.N., for the cover design; Susan Steiner Nash, R.N., and Evelyn Schmit, R.N., Rochester Community College.

We also want to thank Sally Barhydt, McGraw-Hill Nursing Editor, for her dedicated support and Steven Tenney for his careful attention to the quality of the manuscript.

A special thank you is also due our husbands, Myron Smith, Michael Goodman, and Gordon Ramsey, and to our eight children; they all endured the hardship of having the "book" take priority over nearly every other life event. This book could not have been completed without their love and support.

The dedication of this text, "To those who said it was possible, and to all those who made it possible," aptly expresses our appreciation to *everyone* who helped us.

Marjorie J. Smith

Julie A. Goodman

Nancy Lockwood Ramsey

PART I

The Child, Family, Nurse, and Society

1

Child health nursing: a framework for practice*

Upon completion of this chapter, the student will be able to:

1 Identify *child, family,* and *health* as key concepts in pediatric nursing practice.
2 Discuss the central role of the family in the child's growth and development.
3 Explain the importance of health in the child's growth and development.
4 Analyze the role of the nurse as a health care provider for children and their families.
5 Discuss the use of the nursing process as a clinical practice tool for the care of children and their families.
6 Discuss the purpose of quality assurance in pediatric nursing practice.

Within the scope of daily practice, the nurse performs many activities which are designed to promote the health and well-being of the child and the child's family. This role affords nurses the opportunity to establish and maintain therapeutic relationships with children and their families.

THE CHILD AND THE FAMILY

Early life experiences are critical in preparing a child for a self-sufficient role in society. A child is highly dependent on his or her family for many years. Thus the family, or child-rearing unit,† assumes an important role in protecting and promoting the child's growth, development, health, and well-being. The family bears the primary re-

*The editors acknowledge the contribution of Sarah B. Pasternack for material used in this chapter.
†Since there are various forms of "family" in today's society, the terms *family* and *child-rearing unit* are used interchangeably in order to denote a broad meaning of the term *family*.

sponsibility for meeting the child's basic physiological needs, such as for food, shelter, and protection. Love and affection are as essential to the child's growth and development as food, water, and play. Emotional and psychological well-being are influenced by the quality of the child's relationships within the family. The love given a child by parents and other family members assures the child of "belonging" and nurtures feelings of self-worth and self-esteem.

The family serves as a unit of socialization for the child, providing the means through which the child gains self-knowledge, learns about other people, and becomes aware of the world in general. Ideally, experiences within the child-rearing unit afford the child opportunities to cultivate interpersonal relationships, to experience pleasure, and to give and receive affection. The family teaches the growing child how to assume responsibility and provides motivation for achieving personal goals.

HEALTH

Health is a desirable quality of life that enables an individual to experience physical, emotional, and psychological well-being. A dynamic quality, which is difficult to define and impossible to measure, health is different for every individual. A person's health is not static; it changes from moment to moment. A multitude of both internal and external factors influence the individual's health at any given point in time. Health is a necessary prerequisite for optimum growth and development during the period of rapid change that occurs between conception and late adolescence.

During childhood, adequate nutrition, shelter, activity, affection, and intellectual stimulation are effective in promoting health. Measures that prevent communicable diseases and accidental injury are particularly important during childhood. The responsibility for child health promotion and maintenance is shared by the child-rearing unit, health care providers, society, and eventually the individual child. Health may be altered when the child's basic needs are not fulfilled as a result of (1) alterations in body structure, function, or growth and development; (2) traumatic injury; (3) neglect or abuse; or (4) lack of knowledge.

THE NURSE

The nurse has a unique role in relation to the health of children and their families. The nurse's role is different from the role of any other health care provider because the nurse is concerned with the well-being of the child during health and illness. The nurse uses a holistic approach to provide care, comfort, counsel, and teaching for the child and the family. Child health care is given by nurses in the home, school, hospital, clinic, and community. During an acute illness, direct nursing care is of the utmost importance to the child's recovery. The nurse provides emotional support and guidance for the family during the child's illness.

Nursing research, as well as research in other fields, such as medicine, psychology, and family development, forms the scientific basis for the nursing of children. A theoretical knowledge base is the foundation for nursing practice. The nurse's care is guided by scientific principles. A thorough knowledge of growth and development is indispensable for the nurse who provides care to children and their families. The nurse uses a problem-solving approach, the nursing process, to identify children's health problems, including potential problems, and to design a plan of care. The nursing process is used in child health promotion and in meeting the needs of the ill child and his or her family. Keen observation and good interpersonal skills are essential for the nurse who provides care to children and their families. In order to be effective, the nurse must also use sound judgment, set priorities accurately, and collaborate with others.

The nurse has a responsibility to serve as a child-advocate and a family-advocate. In this role, the nurse promotes the health, growth, development, and independence of the child and the family. The nurse assists both the child and the family in becoming knowledgeable health care consumers who are able to assume the responsibility for their own health.

THE NURSING PROCESS IN CHILD HEALTH NURSING

Pediatric nursing is concerned with promoting, maintaining, and restoring the health of children and their families. The *nursing process* is a series of purposeful intellectual and technical activities used by the nurse in providing individualized care to children and their families. The nursing process is based on the problem-solving method, and therefore the steps of the process are taken in a logical order. The *steps* of the nursing process are (1) assessment, (2) nursing diagnosis, (3) planning, (4) implementation, and (5) evaluation and modification. Overall, the nurse takes the steps sequentially: assessment precedes diagnosis, diagnosis precedes making the treatment plan, and so forth. In the reality of daily practice, however, the steps of the nursing process often recur and sometimes overlap while the nurse is caring for any one child. The nursing process is used effectively in providing care to ill children and in promoting and maintaining the health of well children.

Nursing is not a rote activity, and it cannot be practiced in an intuitive or simplistic fashion. The contemporary practice of nursing requires the practitioner to use a scientific knowledge base in order to prevent, minimize, or resolve children's health problems. The nursing process is an indispensable clinical practice tool that enables the nurse to identify and prioritize children's health problems and to plan and evaluate clinical practice.

Nursing care plans

It is essential that the nursing process be communicated, both orally and in writing, to others who participate in the child's care. The *nursing care plan* is the written form of the nursing process. Sample nursing care plans are included in many chapters in Parts 3 and 4.

A nursing care plan documents independent or dependent nursing activities performed on the child's and the family's behalf. It also facilitates continuity of the child's care among nursing staff members. The nursing care plan is often placed in the child's record or in a location which is convenient for the nursing staff. In some states, the nursing care plan is part of the child's legal medical record.

The nursing care plan should always be individualized in order to meet the needs of the child and the family. The length and complexity of nursing care plans vary among children. A child with complex health problems might require an elaborate plan, whereas a child with minor health problems may need only a brief, standardized nursing care plan.

Accountability through the nursing process

Today, consumers are knowledgeable, and they demand quality from those who provide services and products. As health care providers, nurses are no exception. In pediatric nursing, the nurse is *accountable* to both the child and the family for the care given. This means that the nurse is responsible for implementing a plan of care based on nursing diagnoses that will best resolve or minimize the child's health problems.

The nursing process is important because it explains the practice of nursing. It is more accurate, perhaps, than any other description of nursing. It tells the consumer and other health professionals what the nurse *does* in practice. The nursing process serves as the basis for the legal definition of nursing in some state nurse practice acts. Therefore, the nursing process can be used as the *legal standard* against which a nurse's practice may be judged. Many schools of nursing and health agencies evaluate nurses in relation to their ability to demonstrate use of the nursing process in clinical practice.

QUALITY ASSURANCE IN CHILD HEALTH NURSING

As a profession, nursing must be concerned with the quality of care that its members give to consumers. The term *quality assurance* denotes a system by which criteria representing excellence in nursing care may be developed and through which nursing care may continually be evaluated and improved. Students sometimes think that the nursing process and written nursing care plans are merely academic exercises that do not have relevance in daily practice. Quite the contrary is true. The nursing process is the foundation for quality-assurance measures in pediatric nursing.

The American Nurses' Association (ANA) has developed standards enumerating the characteristics of quality nursing practice. These standards are based on the nursing process. The ANA has published the general *Standards of Nursing Practice*,[1] which can be used in any practice setting, and standards for each of the clinical specialties. Included are a rationale to support each standard and specific factors that can be used to evaluate a nurse's ability to demonstrate the ANA standards in practice. The standards have gained acceptance since they were first introduced in 1973, and they are frequently used in quality-assurance programs. Some individual standards of the ANA *Standards of Maternal-Child Health Nursing Practice* are listed in Table 3-4. Two other methods of providing quality assurance are the nursing audit and the peer review.

The nursing of children has changed greatly over the last 100 years. It is changing even faster today. The increased use of high technology forces nurses to learn new skills and work with complex machines. The use of diagnosis-related groups (DRGs) and early discharge lead to more complicated nursing care situations in the home and the clinic. Nurses who are currently working in the home health care and community settings need the knowledge and skills of the acute care nurse as well as those of the community health nurse.

To provide quality care, nurses must bring together all the health care resources to meet the child's and the family's needs. The therapeutic nurse-client relationship continues to be of paramount importance in all pediatric settings.

Reference

1. *Standards of Nursing Practice,* American Nurses' Association, Kansas City, 1973.

2

Susan McKeever Smith
Jean R. Miller

The family

Upon completion of this chapter, the student will be able to:

1. Describe the various types of family structures.
2. Compare the expressive and instrumental functions of the family.
3. Discuss the developmental stages and tasks of families with children.
4. Describe three qualities of the family as a system.
5. Contrast the family roles, characteristics, values, health beliefs, and practices of the Raza-Latina family, the black family, the Asian-Pacific family, and the Caucasian family.
6. Identify at least five contemporary forces that influence family life.

In preindustrial times, most of the work was done in the household. Children were considered members of the work force and were seen as economic assets. Childhood was a brief preparatory period terminated by apprenticeship and the commencement of work, generally before puberty.[1] The family was considered a productive unit that performed all the agricultural, domestic, and social functions. Industrialization caused a transfer of these functions to institutions outside the family. The family retained certain vital functions such as childbearing, child rearing, and socialization of the child.[2] Today, in the postindustrial era, the family is viewed as a consumptive unit that is leisure-oriented. Society expects the family not only to provide for the child's physical needs but also to meet his or her love and emotional needs. Today, the adult role is generally not assumed until the age of 21 or 22.

Definition of family

A *family* may be most simply defined as two or more persons who are related by blood, marriage, or adoption and who reside together in a household. This commonly held perception does not include some of the many alternative arrangements that also exist and, from the nurse's point of view, function as the child's family. A very broad definition of a family is two or more people who interact over time with an intent to nurture. The family's purpose is to meet its members' survival needs as well as their needs relating to cognitive, emotional, and spiritual development.

Overview of family structure and objectives

Structure (the membership and organization of a family group) sets the foundation for the roles and responsibilities of the family as a unit. The structure of the family provides the means for the achievement of family objectives (see Table 2-1). The family functions include giving an identity to its members, educating them for the roles of family life, and preparing them for community interactions. With respect to children, specifically, the family provides training for their becoming social beings able to participate in society.

Historically, a multigenerational household fulfilled the family's objectives. That is, economic support, emotional support, child rearing, homemaking, and the like were shared by grandparents, parents, siblings, and possibly aunts and uncles, living under one roof. More recently, however, the nuclear family has become the most common form of family in western culture. The *nuclear family* is one composed of a mother, a father, and dependent children.

In contemporary society, family structures vary considerably. These variations are not necessarily unhealthy. If a family's structure allows for the achievement of its goals, it is productive and appropriate. Even though the nuclear family is the most prevalent and perhaps most accepted family composition, different forms of family structure may also be viewed in a positive light. Other types of families that exist in today's society include the following: (1) the childless couple; (2) the couple whose children have separated from the family and now have their own families; (3) the single-parent family, in which the adult is widowed, separated, divorced, or unmarried; (4) the commune, or cooperative, family; and (5) the extended family (a nuclear family plus the parents, siblings, and/or in-laws of the adults of that nuclear family).[3] At least one study of four different family types (single-parent families, commune families, unmarried couples, and traditional nuclear families) found that each met the socialization and caretaking needs of children in a similar manner. In all these family types, parents used the parenting practices they were exposed to as children in bringing up their own children.[4] Each of the family structures mentioned has its associated strengths and weaknesses. The extended family, for example, may provide support, but it may also interfere in the mobility of the family by limiting the family's ability to use new means to achieve its goals. The nuclear family, though relatively stable, may not have the resources available to the extended family. Reliance upon one wage earner in the nuclear family can lead to difficulties if that person is incapacitated.[5]

For many people, including some children, the "family" includes people who are not related either by blood or by marriage. Examples include individuals living together who provide emotional support for one another in institutional settings, foster homes, and, in some instances, neighborhood networks. The nurse's assessment must not focus on the structure or the stereotyped perception of "what ought to be," but rather on the achievement of the basic goals of the family. Variations in family structure are discussed later in this chapter.

Table 2-1 Common Objectives of all Families

1. Satisfying the affectional needs of members
2. Satisfying the spouses' sexual needs
3. Socializing and enculturating children
4. Assisting members to relate effectively with social systems, organizations, and agencies
5. Providing an environment conducive to the growth and development of members (such as food, shelter, health care, and economic support)

The child as part of the family

When a nurse provides care to a child, whether in a health care institution or in the home, knowledge of the family and its operations is of prime importance. It is essential for nurses to view the child as part of a family system, noting particularly the family composition, the interactions between the family members, the members' roles, and the family's functions. This *family-oriented approach* helps the nurse conduct an assessment of the family and develop an appropriate plan of care for the child, capitalizing on the family network. This chapter will identify elements of the family system that the nurse must understand and incorporate into pediatric nursing practice.

The family as a child-rearing unit

The family is the environment that helps the child become a functioning adult. Parent-child interactions have an important bearing on the ability of the child to develop emotionally and intellectually (see Fig. 2-1). For example, a lack of positive parent-child interaction, characterized by minimal conversation between the two, may result in impairment of language development and scholastic ability.[6] Children learn about themselves and how to relate with others through their experiences within the family. Consistency, warmth, and dependability of interactions help a child become confident and, eventually, a productive member of society.

The family provides general health care and protection for its children. The well-functioning family ensures that children are immunized, that proper attention is given to food and clothing needs, and that health care is provided.

It is evident that the significance of the family in child rearing relates to the foundation it provides the child. The saying "What is past is prologue" is fitting to describe the relationship of the family to a child's development and later adulthood. What is learned in the family carries over into succeeding generations, perpetuating the system known as *family* for the individual.

FAMILY STRUCTURES

Traditional family structures

Nuclear families Nuclear families have the following three positions: husband-father, wife-mother, and offspring-sibling. Persons in these positions are expected to behave in certain ways and contribute to the emotional gratification of one another. Parents are expected to nurture and socialize their children, and children are expected to behave in ways that meet the norms established by the parents.

Until recently the husband-father was the head of the house and had major decision-making

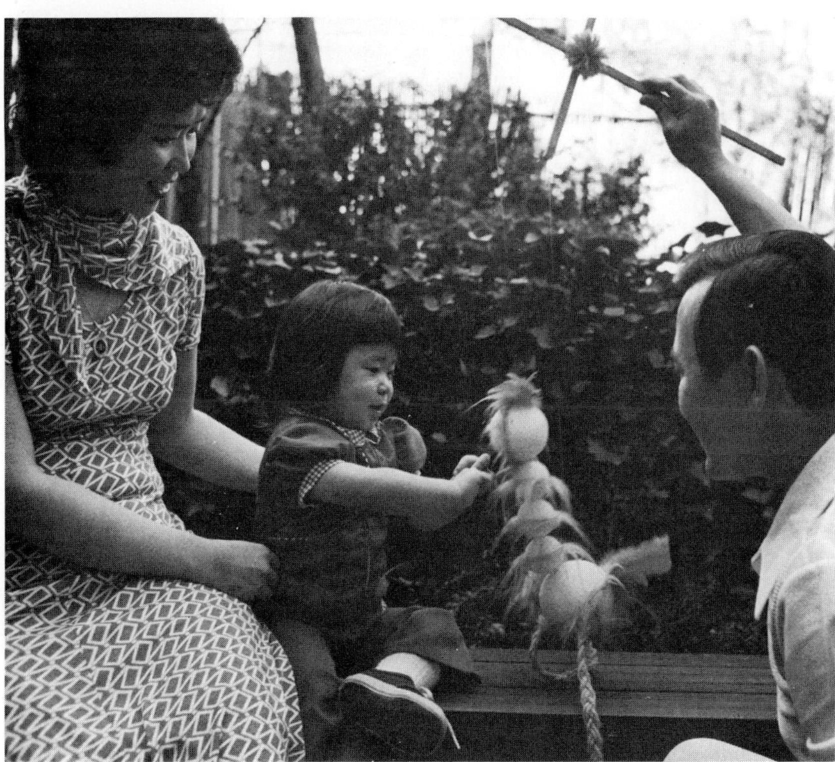

Figure 2-1 The emotional and psychological well-being of a child is influenced by the quality of family relationships. (*Photo by Erika.*)

powers in most households. The wife-mother maintained the household and took care of the children. Only about 10 percent of families fit this pattern today. Today wives and husbands frequently adjust their roles and responsibilities according to their interests and capabilities rather than assuming roles prescribed by society for women and men. The ability to perform a number of different tasks in the home has reduced the chaos which often occurs when a family member becomes ill, dies, or leaves the home, since other members are able to assume the responsibilities of the missing member.

The nuclear family has been viewed as the ideal family type for many years, but the current rate of divorce suggests that the nuclear family is not without its problems. Just as in other types of families, clear and continuous communication between family members is a necessity. Healthy family relationships in all types of family structures require consistent effort in order that all members will be emotionally gratified and will grow to be all they are capable of becoming.

In a growing number of nuclear families both the husband and wife have careers outside the home. The most logical family structure in two-career families is one in which the husband and wife share equally in household tasks and decision making. Many husbands, however, have not been socialized to know what needs to be done in the home or even how to do the tasks if they understand what needs to be done. More often than not, the wife assumes the responsibility of a full-time job outside the home in addition to the responsibilities for maintaining the home. This type of role structure is the beginning of many family problems, since the resultant inequities are irritating and stressful. Healthy family relationships are strengthened when both husband and wife agree on the way everyday tasks can best be accomplished.

Single-parent families Single-parent families consist of one parent, who may be either the mother or the father, and one or more children. Such arrangements are the result of separation, divorce, desertion, or death. Many single-parent families operate successfully, while others do not. Finances are one of the biggest problems among female-headed households. Most single mothers must enter the labor force but often cannot obtain the level of job they formerly held, since their former jobs may not exist or they are no longer prepared for comparable positions. Arrangements for children in either day-care centers or school place another burden on the working single parent. Single parents who play the dual role of mother and father to children often feel frustrated and inadequate. Such arrangements are confusing to the child. Loneliness is a prevalent feeling among single parents, regardless of their socioeconomic class, since American society is oriented toward couples rather than single persons.

Three-generation families Three-generation families usually consist of elderly parents, their adult children, and the adult children's children. When elderly parents live with their children, the structure and roles of the family often need clarification. It is relatively easy for elderly parents to inappropriately assume the parenting role with their adult children or, conversely, to seek parenting from their adult children. Neither type of relationship provides the autonomy and independence that both generations need. Since elderly parents who live with their adult children are usually physically dependent, it is important that they be able to maintain some autonomy through doing physical tasks that are within their capability and making decisions that are related to their own lives. They also can increase their sense of self-worth through interaction with their grandchildren, who readily respond to love and nurturing (see Fig. 2-2).

It is also important in three-generation structures that there be clarity about who assumes the parenting role and who assumes the grandparenting role. One approach is to have the grandparents assume the parenting role when the parents are out of the home but to have them relinquish the responsibility when the parents are home. It is most important that children understand who sets the limits, and at what times. Three-generation family living can be mutually beneficial, but it is one of the most difficult family structures because past relationships influence the enactment of present roles.

Social-support networks Social-support networks include the nuclear family, the kin of every family member, friends, neighbors, work associates, and sometimes helpers from such social agencies and institutions as churches and schools. This network serves as a source of support during easy and difficult times. Furthermore, the support is reciprocal in nature. Members of the

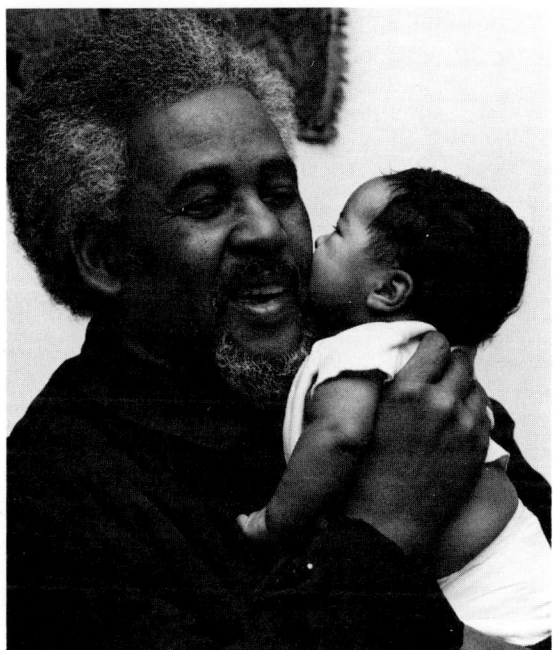

Figure 2-2 A grandparent's loving interaction with a grandchild can be beneficial to both. (*Photo by Erika.*)

network share resources that can be used to solve problems experienced by other members.

The structure of the network changes according to the circumstances and the need for leadership. The intensity, durability, and frequency of interaction within the network also vary for numerous reasons. Crises may bring the whole network together, whereas subgroups may meet together as a matter of routine. The structure within the smaller subgroups of the network is less apt to change, since these tend to be more stable groups, as is the case with various friendship and work groups. The value of social-support networks is that families know there are others beyond the nuclear family to support them, especially in times of trouble.

Emerging family structures

Blended families Blended families, also called *stepfamilies* or *reconstituted families,* consist of a husband and wife who have been married previously and who bring one or more children from a previous marriage into a new family relationship. The former marriage or marriages may have been dissolved through either divorce or death. Decisions about the structure of blended families are no different from the decisions made about structure and roles in first-time marriages. Blended families, however, seem to have additional challenges.

As reported by stepparents and their partners, the major problems can be categorized as follows: (1) problems concerning the children, (2) financial difficulties, and (3) marital misunderstandings and alienation.[7] Problems between stepparents and children are often caused by negative expectations of how new family members will relate to one another and by the tendency to misinterpret various responses as representing rejection. The expectation that there will be instant love and affection between stepparents and children is unrealistic. In the initial stages of the blended family, previous parent-child relationships may be maintained, and the new family members are not allowed to share in the relationship. Gradually, family members become more open, and both parents share in the rearing of each other's children. New family traditions emerge, bonding the family together. Younger children seem to develop a close and affectionate relationship with stepparents more easily than older children.

Family members often are hypersensitive to behaviors that might incorrectly be interpreted as rejection and lack of love. A stepparent may rightfully feel rejected when the stepchild expresses a preference for the biological parent, who may or may not be living in the same household. Time is needed for relationships to grow and mature.

Financial problems may seem less difficult than interpersonal problems, although inadequate finances can cause strains that hinder positive interpersonal relationships. Economic difficulties in blended families are the result of a number of factors, including alimony payments to former partners and a larger number of family members living on the salary of one parent. It is often necessary for both parents to work outside the home.

Marital misunderstandings are common at the beginning of a new relationship between divorced partners, as is also true of first-time married couples. The disadvantage that remarried couples face is that habits formed with the previous partner may not be easily understood by the new partner. This is partly a function of the length of the previous marriage or marriages and the age of the spouses.

Unmarried, single parents The number of unmarried, single parents is rising because unwed mothers elect to keep their children, because of divorce, and because single persons choose to adopt or bear children. In 1984, one-fourth of American families with children under 18 were headed by a single parent. This number will increase to one-third of all families by 1990. Unmarried, single-parent families can be very happy families, although the problems these families face are similar to those experienced by two-parent families. Finances, employment, loneliness, social relationships, role conflicts, child care, and child rearing are some of the problems faced by the unmarried, single parent. In addition, the predominant lack of social acceptance of these arrangements intensifies feelings of alienation.

Unmarried couples The number of unmarried couples is also increasing in American society. Unmarried couples live together for a number of reasons, which include gaining a knowledge about how to live with someone, preparing for marriage, testing a potential marriage relationship, and obtaining a convenient and economical living arrangement. Two general issues that affect the success of the relationship are (1) the responses of the partners' families of origin (the families into which they were born) and of the community surrounding them and (2) the degree to which the couple feel the relationship is permanent.[8] Some unique problems of cohabitation may be guilt due to religious beliefs, instability of the relationships, conflicts, inability to share lives with others, loss of other relationships, different expectations, children, legal problems, and housing difficulties.

Commune families Commune, or cooperative, families are similar to social-support networks except that commune families are countercultural. The members live together, and the group consists of married couples, unmarried couples, single persons, and children. Many members seek the social support discussed in the previous section "Social-Support Networks." Other reasons for living in a commune include wanting personal growth through small group processes, seeking spiritual rebirth, desiring to get back to nature, and wanting to rebel against the establishment. Communes tend to have little or no structure, with very little authority given to any one person. Consequently, there is a certain amount of emotional and financial instability in most commune families. It is difficult in many communes to establish an intimate relationship with any one person, and the numerous relationships tend to be superficial and lack closeness, which is supposed to characterize commune families. Many communes lack privacy, have poor sanitation, provoke conflict with the outside community, and develop legal problems.

There are both advantages and disadvantages to cooperative child rearing. Children have the opportunity to learn cooperation as a part of everyday living. They are exposed to many adult role models who willingly care for them. On the other hand, overly permissive discipline, high turnover and the accompanying instability that often diminishes children's sense of security, and poor education are some of the disadvantages of communal living. The long-range effects on adults as well as children are not known at this time. As is true of all types of family structures, there is much variation within cooperative groups.

Although the popularity of commune families has declined steadily since the 1970s, a different form of cooperation may emerge. Separate households will increasingly share facilities and services as housing arrangements change.

FAMILY FUNCTIONS

Family objectives

A family is expected to be concerned with the needs and demands of the parent or parents as well as with those of the children. These family functions usually fall into three categories: *physical, affectional,* and *social.* Society expects each member to fulfill certain obligations and meet certain demands. The family, therefore, has to mediate the needs and demands of its members with those of society.[9]

Instrumental functions

Tasks

Individual tasks Duvall uses Havighurst's tasks, which arise at or near a certain time in the life of an individual.[10] The successful achievement of these tasks leads to happiness and success with later tasks. Failure leads to unhappiness, disapproval by society, and difficulty with later tasks.

Family tasks *Family developmental tasks* are those basic functions which are specific to a given stage of development in the family life cycle.[11] Specific developmental tasks of the family at each stage of the life cycle will be discussed later in this chapter.

Roles *Roles* are defined as positions in a social structure, a set of expectations associated with a position in a social structure, or a set of behaviors associated with a position.[12] For example, a child may be an older brother (position) in a family. Certain expectations of behavior are associated with this role, such as protecting a younger sibling when walking to school. As another example, the nurse is expected to carry out the physician's orders and be aware of the desired outcome. People have many roles, each of which has certain expectations of behavior associated with it. The brother referred to above also has the position of son in the family and the role of student.

Socialization of children *Socialization* is the process by which individuals acquire knowledge and develop the skills, attitudes, and competence that enable them to function in society.[13] Socialization is an important function of the family.

Health care Health care is a vital and basic family function. Health and illness behavior are learned, and the family is the primary source of health education. The family tends to be involved in decision making and therapeutic processes at every stage, from a family member's state of being well to diagnosis, treatment, and recuperation.[14]

Expressive functions

Communication patterns *Communication* is the means through which family members develop self-worth. If the family environment is one of nurturance, the members will be able to grow and become socialized. Satir states:

> Communication is the largest single factor determining what kinds of relationship he (the human being) makes with others and what happens to him in the world about him. How he manages his survival, how he develops intimacy, how productive he is, how he makes sense, how he connects with his own divinity, all are largely dependent on his communication skills.[15]

There are two main functions of communication: message sending and behavioral guidance for the receiver of the message. Dimensions of message sending include content, representational accuracy, information, and vocal properties.[16] *Content* refers to what is said, while *representational accuracy* is the degree to which the content is depicted accurately or inaccurately. When the content about events, people, or objects is misrepresented, the cause is usually lack of speech specificity, overgeneralization, or other representational inaccuracies. *Information* about a topic reduces uncertainty for the listener, but too much or too little information, or overly redundant or insufficient information, merely confuses the listener. The *vocal properties* of verbal behavior include volume of the message and feeling tones that convey pleasant or unpleasant messages. The person who receives the message affects the sender by his or her response. Sometimes family members inappropriately affect one another's message sending by excessive control, inappropriate control, or ineffective control.

Nonverbal behavior communicates as much as verbal behavior, if not more (see Fig. 2-3). Touch, body positions, and facial expressions all convey messages. For example, shaking hands conveys such messages as acceptance and friendship; feelings of love often are expressed with physical contact. Differences in body position communicate information about how a person is feeling. The way a person sits in a chair or where he or she looks reveals how interested the person is in the subject being discussed. It is of utmost importance that nonverbal behavior be congruent with verbal behavior so that there will not be mixed messages.

Beliefs Those concepts which families feel are worthwhile, desirable, and important are revealed in their beliefs and values. It is these concepts which bind a family together, whether the family members are conscious of this or not. The family is a prime source of the belief systems, value systems, and norms that determine an individual's understanding of the nature and meaning of the world, his or her place in it, and how to reach his or her goals and aspirations.[17] Thus these beliefs are also guidelines for behavior. They are handed down from one generation to another; yet they are never static, but are influenced by many variables. These variables may include the culture, the community, social

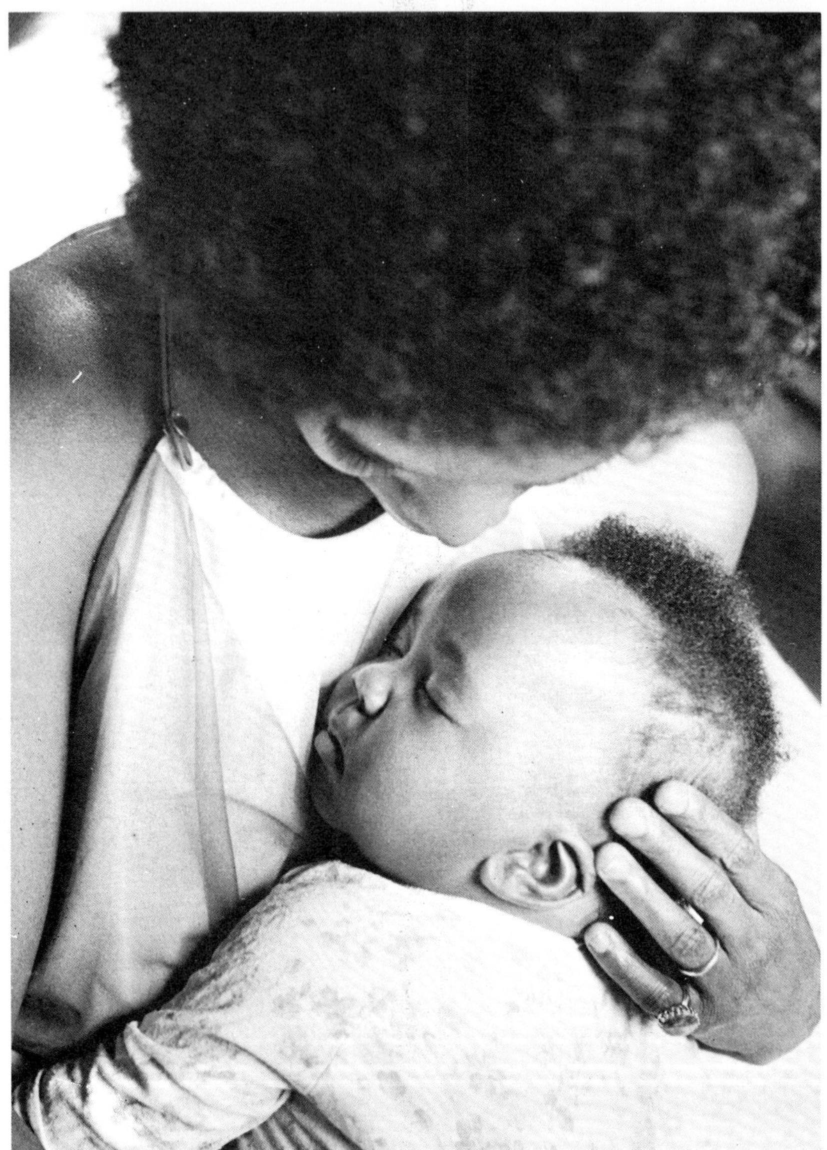

Figure 2-3 The parent's loving touch provides warmth and security for the growing child. (*From D. Papalia and S. W. Olds, Human Development, McGraw-Hill, New York, 1978, p. 31.*)

standing, occupation, religious affiliation, and the stage of individual and family development.

Values and beliefs will be discussed in detail in the section "Cultural and Ethnic Orientation of Families."

The major historical change in family values has been a change from a collective view of the family to one of individualism and sentiment. This shift in values has contributed considerably to the "liberation" of individuals, but it has also eroded the resilience of the family and its ability to handle crises.[18]

Family coping and problem solving Families constantly need to adapt and change in response to developmental and situational stressors. Families' ability to survive, grow, and function on higher levels of wellness depends on how well they adapt or cope. Without effective family coping, the affective, socialization, economic, and health care functions cannot be adequately carried out.[19]

It is important that families learn to become problem solvers so that they can handle problems themselves, rather than always needing professional intervention. The process of problem solving involves the following steps:[20]

1. Clearly defining the problem
2. Determining goals related to the problem
3. Describing existing conditions related to the problem
4. Discussing all possible ways of solving the problem and the consequences of each one
5. Deciding on an approach to try
6. Evaluating the outcome
7. Making future plans.

Parenting styles Parenting styles are the techniques that parents use to discipline their children. Discipline, if used appropriately, not only changes undesired behavior but also teaches appropriate behavior. Children like knowing how to behave. Correct behavior increases their sense of autonomy and security. Discipline is one of the most important ways that parents teach behavior and impart values to their children.[21] Adult behavior, therefore, is usually the result of the parenting style. An open, trusting adult who is eager to take on challenges is the result of one style of parenting, while a hostile, aggressive, underachieving adult is the result of another style.

Generally, three styles of parenting are described in the literature: authoritarian, authoritative (democratic), and permissive. These styles are compared in Table 2-2.

FAMILY DEVELOPMENT

In the family developmental approach, the family is studied throughout its life, from the newly established family (marriage) to the addition of children to the family, to their departure (because of marriage, education, or employment), to retirement, and eventually to the death of both parents. Knowing which stage of the family life cycle a particular family is in makes it easier to predict the developmental crises that the family will face. While each family is unique, there is still a sameness or universality about the stages that families pass through.

Table 2-3 Eight Stages of Family Development

Stage	Family Type	Characteristics
1.	Married couples	No children
2.	Childbearing families	Oldest child: birth to 30 months
3.	Families with preschoolers	Oldest child: 30 months to 6 years
4.	Families with school-age children	Oldest child: 6 to 13 years
5.	Families with teenagers	Oldest child: 13 to 20 years
6.	Families launching young adults	Departure of first child to departure of last child
7.	Families with middle-aged parents	Empty nest to retirement
8.	Families with aging members	Retirement to death of both spouses

The family life cycle

Duvall believes that the family goes through eight stages. These stages are determined by four factors: (1) plurality patterns, (2) the age of the oldest child, (3) school placement of the oldest child, and (4) the functions and statuses of the family before the children come and after they leave.[25] The eight stages are described in Table 2-3.

Family developmental tasks are those basic family tasks which are specific to a given stage of development in the family life cycle.[26] In beginning families, the couple must establish a

Table 2-2 Parenting Styles and Associated Characteristics

Structural Components	Authoritarian Style	Authoritative (Democratic) Style	Permissive Style
Discipline structure	Strict and controlling	Flexible to the child's changing needs	No limits, boundaries, or discipline
Control techniques	Punishment and fear	Praise and positive reinforcement	Vague or nonexistent techniques
The child's role	Compliance	Expanding responsibility as the child grows	No demands or expectations
Goal for the child	To comply with rules	To integrate internal control	To grow freely

Sources: 22, 23, 24

marital relationship, while at the same time separating from their families of origin and establishing new relationships with each set of parents. Families grow and develop as their children do. A family is pushed by its oldest child into new ways of coping, as the child becomes a preschooler, goes to school, and so forth. Younger children enter a different family from that of the firstborn. Launching families—those who are releasing their adult children—need to strengthen their marital relationship, cope with the absence of family members, build new relationships with their children's in-laws, and develop a new role as grandparents.

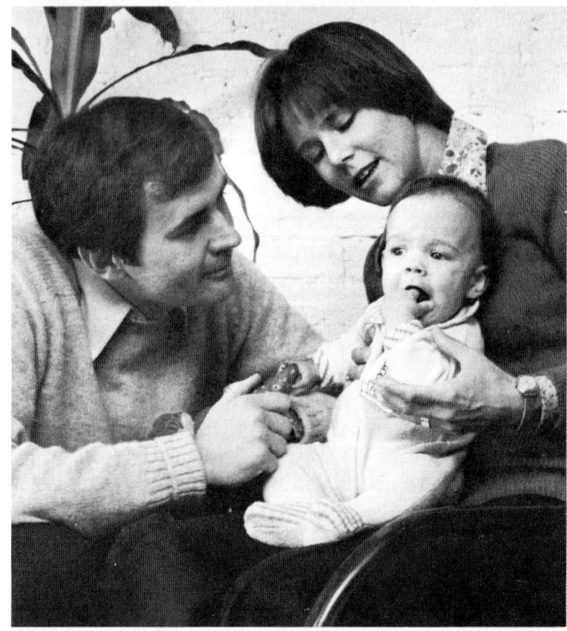

Figure 2-4 Active parenthood begins with the birth of a child and ends when he or she leaves home. However, in a sense, parenthood extends throughout the life of the parents. (*Photo by Erika.*)

Stages of family development

For the purposes of this textbook, only the stages of family development that involve family establishment (stage 1), childbearing (stage 2), and child rearing (stages 3, 4, and 5) will be considered. These are summarized below.[27]

Stage 1: married couples without children This stage begins when the couple marry, and it ends with the birth of the first child. The couple may think of themselves as a family in the making.

Family developmental tasks

1. Establishing a mutually satisfying marriage: finding, furnishing, and maintaining the first home; establishing mutually acceptable personal, emotional, and sex role responsibilities; and maintaining motivation and morale
2. Establishing new relationships with both families of origin
3. Adjusting to pregnancy and future parenthood

Stage 2: childbearing families This stage begins with the birth of the first child and continues until that child is 30 months of age (see Fig. 2-4).

Family developmental tasks

1. Having, adjusting to, and encouraging the development of infants
2. Establishing a satisfying home for both the parents and the infant or infants: adjusting housing arrangements, meeting the financial responsibilities of parenthood, developing mutually satisfying parenting role responsibilities, planning for future children, and maintaining motivation and morale
3. Maintaining relationships with relatives and others

Stage 3: families with preschool-age children This stage begins when the oldest child is $2\frac{1}{2}$ years old and ends when he or she is 6. The oldest child may be joined by one or more siblings.

Family developmental tasks

1. Adapting to the essential needs and interests of preschool-age children in stimulating and growth-promoting ways
2. Coping with energy depletion and lack of privacy as parents: supplying adequate space, facilities, and equipment for the expanding family; assuming more mature roles within the expanding family; rearing and planning for children; and motivating the family members
3. Maintaining relationships with relatives

Stage 4: families with school-age children This stage begins when the oldest child is 6 years old and ends when he or she is 13. The parents' crisis continues to be that of self-absorption vs. finding fulfillment in rearing the next generation. The children become involved with their own outside activities—school and peers.

Family developmental tasks

1. Fitting into the community of parents with school-age children in constructive ways
2. Encouraging the children's educational achievement and socialization: establishing ties for them outside the home and providing for their socialization
3. Maintaining parental privacy and mutuality: staying financially solvent and upgrading communication within the family

Stage 5: families with teenagers This stage begins when the oldest child is 13 years old and ends when he or she leaves home, to attend college or get married, for example. It is characterized by intense upheaval and transition (see Fig. 2-5).

Family developmental tasks

1. Balancing freedom with responsibility as teenagers mature and emancipate themselves
2. Establishing post-child-rearing interests and careers: maintaining the marital relationship and morale
3. Coping with family dilemmas: insisting on firm family control vs. giving teenagers freedom, the parents' assuming all responsibility vs. sharing responsibility with teenagers, emphasizing teenagers' social activities vs. their academic activities, and solving problems stemming from communication styles and patterns

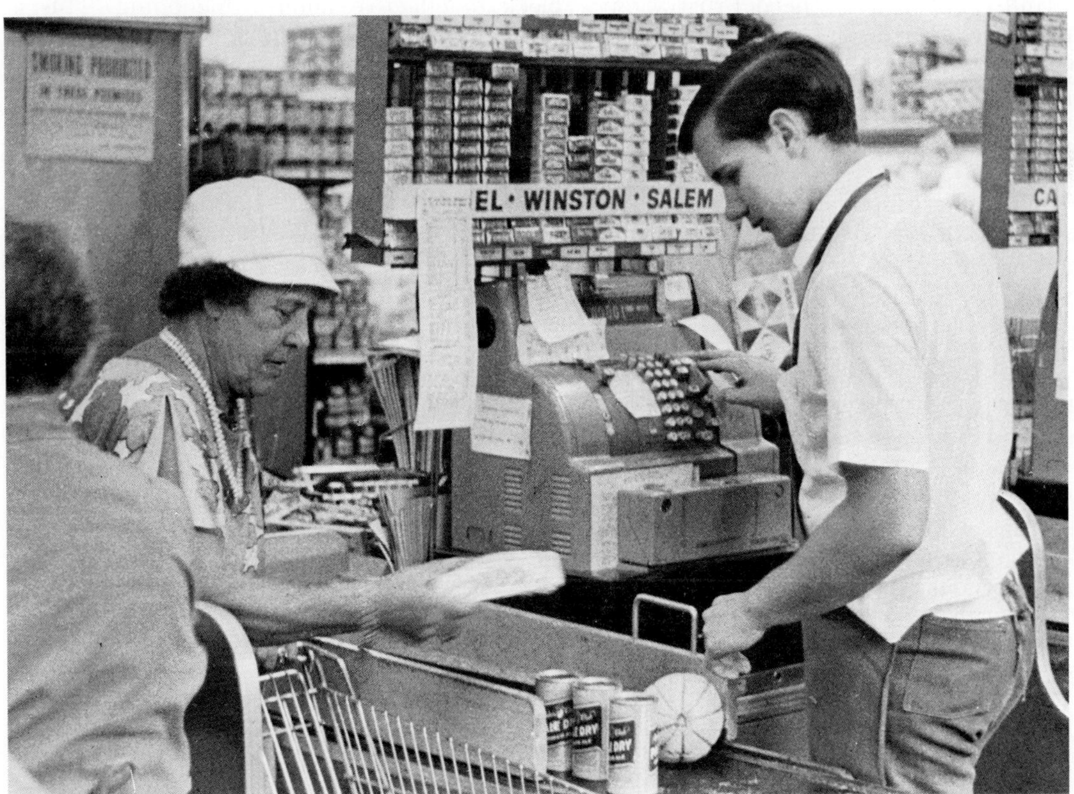

Figure 2-5 The period of adolescence requires alterations of roles and responsibilities within the family as the young person develops independence. (*From D. Papalia and S. W. Olds, Human Development, McGraw-Hill, New York, 1978, p. 271.*)

4. Maintaining the family network: caring for aging parents and bridging the communication gap between generations

The developmental tasks of the family coincide with the development of its members and the family's own increasing maturity. As children become adults and separate from their family of origin, they make lives of their own and establish new families. Eventually the family must deal with the aging and death of the parents—the normal sequence of life.[28]

All these major life stages alter the family structure and involve changes in roles, loyalties, and family membership. During these stages, families also experience unpredictable events, such as miscarriage, illness, divorce, job changes, and even changes in socioeconomic status. Because such events are unexpected, they alter the natural sequence of family life. It is often when such things happen that nurses encounter family members. The family undergoes transition as a member must adapt to a new need. Frustration and turmoil often result, as the needs of one family member collide with those of others. Ideally, the end result is adaptation when a successful solution to the problem is found. Usually the first occurrence of any type of event is the most disruptive, such as the birth of the first child. The birth of subsequent children should be easier. When nurses see that subsequent children cause more than the normal amount of disruption and confusion, they should make careful assessments of the family's concerns and stresses.[29]

THE FAMILY AS A SYSTEM

Families are systems that consist of members who are related to one another in a network of reciprocal causes and effects. Family members relate to one another in a reasonably stable way during any particular period of time. There is continuous interchange within the family as well as with other families and institutions in the community and the larger society. Families vary in terms of their cohesiveness and adaptability and their interaction with the outside world. Family members grow and develop as a consequence of their interchanges with one another and with the outside environment. Healthy families are able to make changes and respond productively to stress and tension. They are able to do this as a system because of their abilities to communicate and solve problems.

An emotionally healthy family is important to all family members, especially to children. The family is the primary place of learning and training; it is where children can test themselves without fear of losing the love of parents and siblings. Children learn to feel good in the family and to accept themselves as they truly are. The family is the source of expectations and beliefs that affect children's behavior and attitudes for the rest of their lives.

Most families, however, are hindered in some way from functioning at optimal levels. Often the parents' beliefs and expectations, which they learned from their families of origin, are in conflict. Beliefs and expectations about how the family should operate often have to be modified in the new family. This can be done only through open communication and acceptance of one another's feelings. However, inability or unwillingness to talk openly to one another is a common block to effective family functioning. This is compounded by family members' not knowing how to handle their feelings and not being able to accept one another's feelings.

The nurse is in an optimal position to assist families with physical as well as interpersonal problems. In many cases, listening and taking a supportive attitude will be all that is needed. With other families, the nurse may assist in assessing and solving problems by using simple logic and suggesting family activities. For instance, one family may decide to set aside one day a week to play together. Another family might decide to keep the television turned off during supper so that the family members can talk and listen to one another better. If the solutions to a family's problems are not so simple, the nurse can refer the family to a psychiatric liaison nurse or a family therapist.

CULTURE AND ETHNIC ORIENTATION OF FAMILIES

Culture

Culture is defined in a variety of ways. It is the heritage of families, and it provides guidelines and directions for families in the areas of language, food, religion, art, health, and relationships. Culture is the learned ways of acting and thinking which are transmitted by group members to other group members and which provide ready-made and tested solutions for serious problems.[30] Culture can also be defined as the knowledge that people use to interpret experience and regulate behavior.

Other concepts are related to culture. *Ethnicity* refers to a shared linguistic, racial, or cultural background.[31] *Race*, on the other hand, has to do with physical characteristics that are transmitted genetically. *Stereotypes* are attitudinal sets that assign attributes to another person solely on the basis of the class or category to which that person belongs.[32]

Acculturation refers to the changes that occur when an individual from a different ethnic background adopts the behaviors of the dominant culture. When the identifying characteristics of the different culture are no longer apparent, the person has been assimilated into the dominant culture.

One of the greatest barriers to effective nursing intervention is ethnocentrism.[33] *Ethnocentrism* is the tendency to use one's own group and customs as the standard for making all judgments about other people. Sensitivity to different beliefs and value systems is essential for nurses who work with children and families from various cultures.

The Raza-Latina family

The term *Raza-Latina* is used here instead of *Latin* or *Hispanic* because it more accurately describes the many Indian and other ancestors of Puerto Ricans, Cubans, Mexicans, Spaniards, and Central and South Americans.[34] *Raza* means "race"; *Latina* means "Latin." According to the Bureau of the Census, in 1980 there were 14.6 million people of Spanish descent in the population. This is the fastest growing minority in the United States.[35] Because of the wide diversity of the Raza-Latina groups, they *cannot* be considered a single, monolithic ethnic group. This culture is united through two powerful forces: language and a strong adherence to Roman Catholicism.[36]

Family characteristics For the Raza-Latina person, the family is the most important social unit.[37] The family's needs are primary, and the individual's needs are secondary. A family member's dishonor or shame reflects on the entire family. Family members' strong sense of obligation to the family unit gives the family strength. Support comes from the family unit and from members of the extended family.[38]

Family roles Roles are clearly defined in the Raza-Latina family. The father is the head of the household.[39] He is viewed as brave and strong and is the decision maker.[40,41]

The woman's role is changing from wife-mother-homemaker to include wage earner as well. This is not viewed positively by the culture. Since family unity is important, family decisions continue to be made primarily by Raza-Latina men, and teaching and health care decisions should be made by them.[42]

Grandparents, uncles, aunts, and godparents are an important part of the extended family. They provide support and transmit cultural history and healing practices to the children. The children are taught to share and to work together. The older children are responsible for their younger brothers and sisters.[43]

Family values The values of the Raza-Latina culture are oriented to the present time.[44] This culture values close family ties and the welfare of the group over that of the individual.[45,46] Second and third generations retain their native language—Spanish—and take great pride in their ethnic music, food, and culture.

Socialization Children are esteemed, and homes are child-centered. There are marked gender differences in child rearing, since different socialization patterns for male and female children begin early.[47] The son–father relationship is a formal, distant one. The son strives to meet the demands and expectations of his father.[48] Mothers pay more attention to their daughters than to their sons. Mothers and daughters work closely together doing household tasks. As a result of this emotional intimacy, the daughters identify positively with their mothers.[49]

Health practices The healing system used by the Raza-Latina consumer will depend greatly on the family's ties to traditional practices. Many Raza-Latina persons first use *remedios caseros* (home remedies) as health-maintenance methods. However, when the *curandero* (folk healer) lives in the community and is accessible, he is often used before western medicine is tried. Traditional healing practices among Raza-Latina people involve the individual's whole psychological, physiological, cultural, and spiritual being.[50] Humans, therefore, are viewed as being in harmony and unity with their natural and supernatural worlds. Illness and disease stem from a loss of homeostasis or balance.[51]

Folk beliefs Margaret Clark, an anthropologist, explains why the Mexican-American people consider folk healers to be vital in meeting their needs:

> Folk healers are not professional in the sense that they have formal training in the art of medicine or earn their living by their practice; they are members of the community who are regarded as specialists because they have learned more of the popular medicinal lore of culture than have other barrio people; use language which patients understand and vocabulary familiar to patients; never dictate what must be done, advise the patient what she or he considers appropriate.[52]

In addition to the *curandero,* family members will initially consult a herbalist *(yerbero),* after using home remedies first. Since this culture believes that illness may be a punishment from God, a *curandero* is consulted, and prayers will also be part of the treatment.[53] Illness may also be thought to have a magical origin. Another folk practitioner is skilled in the use of magic and witchcraft and can cast spells or hexes on individuals, as well as remove those cast by other magicians.[54]

The black family

According to the 1980 census, there are 26,488,218 blacks in the United States. This ethnic minority group constitutes 11.7 percent of the American population.

Family characteristics The development of the contemporary black family is overshadowed by the disastrous legacy of slavery. The matrifocal black family, which had its inception during slavery, does not exist in rural areas to any great extent today. It does exist in cities, where a disproportionate number of black families are headed by women.[55]

The black family has adapted to the larger society in various ways, and the common experience of racial discrimination and economic adversity has played a significant role.[56]

Although the model black family is nuclear (either a single-parent or a two-parent family), its distinctive characteristic is that many more members of the extended family live together than in white families. In working-class and middle-class black families, an older relative often lives in the home to provide child care while both parents work. In poorer families, an older female relative often brings a younger woman and her children into her home.[57] Regardless of social class, religion is important, since it serves political, spiritual, and social needs.

Family roles Since social class is the major determinant of family patterns among blacks, the following discussion is organized according to social class.

Black middle-class families constitute 25 percent of all black families and tend to be nuclear in form, generally consisting of a husband, a wife, and two to three children. Both parents usually work. Because of their dual employment, cooperative work and team effort on the part of the husband and wife are necessary. Thus many family tasks are shared, and there is extensive adaptability to, and flexibility of, roles.[58]

The black working-class family tends to be nuclear and to include four or more children. A relative or boarder is likely to be part of the household. Roles tend to be traditionally assigned, even though the roles of provider and child caretaker may be shared. The mother usually is the social liaison between the family and the school or church.[59]

Black lower-class families constitute about 40 percent of all black families. Poorer black households are much more likely to be headed by a single parent. Extended families—usually consisting of a grandmother, a mother, and the mother's children—are common, and usually there are more children than in the black middle-class family or the black working-class family. There are few shared roles, and the wife and husband pursue separate recreational and outside interests. The husband is expected to be the provider, and even though he is the titular head, he plays a minimal role in family life.[60] The wife assumes the roles of homemaker and child caretaker.

Family values The middle-class black family's value system is congruent with that of the dominant white culture. The family values productivity, achievement, self-reliance, and education.

The black working-class family places great significance on the family. Respectability is very important and is achieved by owning one's home and via the behavior of the children.

The primary feature of the lower-class black family is its low-income status. Because of this, fatalism is a common value. Black lower-class families learn to hope for little and expect even less. Family values are reality-based—a reflection of what families can aspire to and expect in life.[61]

Socialization Irrespective of social class, relatives (grandmothers, aunts, cousins, and older siblings) play a more active role in the socialization of black children than relatives do in the socialization of white children.[62] In the black working-class family, children are taught the skills and behaviors necessary to survive in their world. Young people are encouraged to seek employment as soon as they are old enough, and before that they have household chores to do.

Health practices The poorer black families, both in the South and in crowded urban areas, still use faith healers, spiritualists, and herbalists. Despite the availability of Medicaid and/or Medicare and of health facilities, many of the poorer black families will exhaust home remedies, over-the-counter medications, and friends' advice before seeking professional help. Often they present with serious symptoms of long standing. They see large health facilities as depersonalized and feel strange or uncomfortable in predominantly white clinics. The black cultural philosophy is present-oriented. Planning is done on a day-to-day basis because many problems are so enormous that it is too difficult to think beyond them.[63] Health promotion is not often viewed as a primary need, as food or shelter is.

Folk beliefs Roots, herbs, potions, oils, powders, rituals, and ceremonies have been and continue to be used in many southern communities. In urban areas today there is more reliance on the practices of a black cultural healer (e.g., a priest or priestess or a spiritualist) who focuses more on mysticism and psychological support and less on herbal or root medicine.[64] Most black patients feel that cultural healing remedies help them psychologically in dealing with discomforts; but when these things fail, a physician should be consulted.[65]

Jordon describes three major characters in the black American cultural healing system. First is an old lady, who has a knowledge of common herbs and who functions as a local consultant for those with pediatric, sexual and romantic, or marital problems. Second is a spiritualist, who has received a gift from God for healing incurable diseases or solving emotional or personal problems. Spiritualists are found primarily in urban settings, are well advertised by the black media, and may be male or female. The priest (a voodoo priest or priestess) is the most powerful figure in terms of healing or causing desired events.[66] It should be noted that not all blacks share in the beliefs and practices of the black cultural healing system.

Asian-Pacific families

The Asian-Pacific families discussed below belong to the Filipino, Chinese, Japanese, or Vietnamese culture. It is not the intent of this discussion to minimize the unique differences between these Asian families. The most obvious differences are language and the countries' development as separate nations. But there are similarities between these cultures.

The Filipinos are devout Catholics, while the Japanese have divergent religious beliefs. The Chinese and Vietnamese are strongly influenced by Confucianism, Taoism, and Buddhism. Confucianism has the most pervasive influence because it gives direction for social interactions and stresses ancestor worship. Taoism stresses passivity; followers must not question their unity with the universe. Humans must accept the harmony exemplified in nature by practicing moderation. Buddhists believe that people's present lives predetermine their own and their descendants' future lives. Thus people's past lives also affect their descendants' welfare.[67]

Family characteristics The concept of time is important within the Asian cultures. The family is not time-limited, like the family in the American culture, in which a couple meet, marry, and bear children, who then leave home and start the process all over again. The concept of family in the Asian culture extends both backward and forward. The individual is seen as the product of all the generations of his or her family from the beginning of time. This concept is reinforced by rituals and customs such as ancestor worship and keeping family record books, which trace family members back over many centuries. Personal actions reflect not only on the individual and the nuclear and extended families but also on all the preceding generations of the family since the beginning of time. Individual actions will impact all future generations as well.[68]

In the traditional Asian family, the new wife is absorbed into the husband's family and is relegated to a position that follows that of her husband, his parents, and also his siblings. The choice of a spouse is strongly influenced by both families, except in Asian-American families.

Family roles Traditionally, the father is head of the family, and his authority is unquestioned. He is the primary disciplinarian and provider. Successes and failures within the family are reflections of his leadership. The mother is seen as the caretaker of both the husband and the children. Traditionally, the primary role is one of a nurturant, emotional, devoted individual. Since she is the one who cares for the children when they are sick and who acts as a confidante and as a go-between between them and their father, a strong emotional bond is formed.

When Asian families immigrate, they undergo many transitions that can result in family dysfunction. In Asia the husband-father may have held a prestigious position. When he comes to the United States, his status may change. He may have to do menial work to provide for his family. If his wife must also work, role strain and conflict result.

Traditional Asian cultures value sons more highly than daughters. The eldest son acts as a role model for the younger siblings. These younger siblings are expected to follow the guidance of the eldest son throughout their lives. Upon the death of the father, the eldest son becomes the leader in the family. More recently a change has occurred. If the eldest son is not able to assume this role, either because he chooses not to or because he is no longer living, the role may be assumed by a daughter. The emphasis is on the leadership role, not on the sex of the person who assumes it.

As families have immigrated, the traditional roles of the male as leader and the female as caretaker have changed significantly. As wives share the role of provider with their husbands, the children are seen as an investment in the future. They are sent to school to obtain educations that will prepare them for professional careers. Their success benefits not only them but also the parents, who made the opportunity possible. Household responsibilities are kept to a minimum for these children so that they can devote their energies to achieving their goals.

Family values The values and behaviors of some Asian families are based on their teachings and their beliefs in Confucianism, Taoism, or Buddhism. The salient teachings on social interaction are reciprocity and loyalty; benevolence and righteousness; self-respect, self-reliance, and self-control; and social reciprocity and face-saving.[69] These traditional values conflict with some American values. For example, in the Chinese family submission by the wife and children is highly valued. Respect means total acceptance without questioning. Children must never bring dishonor or disgrace to the family. They are expected to uphold the family's good name and bring honor to it. In contrast, the American culture values independence, equal rights, and freedom of choice. Self-control is expected of Asian children, while American children are encouraged to be spontaneous and informal. Because Asian families value harmony, they will accommodate to situations rather than confront them.

Socialization Socialization, or the rearing of the young, may undergo changes as a culture is assimilated into the larger, dominant culture. Yet some beliefs and values remain to some degree in Asian-American families. Families base their interactions on clearly prescribed roles, duties, and responsibilities. They are characterized by conformity and little social deviance. Behavior is constantly rewarded, punished, reinforced, and reshaped by such parental techniques as emphasis on dependence and ethnic identity; obligation, duty, and responsibility; and the use of shame, guilt, and gossip.[70]

The concepts of shame and loss of face involve not only the exposure of behavior for all to see but also the withdrawal of the family's, the community's, or the society's confidence and support. The fear of losing face is a powerful motivating force for conforming to family and societal expectations.[71]

Health practices All the Asian-Pacific cultures adhere to health practices that are a mixture of eastern and western ideas. Japanese-Americans believe in the germ theory, the surgical removal of diseased parts, and immunization against disease.[72]

As a result of the lengthy Chinese rule, the Vietnamese have incorporated Chinese medicine into their healing practices. When Sino-Vietnamese medicine fails, western medicine may be used.[73]

Chinese-Americans will seek medical care from both physicians and cultural healers. They have found that for acute illnesses, western medicine and antibiotics are more effective. For chronic illness, many prefer to consult cultural healers, who are more familiar with Chinese concepts of health and illnesses.[74]

Folk beliefs The Chinese and the Vietnamese share the concept of medicine based on the complex theory of yin and yang and the five elements. Most do not concern themselves with the abstract theories of "chi" (innate energy) and/or blood or balance between human beings and nature. However, they pay attention to "chi" and blood when something is out of balance. When they do not feel well, they do not have sufficient "chi" and blood. Hot (yang) and cold (yin) are prevalent concepts concerning the body. *Hot* and *cold* are terms that describe certain properties and conditions that are totally unrelated to temperature. From the concepts of deficiency and of hot and cold stems the belief in maintaining harmony and balance. Health practice emphasizes moderation to avoid excesses that bring on illness.[75]

Chinese-Americans will seek health care from both western health practitioners and Chinese herbalists, acupuncturists, and bone setters. Those with chronic illnesses prefer to consult cultural healers, who are more familiar with Chinese concepts of health and illness. The herbalist uses varying amounts of herbs and combines them for a specific problem. These prescriptions are given by trial and error; if there is no improvement, the patient is encouraged to bring back the prescription for revision. Herbs are used to balance the body and prevent illness.[76]

As the Japanese become more acculturated to western society and culture, they tend to be less accepting of Eastern medicine. The Shinto religion teaches that humans are inherently good. Evil is caused by outside spirits who bring retribution to humans because they succumbed to temptation.[77] Treatment consists of purification through cleanliness and the use of natural purgatives. Harmony and balance are important parts of this culture, as they are of the Chinese and Korean cultures. Hence acupuncture, acupressure, and moxibustion are used to restore balance.[78]

The beliefs of the Vietnamese about health and illness reflect their worldviews. Diseases are thought to be caused by natural and physical phenomena or by disruptions of the universal order and of harmony. Since their lives have been predisposed toward certain phenomena by cosmic forces, even the well-educated use physiognomy, astrology, fortune-telling, and divination to determine these cosmic forces.[79] Through physiognomy, which is based on the notion that the body closely correlates with the mind, an attempt is made to determine one's behavior patterns and life adjustment by examining physical characteristics. The use of astrology is based on the belief that, depending on the time, day, month, and year of one's birth, one's life is ruled by the interplay of certain stars. A wise man usually calculates the cyclical changes of these forces and predicts a person's life process. In divination, people visit a temple where they procure divine instruction for problem solving.[80] The Vietnamese also believe that mental illnesses are caused by bad spirits, who must be exorcised by a sorcerer.[81] Even the wandering spirits of the dead, who have not reached nirvana, can cause illness.[82] Because the family regards maintaining the health of its members as its major responsibility, outside aid is not sought until the family resources have been exhausted.[83] The Vietnamese also use special diets to prevent sickness and to promote health.[84]

Caucasian families

Family characteristics Traditionally, throughout history, a man was responsible for supporting his wife and children. The wife was expected to be a homemaker, raise the children, provide regular meals, and care for other dependent members of the family. Her status in the community was dependent on her husband's success and position. This family style is seen less and less. *Dual-career families* is the term used to describe many nuclear families today. As a result of the women's liberation movement and the availability of contraceptives, many women are opting for careers, both for self-fulfillment and for economic reasons. The typical family with two or more children is also seen less and less. In the United States the population growth is zero; couples are barely replacing themselves.

Single people and single-parent families are the fastest-growing segments of the population. The single-parent family may be the result of divorce, death, or the decision to have children out of wedlock. Occasionally the father instead of the mother elects to remain at home and care for the children and the home.

Family roles Many families, particularly lower-middle-class and lower-class families, maintain the traditional mothering and fathering roles. In the low-income family the father is the breadwinner, and the mother cares for the children. The mother tends to be traditional in her outlook on child rearing, emphasizing respectability, obedience, cleanliness, and discipline.[85]

The traditional mothering role requires that the woman maintain the family, offer emotional support based on unconditional love, and keep home strains and stresses under control. She is unquestionably the primary caregiver and does most of the parenting tasks.[86]

Today many couples share the parenting role. They reject the parenting roles of their families of origin because they are no longer viable in today's changing world. In the 1960s fathers moved from the labor and delivery waiting rooms to assume the role of coach during the birth of their children. The advent of the "pill" enabled women to make choices regarding childbearing. The legalization of abortion during the first trimester of pregnancy gave the woman even more choices. The feminist movement has had a considerable impact on women's and men's roles. Advanced technology has created more diversified employment opportunities. Historically, women had limited options; they could become nurses, teachers, clerks, or secretaries. That has changed. More working mothers, more leisure time, smaller family units, and an increasing divorce rate mean that women are no longer committed to the traditional roles of their mothers.

The roles of family members have also become more complex and flexible. Both husbands and wives expect each other to assume the intangible and more demanding roles of understanding companion, stimulating colleague, and loving, sympathetic parent.[87] The child's role requires behaviors that will result in the acquisition of (1) a psychic structure that produces a secure identity and constructive self-esteem, (2) skills for independent functioning, (3) an education, and (4) experience in peer relationships.[88]

Family values The central, unifying theme of the dominant American culture has always been that cluster of values called the *Protestant ethic*, according to which a person's virtue is measured primarily in terms of achieving occupational success for men and being a good wife and mother for women.[89] The most valued role model in the past was the risk-taking entrepreneur, and this is still true to a large extent today. One study done in 1974 and 1975 confirmed the continuity of the Protestant ethic and the importance of the traditional values of family, work, and education.[90] Productivity, a significant value of the American culture, results in success and achievement. The rewards of success and achievement are described as the "American dream": material possessions, approval of others, status, and power. Education is highly valued because it results in productivity. Tied in with this value is the merit of individualism and its associated values of self-reliance and self-responsibility. This is in contrast to the beliefs of many minority cultures who stress or value the family, as opposed to individualism.

Variables affecting a family's value system

Socioeconomic status is a major variable affecting a family's value system. Other variables include cultural heritage or ethnic background, degree of acculturation, and the stage of the life cycle that the family is in.

A family's value system is very much affected by its socioeconomic status. Money and its management also affect marital success. When income is inadequate, basic survival needs are given top priority, and this influences family characteristics, roles, health practices, and child rearing. In 1983, 15.2 percent of the population was below the poverty line; of those, 35.7 percent were blacks, 28.4 percent were Latins, and 12.1 percent were white. This means that 35 million people are struggling to meet the basic needs of daily living. The social and economic gap between middle-class and poverty-level families is expected to increase.

When American and Mexican-American values are compared, one notes the many apparent conflicts. Whereas Americans value individualism, independence, work, and material goods, Mexican-Americans see themselves as part of the family and as working for the family; they work in order to survive and gain status through family and social relationships, rather than through the accumulation of possessions. In the eastern cultures the individual is of secondary importance, and the family and the family reputation are primary. Yet, as in the American culture, education and industry are highly valued.

The members of each succeeding generation of a specific cultural group adopt values of the dominant culture. This acculturation can create conflict within families. In the same way, the members of the younger generation can acquire new values that conflict with those of their families of origin.

CONTEMPORARY INFLUENCES ON FAMILY SYSTEMS

The nurse must be familiar with influences that affect present-day family life. Among the factors impinging on families are ideas about child rearing presented on television, in literature, and in courses and seminars. Some ideas offered to parents are sound; others may need careful examination.

Child-rearing practices

One of the most popular current practices is including the father as an equal participant in the parenting process. It has become acceptable for the father to participate in the childbirth process by supporting his partner during labor and delivery. Following this, the father may share the responsibility for the actual care of the newborn (see Fig. 2-6). Today, many fathers are likely to bathe, feed, and dress their children. Child care has become a mutual endeavor for both parents.

Television

The influence of television on children has been the subject of many research studies. Television viewing greatly influences children's view of the world, their moral beliefs, their sexual relationships, their behavior, and their development.

A relationship between violence shown on television and aggressive behavior in children has been demonstrated.

What kind of moral values does a child learn from television? Strength and carnage are shown to achieve results. Being affluent, seemingly without doing much work, is depicted as a glamorous life-style. Having a number of different marital partners and love affairs outside marriage is also a frequent theme on "soaps." Programs about blacks and black family life are being increasingly shown on major television channels, but programs about other minorities are not, though they are frequently seen on channels devoted solely to ethnic programming.

Television is a passive medium that requires

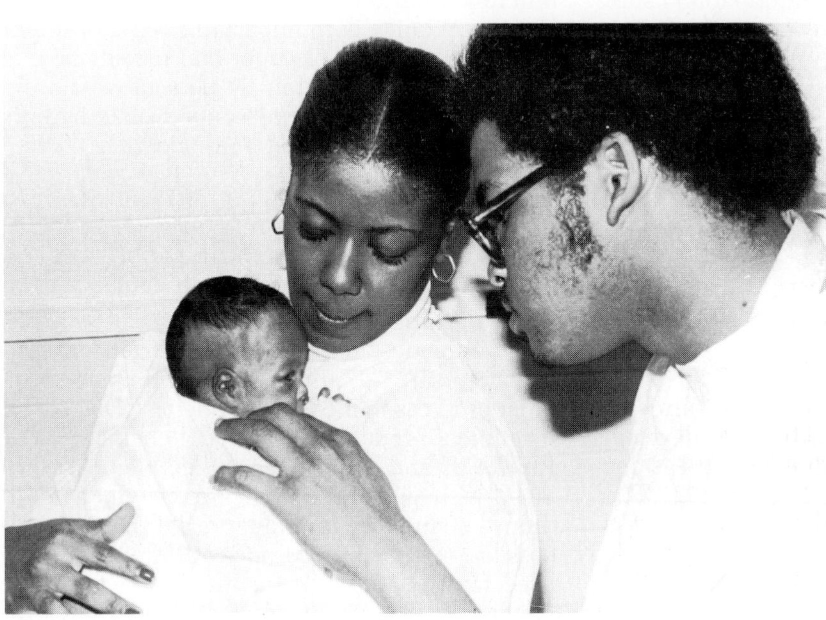

Figure 2-6 Fathers are often eager to be equal participants in the parenting process. (*From G. M. Scipien et al., Comprehensive Pediatric Nursing, 2d ed., McGraw-Hill, New York, 1979, p. 406.*)

no response from the viewer. Although programs such as "Sesame Street" have contributed to children's knowledge, they require no involvement or feedback, and they provide no opportunity to practice reading and writing or motor skills.

Parents should control television viewing by limiting hours watched and by reviewing programs that will be seen and avoiding those whose values do not support family values.

Latchkey children

Latchkey children are children who carry keys to their homes. These children come home at the end of the school day to wait unsupervised for a parent's return. The majority of these children are under 13 years of age, and injury, delinquency, or feelings of isolation can occur during these periods of unstructured and unsupervised activity.[91] Child care is a luxury that many parents cannot afford. With the continuing rise in the number of single-parent families and in an economy in which both parents are frequently employed outside the home, this problem is expected to escalate. Nursing interventions and resources that can be made available to parents include providing quality after-school programs, teaching parents and children basic survival skills, and using a telephone check-in service.[92] PhoneFriend is a community- and volunteer- supported telephone service in southern California that provides information, support, and social contact for any child who might need it.[93]

Day care

Day care or quality child care is more and more essential to today's families. It is difficult to find for infants, and it is unaffordable for many families. Guidelines for selecting a day-care center are given in Chap. 11.

Adoption

For individuals and families there are stresses and adjustments during each new developmental stage. Adoptive families face the same stressors as well as some additional ones. The stress of making the initial decision to adopt is compounded by the fact that it can take years to adopt a child. Factors that affect the length of the waiting period include the agency selected, the number of children the family has, and the desired age, sex, and nationality of the child. Cost can also be an issue. The belief that bonding must occur during a narrow window of time following birth adds to parental anxiety. Establishing a relationship does take work, but with time, patience, and support from health professionals it can be done successfully. Children, depending on their age at the time of adoption, may experience grief related to losing a biological parent, a foster parent, or a social worker or to leaving a home country. Ongoing involvement with parental support groups and health care workers helps the family to adjust and to anticipate future concerns before they arise.

Adoptive parents must face the issue of when to tell the child about the adoption. When preschoolers ask, "Where did I come from?" parents should answer simply and honestly. Children need to know why they were adopted. Feelings of rejection and inadequacy must be expected and dealt with openly.

Adolescence is another period when issues related to adoption may cause strain. Identity formation—"Who am I?"—usually peaks at this time. Issues about why the natural parents placed the child for adoption may surface, along with feelings and fantasies about them. The adolescent may feel guilty for having these feelings when the adoptive parents have been loving and supportive and may also experience sadness because the circumstances of his or her birth were different from those of friends. At a time when peer acceptance is so important, being different may cause feelings of anger and rebellion.

Helpful books written by persons who were adopted are available and can sensitize parents to the feelings associated with adoption.[93a,93b]

Technology

Developed countries are much safer places for children than undeveloped countries because of better housing and nutrition, the use of vaccines and antibiotics, and improved obstetrical and pediatric care.[94] Families also benefit from the great progress in medical technology. Diagnostic machines, fetal monitoring, chemotherapy, RhoGAM, and intensive care techniques, combined with skilled nursing care, give many children a chance for a quality of life that was not possible two or three decades ago. Federal funds used for research and health care services for handicapped and chronically ill children have helped many achieve full mental and physical growth.

Nevertheless, technological change also places increasing stress on families. The explosion of new information creates anxieties and confusion about the pace of change. More family members may abuse drugs and alcohol in an attempt to deal with the stress of everyday life.

The changing status of women

In the preindustrial and early industrial society, women were part of the economic family unit. They not only cared for the children but also worked within the home. The industrial revolution separated the home and the workplace. Since that time, there has been a greater emphasis on mothering and on making the home a retreat from the pressures of the world of work.

According to the U.S. Department of Labor, 39 percent of women were in the work force in 1965, and 52 percent in 1982; it has been predicted that 65 percent of women will be working in 1995. Fields that were traditionally limited to men increasingly include women.

More and more women are the family's primary breadwinner. In 12 percent of families the wife earns more than her spouse; in one-third of families the woman provides the sole support.

Data from the Bureau of the Census released in 1984 showed that many American women delay childbirth until they are in their thirties. The children of these women experience a different home environment from that of children born to younger women. Their mothers usually have completed a year of college, have a higher income, and are more likely to be professional women. Despite this trend, many children are born to single women who live in poverty, and therefore they are born into a less than desirable environment.

The extended family

The influence of the extended family varies, depending on whether the members of the extended family live with the younger family, nearby, or far away. If the extended family is part of a household that includes several generations, its impact may be very strong. Elder family members' ideas about child rearing may be quite traditional. For example, acceptable behavior for family members may be more stringently defined by grandparents than by parents. Members of the extended family who live close to the young nuclear family are usually somewhat influential. If the family boundaries are flexible, there may be a continual exchange of services, communication, and information (see Fig. 2-7). Reliance on members of the extended family may be accepted as the norm, but if they live far away, they are unlikely to influence the family's day-to-day activities.

Increasing dependency on parents

Another factor affecting families is the increasing length of time that a child is dependent on the parents for financial support. The value placed on higher education has pushed dependency upward into the young adulthood years. Previously, children finished high school or college, became employed, and embarked on lives of their own. Preparation for many careers and professions now requires schooling well beyond the twenty-first birthday. Consequently, parents frequently provide economic support for their children until they are well into their twenties.

The "me" generation

Perhaps as an offshoot of increased dependency, many children hold the belief that "someone will always take care of me." A relatively affluent society may contribute to the feeling that the individual is "entitled" to satisfaction of his or her needs. The danger in this is that young adults may not assume the responsibility for their own welfare. Some believe that this phenomenon signifies the family's failure to prepare children for adulthood.

Two-career families

There are many two-career families in today's society. When two parents are employed, arrangements for the care of children and sharing household responsibilities must be made. Support may be necessary from outside agencies or, perhaps, from the extended family. Although both parents may exert a combined effort in family life, parent-child interaction can diminish if both parents are involved in careers.

Economic factors

The economic status of a family affects how the functions of the family are carried out. The health-

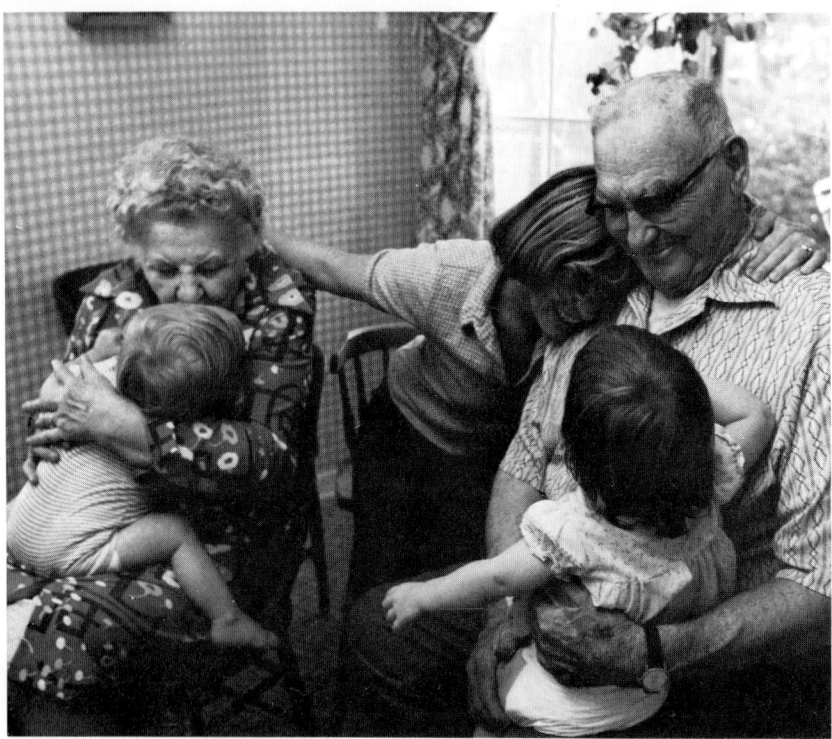

Figure 2-7 The relationship between children and grandparents can be rich and rewarding for both. (*Photo by Erika.*)

promotion function is hard to carry out in the absence of adequate income, and individuals who live in poverty have poor health. In 1984 more than one-half of single-parent families were below the poverty line. It is no surprise that economic security is commonly conducive to a well-functioning family.

Death, separation, divorce, and remarriage

Other influences on the family's interactions include death, separation, divorce, and remarriage. Each of these has a great impact on members in the family system. The effect of a death depends on (1) whether it was anticipated or sudden, (2) when it occurs in the family's development, and (3) the ages of the children involved. There may be a need to reorder the roles of family members, as they take on the family functions of the individual who has died.

Separation and divorce may present similar problems. There may be guilt associated with a parent's leaving a family. Children often feel that they are the cause of the separation or divorce. Bitterness and recrimination between spouses may affect the children's relationships with the parents.

One of the newer developments affecting the family system in relation to divorce is the matter of joint custody. Rather than granting custody to one parent and allowing the other visitation rights, the court assigns a child to both parents. Frequently, children live with each parent 6 months of the year. This allows both parents access to their children. Joint custody works only if both parents have a commitment to it and if consistency is maintained between the two households.[95]

THE NURSE AND THE FAMILY SYSTEM

Until a child is old enough to assume management of his or her own health care, usually in late adolescence, health maintenance and therapy are family matters. Systems theory makes clear two pertinent points: The adequacy of the family's methods of operating directly affects a child's well-being, and the health status of each family member impacts on the family system as a unit as well as on the community, the school, and other environmental systems with which the family interacts.

In both preventive maintenance of well children and intervention for those who are ill, the nurse often has a critical role to play in helping the family system function effectively and in facilitating the family's interactions with the health care system. Assessment of the family is an essential part of pediatric care and enables the nurse to adapt health services to the family system's established ways of operating and to help the family obtain and use supportive input from its environment.

References

1. Hareven, Tamarak, "American Families in Transition: Historical Perspective on Change," in Froma Walsh (ed.), *Normal Family Processes,* Guilford Press, New York, 1982, p. 451.
2. Ibid., p. 452.
3. Sussman, Marvin B., "The Family Today: Is It an Endangered Species?" *Children Today* **7**(2):32–37 (March–April 1978).
4. Eiduson, Bernice, "Child Development in Emergent Family Styles," *Children Today* **7**(2):24–31 (March–April 1978).
5. Sussman, op. cit., p.45.
6. *Task Panel Reports Submitted to the President's Commission on Mental Health,* U.S. Government Printing Office, Washington, DC, vol. 2, 1978.
7. Visher, E. B., and J. S. Visher, "Major Areas of Difficulty for Stepparent Couples," *International Journal of Family Counseling* **6**:70–80 (1978).
8. Kuhn, Kathline, and Ellen H. Janosik, "Establishment of a Family System," in Jean R. Miller and Ellen H. Janosik (eds.), *Family-Focused Care,* McGraw-Hill, New York, 1980, p. 155.
9. Friedman, Marilyn, *Family Nursing: Theory and Assessment,* Appleton Century Crofts, New York, 1981, p. 3.
10. Duvall, Evelyn Millis, *Marriage and Family Development,* 5th ed., Lippincott, Philadelphia, 1977, p. 167.
11. Ibid., p. 177.
12. Hardy, Margaret E., and Mary E. Conway, *Role Theory: Perspectives for Health Professionals,* Appleton Century Crofts, New York, 1978, p. 11.
13. Duvall, op. cit., p. 9.
14. Friedman, op. cit., p. 5.
15. Satir, Virginia, *Peoplemaking,* Science and Behavior Books, Palo Alto, Calif., 1972, p. 30.
16. Thomas, Edwin J., *Marital Communication and Decision Making: Analysis, Assessment, and Change,* Free Press, New York, 1977, p. 11.
17. Friedman, op. cit., p. 172.
18. Hareven, op. cit., p. 456.
19. Friedman, op. cit., p. 244.
20. Johnson, Suzanne Hall, *High-Risk Parenting: Nursing Assessment and Strategies for the Family at Risk,* Lippincott, Philadelphia, 1979, p. 293.
21. Nelson, Gerald E., *The One Minute Scolding,* Shambhala Publications, Boulder, Col., 1984, p. 3.
22. Hurlock, Elizabeth B., *Child Development,* McGraw-Hill, New York, 1972, pp. 386–387.
23. Kaye, Kenneth, *Family Rules: Raising Responsible Children,* Walker & Co., New York, 1984, pp. 5–6.
24. Duvall, Evelyn Millis, *Evelyn Duvall's Handbook for Parents,* Broadman Press, Nashville, 1974, p. 108.
25. Ibid., p. 145.
26. Ibid., p. 177.
27. Duvall, *Marriage and Family Development,* pp. 185–350.
28. Janosik, Ellen H., and Jean R. Miller, "Theories of Family Development," in Debra P. Hymovich and Martha Underwood Barnard (eds.), *Family Health Care,* McGraw-Hill, New York, 1979, pp. 3–16.
29. Thompson, Mary K., "Family Development Theory," *Nurse Practitioner* **9**(6):54–58 (June 1984).
30. Walter, P. A., *Race and Culture Relations,* McGraw-Hill, New York, 1952, p. 17.
31. Werner, E. E., *Cross-Cultural Child Development: A View from the Planet Earth,* Brooks/Cole, Belmont, Calif., 1979.
32. Porter, R. E., "An Overview of Intercultural Communication," in L. A. Samorar and R. E. Porter (eds.), *Intercultural Communication: A Reader,* Wadsworth, Belmont, Cal., 1972, pp. 3–18.
33. Ibid.
34. Monrroy, Lidia S. Adhmada, "Nursing Care of Raza/Latina Patients," in M. S. Orque, B. Block, and L. S. A. Monrroy (eds.), *Ethnic Nursing Care: A Multicultural Approach,* Mosby, St. Louis, 1983, p. 116.
35. Ibid.
36. Friedman, op. cit., p. 81.
37. Murillo, N., "The Mexican American Family," in R. A. Martinez (ed.), *Hispanic Culture and Health Care,* Mosby, St. Louis, 1978, p. 3.
38. Ibid., p. 10.
39. Ibid., p. 11.
40. Ibid., p. 33.
41. Ibid., p. 10.
42. Monrroy, op. cit., p. 135.
43. Ibid.
44. Kluckhohn, Florence R., "Dominant and Variant Value Orientations," in P. J. Brink (ed.), *Transcultural Nursing: A Book of Readings,* Prentice-Hall, Englewood Cliffs, N.J., 1976, p. 70.
45. Garza, R. T., and R. E. Ames, "A Comparison of Chicanos and Anglos on Locus of Control," in C. A. Her-

nancez, M. J. Haug, and J. J. Wagner (eds.), *Chicanos: Social and Psychological Perspectives,* 2d ed., Mosby, St. Louis, 1976, p. 133.

46. Monrroy, op. cit., p. 134.
47. Friedman, op. cit., p. 81.
48. Ibid.
49. Queen, S. A., and R. W. Haberstein, *The Family in Various Cultures,* Lippincott, Philadelphia, 1974, p. 249.
50. Dorsey, P. R., and H. O. Jackson, "Cultural Health Traditions: The Latino/Chicano Perspective," in M. F. Branch and P. P. Paxton (eds.), *Providing Safe Nursing Care for Ethnic People of Color,* Appleton Century Crofts, New York, 1976, p. 6.
51. Friedman, op cit., p. 281.
52. Ibid., p. 282.
53. Dorsey and Jackson, op. cit., p. 59.
54. Ibid.
55. Rainwater, L., "Crucible of Identity: The Negro Lower-Class Family," in J. H. Bracey, A. Meier, and E. Rudwick (eds.), *Black Matriarchy: Myth or Reality?* Wadsworth, Belmont, Calif., 1971, p. 81.
56. Billingsley, A., *Black Families in White America,* Prentice-Hall, Englewood Cliffs, N.J., 1968.
57. Friedman, op. cit., p. 286.
58. Ibid., p. 285.
59. Ibid., p. 286.
60. Ibid.
61. Ibid.
62. Ibid.
63. Stokes, L. G., "Delivering Health Services in a Black Community," in A. M. Reinhardt and M. D. Quinn (eds.), *Current Practice in Family-Centered Community Nursing,* vol. 1, Mosby, St. Louis, 1977, p. 54.
64. Jordon, W. C., "The Roots and Practice of Voodoo Medicine in America," *Urban Health,* **8**:38–41 (1979).
65. Block, B., "Nursing Care of Black Patients," in Orque, Block, and Monrroy, op. cit., p. 94.
66. Jordon, op. cit., pp. 38–40.
67. Orque, M. S., "Nursing Care of South Vietnamese Patients," in Orque, Block, and Monrroy, op. cit., p. 249.
68. Shon, S. P., and D. Y. Ja, "Asian Families," in M. McGoldrick, J. K. Pearce, and J. Giordano (eds.), *Ethnicity and Family Therapy,* Guilford Press, New York, 1982, p. 211.
69. Chen-Louie, Theresa, "Nursing Care of Chinese American Patients," in Orque, Block, and Monrroy, op. cit., p. 201.
70. Kitano, Harry H. L., *Japanese Americans: The Evolution of a Subculture,* Prentice-Hall, Englewood Cliffs, N.J., 1969, p. 66.
71. Shon and Ja, op. cit., p. 215.
72. Hashizume, S., and J. Takano, "Nursing Care of Japanese American Patients," in Orque, Block, and Monrroy, op. cit., p. 226.
73. Hickey, G., *Village in Vietnam,* Yale, New Haven, Conn., 1964, p. 119.
74. Chen-Louie, op. cit., p. 209.
75. Ibid., p. 208.
76. Ibid.
77. Hashizume and Takano, op. cit., p. 225.
78. Le, T. R., "Vietnamese Concepts of Illness and Treatment," International Institute of San Francisco, Indochinese Mental Health Project, San Francisco, 1978, p. 2 (mimeographed).
79. Orque, op. cit., p. 254.
80. Ibid.
81. Ibid.
82. Hickey, op. cit., p. 118.
83. Orque, op. cit., p. 255.
84. Friedman, op. cit., p. 159.
85. Tackett, J. J., "Parenting for the Socialization of Children," in J. J. Tackett and M. Hunsberger (eds.), *Family-Centered Care of Children and Adolescents: Nursing Concepts in Child Health,* Saunders, Philadelphia, 1978, p. 48.
86. Duvall, *Marriage and Family Development,* p. 49.
87. Blanck, R., and G. Blanck, *Marriage and Personal Development,* Columbia, New York, 1968.
88. Friedman, op. cit., p. 173.
89. Flacks, R., *Youth and Social Change,* Markham, Chicago, 1971, p. 20.
90. Friedman, op. cit., p. 194.
91. McClellan, Mary Ann, "On Their Own: Latchkey Children," *Pediatric Nursing* **10**(3):198 (May–June 1984).
92. Ibid., pp. 198–201.
93. Guerney, L., and L. Moore, "Phone Friend: A Prevention-Oriented Service for Latchkey Children," *Children Today* **12**(4):5–10 (July–August 1983).

93*a*. Livingston, C., *Why Was I Adopted?* NACAC, Washington, D.C., 1978.

93*b*. Sorosky, Baran, and Panner, *The Adoption Triangle,* Doubleday, New York, 1984.

94. Lipsett, M. B., "20 Years of Progress in Child Health Research," *Children Today* **12**(4):104 (July–August 1983).
95. Abarbanel, Alice, "Shared Parenting after Separation and Divorce: A Study of Joint Custody," *American Journal of Orthopsychiatry* **49**(2):320–329 (April 1978).

3

Dorothy J. DeMaio

Child health care: history and trends

Upon completion of this chapter, the student will be able to:

1 Identify four societal factors that impeded progress in the delivery of child health care prior to the twentieth century.
2 Describe the historical roots of the nurse as a provider and promoter of sick- and well-child services.
3 List four major governmental activities or programs that significantly influenced the delivery of child health services in the United States.
4 List two documents on child health that reflect U.S. and worldwide concern for children to grow and develop in health.
5 Give examples of the variety of roles and settings in which maternal-child nurses function.
6 Compare child health services in Scandinavia and Great Britain with those in the United States.
7 Discuss the standards of maternal-child nursing practice and their value to practicing nurses and the consumer.

"Maintenance and promotion of health care are the nation's first line of defense in building a healthy society."[1] Finding someone to oppose this statement would be as difficult as finding someone to challenge the belief that health care is the right of every citizen. Yet endless reports from health planners, local and federal health agencies, and consumer health advocates conclude that broad-spectrum health care is lacking for children. A look at history may be helpful in explaining why children in the United States still have problems gaining access to health care.

Child health care in primitive societies

Very little has been recorded about the health care of children in early primitive societies. However, from the evidence it seems clear that, although most children received the physical care essential for survival, some received very different treatment from that received by others. Vitality and strength were often the key to survival. Weak or malformed infants were commonly allowed to die from neglect. In some primitive cultures males were valued, and females, if born in excess numbers, were destroyed.

The advent of child health care

As civilization advanced and humans learned to grow their food, manufacture clothing and tools, and shelter themselves, children became important to the group.

Religious teachings strongly influenced attitudes toward children as individuals and as family members. In ancient Israel the health practices prescribed by Mosaic law improved the quality of life for children. Christianity placed stress on the love of one for another and the need to care for the weak as well as the strong.

Recognition that children have special needs did not become widespread until the sixteenth century, when certain religious orders took as their special mission the care and nursing of children. Vincent de Paul (later St. Vincent) championed the cause of abandoned children and established the Hospital for Foundlings. He was horrified by the way La Couche, the existing institution for abandoned children, indiscriminately gave the children to professional beggars, who sometimes mutilated them to make them more useful in begging. Vincent de Paul founded the Sisters of Charity, one of the earliest nursing orders. The Sisters made the bodily and material needs of children their cause.

In the seventeenth century, the educator John Amos Comenius sought in his writings to aid parents in understanding their children. He provided information on child-rearing practices that fostered emotional health. He believed that in this way the child would find it easier to undertake learning. He also wrote about the importance of age-appropriate sensory stimulation beginning in the home. His important writings included *The School of Infancy* (also known as *The School of the Maternal Bosom*),[2] which was published in 1633 and advocated a healthy relationship between the mother and the child. Jean Piaget considered Comenius one of the pioneers in developmental psychology.[3]

In the eighteenth century, the problem of neglected and abandoned children grew worse. It became common for impoverished mothers to place infants on the doorsteps of the rich or to leave them in the street, where they often died from starvation or exposure.[4] In London between 1730 and 1750, 75 percent of all babies christened died before the age of 5. At times mothers rid themselves of their own newborn children so that they could help support their families by serving as wet nurses for the infants of wealthy women who considered breast-feeding unfashionable. Hospital records of this period show repeated entries noting "death from want of breast milk."[5] In 1761 the educator Jean-Jacques Rousseau attempted in his book *Emile* to persuade mothers to breast-feed and nurture their own infants. Another drawback to the use of wet nurses was the spread of disease from these impoverished women to the children they nursed, further contributing to the high rate of infant mortality.

Child health care in the United States

The nineteenth century was a period of rapid industrialization in the United States. Little thought was given to the special needs of children. In fact, ordinary working people lacked even the basic health services. Children were considered the property of their parents and were often used by them to increase their income.

Children were an essential part of the work force. They were often given dangerous jobs in mines and mills. They also worked on farms and as servants in homes. Parents valued having many children as insurance against the inevitable loss of some family members to disease.

Specialization in the care of sick children

Although educators like Comenius and Rousseau were concerned with the emotional health and the education of children, specialists in their physical health did not emerge until the latter half of the nineteenth century. Of course, great physicians as far back as Hippocrates had reported on diseases peculiar to children, but little interest was shown in the management of childhood illness. It was common for hospitalized children to share a bed with six to eight others or even with seriously ill adults.[6]

In 1855 the first hospital for sick children, Children's Hospital of Philadelphia, was established. In 1860 Dr. Abraham Jacobi opened a clinic for children in New York City and lectured on childhood diseases. In time Harvard University's medical school and others developed children's clinics and educational programs focused primarily on the diseases of organ systems.[7]

The early role of nurses in the care of sick children

Although nurses attended lectures on the care of sick children during this period, the first reference to formal education of nurses in midwifery and the care of sick children occurred in 1798. At New York Hospital, a physician presented 24 lectures on "Early Discovering when the Aid of a Physician Is Necessary and Cautions for Nurses."[8] Were these lectures, by chance, the seed from which the concept of nursing diagnosis grew?

The need for "trained nurses" was first recognized in 1849 when a sanitary commission appointed by the Massachusetts Legislature to develop plans for promoting the health of the public recommended that nurses be educated to care for the sick.[9] The first U.S. nursing school began at the New England Hospital for Women and Children. Lectures were given on medical, surgical, and obstetrical conditions, but none were specifically about child care. In 1903, almost 30 years after the first school was established, nurses were registered by the states. Early boards of nurse examiners refused to register nurses whose training school did not provide a special unit in the hospital for children and relevant education in the care of sick children (Figs. 3-1 and 3-2). This position strengthened the movement to improve hospital care of children.

The early role of nurses in well-child care

Although Massachusetts recognized public health as a governmental responsibility, for a time there was little systematic or organized activity throughout the United States. Special committees and boards of health were set up to deal with specific crises, usually cholera epidemics, but had little to do otherwise.[10] Infant mortality rates were extraordinarily high. In Newark, New Jersey, the third oldest city in the nation, 2 of every 10 babies died within the first year of life. Deplorable living conditions, poor sanitation, bacteria-laden milk, ignorance of the essentials of prenatal and delivery care, and neglectful and ignorant infant feeding were the major causative factors.[11] See Fig. 3-3.

Recognizing the impact of unsanitary conditions on the raging infant mortality rate, citizens' groups, physicians, and nurses established "milk stations." "Pure milk" was distributed by nurses who also visited and instructed in the homes of "improperly fed and sick infants only."[12]

In the early part of the twentieth century the concept of providing maternal and child health services developed in the urban areas. The first governmental unit of any kind devoted solely to maternal and child health services, the Bureau of Child Hygiene in the New York City Department of Health, was organized in 1908.[13] Soon

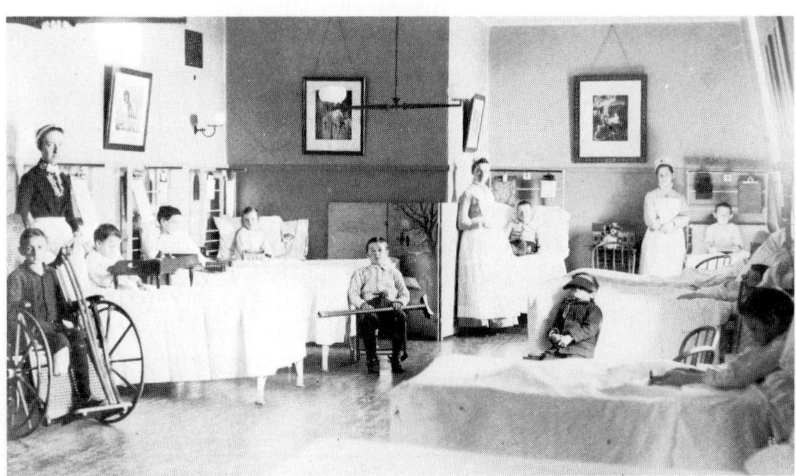

Figure 3-1 Boys' ward, circa 1900. (*Boston City Hospital School of Nursing Alumnae, Boston, Mass. Used with permission.*)

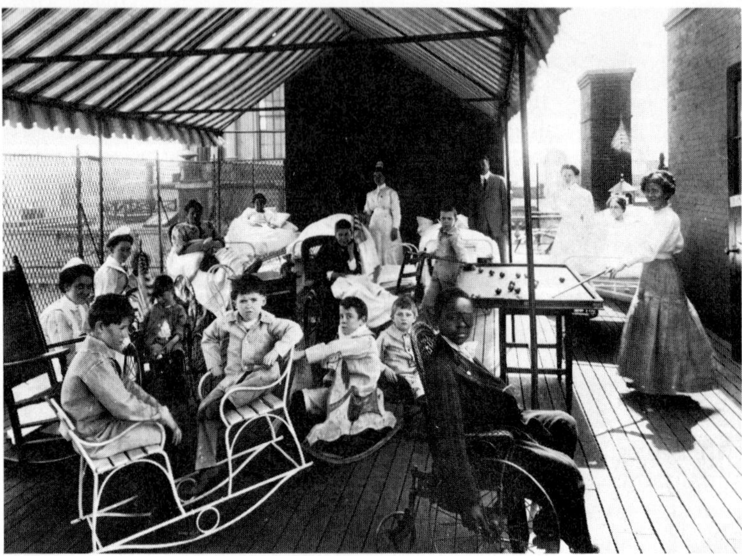

Figure 3-2 Outside on the roof, circa 1915. (*Boston City Hospital School of Nursing Alumnae, Boston, Mass. Used with permission.*)

after, other major cities created divisions of child hygiene within boards of health. Some segments of society had finally come to believe that the welfare of infants and children was the responsibility of the state. Physicians, in general, protested government involvement in the delivery of health services. Those physicians who practiced in the public health sector were very careful to assure other physicians that they would not care for children who had private physicians.

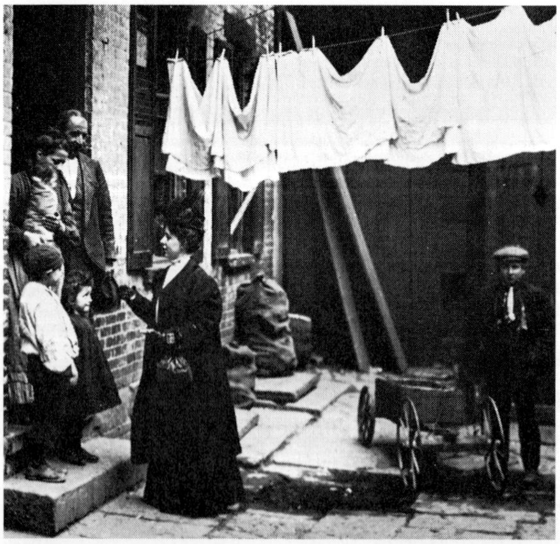

Nurses were integral to the delivery of child health services from the inception of child hygiene bureaus. For example, in the city of Newark graduate nurses were employed to teach infant hygiene and carry out the health supervision of children in the home. Additional activities included casefinding, treating ophthalmia neonatorum, managing all sickly infants delivered by midwives, caring for unmarried mothers, and resolving the problems of housing, sanitation, and poverty. Nurses also supervised hygienic practices of midwives and boarding homes for children.[14] See Fig. 3-4.

The role of nurses in school health was noted in the official records of the Board of Health of the City of Newark. In 1917 the record reported the dismissal of five physicians who provided medical inspection for the children in the 26 parochial schools in Newark. Six graduate nurses were employed to replace the physicians. These nurses were required to perform physical examinations on all the children. Physical examination was fully described in the records and was clearly distinguished from class inspection, which was an examination for cleanliness and open lesions.[15]

The historical literature reflects that child hygiene nurses, public health nurses, and school nurses were the main providers of child health services and, in many instances, the only child

Figure 3-3 A nurse from the New York City Department of Health instructing tenement dwellers about health and sanitation in 1895. (*From Annie M. Brainard, The Evolution of Public Health Nursing, Saunders, Philadelphia, 1922, p. 229. Used with permission.*)

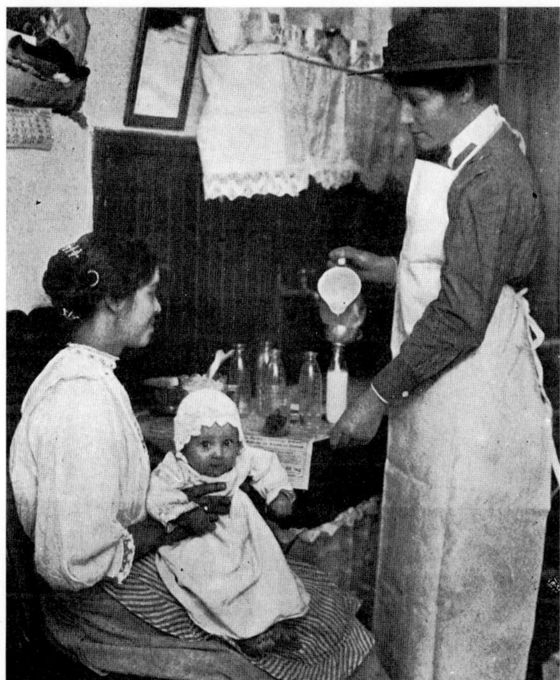

Figure 3-4 The baby welfare nurse. (*From Annie M. Brainard, The Evolution of Public Health Nursing, Saunders, Philadelphia, 1922, p. 230. Used with permission.*)

health care providers.[16] Physicians focused almost exclusively on the care of sick children. In fact as late as 1960, almost 30 years after the American Academy of Pediatrics was organized, there were constant pleas that physicians should "expand" their practices to provide child health services "whether they were completely enthusiastic about them or not."[17]

Federal government concern for child health care

President Theodore Roosevelt initiated the first national effort to address the issues relevant to the needs of children. Known as the White House Conference of 1909, it was an assembly of representatives of consumer groups and federal, national, state, and voluntary human services organizations. Subsequently, White House conferences on the needs of children have been held every 10 years. A concern through all the conferences has been the developmental and physical health needs of children. Recommendations have included changing existing services, providing new services, and reordering the nation's priorities.

Major governmental positions and programs have resulted from the White House conferences. A consequence of the 1909 conference was the creation, in 1912, of the Children's Bureau. By legislative command the Children's Bureau was ordered to study and report on all aspects of child life regardless of social class. Concern for increased and quality health care services for children emerged consistently in the bureau's reports and recommendations. Improvements had been demonstrated in the areas of prenatal care, natal care, infant feeding, and sanitation, but little, if anything, was done for the child surviving beyond infancy. The first legislation introduced in Congress to establish a maternal and infant health program was hotly debated in 1920 and 1921. Known as the Maternity and Infancy Act, or the Sheppard-Towner Act, the bill was scorned by key legislators as "radical, socialistic and bolshevistic" and a departure from "common sense."[18] Counterdebate by Representative Alben Barkley, who endorsed the act, stated that children should have "an equal chance with every child in the world, not only to be born in health and proper environment, but an equal chance to survive after they have been brought into the world." A strong lobbying effort against the bill was made by the American Medical Association.[19]

Although the opposition was intense, the Sheppard-Towner Act was signed into law in 1921. Matching funds were provided to the states, and by 1927, 45 states and the territory of Hawaii were using the funds for a variety of related purposes. These included licensing midwives, sponsoring maternal health conferences, improving the supply of public health nurses, fostering education of doctors and nurses, and creating child health centers. Although a significant number of states established child hygiene clinics, there clearly was no standardized delivery pattern throughout the country.[20]

The Great Depression of the thirties stimulated research in the Children's Bureau on nutrition and child health. The 1930 White House conference had as its theme child health and protection. As a consequence of the disturbing findings, conference participants developed the *Children's Charter,* a document of great importance in the history of child health. The *Children's Charter* recommended that every child be given health protection from birth through adolescence, including periodic health examinations and, where needed, care from specialists and hospital treatment; regular dental examinations and care of the teeth; protective and preventive measures against communicable diseases; and assurance of purity of food, milk, and water. The *Children's Charter* gave direction to the nation regarding the essentials of comprehensive child health care.

However, it was the Social Security Act of 1935 that made the most significant impact on the delivery of child health services. Through this legislation the government pledged support for state efforts to extend and improve health and welfare services for mothers and children.

Title V of the act created a structure to promote maternal and child health, to provide full medical services for handicapped children, to establish a governmental unit for crippled children's services, to develop projects to illustrate innovative and effective ways of providing maternal and child health services, and to expand child welfare services. Frequent amendments of Title V clearly reflect the nation's continuing concern for maternal and child health.[21]

The sweeping provisions of Title XIX (Medicaid) were incorporated in the 1965 amendments that were intended to influence primary care systems to provide comprehensive child health services to children from birth to age 21. Commonly known as *EPSDT* (*e*arly and *p*eriodic *s*creening, *d*iagnosis, and *t*reatment), it was mandated for all Medicaid-eligible children receiving aid to families with dependent children. Guidelines were developed defining the child health services as well as designating time intervals at which care was to be provided. Again the Medicaid-EPSDT program did not achieve the goal of comprehensive well-child care for all eligible children. Although the federal government reimbursed the states 55 percent for EPSDT services, the services were still not being provided because of some states' reluctance to put up matching funds.[22]

In 1969, when the Department of Health, Education, and Welfare (now the Department of Health and Human Services) was restructured, the Children's Bureau became part of the Office of Child Development, and some of its functions were redistributed. Maternal-child health programs are now located in a number of divisions, such as the Bureau of Community Health Services, the Health Services Administration, the Office of Maternal and Child Health, the National Health Service Corps, and the Indian Health Services. Research activities take place in all programs but are the primary focus of the National Institute of Child Health and Human Development, located in the Public Health Service.

More than 75 years have passed since the first White House conference on children. The country still struggles with many of the old problems, and new child health problems continue to emerge.

Great strides have been made in the development of child health care services in the United States, but in spite of medical and technological advances, infant mortality and childhood death rates are still higher in the United States than in many other nations (Tables 3-1 and 3-2). Research shows a difference in the availability and utilization of child health care services for children from different socioeconomic levels. Williams and Torrens report that only 44 percent of children from low-income families have a physician as a regular source of health care, compared with 75 percent of children from high-income families. In addition, 15 percent of all child health care, and 33 percent of child health care in poor urban areas, is provided in hospital emergency rooms.[23] There is also evidence to suggest differences in the health status of children in relation to socioeconomic level. For example, there is a large difference between black and white infant death rates, and the percentage of children with significant eye anomalies is higher in families whose income is less than $5000 than in those with higher incomes.[24,25] As Silver declares, "The evidence is too clear that, in child health, the United States is shamefully behind nearly every other economically and industrially advanced country in the world."[26]

Why do children, the nation's most valuable asset, continue to be deprived of needed health care? Why has this society neglected to create a reasonable, sensible health care delivery system?[27] Borgatta, an anthropologist, points out that "even a fleeting contact with the comparative study of cultures will indicate that accepted ways of doing things do not necessarily exist because of some rational basis or because they are effective."[28]

A WORLDWIDE PERSPECTIVE

The problems in delivering child health care are not unique to the United States. Established na-

Table 3-1 Changing Infant Mortality Rates in 25 Countries: Infant Mortality Rates per 1000 Births

Country	1970–1975	1980–1985*	Change between 1970–1975 and 1980–1985
Sweden	10	7	−3
Iceland	11	7	−4
Finland	12	7	−5
Norway	12	8	−4
Denmark	12	8	−4
The Netherlands	12	8	−4
Japan	12	8	−4
Switzerland	13	8	−5
France	16	10	−6
Canada	16	11	−5
Luxembourg	16	11	−5
Australia	17	11	−6
Belgium	19	11	−8
Singapore	19	11	−8
New Zealand	16	12	−4
German Democratic Republic	17	12	−5
United Kingdom	17	12	−5
Hong Kong	17	12	−5
United States of America	18	12	−6
Spain	22	12	−10
Ireland	18	13	−5
German Federal Republic	22	13	−9
Austria	24	13	−11
Italy	26	14	−12
Israel	23	15	−8

*Estimated.

Source: World Health Statistics Annual—1984, World Health Organization, Geneva, 1984, pp. 32–34.

Table 3-2 Childhood Death Rates by Age in Selected Countries, 1981

Country	Birth to 1 Year	1 to 4 Years	5 to 9 Years	10 to 14 Years	15 to 19 Years
Sweden					
Males	7.3	0.3	0.2	0.2	0.7
Females	6.4	0.2	0.1	0.1	0.3
Norway					
Males	8.5	0.5	0.3	0.3	0.9
Females	6.5	0.5	0.2	0.1	0.3
Denmark					
Males	8.5	0.5	0.4	0.3	0.8
Females	6.7	0.4	0.3	0.2	0.3
United Kingdom					
Males	12.7	0.5	0.3	0.3	0.8
Females	9.4	0.5	0.2	0.2	0.3
United States			(5 to 14 years)		
Males	13.4	0.7*	0.4*		1.6*
Females	10.3	0.5*	0.2*		0.6*

*Estimated.

Source: United Nations Demographic Year Book, 1982, United Nations, New York, 1984, pp. 398, 402, 404, 406.

Table 3-3 Declaration of the Rights of the Child*

WHEREAS the peoples of the United Nations have, in the Charter, reaffirmed their faith in fundamental human rights, and in the dignity and worth of the human person, and have determined to promote social progress and better standards of life in larger freedom,

WHEREAS the United Nations has, in the Universal Declaration of Human Rights, proclaimed that everyone is entitled to all the rights and freedoms set forth therein, without distinction of any kind, such as race, colour, sex, language, religion, political or other opinion, national or social origin, property, birth or other status,

WHEREAS the child, by reason of his physical and mental immaturity, needs special safeguards and care, including appropriate legal protection, before as well as after birth,

WHEREAS the need for such special safeguards has been stated in the Geneva Declaration of the Rights of the Child of 1924, and recognized in the Universal Declaration of Human Rights and in the statutes of specialized agencies and international organizations concerned with the welfare of children,

WHEREAS mankind owes to the child the best it has to give,

NOW THEREFORE

The General Assembly proclaims this Declaration of the Rights of the Child to the end that he may have a happy childhood and enjoy for his own good and for the good of society the rights and freedoms herein set forth, and calls upon parents, upon men and women as individuals and upon voluntary organizations, local authorities and national governments to recognize and strive for the observance of these rights by legislative and other measures progressively taken in accordance with the following principles:

I. The child shall enjoy all the rights set forth in this Declaration. All children, without any exception whatsoever, shall be entitled to these rights, without distinction or discrimination on account of race, colour, sex, language, religion, political or other opinion, national or social origin, property, birth or other status, whether of himself or of his family.

II. The child shall enjoy special protection, and shall be given opportunities and facilities, by law and by other means, to enable him to develop physically, mentally, morally, spiritually and socially in a healthy and normal manner and in conditions of freedom and dignity. In the enactment of laws for this purpose the best interests of the child shall be the paramount consideration.

III. The child shall be entitled from his birth to a name and a nationality.

IV. The child shall enjoy the benefits of social security. He shall be entitled to grow and develop in health; to this end special care and protection shall be provided both to him and to his mother, including adequate prenatal and postnatal care. The child shall have the right to adequate nutrition, housing, recreation and medical services.

V. The child who is physically, mentally, or socially handicapped shall be given the special treatment, education and care required by his particular condition.

VI. The child, for the full and harmonious development of his personality, needs love and understanding. He shall, wherever possible, grow up in the care and under the responsibility of his parents, and in any case in an atmosphere of affection and of moral and material security; a child of tender years shall not, save in exceptional circumstances, be separated from his mother. Society and the public authorities shall have the duty to extend particular care to children without a family and those without adequate means of support. Payment of state and other assistance towards the maintenance of children of large families is desirable.

VII. The child is entitled to receive education, which shall be free and compulsory at least in the elementary stages. He shall be given an education which will promote his general culture, and enable him on a basis of equal opportunity to develop his abilities, his individual judgment and his sense of moral and social responsibility, and to become a useful member of society.

The best interests of the child shall be the guiding principle of those responsible for his education and upbringing; that responsibility lies in the first place with his parents.

The child shall have full opportunity for play and recreation, which should be directed to the same purposes as education; society and the public authorities shall endeavour to promote the enjoyment of this right.

VIII. The child shall in all circumstances be among the first to receive protection and relief.

IX. The child shall be protected against all forms of neglect, cruelty and exploitation. He shall not be the subject of traffic in any form.

The child shall not be admitted to employment before an appropriate minimum age; he shall in no case be caused or permitted to engage in any occupation or employment which would prejudice his health or education or interfere with his physical, mental or moral development.

X. The child shall be protected from practices which may foster racial, religious and any other form of discrimination. He shall be brought up in a spirit of understanding, tolerance, friendship among peoples, peace and universal brotherhood and in full consciousness that his energy and talents should be devoted to the service of his fellowmen.

*As approved by the 14th General Assembly of the United Nations, Nov. 20, 1959.

Source: Children, vol. 7, U.S. Department of Health, Education, and Welfare, Social Security Administration, Children's Bureau.

tions and developing countries the world over face many of the same child health care issues. Developing countries are confronted with different cultural problems, both complex and serious, in providing for child health. There are hundreds of thousands of children who have inadequate food and immunizations and for whom little or no medical care is available.

Developing countries, even those which are rural in nature and are not significantly affected by socioeconomic change, are attempting to improve the standard of living by extending public health programs. The welfare of children is now perceived as a global issue for civilized humankind. The World Health Organization (WHO), historically the first international organization for health, was organized within the structure of the United Nations in 1948. Along with the United Nations Children's Fund (UNICEF) and other organizations, the World Health Organization has provided direction, education, and in some cases financial support to improve health care services for children. The *Declaration of the Rights of the Child* is a substantive document, approved by the United Nations in 1959, that acknowledges the right of every child in this world to have a happy childhood and to grow and develop in health (Table 3-3).

CHILD HEALTH CARE IN SCANDINAVIA AND GREAT BRITAIN*

Some countries have made more progress in child health care than the United States. Examining services that other countries provide can help us identify the gaps in our own services. The following sections describe preventive services, curative services, and social benefits in four sample countries: Denmark, Norway, Sweden, and Great Britain. These countries were chosen because in many ways their pediatric benefits and services are superior to those offered in the United States.

Most nurses who provide child health care services in these countries have completed a 1-year post-basic educational program in either pediatric or public health nursing, depending on the setting in which they practice. The role that is perhaps most interesting is that of the "health visitors" in Denmark and Great Britain. They work primarily with families who have young children, and their educational program focuses on the prevention of physical and emotional illness, the early detection of health problems, health teaching, and the promotion of normal development.[29]

*This section was written and researched by Gay J. Lindquist, R.N., M.S.

Preventive services

All four countries place a high priority on primary health care. Each country's health care delivery system is organized somewhat differently, but each has a type of socialized system and health care clinics located in various districts throughout the country. These clinics are staffed by physicians, nurses, and other health care professionals; the care provided is available either at no cost or for a nominal fee and is funded through national and/or local taxes.

Prenatal care is available to, and utilized by, virtually all expectant mothers in each country. Health visitors or public health nurses visit each family at least once prior to delivery to meet the family and assess the home situation.[30] All births are reported, and infants' records are forwarded to health clinics.[31] Follow-up on these reports varies in the four countries, but at least one home visit to each family is made by a health visitor or a public health nurse. Home visits, by a health visitor, continue throughout the first 2 years of a child's life in Denmark, and then parents take children to their family physician (Fig. 3-5). Health visitors in Great Britain may continue to

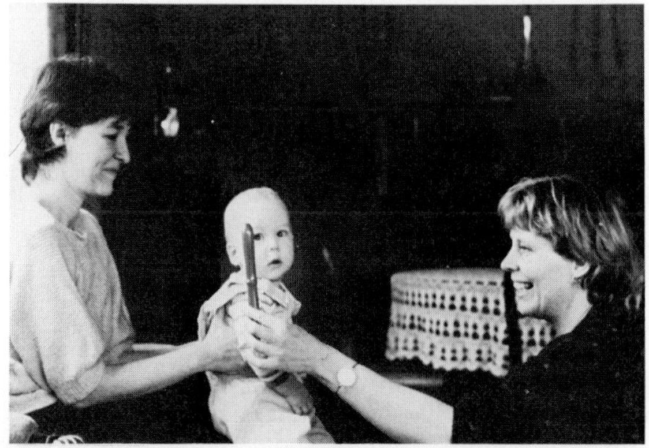

Figure 3-5 A Danish health visitor doing a visual assessment on an 8-month-old child during a routine home visit. (*Photo by Gay Lindquist.*)

make home visits throughout the preschool years or see children at a health clinic. In Norway and Sweden, parents regularly take their young children to health clinics. Statistics show, for example, the following attendance percentages for children of different ages in Sweden: 1 year, 99 percent; 2 years, 98 percent; 3 years, 83 percent; and 4 years, 97 percent.[32] In each country, if parents do not bring children to the clinics, home visits are made.

Health surveillance in each country, whether in the home or in a clinic, includes physical examinations, screening for vision or hearing defects, immunizations, and complete developmental assessments. Most of this is done by nurses, but physicians are also available for routine physical examinations and consultation. Parent and child teaching is done by nurses; this teaching includes information related to the promotion of normal development, good nutrition, safety, health care, and other concerns related to child rearing. The schedule for assessments varies slightly in the four countries, but all children are seen routinely throughout the preschool years. Health and developmental problems are therefore detected early, and appropriate referrals for diagnosis and treatment are made.

Dental care is also an important part of preventive child health care in all these countries. Public dental health clinics or school dentists provide free dental care to all children, beginning at age 3 in Scandinavia and at age 5 in Great Britain. Annual examinations are done throughout the school years.[33,34]

Each of these countries also has a well-organized school health care service that is staffed by general practitioners and public health nurses or health visitors, and other health care professionals are available on a consultative basis. Records from the health clinics are available to the school health service, or, as in Norway, the health clinics are located next to the schools and share the same facilities and staff. Complete examinations are done on each child before he or she starts school. The schedule for additional routine health examinations varies slightly in the four countries, but most commonly examinations are done in grades 1, 3, 7, and 9. In Great Britain, examinations are not done routinely in grades 4 and 7, but health questionnaires are completed by parents and teachers for each child at age 8 and age 12. Children with identified problems are referred to the family's general practitioner or an appropriate specialist. Personnel in the school health care services are also responsible for seeing children with minor illnesses, implementing immunization programs, investigating communicable diseases, and inspecting the hygienic conditions of schools. Nurses in the school health care services are responsible for health education; they cover such areas as physical fitness, sex education, and the prevention of disease.[35]

Curative services

In all these countries, if a child acquires an illness that does not require hospitalization, parents may take the child to their family practitioner or go to a child health clinic to seek care. In Sweden, parents are advised to call a nurse at the child health clinic, who may give advice over the phone or see the child in the clinic. Nurses may also refer parents to the local general practitioner, to a pediatrician, or directly to a hospital. The hospitals themselves provide 24-h pediatric consultation services that parents can use when clinics are closed.[36] Home nursing care is provided, when necessary, by district or public health nurses in all four countries; efforts are made to keep children at home whenever possible.

Acute and long-term care facilities in all these countries are similar to those in the United States, except that family practitioners are not on the hospital staffs and hospital care is supervised by staff pediatricians. Pediatric specialty hospitals are located in different regions throughout each country. There are also pediatric units in most general hospitals, but in some instances, particularly in sparsely populated areas of northern Sweden, children may be cared for on adult wards. It is interesting to note, however, that all hospitalized children in Sweden, whether on a pediatric or an adult ward, have a legal right to play therapy and schooling.[37] Pediatric intensive care units are regionalized in all four countries, and ambulances are available, free of charge, for transport when necessary.

The philosophy of inpatient pediatric care is similar in all four countries; a truly family-centered approach to care is implemented. Cots are available for parents who wish to stay overnight, and in some hospitals special parent units with private bedrooms, lounges, bathrooms, and kitchens are provided free of charge. Generally, parents must pay a nominal fee for meals unless the mother is breast-feeding or their child is critically ill. Both room and board are provided at no cost for one parent when a child is in an intensive care unit, and only a nominal fee is charged for the second parent. Parents are encouraged to be involved in routine aspects of their child's care, such as feeding and bathing, even in intensive care units. In Sweden, if parents live far away and cannot stay with their child, free air transportation is provided weekly for visits. Visits by siblings are also encouraged in each country.

Efforts are made in all these countries to provide as homelike an environment in the hospital as possible. Wards are decorated with bright colors, cheerful posters, and colorful pictures. Children are also encouraged to dress in their own clothes or pajamas whenever feasible.

Great emphasis is placed on therapeutic play for hospitalized children in all four countries.[38] Playrooms are available on all wards and are well equipped with many toys for children of all ages (Fig. 3-6). Children are encouraged to go to playrooms whenever possible, even if they must be moved in their beds. Children who are unable to leave their rooms have toys brought to them. Play programs are supervised by "play teachers" or "nursery nurses." These people have special educational preparation in normal growth and development and therapeutic play. They are well integrated into the staff and sit in on change-of-shift reports in order to become aware of patients' problems and activity restrictions, as well as to discuss children's play needs.

The educational needs of children are also given a high priority in all four countries. Qualified teachers are an integral part of the staff; often they are employed full-time in large institutions and part-time in small hospitals. A schoolroom is usually provided, and teachers communicate with the children's local educational authorities to help them keep up with their schoolwork. There is a trend toward daytime-only hospital care for children who need treatment or diagnostic testing. Separate units, or designated beds on pediatric wards, are utilized for this purpose. These units are staffed with qualified registered nurses and "play teachers." These units are designed to decrease the stress due to hospitalization and separation from the family, as well as to lower health care costs.

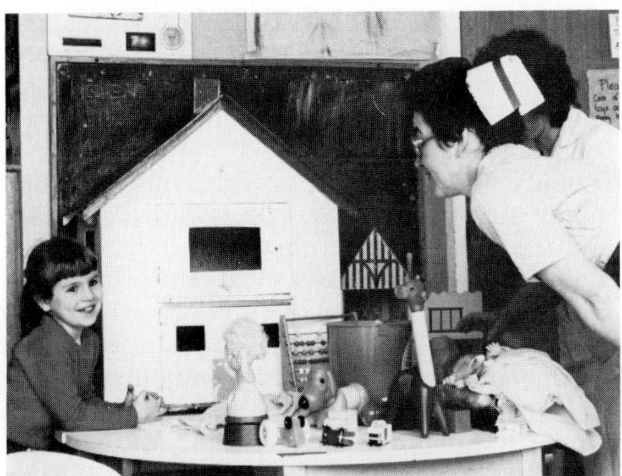

Figure 3-6 A British nurse in a playroom with a hospitalized child. (*Photo by Gay Lindquist.*)

The communication between hospital staff members and health visitors or district nurses is excellent in all four countries. Even in many small hospitals, weekly conferences are held at which hospital and community nursing staff members discuss patients' needs and approaches to care.

A wide variety of facilities and resources are also available for children who have handicaps or chronic illnesses. Many services for these children are provided in centers or clinics located in different regions of each country. For example, Sweden is divided into seven regions, each with a major, central pediatric clinic that has a rehabilitation department for handicapped children. These clinics provide a variety of diagnostic and medical treatment services on both an inpatient and an outpatient basis. They also provide physical therapy, speech therapy, special education, social services, and training in the activities of daily life. In Great Britain, after an initial assessment at a comprehensive assessment center for handicapped children, the responsibilities for providing medical care and educational services are divided between the area health authorities and local educational authorities.[39] National registers for handicapped children exist in each country; they provide a means of following handicapped children and identifying any unusual occurrence of handicapping conditions.[40]

The concept of integration underlies the care and services provided for handicapped children in the Nordic countries. This means that children with any kind of handicap are "integrated" into society and are allowed to lead as normal a life as possible. The concept of integration has three components: *physical integration,* which means that handicapped children attend regular schools; *functional integration,* which means that handicapped children use the same transportation and visit the same places as other children; and, the most comprehensive component of the concept, *social* or *psychological integration,* which means that handicapped children have the same rights, duties, and responsibilities as other children in the society. One can see this concept implemented in many ways. For example, the majority of handicapped children now live in their parents' homes rather than in institutions. A similar concept underlies the care and services for handicapped children in Great Britain.

Various kinds of support services are available to parents of handicapped or chronically ill children in all four countries. These include day-care centers, home nursing care, housekeeping help, and social services. All these services are designed to provide the help necessary to keep children in their homes. There are some residential facilities and special schools available for children who require these services.

Social benefits

Social benefits for families with young children are extensive in all four countries. These stem from a common belief that all people, regardless of age or socioeconomic status, are entitled to a certain standard of living and to the best health care available.

Paid maternity leaves, usually with guaranteed reemployment, are available for working women. These may be shared between mothers and fathers in the Nordic countries. For example, in Norway, a working mother is entitled to 90 days of paid maternity leave. If she returns to work before that time and the father stays home to care for the infant, he may be paid the maternity allowance. If the mother is not eligible for a maternity allowance, she may be paid a lump sum after the birth.[41] In Sweden, at the time of a birth, the father receives 10 days off, with pay, to care for other children in the family.[42]

Many other benefits are available to provide economic support for families with young children in all these countries. One example is a children's allowance paid to parents for each child. Other compensations include rent and/or food subsidies for large families and special allowances for single or widowed parents. Assistance with payment for day care, either in day-care centers or by child-minders in the home, is available for working parents. In Sweden, this means of adjusting income to meet the special needs of families is called *social wages*.[43,44]

Other social benefits are available to children from families with financial need, or in some instances to all children, in all these countries. For example, in Great Britain, such things as free school meals, free milk and vitamins, free travel to school, and grants for school uniforms and clothing are available.[45]

In all four countries, families are also eligible for special benefits when children are ill. Free transportation to hospitals or clinics is generally available if a family has a low income. Prescriptions for medications are filled free of charge. Some countries, such as Sweden, provide paid parental leave, for either parent, so that one can stay home from work to care for a sick child.

Other benefits are available to families with handicapped or chronically ill children. Examples include payment for any special aids necessary for bathing, feeding, or dressing a child; house adaptations, such as ramps and rails; necessary appliances, such as hearing aids; home helpers to assist with housework; and child-minders, so that parents can get out of the home periodically. Necessary home nursing services are also available free of charge. In Denmark, if a child is chronically ill and a parent gives up a job in order to care for the child, that parent can be paid a salary.

Summary

This discussion does not cover all the health and social benefits provided to families with children in these four countries, but it does give examples of many of the benefits available. In all four countries, comprehensive health care is provided to all children, with particular emphasis on preventive health care. The health of children is given a high priority, and a wide variety of benefits and services are provided to support the family structure. As we look toward the future and strive to improve child health care in the United States, perhaps we can learn by examining the child health care services available in countries that have exceeded us in terms of providing health care and social benefits to their younger citizens. Certainly we can agree with them that an investment of time, energy, and money in our children is a worthwhile investment in the future of our nation.

NURSING PRACTICE TODAY: A PERSPECTIVE

The American Nurses' Association (ANA) has provided leadership toward assuring the public of quality nursing services by establishing *standards of practice*. These standards serve as a guide for all practicing nurses in that they assist them in assuring the public of quality nursing care. In addition, the standards establish a baseline for nursing practice for which the nurse must be responsible and accountable when providing nursing care. All nurses must be familiar with, and guide their practice by, the concepts included in the standards. Logically, with time and research, these standards will change. Presently in some states the standards are used as a guide for state boards of nursing in their interpretation of the Nursing Practice Acts.

Standards specific to the specialty of maternal-child health were published by the American Nurses' Association in 1973. The *Standards of Maternal-Child Health Nursing Practice* provide a rationale for each standard and the steps in the process essential to good nursing care. Some individual standards are listed in Table 3-4.

Nursing expertise and services are essential on the total health-illness continuum. Whether the child is in a primary (health-maintenance), secondary (acute care), tertiary (specialty hospital), or long-term health care setting, the nurse needs to synthesize many different pieces of information about the child and the family in order

Table 3-4 American Nurses' Association Standards of Maternal-Child Health Nursing Practice

Standard I
Maternal and child health nursing practice is characterized by the continual questioning of the assumptions upon which practice is based, retaining those which are valid and searching for and using new knowledge.

Standard II
Maternal and child health nursing practice is based upon knowledge of the biophysical and psychosocial development of individuals from conception through the child-rearing phase of development and upon knowledge of the basic needs for optimum development.

Standard III
The collection of data about the health status of the client/patient is systematic and continuous. The data are accessible, communicated and recorded.

Standard IV
Nursing diagnoses are derived from data about the health status of the patient.

Standard V
Maternal and child health nursing practice recognizes deviations from expected patterns of physiologic activity and anatomic and psychosocial development.

Standard VI
The plan of nursing care includes goals derived from the nursing diagnoses.

Standard VII
The plan of nursing care includes priorities and the prescribed nursing approaches or measures to achieve the goals derived from the nursing diagnoses.

Standard VIII
Nursing actions provide for client/patient participation in health promotion, maintenance and restoration.

Standard IX
Maternal and child health nursing practice provides for the use and coordination of all services that assist individuals to prepare for responsible sex roles.

Standard X
Nursing actions assist the client/patient to maximize his health capabilities.

Standard XI
The client's/patient's progress or lack of progress toward goal achievement is determined by the client/patient and the nurse.

Standard XII
The client's/patient's progress or lack of progress toward goal achievement directs reassessment, reordering of priorities, new goal setting and revision of the plan of nursing care.

Standard XIII
Maternal and child health nursing practice evidences active participation with others in evaluating the availability, accessibility and acceptability of services for parents and children and cooperating and/or taking leadership in extending and developing needed services in the community.

Source: Standards of Maternal-Child Health Nursing Practice, American Nurses' Association, Kansas City, 1973. Used with permission.

to provide maximum benefits to them. Nurses must have a substantial knowledge base in order to make the multitude of judgments and decisions required when attending to the unique and highly individualized emotional and physical needs of children.

Rapid technological advances have brought about many changes in nursing practice. Specialization in pediatric nursing is common at the master's level. Increased emphasis is placed on peer review programs, quality assurance, and nursing research. Current continuing education programs in pediatric nursing are broad in scope, focusing on child health maintenance and illness prevention as well as care of the ill child.

Pediatric nurses who wish to validate the quality of their practice may seek certification in nursing of the neonate, child, or adolescent with an acute or chronic illness or a disabling condition. Certification in this area of practice is sponsored by the ANA Division on Maternal-Child Health Nursing Practice. Registered nurses who meet minimum clinical experience requirements and who are currently practicing in a pediatric clinical setting are eligible to apply.

Candidates for certification are required to pass a written examination. They must also submit written documentation and peer references "to provide evidence of the nature and quality of a candidate's clinical practice."[46] Written documentation includes a description of the nurse's practice setting, the individual's personal philosophy of nursing, and a case study which demonstrates use of the ANA standards of practice. Case studies are evaluated anonymously by at least two nurse reviewers who are knowledgeable in pediatric nursing and the nursing process. Nurses who successfully demonstrate the established criteria are awarded certification.

Certification in ambulatory child care nursing practice is also available through the ANA. Only registered nurses who practice in ambulatory settings and who meet certain educational requirements are eligible, however. The process for certification in this area of practice is similar to the one described above.

Providing care to assist children in regaining health is a large part of the contemporary pediatric nurse's role. Nurses prepared at both the technical and professional levels provide care to ill children. As a care-provider, the modern pediatric nurse is responsible for patient counseling and teaching as well as serving as a child and family advocate. Nurses prepared at the baccalaureate and master's levels assume the additional responsibilities of planning and coordinating care and maintaining and promoting child health. Healthy children are the first line of defense in building a healthy society.[47]

References

1. Rogers, Martha, *An Introduction to the Theoretical Basis of Nursing,* Davis, Philadelphia, 1970, p. 122.
2. Benham, David, "A Sketch of the Life of the Author," in John Amos Comenius, *The School of Infancy,* W. Mallalieu, London, 1858, p. 117.
3. Piaget, Jean, "The Significance of John Amos Comenius at the Present Time," in *John Amos Comenius on Education,* Teachers College, New York, 1967, p. 2.
4. Dolan, Josephine A., *Nursing in Society,* Saunders, Philadelphia, 1978, p. 112.
5. Ibid.
6. Stokes, J., *Pediatrics: Choice of a Medical Career,* Lippincott, Philadelphia, 1961, p. 2.
7. Ibid., p. 31.
8. Kalisch, Philip A., and Beatrice J. Kalisch, *The Advance of American Nursing,* Little, Brown, Boston, 1978, p. 72.
9. Ibid., p. 77.
10. Galishoff, Stuart, *Safeguarding the Public Health—Newark, 1895–1918,* Greenwood Press, Westport, Conn., 1975, p. 109.
11. Ibid., p. 110.
12. Waters, Yssabella, *Visiting Nurses in the United States,* Wm. F. Ball, Philadelphia, 1909, p. 166.
13. Schlesinger, Edward R., "The Impact of Federal Legislation on Maternal-Child Health Services in the United States," *Health and Society,* Milbank Memorial Fund Quarterly, Winter 1974, p. 3.
14. New Jersey, City of Newark, Board of Health, *Annual Report,* 1915, p. 177.
15. ———, *Annual Report,* 1917.
16. DeMaio, Dorothy, "Comprehensive Well-Child Care: A Descriptive Analysis of a System in Which Services Were Provided by Physicians and Primary Health Care Nurses/Pediatric Nurse Practitioners," Ed.D. dissertation, Rutgers, New Brunswick, N.J., 1979, p. 46.
17. *Health Supervision of Children,* American Public Health Association, Committee on Child Health, New York, 1960, p. 18.
18. U.S. Department of Health, Education, and Welfare, *Child Health in America,* Public Health Service, Rockville, Md., 1976, p. 29.

19. Ibid., p. 30.
20. Ibid., p. 32.
21. Lesser, Arthur J., *Maternal and Child Health Service Programs,* U.S. Department of Health, Education, and Welfare, Maternal-Child Health Service, Washington, February 1973, Introduction.
22. *A Guide to Screening EPDST,* U.S. Department of Health, Education, and Welfare, Medicaid, Washington.
23. Williams, Stephen, and Paul Torrens, *Introduction to Health Services,* 2d ed., Wiley, New York, 1984, p. 80.
24. Mitchell, Karen, and Richard Harbin, "Our Children: An Economic Priority," *Pediatric Nursing* **11**(2):82 (March–April 1985).
25. Pratt, Margaret, "The Demography of Maternal and Child Health," in Helen Wallace, Edwin Gold, and Allan Aglesby (eds.), *Maternal and Child Health Practice, Problems, Resources and Methods of Delivery,* 2d ed., Wiley, New York, 1982, p. 99.
26. Silver, George A., *Child Health: America's Future,* Aspen Systems, Germantown, Md., 1978, p. 3.
27. DeMaio, op. cit., p. 30.
28. Borgatta, Edgar F., "Research Problems in Evaluation of Health Services," in John B. McKinlay (ed.), *Research Methods in Health Care,* Milbank Memorial Fund, New York, 1973, p. 20.
29. Owen, G. M., "Health Visiting," in Peter Allan and Moya Jolley (eds.), *Nursing, Midwifery and Health Visiting since 1900,* Faber, London, 1982, pp. 96–97.
30. Davies, Brian M., *Community Health, Preventative Medicine and Social Services,* Baillière, London, 1979, p. 186.
31. Peterson, P. Owe, "Aspects of the European and Especially Swedish MCH Services," *Tropical Pediatrics and Environmental Child Health* **24**(2):68 (April 1978).
32. Harker, P., "Child Health Services in Sweden," *Public Health* (London) **94**(3):147 (May 1980).
33. Peterson, loc. cit.
34. Davies, op. cit., p. 151.
35. Wallace, Helen M., "The Role of Maternal and Child Health in a National Health Service," *Children Today* **4**(2):2–6 (March–April 1975).
36. Eastwood, J., "Infant Mortality and Child Care: An Elective Experience in Sweden," *New Zealand Medical Journal* **93**(679):155 (March 1981).
37. Kohler, Lennart, "Chronically Ill and Handicapped Children in the Nordic Countries," *Acta Paediatrics Scandinavia* **73**(2):166 (March 1984).
38. Great Britain Department of Health and Social Security, *Health Services in Britain,* H. M. Stationery Office, London, 1977, p. 22.
39. Ibid.
40. Wallace, p. 218.
41. *Social Insurance in Norway,* National Insurance Administration, Oslo, March 1984, p. 18.
42. Silver, op. cit., p. 208.
43. Ibid.
44. *Social Insurance in Norway,* p. 30.
45. Great Britain Department of Health and Social Security, op. cit., pp. 10–11.
46. American Nurses' Association Division of Maternal-Child Health Nursing Practice, *Guidelines for Written Documentation, Certification in Nursing of the Child/Adolescent with Acute or Chronic Illness or Disabling Condition,* American Nurses' Association, Kansas City, 1980.
47. Rogers, loc. cit.

4

Patricia Crisham

Moral and ethical considerations in child health nursing

Upon completion of this chapter, the student will be able to:

1. Identify moral and ethical issues of concern to the pediatric nurse.
2. Recognize conflicts of rights and responsibilities in specific nursing situations.
3. Recognize the role of the nurse's own values and the values of others in making responses to nursing dilemmas.
4. Use force-field analysis to analyze driving and restraining forces in nursing situations.
5. Examine the nurse's role in facilitating the ethical decision-making process.
6. Analyze nursing dilemmas in terms of selected ethical principles.
7. Plan to implement decisions for resolving moral and ethical dilemmas.

The basic subjects of this book are the child, the family, and health. Interaction between the nurse, the child, and the family potentially enhances health and well-being. The premise of this chapter is that moral and ethical dilemmas, which usually show up as upsetting experiences for individuals and involve a great deal of confusion and struggle, can affect the quality of health care. This chapter considers the possibility that moral and ethical dilemmas in nursing practice are opportunities for nurses, individually and collectively, to rediscover and re-create their commitments in nursing.

Advances in technology and the growing complexity of the health care delivery system, including the enactment of a reimbursement system based on diagnosis-related groups (DRGs), have resulted in increasingly complex moral and ethical dilemmas for the nurse who works with children and their families. The purpose of this chapter is to identify ethical issues inherent in pediatric nursing and to propose a method that nurses can use to analyze the associated dilemmas.

The primary purpose of nursing is to promote optimal health; this is achieved through the nursing process, which is essentially a problem-solving process. The classic nursing process involves the five major steps of assessment, nursing diagnosis, planning, implementation, and evaluation of the significant variables in a nursing situation. While each step involves conscious decision making by the nurse, the end result of the nursing process is a choice of action concerning the continued nursing care of a particular child and his or her family. Value commitments are inherent in this problem-solving process. As nurses participate in decision making about care for a child and the child's family, they are making moral judgments that have an effect on others.

BABY DOE REGULATIONS

Value issues in health care have been highlighted during the past few years. The complex ethical dilemmas that arise in newborn intensive care units have focused national attention on moral issues and points of view. On April 15, 1982, a 6-day-old infant, Baby Doe, died at Bloomington Hospital in Indiana after his parents, with the approval of the courts, chose to withhold surgery, food, and water. Although the facts of the case as reported were inconsistent, the infant was apparently born with a tracheoesophageal fistula. This condition is usually corrected with surgery, but Baby Doe had Down syndrome as well, and it was seemingly for this reason that his parents chose to allow him to die. This case was widely reported in the media and resulted in public controversy and debate about moral points of view.

The controversy surrounding the Baby Doe case, as well as several other well-publicized cases of infants with severe congenital anomalies, resulted in a series of Baby Doe regulations.[1,2] The 1985 regulation contained guidelines to encourage the establishment and operation of infant care review committees. These regulations had shifted from the governmental intervention of the 1982 regulations to support for local infant care review committees that would analyze individual cases and options. These hospital-based committees were described in the March 1983 report of the President's Commission for the Study of Ethical Problems in Medicine and Biomedical and Behavioral Research.[3] The President's commission recommended that the family and the health care provider collaborate in a continuing *process* directed at making decisions that would promote the infant's and the family's best interests in terms of health, well-being, and autonomy.

A broad range of health care associations, including the American Nurses' Association, had taken the position that a collaborative process—which includes ongoing conversations among health care professionals, patients, and their families—is central to the resolution of moral and ethical dilemmas in health care. Numerous health care professional associations had previously endorsed the proposal in the March 1983 report of the President's commission for hospital-based committees as the forum and focal point for efforts to assure that treatment decisions would be informed, thoughtful, and consistent with established standards. Earlier, the American Nurses' Association[4] had passed a resolution calling for the clarification of ethical issues in clinical practice and the development of a process through which nurses could actively participate in ethical decision making.

ETHICAL DILEMMAS IN NURSING

Moral and ethical issues in health care are a worldwide concern. The International Council of Nurses[5] published descriptive statements of nurses from 25 countries identifying ethical problems in nursing practice. Examples of ethical problems, including those involving children and their families, are grouped according to the five main facets of the *Code for Nurses* of the International Council of Nurses: nurses and people, nurses and practice, nurses and society, nurses and coworkers, and nurses and the profession.

Research has begun to identify ethical dilemmas in nursing and to examine nurses' responses to ethical conflict. To systematically document the ethical dilemmas that nurses encounter in their practice and to characterize the ways in which nursing practitioners perceive and respond to these dilemmas, volunteer staff nurses were interviewed.[6] Of the total of 345 nurses interviewed between 1979 and 1985, 85 nurses described dilemmas related to children and their families.

In all the dilemmas, the nurse was in a situation in which it appeared that there was a moral obligation to follow two incompatible courses of action. Such situations raise numerous questions about rights and responsibilities, about who should decide, about criteria to be used in making decisions, and about the primary commitment and loyalty of the nurse. Are nurses accountable to the family, the child, the physicians, themselves, the health care institution, the profession, or society?

A dilemma was classified as a *recurrent nursing moral dilemma* if a minimum of five nurses reported having encountered it. These recurrent moral dilemmas experienced by nurses who worked with children and their families were grouped according to four underlying ethical issues: (1) *deciding the right to know and determining the right to decide,* (2) *defining and promoting quality of life,* (3) *maintaining professional and institutional standards,* and (4) *distributing nursing resources.*

The right to know and decide

Examples of dilemmas associated with the first issue, deciding the right to know and determining the right to decide, include whether a parent has truly given informed consent; whether to correct biased information given to parents and children by a colleague or to say nothing; whether to be an advocate for a child against the wishes of the family or to respect the family's wishes; whether to safeguard a teenager's confidence or to give the information to parents; whether to give information about laboratory tests when the tests have not yet been given or when the information is being withheld; and whether to give information to families about the risks associated with a prescribed treatment.

Quality of life

The second issue, defining and promoting quality of life, includes dilemmas about whether to resuscitate a child; whether to support aggressive nutrition therapy, including hyperalimentation, or drug therapy, including experimental chemotherapy; whether to take a stand on interventions with a newborn with severe anomalies, such as a shunt for congenital hydrocephalus; and whether to give a P.R.N. dosage of medicine that is capable of causing death to a terminally ill teenager.

Maintaining standards

Examples of dilemmas associated with the third issue, maintaining professional and institutional standards, include whether to accept responsibility or delegate authority to other staff members; whether to refuse admission of an infant when the neonatal intensive care unit census is at the maximum; whether to replace an experienced, competent nurse with an inexperienced nurse who is not oriented to the setting; whether to cover for a colleague's negligence; and whether to implement a procedure that would benefit a child but would violate agency policy.

Distributing nursing resources

The fourth issue, distributing nursing resources, results in dilemmas about whether to implement legislative allocation and rationing guidelines for the care of newborns; how to allocate the time of the staff on duty and how to determine who will give direct care to the most seriously ill children; whether to set aside time for patient teaching about health promotion and prevention in a busy, acute care setting; and whether to support legislation to increase expenditures for extraordinarily expensive new medical technology.

How can the nurse create a context in which to experience dilemmas as an opportunity for rediscovering and redefining commitments? Like Socrates, who raised questions when Athenians came to him for advice, the nurse has an opportunity to raise questions when grappling with ethical issues inherent in nursing. It is the nurse's willingness to raise questions that will most significantly facilitate the resolution of ethical conflicts. Ethical dilemmas become an opportunity to "live in the question" and to raise basic questions such as, "What are nursing's reasons for being?" "What is the purpose for which the nursing intervention is used?" "Who am I?" and "What are my commitments?"

A NURSING ETHICAL DILEMMA: INFANT WITH MULTIPLE ANOMALIES

The following Nursing Care Plan illustrates the nursing process as it would be used with an infant with multiple anomalies and with the infant's parents.

As the nurse implemented this plan, the following ethical dilemma emerged. During the afternoon of the day after admission, Mrs. James signed the surgical permit to correct the tracheoesophageal fistula. One-half h later, the nurse

Nursing Care Plan: Infant with Multiple Anomalies*

ASSESSMENT

Mr. and Mrs. James have just become the parents of a son, born at 35 weeks gestation. During the course of the initial physical examination, a strong suggestion of Down syndrome is noted. Cardiac and gastrointestinal anomalies are evidenced by cyanosis, tachycardia, tachypnea, and his rapidly distending abdomen.

The parents are informed of their son's condition. They are visibly upset. Because of the labor and delivery process, both parents are physically and emotionally drained. Now they must deal with their infant's poor condition, mental retardation, and multiple anomalies. The parents must make a decision about surgery to repair the digestive defect. The danger of operating is compounded by the infant's prematurity and cardiac status.

The parents ask to see their son and are taken to the neonatal intensive care unit. The baby is attached to various monitors, has a nasogastric tube inserted, is receiving oxygen, and has an umbilical line. The parents appear extremely anxious and concerned. They ask several times about their child's mental retardation and what can be done to help it. They are also concerned about what the operation will do for their son.

The physical assessment suggests that the James's infant requires comprehensive medical and nursing care. (See the section "Neonatal Care of the High-Risk Infant" in Chap. 17.) The care plan which follows focuses on the parents. Although the nurse is responsible for the physical care of the infant, it is also important that the nurse consider the needs of the parents in planning and providing care for this family unit.

Nursing Diagnosis	Outcome Criteria	Nursing Interventions	Evaluation and Revision
1. Parental grief secondary to birth of defective infant.	☐ The parents will be able to verbalize feelings of anger and sadness (short-term goal)	☐ Provide privacy when talking with the parents. ☐ Help the parents explore their feelings and emotions. ☐ Tell the parents that their reactions are normal; repeat this as much as necessary. ☐ Keep the parents informed of their baby's condition and the care being provided. ☐ Do not wait for the parents to ask questions; provide frequent opportunities for them to discuss their baby.	☐ Day after admission: The parents are confused and bewildered. They keep saying that their son is sick "because of us." Mrs. James can touch the baby with her fingertips, but Mr. James only looks at him. *Revision* (day after admission): ☐ Reinforce that the baby's condition did not occur because of something the parents did or didn't do.

*This nursing care plan was written by Catherine M. Kneut.

Nursing Diagnosis	Outcome Criteria	Nursing Interventions	Evaluation and Revision
2. Parental guilt feelings related to birth of defective infant.	☐ The parents will be able to participate in their son's care (long-term goal).	☐ Encourage the parents to visit the nursery at any time. ☐ Encourage the parents to hold their child. ☐ Allow the parents privacy when visiting their son. ☐ Encourage the parents to participate in their son's care, and increase their participation gradually. ☐ Expect that the parents may direct some of their anger at the nursing staff—do *not* react personally!	☐ Continue to explore the parents' feelings. ☐ Spend time with each parent individually in order to assess personal and unique reactions. ☐ Accept the father's reluctance to touch the infant, but offer positive comments about his visits to the nursery. ☐ Continue nursing actions stated in plan.
3. Impaired decision-making ability related to crisis state.	☐ With the aid of informed consent, the parents will be able to make a decision regarding the proposed operative procedure (short-term goal).	☐ Reiterate the infant's physical problems as necessary to aid the parents' understanding (their anxiety and overload of information may interfere with comprehension). ☐ Explain that the operation will repair only the gastrointestinal defect so that the baby can be fed by mouth. ☐ Answer questions patiently. ☐ Explain the purpose of equipment used in the baby's care. ☐ Clarify what the physician has already told the parents about the infant's condition and the planned surgery. ☐ Tell the parents that the nurses understand that the decision they face is a heavy burden.	☐ Day after admission: Mr. James says he knows that his son is mentally retarded, but he keeps asking how it can be treated. Mrs. James wants to know how retarded her son will be. ☐ The parents seem overwhelmed at the prospect of surgery for so small an infant. *Revision* (day after admission): ☐ Explain that mental retardation is permanent but that many children with Down syndrome can learn to be productive in some way. ☐ Explain that although surgery does pose a risk for the baby, it is the only way he can survive (the parents need to know the consequences if they withhold consent).
	☐ The parents will verbalize satisfaction with the decision they made.	☐ Continue to provide the parents support measures described for Nursing Diagnoses 1, 2, and 3, regardless of their decision.	☐ Continue to update the parents on the baby's condition. ☐ Continue nursing actions stated in plan.
4. Impaired parent-infant interaction related to potential loss of infant and presence of physical defects and mental retardation.	☐ The parents will be able to verbalize feelings about the potential loss of their son (short-term goal). ☐ The parents will progress through stages of grief (long-term goal).	☐ Listen patiently to the parents' fears. ☐ Encourage as much acquaintance with the newborn as they are ready to accept (even with normal infants, this process takes time!).	☐ Day after admission: Mr. James says he knows that he should love his son but he finds it hard because the baby is not what he expected. Mrs. James says: "I am afraid to love him too much. . . ."

Nursing Diagnosis	Outcome Criteria	Nursing Interventions	Evaluation and Revision
		☐ Encourage the parents to engage in caretaking activities, but do *not* push them. ☐ Acknowledge that the baby could die even after surgery. ☐ Continue nursing interventions for Nursing Diagnoses 1, 2, and 3. ☐ Talk to the infant as a person, so that the parents will know the nurses care about them as a family unit.	*Revision* (day after admission): ☐ Acknowledge Mr. James's feelings of disappointment without being judgmental. ☐ Tell Mrs. James that the nurses understand that she is fearful of loving her child and then losing him.

found Mr. James pacing back and forth in the waiting room. He told the nurse that he was opposed to the surgery. He said that his wife was uncertain about what to do but that she felt that the physician wanted to perform the surgery. Mr. James said that he believed he would have confused his wife if he had expressed his point of view. He asked the nurse not to tell others of his strong opposition to the surgery. The nurse wondered whether to share Mr. James's point of view with medical and nursing colleagues or to respect his request not to tell and whether to continue the preparations for the infant's surgery or to initiate action to clarify the decision about the surgery. The nurse faced an ethical dilemma.

The nursing process is an essential tool for making clinical decisions, but it does not facilitate ethical decision making. A nurse faces an ethical dilemma when there is a moral obligation to follow two incompatible courses of action. In the case of the James's baby, the nurse should have respected Mr. James's request not to tell others that he opposed the surgery, but the nurse should also have tried to clarify the parents' decision concerning the surgery. An ethical decision-making model therefore highlights decisions and choices with differing moral points of view. Its focus is not the clinical and technical problems but the questions of one's moral obligation. An ethical decision-making model supplements and expands the third phase of the nursing process, the planning phase.

PROCESS FOR RESOLVING ETHICAL DILEMMAS

The specific process proposed here was designed to supplement the planning phase of the nursing process and to facilitate the resolution of ethical dilemmas in nursing. It will be used to analyze the nurse's dilemma in regard to the infant with multiple anomalies. The model has been previously described[7] and tested with a nursing dilemma involving a terminally ill adult.[8] It is used here with the permission of the author.

The model had an unusual beginning. General hospital staff nurses who had volunteered to describe ethical dilemmas that they had experienced in nursing requested a workable ethical decision-making model as a fair exchange for their participation in the research. Most of the dilemmas that the nurses described in the research had remained unresolved. The nurses anticipated that they would continue to become "stuck" in their dilemmas, to feel unsure about what to do, and to wake up at night wondering about the consequences of their responses. Although the nursing process was useful in making most decisions, it was not helpful in facilitating the resolution of ethical conflicts. In the future, these nurses wanted to be able to formulate a position congruent with ethical principles and to act on their position with some degree of consistency and confidence. They requested an ethical decision-making model which would facilitate this process and which would work in their clinical nursing situations.

William Stockton, a philosopher-anthropologist, and myself have proposed an ethical decision-making model. Numerous groups of nursing clinicians, together with undergraduate and graduate students, have used and tested the model in their analysis and resolution of nursing ethical dilemmas. The model encompasses the steps of the nursing process, but perhaps its usefulness lies in the practical techniques associated with each step; these techniques take into account the nature of nursing ethical conflicts, i.e., being torn between conflicting moral obligations that cannot be fulfilled at the same time.

The major purpose of the model is to facilitate a way to permit nurses to experience moral and ethical conflicts not as dilemmas but rather as opportunities to take committed action. The model makes the decision-making process explicit, facilitates the discovery of the nurse's own implicit moral and ethical rules and principles, relates the nurse's thinking to moral and ethical theories in philosophy and developmental psychology, and links judgment, choice, and action in the nursing experience. It is not a method of determining *the* right answer or of eliminating the inherent conflicting loyalties in ethical dilemmas. Using the model will not yield secure and definite answers, but will raise new questions, new doubts, and new responsibilities. In the end, the nurse will have considered various alternatives in light of moral principles and will have had an opportunity to choose and to take the responsibility for the choice.

As the initial group of nurses who tested the model recommended, there is a mnemonic device for remembering the steps in the process, which explains why it has become known as the *M-O-R-A-L model.* The steps are simply:

M: Massage the dilemma.
O: Outline options.
R: Review criteria and resolve.
A: Affirm position and act.
L: Look back.

M: massage the dilemma

The first step involves creating an image of the ethical conflict that includes all the significant features of the dilemma situation. A "force-field analysis" is a useful technique for graphically describing the forces or considerations in a dilemma situation.[9] Using Fig. 4-1, nurses identify the two incompatible action choices that result in their being stuck in the dilemma and the forces inherent in the health care situation that influence their taking either of these two actions.

Massaging a dilemma is like the process of temple rubbing, in which an intricate pattern is produced on rice paper, or like a child's technique of putting a piece of paper over a leaf and rubbing it with a crayon to get a detailed imprint of the leaf. In the case of a nursing dilemma, the process includes recognizing and questioning whose interests are involved in the conflict, defining the dilemma for the individuals involved, and describing the crunch of conflicting loyalties, feelings, laws, regulations, and so forth.

By completing the force-field analysis, the nurse defines the dilemma and is ready to refocus on the situation from a broader perspective by (1) recognizing the issues that underlie the considerations, (2) formulating a goal in relation to the major issues reflected in the considerations and the nurse's professional commitments, and (3) realigning the forces in relation to the goals.

The major issues inherent in the dilemma will be one or more of the following: (1) deciding the right to know and determining the right to decide, (2) defining and promoting quality of life, (3) maintaining professional and institutional standards, and (4) distributing nursing resources. The major issue in the dilemma involving the infant with multiple anomalies is deciding the right to know and determining the right to decide. Using Fig. 4-2, the nurse specifies the goal or goals and establishes priorities if there is more than one goal in relation to the major issues. To formulate the goal, the nurse determines the desired outcome; i.e., "I would like to act in such a way that. . . ." The focus here is on intentionality and on the question, "What is the possibility that I want to create in this situation?" Fundamental questions about the purpose of nursing emerge. The nurse has an opportunity to clarify primary commitments in nursing and to raise questions about "Who am I?" as a nurse and as a human being. Once the goal is established, the forces are realigned in relation to the goal.

O: outline options

As a result of massaging the dilemma, the nurse has shifted from considering the situation a *dilemma,* requiring two incompatible responses, to defining it as a *problem* of how to reach a goal

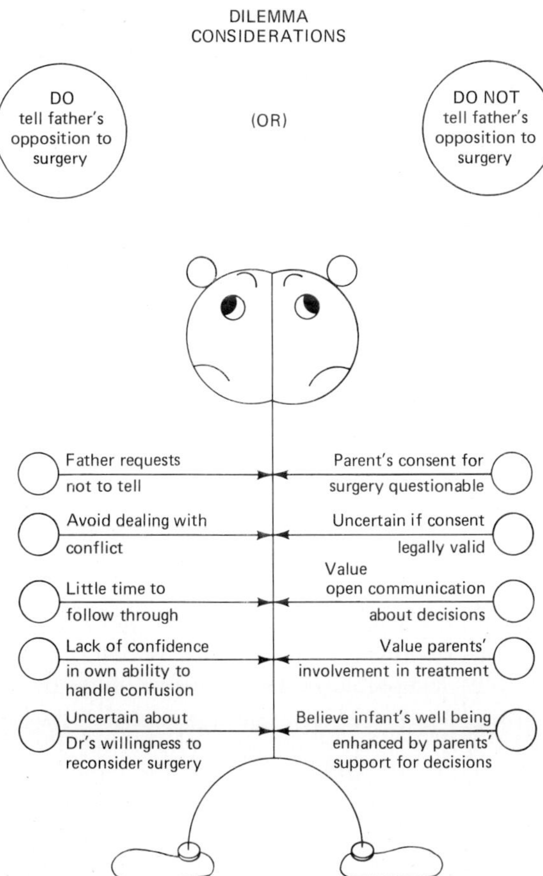

Figure 4-1 Identification of two incompatible action choices and the forces or considerations in the ethical dilemma involving the infant with multiple anomalies. (*Used with permission, from personal sources of P. Crisham.*)

and how to produce results, given the situation. The focus now is on generating several effective alternatives for reaching the goal.

This second step of the model is essentially a brainstorming session to discover alternative solutions to the problem by formulating strategies that will strengthen or add to the driving forces and weaken or eliminate the restraining forces. It is most effective to approach this process in two steps. First, with each of the forces, the nurse asks what actions could be taken to (1) control the force, (2) influence the force, and (3) anticipate the force in the dilemma situation. This process results in numerous specific actions that could either strengthen the driving forces or weaken (or eliminate) the restraining forces. The second step of this process is simply to examine these possible actions and put together selected combinations of actions that are likely to be effective alternatives for reaching the goal. This process usually results in the formulation of three or four general strategies that will be evaluated against selected moral criteria in the next step of the model.

Examples of some of the strategies generated by nurses faced with a dilemma such as that of the James's infant, described earlier, include:

1. Disregard Mr. James's comment about opposing surgery.
2. Inform the physician of Mr. James's opposition to surgery.

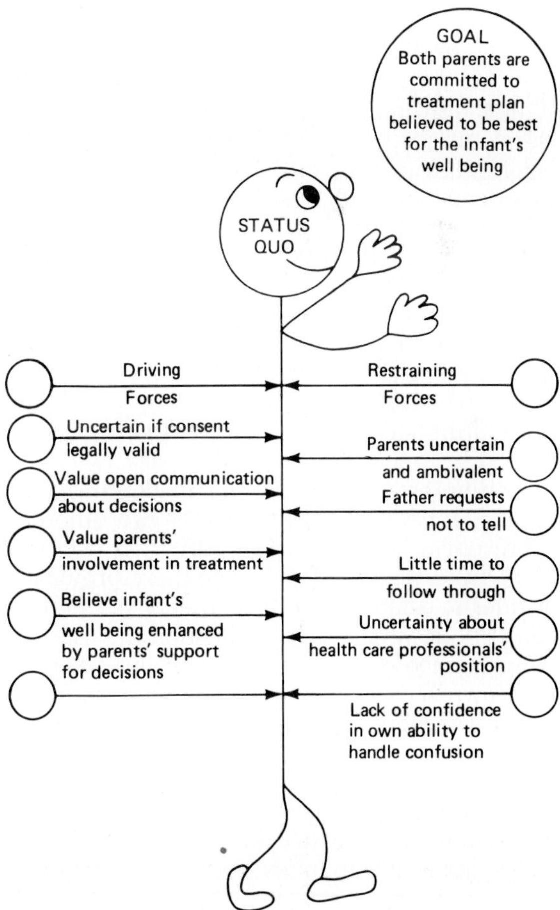

Figure 4-2 Formulation of the goal and realignment of forces in relation to the goal. (*Used with permission, from personal sources of P. Crisham.*)

3. Initiate a conference between the parents, the nurse, and the physician.
4. Inform Mrs. James of her husband's point of view.

R: review criteria and resolve

As a result of outlining options, the nurse shifts from not knowing how to solve the problem to asking which alternative is best. The focus is on deciding in light of ethical principles. The purposes of the "R," the third step in the model, are (1) to identify moral principles or criteria and (2) to select the course of action that is congruent with the criteria. This step, therefore, is crucial to resolving the dilemma and making a moral judgment. It is likewise pivotal in linking the moral judgment to the moral action.

The two phases—identifying the moral criteria and assessing the available options according to the criteria—are often perceived by nurses as complex and difficult. Inexperienced nurses will have the greatest difficulty with this process. A significantly lower tolerance for ambiguity in decision making has been found to exist among beginning nursing students, as compared with experienced practitioners.[10] Experienced nurses also identify themselves as being responsible for a decision significantly more often than undergraduate nursing students when caring for terminally ill adults.[11] Crisham found that nurses who had had experience with dilemmas had significantly higher principled thinking scores than nurses who had not.[12] The following techniques were formulated from Crisham's findings.

Identifying moral principles To identify moral criteria, nurses can use either of two different approaches: (1) they can identify their own implicit principles and then relate these principles or rules to established ethical theory, or (2) they can critique various ethical theories and then attempt to choose and order basic principles to form their own set of principles. Both approaches result in the identification of principles which are thought to be most basic and most important and which will be applied with some degree of conviction and confidence. When this process is repeated with successive dilemmas, a set of principles, applicable to many situations, emerges.

Discovering one's own principles One way in which nurses can facilitate the discovery of their own implicit principles and rules is to take each action suggested with each force in the "O" step of the model and finish the following sentence: "I should—or should not—do [the specific action] because. . . ." The result is a list of implicit "shoulds" which becomes the basis of the exploration and critique of rules and principles.

Nurses can examine their implicit "shoulds" in light of traditional philosophical thinking. Nurses have found it useful, for example, to contrast act and rule utilitarianism, deontological principles of Kant or Frankena, or interrelated principles from various ethical theories. In examining their "shoulds" nurses often have difficulty distinguishing moral "shoulds" from legal, professional, and other types of "shoulds." The distinctions developed by Shweder[13] may be useful during this process. This may also be the time to relate the distinctions between levels of moral judgment offered by Piaget,[14] Kohlberg,[15] and others (see Chap. 5, Table 5-4).

Adopting principles from ethical theory Ethical theory provides a framework for determining morally acceptable positions and actions. In recent years, two major types of ethical theories have been the focus of moral philosophy: teleological theories and deontological theories.

Theories that judge the worth of actions by their *consequences and ends* are described as *teleological theories* (from the Greek *telos,* which means "end"). A feature of these theories is that one's duty and the determining of what is right are subordinated to what is good, because duty and what is right are defined in terms of good or that which will produce good. *Utilitarianism* is an example of a teleological theory that gauges the worth of actions by their consequences. Its central principle asserts that people ought to produce the greatest possible balance of value over disvalue for all persons involved.

Deontological theories (from the Greek *deon,* which means "duty"), on the other hand, assert that the concept of duty is independent of the concept of good and that right actions are not determined by the production of good.[16] Whatever rule of action one adopts, one must act in such a way as to preserve respect for the intrinsic value or dignity of all persons, including oneself. Kant stated: "Act so that you treat humanity, whether in your own person or in that of another, always as the end and never as a means only."[17] According to Kant, this principle must serve as a separate principle against which all other ends or goals are evaluated.

Both deontological and teleological theories address the same question: "What ought I to do?" While they offer different answers to this question, or similar answers with different rationales, they share a common conception: People face ethical dilemmas, and the task of ethics is to spell out moral principles so that people can determine their duties and responsibilities in these dilemmas.

Moral principles To complete the "R" step of the model, the nurse identifies and systematically examines the moral principles involved in the situation. Moral duties are determined by careful examination of, and reflection on, selected moral principles.[18,19,20] Four basic moral principles are autonomy, nonmaleficence, beneficence, and justice.[21]

The duty inherent in the principle of *autonomy* is to respect all persons, including oneself, as autonomous (from the Greek *autos,* which means "self," and *nomos,* which means "governance") beings with a right to their own views and the freedom to act on their judgments. According to the principle of *nonmaleficence,* one's duty is to avoid intending, causing, permitting, or imposing harm or the risk of harm to any person. The principle of *beneficence,* doing or promoting the good, is that one should act to prevent harm, remove harmful conditions, and promote positive benefits for others. *Justice,* in the broadest sense, is giving to each person what is due or owed. To Aristotle, justice meant that equals ought to be treated equally and that unequals should be treated unequally. Justice is concerned with credentialing moral persons and determining the relevant properties or criteria for distributing burdens and benefits. Others believe that justice is determining what is fair.[22]

A decision-making grid, using criteria to determine the action to be taken, is useful in determining which alternative most adequately respects the moral principles. It focuses on moral and ethical criteria, but it allows the nurse to consider professional, technical, and pragmatic criteria. When two or three alternatives seem relatively equal in terms of the moral criteria, the pragmatic considerations become the deciding criteria (see Fig. 4-3).

Although this assessment process cannot be quantified, a number of approaches are useful in helping clarify which alternative to choose. The assessment might focus on whether the moral criterion is met (+), violated (−), or not relevant (0). Another approach is to focus on ranking each alternative with each criterion, giving a rank of "first," "second," "third," or "fourth" to show which alternative met the criterion to the greatest (or least) degree. Individuals may disagree in their assessments of alternatives cho-

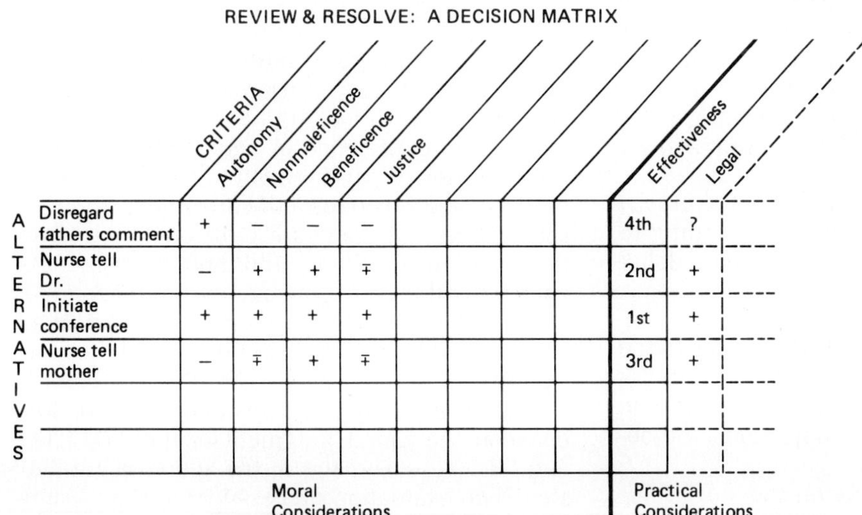
REVIEW & RESOLVE: A DECISION MATRIX

ALTERNATIVES	CRITERIA: Autonomy	Nonmaleficence	Beneficence	Justice	Effectiveness	Legal
Disregard fathers comment	+	−	−	−	4th	?
Nurse tell Dr.	−	+	+	∓	2nd	+
Initiate conference	+	+	+	+	1st	+
Nurse tell mother	−	∓	+	∓	3rd	+
	Moral Considerations				Practical Considerations	

Figure 4-3 A decision-making grid to determine the alternative that most adequately respects the moral principles. (*Used with permission, from personal sources of P. Crisham.*)

sen in relation to the moral criterion used, but each person will be in a position to present the basis of his or her interpretation. What is important is raising the significant questions. Determining the weight and priority of various criteria will bring fundamental issues to light at this point in the process.

A: affirm position and act

As a result of reviewing the criteria, the nurse has shifted from not knowing which alternative is best to making a judgment or decision about which alternative is best according to moral principles. However, a decision or judgment is not a choice. To know which alternative is the best solution is not necessarily to commit oneself to act on that knowledge. The shift that occurs in affirming the position and acting is from deciding to choosing. To decide means "to cut off" (from the Latin *decidere*) the other alternatives, whereas to choose means to take a stand in the full realization that reasonable people could take another stand.

The first three steps of the model result in a moral judgment, namely, a decision that a particular alternative is most congruent with one's specified moral criteria. On the basis of the outcome of the decision matrix, the nurse in the case of the James's baby decides that a conference should be initiated. The "A" step of the model, then, moves beyond gaining cognitive clarity to acting on a commitment. Developing a moral judgment is the essential preparation for taking the moral action; the moral judgment is "necessary but not sufficient" in following through with the process of the model. Affirming one's position and acting calls forth the courage to act out of a choice.

The following heuristic may be helpful in lessening the complexity of acting according to one's moral perspective in the health care delivery system:

A: Anticipate the objections and obstacles to the action.
C: Clarify your position and plan your action to respond to the anticipated objections and obstacles.
T: Test your choice by acting on it.

Psychologists have studied the qualities necessary to act on a resolve—competence, resoluteness, perseverance, and inner strength—in terms of "ego strength." This concept, however, is not well defined. How an individual develops or chooses to use these qualities is not clear at this stage of the research.

The first three steps of the model concentrate on cognitive clarity when delineating a nursing ethical dilemma and identifying the principles that will be used to make a moral judgment. The "A" step—affirm position and act—concentrates on other aspects of morality that influence what nurses ought to do and be: conscience (consciousness of, and reflection on, autonomously accepted action guides), virtue (the acquired habit of doing what is right), and integrity (acting consistently with one's resolve). Numerous contemporary philosophers, in the classical tradition of Plato and Aristotle, have concluded that the fundamental question is, "Who should I *be*?" Morality does not consist in adherence to principles and rules, in their view, but in the expression of conscience, virtue, and integrity internal to oneself.

The "A" step of the model is about choosing, after having deliberated about alternatives and principles, and about taking responsibility for the choice. It is about reversing the trends of apprenticeship and paternalism[23] and about creating, through committed action, a context in which all parties to a dilemma are supported in choosing from their commitments to the health and well-being of the patient.

L: look back

When acting from commitment, the nurse inevitably experiences confusion and doubt, and the shift called for in looking back centers on completing the experience of acting from commitment. As nurses pay attention to their own data—their perceptions of an ethical conflict, their resourcefulness in generating options, their clarification of moral criteria and their assessment of options by these criteria, and their implementation of the resolve—the experience of ethical dilemmas will bring new insights and new responsibilities.

It is useful to focus the evaluation on the link between the moral judgment of the "M," "O," and "R" steps and the moral action of the "A" step. The evaluation process includes an examination of each step in the model. Assessing the "M" step clarifies the most recurrent ethical dilemmas in a particular clinical area of practice. Focusing on the "O" step includes assessing the nature and adequacy of the alternative strategies. Evaluating the "R" step involves reviewing the process of defining the set of basic moral principles, the priority that is consistently given to specific principles, and the effectiveness of the process of using the moral criteria to judge various alternatives.

In summary, advances in technology and the growing complexity of the health care delivery system have resulted in increasingly complex moral and ethical dilemmas that must be faced by the nurse who works with children and their families. The 1983 report of the President's commission, the 1985 Baby Doe regulations, and a broad range of health care associations, including the American Nurses' Association, have taken the position that a collaborative *process* is central to resolving ethical dilemmas in health care.

Nurses who work with children and their families experience ethical dilemmas about the right to know and decide, defining and promoting quality of life, maintaining professional and institutional standards, and distributing nursing resources. In this chapter a situation involving an infant with multiple anomalies was analyzed using a nursing ethical decision-making model. The M-O-R-A-L model, which was designed for use by individuals and groups, begins with the experience of a specific dilemma involving two unacceptable options. It facilitates the formulation of a position by enabling the nurse to compare alternative strategies with specified moral principles, and it creates a challenge to act from commitment and to enhance the quality of health care.

References

1. Medicare, Part A, *Intermediary Letter Transmittal #82-11: Discrimination against the Handicapped by Withholding Treatment or Nourishment,* Department of Health and Human Services, Office of Civil Rights, Washington, May 18, 1982.
2. *Services and Treatment for Disabled Infants: Model Guidelines for Health Care Providers to Establish Infant Care Review Committees,* Department of Health and Human Services, Office of Human Development Services, Washington, Apr. 15, 1985.
3. President's Commission for the Study of Ethical Problems in Medicine and Biomedical and Behavioral Research, *Deciding to Forego Life Sustaining Treatment,* GPO, Washington, 1983.
4. Resolution adopted by the House of Delegates, American Nurses' Association, National Conference, San Francisco, 1980.
5. *The Nurse's Dilemma: Ethical Considerations in Nursing Practice,* International Council of Nurses, Geneva, 1977.
6. Crisham, P., "Moral Judgment of Nurses in Hypothetical and Nursing Dilemmas," unpublished doctoral dissertation, University of Minnesota, Minneapolis, 1979.
7. ———, "Resolving Ethical and Moral Dilemmas of Nursing Interventions," in M. Snyder (ed.), *Independent Nursing Interventions,* Wiley, New York, 1985, pp. 25–43.
8. ———, "MORAL: How Can I Do What Is Right?" *Nursing Management* **16**(4):42–56 (April 1985).
9. Lewin, K., "Quasi-Stationary Social Equilibria and the Problem of Permanent Change," in W. Bennis, K. Benne, and R. Chin (eds.), *The Planning of Change,* Holt, New York, 1969, pp. 235–238.
10. Grier, M., "Decision-Making Process with Undergraduate Nursing Students," paper presented at research conference, University of Minnesota, Minneapolis, Jan. 17, 1983.
11. Eberhardy, J., "An Analysis of Moral Decision Making with Nursing Students Facing Professional Problems," unpublished doctoral dissertation, University of Minnesota, Minneapolis, 1982.
12. Crisham, P., "Measuring Moral Judgment in Nursing Dilemmas," *Nursing Research* **30**(2):104–110 (March–April 1981).
13. Shweder, R. A., "Rethinking Culture and Personality Theory," *Ethos,* **8**(2):60–94 (Spring 1980).
14. Piaget, J., *The Moral Judgment of the Child,* M. Gabain (trans.), Free Press, New York, 1965. (First published in English by Kegan Paul, Trench, Trubner, London, 1932.)
15. Kohlberg, L., "State and Sequence: The Cognitive-Developmental Approach to Socialization," in D. A. Goslin (ed.), *Handbook of Socialization Theory and Research,* Rand McNally, Chicago, 1969, pp. 347–480.
16. Beauchamp, T., and J. Childress, *Principles of Biomedical Ethics,* Oxford University Press, New York, 1983.
17. Kant, I., *Foundations of the Metaphysics of Morals,* Lewis White Beck (trans.), Bobbs-Merrill, Indianapolis, 1959.
18. Beauchamp and Childress, op. cit.
19. Frankena, W., *Ethics,* Prentice-Hall, Englewood Cliffs, N.J., 1973.
20. Muyskens, J., *Moral Problems in Nursing,* Rowman & Littlefield, Totowa, N.J., 1982.
21. Beauchamp and Childress, op. cit.
22. Rawls, J., *A Theory of Justice,* Harvard, Cambridge, Mass., 1971.
23. Ashley, J., *Hospitals, Paternalism and the Role of the Nurse,* Teachers College, New York, 1976.

PART II

Growth and Development of the Child

5

Nancy Lockwood Ramsey

Principles of growth and development

Upon completion of this chapter, the student will be able to:

1 Identify the nine principles of growth and development.
2 Compare the definitions of the following terms: maturation vs. development, growth vs. development, and developmental task vs. developmental milestone.
3 Compare critical periods and stage theory.
4 Describe the three components of consciousness according to Freudian theory.
5 Compare Freud's stages of development with Erikson's stages of psychosocial development.
6 Identify three major ways in which Erikson's theory differs from Freud's.
7 Define the following terms: *cognitive development, assimilation, accommodation, schemata,* and *organization.*
8 Support or refute the following: "Children's cognitive development increases in complexity. A child learns by experience."
9 Identify Kohlberg's theory of four stages of moral development.

The nurse is in a strategic position to help the child and family obtain optimal health.[1] The first step in promoting and safeguarding health is, like the first step of the nursing process, assessment. Only after collecting data can the nurse make accurate nursing diagnoses and plan and prioritize appropriate, individualized interventions. Assessment of every child client includes growth and development.

The assessment of growth and development must be based on scientific knowledge and theory rather than on intuition, habit, or value judgment. The facts and theories nurses use in assessing growth and development come from various biological and psychosocial disciplines, including anthropometry (measurement of height, weight, body proportions, and the other aspects of physical growth), nutrition, physiology, psychology, and sociology (especially as it applies to families and childhood peer groups).

Perhaps the outstanding feature of growth and development during childhood is rapid change. (See Fig. 5-1.) What is normal at one age is often abnormal a short time later. Only by thoroughly

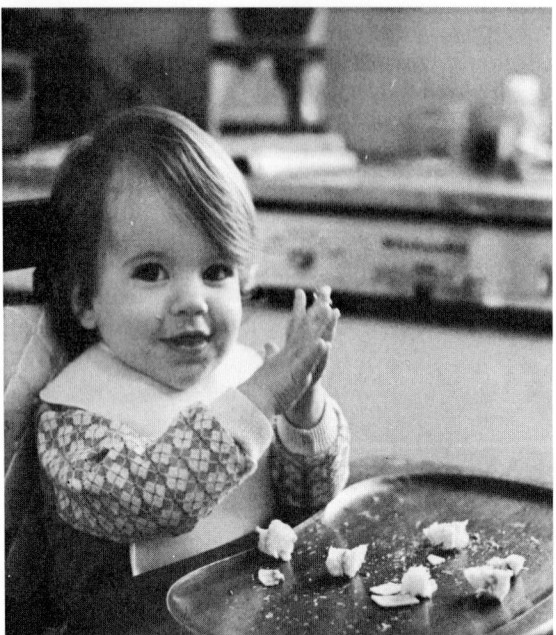

Figure 5-1 Interests and activities that characterize one age are later replaced by other behavioral patterns that are better suited to the developmental tasks of that later period. (*Courtesy of David Carroll.*)

knowing growth and development can the nurse accurately assess the well-being of a child and, equally important, help parents and others in the child's environment anticipate what the child will need to ensure well-being in the next phases of continuing change.

The changes that occur with normal growth and development are both physical and behavioral. Many of the physical changes are obvious even to the unsophisticated observer: the child increases in size, and body proportions change, for example. Other changes are less conspicuous. Internal structural changes take place as growth occurs, and physiological functions are modified as time passes. For example, the ability to digest milk is not well developed until around 3 months of age, when the infant begins to secrete lactase. Metabolic rates are higher in young children than in older ones; this fact accounts for differences in fluid and caloric requirements at different ages, influences temperature regulation, and affects medication dosage and physiological utilization of drugs. Maturation of the myelin sheath influences physiological activity; slow and erratic motor responses, for example, are typical of infants because the immature myelin sheath does not permit efficient muscular control. As the neuromuscular system matures, reflexes and other motor activities expected in young infants become abnormal during later months of infancy. A 2-month-old child does not have good control of the neck muscles that steady the head, but a 5-month-old baby should.

Behavioral changes that accompany growth and development result in part from physical changes. For example, varying maturation of different brain areas is believed to be partly responsible for the toddler's tantrums. Hormonal secretions contribute to the moodiness of adolescents. Increased heart and lung capacities, in addition to improved motor control, enable school-age children to engage in vigorous activities, such as tag and ball games, that are beyond the behavioral capacity of younger children. Behavioral changes that take place as children get older are not caused only by physical changes but are often due to increasing experience and its effect on interests and understanding.

DEFINITIONS

Growth refers to increase in the physical size of the body or a body part. It is usually assessed in units of measurement, such as kilograms, centimeters, inches, or pounds. Growth occurs by two processes: an increase in the *number* of cells, called *hyperplasia,* and an increase in the *size* of individual cells, termed *hypertrophy.* Most, if not all, organs and tissues grow by both processes. Obviously, cell multiplication (hyperplasia) is a very active part of prenatal growth, since new cells are necessary for the creation of all body structures of the unborn child. Hyperplasia depends on adequate nutritional intake, both before and after birth. Hypertrophy often depends on use of the body part. For example, the muscles of the back, buttocks, and legs become larger when the child learns to walk, and the myocardium hypertrophies to an abnormal extent in certain kinds of heart malformations that cause the heart to work hard in its effort to push the blood past a small valve or through a partially obstructed vessel. Cells become *differentiated,* which allows for more mature functioning. For example, lactase-secreting cells mature at 3 months, enhancing the infant's ability to digest milk.

Development refers to a gradual change in function, not size, that results in more complex skills and abilities. These new functions expand the child's capacity for achievement. For example, the school-age child who has progressed to abstract thinking is now able to anticipate and empathize with the feelings of other people and is perfecting fine and gross motor coordination. These developmental changes prepare the child for team play, as they enable the child to compromise for the welfare of the group, to analyze the effects of his or her own behavior upon winning, and to develop the neuromuscular coordination to play the game.

Maturation, a part of development, refers to the attainment of new competencies or characteristics that are transmitted genetically and hence are expected to "unfold" naturally in each member of the species. The word *maturation* is often incorrectly used to mean "growth and development." Maturation is due to genetic endowment transmitted in the cell nuclei, not to practice or learning from the environment. For example, the maturation of the myelin sheath, the attainment of body height, and the secretion of lactase are governed by heredity and maturation, not practice or experience.

A *developmental task* is a global behavioral skill or ability that is best learned or accomplished during a specific period of the child's life. Each particular developmental task occurs at approximately the same age in most children. Mastery of the task prepares the child to deal successfully with later developmental tasks. If the skill or ability is not learned at the appropriate period, the child will probably have greater difficulty mastering it at a later time. Examples of developmental tasks include learning to manipulate symbols (such as letters and numbers used in reading and arithmetic) during the school-age period and becoming able to live independently from parents in late adolescence.

Learning is an increase in understanding or skill mastery as a result of development or experience. Learning may or may not lead to an observable change in behavior. For example, children who have learned to cope with separation from their mothers no longer cry or cling when left at nursery school, but adolescents who have learned about the health hazards of smoking may or may not alter their smoking behavior. Learning is often dependent on maturation; a preschooler cannot learn cognitive skills such as algebra, for example, and toilet training cannot be learned until myelinization makes sphincter control possible. Learning is often made necessary by developmental changes as well as by situational requirements: adolescents learn, for example, to deal with the physical changes of puberty, and they learn how to behave in new social situations, such as dating.

Readiness refers to the child's ability to begin learning a new skill or developmental task. Readiness requires neurological maturity and also involves motivation and prerequisite skills. For example, school readiness is said to be present at age 6, when children have the social and emotional maturity and self-help skills (toileting, eating, etc.) to adapt to being in school and, in addition, the cognitive maturity and motivation to receive teaching in the relatively structured instructional setting. Reading readiness consists of the perceptual maturation to distinguish letters and their associated sounds, the intellectual maturity to see the connection between written words and their meanings, and the motivation to learn to read.

A *developmental milestone* is a specific task, skill, or learned behavior that can be used to assess a child's development at a particular age. For example, children are expected to begin walking at around 12 to 18 months, and failure to do so is a danger signal that calls for more thorough developmental assessment. Infants' developmental milestones are mainly neuromuscular responses to stimuli that reflect neurological maturation. Only gradually do the developmental milestones reflect increasing interactions with the environment.

PRINCIPLES OF GROWTH AND DEVELOPMENT

Researchers in child development have observed a number of common patterns of growth and behavior. These patterns are useful because they identify general principles, or laws, underlying children's growth and development. Most authorities agree on the following principles.

1. Individual rate and style of growth and development

As pertains to growth, for example, some children get bigger than others, some grow faster than others, and some reach puberty earlier than others. Although normative growth charts such as those in Appendix B are of great value in assessing a child's growth, it is important to remember that individual variations among children are entirely normal. Each child's own growth record is in many ways the best standard by which to evaluate his or her present growth data. A child who is relatively small or large in comparison with children of the same age may be experiencing a growth abnormality or may simply be following his or her own appropriate, individual growth pattern. A long-term growth record is invaluable in making the distinction between these two possibilities. That is, a child whose height is at the 25th percentile for children in that age group should not arouse concern if he or she has in the past consistently been near the same percentile on the height chart. A drop from earlier 50th percentile data would be an indication that the child is deviating from the earlier pattern and is in need of further evaluation to rule out some health problem that is being manifested in growth retardation.

Individual differences in behavioral "style" are often evident even from birth. Observation of babies in a newborn nursery reveals that some infants are slower than others to wake up and fall asleep, some are more insistent than others about feedings, some are easier than others to comfort, and so forth. Children naturally differ in their general style of interacting with the environment (alertness, assertiveness, consolability, etc.), as well as many other behavioral traits, with each child following his or her own pattern throughout the various developmental phases for the most part. (See Fig. 5-2.)

Child-to-child variations in growth and development result from both genetic inheritance and environmental influences. Inherited factors that influence growth and development include sex, race, and certain inherited diseases. For example, boys are somewhat larger than girls from birth through the preschool years, after which girls as a group are larger until the boys reach puberty. Boys generally reach the developmental milestones later than girls. Musculoskeletal differences among races are numerous and are generally of little or no practical significance. Such inherited disorders as phenylketonuria, which affects intelligence, or cystic fibrosis, which affects growth as well as general health, obviously have great potential for influencing growth and development.

Environmental influences, such as the amount and consistency of stimulation, religion, ethnic background, education, and discipline techniques, affect the child's rate and style of development. For example, a child who lives with eight other children in a two-room apartment and who is locked in the apartment each day while the parents work may receive inadequate stimulation, education, and nutrition and, as a consequence, may demonstrate developmental delays or distortions.

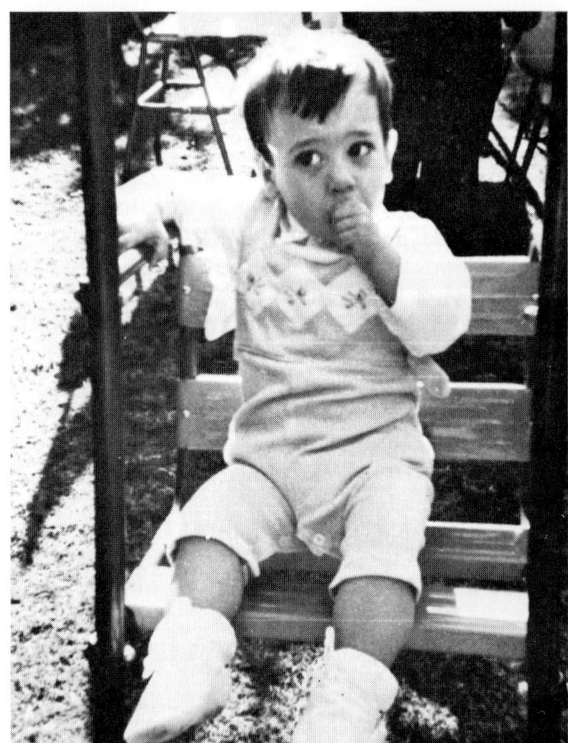

Figure 5-2 One child's usual response to a new or difficult situation may be to sit back and size things up; another might jump right in; still another might seek adult intervention.

2. Growth and development are asynchronous

Different body parts and developmental areas (language, motor skills, etc.) develop at different rates. Each body part has its own time to grow. Brain growth, for example, predominates during early development, for it forms the foundation for later neuromuscular development. During each phase of development, the child focuses intensely on mastering the pertinent developmental tasks and skills. Other developmental areas recede into the background at that time. The toddler concentrates on learning to walk; only after walking is mastered does vocabulary greatly increase. Support for development includes providing toys and muscular activities to stimulate the predominant developmental activity. For example, when an infant is crawling, opportunities should be provided for the child to exercise that skill; perhaps the adult would place a soft blanket on the floor, sit on the floor, and encourage the child to crawl toward toys.

3. Interrelatedness of all areas of growth and development

Growth and development are artificially divided into such subparts as physical, psychosocial, moral, language, and cognitive development to ease investigation. In reality, each area of development is inseparably integrated with every other. Many developmental areas overlap and undergo simultaneous change. For example, providing for the child's basic physiological needs forms a foundation for cognitive and psychosocial development. Language and social development go hand in hand. Physical maturation continually makes new experiences, and hence new learning, possible. (See Fig. 5-3.)

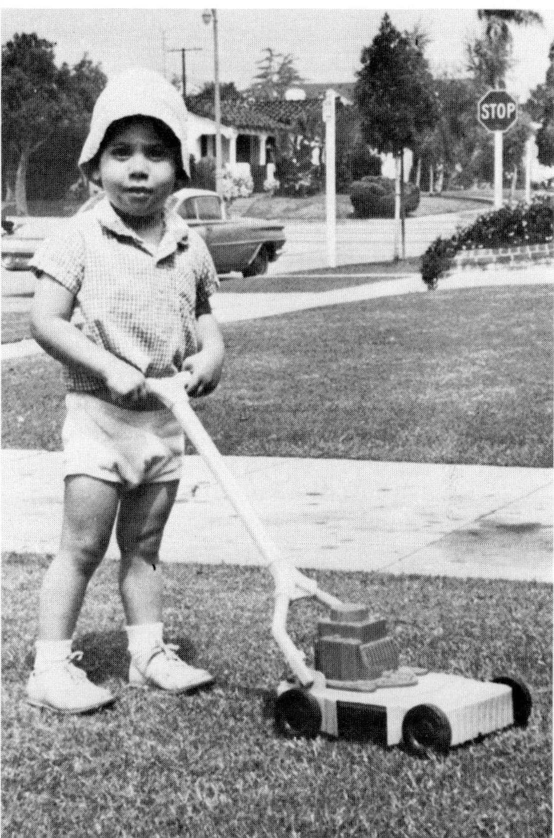

Figure 5-3 Physical, psychological, social, cognitive, and other aspects of development occur simultaneously. This kind of play, for example, involves exercise and motor coordination; cognitive experience in how things work; perceptual learning about colors, textures, and judging distances; and practice in imitating adult roles.

4. Predominance of newly learned skills

The child is preoccupied with practicing and perfecting the current new skill. A majority of the waking hours may be spent practicing the skill. The infant who has recently learned to throw an object for someone else to retrieve, the kindergartner who has just discovered how to whistle, and the school-age child who can make bubbles with bubble gum provide clear examples of the strong drive to repeat and practice newly acquired skills.

5. Orderly sequence of growth and development

Both growth and development are predictable and orderly, not haphazard; develop in sequence; and are approximately the same among most children of the same age. That is why it has been possible to identify developmental milestones. Even children who pass their milestones unusually early or late can be expected to follow the usual childhood developmental *sequence*, and so milestones can be used not only to compare a child with others of a similar age but also to predict what developmental changes will occur next and to provide appropriate stimulation and parental guidance for the next stage. Structured developmental assessments such as can be obtained by use of the Denver Developmental Screening Test (DDST) (see Figs. 14-6 and 14-7) permit the nurse both to identify deviations from normal development and to give anticipatory guidance to parents. In other words, developmental assessments help the nurse to prevent or minimize developmental disability by early detection and to promote optimal wellness.[2]

6. Cephalocaudal progression (head to toe)

This principle is true both before and after birth. For example, the head and upper body portions are relatively large in the fetus and develop before the lower parts. The infant first learns head control, then trunk control, and then control of the legs.

7. Proximodistal progression (midline to periphery)

Body parts near the infant's midline mature and develop before the areas farther away from the midline. Even in utero, the vital organs within the trunk develop before the limb buds form. Arm and hand control precedes finger coordination, so that the infant uses sweeping and raking gestures to acquire a desired object, then a whole-hand grasp to pick it up, and finally a pincer grasp that involves thumb and forefinger.

8. Simple to complex and general to specific development

The child's maturation and development become increasingly advanced and specialized as time passes. For example, development proceeds from simple to complex in utero when the heart—originally a simple, one-chambered tube—evolves into a more complex, four-chambered structure. The child's language also obviously develops from simple to complex. The child forms sounds, syllables, words, short sentences, and then several sentences. An example of general to specific development is the way an infant reacts at first to stimuli with a general response and later with a specific response. A young infant reacts to a noise with the entire body (the Moro reflex); only later does the baby turn the eyes and head toward the noise, a more specific response.

9. Competent behavior

A child has an inherent drive toward normal, competent behavior. Competent behavior includes activities that ensure survival and those which promote independence and self-knowledge. Even a neonate demonstrates competence: the rooting reflex enables the newborn to locate food, and the pleasurable feelings that follow strengthen the quest for food. Recognizing the mother's face and odor promotes attachment, and attachment enhances the child's access to further food and parenting.

Children have a strong drive to overcome genetic and environmental obstacles. Children raised under inadequate circumstances are remarkably resilient and strive toward competency when given even minimal opportunities. Nurses need to remember this. Nurses too often focus on the pathological, the weaknesses, instead of equally emphasizing the child's and family's strengths and competencies. Focusing on strengths builds trust, increases competence, and promotes independence and the expectation of success.

Stages of development

The commonalities among children at specific ages have led developmentalists to classify growth and development into stages. The following stages, based strictly on age, are very commonly used by health professionals, educators, and others who work with children.

Stage	Age
Prenatal	Before birth
Neonatal	Birth to 28 days (1 month)
Infant	1 to 12 months
Toddler	1 to 3 years
Preschooler	3 to 6 years
School-age child	6 to 12 years
Adolescent	12 to 18 years

Stage theories of development Other developmental stages that are not so rigidly based on age are also widely used. For example, the theories of Freud, Piaget, and Erikson classify development into invariant sequential stages that are linked roughly but not precisely to age. Each stage is typified by (and named for) some predominant developmental task or other developmental characteristic that makes it distinctive from earlier and later stages. Each stage builds on the foundations established in previous stages and contains characteristics integrated from earlier stages. The child who succeeds at accomplishing the tasks of a particular stage is prepared to succeed at the next stage. If he or she has failed to master the present stage, success in later stages will be more difficult. At each stage new areas of development become organized and consolidated into orderly patterns of behavior. Each stage consists of two periods: (1) a period of gradual formation, when the child constantly practices the behavior or skill to increasingly organize and perfect it, and (2) a period of competence, when the child has mastered the skill or behavior. During each stage, the child builds more complex activities on old foundations. After the child masters one stage, the next stage begins. The period when one stage merges into the next is called a *transition period*. The child's anxiety increases during this time because of feelings of inadequacy produced by demands of the new stage. A state of disequilibrium exists because older, established behavior patterns and coping mechanisms are no longer effective in solving problems or ensuring feelings of comfort and security. Both physical maturation and environmental influences propel the child toward more mature behavior and into the next stage. The present stage is thus linked to the past and prepares or hinders the child for future development.[3]

Critical periods A *critical period*, also called a *sensitive period*, is a specific period when the child is most vulnerable or sensitive to a particular incoming stimulus. The same stimulus provided before or after the critical period will have less impact on the child.

Critical periods are clearly demonstrated in embryology. A critical period exists for cell specialization. For example, if a brain cell is transplanted to the kidney before the critical period for specialization begins, it will take on the characteristics of a kidney cell. If the brain cell is transplanted after the specialization period, it will not adopt the characteristics of the new location but will continue as a brain cell. The first trimester of pregnancy is the period of initial development (formation) of the organ systems. At this time the embryo and fetus are especially vulnerable to harmful stimuli such as the rubella virus. Unborn infants exposed in the first trimester to the rubella virus may develop cataracts, deafness, cardiac abnormalities, and mental retardation. Exposure to rubella after the critical period, when the body organs are less vulnerable, does not cause such severe defects. Critical periods also exist for visual development and color perception. The neonate must be stimulated with color during the first 2 weeks of life for optimal development of the cones and rods of the eye.

Critical periods also seem to exist for psychological development. Klaus and Kennell[4] believe a critical period exists for mother-child bonding (attachment). Knowledge of critical periods enables the nurse to prioritize nursing care by listing the critical phenomenon at the top of the nursing care plan. If the neonate is in the critical period for attachment, the nurse plans nursing interventions to promote attachment. These interventions include providing skin-to-skin contact in the delivery room; promoting early contact between mother, father, and child; assessing attachment behavior; and providing continuous contact through rooming in and maximum mother-child interaction (see Chaps. 9, 10, and 15). The attachment period used to be designated as ages 3 to 6 months. More recent research indicates that it begins within minutes after birth.

THEORIES OF BEHAVIORAL DEVELOPMENT

A *theory* is an unproven speculation about probable cause-and-effect relationships between a series of events. When a theory is proved, it becomes fact. None of the theories discussed here has been conclusively proved. All are speculative outgrowths of the theorists' observational studies. All the theorists, in turn, were products of their own upbringing, culture, socioeconomic class, and era. Each theorist's conclusions reflect his own "universe" and contain personal biases. The research results were also affected by the research design and method of data collection. For this reason, theories should never be taken as ironclad, eternal rules for normal development. Small portions of theories should not be used to explain a child's total development. No theory explains all behavior, growth, and development, but provides only partial answers.

Freudian theory

Sigmund Freud (1856–1939) was an Austrian physician whose revolutionary ideas about behavior gained popularity in the United States during the 1930s and have had worldwide impact. He founded the method of treatment known as *psychoanalysis*. Freud conceived the following psychiatric concepts: He related increased anxiety to threatened self-image; stated that *all* behavior has meaning; theorized that emotions, thoughts, and strivings originate in the unconscious; defined defense mechanisms; proposed that dreams are communicators of unconscious thought; and conceptualized the unconscious mind and stage theories of sexual development. Freud taught that adult behavior originates in childhood.

The acceptance of Freudian theory today is controversial. Some people consider Freud's theories to be outmoded, constricted by Freud's Victorian society, and nonscientific. Psychoanalytic theory focuses on inner psychic conflicts and ignores the influences of society and culture. Freud believed that the major childhood conflict was sexual; psychologists consider it to be only one of many conflicts. Freud was trained in neurology and treated adult nervous disorders; he did not study children directly. Other people believe that Freudian theory is a sound and fully developed approach to an understanding of behavior. Freud's beliefs are included here because of their familiarity in American life and because they are a basis upon which later theories have been built by others.

Freudian theory focuses upon studying and understanding the person's innermost, personal strivings, thoughts, and experiences. Because adult behavior and mental illness are believed to originate in childhood, parent–child interactions are thoroughly explored to discover the cause of the present behavior. Data are collected through remembering and *free association* (thoughts emerging spontaneously into awareness). Children are observed through nondirective play (see Chap. 15) because the child's innermost thoughts are expressed during play. Thus Freudian theory focuses upon the person's inner motivations rather than on interactions with society and culture.

Freud stressed that anxiety is the major motivation for behavior. Anxiety, which is increased when the person's self-esteem is threatened, has its origins in the unconscious. Freud delineated the *defense mechanisms*, or the unconscious methods used by the person to ward off threats to self-esteem. These mechanisms are used by children and adults to distort reality in order to decrease anxiety. (See psychology books for discussions of defense mechanisms.)

Freud sensed a polarity of opposing instinctual forces in human development: a drive toward pleasure opposing a "death wish," or unconscious drive to destroy oneself and others. Cruelty, hate, aggression, and egocentrism are manifestations of the death wish. Pleasurable feelings result in gratification, reduce anxiety, and are manifested in love, fulfillment, and preservation of life.

Freud's theory can be divided into two main topics: *consciousness* and *personality.*

Consciousness The mind comprises conscious, unconscious, and preconscious portions. The *conscious* portion contains all the thoughts, feelings, actions, and strivings that can be easily remembered. The *preconscious* portion contains thoughts and experiences that are difficult, but possible, to remember. The *unconscious* portion contains thoughts, feelings, and memories that are still more difficult to bring into conscious awareness without special help, as from a psychoanalyst. Even if a person were presented with these unconscious experiences, they would usually not be recognized. Extremely threatening experiences and thoughts are *repressed*, or "buried," in the unconscious. These unconscious thoughts are believed by Freudians to be a major influence on behavior. Dreams, irrational fears, slips of the tongue ("Freudian slips"), selective forgetting, and tics are believed to reveal unconscious wishes when carefully analyzed. The belief that all behavior is meaningful is based upon the conviction that behavior reflects unconscious wishes.

Personality Freud found it useful to imagine the personality as embracing three parts: id, ego, and superego. The *id* is believed to be a seething vortex of life energy, primitive impulses, and passions. It strives for immediate achievement of its goals, no matter what the cost. The id drives take the form of urges to kill, to steal, to enjoy, and to destroy. Thoughts originating in the id motivate one to seek food, to satisfy greed, and to obtain sexual gratification. These feelings are believed to be present in the infant at birth and to be a source of the child's (and adult's) motives and energies.

The *ego* is the reality-based, executive manager of the personality. It mediates the opposing urges of the id and of the superego, the ethical-moral unit. The ego is rational, assesses reality, and enables the individual to react in socially acceptable ways to make gratification possible without overwhelming guilt. It houses personality functions necessary to maintain contact with reality and the environment: memory, intelligence, thinking, analytical problem solving, learning, distinguishing reality from fantasy, and directing body movement. The ego is thought to begin developing during infancy.

The *superego* is essentially the conscience or moral-ethical portion of the personality. It is formed as a result of the child's socialization, as he or she internalizes the parents' values, customs, standards, and beliefs (see Chap. 11). The superego shows in the toddler and preschooler as they learn acceptable behavior. In the pre-

Table 5-1 Psychoanalytical (Freudian) Stages of Development

Stage	Erogenous Zone	Time Frame	Characteristics	Examples of Unsuccessful Experience
Oral	Mouth and lips	Birth to 18 months	Learning to deal with anxiety-producing experiences by using the mouth and tongue	Defenses centered on oral experiences: smoking, alcoholism, obesity, nail-biting, drug addiction, difficulty with trust
Anal	Anus	18 months to 3 years	Learning muscle control, especially that involved with urination and defecation	Defenses centered on holding on and letting go: constipation, obsessive-compulsive personality, fastidiousness, perfection drive
Phallic	Genitals	3 to 6 years	Learning sexual identity and developing awareness of the genital area	Difficulty with sexual identity: transsexuality, difficulty with authority, homosexuality, Oedipus complex (erotic attachment of male child to mother), Electra complex (erotic attachment of female child to father)
Latency	None	6 to 12 years	Quiet stage during which sexual development lies dormant	Defenses centered on inability to conceptualize: lack of self-motivation in school and work
Genital	Genitals	12 years to early adulthood	Developing sexual maturity and learning to develop satisfactory relationships with the opposite sex	Unsatisfactory relationships with the opposite sex: frigidity, impotence, premature ejaculation, serial marriages

Source: Pamela Price Hoskins, "Theoretical Models," in Judith Haber et al., *Comprehensive Psychiatric Nursing*, McGraw-Hill, New York, 1982, p. 49. Used with permission.

schooler, the superego is rigid, tyrannical, and cruel, only later becoming flexible and tolerant. It is the "inner voice" that opposes the id's wishes: "Don't kick your father. He won't like it and will spank you." The superego exercises control by generating guilt.

Freud divided the life span into five stages, listed in Table 5-1. He believed sexual energy to be a main motivator of behavior. He originally called this sexual energy *libido*. It was a broad definition meant to include basic psychic energy, or *life force*, incorporating sexual drive, which directs the person's development.[5] At each stage, the psychic energy is focused upon a body region *(erogenous zone)* that is the main source of pleasure and gratification; each stage is named for the dominant body region. (See Table 5-1.)

Freudian psychoanalysts believe that the personality is essentially formed by the end of the phallic period. The personality develops through the child's response to physiological growth, frustrations, conflicts, and threats.[6] Freud believed that a person who mastered all stages of personality development would be emotionally mature.

Later psychoanalysts have added social and cultural aspects to Freud's basic tenets. These psychoanalysts include Alfred Adler, Karen Horney, Carl Jung, Harry Stack Sullivan, and Erik Erikson.

Eriksonian theory

Erik H. Erikson (1902–1982) was a psychoanalyst who added a new dimension to the work of Freud: society. He considered Freud's work to be a rock upon which later theoretical advances are built. Unlike Freud, Erikson extensively studied children.

Erikson saw development as a lifelong process under the influences of heredity, society, and culture. He believed that the child's hereditary blueprint and social and cultural influences are inseparably intertwined to form the personality.[7] According to Erikson, the child learns to balance inner wishes with outer reality through interactions with the environment.[8]

Erikson divided the life span into eight stages. (See Table 5-2.) Each stage contains a predominant "crisis" to be resolved in order to prepare a firm foundation for success in later stages. The developmental crisis of each stage consists of two

Table 5-2 Erikson's Stages of Psychosocial Development

Stage of Development	Approximate Time Frame	Developmental Tasks	Examples
Sensory	Birth to 18 months	Trust vs. mistrust	Experiences with the nurturing person are the foundations of the level of trust a person will develop.
Muscular	1 to 3 years	Autonomy vs. shame and doubt	The toddler learns the extent to which the environment can be influenced by direct manipulation.
Locomotor	3 to 6 years	Initiative vs. guilt	The child learns the extent to which being assertive will influence the environment. If important others disapprove of beginning assertiveness, the child will experience guilt.
Latency	6 to 12 years	Industry vs. inferiority	Either the child learns to utilize energies to create, develop, and manipulate, or the child learns to shy away from industry, feeling inadequate to the task.
Adolescence	12 to 20 years	Identity vs. role confusion	The adolescent either integrates all life experiences into a coherent sense of self or is unable to integrate these experiences and feels lost and confused.
Young adulthood	18 to 25 years	Intimacy vs. isolation	The young adult is concerned primarily with developing an intimate relationship with another person.
Adulthood	21 to 45 years	Generativity vs. stagnation	The adult is concerned primarily with establishing a family and guiding the next generation.
Maturity	45 years to death	Integrity vs. despair	The life-style gives life meaning, and the person must come to accept his or her life as fulfilling and meaningful. The lack of ego integration results in fear of death.

Source: Pamela Price Hoskins, "Theoretical Models," in Judith Haber et al., *Comprehensive Psychiatric Nursing,* McGraw-Hill, New York, 1982, p. 50. Used with permission.

opposing favorable and unfavorable potential outcomes. Erikson believed that anxiety results from not mastering the crisis of a stage and that unless the favorable alternative is better developed than the unfavorable one, subsequent development will be difficult. Erikson thus retained Freud's stage format and the concept of polarity or opposing forces. Erikson further believed that an inherent drive toward mastery coexists with a desire to regress to an earlier time of comfort and security.[9]

The theories of Erikson differ from those of Freud in three main ways:

1. Erikson believed that the ego, not the id, is the main motivating force in human development. By focusing on the ego, he stressed realistic, healthy behavior; socialization (learning acceptable behavior sanctioned by society); and the ego's relationship with society, culture, and the environment. In contrast, Freud focused upon inner motivations and struggles.
2. Erikson focused on the child's relationship with parents and family within their culture. He believed that the child and family develop together; the action of one influences the other. He addressed social, political, and moral upheavals and the wide diversity of opinions in our society and discussed these pressures on the individual. His theory integrated insights from anthropology, social psychology, the arts, and child development. Freud, in contrast, focused on the drive of psychic energy and an inner, almost mystical, power struggle between id, ego, and superego.
3. Erikson focused upon the healthy personality. In contrast, Freud dealt primarily with psychopathology. Erikson believed that opportunities exist throughout the life span to master a developmental crisis. Each new life phase presents an older crisis in a subordinate position, disguised in new form. His theory was hopeful, for new opportunities are presented to rework older, unmastered crises. The ultimate goal of development was thought

to be a strong identity, a healthy body, and a discerning, creative, and curious mind.[10]

Erikson's theory has been widely adopted by nursing and other health professions. His theory provides a useful pattern for observing behavior. However, Erikson is criticized for not describing the precise behaviors indicating whether mastery of the crisis has been accomplished. With no exact behaviors to assess, further testing and validation of his observations are difficult.

Piagetian theory

Jean Piaget (1896–1980) was a Swiss psychologist who pioneered the study of children's cognitive development. *Cognitive development* is the development of thinking, or the process of knowing. Early in his life, Piaget became very interested in psychoanalysis but preferred to study the normal development of thinking and intelligence. He extensively studied large groups of children throughout the world. The data collected worldwide coincide with the data he initially collected from his own children. Piaget thus studied children in order to discover "how we know."[11] In other words, he studied the development of children's structures of thought and how they are combined to build a child's reality.[12]

Piaget believed that each child has an inherent biological blueprint that outlines his or her intellectual potential. Whether or not the child reaches that potential depends upon stimulation from the environment. He believed that children's thoughts are derivatives of motor actions which began in utero. He stressed that experiences are the roots of all later, more complex thoughts. Children learn by "experiencing their experiences." Thus, experiences, not maturation, are the foundations of cognitive development.[13]

Children are active learners and seekers of new experiences. Piaget believed that each child knows best what he or she needs and is always ready to learn more.[14] Each child seems to have an inherent need to make sense out of the environment. As soon as one problem is solved, the child turns to new experiences.[15] As the child associates thoughts in an organized and increasingly complex manner, he or she learns to deal more effectively with the environment and distinguish reality from fantasy. The child's intellectual capacity depends mainly on the developing cognitive ability to organize the environment.

The following are Piaget's basic concepts:

1. Development is continually evolving and occurs in a predictable, sequential order.
2. New schemata (see below) are introduced within the existing structure and are consolidated, and equilibrium is reestablished. This process repeats continually.
3. Each new developmental phase builds upon previous learning in earlier stages. Piaget thus retained Freud's concept of stage theories.
4. Each new phase has a period of learning and forming, followed by a period of attainment.
5. New organizations of thoughts are increasingly complex and build a hierarchy.
6. Each person will achieve an individual level of development, though all have the same potential.[16]
7. The goal of cognitive development is to attain emotional, biological, and intellectual balance.

There are two important ideas to grasp in understanding the basis of Piaget's theory.* These are what he termed *function* and *structure*. The *process* of interaction between the child and the environment is what Piaget called *function*. There are two major functions or tendencies that govern how a child interacts with the environment: organization and adaptation.[17]

Organization refers to the biological way in which the infant is organized. All levels of thought are organized and are continuously refined. It refers to the tendency to combine two schemata into a more complex schema (see below). Think of the baby's mind as a computer, with the program representing the organizational function or the way in which information is processed by the infant. If the child reaches for a toy, the act of reaching (first schema) is coordinated with seeing the toy (a second schema) and the motivation to get the toy. The child thus integrates, coordinates, and organizes the incoming stimuli.

The second major function governing the child's interaction with the environment is *adaptation*. The adaptation process describes the way in which the child maintains a balanced organization and creates new structures to interact effectively with the environment. There are two parts to adaptation—assimilation and accommodation. According to Piaget, these processes are interrelated and operate simultaneously. *Assimilation* refers to the mental process of taking

*The remainder of this discussion of Piaget is by Ann Sloat.

in new information and interpreting it in light of past experiences. In other words, the child uses old thoughts and actions to understand new events. *Accommodation* is changing earlier ideas or actions (schemata) to better meet or adapt to a new situation or to solve a more complex problem. An example from the biological sciences that might help illustrate this point is the infant's taking in breast milk. The baby's digestive system is functional in that it breaks down the milk into elements that are then assimilated into the infant's body. When we introduce solid foods, however, the infant must accommodate by producing new gastric juices to digest the food. This is very close to what Piaget means when he uses the terms *assimilation* and *accommodation*. The two processes are always going on together. In our example above, as long as only breast milk is given, the infant may be assimilating more than accommodating. When solids are first given, there may be a period during which there is more accommodating than assimilating. The two processes may not always be in balance. Children at play are assimilating more than accommodating. They are acting on information that is already a part of them. When children imitate, they are accommodating more than assimilating. The behavior is new and does not stem from an integration of their own experiences.

Those processes of function (accommodation and assimilation) are constant—are always going on in the same way. (See Fig. 5-4.) Structure, however, is continuously changing, and that change is what accounts for development. *Structure* refers to a structural framework that information must fit into in order to be assimilated. Visualize structure as the structural framework of a building under construction. New information coming into the child must have the potential to relate to past experience or thoughts as the child has organized them, just as new additions to the building under construction must fit onto the basic framework. Think of your own learning, and this may become clearer. Information you learned in a lecture may not be meaningful or "stick" until you are in a situation in which you can see its usefulness. The structure of your thoughts has been organized and reorganized to finally show where the information fits. The same thing is going on with infants' and children's thinking. This organization and reorganization of structure is always in the direction of seeking a balance, or equilibrium. As the structure approaches equilibrium, it becomes sharper and more delineated. As this happens, inconsistencies and gaps of information become apparent, and the child's activities are directed toward filling in the gaps.

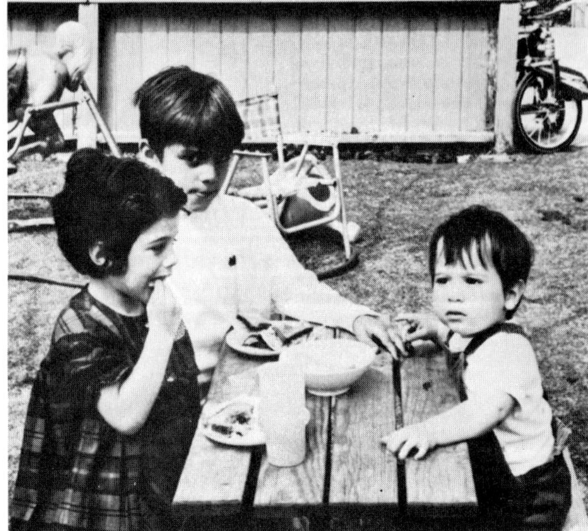

Figure 5-4 Interaction with the physical and social environment is a major source of learning; each child continually influences and is influenced by the surroundings.

Cognitive development, then, consists of a series of changes. These changes are orderly, structural, and directional in that they move toward seeking equilibrium. Piaget used the term *schema* (plural, *schemata*) to describe the units of thought in the structure. A *schema* is an organized pattern of behavior or action (a habit) that displays coherence and order. It is a concept of experiences, the child's way of organizing or classifying earlier sensory events.[18] Each new schema or reorganization of structure incorporates the one before it.

The sequence of development is orderly and recognizable from one child to the next. Piaget described this progression in terms of periods, subperiods, and stages. The basic periods are presented in Table 5-3. Piagetian development is further discussed in Chaps. 9 through 13. Recently, researchers have criticized Piaget's theory of cognitive development. They have shown that children do not always master and use all the cognitive tasks at one stage before progressing to the next. For example, some 4-year-old children are not totally egocentric and sometimes recognize and understand the feelings of others.[19]

Table 5-3 Piaget's Stages of Cognitive Development

Stage (Age)	Summary of Cognitive Characteristics
Sensorimotor phase (birth to 24 months)	
Stage 1: Exercising sensorimotor reflexes (birth to 1 month)	Experiences reflexes in repetitive pattern; uses reflexes to adapt to the world
Stage 2: Primary circular reactions (1 to 4 months)	Uses increased musculoskeletal coordination to practice repetitive actions; is extremely egocentric; attention is focused on body; believes that self causes all events to happen; cannot anticipate result of activity
Stage 3: Secondary circular reactions (4 to 8 months)	Repeats pleasurable behaviors; begins to anticipate results of actions; increasingly focuses on objects in the environment; builds on earlier behavior patterns (imitates sounds)
Stage 4: Coordination of sensory schemata (8 to 12 months)	Refines and coordinates earlier mental associations; object permanence strengthens; behavior or activity is goal-oriented (problem solving begins—combines schemata to reach goal); objects take on symbolic meaning; is increasingly aware of spatial relationships
Stage 5: Tertiary circular reactions (12 to 18 months)	Experiments and observes results of actions (trial and error); recognizes geometric shapes; begins to recognize causality outside self
Stage 6: Inventions of new means through mental combinations (18 to 24 months)	Invents or adapts actions to reach goal (true problem solving); increasingly names and uses symbols; magical thinking continues; symbolic play begins; imitates sex-role behavior
Preoperational phase (2 to 7 years)	
Preconceptual phase (2 to 4 years)	Increasingly uses symbols in language and symbolic play; distinguishes an object from an event; continues to be egocentric; reasons transductively (from particular to part)
Intuitive phase (4 to 7 years)	Centers on one outstanding feature of an object; is irreversible and transductive in thinking; increasingly shows mature use of symbols in language and symbolic play
Concrete operations phase (7 to 11 years)	
Classifies objects according to common features; decenters (focuses on several aspects of an event simultaneously); increasingly uses symbols to organize and manipulate the world; uses seriation to arrange objects; understands conservation	
Formal operations phase (12 to 15 years to adulthood)	
Develops a concept of time; thinks in the past, present, and future; reasons hypothetically (considers all possible outcomes); understands symbolic meaning (understands double meaning of jokes); is egocentric in thinking (personal fable and imaginary audience); reasons inductively and deductively; thinks abstractly	

Cognitive development has prime importance for nurses and all adults working with children. Once an adult knows how children associate thoughts and how they interpret adults' words and events in the environment, the adult can choose words and phrases to best communicate with them. The adult can interpret what a child is really saying. An adult who has studied Piaget's work will never again communicate with children in the same way.

THEORIES OF MORAL DEVELOPMENT

Moral development is defined as the development of a person's sense of justice. It is what guides the person in decisions regarding what is right in terms of relationships with other people and responsibilities toward them. Piaget and Lawrence Kohlberg are two cognitive development theorists who have studied moral reasoning in children.

Piaget believed that children from 3 to 9 years of age reason by a literal interpretation of rules. This first stage, *moral realism,* is characterized by the inability to think about more than one thing at a time or to imagine alternatives or compromises. Children aged 10 and over enter the second stage of moral development—*moral relativism*—when they reach the stage of formal operations. They can consider others when making moral decisions, as well as several possible solutions to a problem, including compromise.[20]

Table 5-4 Kohlberg's Stages of Moral Development

Level and Stage	Summary of Stage	Example
Level I: Preconventional (premoral) Stage 1: Punishment and obedience orientation	Preschoolers decide whether to disobey or not in order to avoid punishment. They are egocentric, cannot appreciate another's viewpoint, cannot anticipate the consequences of disobeying, and cannot analyze thinking; therefore, they have no true moral reasoning. They unquestioningly submit to the power of parents to avoid punishment.	Preschoolers decide not to knock the father's glasses onto the floor because they know that they will be punished.
Stage 2: Instrumental-relativist orientation	School-age children believe that a correct moral choice will be useful to, benefit, and protect them. They recognize the existence of different moral viewpoints but egocentrically believe that correct moral behavior should bring equal reward. Because they are egocentric, they have no true understanding of the abstract concepts of law, fairness, or loyalty.	School-age children's motto might be, "If you scratch my back, I'll scratch yours." They might say, "You must trade me a toy robot that turns into as many cars as the ones I traded you!"
Level II: Conventional (moral) Stage 3: Interpersonal concordance and good boy–nice girl orientation	Preadolescents and adolescents are in the cognitive stage of formal operations and can think abstractly, see another person's viewpoint, analyze their own thinking, and empathize with others. They feel guilty after disobeying, admire authority figures, and are loyal to peers. The teenager obeys rules to be a "good boy" or a "nice girl" and desires approval of authority figures. The adolescent believes that good interpersonal relationships will result in justice.	Most adolescents might say, "You must keep your promise because the other person trusts you." They strive to practice the golden rule.
Stage 4: Society-maintaining orientation (law and order)	Adolescents and adults follow rules, conform to the expectations of their conscience and of society, and recognize that rampant disobedience of laws can lead to the destruction of society. Adolescents strive to maintain good relationships with authority figures to strengthen the community. They examine divergent values but discard them quickly, preferring to associate with persons who have the same values.	Adolescents might say, "If you break the rule, then everyone else will want to." Older teenagers might report a drunk driver or an arsonist in order to protect society.
Level III: Postconventional (principled thinking): achieved in adulthood if it is reached Stage 5: Social-contract orientation, with legalistic overtones		
Stage 6: Decisions of conscience; self-chosen ethical principles		

Kohlberg expanded and validated Piaget's original research by studying children from various cultures. Both Kohlberg and Piaget studied children's intended behaviors, not their actual behaviors. Kohlberg proposes three levels of moral development: preconventional, conventional, and postconventional. Each level is further broken down into two stages (Table 5-4). Although Kohlberg did not link ages to each level, others have assigned approximate ages of 5 to 10 or 12 to level I, ages 10 or 12 to 25 to level II, and ages 25 and over to level III.[21]

Kohlberg believes that children's moral values develop primarily through interactions with parents and peers. Initially the child is exposed to the parents' values. Parental approval of the desired moral behavior causes the child to internalize the value that will subsequently guide behavior. As the child moves into the wider world, peers and other adults stimulate the child to examine and modify his or her existing moral beliefs. It is only by being exposed to people whose thinking is at higher moral levels that one can be stimulated to restructure thoughts and modify existing moral beliefs and thus achieve a higher stage of moral development.

Kohlberg has been criticized for using a sexually biased sample, consisting only of males, and for his stories of moral dilemmas. Like Piaget, he has also been criticized for supporting the concept of invariant stage progression—the concept that a child must go through stage 1 before stage 2, stage 2 before 3, etc.[22]

Nevertheless, nurses should be aware of the stages of moral development in order to assess a child's stage. Nurses can also help parents understand how their child learns moral reasoning and the norms of the culture.[23]

References

1. Hymovich, Debra P., and Robert W. Chamberlin, *Child and Family Development: Implications for Primary Care,* McGraw-Hill, New York, 1980, p. 1.
2. Stangler, Sharon, et al., *Screening Growth and Development of Preschool Children,* McGraw-Hill, New York, 1980, p. 1.
3. Smart, Mollie, and Russell C. Smart, *Children,* Macmillan, New York, 1976, p. 647.
4. Klaus, Marshall H., and John H. Kennell, *Maternal-Infant Bonding,* Mosby, St. Louis, 1978, p. 81.
5. Maier, Henry W., *Three Theories of Child Development,* Harper & Row, New York, 1978, p. 81.
6. Hymovich and Chamberlin, op. cit., p. 5.
7. Maier, op. cit., pp. 79, 81.
8. Ibid., pp. 75–76.
9. Ibid., p. 81.
10. Ibid., pp. 75–76.
11. Ibid., pp. 13, 16.
12. Elkind, David, "Piagetian Psychology and Child Psychiatry," *Journal of American Academy of Child Psychiatry* **21**(5):435–445 (September 1982).
13. Maier, op. cit., p. 21.
14. Ibid., p. 20.
15. Ault, Ruth, *Children's Cognitive Development: Piaget's Theory and the Process Approach,* Oxford University Press, New York, 1977, pp. 12, 13.
16. Maier, op. cit., p. 29.
17. Ault, op. cit., p. 18.
18. Ibid., p. 87.
19. Rest, James, "Developmental Psychology and Value Education," in Brenda Munsey (ed.), *Moral Development, Moral Education, and Kohlberg,* Religious Education Press, Birmingham, 1980, pp. 109–113.
20. McCown, Darlene, "Moral Development in Children," *Pediatric Nursing* **10**(1):42 (January–February 1984).
21. Ibid.
22. Santrock, John W., *Life Span Development,* Wm. C. Brown, Dubuque, Iowa, 1983, pp. 152–153.
23. McCown, op. cit., p. 44.

6

Marjorie J. Smith

Human genetics

Upon completion of this chapter, the student will be able to:

1 Define terms used to describe genetic diseases.
2 Contrast the terms *DNA*, *gene*, and *chromosome*.
3 Compare mitosis and meiosis.
4 Describe the significance of nondisjunction and translocation in chromosomal abnormalities.
5 Diagram the inheritance pattern for (*a*) an autosomal dominant disorder, (*b*) an autosomal recessive disorder, and (*c*) an X-linked recessive disorder in a carrier mother and affected male.
6 List three inborn errors of metabolism.
7 List three polygenic disorders.
8 List four environmental factors that influence genetic expression.
9 Describe the nurse's role in genetic evaluation.

Nurses who work with children and their families are asked many questions about the children's development, characteristics, and illness. In the case of hospitalized children, what is often behind these questions is the concern that heredity is involved in the illness and that in some way the parents are responsible. Recent studies have shown that 30 percent of admissions to children's hospitals and between 40 and 50 percent of deaths occurring in such facilities involve children with genetic disorders or congenital malformations.[1] Nurses must understand the role of heredity in disease. Disease is part of a complex interplay between heredity and the environment. The hereditary (genetic) influence may be great, and the environmental one slight, as in Down syndrome and in many of the conditions discussed in this chapter. The reverse may also be true, as in infections, some congenital defects, and multifactorial disorders. (See Table 6-1.)

Inherited disease can be evident at birth or can appear later in development. Below are examples of inherited characteristics that become

Table 6-1 Terms Used in Describing Inherited Disorders

Congenital Defect
A condition present at birth that may be caused by genetic factors or by such environmental factors as irradiation, infection, trauma, or chemicals

Familial Disorder
Any defect or disorder that appears more often in a family than would be predicted by chance

Genetic Disorder
Any disorder due to:
1. A chromosomal abnormality
2. A single mutant gene (e.g., Mendelian disorders)
3. Multiple mutant genes (polygenic)
4. Multifactorial causes (combination of genetic and environmental factors)

Inherited
Same as genetic disorder. Also called *heritable* or *heredity* disorder. Transmitted by genes from parent to offspring

evident at different stages of an individual's development:[2]

1. Polydactyly (extra fingers and toes): early embryonic stage
2. Eye pigmentation: a few days or weeks after birth
3. Tay-Sachs disease: 6 months to 1 year
4. Duchenne muscular dystrophy: 10 to 15 years
5. Wilson disease: 8 to 20 years
6. Hereditary baldness: 25 to 50 years
7. Huntington disease (progressive mental and nervous deterioration): 30 to 50 years

GENETICS AND INFORMATION TRANSFER

Genetics concerns the flow of biological information from one generation to the next. Humans have always found this subject intriguing. Most often our interest takes the form of deciding which parent contributed to a child's physical features, intelligence, or special skills. Little scientific knowledge was available about genetic information transfer before the development of the microscope in the 1600s. Afterward some curious theories were developed about which parent was responsible for the genetic endowment of the child. Near the end of the century a Swiss naturalist claimed to have seen a miniature human, which he termed a *homunculus,* in sperm cells. This "preformed" adult had merely to grow to become a full-sized human. Others thought that the homunculus existed in the ovum instead.

In the nineteenth century it became clear that fertilization produces a zygote that divides many times, leading to development of the embryo, the fetus, and finally the infant. For a time it was widely believed that the blood carried hereditary factors that somehow entered the fertilized egg. From this notion comes such expressions as "It's in his blood," "blue blood," and "blood brothers."

In 1865 Gregor Mendel, an Augustinian monk, after carefully breeding peas over 8 years and analyzing the results mathematically, announced that inheritance of traits follows a predictable pattern; there are *laws* of heredity. His highly original contribution was neglected until 1900, but then, upon "rediscovery," accelerated the pace of genetic investigations. Since then much has become clear about the physical basis of heredity.

PHYSICAL BASIS OF HEREDITY

Chromosomes: the carriers

The actual units of inheritance, the *genes,* reside on *chromosomes,* the coiled threadlike bodies in the cell nucleus. Because genes are too small to be seen, for a long time their nature could only be deduced from experiments with chromosomes. Using fruit flies and certain plants, investigators, especially after 1900, built up a considerable knowledge of both genes and chromosomes from observable traits.

Information about human chromosomes, which are more difficult to isolate and to visualize, accumulated slowly. Only in 1956 was it determined that the normal human body cell contains 46 chromosomes. Human gametes, the sperm and ova, contain half that number, but in sexual union the male gamete's 23 chromosomes join the female's 23 in the fertilized cell, or *zygote,* which then has the normal complement of 46 chromosomes. The term *diploid* refers to the normal complement of chromosomes in body cells (46), and the term *haploid* to the normal number in mature gametes (23).

After staining, the 46 chromosomes can be grouped by shape into 22 pairs of *autosomes* and two *sex chromosomes*. The sex chromosomes look alike in the female but are unlike in the male. They are symbolized XX in the female, but XY

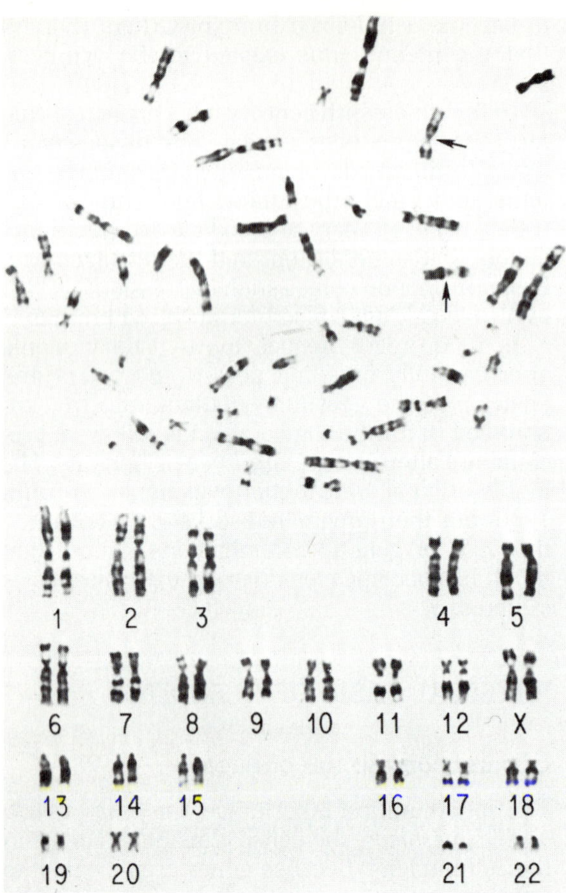

Figure 6-1 Normal female 46,XX. The X chromosomes are marked with arrows. A karyotype is prepared from lymphocytes or fibroblasts cultured from skin, gonad, or amniotic cells. The cells are grown in a nutrient medium and stimulated to undergo mitosis. Colchicine is applied to stop growth in metaphase, when the chromosomes are contracted and duplicated. Chemicals are added to cause swelling and enhance visibility. A photograph is taken of the magnified chromosomes (top half of figure). Then the chromosomes are cut from the picture, matched into homologous pairs, and numbered. The resultant arrangement of homologous chromosomes is known as a *karyotype.* (*Courtesy of Dr. Gordon DeWald, Rochester, Minn.*)

in the male. It is the Y chromosome that determines maleness.

When a photograph of stained chromosomes is cut up and all the chromosomes from a single body cell are arranged by size and shape, the result is known as a *karyotype*. For a normal female it is expressed as 46,XX. Figure 6-1 shows a normal female karyotype and the original picture from which it was prepared. One member of each homologous (matching) pair is from the mother, and one is from the father.

Genes: the units of heredity

Each human being carries 50,000 to 100,000 genes.[3] A single gene is said to reside at a *point* or *locus* on a chromosome. Because chromosomes come in pairs, there is a gene at the corresponding locus on the other member of the pair. Either member of a gene pair can be referred to as an *allele*.

If both alleles are alike, that is, produce an identical trait, the person is *homozygous* for the trait. If they are not alike, the individual is *heterozygous* for the trait.

In a heterozygous person, the allele that is expressed is *dominant;* the unexpressed, nonidentical allele is *recessive*. The latter exists in the *genotype*, the genetic makeup of the person, but not in the *phenotype*, the observable traits. A child's genotype may include a gene for black hair, for instance, and a corresponding allele for blond hair. Because black is dominant, black hair will be part of the phenotype, but the genotype remains a mixture of genes for both black and blond hair. The child would be blond (phenotype) only if he or she were homozygous for the trait, that is, if all alleles were for blond hair. Some traits that display these simple Mendelian patterns are shown in Fig. 6-2. Current information suggests that several genes may determine hair or eye color.

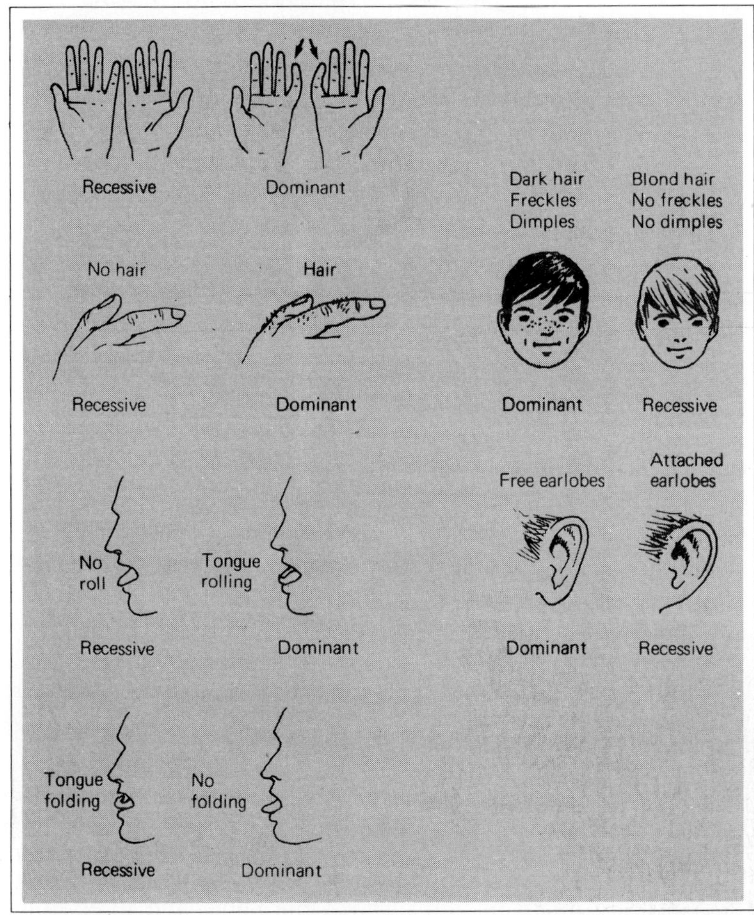

Figure 6-2 Some simple Mendelian traits found in humans. (*From Ana Pai, Foundations of Genetics, McGraw-Hill, New York, 1974. Used with permission.*)

DNA: chemical basis of the gene

Intensive research in the 1940s led to the conclusion that genetic information is stored in the DNA (deoxyribonucleic acid) of the chromosomes. In 1953 Francis Crick and James Watson announced their finding that DNA is actually a double strand resembling a twisted stepladder, a shape that chemists call a *double helix* (Fig. 6-3). The vertical sides are sugars and phosphates; the rungs are small molecules known as *bases*, linked at the middle by hydrogen bonds. Buried in this complex shape in coded form is the cell's genetic message, the information that dictates its nature and serves to regulate and direct its functions.

A gene has been defined as a length of DNA that directs the manufacture of a polypeptide. Long polypeptide molecules are proteins. Protein synthesis is an important task directed by DNA.

Proteins are unique molecules of the body. They may be "structural" (such as keratin, collagen, and elastin) or "functional" (as in antibodies, hormones, and enzymes). Protein synthesis is directed by DNA but employs many other molecules, including amino acids, which serve as building blocks of polypeptides (Fig. 6-4).

A second vital function of DNA is the transfer of the genotype from one cell generation to the next. It does this shortly before each cell division. The double strand of chromosomal DNA comes apart. Each strand acts as a template, or model, on which molecules from the cell are assembled to reproduce the missing strand. This self-reproduction is known as *replication*. Because replication must precede each cell division, it is remarkable that a person's genotype can be carried faithfully through the many thousands of cell divisions that begin with the zygote. It is little wonder that "copying" errors or other changes occasionally take place.

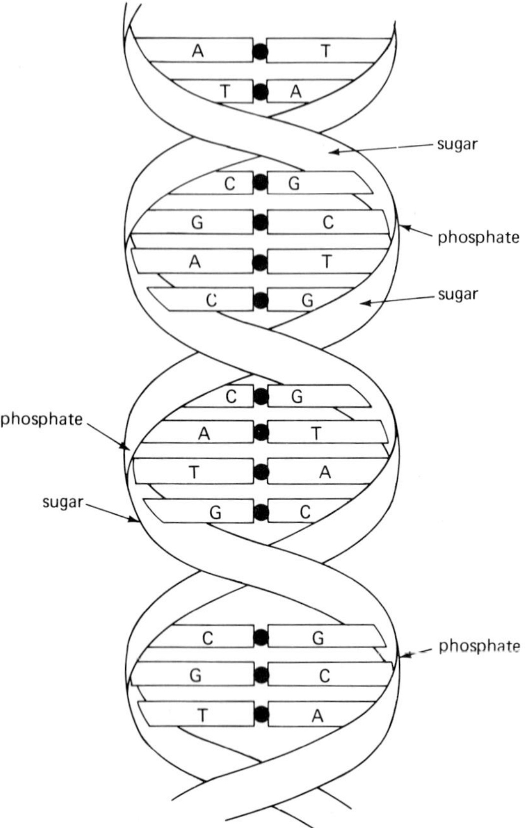

Figure 6-3 The DNA molecule is a double helix composed of sugars and phosphates along the sides. The following bases make up the crossbars: adenine (A), thymine (T), guanine (G), and cytosine (C). (*From E. Dickason and M. Schult, Maternal and Infant Care, McGraw-Hill, New York, 1979. Used with permission.*)

Gene cloning

Methods using restriction enzymes have been developed to cut DNA into specific pieces, or nucleotide sequences, that produce a *restriction map* that is characteristic of the particular piece of DNA being studied.[4] Mutations in a DNA molecule can be detected through this method. DNA fragments can be spliced into plasmids (or phages) and placed in a one-celled organism (bacteria), where they will replicate producing *clones*, or carbon copies, of the DNA piece. This produces enough protein to study gene structure and function. These techniques of recombinant DNA methodology are being used today to isolate the functional or dysfunctional nucleotide sequence of a gene or its mutants and to study it in detail. Isolated genes can be linked to promoters and

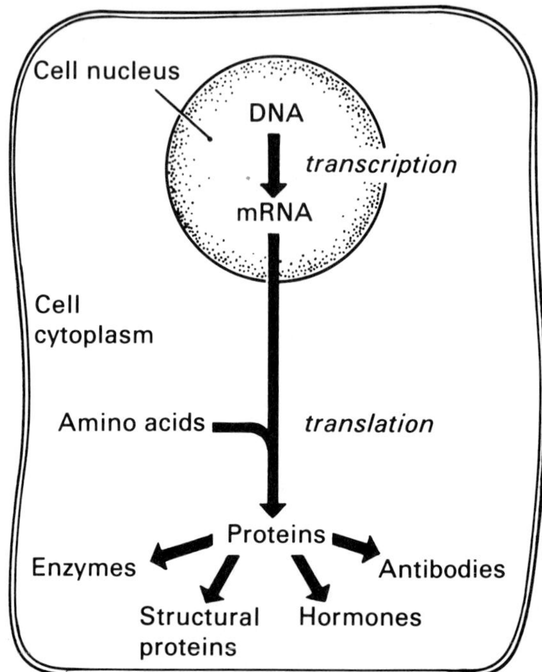

Figure 6-4 Protein synthesis employs messenger ribonucleic acid (mRNA) as the intermediary. In *transcription* mRNA takes the genetic message from DNA in the cell nucleus. In *translation* the message is used to direct protein synthesis in the cytoplasm.

forced to produce relatively large amounts of human insulin, growth hormone, and interferon, for example.[5] Conceivably, genes can be corrected and possibly inserted into humans.

CELL DIVISION

While it is true that cell division is not the only time when genetic changes—or *mutations*, as they are known—occur, the cell engaged in reproducing itself is peculiarly vulnerable to chance occurrences and outside influences. There are two types of cell division: mitosis and meiosis. *Mitosis* is responsible for cellular growth. *Meiosis* is responsible for reproduction and genetic variation.

Mitosis

In all multicellular organisms, dividing cells undergo *mitosis*. Figure 6-5 shows mitosis in a cell that has a diploid number of four chromosomes. During the first step of mitosis, *prophase*, chromosomes in the cell nucleus form a two-

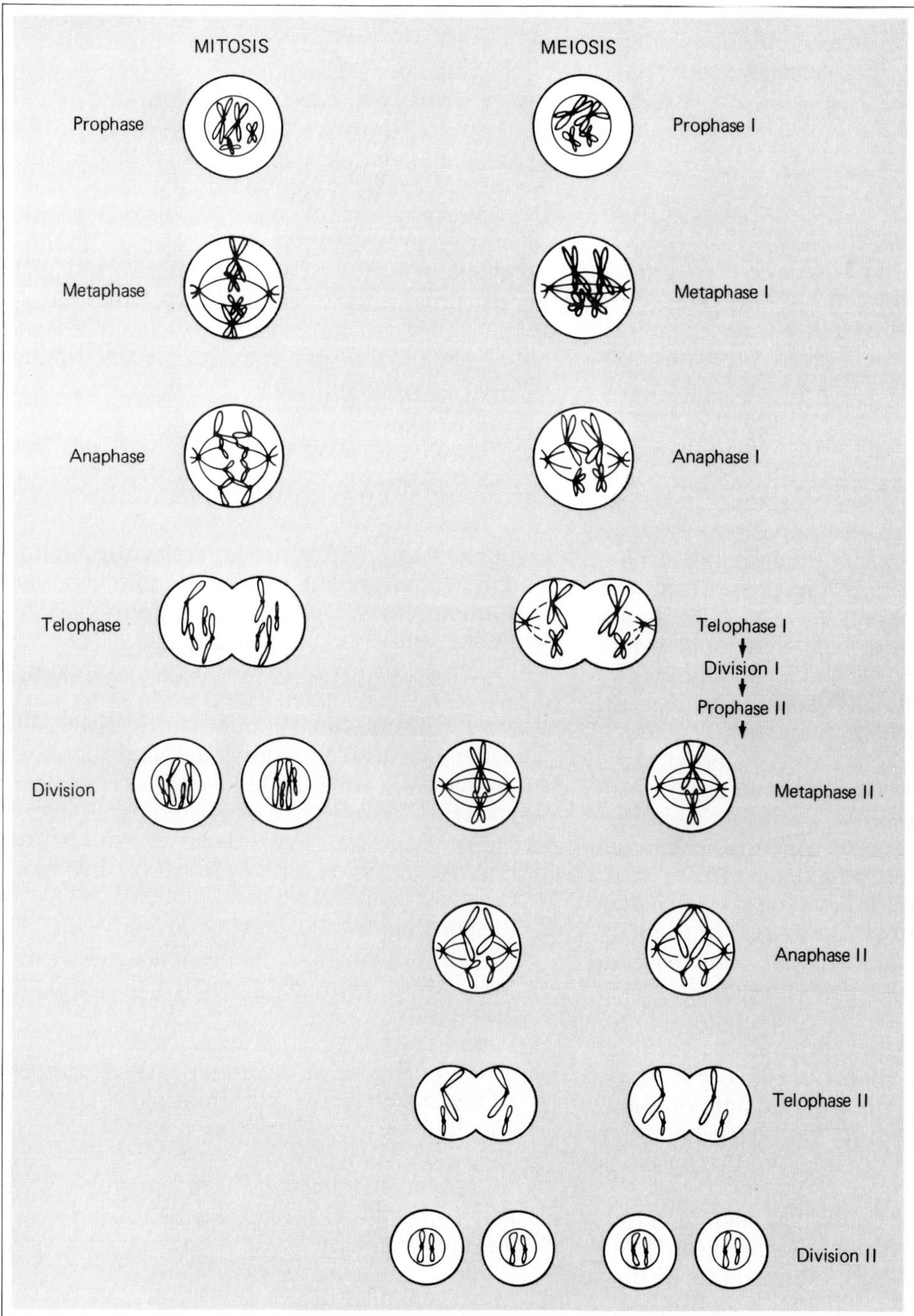

Figure 6-5 Comparison of *mitosis* in somatic cells with *meiosis* in reproductive cells in an organism (fruit fly) with a *diploid number of 4*. (*From Ana Pai, Foundations of Genetics, McGraw-Hill, New York, 1974. Used with permission.*)

stranded coil and take on a short, thick appearance. The constricted portion where the two strands join is called the *centromere*.

During the second phase, *metaphase*, chromosomes line up across the middle of the cell (equatorial plate). *Anaphase* begins when the strands separate at the centromere. Each strand, now itself a chromosome, moves away from its partner toward opposite poles of the cell. In *telophase,* the cell nucleus is reestablished, and the cell prepares to divide. Cell division occurs next. Each resulting cell has a diploid number of four chromosomes that are identical to those of the parent cell.

Meiosis

Production of sperm and ova entails a unique additional step, a reduction division. The number of chromosomes provided by each parent cell is thereby reduced to one-half in the mature gamete. In human beings this means that, while the sex cell begins with 46 chromosomes, the gametes produced contain 23 chromosomes. The overall process is called *meiosis* (Fig. 6-5), of which reduction division is one step.

Meiosis with its reduction division serves an essential purpose. Mitosis without meiosis would leave gametes with 46 chromosomes, and the fertilized egg would begin life with 92 chromosomes. Each cell of the new individual would contain 92 chromosomes. With sexual union the number would be doubled again. Clearly, cell function as we know it would be impossible.

In meiosis, prophase I brings paternal chromosomes opposite homologous maternal chromosomes in a tight pairing known as *synapsis.* The nuclear membrane dissolves, and spindle fibers attach to the centromeres.

During metaphase I the homologous pairs arrange themselves across the middle of the cell. In anaphase I the pairs separate and move to opposite poles. Note that the chromosomes do not split lengthwise at the centromere; therefore, no doubling of the chromosome number occurs as in mitosis. Telophase I is very brief, and the cell completes its first meiotic division, the reduction division, in which each daughter cell contains half the number of chromosomes of the parent cell.

The second meiotic division begins in the daughter cells immediately. In prophase II the pairs condense again, and in metaphase II they line up along the cell's equator. This time the centromere divides, and daughter chromosomes move to opposite poles in anaphase II. In telophase II the nuclear membrane re-forms around the nuclear substance at each pole, and the second cell division follows. This division is not a reduction division; the haploid condition of the parent cell is preserved in the daughter cells. However, there are significant differences between sperm and ova in the details of maturation (Fig. 6-6).

Spermatogenesis begins in the testes at puberty. Sexually mature males continuously produce sperm; however, the lifetime supply of oocytes is present in the female at birth. They remain arrested at prophase I until puberty. Then, as each ovarian follicle matures, meiotic division resumes and is completed at the time of ovulation. The older a woman is, therefore, the older her ova are. There is evidence that, with increasing age, ova are more likely to carry damaged chromosomes that are more susceptible to misdivision or nondisjunction.

CHROMOSOMAL ABNORMALITIES

In a broad sense, *mutation* refers to any change in genetic information, including addition or loss of chromosomes, alterations of chromosome structure, and changes within a gene.

Too much or too little chromosomal material in all or some of a person's cells leads to a clinical disorder. Chromosomal abnormalities have a significant impact on the individual, and therefore on the family of the individual and possibly even on society. Chromosomal alterations are:

1. Present in 6 to 7 of every 1000 live-born infants[6]
2. Responsible for 60 percent of early and 40 percent of late spontaneous abortions[7]
3. Associated with 7 percent of perinatal mortalities[8]
4. Found in at least 10 percent of couples who give a history of *at least two* early abortions, stillbirths, or births with multiple congenital anomalies.[9]

Alterations in chromosomes usually involve either *number* or *structure.* The following types of chromosomal abnormalities are recognized:

1. Abnormal chromosome number—*aneuploidy*
   a. *Monosomy* The absence of *one* of a pair of chromosomes.
   b. *Trisomy* The presence of *three* chromosomes instead of the usual pair (Fig. 6-7).
   c. *Polyploidy* The presence of *extra sets* of chromosomes; a multiple of the haploid number. Polyploidy is common in plants but *lethal* in humans.

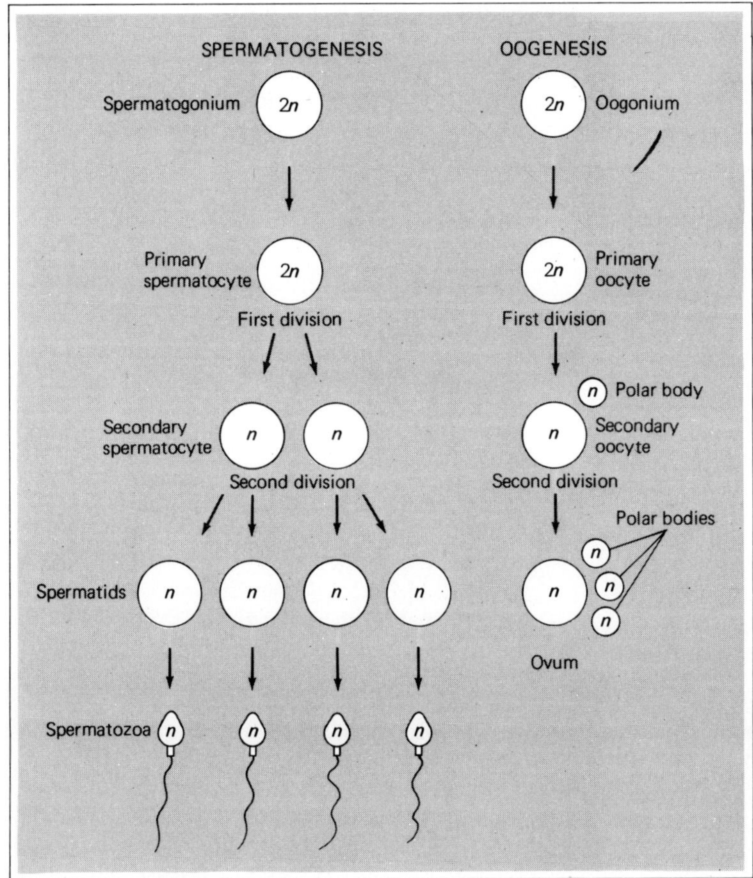

Figure 6-6 Spermatogenesis and oogenesis. In preparation for fertilization sperm and ovum go through the process of meiosis, in which the number of chromosomes is reduced from 23 pairs ($2n$) to $23n$. The four spermatozoa resulting from sperm maturation are all capable of reproducing. Of the four cells resulting from maturation of the ovum, however, three of the nuclei are not supplied with cytoplasm and become polar bodies, leaving only *one* capable of being fertilized. (*Source: Ana Pai, Foundations of Genetics, McGraw-Hill, New York, 1974. Used with permission.*)

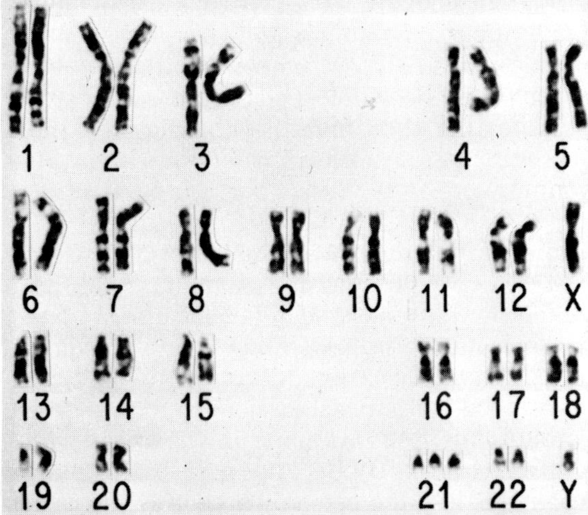

Figure 6-7 Trisomy 21 karyotype from a male with Down syndrome. Note *three* chromosomes No. 21. The shorthand description is 47,XY, +21. (*Courtesy of Dr. Gordon DeWald.*)

2. Abnormal morphology or structure
   a. *Deletions* The absence of part of a chromosome.
   b. *Reciprocal translocations* The *exchange* of chromosomal material between two nonhomologous chromosomes during cell division.
   c. *Inversion* During cell division a section of a chromosome breaks apart, turns end to end, and is reinserted, resulting in the reverse order of the genes.

When there is a net gain or loss of autosomal material, three things happen: growth retardation, mental retardation, and many major or minor malformations.

Mechanisms of chromosome alteration

Nondisjunction Abnormal *numbers* of chromosomes usually result from an error during cell division. The most common cause of monosomy or trisomy is failure to separate, that is, *nondisjunction,* during the first or second division of

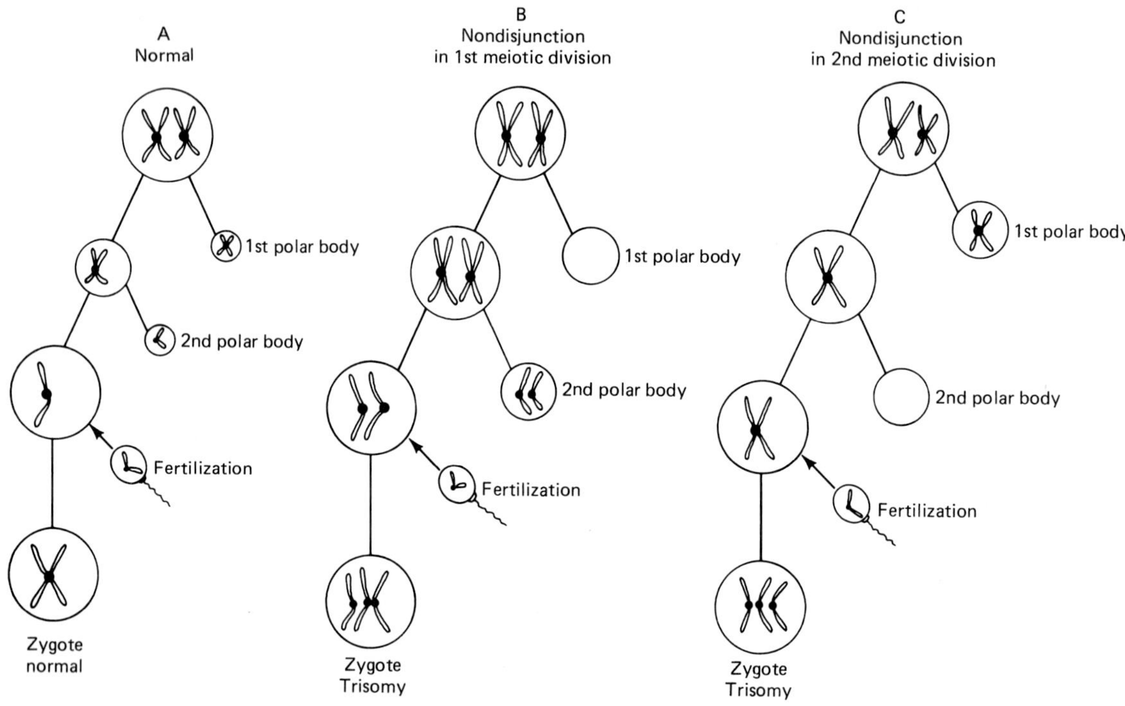

Figure 6-8 (*A*) Chromosome distribution in normal germ cell development. (*B*) Chromosome distribution in nondisjunction during the first meiotic division. (*C*) Chromosome distribution in nondisjunction during the second meiotic division.

meiosis (Fig. 6-8). If an ovum missing one chromosome is fertilized, the zygote, with 45 chromosomes, is said to be *monosomic*. Monosomy of the X chromosome is found both in spontaneously aborted fetuses (9 percent) and in live births. Monosomy of an autosome is lethal and so is found only in spontaneous abortions.

When an ovum with one extra chromosome is fertilized, the zygote, with 47 chromosomes, is said to be *trisomic*. It is also possible for a sperm to be responsible for the extra chromosome. Trisomy occurs in autosomes and sex chromosomes. Trisomy of autosomes 8, 13, 18, and 21 is seen in live infants. Trisomy of the larger chromosomes is usually lethal. (See Table 6-2.) Sixty-five percent of all trisomy 21 conceptions are lost as spontaneous abortions, most in the first trimester. Of the other common autosomal abnormalities, 90 to 95 percent are lost as spontaneous abortions.

Nondisjunction may also occur during mitosis soon after the zygote has been created. This leads to the presence of at least two different cell lines, which is called *mosaicism* (Fig. 6-9). A person can be mosaic and have a normal phenotype or can exhibit some abnormal traits. Most often, a mosaic person shows some signs that would be expected if the whole body were composed of cells bearing the abnormal chromosome number, but is less severely affected than one who is nonmosaic.

Translocation A *translocation* occurs when a part of a chromosome moves and attaches itself to another chromosome. Translocations change chromosome *structure*. They take place during cell division. Occasionally, pieces of two nonhomologous chromosomes join to form a single chromosome. This is known as a *balanced translocation* (Fig. 6-10). Because none of the genetic material is lost, the person whose cells carry such a translocation will appear normal, although the abnormal structure will be revealed in a karyotype. The significance of a balanced translocation appears in the next generation, when a person carrying this abnormal karyotype be-

Table 6-2 Common Chromosomal (Autosomal) Abnormalities*

Autosomal Disorder	Chromosomal Abnormality	Incidence	Characteristic Features	Genetic Significance
Down syndrome	Trisomy 21	1:1000 live births	Mental retardation; congenital anomalies; flat facial features; large, protruding tongue; upward-slanting eyes; prominent epicanthal folds; short, broad, stubby hands with simian crease; hypotonia; usually sterile but some females can reproduce with 50% risk of trisomic offspring	Related to advanced maternal age unless due to translocation (4%); father has been shown to be source of extra chromosome in 24% of cases;† 1% mosaics
Edward syndrome	Trisomy 18	1:8000 live births	Microcephaly; small eyes; deformed ears; small mouth; congenital heart disease; overriding, clenched fingers; 85% die within 6 months; mental retardation; rocker-bottom feet	Related to advanced maternal age, primary nondisjunction; 10% mosaics
Patau syndrome	Trisomy 13	1:6000 live births	Microcephaly; microophthalmos; cleft lip and palate; low-set ears; congenital heart disease; polycystic kidneys; polydactyly; deafness; mental retardation; slanting palpebral fissures	Death occurs in infancy without mosaicism; related to advanced maternal age
Cri-du-chat syndrome	Deletion of short arm of chromosome No. 5	1:15,000 live births	Severe mental retardation; microcephaly; weak, high-pitched cry due to hypoplasia of the larynx; low-set ears; downward-slanting eyes; retarded growth	10 to 15% due to inherited translocation
Warkany syndrome	Trisomy 8	Unknown	Growth and mental retardation; congenital skeletal defects and contractures; urinary tract anomaly; micrognathia; dysmorphic facies	Due to mosaicism or to translocation

*All are detectable in utero.

†L. B. Holmes, "Genetic Counseling for the Older Pregnant Woman: New Data and Questions," *New England Journal of Medicine* **298**(25):1419 (June 1978).

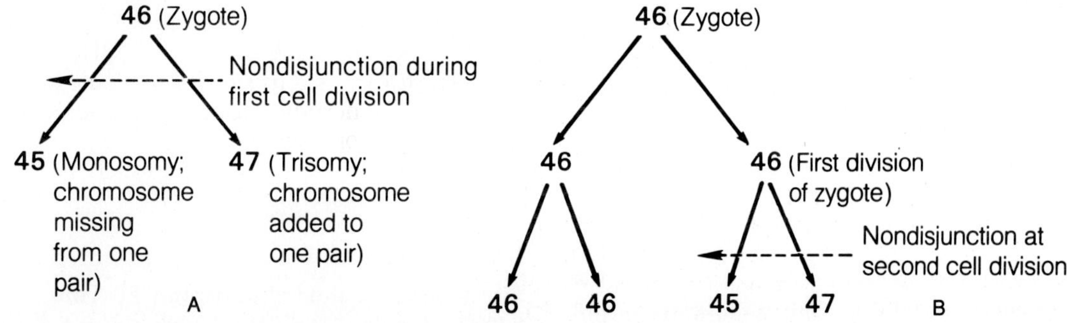

Figure 6-9 Mosaicism due to nondisjunction during mitosis. (*A*) One cell line is monosomic (45). If this involves an autosome, the cell line will not survive. However, a mosaic with a cell line 45,X/47,XXY could survive. (*B*) The cell line 45 will also not survive, but the individual would have two normal cell lines (46) and one with an extra chromosome (47). Survival is then possible if a small autosome or sex chromosome is involved.

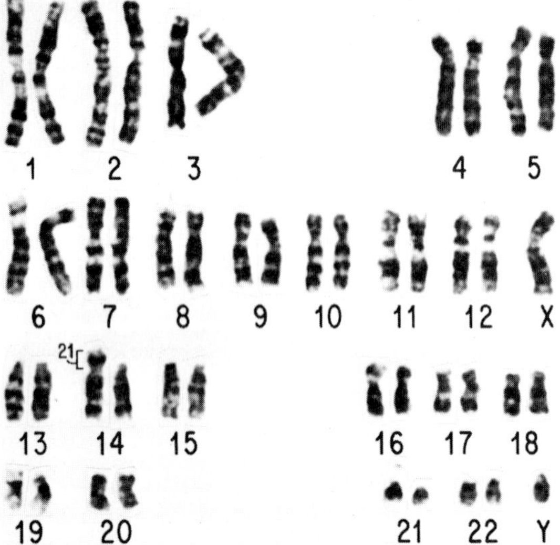

Figure 6-10 Trisomy 21 resulting from translocation of an extra chromosome No. 21 to chromosome No. 14. The father of this subject had one regular chromosome No. 21 and one chromosome No. 21 attached to chromosome No. 14. With only two No. 21 chromosomes the father had a *balanced* translocation and appeared normal. However, during spermatogenesis, the sperm received both the normal chromosome No. 21 and the chromosome No. 21 attached to chromosome No. 14. When this sperm fertilized an ovum containing one chromosome No. 21, the resulting male child received *three* chromosomes No. 21, and is said to have an *unbalanced translocation*. This is written 46,XY, +21. (*Courtesy of Dr. Gordon DeWald.*)

comes a parent. If part of chromosome 21 becomes attached to chromosome 14 in the formation of gametes, both this 14-21 chromosome and a normal chromosome 21 may be passed to the child. If the other parent contributes a normal chromosome 21, the child will be trisomic for chromosome 21.

Deletion Structural defects of chromosomes are best understood as the consequence of breakage. Deletion occurs when one end of a chromosome breaks off and is lost. For example, deletion of the small arm of chromosome 5 results in the cri-du-chat syndrome (Table 6-2). Infants with cri-du-chat syndrome have a distinctive face characterized by microcephaly, hypertelorism, low-set ears, and micrognathia; they also suffer from severe mental retardation, fail to grow normally, and cry like a mewing cat.

Trisomy 21

Trisomy 21 is one of the more common trisomies (Table 6-2). The clinical condition, which includes mental retardation and other defects, is known as *Down syndrome* (DS).

Down syndrome is characterized by mild microcephaly, upward slanting of palpebral fissures with prominent epicanthal folds, small nose and ears, a small maxilla that causes the tongue to protrude, and decreased muscle tone. The hands and feet are short, with incurving of the fifth finger. There is a characteristic single palmar crease, the "simian crease" (Fig. 6-11).

The presence of the triple dose of genes on chromosome 21 is responsible for the characteristics of the DS child. Birth weight and length are normal; growth is also normal until about

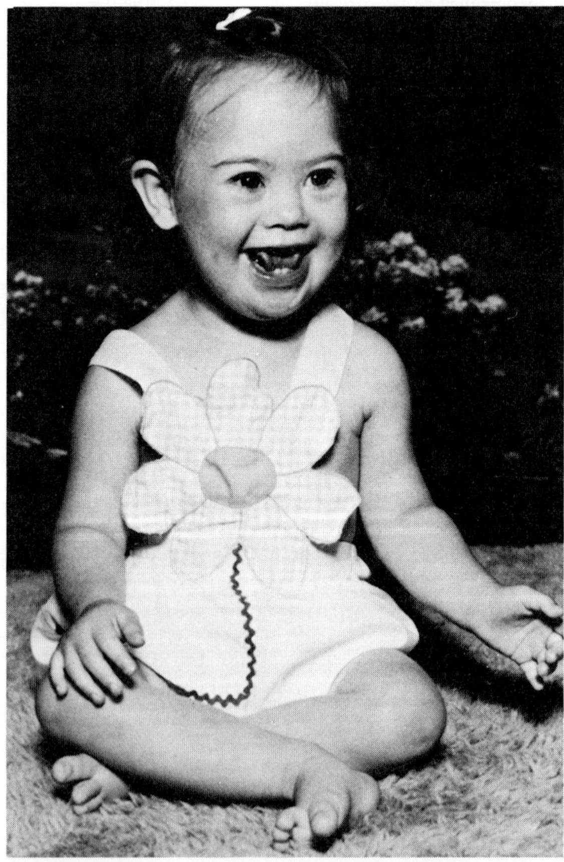

Figure 6-11 A child with trisomy 21. This smiling 18-month-old child shows some of the characteristics of Down syndrome. (*A*) Epicanthal folds on the eyes. (*B*) A prominent tongue. (*C*) A single transverse palmar crease (simian crease). (*D*) A short fifth finger. (*E*) Wide spacing between the first and second toes.

age 4, when it slows. The mean IQ after age 6 is 50, with a range from 15 to 75. Forty percent of these children have congenital heart defects, and they are prone to developing goiters, hypothyroidism, infectious disease, and leukemia (1 in 100).

Demographic changes from 1920 to 1970 caused a trend toward a reduction in the incidence of DS babies.[10] In the 1950s and 1960s, 50 percent of DS babies were born to mothers aged 35 and older. In the 1970s, only 25 percent of DS babies were born to mothers over 35.[11] This was due partly to a decrease in births among older women and partly to prenatal diagnosis and abortion. It is predicted, however, that the number of DS babies born in the United States will increase 35 percent—from 4300 to 5300 per year—by 1990, when it will remain relatively stable.[12] This number could be decreased by one-fourth to one-third if amniocentesis were utilized by 37.5 percent of women aged 30 to 34 and by 75 percent of women aged 35 and older.[13] The incidence of Down syndrome in relation to maternal age is described in Table 6-3.

Holmes[14] reports that the father of the affected baby is the source of the extra chromosome in 24 percent of the cases studied. The risk that the extra chromosome will come from the father is twice as great if he is over 55.[15] Honest genetic counseling of parents who have a baby with Down syndrome may free mothers from feeling solely responsible.

Nondisjunction causes 94 percent of trisomy 21 births. The risk in the general population for an offspring with trisomy 21 is 1 in 1000. If one parent's genotype contains a balanced translocation, however, the risk of a trisomic offspring increases greatly. When the father is the balanced translocation carrier, the chance of having a trisomic baby is 1 in 20, or 5 percent. For a carrier mother, the chance is 1 in 5, or 20 percent. Translocation is responsible for 5 percent of trisomy 21 births; mosaicism accounts for 1 percent.

Table 6-3 Risk of Down Syndrome (Due to Nondisjunction)

Mother's Age	Risk of Down Syndrome	Risk of a Chromosomal Abnormality
15	1:1000	1:450
20	1:1200	1:500
30	1:1000	1:400
35	1:300	1:200
40	1:100	1:70
45	1:30	1:20

Source: Kenneth Garver, "Parental Age in Birth Defects," *Genetics in Practice* **1**(4):3 (Fall 1984).

Balanced translocations in close relatives of an affected child may also serve as a clue to increased risk of Down syndrome.

Example: A 24-year-old female, 6 weeks pregnant, came to her physician concerned about her sister's child with Down syndrome. She wondered if this could happen to her child. Her karyotype revealed a 14-21 translocation. When she learned of the 20 percent risk of having a Down syndrome baby, she decided to have an amniocentesis. When this was performed, at 16 weeks, a fetus with trisomy 21 was revealed. She elected to terminate the pregnancy.

Amniocentesis and karyotyping of fetal cells make it possible to determine whether the fetus is genetically normal, a balanced translocation carrier, or an affected individual with trisomy.

Alterations in sex chromosomes

Sex chromosomes can undergo the same abnormal changes as autosomes; nondisjunction during meiosis plays a major role. Eighteen percent of all chromosomally abnormal abortions are due to abnormalities in sex chromosomes.[16] Sex chromosome abnormalities are present in 0.2 percent of newborns[17] and are manifested anytime from birth to beyond puberty by ambiguous genitalia, delayed onset of puberty, hypogonadism, amenorrhea, infertility, variation in stature, or other congenital anomalies. Table 6-4 describes common sex chromosome abnormalities.

In *all* cells of a 46,XX female one X becomes inactivated in early embryonic development. If this did not happen, the female would have twice as many X chromosome genes as the male. This inactive X, visible at interphase as a dark spot in the cell, is called the *X chromatin* and is also known as the *Barr body* (Fig. 6-12*A*). An XX female has one X chromatin in all cells. An XY male and an X female have *none*. An XXX female will have two X-chromatin bodies. Regardless of genetic makeup, an individual will have only one active X chromosome per cell.

The presence of the Y chromosome can be detected at metaphase when the cell is stained with fluorescing dye, quinacrine mustard. The *Y-chromatin body* is shown in Fig. 6-12*B*. These

Table 6-4 Common Sex Chromosomal Abnormalities*

Chromosomal Disorder	Abnormality	Phenotype	Incidence†	Characteristics
Monosomy X Turner syndrome (gonadal dysgenesis)	45,X (mosaicism possible)	Female	1:2500 female births	Amenorrhea; short stature; webbed neck; lack of sexual development at puberty; hypoplastic nails; sterility
Klinefelter syndrome	47,XXY (most common) 48,XXYY 48,XXXY 48,XXXXY	Male	1:1000 male births 15% mosaics	Hypogonadism; infertility; low birth weight; delayed speech; poor gross motor coordination; variable mental retardation. The more X chromosomes, the more serious is the disease. Often are phenotypically normal at birth, have frequent school problems, gynecomastia, increased height, decreased libido, and decreased testosterone secretion
Supernumerary X (triple X)	47,XXX 48,XXXX 49,XXXXX	Female	1:1000 female births	Often phenotypically normal at birth; one-third may be mentally retarded, have irregular menses, decreased fertility, increased speech and language problems, and a variety of major or minor congenital malformations. Incidence increased with increase in age of parents (offspring have normal karyotype)
XYY syndrome (Superman syndrome)	47,XYY 48,XYYY	Male	1:900 male births	Normal birth weight; phenotypic male; behavior problems; increased height; delayed speech and language development; acne; increase in aggressive behavior (offspring have normal karyotype); 6× more likely to be imprisoned than XY

*All are detectable in utero.

†General frequency of sex chromosomal abnormalities in males is 2.7:1000 and in females is 1.5:1000.

two tests can usually determine the sex chromosome complement of the person from whom the cell was taken without necessitating a karyotype.

SINGLE-GENE DISORDERS

Single-gene defects are due either to a single mutant gene (inherited from one parent) or to a mutant gene pair derived from both parents. Diseases due to mutant genes are classified as autosomal, X-linked, dominant, and recessive. Since the Y chromosome is known to carry only one or two traits, no single-gene disorders have been related to it. Single-gene diseases, though rare, have significant effects on families and children and are responsible for many metabolic diseases.

In the interest of clarity, the following sections describe disorders according to their mechanism of inheritance—autosomal dominant or recessive, X-linked, or inborn errors of metabolism. It is important, however, to keep three things in mind:

1. There are several examples of a clinical phenotype that include autosomal dominant, autosomal recessive, and X-linked forms.
2. Most of the autosomal disorders involve metabolic defects and so could also be considered inborn errors of metabolism.
3. Many of these disorders exist in different forms with varying degrees of severity.

Mendel's laws of inheritance

To understand single-gene disorders, it is helpful to review Mendel's laws of inheritance:

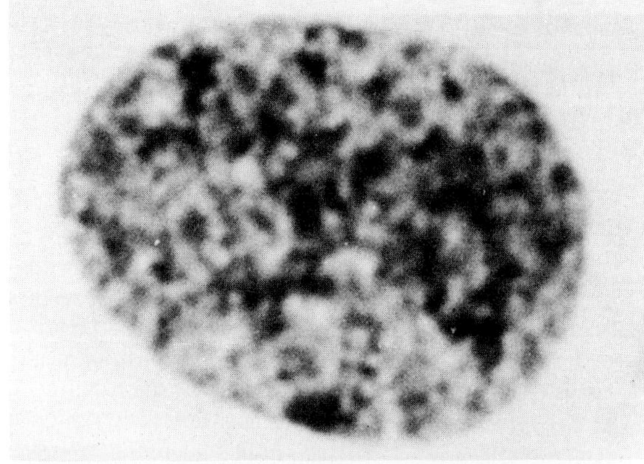

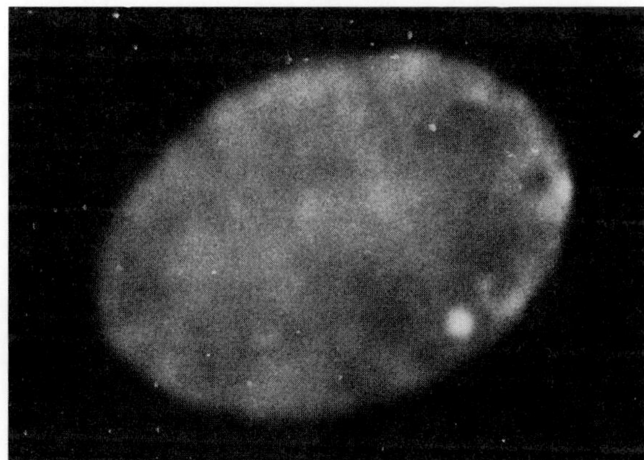

Figure 6-12 (*A*) The dark spot at edge of this cell nucleus is X chromatin and represents inactivated X in the cell with two X chromosomes. (*B*) The light spot in this cell nucleus represents Y chromatin and indicates the presence of a Y chromosome in the cell. (*Courtesy of Dr. Gordon DeWald.*)

Law of dominance and recessiveness When two contrasting genes for a certain trait are paired, one is *dominant* over the other.

Law of segregation When gametes are formed, each gene is *separated from its allele* and passes into a different germ cell (sperm or egg).

Law of independent assortment Different genes segregate independently of one another (i.e., genes are transmitted *independently* of one another).

All genetic traits vary in their *expression,* or the degree to which they are observable in the individual, i.e., whether they are mild, moderate, or severe. *Penetrance* is a statistical term referring to the percentage of individuals with a given gene who express the trait produced by that gene. If only one-half with a mutant gene show its effects, penetrance is 50 percent.

Occasionally two alleles are expressed *equally.* This is true for the major blood groups—A, B, and O. A and B antigens are dominant over O (no antigens). A person with type A blood (phenotype) can be of the genotype AA or AO. When one parent contributes the gene for A antigen and the other parent contributes the gene for B antigen, the offspring will be AB and have both antigens. This is known as *codominance;* i.e., neither gene is dominant over the other.

Autosomal dominant disorders

Autosomal dominant disorders are usually less severe than recessive disorders. They tend to involve defects in the embryo or to have a late onset, as in Huntington disease. The characteristic genetic pattern includes these points:

1. All affected children have one affected parent unless the defect is a mutation.
2. Affected individuals are found in successive generations.
3. Males and females are equally likely to transmit or have the trait.
4. In the long run, half the children of an affected parent will have the disorder.
5. The trait is not transmitted by an unaffected person.

Achondroplasia, or dwarfism, is often the result of a new mutation in the offspring, and so the rule of affected parent may not apply. However, an offspring of an achondroplastic parent has a 50 percent chance of being affected. Some 80 percent of dominant disorders represent new mutations. Figure 6-13 represents the inheritance pattern of an autosomal dominant disorder. Table 6-5 describes selected autosomal dominant disorders.

Autosomal recessive disorders

Because both alleles are mutants in true homozygous conditions, autosomal recessive disorders are often severe. Sickle cell anemia (hemoglobin SS disease) is a well-known example. This disease stems from a genetically defective form of hemoglobin in red blood cells. The red cells are extremely fragile. Fever, anemia, and other symptoms are present (Table 6-6). The infant,

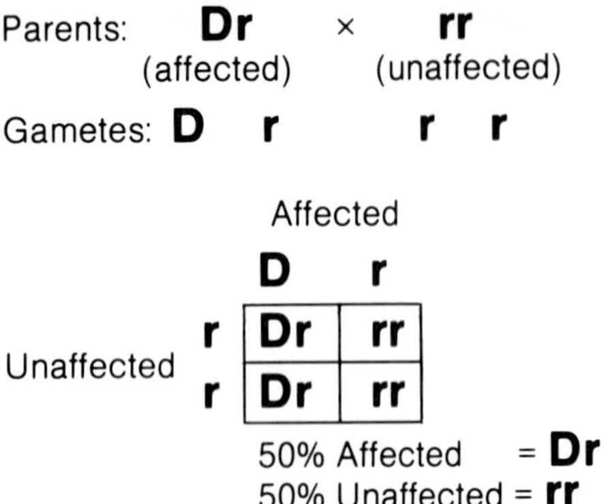

Figure 6-13 The inheritance pattern for autosomal dominant disorder. D is the dominant gene; r is the recessive gene. The Punnett square shows that 50 percent of offspring will be affected and that 50 percent will be unaffected. *Note:* With *each pregnancy* the chance of having an affected child will be 50 percent, whether previous offspring were affected or not.

whose blood until a few months of age contains fetal hemoglobin, is normal; the symptoms usually appear in the first year when fetal hemoglobin is replaced by the adult form. Hemoglobin SS disease is found almost exclusively among blacks.

Everyone carries three to five mutant genes capable of bringing about severe genetic disease. Because these usually are masked by dominant normal alleles, the mutant genes are not expressed. The risk that such mutant genes will be carried in someone heterozygous for the trait increases among parents who have ancestors in common. With such *consanguineous mating* recessive disorders appear more frequently than in the general population. Each person has half his or her genes in common with his or her parents, siblings, and children (first-degree relatives): one-fourth with grandparents, grandchildren, aunts, uncles, nieces, and nephews (second-degree relatives); and one-eighth and one-thirty-second, respectively, with first and second cousins (third-degree relatives). The closer the genetic relationship of the parents, the greater the chance that a child will be born with a genetic defect.

The characteristic genetic pattern for autosomal recessive disease includes these points:

1. Affected individuals tend to group in the same generation.

Table 6-5 Autosomal Dominant Disorders

Disorder	Characteristics
Achondroplasia	Short, thick, tubular bones and dwarfism; bulging cranium with depressed nasal bridge
Apert syndrome	Syndactyly with transverse fusion of distal bones; premature closure of sagittal and coronal sutures, restricting growth of head
Conradi disease	Asymmetric shortening of limbs; dry, scaly skin; scoliosis; alopecia; rounded face; flattening of nasal bridge and face; cataracts
Craniofacial clepostosis (Crouzon disease)	Hypoplasia of maxilla and other deformities of facial bones plus premature closure of sagittal and coronal sutures
Hereditary spherocytosis	Hyperbilirubinemia in neonate; congenital hemolytic anemia; splenomegaly; jaundice; treat with splenectomy; incidence is 1:5000
Holt-Oram syndrome	Congenital heart disease; defects of thumbs
Huntington disease	Adult onset usually after 30 (usually live 15 years after onset of symptoms); choreiform movements; decreasing intellectual function; mental deterioration
Marfan syndrome	Connective tissue disorder; appears in childhood or early adulthood; tall, thin body; long extremities; scoliosis; pigeon breast; mitral or aortic valve insufficiency; retinal tears; incidence is 1:20,000
Neurofibromatosis (von Recklinghausen disease)	Defect in cells of neural crest; 50% of cases represent new mutations; neurofibromas of skin, bone, and central and peripheral nervous systems; kyphoscoliosis; cutaneous pigmentation (café-au-lait spots); predisposed to cancer
Osteogenesis imperfecta	Disorder of connective tissue; osteoporosis with skeletal deformity; blue sclerae; discolored teeth; may also be autosomal recessive

Table 6-5 Autosomal Dominant Disorders (*Continued*)

Disorder	Characteristics
Polycystic kidney disease	Adult onset (usually after childbearing years); cystic disease of liver and kidneys; intracranial aneurysms; incidence is 1:1250
Polysyndactyly	Deformed fingers and toes—webbing; extra digits
Stickler syndrome	Myopia; retinal detachment; deafness; arthropathies; Pierre Robin syndrome may occur in same family
Treacher Collins syndrome	Molar hypoplasia; downward-slanting palpebral fissures; clefts of lower eyelid; malformation of ears and congenital deafness
Bilateral retinoblastoma	Onset in infancy; x-ray therapy *before symptoms appear* has been successful in treating malignancy
Multiple endocrine adenomatosis I, II, III (medullary carcinoma of thyroid, parathyroid, and pituitary)	Other signs include thickened nerve fibers in eyes and benign wartlike changes in tongue. Treat with thyroidectomy. May involve parathyroid and pituitary
Familial polyposis of colon	Adenomatous polyps can become cancerous. Begin screening at 10 years. Observe closely and do resection early
Cancer family syndrome	Familial excess of adenocarcinoma involving colon and endometrium (less frequent in stomach, breast, and ovary), occurring at much earlier ages than in general population

2. Both parents are heterozygous for the disorder and are rarely affected.
3. Both sexes show the trait with equal frequency.
4. For each pregnancy, the chance of having an affected offspring is 25 percent, or 1 in 4.
5. One-half of offspring will be carriers.

Figure 6-14 shows the inheritance pattern for an autosomal recessive disorder. Table 6-6 describes selected autosomal recessive disorders.

Table 6-6 Autosomal Recessive Disorders

Disorder	Characteristics
Oculocutaneous albinism	Failure of normal melanin pigmentation (absence of tyrosine); visual impairment leading to blindness; susceptibility to ultraviolet light; no pigment in eyes, skin, or hair
Congenital adrenal hypoplasia	Impairment of cortisol production causes increased ACTH; ambiguous genitalia; adrenal insufficiency; virilization of female genitalia with normal internal organs; incomplete virilization in males. For girls: high physical energy level and low maternal caretaking behavior. Affected males show advanced somatic and genital growth and tend to have high physical energy levels
Cystic fibrosis	Onset at birth or up to adulthood; disorder of exocrine glands of gastrointestinal tract, pancreas, and respiratory tract; males are usually sterile; incidence is 1:2000
Fanconi anemia	Anemia; thrombocytopenia; leukopenia; small stature with hypoplasia of thumbs; carriers prone to diabetes
Glucose-6-phosphatase deficiency*	Short stature; huge abdomen due to enlargement of liver; flabby, poorly developed musculature; osteoporosis; bleeding tendency; hypoglycemia
Infantile multicystic kidney disease	Renal failure; pulmonary hypoplasia; liver involvement
Meckel syndrome	Microcephaly; encephalocele; cleft lip and palate; congenital heart defects; polycystic kidneys; polydactyly
Sickle cell anemia (and other hemoglobinopathies)*	Fever; anemia; infection; sickle-shaped erythrocytes; infarction of small blood vessels; swelling of hands and feet; pain; splenomegaly; lymphadenopathy
Usher syndrome	Sensory deafness; retinitis pigmentosa; sometimes

*Can be detected in utero.

Table 6-6 Autosomal Recessive Disorders (*Continued*)

Disorder	Characteristics
	mental illness and cataracts
Vitamin D–dependent rickets Type II	Rickets with hypotonia; failure to thrive, tetany; convulsions; rickets
Wilson disease	Degeneration of hepatolenticular system; defect in copper transport; anemia; greenish-brown ring in iris of eyes; cirrhosis; jaundice; neurological defects; joint disorders; presents between 8 and 16 years
Mucopolysaccharidosis I (Hurler syndrome)*	Severe and progressive; usually leads to death by age 10; mental and physical deterioration after 1 year; lordosis; stiff joints; coarse facial features; large head; deafness; enlarged liver and spleen; clouding of cornea

*Can be detected in utero.

X-linked dominant disorders

These conditions are extremely rare. Although X-linked dominant disorders are twice as common in females, their severity is usually much greater in the male because he does not have the normal allele on his Y chromosome to balance the effects of the abnormal gene on his X chromosome. An example of an X-linked dominant disorder is *focal dermal hypoplasia*. It is characterized by digital, oral, and ocular abnormalities, and when it occurs in males, it is lethal. Vitamin D–resistant rickets also fits in this category. The characteristic genetic pattern for X-linked dominant disorders includes these points:

1. Heterozygous affected females transmit to one-half their sons and one-half their daughters.
2. Homozygous affected females transmit to all offspring.
3. Affected males transmit to *all their daughters* but to none of their sons.
4. Both sexes can be affected.

Figure 6-15*A* shows the inheritance pattern for an affected mother, and Fig. 6-15*B* shows the inheritance pattern for an affected father.

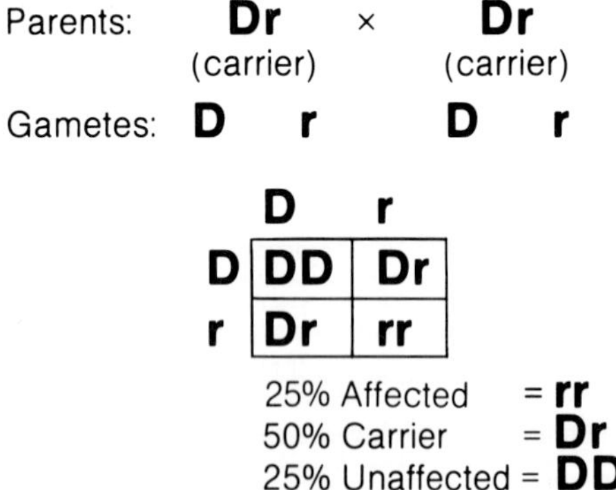

Figure 6-14 The inheritance pattern for an autosomal recessive disorder. Both parents are heterozygous for the recessive gene (*r*). They are unaffected, although they are carriers. With *each pregnancy* the chance of bearing an affected child is 25 percent, the chance of bearing a carrier is 50 percent, and the chance of bearing an unaffected child is 25 percent.

X-linked recessive disorders

Over 150 X-linked recessive disorders have been identified. Males are frequently affected in X-linked recessive disorders because there is no normal allele on the Y chromosome to balance the mutant recessive gene on the X chromosome. In some cases the recessive allele may be partially expressed in females because of the inactivation of their second X chromosome. Therefore, females who are heterozygous for X-linked genes show much greater variation in phenotype than those with autosomal recessive disorders. The characteristic genetic pattern for X-linked recessive disorders includes these points:

1. All sons of affected males are normal (males do not transmit the X chromosome to sons).
2. All daughters of affected males are carriers.
3. One-half the sons of carrier females are affected.
4. One-half the daughters of carrier females are carriers.
5. To be affected, a female must (usually) have an affected father and a carrier mother.

Color blindness is inherited as an X-linked recessive disorder and is present in 8 percent of males. Figure 6-16*A* shows the inheritance pattern for a carrier mother, and Fig. 6-16*B* shows the inheritance pattern for an affected father. Table 6-7 describes selected X-linked recessive disorders.

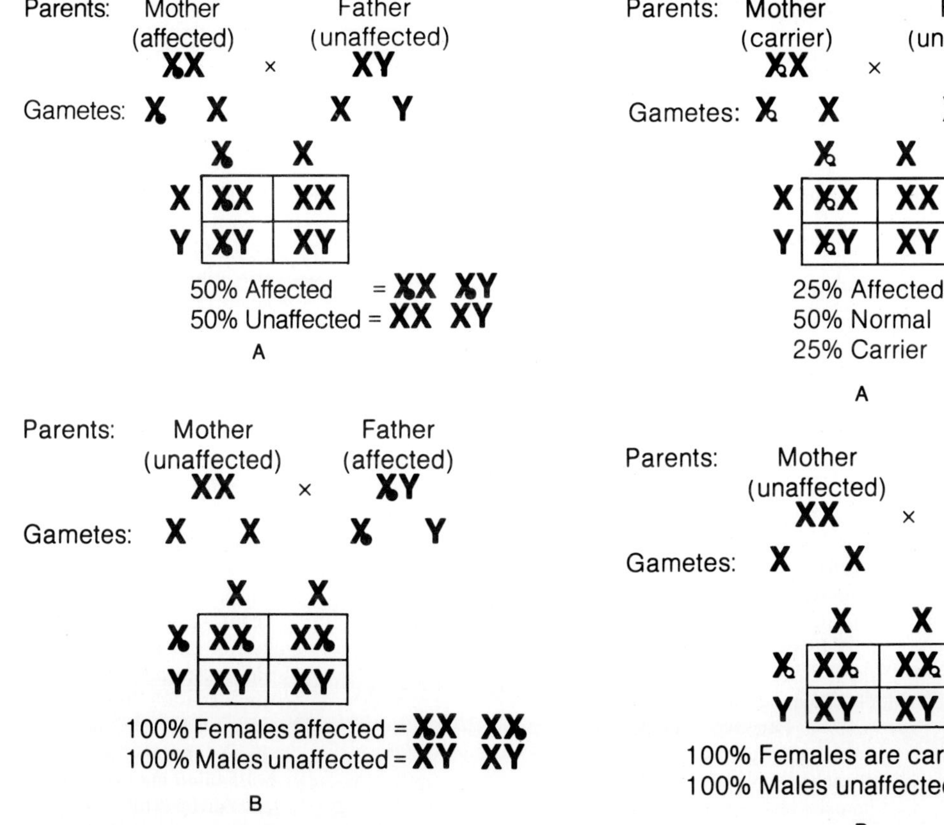

Figure 6-15 The inheritance pattern for an X-linked dominant disorder. (*A*) Affected females transmit the disorder to one-half their daughters and one-half their sons. (*B*) Affected males transmit the disorder to *all* their daughters and *none* of their sons. The risk of having an affected child is 50 percent for each pregnancy when either parent is affected with an X-linked dominant disorder.

Figure 6-16 The inheritance pattern for an X-linked recessive disorder. (*A*) Carrier females transmit the disorder to one-half their sons. One-half their daughters are carriers. (*B*) Affected fathers transmit their affected X chromosome to *all* their daughters and none of their sons. The risk of having an affected child is 50 percent with each pregnancy. (See pedigree chart shown in Fig. 6-18*B*.)

POLYGENIC OR MULTIFACTORIAL INHERITANCE DISORDERS

Many normal traits such as eye color, intelligence, blood pressure, height, and pigmentation of skin are determined by the cumulative effect of several gene pairs. The majority of birth defects are not part of a single gene or chromosomal abnormality but occur as isolated defects due to multifactorial causation. In multifactorial inheritance there may be no major error but rather a number of minor faults that, when combined, produce a birth defect. These disorders can be predicted like other genetic abnormalities. Very often parents of an affected child are normal. When their genes are combined, however, the proportion of abnormal genes is increased to the critical threshold, and a defect is produced. Polygenic disorders are characterized by the following points:

1. They are usually present in one sex more than the other.
2. A *single* organ system is involved.
3. Recurrence risk rises with the severity of the disorder.
4. Recurrence risk increases in proportion to the number of affected first- and/or second-degree relatives. Table 6-8 lists common disorders that can have a polygenic etiology.

Table 6-7 X-linked Recessive Disorders

Disorder	Characteristics
Agammaglobulinemia*	Susceptibility to infection usually appears in second year of life; pain and swelling of joints in one-third to one-half
Anhydrotic ectodermal dysplasia	Absence of sweating; short, fragile hair; misshapen teeth; can be partially expressed in carrier females
Aqueductal stenosis	Hydrocephalus
Fabry disease*	Severe pain; paresthesias of extremities, skin, and mucous membranes; vascular skin lesions; heart and kidney failure; corneal opacities
Duchenne muscular dystrophy*	Onset at 3 to 5 years; progressive loss of muscle strength; contractures; pseudohypertrophy of calf muscles (usually death occurs in twenties and thirties); incidence is 1:7000
Fragile-X syndrome	Mental retardation in males (one of four types of X-linked mental retardation in males); enlarged testes. Female carriers may or may not be retarded
Glucose-6-phosphate dehydrogenase deficiency (G-6-PD)	Hemolytic anemia induced by some drugs (e.g., primaquine and sulfa) because of abnormality in RBC; ranges from mild to severe
Hemophilia A*	Disorder of blood coagulation (factor VIII deficiency); bleeding from wounds and into tissues and joints
Hemophilia B*	Disorder of blood coagulation (factor IX deficiency); not as serious as hemophilia A; incidence of hemophilia is 1:7000
Lesch-Nyhan syndrome*	Progressive nervous system degeneration, incoordination, and spasticity; uric aciduria; mental retardation; compulsive self-mutilation by head-banging and biting lips and fingers (the gene has been isolated and corrected in the laboratory)
Mucopolysaccharidosis II (Hunter syndrome)*	Lysosomal storage disease; progressive with stiff joints, dwarfism, coarse facial features, hoarseness, rosy cheeks, and increasing deafness; severity varies
Testicular feminization syndrome	Failure of embryonic end organs to respond to androgenic steroids despite presence of Y chromosome. 46,XY appears as female with blind-ending vagina, amenorrhea (tubes, uterus, and upper vagina absent). Testes immature or found in groin or labia majora (1 to 2% of girls with inguinal hernias have this syndrome)
Familial vitamin D–resistant rickets	Hypophosphatemia; decreased renal tubular phosphate reabsorption; bowing of legs; rickets

*Can be detected in utero.

INBORN ERRORS OF METABOLISM

Genes produce the enzymes that are the regulators of the many biochemical reactions of metabolism. Each such reaction is under the control of a different gene, and a change in the nature of a gene, that is, a mutation, may alter the ability of a cell to carry out some primary chemical reaction. An inborn error of metabolism is thus created. The immediate consequences may be (1) an accumulation, (2) a deficiency, or (3) an overproduction of a substance produced by the primary chemical reaction (Fig. 6-17).

At birth the child may appear normal. The nurse's first contact with the child may be for hospitalization due to failure to thrive, abnormal laboratory tests, or unexplained drug responses. Once the diagnosis of a biochemical disorder is made, it may not be long before the progressive, diffuse nature of the illness becomes evident. Many inborn errors of metabolism result in a typical pattern that includes liver or spleen enlargement, renal or cardiac involvement, changes in growth, anemia, and a progressive downhill course. Table 6-9 describes selected inborn errors of metabolism.

Fortunately, most genetic mutations have little if any effect on the phenotype. For one thing,

Table 6-8 Common Polygenic Disorders*

Allergies (atopic)	Idiopathic scoliosis
Cleft lip and palate	Pyloric stenosis
Cleft palate	Hirschsprung's disease
Neural-tube defects	Mental retardation (nonspecific)
Hydrocephalus (in isolation)	Urinary tract malformations
Congenital heart disease	Diabetes mellitus (adult onset)
Talipes equinovarus (clubfoot)	Schizophrenia
Congenital hip dysplasia	

*Recurrence rates for first-degree relatives is 2 to 5%.

Source: Vincent Riccardi, *The Genetic Approach to Human Disease,* Oxford University Press, New York, 1977, p. 90.

each person carries two complete sets of chromosomes. Even if an allele on one chromosome is a mutant, its duplicate on the other chromosome is likely to be unaffected and to continue normal functioning.

GENETICS AND CANCER

Analysis of malignant cells often demonstrates chromosomal abnormalities of number and structure. Those changes may represent a premalignant change, such as in Down syndrome, or an altered state of cells after the cancer develops. Burkitt lymphoma cells reveal a balanced translocation between chromosomes 8 and 14. The Philadelphia chromosome, a deleted part of chromosome 22 translocated to chromosome 9, is found in the bone marrow of patients with chronic myelogenous leukemia and represents a similar phenomenon.[18]

Some forms of cancer are heritable, such as bilateral retinoblastoma, a tumor of the retina that usually appears before the age of 2. Thirty percent of cases are inherited.[19] One-third of Wilm tumors are also hereditary. Persons with chromosomal breakage syndromes, such as progeria (premature aging), xeroderma pigmentosa (sensitivity to sun resulting in skin cancers), and ataxia telangiectasia (progressive ataxia of childhood), all have an increased risk of cancer, especially leukemia.

In "cancer families" tumors tend to appear at an earlier age, and affected individuals often have more than one primary tumor. Usually more than 25 percent of individuals are affected. The cancer behaves as an autosomal dominant with about 60 percent penetrance.[20]

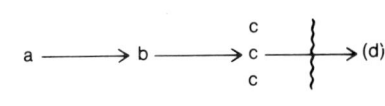

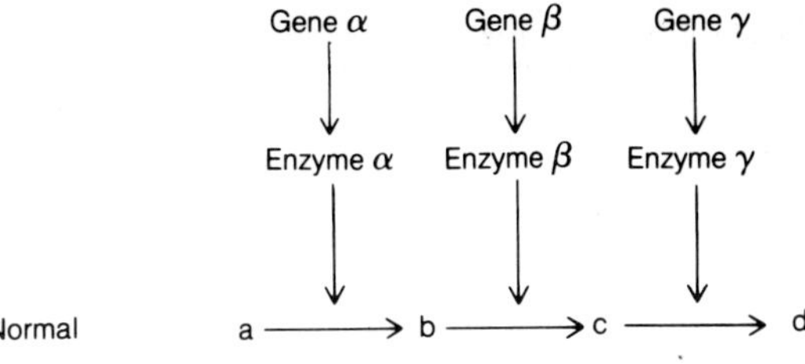

Figure 6-17 Types of metabolic abnormalities resulting from enzyme defects. (*A*) Normal. (*B*) Accumulation of excess substance at the block, as in tyrosinosis and alkaptonuria. (*C*) Lack of the product, as in albinism and cretinism. (*D*) Abnormal metabolites, as in phenylketonuria. *(Adapted from V. A. McKusick (ed.), Human Genetics, 2d ed., Prentice-Hall, Englewood Cliffs, N.J., 1969, p. 69. Used with permission.)*

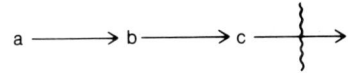

ENVIRONMENTAL INFLUENCES

There is always interaction between genetic and environmental influences in utero. At various times one or the other will dominate. Traits or disorders determined both by the environment and by genes are known as *multifactorial.* A perfect environment will not overcome the effects of an extra chromosome, as in trisomy 21. But a genetically normal infant, born to a mother with untreated phenylketonuria, will show the influence of the uterine environment. The child will have low birth weight, microcephaly, and eventual mental retardation.

Anything that causes change in genetic material is *mutagenic.* When an agent acts to change

Table 6-9 Inborn Errors of Metabolism

Disorder	Characteristic
Errors of Amino Acid Metabolism	
Phenylketonuria*†	Absence of liver enzyme phenylalanine hydroxylase causes excess of phenylalanine in blood, irritability, vomiting, seizures, and mental retardation; incidence is 1:12,000
Maple syrup urine disease*†	Failure to thrive; seizures; sweet-smelling urine (ketoacidosis)
Errors of Lipid Metabolism	
Gaucher disease*†	Deficiency of β-glucoside; excess of glucosylceramide; splenomegaly; thrombocytopenia; bone pain; hepatomegaly; leads to death. Type II, infantile: signs appear before 6 months and death occurs by 2 years. Type III: signs appear later
Familial hypercholesterolemia‡	Elevation in low-density lipoprotein (LDL); xanthomas. Heterozygotes (1:500) develop hypercholesterolemia (350 to 500) with signs and symptoms developing after age 30; homozygotes (1:1,000,000) develop xanthomas within 4 years; coronary heart disease begins in childhood
Errors in Carbohydrate Metabolism	
Galactosemia*†	Absence of enzyme galactose 1-phosphate uridyl transferase; intolerance to lactose; failure to thrive; weight loss; seizures; cataracts
Altered Structural Proteins	
Hemoglobinopathies*†	Disorders of clotting and bleeding—need fetal blood to test for in utero diagnosis; tests not conclusive at present time
Errors of Lysosomal Enzymes	
Farber lipogranulomatosis*	Painful, progressively deformed joints; subcutaneous nodules; hoarseness; leads to death early or later within first few years
Mucopolysaccharidosis (Hurler syndrome, Hunter syndrome, etc.)*	Results from accumulation of acid mucopolysaccharides in the liver, brain, and heart. Coarsening features; cataracts; enlarged head and tongue; mental and growth retardation. Most inherited in autosomal recessive except Hunter syndrome, which is X-linked recessive; incidence in all types is 1:25,000
Tay-Sachs disease (ganglioside storage disease)*	Buildup of hexosaminidase A causes motor weakness at 3 to 6 months; startle response; rapid mental and motor deterioration after 1 year; deafness; blindness; seizures; usually death by 3 years; pale, translucent skin; cherry-red spot on macula; occurs mainly in Ashkenazic Jews (incidence is 1:3000); 1 in 36 Jews is heterozygous for the gene

*Follows autosomal recessive pattern of inheritance.

†Can be detected in utero.

‡Follows autosomal dominant pattern of inheritance.

the structure or function within the fetus during pregnancy, it is known as a *teratogen* (*terato* means "monster" or "anomaly"; *gen* means "causative agent"). The resulting anomaly is said to be *congenital.*

There are four major environmental influences that can act as mutagens or teratogens: physical agents, infection, chemical agents (including drugs), and the maternal intrauterine environment.

Physical agents

Ultraviolet (sun) and ionizing (nuclear and x-ray) radiation and extremes of temperature can damage DNA directly by altering its structure.

Ionizing radiation is by far the most potent mutagen known. Because the effects are cumulative, the risk is proportional to the amount of radiation received. X-rays should be avoided for 12 weeks following conception, unless absolutely necessary. Radioactive iodine (used for diagnostic tests) can become concentrated in the fetal thyroid gland and have a teratogenic effect. The effects of radiation may also become apparent in later life, with an increased likelihood of cancer.

Infection

Viral illness during pregnancy can cause specific congenital syndromes as well as temporary chromosomal breakage. Rubella (German measles) during the first trimester of pregnancy is likely to produce an infant with microcephaly, cataracts, deafness, and mental retardation. The type of defect is related to the gestational age at which the infection occurs. For example, cataracts develop from rubella during the sixth week, deafness during the ninth week, and cardiac defects during the fifth to the tenth weeks.

Other infections known to act as teratogens are toxoplasmosis, cytomegalovirus, *Treponema pallidum* (syphilis), and herpes simplex II virus. Infants infected in utero may have intrauterine growth retardation, microcephaly, anemia, jaundice, ocular defects, mental retardation, and poor motor development.

Chemical agents

Chemical teratogens are eaten or inhaled as drugs or pollutants in air, water, and food. Organic mercurials, often found in fish, can cause neurological defects and blindness. Mustard gas, formaldehyde, and caffeine can produce mutations. The importance of the mutagenic effect of caffeine in humans is still a matter of speculation.

Drugs constitute a significant hazard to the pregnant woman. No drug should be taken unless its benefit *clearly overrides* any harmful effects it might have. Research suggests that the teratogenic effects of agents are more likely to be expressed in genetically predisposed infants. For example, women who take anticonvulsants have a higher incidence of babies with malformations than do their relatives who do not take anticonvulsants.[21] Table 6-10 lists selected drugs and their known or suspected teratogenic effects.

The intrauterine environment

The physiological status and genotype of the mother have a definite effect on the fetus. Most drugs and metabolites cross the placental barrier and affect the fetus. Poor maternal nutrition is associated with a decrease in fertility and infant birth weight. At the present time maternal endocrine imbalance, diabetes mellitus, phenylketonuria, and alcoholism are known to be teratogenic to the fetus.[22] Similarly, exposure of the father to drugs, chemicals, radiation, or viruses can result in damage to the fetus. Factors putting the fetus at risk are discussed in more detail in Chap. 17.

It is helpful for the nurse to remember that

Table 6-10 Drugs with Known or Suspected Teratogenic Effects

Drug	Known Effects	Suspected Effects
Thalidomide	Phocomelia (absence of parts or entire limbs)	
Amethopterin and aminopterin	Abortion; intrauterine growth retardation; cranial and facial abnormalities	
Progestins (birth control pill)	Masculinization of female fetus	Isolated limb defects; increase in abortion
Cigarette smoking		Low birth weight
Anticonvulsants (hydantoins and trimethadione)		Cleft palate; intrauterine growth retardation; congenital heart disease; hypoplasia of fingers and toes
Ethyl alcohol		Growth retardation; mental retardation; microcephaly; distinctive facies

mutations that occur in somatic cells (as in leukemia) will not be passed on to offspring, but will be passed on to all daughter cells. If the mutation occurs in a gamete, the mutant gene or chromosome will be transmitted to the offspring. Since not all gonadal cells may be involved, the risk of producing an affected offspring is calculated on the basis of population frequency of that trait or disorder.

GENETIC SCREENING

Genetic screening programs are an important part of casefinding and health promotion. Newborns are screened for phenylketonuria, galactosemia, and several other amino acid deficiencies. The cost of identifying these diseases is far less than the emotional and economic cost associated with an untreated individual. Heterozygote screening is also useful for selected populations, such as Jews of northern European ancestry (Tay-Sachs disease), or those with sickle cell disease and thalassemia.

GENETIC COUNSELING

Genetic counseling is an important part of health care. It is part of the process by which the affected individual or involved family is evaluated for risk and counseled so that rational decisions can be made about childbearing. In addition, there may be more immediate goals of psychological support, improved management of certain disorders, referral for help in carrying out decisions that the individual or family must make, and casefinding and prevention.

Genetic counseling involves nondirective counseling. The counselor presents information in a variety of ways so that the family has a clear understanding of the genetic basis of the disorder as well as the risks involved for future children. Riccardi has described guidelines for the counselor that include the following:[23]

1. Accurate diagnosis.
2. Communication—useful information regarding diagnosis, risks, and alternatives.
3. Nondirective counseling—the client chooses between alternatives.
4. Respect for, and adjustment to, the family's psychological and emotional turmoil.
5. The focus of health care is the *family unit,* not just the affected individual.
6. A team approach is optional but often helpful.

In one study approximately 60 percent of counselees had improved diagnostic understanding, while 40 percent still misunderstood the disease.[24] Those who were at greater risk remembered information more accurately. Couples seem to construct scenarios of "what will happen if." Then they choose the alternative which involves the smallest loss they can cope with or which entails the smallest burden.[25] *Burden* refers to the total cost to families and society in economic and psychological terms.

COMPONENTS OF A GENETIC EVALUATION

History and pedigree construction

A detailed family history, a pregnancy history, and a postnatal history are essential to genetic counseling. Frequently the nurse can obtain the initial information needed.

Commonly used symbols and a sample pedigree chart are shown in Fig. 6-18. A complete pedigree includes second- and third-degree relatives. Family histories help the geneticist diagnose a heritable disorder, define recurrence risks, and develop an understanding of the possible medical, social, and emotional burdens that the disorder will place on affected and unaffected family members.

The maternal-fetal history should provide information on any infections, drugs, or environmental agents the mother was exposed to during pregnancy. A detailed description of the events at birth and postnatally is an important extension of the history. It is important to elicit the *parents' perception* of significant events, developmental steps, and possible causative factors. Frequently, parents describe events they believe may have caused the problem; they may talk about feelings of guilt. The counselor can correct misconceptions and misunderstandings.

Physical examination

A detailed and precise physical exam is required for a genetic evaluation. Special attention is given to the involved organs and to the reproductive and central nervous systems. The dermal creases

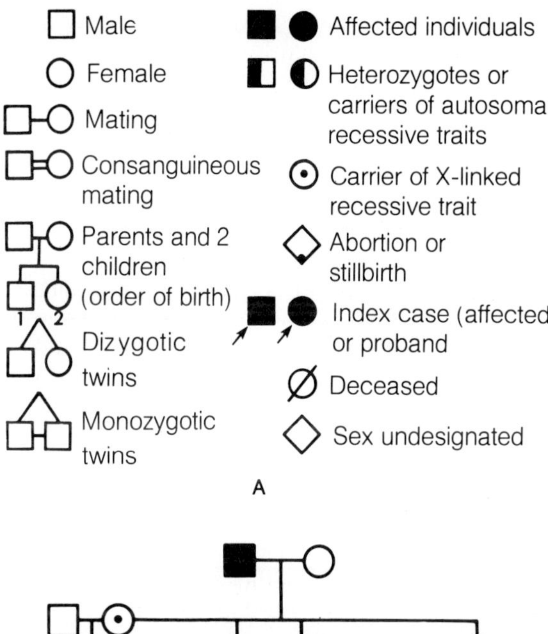

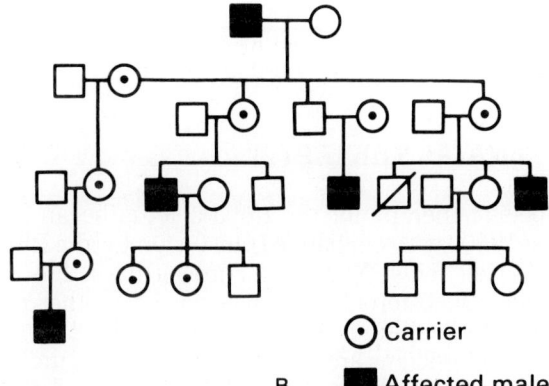

Figure 6-18 (*A*) Symbols used in constructing a pedigree. A pedigree should include all first-, second-, and third-degree relatives of the affected individual. (*B*) A characteristic X-linked recessive pedigree. Males are affected, and they are related through unaffected (or carrier) females. All daughters of affected males are carriers.

and ridges on the hands and feet reveal characteristic patterns in many syndromes. *Phenocopies*, developmental diseases that mimic genetic disorders, must be carefully distinguished from hereditary diseases.

Laboratory data

Routine laboratory tests, specialized tests, and genetic diagnostic tests are the three types of laboratory procedures required for a genetic workup. Specialized lab exams are selected on the basis of presenting symptoms and can include x-rays and biopsies. Specialized genetic diagnostic tests include chromosome analysis and karyotype, enzyme assays, and amniocentesis.

Chromosome analysis Analysis of chromosomes has become extremely important in genetics. Usually lymphocytes from a blood sample or fetal cells in amniotic fluid are grown in a special medium. During metaphase the cell nucleus is photographed after the chromosomes are stained. Special stains allow the identification of each chromosome and its specific parts. Buccal smears (scrapings of the inside of the cheek) are often used for sex chromatin studies.

PRENATAL DIAGNOSTIC TESTING

Prenatal diagnosis of genetic disorders is becoming a very common part of obstetrical care. The techniques used can be classified as noninvasive and invasive.

Noninvasive techniques

Ultrasound is a safe imaging technique that allows visualization of normal and abnormal fetal anatomy as well as moving pictures that show the heart beating and the fetus breathing, swallowing, and moving.

Alpha fetoprotein (AFP), a glycoprotein produced by the fetal liver, is secreted in the fetal urine and is found in the amniotic fluid and the maternal serum. When part of the fetus is not covered by skin, as in an open neural tube defect, the AFP level rises. Because a higher level is also found in multiple gestations and other anomalies as well as in some normal pregnancies, a test of the AFP level is only a screening test.[26] A test showing an elevated AFP level should be repeated, and then a careful ultrasound should be done, followed by an amniocentesis if indicated.

Invasive techniques

Invasive techniques include amniocentesis and fetoscopy. Amniocentesis, which is usually done between 15 and 18 weeks from the last menstrual period, allows the physician to preview the genetic constitution of the fetus. It is usually done as an outpatient procedure after gestational age is carefully calculated. Maternal blood samples are drawn, ultrasound localizes the placenta, and the patient is carefully monitored (vital signs, fetal heart tones) both before and after this sterile procedure. Chromosomal analysis takes 3 weeks, and biochemical assays take 4 weeks, after the amniocentesis.[27]

The National Registry for Amniocentesis Study reported on 1040 subjects at nine institutions who had the procedure.[28] The findings were as follows: (1) There was no significant difference in fetal death between the amniocentesis group (3.5 percent) and the control group (3.2 percent); (2) there were no significant differences in complications of labor, delivery, or infant outcome; (3) the accuracy of diagnosis was 99.4 percent; and (4) maternal and fetal risks are 1 in 200 when the procedure is performed by experienced physicians in large medical centers. Prenatal diagnosis using amniocentesis should be considered in the following situations:[29,30]

1. When the mother is over 35. (The most common reason for doing an amniocentesis is to detect chromosomal abnormality in fetuses carried by women over 35 years of age.)
2. When the mother has had a child with a chromosomal abnormality.
3. When one parent is a balanced translocation carrier.
4. When the mother is a habitual aborter.
5. When a previous child has had multiple congenital anomalies.
6. When there are X-linked recessive disorders in the family. (Even if biochemical diagnosis cannot be made, sex can be determined.)
7. When the child is at risk for inborn errors of metabolism. (It is now possible to identify many rare disorders, such as Fabry disease and Tay-Sachs disease.)
8. When the mother has had a child with a neural tube defect.
9. When the mother has elevated serum alpha fetoprotein.

In fetoscopy, a small fiber-optic scope (the size of a large hypodermic needle) is inserted through a 4-mm incision in the abdomen into the amniotic sac. Ultrasound is used to localize the placenta and fetus, as in amniocentesis. Fetoscopy allows visualizing anatomic defects as well as sampling the placenta and the fetal cord blood, liver, and skin.[31] Defects in blood and enzymes as well as infection can be diagnosed. Antibiotics may be used prophylactically. When the procedure is finished, pressure is applied to the incision site for 2 min, and the fetal heart rate is monitored for 4 h. The risks associated with fetoscopy include infection, hemorrhage, rupture of membranes, and fetal injection. When fetal blood sampling is done, the spontaneous abortion rate is 5 to 10 percent, and there is a premature delivery rate of 10 percent.[32]

Any woman who undergoes prenatal diagnosis experiences a significant increase in anxiety. Sometimes tests are not successful and must be repeated. Prenatal diagnosis involves a slight risk of spontaneous abortion, but even more important is the possibility that the fetus will be found to be abnormal. Decisions concerning amniocentesis and intervention in the case of an affected fetus must be made by the parents. Although most couples choose abortion and would do so again under the same circumstances, they still experience guilt and depression.[33]

PRENATAL THERAPY

Specific therapy for the unborn fetus began in the 1960s with exchange transfusion for the Rh-sensitized fetus. When premature birth is a threat, glucocorticosteroids are given to the mother to promote fetal lung maturity. With prenatal diagnosis, physicians are now contemplating in utero surgical procedures. Some have attempted repair of hydrocephalus and urinary tract obstruction.[34] It is predicted that medication such as thyroid hormone or nutrients could be added to the amniotic fluid for the fetus to swallow. Scientists are using gene mapping and cloning to correct inborn errors of metabolism. Many barriers must be overcome, however, before "corrected cells" can be introduced into an organism to replace defective genes. Fetal therapy raises many legal, ethical, and moral questions.

ROLE OF THE NURSE

Nurses can play a key role in the genetic counseling process by virtue of their specialized training (nurse-geneticists, clinical specialists, or pediatric nurse associates) or their close involvement with families in any nursing setting. They may participate in genetic evaluation by constructing pedigrees, visiting families at home, and helping in clinics. Often nurses are the first ones to be asked about the possible untoward effects of environmental agents during pregnancy. Nurses should be able to construct a simple pedigree chart, obtain a relevant history, understand genetic principles, make appropriate referrals, care for patients who are undergoing prenatal diagnosis, and provide emotional support for families with an affected child.

Referral

Usually referral is made to answer the question, "Will it happen again?" It makes no difference whether the question is asked by the client, family, nurse, social worker, or physician. The question should be asked. The nurse should encourage families to verbalize their concerns and seek answers to their questions. Conditions that call for referral to a clinical geneticist are summarized in Table 6-11.

Once the data base is gathered (history, physical exam, and laboratory data), the geneticist counsels the client and family regarding the risks involved, the *probability* of recurrence, and the probable prognosis of an existing condition. Information is given about available health care, community agencies, and sources of financial support.

Table 6-11 Indications for Referral to a Clinical Geneticist

1. Known or presumed congenital abnormalities
   a. Congenital malformations
   b. Ambiguous genitalia
   c. Mental retardation
   d. Fetal or parental exposure to environmental factors (drugs, irradiation, or infections)
2. Acknowledged familial disorders
3. Known inherited disorders
4. Metabolic or biochemical disorders
5. Known or suspected chromosomal abnormalities
6. Multiple miscarriages or stillbirths
7. Infertility
8. Premarital counseling
9. Consanguinity or incest
10. Prenatal diagnosis
    a. Either parent is a known carrier
    b. Previous child has a chromosomal abnormality
    c. Mother is 35 or older
    d. Inordinate parental concern or anxiety exists
    e. Either parent has a specific metabolic disorder
    f. Mother is a known or presumed carrier for X-linked recessive

Source: Adapted from Vincent Riccardi, *The Genetic Approach to Human Disease,* Oxford University Press, New York, 1977, p. 6

Nursing management

Families who experience the birth of a child who is less than perfect will have feelings of loss and grief. They must mourn for the perfect child they expected before they can come to terms with the reality of the child they have. Nurses can expect reactions that include shock, denial, anger, shame, depression, and alienation. The grief will resolve in time, but it will never disappear completely.

Parents experience profound disappointment and guilt. They may look on the child as punishment for something they did wrong. Grief and guilt can strain a marriage as well as interfere with other family relationships. There is potential for a decline in family self-esteem and a breakdown in communication. Parents may also feel out of control.[35] The nurse can anticipate and recognize these expected effects and explore them with the family as support is given to them.

Parents need to be involved in the care of their child as soon as possible. Seeing, touching, and fondling the infant promote attachment and the development of parenting skills. With acceptance, parents can begin to focus their energy on problem solving. Parents need support as they gather information, integrate facts and feelings, and make decisions regarding the care of their child. See Chap. 17 for further discussion of parenting the high-risk child.

Nurses, too, may experience feelings similar to those of parents. Parents are comforted when nurses participate in their grief. However, parents also look to the nurse's reactions as representative of how others may react to them and their child. They are sensitive to verbal or nonverbal cues that suggest shock, revulsion, or blame. Nurses must examine their own feelings in regard to genetic disorders, prenatal diagnosis, handicapped children, and abortion. A warm, caring, empathic nurse can provide support that will help parents cope with this crisis in their lives.

There are several ways that the nurse can help both the child who has a genetic disease and the child's family:

1. Accept the family's feelings and reactions.
2. Help the family members explore their feelings and work through their grief.
3. Clarify misconceptions.
4. Help the family (and the child, when old enough) identify concerns and questions.

5. Fill in gaps in information.
6. Repeat information as often as necessary.
7. Provide opportunities for the parents and other family members to care for the child.
8. Teach the family members (and the child, when old enough) to provide the care needed.
9. Get the family in touch with other parents or associations of parents who have similar children.
10. Make appropriate public health and social service referrals.
11. Provide written information to the family.
12. Anticipate concerns and problems that the family is likely to experience in the future.
13. Coordinate the efforts of other health team members.
14. Continue care and follow-up.
15. Be very sure that the information provided is correct.

Genetics is a rapidly growing specialty. New techniques and knowledge are added constantly. Nurses have a responsibility to become aware of developments in the diagnosis, treatment, and prevention of hereditary disorders.

References

1. Skinner, R., "Genetic Counseling," in A. Henry and D. Rimoin (eds.), *Principles and Practice of Medical Genetics,* vol. I, Churchill Livingstone, Edinburgh, 1983, p. 1427.
2. Crow, James F., *Genetic Notes,* Burgess, Minneapolis, 1976, p. 77.
3. Stanbury, J., J. Wyngaarden, D. Fredrickson, J. Goldstein, and M. Brown, *The Metabolic Basis of Inherited Disease,* McGraw-Hill, New York, 1983, p. 8.
4. Ibid., p. 29.
5. Ibid., p. 75.
6. Miles, J., and M. Kaback, "Prenatal Diagnosis of Hereditary Disorders," *Pediatric Clinics of North America* **25**(3):593–618 (August 1978).
7. Harrison, M., M. Golbus, and R. Filly, *The Unborn Patient,* Grune & Stratton, New York, 1984, p. 18.
8. Riccardi, V., *The Genetic Approach to Human Disease,* Oxford University Press, New York, 1977, p. 4.
9. Clark, A., and D. Affonso, *Childbearing: A Nursing Perspective,* Davis, Philadelphia, 1979, p. 218.
10. Huether, Carl, "Projection of Down Syndrome Births in the U.S. 1979–2000 and the Potential Effects of Perinatal Diagnosis," *American Journal of Public Health* **73**(10):1186 (October 1983).
11. Ibid., p. 1187.
12. Ibid.
13. Ibid.
14. Holmes, L., "Genetic Counseling for the Older Pregnant Woman: New Data and Questions," *New England Journal of Medicine* **298**(25):1420 (June 1978).
15. Charrow, J., and H. Nadler, "Prenatal Diagnosis," in Henry and Rimoin, op. cit., p. 1475.
16. Thompson, J., and M. Thompson, *Genetics in Medicine,* Saunders, Philadelphia, 1980, p. 163.
17. Skinner, op. cit., p. 1429.
18. Kelly, Thaddeus, *Clinical Genetics and Genetic Counseling,* Year Book, Chicago, 1980, pp. 162–168.
19. Schimke, R., "Cancer Genetics," in Henry and Rimoin, op. cit., vol. II, p. 1401.
20. Ibid., p. 1402.
21. Kelly, op. cit., p. 71.
22. Riccardi, op. cit., p. 148.
23. Ibid., p. 200.
24. Harrison, Golbus, and Filly, op. cit., p. 18.
25. Ibid., p. 19.
26. Harisiades, J., "Maternal Serum AFP Screening: A Programmatic Overview," *Issues in Health Care of Women* **4**(2):26 (February 1983).
27. Golbus, M., C. Loughman, G. Halbasch, J. Stephens, and B. Hall, "Prenatal Diagnosis in 3,000 Amniocenteses," *New England Journal of Medicine* **300**(4):157–163 (January 1979).
28. NICHD National Registry for Amniocentesis Study Group, "Midtrimester Amniocentesis for Prenatal Diagnosis: Safety and Accuracy," *Journal of the American Medical Association* **236**:1471–1477 (1976).
29. Miles and Kaback, op. cit., pp. 597–600.
30. Golbus, Loughman, Halbasch, Stephens, and Hall, op. cit., p. 158.
31. Harrison, Golbus, and Filly, op. cit., p. 125.
32. Charrow and Nadler, loc. cit.
33. Harrison, Golbus, and Filly, op. cit., p. 28.
34. Garver, K., "In-utero Correction of Congenital Malformations," *Genetics in Practice* **1**(2):2–3 (Winter 1984).
35. Brandt, B., "Caring for the Family of an Infant with a Genetic Disorder," *Perinatal Press* **8**(4):55–57 (1984).

7

Marjorie J. Smith

Prenatal development

Upon completion of this chapter, the student will be able to:

1. Define the three stages of human development that occur before birth.
2. Differentiate between menstrual and conceptual age.
3. Describe the timing of events leading to fertilization.
4. Trace the path of the egg from ovulation through implantation.
5. List three functions of amniotic fluid.
6. List three organ systems arising from each germ layer.
7. Identify the period of organ systems' greatest sensitivity to teratogens.
8. List four mechanisms used to transport products across the uteroplacental barrier.
9. Describe the functions of the placenta and its hormones.

Human development is the life process that begins at conception and concludes at death. In this chapter prenatal growth and development are briefly described to provide a basis for understanding later growth and development and arrests in development that lead to birth defects.

The human embryo progresses through stages of development similar to those of other creatures. Development occurs through cell division and growth. At first all cells seem to be alike, but soon they become *differentiated* according to coded information carried within them by genes. Some cells, known as *inducers*, influence other cells around them to develop in a certain way. Because the organism grows in a confined space, and because certain cells grow more rapidly than others, sheets of cells *fold* and *invaginate*. At the same time, other cell groups *migrate* to different areas of the organism.

Development of function and size occurs in a cephalocaudal direction in the embryo and fetus, just as it does in the infant. Growth also occurs from the center, or medial aspect, of the body outward, or laterally.

TIMETABLE OF DEVELOPMENT

The first 14 days of human development are referred to as the *preembryonic stage* or the period of the *zygote* (fertilized egg). During this time implantation occurs; that is, the zygote embeds itself in the uterine lining. The *embryonic stage* begins the third week after conception and concludes at the end of the eighth week. This is the period of major organ system formation. The *fetal stage* encompasses the ninth week through the thirty-eighth week, or to the end of pregnancy.

From birth to maturity, weight increases 20 times, but from fertilization to birth, weight increases 6 billion times.[1] Relative proportions change markedly during fetal development. Figure 7-1 shows the relative proportions of head, trunk, and extremities at different ages.

The gestational age of the *conceptus*, as the product of conception is called, can be calculated from the first day of the last menstrual period, *menstrual age*, or from the time of conception, *conceptual age*. The normal length of pregnancy is 266 days (38 weeks) after conception or 280 days (40 weeks) after the last menstrual period.

THE PREEMBRYONIC STAGE

Fertilization

For pregnancy to occur, healthy spermatozoa, deposited in the vagina at the cervical os, must find their way into a normal, patent fallopian tube at the time when a healthy ovum is present for fertilization.

The fertilization of the ovum usually occurs in the distal part of the fallopian tube within 24 h after ovulation.[2] Once a single sperm penetrates the egg, changes occur in the outer membrane of the ovum that prevent other sperm from entering.

Meanwhile, the second meiotic division occurs (review Fig. 6-7) in the nucleus of the ovum, and the male and female chromosomes come together. Thus the zygote is formed containing a full set of 44 autosomal chromosomes and two sex chromosomes, either XX or XY.

The fallopian tube propels the zygote toward the uterus by cilial and muscular movement. During this time the zygote is dividing mitotically by a process known as *cleavage*. In about 3 days it has become a tiny ball of 16 cells known as the *morula*.

In vitro fertilization Fertilization of human ova in vitro has now been accomplished.[3] The oocyte is recovered from the ovarian follicle with an aspirator just prior to ovulation, when the oocyte is in the late stages of the first meiotic metaphase. It is placed in a culture medium, and sperm is added. The sperm may be from the woman's husband or from a donor. The fertilized egg is allowed to grow to the early blastocyst stage (8 or 16 cells) and is implanted in the uterus.

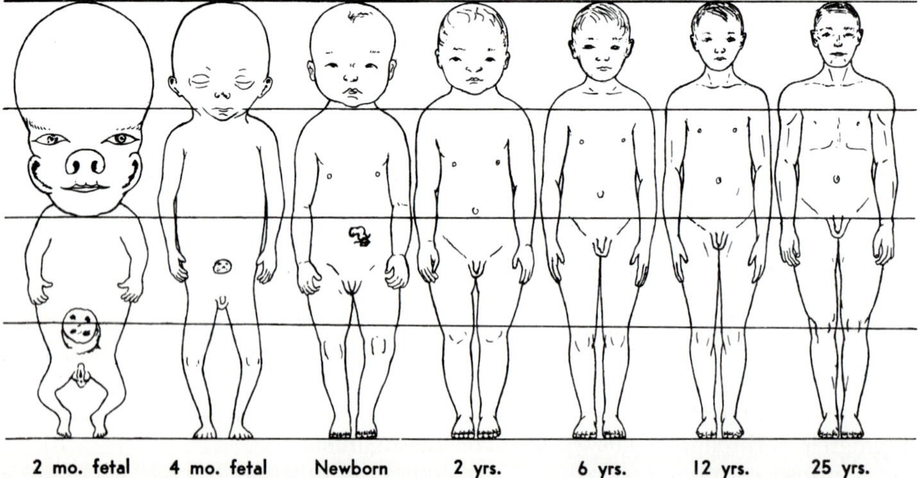

Figure 7-1 Fetal and postnatal stages drawn to same total height to show characteristic age changes in the proportion of various parts of the body. *(From B. M. Patten and B. Carlson, Foundations of Embryology, McGraw-Hill, New York, 1974, p. 13. Used with permission.)*

The blastocyst

When the morula reaches the uterine cavity, it begins to absorb uterine fluid, creating a cystlike space within. The zygote is now known as a *blastocyst* (Fig. 7-2*A*) and is composed of three parts:

1. *Blastocoele* An inner, central cavity filled with nourishing fluid.
2. *Inner cell mass* The *embryoblast*, which will eventually form the embryo.
3. *Trophoblast* (*tropho* means "nutrition") The protective outer-cell coating that invades and digests the endometrium. The trophoblast eventually forms the chorion (outer layer of fetal membranes) and the fetal part of the placenta.

Implantation

On about the fifth day after fertilization the *zona pellucida* (the membrane surrounding the ovum) disappears, and by the sixth day the blastocyst attaches itself to the *endometrium* (the inner uterine lining). The usual site for implantation is the upper posterior or anterior uterine wall.

During the second week the trophoblast continues to penetrate the endometrium. At the same time, two cavities—the amniotic cavity and the primitive yolk sac—appear within the trophoblast. The inner cell mass begins to differentiate into two layers—the *endoderm* (inner layer) and the *ectoderm* (outer layer). This *bilaminar embryonic disk* lies between the amniotic cavity and the primitive yolk sac (Fig. 7-2*C*).

Under the influence of progesterone, the endometrium has greatly thickened. Its glands have become increasingly active and rich in glycogen. The invading trophoblast breaks down the endometrial cells, making nutrients available to the developing embryo until the placenta is formed.

Decidua, meaning "to shed," is the name given the endometrium during pregnancy because it

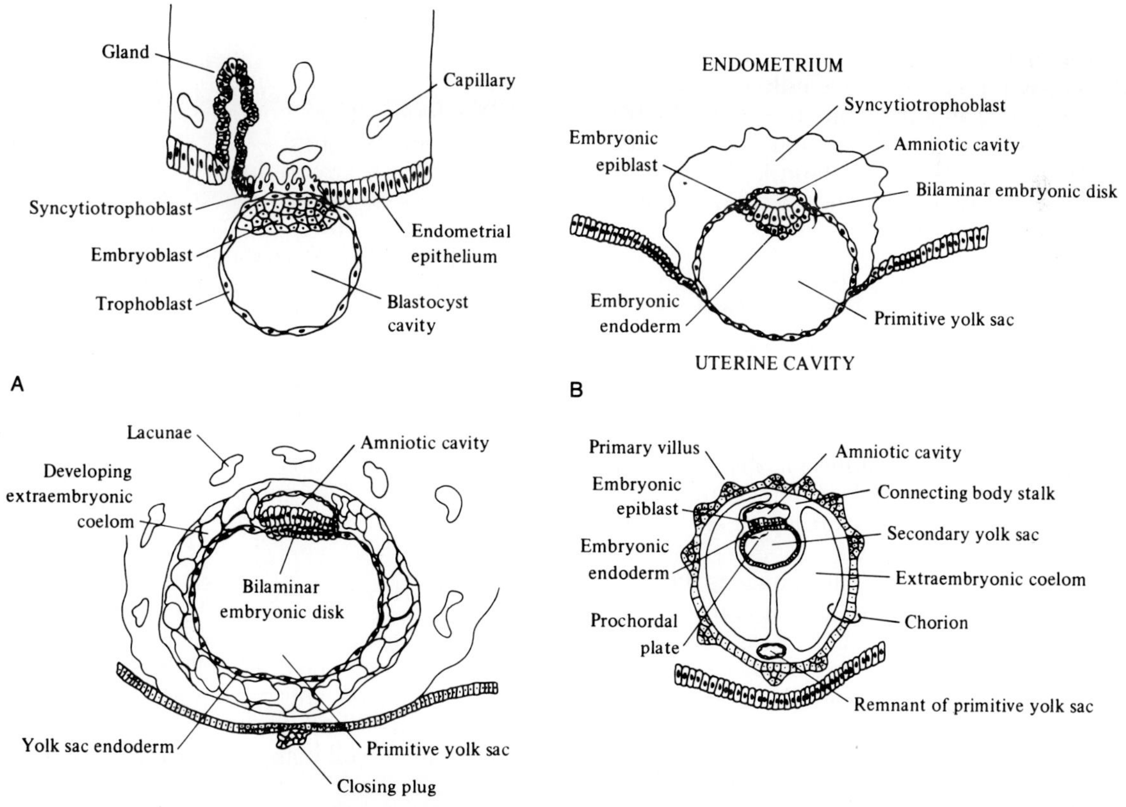

Figure 7-2 Early formation and implantation of the embryo. (*A*) 6 to 7 days: beginning implantation. (*B*) Day $7\frac{1}{2}$: blastocyst embedded in uterine wall. (*C*) Day 12. (*D*) Day 14. (*From M. Tudor, Child Development, McGraw-Hill, New York, 1981, after C. E. Corliss and K. L. Moore, p. 210. Used with permission.*)

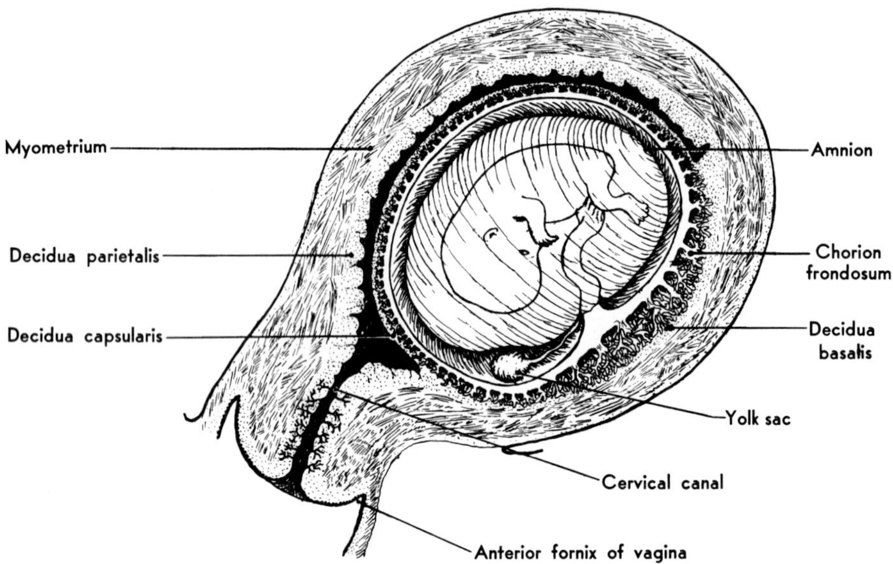

Figure 7-3 The uterus, embryo, and membranes at 8 weeks after conception. (*From B. M. Patten and B. Carlson, Foundations of Embryology, McGraw-Hill, New York, 1974, p. 342. Used with permission.*)

is extensively sloughed and rebuilt after delivery of the baby. The endometrium directly under the blastocyst is known as the *decidua basalis,* and that over the site of implantation is the *decidua capsularis.* The remaining endometrium is called the *decidua parietalis* (Fig. 7-3).

Early development of the placenta

The placenta is the specialized contact between the fetus and the uterus. It develops partly from the invading trophoblast and partly from the endometrium.

By the end of the second week, the blastocyst is usually buried in the endometrium. The trophoblast enlarges, and two layers are recognizable.

The first, the outer layer, is known as the *syncytiotrophoblast.* This layer of cells expands rapidly into the endometrium. Spaces appear in the syncytiotrophoblast and are filled by blood from venules and capillaries of the endometrium.

The second, inner layer of the trophoblast, the *cytotrophoblast,* sends columns of cells into the decidua basalis. About then the trophoblast is renamed the *chorion,* and these fingerlike extensions are *chorionic villi.* Eventually, fetal blood vessels grow into them and the villi become the major surfaces for fetal-maternal exchange. By then, intervillous spaces have formed around the villi and have become pools for maternal blood, which reaches the site by spiral (later uteroplacental) arteries. The chorion is the outer layer of the fetal membranes.

Chorionic villi are originally present over the entire surface of the blastocyst. As it enlarges, however, the decidua capsularis becomes compressed. Circulation to the villi is cut off, and all but those under the embryo atrophy by 4 months. This smooth portion of the chorion is known as the *chorion laeve.* Where the chorionic villi continue to enlarge and proliferate, the surface is called the *chorion frondosum* (*frondosum* means "leafy").

Figure 7-4 shows the anatomic relationship of the fetus and the fetal membranes.

Amnion and amniotic fluid

The fetus develops within the amniotic cavity, which is lined by a layer of cells called the *amnion.* This smooth, shiny membrane secretes a fluid that bathes the fetus. Amniotic fluid is essential for fetal well-being because it provides:

1. A medium for fluid exchange
2. Protection from injury (by cushioning the embryo in fluid)
3. A constant body temperature (by absorbing heat)
4. Prevention of adhesion of body parts

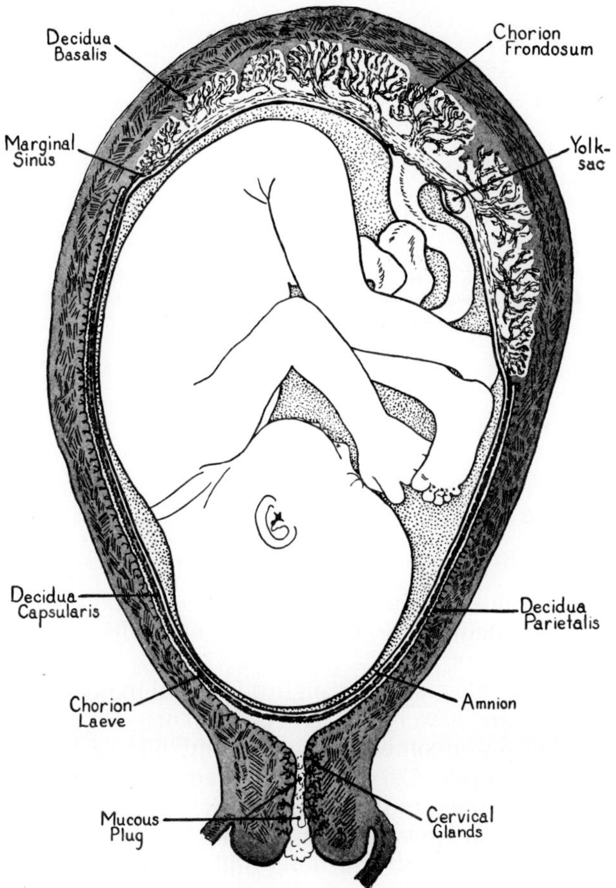

Figure 7-4 The relationships to the uterus of a 5-month-old fetus and its membranes. Amnion is shown as a solid black line, the amniotic cavity is striped, and the chorionic laeve is represented by a broken line. (*From B. M. Patten and B. Carlson, Foundations of Embryology, McGraw-Hill, New York, 1974, p. 348. Used with permission.*)

The amnion produces increasing amounts of amniotic fluid until near term, when 800 to 1000 ml is present. Upon examination, amniotic fluid is found to contain hormones, enzymes, and fetal cells. The fluid can be withdrawn by amniocentesis and examined for genetic diagnosis at 16 weeks and for fetal well-being and maturity near the end of pregnancy.

The umbilical cord

As the placenta develops, the umbilical cord is being formed from a connecting structure known as the *body stalk*. Cells of this structure proliferate into the villi, acting as a core into which the fetal blood vessels penetrate. These vessels extend along the body stalk to form the two umbilical arteries and single umbilical vein that connect fetal circulation to the placenta. In some ways fetal circulation resembles extrauterine circulation to the lungs. Oxygen-depleted blood circulates to the placenta through the two umbilical arteries, and oxygen-enriched blood returns to the fetus through the umbilical vein.

THE EMBRYONIC STAGE

The beginning of the embryonic stage, the third week after conception, is signaled by the development of the third, or middle, cell layer—the *mesoderm*—between the ectoderm and the endoderm. These three germ layers form the basis for differentiation and specialization of different body parts. Figure 7-5 shows the various parts of the body derived from each germ layer.

During the third week the primitive streak, formed from ectoderm, develops in the posterior midline of the embryo. The streak thickens, the embryonic disk elongates, and the neural plate forms. The neural plate then folds inward, creating the neural tube, forerunner of the central nervous system.

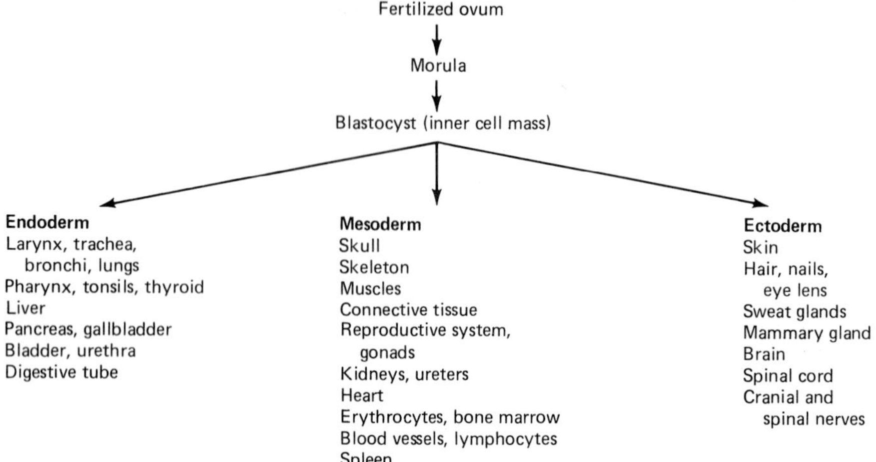

Figure 7-5 The derivation of various body parts from the three primary germ layers.

Thickened groups of mesodermal cells, called *somites,* begin to form in pairs alongside the neural folds. The somites eventually give rise to the skeleton and skeletal muscles.

Also by the third week the heart tubes and a simple vascular system have developed sufficiently to begin circulating the early blood cells that are formed in the yolk sac.

The body of the 4-week-old embryo is C-shaped. The embryo has folded longitudinally, pinching the yolk sac from the gut and thereby hastening the formation of the umbilical cord. Transverse folding causes incorporation of the embryonic coelom, leading to the formation of the peritoneal and pleural cavities.

Thickened areas of tissue, called *placodes,* appear in the cephalic end of the embryo, where the eyes, ears, and nose will develop. Tiny arm and leg buds appear.

During the fifth week the greatest development continues at the head of the embryo. The brain grows rapidly and is composed of five vesicles. Facial features move closer together. All 44 pairs of somites are now present. Septa begin to develop within the heart while the primitive umbilical cord is developing from the body stalk.

By the middle of the sixth week the face is more identifiable, and the arm and leg buds resemble paddles (Fig. 7-6). Cartilage centers develop, and tooth buds form. The trachea enlarges and bifurcates (forks) to form lung buds.

During the seventh week the limbs continue to develop. The fingers are evident, and the limbs move laterally, causing the palms and soles to face toward the middle of the body. The gonads are beginning to differentiate internally, to form ovaries or testes.

By the end of the eighth week all major organ systems have begun their development. The heart has four chambers and is beating 40 to 80 times per minute. The head is one-half the body length and is more rounded and less flexed than before. The embryo has grown 10 mm during this week and is now 30 mm long and weighs 1 to 2 g. The mother has missed two menstrual periods and probably suspects she is pregnant. It is during this crucial embryonic period, while the organs are forming, that the unborn child is most vulnerable to insults that can cause congenital anomalies. Table 7-1 lists the time periods dur-

Table 7-1 Sensitivity of Fetal Organs to Teratogens (Periods of Development in Weeks)

Organ	Most Sensitive	Less Sensitive
Central nervous system	3 to 5	6 to 38
Heart	3 to 6	6 to 12
Eyes	4 to 8	8 to 38
Ears	4 to 9	10 to 20
Arms	4 to 8	8 to 12
Legs	4 to 8	8 to 12
Palate	6 to 9	9 to 16
Teeth	6 to 9	9 to 20
External genitalia	7 to 16	16 to 38

Sources: Adapted from Seymour Romney et al., *Gynecology and Obstetrics: The Health Care of Women,* McGraw-Hill, New York, 1975, p. 71; and Keith Moore, *The Developing Human: Clinically Oriented Embryology,* Saunders, Philadelphia, 1982, p. 152.

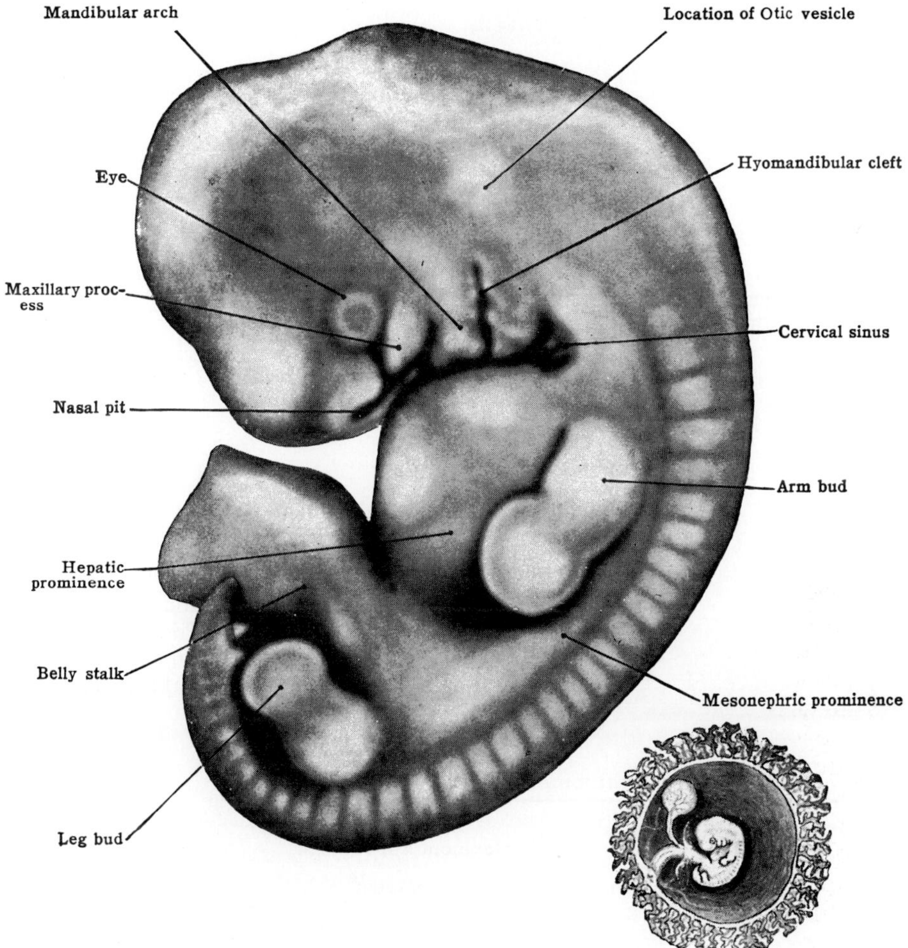

Figure 7-6 A human embryo at about the middle of the sixth week after conception. The small sketch at the lower right shows the *actual size* of the embryo and its chorionic vesicle. (*From C. E. Corliss, Patten's Human Embryology, McGraw-Hill, New York, 1976, p. 57. Used with permission.*)

ing which various organs are most sensitive to teratogenic influences (factors causing birth defects).

THE FETAL PERIOD

From 9 weeks until birth the fetus grows rapidly in length and weight. At 16 weeks there is hair on the head and body, and the mother feels the fetus move (Fig. 7-7). By 24 weeks the fetus looks like a shriveled old man with red, wrinkled skin. By 30 weeks fat is beginning to accumulate. From then on the fetus continues to gain weight, and the body systems mature to enable the baby to survive in extrauterine life.

Embryonic development and fetal development are outlined in Table 7-2. Later chapters describe the embryonic development of each body system in more detail.

PLACENTATION

Structure

As the placenta becomes established, the anchoring villi enlarge and divide it into 15 to 30 segments, or lobes, known as *cotyledons*. Each lobe is composed mainly of a single large main stem villus and its surrounding branches. Each cotyledon is bathed by the blood from a single

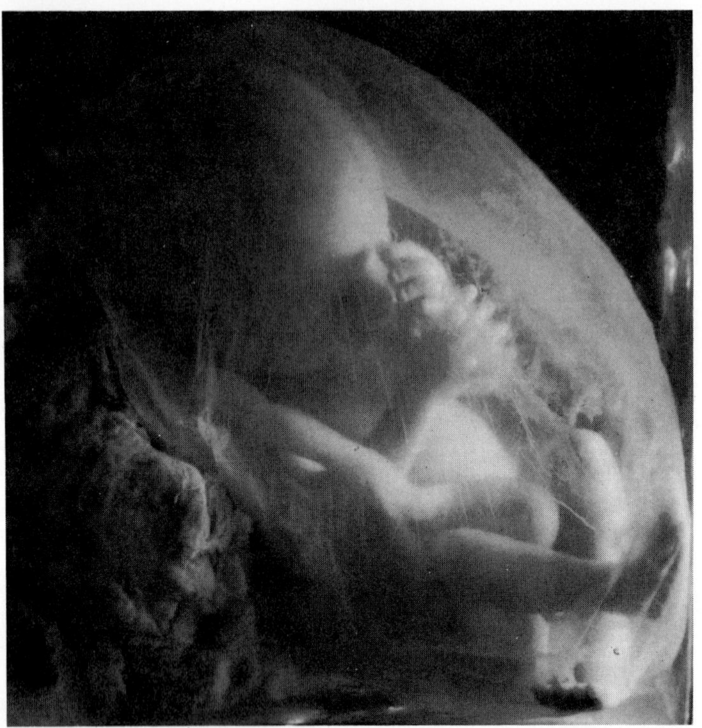

Figure 7-7 A 4-month-old fetus with intact membranes and attached placenta. (*From E. Page, C. Villee, and D. Villee, Human Reproduction, Saunders, Philadelphia, 1972, p. 209. Used with permission.*)

Table 7-2 Overview of Embryonic and Fetal Development

Age, weeks	Length, cm (crown to rump)	Weight, g	Development/Appearance
2			Three germ layers are present
3	0.2		Primitive streak and notochord are present Neural tube forms from closure of neural groove Oral cavity forms Digestive tract forms Liver function begins Embryonic blood begins circulating Primitive kidneys form Somites develop in cephalocaudal direction
4	0.4	0.4	Heart tube fuses at 22 days and beats at 24 Anterior end of neural tube closes to form brain; posterior end closes to form spinal cord Esophagotracheal septum begins division of tubular esophagus and trachea Limb buds are present Stomach forms Intestine becomes tubular Auditory pit is enclosed Head is one-third of total body length
5	0.8	1	Embryo is C-shaped Brain is differentiated into five areas Ten pairs of cranial nerves are present

Table 7-2 Overview of Embryonic and Fetal Development (*Continued*)

Age, weeks	Length, cm (crown to rump)	Weight, g	Development/Appearance
			Division of cardiac atria occurs Permanent kidneys begin to form Optic cups and lens vesicles of eyes form Somite formation is complete
6	1.3	1.5	Tracheal bifurcating begins lung formation Primitive skeletal shape forms Muscle and cartilage begin to form Upper lip is formed; upper and lower jaw are recognizable; tooth buds form Ear formation continues Liver is forming red blood cells Tail is still present but is beginning to regress
7 to 8	2 to 3	2	Eyes, ears, nose, and mouth are recognizable Inferior vena cava and valves form Heart is basically developed and beats 40 to 80 times per minute Differentiation of sex glands into ovaries or testes occurs Optic nerve is formed; eyes are converging; eyelids are forming Diaphragm separates abdominal and thoracic cavities Muscle development continues and ossification begins Fetal movements begin Bladder and urethra separate from rectum Stomach attains final form Digestive tract rotates in midgut All components of reflex arc are present
10	6	14	Palate fuses; face and mouth develop Nail growth begins Formation of tooth enamel begins Basic division of brain is present Intestines are enclosed in abdomen Bladder sac forms; urine forms Testes can form testosterone Responds to tactile stimulation Bone marrow forms and functions Eyelids fuse
12	9	45	Palatal fusion is complete Respiratory motion is visible Swallows in response to thumb-sucking Distinctive external genitalia are present Head is one-half the size of fetus Human growth hormone is produced in pituitary Movement is more pronounced in lower trunk
16	14	200	Phase of rapid growth; looks more human Bladder assumes adult form Ossification of bone will show on x-ray Meconium is present in intestines; anus is open

Table 7-2 Overview of Embryonic and Fetal Development (*Continued*)

Age, weeks	Length, cm (crown to rump)	Weight, g	Development/Appearance
			Lanugo is growing on body; hair is growing on head Differentiation of hard and soft palates Cerebral lobes are delineated General sense organs are differentiated Vagina is open Nipples appear
16 to 20			Fetal heart tones can be heard by fetoscope Mother feels movement (quickening)
20	19	400	Sucking reflex is present; swallows amniotic fluid First patterns (rhythms) of respiratory movement begin Vernix caseosa begins to form Eyelashes and eyebrows form Myelinization of spinal cord begins Brown fat begins to be formed
24	23	820	Skin is red and wrinkled Vernix is present Alveolar ducts and sacs are present Testes are at inguinal ring Eyes are structurally complete
28	27	1300	Body is lean and less red Surfactant forms on alveolar surfaces Cerebral fissure and convolutions appear Pupils react to light Movements are poorly sustained
32	30	1700	Lecithin/sphingomyelin ratio (L/S ratio) is 1.2 to 1 Testes are descending Lanugo is beginning to be shed Subcutaneous fat is beginning to collect Skin is pink and smooth Movements are sustained Moro reflex is present Hunger cry is present Primordia of permanent teeth form
36	34	2900	Skin is pink, and body rounded L/S ratio is 2 to 1 or greater Spinal cord ends at L3 Lanugo is disappearing Good hunger cry is present
38	36	3400	Skin is smooth and covered with vernix Pulmonary branching is two-thirds complete Myelinization of brain begins Testes descend into scrotum Lanugo exists on shoulders and upper body only Sucking reflex is strong Lifts head in prone position Cartilage is present in nose and ears

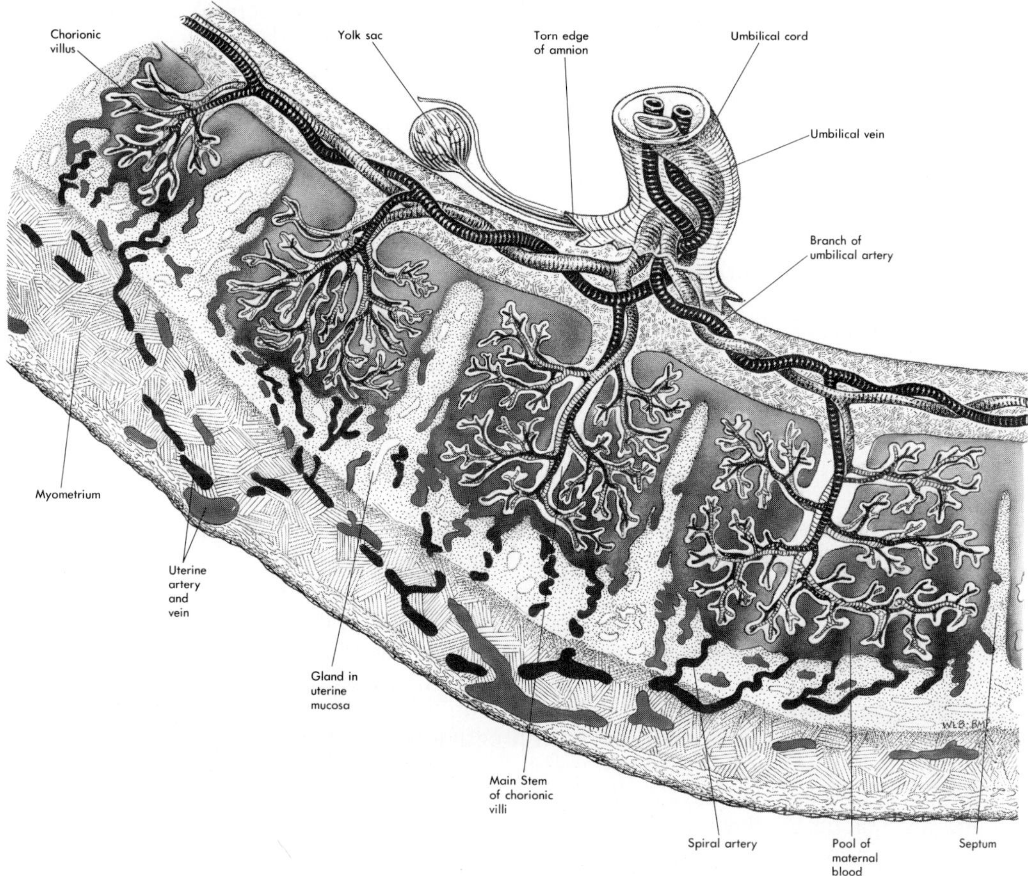

Figure 7-8 The interrelationships of fetal and maternal tissues in formation of the placenta. Chorionic villi are represented as becoming progressively further developed from left to right across the illustration. (*From B. M. Patten and B. Carlson, Foundations of Embryology, McGraw-Hill, New York, 1974, p. 344. Used with permission.*)

uteroplacental artery[4] (Fig 7-8). By 6 weeks the placenta covers one-sixth of the uterus; by 20 weeks it covers one-half. At 8 to 10 weeks after conception the placenta has achieved its definitive form, and no new lobules are added after 12 weeks. Placental growth then occurs in depth rather than in size through the addition of new peripheral villi to the stem villi.

By the end of pregnancy the placenta weighs approximately 500 to 600 g (one-sixth as much as the fetus) and measures 15 to 20 cm by 2.5 to 3 cm. The fetal surface is shiny and slightly grayish. The umbilical vessels that enter the cord look like a branching root system just beneath the amnion and chorion. The maternal surface is dark red, rough, and liverlike. The cotyledons can be seen, divided by shallow clefts.

The placenta as an organ of homeostasis

The placenta is the main organ of homeostasis for the fetus. It functions as an immunological barrier and as an organ of respiration, excretion, endocrine production, and alimentation.

Maternal and fetal blood do not normally intermix. The two circulations are separated by (1) fetal capillary endothelium, (2) connective tissue of the villous core, and (3) trophoblastic cells covering the villi.

Numerous substances cross the uteroplacental barrier by several mechanisms:[5]

1. *Passive diffusion* Water, electrolytes, drugs, oxygen, and carbon dioxide move from an area

of high concentration to one of low concentration.

2. *Facilitated diffusion* Glucose is transferred to an area of lower concentration by means of a carrier system.
3. *Active transport* Amino acids, water-soluble vitamins, and calcium and iron ions (Ca^{2+} and Fe^{2+}) are transferred by metabolic energy.
4. *Pinocytosis* Cells of the syncytiotrophoblast engulf serum proteins and antibodies, transferring them from maternal plasma to fetal circulation.
5. *Bulk flow* Rapid transfer of water and electrolytes occurs through submicroscopic channels in the placenta.
6. *Breaks* Accidental breaks in the fetal capillary wall and villous covering permit passage of maternal and fetal blood cells. Usually this occurs at the time of delivery and placental separation, but it can happen earlier, around 28 weeks. This process accounts for the production of maternal antibodies by an Rh-negative mother against an Rh-positive fetus.

Uteroplacental blood flow is of prime importance in the maintenance of maternal-fetal exchange. It increases 10 to 12 times over the course of a normal pregnancy, reaching a flow of 500 to 600 ml/min near term.[6] Uteroplacental blood flow decreases under severe stress, during labor, and when the mother has a chronic disease. As the placenta ages near term, it becomes less effective. This places the postterm fetus at risk.

Any chronic disease, fetal abnormality, or maternal infection is likely to affect placental functioning and result in growth retardation in the fetus. When vascular disease, such as maternal hypertension or preeclampsia, is present, the placenta is small and thin and often functions poorly. As a result, fetal growth is impaired. Maternal diabetes produces a hypertrophied, edematous placenta.

If placental insufficiency develops rapidly, as it might in the case of diabetes or early separation of the placenta from the implantation site, the fetus can die quickly from hypoxemia and acidosis.

The placenta as an endocrine organ

Human chorionic gonadotropin (HCG) Besides functioning as an organ of homeostasis for the fetus, the placenta produces hormones essential to the continuation of the pregnancy. During the first 3 months of pregnancy, almost all necessary steroid hormones (estrogen and progesterone) are supplied by the corpus luteum of the ovary. Corpus luteum degeneration is prevented by a hormone produced by the trophoblastic cells that is known as *human chorionic gonadotropin*. HCG secretion increases rapidly during early pregnancy, reaching a peak 60 to 80 days after the last menstrual period. HCG forms the basis for pregnancy testing. The decrease in HCG is associated with an increase in placental production of estrogen and progesterone during the last 6 months of pregnancy (Fig. 7-9).

Human chorionic somatomammotropin (HCS) Trophoblastic cells also produce *human somatomammotropin*, or human placental lactogen. HCS is similar to human pituitary growth hormone. It stimulates certain maternal metabolic adjustments that increase the availability of protein and glucose to the fetus and free fatty acids for the mother. Because it counteracts the action of insulin, it is known as the *diabetogenic factor* in pregnancy.

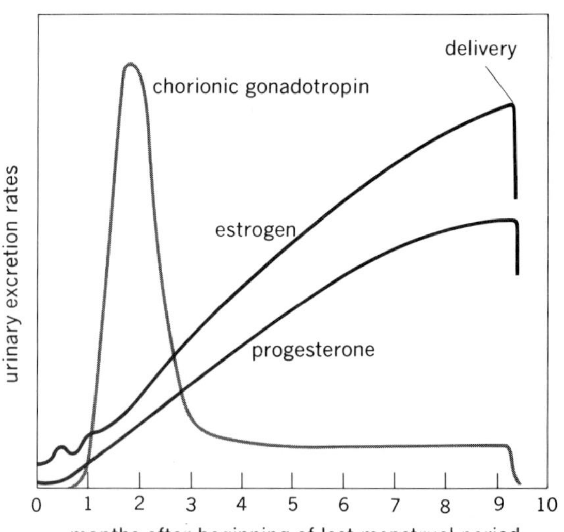

Figure 7-9 Urinary excretion levels of estrogen, progesterone, and human chorionic gonadotropin during pregnancy. Urinary excretion rates reflect blood concentrations and actual production. *(From A. Vander, J. Sherman, and D. Luciano, Human Physiology, 3d ed., McGraw-Hill, New York, 1980, p. 508. Used with permission.)*

Progesterone Progesterone is essential for the continuation of the pregnancy, especially during the early months. It reduces the contractility of uterine smooth muscles and other smooth muscles, maintains the endometrium, and prepares the breasts for lactation.

Estrogens The placenta, using essential precursors from the fetal adrenals, synthesizes estriol. It also produces other estrogens—estradiol and estrone. Placental estrogens increase markedly during pregnancy, causing growth and enlargement of the uterus and breasts and an increase in uterine blood flow. The level of maternal urinary estriol is indicative of fetal well-being and uteroplacental functioning. Estrogens continue to increase until just before delivery. They appear to promote mothering behavior at term.

References

1. Corliss, Clark Edward, *Patten's Human Embryology,* McGraw-Hill, New York, 1976, p. 112.
2. Langman, Jan, *Medical Embryology,* Williams & Wilkins, Baltimore, 1981, p. 22.
3. Ibid., p. 26.
4. Martin, Chester B., and Barbara Gingerich, "Uteroplacental Physiology," *Journal of Obstetrics-Gynecology Nursing,* suppl., September-October 1976, p. 17.
5. Ibid., pp. 19, 20.
6. Ibid., p. 21.

8

Nancy A. Coulter

The newborn

Upon completion of this chapter, the student will be able to:

1. Describe the physiological changes necessary in the transition from fetal to neonatal life.
2. Identify the special needs of the newborn immediately after birth.
3. Describe nursing actions to meet the special needs of the newborn.
4. Describe the characteristics of the normal newborn.
5. Correlate nursing interventions in the hospital nursery with the goals of nursing care of the newborn.
6. Teach parents about their newborn infant's characteristics and needs.
7. Identify nursing actions to assess and facilitate the process of parent-infant bonding.
8. Describe the newborn's ability to interact with and affect the environment during attachment.
9. Assess the parents' readiness to assume the care of their newborn infant.
10. Provide the parents with anticipatory guidance to maximize the newborn's developmental potential.

The neonatal, or newborn, period is the first 28 days of life. It is a period of great change, during which the infant must recover from exhaustion brought on by the birth process, undergo physiological changes for adaptation to independent functioning, and begin the lifelong process of psychological adaptation to life experiences.

The nurse must understand these physiological and psychological processes in order to be able to meet the newborn's nursing care needs. Clark and Affonso[1] have identified the goals of care for newborns as *assessment, protection, nurturance,* and *stimulation;* these four goals will be discussed throughout this chapter. The nurse has a primary role in parent teaching and should translate these nursing goals to parenting goals for care of the newborn. Expert neonatal management and parental guidance during this 28-day period lay the foundation for healthy parent-child development.

THE INFANT AT BIRTH

Transition to extrauterine life

Perhaps the most important adjustment that a human being must make during his or her lifetime is the transition from fetal-placental circulation to independent cardiopulmonary functioning. The first few minutes and hours of life are a critical time of dramatic adjustment.

Initiation of respiration The change that takes place immediately after birth is the onset of breathing. During passage through the birth canal, the neonate experiences pressure on the thoracic cage that can force out as much as 5 to 10 ml of tracheal fluid. Most of the liquid remaining in the infant's airway at birth is removed by the pulmonary circulation. The rest is removed by the pulmonary lymphatics or is expelled through the infant's nose and mouth when the face is exposed to atmospheric pressure. Following delivery, the chest walls recoil to the position they were in prior to labor, drawing in air to fill the airways.[2] The alveolar surfaces of full-term infants are covered by a substance called *pulmonary surfactant,* which diminishes surface tension during expiration, thus allowing the alveolar sacs to remain partly open. The second breath requires much less effort than the first, because the sacs are already open, and successive breaths require even less effort.

In addition to these mechanical processes, there are sensory and chemical stimuli which aid in the initiation and maintenance of respiration. Birth is potentially an asphyxiating process because it stimulates chemical changes that lead to the following conditions in the blood: increased carbon dioxide, lowered oxygen, and lowered pH. These conditions stimulate the respiratory center in the medulla, either by acting on it directly or by affecting chemoreceptors in the carotid artery or aorta, thus initiating respiration. However, if asphyxiation and these altered blood conditions are prolonged, respiration will be inhibited rather than stimulated.

At birth the neonate passes from an environment that is relatively devoid of sensory experiences to one in which the infant is bombarded with sensations of pressure, pain, noise, light, and cold. Chilling may act as a stimulus to sensory receptors in the skin. Nerve impulses are then transmitted to the respiratory center in the medulla, thus stimulating respiration. In animal studies on thermoregulation, it has been found that chilling stimulates breathing even when fetal-placental circulation is still intact and the level of blood gases is unchanged, and that respirations are inhibited by a heat stimulus. However, excessive cooling interferes with respiration by increasing the need for oxygen and by producing acidosis. The practice of slapping the baby on the backside or feet to induce respiration is essentially a misuse of precious time if initiation of respiration is delayed.

Transition from fetal to neonatal circulation At the same time that respiration begins, critical changes from fetal to neonatal circulation must be made. Fetal circulation is discussed in detail in Chap. 22 and is only briefly reviewed here (Fig. 8-1). Oxygenated blood leaves the placenta and enters the fetal circulation via the umbilical vein. This oxygenated blood mainly bypasses the fetal liver via the *ductus venosus* and then empties into the inferior vena cava. The majority of the blood entering the right atrium from the inferior vena cava crosses directly to the left atrium via the *foramen ovale* ("oval window") and then follows the normal route through the left ventricle and out the ascending aorta to the head and upper extremities.

Most of the deoxygenated blood entering the right atrium from the superior vena cava passes through the right ventricle and then out via the pulmonary artery. There is no functional need for this blood to pass through the pulmonary system. Because of high fetal pulmonary vascular resistance, most of this blood bypasses the lungs via a third fetal shunt, the *ductus arteriosus.* The ductus arteriosus connects the pulmonary artery and the aorta. Blood passing through the ductus arteriosus enters the descending aorta, mixing with some oxygenated blood from the left ventricle. Some of this pool of blood supplies the lower extremities and visceral organs, but most of it returns to the placenta, via the two umbilical arteries, for reoxygenation. Only about 12 percent of the blood in the fetal circulation actually reaches the pulmonary vascular beds.

Increases in systemic and decreases in pulmonary vascular resistance at birth serve to close these fetal blood shunts. It is important for the nurse to realize that closure of these structures at birth is not absolute. The ductus arteriosus closes gradually over the first 3 to 4 days of life. Functional heart murmurs are not uncommon

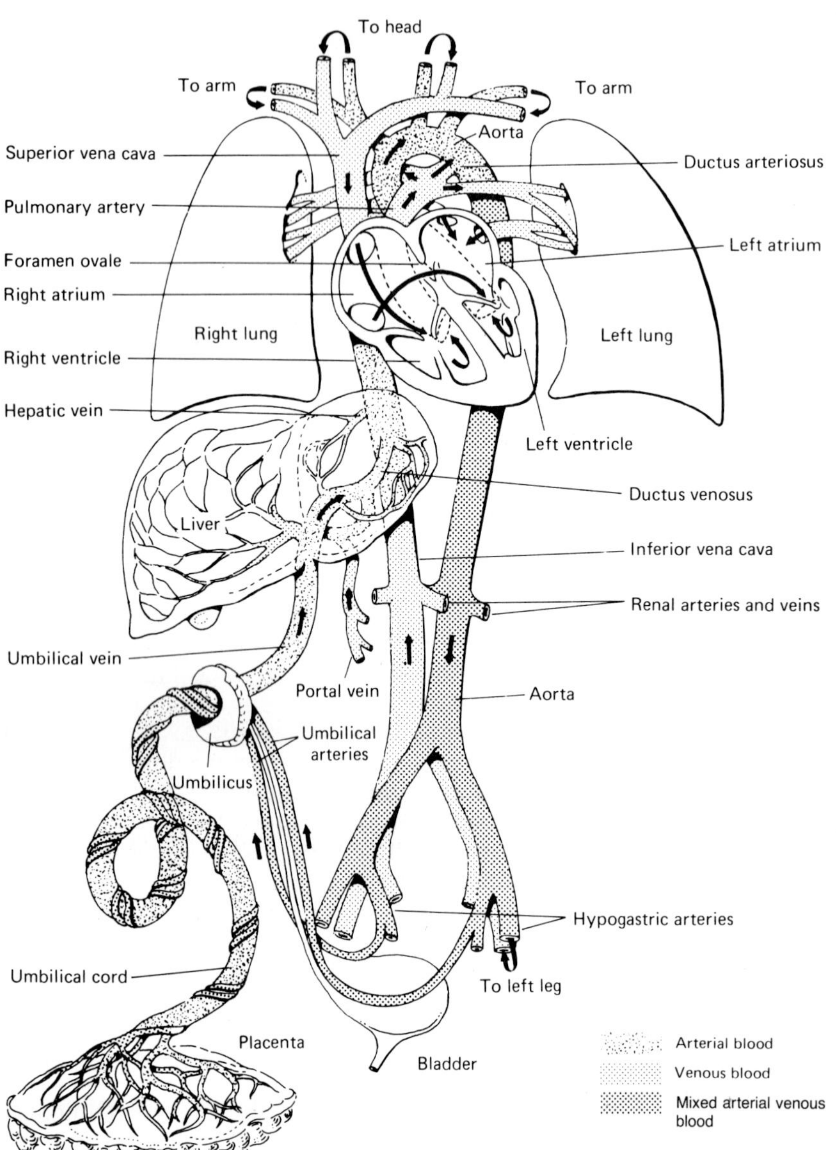

Figure 8-1 Fetal circulation. (*Clinical Educational Aid No. 1, courtesy of Ross Laboratories, Columbus, Ohio.*)

during this period. Likewise, closure of the foramen ovale is not absolute during the first few days of life. Situations such as stress or crying increase pressure in the venae cavae and right atrium and may cause shunting of unoxygenated blood across the foramen ovale to the left side of the heart. This results in transient cyanosis in the newborn.

Nursing management of the neonate in the delivery room

Nursing care of the neonate in the delivery room should be consistent with meeting the previously stated goals of assessment, protection, nurturance, and stimulation.

Initial assessment: the Apgar score Because of the extensive physiological changes that the neonate undergoes during the first few minutes after birth, it is important that caretakers make astute and systematic observations of the neonate. The most uniform criterion used to evaluate the neonate in the delivery room is the Apgar scoring system, developed by Dr. Virginia Apgar in 1952. This method of assessing the cardiopulmonary status of the neonate is based on five evaluative criteria: heart rate, respiratory ef-

Table 8-1 The Apgar Scoring System

Sign	0	1	2
Heart rate	Absent	Slow (below 100)	Over 100
Respiratory effort	Absent	Slow and irregular	Good crying
Muscle tone	Flaccid and limp	Some flexion of extremities	Action motion
Reflex irritability	No response	Grimace	Cough, sneeze, or cry
Color	Blue and pale	Body pink, and extremities pale	Completely pink

fort, muscle tone, reflex irritability, and color. Each criterion is given a score of 0, 1, or 2; then these individual values are totaled to yield the actual score. The Apgar score is usually obtained at 1 and at 5 min of age (Table 8-1).

The *heart rate* is the most valuable indicator of the effects of asphyxia associated with the process of delivery. It is most reliably counted for at least 15 s, with a stethoscope. Palpation or visualization of pulsations in the umbilical cord, at the abdominal junction, is an acceptable assessment technique. A rate of less than 100 beats per minute indicates severe asphyxia, and the need for immediate resuscitative efforts.

Respiratory effort, an indicator of adequate ventilation, can be assessed while the heart rate is being checked.

Muscle tone refers to the degree of flexion and resistance offered by the infant when the examiner attempts to straighten the extremities. A score of 2 is given if the infant actively resists alteration of the normally flexed position, a score of 1 is given for less vigorous resistance, and a score of 0 is given if the infant is limp and therefore offers no resistance.

Reflex irritability may be evaluated by either (1) eliciting a grimace or gag reflex when suctioning the nostrils or (2) slapping the soles of the feet with the examiner's hand. The normal, healthy infant will respond to either of these stimuli with a loud cry; the moderately depressed infant will respond with a facial grimace; and the severely depressed infant will exhibit no reaction.

Color is indicative of peripheral tissue oxygenation and is the least significant of the five criteria. Few infants are completely pink at birth; most will manifest some blueness of the extremities (*acrocyanosis*). Generalized pallor and cyanosis indicate a severely asphyxiated baby. Reliable techniques for assessing color include inspection of the mucous membranes of the mouth and inspection of the lips, the palms of the hands, and the soles of the feet.

The Apgar score is of particular value for two reasons: First, it is a uniform assessment scale for use in a variety of delivery settings, and second, and perhaps of greater significance, it allows anticipatory planning in the management of newborns. The clinical management of infants with a 1-min Apgar score can be summarized as follows:

Apgar 0 to 2 These infants require immediate endotracheal intubation and positive-pressure ventilation with oxygen.

Apgar 3 to 6 These infants will frequently respond to gentle suctioning and receiving oxygen supplied by mask. If they do not promptly improve or if signs of deterioration occur, immediate endotracheal intubation should be performed.

Apgar 7 to 10 These infants will rarely need any resuscitation, unless the Apgar score suddenly drops several minutes after birth. Appropriate management should be instituted if any danger is imminent.[3]

The severely asphyxiated infant may be recognized, and resuscitation begun, *before* determination of the 1-min Apgar score. (See Chap. 17 for additional information regarding assessment and clinical management of the high-risk neonate in the delivery room.)

Protection against airway occlusion The neonate is subject to airway occlusion for a variety of anatomic and situational reasons:

1. The newborn is a nose breather and has very narrow nasal passages, which are easily occluded.
2. The tongue is large, and the trachea and glottis are small.

3. The respiratory tract of the neonate is especially susceptible to edema.
4. Pressure exerted on the thoracic cage during delivery expresses fluid via the mouth and nose.
5. Excessive amounts of mucus are produced during the first few hours of life.

For these reasons, it is of utmost importance that the nurse pay careful attention to maintenance of a newborn's airway. The oropharynx and nostrils are cleared with a bulb syringe as soon as the head is delivered to prevent aspiration of secretions into the bronchi. For most healthy newborns, a bulb syringe is both adequate and the preferred instrument for suctioning the oropharynx and nose. If there is need for additional suctioning, a DeLee or mechanical suction apparatus is used. The nurse must exercise care and careful judgment in selecting a catheter of the appropriate size and the correct suctioning technique. It is important that only gentle suction, for periods no longer than a few seconds, be used; vigorous or prolonged suctioning can cause bradycardia and cardiac arrhythmias, which are the result of vagus-nerve stimulation and laryngospasm. During and after suctioning the infant should be placed in a position which facilitates drainage of fluids from the airway. Usually this position is achieved by placing the infant on his or her side with the head slightly lower than the chest.

Protection against heat loss Heat loss by the neonate occurs through four distinct mechanisms: evaporation, conduction, radiation, and convection. *Evaporation* of amniotic fluid from the skin surface immediately after birth is a major cause of heat loss. Immediate drying of the skin and hair and placement of the baby in a warmed environment are essential nursing actions to minimize heat loss by evaporation. The warmed environment may be created by a warmed blanket, which is wrapped around the baby, or by a radiant heater, under which the infant is placed. For most full-term infants, the relatively simple procedure of immediately drying and wrapping the infant in a warm blanket is nearly as effective as using a radiant heater.

Heat loss also occurs by *conduction;* that is, when the neonate's skin is in direct contact with a cooler solid object, heat is conducted away from the body to the cooler object. Placing the baby on a padded, warm surface, as opposed to a cold examining table, and warming all examining devices that come in contact with the baby are some ways to avoid heat loss by conduction.

Infants also lose heat by *radiation;* that is, heat in the form of radiation is emitted by the body and absorbed by objects in the room. Heat loss by radiation increases as the cooler objects are brought nearer to the baby, regardless of the temperature of the surrounding air. A critical point for the nurse to remember is that even though the ambient (surrounding) air may be at an optimal temperature for the infant, heat loss can still occur by radiation. A key factor in preventing heat loss by radiation is keeping the infant in the center of the room, preferably near the mother and as far away from cooler external walls as possible.

The last major way in which heat loss occurs is by *convection,* in which body heat is lost to surrounding cooler air. This can be minimized by increasing the temperature in the delivery room, keeping infants away from air currents (drafts and air-conditioning), and placing newborns in recessed cribs to shield them from cross-ventilation during examinations.

Protection against infection Newborns are routinely given treatment against *Neisseria gonorrhoeae,* which can cause blindness in a baby born to a mother who harbors gonorrhea in her birth canal. The most commonly used prophylaxis is 1 drop of silver nitrate (1%) placed in each eye. The drops should be carefully placed on the inner aspect of the conjunctival sac and allowed to flow laterally. The practice of irrigating the eye with normal saline following instillation of silver nitrate is no longer recommended, as it dilutes the drug and decreases its potency. Care must be taken, however, during the administration of silver nitrate since chemical conjunctivitis may occur if too much is used or if the infant is sensitive to it. Erythromycin and tetracycline ophthalmic products are less irritating and can be used effectively in place of silver nitrate. Erythromycin has the additional advantage of providing antimicrobial activity against *Chlamydia trachomatis.*[4] Prophylaxis against ophthalmia neonatorum is required by law in 47 states; the nurse should be acquainted with local public health department regulations regarding this treatment.[5]

Protection against bleeding Newborn infants are susceptible to bleeding disorders because they lack adequate supplies of vitamin K during the first 3 to 4 days of life. This is because vitamin K is normally produced by bacterial action in the large bowel, and infants have sterile bowels at birth. Vitamin K is used mainly in the production of prothrombin, which is necessary for the clotting process. Diminished amounts of vitamin K interfere with the coagulation process. A single dose of a water-soluble vitamin K preparation, 0.5 mg vitamin K_1, is given intramuscularly in the anterolateral aspect of the thigh.[6] The drug should be given shortly after birth, either in the delivery room or upon admission to the newborn nursery to prevent hypoprothrombinemia.

Protection through identification Every mother and baby must be properly identified before either of them leaves the delivery room. This is accomplished by the use of matched identification bands: one on the mother's wrist and two on the infant (one on the wrist and one on the ankle). The bands should include the mother's full name and hospital number, the infant's sex, the date and time of birth, and a code number. The nurse in charge of the delivery room is responsible for preparing and securely fastening the identification bands.[7] Care must be taken in attaching the bands to the infant; if they are too tight, they can impede circulation; if they are too loose, they may fall off. The possibility that they will fall off is the reason for placing *two* bands on the infant. Some hospitals also take a footprint of the baby and a fingerprint of the mother, using a special form that remains a part of the baby's medical record. If taken carefully, a footprint provides a means for making positive identification of the infant, since the arrangement of ridges on each infant's soles is unique. Nurses responsible for this procedure should carefully study the instructions for the particular material used (Fig. 8-2).

Final delivery room assessment Before the infant leaves the delivery room, a cursory physical examination should be done. In addition to making a cardiopulmonary evaluation by using the Apgar score and inspecting the infant to determine whether birth trauma is present, the American Academy of Pediatrics recommends that the following screening tests be made before the infant leaves the delivery room to determine whether he or she has congenital anomalies:[8]

1. A brief appraisal of total body appearance and size relationships of various parts of the body
2. Palpation of the abdomen for masses
3. Observation of breathing to see whether the infant can breathe with a closed mouth (to rule out choanal atresia)
4. Passage of a soft tube through the mouth to the stomach (to rule out esophageal atresia)
5. Aspiration and measurement of gastric contents (since more than 15 to 20 ml of gastric content could suggest high intestinal obstruction)

These guidelines are modified by many hospitals to include other maneuvers, such as palpating the palate to rule out cleft palate and counting the number of vessels in the umbilical cord. There should be two arteries and one vein. A single umbilical artery, found in 0.7 percent of all single births, may indicate other congenital anomalies.[9]

Nurturance The decision to breast- or bottle-feed the newborn is central to every new mother's thinking; factors influencing this decision are discussed later in the chapter. If a woman has made the decision to breast-feed her infant, the nurse can enhance breast-feeding by helping the mother and baby begin a feeding as soon after birth as possible. This may begin in the delivery room or, if more appropriate, in the recovery room. It is important for the nurse to realize that breast-feeding is not instinctive with humans, as it is with some lower animal species. Mothers require assistance with this process. Although this is especially true of mothers who are breast-feeding for the first time, the nurse must also carefully assess the teaching and support needs of mothers who have breast-fed other infants. For successful breast-feeding, mothers who choose to nurse should begin as soon as possible, preferably within the first hours following delivery.

Stimulation and bonding Facilitating optimum stimulation for the infant is one of the most important and rewarding of the nurse's goals. During the first 30 min to 1 h after birth, the infant is usually alert, with open eyes, and appears very interested in the environment. The nurse should capitalize on this state by allowing the parents uninterrupted time with their infant.

Klaus and Kennell, pioneers in the field of parental bonding, state: "Immediately after birth

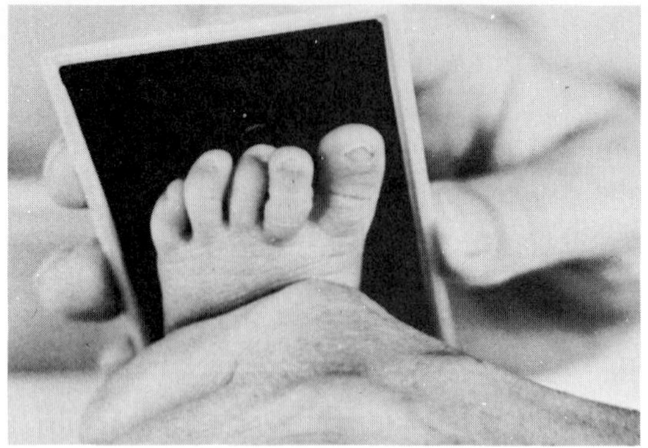

A

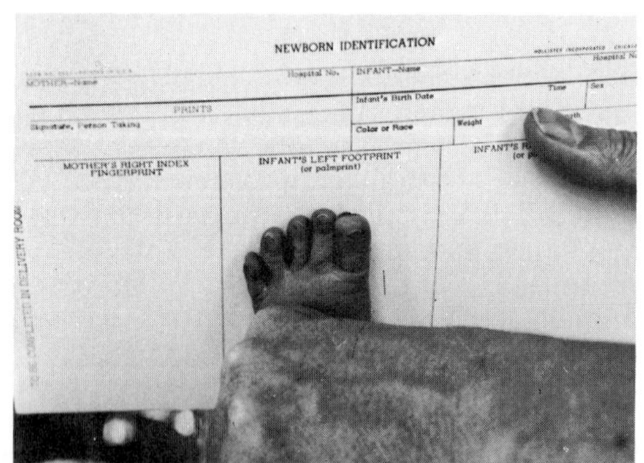

C

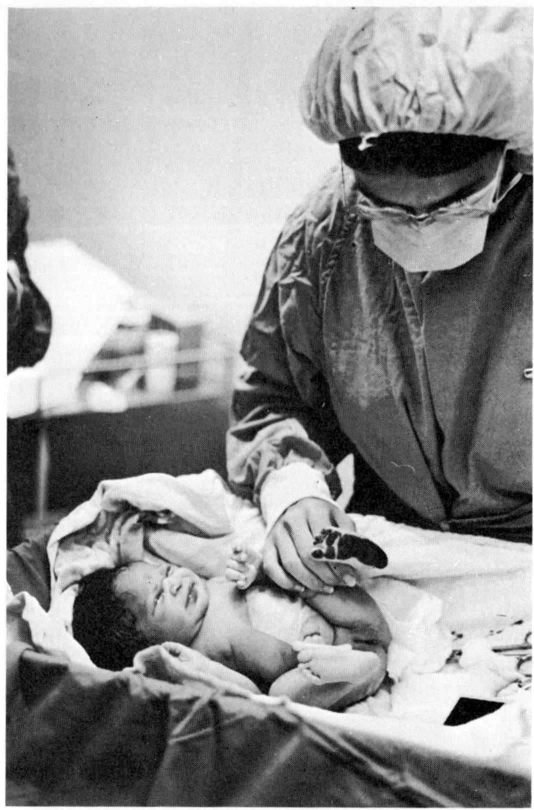

B

NEWBORN IDENTIFICATION

FORM NO. 5821—PRINTED IN U.S.A. HOLLISTER INCORPORATED CHICAGO 60611

MOTHER—Name	Hospital No.	INFANT—Name		Hospital No.
PRINTS		Infant's Birth Date	Time	Sex
Signature, Person Taking		Color or Race	Weight	Length

MOTHER'S RIGHT INDEX FINGERPRINT	INFANT'S LEFT FOOTPRINT (or palmprint)	INFANT'S RIGHT FOOTPRINT (or palmprint)

TO BE COMPLETED IN DELIVERY ROOM

D

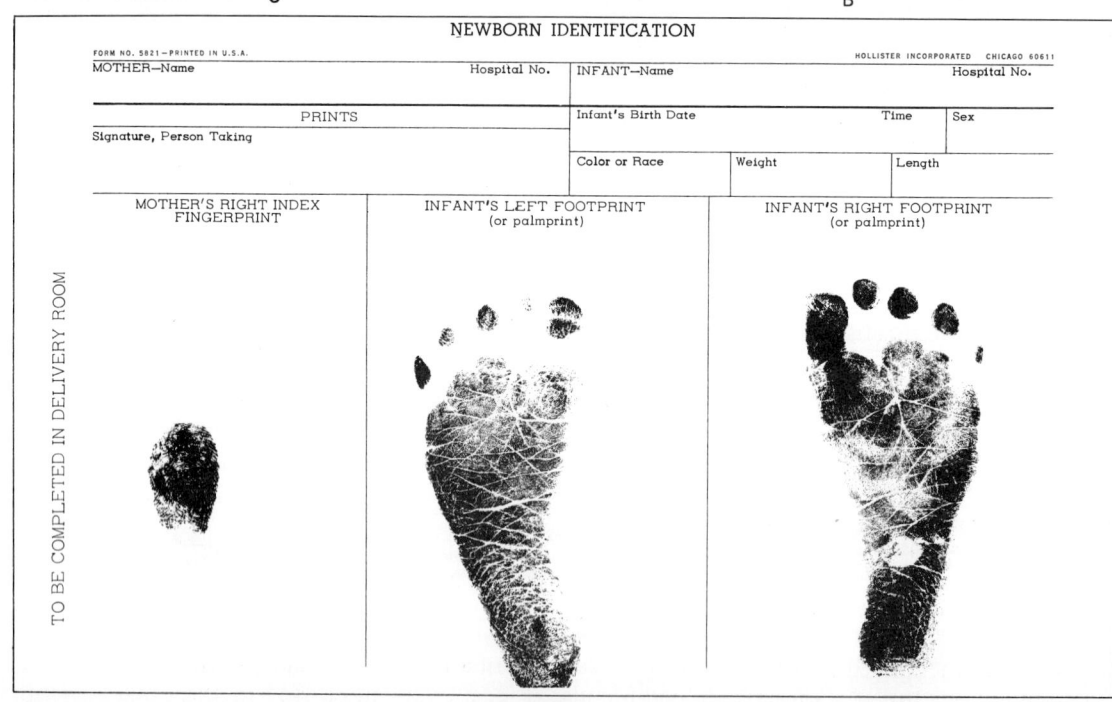

Figure 8-2 The identification process. (*A*) A footprint pad. (*B*) An inky foot. (C) Printing. (*D*) The mother's right index fingerprint. (*From Elizabeth J. Dickason and Martha D. Schult, Maternal and Infant Care, 2d ed., McGraw-Hill, New York, 1979. Used with permission.*)

the parents enter into a unique period during which events may have lasting effects on the family. This period, which lasts a short time, and during which the parents' attachment to their infant blossoms, we have named the *maternal sensitive period*."[10] Mothers who are left alone with their infants shortly after birth exhibit specific bonding behaviors. Perhaps the most notable is touch. In Klaus and Kennell's research, when nude infants were placed next to their mothers shortly after birth, most mothers touched them in a progressive pattern that began with placing the fingertips against the infant's extremities, from where they proceeded to use the palm to massage, stroke, and encompass the trunk. Actual eye-to-eye contact, or at least an intense desire for it, was expressed by 70 percent of the mothers. Many assumed the *en face* position.[11] *En face* is the position in which the mother's face is rotated so that her eyes and those of the infant meet fully in the same vertical plane of rotation.[12] Mothers speak to their infants in a higher-pitched voice than they use in normal conversation, which appears to alert and attract the infant.[13] Fathers exhibit specific behaviors during the first few minutes after birth. They hover over, point at, look into the eyes of, gaze at, and present their faces to their infants.

Moments after birth, neonates exhibit a large repertoire of behaviors. Their eyes are wide open and alert. They turn their heads toward voices in the delivery room, looking for the sources of the voices. They move their arms and legs in synchrony with rhythms of human speech. Most important, they are particularly attentive to human faces, seeking eye-to-eye contact with their caregivers.[14] Such behaviors stimulate further parental response and thus enhance the bonding process. Hence, the nurse must realize that the initial bonding process is one of mutuality, in which each party plays a unique role. Parents and infants who are allowed time for this acquaintance process ultimately demonstrate healthier parent-child relationships than those who are separated at birth.

Nursing actions that may facilitate parent-child bonding include:

1. Placing the infant on the mother's abdomen or chest immediately after birth
2. Providing the parents privacy with their infant for 30 to 40 min shortly after birth
3. Allowing the mother to have the baby in bed with her
4. Encouraging the parents to unwrap and examine the infant (a radiant heater may be necessary to prevent chilling)
5. If the mother plans to breast-feed, encouraging the initiation of nursing
6. Withholding the application of silver nitrate to the eyes for 1 h to allow maximum eye-to-eye contact
7. Accurately recording observed behaviors and responses

Dr. Frederick Leboyer, a French physician, incorporates many of these guidelines into his conceptual approach to childbirth, commonly referred to as "birth without violence." This physician demonstrates unusual sensitivity to the infant as a sensitive and unique human being. Some of his practices are unconventional by American standards. All unnecessary stimuli in the delivery room are minimized. The delivery is conducted either in silence or to the sound of soft music. Lighting is lowered; only the amount of illumination necessary for initial assessment of the newborn is used. The delivery progresses naturally. The cord is tied when pulsations cease. The infant is then placed on the mother's abdomen for 3 to 6 min and is given a gentle back massage. The infant is then transferred to a warm bath for another 3 to 6 min, with his or her head carefully supported out of the water, and is allowed to move freely. Dr. Leboyer feels that this bath simulates the amniotic-fluid environment, to which the infant is accustomed, and therefore reduces stress. Following the bath, the infant is dried, diapered, wrapped in a warm blanket, and given back to the mother for extended contact.[15]

The Leboyer method of childbirth, although controversial, obviously facilitates early bonding. There is a planned time for increased skin contact. The diminished lighting in the delivery room stimulates the infant's eyes to remain open for longer periods of time, thus allowing for maximum eye contact. In addition, the low-key, nonthreatening environment allows parents to "take in" all infant behaviors and generally to respond to them without inhibition.

Signs of the newborn's transition

The infant undergoes intense physiological and psychological adjustment during the first 24 h of life. Extensive research on the newborn during this transition period resulted in findings of two distinct periods of activity: the first and second periods of reactivity. The *first period of reactivity,* which begins with birth, is normally characterized by short periods of random movements interspersed with short quiet periods of inactivity. During this period, there may be transient flaring of the nares, retracting of the chest, and grunting upon expiration. The respiratory rate is rapid and can reach up to 80 breaths per minute during the first hour, before decreasing to 35 to 60 breaths per minute. Tachycardia is initially present, reaching a maximum of approximately 180 beats per minute at 3 min of age and falling gradually to 120 to 140 beats per minute at 30 min of age. Following this period of intense activity, the infant becomes quiet, relaxes, and usually falls asleep. The average age at which the infant falls asleep is 2 h, with sleep lasting from a few minutes to 2 to 4 h.

Upon awakening from this sleep, the infant enters the *second period of reactivity.* During this time, the infant may be hyperresponsive to all stimuli. The heart rate fluctuates appropriately with stimulation, and there are marked changes in color. The appearance of increased oral mucus is frequently a problem during this period and may cause gagging, swallowing, vomiting, and occasionally choking. The second period of reactivity lasts for varying periods of time; when it is over, the infant becomes relatively stable.[16]

NORMAL PHYSICAL CHARACTERISTICS OF THE NEWBORN

General appearance

The neonate is differentiated from the older infant by specific structural and physiological characteristics. The head of the neonate is relatively large, accounting for approximately one-fourth of the total body length; the limbs are short; and the abdomen is prominent. The predominant posture of the neonate is one of flexion, or persistent fetal position. The neonate should demonstrate symmetry in size and movement.

Weight and length

The average weight, at sea level, of a full-term Caucasian infant is approximately 7 lb 8 oz (3400 g) for the male and 7 lb (3200 g) for the female. The average weight of full-term non-Caucasian infants (black, Oriental, or Indian, for example) is usually slightly lower. Ethnic differences in weight, however, depend most significantly on differences in levels of malnutrition and the incidence of infectious disease in different parts of the world.[17] Approximately 95 percent of all full-term infants weigh between $5\frac{1}{2}$ lb (2500 g) and 10 lb (4600 g).[18]

The average length of a full-term infant is 20 in (51 cm); approximately 95 percent of full-term infants have lengths from 18 to 22 in (45 to 55 cm).[19] Male infants tend to be slightly longer (0.8 in, or 2 cm) than female infants.

The head

The head circumference of the full-term infant is almost invariably between 13 and 15 in (33 and 37 cm). The skull is composed of six bony plates, joined loosely by membranous suture lines (Fig. 8-3). The junction of several sutures forms an irregular space. These spaces are enclosed by a membrane and are called *fontanels,* the two most important of which are the anterior fontanel and the posterior fontanel. The *anterior fontanel,* located between the sagittal and coronal sutures, is diamond-shaped and varies in size up to approximately 5 cm (2 in). This fontanel closes by approximately 18 months of age. The *posterior fontanel,* located between the sagittal and lambdoid sutures, is triangular in shape and much

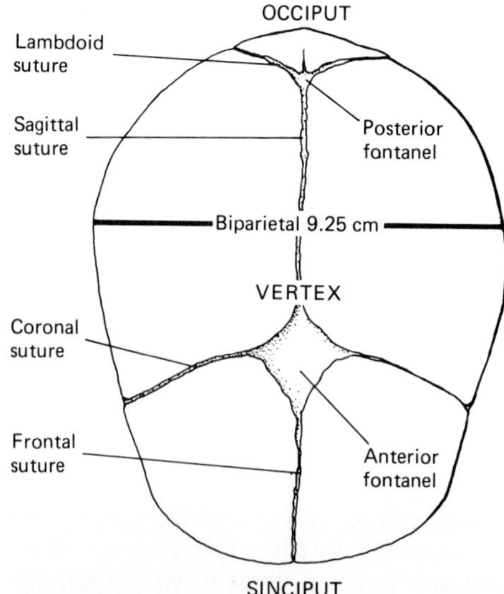

Figure 8-3 The anterior and posterior fontanel. (*Clinical Education Aid No. 13, courtesy of Ross Laboratories, Columbus, Ohio.*)

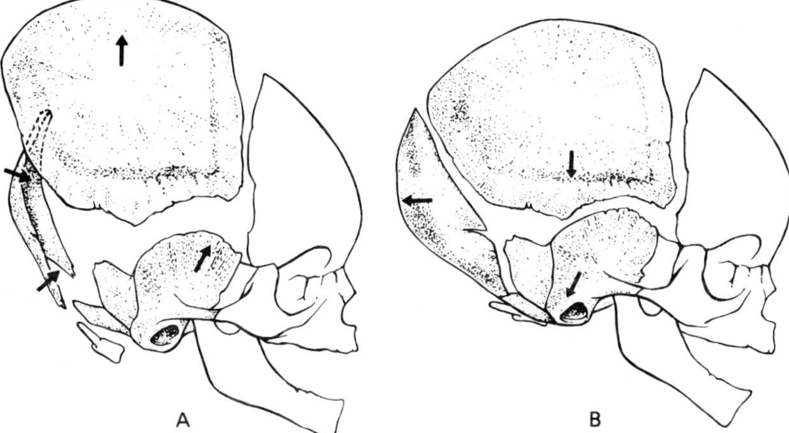

Figure 8-4 The molding of the bones of the head; overlapping is caused by the normal process of compression during passage of the head through the birth canal. By the third day of life, the bones have returned to their normal position. (*Courtesy of Meade Johnson Company.*)

smaller than the anterior fontanel. It may actually appear, upon palpation, to be nearly closed at birth and usually closes by 2 to 3 months of age. A third fontanel, located between the anterior and posterior fontanels along the sagittal suture line, is found in some normal neonates. A much more important consideration than size is the tension exhibited by the fontanels. A bulging fontanel may indicate increased intracranial pressure, while a depressed or sunken fontanel is indicative of dehydration.

Molding The fact that the bones of the head are not fused, but rather held together by these membranous sutures, allows the cranium to change shape in response to the external pressure exerted on the head during labor and delivery (Fig. 8-4). This process is termed *molding* and may result in an elongated head at birth. This distortion diminishes rapidly, and the head assumes its normal shape within 1 week.

Caput succedaneum Profuse edema caused by pressure on the presenting part of the head during vertex deliveries is termed *caput succedaneum.* This edema, which crosses suture lines, usually subsides by 2 to 3 days of age.

Cephalhematoma Occasionally a neonate will develop a cephalhematoma, caused by bleeding from a ruptured blood vessel between the surface of a cranial bone and the periosteum covering that bone (Fig. 8-5). This will appear during the first few hours of life as a swelling confined to the area over the cranial bone involved; it will not cross suture lines. It is possible to have a cephalhematoma over more than one cranial bone simultaneously. A cephalhematoma will disappear spontaneously, but may take up to 6 weeks to do so. Since the cephalhematoma is a collection of blood, significant amounts of serum bilirubin may result as the blood breaks down and is absorbed (Fig. 8-6).

The face

The nose and mouth Proper anatomic and physiological functioning of the nose and mouth is of utmost importance in the neonate. Since neonates are primarily nose breathers, any obstruction of the nasal passages is of extreme significance.

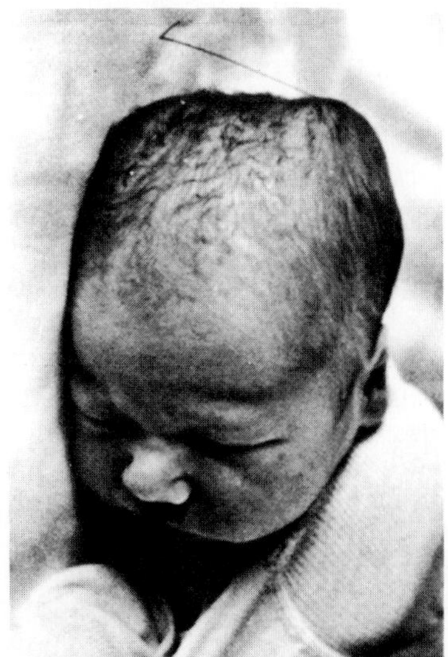

Figure 8-5 Cephalhematoma. (*Courtesy of Meade Johnson Company.*)

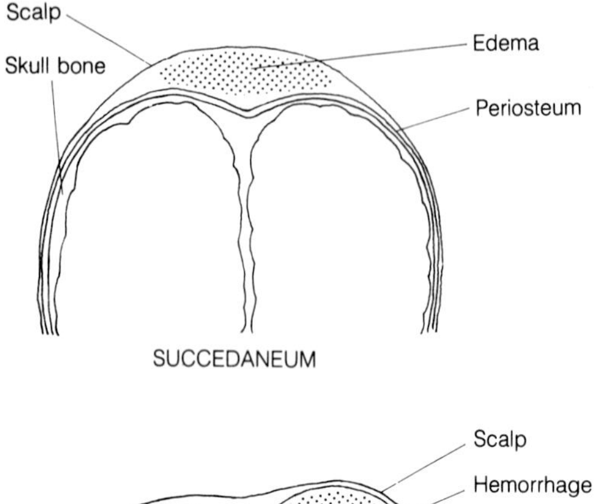

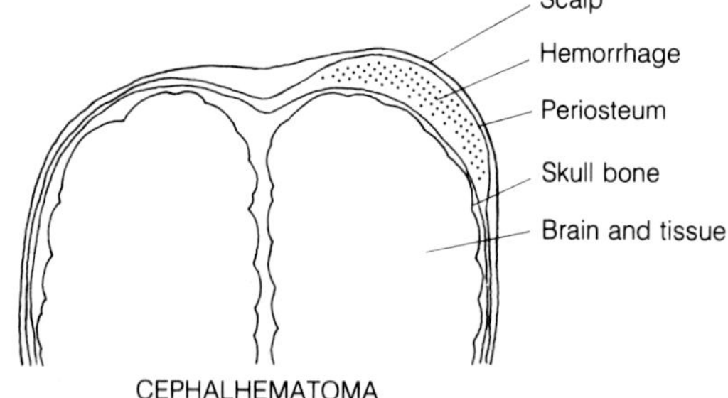

Figure 8-6 Comparison between caput succadaneum and cephalhematoma. (*From Elizabeth J. Dickason and Martha D. Schult, Maternal and Infant Care, 2d ed., McGraw-Hill, New York, 1979. Used with permission.*)

The neonate normally exhibits a *sneeze* reflex in response to obstruction or irritation of the nasal passages. This should persist throughout life. In addition, the neonate has the ability to *differentiate odors,* although the precise developmental sequence of this is unknown. Neonates are able to distinguish between various olfactory stimuli.[20]

When the *tongue* is touched, the neonate responds by forcing it outward. This *extrusion reflex* normally disappears by 4 months of age. The tongue is attached to the floor of the mouth by the frenulum, which is short and inelastic. This structure occasionally appears to limit the mobility of the tongue. This condition is termed *tongue-tie,* and is frequently accused falsely of causing feeding difficulties in the neonate. Since it is recognized that limited tongue protrusion is needed for the activities of the normal newborn, intervention is seldom indicated. The short frenulum will lengthen in the course of normal development, thus increasing tongue mobility.[21]

The neonate is known to have a discriminating sense of *taste,* demonstrating differing responses to sugar, salt, quinine water, and citric acid solutions. There is increased sucking in response to sweets and decreased sucking in response to other tastes.[22] The tongue of the neonate is not controlled well enough to propel food from the lips to the pharynx; therefore, food must be delivered to the back of the tongue before swallowing is possible.[23]

The neonate is equipped with deposits of fatty tissue, called *sucking pads,* in each cheek. These assist the sucking and feeding process by preventing the pulling in of the cheeks during the sucking process. Even in the presence of malnutrition, these sucking pads remain intact until sucking ceases to constitute a major portion of the infant's way of getting nutrition.

Approximately 80 percent of neonates have small inclusion cysts visible at the junction of the hard and soft palates. These are called *Epstein's pearls* and are of no significance. It is estimated that 1:5000 to 1:10,000 neonates are born with, or experience the eruption of, *teeth.* These are commonly termed *natal teeth,* and if their roots are inadequate, they should be pulled to prevent their being aspirated or ingested.[24]

The eyes The neonate's eyes appear slightly large when compared with the rest of the body. The eyeballs should be equal in size. The irises of all neonates are blue, blue-gray, or blue-brown. Pigmentation of the iris, which will determine permanent eye color, may begin to be evident at 3 months of age but is not complete until 6 to 12 months of age. The sclerae of the neonate appear to be slightly bluish gray because they are thin. Any yellow tinge in the sclerae is indicative of jaundice and warrants further investigation.

Most neonates exhibit *pseudostrabismus,* commonly known as *cross-eye,* because they seldom make attempts at visual accommodation. A wide, flattened bridge of the nose in some newborns also contributes to the cross-eyed appearance. This is a normal finding and requires no intervention.

Subconjunctival hemorrhage A bright red, crescent-shaped band located on the eyeball near the iris may be evident at birth. This is due to pressure on the neonate's face during delivery. This subconjunctival hemorrhage is of no long-term significance and disappears during the first few weeks of life.

Ophthalmia neonatorum Many infants exhibit ophthalmia neonatorum, or an acute conjunctivitis of varied etiology. A *chemical conjunctivitis* secondary to prophylactic treatment with silver nitrate is frequently seen. This condition manifests itself by profuse edema and redness of the eyelids, frequently accompanied by copious amounts of purulent drainage. This inflammation may appear 2 to 4 h after the instillation of silver nitrate and should subside without sequelae by the fifth or sixth day of life. Perhaps the most significant problems posed by chemical conjunctivitis are that it interferes with parent-infant eye contact, and thus bonding, and that it makes the eye itself inaccessible to examination during this period.

In the past, the term *ophthalmia neonatorum* usually denoted an eye infection secondary to a gonorrheal infection. In spite of preventive measures, ophthalmia neonatorum caused by *Neisseria gonorrhoeae* continues to be seen. Gonorrheal conjunctivitis usually appears on the second or third day of life. Untreated, this condition progresses rapidly with symptoms similar to those of chemical conjunctivitis and with a constant discharge of *green* purulent material. Without proper treatment, ocular involvement progresses to blindness.

Fortunately, since the advent of widespread prophylaxis against this organism, most neonatal conjunctivitis is caused by a variety of other organisms. Once identified, these may be treated appropriately.

Eye reflexes Three reflexes are noted when the eye is examined. The first is the *blinking,* or corneal, reflex, in which the infant blinks at the sudden appearance of a bright light or object. This is a protective reflex and should continue throughout life. The second is the *pupillary response,* in which the pupil of the infant constricts when a bright light is shone toward it. This also persists throughout life. The *doll's eye reflex* is seen only early in life. It is demonstrated by moving the infant slowly to the right, to the left, or vertically. The neonate's eyes remain in a fixed position. This reflex disappears as fixation develops.

The ears

The ears of the full-term neonate should be of normal shape, with some palpable cartilage on examination. Preauricular skin tags are not uncommon. Placement of the ears is of utmost significance. Low-set and malformed ears are associated with kidney or chromosomal abnormalities.[25] The pinna of the ear should arise from a point above the level of the inner canthus of the eye (Fig. 8-7*A* and *B*). Neonates have a well-developed sense of hearing and are able to discriminate between high- and low-pitched voices.

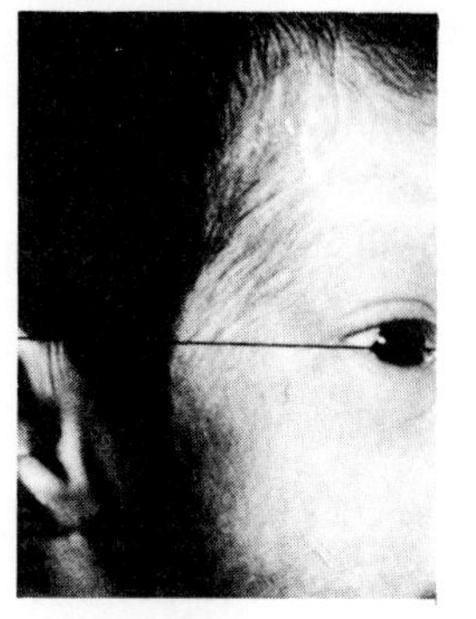

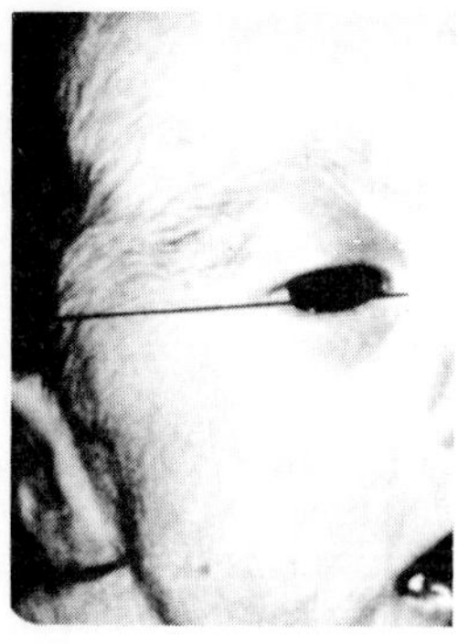

A B

Figure 8-7 Position of the ears. (*A*) The normal position. (*B*) True low-set ears. In the normal infant the insertion of the ear falls on the extension of a line drawn across the inner and outer canthus of the eye. (*Courtesy of Meade Johnson Company.*)

The skin

Color The skin color of a neonate is an important indicator of overall status. The skin often looks slightly bluish red because of the visibility of the capillary bed through the thin epidermis. Central cyanosis, evidenced by blueness of the mucous membranes, and/or circumoral cyanosis is indicative of inadequate general oxygenation. *Acrocyanosis,* or cyanosis localized in the hands and feet (and occasionally also in the nose), is a normal finding which usually disappears during the first few days of life. Pallor of the skin, mucous membranes, and nail beds is indicative of shock and necessitates further assessment and intervention. *Cutis marmorata,* or mottling, is seen most often in preterm babies, but also in some full-term babies, as a response to chilling. It is due to immaturity of the neonate's vasoconstrictive ability and disappears with increasing maturity.

Jaundice, or yellowness of the skin, is frequently seen during the first week of life. The normal finding, termed *physiological jaundice,* is due to two major factors: (1) There is an increased rate of red blood cell breakdown during the first week of life because of the increased number and shortened life span of fetal red blood cells, resulting in increased amounts of bilirubin to metabolize, and (2) the immature neonate liver has a limited capacity to conjugate bilirubin. These two factors combine to result in serum bilirubin levels above the normal value (0.2 to 1.4 mg per 100 ml) in nearly all full-term infants. Only about 50 percent of all neonates demonstrate observable jaundice. It is interesting to note that bilirubin levels must exceed 5 mg per 100 ml of serum before jaundice is observable in the skin or sclera. In full-term neonates, physiological jaundice appears *after* the first 24 h of life and usually peaks by the second or third day. At this time, the bilirubin level averages 6 mg per 100 ml and then rapidly declines to normal levels by the seventh to the tenth day of life. See Chap. 17 for a discussion of pathological jaundice and phototherapy.

Common variations The skin of the neonate manifests several variations specific to this age. *Vernix caseosa,* a non-water-soluble white cheesy substance, is formed on the fetus during the fifth lunar month. It is present to some degree on the skin of most neonates to protect their skin from the amniotic fluid. It is seen in abundance in premature infants, but may be noticeable primarily in skin creases in full-term infants. *Lanugo,* a fine downy hair which forms during the fourth lunar month of gestation and starts to disappear during the eighth month, may still be present to some degree in the full-term infant. *Milia* are tiny white epidermal inclusion cysts (plugged sebaceous glands) which appear mainly on the face, primarily on the nose and chin. They are a normal finding, require no treatment, and usually disappear within a few weeks.

Erythema toxicum, or the typical newborn rash, affects many full-term neonates. The rash usually develops during the first or second day of life and disappears spontaneously by the end of the first week of life. It appears on all parts of the body as small papules surrounded by areas of redness and resembles insect bites.

Desquamation, or the flaking off of skin, is normally seen in the neonate. This usually begins on the second or third day of life and continues through the second or third week. During this period, the skin may appear to be dry, and there may be fissures in the skin folds of the ankles and wrists. This is a normal, transient occurrence. Excessive desquamation may be indicative of postmaturity. *Harlequin color change,* not to be confused with a different disorder called *harlequin fetus,* is sometimes seen in neonates, especially during the first 4 days of life. It is characterized by blushing of one-half of the body, with simultaneous blanching of the other side. It is assumed to be related to the immaturity of the neurovascular control of the neonate, is of no physiological significance, and in most cases disappears by the third week of life.[26]

Skin trauma It is not uncommon for the newly born infant to have evidence of trauma secondary to labor and delivery. General *abrasions,* and those associated with the application of obstetrical forceps, usually heal without incident. *Ecchymoses,* appearing as black and blue areas, may be associated with trauma during the delivery process. *Petechiae,* or minute subcutaneous hemorrhages, are frequently noted after delivery, particularly in the head and trunk areas. They are due to rupture of capillaries too fragile to withstand the pressure exerted by the labor and delivery process. Ecchymoses and petechiae secondary to birth trauma usually disappear by the second day of life; persistence is worthy of investigation for pathological etiology.

Birthmarks The neonate frequently has a variety of "birthmarks." Perhaps the most common of these are telangiectatic nevi, more commonly known as *nevus flammeus*. These are typically flat and pale red and are found most often over the eyelids, between the eyes, and at the base of the skull. Because of the location at the base of the skull, these lesions have come to be referred to as "stork's-beak marks" or "stork bites." These are a normal finding and tend to fade with age. However, nevi on other areas, such as the cheeks, do not fade, but develop a purplish coloration. This gives them the common name "port-wine stains." These frequently cause cosmetic difficulties later in life.

Strawberry hemangiomas may be present at birth or may develop during the neonatal period. These small red lesions grow outwardly and become raised, acquiring a strawberry-like texture—hence the name. Most of these lesions disappear spontaneously during childhood. *Cavernous hemangiomas,* benign vascular tumors, can cause difficulty because they sometimes impinge on specific structures; if this is the case, intervention is indicated. However, the vast majority of these also remit spontaneously.[27]

Mongolian spots are deep brown to greenish or blue-black pigmented areas of varying shape and size. They are located most often over the lumbosacral area and/or the legs and are found most often in infants of Asian, African, or Mediterranean descent. These lesions are a normal finding and bear absolutely no relationship to Down syndrome, formerly referred to as *mongolism*. They fade or disappear by early childhood, although some remain as slate-gray discolorations.

The neurological system: major reflexes

The infant is born with a repertoire of basic reflexes that are important to note as evidence of normal development. Their presence or absence, time of appearance and disappearance, and character yield valuable information regarding the general neurological status of the newborn.

The Moro reflex The Moro reflex is an important indicator of neurological status, since it requires activity of both the central and peripheral nervous systems. It is best elicited, with the infant in the supine position, either by lifting the head approximately 2 in and releasing it abruptly or by pulling the infant up slightly with both hands and then releasing them. The baby first stiffens and then throws both arms out and brings them forward, as though he or she were embracing something. It is usually noted that the infant extends the third, fourth, and fifth fingers of each hand and frequently will end the response with crying (Fig. 8-8). The Moro response should be present in all full-term infants and will gradually diminish and disappear by 3 to 4 months of age. Retention of this response after that age is an abnormal finding.

The asymmetrical tonic neck reflex In the asymmetrical tonic neck reflex (ATNR), often referred to as the "fencer's position," the turning of the baby's head to one side will result in partial or complete extension of the arm and leg on the side to which the head is turned and in flexion of the opposite leg. The infant normally is able to break this posture after a few seconds; any infant who sustains this position for prolonged periods is demonstrating an abnormal response. This developmental reflex should disappear by 2 to 3 months of age (Fig. 8-9).

The grasp reflex The neonate has grasp reflexes present in both the hands and the feet. In the *palmar grasp reflex*, the fingers will flex around anything placed in the palm of the hand. This should diminish by 3 months of age and be replaced later by voluntary action. The *plantar grasp reflex* is elicited by pressing something against the balls of the feet, which will cause the toes to curl around the object. The plantar grasp lessens by 8 to 10 months of age.

Feeding reflexes Basic reflexes aid the infant in the feeding process. The baby seeks food by use of the *rooting reflex*, which is elicited whenever the cheek is touched by the mother's breast, a hand, or any other object. The baby will respond to this stimulus by turning the face toward the stimulus and opening the mouth in the anticipation of food. The *sucking, swallowing, coughing*, and *sneezing* reflexes should be adequately developed to allow safe and effective feeding.

Placing, stepping, and crawling reflexes Responses that occur when the baby is in the upright position include *placing* and *stepping*. When the infant is held so that the top of the foot lightly touches the edge of a surface, the foot will normally lift onto the surface. This is placing. Likewise, when the infant is lowered so that the soles of the feet lightly touch the surface of a table or bench, the infant's legs exhibit an alternating stepping motion (Fig. 8-10). These two reflexes normally disappear by 4 weeks of age. Full-term babies will make *crawling* movements when placed on the abdomen. This should disappear at 6 months of age.

The Babinski reflex This reflex should be present and is elicited by lightly stroking the sole of the foot from heel to toe. This should result in dorsiflexion, or extension, of the great toe and spreading of the smaller ones. Persistence of this reflex beyond 1 year of age indicates a pyramidal tract lesion.

The gastrointestinal tract

The mouth and its characteristics, senses, and reflexes have been discussed earlier in this chapter. General characteristics of the gastrointestinal tract of the neonate include the following:

1. The intestinal tract of the neonate is relatively longer than that of an older child or an adult.
2. The musculature of the intestinal tract, including the sphincters, is underdeveloped.

Figure 8-8 The Moro reflex. (*A*) The infant is at rest prior to testing for the Moro reflex. (*B*) The first stage in the Moro response. Note the abduction of the arms and fanning of the fingers. (C) The second stage in the Moro response. (*From Joy P. Clausen et al., Maternity Nursing Today, 2d ed., McGraw-Hill, New York, 1977. Used with permission.*)

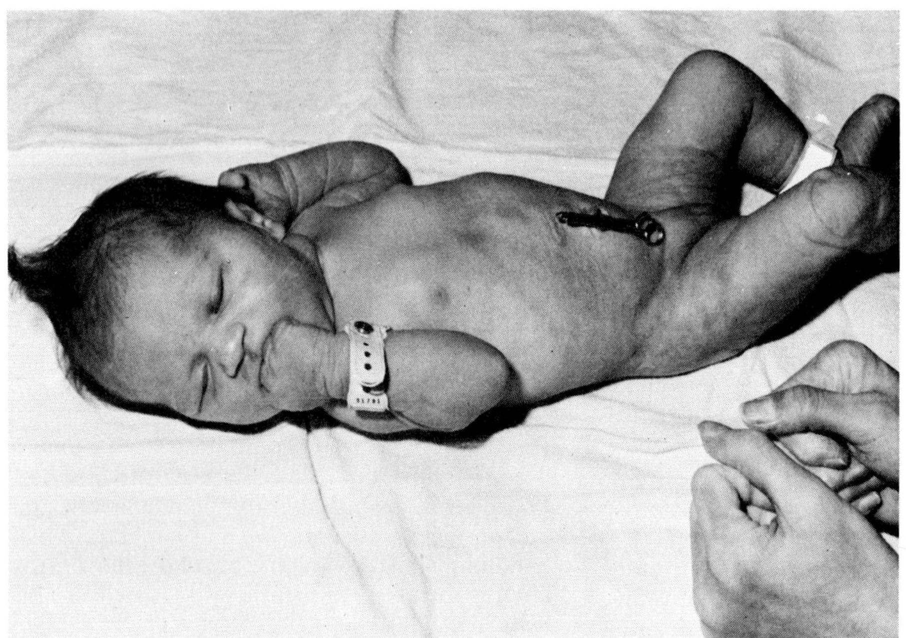

A

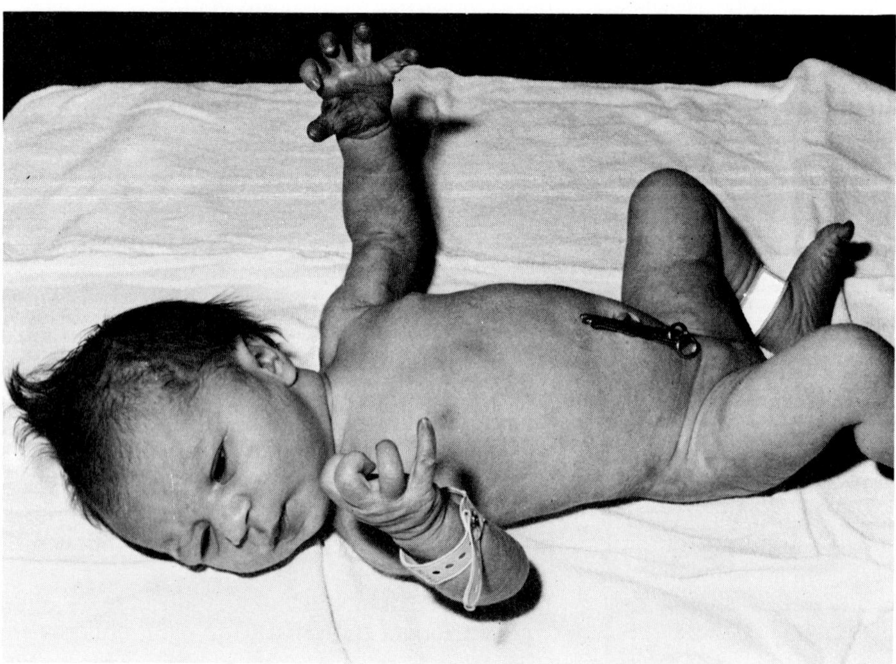

B

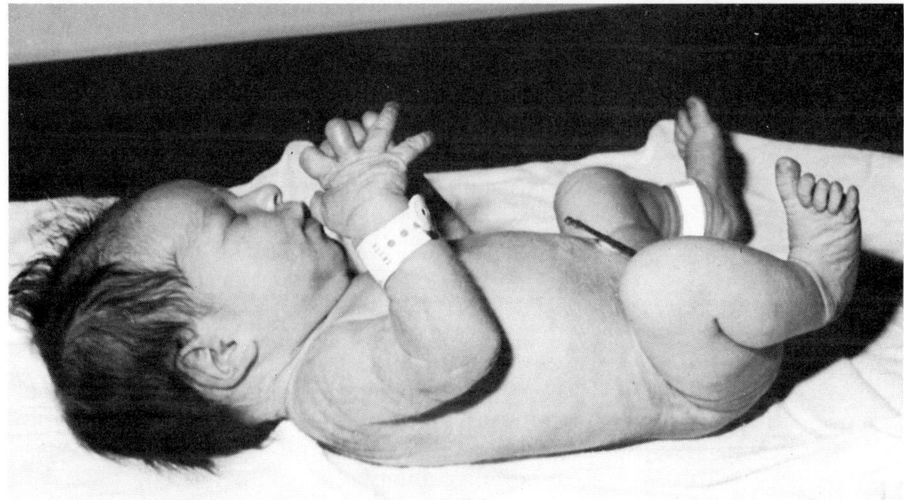

C

3. There is a deficiency of elastic fibers.
4. The digestive and absorptive surfaces of the intestine are almost completely developed.

The stomach The stomach capacity of the full-term neonate is approximately 90 ml at birth and reaches approximately 150 ml by the end of the first month of life. The infant normally swallows a considerable amount of air when eating and especially when crying. Peristaltic movements occur less frequently in the neonatal period than later in life, but reverse peristalsis is common. This, coupled with an immature and relaxed cardiac sphincter, frequently results in regurgitation. Regurgitation is the backflow of a small amount of milk from the stomach. It is spitting up, not vomiting.

Stomach emptying and intestinal transit times during the neonatal period differ from those found in the older child. The first part of the meal reaches the pylorus 1 to 2 min after ingestion (when the infant is lying on his or her right side).

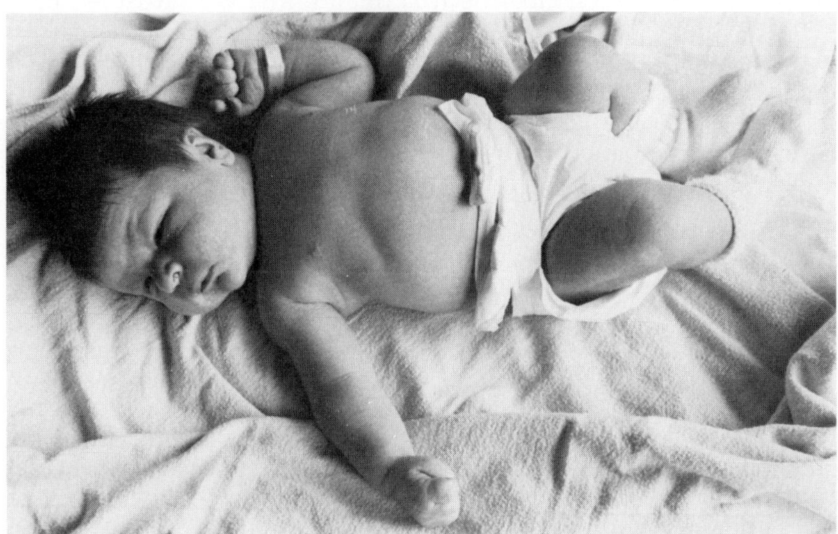

Figure 8-9 The asymmetrical tonic neck reflex (ATNR), or "fencing position." *(From M. Tudor, Child Development, McGraw-Hill, New York, 1981, p. 338. Used with permission.)*

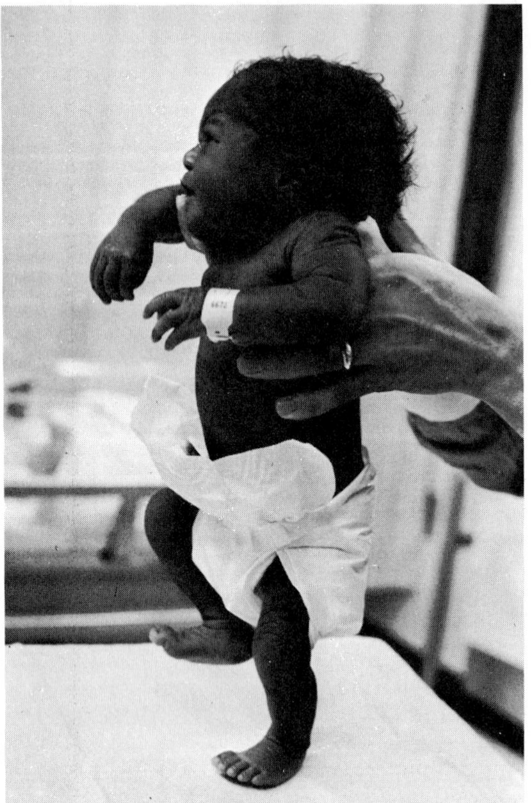

Figure 8-10 The stepping reflex. (*From Elizabeth J. Dickason and Martha D. Schult, Maternal and Infant Care, 2d ed., McGraw-Hill, New York, 1979. Used with permission.*)

The stomach *empties* more slowly during the neonatal period than at any other time of life. Although the major portion of the meal leaves the stomach in 3 to 4 h, a considerable amount may remain for up to 8 h. Human milk passes through the stomach more rapidly than cow's milk. Stomach contractions due to hunger have been detected 2 to 4 h after eating, frequently before the stomach has emptied. These waves do not necessarily mean that the infant needs more food and are not regularly a cause for crying or waking.

The intestines Food enters the cecum approximately 3 to 6 h after reaching the stomach, and the first part of the meal appears in the stool in a little over 8 h from the time ingested. The normal full-term neonate appears to possess the conditions and enzymes necessary for the digestion of nutrients commonly fed during this period. However, there is a deficiency in pancreatic amylase, which impairs the utilization of complex carbohydrates, and of pancreatic lipase, which limits the absorption of fats.

The stools undergo major changes during the neonatal period. The first stools are *meconium*. Meconium begins to appear in the fetal intestine toward the end of the fourth month of gestation. Meconium is a black, odorless, sticky substance. It contains vernix caseosa and lanugo (which have been swallowed in the amniotic fluid), digestive secretions, desquamated epithelium, mucus, and bile pigments. Passage of the first meconium stool is frequently preceded by a meconium "plug," which is usually grayish white in color and 3 to 5 cm long and has the consistency of rubber. Meconium may be passed in utero, in response to hypoxia, or as a result of a breech presentation. Some meconium should be passed during the first 24 h of neonatal life. If this does not occur, concern regarding the possibility of intestinal obstruction arises.

The character of the stools changes rapidly during the first week of life. During the first day of life, meconium stools will vary from black to blackish green in color. From the second through the fourth days, stools contain some mucus and are greenish brown, brownish yellow, or greenish yellow. These are appropriately called *transitional* stools.

From about the fifth day on, the characteristics of the stools will depend largely on what the infant is fed. Infants who are breast-fed have soft, yellow stools which change to a pasty golden yellow and have a characteristic sour odor. The stools of infants who are fed cow's milk formula are somewhat drier and more formed, are paler in color, and have a foul odor.

The liver The neonatal liver has a decreased or limited capacity to conjugate bilirubin. Unfortunately, this enzymatic deficiency occurs at a time when the increased red blood cell breakdown and resulting increased serum bilirubin levels place high demands on the system. This limited ability to conjugate bilirubin results in physiological jaundice.

The neonatal liver also has a decreased ability to form plasma proteins. The subsequent decreased plasma protein concentration may contribute to the generalized edema seen in the neonate. Another very important hepatic deficiency is that of adequate gluconeogenesis, frequently resulting in low blood sugars. For this reason, early feedings are advisable.

During this period the liver is unable to form adequate amounts of prothrombin and other substances necessary for adequate blood coagulation. As has been discussed earlier in this chapter, the newborn lacks vitamin K, which is necessary for the clotting process, and therefore is given a supplement of this vitamin shortly after birth.

The chest and abdomen

At birth the infant's chest circumference is 1 or 2 cm less than the head circumference. The normal chest is approximately cylindrical and symmetrical. Breath sounds should be equal on both sides, as should the chest wall movements that occur with respiration. Neonates are "abdominal breathers"; that is, the abdomen rises and falls more noticeably than the chest expands and contracts with each breath.

As a result of the influence of maternal hormones, the breasts of babies of both sexes may be enlarged. A milky fluid called "witch's milk" may be secreted from the swollen breasts. Engorgement and secretion diminish rapidly after the first week of life and should disappear by 1 month of age.

The abdomen of the neonate is normally cylindrical in shape. Bowel sounds should be audible within a few hours after birth. If meconium is not passed during the first 24 h, the anus should be examined for patency.

An *umbilical hernia,* or skin-covered protrusion at the umbilicus, is not an unusual finding, especially in black children and premature infants. It results from weak abdominal muscles, normally requires no intervention, and usually disappears early in childhood. An umbilical hernia cannot be corrected by applying a bellyband or taping a coin over the umbilicus, which are common practices among some cultural groups.

The *liver* is palpable 2 to 3 cm below the right costal margin. The tip of the *spleen* is normally felt in the lateral portion of the left upper quadrant. Deep palpation is necessary to locate the *kidneys,* which are felt as small oval structures between the examiner's thumb and index finger. The lower pole of each kidney shoud be 1 to 2 cm above the level of the umbilicus; if felt below this level, the kidneys may be enlarged, warranting further investigation.

The genitourinary system

The kidneys The kidneys of the full-term neonate are anatomically well developed and capable of basic and essential excretory functions. The neonate's kidneys are functionally immature. They are limited in their ability to excrete some metabolites, in their buffering capacity, and in their ability to control sodium excretion. The newborn's kidneys are unable to conserve water in response to dehydration.

The neonate has an average of 6 ml of urine in the bladder at birth. Studies have shown that as many as 17 percent first void in the delivery room. Approximately 90 percent void in the first 24 h of life.[28] Average urine output increases from 20 ml during the first days of life to 227 ml on the seventh day. The neonate voids two to six times per 24 h during the first few days of life; voidings then increase to 10 to 20 per day.

The urine of the neonate has very little odor and is normally clear. There is an increased excretion of uric acid, which may crystallize and be seen as red spots on the diaper. These spots are frequently mistaken for blood. Concentration of urine *may* be slightly elevated during the first 2 to 3 days of life—a condition secondary to low fluid intake. After the baby is about 3 days old, urine normally has a low specific gravity, rarely reaching 1.025. Infants who are breast-fed have urine with an unusually low specific gravity, averaging 1.008 after the third day of life. Protein is normally present in small amounts (under 10 mg per 100 ml). Excessive proteinuria may occur in pathological situations, such as neonatal asphyxia, and warrants further investigation.[29]

The male genitalia The *scrotum* of the full-term male infant frequently appears unusually large and may contain some fluid at birth. This fluid disappears during the first few days of life. The *testes* have descended into the scrotal sac in approximately 96 percent of full-term male infants. They are approximately 1 cm in diameter and should be easily palpable. The testes of most neonates who have undescended testicles, or *cryptorchidism,* will descend spontaneously during the first year of life.

The urinary meatus is normally at the tip of the penis. The foreskin covers the glans penis completely and is usually seen extending somewhat beyond the tip and narrowing to leave a small opening. During the neonatal period the foreskin is relatively inelastic and adherent to the glans. It cannot be retracted without trauma until about 3 years of age. In *phimosis,* the foreskin is so tightly fitted over the glans of the penis that it cannot be retracted. This is a normal finding in the neonate and becomes abnormal only if present after 3 years of age.

Circumcision of the male infant Circumcision, or the surgical removal of the foreskin, continues to be widely practiced in this culture. There are three basic methods for performing a circumcision. The first, and simplest, is the "dorsal-slit method," in which a small incision is made in the foreskin to allow complete retraction without the actual removal of the foreskin. The second is the clamp method (Fig. 8-11). In this method the glans and prepuce (foreskin) are separated, the glans is covered, and the prepuce is amputated by cutting. The third method involves the use of the *Plastibell* (Fig. 8-12). In this method, a small plastic bell is placed over the glans, and the prepuce is draped over it. A suture is then tied tightly around the prepuce and bell. This is left in place, and the foreskin drops off in 1 to 2 weeks; thus no cutting is required.

Circumcision is performed on the eighth day of life, as a religious rite, by Orthodox Jews. On other babies it is usually done on the day before discharge from the newborn nursery; if the procedure is contraindicated at that time, it may be done later on an outpatient basis.

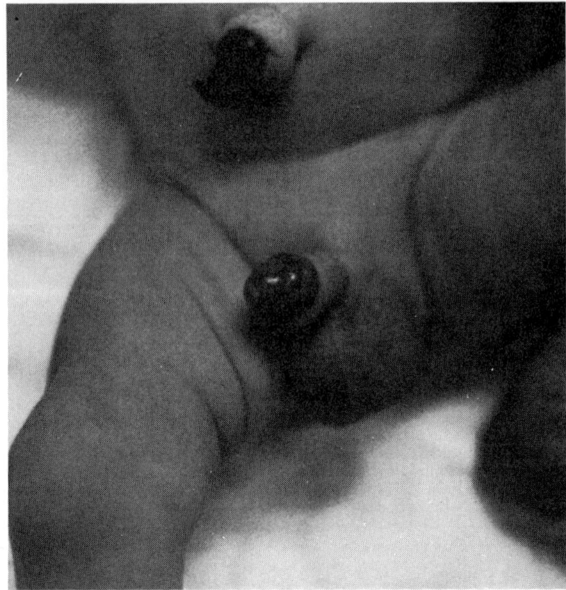

Figure 8-11 The penis of an infant after circumcision with a Gomco clamp. (*From G. Scipien, Comprehensive Pediatric Nursing, 2d ed., McGraw-Hill, New York, 1979. Used with permission.*)

Although few would argue the relevance of circumcision when performed as a religious ritual, the medical value of the procedure is very controversial. Proponents of circumcision argue that it promotes the following: (1) the prevention

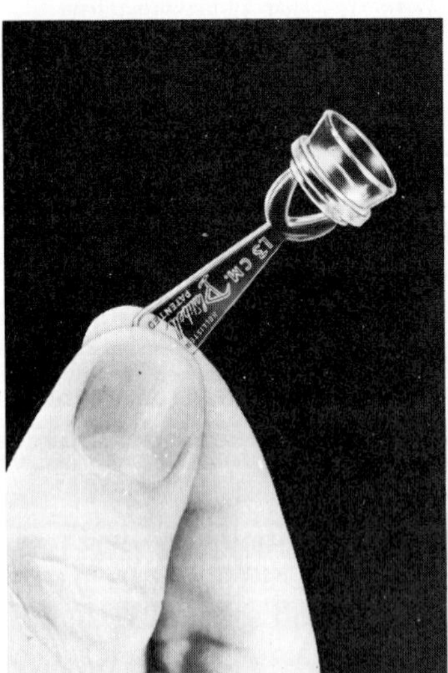

A

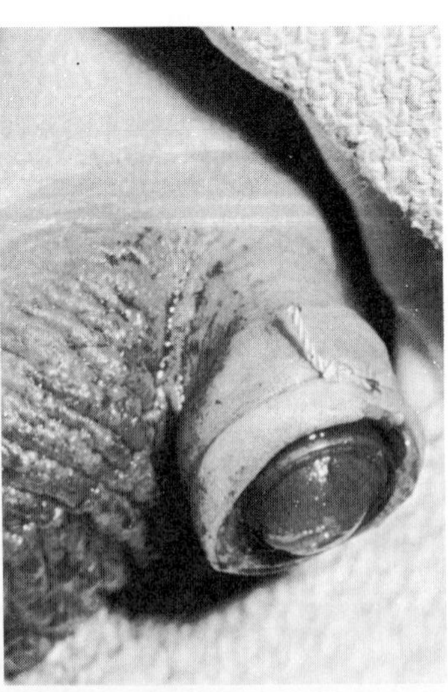

B

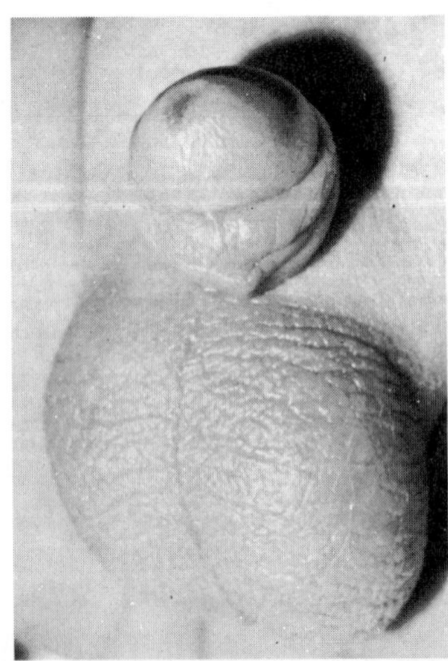

C

Figure 8-12 Circumcision. (*A*) The Hollister Plastibell. (*B*) The suture around the rim of plastic controls bleeding. (C) The plastic rim and suture drop off in 7 to 10 days. (*Courtesy of Hollister, Inc. From Elizabeth J. Dickason and Martha D. Schult, Maternal and Infant Care, 2d ed., McGraw-Hill, New York, 1979. Used with permission.*)

of permanent phimosis; (2) greater cleanliness because it eliminates a blind pouch in which smegma, a cheeselike substance, can collect, with ensuing infection; (3) avoidance of the potential trauma of pulling or tearing a nonretractable foreskin during sexual intercourse; and (4) a possible reduction in the risk of cancer of the penis in men and uterine cancer in their mates.

Opponents of circumcision as a routine procedure cite the following reasons for their disapproval: (1) hemorrhage secondary to the procedure; (2) infection at the circumcision site, which may escalate to generalized sepsis; (3) the fact that removal of the prepuce leaves the glans exposed and liable to injury or ulceration, frequently leading to meatal stenosis; (4) reports of complications, including gangrene, with use of the Plastibell; (5) mild distortion of the penis secondary to scarring, which may lead to physical and psychological trauma; and (6) the fact that constant exposure of the glans to air may cause it to lose some tactile sensation, decreasing pleasure during intercourse.[30]

Although the pros and cons regarding circumcision continue to be argued vehemently by those concerned, perhaps the most important considerations regarding circumcision concern its relationship to cancer. Attempts have been made to demonstrate a decreased cancer rate both in circumcised males and in their sexual partners, but the results of such studies continue to be controversial.

The female external genitalia The labia and clitoris of the female neonate are unusually edematous because of maternal hormonal influences. The labia minora are more fully developed than the labia majora, and because of this the latter seem to be somewhat separated when compared with those of the older child. Vernix caseosa is found between the labia of the newly born infant.

The urinary meatus is frequently difficult to see. The vaginal opening is seen without difficulty. From it there frequently is the protrusion of a hymenal tag. The female infant usually has a mucous discharge from the vagina, sometimes blood-tinged, during the first week of life. This is also due to the influence of maternal hormones and is called *pseudomenstruation*.

The cardiovascular system

The transition from fetal to neonatal circulation has been discussed earlier in this chapter. Once this transition has been adequately accomplished, the circulatory pattern of the neonate is like that of the older child and adult.

The heart The neonatal heart is proportionately larger than that of the older child and therefore occupies proportionately more space within the thoracic cavity. Because the heart assumes a more lateral position at this age, the maximum impulse is heard at the third to fourth intercostal space, lateral to the midclavicular line.

The apical pulse rate changes markedly in the neonatal period. At birth, or shortly thereafter, it may reach as high as 180 beats per minute, typical of the first period of reactivity. As the neonate progresses through the period of transition, the rate will vary. By the second day of life the rate should have stabilized, and it is most often heard in the range of 120 to 140 beats per minute. However, it may range from 100 to 160 beats per minute, depending on activity. Soft systolic murmurs are often heard, caused by incomplete closure of the fetal shunts. These usually are of no significance and disappear by the end of the first month of life.

Hematologic values The blood volume of full-term infants varies from an average of 99 ml/kg for those infants who have received a placental transfusion to 86 ml/kg for those who have not. *Placental transfusion* refers to the baby's receipt of 50 to 100 ml of blood from the placenta, which occurs if the umbilical cord is allowed to stop pulsating before it is clamped. Obstetrical practice in this regard varies. The corresponding hematocrit values are an average of 59 percent for the transfused group and 46 percent for the others.[31] The white blood cell count varies from a value of 9000 to 30,000 per cubic millimeter at birth, rising to 13,000 to 38,000 per cubic millimeter at 12 h of age and then declining to 5000 to 20,000 per cubic millimeter by 14 days of age.[32]

Respirations

Initiation of respirations was discussed earlier in this chapter. The normal respirations of the neonate are usually between 30 and 60 per minute, are irregular, and are more abdominal than thoracic. Neonates experience both apnea and periodic breathing.

A 1977 study revealed that *apnea* (cessation of breathing exceeding 6 s) is a normal phenomenon in the normal full-term infant. The study found that the incidence of apnea is highest during the newborn period, when some periods of apnea exceed 15 s. Periodic breathing, or the cessation of breathing for periods shorter than 6 s and occurring twice within a 24-s period, is common throughout the first 6 months of life.[33] More detailed information regarding evaluation of respiratory status is given in Chap. 17.

The musculoskeletal system

The skeletal frame of the neonate is soft because it has relatively low amounts of mineral deposits and contains a large amount of cartilage. These facts, coupled with the increase in mobility of the joints during this period, make the body of the neonate extremely flexible. The neonate's trunk is disproportionately long, the extremities disproportionately short, and the head disproportionately large when compared with the same structures of older infants and children.

The legs normally appear so bowed that the soles of the feet may seem to meet. The spine is normally straight, with no dimples or sinuses.

The normal neonate has good muscle tone and prefers to flex the extremities. This is demonstrated when an extremity is pulled to an extended position. The neonate will attempt to return it to the flexed position.

When being picked up, the baby should have head and back support. When prone, the neonate is able to lift the head momentarily and rotate it from side to side.

Body defenses

At the moment of birth, the neonate passes from an environment that is essentially sterile to one laden with pathogens. The nurse should understand what mechanisms are available to the baby to cope with this changing situation. The skin, traditionally considered the body's first line of defense, provides an effective barrier to pathogens. The reticuloendothelial system, the second line of defense, is capable of mobilizing phagocytes, such as neutrophils and monocytes. However, for reasons not fully understood, its phagocytic action does not reach full strength in the neonate. The inflammatory response, which is so important in dealing with pathogens that succeed in penetrating the skin, depends in large part on the activity of phagocytic cells. Therefore, the inflammatory response is less vigorous in the neonate than in older infants, in children, and in adults.

Immune responses, the third line of the body's defenses, are of mixed value to the neonate. There are two kinds of immune responses: cell-mediated responses and antibody-mediated responses. Cell-mediated responses depend on encounters between pathogens and certain prepared lymphocytes. These encounters can begin only at birth and for a time are unable to set off a fully effective counterattack against pathogens. Thus cell-mediated immune responses are deficient. Cell-mediated responses are ordinarily effective against fungi, cancer cells, parasites, and certain viral infections.

Antibody-mediated immune responses provide mainly protection against such bacteria as pneumococci, streptococci, and staphylococci. Antibodies may provide some initial protection against certain viruses. Antibodies are serum proteins that are better known as immunoglobulins (Ig). Immunoglobulins G (IgG) and M (IgM) are the most important in the neonate. IgG crosses the placenta, and throughout neonatal life the bulk of the infant's IgG is that received from the mother in the fetal period. IgG provides protection against such bacterial toxins as diphtheria and tetanus; viruses that cause such diseases as measles, rubella, and chickenpox; and some gram-positive bacteria, notably staphylococci, streptococci, pneumococci, and *Haemophilus influenzae*. The nurse should recognize that no protection is available for the enteric gram-negative organism *Escherichia coli,* which frequently invades the newborn child.[34]

IgM does not cross the placenta but is made by the fetus beginning in the twentieth week of gestation. IgM is produced in response to such infections as syphilis, toxoplasmosis, rubella, cytomegalic inclusion disease (CID), and herpes simplex. These five diseases are commonly abbreviated as STORCH, and the last four as TORCH, infections. Because the fetus responds to the presence of these pathogens by producing IgM, a cord blood level of IgM greater than 20 mg per 100 ml is probably a sign of intrauterine infection. (The normal cord blood IgM is 11 mg per 100 ml.)[35]

Immunoglobulin A (IgA) does not cross the placenta. It is detectable in the serum by the end of the first month after birth, but normal adult levels are not reached until adolescence.[36] IgA can neutralize some viruses, especially influenza and polio. It is not active against bacteria.

Immunoglobulin E (IgE) does not cross the placenta. It is responsible for allergic skin reactions. Since the neonate's level of IgE is only about one-tenth that of the adult, one can safely assume that skin problems in the neonate are not allergic in nature.

In summary, although the neonate is not without some ability to combat pathogens in his or her new environment, the nurse must take care to offer protection against known pathogens, to recognize the presence of infection immediately, and to take appropriate actions to combat an infection.

HOSPITAL NURSERY CARE OF THE NEWBORN

Admission to the newborn nursery

When the newborn is transferred to the nursery, effective communication between delivery room nurses and nursery nurses is critical. During this time, nursing actions generally revolve around meeting the goals of protection and assessment.

The neonatal nurse first acts to protect the newborn by verifying the infant's identification tags with the delivery room nurse and with the medical record. The record is checked to confirm that prophylactic treatment for *Neisseria gonorrhoeae* has been administered. If vitamin K has not been given in the delivery room, the nursery nurses will administer it as ordered.

The nursery nurse should carry out the assessment of the newborn by proceeding in an orderly and systematic manner.

Obtaining an accurate history The nurse in attendance in the delivery room should report to the nursery nurse, who now assumes responsibility for care of the neonate. From direct knowledge or by notation on the medical records, the nurse provides the following information:

1. A history of genetic conditions in the mother's or father's family.
2. The estimated date of confinement (EDC).
3. The mother's blood group and Rh type and evidence of sensitization and/or immunization (such as the administration of RhoGAM after previous deliveries). This subject is covered in more detail in the discussion of erythroblastosis fetalis in Chap. 17.
4. The results of tests for syphilis (including dates performed).
5. The number, duration, and outcome of previous pregnancies, with dates.
6. Any maternal disease (diabetes, hypertension, preeclampsia, infections, etc.).
7. Smoking or drugs taken during pregnancy, labor, and delivery (with time of administration if during labor and delivery).
8. The results of measurements of fetal maturity and well-being.
9. The duration of ruptured membranes and of labor.
10. The method of delivery, including indications for operative or instrumental intervention.
11. Any complications during labor and delivery.
12. A description of the placenta, including the number of umbilical vessels.
13. The estimated amount and a description of amniotic fluid.
14. The Apgar scores at 1 and 5 min, the age at which respirations became spontaneous and sustained, and a description of any resuscitative measures employed.
15. The results of any screening tests done, with a description of any observed anomalies.
16. A summary of parental involvement during labor and delivery, with nursing observations about bonding behavior. Nursing observations of parental responses have long-range implications for bonding and for the establishment of positive parenting patterns. This information allows the nurse to deliver comprehensive psychological care to the new family. On the basis of observations, the nurse can give anticipatory guidance.

Initial physical assessment of the newborn If the infant appears stable on admission to the nursery, assessment is begun by obtaining an accurate weight and checking vital signs.

The nurse then briefly examines the infant for congenital anomalies and assesses the general physical status of the infant. The nurse takes the infant's temperature, wraps the infant in a warmed blanket, and places him or her in a side-lying position in clear view of the nursery nurse. If the temperature is below 35.5°C (96°F) on admission to the nursery or fails to rise and stabilize with wrapping, warming lights or an incubator may be indicated. Many institutions routinely lower the head of the bassinet to facilitate drainage of mucus.

If the infant appears to be stable at this point, it is wise to provide a time for rest and recovery from the birth process before continuing to meet the goals of assessment, protection, nurturance, and stimulation.

Assessment

A basic understanding of the characteristics of the normal newborn, as discussed earlier in this chapter, is essential background knowledge which enables the nurse to systematically assess the neonate. Assessment began with interpretation of data regarding the history of the family, pregnancy, labor and delivery, fetal status, and status of the newborn in the delivery room. This information was obtained on admission of the infant to the nursery and was augmented by the brief physical inspection done by the nursery nurse. Comprehensive, ongoing assessment of the newborn is the responsibility of the neonatal nurse.

Physical assessment A detailed and systematic physical examination of the newborn should be carried out by the nurse or physician. A neonatal assessment is done for the following purposes:

1. To determine whether the infant has made a successful transition from intrauterine life to being an air-breather
2. To determine whether congenital anomalies are present
3. To collect baseline data against which future findings may be assessed
4. To learn things about the baby's unique qualities that can be used in providing the parents with appropriate anticipatory guidance in the care of their newborn

Guidelines for assessing newborns There are some basic guidelines to consider when undertaking a physical assessment of a newborn. Chilling must be avoided. It is wise to take the infant's temperature prior to the examination, and to defer the procedure if the temperature is below 36.1°C (97°F). The examination should be done in an environment which will minimize heat loss.

The assessment should proceed in an orderly cephalocaudal (head-to-toe) progression. However, it is advisable to begin the examination by listening to the heart, lungs, and abdomen. Undressing and manipulating the infant may lead to crying, making these important observations impossible or inadequate. The nurse must use the techniques of inspection, palpation, percussion, and auscultation to obtain data. The guidelines for physical assessment of the neonate (Table 8-2), used in conjunction with the previous section "Normal Physical Characteristics of the Newborn," will provide the nurse with direction in this phase of assessment of newborns.

Vital signs Regular measurement of the neonate's vital signs will provide valuable information regarding physical status. Because these measurements may fluctuate markedly with activity, the nurse increases the accuracy of their interpretation if the activity, or behavioral state, of the infant is recorded at the time the measurement is made. Behavioral states (deep sleep, active sleep, and so forth) are explained below.

Temperature Axillary temperatures are safest and hence preferable. The use of a rectal thermometer involves risk; inserting it more than 2 to 3 cm into the rectum can cause severe damage, not the least of which is perforation of the bowel. However, many institutions routinely take the *initial* temperature rectally to rule out imperforate anus. If the nurse does this, great care must be exercised. Since studies have indicated that there is a high correlation between axillary and rectal temperatures, taking axillary temperatures is recommended for newborns.[37] At delivery the newborn has an average rectal temperature of 37 to 37.8°C (98.6 to 100°F), and a decrease of 1 to 3°F is not unusual before the infant leaves the delivery room, despite the use of measures to minimize loss of body heat.[38] The infant's temperature should be monitored hourly for the first 2 h following transfer to the newborn nursery and then at least every 8 h. Once stabilized, the usual axillary temperature for the normal full-term infant ranges from 36 to 37°C (96.8 to 98.6°F), and the corresponding rectal temperature is 0.4 to 0.5°C (1°F) higher than the axillary temperature.[39] It is important for the nurse to realize that thermoregulation in the neonate is a complex process and that optimal body temperature may vary with each infant.

Heart rate The neonatal heart rate varies greatly with activity within a range of 100 to 140 beats per minute. Some authorities cite acceptable ranges as low as 90 during deep sleep and as high as 180 when the infant is active.[40] The usual range is between 120 and 140 beats per minute. When obtaining the apical pulse, it is

Table 8-2 Newborn Assessment Guide

Manifestation and Normal Findings	Minor Abnormalities and Common Variations	Major Abnormalities and Signs of Potential Problems
Measurements		
Length—45 to 55 cm (18 to 22 in) Weight—2500 to 4600 g (5½ to 10 lb) Head circumference—33 to 37 cm (13 to 15 in)* Chest circumference—30 to 33 cm (12 to 13 in)	Neonate normally loses 10% of birth weight by 3 to 4 days; regains it by 10 days	Head circumference more than 4 cm greater than chest (may indicate hydrocephaly) Head circumference less than chest (may indicate microcephaly)
Position and Movement		
Assumes "fetal position"; head is flexed, and extremities rest on chest and abdomen Size and movement of body parts should be symmetrical	Frank breech—abducted, externally rotated thighs; extended legs and neck	Hypotonia (limpness); extension of extremities
Skin		
Is pink in color Epidermis is red, soft, smooth, and delicate at birth; by third or fourth day becomes dry, flakes, or peels Vernix caseosa is present Lanugo is present Skin turgor is good	Jaundice after first 24 h Acrocyanosis Milia Erythema toxicum (newborn rash) Harlequin color change Mongolian spots Cutis marmorata (mottling) Telangiectatic nevi ("stork bites") Petechiae or ecchymoses caused by birth trauma	Jaundice during first 24 h of life Generalized, central cyanosis Excessive vernix caseosa (may indicate preterm) Absence of vernix caseosa (may indicate postterm) Poor skin turgor Persistent and/or generalized petechiae
Cranium		
Anterior fontanel is diamond-shaped (to 5 cm) (2 in) Posterior fontanel is triangular (0.5 to 1 cm) (0.2 to 0.4 in) Fontanels should be flat, soft, and firm	Third sagittal fontanel Caput succedaneum Cephalhematoma	Bulging or depressed fontanels Fused suture lines
Eyes		
Eyes are usually closed—strong blink reflex Lids are frequently edematous Color is usually gray-blue or blue-brown Sclera usually has a bluish tint Fixes on bright object; has ability to follow to midline	Chemical conjunctivitis Subconjunctival hemorrhage Pseudostrabismus	Purulent discharge Congenital cataracts Mongoloid slant Inability to follow
Ears		
Top of ear should be at level of eye Some cartilage should be palpable	Lack of cartilage is indicative of preterm infant	Low-set ears (may indicate chromosome abnormality and/or renal disorder)
Nose		
Both nares are patent Thin, white mucous discharge is present		Nonpatent nares Unusual nasal discharge Nasal flaring
Mouth and Throat		
Palate is intact Salivation is minimal	Inclusion cysts (Epstein's pearls) Natal teeth Thrush	Cleft lip and/or palate Inability to pass nasogastric tube Large, protruding tongue Excessive salivation

Table 8-2 Newborn Assessment Guide (*Continued*)

Manifestation and Normal Findings	Minor Abnormalities and Common Variations	Major Abnormalities and Signs of Potential Problems
Neck		
Full lateral (side-to-side) and anterior-posterior range of motion is possible Neck is short and thick		Excessive skin folds Webbing Restricted movement Hyperextension
Chest		
Ribs should be flexible Xyphoid process is observable	Supernumerary (extra) nipples Breast enlargement Secretion of "witch's milk" from nipples Funnel chest (pectus excavatum)	Marked retraction of chest and intercostal spaces with respirations Asymmetrical chest expansion Redness around nipples Depressed sternum Widely spaced nipples
Lungs		
Bilateral breath sounds are audible Respiratory rate is 40 to 60 breaths per minute Abdominal breathing is present Respirations are irregular	Apnea of 6 to 15 s Periodic breathing Rales shortly after birth	Reduced or asymmetrical breath sounds Apnea exceeding 15 s, dyspnea, tachypnea, grunting
Heart		
Rate is 120 to 140 beats per minute Rhythm is regular Apex is near fourth intercostal space on left, lateral to midclavicular line First and second sounds clearly discernible	Murmurs Rate: 100 to 120 beats per minute Rate: 140 to 180 beats per minute with activity	Apex abnormally placed Obvious enlarged heart Tachycardia Bradycardia
Abdomen		
Is cylindrical with slight protrusion Umbilical stump: at birth, is blue-white and shiny; by 24 h, is yellow-brown, dull, and dry; eventually turns black-brown; shrivels and falls off in 7 to 14 days Liver is palpable 2 to 3 cm below right costal margin Spleen feels like slight mass in lateral aspect of left upper quadrant Kidneys are palpable 1 to 2 cm above the umbilicus Femoral pulses should be palpable and equal	Umbilical hernia Visible peristalsis in thin infants Bladder distention—firm globular mass felt in suprapubic area	Distention Localized bulging at the flanks Red, oozing, and/or malodorous umbilical stump (or area) Any abnormal mass Persistent bladder distention after voiding Absent, diminished, or unequal femoral pulses
Male Genitalia		
Both testes are palpable in scrotum Urethral opening at tip of penis is present Smegma is present Foreskin is adherent to glans; is difficult to retract	Testes palpable in inguinal canal Inability to retract foreskin Hydrocele Small scrotum Inguinal hernia Penile erection	Testes nonpalpable Hypospadias Epispadias
Female Genitalia		
Labia minora are larger than labia majora	Pseudomenses (blood-tinged mucous discharge from vagina)	Fused labia No vaginal opening

Table 8-2 Newborn Assessment Guide (*Continued*)

Manifestation and Normal Findings	Minor Abnormalities and Common Variations	Major Abnormalities and Signs of Potential Problems
Vernix caseosa exists between labia folds		
Labia and clitoris are edematous		
Urinary meatus is difficult to visualize		
Hymenal tag is present		
Anus		
Anal opening is patent		Imperforate anus
Anal opening is normally placed		
Musculoskeletal System		
Spine is intact with no prominent curves, masses, or openings	Pilonidal dimple in coccygeal area	Spina bifida
Has full range of motion, including hips	Simian crease in palm	Pilonidal cyst or sinus
Soles are usually flat	Occasional momentary tremors	Polydactyly (extra digits)
Extremities are symmetrical		Syndactyly (webbing or fusion of digits)
Head sags while sitting but is momentarily able to hold head erect		Dislocated hip—symptoms: 1. Limitation in abduction 2. Audible "click" on abduction 3. Unequal leg length 4. Unequal gluteal or thigh skin folds
Is able to hold head in horizontal line with back when held prone		Hypotonia
Is able to turn head from side to side when prone		Paralysis
Extremities maintain some degree of flexion		Marked head lag
		Tremors, twitches, and myoclonic jerks
Neurological system		
Reflexes are present: blinking, pupillary, sneeze, suck, gag, rooting, extrusion, yawn, cough, grasp, Babinski, Moro, tonic neck, crawling, stepping	Response will vary depending on state	Absent or asymmetrical reflexes
Doll's eye response is present	See text	Constant tongue protrusion

Head circumference should exceed chest circumference by 2 to 3 cm.

important to use the appropriate stethoscope and to count the rate for a full 60 s.

Respiratory rate The rate at which a neonate breathes, like the heart rate, varies with activity. The normal range is 30 to 60 breaths per minute. Because the newborn normally has an extremely irregular breathing pattern, it is especially important to monitor respiration for a full minute.

Blood pressure The blood pressure of the normal full-term newborn ranges from 64 ± 10 mmHg systolic and from 41 ± 8 mmHg diastolic.[41] For an accurate reading, the appropriate-sized cuff (2.5 to 4 cm) must be used. The pressure may be obtained by auscultation, palpation, or the flush method. See Chap. 16 for a discussion of methods of measuring blood pressure. It is the practice of many hospitals to omit routine blood pressure monitoring in the normal, healthy full-term newborn, since standards for normal blood pressure readings of neonates are not well established. In general, treatment for hypotension is required for (1) full-term infants with a systolic blood pressure less than 54 mmHg, (2) large preterm infants with a systolic blood pressure less than 50 mmHg, and (3) infants with a systolic blood pressure less than 40 mmHg.[42]

Laboratory tests Biochemical and other laboratory screening tests are used to supplement data obtained through the history and the physical examination. Which of these tests are routine and which will be done only when specifically indicated vary greatly from institution to institution.

Tests on cord blood The newborn has one thing that he or she will not have during any other period of life: a ready-made blood sample. Blood obtained in the delivery room from the umbilical cord can be used to gather valuable diagnostic data. The baby's blood type and Rh factor are determined from this blood source. The Coombs' test is performed to detect sensitized red blood cells in hemolytic disease of the newborn. A weakly positive Coombs' test is indicative of mildly low levels of antibodies, most likely causing only mild hemolysis, while a strongly positive (3^+ to 4^+) Coombs' test result indicates the presence of high concentrations of antibodies and, most likely, ensuing severe hemolysis. In many hospitals cord blood is tested for the presence of syphilis. Blood cultures are done if infection is suspected. Several other screening and diagnostic tests may be performed if indicated. It is wise for the laboratory to retain a sample of each infant's cord blood until the baby is discharged.

Blood and urine tests Depending on the nursery policy, routine tests of hematocrit and hemoglobin and a urinalysis may be done on all infants. Other services are of the opinion that these tests should only be carried out if the history and physical assessment of the infant yield abnormal or suspicious findings.

Cultures Most nurseries do not culture each infant routinely, although some institutions do culture the rectum, cord stump, and nasopharynx. The nurse should be aware of the severity and rapidity of progression of sepsis in newborns. If an infection is suspected, the appropriate culture should be taken.

Screening tests Screening tests for several congenital and inherited disorders may be done, either before the infant leaves the hospital or on an outpatient basis. For detailed information regarding testing, refer to Chap. 14.

Behavioral assessment The behavioral evaluation is perhaps the most recent component of infant assessment. Little more than a decade ago, newly born infants were regarded by most professionals as passive beings, with no capacity to react to or affect their environment. We are becoming more and more aware that this is far from the truth. The Brazelton Neonatal Assessment Scale was developed by Dr. T. Berry Brazelton.[43] This tool evaluates a baby's behavior toward, and responses to, stimuli in the environment and the way in which this young individual attempts to control his or her environment.

The Brazelton Behavioral Assessment Scale scores babies on 27 behavioral and 20 neurological responses. The behavioral portion of the evaluation tests and documents the infant's behavioral states (deep sleep, active sleep, etc., described just below) and responses to external cues administered by a caretaker. Behavioral state is plotted throughout the examination. The ability of an infant to vary his or her behavioral state directly relates to the infant's capacity for self-organization. The neurological items included in the examination act as a screening test for neurological adequacy. Dr. Brazelton advocates a complete neurological examination if there is any reason to question the neurological status of the infant.

The test is relatively sophisticated. To achieve an acceptable level of reliability, which is necessary before data collected from different samples of neonates can be compared, observers must undergo an intensive 2-day training period. Although this test was developed as a research tool, it is easily used as part of the nurse's clinical assessment.

Recent studies have indicated that neonatal behavioral assessment may be extremely useful for identifying infants at risk for developmental delays. Brazelton states that early identification of developmental deficits can lead to early intervention and that early intervention in an optimum environment can possibly increase the recovery of function in the damaged central nervous system.[44] The Neonatal Behavioral Assessment Scale can be employed to identify infant–caregiver–environment combinations, which may allow researchers and clinicians to predict different developmental outcomes and may also allow early intervention in cases of developmental deficit.[45] (See Chap. 14 for a further discussion of the Brazelton test and Table 14-8 for developmental screening tests suitable for the newborn.)

An infant's responses elicited during the Brazelton exam should be shared with parents to increase their awareness of the reciprocal effects of their own and their baby's behavior and responses. Nurses interested in utilizing all or portions of this scale in their newborn assessments should seek out and study the original test.

The neonate demonstrates distinctly different behavioral states. The six states used by Brazelton and many others are described below.

The cycle of these states of sleep is highly variable and heavily influenced by environmental stimuli. It is therefore extremely helpful for parents to understand the characteristics of the states and the methods for altering them. For instance, wrapping an infant will usually promote drowsiness, and feeding will usually terminate crying if the cause of the crying is hunger. In addition, observation of the neonate in various states assists the parent in appreciating the individuality and potential of the infant. See Chap. 9 for a further discussion of ways the nurse can apply knowledge about behavioral states to support infant development and foster parent–child relationships.

Deep sleep In this state, the infant has closed eyes and regular respirations. There is no spontaneous activity except for startles or jerky movements at regular intervals. External stimuli produce startles with some delay, but these are rapidly suppressed. There are no eye movements. State changes are less likely from deep sleep than from other states.

Active sleep Although the eyes are closed in this state, rapid eye movement (REM) can be detected under the lids. For this reason this state is also known as *REM sleep*. There is little activity except random movements and startles. Movements are less jerky than in deep sleep. Respirations are irregular; sucking movements occur sporadically. The infant responds to stimuli with startles, often resulting in a change of state.

Drowsiness In this state, the eyes may be open or closed, with the eyelids fluttering. The activity level is less variable, with mild startles interspersed. Although the infant is responsive to sensory stimuli, the response is often delayed. Movements are usually smooth. There is frequently a change of state after stimulation.

Alert inactivity In this state, the infant appears to focus on some source of stimulation (e.g., a visual or auditory stimulus). Impinging stimuli may break through, but with a delay in response. There is a minimum of motor activity in this state.

Alert activity In this state, the eyes are open. There is considerable motor activity with thrusting movements of the extremities. Spontaneous startles may be seen. The infant reacts to external stimuli with increased startles or motor activity. However, because of the high activity level, discrete reactions are difficult to discern.

Crying This state is characterized by intense crying which is difficult to break through with stimulation.

Protection against infection

Because newborns have diminished capacities to ward off infection in the neonatal period, careful attention must be paid to protecting them against pathogens in the environment. The nurse must act as infant advocate in this regard.

Control of infections in the nursery includes measures directed toward personnel, the physical environment of the nursery, and the infants, particularly identification and management of infants with a proven or potential transmissible infection.

Personnel The nursery techniques and health status of personnel caring for infants are the most important factors in infection control. The number of people coming in contact with the newborn should be limited to those directly involved in neonatal care. Nursery personnel and others who have contact with the newborn should be free of transmissible diseases. The American Academy of Pediatrics suggests that all personnel assigned to newborn infant services should have at least an annual health assessment, including screening for tuberculosis. Nurses who have a respiratory or skin infection, mucocutaneous (especially herpes) lesions, an intestinal infection, or other transmissible infections are a clear threat to newborn infants. Infected personnel should be excluded from working with infants and should not return to work until the infection has subsided. It is recommended that personnel health policies be instituted in such a way that staff members will feel free to report infections without fear of loss of income.[46] Unfortunately, this is not always the case. Neonatal nurses must exercise sound ethical judgment regarding their own health status and that of other hospital staff members, parents, and visitors to ensure that none of these people, perhaps unknowingly, harbor infections which might affect the neonate.

After individuals have been screened and it is considered safe for them to come in contact with the newborn, the foremost guard against the transmission of infection is thorough hand-washing. All persons caring for newborns should carry out a 2-min scrub at the beginning of each shift. This is most effectively done with an antiseptic agent, such as hexachlorophene or iodophor. Table 16-11 details hand-washing techniques. Following the initial scrub, the hands should be thoroughly washed *immediately* before and after handling each infant. Even more specifically, the nurse should be conscientious about washing hands if he or she plans to examine or feed an infant. This should also be done following a diaper change. Following hand-washing, touching any part of one's own body (face, hair, nose, etc.) will contaminate the hands, necessitating rewashing. Nurses must develop an unceasing awareness of this aspect of infection control, since touching the head is an unconscious habit that many people have. In general, jewelry should not be worn while caring for the newborn, as it provides a harbor for pathogens. The one common exception to this is a flat wedding band.

Caps and masks are no longer considered necessary for routine nursery care. Long hair must be tied back so that it will not come in contact with the infant or equipment during examinations or treatments. To facilitate the scrubs and hand-washing, nurses caring for neonates should wear short-sleeved garments. Hospital staff regularly assigned to the nursery should wear short-sleeved gowns to cover their clothing and to facilitate scrubbing to the elbow. Some nurseries also require this of regular staff, but many policies state *only* that it is necessary that a "barrier" be provided between the nurse's body and the infant during care. "Barrier" may be interpreted as a cover gown, in the case of extended nurse-infant contact, or merely an infant blanket placed against the nurse while the infant is being held to the nurse's body. If a gown is worn, it should be changed after each use. Parents and others who might touch the infant should be instructed in hand-washing and gowning techniques before handling the infant.

The physical environment Another very important aspect of protecting the neonate from infection is maintaining a safe physical environment. Each infant's bassinet and equipment should be thought of as an "island." Nothing contaminated should come in contact with this island, and everything leaving it should be considered "dirty" and be disposed of or cleaned appropriately. Each nursery should have a manual describing the policies for care of the physical environment, and the nurse should be aware of these policies and procedures. This should include approved materials for cleaning, disinfecting, and sterilizing equipment, as well as for taking care of the bassinet itself.

Common scales and examining tables should not be used unless they are protected with a cloth or paper barrier or are properly disinfected after each use.

Parents should be taught the importance of hand-washing and infection control while they are in the hospital and encouraged to continue these practices at home.

Infections transmitted from other infants The third major factor in infection control within the nursery situation is preventing the spread of infection from one infant to others. Obviously, good techniques relative to the first two points—control of personnel and the physical environment—will greatly reduce this danger. Despite conscientious care in these other two areas, once a neonate becomes infected, that infection may spread rapidly from infant to infant, with devastating results. For this reason, the nurse has a responsibility in the early identification of infected infants. Many of the symptoms of generalized infection in the neonate are subtle and subjective, such as hypothermia, lethargy, irritability, a general change in behavior, a change in feeding habits, and jaundice. Because the nurse is the one professional person most aware of the norms for any particular baby, the nurse is best equipped to detect possible infection. In addition to these generalized signs, the nurse should be alert for symptoms such as any pustules, an obviously inflamed or infected skin lesion, and diarrhea. If a mother develops an infection of unknown origin during the postpartum period, the infant should also be suspected of harboring the infection.

Infants who have, or are suspected of having, any infection should be cultured and separated from the others. This may involve placing them in a separate nursery, to be closely observed, or maintaining the infant in the mother's room. The nurse should ensure that the parents have adequate instructions concerning the indicated precautions (putting on a gown, a mask, or gloves) so that contact with the baby will continue. The nurse must always be aware of the significance of uninterrupted contact during the bonding process.

Protection through physical care

The newborn is also protected by the nurse's appropriately meeting the infant's physical care needs.

Protection against heat loss Since the infant is frequently admitted to the nursery in a slightly hypothermic state, great care must be taken to stop further heat loss. On admission to the nursery, the infant's temperature should be measured. Further procedures, such as bathing or making a formal and complete assessment, should be delayed for at least 2 to 6 h, or until the temperature has stabilized. The nurse should then utilize the concepts of care related to thermoregulation as they were discussed earlier relative to nursing care of the newborn in the delivery room.

Bathing The initial bath should be given in the nursery, after the temperature has stabilized. The bath is frequently given with warm water, using a mild soap. However, the "dry technique" is preferred by many authorities for the following reasons: (1) It reduces heat loss by exposure, (2) it diminishes skin trauma, (3) it does not expose the infant to agents with known or unknown side effects, and (4) it requires less time.[47] In the dry technique, cotton balls or a washcloth are soaked with water (a mild soap may be used also) and used to remove blood from the face and head and meconium from the perineal area. The rest of the skin is not touched, unless grossly soiled. During the remainder of the hospital stay, only the diaper area is cleansed. Bathing the infant also provides an opportunity for ongoing assessment. There are many other acceptable "wet" and "dry" techniques for bathing the newborn.

Diaper care The perineal and anal area should be thoroughly cleansed of any urine or fecal material. This may be done with plain warm water or with mild soap and water; cotton balls or a soft cloth should be used. The area should then be dried well, because a warm, moist environment promotes the growth of bacteria. Diapers are always applied and removed in a front-to-back motion, to avoid contamination of the urinary tract with fecal material. Diapers should be fastened with the back overlapping the front so that hip flexion is not inhibited. Cloth diapers are folded in such a way as to provide extra thickness in the front for the male infant and in either the front or the back for the female infant, depending upon her lying position. The nurse should discuss with the parents the relative cost and convenience factors of using cloth diapers laundered at home, a diaper service, or disposable diapers. If cloth diapers are used, great care must be taken to prevent injury to the infant through contact with open pins. The safety pin should be placed in the diaper with the pin pointing to the rear of the infant; if the pin accidentally opens, there is less danger of damage to the abdomen, thighs, or genitalia. In addition, during diaper changes, all pins should be closed and kept well out of the active grasp reflex of the baby.

Diaper rash results from inadequate cleansing and may lead to excoriation of the area and a secondary bacterial or yeast infection. When redness or rash appears in the area, the buttocks or groin should be left exposed to the air. This simple treatment is most effective if done faithfully. A mild ointment may also be used to protect the skin. Plastic pants should not be used on infants with this condition; they promote the rash by increasing warmth and decreasing air circulation. Cloth diapers should be soaked in an agent designed to reduce ammonia, washed with soap, and rinsed well. Disposable diapers may cause a reaction similar to that caused by plastic pants in some infants. The ability to properly attend to the infant's diapering needs appears to play an important role in the achievement of the tasks of parenting. Nurses should not underestimate the importance of parental guidance in this matter.

Umbilical stump care Careful attention must be paid to the care of the umbilical stump. It is essentially an open wound. After the baby is bathed and inspected for potential signs of infection, such as redness, induration, or oozing of foul-smelling drainage, alcohol or an antiseptic agent may be applied to the stump. The diaper should be kept below the cord to promote drying.

Circumcision site care Following a circumcision, the glans is covered with a gauze petroleum dressing, and the diaper is applied loosely. The nurse should observe the infant carefully for bleeding from the site and check voiding to ensure that the procedure did not cause edema of, or trauma to, the urethra. The initial gauze dressing may be left in place until it falls off, or it may be removed by moistening it with water or hydrogen peroxide. Any attempt to forcibly remove it may lead to bleeding. Once this dressing is off, the circumcision site appears as a raw, reddened, and sensitive area. Petroleum jelly should be applied after each voiding for a few days or until the circumcision appears healed. Following a circumcision, the nurse should instruct the parents in proper care of the site and also in wiping stool from front to back, when diapering, to avoid contamination. The penis should be examined regularly, and any sign of infection or bloody urine should be reported to the surgeon immediately.

Protection through identification

In the section of this chapter dealing with care of the neonate in the delivery room, an explanation of the technique and importance of adequate mother-infant identification was given. Caution should be continuously exercised. The neonatal nurse has the responsibility of ensuring that each infant has two coded identification tags on at all times. Before placing a baby with the mother, the nurse should ask the mother to read the code numbers on her bracelet. The nurse then verifies that the baby belongs to this woman. The nurse also has the responsibility of monitoring other personnel to ensure that they also can verify the infant's identification.

Protection through nurturance

It is imperative that the nurse maintain an awareness of the traditional role that feeding has played in the development of positive maternal self-esteem. A mother who can successfully, comfortably, and satisfyingly manage her newborn infant's feeding needs has mastered one of her most basic mothering tasks. Positive reinforcement from the nurse will have a sustaining effect on the mother's ability to progress to other tasks of motherhood.

The question, "Do you plan to breast-feed your baby?" is one that is frequently asked of pregnant women. Many factors will affect her decision—her cultural background, her own general attitude concerning nursing, the feelings of her husband or other people important to her, and her previous experiences with breast-feeding. The nurse should support the mother in *her* decision regarding breast- or bottle-feeding and give her guidance and support to make feeding pleasurable and successful.

Breast-feeding Human breast milk is the most nearly perfect food for babies. In addition, breast-feeding offers certain advantages to both mother and infant. Perhaps the most striking of these is the promotion of a close mother-infant relationship. During the feeding the infant is nestled close to the mother's body, can sense her warmth, can hear her heart beat, and appears to develop a sense of security. This response by the infant frequently has a reciprocal effect on the mother, who has her nurturing role reinforced.

In addition to the psychosocial aspects of breast-feeding, there are physiological advantages. Colostrum, which is secreted from the breasts during the first 2 to 3 days after birth, contains many antibodies in which the newborn is deficient, thus affording the infant passive immunity against some infections.

Colostrum and breast milk appear to have a laxative effect, helping the infant avoid the problem of constipation and speeding meconium passage.

Breast milk is always available, sterile, and at the appropriate temperature. It is the most economical form of infant feeding, although not actually free: the nursing mother must have a high-protein, high-calorie diet. There appears to be less overfeeding and subsequent obesity in breast-fed infants because they are not encouraged to "finish their bottle."

Breast-feeding is inadvisable only in rare circumstances. Debilitating or infectious diseases in the mother, such as tuberculosis, AIDS, severe heart or kidney disease, or advanced cancer, may prevent the mother from nursing. Mothers who have inverted or cracked nipples may experience difficulty, but with proper support and guidance, the mother who truly wants to breast-feed her infant usually succeeds.

Perhaps the most common deterrent to breast-feeding for some mothers is the amount of time it takes. In our society today many mothers return to a career shortly after delivery and therefore must be away from their infants for extended periods of time. It is important to communicate to these mothers that they can pump their breasts every 3 to 4 h while away from their infants to sustain lactation and that either this breast milk or formula may be given by bottle for one to two feedings each day. This method is not ideal and can cause frustrations, but is a viable option for the working mother who wishes to breast-feed her infant. Breast milk can be refrigerated in a clean bottle or other container and used within 24 h. If longer storage is desired, the milk can be frozen in a plastic container ("self-zipping" bags are ideal) for up to 6 months. All milk to be used within 24 h should be labeled with the time it was collected; frozen milk is labeled with the date.

There are known advantages to nursing the infant as soon after birth as possible. From that time on the mother and infant will develop a rhythm, a signaling system, and a unique pattern for feeding. Breast-fed infants tend to be hungry every 2 to 3 h and, since lactation depends only on the stimulation of sucking, can and should be fed at these times. The nurse must remember that the breast-feeding mother needs a tremendous amount of teaching, guidance, and psychological support. However, the success that a mother experiences in breast-feeding will be due largely to her desire to nurse her baby.

An analysis of the components of breast milk, necessary supplements, and a comparison with cow's milk formula are covered in the section "Nutritional Needs of the Newborn" at the end of this chapter.

Bottle-feeding Bottle-feeding is the most popular method of infant feeding used in the United States today. Many commercially prepared cow's milk formulas closely resemble human milk and provide adequate nutrition for the healthy neonate. Refer to Chap. 9 for further discussion of bottle-feeding.

If a mother chooses to bottle-feed the infant, she should of course be supported in her decision. Support includes teaching both feeding techniques and formula preparation. The emphasis on teaching nursing mothers proper breast-feeding techniques is so great that teaching bottle-feeding mothers is sometimes overlooked.

The age at which the first bottle-feeding is given is largely dependent on the neonate's condition. If the baby appears to be awake and alert and does not have excessive mucus, feeding may begin within 1 or 2 h after birth. Bottle-fed babies should be allowed to adjust to a "demand" feeding schedule. Newborn infants usually require six to eight feedings per 24 h.

Stimulation Little more than a decade has passed since the days when it was assumed that newborn infants were only passive individuals, unable to react to or affect their environment. It is now a recognized fact that this is not the case. The nurse has a tremendous opportunity and responsibility to ensure that the infant receives appropriate stimulation and that parents recognize the importance of their role in this regard.

Provision of a stimulating environment In the process of developing behavioral assessment scales, much has been learned about infant stimulation techniques. Sharing this information with parents can serve to enhance their relationship with the child as well as enhance the infant's development. Parents must be aware that *touching* not only plays an important role in bonding but also is a stimulating activity for the baby. *Visual interaction* and stimulation are also important parts of a healthy newborn's environment. The ability of an infant to follow a bright object and to fixate on a face should be demonstrated to parents. *Verbal interactions* play an essential role in infant development. The nurse should act as a role model, interacting verbally with the newborn, to alleviate any feelings of "foolishness" that the parents might have about conversing with so young a being. The infant's varying responses to different noises and tones should be explored.

Promotion of bonding This process of parental attachment, or "the unique relationship between two people (infant and parent) that is specific and endures through time,"[48] begins in the prenatal period. We have discussed the importance of encouraging activities to promote the bonding/attachment process, beginning with the moment of birth. The nurse may continue to facilitate this process by allowing the parents and infant as much uninterrupted contact as possible (Fig. 8-13).

Each individual infant, mother, and father plays a vital role in the development of the parent-child relationship. Newborns respond differently to their parents from the way they respond to others in their environment, and immediately begin to behave in a special way with them. When interacting with their mothers a few weeks after birth, newborns move their bodies in a smooth and cyclical manner and have a long attention span; with their fathers they are more wide-eyed and playful. They interact with their fathers in

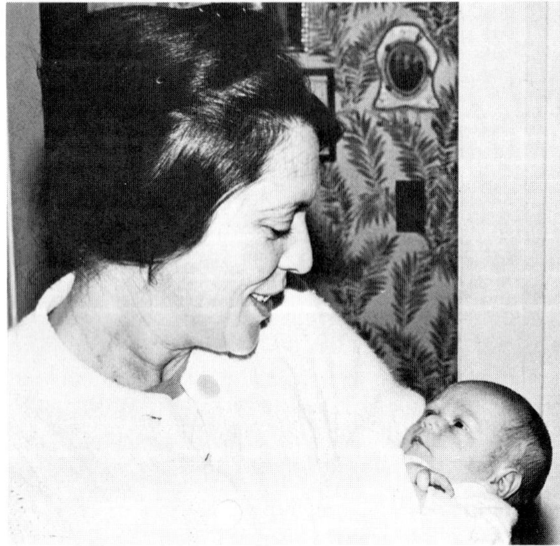

Figure 8-13 Allowing the mother and the infant time to become acquainted will facilitate the bonding process. Note the *en face* position.

a more active, intense manner than they do with their mothers.[49]

The formative stages of the maternal-child relationship have been described by Reva Rubin as a process of "binding-in." Binding-in occurs throughout the pregnancy and during the first 6 months after the infant's birth; it consists of three phases: (1) polarization, (2) identification, and (3) claiming. The mother must first polarize, or separate herself from the infant as part of herself, so that she can accept the infant as a separate being. The infant provides the initial stimulus for this maternal binding-in by his or her physical presence and movements. The physical reality of the infant's existence after birth presents the mother with a compelling need to identify the baby as her own, unique infant. Holding the infant enhances the identification process. The process of identification is usually complete after 4 weeks. At this time the mother can sense when the infant is hungry or satisfied and comfortable or uncomfortable by his or her appearance and cries. As others in the social environment claim and accept the infant, the mother's binding-in is complete.[50]

The father also develops a particular bond to his newborn. This process, called *engrossment*, is influenced by the newborn's reflexive behavior. After the birth the father is absorbed in, preoccupied with, and intensely interested in the infant. He is extremely aware of the newborn's physical characteristics and perceives the infant as perfect. He feels attracted to the newborn and focuses his attention on the infant. The father experiences a sense of elation, or a "high," and a feeling of increased self-esteem.[51] This high level of paternal involvement with the newborn is not always sustained when the family returns home. Although mothers and fathers seem to be increasingly aware of the need for both parents to participate in infant care, nursing interventions to enhance paternal involvement are essential. The nurse can encourage the father to come to follow-up pediatric visits, include the father in postpartum infant care classes, discuss with him the difficulties inherent in sharing the responsibilities for infant care, and help the parents develop a plan for sharing infant care.[52]

During this period, it is important that the nurse allow the parents control over the care and handling of the infant; the nurse should act as a "consultant" rather than "manager" in the relationship. The nurse may point out to the parents the unique capabilities of an infant by helping them identify the infant's various behavioral states and by helping them learn how to interact with these states. Parents who have an awareness of the behavioral and neurological capabilities of their own infant will cease to regard the infant as "a" baby and begin to know "their" child.

During the time spent with the parents, the nurse should capitalize on the positive aspects of the observed parenting role. Positive reinforcement will increase the parents' self-esteem and confidence, and they will be open to learning new concepts. By gaining an awareness of the unique behaviors of each infant and by sharing these sensitivities with the parents, the nurse has a special opportunity to have a lasting impact on the eventual quality of the parent-child relationship.

As caretakers, nurses do not always allow parents and their infants as much contact as they should; many institutional practices tend to separate parents from their infants. Dr. T. Berry Brazelton states:

1. As physicians and nurses, we basically like to help people depend on us. If we allow them too much choice or autonomy, our rewards are minimized.
2. To do this most effectively, we must push a pathological model, one in which childbirth and neonatal care are based on treating pathology, rather than reinforcing for strengths

> that are present in most people and for the odds that are enormously in favor of a good outcome.
>
> 3. All adults who care about babies are competitive with all other adults, and each of us would like to be the primary caretaker of the attractive helpless infant. *Unconsciously,* we devaluate the role of parents to fulfill our own role as *the* important caretaker of this new infant. No one would ever admit this drive, but it is universal.[53]

This is a strong and disturbing statement and one which all neonatal nurses should consider in light of their own feelings and activities. The role of the nurse is to unite and strengthen the family unit, not to come between its members.

Klaus and Kennell suggest that every parent and infant be allowed 30 to 60 min of contact in private during the early, sensitive period. There are not yet any reliable studies to indicate how long this contact should last or exactly when it should take place in the neonatal period to produce optimum parent-child bonding. Some evidence suggests that this contact can be beneficial either immediately after birth or within the first few days after birth, depending on the infant and the parents.[54]

In addition to facilitating and promoting attachment behavior, the nurse must assess and document the progression of this process. Criteria for assessing positive parent-infant bonding include the following:

1. The parents understand the infant's states and react appropriately.
2. The parents derive pleasure from interacting with their infant and performing caretaking tasks.
3. The parents refer to the infant by name and demonstrate an awareness of his or her unique personality and potential.
4. The parents' discussions of future plans include the infant as a positive factor.

There are exhaustive lists of criteria and evaluating tools available regarding assessment of bonding; these are a sample of points to consider. Likewise, there are behaviors that are exhibited when parents are not bonding adequately. These center around general displeasure regarding the infant; disgust caused by such normal infant activities as drooling, defecation, urination, and regurgitation; abnormal or unfounded fears that the infant has an abnormality or serious illness; and inappropriate response to the infant's needs. A parent who exhibits these behaviors usually fails to demonstrate the behavior seen in the normal progression of the bonding process. The parent may not have eye-to-eye contact with the infant, may not hold the infant close, or may refer to the infant as "it," rather than by name. Early assessment of this process is essential if crisis intervention is to be effective.

Discharge from the nursery

Many mothers and infants leave the hospital when the infant is 2 or 3 days old, and the trend is toward even earlier discharge. This practice leaves little time for the nurse to meet the goals of neonatal care while the mother and infant are in the hospital. The nurse must use every opportunity to fulfill these goals during hospitalization and then appropriately plan for ongoing care at home.

Preparation for discharge from the hospital should begin with the newborn's admission to the nursery. The ongoing assessment of the infant and of the parent-infant interaction gives important clues as to the readiness of the family to function as an independent unit, outside the confines and security of the hospital setting. Infants are usually discharged on the third or fourth day of life, although some may leave earlier if stable.

The physical examination Within the 24 h preceding discharge, the neonate should have a complete physical examination by a physician or, in some cases, a pediatric nurse practitioner. Significant maternal, fetal, and neonatal observations and treatments should be summarized in writing so that they can be made available to health care workers who will provide follow-up services. The examination should include consideration of any laboratory tests done on the neonate.

Evaluation of parental readiness By the day of planned discharge, the nurse should have completed the evaluation of the parents' readiness to assume independent care of the infant. This should include evaluation of bonding behavior, skill in infant care, and demonstration of appropriate judgment regarding the needs of the infant. Any uncertainty that the nurse feels regarding the parents' ability to cope in any of these areas should be sufficient reason for postponing discharge.

Home preparations The nurse should explore with the parents the home preparations for the baby, discussing the *physical environment*, such as the temperature in the home. If it is cool, the nurse should emphasize the importance of keeping the baby warmly dressed and of placing the bassinet or crib away from outside walls.

The nurse should determine the answers to the following questions and provide appropriate intervention when indicated: Do the parents *have* a bassinet? If the infant is bottle-feeding, do the parents have the formula or ingredients for the formula and directions and equipment for preparing it? Does a breast-feeding mother know how to prepare glucose water or formula in the event that she must use an alternative feeding method? Is there anyone in the household with a transmissible infection, such as a severe cold, a skin infection, or diarrhea? If there are other children, have the parents considered their response to a new family member? Will the new mother have adequate support services for home and child care so that she may fully recover from the labor and delivery experience? All these, and in some cases many more, issues should be addressed when the nurse is evaluating home preparation.

Birth registration The registration of the baby's birth is of utmost importance and should be done before the infant leaves the hospital. The law requires that the birth attendant submit notification of the birth to the local registrar, with specified information about the infant's name, date of birth, and parents. Each state has its own certificate standard, and these records are legal documents filed permanently with the state bureau of vital statistics. The parents should be aware that a copy of this certificate will be made available to them.

Preparations for follow-up care Plans for medical supervision of the newborn should be made. Appropriate referral should be made if the infant will be transferred to a different caregiver. Contact should be made with the clinic or private physician to arrange for the first pediatric visit and to establish contact for emergency care or intermediate guidance. If the neonatal nurse feels it advisable, a referral to a visiting nurse should be completed, and the agency contacted by phone to ensure immediate follow-up care.

HOME CARE OF THE NEWBORN

Although the newborn has undergone the most dramatic changes during the first few days of life, the remainder of the first month continues to be a dynamic period during which the incorporation of the infant into the family system becomes more solidified. *Adaptation* may best describe the task of each participant.

Although it is hoped that the new parents have had adequate instruction regarding infant care while in the hospital, they need to be aware of modifications in this care after discharge from the hospital.

Bathing

The newborn should continue to have sponge or dry baths until the umbilical cord has fallen off and the site is completely healed, at about 1 to 2 weeks, at which time tub baths may be started. The first bath may consist merely of placing the baby in a tub of warm water in order that he or she can adjust to the new experience. Parents need to learn to hold and support their baby in the tub, with one arm and hand, while leaving the other hand free. There is no reason for the baby to be bathed daily, unless it becomes a stimulating and enjoyable experience for both infant and parents. A mild soap should be used, and afterward rinsed off carefully to avoid excessive dryness of the skin.

The hair and scalp should be shampooed twice a week. Active sebaceous glands lead to sebum on the scalp, frequently causing a "cradle cap," or a crusting of these secretions. If cradle cap does occur, it is helpful to rub mineral oil into the skin of the scalp the night before the shampoo is to be given.

Cotton-tipped applicators should not be used to cleanse either the nose or ears, as they may cause damage to delicate tissues; it is adequate to gently wipe away obvious mucus with the twisted end of a washcloth or a cotton ball. Parents may feel that they want to moisturize the baby's skin, which frequently appears to be dry during the first few weeks. Lotion should be used rather than oil, as the latter clogs skin pores.

Bath time provides an excellent opportunity for parents to utilize their skills in assessment and stimulation. A pleasant bath experience can play an important role in the parent-infant bonding process.

Cord care

If the umbilical cord is still on, parents should be instructed to keep it clean and dry. It is important to apply the diaper in such a way that the stump is exposed. When the cord dries and falls off, a small amount of serous drainage, occasionally blood-tinged, is normal. At this time it is helpful to cleanse the area with alcohol three or four times a day. Parents should be advised that if there is a large amount of drainage or bleeding, a foul odor, or reddening or swelling of the skin around the umbilicus, the doctor should be notified immediately. The use of belly-binders is discouraged because they hinder the healing process.

Clothing

Clothing should be considered in relationship to family finances. This is an exciting time for most parents. Enthusiasm leading to the purchase of expensive wardrobes may need to be tempered with the reality that the baby will grow rapidly during the first few weeks and months of life and has a limited need for "special outfits."

The infant will need about two to three dozen cloth diapers if disposable diapers are not used. Since neonates are "droolers," parents should be advised that they will need an adequate supply of tops. A few nighties, receiving blankets, caps, and a bunting may be needed, depending on the weather and climate. It is sometimes helpful for parents to know that they should dress their infants in approximately the same amount of clothing that is comfortable for other members of the family in the same environment. Any new clothing should be laundered before the baby wears it, since it is often fuzzy and contains sizing, which is very irritating to the infant's delicate skin.

Crying

Few parents leave the hospital prepared for how disturbing their own infant's *crying* is, nor do they realize that young infants spend much of their waking time crying. It may be helpful to point out that the infant's cry is an effort to communicate; by trial and error, the parents will learn to differentiate what a specific cry means within 1 month.

Comforting Parents need to be told that if rocking, holding, walking, or talking to the neonate appears to be comforting, they should not be concerned about "spoiling" the infant. Infants derive a great deal of comfort from sucking; use of a pacifier is acceptable, and it may be gradually withdrawn as the infant gets older.

Colic *Colic* is described as paroxysmal abdominal cramping accompanied by loud crying and drawing of the legs up to the abdomen, as if in pain. In spite of this, the infant appears to tolerate the feeding and gains weight. Many theories related to the type, amount, and technique of feeding have been investigated. The effect of emotional stress between parent and child has been explored as a causative factor. Generally, colic is thought to be caused by excessive fermentation and gas production in the intestines. Regardless of the etiology of the problem, a crying, irritable baby with colic creates great stress and feelings of inadequacy in the parents. Occasionally, the reason for the problem is discerned, and nursing intervention is successful. More often, the most helpful role the nurse can play is to provide support for the parents during this difficult period, assuring them that in the normal growth and development process infants do outgrow these spells.

Sleeping

Parents also have questions regarding how much time they can expect their baby to *sleep* when at home. The neonate rarely sleeps more than 3 to 5 h without waking to be fed. Although parents should be encouraged to allow their healthy newborns to sleep as much as possible at night, the new mother should attempt to sleep several hours during the day. She will lose several hours of nighttime sleep during the first 4 weeks of her baby's life. It is helpful to know that as babies get older, the amount of time they spend sleeping at night gradually increases.

Adjustment to the new infant

Just as the infant undergoes a series of adaptations during the neonatal period, so do other members of the family. They need to adjust to the newcomer. If the infant is a firstborn, parents undergo phenomenal psychological adjustments to their new roles as a mother and father. The role changes of parenthood produce stress. There are few role models available for new parents, and they must define their roles themselves. The demands of a new infant, who is totally dependent, decrease the amount of time the parents spend with each other and drain them of energy. The costs associated with the infant, and possibly the loss of the mother's income, can create financial burdens, making the period of adjustment to the new infant a time of family stress and crisis.[55]

If there are other children, they now must adapt their lifestyle to include someone they may see as a "stranger," perhaps even an unwanted stranger, in their lives. Sibling rivalry needs to be recognized and dealt with openly. (See the section "Sibling Rivalry" in Chap. 9.) The nurse should assess adaptive behavior within the family structure and intervene if this is indicated; provide guidance and support for family members in their changing roles; and, if indicated, refer the family that is experiencing difficulty to family counseling.

Socialization of the newborn

The neonate actively participates in a socialization process as he or she attempts to become acquainted with the environment and to develop a social relationship with others. The newborn is well equipped to begin this process. The newborn can see, hear, smell, and feel from the moment of birth. By processing external stimuli through these senses, the infant begins immediately to interact with the environment. Specific neonatal actions and reactions observed in behavioral assessments demonstrate that the infant's responses to stimuli vary greatly with her or his behavioral state. At a very early age the neonate is able to control the effect of the environment and stimuli by moving from one state to another, thereby "shutting out" unwanted stimuli.

Studies of maternal-infant bonding show that each infant, through behavior, modifies markedly how much interaction and stimulation he or she elicits.

During the first 4 weeks of life, the infant becomes increasingly active in the socialization process. This is a great joy to parents as they watch their baby develop into a unique person.

Infant temperament Each newborn infant has a particular style of behavior or method of reacting to the world that is characteristic of his or her individual temperament. The characteristics of an infant's temperament include (1) level of motor activity; (2) regularity or rhythmicity of biological functions, (3) approach to, or withdrawal from, new stimuli or situations; (4) ability to adapt to new situations after the initial stimulation; (5) threshold of responsiveness to stimulation; (6) intensity of reactions; (7) quality and variability of mood; (8) ability to be distracted from one activity to another; and (9) attention span and persistence in continuing with an activity even when it is difficult.

Infants can be classified into three different groups on the basis of temperament: (1) the easy child, who is regular in behavior, positive in approach, and adaptable; (2) the difficult child, who is irregular in biological functions, negative in approach to stimuli, and slow to adapt; and (3) the slow-to-warm-up child, who is variable in behavior and combines mildly negative responses with moderate adaptability and some irregularity in biological functions.[56]

A recent study has demonstrated that there is a positive relationship between the parents' coping behaviors and functioning and the infant's temperament and that parents respond reciprocally to their infant and the infant's behavior.[57] Parents can be taught about the variations in individual temperament during the neonatal period and helped to recognize their infant's individual characteristics and strengths early in the parent-infant bonding process. The nurse can then help them plan a method of raising their child that is comfortable for them and appropriate in terms of their infant's temperament.[58]

Communication Infants strengthen their attachment to their caregivers through various means of communication. They communicate with others in the environment to bring them in close proximity as a means of ensuring their safety. They do this through three specific types of behavior: (1) orienting, (2) making physical contact, and (3) signaling. Orienting behaviors include gazing (especially at faces), fixating on objects, and tracking with the eyes and head. Rooting and sucking reflexes are two other behaviors that orient the infant to the mother and help promote mother-infant contact. Active physical contact such as clinging and grasping are used by the infant to secure contact with the caregiver. The newborn also signals his or her needs to the caregiver by smiling, vocalizing, and crying.[59] Neonates smile in response to stimuli as early as 2 weeks of age. By the fourth week the newborn is sophisticated enough to smile when eye-to-eye contact is made with a caretaker. The neonate also employs many different sounds in an attempt to interact with the environment. These range from miscellaneous noises at birth to a well-organized ability to respond with gurgles and "coos" by the end of the first month.[60] Both smiling and cooing are attempts by the infant to communicate or relate to others. In addition to these signals, the cry of the neonate becomes increasingly differentiated during this period. Parents learn to recognize these cries and respond to meet their baby's needs.

Play Appropriate toys add necessary stimulation to the neonate's life. It is important that all the senses through which the infant perceives stimuli be considered and that toys that will stimulate as many of these senses as possible be provided. Rattles and mobiles are particularly good selections for the 1-month-old. If mobiles are used, they should be safe and designed with the infant's age in mind. Dr. Burton White suggests the following guidelines for making a mobile for a 3- to 8-week-old infant:

1. A mobile should be placed where the infant tends to look. Since infants of this age prefer to look either to the far right or far left, mobiles should be placed to the side of, rather than above, the infant.
2. A mobile should be placed at a distance the infant prefers—at this age, about 12 in from the head.
3. In designing a mobile, one should keep in mind what the baby sees while lying in the crib.

Safety measures

Parents need guidelines for providing a safe environment for their rapidly developing infant. At 1 month of age the infant retains much of the vulnerability of the first week of life but is gaining new motor skills that endanger his or her safety.

Parents should have a plan for medical emergencies in the home and know where the nearest medical facility is. Because the neonate, even at 4 weeks, is still immunodeficient, crowds and exposure to infectious diseases should be avoided. Parents need to be thoughtful of surfaces, such as countertops, beds, and bath tables, from which the infant may roll. The parents should not leave the infant unattended on high surfaces or even in infant seats. Cribs and playpens should be checked to ensure that the bars are spaced so that the infant's head cannot get caught. Also, since automobile accidents are a leading cause of death during the first year of life, parents should be encouraged to put their infant in an approved infant seat while driving.[61] Infants should not be held in a passenger's (or the driver's) lap. Many states now require car seats for children under 4 years of age or up to 40 lb.

Anticipatory guidance is necessary on a frequent and regular basis in order to guide parents in accident prevention as the infant passes through the forthcoming developmental stages.

THE NUTRITIONAL NEEDS OF THE NEWBORN

During the first few months of life, the growth rate of the infant exceeds that of any other time during life. Therefore, careful attention should be given to providing the infant with nutrients necessary for healthy development. Unfortunately, health care professionals frequently overlook the role of nutrition in the maintenance of a healthy neonate.

Nutritional requirements

The nutrients that a full-term infant needs for healthy development are based on body weight. Since the weight is constantly changing, so are the nutritional requirements. Dietary allowances are expressed in daily requirements unless otherwise indicated.

Caloric needs The infant from birth through 6 months of age requires 117 kcal per kilogram of body weight, or about 54 kcal per pound. To calculate the daily caloric requirements, the nurse simply multiplies the infant's weight in kilograms by 117. For instance, an infant weighing 3.2 kg would require 3.2×117, or 374 kcal each day.

Fluid requirements The amount of fluid an infant needs is related to his or her caloric requirements and is approximately 1.5 ml for each kilocalorie required. Fluid requirements can also be calculated, like caloric requirements, directly by the infant's weight. The infant should receive 165 ml per kilogram of body weight per day. Thus, a 3.2-kg infant should have 3.2×165, or 528 ml of fluid per day.

Vitamins and minerals Recommended dietary allowances vary somewhat; see Appendix C 4 and 5 for a summary of average values.

Feeding

Following the establishment of feeding patterns during the hospital stay, parents need continuing guidance and support to gain maximum satisfaction for both themselves and their infants during feeding.

Position during feeding *Nursing* mothers find a variety of positions comfortable for breast-feeding. Soon after delivery, many mothers find the side-lying position—placing the infant in a horizontal plane beside them—most comfortable. Others may sit upright in bed to nurse. By the time of discharge, most mothers find sitting most satisfactory. Far more important than the general position of the mother and infant is the specific position of the child's mouth in relation to the areola. For successful nursing, the infant must have the nipple well back in the mouth. The gums are then able to press on the areolar surface, and the lips can close tightly around the breast tissue to permit suction (Fig. 8-14). In this position, the infant is able to apply pressure to the lactiferous sinuses and obtain milk by a process of compression and suction. The mother who, for one reason or another, experiences difficulty with breast-feeding becomes very frustrated. This frustration and tension then interfere with her "let-down" reflex and create a cycle that may set both mother and infant up for failure in nursing. Prompt nursing assessment and intervention may alleviate this problem.

Bottle-feeding is the most common infant feeding method used in the United States. Yet mothers may not know how to bottle-feed their infants. Many mothers may need as much teaching and support as those who are nursing. It is important to stress to mothers that thoughtful bottle-feeding allows a mother and infant a time for intimacy, much as breast-feeding does. Holding the infant closely and cuddling help ensure the realization of the emotional component of feeding. Parents should be encouraged to position the infant close to their bodies to allow eye contact. Although newborns will accept cold formula, most parents warm it to body temperature.[62] Parents should be cautioned to avoid overheating formula in a microwave oven. The bottle should be kept tipped to keep the nipple filled with milk. This will decrease the amount of air consumed with the feeding. Propping the bottle should be very strongly discouraged, as it denies the infant parental contact and may result in choking and aspiration.

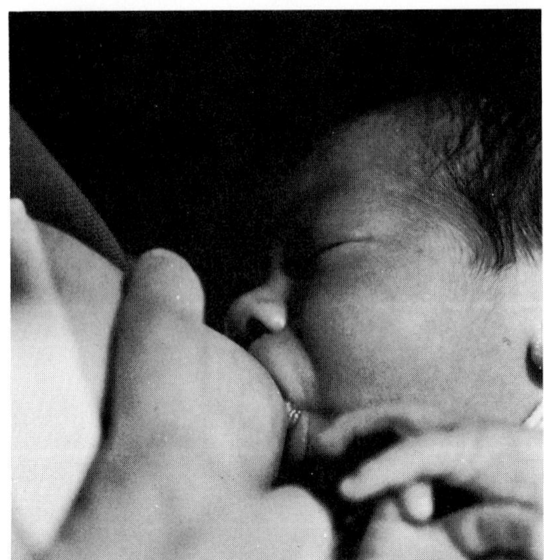

Figure 8-14 The proper position of the infant's mouth on the breast during breast-feeding. (*Clinical Education Aid No. 10, courtesy of Ross Laboratories, Columbus, Ohio.*)

Bubbling During the process of feeding, particularly bottle-feeding, infants ingest varying amounts of air. Periodically "burping" them, allowing them to expel this air, will reduce the possibility of vomiting. During burping all babies regurgitate small amounts of breast milk or formula. Mothers usually refer to this as "spitting up" and come to view it as a normal occurrence.

Techniques for bubbling a baby vary. The traditional method is for the parent to place a diaper or cloth on the shoulder and then hold the infant against his or her chest and gently rub the baby's back. This is a comfortable position for both infant and parent. However, during the first few weeks of life there is some advantage in bubbling with the infant sitting on the parent's lap. If the infant is leaned slightly forward and the head and face are supported with one hand, the parent is free to gently rub the back with the other (Fig. 16-19). This position allows greater visibility of the infant and is especially preferred when caring for babies who tend to regurgitate particularly large amounts of formula or breast milk.

Position after feeding Following the feeding, the infant should be placed on the right side or stomach. Positioning on the right side will permit the feeding to flow toward the lower end of the stomach and will allow any excess air to rise above the feeding and escape via the esophagus, thus preventing vomiting and abdominal distention. A rolled blanket may be placed behind the back to keep the infant from changing position. Parents should be cautioned *never* to place the infant on his or her back after feeding, since regurgitation may lead to aspiration.

Feeding problems

The normal full-term infant encounters few feeding problems. However, it is important for the nurse to recognize them in order to intervene appropriately.

Overfeeding In the case of breast-feeding mothers and infants, it is the *infant* who decides how much milk will be drunk; sucking continues until the baby's needs are met. The mother actually does not know how much fluid the infant has consumed. Therefore, overfeeding is rarely a problem for the breast-fed infant. Conversely, overfeeding is the greatest nutritional hazard of bottle-feeding. Parents frequently encourage their infants to "finish the bottle" and see the infant's compliance with this wish as a demonstration of love. There is much research currently being conducted to determine a relationship between early feeding in infancy and obesity in later life. (See the section in Chap. 9 on overfeeding.) The mother who is bottle-feeding her baby needs much guidance and encouragement to let her infant signal her when satisfied.

Feeding prepared formula The infant who is breast-fed has the advantage of always receiving food that is suited to meet his or her physiological needs. Unfortunately, the use of formula leaves room for human error. It is not uncommon for mothers unknowingly to prepare formula incorrectly. In such cases, the infant may receive a feeding so rich that the baby cannot process it or one so diluted that the infant receives inadequate nutrients per fluid ounce.

Drug companies are currently under scrutiny for promoting the use of commercially prepared formulas in low-socioeconomic communities in this country as well as in underdeveloped countries throughout the world. When bottle-feeding replaces breast-feeding in these areas, it presents two basic problems. The first is one of contamination. Mothers from these environments may have difficulty understanding or applying principles of asepsis relative to preparation of the feeding and also frequently have inadequate refrigeration available for safe storage. Second, these mothers, many of whom do not understand written instructions and have limited resources to purchase formula, overdilute the mixtures to gain the volume their infants need. Obviously, the end result of such a continued practice is severe malnutrition. These infants would be far better served if resources spent on purchasing formula were spent to improve nutrition of breast-feeding mothers. Formula allergies are discussed in Chap. 9, as is the nutritional value of breast milk as compared with that of formula.

Formula preparation

The composition of unmodified cow's milk makes it unsuitable for young infants' nutrition. Therefore, careful consideration of formula composition is necessary so that infants who are not breast-fed will have their nutritional needs met.

Evaporated milk formula Cow's milk formula may be easily prepared at home. Evaporated whole milk is usually modified to meet the specific needs of the infant. Care must be taken not to confuse evaporated milk with either canned condensed or skim milk. Condensed milk is a form of evaporated milk that has large amounts of sugar added to it; it is disproportionately high in sugar and low in fat and protein, making it inappropriate for infant feeding. Skim milk should not be given to infants because it has a low caloric concentration, deprives the body of essential fatty acids, and places increased demands on the kidney.

One evaporated milk formula is prepared by mixing 13 oz of evaporated milk with 18 oz of water and adding 2 tbsp of corn syrup. This formula yields approximately 20 kcal/oz. Errors in the preparation of evaporated milk formula are usually of two kinds: (1) parents reverse the proportion of milk to water, and (2) they confuse tsp (teaspoon) with tbsp (tablespoon). The nurse should be aware of the potential problems and incorporate appropriate instructions into the teaching plan.

Infants receiving evaporated milk formula should receive supplements of vitamin C and iron. Fluoride may be recommended, depending on whether it is present in the water supply. This should be discussed with the pediatrician at the first visit.

Commercially prepared formulas These prepared formulas, such as Similac, Enfamil, and SMA, have a cow's milk base and have been modified to closely resemble human milk. They are available in three forms: (1) a powdered form, which must be diluted according to the manufacturer's directions; (2) a concentrated liquid form, which must be diluted with an equal amount of water; and (3) a ready-to-feed form, available in either cans or bottles. The manufacturers of these products supply explicit directions for their use, but the major problem encountered in their use is either underdilution or overdilution.

Each type of preparation varies and needs to be understood by parents. These prepared formulas offer the busy parent much-appreciated convenience. They are considerably more expensive than an evaporated milk formula. Most of these formulas are fortified with vitamins D and C and iron.

Calculation of caloric and fluid requirements

The information given thus far should enable the nurse to easily calculate the amount of formula that an infant must consume each day to fulfill caloric and fluid requirements.

Caloric requirements To calculate the number of ounces of formula needed by an infant each day, the following formula should be used:

$$\frac{\text{Weight (kg)} \times 117\ \text{kcal/kg}}{20\ \text{kcal/oz}} = \text{total number of ounces per day}$$

If this formula is used to calculate the number of ounces of formula that a 3.2-kg infant needs each day, the results are as follows:

$$\frac{3.2\ \text{kg} \times 117\ \text{kcal/kg}}{20\ \text{kcal/oz}} = 19\ \text{oz}$$

Fluid requirements To calculate the daily fluid requirement for an infant, a simple calculation is used:

$$\text{Weight (kg)} \times 165\ \text{ml} = \text{total milliliters needed per day}$$

If this formula is used to calculate the number of ounces needed by the infant each day, results are as follows:

$$3.2\ \text{kg} \times 165\ \text{ml} = 528\ \text{ml}$$

To convert 528 ml to ounces, divide by 30 (30 ml = 1 oz):

$$528\ \text{ml} \div 30\ \text{ml/oz} = 14\ \text{oz}$$

Therefore, by doing these two calculations, the nurse finds that 19 oz of formula will supply the caloric requirements, plus 5 oz of fluid more than the baby requires.

Prevention of contamination

Great care must be taken in the preparation and storage of formula to prevent contamination. There are several different ways of preparing and storing formula.

The terminal heating method Bottles, nipples, caps, and utensils used for preparing the formula should be clean. The formula is prepared and poured into the bottles. The nipple, turned downward, is put into the mouth of the bottle. Caps are applied loosely to allow steam to escape. The bottles are placed in a sterilizer, or deep kettle, and water is poured into the container until it covers the lower third of the bottles. A tight cover is applied to the sterilizer or kettle, and the water is boiled for 20 to 25 min. After the boiling period, the sterilizer should be allowed to cool slowly. When the bottles are cool enough to handle, the caps are tightened, and the bottles are placed in the refrigerator.

The aseptic or modified method All equipment is washed before starting the procedure, as in the terminal heating method. Then the bottles, nipples, and utensils (including measuring cups) needed for formula preparation are boiled for 5 min. Next, water to be used in mixing the formula is also boiled for 5 min (allowing a few extra ounces for evaporation). In actually mixing the formula, water should be remeasured to the exact amount needed, and the other ingredients added. This is then poured into the presterilized bottles. Care should be taken not to touch the inner surfaces of caps and nipples when they are put on and tightened. The formula may then be refrigerated.

Note: Except for premature infants or others who for some reason need protection from bacteria normally tolerated by infants, families who use city water or tested well water can simplify the preparation of bottle feedings by using a dishwasher, if one is available. In this method, the bottles, nipples, and caps are washed in the hot-water cycle of the dishwasher. The formula, which has been prepared with unboiled water, is then poured into the bottles. Bottles are capped and refrigerated until used. No terminal heating or other sterilization is used in this method. An even simpler method is to premeasure dry formula powder into clean bottles when they are taken from the dishwasher; the bottles are capped and stored at room temperature, and tap water is added at feeding time.

Disposable bottles Several companies market plastic bottles with disposable bag liners, into which the sterile formula is placed. Many families prefer that convenience. If this method is used, directions given by the manufacturer of the product used should be followed.

References

1. Clark, Ann L., Dyanne D. Affonso, and Thomas Harris: *Childbearing: A Nursing Perspective,* 2d ed., Davis, Philadelphia, 1979, pp. 564–565.
2. Behrman, Richard E., and Victor C. Vaughan (eds.), *Nelson Textbook of Pediatrics,* 12th ed., Saunders, Philadelphia, 1983, p. 364.
3. *Standards and Recommendations for Hospital Care of Newborn Infants,* 6th ed., American Academy of Pediatrics, Evanston, Ill., 1977, pp. 53–54.
4. Bryant, Bobby G., "Unit Dose Erythromycin Ophthalmic Ointment for Neonatal Ocular Prophylaxis," *Journal of Obstetric, Gynecological, and Neonatal Nursing* **13**(1): 83–87 (February 1984).
5. American Academy of Pediatrics and American College of Obstetricians and Gynecologists, *Guidelines for Perinatal Care,* American Academy of Pediatrics, Evanston, Ill., 1983, p. 85.
6. Perez, Rosanne H., *Protocols for Perinatal Nursing Practice,* Mosby, St. Louis, 1981, p. 244.
7. Ibid., p. 245.
8. *Standards and Recommendations for Hospital Care of Newborn Infants,* pp. 57–58.
9. Avery, Mary E., and William H. Taeusch, *Shaffer's Diseases of the Newborn,* 5th ed., Saunders, Philadelphia, 1984, p. 20.
10. Klaus, Marshall H., and John H. Kennell, *Parent-Infant Bonding,* Mosby, St. Louis, 1982, p. 39.
11. Ibid., p. 74.
12. Ibid., p. 171.
13. Ibid., p. 75.
14. Restak, Richard M., "Newborn Knowledge," *Science* **82** (3):60 (January–February 1982).
15. Leboyer, Frederick, *Birth without Violence,* Knopf, New York, 1975, p. 77.
16. Klaus, Marshall H., and John H. Kennell, "Pregnancy, Birth, and the First Days of Life," in Melvin D. Levine, William B. Carey, Allen C. Crocker, and Ruth T. Gross (eds.), *Developmental Behavioral Pediatrics,* Saunders, Philadelphia, 1983, pp. 67–68.
17. Behrman and Vaughan, op. cit., p. 8.
18. Ibid., p. 13.
19. Ibid.
20. Tudor, Mary, *Child Development,* McGraw-Hill, New York, 1981, p. 337.
21. Keay, A. J., and D. M. Morgan, *Craig's Care of the Newly Born Infant,* Livingstone, Edinburgh, 1982, p. 240.
22. Tudor, loc. cit.
23. Keay and Morgan, op. cit., p. 127.
24. Ibid., p. 115.
25. Powell, Marcene L., *Assessment and Management of Developmental Changes and Problems in Children,* 2d ed., Mosby, St. Louis, 1981, p. 42.
26. Behrman and Vaughan, op. cit., p. 1666.
27. Ibid., p. 1670.
28. Avery and Taeusch, op. cit., p. 395.
29. Keay and Morgan, op. cit., p. 446.
30. Avery and Taeusch, op. cit., p. 402.
31. Avery, Gordon B., *Neonatology: Pathophysiology and Management of the Newborn,* Lippincott, Philadelphia, 1981, p. 233.
32. Behrman and Vaughan, op. cit., p. 14.
33. Ibid., p. 365.
34. Avery and Taeusch, op. cit., p. 721.
35. Behrman and Vaughan, op. cit., p. 498.
36. Ibid.
37. Schiffman, Rachel F., "Temperature Monitoring in the Neonate: A Comparison of Axillary and Rectal Temperatures," *Nursing Research* **31**(3):274–277 (May 1982).
38. Behrman and Vaughan, op. cit., p. 337.
39. Ibid., p. 336.
40. Ibid., p. 334.
41. Weidman, W., "Standards for Blood Pressure," in *Children's Blood Pressure,* Report of the Ross Conference on Pediatric Research, Columbus, Ohio, 1985, pp. 14–15.
42. Haddock, Nancy, "Blood Pressure Monitoring in Neonates," *American Journal of Maternal-Child Nursing* **5**(3):134 (May 1980).
43. Brazelton, T. Berry, *Neonatal Behavioral Assessment*

Scale, Clinics in Developmental Medicine, No. 50, Lippincott, Philadelphia, 1973.
44. ——— and Barry M. Lester, *New Approaches to Developmental Screening of Infants,* Elsevier, Amsterdam, 1983, p. 4.
45. Ibid., p. 48.
46. *Standards and Recommendations for Hospital Care of Newborn Infants,* p. 110.
47. Ibid.
48. Klaus and Kennell, *Parent-Infant Bonding,* p. 2.
49. Restak, op. cit., p. 59.
50. Rubin, Reva, *Maternal Identity and the Maternal Experience,* Springer, New York, 1984, pp. 133–136.
51. Greenberg, Martin, and Norman Morris, "Engrossment: The Newborn's Impact upon the Father," *American Journal of Orthopsychiatry* **44**(4):520–531 (July 1974).
52. Kunst-Wilson, William, and Linda Cronewett, "Nursing Care for the Emerging Family: Promoting Paternal Behavior," *Research in Nursing and Health* **4**:208 (April 1981).
53. Klaus and Kennell, *Parent-Infant Bonding,* p. 88.
54. Klaus and Kennell, "Pregnancy, Birth, and the First Days of Life," p. 73.
55. Wheeler, Kathy, "The Crisis of the First Child," in Peggy L. Chinn and Kathy B. Leonard (eds.), *Current Practice in Pediatric Nursing,* vol. III, Mosby, St. Louis, 1980, pp. 22–25.
56. Chess, Stella, and A. Thomas, "Dynamics of Individual Behavioral Development," in Levine, Carey, Crocker, and Gross, op. cit., p. 166.
57. Ventura, Jacqueline N., "Parent Coping Behaviors, Parent Functioning, and Infant Temperament Characteristics," *Nursing Research* **31**(3):273 (May 1982).
58. Chess, Stella, "Temperamental Differences: A Critical Concept in Child Health Care," *Pediatric Nursing* **11**:168 (May–June 1985).
59. Jenkins, Ruth L., and Nina Kelsey, "The Nurse Role in Parent-Infant Bonding: Overview, Assessment, Intervention," *Journal of Obstetric, Gynecological, and Neonatal Nursing* **10**(2):114 (February 1981).
60. Tudor, op. cit., p. 350.
61. Krozy, Ronna E., and James J. McColgan, "Auto Safety: Pregnancy and the Newborn," *Journal of Obstetric, Gynecological, and Neonatal Nursing* **14**(1):11 (January 1985).
62. Pipes, Peggy L., *Nutrition in Infancy and Childhood,* Mosby, St. Louis, 1985, p. 114.

9

Ann R. Sloat

The infant

Upon completion of this chapter, the student will be able to:

1. List at least four characteristics of infant growth and development.
2. Describe four or more factors that contribute to positive parenting.
3. Describe at least three methods the young infant uses to communicate with adults.
4. Select appropriate stimulation (e.g., toys) for the infant on the basis of the infant's age.
5. Describe a schedule for introducing solid foods to infants.
6. Describe the physical growth and function of the infant's body systems.
7. Describe Erikson's psychosocial stage of trust vs. mistrust.
8. Identify at least four caretaking measures that promote the development of a sense of trust in the infant.
9. Summarize each of the three stages of the infant's attachment behavior.
10. Identify the characteristics of each of the four stages of the infant's cognitive development.
11. Identify essential nursing interventions in infant care with regard to diapering, diaper rash, teething, weaning, the feeding schedule, introducing solid foods, and taking safety precautions.

This chapter discusses the child between the ages of 1 month and 1 year, the period termed *infancy*. During this period the infant experiences very rapid growth and accomplishes an impressive repertoire of developmental tasks. Within a brief year, the infant begins to learn language, becomes mobile, develops obviously purposeful and controlled behavior, and becomes physiologically much more capable of flourishing. This rate of growth and development will not be equaled, let alone surpassed, during the rest of the individual's lifetime.

DEVELOPMENT: EXPECTATIONS AND REALITY

The growth and change that infants experience are patterned and predictable. Being able to predict the general pattern of development has distinct advantages. The infant's environment can be enriched to provide opportunities to practice whatever developmental adventure the infant is ready for. It is important to allow time for practice and not to push the infant ahead of his or her own timetable.

Infants give cues when they are ready to do something new. An observant parent will tune in to the infant's messages, but may sometimes need a little help. A 2-month-old may "tell" the parent that he or she is ready to practice grasping objects by attending to, and reaching toward, the parent's earring or tie. If the playpen and crib lack attractive and reachable playthings or if the infant spends much of the day in an infant seat, then no one is hearing the message. The nurse can point out the baby's emerging capabilities. It is helpful for the nurse to teach the parents about developmental expectations and to suggest ways of encouraging new endeavors and enriching the infant's environment. The parents and other family members are best able to provide stimulation for the infant. Additionally, this knowledge helps the parents be prepared for, and realistic about, the demands of parenthood. Knowing what to expect of the infant increases the enjoyment that the parents and other family members experience in living with the child.

Characteristics of infant development

Babies are individuals. They have their own personalities from the very beginning. They all express themselves somewhat differently as they progress in their own way through the first year. One of the differences between infants is the timing of the developmental sequence. While the pattern of developmental milestones is predictable, the rate at which each child progresses varies. One infant sits unsupported at 6 months, and another not until 8 months. These differences are not indications of the child's later abilities. Healthy infants are simply expressing their own timetables. They will remain consistent with themselves. For example, a late crawler will probably be a late walker as well.

All areas of the infant's growth and development are *interdependent*. A cognitive achievement such as removing a barrier to find a toy may be dependent on a motor skill such as the ability to crawl and grasp. This in turn is dependent on visual maturity, and so on. Not only is the whole process interdependent, but it is *interrelated* as well. Language development, for example, not only is dependent on some degree of neurological maturity but also is interrelated with cognitive and psychosocial development.

Another characteristic of development is that it does not always progress in a smooth, forward movement. There are spurts and stops and regressions. An infant may seem to concentrate on one certain skill while everything else waits in the wings for its time on stage. Infants may master a skill and then seemingly lose it, only to have it reappear later. Regressions frequently occur, especially as a response to stress.

The pattern of infant development is from the head downward. Infants can control their heads before they can control their arms or legs. They can use their heads to look about before they can crawl or walk. Development also progresses from the *main axis outward*. This means that they are able to move their arms about before they develop the ability to pick up objects with their fingers. In this way, development follows the pattern of neurological maturation.

Individual differences

Infants are active participants in their growth and development. The process they are experiencing is not something that simply happens to them. They engage in activities that in many ways make it happen. They are *active stimulus seekers*. The amount of stimulation babies seek depends on their own temperament and other individual differences. (See the section "Infant temperament" in Chap. 8.) Some infants have higher stimulus thresholds than others. This means that they can tolerate more intense or greater levels of stimuli. When stimulation becomes too intense, however, infants are able in some measure to block it out. Thus they are able to regulate the stimulation they need to foster their growth and maturation.

Another observable difference between infants is the *amount* and *intensity* of stimulation that each will comfortably tolerate. Infants in general need a moderate level of stimulation in order to keep their attention. They lose interest in, or do not attend to, stimulation that is low in intensity. They withdraw (by avoiding or crying) from overly intense stimuli. The type of stimulation, as well as its intensity, must be varied to keep the infant interested. The complexity of stimulation needed differs among infants and among children of different ages as well.

Some infants respond to stimuli more slowly than others. These infants will not show the same degree of vigor in their response as a baby who reacts strongly and rapidly. They may also have less activity in general. Some infants seem to be always moving and on the go. Others are content to sit back, watch, and think things over.

Most babies have periods of fussiness, especially during the first few months. These periods generally follow a daily pattern and often occur, much to parents' displeasure, at about dinnertime in the evening. Some babies carry fussiness to extremes, however. These same infants are often the more active, responsive ones. They can be more difficult to console than their less fussy peers.

Cuddliness is another way in which infants differ significantly. Some infants mold to the adult's body when picked up and cuddled. They give the impression of relaxation and pleasure when held. Other infants simply are not that fond of being held. They are stiffer in the adult's arms and may push away. They are not content, as others are, to snuggle in.

Influence of the family on development

Parents come in all sizes and shapes and have varying degrees of skills. They come in pairs or as singles, with extended supports or with no supports. Whatever their circumstances, temperaments, and experience with the parenting role, they are a critical factor in the infant's development. Besides meeting basic physiological needs, which include nutrition, protection, nurturance, and stimulation, parents also carry out more complex tasks and responsibilities. The infant must learn about being human within a society of other humans. His or her beginning self-concept, ability to learn to interact with others, and incorporation of the values of the culture will depend a great deal on the parents' abilities in child rearing and their attitudes toward it.

Conditions of good parenting

Good parenting is not just a matter of instinct. Though the importance of good parenting is well established, we really do not know what conditions make it possible. The following list will no doubt be expanded and refined as research increases our understanding. It is offered as a basis for nursing assessment.

1. *Manageable stress* There are limits to the individual parent's coping ability. Stress, which we all experience in some degree, should be within the individual's ability to effectively manage. We know that such highly stressful conditions as poverty and severe illness are detrimental to positive parenting.
2. *Healthy state of mind* Parents need the capacity to get out of themselves and sometimes put their children first. Depression or other psychiatric conditions limit this ability. Acute grief may in some instances also have this effect, though its influence should be temporary.
3. *Positive childhood experience* Parents whose own childhood experience was enriching and nurturing have a better base to build upon than those who were less fortunate. Being loved as an infant and child builds in the capacity for love and makes possible the positive reciprocal relationship we call *good parenting*.
4. *Reasonable health* Good health allows the parent a full range of responsiveness. Chronic poor health can limit or influence the ability to be responsive and positive toward the child.
5. *Early bonding opportunity* There is evidence that early bonding has an influence on the parent-infant relationship. Many hospitals are adjusting their policies to allow for extended contact between the newborn and both parents to facilitate this parent-infant attachment. (Refer to Chap. 8 for a discussion of bonding.)
6. *Adequate knowledge about children* Parents who have had experience with young children are more able to accurately interpret their infant's behavior. They are likely to be more skilled in such parenting activities as feeding, diapering, bathing, and generally communicating with their infants. Unfortunately, many parents of this generation may be lacking in this experience. The decrease of size and the increased mobility of nuclear families and the subsequent loss of supportive contact with extended families have reduced exposure to infants and small children.

THE INFANT AND THE ENVIRONMENT

Communication in infancy

One-month-olds are awake more than one-third of the day. Most of their time awake is during daylight hours, giving them a significant amount of time to interact with people in their environment. Additionally, they are perfecting the use of basic equipment that they were born with and are developing new skills that aid them in communicating.

Infant-to-parent communication One of the most potent communication tools that infants have is *gaze*. They have the ability at birth to follow and fixate on an object, but this is limited by a visual field of about 8 to 10 in (a perfect distance for viewing a mother's face while nursing or being held). At 3 months infants can fixate on the mother's face and follow an object almost as well as an adult. They can follow the mother visually as she moves about the room and let her know of their interest. Infants communicate with their gaze. They "hold" onto the caregiver's eyes and brighten with excitement. This kind of stimulation given by the infant elicits a good deal of social behavior from the parent. (See Fig. 9-1.)

Infants aged 3 to 4 months have the ability to determine how much eye-to-eye communication they are willing to engage in. They can seek out eye contact or look away. Their movements are under control, and they can turn their heads to facilitate seeking or disengaging. This puts them on equal footing with the adult. They have become true partners in the interaction.

Facial expressions, of an impressive variety, are another means that infants use to communicate with adults. The smile is present at birth, but is most often seen when the infant is in a drowsy state or REM sleep. At about 6 weeks infants smile in response to tickling, a happy voice, a human face, or a gaze. By about 3 to 4 months infants use the smile to elicit a response from someone else. They have enough control over facial expressions to mix the smile with other gestures, communicating such complex feelings as ambivalence by just 4 to 5 months. (See Fig. 9-2.)

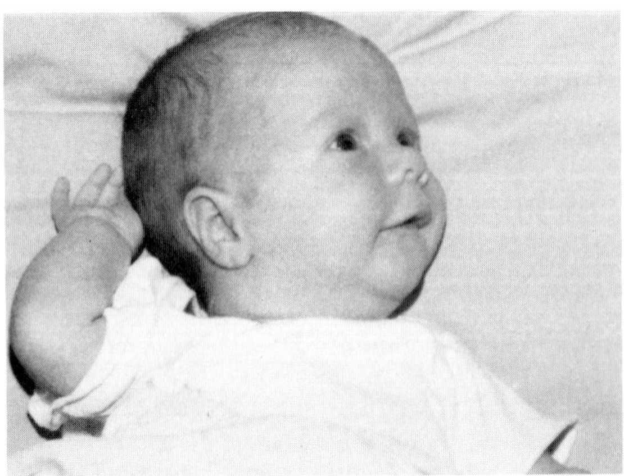

Figure 9-1 This baby girl is looking directly into her parents' eyes; observe her readiness for interaction, which is communicated by her gaze.

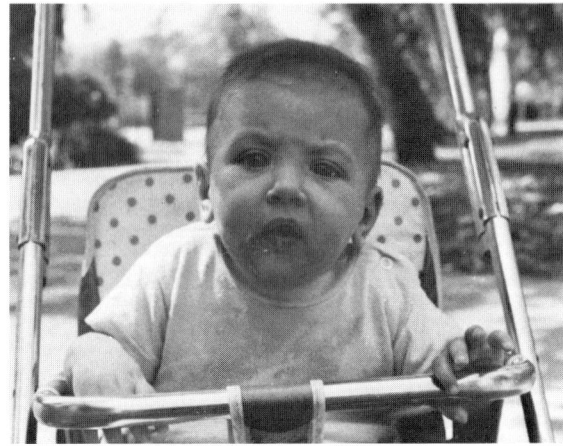

Figure 9-2 Complex facial expressions are the infant's means of communicating.

Laughing, another means of communication, appears between the fourth and seventh months. Laughing is first a response to tactile stimulation, such as tickling or playing patty-cake. Soon the infant begins to laugh at visual or auditory stimulation and then learns to utilize laughter to initiate an interaction or get a desired response from a caregiver. Crying and pouting are methods that infants use to communicate displeasure. The infant learns to expand on all the behaviors leading up to a cry to express varying degrees of unhappiness. A sober face and then a frown may be all that is needed in some situations. The full-blown cry is a call for some action.

Sensitivity of the infant to feeling tones Infants are very sensitive to the mood or tone of the environment around them. If the mother is relaxed, they are likely to be relaxed as well. If there is tension, the infant will probably show it in his or her behavior. The baby may respond with an increase in restlessness or fussiness or may be difficult to comfort, especially by the tense or upset caregiver. There may be a decrease in willingness to play or engage in playful interactions. Whatever behavior is displayed, the infant shows that he or she is a part of, and is sensitive to, the activities of the family and the immediate surroundings.

The infant's behavioral states The concept of behavioral state is included here because of its importance in understanding the relationship of the infant to the environment. In the last few years there has been considerable research looking at aspects of this relationship. Most descriptions of infant states identify the following clusters of infant behaviors:

Deep sleep state Breathing is deep and regular, the eyes are closed, and there are no movements except occasional startles.

Active sleep state Breathing is irregular, the eyes are closed and rapid eye movements are evident, and there are small muscle movements.

Drowsiness The eyes open and close but seem unfocused, there is little activity, and responses to stimuli are slowed.

Quiet alert, or alert inactivity, state The eyes are open, and there are no large movements.

Active alert, or alert activity, state The eyes are open, and there is diffuse movement and irregular breathing.

Crying state The eyes are usually closed or partly closed, and there are large movements and vigorous crying.

For the first 6 months and perhaps longer, the state of the infant at any given time influences his or her reaction to stimuli from the environment. A major part of the caregiver's task is to recognize the state and accordingly modify the stimulation the infant receives. A playful tickle when the infant is asleep may have little effect (unless of course it is quite vigorous, in which case it may bring the baby from deep sleep all the way to crying). The same tickle may be thoroughly enjoyed in an active alert state. It may aggravate the baby in a crying state and make the infant even more difficult to console. The mother's ability to approach the infant according to his or her state is very important in their developing relationship. How the mother perceives her infant's state will determine what she does and the kind of stimulation she provides. Conversely, what state the infant is in will determine his or her readiness for interaction and receptiveness to types and levels of stimulation.

Infant states can be modified by the caregiver and by the infants themselves. Some infants seem to have better inner resources and can keep themselves from reaching a crying state by self-consoling measures. Thumb-sucking, for instance, is a calming tactic employed by some infants. Picking an infant up is one method that mothers use to bring an infant from crying to a quiet alert state. Holding the infant upright, bouncing, swaying, or other vestibule-stimulating movements (such as rocking) are methods that mothers seem to use naturally.

The quiet alert state is the time when the infant is ready to interact by gaze. It has already been mentioned how significant this behavior is in terms of attracting and maintaining social interaction with the caregiver. If parents are not tuned into the readiness of their infant, their efforts to communicate may be frustrating and misleading. Insensitivity to state can lead to misinterpretation of the infant's behavior as dislike or rejection. For example, the infant's response to a friendly peek-a-boo game when in a drowsy state may be interpreted by the parent as boredom. Parents need to feel that the infant is responsive to the care and love they give. Parents need positive feedback from their infant to maintain the kind of mutual relationship that is so beneficial for growth and development.

Assessment of the infant's state and the parents' sensitivity to it is an important nursing intervention. Parents can be taught how to observe their infant, what to look for, and what approach might be best. They can also be taught how to bring the infant into an alert state from crying or sleeping. No parent and infant pair will be perfectly in tune all the time. Neither will all the techniques they learn work every time. The quality of reading each other's cues and being sensitive to each other's signals is a vital characteristic of healthy parent-infant interaction. Sometimes it takes a few months to establish this kind of harmony. The nurse who is involved with parents and infants throughout this first year should consider the quality of interaction a priority for assessment.

Parent-to-infant communication Parents hold, handle, stroke, cuddle, rock, sing, talk, play, and make faces when communicating with their infants. Adults, even those who are not parents, will automatically alter their interaction style to the infant. Mothers tend to be more gentle and comforting; fathers are more playful. If one characteristic stands out, it is *touch:* Touch is an important component of almost all parent-to-infant communication.

The timing of parent-to-infant communication is one of the most crucial variables. Communication, along with the intensity and type of stimulation offered to the infant, should be within the context of affection for, and interest in, the child.

The function of play

Ask a mother why she plays with her infant. The answer may well be something like: "Because I like to; it's fun!" Daniel Stern, in his book *The First Relationship: Infant and Mother,* expressed this by writing:

> The immediate goal of a face-to-face play interaction is to have fun, to interest and delight and be with one another. During these stretches of purely social play, there are no tasks to be accomplished, no feeding or changing or bathing on the immediate agenda. . . . We are dealing with a human happening, conducted solely with interpersonal "moves" with no other end in mind than to be with and enjoy someone else.[1]

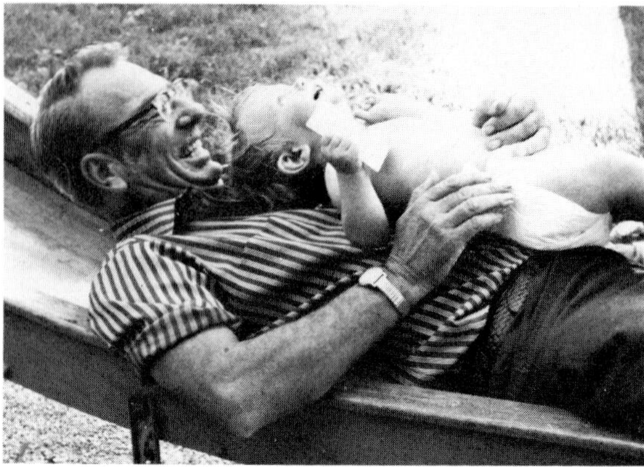

Figure 9-3 This grandfather and grandson are enjoying each other through sharing playful moments.

This kind of experience is invaluable for the infant. Learning is not the goal of playful interaction of this type, but of course learning is going on. The infant experiences how to be with another individual and how to share moments in his or her life. (See Fig. 9-3.) Appropriate toys

Table 9-1 Toys and stimulation for infants

1 month Pacifiers Lullabies Tape recordings of heartbeat Rocking chair Small, textured toys to clutch Mobile Large, bright pictures Your face close by	**7 months** Floating bath toys Kitchen objects String Soft rubber squeeze toys Small, soft, washable toys to clutch
2 months Music box Mobiles, dangling toys for crib Your smile	**8 months** Nested cups Roly-poly toys Space to creep Toys to bang together Big soft blocks Activity center for crib or bath
3 months Rattles (ring or dumbbell shaped) Music	**9 months** Toys tied to high chair Mirror (unbreakable) Jack-in-the-box Soft balls
4 months Crib or playpen gym Bells tied to crib Plastic disk on chain	**10 months** Pegboard Cardboard or cloth books Push-and-pull toys without handle Kitchen objects
5 months Suction toy for surface Toy to kick Interlocking plastic rings	**11 to 12 months** Stacking disks Large crayons Small items to place inside container Own drinking cup Bright, medium-sized ball
6 months Household objects to bang and throw Cups, spoons, pot lids, plastic containers Teething rings Squeaky, clutch toys Walkers and bouncers	

and other stimulating objects for infant play are listed in Table 9-1.

Playful periods are framed within the optimal stimulus level for the infant. If the mother and the infant are enjoying each other, then the stimulation being directed toward the baby is at the right level of intensity and is novel enough to maintain the infant's interest. At the same time, the infant is giving the mother positive signals, which is gratifying to her. (See Fig. 9-4.)

Mothers and infants are not the only playful pairs in the family. Fathers and babies play, too. In fact, fathers often take on the play role—especially the more rough-and-tumble type—within the family. When the father comes into view, the baby may anticipate this play and be ready and in an alert and aroused state.

Siblings also provide playful stimulation for the infant. Having a sister or brother is a very enriching factor in the infant's environment. Eye-to-eye playful interactions may be shorter in duration than with an adult or an older child and the infant. The enjoyment of being in each other's company and the acceptance that small children demonstrate for each other can help create a very positive atmosphere. The function of this play among all members of the caregiving unit is to deepen the affectional relationship they share with one another. (See Fig. 9-5.)

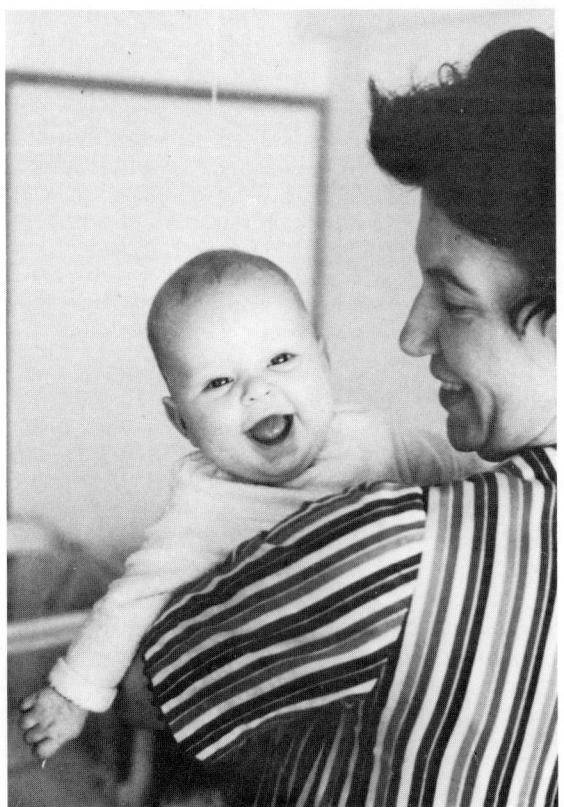

Figure 9-4 This infant is giving her mother positive signals.

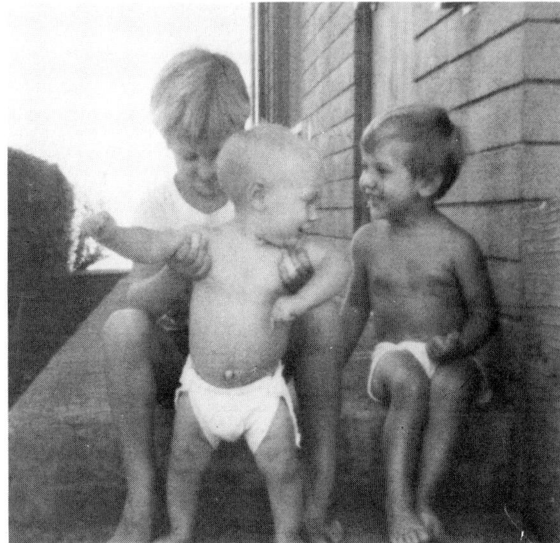

Figure 9-5 Siblings offer stimulation and learning opportunities for one another.

NUTRITION IN INFANCY

The relationship of nutrition to growth and development

The healthy infant grows at a very fast rate. Parents will claim that their son or daughter seems to get bigger right before their eyes. This is not far from fact. Normally, the birth weight is doubled by 5 months and tripled by 1 year. During this time the infant is gaining an average of 30 g a day.

The nurse must understand the special needs of the infant's immature body in order to understand the infant's nutritional needs for optimal growth and development. The infant's growth is a sensitive measure of his or her nutritional status. The human body uses nutrients first to maintain itself and then to support growth. The infant normally is very active and has high energy needs for maintenance. Because the organs and tissues of the infant are growing rapidly, the need for a constant supply of raw materials, or nutrients, is of paramount importance.

Consequences of inadequate nutrition

The infant under 1 year of age is particularly vulnerable to inadequate nutrition. Inadequate nutrition may take several forms. First, the infant may not get enough of the calories or nutrients needed to support both maintenance requirements and growth. Consider the consequences if this happens at a time when an organ or body part is growing by increasing its number of cells. The optimal number of cells for that infant's organ or tissue will simply not be produced. The size in terms of cell number is then fixed when this stage is completed.

Underfeeding of infants is a major cause of growth retardation and infant mortality in developing countries and those which experience famine and drought. Even in poor families in the United States, infants are at risk. The nurse should be aware that according to the 1983 census, one in every four children in the United States lives in poverty. The number of poor children from ethnic minorities is even more alarming, approaching one in two.[2]

The infant may have adequate caloric intake but lack specific necessary nutrients. An example of this might be inadequate iron ingestion or absorption, with resultant anemia.

Inadequate nutrition can also occur when the infant ingests too much of certain nutrients. Cow's milk, for instance, given undiluted to the young infant would be harmful because of the higher protein concentration. The young infant lacks the enzymes necessary to convert the type and amount of protein in cow's milk until about 1 year of age. The extra protein puts a burden on the immature kidneys. In addition, milk proteins cause injury to the intestinal mucosa of the infant, thereby causing small amounts of blood to be lost through the infant's stool. This compounds the possibility of anemia through loss of iron.

Malabsorption is another cause of inadequate nutrition in infancy. Malabsorption occurs when the infant's intake is adequate but the absorption of nutrients from the gastrointestinal tract is insufficient to meet energy and growth requirements. (Refer to Chap. 19 for a discussion of gluten-related malabsorption.) Allergies (cow's milk and milk-based formulas are often implicated) and intolerances to specific substances, such as lactose, can also cause malabsorption. Infectious diarrhea and parasites, which are common problems worldwide, also deprive infants of the benefit of the nutrients they consume.

The result of inadequate nutrition is, very broadly, the inability of the human body to function optimally. For the infant this may include growth retardation, problems in development, or both. It may also include a weaker body system that is unable to fight against pathogens and thus greater susceptibility to infection and disease. Severe forms of inadequate nutrition such as marasmus and kwashiorkor are rarely seen in the United States. These do exist in developing countries, during famine years particularly. Infants under 1 year are always the group most affected by lack of food or starvation. The morbidity and mortality rate worldwide is still high for nutrition-related causes.

Overnutrition may be considered inadequate nutrition because it is not optimal for the infant's health and well-being. There has been much speculation that overfeeding produces chubby infants, who then grow up to be obese adults. Recent research has not supported the belief that overfeeding in infancy results in fat cells that expand permanently, causing obesity in adulthood.[3] The psychosocial consequences of obesity in infancy and childhood are significant. Obesity that begins in childhood and continues into the adult years is very resistant to treatment.[4] The habit of overeating is formed early in childhood and is difficult to break. It is therefore important for the nurse to teach mothers not to overfeed their infants.

The nurse should teach mothers not to introduce solid foods before 6 months in order to prevent excessive caloric intake. In one study, feeding solid foods in infants under 3 months of age was found to result in caloric intake that was 125 percent of the recommended daily dietary allowance.[5] The mothers who introduced solid foods early had less knowledge of infants' nutritional needs and relied on their own mothers for advice. Less than 10 percent found the doctors' and nurses' advice helpful. They interpreted any crying and fussiness as indicating hunger.[6] Mothers need to understand the reasons for later introduction of solid foods and to be helped interpret their infants' crying.

Breast milk vs. formula

There is no doubt that breast milk is the optimum food for infants. Health professionals have sound reasons for encouraging mothers to nurse

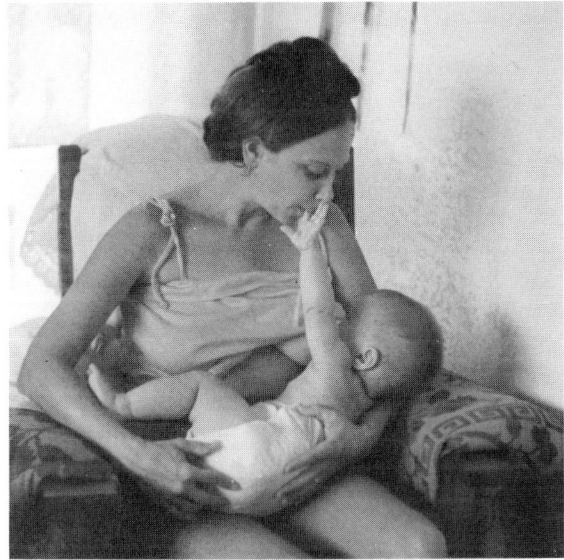

Figure 9-6 Breast-feeding is the preferred method of infant feeding. This infant is 8 months old.

their babies. An increasing percentage of women are now choosing to breast-feed. This increase follows a general decline in breast-feeding in the industrialized countries that began about 50 years ago.

Until dramatic improvements in sanitation practices came about in this century, non-breast-milk feedings were associated with very high infant mortality rates. Even today, in developing countries and among disadvantaged people in the United States, breast-feeding continues to confer an advantage in terms of infant health as compared with feeding formula. This advantage is most evident in the lower incidence of gastrointestinal diseases and in better growth patterns during the first 6 months of life among babies who are breast-fed.[7]

Most commercial formulas use cow's milk and have been made to resemble human milk in nutritional composition. Generally speaking, infants do well on these formulas. For mothers who choose not to breast-feed or for whom breast-feeding is contraindicated, these formulas offer very acceptable alternatives.

Nutritional comparisons *Protein* Current research indicates a need to reassess the protein requirements of infants. Recent studies have shown that infants fed with formula have metabolic changes indicating that they are receiving more protein than they require (most formulas contain 15 g of protein per liter).[8] Mature breast milk of well-nourished mothers contains about 7 g of protein per liter. The mean intake of protein of the breast-fed infant in the first few months of life, which can be used as a standard, is about 1.3 g/kg per day. Formula-fed infants take in approximately 2.2 g/kg per day, which is substantially more than their breast-fed counterparts get. Unmodified cow's milk must be diluted before it is safe for young infants because the protein content is 3 times higher than that of breast milk.

The most predominant proteins in breast milk are *casein* (curd protein) and *lactalbumin* (whey protein). The ratio of casein to lactalbumin in breast milk is approximately 35 to 65; the ratio in cow's milk is 90 to 20. These are significant differences in amount and kind of protein. The relatively low concentration of casein in breast milk makes it more digestible. Some infant formulas are modified in protein composition to increase the prominence of whey; altering the amino acid composition enables formula to compare more favorably with breast milk.

Breast milk is low in amino acids such as phenylalanine, which is detrimental in large quantities, and is high in cystine and taurine, which the infant cannot synthesize well. While the action of taurine in the infant is not well understood, it is found in the retina, it plays a role in the integrity of the cell membranes and in bile acid conjugation, and it may act as a neuromodulator. Cow's milk contains little taurine; the plasma taurine concentration is lower in formula-fed babies than in breast-fed babies.[9]

Enzymes present in the whey protein of breast milk may also protect against certain gastrointestinal tract infections. Lactoferrin is iron-binding and inhibits the growth of some iron-dependent bacteria, such as staphylococci, *Escherichia coli*, and *Candida albicans*. Immunoglobulins are also present in breast milk; IgG and IgA are the major types. Breast milk also contains leukocytes, which stimulate the maturation of the intestines and can prevent bacterial colonization and antigen penetration.

Carbohydrates Lactose is the major source of carbohydrate calories in milk. It constitutes 7 percent of breast milk, as compared with 4.8 percent of cow's milk. In addition to providing energy, this carbohydrate enhances the absorption of amino acids and minerals and the synthesis of B vitamins. Lactose promotes normal intestinal flora and discourages the growth of undesirable bacteria.

Breast milk contains a higher amount of lactose than cow's milk. When cow's milk is diluted to reduce the protein concentration, the lactose content is reduced as well. Milk-based formulas must be fortified with sugar in order to meet the caloric requirements of the infant. The fortification should be with lactose, since sucrose (table sugar) and corn syrup contain no galactose. A galactose deficiency can be damaging to the growing and developing infant.

Lipids A high percentage of the infant's weight gain during the first 4 months is fat (75 percent). This percentage continues to be high (44 percent) during the first year and then declines rapidly. In these first few months of life, the infant builds up a store of reserves. The infant with adequate fat reserves is better able to withstand infections and regulate body temperature and draws upon these reserves for energy as well.

Breast milk fat differs from that of cow's milk in several ways. It contains fewer total saturated fatty acids and 3 times as much polyunsaturated fatty acids as cow's milk. Infants digest and absorb fat from breast milk better than that from cow's milk. This in part is due to the fatty acid composition. Polyunsaturated fatty acids perform another important job for the infant. They are incorporated into cell membranes and help make hormone-type substances. These substances help regulate the transmission of nerve impulses and help control blood pressure and digestion. Breast milk fat also has antiviral properties.

Vegetable oils have replaced butterfat in many of the infant formulas because they improve fat absorption. Average breast milk is about 14 percent polyunsaturated fatty acid. Formulas with vegetable oil are higher by 2 or 3 times that amount. The effect of the higher levels of polyunsaturated fats on the infant is not yet known. There is a possible danger of vitamin E deficiency, however. This replacement of butterfat with vegetable oils has removed cholesterol from most formulas. Breast milk is a rich source of cholesterol. There is some thought that the cholesterol in early feeding may stimulate the body to produce enzymes that help in metabolizing cholesterol later in life. Cholesterol may also be important in the formation of nerve tissue.

Vitamins All vitamins except vitamin D are present in the breast milk of a well-nourished mother. Vitamin D is supplied by exposure to sunlight. Infant formulas are fortified with vitamins A and D.

Minerals Infants need the right amount of minerals in their diet. Salts are needed for bone growth and tissue growth, in conducting nerve impulses, and in muscle movement. Breast milk contains the right amount for humans. Cow's milk contains 3 times as much calcium and 6 times as much phosphate. These higher concentrations of minerals overwork the infant's immature kidneys. The undesirable ratio of calcium to phosphate can result in convulsions in the infant. This is another reason why cow's milk must be diluted, modified, or both when fed to young infants.

Zinc is an important element needed by the infant. Cow's milk contains more zinc than breast milk. Breast milk, however, contains a special zinc-binding protein that makes it possible for the infant to absorb zinc more readily. The infant therefore absorbs more zinc from breast milk. The bioavailability of iron and zinc is greater in breast milk than in cow's milk. Absorption of iron from breast milk is 50 percent or greater, whereas absorption from cow's milk is 10 percent; absorption from iron-fortified formulas is only 4 percent.[10]

Body defense systems There is a complicated system of defenses against penetration of the developing mucosal barrier by infection. Besides those previously mentioned, infants receive maternal antibodies that protect them against infection. Breast milk contains white cells, macrophages, and lymphocytes. Macrophages ingest and digest pathogenic bacteria. Lymphocytes, when suitably stimulated, can produce antibodies against bacteria. Breast-fed babies also receive protection against respiratory tract infections and otitis media. Breast milk prevents the attachment of certain bacteria—specifically, pneumococci and *Haemophilus influenzae*—to the pharyngeal cells.

Other disease fighters are friendly bacteria which discourage the growth of pathogens. Breast milk encourages the growth of these friendly organisms in the infant's intestine. In addition, it helps prevent allergies by providing antibodies that coat the intestine and prevent allergens from being absorbed. Breast milk is in itself nonallergenic.

Feeding patterns

No single feeding pattern or schedule will fit every mother-infant pair. Mothers and infants seem to adapt to each other's schedules and find the most satisfying and convenient times for feeding. Most infants will establish a pattern of feeding that is predictable before the end of the first month.

A *demand feeding* schedule is the term used to indicate that infants are fed whenever they are hungry. Most health care workers advocate feeding on demand. This is based on the belief that infants create their own schedule that is best for meeting their nutritional and psychological needs. For many years, however, scheduled feedings were advocated—usually every 4 h. Strict scheduling of feeding times does not meet the individual needs of the child and is rarely suggested today.

Parents have many concerns and anxieties regarding infant feeding. Many of these could be relieved if parents knew what to expect of their infants. Breast-fed infants, for example, may require feeding every 2 to 3 h during the first weeks. If mothers have not been prepared for this, they may think something is wrong with the infant or themselves. New mothers, especially, are sometimes apprehensive about their mothering skills and their ability to provide for their infant. They may fear that the infant is not getting enough milk and assume that their milk supply is inadequate. This uncertainty leads to discouragement.

After this first few weeks, infants usually require between five and nine feedings a day. This gradually decreases, until at 2 years they have adapted to the cultural feeding practices of the family. For most infants in western culture, that would be three meals a day, possibly supplemented with milk at naptime or before bed.

Infants differ greatly in their need for night feedings. Most infants are sleeping through the night by 2 months. Some lucky parents may get a relatively complete night's sleep by 3 weeks. It is not unusual for an infant to wake for night feedings until 10 or 11 months. Parents need to know that this is normal.

Breast-fed infants will regulate the amount of milk they take in to meet their needs. Bottle-fed babies must depend on the person feeding them to be sensitive to the cues they give that they are done. There is a tendency to overfeed formula-fed infants. The mother may think the meal is over when the bottle is empty, rather than when the infant signals that he or she is full. A pattern of constant overfeeding may be detrimental to the infant in that it may form habits that persist into adult life.

Parents are sometimes tempted to use the bottle as a pacifier. This practice has some inherent dangers, as does going to bed with a bottle. Young infants should *never* be left with a bottle propped. Most babies can begin to handle the bottle themselves by about 6 or 7 months. By this time they are mobile and adept enough to avoid the dangers of aspiration. However, these infants are erupting their first teeth. When an infant goes to sleep with a bottle in his or her mouth, milk or juice remains in the mouth. This gives rise to a condition called *nursing bottle mouth*. Bacteria in the mouth convert the carbohydrate in the milk to acid products which cause the teeth to decay. If the fluid in the bottle contains sugar or any freely fermentable carbohydrate, as is true of soda pop, punch, and juice, the decay and damage to the teeth increase. Babies who are breast-fed to sleep do not develop this syndrome if held in an upright or semiupright position (the usual nursing position). It is very important for parents to know about this easily preventable problem.

Weaning Mothers sometimes ask when they should wean their babies. There is no magic time when this should be done. In general, the mother should be encouraged to breast-feed for as long as she and the infant gain satisfaction from the experience. In the past, breast milk was an economically and nutritionally significant element in the infant's diet well into the second and third years. This is still true today in many traditional societies. In the more recent past, societal pressures have seemed to discourage all but the most single-minded mothers from breast-feeding beyond a few months. Today, however, there is growing acceptance of breast-feeding for longer periods of time.

Many infants gradually wean themselves. The pattern is generally from several feedings per day to one a day to several per week. The process may take a month or two to complete. The same pattern can be followed for weaning older infants from the bottle. It is a good idea to wean bottle-fed infants by 1 year in order to help prevent nursing bottle mouth.

Parents should be cautioned not to attempt to wean their infants during periods of disequilibrium for the family. A family vacation, a move, or any other change in routine may increase the infant's dependency on the bottle or breast. Parents should be sensitive to this when it is pointed out and wait for better timing.

The eruption of teeth is not a reason in itself for weaning a child from the breast. Infants may try their new teeth out on their mother's breast, but can be taught that this is not in their best interest. Simply stopping the feeding immediately when the infant bites will usually get the message across. Nutritionally, it is sound practice to continue breast-feeding through the first year or longer.

Introducing solid foods *Beikost* is the term used for foods other than milk or formula that are introduced into the baby's diet. In the past, the suggested age at which beikost should be introduced has been based more on opinion than on a sound understanding of infant physiology. Recent information suggests that there is no physiological advantage to introducing solid foods before 6 months. In fact, the liquid diet is best suited to the infant's physiological needs throughout the first year of life. (See Table 9-2 for feeding guidelines during infancy.)

Until very recently beikost has been introduced early, usually beginning with rice cereal as early as 2 to 3 weeks. This may have been encouraged because infants seem to tolerate these feedings without obvious distress. There are dangers, however. Introducing solids before 4 or 5 months may cause food allergies. Furthermore, if solids such as cereal are given in place of a formula or breast-feeding, the infant may not receive enough calories to maintain energy requirements and grow. If solids are given in addition to the formula, breast milk, or both, the infant risks being overfed, with resultant overweight by 3 to 6 months of age. In addition, the high-solute load of beikost creates a problem of hyperosmolarity. This, among other things, compounds the problem of obesity in infants.

There are natural compounds in food which can be harmful to the infant. These include sucrose, gluten, salt, and nitrates. And of course food additives, which may be harmful to all of us, are particularly dangerous to the more vulnerable young infant. The ingestion of food additives and contaminants can be reduced by preparing baby foods in the home and carefully reading the labels on commercially prepared baby foods.

The currently suggested age for introduction of beikost is between 4 and 6 months. It may be difficult to convince parents to wait this long. Parents are open to good information and advice, however. According to a Ross Laboratory survey, between 40 and 50 percent of mothers seek information about infant feeding from health professionals—the physician and the nurse.[11]

When semisolid foods are introduced, the usual order is cereal, fruits, vegetables, and finally meats. Variations in this order are common and depend on the preference of the family and the advice they receive from health professionals and friends. The order is not critical, but there are some ground rules that should be carefully explained to parents and reinforced as the infant begins solid foods.

First, new foods should be introduced one at a time in a small amount (1 tbsp), and not more often than every 1 or 2 weeks. The infant should then be carefully watched for intolerance of the food. This intolerance would most likely take the form of a food allergy. A symptom indicating a food intolerance might be rash, colic, gas, diarrhea, or vomiting.

Second, if there is a history of allergies in the family, foods that are potentially highly allergenic should be avoided. Egg whites and orange juice are examples of foods that are likely to produce allergic responses in susceptible infants.

Third, it is important to be sensitive concerning the right time to introduce foods. Infants show a readiness to accept beikost as the neuromuscular physiology of their mouths develops. The *extrusion reflex* (pushing food out with the tongue) begins to disappear at about the third or fourth month of life. Infants can then accept food on their tongues and swallow without most of it ending up on their chins. Infants begin to chew with a lateral motion of their jaws at about 6 or 7 months and can handle foods with more texture at this time.

When the infants' erupting teeth urge them to bite, junior (lumpy) foods should be introduced. Parents should be instructed to simply mash table foods for the baby; to use bite-size pieces of food, such as bananas or other soft-cooked fruits and vegetables; to give the child a few pieces of food and replenish them as necessary; and to allow the child to put his or her hands in the food—infants accept food better when allowed to explore and play with it. The floor should be protected with newspapers or towels. Then the child can hold a graham cracker, for instance, and enjoy practicing this skill, eating at his or her own pace.

At 9 months the spoon is introduced, and the child is allowed to continue finger-feeding. The

Table 9-2 Feeding guidelines for infants 6–12 months old

Age	0–2 months	2–4 months	4–6 months
Formula	Breast milk or iron-fortified formula	Breast milk or iron-fortified formula	Breast milk or iron-fortified formula
Total feedings per day	5–9	4–7	4–6
Each feeding	3–4 oz	5–7 oz	7–8 oz
Total intake per day	16–32 oz	20–36 oz	24–40 oz
Foods to add			Single-grain infant cereal (rice, barley, oatmeal) Fruit juice from cup (apple)
Foods to avoid	Honey (carries botulism spores)		Wheat and mixed cereals (allergy-producing) Citrus juices are acidic and particles cause choking
Guidelines	Hold nursing or bottle-fed infant securely in upright position. Never leave infant unattended or with propped bottle. Human milk can be hand expressed or pumped and frozen for later use. Formula should be tepid or cold. Plain water may be given.	Warm formula or breast milk by heating in pan of water (avoid microwaving)	Iron-fortified dry, boxed cereals are better source of iron and protein. Mix 1–2 tbsp dry cereal with breast milk or formula. Use spoon (not infant feeder, not mixed in bottle) to feed infant, which stimulates tongue development. Cereals are easily digested and low in protein

Age	6–8 months	8–10 months	10–12 months
Formula	Breast milk or iron-fortified formula	Breast milk or iron-fortified formula	Breast milk or iron-fortified formula
Total feedings per day	3–5	3–4	3–4
Each feeding	8 oz	8 oz	8 oz
Total intake per day	24–32 oz	16–32 oz	16–32 oz
Foods to add or continue	Strained or mashed fruits (applesauce, bananas, pears, peaches) Strained or mashed vegetables (carrots, green beans, squash, sweet potatoes) Toast, crackers, soft finger foods with increasing texture Fruit juice from cup	All infant cereals and adult-type hot cereals Mashed table vegetables Soft, peeled fruit (banana, pear, peach, apple, papaya) Strained meats (chicken, turkey, veal, liver, lamb, beef) Egg yolk, tofu, cottage cheese, sieved legumes Fruit juice from cup	Cereal, bread products, rice, pasta Cooked and raw vegetables Peeled, cup-up fruit Canned fruits (no added sugar or sweetener) Small pieces of tender meat, whole egg, peanut butter (smooth), mashed, cooked dry beans Fruit juice from cup
Foods to avoid	Foods with seasonings and sweeteners Corn, tomatoes	Fish, shellfish Continue to avoid foods with seasonings and sweeteners.	Foods which may cause choking (grapes, hot dogs, cocktail sausages, nuts, popcorn, carrot sticks)
Guidelines	Infants will take 6–9 tbsp of solids per meal on average. Fresh fruits and vegetables are best. Add textures as eye-hand coordination develops. Whole grain bread products have less sugar than teething biscuits.	Slowly introduce infant to table foods. Cut foods into bite-size pieces. Encourage self-feeding. Add foods with new textures.	The formula-fed infant can be weaned from the bottle and drink from the cup by 1 year. Continue to encourage self-feeding and table foods.

Sources: "Current Issues in Feeding the Normal Infant," *Pediatrics Supplement* 75(1), January, 1985; Furuno, Setsu, et al.: *Hawaii Early Learning Profile (HELP) Activity Guide*, VORT Corp., Palo Alto, 1979; Howard, Rosanne B., and Winter, Harland S. (eds.): *Nutrition and Feeding of Infants and Toddlers*, Little Brown, Boston, 1984; Perry, David G., and Kay Bussey: *Social Development*, Prentice-Hall, Englewood Cliffs, N.J., 1984; "Report of the Task Force on the Assessment of the Scientific Evidence Relating to Infant-Feeding Practices and Infant Health," *Pediatrics Supplement*, 74(4), October 1984.

child should be encouraged to practice drinking a small amount of liquid from a cup. Junior foods should be eliminated by 12 months, and finger foods from the family dinner should be used.

Caution and common sense should go together when determining what foods are appropriate for the infant. Nuts, raisins, small candies, corn, and other small foods are difficult to manipulate in the mouth and impossible to chew with the infant's limited teeth. They can cause choking and are therefore dangerous. In addition, it is amazing how often peanuts, in particular, find their way into even the older child's nostrils and ears. Parents can be warned about these hazards. (See Table 9-2 for guidelines for introducing new foods.)

Preparing baby foods Improper formula preparation is a common problem leading to nutritional disorders in infants. Overdiluted formula supplies too few nutrients and results in a decrease in, or cessation of, growth. If the formula is too concentrated, with insufficient water added, dehydration, hyperglycemia, acidosis, and other metabolic abnormalities develop. Severe fluid and electrolyte imbalances are usually corrected with intravenous feedings, and oral feedings of normal strength can then be reinstituted. Once the improper formula preparation is discovered, an important function for the nurse is parent education. Directions for preparing concentrated liquid and powder formulas are printed on the can. (Refer to Chap. 8 for a discussion of formula preparation.) The nurse reviews these directions with the parents. Measuring cups should be used when demonstrating correct water-measuring and formula-mixing techniques. It is important that the nurse ask the parent to repeat and demonstrate the correct procedure for formula preparation. If the parent is unable to read the directions on the can, then other directions should be obtained. This may mean that the directions have to be translated into the parent's language or into pictures. The community health department is an excellent resource for obtaining printed material on infant nutrition.

There are many commercially prepared baby foods on the market. These foods have no nutritional advantages over those prepared at home. The primary advantage is that of convenience. (See Table 9-3 for guidelines for buying commercially prepared baby foods.)

Home preparation of baby foods is easy and economical. A blender or food processor is helpful, although not absolutely necessary, if the parents are planning to do most of the preparation themselves. Fresh fruits and vegetables should be used whenever possible. Cooking techniques which preserve the nutrients in the foods should be used; it is best to steam vegetables, use minimal amounts of water, and avoid overcooking and frying. Canned foods packed in their own juices and without added salt are the next best alternative. Home preparation of baby foods helps reduce the amount of food additives, sugar, and salt that the infant ingests.

Table 9-3 Guidelines for buying commercial baby foods

1. Meats are vastly superior to meat combinations. High-meat dinners contain one-half the protein of whole-meat dinners.
2. Fruit juices with added sugar should be avoided.
3. Baby desserts are high in calories and low in nutrients and usually contain additives.
4. Labels on different brands of food should be compared for the best nutrition.
5. Foods with water listed first or foods with added salt, sugar, or starches should be avoided.
6. Lids should have an unbroken seal with no debris between the jar and the lid.
7. Food should be removed from the jar before being warmed and fed to the infant. When the baby is fed from the jar, the enzymes from the saliva may spoil the remaining food.

Source: Catherine DeAngelis et al., "Introduction of New Foods into the Newborn and Infant Diet," *Issues in Comprehensive Pediatric Nursing* 22–33 (April, 1977).

Baby foods can be prepared ahead of time and frozen in ice-cube trays; then a food cube is reheated when needed. The nurse should stress to parents the importance of scrupulously clean hands, utensils, and working surfaces to reduce the chance of food-borne diseases. Prompt refrigeration of home-prepared and opened commercially prepared food is necessary. Food should be frozen if it is not going to be used within 24 h.

Many babies are fed foods from the table that are part of the family's cultural eating patterns. Pacific Island infants are fed poi (made from taro root), while mashed potatoes or beans might be given to other infants, depending on the family's preference. In general, infants accept semisolid foods well and will express individual likes and dislikes, just as any other member of the family will.

Food supplements The breast-fed infant of a healthy woman receives all the vitamins necessary for growth. Vitamin D supplements are recommended for breast-fed infants if they do not have adequate exposure to sunlight or if the mother's diet is low in vitamin D. Commercially prepared formulas are enriched with vitamins, and almost all strained commercially prepared baby foods and junior foods also contain vitamin supplements. Many infants are given daily vitamin supplements. Three vitamins—A, D, and K—are potentially toxic if given in excessive amounts over a long period of time. The toxic effects of vitamin oversupplementation are discussed in Chap. 19. The need for supplemental vitamins should be based on an assessment of the family's and the infant's eating habits and the nutritional soundness of their diet. (See Appendix C-2, C-3, and C-4 for a list of the recommended daily dietary allowances of essential nutrients for infants.)

Fluoride strengthens the enamel of the teeth and increases their resistance to decay. This is particularly important in infancy and early childhood, when the teeth are being formed. Fluoride appears naturally in the water supply of some areas and in many vegetables grown where fluoride is in the soil or the water used for irrigation. Some cities and counties routinely add fluoride to the water supply. Fluoride supplements are recommended for infants even if they live in areas where fluoride occurs naturally or is added. The reason for this is that most infants do not drink water in quantities large enough to provide them with all the fluoride they need.

PHYSICAL GROWTH AND MATURATION

Why study growth?

Infants' growth patterns and the rate at which they progress toward maturity provide essential information about their health status. Comparing their progress with that of others of the same age, sex, and race and with their own progress over time provides the data needed to monitor growth. The usefulness of this information is based on several known characteristics of growth itself. First, human growth proceeds in an overall pattern that is similar in all healthy individuals. Second, this overall pattern is consistent over time. There are wide variations in individuals when it comes to actual size and rate of growth. The pattern remains consistent, however, and the individuals remain consistent with themselves.

The measurement of growth

Growth is measured by length or height, weight, volume, and tissue thickness. The most common measurements made of the growing infant are of length and weight. Newborn infants, tiny as they may seem, are almost one-third their adult height. If all is going well, they will increase in length to about half their adult height in the first 2 years. Along with this rapid early gain in height comes an equally impressive weight gain. Infants can be expected to triple their weight by the end of the first year of life.

Skeletal growth

Bone tissues serve a number of important purposes for the infant and child. The first that usually come to mind are the mechanical support, the mobility, and the protection provided by bones. The bones also store minerals that the body can draw upon to maintain a proper balance. The body manufactures blood cells in marrow tissues which help maintain the blood supply. Infants have blood-producing marrow throughout most of their skeleton. During childhood some of this marrow is replaced by fatty tissue.

Skull growth Infants' heads are larger in proportion to the rest of their bodies, as compared with adults' heads. At birth the infant's head is one-quarter the length of the body, while the adult's head is only one-eighth the length of the body. The head is one of the more rapidly growing body parts; it reaches adult size by the time the child is about 6 years of age.

Skull growth closely parallels brain growth. Measurements of head circumference and assessment of fontanel status are the methods that health professionals use to monitor this growth. The posterior fontanel usually closes by 3 months. The anterior fontanel remains open throughout the first year, closing between 18 and 24 months.

Facial skeletal growth The facial skeleton does not grow as fast as the skull. While the skull will be about adult size by age 6, the facial skeleton grows into late adolescence. If one looks closely at an infant, one can see that the eyes are about in the middle of the face, dividing the face equally from top to chin. As the facial skeleton grows, the facial proportions change. The largest amount of growth is in the lower portion of the face. The respiratory passages are increased, and the jaws develop to accommodate the permanent teeth.

Dentition

Teeth begin to form during the third fetal month. Usually the first teeth emerge through the gum when the infant is about 6 or 7 months of age. There is wide variation among infants, however; some infants show teeth as early as 3 months, and others not before a year. These first teeth are called the *primary* or *deciduous* teeth.

The teeth developed in the upper jaw, or maxilla, are called the *maxillary teeth*. The lower teeth, those developed in the mandible, are called the *mandibular teeth*. The infant's first two teeth are usually the lower central incisors. Next to emerge are usually the upper central incisors, followed by the upper lateral incisors. These six teeth are what the infant of 1 year of age usually sports as basic equipment. (See Fig. 14-9.)

Each infant responds differently to *teething*, the process of erupting the first teeth. Some babies become fussy and irritable during this time, and others have little discomfort. Most babies drool what seems like cupfuls. The salivary glands are active at this time, and teething stimulates them to produce. The infant has not yet developed the habit of swallowing saliva, and so it simply comes out of the mouth. While they are teething, infants also gum or bite whatever is in reach.

Some infants have diarrhea, refuse food, or have "cherry cheeks," or a teething rash around the mouth. Symptoms of an upper respiratory tract infection are often caused by the erupting teeth. The erupting tooth ruptures blood vessels and causes pain. This kind of behavior can go on for several weeks until the tooth emerges.

Teething can be stressful for parents because of the difficulty they have in consoling their infants. Rubbing analgesic ointment on the gums, providing a chilled teething ring, or giving the infant a frozen banana to bite on may effectively numb the gums and offer the infant relief.

Neurological maturation

Neural tissue grows faster than other tissues or organs of the body during infancy. In many ways the neurological system provides both the foundation and structure upon which the child grows and develops. This system, unlike other body tissues, experiences only one growth cycle. This cycle begins in the embryonic stage and continues at a rapid rate through the first year of life.

Myelinization *Myelinization* is the process whereby a fatty substance called a *myelin sheath* surrounds or coats the axon portion of some nerves. This seems to serve the same kind of function as insulating an electric wire. It helps the nerve impulse travel more rapidly and with less expenditure of energy.

The process of myelinization begins before the infant is born. By the time of birth the pathways of sensation and equilibrium are already myelinated in the brain. Most of the afferent (sensory) nerves are myelinated as well. This is very important when one considers the capabilities of the newborn and young infant. Many of these capabilities, such as sense of smell, are used in establishing the initial attachment with the mother.

Myelinization continues at a rapid rate for the first 2 years. Just after birth, there is a lot of activity in the cerebral cortex. The descending motor fibers (efferent nerve fibers) are myelinated from the head downward and correspond to the infant's developing capabilities.

Brain growth Before birth the brain develops by hyperplasia—an increase in cell numbers by cell division. From about the time of birth to 10 or 12 months of age, the brain grows by both hyperplasia and hypertrophy—an increase in cell number and size. After 1 year and until maturity, the brain grows by hypertrophy only.

Most brain growth occurs while the infant is still in utero, but the brain still develops rapidly until about age 2. At 2 years of age the brain is two-thirds the adult size. The importance of nutrition for the pregnant mother and the infant *cannot be overemphasized*. All this rapid growth is compromised if the necessary nutrients are not present and available.

A continuous supply of adequate oxygen is also necessary for the infant's brain development. Hypoxia results in nerve cell death and thus compromises brain growth. Like malnutrition during this critical period, hypoxia may leave brain development permanently retarded.

Reflexes Reflexes begin diminishing as voluntary muscle control develops and the cortex matures. Rooting, sucking, and swallowing come under voluntary control fairly rapidly as the infant refines these reflexes into well-organized, complex behaviors. Other reflexes, such as the survival reflexes, similarly disappear as voluntary behavior makes them unnecessary. Health professionals use the character and disappearance of reflexes to assess the neurological maturation of the infant. (Refer to Chap. 8 for a discussion of the infant's reflexes.)

Muscle growth

Muscles also grow rapidly during infancy. Muscles are developed and innervated early in uterine life, making movement possible. The newborn infant's body is about 20 to 25 percent muscle tissue. As the child grows, this percentage will increase until the muscle mass is comparable to that of an adult, or about 33 percent.

Probably the number of muscle fibers does not increase much after 1 month of age. By this time, the period of hyperplasia is over, and from early infancy the predominant growth is from an increase in muscle fiber size. The muscle growth rate throughout the first year is about twice that of bones.

Muscle growth is influenced by a number of factors, including nutrition, exercise, general health, and hormones. The hormones most influential during this period are the pituitary growth hormone, thyroid hormones, and insulin.

Gross and fine motor development

Motor development refers to the process by which the infant or child gains control over his or her body. The infant must practice in order to gain skill and strength. An alert, healthy infant is engaging in this process almost constantly.

Gross motor development refers to the development and maturation of the large muscles involved in the infant's sitting, crawling, standing, walking, and head control.

Motor development progresses from reflexive and generalized movement of the entire body to a more purposeful, differentiated movement in the infant. The head and neck muscles are the strongest and most developed at birth. By 3 months, infants are able to lift their heads to look around when lying on their stomachs, and they have some amount of head control when pulled to a sitting position or when held upright. Development progresses from the head downward and from the main axis outward. The trunk of the infant is the next area of increased strength and differentiation. Infants demonstrate this by coordinating the head, neck, and trunk to turn themselves over. As gross motor behaviors become mastered and integrated into more complex behaviors and as myelinization continues, infants learn to sit, crawl, and then pull themselves to a standing position. Table 9-4 presents gross motor developmental milestones of the first year of life.

Fine motor development requires use of the hands, the fingers, and the smaller muscles of the legs and feet. Fine motor development follows gross motor development. Infants can support their weight on their legs before they can develop the skill necessary to balance and step in order to walk. Table 9-5 shows the fine motor developmental milestones of infancy.

The digestive system

The infant's digestive system is so well developed that it can swing into action at the moment of birth. It is ready to digest and assimilate breast milk or a suitable substitute. Even the structure of the mouth is ready to assist the infant in supplying nutrients to his or her own body.

For the first 6 months of life infants swallow differently from the way they do later in life. They have some built-in safeguards to prevent choking while sucking and swallowing. The posterior portion of the tongue is raised against the soft palate while the infant sucks. This separates the mouth from the throat and provides a place to hold the milk. In this way the infant can suck and breathe at the same time. When swallowing, respiration is inhibited briefly while the epiglottis closes and the milk goes into the stomach. This whole process is aided by the infant's anatomic structure. The infant has a longer posterior soft palate than the older child or adult to assist in holding milk. Additionally, the passageway from the mouth to the pharynx is smaller.

The infant's taste buds are present at birth, but taste discrimination is not fully developed until about 3 months of age. Infants are fast learners and can tell differences in tastes and textures of food quite well by the time beikost should be introduced into their diets.

Intestinal flora are introduced through the infant's mouth almost immediately after birth. By 2 days they are well established. These bacteria are essential in the digestive process and also help protect the infant against infection.

Table 9-4 Developmental milestones: Gross motor development*

1 month	2 months	3 months	4 months	5 months	6 months
Reflexes					
Reflexes govern all movements Rooting, Moro, tonic neck, walking, and grasp reflexes are strong	Tonic neck and Moro reflexes still strong	Movements becoming voluntarily controlled Tonic neck, Moro, and walking reflexes are fading	Voluntary movements predominate Tonic neck, Moro, rooting, and grasping reflexes disappear		Swimming reflex disappears
Head					
Head sags unless supported Turns head side to side when on stomach Lifts head momentarily	Head sags forward when held in sitting position Lifts head momentarily at 45° angle when on stomach	Head sags minimally May lift chest off surface for 10 s when on stomach	Head erect. Turns head in all directions. Briefly holds head erect Raises head and chest off surface when on stomach. Bears weight on arms	Head held erect when sitting or pulled up to sitting position Helps to pull up body Balances head well Lifts head and shoulders when on back	
Sitting					
		Sits supported, back rounded, knees flexed	Sits with minimal support, if propped for 10 to 15 min. Back less rounded. May flex legs to lift hips when on back	Sits for longer periods (30 min) when well supported	Sits with slight support, pulls self up to sitting position. Sits well balanced in chair

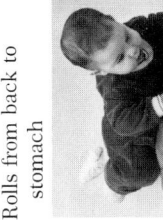

Kicking and rolling Straightens out arms and legs when playing Rolls side to back partway	Kicks well when excited or playful	Rolls from side to side May roll from stomach or side to back 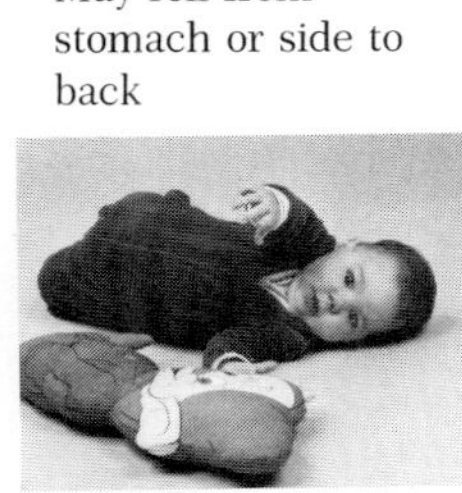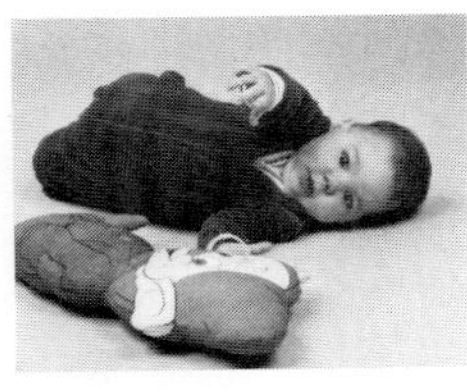	Rolls from stomach to back	Rolls from back to stomach Turns and twists toward all directions.
Crawling Makes crawling or swimming movements when on stomach	Moves arms and legs together on one side of body, then the other		Pushes on hands and flexes knees when on stomach	Crawls
Walking		Stands briefly with feet on surface when held in position	Stamps foot and supports most of weight in standing position 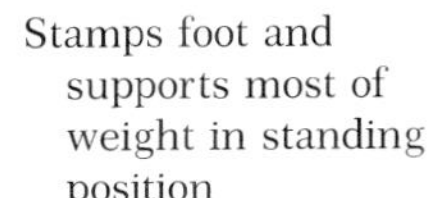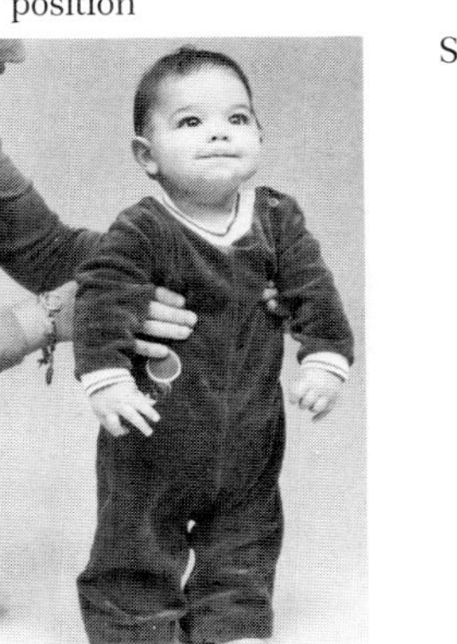	Stands with support

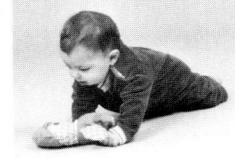

Table 9-4 (*Continued*)

7 months	8 months	9 months	10 months	11 months	12 months
Reflexes					
	Parachute and plantar reflexes disappear				
Sitting					
Sits alone steadily and briefly. Pushes self into sitting position	Sits alone steadily and bounces	Sits alone for long periods	Lowers self to sit		Lowers self to sit
Crawling					
Rocks in crawling position	Creeps 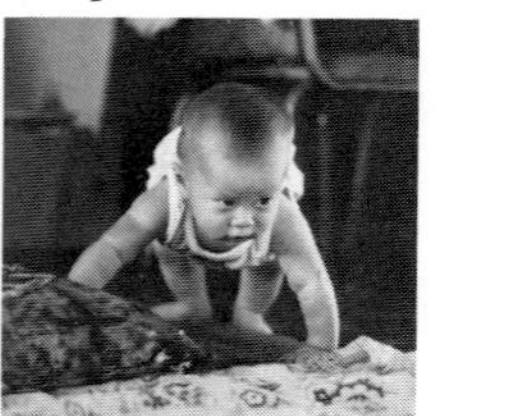 Pivots on stomach	Crawls and creeps instead of hitching (often backward at first)	Creeps forward Creeping and crawling are well coordinated		Prefers to crawl

Walking

Hitches Bounces and supports weight when held in standing position	Supports weight well when standing Stands leaning on furniture. Pulls self up on furniture	Cruises Pulls self to feet with help Stands alone briefly Stands holding onto furniture	Stands with little support Walks holding two hands	Cruising continues Pulls self to stand Lifts one foot while standing Walks with help	Stands by self Walks around small objects

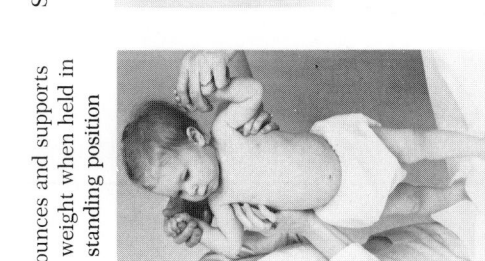

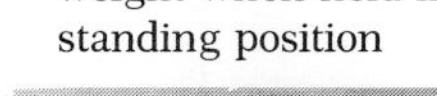
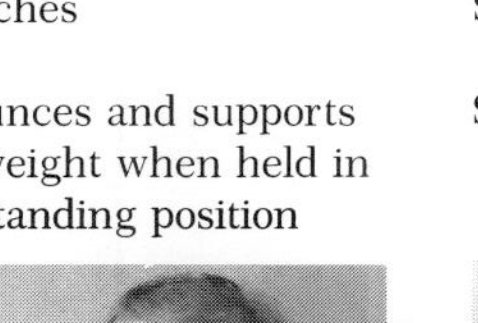
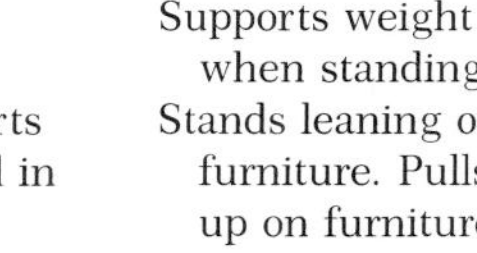
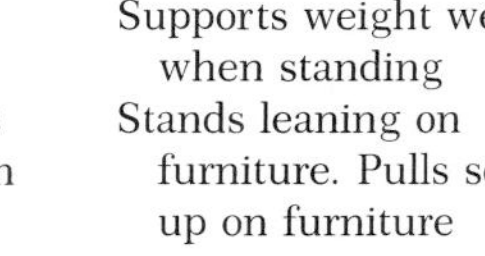
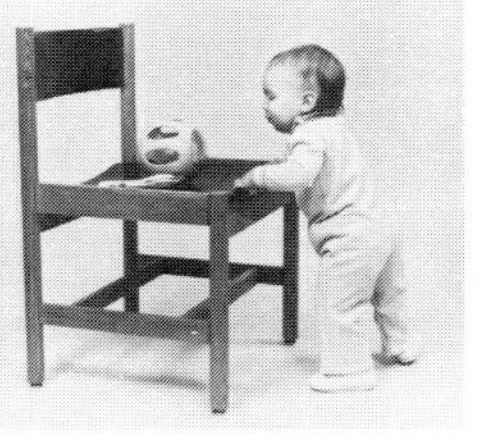
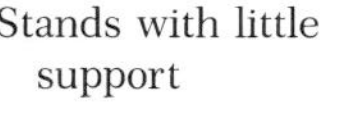
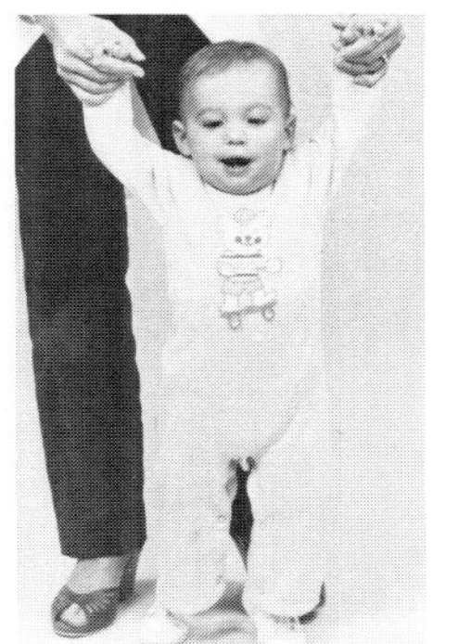
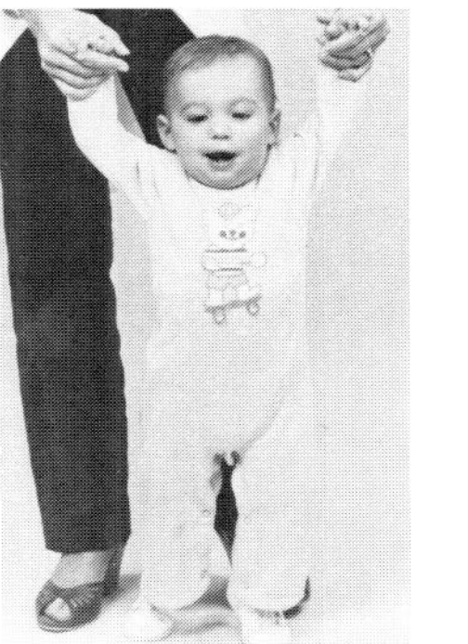

*Compiled by Nancy L. Ramsey.

Table 9-5 Developmental milestones: Vision and fine motor development*

1 month	2 months	3 months	4 months	5 months	6 months
Hand					
Immediately drops object placed in hand	Holds object momentarily (voluntary movement replacing grasp reflex)	Holds objects placed in hands	Grasps, holds objects, has better coordination Puts objects in mouth	Picks up object at will; often misses Holds one block; drops it to pick up another	Picks up object well Turns wrists to examine object Holds object well (bottle)
Fists usually clenched (grasp reflex)	Hands often open (grasp reflex fading)	Hands open (grasp reflex absent) Begins to hit at and often misses objects by large distance Begins to reach for object with closed fist Explores own hands and feet	Hits at objects; still misses Picks up object with entire hand; often misses it Plays with small objects and hands	Immediately puts object in mouth Begins to use thumb when picking up object Reaches for object with two hands. Pulls paper off face. Plays with toes. Plays with rattle in hand	Transfers toy from one hand to another Holds block no. 1, reaches for block no. 2, looks at block no. 3 Reaches with one arm
Vision					
Follows light with eyes up, down, and sideways Stares at objects	Follows moving light from outer edge to past midline Coordinates eye movements in circle	Follows object 180° Looks toward sound Looks from one object to another	Follows moving objects well Binocular vision coordinated Has increased eye-hand coordination	20/20 vision develops Stares at small objects Eye-hand coordination improving	Moves body to better view object Examines objects upside down to change perspective
Prefers pattern to color	Begins to focus on close object (8 to 10 in)	Focuses on objects throughout the room	Sees in color Looks at and grabs objects Perceives depth and distance		Eye movements coordinated and mature

Table 9-5 *(Continued)*

7 months	8 months	9 months	10 months	11 months	12 months
Hand					
Holds 2 to 3 blocks Picks up small objects; bangs objects on table Searches for dropped object Lifts cup by handle	Holds objects for 3 min Begins to use pincer grasp to pick up objects Reaches for toys Rakes at objects Releases objects	Plays with two objects held at same time; hits them together Hand preference obvious Pokes with index finger	Holds two objects in one hand	Holds crayon to mark on paper	Reaches for objects without looking
			Pincer grasp is well coordinated Finger-feeds self May build two-block tower	Places several objects in container Finger-feeding is better coordinated Pushes toys	Pincer grasp is complete Places tiny objects in bottle Removes covers of containers Turns book pages
				May pull off socks and untie shoes	Feeds self with spoon May undress self
Vision					
Stares at tiny objects Depth and space perception begins Searches for fallen objects	Looks before reaching for object	Depth perception is more acute	Reaches for unseen objects		

*Compiled by Nancy L. Ramsey.

Parents are often distressed if their infant spits up frequently. Many infants do this on a regular basis. Unless the amount is substantial (in which case it is more like vomiting than spitting up), there are no ill effects. Infants will grow out of this by 6 or 7 months as the digestive system matures. Holding the infant in an upright position after feeding and burping may help.

The small and large intestines Milk is held in the stomach and released slowly into the small intestine. In the infant, the stomach is usually emptied within 3 h after a meal. The rapidity with which the stomach is emptied can vary depending upon the type of food ingested. Breast milk leaves the stomach at a faster rate than formula.

Most of the actual digestion occurs in the small intestine. Bile and pancreatic secretions join with the food to break it down into usable nutrients. These nutrients are then absorbed into the bloodstream from the small intestine. What is not absorbed, plus the waste, continues on to the large intestine.

The composition of the infant's bile is not mature until about 6 months of age. Bile and pancreatic lipase, which is being secreted adequately by about 3 months of age, are necessary for the digestion of fats. The infant is not capable of digesting all fats until about 1 year of age.

The large intestine absorbs water into the bloodstream. Infants' stools are usually watery and frequent, partly because food is passed swiftly through the large intestine and there is not enough time for water absorption. Another reason is that the infant simply does not absorb water as well as an older child because his or her system is relatively immature. More residue remains in the intestine, which in turn keeps more water from being absorbed. By the time the infant is 1 year old, the large intestine is more efficient, and the stools are firmer and less frequent.

Liver function related to digestion The liver performs a great many functions in the body, some of which are directly related to digestion. Besides producing bile, the liver helps metabolize proteins, fats, and some vitamins. It acts as a storage center for iron, supplying the infant with this needed mineral for several months. The liver converts glucose into glycogen and stores it in order to keep a relatively stable blood sugar. Though the infant's liver is immature, it performs these functions well, increasing in efficiency as the child grows.

The excretory system: kidneys and bladder

The newborn infant's kidneys are quite immature. They are equipped to handle breast milk. Increased amounts of fluids or foods with a high solute load (e.g., cow's milk) endanger the infant by overtaxing the kidneys. The kidneys mature at a rapid rate during the first few weeks of life. Specifically, there are maturation changes in the tubules and in the Bowman's capsules. The tubules become longer and wider, and the epithelial membranes of the Bowman's capsules become thinner and better able to filter. By 6 months, the kidneys have become better able to adapt, and renal function is markedly improved. Because of the relative immaturity of the kidneys, infants are especially vulnerable to fluid and electrolyte imbalance.

During early infancy, the bladder empties automatically when it contains about $\frac{1}{2}$ oz of urine. The amount of urine the bladder can hold increases by small amounts over the first year. The infant is not ready for voluntary bladder control. The child develops an awareness of a full bladder after 1 year of age.

The immune system

Infants begin life protected against infection by antibodies provided by the mother through placental transfer. Shortly after birth, they begin to develop their own antibodies through their own immune systems. (See the section "Body Defenses" in Chap. 8.) At first this immature system is sluggish and responds slowly or not at all. With more antigenic stimulation the infant begins to respond more quickly in making antibodies. By about 5 months of age the infant's immunoglobulin level is based almost completely on antibodies made by his or her own system. It takes the entire first year to approach levels similar to the older child's or adult's, however. Even then, not all types of immunoglobulins are being produced at the same level as by an adult. Immunoglobulin A (IgA), for instance, found in saliva and secretions of the respiratory tract, does not reach adult levels until adolescence.

The thymus is the most important of the infant's lymphoid structures. It has a particularly important function for the young infant and child.

The thymus secretes a hormone called the *thymic factor*. It is believed to be essential for production by the thymus of T lymphocytes, which are important in cell-mediated immune reactions. Normal functioning of the infant's immune system is dependent on a healthy thymus.

Other lymphoid tissues include the tonsils, adenoids, spleen, and lymph nodes throughout the body. Certain lymphoid tissues are responsible for producing activated lymphocytes in the course of an immune response. The nodes and other lymphoid tissues also act as filters to trap pathogens before they enter the bloodstream so that phagocytic cells can attack them. Because the ability to make antibodies is not well developed in infancy, this filtering system is especially important. The lymphoid tissues grow rapidly during infancy and reach peak volume at about 12 years.

Vision

Vision does not depend strictly on the maturity of the eye. The infant must learn to utilize the eye and all its properties and to interpret what he or she sees. Much of this process is cognitive in nature.

Vision is dependent on a number of capabilities that the infant must develop. *First,* the infant must focus the image on the macula while adjusting to differences in distance. *Second,* both eyes must function together. This is accomplished by control of the extraocular muscles. Most infants coordinate their eye movements well by 3 months, and by 6 months this function is mature.

Third, the infant must develop the capacity to perceive differences in color and brightness. The macula is mature at about 6 months of age. The rods are probably well developed by birth. The cones, however, take longer and mature as the macula develops. Color vision then follows brightness discrimination. Infants seem to begin to respond to specific colors by 1 or 2 months. Maturation of the macula also allows the infant to see smaller items in detail.

Fourth, the infant must learn to perceive depth. This is dependent on being able to focus the image on the macula in both eyes simultaneously. The image seen with each eye is slightly different because of the different angle and distance of each eye from the object. These images must be fused in the brain to get depth perception. Crawling infants avoid steps and steep drops. Because of this, it can be assumed that depth perception is developed in the infant by crawling age—6 to 9 months. Table 9-5 shows visual development throughout the first year of life.

Hearing

Hearing is one of the better-developed senses in the infant. The fetus can hear in utero and responds to loud sounds. The newborn can distinguish sound frequencies and will turn toward a voice or other sound. Newborns may even already be familiar with the mother's voice. By just a few months of age babies can locate the mother by her voice even in a crowded or noisy room. The progressive development of the infant's hearing is outlined in Table 9-6.

PSYCHOSOCIAL DEVELOPMENT

Building a sense of trust

Erik Erikson's work has had an enormous impact on the study of children. He offers the hypothesis that there are eight stages of social development, each with a task that must be mastered before a stage is achieved. The task of infancy is development of a sense of *trust.* The counterpart of trust is mistrust. Establishment of this basic sense of trust or mistrust will determine how the child approaches all the future stages of his or her growing identity. If infants establish a basic trust in other people, themselves, and the environment, they will have a healthy beginning. Future relationships will be characterized by this trust, allowing for deeper commitment and intimacy.

Factors influencing the establishment of trust

Gratification of basic needs Need gratification is an important part of the establishment of basic trust. Infants make valiant attempts to communicate their needs—often by crying—but are dependent on the willingness and sensitivity of those around them to respond appropriately. Infants are in the best possible position to grow and develop when their needs are consistently met.

Sucking can be considered a basic need in the infant. Sucking has a specific function, that of getting nutrients into the body. Apart from the need to obtain food, however, babies seem to need to exercise their ability to suck. Here again there

Table 9-6 Developmental milestones: Hearing and language*

1 month	2 months	3 months	4 months	5 months	6 months
Hearing					
Is startled by sounds (Moro reflex) Quiets when hears voice	Turns head toward close, familiar sound Listens to bell	Turns head toward sound; searches for it in room Stops sucking to listen		Locates sounds below ear	
Crying					
Cries and makes throaty sounds	Crying predominates Crying becomes differentiated; pattern, pitch, and intensity vary	Cries less	Cry increasingly varies in volume, tone, and duration		
Laughing					
		Chuckles; squeals with pleasure when talked to by parents or when happy	Laughs aloud Smiles, gurgles, and grunts "Talks" with pleasure for 20 min	Still squeals	Belly laughs Laughs and squeals Babbles (one syllable) with pleasure Enjoys listening to own voice
Talking					
Responds to voice Begins to coo	Coos; still makes throaty sounds "Talks" to family members	Babbles and coos "Talks" when spoken to	Cooing changes pitch and volume Talks more to face than objects Is "talkative" "Talking" varies with moods Begins consonant sounds: H, N, K, G, P, B	Makes vowel sounds (ee, ah, ooh) Consonant sounds increase Attempts to imitate sounds	Combines vowel and consonant sounds (ee, ka) Imitates sounds; varies pitch and rate "Talks" to toys and image in mirror Calls for help

Table 9-6 *(Continued)*

7 months	8 months	9 months	10 months	11 months	12 months
Hearing					
Reacts to changes in music volume	Recognizes familiar words; responds to familiar sounds	Listens to talking Understands and responds to one or two simple commands	Listens to common words	Begins to differentiate between words	
Talking					
Makes four different vowel sounds Combines syllables (da-da, ma-ma) "Talks" with adultlike inflections when others are talking	Shouts for attention Talking shows emotion Responds to "no, no" and "bye-bye" May label object with sound (kitty, meows)	Says "ma-ma" and "da-da" meaningfully "Talking" increasingly shows emotions Initiates coughing Intonation becomes patterned	Says one word ("hi," "no") Combines consonants Understands and responds to own name and "bye-bye" Associates action with word (waves); says "bye-bye" Understands simple commands ("Come here")	Says two or three words with meaning; uses jargon Uses few definite speech sounds Continues to imitate intonation and expression Recognizes word as symbol for object	Says three words with meaning Enjoys jabbering expressively, in short sentences Vocalization decreases when walking Comprehends meaning of word before speaking Understands commands ("Go get my shoes") Knows own name May have one word for a whole class of objects

*Compiled by Nancy L. Ramsey

are individual differences. Some babies seem to experience a great deal of need gratification from sucking, both when feeding and when using a pacifier. These babies use this mechanism to help establish a state of quiet and comfort, allowing them to devote more of their energies to the task at hand—developing basic trust.

Another need that must be gratified in the infant is relief from *hunger*. Hunger may be one of the most intense need states that the infant experiences. If infants' need for food brings a quick response, they are likely to perceive the environment as trustworthy. They learn to rely on the primary caretaker, who is usually the mother. Infants who are deprived of food or who receive an inconsistent response are at risk for viewing the world with distrust.

Infants need to be kept warm. Very young infants, because of their relatively low proportion of body fat, large amount of body surface area, and physiological immaturity, cannot adequately regulate their temperatures. By providing *physical warmth,* caregivers help infants maintain some physiological equilibrium and thus help them conserve energy. When infants are comfortable, their behavior is much better organized, their development is enhanced, and their physical recovery is faster. Comfort helps establish a sense of trust.

Psychological warmth is just as important to the infant as physical warmth. Psychological warmth is difficult to look at in isolation because it is related so closely to stimulation and affection. Infants need to be in close human contact. They need to be held, enveloped, and cuddled. They need to be *touched*—skin to skin and with gentleness and warmth.

Infant carriers of the type pictured in Fig. 9-7 are excellent aids for providing this close human contact to young infants. They allow the mother or caregiver to spend more time with the infant while attending to daily tasks. The alternative is for the infant to spend this time in a crib, stroller, or infant seat, none of which provide the same mobility or person-to-person contact. The mother is in close contact and is better able to anticipate changes and respond to the baby's states or needs.

Infants need *stimulation* to maintain their growth both physically and psychosocially. Stimulation that is appropriate for the individual child in amount, intensity, and timing characterizes the loving and responsive relationship and helps to establish the infant's basic trust.

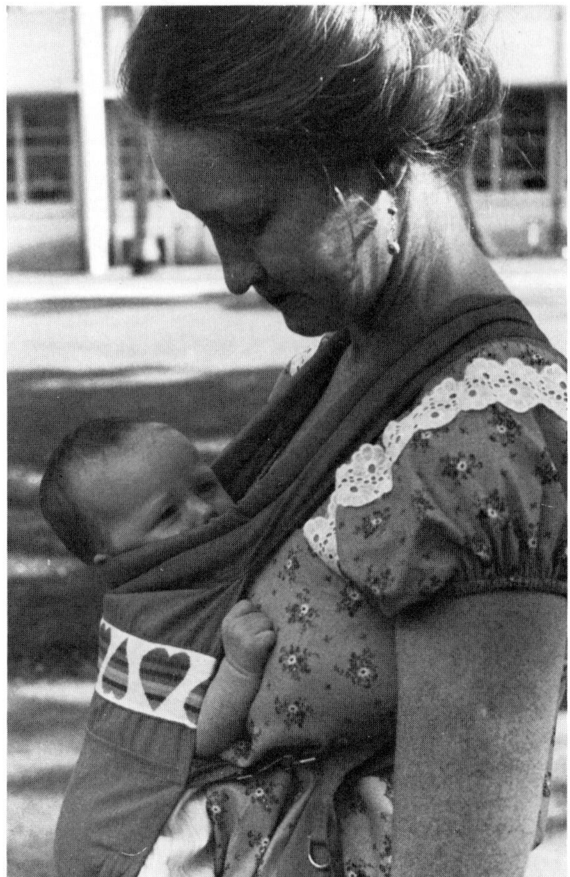

Figure 9-7 Using an infant tote is an excellent way of maintaining close contact with the infant and promoting the infant's trust.

Predictability Part of developing trust is dependent on the infant's ability to predict what will happen in his or her environment. Some families have very well-established routines, while the life-styles of others are not, at least on the surface, so well organized and patterned. Generally, babies are very adaptive and can pick out those consistencies and people they can rely on. Difficulties arise, however, when events such as illness and hospitalization make it impossible for the infant to predict what will happen. Such events should be viewed as grave threats to the infant's ability to establish trust. Every effort should be made to restore a sense of normalcy and predictability to the infant's life.

Interpersonal relationships The quality of the *interpersonal relationships* that the infant is engaged in is of utmost importance in developing trust. There are several characteristics the nurse can look for when assessing these relationships. First, the response the infant receives should be related to his or her behavior. Something should happen as a result of what the baby does. It is confusing if the infant smiles at his or her mother in a face-to-face position and nothing happens. The infant must learn what effect he or she has had on the environment. Much of this contingency is dependent on the caregiver's ability to respond to and interpret the infant's cues (Fig. 9-8).

The relationship should be characterized by *affection* and *nurturance*. The caregiver is genuinely interested in the well-being of the child and emotionally involved in the interaction. The emotional involvement may include elements of protectiveness and possessiveness. There is identification with the infant as well. When the infant gets an immunization injection, the mother may shed tears right along with the child. As a whole, the relationship is loving and responsive.

It is a normal part of the infants' experience to encounter new situations. Because of their rapid development, their world expands almost continually. The parents' function is (1) to make sure that the new encounter is not needlessly stressful, overwhelming, or dangerous and (2) to provide a base from which the infant can try out short periods of independent exploration. Children who face new encounters with the support of a loving adult establish trust and maintain their curiosity and openness to the world and events around them. Table 9-7 summarizes the psychosocial developmental milestones of the first year of life.

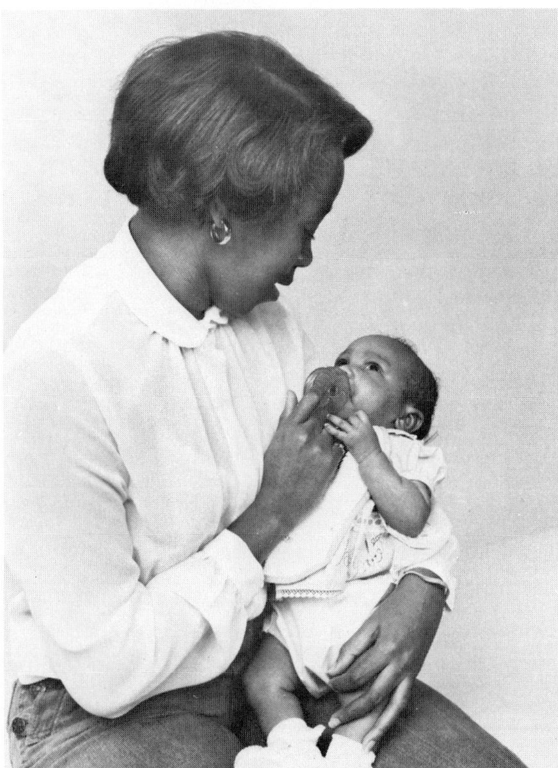

Figure 9-8 The caregiver's response to an infant is important in promoting trust.

Attachment behavior indicative of trust Babies become attached to their primary caregivers. The quality of this attachment is important in the establishment of basic trust. It is also a major determinant of how an infant will face new situations or tolerate and enjoy independent exploration.

In order for infants to show attachment behavior, several skills related to their cognitive development must be evident. First, they must be able to differentiate the mother or other primary caregiver from other individuals. To do this, they will first have to develop the ability to view themselves as separate from the environment and to distinguish between objects and people and finally between the mother and other people. Infants become aware of themselves as separate from, but dependent on, the environment (Fig. 9-9). As they experience contingent relationships, they sense their own power to control what happens to them. If they cry when hungry, they bring the mother to the rescue. Their interactions help them become more differentiated from the environment and focused in their responses.

Next, infants must develop a set of expectations for the mother or primary caregiver. This requires even more cognitive skill, for they must anticipate the mother's behavior on the basis of what they know of her. They have then developed a concept of mother that requires both memory and object permanence. These expectations reveal the quality of the trusting relationship.

Infants seem to progress through three very broad stages in developing attachments. In the first stage very young infants are undifferentiated in their attachment behavior. They prefer people over inanimate objects but will respond to all adults who give them appropriate social stimulation. Infants smile and brighten as a re-

Table 9-7 Developmental milestones: Psychosocial development*

1 month	2 months	3 months	4 months	5 months	6 months
Interaction					
Watches parent's face Establishes eye contact	Follows movement of caregiver around room Prefers people to objects Sucking need continues to be maximal	Watches environment, alert up to 45 min Recognizes mother Recognizes and distinguishes between family members	Has increased interest in mother; shows trust—knows mother Discriminates among faces; adjusts responses to people	Distinguishes self from mother Begins to explore mother's body; is playful Lifts arms to be picked up Clings when held Is interested in other family members; distinguishes adults from children Shows emotions of fear and anger Protests when toy is removed Delays gratification Begins to smile at self in mirror	Knows parents; begins to stop indiscriminate socializing with adults; begins to show stranger anxiety Imitates parents' behavior Smiles at self in mirror Plays peek-a-boo
Molds and cuddles when held; interested in mother Intensely needs to obtain satisfaction and comfort through sucking and being held, rocked, and touched	Shows satisfaction and delight in response to pleasurable stimuli Smiles and "talks" to family members	Social stimulation is more important Moves entire body and changes facial expression when stimulated	Demands social attention; becomes fussy and bored if left alone Enjoys attention		
Play					
Becomes excited when sees parent or toy	Excitedly anticipates movement of objects	Smiles immediately	Chuckles, laughs, and "talks"; talks more to face than object Entire body shows excitement	Plays with rattle Pats mother's breast	Plays with feet

Table 9-7 *(Continued)*

7 months	8 months	9 months	10 months	11 months	12 months
Cries					
Cries for attention, help, or when distressed. Cries are result of inner needs, not reaction to environment Quiets when picked up or watching parent's face	Crying differentiated; volume, pitch, and strength vary with inner need Shows distress Sucks to quiet self	Crying decreases markedly; stops crying when parent enters room and holds child Is awake for longer periods without crying Squeals when frustrated Quiets quickly when concentrating on a face	Has mood changes Responds to "No!" Wails when pleasurable activity interrupted Quiets self Is quieted by music		
Interaction					
Stranger anxiety increases; cries when mother leaves Wants to be included in family's social interaction Distinguishes between angry and happy voices Mood swings increasing; shows humor; bites; mouths objects aggressively Resists unwanted objects and food Pats image in mirror	Stranger anxiety is at its height Separation anxiety is increasing; fearing separation, follows mother around house Resists and avoids isolation or confinement Continues to reject unwanted objects Kisses image in mirror	Perceives mother as separate being Anticipates feeding by mother Performs for family members if rewarded Plays out fears and problems Begins to evaluate moods	Tenderly cuddles toy Begins sexual identity Is jealous if other child receives attention Still shows emotions: happy and sad Is increasingly aware of approval or disapproval	Is increasingly dependent on mother Asserts self among family members Seeks approval; avoids disapproval Shows guilt	Separation anxiety increases Prefers certain people, especially women Fears strange people and places Expresses all emotions; has sense of humor and is affectionate Is negative; refuses toys, meal, etc.
Play					
Chews feet, explores body Excitedly anticipates play Plays with toys	Constantly reaches for toys Loves play	Imitates play Chooses a specific toy Plays ball and pat-a-cake	Enjoys music	Engages in parallel play Imitates other children's play	Plays games

*Compiled by Nancy L. Ramsey.

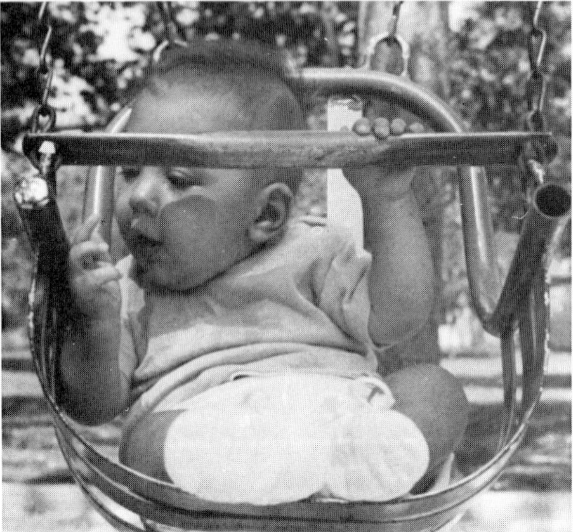

Figure 9-9 Looking at the hand is an indication of the infant's growing awareness of himself or herself as separate from the environment.

sult of face-to-face attention and show general arousal. They may show a preference for their mother by visually pursuing her and looking at her when there is a choice, but they are happily responsive to all people around them. In the second stage, between about 4 and 8 months, infants progress to an exclusive or single attachment to the caregiver, usually their mother. At this time infants show a definite preference for their mother. They clearly want to be in her presence and show this in no uncertain terms. They brighten when she comes into view, reach up to be held, and follow her both with their eyes and to the extent of their mobility. Early in this stage infants are still relatively friendly to strangers, though they definitely prefer their mother.

From 6 months through toddlerhood, babies' attachment to their mother and significant others is intense and is clearly a source of emotional security. They will allow only attachment figures to console them, especially when very distressed. They protest separation from their mother with great vigor.

The infant begins to show some degree of fear of strangers soon after this single attachment becomes evident. This behavior is called *stranger anxiety* and is typically very strong at 8 months. At this time the infant does not respond happily to all people. Social stimulation from a stranger is likely to elicit a sober face from the attached infant. The amount of stranger anxiety displayed is different for each infant. The familiarity of the setting, whether the mother is present or not, the behavior of the stranger, and possibly the behavioral state of the infant will all have an effect.

Stranger anxiety is sometimes considered an indication of attachment because it clearly shows that the infant has a preference for the mother. Infants have different strategies for responding to the approach of a stranger, however, which might not be related to the firmness of their attachment. Some infants scrutinize the stranger for a few moments before showing a fear response and then use gaze aversion or look away in order to control their exposure to the threatening situation. These infants seem to have developed techniques to help them pace their responses. Other infants become intensely distressed and overwhelmed when confronted with the task of socializing with a stranger. Sometimes this behavior is elicited if the stranger approaches rapidly, loudly, or directly, for example, giving the infant little opportunity to cope effectively.

The third stage of attachment formation is an expansion to multiple attachments. Here the infant adds the father, siblings, and grandparents and other significant and constant people in the environment to his or her little social group.

Babies differ not only in the age at which they develop the foregoing attachment behaviors but also in the intensity and strength of the attachment. The quality of attachment depends on the quality of the mother-infant relationship. Infant-mother pairs who are adept at reading each other's cues and responding to each other's needs could well be those whose interpersonal bonds are firmer and less ambivalent. These infants may show very strong attachments. The behavior of firmly attached infants is most indicative of trust. These babies expect their mother to be there to meet their needs. They can delay gratification because there is no doubt in their minds that whatever they need is forthcoming.

Assessing infants' attachment to their primary caregiver is an important function of the nurse. This relationship is critical for babies and represents their main source of security. Infants demonstrate their attachment with specific kinds of behaviors that the nurse can observe. These behaviors vary in intensity among infants and are affected by the environment. When placed in a strange environment, infants may show more disturbance and stronger dependence than when placed in familiar surroundings.

Infants demonstrate individual differences in their response to brief or prolonged separations. The firmly attached, trusting infant is more able to tolerate periods when the mother is absent. When the mother returns, the infant shows delight in greeting her and has an immediate rapport with her. The infant who is ambivalent tolerates the experience less well. He or she may show more *separation anxiety*—crying, general distress, or possibly a decrease in animation and ability to play. When reunited with the mother, there is not always immediate rapport. The infant may respond by crying or by wanting to be held, but without experiencing the comfort and delight that being held usually elicits. (Refer to Chap. 15 for a discussion of separation anxiety.)

Parents sometimes have concerns about separation anxiety. The nurse can help by assuring them that this phenomenon is normal and common among infants. It can be lessened by simple measures of keeping the surroundings as familiar as possible when separations are anticipated. Such suggestions as having the mother and infant spend some time together with a new babysitter before the mother leaves may be very helpful. Most important, parents and health care workers should realize that the mother's presence is very necessary to the infant who is hospitalized or undergoing unusual stress of any kind. Maintaining the integrity of this relationship should be a priority goal.

Sex role identification

There are differences in male and female infants besides the obvious one of anatomy. Male babies are on the average larger and have proportionately more muscle mass at birth. Female infants are generally smaller in size but physiologically more mature at birth than males and are less vulnerable to stress. Differences in activity level, cuddliness, and so forth, are not due to gender, however. Such differences are more likely to be the result of temperament than of sex.

Sex differences are usually reinforced very early. Little girls are dressed in ruffles and lace, and little boys in overalls and baseball caps. Stereotyped male or female behavior is encouraged as well. Because of this, it is difficult to know how much femaleness and maleness is due to true gender differences and how much to learning. What is known so far suggests that behavioral and aptitude differences are not gender-based. Children do not identify themselves as male or female until after the infancy period. Their play and choice of toys does not take on gender identity until early childhood.

Cognitive development

The newborn infant is something like a computer which has already been programmed to sort and process data. He or she is born with many abilities and built-in methods of interacting with the environment. Jean Piaget, a prominent theorist in the area of cognitive development, established a framework for explaining how children develop thinking, or cognition.

Piaget maintained that the sequence of cognitive development is orderly and recognizable from one child to the next. He described this progression of thinking ability in terms of periods, subperiods, and stages (see Chap. 5). The following section focuses on the *sensorimotor period* to provide a better understanding of the infant's cognitive development.

The sensorimotor period There are six stages in the sensorimotor period. It is important to remember that these stages are sequential and that each is built on the previous one. The first four stages generally occur during the first year of life. The last two are discussed in Chap. 10. The ages assigned to the stages are meant only as guidelines, since children progress at different rates.

Stage 1: Exercising sensorimotor reflexes (birth to 1 month) The infant comes equipped with a group of behavioral activities called *reflexes*. (Refer to Chap. 8 for a listing of these reflexes.) Piaget felt that the sucking and palmar grasp reflexes are particularly important. The infant practices these reflex patterns during the first month. The infant becomes better at finding the nipple and sucking after a few days' practice and may soon find his or her thumb and suck that. Infants thus begin to experience these basic reflexive behaviors in a pattern. In order to suck their thumbs, they must coordinate arm and hand movements with their mouths. This goes beyond reflex behavior.

Stage 2: Primary circular reactions (1 to 4 months) During this stage infants assimilate more and more information into the sensorimotor schemata. (Schemata are discussed in Chap. 5.) What they see becomes related to what they hear, grasp, mouth, and touch. They learn to stop crying when they see the mother approach with the bottle. They begin to show preference for some things over others and to develop more pattern to their behavior (similar to habits). Their increased neuromuscular development is an important factor in this stage. They are capable of repeating behaviors that they find interesting and of abandoning those which are no longer gratifying or helpful. There is no evidence that children at this stage have any notion of time or space. For them, there are only events, and these events are related to their own functioning. There is also no relationship between the means and the end. Infants of this age do not seem to have an end in mind when they begin an activity (Fig. 9-10).

Stage 3: Secondary circular reactions (4 to 8 months) In this stage babies begin to identify the means to an end. For instance, if there is a mobile over the crib with a cord hanging down that they can grasp and pull to make the mobile move, they figure out this relationship and purposely pull the cord. If another toy is placed above the crib, they look for the cord. At the beginning of this stage, they are very actively grasping everything they can get their hands on. They are building on the patterns of behavior they developed earlier (that is why this stage is termed *secondary*), and their behaviors are repeated over and over because they derive pleasure from them (which is why the term *circular* is used). They are interested in the results of their actions and in prolonging them. Piaget described infants in the early part of this stage as being on the threshold of intelligence. They are beginning to link vision with prehension (Fig. 9-11).

During this stage, infants also begin to de-

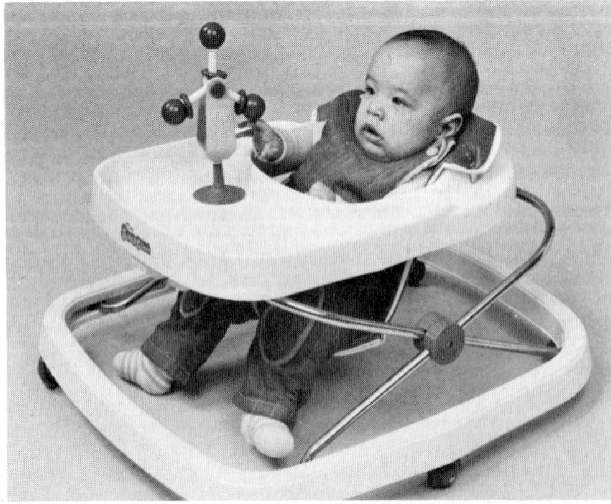

Figure 9-10 At this age an infant does not yet seem to have an end in mind when beginning an activity.

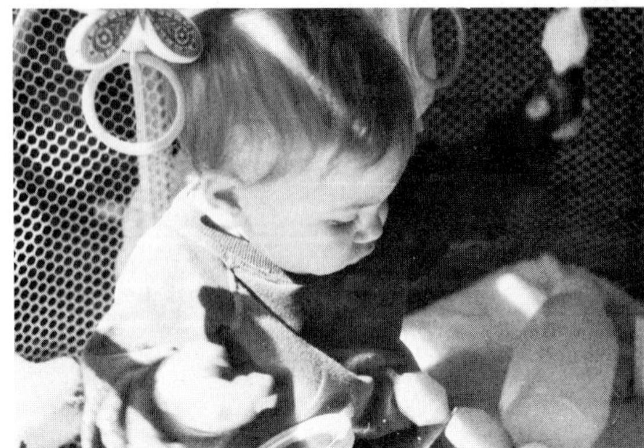

Figure 9-11 This 7-month-old child has toys that can be put together and pulled apart. Manipulating these objects will help the child practice means-to-end relationships.

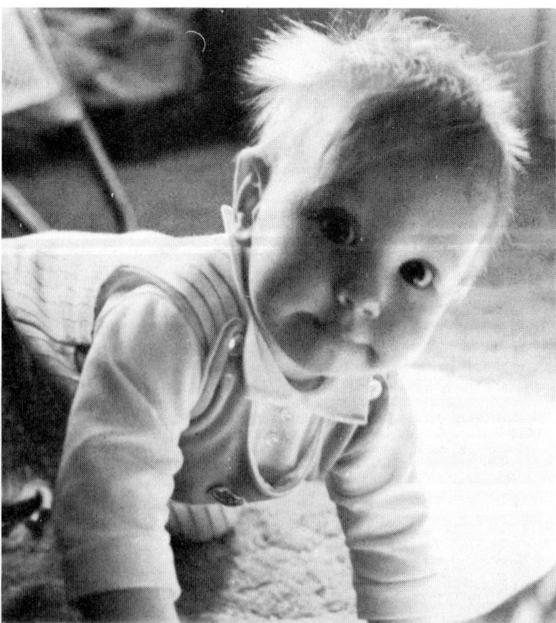

Figure 9-12 This 8-month-old infant is beginning to become mobile by creeping. Increased mobility aids development of object permanence. The infant can actively seek objects that he or she thinks about.

velop what is called *object permanence*. Before this time, if an object was removed from the infant's vision or grasp, he or she would focus on something else. Now the child will look for the object (Fig. 9-12). This has implications for the onset of separation anxiety; the child can think about (remember) the parents even if he or she cannot see them.

Stage 4: Coordination of secondary schemata (8 to 12 months) In this stage infants refine those behaviors and mental associations which were begun in stage 3. There is now a clear difference between the means and the end goal. Infants may try several ways to get at their goal in spite of barriers. Object permanence continues to develop in this period and is related to the child's beginning knowledge of space. It is in this period that objects begin to take on symbolic meaning for children (Fig. 9-13). They can begin to experience an event or object by watching it, without having to touch it.

In summary, Piaget described how he believed infants progress from essentially reflex behavior to the ability to use symbols in thinking. Infants develop from a very narrow conception of reality which is limited to the experience of their own actions to a beginning understanding of causality, space, time, and object permanence. They are very active in bringing about this process. They act on their environment, and it in turn acts on them as they assimilate new information and accommodate to new situations. Cognitive development during infancy is summarized in Table 9-8.

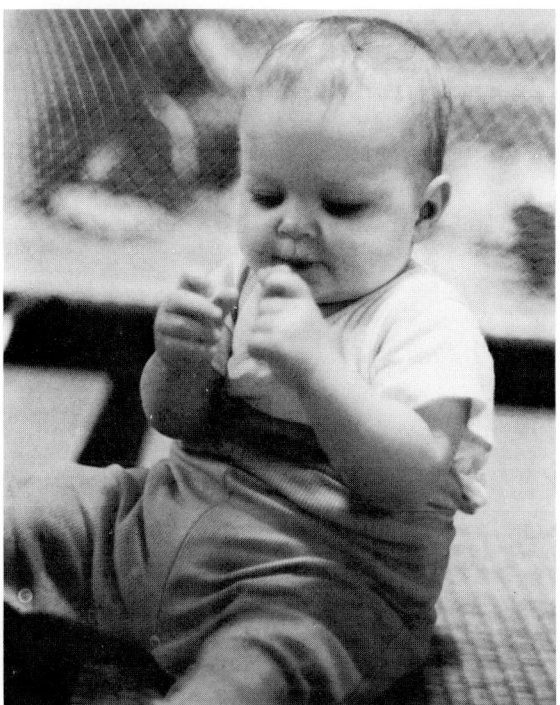

Figure 9-13 This infant is able to transfer objects from hand to hand. An increase in motor skills is closely related to the development of cognition.

Language development

Infants make almost incredible progress in developing language during the first year of life. They go from crying as their only vocal sound to the beginnings of patterned speech in just 12 short months! The nurse can observe what children do and can identify the general rules that seem to govern language development. Deeper questions concerning the hows and whys of language development are more difficult. There are a number of theories, but none are very complete. Current thoughts suggest that infants may be born already programmed to develop language. They may already be tuned in to sorting and analyzing language in terms of specific rules. It may also be that language, as opposed to production of sounds, depends on cortical development. Development of the two seems to coincide in the second half of the first year of life. Table 9-6 includes milestones of language development throughout the first year.

Stages of prelanguage development

Stage 1: Crying Newborns' only vocal sound is crying. They may vary the intensity, pattern, and duration of the cry, but crying it still is. Even at this early stage the infant is positively responding to voice sounds. Listening skills and attentiveness are important in overall language development and can be encouraged even during the first month.

Stage 2: Cooing Infants begin to make cooing sounds by about 1 month of age. Cooing sounds are noncrying, voluntary sounds. Usually infants make these sounds when they seem contented and happy. Parents can be instructed in how to listen for these first sounds. When the infant is cooing, it is an opportune time for "conversation" between parent and child. Saying the sounds

Table 9-8 Developmental milestones: Cognition*

1 month	2 months	3 months	4 months	5 months	6 months
Memory					
Remembers existence of object for 2 to 3 s		Is alert up to 45 min Memory is obvious	Memory span is 5 to 7 min Recognition of strange places indicates memory	Remembers own actions in immediate past	Is alert for $1\frac{1}{2}$ to 2 h
Causality: repeated behavior causes same response					
Expects feedings at specific, routine times Daily responses to activities are disorganized	Anticipates movement of objects	Anticipates feedings (a reward)	Shows anticipation and excitement	Anticipates entire object when sees part Anticipates; searches for dropped or fast-moving objects	Reaches quickly for things seen and desired
Separation of self and others from environment					
Perceives self and parent as one Is totally self-centered Does not recognize objects in environment	Discriminates between people, voices, and objects	Begins to be aware of self Differentiates between family members Explores body parts with hand; begins to realize they are part of self	Becomes aware of self as separate from environment and external objects Begins to separate act from result Distinguishes between strange and familiar places	Recognizes objects external to self	Recognizes mother in other clothes and places
Reflexive or voluntary movement					
Movements are reflexive, not voluntary (initiated by infant) Repeated reflex movements establish a pattern of experiences Relates to world by touch and orally (not verbally)	Repeats reflex movements May associate action with people (bottle with mother)	Still repeats actions for pleasure, more than result May associate action and result Becomes bored with repeated sounds or images Begins to coordinate body movements and vision Begins to combine reflexes and voluntary actions	Combines behaviors to vary them or to reach goals Plays with favorite toys and games; shows discrimination	Voluntarily begins movements in pattern, or order Repeats actions to make environment interesting	Manipulates objects to change their position Senses relationship between hands and objects being manipulated Is interested in movement and action

Table 9-8 *(Continued)*

7 months	8 months	9 months	10 months	11 months	12 months
Memory					
Concentrates more Is interested in detail Remembers series of events only if involved	Remembers series of events even if not involved Remembers time sequence Imitates behavior of people by memory	Remembers series of actions and ideas Remembers event of past day			Remembers events for increasingly long periods
Causality: repeated behavior causes the same response					
Expects events to be repeated Searches for object he or she sees being hidden; believes it remains in last place seen Remembers part of series of behaviors; knows it represents the entire series of behaviors Is interested in results of own behavior Realizes goal only after attaining it Distinguishes between near and far	Recognizes objects as separate from self Begins to learn, combines behaviors; solves problem to obtain toy Further separates action from result Begins to differentiate one object from several objects Uses hands to learn concepts of in and out	Anticipates return of person or object Uncovers hidden toy Plays out solution to problems (shows use of symbols) Is bored by repetition of same stimuli Explores toys; pokes finger in hole; mouths, sucks, and chews Compares size, similarities, and differences of objects Fears height	Searches for hidden object in several places Experiments and changes actions to attain goal; changes old actions by trial and error Sees objects as increasingly distinct; explores and manipulates toys Begins to match similar objects	Is aware of results of some actions Associates sounds with object (barks for dog) Separates action from object Explores boxes; inserts objects in container and removes them Symbol recognition is developing (enjoys books)	Perceives objects as separate and used for play Perceives self as different from other objects Finds new solutions and removes barriers to problems Continues to associate symbols with events and objects; classifying is based on own experience Experiments with object displacement: removes objects from container, turns them, and inserts them in container Visualizes actions before acting them out in play

*Compiled by Nancy L. Ramsey.

back to the baby and attending to his or her efforts can be stimulating and rewarding.

Stage 3: Babbling By about 6 months (the range is wide: 3 to 7 months) the baby is babbling. Babbling sounds are often consonant sounds combined with a vowel repeated several times (e.g., "da da da da da da"). The infant uses many sounds and seems to play and experiment with them. Babbling may take on similar rhythms and intonations. One predominant characteristic of babbling is that babies do it a lot.

There is not a clear understanding of the relationship between babbling and true language. Babbling does not seem to have the same intent as the infant's first words or language—that of communicating. It is interesting to note that all infants babble with the same sounds. When they begin to speak words, different sounds are used, depending on the language spoken in their environment.

Stage 4: Patterned speech The infant's first words appear sometime between 9 and 14 months of age. These words are usually in the form of sounds used consistently to mean particular objects, people, or whatever. Often they are invented words created by the infant. Parents become adept at interpreting the meaning of the words used by the infant. One word may convey variations of meaning, depending on the context and tone in which it is used. For example, the infant may say "Ball," meaning "There is my ball," and expressing delight at discovery. Another time the infant may say "Ball," meaning "Play ball with me" or "I want my ball."

Babbling continues during this fourth stage but becomes less repetitive and more like regular speech. This later type of babbling is termed *jargon*.

One thing is certain: Infants can understand language and follow simple instructions before patterned speech develops. "No-no" is generally responded to before the child is 9 months old. Infants also respond to their own names by this time. They are likely to be able to wave "bye-bye" when requested to do so or when they want to leave.

Factors influencing language development Although it is not clear how and why children learn language, there are observations that can be made about the *way* they learn. Imitation of adult speech by the child cannot constitute a full explanation of language development. Children do not put words together the way adults do, as would be expected if they were learning by imitation alone, although imitation must have some role. Children do learn the language spoken in their environment. It can be assumed that some aspects of language are at least in part learned by imitation of words they hear. Similarly, reinforcement for words spoken cannot account for the actual development of language. It may, however, play an important role in how much infants vocalize and the rate at which they progress with language. An infant who is given attention and praise for attempts at language may vocalize more than one who is ignored.

Parents play a significant role in language development. It is interesting to note that there are similarities across cultures in the way parents talk to infants and young children. Adults raise the pitch of their voice when speaking to infants. They also exaggerate speech with pitch, tone, intensity, and facial expression. A conversation of an adult to an infant is much richer and more varied with respect to these qualities than a conversation between two adults. Vowel sounds are often elongated, and the pace is slower, with longer pauses between vocalizations. The mother and father tailor their speech to the infant as he or she progresses. They lead the infant, in a way, by slowly increasing the complexity of their sentences as the infant keeps pace with his or her own language development.

The amount the baby is talked to also makes a difference in overall development. Infants from culturally deprived environments do not score as high on tests of language or cognitive skills as those from culturally richer environments. Talking to the infant probably does not speed up language acquisition. It does, however, broaden the repertoire of the young child and has a positive overall effect on his or her development.

HEALTH MAINTENANCE

It is the nurse's role to assist the parents in promoting the health and well-being of their infant. In order to do this, the nurse must understand and appreciate what is involved in the daily care of an infant. Many times it is the "small" things that occur during a normal day that disturb and worry parents the most. It is also these same routine occurrences that can blow up into major threats to the well-being of the infant and the family. Nurses must be sensitive to the cues parents give. Listening skills are of paramount importance here. Often parents feel uneasy about asking what they view as simple or trivial questions of the health professional.

The nurse should use interviewing skills to open up areas of conversation concerning the infant's home routine. Specific information can be asked for to help the nurse assess the care and environment of the infant. This also provides an opportunity to encourage the mother or other caregiver. Mothers need to know they are doing a good job.

Daily care

Safety Accidents are a tremendous threat to the child's health. As the infant becomes mobile, the hazards increase. The nurse should instruct parents to do the following in relation to the more common hazards discussed below.

1. Never leave an infant unattended on a changing table, on an examining table, in a crib with the siderail down, or in another area where he or she might fall off. It is a good idea when working with the infant to place a hand on the body when turning or looking away.
2. Remove all small items—including safety pins (which, of course, are always kept closed)—from the infant's reach. Infants put virtually everything in their mouths. This is especially important for the infant who is creeping. A particularly hazardous item is a plugged-in extension cord on the floor; these should be removed.
3. Keep all soaps, cleansers, lotions, insecticides, and the like, locked up or out of baby's reach. Kitchens, porches, and bathrooms are particularly dangerous areas because of low cupboards and storage areas. Hospitals are full of dangerous solutions, as well, which sometimes find their way to the bedside table.
4. Never leave an infant unattended in a bathtub or other water, such as a wading pool.
5. Be especially careful of medicines. Child-proof caps should be used but not depended on to do any more than slow the child down. The aspirin in mother's purse or the vitamins on the table are sometimes overlooked in a routine safety check and remain accessible to the infant.
6. Use infant car seats that have been tested and approved for safety. Automobile accidents are the number one cause of injury and death in childhood. Even a sharp curve or sudden stop can cause injury to an infant who is lying or sitting unrestrained on the seat. Parents should be cautioned not to hold infants on their laps—especially in the front passenger seat—as an alternative to a safe car seat. Parents may feel that they can protect the infant if an accident occurs, but this has not proved to be the case (Fig. 9-14).
7. Never leave small children alone in automobiles. Cars are filled with hazards. Automobiles can become very hot when left parked in the sun. This can be very dangerous to the infant.

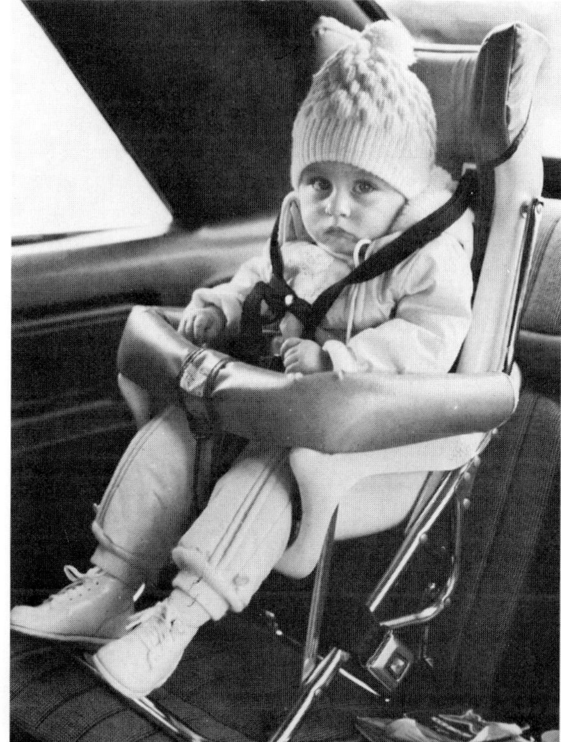

Figure 9-14 Putting children in an infant seat is the safe way to transport them in a car.

Feeding Mealtime for the infant should be unrushed and as free from distraction as possible. If the mother is nursing the infant, this is a good opportunity to get in a comfortable position and rest. Whether nursed or bottle-fed, the infant should have an enjoyable and satisfying experience. Beginning the infant on beikost may take some patience and skill. Mothers will find it easier to use an infant-sized spoon with a long handle. Having what is needed ready and in position helps. Placing the infant at eye level, directly in front of and facing the person doing the feeding, will allow for the best visibility and control. If the bowl of food is within reach, it will likely be explored by a tiny fist and end up on the floor.

Infants enjoy being with their families at mealtime. Nine- or ten-month-old babies are capable of sitting in a high chair or feeding table and eating some finger foods unassisted.

Constipation Constipation (the passage of dry, hard stools) in infants is usually caused by inadequate water intake or by iron supplements added to the diet. It can also occur when the infant's diet is changed, such as when breast milk is replaced with formula.

Young infants who are fed exclusively breast milk or formula normally take in enough water to avoid constipation. Infants who have progressed to solid foods may need to be given water to drink, especially in the summertime or when they are likely to lose fluids through perspiration. Caregivers frequently do not offer water to infants. Mild constipation can be treated by giving the infant a glass or a bottle of water containing 1 tsp of corn syrup or molasses (not honey, which can carry the spores of infant botulism). The sugar pulls fluids from the gut into the stool. (Refer to Chap. 18.) Offering the infant diluted prune juice and adding more fruit to the diet may also solve the problem. The infant should be referred to a physician if the abdomen is distended or if constipation persists for more than 3 days.

Sleeping Infants need a lot of sleep, especially in the first few months. This is good because so do mothers. Mothers should be encouraged to take rest periods when the baby naps instead of trying to "get everything done" then.

Infants differ in their ability to sleep in the presence of noise and other activity. Very young infants are able to block out some stimulation, but as they grow older, they may require a quieter environment. Some infants drop off to sleep easily and seem to prefer the crib. Firstborn children have more difficulty and may want to be rocked or sung to sleep.[12]

Infants have sleep cycles during the course of a nap or the night. They may go from deep sleep to active sleep and back to deep sleep again several times. Parents should be instructed to be sure that infants are ready to wake up before disturbing them. A stretch and a change of position may not be the signal for waking.

The infant should be kept warm when sleeping but not restricted by bedclothes. A blanket sleeper or "sleeping sack" may be appropriate for cool climates. Plastic pants on the young infant, especially for overnight wear, should be avoided. They hold in the moisture, which is not good for the baby's skin. A double diaper and a cotton-backed waterproof sheet may be adequate for use overnight.

Diapering It is a good thing that infants are small and relatively easy to diaper, because parents need time to practice. Diapering an 8-month-old can be a real challenge if one is not fairly skilled and swift. Diapering is discussed in Chaps. 8 and 16.

Diaper rash Diaper rash may exist until the infant is toilet-trained. Most infants, in spite of their mothers' best efforts, occasionally develop diaper rash. If the rash stubbornly persists, the following should be assessed: (1) How often does the mother change the diapers? Is the child double-diapered? Urine continuously contacting the skin irritates it. The double thickness of the diaper absorbs the urine and draws it away from the skin. (2) Are the diapers rinsed twice? If the diapers are washed in a laundromat, rinsing them twice is more difficult and expensive. (3) Are irritating substances being added to the water? Harsh detergents, water softeners, and bleach irritate the skin. (4) Are the feces being completely washed off the skin before a non-water-soluble ointment is applied? Water is not an adequate cleanser for rinsing feces off the skin. A mild soap or cleansing lotion (without alcohol), followed by a rinse with a soft cloth, removes the irritating feces and bacteria. (5) Is the mother using adequate amounts of a non-water-soluble ointment to protect the skin? Petroleum jelly is one of the most economical products. (6) Can the mother remove the diaper for a period of time each day to allow air and sunlight to reach the rash? (7) Is the child wearing plastic pants? If so, the mother should be instructed to remove them. Plastic encourages a bacteria-supporting environment: airless, warm, and moist. (8) Is the child allergic to disposable diapers? (9) Do the diapers have an ammonia odor? Ammonia, which is formed by the bacteria on the diapers and by urea, irritates the skin. The mother should be instructed to add 1 cup of vinegar to the rinse water or an antiseptic to the wash water. (10) Does the choice of diapers fit the parent's lifestyle and budget? Disposable diapers are more expensive but very convenient. A diaper service is approximately one-half the cost of disposable diapers. Cloth diapers are most economical. The mother's knowledge of diaper care should always be assessed. Having a baby with a persistent diaper rash can be detrimental to a mother's self-concept.

Bathing Babies are slippery when wet. It is very important to have the infant well supported and to have everything that is needed within easy reach. The water should be warm, and care taken not to chill the infant if the air temperature is cool. Bathing is discussed in Chap. 16.

Shampooing the hair helps remove *cradle cap* from the infant's scalp. Cradle cap is common in young infants. It looks like yellowish, crusty, scaly patches on the scalp. The patches are unappealing in appearance, may cause the baby discomfort, or may contribute to inflammation or infection. Applying petroleum jelly or mineral oil to the infant's scalp several hours before shampooing will help soften the crusts so that they may be removed.

Cleaning the infant's head and scalp is often the last part of the bath. Young infants can be wrapped in a towel and held securely under one arm, with the hand supporting the head (like a football hold). This leaves the caregiver with one hand free to wash the scalp, and it makes the baby feel secure. Most infants enjoy this procedure. A bath often relaxes the infant and provides an especially good opportunity for interaction between the baby and the caregiver. Parents should be instructed *never* to leave the infant alone in the bath.

Baby powder should be used sparingly. Inhalation of large quantities of powder containing talc dries the mucous membranes of the respiratory tract, decreases the function of the cilia, and can lead to complete airway obstruction and death. The infant who has aspirated talc has the characteristic symptoms of dyspnea, tachypnea, wheezing, cyanosis, and fever.[13]

If committed to using baby powder, parents should be instructed to apply small amounts to their hands, keeping them away from the baby's head. Lotions and non-water-soluble lubricants should be substituted for baby powder.[14]

Clothing The infant's clothing should be nonconstrictive. Babies grow rapidly, and clothing quickly becomes too small. Many mothers swap baby clothes with friends or family members. Others discover thrift shops or simply buy larger-sized clothes that the infant can wear for a longer period. Strings, ribbons, and reachable buttons on clothing should be avoided. All these things can present a hazard. Soft, comfortable garments that allow a full range of motion for the infant are appropriate.

Well-baby health care The well-baby visit to the pediatrician or nurse practitioner provides the opportunity for effective health care maintenance. A physical and developmental examination is performed, and an assessment of the infant's overall health status is made. This is also an excellent opportunity to assess and support the positive interaction between the infant and the caregiver. Astute observations are critical at this time. A positive outcome for the infant may depend on the identification of problems or potential problems and the initiation of early intervention.

At this time, the infant's growth and development are monitored. Nurses can use their knowledge to point out specific gains the infant is making. Suggestions concerning things the parents can do to foster their child's progress can be made. The nurse can also encourage the parents by letting them know that the things they usually do with their infant—singing, rocking, and playing—are critical to his or her development. Parents are not always aware of the importance of their actions.

This is also the time to take preventive health care measures. Immunizations should be started (see Table 14-2). Health teaching, including preventive guidance about avoiding accidents, should be ongoing. Instructions for handling common illnesses at home are especially important. The nurse should make sure that parents know how to use a thermometer safely, how to recognize illness in a child, and when to call on professionals for help.

A major part of the role of the nurse is anticipatory guidance. Parents should be informed about what to expect of their infant and, just as important, what to expect of themselves. Letting the parents know that they may sometimes feel anger and frustration at the infant can be very helpful. Parents can experience a sense of guilt because of feelings that are naturally associated with the strain of having an infant in the home.

In summary, the first year of life is a critical

period. The child's rapid development and the far-reaching implications of environmental influences on the child's potential underline the reason for concern. The nurse, the physician, the family, and even the child all have a role in ensuring the child's well-being.

REFERENCES

1. Stern, Daniel, *The First Relationship: Infant and Mother,* Harvard, Cambridge, Mass., 1977, p. 71.
2. U.S. Bureau of the Census, *Current Population Reports,* ser. P-60, no. 147, "Characteristics of the Population below the Poverty Level: 1983," GPO, Washington, 1985.
3. Golden, M., "An Approach to the Management of Obesity in Childhood," *Pediatric Clinics of North America* **26**(1):187–197 (February 1979), p. 190.
4. Hammer, S., *Obesity: Early Identification and Treatment in Childhood Obesity,* Acton Publications Sciences Group, 1975, quoted in Winkelstein, Marilyn L., "Overfeeding in Infancy: The Early Introduction of Solid Foods," *Pediatric Nursing* **10**(3):204–236 (May–June 1984).
5. Ibid., p. 206.
6. Ibid., pp. 206, 208.
7. "Report of the Task Force on the Assessment of the Scientific Evidence Relating to Infant-Feeding Practices and Infant Health," *Pediatrics Supplement* **74**(4):136 (October 1984).
8. Ibid.
9. Worthington-Roberts, Bonnie S., et al., *Nutrition in Pregnancy and Lactation,* 3d ed., Times Mirror/Mosby College, St Louis, 1985, p. 263.
10. Ibid., p. 272.
11. Winick, Myron, "The Physician's Role in Nutrition Counseling," in *Year One: Nutrition Growth Health,* Ross Laboratories, Columbus, Ohio, 1975.
12. Edgil, Ann E., et al., "Sleep Problems of Older Infants and Preschool Children," *Pediatric Nursing* **11**(2):87–89 (March–April 1985).
13. Wagner, Timothy J., and Michelle Handi-Alexander, "Hazards of Baby Powder?" *Pediatric Nursing* **10**(2):124–125 (March–April 1984).
14. Ibid., p. 125.

10

Nancy Lockwood Ramsey

The toddler

Upon completion of this chapter, the student will be able to:

1 Summarize the toddler's physical maturation within the following areas: changes in body size, vision, teeth, and musculoskeletal, nervous, and respiratory systems.

2 Identify the toddler's nutritional requirements and use interventions to cope with food jags, food refusal, and eating rituals.

3 Describe the development and characteristic behaviors of Erikson's developmental task autonomy vs. shame and doubt.

4 Relate the impact of parental methods of, and attitudes toward, toilet training to the toddler's attainment of autonomy or feelings of shame and doubt.

5 Cite key steps in toilet training a toddler.

6 List guidelines for disciplining a toddler and relate these guidelines to socializing the toddler.

7 Identify the cause of, and interventions to cope with, the following behaviors: temper tantrums, negativism, dawdling, and ritualism.

8 List five functions of the toddler's play and state an example of each function.

9 Describe the toddler's cognitive development in stages 5 and 6 of the sensorimotor period.

10 Cite several accidents a toddler may have and describe methods of preventing each one.

The foundations for the toddler years are built in infancy. Infants learn to trust their parents and to perceive the world as safe to explore and able to fulfill their needs. They gradually begin to separate from their mothers and to learn that they have a predictable effect on others.

The toddler years, which last from 1 to 3 years, are an age of discovery and exploration. The boundless energy and maturing neuromuscular system of toddlers support an insatiable need to explore and to master skills. With walking, toddlers enter a new world. They explore everything in sight and are in perpetual motion. They curiously investigate objects, using more senses than they did as infants: mouthing, shaking, poking, and smearing. By exploring, toddlers learn new skills, feel new sensations, and learn about the environment.

Toddlers gradually separate themselves from their mothers and learn to tolerate their mothers' absence. Toddlers want to be in control, to do things alone, and to be independent. To be independent, they must begin to learn self-control and self-care. They struggle with emotional control, caught between following their wishes and their parents' demands. Temper tantrums, negativism, and dawdling have helped earn this period the label "the terrible twos." Toddlers learn to care for themselves, dress, eat, toilet, and talk. They want and seek discipline to help them behave acceptably. Their autonomous behavior eventually results in accomplishment and mastery. They experiment, solve problems, and think using symbols. They imitate sex role behavior. Their play includes fantasy and imitation.

The nurse who cares for the toddler and the family unit must understand the growth and development that take place at this exciting age. Knowing what is normal at this age enables the nurse to understand the toddler's behavior, anticipate problems, counsel parents, and design age-appropriate nursing care plans.

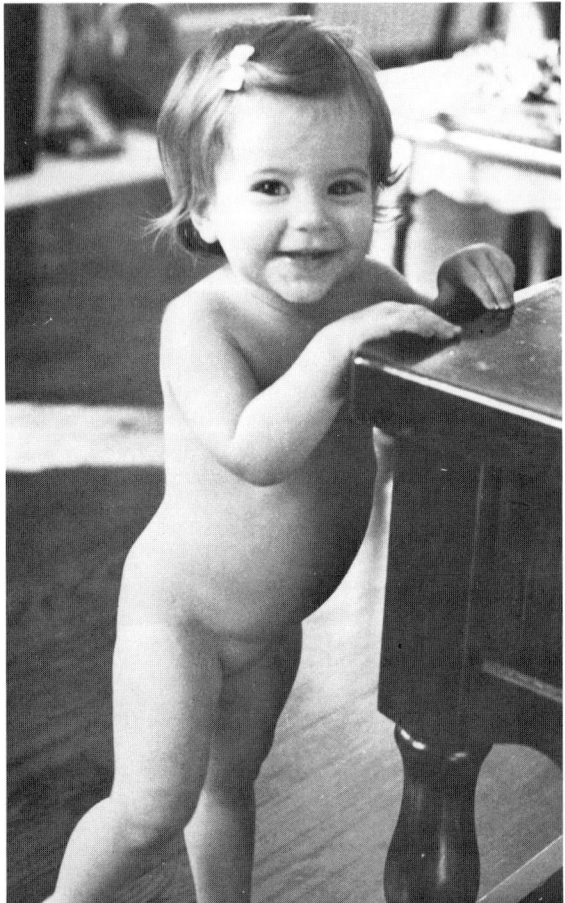

Figure 10-1 Toddlers have proportionally large heads and protruding abdomens. (*Photo courtesy of David Carroll.*)

PHYSICAL MATURATION

Changes in body size

The toddler's height and weight increase, although the growth rate slows in comparison with that of the infant. The toddler gains more height in proportion to weight. Height increases from 3 to 5 in per year, in comparison with the infant's growth of 4 in during the first 3 months. Boys tend to be taller than girls, although the difference is very small. Adult height can be estimated by multiplying the child's height at 2 years by 2. (Refer to Appendix B for growth charts.)

The toddler's rate of weight gain declines sharply because of decreased appetite, reduced metabolic rate, and a resulting loss of subcutaneous fat. A newborn gains 7 oz per week; a toddler gains approximately 7 oz per month. A toddler gains 5 to 6 lb per year and begins the second year weighing 20 lb and the third year weighing 30 lb. Weight gain is steplike rather than smoothly continuous, and weight gains occur in spurts.[1]

Toddlers appear top-heavy when they begin to walk. Their legs are relatively short and stublike, and the trunk is long and "potbellied" (see Fig. 10-1). The chest, after the second year, is larger than the head in circumference. The abdomen protrudes because of an immature musculature and a relatively large liver. The arms and legs grow faster than the trunk because of the rapid ossification and growth of epiphyseal centers in the legs. Toddlers begin to lose their chubby appearance as walking improves their musculature, fat storage is altered, and increased muscle development replaces baby fat. The legs often appear bowed (tibial torsion), and the feet flat, as a residual of the intrauterine position. This appearance gradually changes as the muscles strengthen. The toddler's arch develops and becomes noticeable, and walking causes the fat pads on the soles of the feet to disappear.

Vision

The toddler's vision is well developed by 2 years and reflects neuromuscular maturation. (See Table 10-1.) During childhood the eyeball becomes increasingly rounded rather than short, as in infancy. The rounded shape causes the far-

Table 10-1 Visual Development

12 to 18 months
Identifies forms
Displays an intense interest in pictures
Scribbles on paper
Convergence becomes well established
Has crude depth perception
18 to 24 months
Accommodation is well developed
Has 20/40 vision
Discriminates between simple geometric shapes
2 to 3 years
Convergence is smooth
Fixes on small objects or pictures for 50 s
Recalls visual images
Has 20/30 vision

Source: Adapted from Peggy L. Chinn, *Child Health Maintenance*, Mosby, St. Louis, 1979, p. 871.

sightedness of infancy to decrease. Perception of light and dark, color, and detail is developed by 8 months. Visual acuity is approximately 20/40 at 2 years. The toddler needs large objects and pictures in order to make clear distinctions between objects. Binocular vision, the fusion of images, is developed at 1 year. Distance focusing remains poor; the toddler needs to be within a 6-ft range to see an object clearly.

Teeth

The development of teeth begins in utero and ends at approximately age 10. The eruption of *deciduous teeth*, or baby teeth, is completed by $2\frac{1}{2}$ years. The lower lateral incisors appear at 12 to 18 months. Both cuspids appear at 18 to 24 months. Both first molars appear at 12 to 18 months. Second molars appear at 24 to 30 months. (See Fig. 14-9 for the tooth eruption schedule.) See the "Child Health Maintenance" section later in this chapter for prevention of caries.

The musculoskeletal system

The rate of skeletal growth decreases during the toddler years. Bone ossification continues. The height increase is primarily a result of growth of the legs. More than 25 new ossification centers appear during the second year.[2] Brain and skull growth rates also decrease. The anterior fontanel closes by 18 to 24 months, and the posterior fontanel closes by 2 to 3 months because brain growth slows and rapid skull growth is no longer necessary. Rickets or hypothyroidism may delay fontanel closure.[3] The infant's head circumference increases 4 to 5 in during the first year. In contrast, the 2-year-old's head circumference increases less than 1 in per year, and the 3-year-old's less than $\frac{1}{2}$ in per year. Appendix B shows head circumference norms.

Muscle size increases in response to hereditary predisposition and increased use. The child's strength increases as the muscle mass increases. Greater strength is needed to support the more complex muscular functions needed to explore the world, such as walking, climbing, and running.

The nervous system

The brain increases from an average of 350 g at birth to 1000 g at 2 years[4] and reaches two-thirds of adult size at 2 years. The nervous system's development and function become more refined during the second and third years because of increased *myelinization*. Growth of the myelin sheath continues for many years and is not completed until late adolescence. At 2 years the myelinization is complete enough to allow for most general movements. The myelinization proceeds cephalocaudally, as evidenced, for example, by children's ability to grasp a bottle with their arms before learning to walk. Completion of myelinization ensures that nerve impulses speedily reach their destination. When the myelin sheath is incomplete, the slower impulse may not reach the destination. For example, if a 14-month-old toddler has a fever of 40.3°C (104.5°F) and the fever is not reduced within 20 min of a tepid water bath and administration of an antipyretic drug, the incomplete myelinization may have caused the delayed response.

The limbic system controls temperament and emotional control of behavior and also sleep and wakefulness (arousal). Feelings are monitored by this system. While young children function by feelings, not logic, the immature limbic system cannot associate the feelings in a mature, rational pattern; this is thought to be a factor in toddlers' inability to control their emotions.[5]

The various areas of the cerebrum develop differently and correspond to the development of the child's intellect. The integration of these areas is intricately complex; the immature development of some areas is believed to limit the child's attention span. Because the nervous system cannot handle more than one incoming stimulus at a time, the introduction of another, second stimulus will intensify and prolong the action resulting from the first stimulus. For example, when a toddler is slapped for touching a forbidden object, the child's grasp (a result of the first stimulus) momentarily tightens or is prolonged. The child's inability to respond immediately to the parent's command is physiological, not a refusal to cooperate.

The brain also requires its largest supply of oxygen in early childhood: 5.21 ml per 100 g.[6] The prevention of anoxia is therefore vitally important.

Stimulation of the nervous system is crucial for organ development. For example, untreated strabismus in toddlerhood causes the affected eye not to be stimulated, and the capacity for vision in that eye is lost as a result of inadequate stimulation. Physical maturation, changed body proportions, advanced neural development, and increased muscle strength are far more crucial than practice in determining the child's neuromotor progress.[7] For example, the overly zealous mother who toilet trains her child by repeatedly placing the child on the potty chair before he or she is walking is training herself, not the child. All the practice in the world will not toilet train the child if the myelin sheath has not matured far enough down the spinal cord to permit sphincter control. When the child can walk, the myelin sheath is sufficiently mature to transmit the messages to voluntarily empty bowel and bladder.

The gastrointestinal system

Food travels more swiftly through the toddler's gut than through the infant's. The acidity of the digestive juices increases, and their composition compares with that of the adult's digestive juices. The salivary glands mature by age 3.[8]

The endocrine system

The functioning of the toddler's endocrine system is minimal and is not completely understood. However, it is known that insulin and glucagon production is limited and erratic.[9]

The respiratory system

The lungs grow and expand to hold a greater volume of air. The anatomic portions of the respiratory tract are farther apart, which decreases the incidence of infection. However, the adenoids and tonsils increase in size.[10] The middle ear and eustachian tube are short and horizontal, which provides easier access of nasal bacteria to the ear. These changes, coupled with entering day care or nursery school, contribute to the numerous upper respiratory infections of the toddler.

Nutrition

The toddler's appetite decreases at approximately 2 years. If toddlers continued to eat and to grow at the same rate as during infancy, they would weigh over 200 lb by the time they reached the age of 10 years.[11] (The "finicky, birdlike appetite" of toddlers is a major parental concern.) To offer more calories than the toddler needs increases the risk of food refusal. The growth and metabolic rates of toddlers have slowed; they no longer require so much food. Their short attention span and fascination with the environment distract children from eating.

Nutritional requirements Toddlers need a well-balanced diet that meets their nutritional requirements for maintenance and growth of body tissue and supports their large expenditures of energy. The diet should include essential nutrients from the four food groups to meet the minimum daily requirements. Toddlers need three regularly timed meals and several nutritious snacks each day. (Serving sizes and the recommended daily dietary allowances of proteins, fats, carbohydrates, minerals, and vitamins are given in Appendix C.)

The toddler's total amount of body water has decreased, and the amount of cell water has increased. Fluid intake needs are now 100 to 125 ml/kg per day, except in the case of illness, increased temperature, or hot weather. Average calorie, protein, and water requirements of the 1- to 3-year-old are given in the table below.

Calories	Protein	Water
100 to 120 kcal/kg per day or 45 kcal/lb per day	3.5 g/kg per day	100 to 125 ml/kg per day

The toddler's skeletal growth rate has slowed, but more minerals are deposited in the bones for weight-bearing support. Calcium and phosphorus are also needed for tooth development. Two to three cups of milk per day are adequate; allowing the child to drink larger amounts of milk decreases intake of other essential foods.

Psychological and cultural factors influence food intake. To say, "Clean your plate; many children in the world are starving" is to impose unnecessary and meaningless anxiety on any child. Adults must know that toddlers can choose adequate foods in the amounts needed. In many subcultures, children who do not eat heartily and are not enjoying food are thought to be ill, unhappy, or manipulative of the caregivers. Some people equate health, beauty, and prosperity with hearty eating. Greeks, Italians, Germans, and Jews often associate food consumption with love and excellent parenting. Often, the family unit is knit around festive or large daily meals.

American parents have unknowingly encouraged poor food habits in their children by demanding that they clean their plates; giving their children huge, adult-sized portions instead of tiny, toddler-sized portions; providing snacks with a high sugar content; and using desserts as bribes for desired behavior. Dietary trends today encourage high-protein, nutritious snacks, which prevent tooth decay and maintain the blood sugar at higher levels and for longer periods than refined-sugar snacks. Nurses should instruct parents to offer their children snacks of cheese, peanut butter and jelly sandwiches, fruit juice, and homemade juice popsicles instead of cookies, chips, or colas. Toddlers should be given small portions. When they eat all their food, they feel proud, powerful, and in control and can request second helpings.

Food jags Toddlers frequently go on *food jags*, or "binges," on several foods for a few days, excluding other foods. If given a nutritious, well-balanced selection of food, toddlers will choose a balanced diet over approximately 1 month. Many children change preferred foods on a 3- to 4-day cycle; knowing this calms the parents' fears. Parents who are worried that their toddler is not getting a complete diet may be advised to keep a food diary for a few weeks and to record what the child eats. This record generally shows that the quantity and variety of food intake are greater than the parent had supposed.

Food refusal Toddlers frequently refuse food and often imitate the food dislikes of parents or siblings. A child should *not* be forced to eat. Parents should ignore poor eating and praise healthy eating and should allow the child to avoid disliked foods. Food can be introduced in minute portions or disguised in other foods. Parents should allow the child to eat foods in his or her preferred sequence.

When a toddler says "No!" to a certain food, the parent should avoid reacting to the refusal to eat and distract the child to another food. A child may test the parents and will feel more secure with specific food choices, such as, "Do you want the potato or the beans?" Negative behavior at suppertime may be caused by fatigue from play or by being too hungry. A short rest period or nutritious snack 1 to $1\frac{1}{2}$ h before a meal may increase the toddler's cooperation. Most toddlers enjoy eating attractive, small portions of food served in a relaxed, pleasant atmosphere. (See Fig. 10-2.)

"Milk babies" are infants or young toddlers who primarily drink milk and refuse most solid food. These children are obese and pale and have low levels of hemoglobin. They are anemic because milk contains inadequate amounts of iron. Taking the bottle away (out of sight) until the child becomes hungry enough to accept solids

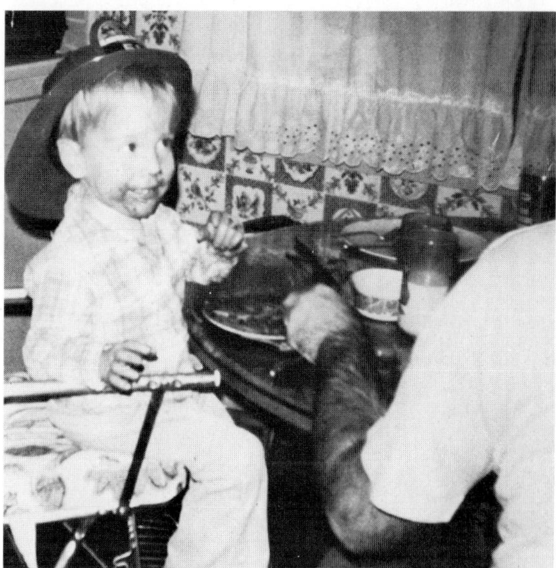

Figure 10-2 Toddlers enjoy mealtimes if permitted to feed themselves in their own way, which is messy because hand and arm control are not well developed. Pleasant social interaction is an important aspect of eating and of social learning. Excessive adult interference can easily lead to parent–child conflict and eating problems that may last for years.

works well. Milk in a glass is then offered after the meal. The child will cry for milk, and parents need reassurance of the need for solids and of the fact that retraining will take only a few days if they do not give in.

Eating rituals The toddler is object-oriented and attempts to control the environment by manipulating objects in a rigid pattern. The toddler cannot rationally relate actions and events and so establishes many ritualistic behavior patterns, some of which have to do with eating.

The child should be fed small portions on the same unbreakable plate and given child-sized utensils and a wide-bottomed cup. It is best that the child be fed at the same place and the same time. The child can be given favorite foods initially, and gradually and inconspicuously new foods can be introduced.

Toddlers' interest in objects, coupled with their short attention span, makes them easily lose interest in eating. Parents can encourage a child to eat in "one place" and not to run throughout the house eating. Having one place to eat teaches the child that sitting on his or her chair has one meaning: It's time to eat. The child should not be made to wait at the table until adults are finished. If the child loses interest in eating, appropriate play activities can stimulate eating. (See Fig. 10-3.) For example, the parent can feed the teddy bear, saying, "Yum! I love this. It's good. I want more!" The child will often immediately begin eating. Parents should serve colorful, attractive food; children enjoy pancakes made in the shape of a face, a face on cottage cheese made with raisins and peaches, or a cheese "sail" in a potato "boat," for example.

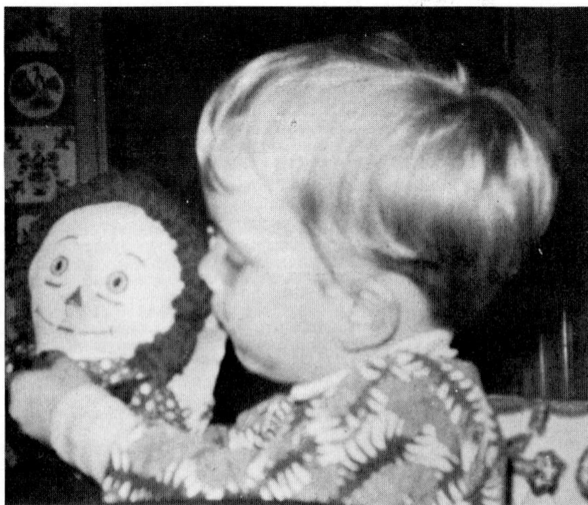

Figure 10-3 Pretending to feed a doll may increase a finicky eater's food intake and willingness to take time for eating.

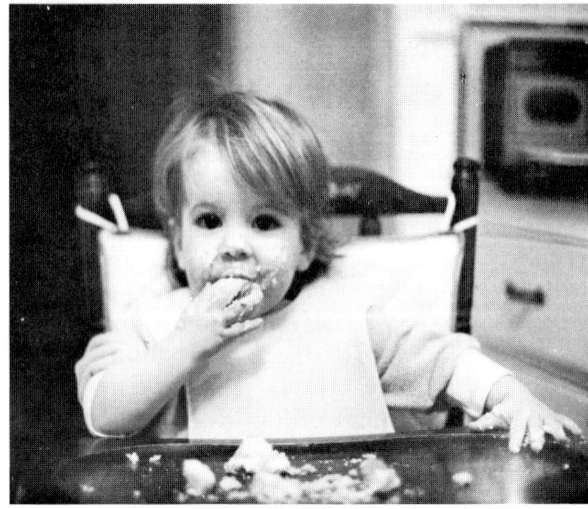

Figure 10-4 Self-feeding skills are initially quite primitive; toddlers eat with their hands before they learn to use utensils. (*Photo courtesy of David Carroll.*)

Toddlers should be allowed to feed themselves, although they are clumsy, and to choose the foods they prefer. Toddlers love *finger foods*—small, bite-sized pieces of food that do not require use of a spoon. They prefer raw vegetables to soft, cooked ones. Cereal or raisins will stimulate fine motor development. Spilled foods are to be expected. The floor can be covered with newspapers or large towels, and the toddler should wear a bib. An absorbent cloth should be kept at the table. Young children develop creativity and learn about foods by touching, tasting, and playing in them (Fig. 10-4).

Motor development

The toddler's maturing neuromuscular system, including the myelinization of the spinal cord, readies the child for walking and exploring. The majority of the motor movements of toddlers have been learned by 2 years; the remaining toddler and preschool years are spent perfecting these skills. Toddlers have an insatiable, inherent need to perfect new skills. They spend long hours repeatedly practicing and refining these skills during play (see Fig. 10-5). Their repetitious practice is directed toward new skills; it is selective

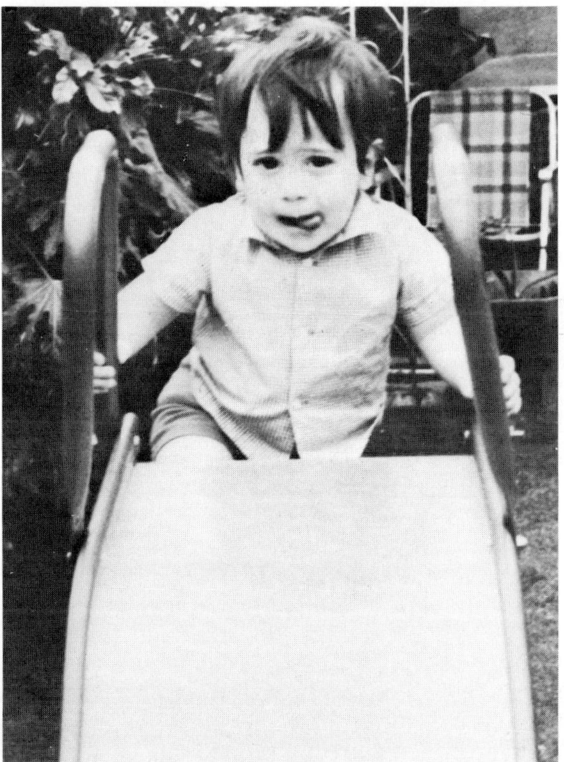

Figure 10-5 The toddler shows great determination in perfecting new skills and mastering the environment.

and persistent, and it satisfies an intrinsic need to deal with, and learn about, the environment.[12] For example, a child may repeatedly climb upstairs until he or she drops from exhaustion. A toddler who becomes excessively frustrated learning a new skill retreats to an old, favorite activity to increase his or her sense of competence and self-esteem.

The toddler's motor development is the most accurate criterion for assessing developmental level until verbal skills increase. If the child has not learned to walk by 20 to 22 months, he or she should be referred to a physician for a thorough pediatric and developmental assessment. Failure to walk may be a symptom of inadequate stimulation or mental retardation.

Gross motor development In order to walk, the toddler must first be able to hold head and shoulders erect, sit up, stand, and make stepping movements.[13] Cruising (walking while holding on to furniture) develops the infant's walking skills. Most toddlers walk alone by 15 months, walk backward and run by 18 months, and climb up stairs and kick a ball by 2 years. By $2\frac{1}{2}$ years the child walks on tiptoe and walks up and down stairs on alternating feet (see Table 10-2). The age at which the toddler masters these skills depends upon personality, stimulation in the en-

Table 10-2 Gross Motor Development

Behavior	15 months	18 months	24 months	30 months
Walking	Walks alone (usually since 13 to 14 months) Loses balance with sudden stops	Walks sideways and backward Walks pulling pull toy Pushes furniture around room	Walks steadily	Tiptoes a few steps
Standing	Stands up alone			Stands on one foot momentarily
Running		Runs awkwardly; falls often	Runs well with wide base of support; rarely falls	
Jumping	Jumps in place; falls forward often		Jumps with both feet in place	
Climbing	Creeps up stairs	Walks up stairs while holding onto rail Creeps downstairs	Goes up and down stairs, placing both feet on same step	Walks up and down stairs, one foot on a step
Sitting		Sits down on chair alone		
Throwing and kicking	Falls when throws ball	Throws ball overhand; does not fall	Kicks ball forward with good balance	Throws large ball 3 to 4 ft
Riding				Rides in toy car

vironment, and heredity. For example, the trusting child eagerly forges ahead into the new environment and learns to walk faster than the more cautious child, who is hesitant to explore the environment. Children who have received inadequate sensory input will not reach out to interact with the environment, and their developmental skills will be delayed (see Chap. 15). The toddler with athletic parents will probably walk earlier than the child of more sedentary parents.

The toddler who is beginning to walk has an unsteady gait, points the toes outward or inward, toddles with flat feet, and places the feet far apart to gain a wide base of support and improve balance (see Fig. 10-6). Practice steadies walking. Parents can promote the development of strong foot, ankle, and leg muscles by permitting the toddler to walk barefoot. Shoes should be soft and pliable and should not brace the foot or ankle. (See the section "Shoe Selection" later in this chapter.)

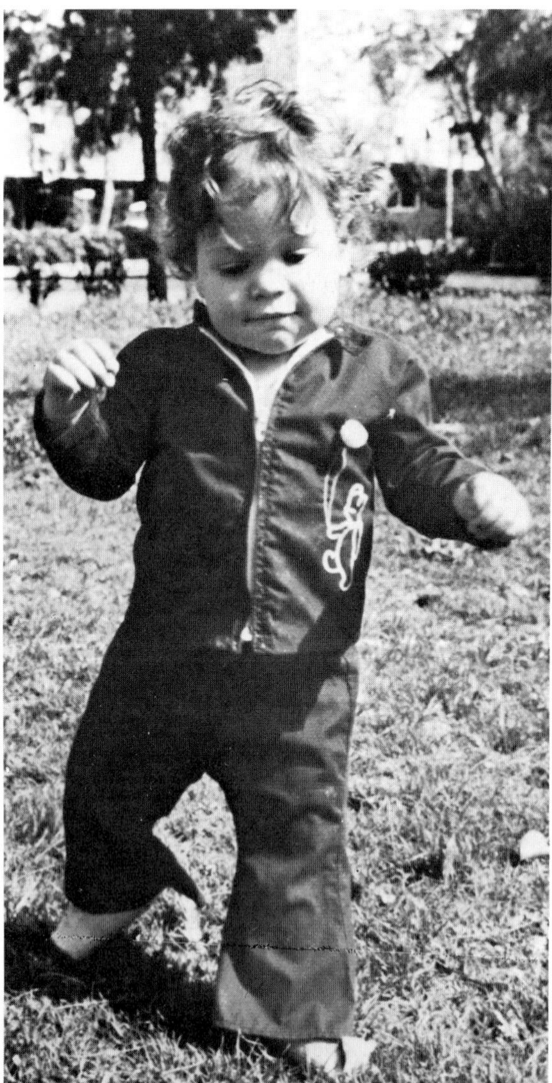

Figure 10-6 The toddler walks and runs awkwardly at first, with the feet apart and the arms held out for balance.

Toddlers' increased competence in walking, climbing, and opening doors gives them the confidence to explore the fascinating world. Because children have no earlier experience with new and occasionally dangerous objects, it is *absolutely imperative* that the parents constantly supervise children and provide a *safe indoor and outdoor* world to explore. (See the section "Accidents" in this chapter.)

Fine motor development The increasingly refined fine motor development of toddlers is illustrated by their ability to move a single muscular group instead of a larger, less differentiated group of muscles. For example, the infant picks up a pencil with an entire-hand grasp, whereas the toddler uses a perfectly refined pincer grasp. At 15 months toddlers can grasp a cup but cannot scoop up food. They turn a spoon upside down when bringing it close to the lips. The 18-month-old child fills the spoon but spills the food when turning it upside down. At 24 months the child eats with a spoon correctly. By 30 months the child can pour from a pitcher. The 15-month-old builds a two-block tower; the 24-month-old builds a five- to six-block tower (see Table 10-3).

PSYCHOSOCIAL DEVELOPMENT

Developmental task: autonomy vs. shame and doubt

The psychosocial developmental task of toddlers is to achieve a feeling of autonomy instead of shame and doubt. This stage lasts from approximately 18 months to 3 years. Toddlers must attain a sense of *autonomy*, or develop a sense of selfhood, i.e., a sense of being separate from others. Autonomous children feel competent and are able to assert their will and to do things independently. Toddlers who don't achieve autonomy experience *shame and doubt* and feel small, dependent, and worthless. These opposing forces are discussed in detail in this section.

Table 10-3 Fine Motor Development

Behavior	15 months	18 months	24 months	30 months
Building	Builds tower of two blocks	Builds tower of three blocks	Builds tower of five to six blocks Makes train of cubes	Builds tower of seven to eight blocks
Opening	Opens small boxes	Closes small boxes	Opens doors by turning knob Unscrews lid of jar	
Poking and turning	Pokes fingers in holes	Picks up small objects and places them in box Puts blocks in hole Turns book pages		
Feeding	Grasps cup but frequently spills when tipping cup Grasps empty spoon; cannot scoop up food; turns spoon upside down when bringing it to mouth	Drinks well from cup Fills spoon but spills often when bringing it to mouth Turns spoon upside down in mouth	Drinks well; holds glass in one hand Puts filled spoon in mouth without turning it over	Pours from pitcher; spills often
Drawing	Scribbles	Scribbles; tries to draw straight lines	Scribbling is more controlled; copies vertical and circular strokes	Draws horizontal and vertical lines; makes two lines for cross Holds crayon with fingers rather than entire hand
Self-care	Pulls shoes and socks off; sticks out arm or leg to help dressing	Removes own mittens; helps pull off shirt; helps unzip clothes	Removes most of own clothing; puts on own shoes, socks, and pants (inside out and backward)	

Autonomy The toddler's burgeoning sense of autonomy originated during infancy and strengthens to dominate the toddler's behavior (see Table 10-4). The infant complied with the mother's wishes in order to develop trust but probably protested being returned to bed by screaming and resisted being diapered by rolling away. Feelings of self-assertion began as the infant learned to influence the environment and make it respond to meet his or her needs. Trusting infants learned that the world and its caregivers were dependable and would meet their needs; the world became a safe place to explore. The toddler's readiness for becoming aware of selfhood, for being in control, and for influencing the world began in infancy.

The achievement of autonomy is based upon mastery of four concepts learned during infancy: (1) permanence of objects, (2) discrimination between inner and outer worlds, (3) recognition of the self as separate, and (4) gaining control over the body and the environment.[14] Each of these concepts will be discussed and related to the development of autonomy.

The infant learned that objects (people and toys) are permanent and exist when out of sight. This meant that the infant was developing a memory (could remember the lost toy), thought symbolically (mentally visualized the out-of-sight toy), and recognized the toy as separate from self. The child must discriminate between inner and outer worlds; without this distinction, there would be no outer world to control. The toddler's awareness of being separate from others increases the inner need to control the environment.

The toddler's need to autonomously control the environment and "to do things my way" per-

Table 10-4 Psychosocial Development

Behavior	18 months	24 months	30 months
Ritualism		Ritualistic behavior begins; is upset by changes in routine	Ritualistic behavior peaks
Imitation	Imitates parents' behavior; focuses on actions.		Imitates adult behavior, such as sex role behavior
	Imitates actions during play		Imitation is increasingly symbolic
Exploration	Explores drawers, house, everything	Explores constantly; resists restrictions on exploring	
Autonomy	Autonomous behavior is increasing, but is still dependent on mother	Is increasingly independent when away from mother	Independent behavior continues; is reluctant to go to bed
	Temper tantrums begin	Temper tantrums continue	Temper tantrums decrease
		Negativism increases; focuses on own wishes	Negativism continues
		Dawdles	Dawdles
Separation anxiety	Recognizes strangers but has less fear of them	Separation anxiety is at height; fears parents' leaving	Separation anxiety is still at peak; begins to learn to cope with separation anxiety
	Sucks thumb for comfort	Thumb-sucking decreases	Begins to use transitional object (security blanket or favorite toy) for comfort
Toileting	Is increasingly ready for toilet training; will eliminate in potty-chair; fecal smearing is common	Begins to cooperate in toilet training	Has mastered daytime bladder control; is beginning nighttime bladder control. "Accidents" are common
Play	Solitary play predominates	Parallel play begins	Parallel play continues
	Possessiveness begins	Cannot share toys; is still possessive	
Attention span	Has short attention span; shifts rapidly	Attention span is longer	

meates all aspects of development. *Negativism*—saying "No!" to most requests—is an automatic response of this age group. For example, a toddler will respond "No!" when offered a cookie. The response has little meaning for the toddler, who then immediately grabs the cookie and gobbles it. Such negative toddlers are simply asserting their will and testing their power to control other people. Negativism is the observable aspect of toddlers' inner need to assert autonomy.

The physical maturation of toddlers prepares them to assert their will and to control their actions and pushes them toward selfhood. The refining neuromuscular maturation of toddlers enables them to begin exploring the world. Fine and gross motor coordination mature. Toddlers can open the lids of jars to touch and taste the contents and can turn doorknobs to explore the outside world. They can run and may chase a ball into the street. Increased physical and psychological energy is needed to support these explorations. The increased energy levels of toddlers coincide with the development of increased ego growth.[15] Myelinization of the central nervous system readies toddlers to control elimination. A greatly expanding vocabulary allows them to express their needs and wants.

Gaining control over elimination, feeding, and dressing increases toddlers' feelings of self-control and autonomy (see Fig. 10-7). The toddler period corresponds to the anal stage of psychosexual development. The child must learn "to hold on and to let go." The child must let go of an inner wish to hold on to the stool and defecate when and where he or she wishes. Instead, the child must defecate when and where the parent decides. The toddler learns self-control and compromise. The toddler is also proud of the ability to eat and dress almost alone.

Self-control and compromise are two key components of *socialization*. Socialization is the

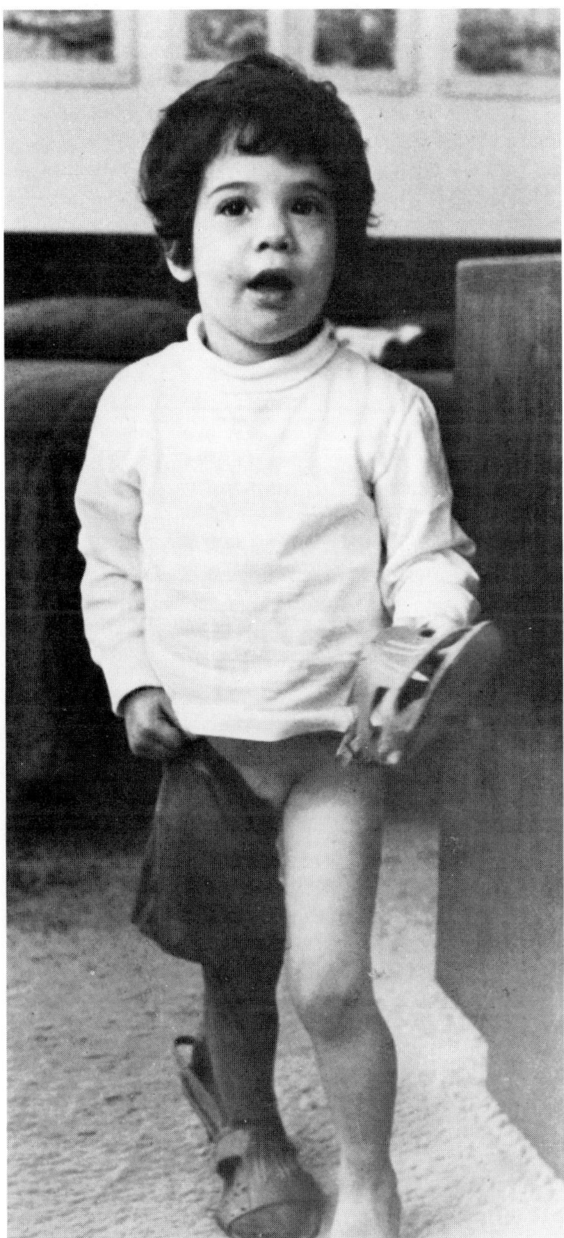

Figure 10-7 This child has partially undressed herself and has attempted to put on her mother's stockings and shoes. Toddlers learn to remove their clothing early, but they lack the perceptual and motor skill to get dressed without help.

learning of behavior needed to function successfully in a society: table manners, social conduct, and modesty, for example. Parents devote large amounts of time to the socialization of toddlers and preschoolers. The toddler must learn self-control and give-and-take. If children are always allowed to have their way and believe they can always dominate others, they will not learn to compromise. Awareness of the needs and wishes of others must begin in toddlerhood in order to assure future adaptation. Toddlers must learn to tolerate frustration of their own wishes to control others and to remain in emotional control.[16]

Shame and doubt Toddlers who do not achieve autonomy learn to feel shame and doubt. Shamed children feel small, self-conscious, dependent, worthless, and incompetent. While they feel increasingly in control, toddlers also recognize their inability to control everything and are aware of their dependency upon parents. These feelings plant the seeds of self-doubt. Toddlers recognize that their emotional outbursts may result in parental disapproval. When parents consistently restrict a toddler's attempts to manipulate objects, the child feels ineffectual, thwarted, and unable to learn about the environment. Overprotected children (see Chap. 34) are classic examples of children who feel shame and doubt. They are kept dependent upon parents and have difficulty achieving their potential. It is important that children avoid experiencing shame and doubt, for feelings of viciousness and hostility seem to result from a sense of worthlessness.[17]

Sex role distinction

Toddlers learn the appropriate sex role behavior by observing and imitating the behavior of same-sex models within the family. Sex roles are learned by age 3 (see Fig. 10-8). Toddlers imitate the same-sex parent's gestures, actions, tasks, posture, body movements, verbal expressions, and emotional control. For example, boys pretend to smoke pipes like their fathers, and girls apply makeup and wear jewelry like their mothers. The depth of an older toddler's learning of a sex role is obvious in his or her play. The toddler frequently copies the parent's exact movements, posture, actions, word choice, and inflection of voice. Parents are often surprised to see and hear a child-sized replica of themselves punishing a doll during play!

Children imitate their parents' behaviors that produce social and material rewards. They appreciate their parents, and they want to be like the same-sex parent and gain their parents' approval. Children will not imitate behavior that is

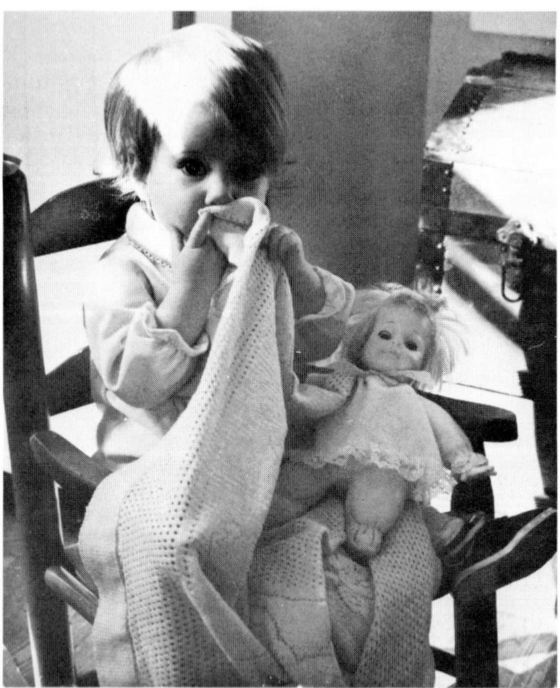

Figure 10-8 Play and imitation promote sex role learning. (*Photo courtesy of David Carroll.*)

punished.[18] If a child sees a same-sex parent repeatedly demeaned or abused, the child may avoid learning the sex role behavior to avoid punishment.

Despite the loosening of sex role stereotypes that has taken place recently, most parents expect different behavior from boys than from girls. This molding of the child's sex role behavior began during infancy and continues throughout childhood. Girls generally are allowed more emotional expression than boys. They are allowed to cry, pout, and whine longer than boys. Boys are traditionally expected to act stoically and are told, "Boys don't cry!" Girls are expected to be quieter and cleaner than boys. Boys are expected to show more aggression and physical exertion, as in rough-and-tumble play.

Parents' expectations of appropriate sex role behavior differ according to their cultural backgrounds. For example, boys in the United States are not encouraged to hug, kiss, or hold hands. In Middle Eastern cultures this behavior is acceptable. If the two parents have different expectations for behavior, the child will be confused about expected behavior and will have difficulty learning a sex role. The parents should discuss their different expectations, compromise, and present the child with consistent expectations.

Boys may have more difficulty learning their role than girls. This occurs because a boy is physically close to a role model of a different sex—the mother—for extended periods of time. He must then copy the behavior of a frequently absent parent. In order to clarify sex role differences and sexual identification, children of both sexes need role models of both sexes. Fathers should participate in child care, play with their children, and be physically present during the early years of childhood. Male teachers in nursery schools and male nurses in hospitals will strengthen children's sex role learning.

Young toddlers normally mix up sex role behavior because they are only beginning to distinguish between the sexes. Boys experiment with wearing lipstick and jewelry; girls experiment with shaving. This normal behavior does not indicate future homosexuality but rather demonstrates the child's learning about the world.

Toddlers begin to develop a sense of body awareness and a sense of body image. Toddlers are determining the outer boundaries of their bodies. The parents' sense of comfort or anxiety with their own bodies is easily transmitted to toddlers. Toddlers will imitate the parents and easily integrate feelings of shame about their bodily parts. A child learns shame if the parents exhibit shame, disapproval, or cover-up behavior when the child runs outside naked or touches the genitals. The child is *not* expressing precocious sexual urges but is simply learning about the body by touching it. Masturbation is normal and is universally practiced by both sexes. A child should not be shamed or slapped for this. Ways for helping parents deal with masturbation are discussed in Chap. 11.

Dolls that have genitals do not develop precocious sexual feelings in a child. The toddler's hormonal secretions are *not* mature enough to awaken sexual feelings. The child identifies with the doll and is pleased by their similar bodies. One mother bought her toddler a boy doll with genitals when his toilet training had slowed after hospitalization. The boy undressed the doll and excitedly exclaimed, "Mom, he looks just like me!" He then immediately rushed to the bathroom and "toilet trained" the doll. From then on, the child's toilet training progressed smoothly.

The feminist movement has altered the traditional sex roles. Toddlers should be allowed to

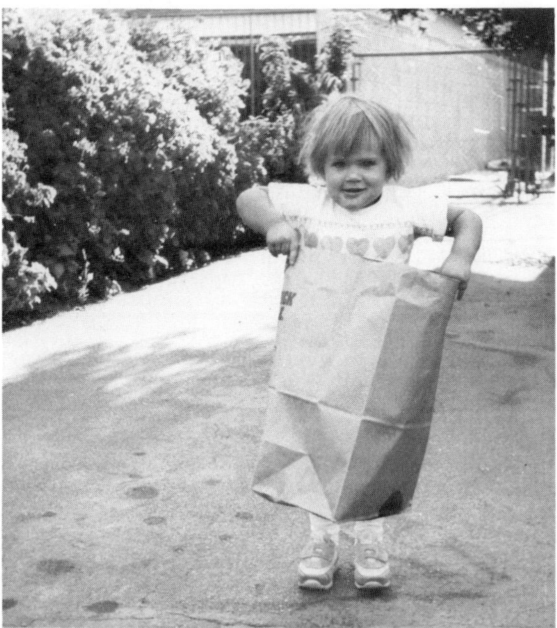

Figure 10-9 Toddlers are not sex role traditionalists: they enjoy experimenting with adult roles of all kinds.

play with toys they prefer. Girls can use tools and garden, and boys can learn parenting skills and express emotion by practicing on dolls. By having a variety of play experiences instead of being restricted to traditional boy or girl toys, children will learn more about the world and its people. (See Fig. 10-9.)

Toilet training

Toilet training is a main task that a toddler must master. *Toilet training* refers to the learned process of eliminating in a place and manner sanctioned by society. Attitudes toward toilet training vary among cultures. In many poorer socioeconomic classes of the world, infants and toddlers run through the house and yard eliminating at will. Parental attitudes toward toilet training are thus more lenient, and the children may essentially train themselves. In the United States, children are trained earlier, and the excreta is confined to bathrooms.

The parents' methods of, and attitudes toward, toilet training will influence various aspects of the toddler's present and future life. They will affect the child's feelings and attitudes toward the body, sexuality, cleanliness, generosity versus miserliness (the ability to give and receive), self-esteem, and achievement of autonomy or feelings of shame and doubt.

Toilet-trained toddlers are increasingly autonomous and able to care for themselves, and they take pride in their independence and ability to please their parents. If children are shamed, perhaps for fecal smearing, they feel inadequate and incompetent, and their self-esteem will be lowered. Children learn to associate these negative feelings with the body. A toddler perceives his or her body with indefinite boundaries, is establishing separate identity, and may label the entire body as negative. In an attempt to avoid parental displeasure, a child may try to overcontrol toileting and may even avoid it.

Freud placed prime emphasis on toilet-training methods as indicators of later adult adjustment. He believed that the adult personality trends of generosity versus miserliness (to hold on versus to let go) were outgrowths of toilet training during toddlerhood. Research suggests that emotional problems in older children are related to premature bowel training with the use of coercive methods. Children whose parents used such methods may exhibit restlessness, tics, body manipulation, speech disturbances, psychosomatic ailments, or school failure despite adequate intelligence. Other symptoms include compulsiveness, aggression, negativism, fearfulness, timidness, overconformity, and inability to make decisions.[19]

Toilet training is an area in which an early mother-child contest of wills takes place. The mother requires the child to become socialized—to eliminate in a certain place and at a certain time. By following inner urges to defecate when and where he or she wishes, the child risks disapproval. The toddler wants to retain the mother's approval and so bows to her wishes. This submission in order to obtain later gratification of wishes is one area in which the toddler learns compromise, an essential ingredient of successful adult relationships.

Timing Children should not be rushed or forced into toilet training until the age of 18 to 24 months, when voluntary sphincter control develops.[20] Toddlers simultaneously learn bowel and bladder control. They achieve daytime bowel and bladder control at 27 to 29 months,[21] and nighttime bladder control by 3 to $4\frac{1}{2}$ years. Almost 50 percent are still bed-wetting at 4 to 5 years. There are several reasons why bowel control is sometimes mastered first. Bowel movements are more regular, easier for parents to predict, and fewer in number than urinations. Bowel movements also cause a stronger sensation and urge; it is easier for the toddler to associate these feelings with defecation. Girls toilet train earlier than boys. This is believed to be due to boys' slower development in general.

Readiness There are several prerequisites that must be met before a toddler is ready to be toilet trained. The child must have the neuromuscular maturity to walk to the bathroom, pull down clothing, and recognize the urge to urinate or defecate, as well as the sphincter control to hold in the urine or stool until he or she is on the potty. The child must be able to communicate his or her need to defecate by words, actions, or facial expression. The mother must be alert to the child's nonverbal behavior indicating a need to eliminate because the child has limited verbal ability (see Fig. 10-10). The toddler must recognize the sensation of the urge to defecate and associate it with releasing the stool on the potty.

In order for the child to learn bowel and bladder control, the central nervous system must be fully myelinated. Myelinization ensures that the brain's message will speedily reach the bladder or rectum. Only then can the child hold in and excrete voluntarily. Toilet training should begin after the child walks. (See Table 10-5 for readiness behaviors and training procedures.)

Fecal smearing Most toddlers smear feces, commonly between 15 and 18 months. Toddlers have not learned that stool is dirty and should be avoided. To them, it is not shameful but is something warm and smearable that they have produced. They are proud of this product and smear it to learn about it. Parents should not shame a child for fecal smearing. They should instead tell the child not to play with the stool and offer clay, paste, finger paints, or another, more acceptable substance that allows smearing. (See Fig. 10-11.) The toddler thus learns a new method of handling this urge to smear.

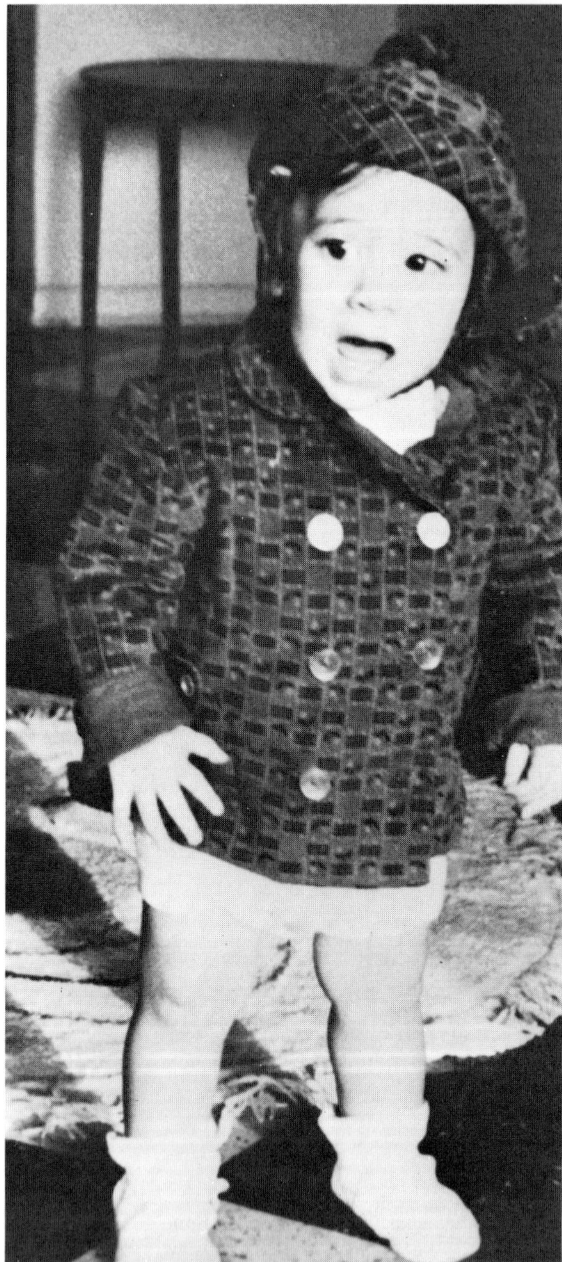

Figure 10-10 Toddlers indicate their toileting needs through gestures and facial expressions before they learn to use words for that purpose.

Wetting accidents "Wetting" accidents occur among all children *throughout* the preschool years. Parents need not be overly concerned about wetting. Toddlers frequently are so absorbed in play that they do not feel or heed the urge to urinate until it is too late. If a child wets the bed several times a week, a casual wait-and-see attitude after a negative physical examination is best. The child should not be punished. Parents should preserve the child's self-esteem by saying, "It's okay. Next time I bet you'll come in earlier to pee." Excessive spanking reinforces the unwanted behavior; ignoring the behavior weakens it.

Table 10-5 Guidelines for Toilet Training

1. Indications that child is ready for training	Rationale
Walks	Indicates myelinization of spinal cord to bladder and anus
Is dry for 2 h or awakens from nap dry	Bladder size will expand to hold urine
Indicates neuromuscular maturity. Can walk to bathroom, can pull down pants, and attempts to hold in urine or feces (may not succeed at first)	Child has sufficiently mature nervous and musculoskeletal system and is ready for more self-care and toileting
Indicates wish to be trained. May pull down diapers, point to puddles on the floor, or bring dirty diapers to parent	Child feels uncomfortable in wet diapers; wants to control elimination
Has characteristic behaviors before defecation; grunting, glassy stare, or red face	Each child has individual behaviors which the mother can "read" to help predict defecation

2. Training procedure	Rationale
Record time of child's elimination for several days	Child will train more easily on own schedule than on parent's schedule
Do not start training if child is under stress caused by illness, hospitalization, or divorce, or has a new baby sitter or new sibling	Child needs to deal with present stress; learning new task during stress will take longer and be less successful
Approach child with nurturant, nonthreatening, and expectant attitude	Parent is setting up expectancy to succeed, not fail
Tell child in simple words what to do. "This is your potty-chair where you sit down and go poop." Use the family term for excreta	Child needs to be told clearly what is expected in simple words
Use potty-chair or toilet seat. Set child on it for 10-min periods at usual time for defecation or about 1 h after meals	Chair feels more secure to child than adult's toilet; extremely long time periods will cause child to reject potty-chair
Stay with child	Child left alone may feel abandoned
Place potty-chair in bathroom in one place	Toddler must know there is *one* place to defecate. Moving potty-chair may tell child it is okay to defecate in several places
Do not allow toys while child is on potty-chair	Child needs to know there is *one* reason to sit on potty-chair. Toddler's attention span is short, and toys will distract them from defecation
When child defecates, give a reward: "That's great! You went in the potty-chair."	Rewarding the desired behavior strengthens it. This statement increases child's self-esteem and emphasizes the achieved behavior
Toddlers frequently wet pants accidentally going to the bathroom or while playing. Ignore the accident and do not punish child	Accidents usually occur. Child has not perfected sphincter control and does not heed elimination urge while playing until too late
Dress child in training pants or "fancy" pants	Training pants are associated with "big girls and boys," whereas diapers are associated with babies
Provide slacks with elastic waistband	Elastic waistbands are easy to pull down and encourage self-care
Have children of both sexes sit to void at beginning. If boy stands to urinate, be certain toilet seat will not fall and hit penis	Toilet seat may injure penis. Pain associated with toilet may delay training
Have child with same-sex adult in bathroom each day	Child will imitate parent's behavior
Child is ready for night training when dry the entire day. Protect mattress with plastic	Bladder is storing urine for larger periods. Mattress protector decreases the mother's anxiety and work

Ill or anxious children regress, and toddlers usually regress by losing their newly acquired toilet-training skills. They regain control when the stress is relieved. Additional nursing interventions are listed in Chap 11, and regression is discussed in Chap. 15.

Learning self-control

Toddlers must learn to control primitive, emotional outbursts and learn more constructive methods of emotional control. Learning emotional self-control and balance is not easy. Many

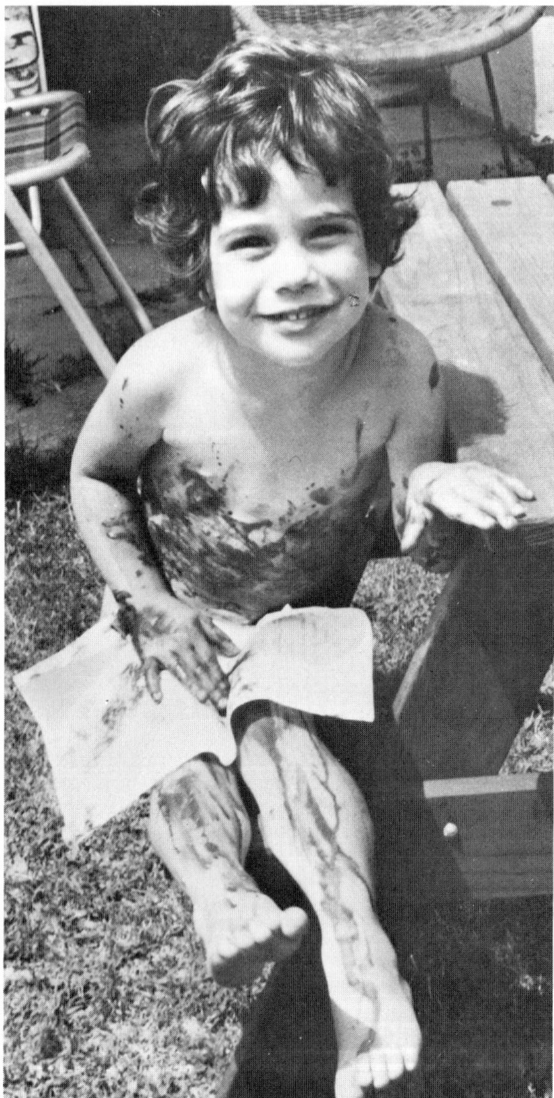

Figure 10-11 Toddlers like to play with mud and finger paints. Smearing is a natural way of enjoying and learning at this developmental stage.

people do not achieve emotional self-control until adulthood. In order to develop self-control, toddlers must recognize their own actions in a situation, want to copy the behavior of a role model, and imitate the role model's behavior while trying to control their behavior.[22]

Discipline *All* children need and want discipline. The goals of discipline are to help the child learn (1) how to gain self-control, (2) how to comply with the behavior approved by the parents and society, and (3) how to get along with others. Each goal will be discussed in this section.

Punishment and discipline are not synonymous. Discipline includes both power-assertive (punishment) and love-oriented techniques. Punishing helps the punisher feel better, appeases the punisher's anger, and may prevent a recurrence through fear. Punishment makes the child feel powerless, forces submission, does not teach acceptable behavior, and lowers the child's self-esteem. Love-oriented techniques, discussed later under "Guidelines," correct behavior. They increase motivation to behave by building on the child's inherent wish to please the parents and increase self-esteem.

Children must learn respect for authority. Parents are the first teachers of authority, and the parent-child relationship is the model for all later relationships. If parents want to be respected during the teen years, they must be worthy of and establish respect during the preschool years.[23] For example, a parent can establish authority during a fight by bodily removing a biter or kicker from the victim and using spoken words to reinforce the physical command: "Stop biting Johnny now. It hurts." Children become respectful and responsible as a result of love and discipline.[24]

Discipline helps children learn self-control. Toddlers intensely feel the emotions of love, hate, and aggression. Only with the parents' limit setting will they learn to control these emotions, to channel them in constructive ways, and to learn new methods of coping.

Discipline is an essential component of accepting the self and successfully interacting with others. Many parents are afraid that discipline will squelch a child's development. This is one of the most widespread fallacies about discipline. One child psychologist writes, "The greatest social disaster of this century is the belief that abundant love makes discipline unnecessary."[25] Discipline *is* necessary. Children do *not* know how to act and must be told how to behave. Each neighborhood has an "obnoxious kid" or a "holy terror" who causes parents to cringe when he or she arrives. This child, who has not learned the rules of society's "game plan" through discipline, begins life and school at a disadvantage. He or she must later learn the rules from strangers, with a greater risk of rejection, disapproval, and even ostracism. Discipline helps children learn to live within the rules of their society and sociocultural group.

Limit setting may cause temporary anger but will make the child feel secure. The toddler's limit testing indicates a need for consistent limits and help in controlling primitive impulses. For example, 2-year-old John has broken the television and has been told not to "touch or kick the TV." John touches the TV, is told "No," and reaches toward the TV again while looking at his mother's face for disapproval. The mother again says, "John, don't touch it. No." John withdraws his hand, slaps it as if to reinforce his mother's command, and says, "John, no touch!" The mother was patient, repeated the instructions several times, and used action-oriented words ("kick" and "touch") instead of abstract terms ("Don't go near it" or "Cool it!"). John illustrates the toddler's reaching out for consistent discipline.

Discipline is necessary to prevent accidents. Toddlers do not know the consequences of their actions and are often on the brink of an accident. (See Fig. 10-12.) Eventually, children learn to trust parents' words—that the iron *is* hot, that injuries *do* result from unsafe play. They listen to parents' warnings and feel more comfortable, self-assured, and secure.

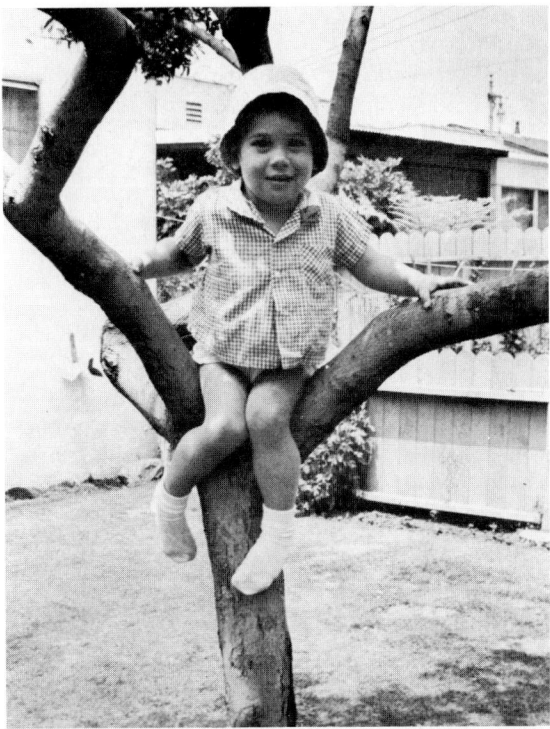

Figure 10-12 Toddlers develop the curiosity and motor skills to get into unsafe situations, but they lack the experience and judgment to avoid hazards. Discipline and safe, supervised play settings are essential to prevent accidents.

Guidelines While there are many theories of, and approaches to, disciplining children, the following are the essential components of all techniques:

1. Discipline must be *consistent*. If toddlers receive different responses when they break rules, they become confused and unsure about how they are expected to act and insecure, anxious, and doubtful of their self-control. Toddlers need consistency in order to predict responses to their actions.
2. Discipline must be *immediate*. Toddlers have a very short attention span and are easily distracted. If forced to wait for discipline, toddlers will forget what they did wrong and the discipline will have no meaning. Some mothers "wait until Daddy gets home" to discipline. Some theorists believe this practice allows the mother to project her anger onto her husband, forcing him to be the "bad guy." Discipline should be *jointly* practiced by all caregivers.
3. Discipline must be *related* to the incident. When a toddler is caught digging up a neighbor's flowers, for example, the child should be led firmly away from the neighbor's garden and directed to his or her own sandbox or garden to dig. The parent should tell the child, "You cannot dig in Mrs. Clark's garden. You can dig here in your sandbox." Preventing the toddler from watching television is not related to the incident, does not tell the child how to act, and will have less impact on the child.
4. Instructions should be *repeated* many times. Toddlers should not always be expected to respond after being told something one or two times. It takes several repetitions for many adults to learn a procedure, and so it is unrealistic to expect a small child to learn quickly.
5. Toddlers must be given time to respond to instructions; an immediate response cannot

be expected. The toddler's nervous system is immature and cannot process two messages at the same time (see the earlier discussion of the nervous system). The child may be physiologically unable to respond immediately. Toddlers should be given time to weigh following their inner urges against minding their parents. They must be given the *time* to learn self-control.

6. If the toddler does not mind, he or she probably *did not understand* the parent's directions. Parents often give instructions using colloquial or abstract terms. The toddler thinks concretely and does not understand the parent's slang words. If a parent says, "Bug off," "Simmer down," or "You're cruisin' for a bruisin'," the child thinks concretely and may visualize a bug or simply be confused. To the child, such statements are not clearly related to the broken rule. Parents should use action-oriented words and focus on feelings. For example, "Billy, don't touch the waffle iron. It's hot and will hurt!"
7. Adults should *not* expect each detail of a toddler's behavior to be correct. This expectation is incompatible with the toddler's development and imposes adult standards on a small child. Even most adults do not have perfect behavior. An adult who expects a toddler to act perfectly is setting the child up to fail.
8. Behaviors to be disciplined should be *prioritized*. The highest-priority behaviors needing discipline are usually potentially *unsafe* activities, such as running into the street, playing in a parked car, or exploring medicine cabinets or shelves under kitchen sinks. Both parents should jointly decide which behaviors to focus on. When these are mastered, new behaviors can be addressed. The toddler will be overwhelmed and shamed by a burden of many behaviors to control simultaneously.
9. Children must be given *clear limits*. They must be told exactly what behaviors will not be tolerated. Their energies should be redirected to acceptable outlets. Clear instructions will tell a child exactly what is expected. For example, 3-year-old Alice is chasing a playmate, shouting, "I'll kill you! Go away," and is swinging wildly, attempting to hit her playmate on the head with a large board. Her mother should take the board away and say, "Alice, you *cannot* hit Mary on the head with a board. It will hurt her." Then she should redirect the child's energy to an acceptable outlet—such as a beanbag toss. The child should also be told how to act: "Alice, when you get so angry next time, come and tell me, and we'll toss the beanbag."
10. If a child is out of control, is unsafe, or is harming another child, *soft restraint* should be employed. For example, the mother can hold the child in her lap while calmly and quietly saying, "I will hold you to help you be calm and quiet. You cannot pull the cloth off the table." While continuing to hold the child, the mother should speak softly until the child regains control. The mother should then tell the child what behavior is acceptable and choose an activity to help the child express aggression.
11. Withdrawal of love should *not* be used as a punishment. Saying, "If you don't mind me, I won't love you anymore," establishes distrust and insecurity in the child. Loss of parental love is the toddler's greatest fear. If toddlers cannot trust their parents, it is difficult for them to achieve autonomy and may adversely affect their later relationships. Instead, the *action* should be focused on, not the love. For example, "John, I love you, but you *cannot* poke the dog's eye." This statement separates the love from the action. Children need to *know* they are loved in spite of their wrong actions.
12. Extensive explanations and arguing should be *avoided*. The toddler cannot think logically and cannot understand the adult's point of view. Valuable time is wasted on explanations of why the adult is correct.
13. The child must have a *reason* for minding. "Do it because I said so" communicates only anger and power and does not provide a basis for learning. Toddlers believe there is a reason for everything, and they understand (although they may not like) such a simple reason as "because Grandmother would be sad if you broke her dish."
14. *Bribing* must be avoided. Bribing statements such as, "If you stop screaming, I'll buy you a new toy," establish child-parent manipulation. The screaming behavior is rewarded with a new toy, and the child will use it again. Instead, parents should imply

that compliance is *expected:* "Jane, it's time for your bath now. After your bath, do you want to play paper dolls or something else?"

Techniques Ideal discipline techniques for the toddler are time out, reward, and diversion and are discussed in Chap. 11. Doll play is an ideal, pleasurable method of disciplining and communicating with children (see Chap. 15).

Temper tantrums A *temper tantrum* is a violent outburst of emotional and physical energy in response to anger (see Fig. 10-13). Toddlers express anger and frustration by falling to the floor, screaming, kicking, biting, and even holding their breath until they faint. Tantrums are a notorious cause of the label "the terrible twos," and parents frequently seek a nurse's counsel.

Toddlers have limited methods of expressing frustration when their wishes are thwarted. They have limited verbal ability and so have difficulty expressing their wishes and their increasing frustration. They have not learned emotional control. They cannot solve problems, cannot delay gratification, cannot anticipate the consequences of the tantrum, and cannot see the parent's increasing anger. Instead, they are immersed in feelings of rage and frustration.

When toddlers have temper tantrums, it is very important *not* to give in and let them have their way. Rewarding the behavior (giving in to a toddler's wishes) strengthens the tantrum behavior. Toddlers then use tantrums increasingly to control their parents, even in markets or restaurants. Toddlers will stop using tantrums to control others when the tantrums do not help them achieve their goals. Wise parents give negative reinforcement by *ignoring* the behavior. Toddlers quickly stop screaming when the audience (the parent) leaves the room. Toddlers' breath holding should also be ignored. Even if the breath is held until fainting is induced, breathing (driven by carbon dioxide buildup) resumes automatically.[26]

The disciplinary methods of bribing, screaming, and spanking are less effective than ignoring. Bribing a child sets up child-parent manipulation. Screaming at a child or comparing the child's behavior with that of a "bad" sibling or a

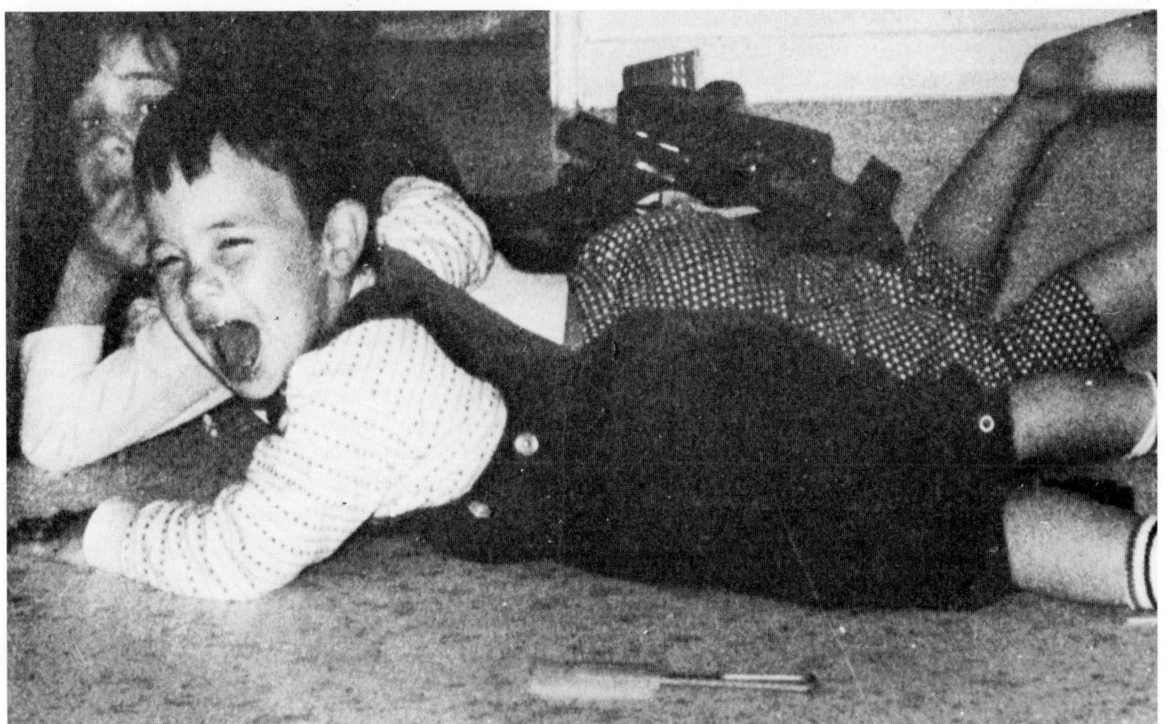

Figure 10-13 Temper tantrums are common reactions of toddlers to the frustration of being either unable or forbidden to do as they wish.

television tyrant is ineffective. Toddlers are self-centered and cannot compare their behavior with that of other children.

Ignoring tantrum behavior works well. After the toddler has calmed down enough to listen, the parent should do the following: (1) Label the child's feeling: "Jill, the way you feel now is called angry or mad." (2) Teach the child a more socially acceptable method of expressing anger: "Jill, instead of screaming, say, 'Mom, I'm angry,' and hit the punching bag as hard as you can!" (3) Offer the child alternative play materials on which the child can take out the anger: punching bags and gloves, hammer and peg sets, beanbags, stuffed animals or pillows, or clay. Many toddlers are reluctant to express aggression and at first hit the toys gingerly. The parent should approve of the child's expression of anger, saying, "Jill, that's it! Hit it harder! Harder! It's OK. Hit the punching bag when you're mad!" (4) Reassure the child that he or she is loved. Toddlers' loss of self-control makes them feel insecure. Egocentric toddlers think that everyone thinks as they do; they assume that the parent hates them as they hate the parent. They are therefore afraid of the parent's hate and possible withdrawal of love. Verbal approval can be reinforced with touch, perhaps a hug or a pat. (5) Offer a task which the toddler can do. This will encourage feelings of competence and decrease the shame and insecurity caused by the loss of emotional control and the parent's disapproval. (6) Use star charts and time out to reinforce approved behavior (see Chap. 11).[27]

Negativism *Negativism* refers to the toddler's "No!" given in response to almost every request. Negativism is the observable behavior resulting from children's inner need to assert their will and their wish to dominate others. Parents frequently need assurance that the toddler's "No!" is an automatic response and is not a defiant testing of their authority. Toddlers are egocentric, believe that everyone thinks as they do, and cannot imagine what adults are thinking.

Nurses can instruct parents to use several methods of handling negativism. Parents should be instructed not to overreact by spanking, but instead offer the toddler safe, alternative choices. Choices give children an opportunity to assert their will within reasonable limits that are acceptable to parents. For example, a parent should say, "It's time to eat dinner now. Do you want to eat the meat or the vegetables first?" This does not encourage a "No!" answer and gives the toddler an opportunity to make a choice and assert his or her will. Parents should be urged not to ask questions such as, "Do you want to go to bed now?" because they will always elicit a "No!" response. Instead, the mother can use a clear, action-oriented statement about her expectations and then allow a choice: "You must go to bed now. Which doll do you want to take with you?" A parent can easily divert a toddler's attention to another object, and the toddler will quickly forget the "No!" Finally, the toddler should not be given a time-consuming choice when the parent is in a hurry. This increases the parent's frustration and promotes dawdling.

Destructiveness Parents should be instructed to avoid constantly saying "No" to a toddler. This will stifle the child's development, thwart exploration, promote shame and doubt by making the child feel powerless and incompetent, and decrease the child's creativity and independence. When a parent constantly says "No," the child stops hearing it. "No" should be reserved for times when the child's safety is endangered.

Toddlers have limited self-control and cannot be expected to leave their parents' treasures alone indefinitely. Therefore, breakable, valuable objects should be moved to high places, and toddlers can be given their "own" drawer in the living room or kitchen. Toddlers must be given the opportunity to make choices and explore safely. Otherwise, they will not learn to assert themselves and will have difficulty becoming separate, autonomous people.

Dawdling *Dawdling* occurs when toddlers resist their parents' requests and do nothing. Dawdling reaches its height during toddlerhood, when children are caught in an ambivalent conflict, choosing between their own wishes and their parents' requests. They do nothing while making a decision. Toddlers can be affectionately helped to make decisions and to act by being told, for example, "I will help you put your jacket on this time. Next time perhaps you can do it alone." Such guidance helps children obey and establishes the expectation for cooperating in the future.

Ritualism Rituals give the toddler control over the environment and nurture feelings of security. The toddler relies on the sameness of all minute objects to maintain consistency and security in the environment. Field dependence, a characteristic of cognitive development, causes the toddler to believe that the entire environment is changed if one small object is altered. This accounts for the toddler's occasional hysterical, anxious overreactions when given a different cup, when two foods touch on a plate, or when the security blanket is missing.

The understanding parent encourages security in the toddler and avoids tantrums and frustration by catering to the child's need for rituals. Favorite times for rituals are mealtimes and bedtime. The toddler therefore needs the same cup, plate, and silverware and the same bedtime sequence of a quieting-down time, a story, a lullaby, prayers, and a favorite doll or stuffed animal.

Sleep Toddlers are reluctant to go to bed, they have nightmares, and they often disrupt their parents' sleep. Parents frequently seek a nurse's advice. The toddler's need for sleep decreases to 12 to 14 h a night. Toddlers gradually relinquish the morning nap, but most need an afternoon nap of 1 to 2 h. REM (rapid eye movement) sleep, during which dreams occur, constitutes 25 percent of sleep at age 2 and 20 percent between ages 3 and 5. NREM (non-rapid eye movement) sleep increases from 75 percent of sleep at age 2 to 80 percent between ages 3 and 5.

Toddlers are extremely reluctant to go to bed and will try every excuse and delay tactic to stay up. They seem to be afraid of missing some excitement while sleeping. Nightmares peak at 2 to 4 years. Toddlers need parents' support and consistent limit setting to obtain adequate rest and sleep. They should be placed in bed for a nap or a rest and kept there for a "rest time" even if they resist sleep. The child may take one favorite cuddly toy, but several toys divert the child to play, not sleep. Specific interventions for putting a child to bed and dealing with nightmares are discussed in Chaps. 11 and 15. Toddlers need adequate sleep to avoid frequent infections, irritability, and dulled intellectual functioning. The toddler who gets enough sleep can get up in the morning; is relaxed and happy; has a good appetite, bright eyes, erect posture, and vibrant skin; is curious and enthusiastic; and has sufficient energy for active play.[28]

Play Toddlers would rather play than do anything else. They spend most of their time at play. (See Tables 10-6 and 10-7.) Play is not wasted time but is serious business, i.e., the child's *work*. Toddlers work very hard to master tasks and seem to concentrate their entire being on gaining proficiency. When they master a skill, they integrate it into other movements and play activities. For example, at first, children run slowly and falteringly, and then faster and more assuredly. Soon they run up stairs, backward, in circles, and in short spurts, making fast stops. Eventually, they master running. Then the reciprocal leg motion is adapted to riding a kiddie car.

Table 10-6 Content of Play

Content of play	Examples
Social play. Toddlers receive pleasurable stimulation and learn social skills as they relate to others. They learn slowly to play with others (Fig. 10-14).	Playing alongside others. Nuzzling, playing pat-a-cake, smiling, teasing siblings
Sense pleasure play. Stimulation from both animate and inanimate objects brings pleasure. Toddlers reach out for stimulation.	Finger painting (smearing), pounding pegs, sand play, masturbation, bouncing to music, fondling a soft blanket, feeling the heat of the sun, smelling flowers
Skill play. Toddlers reach out for stimulation by an object. This involves more than one sense. They repeat skills to master them.	Playing with blocks, throwing a ball, playing with a push-pull toy, stair climbing, tricycle riding, dressing dolls, running
Dramatic play. Toddlers imitate or copy everyday events or scenes, usually within the family. This introduces sex roles and socialization.	Putting on lipstick and pretending to shave (copying the same-sex parent)

Source: Adapted from L. J. Stone and J. Church. *Childhood and Adolescence,* Random House, New York, 1973, pp. 235–238.

Play is a crucial part of physical, cognitive, and psychosocial development. The purposes of the toddler's play are to:

1. Refine fine and gross motor skills, eye-hand coordination, and spatial orientation (Fig. 10-15). Muscular strength and coordination are increased by banging drums, throwing balls, hammering nails, and feeding dolls.
2. Gain independence and differentiation of self. Play allows once-dependent toddlers to explore all objects in a search for new stimulation. Ambulation increases their exploration to new vistas. Exploration of each object brings

Table 10-7 Play Activities

Type of play	18 months	2–3 years
Gross motor play	Large hollow wooden blocks Low slide Low swing with arms and back Large riding toys (car, fire engine, etc.) Rocking chair Small table and chair Push and pull toys	Sand box, mud Large blocks, cardboard boxes Interlocking block trains Wagon, shopping cart Soft balls Punching bag
Creative play	Nesting blocks Hammer boards Toys with shaped openings to receive different shaped blocks Wrist bells	Large beads to string Braided strings with rigid tips to lace Wooden puzzles Fingerpaints Clay Colored construction paper Blunt scissors
Dramatic play	Wooden train Sand toys (pail, shovel, sieve) Stuffed toys	Strong vehicles (car, truck, etc.) Toy telephone Housekeeping toys (mixer, iron, broom) Carriage, doll bed, and high chair Washable doll to bathe Baby doll
Quiet play	Fingerpaints Clay Water play Blowing bubbles	Wooden shoe to lace Paint Large crayons Cloth or cardboard books Cloth boards to lace with string Toys for water play (sponge, soap, rotary beater, sieve) Simple puzzles

Source: Adapted from Ruth E. Hartley and Robert M. Goldonson, *The Complete Book of Children's Play,* Thomas Crowell, New York, 1957, pp. 39–67, 399–400, and Ruth B. Roufberg: *Today He Can't, Tomorrow He Can! Your Child from Two to Five Years,* vol. 2, The Learning Child, New York, 1971, and Sandra Streeply: *Today He Can't, Tomorrow He Can! Your Child from Birth to Two Years, A Comprehensive Guide to Educational Materials,* vol. 1, The Learning Child, New York, 1971.

new sensations and a realization of self as separate from the object.

3. Gain self-esteem. Toddlers learn that they initiate an action and have power to affect movement, and they study the results (Fig. 10-16). How powerful they must feel being able to manipulate objects and cause something to happen! When they are disciplined for misbehaving and their self-esteem is lowered, they retreat to the small, safe harbor of toys. They manage these toys, practice solutions to the problems, and once again feel powerful and autonomous.
4. Learn to control inner urges within the limits set by parents and begin socialization. Toddlers cannot play with medicines, cross the street unescorted to retrieve a ball, or hit the dog with a hammer. They practice emotional control by projecting feelings onto toys, especially dolls, and playing out emotions. They practice controlling these emotions and expressing them during play.
5. Learn sex role identification. Young toddlers begin to adopt a sex role, and frequently they become confused. A boy may parade around in his mother's jewelry and makeup, and a girl may pretend to shave and smoke her father's pipe. With parental feedback, toddlers quickly adopt traditional sex roles. Young toddlers spend long hours pretending to do household chores: washing dishes, mowing, and cooking.

Toddlers have progressed from the solitary play of infancy to *parallel play.* In parallel play, two or more toddlers play side by side, even in the same sandpile. They are too egocentric to play together. Toddlers frequently grab each other's

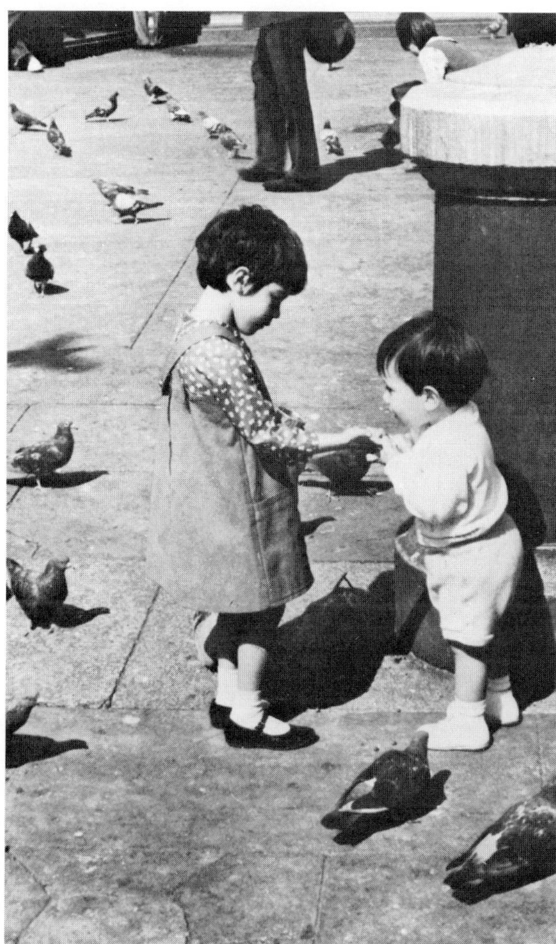

Figure 10-14 Toddlers are attracted to other people and, with experience, gradually learn the rules of social give-and-take.

toys and are very possessive. They hit and fight to obtain the coveted toy, not to hurt the other child. They do not realize that they are hurting the other child because they are self-centered and they are not hurt. They feel no shame because no conscience has yet developed.

Toddlers still function in a sensorimotor modality. They learn about objects by exploring and manipulating them. (Fig. 10-17). For this reason, play that stimulates the senses is especially beneficial for toddlers: sandboxes with strainers, buckets, shovels, funnels, and spoons; water play with cups, boats, bubbles, colanders, plastic cups, and eggbeaters; mud pies; and finger paints.

Play is a superb method of encouraging socialization and teaching a child. Many child care activities are made fun and educational through play. Favorite dolls are bathed; bath toys encourage fun and new sensations; cutting out cookies teaches geometrical shapes. Doll play reflects the feelings of the child and is an excellent method of eliciting the child's thoughts. (See Chap. 15.)

Parents should be observers of play, guardians of safety, and arbitrators of fights. Toddlers need freedom to explore in a safe environment. The yard and house must be child-proofed *daily.* Toys must be safe, strong, and too large to swallow or insert in an ear. Parents must lock up medicines and tools and put away household breakables; they must use caution when they allow the child to explore the yard or neighborhood. They must also firmly forbid crossing the street without an adult for any reason and provide close supervi-

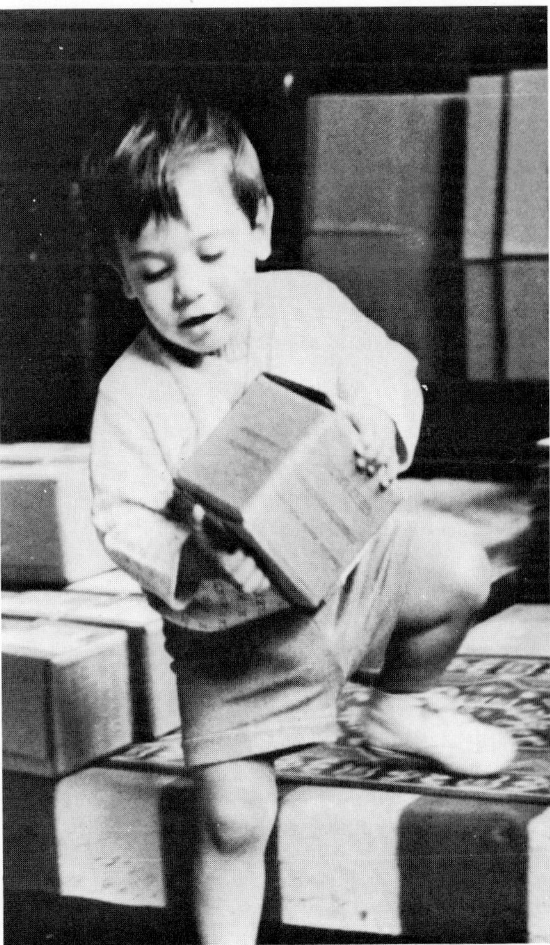

Figure 10-15 Play activities develop toddlers' balance, perception, learning, and control of large and small muscles.

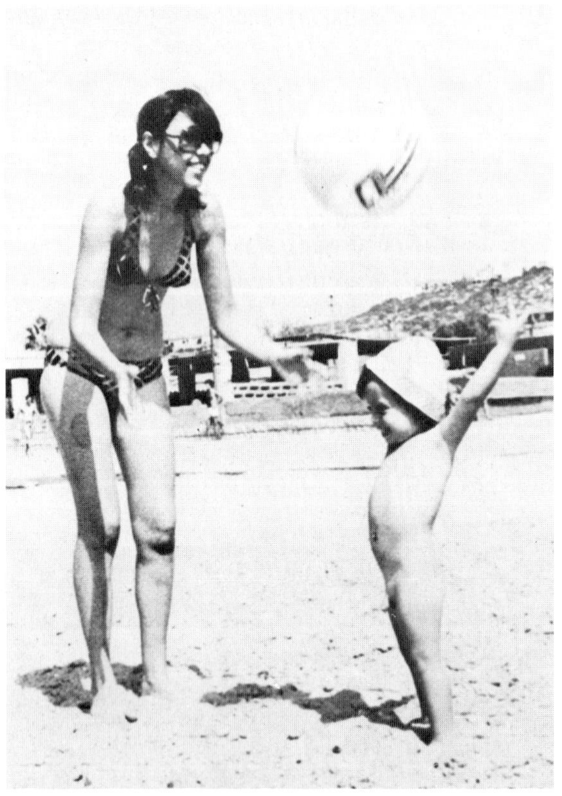

Figure 10-16 Toddlers take great delight in physical activity and in their abilities.

sion to enforce this rule. In unsafe situations, instructions should be simple and authoritarian in tone, and no choices should be given.

Parents should allow toddlers to choose from among their toys without interfering. Child development theorists believe that a child will instinctively choose the most healing, beneficial toy. A toy selected by the parent meets the parent's needs. Further discussion of the nurse's role in play appears in Chap. 15.

Fear and anxieties *Separation anxiety* The greatest fear of toddlers is losing their parents. Toddlers who are separated from their parents progress through a series of grief reactions called *separation anxiety.* Children attached themselves to their parents during infancy and learned that unseen objects still exist. Paradoxically, the urge of toddlers to separate from their parents intensifies the fear of losing them. They want to do things alone, but realize that they are dependent on their parents and want their attention and care. These ambivalent feelings increase feelings of insecurity and foster separation anxiety.

One of the main tasks of toddlerhood is to master separation from parents for short periods. Games such as peekaboo and hide-and-seek help toddlers master separation. Toddlers gradually learn that parents leave for work and then return home, and they associate the return with a meaningful activity, such as dinnertime. However, toddlers have no true concept of time. An hour may seem like an eternity, which increases a child's feelings of vulnerability.

Parents can decrease a toddler's separation anxiety by having the same baby-sitters. A new sitter should be introduced gradually to the child. If the sitter visits several times in the home and

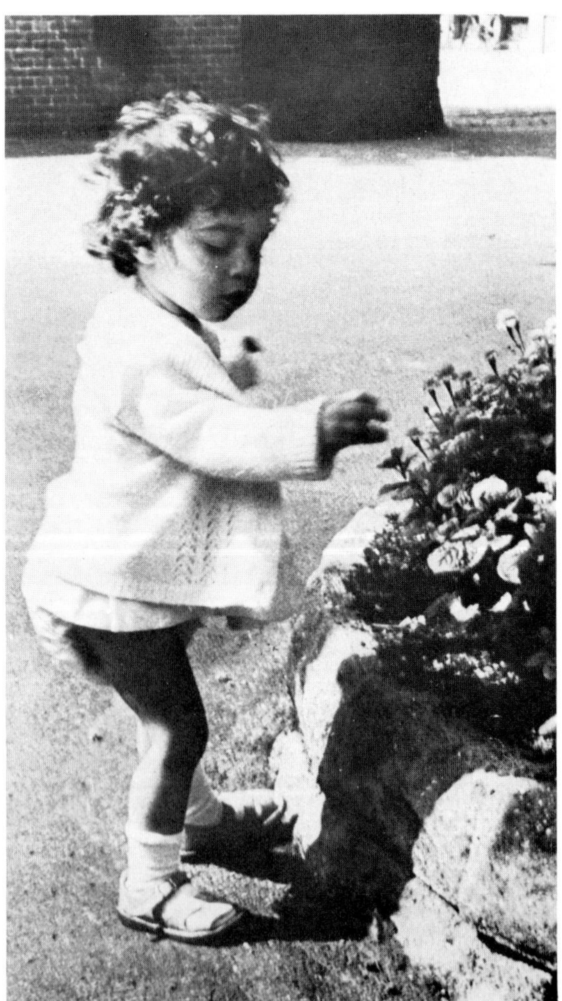

Figure 10-17 The toddler's learning depends on having experiences that involve the senses: touch, smell, vision, and hearing.

interacts with the parents and the child and if the child sees the parents' approval of the sitter, the child will accept the sitter more easily. Parents should leave behind some object that is associated with them, such as keys, a wallet, a purse, or jewelry. The toddler is object-oriented and will feel reassured that the parents will return for the object. Toddlers also cling to a *transition object*—a security blanket or favorite toy that represents the home and is used for self-comfort. Finally, parents should relate their return to an activity, not time: "We'll be back after you eat lunch." (See Chap. 15 for a detailed discussion of separation anxiety.)

Reality vs. fantasy The distinction between reality and fantasy is totally unclear to toddlers. They engage in *magical thinking*; i.e., they believe that whatever they think is real and that whatever is in their minds will become true. Their tendency to focus on one feature of an object at a time and their self-centeredness distort reality. For example, a toddler fearfully focuses on the great size of a television monster, while overlooking the monster's good deeds. Egocentricity makes toddlers believe that the monster is after them. Cartoons in which people or animals are killed and immediately recover further distort reality.

Young toddlers will kick or slap a monster on television, expecting it to leap out of the television as a real person. Parents should help a child distinguish between reality and fantasy by saying, "Look, that is a TV picture of a monster. It is not real. It is a picture of a man dressed up in a green suit." When children are afraid of pictures in books, parents can draw a picture, saying, "This is drawn with crayons. It is not real, doesn't move, and will always be a picture." Parents can help a toddler in make-believe play distinguish reality from fantasy by saying, "That's a wonderful make-believe animal story. It's fun to pretend that animals really talk, but real animals don't talk."

COGNITIVE DEVELOPMENT

The toddler years encompass two phases of cognitive development. From 12 to 24 months, the toddler is in Piaget's *sensorimotor phase*, classified as part of infancy; the toddler then proceeds through the *preconceptual phase*, from 2 to 7 years (see Table 10-8; see also Chap. 11).

Table 10-8 Cognitive Development

Behavior	12 to 18 months	18 to 24 months
Experimentation and inferring	Uses trial-and-error experimentation to reach goal; varies activities to observe result; learns about object by experiencing it; uses tools to reach goal	Invents new methods, through trial and error, to solve a problem; infers cause from observing event and predicts result from observing cause
Causal relationships	Begins to sense causal relationship between objects being manipulated	
Object permanence	Is increasingly aware of object permanence; searches briefly for hidden object; ventures further away from parent for longer time	Is more aware of object permanence; will search several places for longer time for hidden object
Spatial awareness	Spatial awareness begins; recognizes different shapes	
Memory	Memory is beginning	Memory increases
Time sense	Can enter into middle of series of actions without returning to beginning	Anticipates events; waits for brief period before anticipated event
	Is beginning to have a sense of time and to anticipate events	Begins to have knowledge of past, present, and future
Symbolic thought	Is capable of concrete thought	Symbolic thought begins; can "pretend"; begins to think about own behavior; imitates nonpresent behavior or objects
Characteristics of thought	Egocentrism Irreversibility Ritualism Global organization Magical thinking	

The sensorimotor period

Stage 5: Tertiary circular reactions (12 to 18 months)* The same processes that are going on in stage 4 (see Chap. 9) continue in stage 5, but at a higher level. In stage 5, children actually experiment much as scientists do by varying their activities and changing the environment in order to see the different results. In this way they learn to separate the means of achieving a goal from the goal itself. Space perception and time perception continue to develop in relation to object permanence. Children begin to recognize different geometric shapes and to investigate relationships between them. They learn to use tools to help them reach their goals. For instance, a toddler may use a stick to push a toy off the table in order to get at the toy. The child has learned about and has understood the event by experiencing it. Using a stick to get the toy indicates that an understanding of causality is developing: the toddler is aware of a causal relationship between the action and the resultant accessibility of the toy. Toddlers are very systematic in accommodating to new situations, and their actions become very deliberate and efficient. However, they cannot transfer information from one event to another and must repeatedly reinvestigate the situation. They are curious and are seeking out new experiences.

Stage 6: Invention of new means through mental combinations (18 to 24 months)* This is truly a transitional stage to the next period. Infants are capable of mentally putting together schemata (discussed in Chap. 9) through the process of assimilation to develop new ways or behaviors to reach their goals. In the first stages they apply familiar schemata to new situations and then modify these schemata. Toddlers invent new ways to do things, developing insight into the problems they are solving. Their muscles may involuntarily do the same things they are thinking about as the solution to a problem. For instance, a child's hand or mouth may open and close before he or she tries to open a box to get something (adults do this too). At this stage toddlers can also infer causes from observing events and can predict the results by observing causes.

Children's ability to imitate has changed considerably by stage 6. Earlier imitation was limited to mimicking certain actions, such as another's laughter. Imitation now has deeper meanings, as children begin to imitate sex role behavior. They are now able to imitate models that are not physically present at the moment. They have a beginning sense of time. They think about out-of-sight objects, past events, and events in the immediate future. They think about what they are going to do before they do it. This ability is very important in the development of play. Children in stage 6 no longer play by simply manipulating objects, experimenting with them, and focusing on their actions. They are now able to visualize an event in their minds and to make believe. Their play is truly symbolic at this stage.

At this age children's thoughts are *egocentric*, or self-centered. Toddlers view themselves as the center of their world; they believe that they have caused all outer events to happen and that the events happen for the purpose of bringing them pleasure or causing them frustration. They believe that their opinions are the only ones that exist. Egocentrism predominates all aspects of toddlers' behavior, as illustrated by the following quotation:

> The magician is seated in his high chair and looks upon the world with favor. He is at the height of his powers. If he closes his eyes, he causes the world to disappear. If he opens his eyes, he causes the world to come back. If there is harmony within him, the world is harmonious. . . . His wishes, his thoughts, his gestures, his noises command the universe.[29]

Magical thinking also predominates during these years. Toddlers believe that their thoughts have the same far-reaching power as an action. Toddlers feel supremely powerful and responsible for events but are also vulnerable to feelings of guilt and remorse. A classic example is that of a child who wishes his or her mother dead and whose mother dies; the child believes that he or she caused the death. Adults need to help children distinguish between reality and fantasy, but confusion will continue through the preschool years.

Language development

Language develops very markedly during the toddler period (see Table 10-9). Language varies greatly according to subcultures, experience in

*The author thanks Ann Sloat for writing most of the discussion of stages 5 and 6.

Table 10-9 Language Development

Behavior	15 months	18 months	24 months	30 months
Word usage and sentence length	Expresses self with jargon; combines two to three words in a sentence	Imitates adult words; uses short phrases with adjectives and nouns	Combines three to four words to form short sentences; uses short sentences	Uses plurals Talks constantly
Communication	Points to desired objects; responds with "No" to all requests; understands simple commands	Uses few words to communicate need; points to some objects when named; uses gestures and few words to communicate needs	Uses "telegraphic" speech; refers to self using pronouns ("I" and "me") or by own name; names familiar objects	Speech is "telegraphic" and a monologue; knows first and last name; knows one color
Communication		Follows directions; understands simple requests	Vocalizes needs for food, drink, or potty-chair; understands and obeys simple commands	
Vocabulary size	20 words	25 words	275 words	900 words

hearing others speak, involvement in sensorimotor skills, sense of self-esteem, and stimulation to acquire language. Some children are reluctant to speak when there is (1) a problem with interrelationships with parents and siblings, (2) lack of stimulation, or (3) overstimulation, all of which generally lower the sense of self-esteem. The child then withdraws. In an overstimulating home, the child "turns off" the stimuli.

The development of language is closely associated with the expansion of cognition (thinking). Delay in one area causes delay in the other. Verbal ability enhances thinking, problem solving, and autonomy.

There are differences in the speed of language acquisition. Girls develop language faster than boys, who catch up in midchildhood. Crowded ghettos and institutions result in slow acquisition of speech. Seemingly, this is due to sensory overload or understimulation or to emotional and intellectual deprivation. Role models may not be available to imitate. Bilingual children acquire language more slowly. (See the section "Sensory Deprivation" in Chap. 15.)

Children imitate sounds and words and are rewarded for correct usage. They may create sentences without ever hearing them before. The acquisition of grammar may be controlled by special programmed neural structures in the brain that spew out correct grammar. Only a small number of errors occur in relation to the amount of words spoken by toddlers. There is no satisfactory explanation for the phenomenally rapid acquisition of grammatical structure at this time.[30]

Toddlers understand more words than they express. The average vocabulary is about 20 words at 15 months, 25 words at 18 months, 120 words at 21 months, and 275 words at 24 months. By age 2 toddlers use sentences of two to three words, and at age 3 they use about 900 words.

Children of all races proceed through language development at the same rate. Stuttering (see Chap. 37) and hesitation in speaking are common. Listening to people read stories exposes a child to language and speeds acquisition. At 1 year, stories with simple pictures and one-word explanations of each picture are best, and at age 3, paragraphs with pictures are appropriate. Children's readiness for various kinds of stories is indicated by their sentence structure. When two or more words are used in an expression, books with captions of two or more words are appropriate for the toddler's short attention span. Toddlers learn nouns first, such as *baby, milk, banana.* and *cookie,* and they use subjects, objects, and verbs by age 3, for example, "Mom go store" or "Suzie want cookie." They are also capable of learning numbers and colors.

Parents should talk often to a child, explaining reasons for objects and occurrences and expanding the child's one- to two-word phrases such as "See doggie?" to "See the big doggie? He has long hair and is brown. He says woof woof." This helps stimulate speech and cognitive development. If a child is not speaking by age 3, he or she should be seen by a physician or speech therapist for diagnosis and referral.

CHILD HEALTH MAINTENANCE

Accident prevention

Accidents are the leading cause of death among toddlers. Accident prevention is extremely important, and the nurse's role in prevention can be critical. The nurse can counsel parents, neighbors, and friends to help the parents control the child's behavior to prevent accidents, understand the child's level of cognitive development, and point out potential safety hazards for this age group.[31] The accidental causes of death and measures for preventing them are discussed in Chap. 11.

Toddlers have an insatiable need to explore, and their ability to climb, crawl, and walk greatly increases exposure to potential safety hazards. Toddlers cannot reason and cannot anticipate accidents that may result from exploration. They are egocentric. A toddler can be immersed in the joy of chasing a ball into the street and be totally oblivious to an oncoming car. For these reasons, parents of toddlers must be committed to maintaining a safe environment. Safety locks must be secured on cabinet doors, all medicines must be locked away, and covers for electrical outlets should be installed. All caustic substances should be removed from below sinks and placed in locked cupboards because toddlers can climb and sit on top of counters. It takes only one taste of a drain opener to injure a child's mouth and esophagus. Dishwasher soap is also caustic, and a toddler should not be allowed to play with it. Many poisonings occur from 4:30 to 6:30 P.M. when the mother is busy cooking dinner and is unable to watch the child. The mother should consider placing the child in a playpen or turning on a favorite television program to increase safety during these hours.

The garage, yard, and car must be childproofed. Poisonous substances should never be stored in drink bottles or food containers. Caustic substances, sharp tools, and ladders should be safely stored. Ladders should not be left upright, ready for a toddler to climb. Toddlers should not be allowed to play in cars because of their urges to move the gears and "drive" the car. They should not be allowed to lie under the car's rear window or scramble around in the car. Toddlers should always sit in car safety seats. In a collision, unrestrained toddlers become projectiles flying at several miles per hour. Additional safety precautions are given in Table 10-10 and discussed in Chap. 11.

Vision

Vision should be tested at 3 years. Obvious eye problems such as nystagmus or strabismus ("cross-eyes") must be referred to a physician. Untreated strabismus results in amblyopia ("lazy eye") and vision suppression in the affected eye. Such subtle behavior changes as spatial discoordination, evidenced by missing a step, reaching unsuccessfully for a toy, squinting excessively, or being unable to fix the gaze on objects, should be reported to a physician. See Table 10-1 for milestones in visual development. Since language and thought processes are very simplistic and self-oriented at this age, it is difficult but possible to test for visual impairments. Early diagnosis and treatment of eye problems will prevent future reading problems and alterations in the musculature of the eye.[32]

Dental care

Preventive dental care is an important health teaching concept to be emphasized to the toddler's caregiver. Tooth decay results when bacteria act on carbohydrates on the surfaces of the teeth. An acid environment is produced, resulting in destruction of the enamel. Frequent snacks, sticky foods, and bedtime bottles cause caries. Bottle caries result from the constant contact of the child's teeth with liquid containing sugar, such as milk, juice, and carbonated beverages. Fluoridated water at 0.7 to 1.2 parts per million or fluoridated vitamins are optimal for caries prevention. Health departments can recommend dosages of fluoride drops to the teeth if water fluoride levels are not optimal and will notify consumers of fluoride levels in different localities. Thumb-sucking beyond the age of 4 or 5 years can result in significant malocclusion, and referral to a dentist is appropriate. The parent can clean the infant's and toddler's teeth by gently wiping them with a washcloth. As toddlers' fine motor coordination becomes more refined, they can brush their teeth. Their toothbrushing should

Table 10-10 Accident Prevention (ages 1 to 3 years)*

Dangers at home

Gravity

Falls from one level to another

Falls on dangerous surfaces or objects

Water

Tubs, pools, puddles, and toilet bowls

Heat

Stoves, fireplaces, hot foods or liquids, matches and lighters

Poisons

Medicines, caustics, cleaning compounds, paint thinner, bleaching fluid, etc.

Machines

Electrical machines, cars and lawn mowers

What they do

They are in perpetual motion. They are curious about everything. They run almost as soon as they walk.

They put things in their mouths whether these things are edible or not.

They pull on everything they can reach.

They crawl into boxes and cupboards and behind and under furniture.

They climb. They can go up more easily than they can get back down.

They play alone and will wander away from a group.

They are fascinated by fire.

They may fear animals or chase dogs and cats, often provoking them.

They have no fear of water.

They are big operators who leap before they look.

How they protect themselves

At 1 year they have not learned anything to protect themselves. Their locomotion makes them more susceptible than before.

At 3 they may know that stoves and fire are hot, but they cannot be depended on to remember this.

They act largely without previous planning and cannot anticipate danger.

What they need

They need protection; safety education and discipline must begin.

They need good examples to imitate.

They need a happy but orderly home in which to grow and learn how to behave safely.

What the family can do to protect them

Anticipate their activities in the home environment. Remove potential hazards. Look around for "attractive nuisances." Demonstrate safe living. Integrate education for safety into daily living, showing "why."

Improve housekeeping—avoid keeping poisonous substances or bottled or packaged nonfoodstuffs anywhere they can reach them or climb for sampling.

Provide a place for toys and a place to play on the floor. Remove destructible bric-a-brac and loose scatter rugs. Teach the meaning of "hot," "hurt," and "tastes bad," rather than "don't".

Unless they are in playpens or closed-off areas, keep crawling babies and toddlers out of the kitchen and traffic areas. Place playpens or high chairs as far away from stoves or other potential hazards as possible.

Put a fence around pools and ponds, and *never* allow a potential crawler or toddler to be alone near water wherever it may be. Even an empty bathtub or sink, or 2 to 3 in of water in a plastic pool, is dangerous.

Check bed and sleeping room for potential hazards, including inviting places to put the head.

Assume that toddlers are in danger unless they can be seen. Danger may be most imminent when they are quiet; they have probably found something new to try.

Be sure child can be seen before moving the family car or driving over empty packing cases.

*Written by Hope Ecklund, R.N., R.H.N., M.P.H. Used with the permission of the city and county of San Francisco, Department of Public Health.

be closely supervised by the parents. Daily brushing and flossing, the latter performed by an adult, are recommended by dentists. Parents can encourage toddlers to practice brushing a doll's teeth and other household objects.

Shoe selection

Regular monitoring of shoe size is important because during periods of rapid growth, children may need shoes every other month. The child's shoes should be $\frac{1}{2}$ to $\frac{3}{4}$ in longer than the feet when the child is standing. Parents can press the thumb on the edge of the shoe to estimate the space between the longest toe and the end of the shoe. Shoes should be soft and flexible, have a strong sole, and protect the feet. High-topped leather shoes are no longer the only shoes recommended. Tennis shoes have cloth uppers that provide good ventilation. They protect well, dry easily, and are flexible, which provides for maximal development of the muscles of the feet and legs. Primitive people who do not wear shoes have very strong muscles; for this reason, orthopedists today recommend more flexible shoes and believe that high-topped leather shoes are not necessary and may actually retard muscular development. If a child cries when standing or walking or if he or she sits down when trying to walk, the shoes may be too small.

REFERENCES

1. Thorp, Isobel, et al., "The Toddler, 1–3 Years," in G. Scipien, M. U. Barnard, M. A. Chard, J. Howe, and P. J. Phillips (eds.), *Comprehensive Pediatric Nursing*, 2d ed., McGraw-Hill, New York, 1979, p. 234.
2. Whaley, Lucille, and Donna L. Wong, *Nursing Care of Infants and Children*, Mosby, St. Louis, 1979, p. 511.
3. Waechter, Eugenia, and F. Blake, *Nursing Care of Children*, Lippincott, Philadelphia, 1979, p. 373.
4. Mussen, P., J. Konger, and J. Kagan, *Child Development and Personality*, Harper & Row, New York, 1969, p. 244.
5. Chinn, Peggy L., *Child Health Maintenance: Concepts in Family Centered Care*, Mosby, St. Louis, 1979, p. 319.
6. Watson, Ernest H., and George H. Lowry, *Growth and Development of Children*, Year Book, Chicago, 1967, p. 219.
7. Mussen, Konger, and Kagan, loc. cit.
8. Chinn, op. cit., pp. 320–321.
9. Ibid., p. 321.
10. Ibid., p. 320.
11. Homan, William E., *Child Sense*, Basic Books, New York, 1969, p. 94.
12. White, R. W., "Motivation Reconsidered: The Concept of Competence," *Psychological Review* 66:297–333 (1959).
13. Smart, Mollie, and Russel C. Smart, *Children: Development and Relationships*, Macmillan, New York, 1977, p. 113.
14. Waechter and Blake, op. cit., p. 385.
15. Maier, Henry W., *Three Theories of Child Development*, Harper & Row, New York, 1978, p. 85.
16. Thorp et al., op. cit., p. 237.
17. Stone, Joseph L., and J. Church, *Childhood and Adolescence*, Random House, New York, 1973, p. 243.
18. Johnson, Ronald C., and Gene R. Medinuss; *Child Psychology, Behavior, and Development*, Wiley, New York, 1969, p. 381.
19. Mussen, Konger, and Kagan, op. cit., p. 264.
20. Brazelton, T. B., "A Child-Oriented Approach to Toilet Training," *Pediatrics* **29**(1):121–128 (January 1962).
21. Ibid.
22. Thorp et al., op. cit., p. 229.
23. Dobson, James, *Dare to Discipline*, Tyndale House, Wheaton, Ill., 1974, p. 12.
24. Ibid., p. 7.
25. Ibid.
26. Whaley and Wong, op. cit., p. 522.
27. Melichar, Marshelle M., "Using Crisis Theory to Help Parents Cope with a Child's Temper Tantrums," *American Journal of Maternal-Child Nursing* **5**(3):181–185 (May–June 1980).
28. Smart and Smart, op. cit., p. 209.
29. Fraiberg, Selma, *The Magic Years*, Scribner, New York, 1959, p. 107.
30. Mussen, Konger, and Kagan, op. cit., p. 254.
31. Thorp, op. cit., p. 238.
32. Watson and Lowry, op. cit., p. 222.

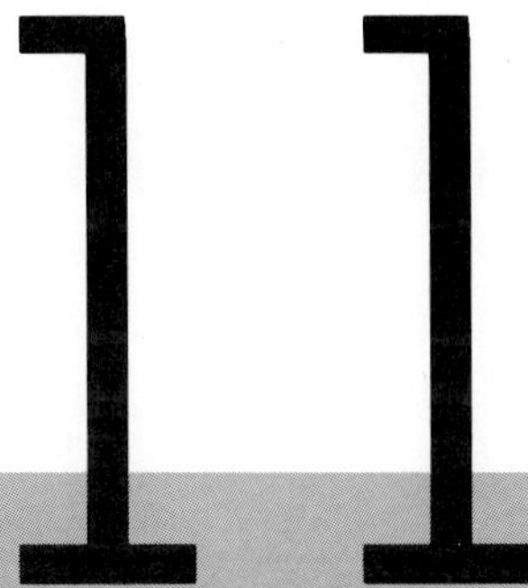

Phyllis Nie Esslinger

The preschooler

Upon completion of this chapter, the student will be able to:

1 Describe the physiological development of the preschooler in the following areas: body proportions, weight gain, brain size, metabolic rate, vision, and neuromuscular development.

2 Summarize the preschooler's nutritional needs and problems: caloric, protein, mineral, and milk needs; food jags; food intake; and serving size.

3 Summarize the preschooler's characteristic behavior with respect to Erikson's initiative vs. guilt stage of psychological development.

4 Relate the following concepts to the preschooler's sex role development: identification, child-rearing practices, and sex role stereotypes.

5 List four guidelines for educating the preschooler about sex.

6 Compare the following types of play: cooperative, creative, dramatic, and quiet.

7 Define socialization and describe how the following types of learning socialize the preschooler: learning by insight and unfolding, conditioning, positive reinforcement, and negative reinforcement.

8 Identify the characteristics of the preschooler's cognitive development in the preconceptual and intuitive phases and illustrate each with an example.

9 Summarize Kohlberg's stage of moral development for the preschooler.

10 Identify eight criteria for selection of a nursery school.

11 Describe methods of preventing the three most common accidents among preschoolers.

The preschool period, from age 3 through age 5, is delightful—a period of enthusiasm, energy, activity, and creativity. The preschooler is an autonomous, discerning little individual who can run, jump, skip, ride a tricycle, and enjoy moving rapidly through space. Control over many bodily processes has been achieved; the child has much pride in these accomplishments.

The preschooler is highly social and independent. He or she is now beginning to know right from wrong and is developing a conscience. Play often takes the form of imitation as the child assumes appropriate sex roles and dresses or acts like the mother or father. The preschooler constantly asks "Why?"—evidence of a burgeoning vocabulary. The preschooler volunteers much information peppered with continual expressions of likes and dislikes.

This period is one of rapid learning in which the child is naturally curious and pushes out into the world (Fig. 11-1). The preschooler needs to have freedom to explore, to test, and to control his or her individual actions as well as the actions of others. The child needs to know what

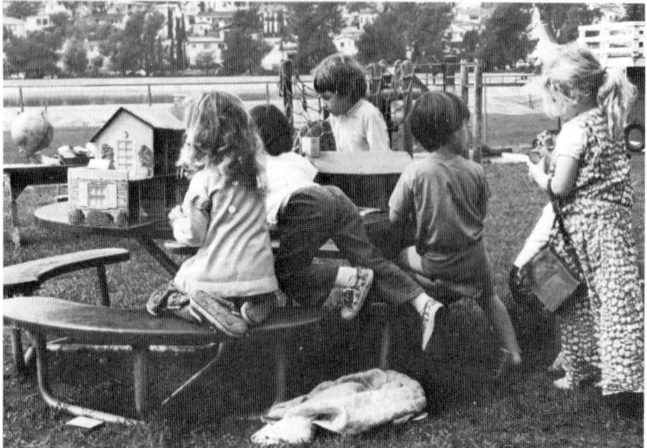

Figure 11-1 Preschoolers are highly social and curious beings who love to play and explore.

makes things tick—what things look like inside and how they work and why. This insatiable curiosity often gets the little preschooler in trouble, when he or she plays with Mama's watch, Daddy's tools, or things in the medicine cupboard. The child curiously explores his or her body and its functions and the bodies of others. What the child lacks in knowledge is made up through fantasy or magical thinking. Observation is keen; the preschooler sees, hears, and feels every detail of the environment.

This is a vital time in the development of the child, since so much of the personality is being molded. Children need love, adequate role models, attention, and consistent guidance. They also need a safe, stimulating place where they can explore their own attributes, satisfy their curiosity, and master skills. To provide a more expansive world for preschoolers, their families often put them into nursery schools. Here they can expand their social and play world under the supervision and guidance of trained personnel. Nursery schools provide safe equipment to foster stimulation, curiosity, and activity in an environment that is tailored for preschoolers.

Health professionals must be aware of the preschooler's activity and curiosity and of the necessity of providing a *safe environment*. This need is reflected in the fact that accidents are the leading cause of death in this age group. Approximately one-third of all deaths among preschoolers are attributed to accidents, most of which are preventable. The next leading causes of death include congenital malformations, influenza and pneumonia, and malignant neoplasms.[1]

PHYSICAL DEVELOPMENT

The preschooler, unlike the chubby toddler with a protuberant abdomen, is a sturdy child who stands straight and appears tall and thin (Fig. 11-2). Physical development during this period is slow and follows an orderly sequence at a rate that is unique for each individual child.

Physical maturation

The child grows relatively more in height than in weight during these years, gaining about 2 to $2\frac{1}{2}$ in in height and approximately 5 lb in weight per year.[2] Changes in body proportion occur because there are relatively large increments of growth in the trunk and legs. The head slows in growth rate as the brain approaches adult proportions. There is little difference in growth rate

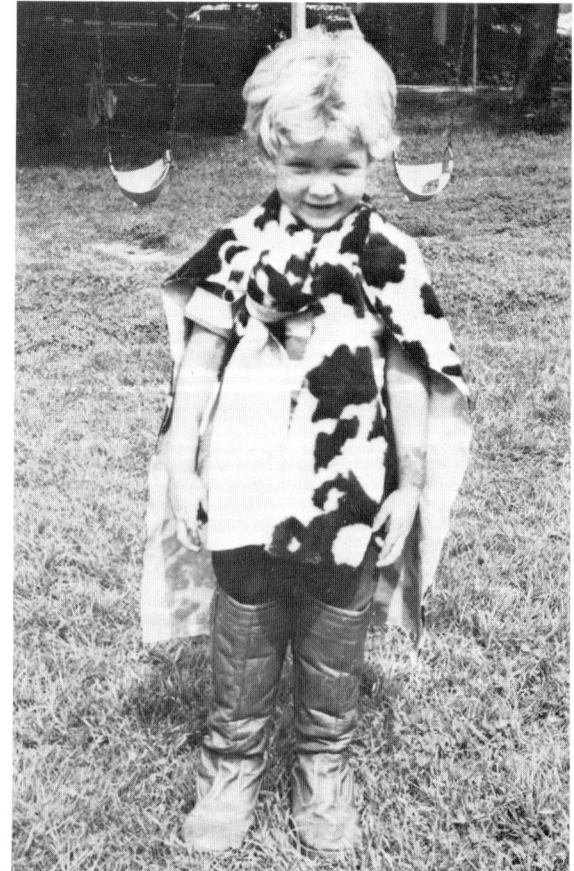

Figure 11-2 Preschoolers are thinner and stand taller than toddlers.

or size between boys and girls. (See Appendix B for growth charts.)

The preschooler's metabolic rate decreases from that of the toddler period. This decrease is reflected in the lowered vital signs. (See Tables 16-18 through 16-20 for normal ranges of the preschooler's vital signs.) Elevated vital signs in the preschooler often indicate stressful circumstances, such as extreme physical activity or infections. Exposure to upper respiratory infections and childhood diseases increases during this period, if the child starts nursery school and has not yet developed immunity through frequent exposure. The eustachian tube is nearly horizontal at this stage, and this causes more susceptibility to ear infections. A significant increase in respiratory rate or pulse rate is the first evidence of an elevated temperature due to infection.

The preschooler's body systems undergo gradual development at varying rates. The most conspicuous development during the preschool period is related to the neuromuscular system.

Neuromuscular development Some of the most exciting behavioral changes or milestones in the physical development of the preschooler are related to the ability to control and coordinate the small and large voluntary muscles and to maintain visual attention.[3]

Development of the corticospinal tract is advanced enough to permit most movements, but full control does not occur until later adolescence. By 4 years of age, the child is clearly right- or left-handed.[4] Left-handed children may need encouragement and extra help in accomplishing such tasks as cutting with scissors or tying a shoelace. Parents should allow children to utilize the dominant side; this will lead to better fine motor coordination and prevent many emotional upsets.

Visual development continues throughout the preschool period. The child of 4 has approximately 20/30 vision. The 4-year-old is usually ready to read, but since farsightedness (hyperopia) is normally present, print must be large to prevent eye strain. During this period referral to an ophthalmologist is indicated when strabismus is present or if the eyes cross when the child is ill or fatigued. If strabismus is not corrected, amblyopia (dimming of vision and possibly loss of sight) can occur (see Chap. 31).[5]

Gross and fine motor development When visual development and neuromuscular development are proceeding normally, gross and fine motor development can be assessed (see Tables 11-1 and 11-2). *Normative* (average for age) behaviors are helpful guidelines for determining a child's level of functioning. Decisions about the

Table 11-1 Gross Motor Development

Activity	3 years	4 years	5 years
Walking and running	Tandem walks a line without watching feet	Heel-to-toe walking	Backward heel-to-toe walking
	Walks backward		
	Runs with smoothness, turns sharp corners, and stops suddenly	Runs easily	Runs with skill, speed, and agility and plays games simultaneously
		Skips clumsily	Skips
Stepping	Climbs upstairs alternating feet	Climbs downstairs alternating feet	
		Climbs without holding rail	
	Hops down three stairs on one foot	Hops on one leg	Hops well
		Hops down four to six stairs on one leg	
	Balances on one foot for 1 s	Balances on one foot for 5 s	Balances on one foot for 10 s
Throwing	Throws ball overhand		Throws and catches ball
	Catches ball with arms fully extended one out of three times	Catches ball thrown at 5 ft two to three times	Uses hands more than arms to catch ball
Jumping	Jumps from low step		Jumps three to four steps
	Jumps in place		Jumps rope
Other	Pedals tricycle	Climbs jungle gym	Roller-skates
	Swings		

Table 11-2 Fine Motor Development

Activity	3 years	4 years	5 years
Dressing	Undresses self; helps dress self	Dresses and undresses self except tying bows, closing zippers, and putting on boots	Dresses self without assistance
	Undoes buttons on side or front of clothing	Undoes buttons	Ties shoelaces
		Laces shoes but cannot tie bow	
		Distinguishes front	
Self-care	Washes hands and feeds self	Brushes teeth alone	Washes self without wetting clothes
	May brush own teeth		
Writing and drawing	Recognizes and draws a complete circle	Recognizes and draws a crude square	Copies triangle or diamond
			Prints a few letters or numbers crudely
	Draws a crude cross	Combines two simple geometric forms	Can combine more than two geometric forms
	Tries to draw a picture and name it	Draws a crude three-part man	Draws a six-part man
	Scribbles	Form and meaning in drawings are apparent to adult	Draws clearly recognizable life-like representations; differentiates parts of drawings
			Prints some letters correctly
			Prints first name
			Knows there is a right and a left side but cannot distinguish
			Has a definite hand preference
Play	Pours fluid from a pitcher, with occasional spills	Likes water play	Likes water play
	Hits large pegs on a board with a hammer		Uses a hammer to hit a nail on the head
	Begins to use scissors	Uses scissors without difficulty	Uses scissors and tools, like screwdriver, well
	Strings large beads	Enjoys fine manipulation of play materials	Folds paper diagonally
	Does puzzles by trial and error	Surveys a puzzle before placing pieces	Does simple puzzles quickly and smoothly
		Matches simple geometric forms	
		Has poor space perception	
	Builds a tower of 9 to 10 blocks	Builds complicated structures extending vertically and laterally	Builds things out of large boxes
	Builds a three-block gate	Builds a five-block gate	Builds complex three-dimensional structure
		Notices missing parts—requests to fix	Disassembles and reassembles some objects

child's individual needs, play equipment, and health assessment can be based on these guidelines. Children who deviate significantly from average behaviors should be referred for workup and assistance. Chronological age by itself can be misleading as a basis for identifying deviations. To assess development, many aspects of gross and fine motor coordination are considered as well as the child's overall developmental pattern. Some children develop faster than others, and some at a slower pace than the average. The pace depends on inherent factors and the extent to which these factors are stimulated by the environment.

Different types of movement occur as a child develops. Much of a young child's movement is expressive; that is, the motor activities express emotions and needs. The young child expresses curiosity by direct involvement with objects; for example, a 3-year-old might poke or pull at the nose or eyes of a doll to see what it is all about. To relieve frustration, a preschooler enjoys

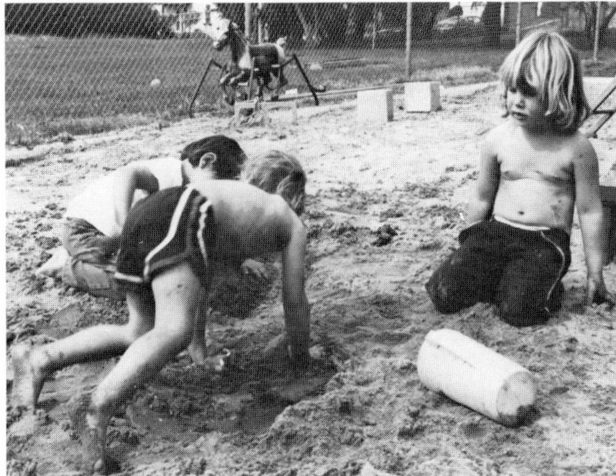

Figure 11-3 Large-muscle activities express emotions and "let off steam" in the preschool period.

pounding on a pegboard, molding play dough, swinging intensely, and engaging in other kinds of vigorous activity (Fig. 11-3).

As hand-eye coordination becomes more precise and as fine muscles are better controlled, the child becomes involved in *instrumental* movement, in which he or she learns to use instruments and tools. For example, a 3-year-old is usually unable to hammer a nail, while a 5-year-old can use a hammer to hit a nail on the head.

PHYSICAL HEALTH MAINTENANCE AND PROMOTION

Because of the high activity level of the preschooler, it is especially important to prevent accidents and ensure good nutrition, exercise, and sleep to maintain adequate growth patterns and health. Signs of pathophysiology should be watched for, since the child is often too busy to complain. Yearly visits should be made to the physician for preventive health examinations and immunization (see Table 14-12 for an immunization schedule). Dental examinations should begin.

Accident prevention

Accidents are the leading cause of death of children between the ages of 2 and 5. One-third of preschool children suffer injuries requiring medical assistance, and many children develop permanent disabilities. Two-thirds of these serious accidents occur in the home. The leading types of accidents are injuries from motor vehicles, drowning, and burns. Other major causes include poisons; machinery, such as power tools and electric equipment; projectile toys, such as darts, bows and arrows, and guns; old refrigerators and freezers; and ditches.

Preschoolers who are under the age of 4 or who weigh less than 40 lb should be placed in car seats recommended by the National Safety Council. After the age of 4, lap safety belts should be used to prevent serious injury in case of an accident. This should be emphasized to parents, since these children resist restraint; this often causes the parents to become lax. Children in this age range are more frequently in pedestrian-vehicle accidents than in within-vehicle accidents because of their spontaneity, well-developed gross motor abilities, and inability to recognize immediate dangers. Preschoolers never seem to hesitate to chase a ball into the street, run a tricycle down a driveway, or play between parked cars. They climb fences, open gates, and unlock doors in order to gain access to the street.

The child, who is now old enough to understand simple explanations, should be taught to look both ways before crossing a street, to recognize pedestrian crossings, and to differentiate between red and green traffic lights. Explanations are not enough; good examples must be set by the parents. This is the age of imitation.

Household accidents should be prevented by removing dangers in the environment, providing adequate adult supervision, and teaching the child to understand potential dangers. Parents should be advised to make a complete inspection of the home and yard daily to identify and remove possible dangers before accidents occur. Caustic materials and medicines should be placed in locked and inaccessible cabinets; electrical equipment, machinery, and appliances should be put out of reach of children; dangerous toys should be removed or repaired; pools should have high fences and locked gates; and unused equipment such as refrigerators and freezers should have the doors removed or be taken from the premises (see Table 11-3).

Adequate adult supervision is still essential during the preschool period. Children this age do not have the ability to judge dangers. Because of their inquisitiveness, imagination, and physical activity, they can get into dangerous situations quickly. A preschooler must *never* be left alone and unsupervised, and it is certainly ill-advised to leave a preschooler in the care of an

Table 11-3 Accident Prevention for Preschoolers*

Dangers at home	How they protect themselves	What they need	What the family can do to protect them
Falls From windows, roofs, and trees **Burns** Food and caustics **Fire** Matches, lighters, and inflammable clothing **Poisons** Liquid medicines, pills or colored particles, fluid in bottles, caustics, plant sprays, and insect paste **Water** Bathtubs, pools, ponds, and streams **Machinery** Wringers, lawn mowers, power tools, and automobiles **Electricity** Electric outlets and TV sets **Toys** Projectile toys, guns, bows and arrows, darts, toys with points or sharp edges, and cap guns **Odds and ends** Old refrigerators, old wells and ditches, and sharp	They have better muscles and coordination and are less likely to fall on stairs, etc. They may have learned that stoves are hot and that fire burns. They begin to get out of the way of objects moving toward them. They may have developed a fear of water. They begin to reason and remember what has been taught. They begin to have a better concept of time and distance but have a long way to go.	They need kindness and affection. They need education integrated with protection and discipline for self-reliance and ability to perform safely. They need good examples of safe, orderly, and kind behavior from adults. They need exposure to new experiences and weaning from complete protection to be able to make decisions for themselves. They need to learn that limmitations and rules are for their protection as well as for the rights of others. They need to share and to take turns. They need the basis for the kinds of attitudes and actions which will last them the rest of their lives.	Think ahead. Make plans and carry them out. Learn the common developmental sequences which all children reach sooner or later. Anticipate the subtle as well as obvious hazards which children will be exposed to or will seek on their way to learning what life is all about. Survey the home and eliminate danger spots. Do this *before* an accident happens, not after. Educate—show and explain over and over again (sometimes 10 times a day) *how to do things safely.* Concentrate on "how" and "why" rather than "don't." Provide experience rather than limiting activity. Provide *planned* play equipment, including large packing boxes, large blocks or construction toys, coloring books and art materials, dolls, simple toys that do things, and housekeeping toys. Expect them to do as you do—not as you say. Demonstrate respect for law

older sibling unless the sibling is a responsible teenager who can make mature decisions and take aggressive action should danger occur. *At no time* is a preschooler to be left unattended around a swimming pool, even if the child is able to swim. A child's swimming abilities are often overestimated, and the child may not recognize the potential danger.

Children cannot be protected against all dangers and must gradually learn to live in the world around them. Preschoolers are ready to learn to use simple equipment safely. Learning to saw, to use the stove, to carry scissors, to turn on the TV, or to plug in a lamp can all be accomplished safely with simple explanations and praise. Encouraging preschoolers to help around the home and introducing them to new experiences help them learn the appropriate use of equipment and toys. Rules of safety for daily living must be learned: how to cross a street, how to behave in a swimming pool area, how and when to approach animals, and how to react to strangers. Nurses can help parents teach their children and can help them understand that their children need to be shown how to do things and need to be given simple explanations. Often explanations must be repeated over and over again before they take on meaning and become part of a child's behavioral pattern. Children should be *praised* when they do things safely and well. In addition, parents should not approach children with "Don't" but should concentrate positively

Table 11-3 Accident Prevention for Preschoolers* (*Continued*)

Dangers at home	How they protect themselves	What they need	What the family can do to protect them
garden and household knives and tools			and order and the need to be considerate of the rights and feelings of others. Set limits and explain "why." Let them make choices, but don't expect them to make decisions which are beyond them. Let them help with every task that is within their ability, and help them use their mind and muscles. Give them "on-the-job" safety education. Teach them to do things and to use tools and toys. Teach them how to swim, how and when to cross the street, who they are and where they live, situations in which they must ask permission, and manners. Plan with them and arrange for them to visit friends after school and to be away from the family for several hours or overnight. Teach them to be courteous, but not to accept favors or rides from strangers.

*Compiled by Hope Ecklund, R.N., P.H.N., M.P.H.

Source: Accident Prevention through Growth and Development Patterns, San Francisco Department of Public Health, San Francisco.

on *how* things are done safely and *why* things are done in certain ways to prevent accidents. Preschoolers are usually willing learners, enjoy assuming more responsibilities, and like receiving praise.

Nutrition

The preschooler's appetite fluctuates continually. Periods of overeating or refusing certain foods occur but do not persist. Food fads and strong taste preferences, common in the toddler period, also occur among some young preschoolers. Around the age of 4, finicky eating is not unusual. The short attention span of 3- and 4-year-olds often prohibits them from sitting quietly through a family meal. In contrast, 5-year-olds are more open to the introduction of new foods because of their maturity level, acquisition of new interest in taste, lengthened attention span, and sociability.

Parents should be made aware of this fluctuation to prevent overconcern, which can readily lead to conflict between the parents and the child. Generally speaking, the child who is offered an adequate diet in small portions, including foods from the four major food groups, will over a period of time (1 month or longer) be eating an adequate diet. Parents' concern regarding food "jags" can be eased by having them keep a daily log for several weeks of the amount and type of food consumed by the child. It is comforting for the parents to see the actual quality and amount of food consumed over time and the gradually diminishing food jag. Parents should know that it is the quality of food consumed, not the quantity, which is of primary importance and that the appetite will improve as school age approaches and the growth rate increases.

Preschoolers need approximately 1400 to 1800 cal per day (90 cal/kg or 40 cal/lb). Of the total caloric intake, the child should receive about 1.0 g of protein per pound of body weight, half of which should be from animal origin to ensure adequate intake of amino acids, B complex vitamins, vitamin D, and such minerals as calcium and iron. During this period there is an increase in the deposit of minerals in the bones. Specifically, calcium and phosphorus are necessary for bone and tooth mineralization. The American Heart Association has recommended dietary guidelines for healthy children over 2 years of age. (See Table 11-4.)

Preschoolers eat only a little more than toddlers. Servings for the preschooler are about half the size of an adult serving. An adequate daily diet for the preschooler includes approximately $1\frac{1}{2}$ pints of milk, four or more servings of vegetables and fruits, two servings of meat or meat substitutes, and four servings of bread and cereal. Refer to Appendix C4-5 for nutritional guidelines for the preschooler. Three meals daily—plus a midmorning, midafternoon, and evening snack—should be provided because of the child's high activity level and inability to sit for long periods at a meal. Parents should choose snacks that augment the daily diet and should avoid such "empty calorie" foods as potato chips, candy, and carbonated drinks. Snacks may include milk, juice, ice cream, raisins, cut-up fresh vegetables and fruits, cheese, and peanut butter with crackers. Such a diet begins to establish good eating habits, provides adequate nutrition, and prevents health problems associated with a poor diet, such as malnutrition, dental caries, and anemia.

Table 11-4 Recommended Dietary Guidelines for Healthy Children over 2 Years of Age (American Heart Association)

1. Diet should be nutritionally adequate, consisting of a variety of foods.
2. Caloric intake should be based on growth rate, activity level, and content of deposits of subcutaneous fat so as to maintain a desirable body weight.
3. Total fat intake should be approximately 30% of calories, with 10% or less from saturated fat, about 10% from monounsaturated fat, and less than 10% from polyunsaturated fat. The emphasis should be on reducing total fat and saturated fat intake rather than on increasing polyunsaturated fat intake.
4. Daily cholesterol intake should be approximately 100 mg of cholesterol per 1000 cal, not to exceed 300 mg. This allows for differences in caloric intake in children in various age groups.
5. Protein intake should be about 15% of calories and should be derived from varied sources.
6. Carbohydrate calories should be derived primarily from complex carbohydrate sources to provide necessary vitamins and minerals. Thus, the total amount of calories from carbohydrates would be about 55%.
7. Excessive salt intake may be associated with hypertension in susceptible persons. On the whole, American diets contain excessive amounts of salt. Therefore, limiting intake of most highly salted processed foods and sodium-containing condiments and not adding salt at the table are recommended.

Source: W. Weidman, P. Kwiterovich, M. J. Jesse, and E. Nugent, "Diet in the Healthy Child," *Circulation* **67:**1411A (1983).

Children should eat with their families. The family mealtime is an important aspect of the socialization process and ideally is a happy, warm, and accepting part of the daily routine. Children learn social customs, language skills, and the family's standards of behavior through interaction and identification with their parents and older siblings. Table manners should not be emphasized, since this may lead to rebellion. Children learn adequately by example, but they do make mistakes and have accidents. Compliments on good behavior reinforce good table manners, but negative comments are to be avoided.

To encourage children to eat new foods or increase food consumption, no snacks should be allowed during the hour before a meal. Other suggestions include having the child assist in meal preparation, providing a quiet time before meals, providing a chair that is high enough and utensils that are small enough for the child, allowing the child sufficient time to eat, and allowing the child to leave the table when he or she appears restless. During meals, parents should avoid making food an issue through coaxing, bribing, or threatening, since this is the root of many later eating problems.

Children's plates embossed with Big Bird or the current TV favorite do wonders for the appetite. Large servings tend to "turn off" the appetite. If the child wants to, he or she can ask for more; this promotes a feeling of achievement in the child. When preparing foods, flavor, texture, form, and color should be considered. Foods should be mildly flavored and presented attractively; where possible, different foods should be served individually rather than in such mixtures as casseroles, stews, and salads. Preschoolers prefer meat, cut up in bite-sized pieces, and fruit. They are resistant to vegetables unless the vegetables are uncooked and cut into bite-sized pieces that can be picked up with the fingers. New foods should be introduced gradually. Parents should not insist that new foods be eaten. Children will eventually experiment with new foods if exposed to them often enough.

The exact amount of food intake must be determined before a conclusion is made that a child is eating insufficiently. If the child is eating poorly, the following causes should be explored: (1) poor eating habits, such as excessive snacking, unavailability of adequate varieties and quantities of foods, and foods that are too highly seasoned; (2) poor mealtime socialization, such as an irregular family meal schedule, an unhappy and argumentative or confusing mealtime atmosphere, excessive parental expectations, force feeding, or nagging; (3) physical problems, such as illness, overfatigue, or tooth decay; and (4) emotional disturbances, such as phobias, fears, or sibling rivalry. Specific causes must be identified, and when necessary the child should be referred for further evaluation and intervention before physical or psychological damage occurs.

Exercise, rest, and sleep

Exercise promotes gross and fine motor development and provides an outlet for pent-up energy, tension, and aggression. It also enhances language development and social skill, as preschoolers learn to play together. Each preschooler therefore needs to have daily exercise. Since this is a period of great activity and energy, there usually is little need to be concerned about exercise. If a child is "glued" to television or prefers other passive activities, outside play should be encouraged, and television watching limited. One or two hours of selected television programs are more than adequate each day. Family outings and nursery school encourage physical activity.

For the normally active child, activity periods should be alternated with periods of rest or quiet (Fig. 11-4). Quiet times may include a rest or nap period after lunch, a reading time with the mother or father, or perhaps watching "Sesame Street" on television. Without adequate rest periods during the day, the child can readily become fatigued, which may lead to irritability, poor resistance to infections, and restless nighttime sleep. A 3-year-old may not sleep at naptime but will usually rest quietly for at least 1 h. Four-and five-year-olds usually do not need naps if they get adequate sleep at night. Nevertheless, a quiet time is still important for reducing fatigue.

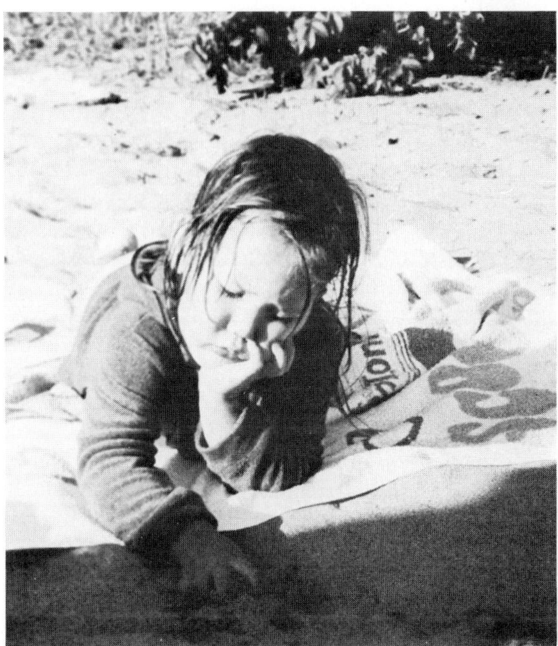

Figure 11-4 Care must be taken to alternate preschoolers' periods of activity with rest periods.

Nighttime sleep decreases for the preschooler to 10 to 12 h. However, children vary widely in the amount of sleep they need. Some function well with as little as 8 h of sleep, while others require 14. Parents need to understand this variation and provide for a period of uninterrupted sleep in a conducive environment. Bedtime around 8 P.M. will provide for a long enough sleep period during the night.

Since it is a common practice for children to watch television in the early evening hours, parents should select programs that are appropriate for a preschooler. High-action, bizarre, and violent programs should be avoided since they tend to overstimulate the child and promote nightmares or difficulty settling down to sleep. Ideally, watching early evening television is a family affair; parents and children view carefully selected programs together, and the parents discuss them with their children. Not only are the children participating with adults in a mutually enjoyable experience, but they are also being provided with an excellent learning experience. In addition, parents can monitor their children's reactions to the content of programs and can prevent misunderstanding and overstimulation by providing simple and logical explanations.

If possible, a child should sleep in his or her own room and in his or her own bed. The room should be located away from noise and other distractions, such as television and the dishwasher. Frequently, siblings share rooms; it is helpful to place children with similar sleep patterns in the same room. Sleeping conditions should be carefully assessed. Poor sleeping patterns are related to physical illness, parental overpermissiveness, and poor learning performance. Some children from large families in the lower socioeconomic levels sleep on the floor or in the same bed with several siblings—a practice which is not conducive to good sleep. Each child should have his or her own "space" to sleep in at night.

Although they like to postpone going to bed, preschoolers are quite ritualistic about bedtime and respond well to routines and a specific hour for bedtime. There should be a quieting-down period before bedtime, which may include bathing, reading, listening to records, and saying prayers. This is a prime time for the preschooler to spend with parents while slowly unwinding from the activities of the day and gradually moving toward bedding down. Some preschoolers still feel more secure if they take a favorite toy or blanket to bed with them. Parents should be instructed to allow this. This *transitional object*, the favorite blanket or teddy bear, is something special. It represents security and familiarity, which helps the child separate from mother and the active household and enter the quiet and seclusion of his or her own room.

Three- and four-year-olds may wake up during the night to urinate, and most still have an occasional "accident." Often these accidents are associated with dreams and nightmares, a normal occurrence in this period. When awaking from a dream, a child is often extremely fearful and upset. It is difficult for the child to separate reality from the dream or fantasy world. The preschooler's active imagination can lead to terrifying experiences. The curtains become moving monsters in the dark, the unlit lamp is a lurking vulture, and the electric cord is a snake! Parents should reassure a child who awakens from a dream by turning on the light and gently talking. The child should be reassured that there are no monsters, and what is actually being seen should be explained. This helps the child distinguish reality from fantasy. Rocking in a chair, gently stroking the back, and singing lullabies often calm the child. If these measures are not sufficient to get the child back to sleep, it may be well to sleep with the child for a few hours. Allowing the child to crawl in bed with the parents frequently can lead to a habit that is most difficult to break. It is best to sleep with the child in his or her own room. Parents should be cautioned not to make a *habit* of sleeping with the child, since some children may use night fears as a way of gaining attention from the parents.

PSYCHOLOGICAL HEALTH AND DEVELOPMENT

The development of a healthy personality is as important as physical development. Healthy psychological and emotional development is critically important throughout the preschool years. Hereditary, physical, environmental, and social factors play a significant role in the development of a healthy personality. The influence of methods of socialization on personality development is discussed in the following section.

Freud first identified the preschool period as the *Oedipal stage* of development, emphasizing heredity (gender) as the prime factor in development. He recognized that sexual identification and development of the superego (conscience) occur between the ages of 3 and 5. Later, Erik Erikson, who expanded Freud's stages and included the importance of socialization, posited that the child gains a sense of *initiative* during this period as a result of adequate environmental stimulation and support from family members and other significant adults.

Initiative vs. guilt[6]

Initiative is the channeling of energy to plan and undertake activities or attack problems. That is, preschoolers learn to give direction and purpose to activities by *making things* and by *making like* or imitating other people in their play. For example, little boys love to build castles in the sand or wooden rockets that will fly to Mars and to pretend that they are astronauts or firemen. Little girls love to make mud cakes, dress dolls, and dress up like admired adults. The preschooler's high energy level, motor development, cognitive development, curiosity, and imagination motivate the child to seek activities involving assertion and aggression tempered with some judgment and self-confidence. To accomplish a sense of initiative, the child must have a safe but stimulating environment where exploration can be *freely* carried out under *adult supervision.* The child must have the opportunity to explore the wonderful world of people and the fascinating world of things (Fig. 11-5). The supervising adult should praise appropriate behavior and encourage imagination and creativity. Discipline should be restricted to acts which are morally wrong, socially unacceptable, destructive, or harmful to the child or others. When discipline is necessary, the child needs to have a simple explanation of why the behavior was inappropriate and must be guided to more constructive activities. For example, the nurse might say, "You must stop hitting Johnny because it hurts him the way it hurts when someone hits you. You feel angry and want to hit. Maybe if you pound this clay you will feel better." In this way, a true sense of initiative can be developed. As part of the process, the child is also learning self-confidence, sex and social role identification, social behavior and self-control, and moral and ethical values.

A child who does not develop a positive sense of initiative develops a sense of *guilt*. The child feels defeated, angry, afraid of attempting projects, accountable for things he or she really is not responsible for, and generally guilty. Such children are often timid about people and new experiences and lack interest in other children or adults. The sense of guilt develops from a lack of positive recognition for achievement, repeated punishment for exploratory behavior, stifled initiative because an adult does things for the child, lack of opportunity to try out new things, and limited playtime to fantasize and interact with other children. Criticism, too, can cause feelings of guilt in children. Too often, one can hear adults saying to a preschooler, "That's nice, but you could do it better if . . ." or "Try it again, that's not good." Such comments cause the child to become anxious, frightened, and reluctant to attempt new tasks. The child should be approached more positively with comments such as, "You really worked hard."

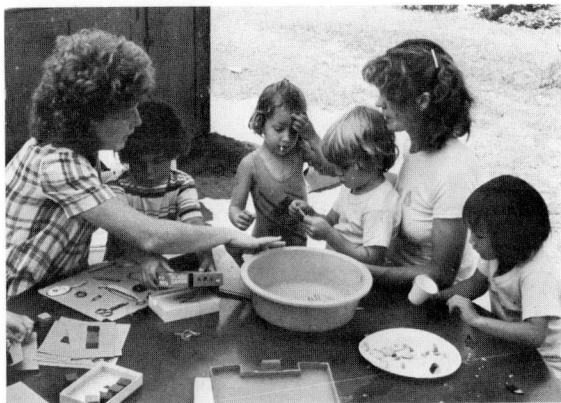

Figure 11-5 The preschooler must be provided with a safe and stimulating environment in which there is adult supervision.

A sense of guilt is frequently evident in a passive child, who will become an inhibited and dependent adult, avoiding new experiences and responsibilities. Some symptoms of serious disturbances in personality development during this period include enuresis (see Chap. 37), nonspeaking, inappropriate play, withdrawal from peers, assaultiveness, destructiveness, night terrors, and persistent fears.

Sex and social role identification

The preschooler's insatiable curiosity, awareness of himself or herself as different from others, increased sense of balance and spatial orientation, development of cognitive and language skills, and increased neurological maturation lead to the development of *body image*, i.e., what the child believes his or her own body to be. One aspect of body image is gender. Children examine themselves, compare their own physical attributes with those of others, and soon become aware that there are sexual differences. Playing "doctor" and hiding in the bathroom with a friend are both normal behaviors at this age. The child is simply learning about his or her body; this does not indicate later homosexuality. Parents should avoid shaming children and instead distract them to another activity. By age 3 or 4, the child has developed an awareness of gender and is becoming increasingly aware of the physical attributes of the two sexes. Boys know they are boys; girls know they are girls.

Sex roles—the roles that society considers appropriate for males and females—involve behaviors as well as feelings, attitudes, motives, and beliefs. A child's actual behaviors, feelings, attitudes, motives, and beliefs become part of the child's personality and determine that child's *sex role identity*. The process by which the child develops sex role identity is *identification*[7] (see Fig. 11-6).

Identification is the process whereby the child imitates and acquires some of the attributes of parents, siblings, and others. Freud, who introduced the concept of identification, believed that girls identify with their mothers, and boys with their fathers. Research has shown that a child actually identifies with a person or persons who have certain qualities that the child *values*. A child will identify with a person who (1) is physically or psychologically similar to the child, (2) is nurturant to the child, and (3) has something desired by the child, such as a special power, the love of others, or task competence.[8] A child may identify with people other than the same-sex parent. Identification is strongest when the child identifies for all three reasons listed above. For example, Jimmy's father is a loving person, gives him much attention, and is a well-known football player. Jimmy senses his father's concern for him and is impressed with his father's fame and physical prowess. He wants to be like him. Jimmy begins to walk and talk like his father and even has his own football uniform, which he wears constantly—Jimmy is identifying with his father.

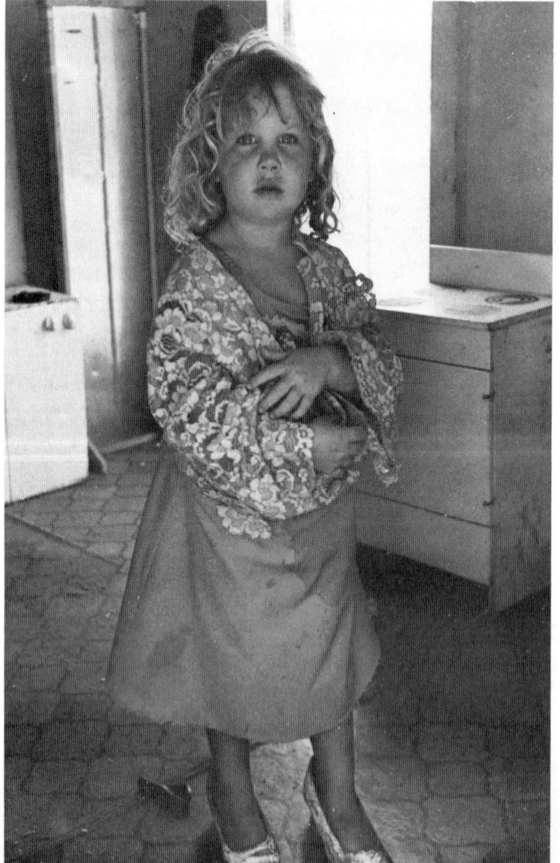

Figure 11-6 Preschoolers learn sex role identity by identifying with and imitating their same-sex parents.

Our society traditionally considers masculine attributes to include aggressiveness, independence, and emotional control; feminine attributes are passiveness, nurturance, poise, and attractiveness.[9] A child who adopts the sex role behaviors that are approved in his or her social group is likely to be accepted by peers because he or she behaves the way a boy or girl is expected to behave. Conversely, a child who does not behave as expected by society may have difficulty being accepted by peers during later childhood.

Five-year-old Erica, for example, whose family consists of a passive father, a mother who is aggressive and independent, and three older brothers, has identified with her mother and to some extent her oldest brother, who is the family favorite. Erica's nursery school teacher reports that Erica is frequently involved in fighting, uses foul language, and takes little part in cooperative play. Erica is not playing the role that is expected by society. Erica will probably be pressured to adopt traditional feminine roles at puberty.

To prevent serious personality disturbances, especially those associated with sex role identity, children must be exposed to adequate female and male role models. This is not always easy to do because of the many different family structures in our society. One-parent families may not provide adequate adult role models for a child to imitate and identify with. A parent who is raising a child alone needs to provide an opposite sex figure from whom the child can learn sex roles. Relatives or "big brother" organizations often provide positive, substitute relationships.

Although it is extremely important, identification is only one aspect of learning sex role behavior.

Child-rearing practices also play a significant part. The parents' method of rewarding a child for specific male or female behaviors and their attitudes toward, and expectations of, the child help the child adopt the appropriate sex role. Parents' expectations are continually displayed.

Until World War I, sex roles were strictly defined and were handed down from generation to generation. These sex roles, often described in "gothic" novels, were traditional sex role stereotypes. Sex role stereotypes are less rigid today but continue to exist. The blend of sex role stereotypes learned by the child depends upon the family's orientation and socioeconomic class. Parents from lower socioeconomic classes tend to have more traditional sex role stereotypes; the mother cares for the home without the father's help, and the father is the breadwinner. These fathers nurture their children less and display less affection. The expectations of middle-class parents are more flexible. Middle-class fathers nurture their children more, express affection more openly, and encourage more emotional expression. Middle-class parents allow their children to play with toys for either sex until age 6 or 7. Parents from lower socioeconomic classes limit their children's toys to those appropriate to the traditional sex role at an early age.

Sex role adoption begins with learning to act the appropriate sex role. The child learns which objects are appropriate for his or her role. Parents choose toys, books, and clothes that they consider suitable. Though both sexes may today wear jeans, many parents would disapprove of their son's repeated application of lipstick. They would probably substitute a traditionally appropriate razor. Since sex role learning is a gradual process, the child next adopts the attitudes of parents and society toward that role. Even today, girls are often protected from injury, restricted from frequent fighting, kept closer to home, and encouraged to cry and to express emotions. Boys are often expected to express aggression, fight more, be dirtier than girls, and not be "crybabies." A parent may typically scold Bobby for kicking Jenny but tell Bobby, who was kicked and beaten by another boy, "Go out and kick him harder, and don't cry!" Parents use these responses almost automatically and are not always aware of their influence on molding sex role behavior.

Even with the feminist movement, traditional sex role stereotypes remain. Because girls receive conflicting messages and because male sex role behavior is more strictly defined, girls, such as Erica, discussed above, often have more difficulty than boys in adopting the socially expected sex role attitudes and behavior.

All children seek approval, and approval is one of the most common and powerful motivators of behavior. When approval is given consistently and repeatedly for a specific sex role behavior, such as bravery or gentleness, children usually adopt the behavior to gain approval.

The preschooler is in the phallic stage of Freudian psychosexual development. During this stage the child's instinctual (libidinal) energy is focused on the genitals. The preschooler's behaviors seem to substantiate these beliefs; masturbation and sexual play frequently occur. Masturbation gives pleasurable feelings to the child and strengthens the behavior. The child uses these bodily sensations to establish the boundaries of his or her body.

Children unconsciously want to "own" and intensely love the opposite-sex parent and hate and want to destroy the same-sex parent. Freud called these ambivalent conflicts the *Electra complex* in girls and the *Oedipus conflict* in boys. (In Greek myth, Electra urged her brother to kill their mother, who had murdered their father, and Oedipus unknowingly killed his father and married his mother.) The preschooler frequently crawls into bed between the parents, seeking to separate them or force one out of the bed.

Preschoolers' love-hate ambivalent attitude toward the same-sex parent causes strong emotional feelings which they find difficult to control. Their thinking is magical and egocentric (self-centered). They believe that thoughts are as powerful as actions—that the urge to destroy the father, for example, will actually kill him. Preschoolers recognize their dependence on parents and gradually learn that the wish to possess a parent cannot come true. These unacceptable urges are then repressed, and the child is ready to enter the next (latency) phase of psychosexual development.

Sex education

Parents' attitudes toward, and approach to, sex education also influence the child's feelings and beliefs about sex roles. Because of their curiosity and developing sexual identity, preschoolers invariably are interested in "where they came from" or "how babies are made." For such information they must rely almost exclusively on parents. If parents refuse to give answers, appear highly anxious when discussing sexual matters, or imply that the subject is "taboo" or "dirty," children often develop similar attitudes. When approached with questions about sex, parents tend either to close communication or to overwhelm the child with information. Four helpful guidelines for parents answering preschoolers' questions are: (1) Remain calm—do not show anxiety, confusion, or concern over the question; (2) find out from the child *why* he or she is asking the question; (3) find out *what* the child *knows* about the subject in question; and then (4) provide the child with a *simple, honest* answer.

Parents should be advised that these questions will come up during the preschool period. In this way the parents can be prepared with appropriate information and can provide their children with objective answers. This will also prevent the transference of anxiety or negative attitudes. Asking *why* a child asked a question will help the parent understand what type of answer the child expects. For example, 4-year-old Sandy asks, "Mommy, where did I come from?" The mother replies, "Why do you ask?" The child responds, "Because Riza came from New York. Did I too?" Using this approach, the mother discovers that the child did not want sexual information at all, which is often the case.

Now assume that the mother's question elicited the following question from Sandy: "Well—how did you make me?" In order to respond adequately, the mother needs to be aware of what the child actually knows; then she can provide a simple answer or correct any misconceptions. Preschoolers often have strange ideas about procreation as a result of misinformation, their inability to think logically, and their absorption in the world of fantasy. Mother may now ask, "Sandy, how do you think I made you?" Sandy will now tell mother what she needs to know: "Well, I thought I grew in your stomach, but my food goes there!" Now the mother knows that the child needs to know the difference between the stomach, abdomen, and uterus. The child wants only one short explanation, a *simple* answer that she can comprehend. Honest, simple, and factual information is best given using anatomic terms, which build a pathway for further knowledge. If the child does not comprehend at first, or forgets or misinterprets the explanation, factual material can be restated when the child is able to absorb the information. When the child is ready for further information and is able to handle more complexities, questions will follow about eggs, sperm, or how the baby "gets in" and "comes out." Questions should be answered one at a time.

Often, pictures help answer questions, and parents may need this assistance in providing adequate explanations to children. There are many excellent sex education books that help parents meet the needs of the preschooler.[10] Parents should review books before presenting them to children so that they will be comfortable and familiar with the material.

Conscience and moral development

Moral development, which Freud called *superego* or *conscience development,* has strong roots in the preschool years. *Moral development* is the adoption of cultural standards of social behavior. (See Chap. 5.) The child is learning what constitutes "right" and "wrong" and "good" and "bad" behavior. The preschooler begins to behave morally to avoid feelings of guilt and is beginning to use self-control to resist temptation.

Kohlberg, expanding on Piaget's developmental stages of cognition, has developed a theoretical framework of moral development.[11] Kohlberg studied the moral reasoning of children throughout the world for 20 years and found that most preschoolers were in stage 1 of moral development.

Level I: Preconventional (premoral)

Stage 1: Punishment and obedience orientation The preschooler is extremely egocentric (self-centered) and has no true moral reasoning. This self-centered child is unable to see another's viewpoint, anticipate the consequences of an action, or analyze his or her thinking or that of another—all of which is necessary to solve a moral dilemma. The preschooler decides whether to break a rule on the basis of the amount and type of physical punishment that will result. Parents are viewed as all-powerful, and rules are thought to be rigid and unbreakable. The preschooler unquestioningly submits to the superior strength and power of adults, modifying his or her behavior to avoid punishment.

Moral development is an outgrowth of identification and of child-rearing practices, especially those associated with reward and punishment. Through identification the child begins to imitate the parents by following social rules such as eating with a fork rather than a knife, not pushing or shoving others around, and answering honestly when asked a question. At the same time, parents acknowledge the child for "obeying the rules" by approving and disapproving. For example, if a child lies, the parent may respond, "Don't tell lies; people won't like you if you do," or "Lies will get you in big trouble." If the child is truthful, a response from the parent may be "I am glad you told the truth; that makes me feel really good." Consistent rewards for good behavior and punishment for bad behavior help children develop a conscience. They begin to accept the rules and to feel guilty when they do not follow the rules, even when an adult is not present to reprimand them. Guilty feelings are highly uncomfortable, and so children try to avoid breaking the rules in order to prevent discomfort. Children avoid breaking the rules by self-control or the postponement of desires. For example, 5-year-old Traci just loves her friend's little doll lying on the table and wants it very badly. No one is in the room at the moment, and so she picks it up and is tempted to put it in her pocket. Suddenly Traci feels very uncomfortable and can almost hear her mother say, "You must not steal." She puts the doll back on the table.

Conscience development is dependent on a *warm, consistent* relationship with adults, especially the parents. If the child perceives the parents as loving, wants to please them, and is fearful of losing the parents' love by displeasing them, the child will develop a healthy conscience. However, if the child feels greatly threatened by the parents, especially with regard to the loss of parental love, initiative and creativity can be inhibited. That is, the "overdeveloped" conscience can prevent the child from becoming involved in new activities or social situations simply because there is a fear of not performing well enough to please the parents. This can be avoided if the parents do not demand more than the child is capable of and if they use punishment wisely. When the child is reprimanded for poor behavior, an explanation of *why* the behavior was unacceptable should be given. The focus should be on *the behavior itself* rather than on the relationship between the parent and child. For example, the parent might say, "I don't like to hear the language you are using," not "I don't want you around me when you are talking that way" or "You're a bad boy for talking that way."

Lack of a consistent, warm relationship with a parent can result in the child's developing a weak conscience. This can occur in families in which the parents are too busy to bother with their children. The child does not internalize the social rules and does not feel guilty about breaking the rules. Such children appear unruly and mischieveous and may later become delinquent. They are unable to follow the social and moral standards of society.

SOCIALIZATION AND THE LEARNING PROCESS

Socialization, the eventual transformation of a child into an adult participant in society, begins actively in the preschool years. At this time the child moves beyond the home environment and out into a social world. Rules of behavior are learned and enforced, and social roles are defined, practiced, and learned.

A child is socialized by formal and informal means. Formal social learning (socialization) is the deliberate and controlled attempt to mold children into specific social roles by such social institutions as schools and churches. The young child is socialized informally primarily through exposure to parents and family. The preschool years are significant; very few demands can be made of the infant or toddler, but the preschooler must learn to adapt to society. Informal types of social learning include insight and unfolding, imitation and identification, reinforcement and conditioning, and guidance and discipline.

Learning by insight and unfolding occurs as a result of the child's maturation. *Natural unfolding* refers to the child's spontaneously becoming able to carry out a behavior when the physiological capacity is present. For example, a child may suddenly learn to skip without ever having seen another person skip. *Insightful learning* occurs when a child realizes a relationship of some significance during play, exploration, or experimentation. Reinforcement, conditioning, guidance, and discipline are modes of teaching. How these modes are utilized by parents is termed *child-rearing practices*.

Reinforcement and conditioning

So much must be learned by the child during the preschool years, and so much must be taught by the parent: how to behave toward adults and peers; how to bathe, dress, and tidy up the bedroom or playroom; how to behave at the table or in the living room; and so on. Much of this learning is achieved during the preschool years through the use of reinforcement and conditioning. Parents value certain behaviors and may not accept others. Almost automatically or unconsciously, parents reward or punish their children until the "right" behavior is finally carried out. This is called *conditioning*, a form of learning in which the frequency of a certain behavior is increased or decreased by a system of rewards or punishment to influence the behavior. *Reinforcement* has occurred when the behavior has increased because of the reward. For example, mother wants Janie to wash her hands before every meal. Each time Janie washes her hands before a meal without being told to, mother rewards Janie's behavior with a hug and the comment, "It makes me so happy that you remembered to wash your hands." After a time, Janie washes her hands before every meal (reinforcement has occurred).

Rewards—parental actions which show approval or give the child pleasure—are most influential in leading the child to learn and adopt the rewarded behavior. Behaviors which result in disapproval or punishment or which elicit no reaction from the parents tend to be abandoned. Therefore, how the parents or other significant adults react to the child's behavior determines which behaviors will be learned.[12]

Reinforcement not only helps explain the social development of the child but also is an important tool with which to improve a child's behavior. To teach a child a set of behaviors, the desired behaviors must be identified, and only one small behavior change must be required at a time. Too much cannot be expected of the child. Once parents are aware of the behavior they wish to encourage, they should be advised to show *consistent* approval of the behavior when it occurs. The reward must be given right after the behavior occurs if it is to be effective, and it must be given each time the behavior occurs over a period of several weeks. This can be a most effective method of teaching a child how to behave appropriately in the social world. (See also Chap. 10.)

Guidance and discipline

The preschooler must learn to understand and obey the rules and get along with others. *Discipline*—guidance in helping the child understand and follow social rules and behave appropriately—is essential to the attainment of this goal. Preschoolers are struggling to gain control over inner impulses, and they need, first of all, to have limits set on their behavior.

Setting limits for the child provides a frame in which the child can function with freedom and safety. For example, the preschooler may be told to play in the backyard and not on the street or not to hit or shove. If the child goes beyond these limits, disciplinary action is taken. Children of all ages need to have established limits; limits are essential for the adventurous and ever-curious preschooler. The establishment and enforcement of limits provides the child with a clear definition of what he or she can and cannot do and ensures a safe environment. This gives the child a feeling of security. When limits are set, they must be clearly explained to the child. Limit setting and disciplinary action must be consistent in order to be effective. If a rule is in effect one day, it should also be in effect the next day, and if disciplinary action has been suggested to the child, it should be immediately carried out. Being consistent prevents confusion and anxiety in the child. However, limits must have some flexibility since extenuating circumstances do arise.

Disciplinary measures which are most effective with preschoolers include time out, diversion, and offering restricted choices. *Time out* consists of removing a child from a situation for a short period. For example, 4-year-old Scotty and Tony are suddenly pounding each other and pulling each other's hair. Mother asks them to stop, but the fight continues. Mother picks up kicking Scotty and removes him to his room, where he must remain for several minutes until he settles down. She then offers Scotty an explanation. A few minutes alone seem like an eternity to the preschooler who has no sense of time, and have an amazing calming effect.

Diversion is most effective when used with a child who repeats unacceptable behavior. This technique consists of diverting the child to another activity and giving an explanation. For example, Karen persists in throwing sand at her playmates. She is asked to stop but refuses. The teacher then states, "You must stop throwing sand—it may get in someone's eye. Here, let's throw the big red ball instead." Karen takes the ball and throws it to her teacher. She has been diverted from an unacceptable behavior to one that is acceptable. Preschoolers are quickly interested in, and diverted to, another activity because of their short attention span.

Offering restricted choices is a helpful technique when there is some danger involved in a child's activity. It is an alternative to repeating, "Stop it." This technique consists of allowing the child to continue the activity, but in a modified way. For example, Jackie and his 4-year-old friends are furiously and continuously riding their big wheels down the driveway toward the street. Jackie's mother is worried that they might go into the street and requests a change in the activity: "You may ride your big wheels, but you will have to do it in the backyard. It would be dangerous if you accidentally went into the street." Here the children have the choice of continuing to ride if they go to the backyard or of ceasing the activity.

Play and socialization

Play, often referred to as the *child's work*, is one of the major modes of learning during the preschool years. Play enhances physical and cognitive development by providing opportunities for coordination of fine and gross motor development and development of depth perception, spatial relationships, and other sensory experiences. Play also stimulates curiosity, creativity, and the development and use of vocabulary.

Play nurtures psychological and social development by providing situations in which the child can imitate and practice adult roles to learn sex role identification. Social behaviors and rules are developed and practiced in social play. Play also helps children overcome the feeling of powerlessness in the big world of adults, as they exercise control over the small world of manageable toys. Through the medium of play, the child is able to work out such negative feelings as anxiety, fear, aggression, and anger in a relatively nonthreatening and socially acceptable manner. (See Chap. 15 for a discussion of play and the hospitalized child.) If a child is angry, a ball can be kicked, a hammer pounded, or a doll spanked without punishment. The child thus repeats a play situation until feelings are assimilated and fears are mastered.

A child can play alone, with peers, or with adults. Preschool children especially enjoy playing with peers and adults. They are very social. For this reason, parents should be encouraged to seek opportunities for children to socialize with other children their own age and to find time to play with their children on a daily basis. Parental involvement in play activities is considered "prime time" for learning and establishing relationships. Games and activities are taught and learned that otherwise might not be, and warm relationships are developed through mutual pleasure and enjoyment. Also, a mutual appreciation of parent and child as individuals is developed.

The preschooler's tremendous drive for social involvement sometimes leads to having an *imaginary playmate*. The adoption of an imaginary playmate is directly related to the child's ability to fantasize and is a normal behavior at this age. Imaginary playmates serve several purposes: They provide companionship in times of loneliness, are patient and understanding about accomplishments and failures, are sympathetic about problems that no adults seem to comprehend, and always play what the child wishes. Children soon give up the imaginary playmate as they become more involved with real friends and activities and as they approach school age.

Solitary and parallel play, most frequently seen in the toddler period (see Chap. 10), persist in the preschool years, when the child feels a need to withdraw from the group or be alone. However, preschoolers are very social, and their predominant forms of play are associative and cooperative play. *Associative play* occurs when children engage in a common activity with only loosely established rules (Fig. 11-7). No child is the leader, there are no goals, and there is no division of functions. An example of associative play is two children playing in a sandbox next to each other. They pass each other shovels, strainers, and other toys and carry on a conversation about their activities. They play in association with each other.

In *cooperative play*, children cooperate in activities such as games, playing house, and building a spaceship. They assume specific functions and roles, such as mother, father, or fire chief. Rules are established for play, and there is a feeling of belonging to the group. The group is structured; there are definite leaders and follow-

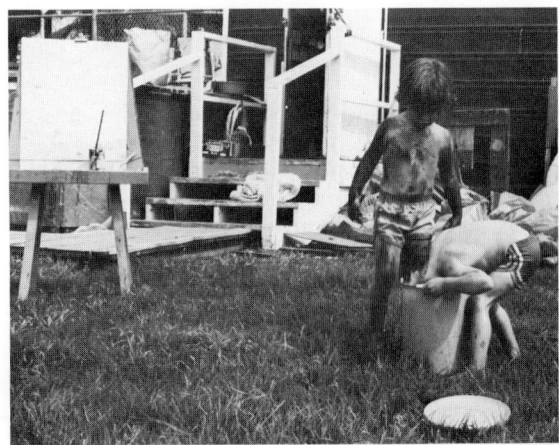

Figure 11-7 Associative play occurs when children engage in a common activity in which the rules are loosely established.

ers, and one or several children assume the leadership and direct the activity.

Children, however, are not always involved in direct social interaction. A child who feels insecure about joining a group or who is tired may become an *onlooker*. The onlooker may not be actively participating in an activity but is passively involved by observing and learning. This type of play is normal, but if it is prolonged it may also suggest that the child needs adult assistance in entering a group. Onlooker behavior must be differentiated from withdrawal behavior, which is a symptom of psychological disturbance. The withdrawing child shows little interest in what is going on and manifests this behavior in much of the daily routine. When withdrawal is a pattern of behavior, referral for assessment and treatment is necessary.

Children who actively socialize with their peers need constant adult supervision. Parents must provide adequate opportunities for play, stimulating and safe play equipment and materials, and a safe environment and safety rules before play begins. Children should be allowed to develop their own play activities, try things out for themselves, and work out their own differences whenever possible. Structuring activities limits children's interest and curiosity. They should be allowed to play freely with little adult interference, unless they need help or the play is unsafe. When children cannot work out their problems, they should be diverted, or another activity substituted. An adult should join in the play only when asked; these occasions provide wonderful opportunities for the adult to view the fascinating world of children.

Play activities, equipment, and materials should provide for gross motor play, creative play, dramatic play, and quiet play. *Gross motor play* provides opportunities for the development and refinement of motor skills, such as running, jumping, climbing, and tricycle riding. *Creative play* promotes fine motor coordination, self-expression, and practice in manipulation and construction. Creative activities include painting, pasting, cutting, manipulating carpentry tools, playing with musical toys, and building with small blocks. *Dramatic play* enhances the process of identification and the learning of social roles by providing an opportunity to imitate and pretend to assume future adult roles. This type of play is most characteristic of the preschooler. Playhouses, dress-up clothes, housekeeping toys, dollhouses, farm sets, trucks, little cars, planes, and dolls are all materials with which to carry out dramatic play. *Quiet play* occurs primarily when activity is very limited or when the child is passively involved. Quiet play includes looking at books, listening to stories, being read to, listening to records, and watching television. Some aspects of creative play may also be considered quiet play (see Fig. 11-8), such as doing puzzles or making simple handicrafts. All children need periods of quiet play to wind down from more strenuous activities before mealtimes and bedtime. Quiet play is also important when children feel tired or are ill.

Play activities and equipment should be selected in accordance with the developmental level of the child and the desired goals (see Table 11-5). Goals may include providing a specific learning experience, an opportunity for socializing, a chance to release energy, or a moment of relaxation. Toys must be durable, since damage occurs from use and experimentation. Toys that will cause family disturbances if lost or damaged must not be purchased. The preschooler is not able to appreciate the value of toys and cannot be responsible for all his or her actions. A great many play materials are inexpensive (see Fig. 11-9). Children love cuddly handmade rag dolls, dollhouses built out of wooden boxes, old clothes from the parents' closet, homemade play dough, large cardboard boxes, and spare wood, nails, and

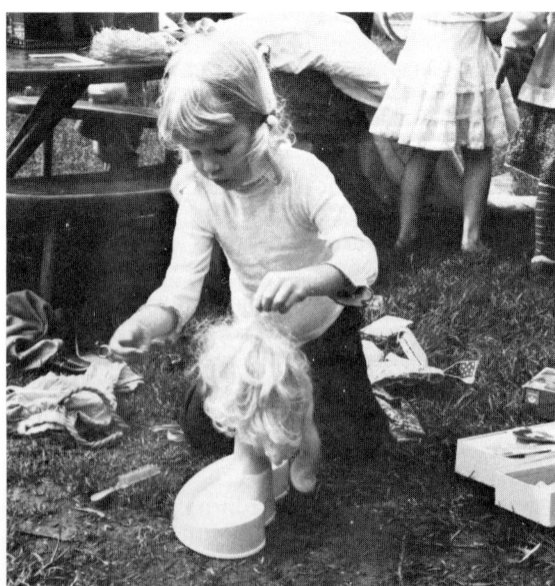

Figure 11-8 A child may need time out from group activities to engage in quiet play.

Table 11-5 Suggested Toys and Play Activities for the Preschooler

	3 years	4 years	5 years
Gross motor play	Swings Slides Tricycles Sandbox Wading pool Wagons	Rope ladders Jungle gym Swimming Trapeze	Roller skates Ball playing Bicycle with training wheels
Creative play	Sand play Water play Play dough and clay Finger painting Large blocks Musical toys	Crayons and chalk drawing Easel painting Rhythm band Simple puzzles Markers Stamp pads Scissors	Cutting pictures Carpentry tools Simple sewing and handicrafts Puzzles
Dramatic play	Block building Farm animal toys Dolls Dollhouses Trucks, cars, planes Toy phones	Dress-up clothes Group play Housekeeping toys Store play toys Nurse and doctor kits Wooden boxes	Paper puppets Handkerchief puppets Large wooden and cardboard boxes Pedal cars and trucks
Quiet play	Books—fairy tales Nursery rhymes and stories Children's records	Books—fairy tales and adventures Design construction sets	Books about real adventures of people and animals Selected television programs
Games	Where is Thumbkin? Mulberry bush Clapping games Eentsy-weentsy spider Lotto cards Match-ups or put-togethers	Simon says Dog and bone Two little blackbirds Candyland Sequence cards, visual games	Beanbag throwing Skip tag Ball play Hide-and-seek

hammers. Jungle gyms, playhouses, and furniture can be made from poles, ladders, pipes, large boxes, and wood. Sandboxes can easily be dug in the yard. Pieces of cloth, beans, macaroni, sticks, leaves, and paper and glue are good, inexpensive creative materials. Puppets can be made from peanut shells, paper bags, or discarded toilet-paper rolls. Plastic jars, boxes, and discarded juice containers are perfect toys for sand and water play. For the preschooler, some of the best things in life to play with are free and easily accessible.

NURSERY SCHOOLS AND DAY-CARE CENTERS

Because parents have become more aware of their children's social needs and because more mothers have joined the work force, increased numbers of children are attending nursery schools. There has recently been an upsurge of nursery schools called *day-care centers*, which provide care over extended periods. The intent of day-care centers is to provide complete child care for children whose parents work or attend school. In the past, nursery schools focused primarily on providing the child with supplemental social and learning experiences.

The more time a child spends in nursery school, the greater the influence the school will have on the child's social and psychological development. Careful selection of a nursery school is very important. A nursery school or day-care center should meet the following criteria:

1. The nursery school or day-care center must be licensed by the state. This establishes minimum standards for safety and care.
2. The staff must include several members with 1 or more years of academic preparation in early childhood education or child development. One staff member to every four children is considered a safe ratio in terms of supervision. The staff should be stable, qualified, and able to provide references.

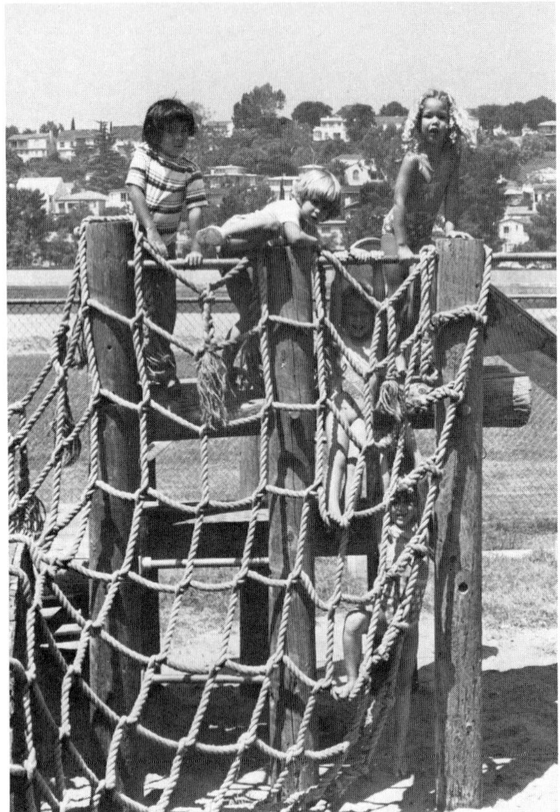

Figure 11-9 A nursery school jungle gym built entirely of discarded materials found in the community.

3. The facilities must include a safe environment for both indoor and outdoor play, including appropriate play equipment for gross motor, creative, dramatic, and quiet play.
4. Parents should know and agree with the philosophy of the staff regarding education, child rearing, and discipline.
5. The facilities must include adequate meal services, bathrooms, areas for rest, and individual places for each child's personal belongings.
6. Health services may not be provided, but health histories and emergency information must be on file, and adequate health policies established.
7. Food services must include a nutritious noon meal and healthful snacks.
8. Routines for play and rest periods must be established but flexibly administered.

When selecting a nursery school, parents must consider price, closeness to the home, and obligations that they might have to the school. Many nursery schools require parents to participate in activities such as fund-raising, administration, or actual child care. Before a final decision is made, it is imperative that the parents and the child visit the nursery school. There is no better way for the parents to evaluate the quality of child care than through direct observation. They should ask themselves the following questions: Is the staff competent? Are the staff members warm and attentive toward the children? Do the children appear happy—and are they working and playing with one another? Does the program *actually* provide stimulation and the freedom to explore? Is the food adequate, and the environment safe? The visit to the nursery school will introduce the child to the new environment, the teachers, the other children, and the program.

Once the selection of a nursery school has been made, the child needs adequate preparation. Parents can tell the child what to expect in a simple, direct fashion. If the child wants to attend the nursery school or has friends who go there his or her adjustment will be facilitated.

A parent should be encouraged to accompany the child on the first day and remain until the child feels secure enough to let the parent go. The process of separation may take several hours, days, or weeks; moving at the child's pace will prevent the trauma associated with separation anxiety. Parents also feel anxious about leaving their child for the first time. When they recognize the security of the nursery school, separation from the child becomes much easier. Parents need to inform the child exactly who will pick the child up, and when. When the parents and the child feel secure and confident about the nursery school, a wonderful learning and socializing experience is their reward.

INTELLECTUAL AND LANGUAGE DEVELOPMENT

Preoperational stage

The preschooler makes tremendous advances in cognitive development. These strides lead to readiness for formal schooling. Progress results from maturation, experience, and social interaction.[13] (See Fig. 11-10.) Preschoolers between

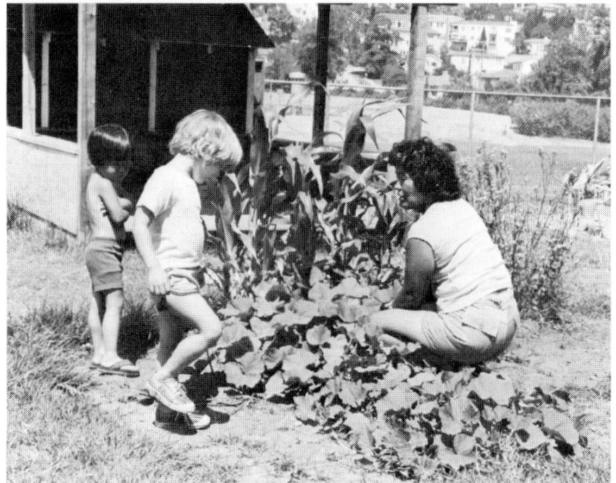

Figure 11-10 Much of the preschooler's learning comes from experience and from association with significant adults.

the ages of 2 and 7 are in Piaget's *preoperational stage* of cognitive development. This stage is divided into two phases: the *preconceptual phase* (2 to 4 years) and the *intuitive phase* (4 to 7 years). The preschooler's greatly expanding language skills are an outgrowth of the child's cognitive development. (See Table 5-3 for a summary of cognitive development.)

The preconceptual phase During the *preconceptual phase* the child begins to use symbolism. The child can now discriminate an object from an event. He or she recognizes that a high chair is not a part of the eating process but something to sit upon. Preconceptual thought is characterized by egocentrism, distortion of reality, lack of generality, and transductive reasoning.

Preschoolers continue to think egocentrically and view themselves as the center of the universe. From the perspective of preschoolers, all events are either occurring to them or happening because of them. Such statements as "I got sick because I was bad" and "He fell down because I wanted him to get hurt" reflect such thought.

Symbolism, the ability to let one thing stand for or represent another thing that is not there, is developing throughout these years. It is the foundation for logical thought. Mental symbols allow the 3-year-old to remember the past and act on it. The child knows about "Grandmother's house" because he or she has learned the words and can associate them with past visits to Grandmother's.

Symbols allow the child to "remember." With symbolic words the preschooler can describe something that happened in the past or ask for something that is not present. The preschooler does not have a true concept of time, and so explanations regarding time should be related to events *known* by the child. For example, a child should be told that "your mother is coming to pick you up from the nursery school when you have finished lunch"—not "at twelve o'clock"—since lunch, not twelve o'clock, has meaning for the child. Objects are used symbolically in make-believe play. Play dough can be transformed into food for a tea party, a box on a cart can become a tank or a bulldozer, and a blanket over a table can become a house.

In *animistic thought,* objects are endowed with qualities that adults reserve for other human beings and for animals; thus a teddy bear talks or protects the child from the dark, or a doll becomes a real friend or a crying baby. This type of symbolic play is vitally important for both cognitive and emotional development. If children are feeling overpowered by the adults around them, they may regain a sense of power and well-being by pretending that a doll is alive or that a toy lion is ferocious. After a traumatic experience, a child may work out his or her feelings through symbolic play, or imagination. Four-year-old Susie left the doctor's office very angry after being given a shot. Susie worked out her feelings at home by pulling out her doctor bag and "shooting" her doll many times.

Distortion of reality is caused in part by *transductive reasoning*. Adults reason from particular to general, or vice versa, but the preconceptual child reasons from particular to particular, or transductively. This kind of reasoning assumes relationships that do not exist and results in marvelous distortions of reality. A 3-year-old asked her father, "Why are you giving the dog a bath?" The father replied, "To wash the dirt and grease away." The child then asked, "What is grease?" "A fatty substance," responded the father. After a pause the child answered, "Oh, then if Grandma took more showers, she wouldn't be so fat!" This type of reasoning is accompanied by the inability to view the whole in relation to its parts or to reverse the thought process.

Preschoolers also have difficulty focusing on the important aspects of a situation. To a child, everything is important and interrelated; this kind of thinking is called *field dependency*. For example, a preschooler might have difficulty going to sleep if one night the parent fails to read the usual bedtime story. To the child, this is as important as closing his or her eyes in order to get to sleep. Objects, people, and routines are equally important. Because of this, the preschooler has a great need for sameness and routine.

Preconceptual thought lacks generality and individuality; the child cannot form true and stable concepts or classes. If the child sees a dog and later sees another dog, the two dogs may be considered the same dog rather than members of the same class of animal. Because the preschooler's thought lacks generality and the child cannot yet form true concepts, classifying is inconsistent. For example, Janie is collecting shells at the beach when suddenly she adds a rock to her collection because "it was pretty too."

The combination of the elements of preconceptual thought (symbolism, egocentrism, transductive reasoning, and the associated distortion of reality) leads to the wonderful world of fantasy and magical beliefs of preschool children, to whom Puff the Magic Dragon is under the piano and whose cape will transport them to Mars!

The intuitive phase The *intuitive phase* spans the ages from 4 through 7 and is still dominated by the child's perceptions rather than by logic. Characteristics of this phase are centration, a static quality, and lack of reversibility. *Centration* is the child's tendency to *center* or focus on one part of a problem and ignore the other parts. The child therefore fails to consider the relationship between the parts or between parts and the whole. For example, a child may have difficulty doing a relatively complex puzzle because he or she is determined to match colors, when the shapes of the pieces and the picture are also important. However, the child can now form true classes and hierarchies. For example, blocks can be sorted into groups according to shape or color. The child groups objects on the basis of one outstanding feature.

The child's thought has a static quality; that is, the child may focus on the *state* of an object rather than on the transformation of one object into another. For example, a ball of clay is made into a pie. Once the pie is made, the child is unable to recognize that the ball and the pie contain the same amount of clay. The child focuses only on the shape of the clay.

The child in the intuitive phase lacks *reversibility* in thought. A 4- or 5-year-old might correctly perceive that two identical glasses contain the same amount of water; if the water in one glass is then poured into a third glass of a different shape, the child will believe that the third glass contains a different amount of water. The child under 7 does not realize that if the water is poured back into the original glass, the glass will contain the same amount that he or she had to begin with. This demonstrates lack of reversibility. Another example is simple addition and subtraction; a 5-year-old might add 1 and 1 and get 2, but to reverse the problem ($2 - 1 = 1$) would be too difficult.

When the child's thought becomes decentered, when the child is able to focus on transformations, and when reversibility occurs, the child then enters the stage of concrete operations—the age of reason—and is ready for academic work and school. Understanding a preschool child's way of thinking helps not only in assessing developmental level but also in communicating. By being aware of poor conceptual abilities, transductive reasoning, distortion of reality, centering, and lack of reversibility, the knowledgeable nurse understands that when children ask "Why?" they need simple, concise answers. Since the preschooler's thought has a magical and fantastic quality, it is all right to believe in Santa Claus and the Tooth Fairy at this age. Reality comes later, as the child moves into the age of reasoning and of understanding cause-and-effect relationships. But it is important that parents help preschoolers distinguish what is *pretend* from what is *reality*. A parent might say, "I see you are pretending you are Superman today," not "Here comes my little Superman." Adults should become concerned only when a child withdraws into the fantasy world, forsaking relationships with peers and the spontaneity and driving curiosity that are so much a part of the normal behavior of this period.

Language development

Language development parallels the rapid intellectual development of the preschool period. The child's vocabulary increases by approximately 600 words a year. The preschooler's constant activity is reflected in his or her vocalization. Four- and five-year-olds constantly talk and tend to boast, exaggerate, and playfully use silly language. Speech is used as an aggressive behavior by the 4-year-old, who now uses full sentences. Little girls, especially, tend to be verbally aggressive toward each other at this age, and children of both sexes may use profanity to get attention. Such behavior will usually disappear if ignored, as will the tendency to mix fantasy with reality, which the adult may perceive as lying. It is most helpful if parents understand that this verbal behavior is normal at this age.

Language is used as a part of the learning and socialization process to get information, seek meaning about experiences, gain attention, and relieve anxiety. Language development involves the *expressive capacity*, or the actual vocalization of the child, and the *receptive capacity*, or the comprehension of the language. Reading and writing at this age, as part of language development, would indicate that the child was exceptionally bright. The child's receptive capacity exceeds his or her expressive capacity; that is, the child understands words and phrases which are not yet part of his or her daily talking. The development of language depends on the child's ability to learn the language, the quality and amount of language used in the home, the opportunity the child has to express himself or herself, and the amount of exposure to language outside the home. Without exposure to language, whether the child is partially deaf, deaf, or isolated, language development will be limited. Exposure of the child to talking is extremely important. It is during the preschool period that normal children acquire and master the basic syntactic structure of their language. Children learn to express themselves like the adults in the environment (although vocabulary and refinement of sentence structure will continue to grow throughout life). Children gradually learn to speak in full sentences.

The preschooler constantly asks "Why?" "What?" "When?" "Where?" and "How?" in an effort to explore the world. Adults should readily respond with simple, short, and honest answers. Language is learned through direct communication with others, through reading, and through television. Parents should be encouraged to discuss things with their children, since verbal explorations are essential to learning. Adults must be attentive and show that they care about what the child is saying.

Some helpful modes of communicating with children include the following:

1. Be positive, and provide no alternatives if the child must conform to a request. For example, a parent should say, "You must eat now," not "Would you like to eat?"
2. Use positive phraseology, since preschoolers tend to respond to this more readily than to "Don't do that," for example. Be instructive, telling the child what to do and what the choices are, and point out the consequences. For example, "You will need to hold your arm still so the doctor can get the bandage on evenly and fast," not "Don't move your arm."
3. Give praise for good behaviors. Praise is recognition of achievement. Avoid evaluative phrases and words such as *good, bad, nice,* and *naughty*. Acknowledge specific acts and efforts. For example, "You have learned how to do that very well; thank you for helping," not "What a big boy you are; that is nice." Immediate praise and reward foster the child's learning.
4. When a child appears upset, precede statements of advice or instructions with a statement of understanding of how the child feels. For example, "I understand that you are angry because your mother left you, but she will be back at lunchtime," or "I know that shot hurt you, but now wouldn't you like to go back to the playroom?" This also helps the child label his or her feelings and builds adult-child trust.
5. If a child has an anger outburst, stay with the child until calmness is regained. The child may need to be picked up and comforted, though not all children will respond to this or accept it. The parent might say, "That was a painful thing to happen to you. The way you feel is called angry. I think you'll be ready to play again."
6. If a child has an anger outburst following interference or physical restraint by an adult, try bodily contact. The parent might say calmly, "I can help you hold still so you can stop and listen. You're angry now. Soon you can go back and play with Jane." Undue attention, however, should be avoided.
7. Warn children of impending changes in activities in order to prepare for them. For example, "In a few minutes, it'll be lunchtime. Finish what you are doing." "Time in the

playroom will be over in a few minutes, and you need to get ready to go back to your room."
8. Do not make promises unless you can keep them. Children feel insecure with adults who do not fulfill promises.

Table 11-6 presents a summary of the cognitive and language skills of the 3-, 4-, and 5-year-old.

DEALING WITH COMMON PROBLEMS

Maintaining and promoting optimum physical and mental health is the goal of all nurses. This goal is achieved by providing education, counseling, and anticipatory guidance. Education is the communication of information to the parents, with the goal of changing their behavior. Counseling helps parents identify problems and find alter-

Table 11-6 Cognitive and Language Skills

3 years	4 years	5 years
Much egocentrism Knows own sex Knows he or she is a separate person Uses "me" and "I" frequently	**Less egocentrism** Sees self as an individual in a group Uses "I" frequently	**Little egocentrism** Is aware of cultural differences Knows name and address
Much distortion of reality Is imaginative Talks to self Does not care if another is listening Makes some inappropriate answers	**Less distortion of reality** Is highly imaginative Talks with imaginary playmate Tells family secrets Exaggerates, boasts, and tattles Tells stories mixing reality with fantasy	**Little distortion of reality** Is less imaginative Can tell a story accurately May use fantasy in stories but is aware of the distortions made
Weak concept formation and symbolism Has a vocabulary of 900 words Uses language experimentally Talks in simple sentences (using some adjectives and verbs) of three to four words Needs simple explanations May repeat several numbers by rote Has an attention span of 10 min	**Concepts weak but improving in accuracy** Has a vocabulary of 1500 words Uses concrete speech Uses more complex sentences (uses prepositions and plurals) Defines simple words Knows one or more colors Understands concepts of 1, 2, and 3 Counts to 5 Has an attention span of 20 min	**Symbolic thought and concepts improved** Has a vocabulary of 2100 words Uses language correctly—full syntax Uses meaningful sentences Can follow plot of a story Knows four or more colors Counts to 10 Begins to understand money Has an attention span of 30 min
No generalization Has slight understanding of past and future	**Some generalization** Understands concept of time of day Knows days of the week	**Generalizes** Knows days of the week Knows the month and year Has a sense of time and duration
Transductive reasoning Thinks illogically Understands very simple reasoning	**Some logic with crude comparison** Begins to organize experiences Asks "why?" frequently	**Begins to reason logically** Grasps some cause-and-effect relationships Likes to know how to use objects Frequently asks "How?" "When?" and "Where?" Knows meanings of words
Field dependency Thrives on routine Lacks reversibility Has little awareness of feelings of others when talking Desires to please; is friendly Needs directions	**Centration** Focuses on one thing at a time Lacks reversibility Has some awareness of feelings of others when talking Bosses and criticizes others Uses profanity to get attention	**Centration** Lacks reversibility May do simple addition Is unable to subtract Is aware of others' feelings and differences Is increasingly independent

native approaches to child rearing. Anticipatory guidance assists parents in preparing for future developmental behaviors. Education and anticipatory guidance are preventive approaches to health promotion and maintenance. Anticipatory guidance will help prevent undesirable habits and feelings, conflicts, and frustrations. Nurses should explain normal behaviors and milestones of development to parents, make an assessment of the family, and anticipate situations and behavior for parents and explain them before they occur. Through understanding, parents will be able to take a healthy attitude toward their children's behavior and use desirable methods of dealing with it. Parents need to be informed of the common, normal behaviors of children in each age group; although these behaviors may cause parental concern, in reality they are not problems and, if ignored, usually pass (are extinguished) when no mention (reinforcement) is made of them. Some normal behaviors in the preschool period which cause parental concern include masturbation, messiness, stuttering and stammering, temper tantrums, and short-lived unreasonable fears (see Table 11-7). It is only when behaviors become *persistent* and *interfere* with the normal daily routine of the child that they may be considered symptoms of physiological or psychological disturbances. To determine whether a child's behaviors are interfering with normal development, it is necessary to observe the child in his or her own environment. The nurse should observe the child's toileting, speech, play and peer relationships, sibling relationships, eating patterns, fears, and other general behaviors. Children with problems should be examined by a pediatrician; other referrals (e.g., to a speech pathologist or a psychologist) may also be necessary.

Sibling rivalry

Sibling rivalry involves one child's negative feelings toward a sibling because of competition or

Table 11-7 Anticipated Behaviors of the Preschooler

Areas of observation	Normal behaviors	Behaviors which are not typically problems	Behaviors which are signs of disturbance
Toileting	Successful toilet training (2 to $2\frac{1}{2}$ years)	Occasional soiling and wetting	Persistent soiling past 5 years—enuresis and encopresis
Speech	Creative use of speech (3 to 4 years)	Stuttering and stammering Aggressive speech—some swearing and lying Talking to self ($2\frac{1}{2}$ years)	Nonspeaking beyond 2 years Persistent lying
Play and peer relationships	Associative play (3 years) Cooperative play (4 years)	Aggressive and possessive play Messy play Refuses to put things away	Inappropriate play (involving death or torture) Withdrawal from peers Assaultive and destructive behavior
Eating	Food preferences Occasional finickiness	Refuses to try new foods	Persistent eating problems
Sibling relationships	Some sibling rivalry (3 years)	Some conflict between siblings	Persistent signs of jealousy or assaultiveness
Sleep	Bedtime ritual (including transitional object)	Has some dreams	Persistent signs of disturbed sleep, night terrors, or excessive body-rocking
Fears		Has short-lived and unreasonable fears	Persistent fear of the dark, ghosts, or burglars
General behaviors and daily routine	Sexual curiosity Aggression; stubbornness Willingness to accept reasonable limits (2 to $2\frac{1}{2}$ years)	Masturbation Finger-sucking Temper tantrums Wants own way Regressive behavior with stress	Shyness Tics

jealousy. Rivalry occurs when the child's need to feel worthwhile is frustrated. It usually is directed toward an older sibling or occurs when a child tries to do better than a sibling. Jealousy occurs when the child's need to be loved and to love is frustrated; it is commonly directed toward younger siblings. Behaviors characteristic of sibling rivalry may include acting out the negative feelings through fighting and verbal aggression or expressing the feelings in such regressive behaviors as bed-wetting, nail-biting, or having nightmares. Although there is often a quiet period of sibling truce around the age of 4, sibling rivalry occurs during the preschool period, since this is a time when aggressive behaviors are common. Fighting with an older sibling or one close in age can readily disrupt a household, while fighting with, and aggression toward, a younger sibling can lead to injury.

Although some sibling rivalry is normal, severe symptoms can be prevented by preparing the preschooler for the arrival of a new baby and by recognizing each child in the family for individual accomplishments. Parents should be instructed to provide the preschooler with *his or her own time* of love and affection, to let the preschooler help care for the infant, and to treat the preschooler as an individual. Parents should also be instructed to praise the preschooler each time visitors praise the baby, to give the preschooler an inexpensive present when the baby receives one, to encourage the child to voice any negative feelings without judgment, and to channel aggressive behavior in other directions.

If the regressive behaviors associated with sibling rivalry interfere with the child's daily routine and are persistent or if the aggressive verbal or physical behavior seems to be inflicting psychological or bodily harm on the sibling, referral should be made for psychological counseling.

Fighting, which is the most common symptom of sibling rivalry and one that few families avoid, is most effectively reduced by the use of time out. The children are placed in separate rooms or are told to sit on a chair for a short time.[14] This cooling-down period may be as short as 2 min but must not be more than 10 to 15 min. The parent should make no attempt to determine who was to blame for the fight. Siblings are then discouraged from arguing with the parent or from baiting each other into starting another fight. To be effective, this approach must be used consistently and be coupled with praise and attention when the siblings are playing cooperatively together.

Thumb-sucking

Thumb-sucking is reported in approximately 46 percent of children between birth and 16 years of age.[15] Although it may cause social embarrassment to both the child and the family, it has little significance before the age of 4. If it continues when the permanent teeth appear, it contributes to malocclusion. It is desirable to extinguish the habit between the ages of 4 and 5, before the child starts school. Suggested causes of thumb-sucking include strong instinctual drives for sucking, regressive behavior, and a need for security when the child is under stress. If the behavior is ignored, it usually disappears. When this is not the case, action must be taken. Home management techniques and interventions that have been used with varied success include having the child wear special mittens or restraints, applying bitter-tasting chemicals to the thumb, and rewarding good behavior (positive reinforcement). Rewarding good behavior is often successful with young children if done consistently over a period of weeks. For example, a mother might say that every morning her 4-year-old daughter wakes up with a dry thumb, the child will receive a gold "big girl" star on a chart, and that at the end of the week, if there is a gold star for each day, she can have a party or other reward. Success with this approach depends on the mother's remembering to reward the child *every day* with the star. Each star and unsucked thumb *must* receive lavish praise, while the child's failure is ignored. However, parents must be informed that the unwanted behavior will become stronger before it is extinguished.

Thumb-sucking is often associated with an object such as a security blanket. The child picks up the blanket when watching TV, resting, or going to bed; this blanket usually has been a treasured object since infancy. Interestingly, if the blanket is slowly reduced to nothing (the mother washes it until it falls apart), the thumb-sucking may also disappear.

If the problem persists beyond the age of 4, referral should be made to an orthodontist, who may intervene with the use of dental devices to prevent malocclusion. Such intervention has proved quite successful.

Sexual curiosity and masturbation

A child's sexual curiosity and masturbation rank among the top concerns of parents during this period, and yet they are *normal* behaviors if not carried to excess. Both behaviors are triggered by the child's developing sexual identification and also result from the child's insatiable curiosity about his or her own body and the world.

Preschoolers manifest sexual curiosity by asking many questions about sex (see the section "Sex Education" earlier in this chapter) and in their play activities. Preschoolers are commonly found in the bathroom or playhouse engaging in mutual exploration while playing "doctor," "nurse," "mother," or "father." The preschooler frequently "peeps" around or under the bathroom door. Peeping behavior is usually quite limited in children who receive adequate answers to sexual questions at home and in children who are exposed to siblings and parents who comfortably accept their own sexuality. Sexual curiosity seems more intensified in children when parents are overly modest or when there are no siblings whose bodies preschoolers can compare with their own.

When parents are confronted with these behaviors, the problem is more one for the parents than for the child. Parents need to know that most children exhibit this type of sexual curiosity during the preschool years, and they should be prepared to handle the situation. The most effective approach to the child's sexual explorations with others is to actually intrude on the activity, suggesting some diversional activity, while avoiding embarrassing the child in front of others. Later, when the child is alone, the parent can explain that undressing and touching another's genitals is not acceptable behavior and can suggest that the child ask any questions that he or she has.[16] A calm and rational approach will limit sexual experimentation without damaging the child's interest in the body or sex.

A calm, rational approach is also necessary in the management of the child who is masturbating. Masturbation is more common in boys than in girls during the preschool period, probably because of the anatomic availability of the penis. Children frequently masturbate in bed; some do so openly in public. It is not unusual to see a 5-year-old walking about holding his penis in public. Such behavior, though harmless, can cause the parent embarrassment and anxiety. Parents should be reassured that the practice is normal during the preschool years and is absolutely harmless.

A small number of children use this form of self-gratification to retreat from relationships with parents and peers. Normally, children receive gratification primarily from interpersonal relationships. Excessive masturbation is usually indicative of some difficulty, such as loneliness, boredom, or rejection.[17] Ignoring the behavior completely, therefore, is not beneficial to the child. Children must be told that it is not appropriate behavior in public. More attention and praise from the parents, more structured activity, and more involvement with peers are beneficial. Parents should set aside an hour or two a day to give personal attention to the child and, perhaps, enter the child in a nursery school to increase activities and widen peer associations. With such an approach, as the child passes through the preschool period, normal masturbatory activity subsides.

Bed-wetting and soiling

Bed-wetting and soiling of underwear with urine or feces are common problems during the preschool years. It is estimated that 19 percent of normal 5- and 6-year-olds wet the bed at night (nocturnal enuresis) and that 1.5 percent soil their pants (encopresis).[18] These problems occur more frequently in boys than in girls. These behaviors tend to disappear by school age, and so no treatment is usually initiated before the age of 5. Differentiation between occasional episodes and actual lack of control of bladder and/or bowel must be made. Total or partial lack of control is often a symptom of serious physical or psychological disturbances. Assessment of the problem is made over a period of several weeks by actually counting the number of accidents a child has had. One or two episodes a week is not considered significant. If bed-wetting or soiling occurs more frequently and persists past age 5, a physician's examination is necessary to rule out a pathological basis for the symptoms.

Almost *all* preschoolers under the age of 5 have occasional "accidents" both during the day and at night. During the day the child is often just too busy to go to the toilet. Overfatigue, illness, dreams, and disturbances may trigger nighttime accidents. Occasional accidents are to be expected, and no significance should be attached to them. Soiling during the preschool period causes greater concern to parents than to children. The parents frequently feel they have failed at toilet training or are inconvenienced when they must change clothing or bed linens.

When accidents occur, clothing or beds are changed, with recognition of the occurrence but *without* recrimination. Parents might say, "I know you are uncomfortable; let's quickly change your clothes." The less made of the accident, the better for the child, since *it is indeed an accident.* Some measures that are helpful in limiting enuresis or encopresis are (1) to encourage children to use the toilet following meals and before midmorning and midafternoon snacks so that they will not have to interrupt play; (2) to encourage using the toilet before going to bed; (3) to restrict the intake of fluids 1 h before naptime and 2 h before going to bed; and (4) to avoid serving meals too close to bedtime. If a child wets the bed frequently, it may be helpful to awaken the child once during the night for toileting. With patience and understanding, accidents will subside—they are a part of development.

Temper tantrums

Temper tantrums are violent outbursts of anger characterized by complete loss of control, screaming, and kicking. Occasional temper tantrums, although most common around the age of 2, continue to be normal in the 3- and 4-year-old. Tantrums are the only way some children have of coping with an emotional crisis.[19] Children often have tantrums when they face a frustrating situation. Tantrums that occur frequently (e.g., daily) and tantrums in children over 4 years old are indicative of psychological disturbances. Referral for counseling is made, since standard procedures for handling tantrums in younger children may have little effect or may even be damaging.

Temper tantrums are greatly distressing to parents since tantrums arouse feelings of helplessness, fear, and lack of control. It is extremely frustrating to see 3-year-old Laurie throw herself on the floor screaming, kicking, and holding her breath until she is "blue." There is no reasoning with the child and no way to stop the tantrum immediately. As a result, the parent gives in to the child's demands or desires, which reinforces the tantrum behavior. Laurie knows that she gets what she wants.

The lesson the child must learn is that of *frustration tolerance*, or the ability to put off desires and handle disappointment; this is a very important aspect of personality development. Frustration tolerance is learned and temper outbursts disappear when limits are enforced through methods such as time out.[20] When the child throws a tantrum, providing there is no danger, he or she is left alone, and *no* attention whatsoever is paid to the child's actions until the tantrum has passed. The parent must stand firm and under no circumstances concede to the child's wishes. Coupled with this approach, the child is consistently rewarded (praised) for appropriate behavior. An example might be Laurie, who always interrupts adult conversations with her own wishes. If she is asked to wait, she has a tantrum. Today she approaches her mother, who is talking to a neighbor. She wiggles with impatience but does not interrupt. Her mother acknowledges the child when her conversation is over, saying, "I'm so happy you waited until I was through talking—what do you want, Honey?"

Parents should be informed of the necessity of carrying out this approach consistently and over a period of several weeks or months if it is to be successful. They should be told that the task of ignoring a child's behavior is most difficult but that the reward is the child's own psychological growth and family peace.

Lying and stealing

Between the ages of 3 and 5, lying and stealing are common. Both behaviors are consequences of cognitive and moral development and should be approached as learning experiences for the child.

Lying occurs for two reasons: (1) It is an attempt to avoid punishment for an act which the child knows is wrong, or (2) it is an attempt to have something in fantasy which is lacking in reality. In either case, the preschooler is *not* deliberately being dishonest. Dishonesty, however, can be encouraged if the child consistently needs to tell a lie in order to avoid punishment. In this case, lying brings the reward of avoiding discipline. On the other hand, when the child does tell the truth about some wrongdoing, parents initiate punishment, not recognizing that it is painful enough to admit guilt and tell the truth. Parents should be advised to approach lying as an opportunity to encourage growth. If the parent knows that Johnnie broke the vase or that Susie robbed the cookie jar, the parent can assist the child in telling the truth by verbalizing the problem. "Johnnie, I see my new vase is broken. I am very unhappy about it. It really was my favorite one." After the child admits guilt, the parent may say, "I am so happy you told me the truth. I will not punish you." This statement not only aids the child in being truthful but also affords a feeling of parental understanding. No further discipline is necessary, since displeasure with the child's action has already been made clear.

Fantasizing something the child desires is part of the wonderful world of the preschooler. When a little girl says she is going to star on television next week or when a little boy says he got a motorcycle for his birthday, the child is revealing wishful fantasies. This is an excellent opportunity for the adult to help the child distinguish between wishful thinking and reality. The parent should avoid confronting the child with "That's not true" or labeling the child with "You are a liar!" Instead, the parent should say, "You wish you could star on television; you wish you were all grown up. Maybe someday you will be a big star."

Stealing during the preschool period is also a form of fulfilling desires. At this period moral development is just beginning; the child is not always in control of his or her own actions. When a "theft" is discovered, the parent should approach it directly. The theft is verbalized by the adult, and restitution is demanded. If the child stole a little car from nursery school, the parent says, "You took the car, but it is not yours. You must return it to the nursery school. It belongs there." The car must then be returned. If the child has difficulty giving up the object, it is important that the parent either guide the child through the process of returning the object or secure the object from the child and return it. The parent does the latter in the presence of the child and thus provides a role model for the child.

The act of returning an object is often enough punishment in itself. The use of a statement of disapproval may emphasize the seriousness of the situation to the child and foster learning. The mother says, "You took Janie's doll dress, when I told you not to. I am really disappointed."

Whatever the cause for lying, distortion of the truth, or stealing, parents should be advised to be calm, understanding, factual, and realistic. These behaviors are an inherent part of the developmental process and provide experiences that are necessary for learning.

Fears and phobias

Although fantasy, magical thought, and transductive reasoning lead to many exciting adventures in the mind of the preschooler, they also lead to the production of fears. *Fears* are negative emotions caused by the anticipation of danger. No other period in the development of the child is so laden with fears. They are reflected in the child's daily behavior and in dreams. Common childhood fears include fear of the dark, solitude, heights, animals, monsters, bodily injury, and strange sights and sounds. Little girls tend to be more fearful of strange sights and sounds, of being alone, and of small crawling things like spiders and bugs. Little boys tend to be more fearful of body injury. These fears can be managed by the parent if approached realistically; they tend to disappear by the age of 5. If a fear is irrational and becomes persistent—a *phobia*—and disrupts the child's daily patterns, professional assessment and treatment must be sought (see Chap. 37).

Informed parents will anticipate fear behaviors in their children and will be prepared to recognize fear when it occurs. Parents should be instructed that fear is *very real* to the child and that they should never ridicule or tease a child when fear is expressed, since this causes concealment of feelings. Parents should be encouraged to talk with the child about the fears and to express them. Both communication techniques are important in reducing tension and anxiety. They also assist in exploring the fear with others who can point out the irrationality of the fear and give explanations. An example of this would be the little boy who sees "spiders" moving on the dark, shadowy wall of his room. He screams with fear. The parent identifies the fear and then reassures the child that nothing is there—that it is just the shadows from the moving trees outside the window. The child has an opportunity to explore the situation and to ask questions, which in turn reduce the fear.

Once a fear is identified, a child must *not* be forced to confront it directly. This may only intensify the fear. Four-year-old Felissa expressed fear of water and heights. Thinking that facing the problem directly would help, her father held her out over a bridge. Felissa became terrified! Felissa never learned to swim, nor would she ever fly! Her fears became phobias.

Several approaches may help reduce a child's fear. One is providing the child with an opportunity to observe a nonfearful model in the fearful situation. Three-year-old Sara had a great fear of dogs. Her little playmate Traci had a large, friendly dog with whom she continually played in the yard. Arrangements were made to have Sara play at Traci's house several times a week, where playful interactions between Traci and her dog were observed. After a period of 6 months,

Sara was able to approach and pet Traci's dog without fear. Subsequently, she made friends with many dogs and was able to have one of her own.

Another approach is that of *desensitizing* the child through indirect exposure to the fearful situation. Kevin, 4 years old, was terrified of being examined by the doctor but had to visit the doctor frequently to receive allergy treatments. A plan was developed to introduce stories and books about doctors, followed by providing Kevin with a doctor's kit so that he could manipulate the play equipment and, through play, confront the doctor's visits without the actual threat of the doctor's office. The child was encouraged to tell stories about the doctor's office. After Kevin was exposed to this routine for several weeks, his fear was reduced significantly.

Parents should be helped to recognize that the process of reducing fear takes much time and patient understanding. Children do not readily comprehend the cause of their fears. They must learn to connect the object of their fear with safe and positive events. As children learn to handle themselves with safety and to think more logically, their fears are slowly conquered.

REFERENCES

1. Wegman, M. E., "Annual Summary of Vital Statistics—1983," *Pediatrics* **72**(6):755–765 (December 1983).
2. Pipes, Peggy, *Nutrition in Infancy and Childhood,* Mosby, St. Louis, 1981, pp. 12–16.
3. Hill, Patty, and Patricia Humphrey, *Human Growth and Development throughout Life,* Wiley, New York, 1982, pp. 194–196.
4. Menkes, J. H., "The Neuromotor Mechanism," in R. H. Cooke (ed.), *The Biological Basis of Pediatric Practice,* McGraw-Hill, New York, 1978, p. 267.
5. Chow, Marilyn, B. Durand, M. Feldman, and M. Mills, *Handbook of Pediatric Primary Care,* Wiley, New York, 1984, p. 656.
6. Erikson, Erik, *Childhood and Society,* Norton, New York, 1963, pp. 255–257.
7. Kagan, Jerome, "Acquisition and Significance of Sex Typing and Sex Role Identity," in A. Hoffman and L. Hoffman (eds.), *Review of Child Development Research,* vol. 2, Russell Sage, New York, 1964, pp. 144–146.
8. Kagan, Jerome, "The Concept of Identification," *Psychological Review* **65**:296–305 (1958).
9. Kagan, "Acquisition and Significance of Sex Typing and Sex Role Identity," pp. 141–144.
10. Stein, Sara, *Making Babies,* Walker, New York, 1984.
11. Kohlberg, Lawrence, "Moral Development," in *International Encyclopedia of the Social Sciences,* Crowell Collier & Macmillan, New York, 1968.
12. Sears, R. R., "Social Behavior and Personality Development," in T. Parsons, and E. A. Shils (eds.), *Toward a General Theory of Action,* Harvard, Cambridge, Mass., 1951, p. 465.
13. Ginsberg, H., and S. Opper, *Piaget's Theory of Intellectual Development,* Prentice-Hall, Englewood Cliffs, N.J., 1969.
14. Schaefer, Charles, and Howard Millman, *Therapies for Children,* Jossey-Bass, San Francisco, 1977, p. 252.
15. Schaefer and Millman, op. cit., p. 253.
16. Chow, Durand, Feldman, and Mills, op. cit., p. 384.
17. Ibid., p. 385.
18. Schaefer and Millman, op. cit., p. 177.
19. Ibid., p. 267.
20. Ibid., p. 271.

12

Janet L. Wilde

The school-age child

Upon completion of this chapter, the student will be able to:

1 Identify the school-age child's growth and developmental changes within the following areas: height, weight, physique, and organ development.

2 Describe Erikson's developmental task of industry vs. inferiority.

3 Identify four functions of the peer group.

4 Describe the attributes of the ideal school and teacher.

5 Describe the school-age child's characteristic behavior related to mealtimes, snacking, and school lunches.

6 Analyze the reasons for the school-age child's rigid behavior.

7 Compare Piaget's stage of cognitive development (concrete operations) with cognitive development in the preschooler and adolescent.

8 Illustrate each of the following characteristics of cognitive development with an example: conversation, classification, ordering, and syncretic thinking.

9 Compare the characteristics and functions of the following types of play: cooperative, aggressive, and dramatic.

10 Identify the nursing interventions to prevent the two most common accidents in school-age children.

11 Summarize Kohlberg's stage of moral development in the school-age child.

The keynote themes of the school-age years (ages 6 through 12) are *freedom* and *expansion*. At no other developmental stage does a person have such freedom and lack of responsibilities. School-age children's freedom and inexhaustible energy enable them to explore the boundless expanses beyond the home.

Several factors are responsible for the school-age child's readiness to explore the world. One factor is mastery of the earlier stages of psychosocial development. Having learned trust during infancy, children expect the world to be safe and meet their needs. Having mastered autonomy as toddlers, they have learned to believe in themselves and to separate from their parents. From having mastered initiative as preschoolers, they have enough self-confidence to begin new activities independently without the need for excessive parental approval. A child who has not mastered a previous stage of development will be psychologically handicapped. He or she will lack one of the earlier psychological building blocks supporting the present stage. However, there is hope for such a child, since each psychosocial stage is reworked in later stages.[1]

Children's maturing cognitive development also prepares them to explore the world. Learning to think logically, classify information, use symbols, remember a series of past events, and tell time readies the school-age child for gathering new information. The child encounters new, differing opinions and value systems from schoolmates and teachers, during overnight visits to friends' homes, and while camping, scouting, shopping, etc. The parents' role diminishes, while the role of other important adults increases. The school-age child is learning acceptable behavior within different parts of society. Through significant adults the child learns the roles and technical skills necessary to function as a competent adult in society. This preparation for adulthood is called *socialization*. The school-age child becomes socialized within society, whereas the preschooler learned socialization within the family.

PHYSICAL MATURATION

Weight and skeletal development

The rapid height and weight gain of earlier years decreases significantly during the school-age period. Physical growth at this age is slow and steady (see Appendix B for growth charts). The average weight gain is 2 to 3.5 kg (5 to 7 lb) per year. This increase in weight is more noticeable in late summer and autumn.[2] The school-age child grows an average of 6 to 7 cm (2.5 to 3 in) per year. Boys are generally taller than girls until 10 years of age; then girls are taller until approximately age 14. A growth spurt occurs by age 11 to 13 in girls and by age 14 to 15 in boys. Head circumference increases much more slowly during the school-age years than earlier, from about 51 cm (20 in) to 53 or 54 cm (21 in). The brain and skull grow slowly because 90 percent of brain growth has already occurred by age 5 or 6. At the end of the early school-age years, the brain has achieved virtually adult size.[3] The child's facial appearance changes because the face lengthens and grows faster than the skull.

Height increases more slowly because the skeletal system is delayed in its general growth pattern. The long bones lengthen, and the child may appear taller and thinner. The bones are largely cartilaginous and soft in early childhood. These cartilage cells are ultimately replaced by bone as growth proceeds. (See Chap. 29 for a detailed discussion of skeletal development.) Physical activities for the school-age child must be planned accordingly, with "close supervision to detect any complaint of injury to any bone or joint."[4]

During the last 15 years there has been an increased attempt to detect potential scoliosis cases. Scoliosis is a lateral curvature of the spine. Routine screening programs for children in this age range will not only uncover cases early enough to avoid surgery but also will ensure greater success in cases requiring surgery. The nurse's role in bringing this important information to local school communities and in assisting with the screenings is invaluable.[5]

The school-age child often complains of leg pains. It is common but erroneous to call these "growing pains" because growing itself is *not* painful. The cause of leg pains may be overexertion, bruising, or injury. Pains in the knees with no exertional signs are also common in school-age children. Such pains, especially if they occur late in the day or night and disappear in the morning, are usually not significant. This is true even if the pains are fairly severe.[6] Children with persistent leg pains should be referred to a physician.

The school-age child looks slimmer, more graceful, and better coordinated than the preschooler. Posture improves, the legs are longer, and the preschooler's potbelly and "baby fat" have disappeared. The child appears increasingly in control and has far fewer collisions and falls. Movements appear increasingly skilled and precise.

Fine and gross motor development

The reduced growth rate allows time for refinement and expansion of newly developed motor coordination. School-age children learn to refine skills by practicing specialized games. Their muscular strength doubles; they can play games for longer periods of time. However, their strength is not comparable to an adult's. They are increasingly able to concentrate and play as team members. School-age children need regular exercise and should spend time each day engaged in games and activities such as tag, jump rope, basketball, swimming, skating, soccer, or football. Regular exercise develops new muscle groups necessary to perform these activities. (See Fig. 12-1.)

Fine motor coordination and creativity develop as the child refines printing and writing skills. The preschooler's gross motor skills of running and climbing give way to these finer motor skills. Children enjoy writing plays and stories and publishing neighborhood newspapers. Artistic talents blossom as children develop skills at drawing, ceramics, embroidery, or macramé. Refinement of fine motor skills is dramatic, for example, in the 9-year-old child who was unable to color within the lines when a preschooler but who can now paint a landscape. Other children excel at music. School-age children commonly enjoy composing songs, playing in orchestras, singing in concerts, and studying ballet.

Organ growth and development

The school-age child's body is physiologically more mature than the preschooler's. The myelinization of the school-age child's central nervous system is complete; hence physiological responses are more stable. The child's bladder capacity increases, and the kidneys are better able to filter and concentrate urine. The gastrointestinal tract is also more stable. The school-age child can go without food for longer periods than a younger child and experiences diarrhea and vomiting less often. The eyes mature and achieve 20/20 vision at 7 or 8 years of age. The immunological system responds faster than before to antigen invasion. The antibody response is faster, and antibody levels are higher. The school-age child therefore catches fewer childhood diseases and is sick less often.

The heart grows at a slow rate during the school-age years. Only after the growth spurt of puberty will it grow rapidly and double its weight, to reach adult size in the middle to late teens.[7] During the school years the heart is smaller in relation to body size but must continue to supply the needs of metabolism, rapid growth, and physical activity. For this reason, sustained physical activity is not desirable. No damage to the heart will result, but the young child is not yet capable of the same athletic performance as an older child. Evidence of this can be seen in the young school-age child who can seemingly play all day with friends, only to collapse in a tired bundle at the dinner table,[8] or say, "Mom, I'm tired. I need a nap." Knowing the physiological reasons for fatigue will enable parents to understand rather than criticize this behavior. School-age children's vital capacity increases, which enables them to engage in sports such as swimming and diving (Fig. 12-2). The school-age child's vital signs approach adult levels. The blood pressure increases, and the heart and respiratory rates decrease (see Tables 16-18 through 16-20).

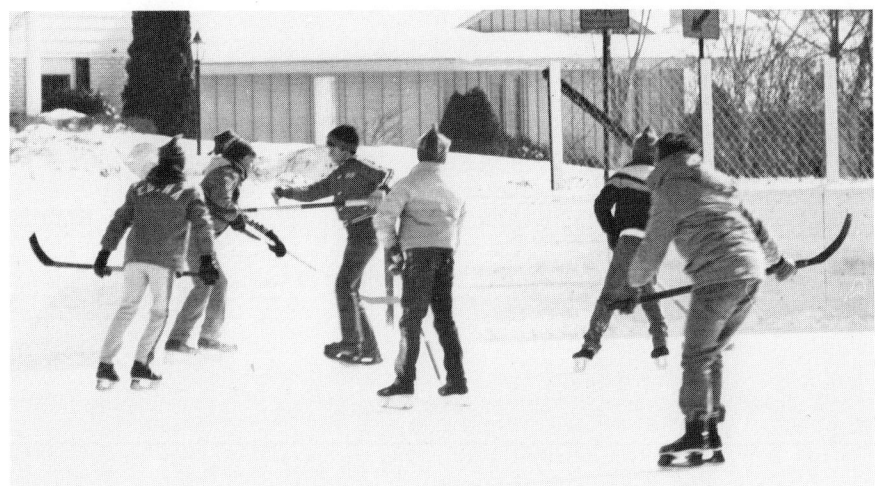

Figure 12-1 Playing hockey at a local grade school. (*Photo by Janet Cardle.*)

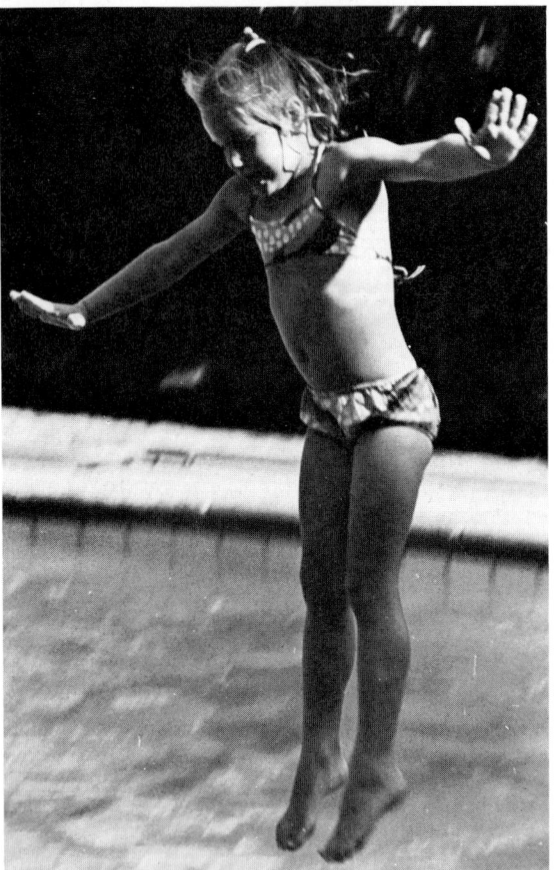

Figure 12-2 This school-age child is practicing swimming skills and refining gross motor coordination.

Perceptual development

Perceptual development is crucial for the development of body image and coordination. Directional and positional skills (i.e., up vs. down; right vs. left; behind vs. in front of) are also learned at this time. All these aspects of development are precursors to the ability to read from left to right, to follow directions, and to generally begin to conceive of oneself within one's surroundings.

Dental development

Dentition changes are readily apparent in the school-age child. The 6-year molars, which erupt at age 5 or 6, are the first secondary (permanent) teeth to appear. These teeth serve as the focal points in the dental arch. They determine to a large extent the spacing of the other secondary teeth and the ultimate shape of the jaw. For this reason, children who are evaluated for braces are often not fully evaluated until all four 6-year molars have come in (see Fig. 14-9 for a tooth eruption schedule).

Nutrition

Nutritional needs change with the age of the child. During periods of rapid growth, caloric needs are particularly high. During the school-age years, caloric, protein, vitamin A, carbohydrate, and calcium needs particularly increase. (See Appendix C for daily requirements.) The later school-age years are a period of preparation for the rapid physiological changes of puberty; consequently, caloric needs increase.

The caloric needs of the school-age child, though not as high as those of the infant, are still approximately *double* the average adult's requirements per kilogram of body weight. A 7- to 9-year-old requires 80 cal and 2.8 g of protein per kilogram of body weight. The 10- to 12-year-old requires 70 cal and 2.0 g of protein per kilogram of body weight.[9] Maintenance of the basal metabolism of the 6- to 12-year-old uses 50 percent of the caloric intake. Physical activity uses 25 percent of the caloric intake. The other 25 percent is divided between growth (12 percent), specific dynamic action of food (5 percent), and loss through feces (8 percent).[10]

Mealtime and discipline Mealtime is more than just a time for eating. It is an ideal time for family interaction and the child's learning of social skills. It may be the only time of the day when the whole family is together. Mealtime can be a time of great satisfaction for individual family members as they relate the day's achievements or have an opportunity to ask questions or voice opinions about items of interest to them. This is an ideal time to praise the accomplishments of individual children.

Often, however, mealtime becomes a time of conflict instead of fellowship. Too often parental concern over table manners and the picky eating habits of children this age is so overemphasized that the restful, pleasant atmosphere is lost. A power struggle then results between parent and child. The child's eating habits will improve as the child grows older. The 6-year-old who stuffs her mouth, grabs for food, and is an active talker at mealtime will gradually become a 10- or 12-year-old who eats like the adults around her.

The dinner table is not the appropriate place for discipline. If discipline during meals is necessary, it should be kept to a minimum. When mealtime becomes a time of stress, digestion does not occur as readily. Poor eating habits or a temporary aversion to food can result from tense situations or from periods of great excitement.

As the school-age child's world expands, he or she may visit friends for meals and eat new foods or observe other people's eating habits. A favorite friend's food likes and dislikes may be copied. The child may refuse a new food or method of preparation at home by saying, "Betsy doesn't eat that." Understanding why the child responds in this way, insisting that "one bite" be tried before a decision is made, and pointing out favorite foods that contain the rejected item will help the family through the situation in a positive manner. This will also set a precedent for other family members.

School lunches As the child's desire to be liked by peers increases, the kind of lunch preferred often depends on whether friends take lunch to school or eat the food served in the cafeteria. Whether the food comes from home or is prepared at school, the school-age child often trades lunches or parts of lunches with members of the peer group. As a result, portions of well-planned meals may not be eaten.

If the school is located near a shopping center, the older school-age child will sometimes save the money for a cafeteria lunch until after school, when the peer group goes to the local store to buy "junk" foods (foods without nutritional value). If vending machines are located in the school, a source of nonnutritional food is readily available. To combat this, some parent groups are working to eliminate vending machines or, at least, to have nutritional snacks, such as oranges and food bars, replace the traditional candy bars and soft drinks.

School cafeteria lunches are regulated by federal and state standards when the school is part of the National School Lunch Program. Lunch must provide approximately one-third of the daily food requirements of the school-age child. However, because the food may be prepared in unfamiliar styles or served in portions too large for the child to eat, lunches that are paid for are often not eaten.

Nutritional status The situations just described are common in the life of today's school-age child. Parents need to be aware of these possibilities and make up for the deficiency at breakfast and dinner. The school-age child usually eats well and has fewer food fads than in earlier years. At home, eating problems are more apt to be related to a disrupted mealtime environment (distraction by friends or television) than to specific food dislikes.

After-school snacks can help make up for lack of food at the noon meal and can satisfy the hunger usually experienced when the child returns home. Snacks eaten 1 h or more before meals will not diminish food intake at mealtimes. Milk, cheese, fresh fruits and vegetables, peanut butter, unsugared nuts, yogurt, and fruit juices are desirable snacks both for general nutritional needs and for good dental health. Minimizing sugar intake will protect against dental decay.

The school-age child's increased responsibility can be extended in the home to the area of nutrition. Children can be encouraged to "work as a team" and help at mealtime to prepare food. They can help plan menus, shop for the food, prepare some of the simpler foods, set the table, and wash the dishes. They thrive on mastering these tasks. However, the amount of participation should not be so great as to reduce time spent in the necessary outdoor play. Working parents should not leave cooking to school-age children. Children need specific foods set out in front of them to eat.

The school-age child usually learns about the basic four food groups in school. The child should be encouraged to use this information and share it with other family members. This becomes a link between home and school, as information learned in the classroom is demonstrated and discussed at home for everyone's benefit (Fig. 12-3).

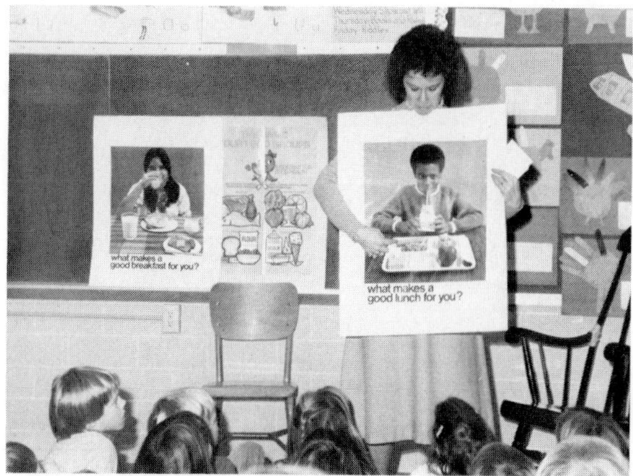
what makes a good breakfast for you?
what makes a good lunch for you?

Figure 12-3 This school nurse is teaching children about the four basic food groups and about foods that are appropriate for lunch. (*Photo by Janet Cardle.*)

PSYCHOSOCIAL MATURATION

Developmental task: Industry vs. inferiority

The basic psychosocial maturational task of the school-age child is to develop the sense of industry vs. inferiority. According to Erikson, it is during this stage that the child "must begin to be a worker and a potential provider."[11] The child now "becomes ready to apply himself to given skills and tasks"[12] and thus "learns to win recognition by producing things."[13] It is common to see children repeatedly practicing motor skills on the baseball diamond or math and spelling skills in the classroom.

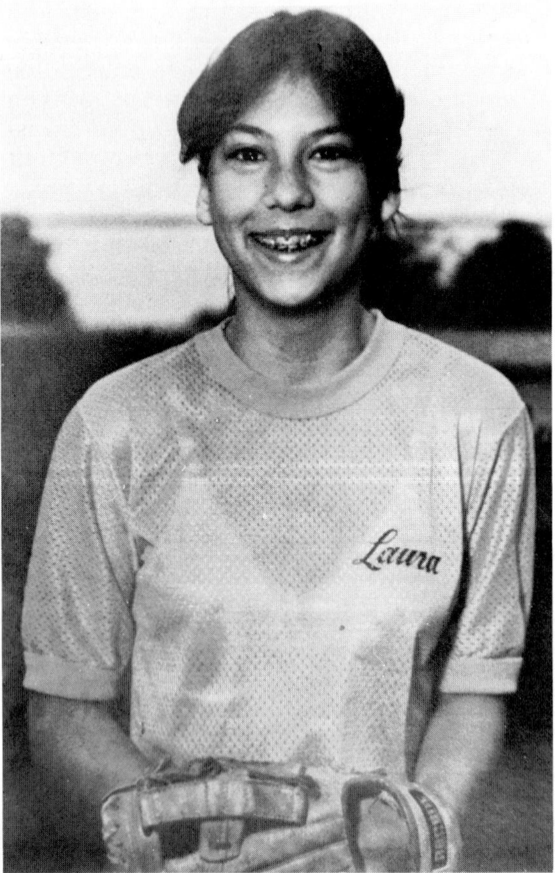

Figure 12-4 Being praised for perfecting her skill at baseball increases this girl's self-esteem. Note her choice of baseball, a nontraditional sex role activity.

Achievement vs. failure Children who are skilled on the playing field, in the classroom, or in the neighborhood will receive praise and recognition from peers and adults for a job well done. This praise makes them feel good about themselves and helps them see that others also consider them worthwhile, competent individuals. (See Fig. 12-4.) These are the children who are frequently seen surrounded by peers in play and who are "everyone's first choice for the team." But the situation is different for children who fail or are not readily able to master skills such as reading or playing ball. These children will view themselves as poor performers who cannot compete or who will not be sought after as valued persons. For example, a boy who is consistently rejected for the football team begins to see himself as a failure, unwanted, and inferior; his self-concept is tarnished. Such a child is in danger of developing a "sense of inadequacy and inferiority."[14]

Children who feel inadequate may despair of their skills or their status among peers. Self-esteem suffers, and they may be unable to identify with others who do succeed in the world of skills and tools.[15] They often sit quietly and unnoticeably in the back of classrooms or stand at the back of a group, not participating unless coaxed over and over to do so. These children fear exposing themselves to laughter and criticism. They rarely ask questions or seek explanations. They need the help of significant adults or peers to find meaningful roles in which they can succeed. Although they do have skills to develop and contribute, often these children drop out because no one takes the extra time necessary to start them on the way to experiencing recognition for skills they *can* master.

Hobbies are common among school-age children and can play an important role in the accomplishment of developmental tasks, including acquiring a sense of achievement. By learning everything he or she can about a subject, such as sewing, painting, soccer, or electronics, a child acquires new skills. These skills help perfect gross and fine motor coordination, and new information is gained for successful functioning as an adult. Organizations for children, such as the Girl Scouts of America, Boy Scouts of America, Camp Fire Girls, and 4-H, also provide opportunities to develop the skills of children in this age group. In addition, these organizations provide opportunities to develop skills that will help them function in their respective sex roles.

Self-esteem As new skills are learned and as new thought processes develop, self-esteem becomes increasingly important. *Self-esteem* is self-respect or appreciation of one's own worth. The "primary antecedents for fostering self-esteem seem to be: (1) a high degree of acceptance by parents and others; (2) clear and consistent limits; and (3) flexibility within those limits to permit individual actions."[16]

The child with high self-esteem accepts criticism, states his or her beliefs even if they challenge authority, and feels competent. The child enters new situations confidently. Because nothing succeeds like success, he or she usually succeeds. This repeated achievement increases self-esteem.[17] (See Fig. 12-5.)

Popularity results from many aspects of a child's personality. School-age children who feel confident that others accept them share freely with others and set aside some of their own desires, while contributing to the good of other people and the group as a whole. The intellectual growth at this age enables school-age children to cooperate with others and to understand and respect others' thoughts and opinions. They are ready for team activities. They now feel empathy for others who experience happiness and sorrow.

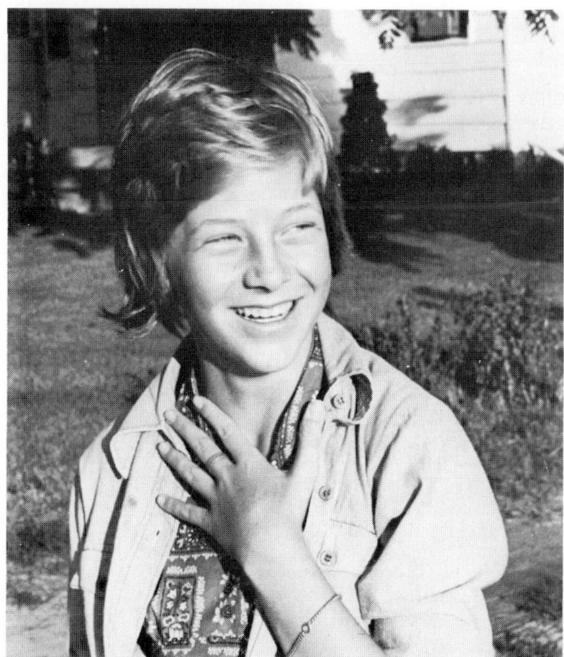

Figure 12-5 The school-age child with high self-esteem feels accepted by others, accepts criticism, states his or her beliefs, and feels competent.

Children with low self-esteem often withdraw from new situations; it is easier than failing again. They may destroy other people's possessions, not try hard, have psychosomatic pain, and worry whether their actions are correct. They may go to extremes to please adults and receive their approval.[18]

School-age children receive messages about self-worth from many sources: parents, teachers, classmates, and team members. They perceive their parents as all-powerful. They judge their performance by their parents' comments and by comparing these with an inner vision of their ideal selves. Therefore, teachers and parents need to establish activities that promote success.

School-age children need to experience success in the task they master *and* to receive recognition for those achievements. This recognition is as important to the child who is able to recognize all the letters of the alphabet for the first time as it is to a 10-year-old who writes a short story for the first time. It cannot be assumed that children know they have done well because the way children view themselves is a reflection of the way they perceive that others feel about them.[19] Each new achievement should be praised, no matter how small.

School

The main function of school is to transmit the society's cultural mores and values, technological information, and basic academic skills to children. The average child spends 14 years in school; school is thus a major influence on the child's development. In school the child must learn to relate to authority figures other than his or her parents, to develop independence, to interact with other children, to grow cognitively, and to think analytically. Schools also strive to develop self-esteem in children because a child must learn independence and social competence and must develop self-esteem before he or she can learn basic facts.[20]

Two major educational philosophies have developed in the United States: traditional and progressive. *Traditional education,* which is based on English classical education, stresses basic academic skills. The teacher imparts information to the students, is authoritarian and dominant, and stresses conformity. *Progressive edu-*

cation reemerged in the late 1960s as a protest against the alleged dictatorial nature of traditional education. Progressive schools emphasize individualized education, positive socialization experiences for children, humanistic values, and pleasurable educational experiences. However, no studies have thus far proved conclusively that either type of education is superior.

Regardless of the educational philosophy, all excellent classrooms have the same characteristics. Instruction is tailored to individual students' differences, and students learn to respect and trust one another because the teacher treats them with respect and trust. Students develop cognitively through many "hands-on" learning experiences, which teach them the joy of discovery. The classroom atmosphere is characterized by responsibility, self-discipline, respect for others, and freedom to learn (Figure 12-6).[21]

School readiness Children who have successfully completed prior stages of emotional maturation will be better prepared to begin school and to accomplish its many social and educational tasks. Those who have experienced encouragement and support of normal curiosity, exploration, and manipulation (investigation of their own bodies, of toys, and of other objects); recognition of success in physical and mental endeavors (first steps or the first recitation and/or recognition of the alphabet); and maximum stimulation and life experiences in earlier years (trips to the zoo or beach and interactions with other children and adults) will be more ready and eager for the further development of intellectual skills in a more formal setting. These positive experiences of the past will decrease anxiety and allow these children to concentrate more easily on the tasks of this period.

Reading is a primary focus of the school-age years. But reading does not just happen. Many skills and developmental tasks must be mastered before reading can occur. Visual motor skills (drawing shapes), gross motor skills (jumping and hopping), recitation, sequencing (ordering), and perceptual skills such as alphabet recognition all contribute to readiness for reading. Studies have even established crawling as a precursor to reading readiness. If crawling did not actually occur in the developmental sequence of events, the child may have been taught to crawl. Usually, the development of this skill will result in an improvement in reading ability.

A variety of life experiences, verbal fluency, and exposure to books (including manipulation of them) also contribute to reading readiness. Adequate functioning of the auditory and visual systems is essential for a child to learn to read.

School-age children live largely in a visual mode. Many new tasks and concepts must be visually seen and manipulated in order to be understood and assimilated. The cognitive system of children this age is now at a level which allows them to organize and control the environ-

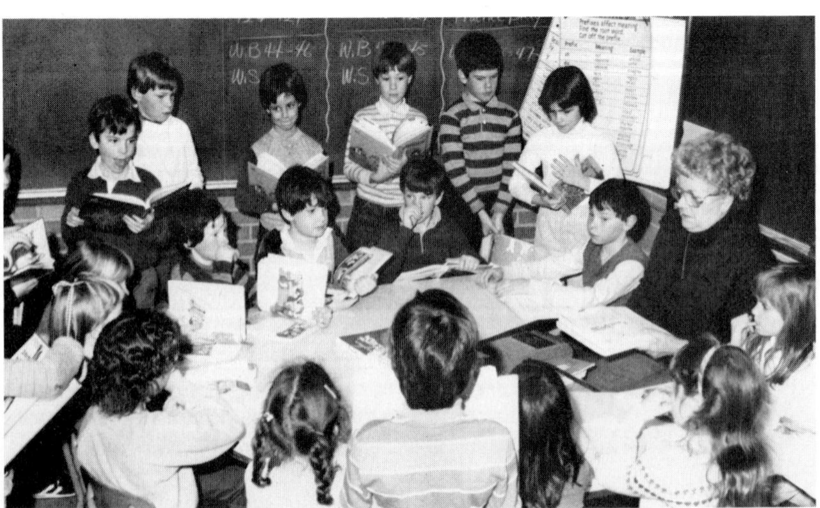

Figure 12-6 A typical elementary school classroom. (*Photo by Janet Cardle.*)

ment in order to understand it. They are better able to understand something if they can concretely experience it through handling, seeing, or hearing it.

As children progress through the school years, it becomes less necessary for an object to be present for them to understand and experience it. That is, conceptualization gradually replaces the earlier reliance on sensorimotor learning. Thus the ability to use symbols when thinking increases.

The teacher Next to parents, the teacher is the most powerful and influential adult in the school-age child's life. The teacher affects the child's attitudes toward adult authority, school, and society. Through the teacher, the child learns more about society and how to obtain the knowledge and skills necessary to live in it successfully.

Children want a teacher to resemble the ideal parent. In the early years the teacher takes on the role of parent by helping the child to go to the bathroom, conform to the group, and control aggressive impulses. The ideal teacher is warm, nurturant, kind, and enthusiastic; is a consistent, fair disciplinarian; and is sympathetic, attractive, and understanding. Children do not want a teacher who yells, has unbending expectations, and uses ridicule and sarcasm to control students.

Children strive to fulfill the teacher's expectations and avoid disapproval. They want to be regarded as valuable human beings, capable of individual learning. Teachers are obviously extremely important in molding children's self-esteem (Fig. 12-7).

Parents often seek the advice of their child's teacher to help them find solutions to the problems they have in understanding or dealing with their child. School-age children gain new ideas from adults such as teachers, television performers, parents of friends, and authors of textbooks. Often these ideas and attitudes conflict with those of the parents. Ideally, the parents and the teacher should communicate well and have compatible ideas about both the child's strengths and areas needing improvement.

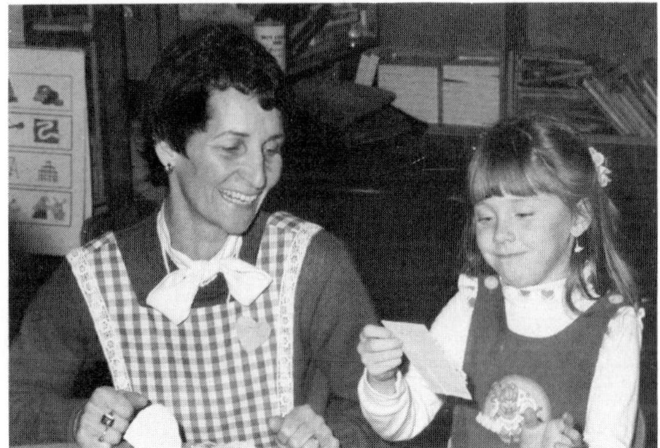

Figure 12-7 This teacher shows warmth and approval of the child as well as of her Valentine. (*Photo by Janet Cardle.*)

The peer group

The school-age child spends more and more time with, and relies increasingly on, his or her *peer group*, a group of friends of similar age. Societies throughout history have described special subcultures of children. All subcultures require strict conformity to rules. This increases the group's security and isolates it from other groups—in this case, adults. School-age gangs have characteristics of a primitive society: oral communication of traditions, rituals, and magical incantations. School-age children have secret clubs and teach one another secret languages like pig latin, passwords, and jingles. Superstitious rituals represent children's attempts to increase power over the future: "If you step on a crack, you'll break your mother's back."

Prospective members of the peer group are closely examined and are admitted or rejected on a pass-fail basis. They must conform to the group's standards of acceptable behavior. The rules become increasingly rigid as children grow older. Children are admitted on the basis of physical development, strength, height, weight, athletic ability, dress, and skills benefiting the group. Conformity to the group is healthy: the accepted child feels satisfied, secure, and comfortable.

The peer group has several functions:

1. It provides a mirror into which the child looks to examine and evaluate himself or herself. By receiving group feedback, the child practices behavior and skills in order to conform to the group's standards. This feedback increases the child's security and self-esteem.
2. It socializes the child. Members must conform to the group's rules. Children learn acceptable behavior and learn to compromise individual needs for the total group's benefit.

Because groups usually consist of neighborhood friends and because most neighborhoods are grouped by socioeconomic class, the group helps the child learn the standards of the socioeconomic class.

3. It encourages sharing of information. Members expose one another to differing value systems and opinions and evaluate their own thoughts. They learn that acceptable behaviors vary within different parts of society. This sharing, which is enhanced by television, decreases the child's self-centeredness.
4. It provides an environment for practicing sex role behavior. Friendship groups during the school-age period are sexually segregated. Within these same-sex clubs the child practices skills and actions needed to solidify his or her sex role. Best friends are inseparable, sharing secrets, jokes, clothes, and family gossip. They buoy up one another in times of stress. Occasionally they fight, learn to solve their conflicts, and reunite. These secret club friendships strengthen the child's sex role learning in preparation for boy-girl relationships during adolescence. (See Fig. 12-8.)

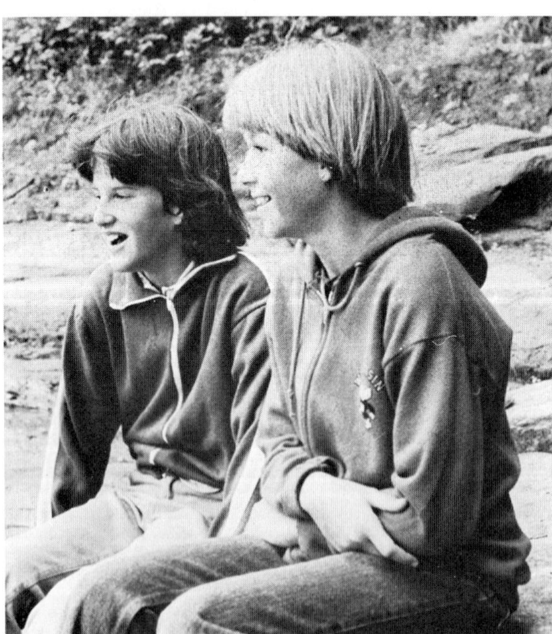

Figure 12-8 Friendship helps school-age children evaluate themselves, share information and ideas, and learn sex roles and acceptable behavior.

Rigid behavior

Rigid behavior pervades many aspects of the school-age child's life, in rules followed, in thinking, in rituals, and in learning new roles. This strong rigidity results in a driving desire to complete such tasks as games, sewing projects, and building with an erector set. This rigidity is seen, for example, in a 10-year-old who is doing a homework assignment and cannot write a sentence for the second word on the list until he or she has thought of one for the first word.

Though certain behavioral expectations are necessary within the family setting, clear and consistent limits are more important than rigidity. Rigidity not only adds to the rigidity that is self-imposed by the child, but also does not allow for flexibility and development of individuality. Too many rigid rules discourage children from trying to solve problems by themselves as they develop their sense of initiative.[22]

New roles Taking on new roles also entails rigid, concrete behavior. Any new role or situation is learned and experienced in a very precise, rigid manner so that the child will successfully master feelings of inferiority and anxiety. Unless children perfectionistically practice the actions of the role, they fear that they may be unable to win the approval of peers and the important adults in their lives. For example, a 10-year-old girl may be seen making precise work out of cleaning her desk at school. She may actually appear to be moving in slow motion as she completes this task.

Bedtime rituals An extension of rigid behavior is the nighttime routine. In earlier stages, the fear of death was expressed in the child's fear of the dark and fear of going to sleep in the dark. Now the school-age child's thinking becomes more concrete. The child begins to conceive of death as happening to others but is unable to accept it as a part of his or her own life. When logical thinking occurs about 9 or 10 years of age, the child begins to view death as final and inevitable. While emotional capacity grows with experiences related to dying (seeing a dead bird, pet, or fish), an unconscious fear of death often continues to exist. Children often attempt to control their fear of death by being good, which they hope will keep death away. They may project their fears onto others or onto inanimate objects, like a stuffed animal, skeletons, witches, or vam-

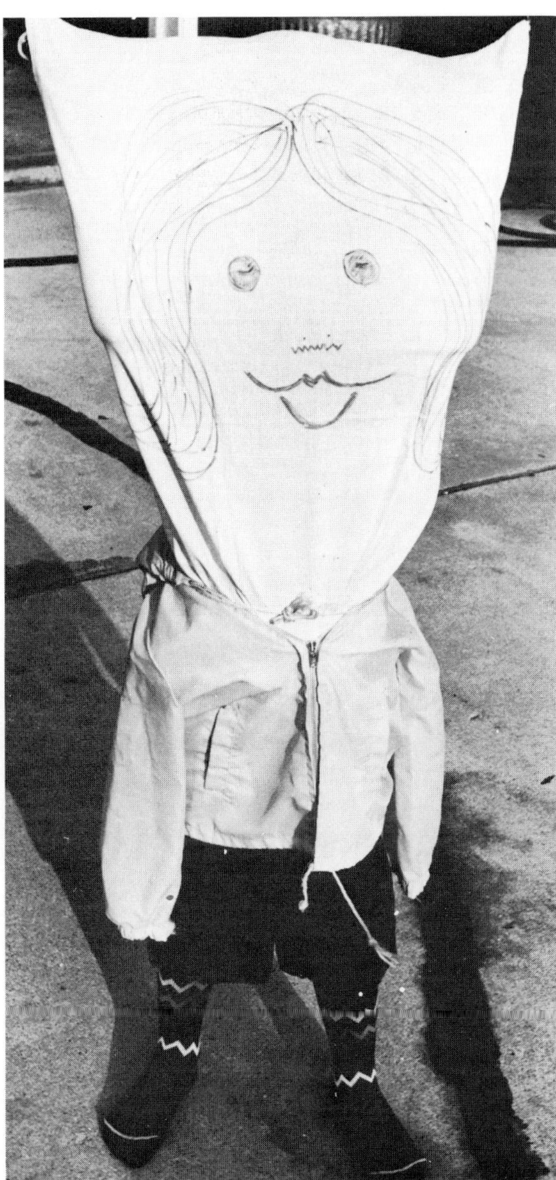

Figure 12-9 Children project their fears onto inanimate objects and fantasy characters. Play—in this case, dressing up at Halloween—is used to help work through fears.

pires. (See Fig. 12-9.) They believe that maintaining a routine makes things predictable. This allows less anxiety to surface. The rituals of the age are normal unless the child becomes so obsessed that he or she is no longer able to function without them.

Play

Play for the school-age child revolves around social interaction. The child now seldom plays alone, but in organized and unorganized groups. Group acceptance and the need for friends with whom to share experiences and thoughts take on great urgency. Groups and their opportunities for socialization give the child the opportunity to feel secure while slowly becoming less dependent on the family.

The 6-year-old at play displays endless energy and constant activity, often overdoing in the process. Children in this age group are self-centered, and conflicts erupt because of their tendency to show off and be bossy while trying to dominate a situation. Boys and girls play together in a rough-and-tumble manner. Inhibitions are weak; aggressive thoughts are acted out in kicking, hitting, and even biting. Hand coordination allows for printing of large letters and gross motor hand skills like hammering nails. Six-year-olds are able to bounce and throw a ball, jump and run in games, and do elementary stunts on a bar. Athletic endeavors are still at a beginning performance level.

The 7-year-old takes a more cautious approach to activity and is less demanding in terms of desires and opinions. Thus the 7-year-old is easier to deal with. Gross motor skills are improving. Children can catch now, throw a ball, and may try to use a baseball bat. If not already riding a bicycle, most will want to learn. Pencils are now preferred over crayons, and printing is not only smaller but also easier to do. Fine motor development is improving.

Muscle movement is becoming smoother and more coordinated in the 8-year-old. Boys prefer soccer and baseball and may even try skateboarding. Girls now play jump rope and roller-skate. Printing is now slowly replaced by cursive writing.

Perfection of skills already learned at a younger age can be seen in the 9-year-old. Differences between the abilities of those who are increasing their skill levels and those who are not become more noticeable.

During the rest of the school-age years, children of both sexes develop increasing physical strength and endurance, but boys are stronger than girls. Many late school-age children come close to adult levels of proficiency as they perfect individual skills.

Table 12-1 Toys and Play Activities

Purpose or function	Age 6	Age 7	Age 8
Gross motor development	Bicycle Skates Baseball bat and mitt Rough-and-tumble play Relay races, tag, and hide-and-seek Swimming	Baseball Pogo stick Football equipment Flying planes Kite Bouncing balls Jump rope Skating	Badminton Basketball and hoop Bicycle Tennis racket Swimming Ping-pong
Fine motor development	Puppets Rhythm instruments and the piano Bead jewelry-making sets Coloring books and crayons Clay Painting and drawing Paper dolls Hammer and pliers	Yo-yo Checkers Chinese checkers Dominoes Collages Clay Puzzles Magic tricks	Making and building objects Interlocking small plastic brick set Dart set Leathercraft set Watercolor paints and brush Recorder
Sex role establishment	Cooking sets Fishing tackle Large trucks and machinery toys Sewing machines Toys for playing store Dress-up play Household furniture	Costumes Household play Brownies, Cubs, and Blue Birds	Performing dramatic shows Dolls
Collections and completion of tasks	Raking leaves Collecting insects Collecting minute objects ("odds and ends") Games (simple) Small play sets	Parcheesi Erector set Quiz and puzzle sets Simple games Magic tricks	Coin books Interlocking small plastic brick set Group games
Quiet play	Card games Stories Darts (magnetic)	Reading Comics Robots	Books Comics Videogames

Source: Adapted from Ruth E. Hartley and Robert M. Goldenson, *The Complete Book of Children's Play.* Thomas Y. Crowell, New York, 1957, pp. 402–405.

Table 12-1 lists common, appropriate play activities for school-age children and groups those activities according to some of the purposes or functions they serve, such as development of gross motor skills. The age categories are useful guidelines but are not absolutes.

Cooperative play *Cooperative play* (playing together and sharing, as when two children build together with an erector set) now predominates, as solitary and parallel play did in earlier years. Cooperative play and the maturity level that allows sharing between more than two children at one time now offer the opportunities to experiment with life in group situations. Children now cognitively differentiate themselves from their environment. This gives them the capacity to see and respect another's point of view. It makes them capable of true cooperative play and allows them to become valued members of a group or team.

In cooperative play, children learn to relinquish their own needs for the overall good of a team. The group members learn to work together and to rely on one another. Each member has a specific role; the members learn to combine their efforts and win. Through group play

Table 12-1 Toys and Play Activities (*Continued*)

Purpose or function	Age 9	Age 10	Ages 11 and 12
Gross motor development	Rough-and-tumble activities Baseball Swimming Skating Dancing: ballet and tap Hiking All competitive sports Wrestling	Bicycles All gross motor activities Out-of-door games Sliding Climbing Running	Bicycle (large) Archery sets Swimming Horseback riding Skateboard
Fine motor development	Practical jokes and tricks Steam engine Radio-controlled vehicles Wood-burning set	Tool set Dart set Electrical model kits Typewriter Assembling models	Electric train set Chemistry set Model cars with engines Shell jewelry sets Wire cutters Papier-mâché Weaving Woodworking Knitting and sewing
Sex role establishment	Little-girl dolls Male role-model dolls		Boy or Girl Scouts
Collections and completion of tasks	Collections of objects Doll collections Card games	Card games All collections Erector set with motor Stamp album Computer games	Various aids for collections of objects and mementos ("movie stars") Perfume-making set Model cars with engines Computer games
Quiet play	Table games Reading books Robots (moveable)	Books Games Videogames	Electric table games Portable computer games

the school-age child learns to compete successfully and to handle feelings of anger, disappointment, loss, and success.

A desire to play games with rules emerges at about 7 years of age. The peer group members now have the ability to agree on rules and adhere to them and to compete with and control one another for the benefit of the entire team. Games with rules range all the way from table games to football and baseball; red light–green light and statues are familiar examples of games that illustrate the young school-age child's strict adherence to rules.

Rules for games give everyone who plays specific guidelines. Rules also reduce the child's anxiety about a new situation. Conforming to rules promotes peer acceptance, while nonconforming, "different" children are excluded. Rules also give children an opportunity to measure themselves against an external standard (the rules). After children have become familiar with the rules, they may modify them by group consent.

As a member of the team or play group, a child who successfully competes (by winning or by playing by the rules) experiences increased self-esteem. The child's skills give group status, con-

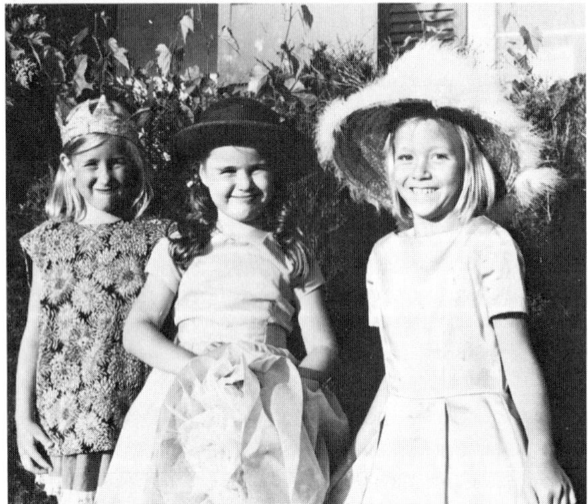

Figure 12-10 These girls are playing *dramatically*, dressed up as they would be in real-life situations. Dramatic play helps children feel in control, learn solutions to problems, and reduce anxiety.

fidence about competency, and feelings of control. Successfully creating something, following instructions, and completing a task, such as painting a picture or assembling a model car, also increase self-esteem. It takes some children longer to learn and follow rules or instructions. They may choose to give up without making much effort to complete a project. For these children, encouragement and support are necessary so that decreased self-esteem will not result.

Dramatic play Children enjoy *dramatic play* in the early school-age years. (See Fig. 12-10.) They create plays about real-life situations and enjoy presenting them to adults. They jointly develop a set of rules (script), entertain, and gain approval from others. They express emotions, such as anger and sadness, and use their imaginations to play through problems to find solutions. They learn to master their anxiety over a situation while expressing creativity within a group. They need to feel in control and powerful over their foes. Older children often wish to take a drama class.

Aggressive play *Aggressive play* is more common among boys than among girls in this period. All children need room to run, jump, skip, and express pent-up hostility and tension. Aggressive play involves expressing hostility and boldness. (See Fig. 12-11.) It represents a symbolic way of conquering an enemy and may be accompanied by squeals of delight. Watching westerns, space programs, or competitive sports on television can be a vicarious means of mastering the enemy. Television, however, is *not* a substitute for active or creative dramatic play.

Parental approval Many children need parental approval before they can make their "own" choice of games and activities. The Oedipus conflict of the preschool years has been resolved. Children love and respect both parents and imitate the parent of the same sex. They strengthen their sex role identity by imitating that parent's actions and verbalizations. What the parent of the same sex likes or approves of thus has a great influence on the child's choices.

Sex role identification

The preschooler began to assume behaviors characteristic of sex role identity and to turn his or her interest to the parent of the opposite sex.

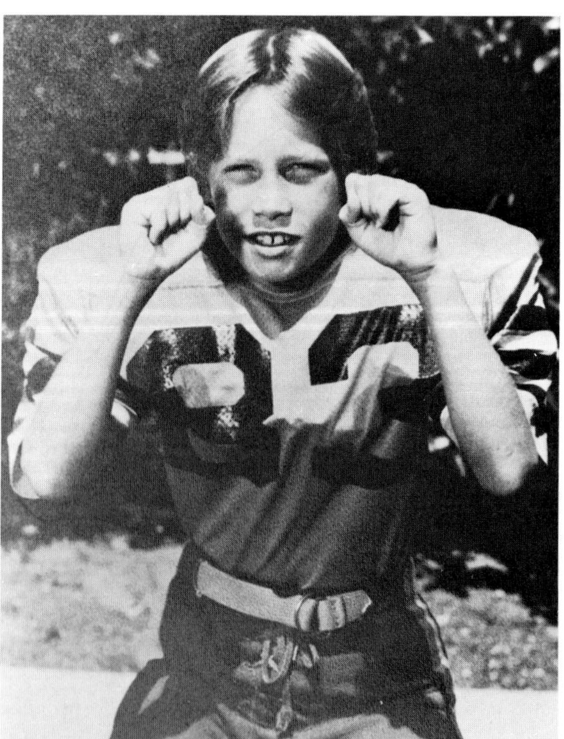

Figure 12-11 Aggressive play allows children to express hostility and boldness, releases tension, and provides an opportunity to be the "enemy." Note this boy's traditional sex role activity.

The school-age child becomes more interested in, and identifies with, the parent of the same sex. The school-age child associates with a same-sex group to reinforce sex role identity and to practice the sex role which will be assumed later in life. By focusing on the same sex and its role, the child submerges earlier feelings of anxiety, anger, and conflict surrounding feelings about the opposite sex for a few years. This liberates psychological energy that the child uses to learn, explore, and develop new skills, free from sexual conflict. Once the important skills of this period are mastered, the child will be better prepared to cope with heterosexual relationships in adolescence.

The school-age child also learns his or her sex role by participating in same-sex peer groups. These may be formal organizations (the Boy Scouts of America, Blue Birds, Blue Jays, etc.) or informal neighborhood groups and secret clubs. (See Fig. 12-12.) The peer group activities also enable children to explore sex roles through choice of toys and activities. Girls may still learn crafts, cook, play with dolls, and play house. Boys are more concerned with developing some physical prowess within the play group and/or on the athletic field. Because of the feminist movement, the traditional sex roles have become blurred. Today, children of both sexes explore areas and choose toys once reserved for one sex. Boys play with dolls (often exploring the male role in child rearing), cook, and clean the house. Girls compete on athletic teams and take carpentry and fix-it classes. By learning these roles, children will perhaps be increasingly self-reliant as adults and may also better understand people of the opposite sex.

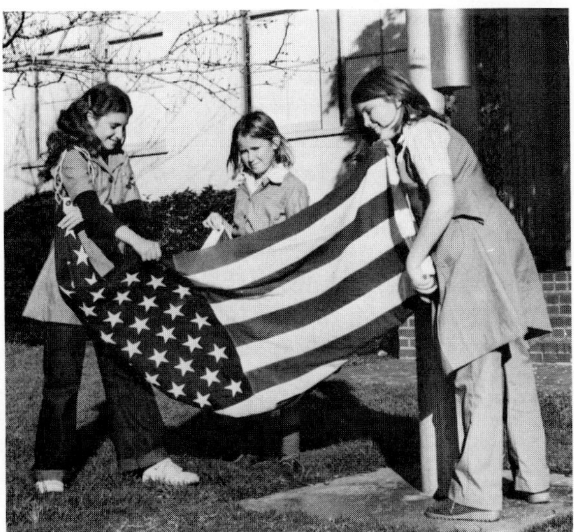

Figure 12-12 The school-age child learns his or her sex role by joining same-sex clubs, such as the Girl Scouts.

The child learns the actions of new roles before the symbolic meanings. The girl learns the mother's sex role actions—cooking, giving first aid, doing housework, etc.—before she understands the concept of mothering.

The school-age child is in the latency period of Freudian psychosexual development. The preschooler's major area of sexual conflict, the Oedipus or Electra complex, has been resolved. The older preschooler realized that the wish to possess the opposite-sex parent was impossible and focused his or her instinctual energy on more potentially successful areas. (See the section "Freudian Theory" in Chap. 5 for a discussion of instinctual energy.) The school-age years are quiet, or latent, with few sexual conflicts. This frees the libidinal energy to focus on learning the vast amounts of information needed to function in society.

The school-age child does, however, have sexual feelings. These feelings are expressed through masturbation and sexual curiosity. A child's rigid conscience and urge to obey rules allow tight control of sexual feelings.

Sexuality Many school-age children are increasingly interested in sex within the peer group and are often involved in sex play. Curiosity about sexual differences intensifies, partially as a result of the media's emphasis on nudity and sexual behavior. Many children explore their own bodies and those of peers. This is due to curiosity, not sexual urges. Secret conversations commonly involve sharing information (often incorrect) learned from books, magazines, or television. The child may view a television program and tell a parent about the scene "where the man tore all her clothes off" rather than the story of the whole program.

Sex education Early in the preadolescent period, the child may be eager to learn biological facts and can do so with relative comfort, since sexual feelings are not yet causing anxiety. But later, conflicts about sex become heightened, and therefore information about sex is received with apprehension as well as interest. Preadolescents sometimes test adults' reactions to "touchy" subject matter. By such testing, the child learns whether a particular adult will discuss emotional or controversial subjects, such as sex.

Sex education, although controversial, is included in many school curricula. The information may, however, be incompletely understood or quickly forgotten. Answers to questions should be honest and at the child's level of understanding, and information should be given when the child seeks the knowledge. Sex education may include the information that sex is necessary for the survival of all species; drawings about anatomic differences; a discussion about body changes common to all children and their effects on skin care, nutrition, and the need for rest and exercise; information for girls about personal care during the menses; general information about voice changes in boys; how twins are conceived; marriage and sex as an expression of love and sensitivity; communications; and other items of general interest to children in this age group. An objective approach provides emotional distance that encourages group participation.

Preadolescents are also becoming aware of many ambivalent and conflicting aspects of sex in our society. On the one hand, they learn about cultural prohibitions and disapproval of sexual activity, while on the other hand, they witness the mass media's emphasis on sexuality. Parental reluctance to discuss sex can confuse children, blocks communication, and leads them to turn to peers for information. School-age children obtain most of their information about sex from peers. Misinformation and misconceptions acquired from peers may increase anxiety and prevent understanding of body functions. Misinformation can lead to difficulties later in life when attempting to handle the social and emotional aspects of sexuality as an adult.

Absence of the same-sex parent For the child whose same-sex parent is absent from the home as a result of death, divorce, or other cause, learning the sex role may be difficult. In the case of a boy, "big brother" programs, a grandfather, or a favorite uncle can provide a male role model. For girls, a grandmother, aunt, or concerned "big sister" may be appropriate. Relationships with adults of their own sex are crucial, since children need a sex role model to copy and a same-sex adult who will share and clarify new experiences.

For the older school-age child (10 to 13 years), the beginnings of interest in the opposite sex result in an increased effort to become more closely related to members of the same sex. If the parent of the same sex is absent from the home, the increased anxiety of children in this age group may further increase unless they have developed a trusting relationship with a surrogate parent. As much as a single parent tries to be both parents to the child, the youngster needs close ties with adults of both sexes to learn to understand people and develop his or her own sex role.

Role unification Feminist life-styles of recent years have contributed another dimension to child rearing. Children whose families have adopted these life-styles are raised in nonsexist ways. From a very young age, they experience and observe that roles played by men and women need not be strictly linked to one of the sexes. Men cook, clean house, and participate in child rearing, just as women go to work to earn money and to seek self-fulfillment.

It remains to be seen, but children raised in a nonsexist environment may grow up to be more self-reliant and to share roles even more easily than their parents. Reduced sexual stereotyping may cause them to be more tolerant, loving, and understanding of other people of both sexes.

Hero worship For the preadolescent, an older friend of the same sex becomes a "worshiped" hero who provides support as parental ties are gradually loosened. This hero is usually an older teenager or young adult who is viewed as protective, warm, and someone the preadolescent wishes to be like.

Hero worship softens the child's previous dependence on parents and helps in the transition to the adolescent's developmental task of establishing greater self-reliance and interdependence with nonparent adults. The child who has a hero commonly is quite critical of the same-sex parent, who is perceived as not comparing favorably with the admired person. This can become a potential source of friction in the home, especially between girls and their mothers. However, if the parent maintains stability in the face of these expressions of contempt, it will serve to prevent the preadolescent from becoming overly anxious or rebellious about split loyalties. The child does not actually hate the parents, but is moving toward appropriate independence from them and from home.

Boys usually experience less intense hero

worship than girls, probably because our society tends to frown on strong attachments between males. Boys may master their fear of continuing dependence on parents by becoming heavily involved in a sport or by looking for a job outside the home.

The family

While the child's world expands beyond the home, the family stabilizes his or her total development. Whenever they feel vulnerable, school-age children need to retreat to their families. Here they can recharge their emotional energy, discuss topics, find solutions to problems, and experience companionship, affection, comfort, and stimulation for their emotional and moral growth.

The family also enhances the child's intellectual development and teaches the basic skills necessary to function as a valued, competent adult. Parents help children develop intellectually by having high expectations for them, being interested in their activities, praising their efforts, and encouraging their curiosity and explorations.

School-age children, at least until preadolescence, usually consider themselves closer to the same-sex parent. They also see the same-sex parent as more punitive. Even when the mother works, they tend to view her as the homemaker who nurtures them and pays attention to their feelings and needs. Fathers are seen as the breadwinners—stronger, bigger, dirtier, and more menacing.

Social class affects children's perceptions of their parents. Middle-class parents tend to reason with their children, accept their behavior, and give them attention. Lower-class fathers are more apt to be authoritarian and often punish physically; middle-class fathers are more often companions and are interested in their children's school activities and in promoting a positive self-concept.

Parents As the school-age child progresses developmentally, the parents often need support and knowledge of normal growth and development to help them adapt to the changes in their child. This is particularly true of parents who have not dealt with a school-age child before. The ease with which the parents adapt to their child's travels away from them depends on their ability to accept the child's new image and the child's new, more realistic view of them. Often parents say, "What a big girl she is now! She's in school and doesn't need me much anymore."

Children this age see their parents more realistically than they did as preschoolers. They become independent of their parents in most daily activities and question their expertise and their standards. This behavior threatens the parents. They may feel inadequate and disappointed. Both the parents and the child may feel hurt and angry and may reject each other. The nurse can ensure that this rejection will be temporary by educating the parents about the causes of these feelings, what to expect, and how to recognize the former strengths that still exist in their "new" child. Parents need reassurance that even the most critical children will *not* tolerate any criticism of their parents by others.

Siblings Siblings generally experience the same basic child-rearing patterns, but parent and child personality characteristics modify the parenting styles. For example, a parent may be warmer toward one child than another, even while being restrictive toward both in the same situation. This results in one child's appearing to be more socialized, self-confident, and friendly than the other child. Likewise, one parent may relate better to some children in the family, and the other parent may relate better to other children. Parents should share responsibilities to ensure that each child receives equal affection, attention, and discipline.

COGNITIVE DEVELOPMENT

Concrete operations

School-age children, beginning at approximately age 7, are in the concrete operations stage of cognitive development. Their primary intellectual goal is to learn the logical relationships between objects encountered in the world. They therefore organize, order, and classify objects that can be concretely experienced (hence the label *concrete operations*) through the senses of taste, smell, and hearing. School-age children are able to use symbols to organize their thoughts (mental activities or operations) and manipulate the world around them. The preschooler had to experience an object physically before he or she could think about it (concrete thinking). The

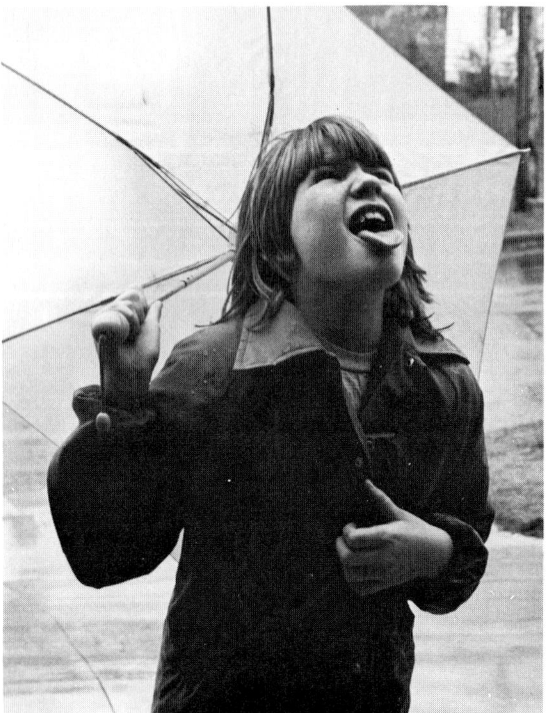

Figure 12-13 School-age children think symbolically. This girl is tasting raindrops (a concrete experience) and will later think symbolically by remembering the mental image of the raindrops.

school-age child can experience an event *without* touching or seeing it. (See Fig. 12-13.) For example, the child can "taste" a chocolate cake by thinking about it (symbolic thinking). The child can think about the past, present, and future and can use parts of past experiences to help understand the meaning of the present. He or she gradually becomes less self-centered and is able to see another person's point of view. The child is gradually moving toward the abstract thinking of the adolescent and the adult. (See Table 5-3 for a summary of cognitive stages.)

Conservation A characteristic of the school-age child is the ability to *decenter,* or focus on several aspects of a situation simultaneously. Children in this stage are also sensitive to *transformations* (for example, they know that the amount of liquid remains the same even when it is poured into different-sized containers with varying fluid levels) and can *reverse* their thinking (if half the contents of a 2-cup container is poured into a second cup, they know that the first cup will again contain 2 cups when the second cup is emptied back into the first cup). Piaget believed that these three aspects of cognition (decentering, transformation, and reversibility) are interdependent and not able to exist individually. These three characteristics form the basis for the development of the characteristic of conservation. *Conservation* is the ability to be aware of the constancy of the properties of objects as they undergo transmutations (e.g., conservation of volume: the amount of liquid remains constant even though it is poured from a tall, thin glass into a short, fat one).

Classification The school-age child gathers information, sorts it by defining properties, understands relations between classes and subclasses, and moves closer to the abstract thought of the next cognitive stage. The child may collect stamps or shells, separate them into groups, and classify them in any number of ways (for example, by size, color, or place of origin). In the process, new relationships between the objects may be discovered, and new ideas generated.

By gathering, sorting, and classifying information, school-age children determine the cause or reasons for events in their lives. They delight in learning and collecting all the facts about things of interest to them, such as airplanes, and in learning about what will happen to them during a medical procedure, for example. They manipulate symbols and information to order, interpret, and understand their world. In this stage they collect all information on a subject. Later, when abstract thought is possible, the adolescent will judge a subject's merits and form conclusions.

Ordering *Ordering* of information also demonstrates the child's inability to think simultaneously about several aspects of a situation. The child is able to determine, for example, that a city is part of a larger whole (Los Angeles is in California). But when questioned, he or she is unable to see that people who live in Los Angeles are Californians. The child sees the part and whole separately, as if they were unrelated.

Seriation After age 8, the child is able to rank objects in a hierarchical order according to one common characteristic. For example, an 11-year-old classifies animals as either vertebrates or invertebrates.

Symbol manipulation The cognitive system of school-age children enables them to organize and manipulate the surrounding world. They do this by starting with what is immediately present or concrete. They can think of future events or possibilities only to a limited degree. This use of manipulation consists mainly of simple generalizations of the immediate present leading to new content. The child will take several math symbols and create new problems and relationships with them. In the process, he or she may discover simple truths about higher levels of math, but is not yet able to appreciate their scope.

Time recognition By age 7, the child is becoming more oriented in time and space. The ability to recognize time relationships, to place events in successive order, and to understand time intervals between events enables the child to begin to understand time in relation to a clock. Seasons and months are known, especially those involving something of special interest—birthdays, Halloween, etc.

Conscience development

The conscience, which Freud called the *superego*, evolves as a part of cognitive development. As the child approaches the late preschool years, the conscience strengthens as the child incorporates the same-sex parent's moral values into his or her personality and behavioral patterns. (See Chaps. 5 and 11.) These values, which previously were communicated by the parent in terms of "Thou shalt" and "Thou shalt not," are now perceived in terms of "I must and "I must not." This arouses feelings of guilt, and the child now uses various defense mechanisms (rationalization, regression, etc.) to reduce the guilt.

Initially, the school-age child's conscience is tyrannical and rigid. (See the section "Moral Development" in Chap. 11.) This is demonstrated in the moralistic school-age child who learns and applies rules of right and wrong in a rigid, strict, absolute manner that makes no allowances for extenuating circumstances. For example, a young school-age child might think that losing one's shoes or stealing cookies is an offense as serious as a crime. This unyielding standard of right and wrong leads children to be highly condemning of others' behavior and even of the unfairness of uncontrollable events. For example, a planned trip to the beach may be cancelled for one group of children and not for another. Despite explanations that seem clear and reasonable to an adult, the group unable to go continues to protest. It is not unusual to hear "It's not fair" in protest against being denied a wish. Having been told they live in a free country makes it hard for children to understand why they cannot do what they want to do when they want to do it. This literal translation of right and wrong will gradually become more flexible. Children will become less harsh in judging themselves and others and will learn to allow for extenuating circumstances.

The majority of 10-year-olds are in stage 2 of moral development, which is discussed below.[23]

Level I: Preconventional (premoral)

Stage 2: Instrumental relativist orientation The young school-age child, aged 10 and under, believes that a fair and honest moral choice will bring mutual benefits. The motto of the child might be, "If you scratch my back, I'll scratch yours." Children aged 10 to 12 judge a correct moral choice according to how well the results will meet their inner needs and benefit and protect them. While they recognize that people have different viewpoints, they judge others' behavior by its usefulness to them—an egocentric viewpoint. The school-age child recognizes the intent of laws and the consequences of disobeying them, but obeys laws to avoid personal discomfort—another self-centered viewpoint.[24] The child has no true understanding of the abstract concepts of fairness, gratitude, loyalty, or laws.

Cheating and lying

Kohlberg found that all children, including school-age children, cheat and that cheating increases with pressure to succeed. The amount of cheating and the amount of energy expended to cheat again vary with the need to achieve. Young school-age children unquestioningly submit to adult authority and view rules as rigid and unbreakable. They believe that they pay for their mistakes by being punished and that punishment appeases adults.[25] The 6- to 7-year-old may blame others for a misdeed to avoid punishment.[26] This is normal behavior and is not a deliberate, premeditated lie. (Refer to Chap. 11 for additional information on stage 1 of moral development.)

The 8- to 9-year-old is moving into stage 2 of moral development. He or she views rules in terms of their intent, seeks to conform to external rules, and strives to maintain good relationships with family members, the teacher, and the peer group. The peer group now punishes members for disobeying its rules. By age 10 to 12, the child differentiates feelings from motives, becomes self-critical of misdeeds, and experiences guilt. The older school-age child's intense need for peer group membership and for approval from authority figures lessens lying and cheating. The 11- or 12-year-old may lie to protect a friend, but lies less frequently because of the need for self-approval.[27] The older school-age child's need for self-respect is thus stronger than the urge to lie or cheat.

When a child cheats or lies, the parents should show displeasure; explain the possible consequences of the cheating or lying; briefly instruct the child in correct, socially acceptable behavior; and emphasize the importance of telling the truth. When the child does tell the truth about a misdeed, the parents should praise the child for telling the truth, hug the child, and reassure the child of their love. Children should not be punished after admitting the truth because this will teach them that telling the truth results in punishment. A calm, supportive, open environment in which parents and children can discuss these moral dilemmas and alternative solutions will best promote moral development.[28]

Discipline

Piaget pointed out two main characteristics of the child's moral judgments. The first of these is termed *moral realism* and involves the assumption that moral rules exist in their own right (similar to the idea of natural law). The second is the idea that misdeeds have their own built-in punishments. For example, a child may cheat on a test unknown to the teacher, and receive a failing grade. The child is convinced that the failing grade was a punishment for the misdeed.

School-age children actually judge themselves and one another more stringently than adults would and are likely to suggest punishment that sounds tantamount to an execution. It is possible, in terms of Freudian theory, that this behavior represents their attempts to maintain control over their impulses. School-age children need realistic and consistent limits on their behavior, even while they are protesting and testing the rules. They need help in controlling their outbursts. These children respect and feel secure with the adult who establishes consistent rules and discusses the issues involved. Children who "run wild" without realistic parental controls feel insecure and are begging, by their misdeeds, for help in controlling their behavior.

Because school-age children are in such a rigid stage of morality, the adults around them must help them understand the reasons for punishment and what distinguishes right from wrong. It is most important to help school-age children understand that they are punished because of *deeds* they have done and not because they personally are not liked. A child's self-concept must be preserved and positively supported as he or she is being punished. For example, saying "I'm angry at what you did to your sister" instead of "I'm angry at you" separates the child's unacceptable action from the still accepted child and preserves the child's self-concept.

All children learn, as they grow older, which behaviors bring positive or negative results in which circumstances. Punishment (withdrawal of love, isolation, or spanking) is not the only aspect of discipline that teaches a child the consequences of misbehavior. It has been hypothesized that the parent who *talks* and *reasons* with a child about misbehavior is more likely than one who simply punishes to give the child a clear idea of what he or she did wrong. This allows the child's anxiety about misbehavior to be connected to the right cues. Explanations and reasons also give children internal resources for evaluating their own behavior and give them specific training in making moral judgments about their behavior. In the case of children whose parents do not talk about misbehaviors but only punish them, anxiety may continue to exist but not be related to the specific consequences of misbehavior.

All children's moral behavior depends on the degree to which their family environment has taught them moral behaviors and judgments which conform to the moral codes of their socioeconomic class and culture. Fair rules and good role models will help children internalize desirable societal values. As they move toward a more democratic morality and as their own sense of right and wrong develops, they will begin to experience guilt after breaking a rule and will worry about the type and timing of punishment. A child who has learned that punishment is consistent, immediate, and appropriate to the nature of the infringement will experience less anxiety and feel more secure in relating to others. He or she will be less unsure about what constitutes acceptable and unacceptable behavior.

HEALTH MAINTENANCE

Safety

Motor vehicle accidents are the most common cause of accidental injury and death among children between the ages of 6 and 12. Injuries occur not only while children are riding in cars but also while they are walking between parked cars, crossing streets against the light, or riding bicycles or skateboards.

Statistics continue to support the use of appropriate automobile seat belts as the best way to prevent severe injury or death. School-age children should be strapped into seat belts and not allowed to sit in the back of a station wagon or climb boisterously around a car.

Drowning is another major cause of death among children in this age group. Water safety and survival skills should be taught along with basic swimming skills at an early age. Pools should be locked and fenced with unclimbable materials.

Many nurses give counseling regarding smoke detectors during their visits with parents. Smoke detectors are effective in preventive injury or death due to fires. A family-designed fire escape plan should be initiated and practiced one or two times a month. Burns among children also frequently result from curiosity and fascination with matches and fire.

Accidents frequently occur while children are playing, skating, or riding school buses. Children of this age are energetic and in almost constant motion. In their activities, they are not aware of potentially harmful situations. Thus burns, bumps, bruises, sprains, and even eye injuries may result. Accident prevention should be taught and enforced in schools and homes, and nurses need to promote safety by helping parents and children identify and avoid hazards. Skateboard, "3 wheeler," and motorcycle enthusiasts should use helmets and knee and elbow pads to prevent serious injury and possible death. Parents should be encouraged to enforce strict safety rules before children are allowed to participate in these dangerous sports. When a child does become injured, treatment should include being helped to identify the reasons for the accident and planning clear-cut methods for preventing subsequent accidents.

As children spend increasing amounts of time away from parental supervision, new aspects of safety become important for their well-being. At this age they must be taught to refuse to accept things from, speak to, or ride with strangers. This concept is often integrated into the classroom teaching of the preschooler and then is reinforced in kindergarten and elementary school. If safety measures designed to prevent accidents are emphasized early, school-age children can increasingly avoid common accidents.

Sleep disturbances

Nightmares and sleep disturbances are common during the early school years. One reason for this is that these children have reached a stage of mental development in which they have a concept of death. At home, the bedtime hour should be a quiet time of sharing and support between parent and child. It is an optimal time to exchange experiences, explore and answer questions, and have quiet talks. The consistent routines of prayers and preparing for bed can be a source of comfort and ritual for the child who is frightened of the dark or of going to sleep.

Fears of death and mutilation are very real for children this age. Television movies (especially violent ones), catastrophic news events, discussions with friends, and pictures in books can provoke anxiety and cause reluctance to go to bed, fear of the dark, and bad dreams. This anxiety may seem unreasonable to an adult, but it is a reflection of a child's feelings of powerlessness and fear of death. An adult whom the child trusts can, through his or her presence and support, strengthen the child's coping and alleviate at least some of the fears. Empathetic adults also understand that pretenses of independence and bravado are actually defenses to cover up the child's feelings of helplessness and fear.

Parents can reassure a fearful child by maintaining as much bedtime ritual as necessary to make the child feel secure. Nightlights, authoritative reassurances that the child's fears will not come true, and assurances that the parent will be in the next room, if needed at all during the night, often reduce fears and improve sleep.

Self-care and hygiene

School-age children are eager to learn about their bodies and to become self-reliant in caring for themselves as they grow older. The school can assist the family in health education. As children grow, they should assume responsibility for more aspects of self-care. This gradual process is reinforced by the three main influential groups: parents, teachers, and peers.

The health curriculum within the school setting reinforces the importance of good, basic self-care habits, such as bathing, washing hair, using only one's own comb and brush, eating nutritious foods, and getting exercise and adequate rest each day. Each of these content areas should be included in the health curriculum and presented in interesting and creative ways. Class projects can be used. For the child approaching adolescence, a knowledge of basic hygiene will help eliminate peer group rejection that can result from body odor, unbrushed teeth, and dirty hair. The peer group influences the older child's conformity to hygiene standards.

Dental care

Dental decay is the single most prevalent health problem during the school years. Ninety-five percent of school-age children are affected by dental caries. By age 16, the average person has had seven teeth and fourteen tooth surfaces attacked by decay. This is unfortunate; dental caries are completely preventable. Parents and children should be taught to exercise good oral hygiene habits (brushing and flossing) at least twice a day; to maintain good nutrition; to use fluoride toothpaste; to avoid sticky, sweet foods or at least to brush immediately after eating them; and to have regular 6-month dental checkups.

Many children of school age wear braces. In some schools and neighborhoods braces are well accepted or are even considered to increase one's social status, but some children experience teasing by peers. Comments such as "railroad tracks" or "tin grin" are commonly heard. Group conformity is important during the school-age period. Any slight difference will increase group pressure to conform and will increase the "different" child's anxiety level. A trusted adult can give support to alleviate the child's anxieties and can discuss feelings and attitudes with others in the group, who may realize that it is all right to be different, especially when it leads to self-improvement.

Drug use

Parents frequently feel uninformed about drug use and are hesitant to approach their children about drugs; many believe in delaying the discussion of alcohol and other drug abuse until their children are over 12 years of age. Parent and child denial of substance abuse is widespread. Parents should be encouraged to discuss topics as general as feelings about oneself in relation to others and peer pressures and how to deal with them. As role models, adults can serve to initiate some thinking and discussion with children before they reach upper grades, where all kinds of experimentation is common. (See Chap. 39 for a discussion of substance abuse.)

Child abuse

The increased reporting and awareness of child sexual and physical abuse indicates a growing need for parents to educate their children about this subject. Preventive education about child abuse is being increasingly integrated into classrooms at all grade levels across the country. (See Chap. 38 for additional information on child abuse.)

The handicapped child

Current education laws are increasing the "mainstreaming" of physically and emotionally handicapped children into the regular classroom. This requires many school nurses to use acute-care nursing skills in their daily work. They act as resources to school staffs and as liaisons between the school, the family, and health care professionals. (See Chap. 34 for a discussion of the chronically ill child.)

Mental health

Mental health is of overriding importance to children's well-being and positive views of themselves. Parents and other adults can support mental health by (1) taking time to share themselves and not just things with children; (2) being good listeners, which makes children feel worthwhile; and (3) directly telling children the good things about them. The adult who can be genuine and is not afraid to apologize and who lives a life worthy of respect sets a positive mental health example.

DEVELOPMENTAL MILESTONES*

Six-year-olds

Six-year-olds are self-centered, opinionated, "know-it-alls," bossy, and easily hurt by criticism. Their boundless energy allows them to explore the world. They have an insatiable appetite for new experiences and are easily distracted by fascinating objects.

Fine and gross motor development Six-year-olds are whirlwinds of constant motion: jumping, hopping, rolling on the floor, and wiggling while sitting on a chair. Their gross movements are awkward at times. Their skill increases while practicing skating, skipping, running, bicycling, and jumping rope. Fine motor coordination is less developed than gross muscle coordination. Six-year-olds cut with scissors, hammer, tie shoelaces, and dress themselves. They print unevenly and frequently reverse letters (Fig. 12-14).

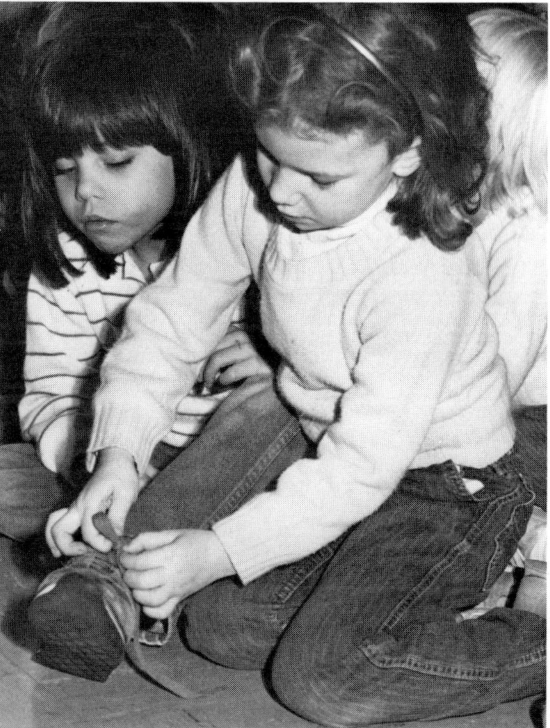

Figure 12-14 This 6-year-old is showing her friend how to tie her shoelaces. (*Photo by Janet Cardle.*)

Family and social relationships Six-year-olds' relationships with their parents vary widely. One moment they seek affectionate hugs and kisses; the next moment they defy a parent's request, blame the parent for everything, whine, argue, and dawdle when hurried. They want to accept full responsibility for tasks or projects, but frequently lack the experience and attention span to complete them.

Six-year-olds are in emotional upheaval. They are innocent, charming, and affectionate, but also tense and upset. They frequently return briefly to earlier patterns of tension-reducing behaviors: chewing on fingers or thumb-sucking. As they leave home, separation anxiety briefly recurs. When they go to a new school, they need praise and consistent home routines. They frequently vacillate between acting like babies and like older children. The 6-year-old is fearful of strange noises, witches, skeletons, fantasized persons, and the elements of wind, fire, and rain.

Six-year-olds seek out a same-sex play group (Fig. 12-15). They are too self-centered, expecting people to adapt immediately to their wishes, to be truly team members. Six-year-olds play together, but their play is often independent. Group play frequently ends in brawls because they do not know when to withdraw to avoid getting hurt.

School Six-year-olds' days center on school. Their language is well developed; it shows thought and gives them pleasure. They can read, count to 20, and define shapes. They are beginning to understand the abstract concepts of afternoon, morning, and tomorrow. They define objects by their use and are interested in religion, including the concepts of heaven and God.

Self-care Six-year-olds play in the tub but resist getting washed. They must be reminded to wash before dinner, but dress and undress alone. They drop toys on the floor and leave their clothes wherever they were removed. They go to the bathroom alone.

*This section was compiled by Nancy L. Ramsey.

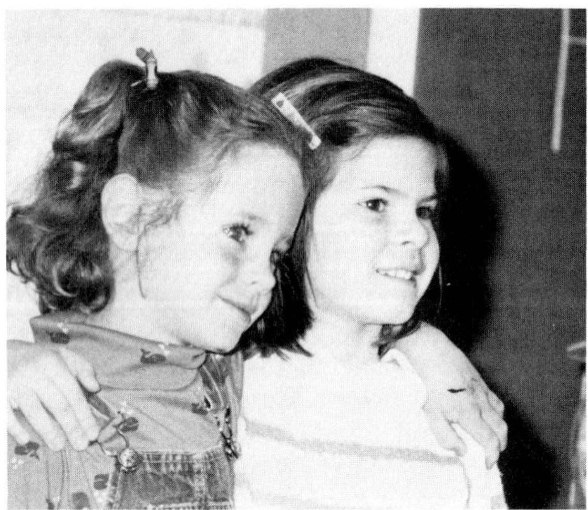

Figure 12-15 The first grade classroom is a good place to make new friends. (*Photo by Janet Cardle.*)

Seven-year-olds

Seven-year-olds are quiet, pensive, and reflective. They are consolidating past life experiences into an understandable whole. Seven-year-olds are less satisfied with themselves and the world. They demand perfection from themselves and their families, they are conscientious, and they value the opinions of others. Mood swings range from exuberance to anger when family members do not fulfill their expectations.

Fine and gross motor development Seven-year-olds are more cautious than boisterous 6-year-olds. Their activity level is lower. They practice skills to perfect them. They swim, bicycle, skate, and enjoy reading and quiet games.

Family and social relationships Seven-year-olds' relationships with their parents are closer than those of 6-year-olds. They want to be liked by family, peers, and teachers. They are eager to cooperate and please these people and are sensitive to their opinions of them.

Children this age enjoy teasing others but tolerate criticism and teasing poorly. They may feel "picked on" and may threaten to run away when feeling mistreated. They know right from wrong and establish very high standards for themselves and their families. Even tiny failures to reach these high standards may make them feel inferior, withdraw, act shy, or be angry.

Fears of the dark, robbers, and ghosts and of feeling inadequate in a new situation continue.

School Seven-year-olds enjoy school and seek the teacher's approval. They can tell time and know the day, month, and season. They understand the basic concepts of addition and subtraction. They print several sentences and reverse letters less frequently.

Seven-year-olds are less egocentric, are able to see another person's point of view, and can identify with and feel another child's emotion (such as hurt). They have a more realistic understanding of cause and effect.

Self-care Children this age need less help from parents in caring for themselves. They can dress and undress alone, brush their teeth, scrub themselves clean, brush their hair, and go to bed alone. However, they still need reminding to wash before meals. Like 6-year-olds, they dawdle during self-care activities and drop their clothes on the floor.

Eight-year-olds

Eight-year-olds are more self-confident, enthusiastic, and friendly. They curiously explore the "whys" of new experiences in the world. Eight is an age of creative intellectual expansion. These children enjoy learning about science and nature. They excitedly begin new activities but have difficulty completing them.

Fine and gross motor development Eight-year-olds perfect their skills, whether playing jump rope or wrestling. Their body movements appear more graceful and coordinated.

Family and social relationships Eight-year-olds' relationships with both parents are closer and more sensitive. They want their parents' approval. They are interested in adult activities and closely scrutinize the adults around them. They are less self-centered and listen to and try to understand their parents' explanations.

Children this age increasingly merge into a same-sex peer group's activities. They want to join the group rather than play alone. They often have a love-hate relationship with friends of the opposite sex. Boys tend to be secretive about a girlfriend. They may have a best friend of the same sex, and hero worship begins at this age. Eight-year-olds are truthful and lie less. They more clearly distinguish reality from fantasy and have fewer fears than younger children.

School Eight is a year of intellectual expansion, growing from the child's explorations of the world. Eight-year-olds' memory increases, and as memories increase their vocabulary expands. They are learning to write rather than print. They can categorize objects by both similarities and differences. They enjoy studying rocket ships and science.

They are proud of their accomplishments, fear poor grades, and want to be praised by both teachers and parents. They are friendly and enjoy playing with friends at school.

Self-care Eight-year-olds dress themselves completely. Their social manners are better. They eat food more reasonably, no longer grabbing and cramming it into their mouths. They still enjoy being tucked into bed with a consistent routine. They should have the responsibility for completing a list of chores, and they enjoy being paid for their work.

Nine-year-olds

Nine-year-olds play hard and work hard. They are very interested in all group activities, both the team play of friends and the activities of their families. Their behavior appears more mature, refined, and independent. They are less restless than 8-year-olds.

Fine and gross motor development Nine-year-olds' eye-hand coordination is almost perfected. Children this age enjoy activities that develop this coordination: writing, sewing, knitting, and model building. They also spend long hours perfecting gross muscle skills, such as those used in basketball. Their muscular control and timing show more expertise.

Family and social relationships Nine-year-olds are more interested in their friends than in their parents. However, they enjoy taking part in family decisions. They like helping their mothers with housework and running errands. They are easier to discipline and begin to take responsibility for their actions. They have fewer fears and know that Santa Claus is not real.

If the peer group's and the parents' wishes collide, nine-year-olds will follow their friends. They are more empathetic, sympathetic, and loyal. These attributes enable them to become valued team or group members. They still prefer same-sex friends. They are loyal to peers, and the group increasingly dominates their behavior. Hero worship intensifies; crushes on teachers are common. Nine-year-olds, however, do occasionally chase members of the opposite sex around the playground.

School Nine-year-olds' attention span is longer. They are increasingly interested in the subject rather than the teacher. They understand explanations and strive to follow the teacher's directions. They now enthusiastically complete tasks. Children this age describe the characteristics of objects, rather than simply defining them in terms of usage. They multiply, divide, and recite five numbers in reverse order. Nine-year-olds love historical sagas, reading, constructing projects, and winning at team sports. Good students are accepted by classmates, while superior students are rejected. At this age, girls are usually intellectually superior to boys.

Self-care Nine-year-olds can care for themselves completely. They have good table manners but often need reminding to brush teeth. Boys are unaware of dirty clothes, while girls are interested in cleanliness and clothes. Nine-year-olds clean their rooms and take care of their toys. They are still reluctant to go to bed.

Ten-year-olds

Ten-year-olds are on a peaceful plateau. They are at peace with themselves and the world. They are happy, confident, serene, and content. Their behavior is more predictable and consistent, since they have more control over their emotions and behavior and over the environment. They are courteous to adults outside the home.

Fine and gross motor development Ten-year-olds have greater muscular strength, stamina, and coordination. They thoroughly enjoy all physical activity: climbing, jumping, and skating. Fine motor development is perfected. Children this age spend hours practicing skills, such as playing the clarinet, since their talents are becoming increasingly obvious. Girls begin the pubertal growth spurt and tower over boys, whose height varies widely.

Family and social relationships Ten-year-olds are closer to their families than 9-year-olds and have a better relationship with their mothers. They enjoy attention from their fathers and want to join their fathers in activities.

Ten-year-olds are more relaxed and more easily express affection toward their parents. They adapt more easily to rules, tolerate frustration better, and live more harmoniously within the family. They explosively but briefly express emotions, ranging from impulsive hugs and kisses to crying and depression. They get angry but do not hold grudges.

Ten is the age of intense peer group memberships. Children this age desperately want to join clubs and teams. They delight in competing and in winning at competitive games. They often love and praise a best friend. Hero worship intensifies. The 10-year-old is a successful group member.

School Ten-year-olds reason by cause and effect but have difficulty visualizing abstract relationships (combining facts and seeing the relationship). They ponder solutions to the world's social problems. Children this age believe in fairness and stern punishment for misdeeds. They focus on the wrong more than the right.

Ten-year-olds enjoy learning in school. They write clearly and fast. They relish detective and adventure stories and magic tricks. Ten-year-olds manipulate fractions and numbers over 100. They memorize longer material. However, they are impulsive and, although they work hard, perform better when following a schedule. They would rather listen and play than work.

Self-care Ten-year-olds neglect self-care. They hate and masterfully avoid self-care activities. Their rooms are messy, and they drop their clothes on the floor throughout the house. They hate to change into clean clothes and need prodding to take a bath.

Eleven-year-olds

In contrast to the happy, serene 10-year-old, the 11-year-old gives his or her parents a glimpse of adolescent mood swings. Eleven-year-olds are resentful and critical of adults in authority. They rebel against instructions and rules. They are often moody, unhappy, and in turmoil.

Eleven-year-olds want to be independent. They thrive on exploration and adventure, through which they learn about the world. Children this age are highly moralistic, are interested in religion, and attack injustices in the world. They expect fairness and believe in unyielding punishment for misdeeds. However, they want friends to lie to protect them from punishment.

Eleven is a fearful age. The 11-year-old worries about everything—school, parents, money, and illness.

Fine and gross motor development Eleven-year-olds are active and energetic. They enjoy outdoor activities and love sports. They are agile at sports, but because of their rapid body changes, they may be clumsy at home. The body changes of puberty become more noticeable. Girls are more interested in their body changes than boys are.

Family and social relationships Eleven-year-olds are constantly with their families and enjoy family activities. They scrutinize how adults (and parents) treat one another. Their emotions are ambivalent: one moment sneaking affectionate hugs and the next moment criticizing and rebelling against their parents. However, their behavior away from the parents is courteous and considerate.

Eleven-year-olds are cheerful and kind when with their friends, as contrasted to the way they behave when with their parents. They want their friends' approval and acceptance. They confide innermost secrets to them, not to the parents. They often work together with other young people in a group effort to improve the community. They want to be financially independent and seek part-time jobs after school.

School Eleven-year-olds are excited about learning and constantly ask "Why?" and "How?" They resist doing, and complain about, homework. These preadolescents begin to describe abstract things, such as peace and justice. They want the teacher, and the peer group, to challenge their learning.

Self-care Eleven-year-olds are capable of completely caring for themselves. However, they rebel against all rules and authority. Therefore, they need urging to wash their necks and behind their ears and to shampoo their hair. Eleven-year-olds still resist going to bed and arising in the morning.

Twelve-year-olds

Twelve-year-olds are more cooperative, friendly, and even-tempered. They are more self-reliant and independent. These preadolescents are more satisfied with themselves and the world. They are less tormented and are obviously growing up. They misbehave less because they think abstractly and can analyze the consequences of their behavior. They will lie to protect a friend.

Fine and gross motor development Twelve-year-olds thrive on frantic, intense activity, at which they persist until collapsing. They enthusiastically enjoy all gross motor activity.

Both boys' and girls' interest in sex increases. Girls' height and weight gain is at a peak. Breasts develop, and axillary hair appears. A girl at 12 may flaunt her developing body or be embarrassed by it and hide it. She comfortably discusses sexuality and masturbation with an older female friend. Boys are increasingly interested in their own sexual development. Discussions with friends often center on sex. Boys masturbate and have frequent erections.

Family and social relationships Twelve-year-olds relate to their parents better but are less affectionate. They expect parents to respect their privacy. Although they test limits, 12-year-olds want consistent limits.

The 12-year-old's peer group decreases in size. He or she often pairs off with a best friend and appears constantly accompanied by one or more friends. At school, interest in the opposite sex intensifies. Girls talk about boys, and both girls and boys play games involving close accidental contact with one another.

School Twelve-year-olds learn quickly. They enjoy collecting facts, doing math, playing sports, and reading about travel, science, home, and nature. Girls prefer romantic novels, while boys prefer adventure and mystery stories.

Twelve-year-olds ask many questions. They want to excel at school and be liked by teachers and classmates.

Self-care Twelve-year-olds are more concerned with their appearance. Boys bathe more frequently and change into clean clothes more often. Girls are intrigued by makeup and stylish clothes. Both boys and girls are still reluctant to go to bed at night, but arise more easily in the morning.

REFERENCES

1. Erikson, Erik H., *Childhood and Society,* Norton, New York, 1950, pp. 219–234.
2. Nemir, Alma, and Warren E. Schaller, *The School Health Program,* Saunders, Philadelphia, 1975, p. 16.
3. Vaughn, V. C., and R. I. McKay (eds.), *Nelson Textbook of Pediatrics,* Saunders, Philadelphia, 1975, p. 30.
4. Ibid., p. 21.
5. *Why Is Your Child Being Screened for Scoliosis?* Children's Hospital of Los Angeles, 1979, p. 77.
6. Vaughn and McKay, op. cit., p. 77.
7. Ibid., p. 21.
8. Ibid., p. 254.
9. Ibid., p. 109.
10. Ibid., p. 109–110.
11. Erikson, op. cit., p. 226.
12. Ibid., p. 227.
13. Ibid., p. 226.
14. Ibid., p. 227.
15. Ibid., p. 22.
16. Sieman, Mari, "Mental Health in School-Aged Children," *American Journal of Maternal-Child Nursing* **3**(4):215 (July–August 1978).
17. Papalia, Diane, and Sally W. Olds, *Human Development,* McGraw-Hill, New York, 1978, p. 236.
18. Ibid., p. 237.
19. Sieman, loc. cit.
20. Edwards, E., "Kindergarten Is Too Late," *Saturday Review* **51**:68–80 (June 1968).
21. Nyquist, E. D., and G. R. Hawes, *Open Education: A Sourcebook for Parents and Teachers,* Bantam, New York p. 2.
22. Sieman, loc. cit.
23. Colby, Anne, and Lawrence Kohlberg, "Relationship of Moral Judgement to Age," in "Invariant Sequence and Internal Consistency in Moral Judgement," in William M. Kurtines and Jacob Gewirtz (eds.), *Moral Behavior and Moral Development,* G. Allen, London, 1984, pp. 47–64.
24. Wilcox, Mary M., *Developmental Journey—A Guide to the Development of Logical and Moral Reasoning and Social Perspective,* Abingdon, Nashville, 1980.
25. Schuster, Clara S., and Shirley S. Ashburn, *The Process of Human Development: A Holistic Approach,* Little, Brown, Boston, 1980, pp. 542–548.
26. Ginott, Haim G., *Between Parent and Child,* Macmillan, New York, 1971, p. 58.
27. Wilcox, op. cit., p. 105.
28. Kohlberg, Lawrence, "Cognitive-Developmental Approach to Moral Education." in Peter Scharf (ed.), *Readings in Moral Education,* Winston, Minneapolis, 1978, p. 4.

13

Sally Winn Nicholson

The adolescent

Upon completion of this chapter, the student will be able to:

1 Define the terms *adolescence* and *puberty.*
2 Describe the nutritional requirements of an adolescent.
3 Describe the psychological development task of identity vs. role confusion.
4 Describe the adolescent's body-image changes.
5 Identify the functions of peer groups in adolescence.
6 Describe the adolescent's cognitive development.
7 Describe moral development during adolescence.
8 Describe accident prevention for adolescents.
9 Identify five guidelines to facilitate communication with teenagers.

Adolescents are the focus of a lot of public attention. It is unfortunately often true that the most conspicuous teenage activity is that which "causes problems" of one kind or another. Until there is trouble, people often do not notice what adolescents do, and a great deal of positive behavior goes unrecognized and unrewarded. Bandura[1] has suggested that a self-fulfilling prophecy may take place: Adults, having been brainwashed to expect trouble from adolescents, may unintentionally act in ways that foster problematical behavior.

No one exists in a vacuum, and this is perhaps most true of adolescents. They are subjected almost daily to a barrage of sexually stimulating books, magazines, and advertisements, and yet the reason behind their early sexual activity is questioned. Violence is glorified by television and movies, and yet when young people behave violently or commit crimes, people wonder why. Adolescents reflect the society in which they grow up; adults often lose sight of this fact.

Since World War II, teenagers have had to deal with threats unknown to previous generations: technological "advances" that make possible the destruction of the world or its inhabitants, pollution that makes the quality of life in some areas questionable, energy shortages, radical religious cults, and brainwashing and deprogramming. Little wonder, then, that an adolescent's attitude may be one of "live for today."

Our incredible technological advances also hold little for the teenager. A modern technological society cannot avoid alienating its young people from adult value systems.[2] Western technology and society have become so complex that it is increasingly difficult for adolescents to obtain the qualifications for entry into the adult world of work, economic independence, and social position. Advanced technology also fosters a relatively demanding, specialized, and impersonal approach to living that does not inspire much enthusiasm or commitment among young people. They often feel that western society has worshiped technological advances and has forgotten the humanistic and spiritual aspects of human development.

A further difficulty for adolescents is that there are few, if any, clear-cut landmarks to signify to them and others *when* a child has entered adolescence or when an adolescent has become an adult. In primitive societies, *rites of passage* mark these transitions and make each person's status as child, adolescent, or adult clear to everyone. In our own social practices, there are no universally recognized milestones into or out of adolescence, although Christian confirmation, the Jewish bar mitzvah and bat mitzvah, and marriage signify adolescent and adult status to some extent within some social subgroups. One important outcome of the uncertainty about when adolescence begins and ends is that many people, including adolescents themselves, have conflicting expectations about how "grown up" teenagers should be in various situations. One may be considered old enough to date but not old enough to drive a car on a date, for example, or old enough to choose to have an abortion but not old enough to sign a legal contract. Until a few years ago, young people could join the armed forces several years before they could vote. Adolescents often feel that they are expected to act like adults without receiving the privileges that accompany adulthood.

STAGES OF ADOLESCENCE

Adolescence is a roughly defined period that begins with puberty and ends with maturity. At puberty, one first becomes physically capable of reproduction. It is characterized by growth and maturation of the genital organs and by the appearance of secondary sex characteristics. Adolescence can be thought of as the period during which one adapts to these changes and incorporates them into one's self-concept.

While specific age groupings may not be applicable to a particular individual, they do make it easier to discuss characteristics in general. The age divisions used for the stages of adolescence are only guidelines for assessing adolescents, not absolutes. Each adolescent has her or his own developmental pace and schedule.[3]

Early adolescence

Early adolescence, usually from about 11 to 13 years of age in girls and from about 12 to 14 in boys, is characterized by the rapid physical and psychosocial changes that terminate childhood. Physical changes are pronounced, as will be described later, and the young adolescent is preoccupied with them and worries whether the changes are progressing normally and will "turn out all right." Early adolescents form strong loyalties to friends who are in about the same stage of physical maturity; childhood friendships tend to dissolve if some members of the friendship group begin their pubertal changes earlier than others. Family relationships become strained, especially between girls and their mothers, and fathers and their sons, as the young person begins the necessary but awkward process of loosening ties to parents and strengthening alliances with peers and adults outside the family. Most early adolescents decrease their involvement in family activities and tend to "put down" parents and resent parental criticism. Although early adolescents are not as strongly tied to the family as before, they also are not as firmly allied with the peer group as they will be in middle adolescence, and they move freely between the two.

Early adolescent males, because of their rapid growth, are often clumsy, lazy, and uninterested in their appearance. They may have to be reminded frequently of the need for good hygiene. Boys are acutely aware of the change in their genitals. They need to be reassured that masturbation is engaged in by virtually all teenage males and that it is normal—it will not cause hair to grow on their palms! Boys assess their masculinity primarily in relation to other boys by comparing their chest, muscle, and genital size and their capacity to ejaculate. Involvement in an all-male peer group provides support and a needed sense of security. Masturbation and other sexual experimentation with friends of the same sex is common, especially among boys, and at this age is not predictive of a homosexual orientation in later life. Seminal emissions, or "wet dreams," should be explained to boys, and when they occur, the vulnerable adolescent male should not be teased. Likewise, *gynecomastia*, the development of breast tissue in early adolescent males, should be explained as a normal consequence of temporary hormonal imbalances so that the young man does not suffer needlessly from doubts about his masculinity. Both boys and girls at this age are extremely sensitive to the opinions of others, and even gentle teasing can be very distressing.

Early adolescent girls may become intensely preoccupied with their physical appearance very early in puberty and often feel that, in a society that places such a premium on beauty, they do not measure up. The new stresses of becoming an adolescent, combined with hormonal fluctuations and imbalances, often cause them to be moody and tense. Girls compare breast size and menstrual function with one another but use boys to assess their femininity.

The young girl is vulnerable to sexual exploitation. If she is to develop a healthy sense of her sexuality, it is important that there be men in her life who care about her and do not view her as a sexual object. Fathers are often uncomfortable with their daughters as they begin to develop sexually. As a result, they may rebuff the girl's attentions and say, "You're too old to sit on my lap or hug or kiss me." The young adolescent is unable to perceive that her father is having difficulty dealing with the fact that she is growing up, and she often blames his changed behavior on herself. In extreme cases this misunderstanding may lead to embarrassment about, and dislike of, her developing body and make her journey through adolescence more difficult.

Girls, like boys, need accurate information about physical changes to expect during puberty. The young girl who has her first menstrual period without having received information beforehand will imagine that she is going to bleed to death or that she is terribly ill or injured. Even girls who have been adequately prepared for menstruation routinely call it "the curse." Often well-meaning parents make menstruation even more difficult to accept by insisting that the young girl curtail her activities, thereby making her feel that growing up is hampering her life.

Early adolescent girls often form intense attachments with a best friend of the same sex. Usually the attraction is based on complementing each other—one is looking to the other for some trait she would like in herself, and vice versa. By forming a close relationship with one who possesses this trait, it is almost as if she has it herself. She can examine her dress, behavior, and values through her friend's feedback. These early adolescent best friends are often inseparable and tend to dress, talk, and think alike. Hours are spent analyzing the minutest detail of behavior. The friendship usually does not stand the test of time well, however, for eventually one girl fails to live up to the standards the other has set, and the relationship crumbles. These intense relationships are replaced by peer group relationships in middle adolescence.

Girls are usually about 2 years ahead of boys the same age, not only in physical maturity but also in their capacity for imagination and abstract thought, in their ability to perceive the feelings of others, and in their tolerance for frustration. Girls often are quite creative and record their deepest thoughts and feelings in diaries, a prelude to the journals kept by adults.

Toward the end of early adolescence, both boys and girls begin fuller participation in their peer groups. At this time, while complaining about parental restrictions, they eagerly take on the restrictions imposed by the peer group. As they move away from the family, they have a new sense of belonging within the peer group.[4]

Middle adolescence

Middle adolescence is the period from about 13 to 16 years of age in girls and 14 to 17 years of age in boys. The period of most rapid physical change is past, and the adolescent now focuses somewhat less on growth and other body changes and becomes absorbed in personal identity: "Who am I?" "What will I do with my life?"

As a necessary part of developing a strong, personalized sense of self, middle adolescents typically become rather harsh critics of parents and other authoritative adults and of their attitudes and values. As they "declare independence" from their families, they become intensely involved in their peer groups and the adolescent subculture. Adolescents mimic peers and other acquaintances and public figures they admire,

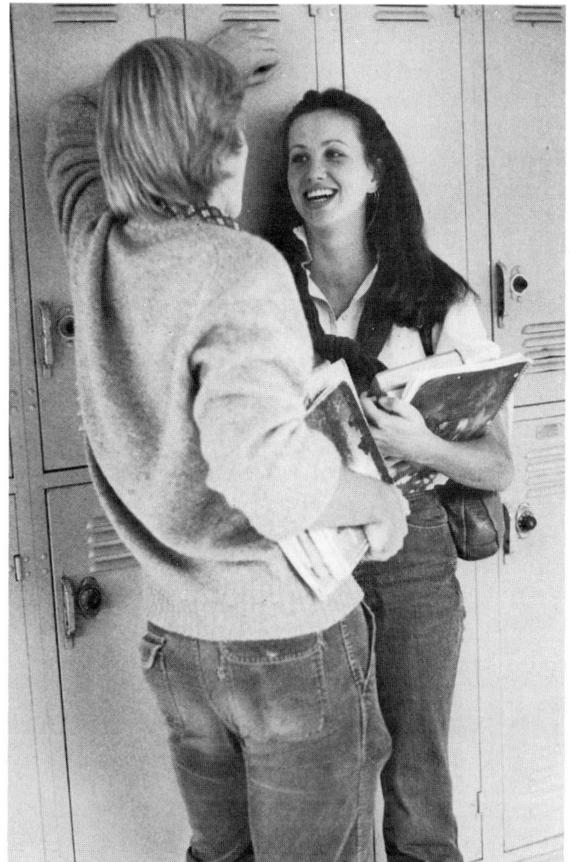

Figure 13-1 Intense boy-girl relationships are part of middle adolescence.

borrowing portions of the behavior and opinions of these people as part of the process of establishing who they are and what they want to be like. Some career planning takes place at this age. Dating is usual, and romantic and sexual interests or activities are a preoccupation for many middle adolescents (see Fig. 13-1).

Late adolescence

Late adolescence usually lasts from about age 16 or 17 to age 21. Physical changes are far less apparent than earlier, as the growth process draws to a close. In late adolescence young people step up their preparations for living an adult life-style. They must now make career choices, an important step toward financial independence.

Intimacy and maintaining an intimate relationship with another person are developmental goals of late adolescence. The large peer group often is replaced by a smaller group of closer friends, and dating activities commonly become narrowed to one or a small number of dating partners; many adolescents marry or form other exclusive love relationships during this period. Before adolescents can engage in genuine psychological intimacy with others, they must have a fairly firm sense of personal identity. Intimacy requires sharing one's inner self, and they cannot share what they do not yet have; moreover, such self-exposure causes anxiety until identity is secure.

Relationships with parents are far less stormy as young people become increasingly confident about their independence and therefore find adult guidance and advice less threatening. Parents and adolescents begin to develop a new relationship in which they enjoy one another as adults.

Late adolescents also typically become involved in issues that have to do with their concern about the future of the society in which they are about to take their place as adults. They devote much energy to the issues of peace, ecology, population control, and racial harmony.

In summary, late adolescents are involved in applying the psychosocial development that has built up during childhood and the earlier adolescent years. They are putting the final touches on their readiness to function as adults. Maturity in late adolescence is characterized by the capacity to be loving, to put the welfare of others before one's own pleasure, to wait for emotional gratification, to control aggression and impulsivity, and to plan for the future.

PHYSICAL DEVELOPMENT

Adolescence causes pronounced changes in body size, structure, and shape. One-fourth of adult height is acquired during the adolescent growth spurt, which begins at about age 10 in girls and at about age 13 in boys. Children of both sexes approximately double their weight between 10 and 18 years of age. The extremities grow first; this fact is responsible for the young adolescent's characteristic "leggy," gangly appearance and large hands and feet. The hips, chest, and shoulders widen next, and finally the trunk and spinal cord lengthen so that adult height is reached. Girls usually achieve their full height by 17, and boys by 21. The longer growth period of males results in their usually having greater height, larger muscles, a larger heart and larger lungs, bigger skeletal frame, and a larger oxygen-carrying capacity of the blood at maturity than most females.

If the nurse were to observe a group of 13-year-old boys and girls, marked differences in stage of physical maturity would be apparent. Some of the young adolescents would be *prepubertal* children (not yet beginning puberty), some would be just starting their pubertal changes, and others would be close to their adult height and weight.

The triggering mechanism by which puberty occurs is unknown, but it is clear that hormonal changes play a central role in producing the increased growth rate and sex differences that take place in early adolescence. An increase in the production of gonadotropin-releasing factor (GnRF) from the hypothalamus causes increased pituitary secretion of gonadotropins (follicle-stimulating hormone [FSH] and luteinizing hormone [LH]), and these hormones in turn cause the gonads to increase their production of estrogen and testosterone, as shown in Fig. 13-2. Estrogen and testosterone are responsible for the maturation of the genital organs and the development of the secondary sex characteristics (voice changes, breast development, and growth of pubic, facial, and axillary hair). Under the influence of the pubertal hormone changes, females acquire a characteristically rounded body. The hips widen to accommodate childbirth, the breasts enlarge, and adipose tissue is laid down in the breasts, hips, and thighs. Estrogen also stimulates uterine endometrial and vaginal growth and accelerates linear growth and skeletal maturation. In males, testosterone stimulates the growth of pubic, axillary, and facial hair; accelerates skeletal growth and maturation; produces the male characteristics of broad shoulders, large chest, and narrow hips; and increases the number and size of muscle cells. The sexual development of adolescents of both sexes is further described below.

Female physical development

Pubertal changes in females are assessed according to breast development and pubic hair growth. In American girls the average age of *thelarche* (initial breast development) is 10.8 years. *Pubarche* (first appearance of pubic hair) follows soon after, at the average age of 11 years. *Menarche* (first menstruation), which is widely used as the indication that adolescence has begun, is

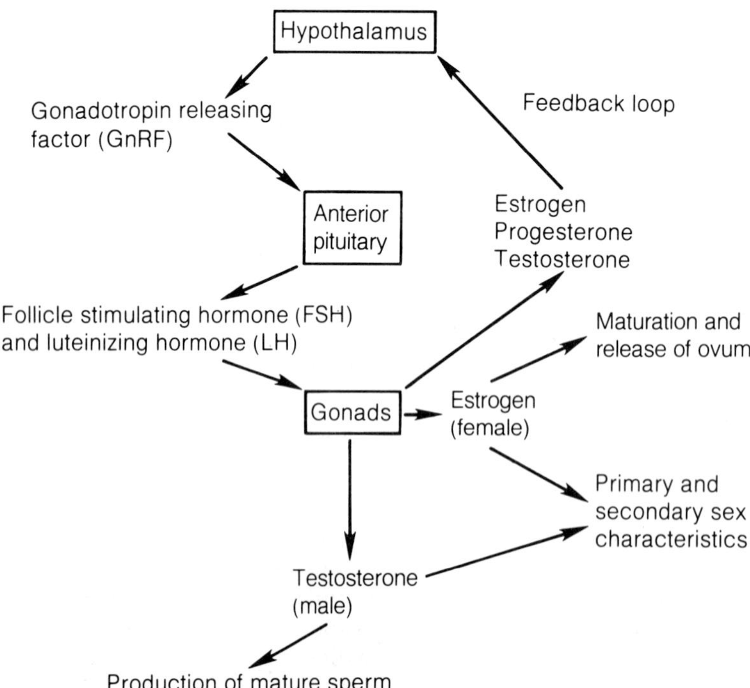

Figure 13-2 Hormonal interactions of sexual maturity.

actually a rather late event in puberty and does not occur until the average girl is within 3 or 4 in of her adult height. The average age at menarche among American girls is reported to range between 12.6 and 12.9 years, but it is not unusual for menarche to take place as early as 10 or as late as 16. Over the past century or so, the age at which girls first menstruate has declined. This earlier maturation may be due to better nutrition, better medical care of children with severe illness, and other environmental factors. A direct relationship may exist between height, weight, and onset of puberty; i.e., it may be that when a "critical" weight for a given height is attained, adolescent maturation begins. In the United States, menarche occurs at an average height of 158.5 cm and a weight of 43 kg (ranging from 32 to 60 kg).

J. M. Tanner[5] has developed a standard method of assessing and classifying physical development in adolescence. Tanner's five stages of female maturation are reviewed in Table 13-1. Figure 13-3 shows the average ages at which the stages are reached.

Other aspects of physical development can be expected to occur in conjunction with certain of Tanner's stages. For example, the adolescent height spurt begins in stage 2. Total body fat increases, the hips widen, and, with breast enlargement, the adult female form begins to emerge.

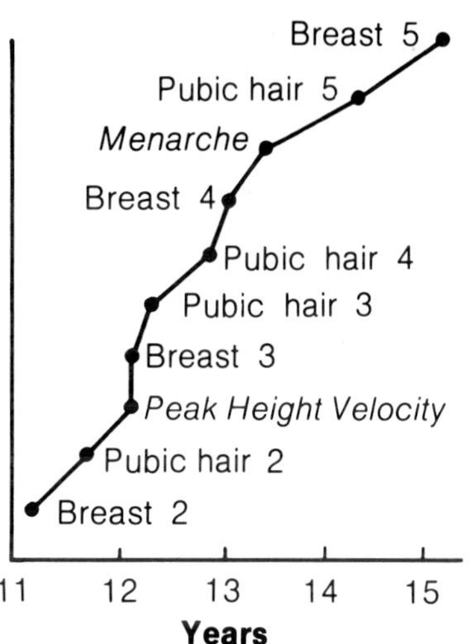

Figure 13-3 The sequence and mean ages of pubertal events in females. *(Adapted from the data of Marshall and Tanner. The numbers refer to Tanner's growth stages, described in Table 13-1. From A. Root, "Endocrinology of Puberty," Journal of Pediatrics* **83***(7):1–19 [July 1978].)*

Table 13-1 Stages of Female Maturation

Stage	Breast	Pubic hair
1	Only the papilla shows elevation	None
2	Breast bud appears as a small mound formed by the elevation of the breast and papilla. Areola increases in diameter	Sparse, long, slightly pigmented, downy. It is straight or only slightly curled, primarily along the labia
3	Further enlargement of breast and areola with no separation of their contours	More widespread, darker, coarser, curlier
4	Areola and papilla may rise to form a secondary mound above the level of the breast	Adult in type but not as widespread
5	Areola has recessed to general breast contour. Breast is now mature	Adult in type, quantity, and distribution pattern

Source: J. M. Tanner, *Growth at Adolescence*, Blackwell, Oxford, 1962.

In stage 3, the vagina enlarges, and the vaginal epithelium, under estrogen stimulation from the ovaries, increases in thickness. *Döderlein's bacillus*, which is actually a group of microorganisms that produce lactic acid, appears in vaginal mucus, making the vaginal environment acidic and thereby protecting it against pathogenic bacteria. The height spurt reaches its peak late in stage 3.

If menarche did not occur late in stage 3, it occurs in stage 4. Axillary hair appears just before or just afterward. Ovulation during the first few menstrual cycles is rare; hence most early adolescent girls are infertile.

Male physical development

Pubertal progress in males is measured according to genital growth and pubic hair development. In the United States, pubic hair appears in males between 11.5 and 11.8 years of age on the average. The pubertal growth spurt is accompanied by an increase in number and size of muscle cells, which leads to the greater muscular strength of the male.

Tanner's classification of male maturation is reviewed in Table 13-2. Figure 13-4 shows the

Table 13-2 Stages of Male Maturation

Stage	Genitalia	Pubic hair	Facial hair
1	Penis, testes, and scrotum are of childhood size	None	Like that in childhood
2	Scrotum and testes enlarge, but not penis. Scrotal skin reddens	Sparse, long, slightly pigmented, downy. It is straight or slightly curled, primarily at base of penis	Little change
3	Continued growth of scrotum and testes. Penis grows mainly in length	Darker, coarser, curlier, spreading sparsely over the junction of the pubes	About 50% of males show a small amount of short, lightly pigmented hair at corners of upper lip and on sides of face in front of ears
4	Continued growth. Penis grows mainly in width	Adult in type but not as widespread	Moderate amount of short, lightly pigmented, coarse down on upper lip; also long, fine unpigmented hair on cheeks and occasionally along borders of the chin
5	Adult in size	Adult in type, quantity, and distribution pattern	Conspicuous growth on upper lip. Longer, more pigmented hair on sides of face

Source: J. M. Tanner, *Growth at Adolescence,* Blackwell, Oxford, 1962.

average ages at which Tanner's stages are reached. The rapid gain in weight and height begins in stage 1. There is also an increase in body fat. These trends continue in stage 2, and the male physique begins to appear. The height spurt continues through stage 3. The shoulders broaden, and muscle mass increases in proportion to fat. The cartilage of the larynx enlarges, and the voice begins to deepen. In stage 4, axillary hair appears, the voice deepens, and the boy may experience ejaculation. There is a distinct enlargement of the breasts with a slight projection of the areola. The conspicuous breast enlargement (gynecomastia) ends in stage 5 as hormonal balance is established and the body reaches adult form.

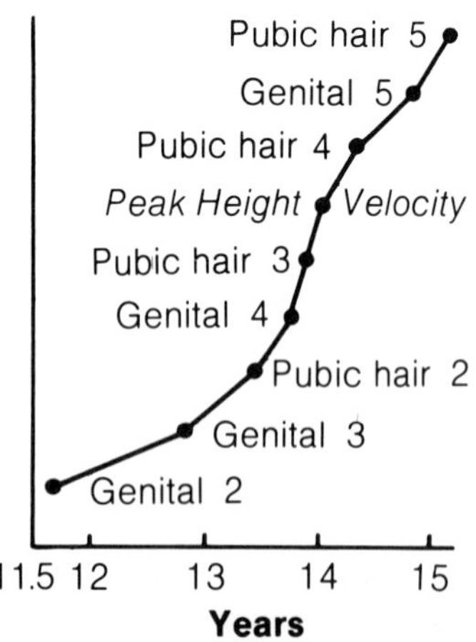

Figure 13-4 The sequence and mean ages of pubertal events in males. (*Adapted from the data of Marshall and Tanner. The numbers refer to Tanner's growth stages, described in Table 13-2. From A. Root, "Endocrinology of Puberty," Journal of Pediatrics* **83***(7):1–19 [July 1978].)*

PSYCHOSOCIAL DEVELOPMENT

Emotional characteristics of adolescents

The emotional status of adolescents is often unpredictable and labile (changeable). Teenagers live enthusiastically in the present, reaching emotional heights (see Fig. 13-5). They may quickly then plunge to the depths of moodiness and depression. These emotional outbursts may be precipitated by what seem to be minor events to parents but are interpreted as major crises by teenagers.

All teenagers occasionally lose control of themselves in an emotional outburst; this outburst releases accumulated anxiety. They then feel guilty, fear future loss of control, and retreat to reassess their behavior. They plan methods of maintaining self-control in the future, and later they reassert themselves. Teenagers may daydream deeply, not hearing others talking to them. The unstable emotions or behavior of adoles-

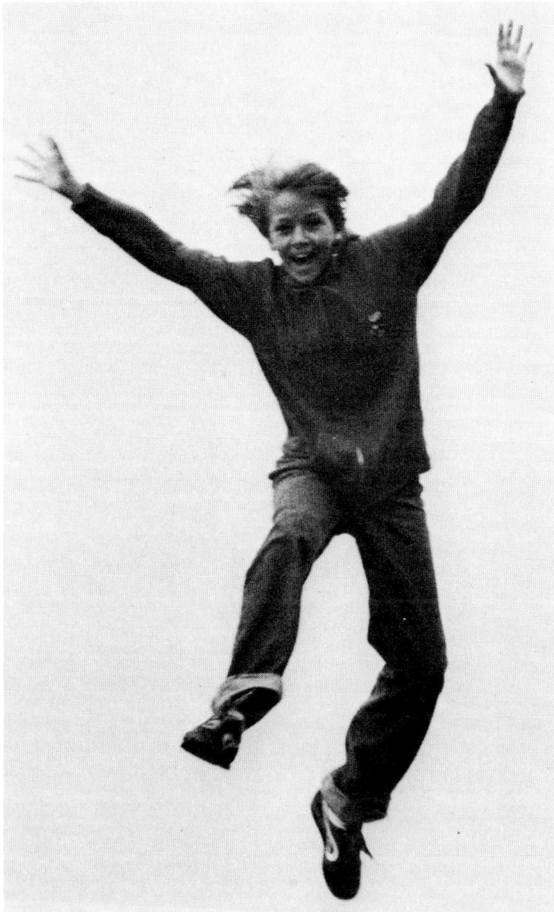

Figure 13-5 The teenager enjoys life to the fullest.

cents should not be ridiculed. Parents should be advised to allow teenagers time to be alone. Parents should accept their feelings, saying, "It's okay to be angry," and then discuss other ways to express anger the next time: "What else can you do when you're so angry?" They should avoid immediately criticizing the outburst of behavior, since teenagers will usually quickly regain self-control; they should be praised for this.

Developmental task: Identity vs. role confusion

Before puberty, school-age children have a well-developed self-identity. From infancy on they have developed their sex role identity, their moral standards, and their various roles as members of their families, neighborhoods, and school groups. They know how other people feel about them (a C student, shy, good-looking, athletic, etc.), and they are fully familiar with their own bodies and abilities. But adolescence brings many extensive changes that put the childhood sense of self out of date; one cannot be the same at 15 as one was at 10 or 12. By the end of adolescence one must be a worker or homemaker (or both), not a schoolchild. One must be a person who makes provisions for day-to-day needs, not one who is taken care of by parents. Adolescents must make some satisfactory adaptation to their new sexual maturity. They must develop their own standards of behavior, which necessarily vary from their childhood beliefs.

Adolescence, then, is dominated by the process of becoming someone rather different from the person one was as a child. Accordingly, the main developmental task of adolescence is to build a new sense of personal identity, and adolescent psychosocial development is directly related to accomplishing this task. Erik Erikson[6] has described the sense of *identity* as the feeling that one's self (personality) has continuity (consistency and predictability) and that one's self-appraisal is essentially the same as the views other people have about one. According to Erikson, failure to accomplish the adolescent developmental task of achieving identity is *role confusion,* in which adolescents lack a firm sense of inner sameness; they feel they are not who people think they are, and they have chameleon-like fluctuations in life goals, personal beliefs, or ways of relating to others. It must be understood that identity is not attained all at once and that a firm sense of identity is not to be expected before the end of the adolescent period.

During adolescence the earlier developmental tasks are reworked so that adolescents can master them in an adult way rather than in the earlier ways that were appropriate to childhood. They now reestablish trust, not with the mother, but within peer friendships, relationships with non-parent adults, and, eventually, intimate heterosexual relationships. Their struggle for autonomy now centers not on resisting the control of the mother but on establishing themselves as individuals whose activities and beliefs are under their own control, rather than dominated by the family. Initiative is tested anew as adolescents put themselves into dating situations and other unfamiliar experiences. Industriousness now focuses on entering or preparing to enter the competitive arenas of employment or post-high school education.

While establishing who they are, adolescents

experience periods of self-doubt. Several factors contribute to this inner uncertainty. These young people no longer feel in control of their bodies or know just what to expect from them. The growth spurt produces a larger, unfamiliar, and sometimes awkward and displeasing body. New thoughts about oneself and changing attitudes toward parents are confusing and upsetting. Sexuality is something new and must be dealt with in some way. The peer group on which adolescents rely for a sounding board is itself quite changeable and uncertain. As social experience expands into new arenas, young people have to learn new roles and adapt to new expectations. They are frequently dissatisfied with their own performance and feel pessimistic about ever becoming the kind of persons they would like to be. Society, itself changing, offers little in the way of clear, universally approved standards for behavior or goals for the future.

Incorporating physical changes into identity Adolescents experience changes in height, weight, body build, and secondary sex characteristics. Because so many changes occur at once, the early adolescent's body often does not feel like his or her own. A boy's body may also betray him by its awkwardness, sudden changes in voice, or an embarrassing sexual response. Breast development and the onset of the menses often occur before a young girl feels she is ready to cope with them.

Teenagers believe that their bodies are the main criterion by which others will accept or reject them, and therefore they become acutely aware of their bodies. They spend hours inspecting themselves for a blemish or imperfection. In a society that idealizes the perfect beauty, one pimple can cause the adolescent to despair. The teenager's body must meet peer group standards. The tall girl, the short boy, or the obese or handicapped teenager of either sex will have a difficult time winning peer acceptance. Illnesses that impair the development of primary or secondary sexual characteristics may have serious psychological and social consequences. An 18-year-old male who looks age 12, a girl of 11 who has fully developed breasts, and a young woman of 18 whose breasts have not fully developed may suffer greatly from real or imagined unacceptance by peers.

An important aspect of identity is *body image*, the mental picture one has of one's own body. When physical changes occur, the body image must be revised to incorporate the changes. Revising the body image takes time, as anyone can attest who has gotten a new hairstyle and is surprised for a few days when looking in a mirror. The rapid physical changes of early adolescence take time to incorporate into the body image. This lag between body configuration and body image accounts in part for the young adolescent's awkwardness; for example, a teenage male may bump into objects because he has not become accustomed to his new size. The desire to update one's body image in order to feel familiar with one's body is one reason why adolescents, especially young ones, are so preoccupied with their appearance and with examining themselves in photographs and mirrors.

All people are critical of their own body image, but adolescents are especially so. Teenagers are renowned for thinking they are too fat, too tall, too thin, too short, or in some other way not built satisfactorily. Adults need to refrain from giving verbal reassurance. Adolescents need acceptance and recognition that these feelings are real. This helps them move toward self-acceptance.

Development of independence: Relationships with parents In order to become people who will, as adults, make their own decisions and provide for their own needs, teenagers have to reduce drastically their childhood reliance on parents. Both teenagers and parents usually experience considerable stress and strain in making the necessary role realignments. Parents feel uneasy about turning over their previous functions as supervisor, protector, adviser, and decision maker to teenagers, who are inexperienced and whose judgment is relatively untested. Adolescents are often awkward and ambivalent about making the transition toward independence. Early and middle adolescents may protest that almost any parental interaction is "interference," but they may fluctuate between insisting that they are grown up and then at times behaving quite childishly or expecting parents to do things they can do for themselves.

Middle adolescents refight the battle of the preschool period: ambivalence toward the same-sex parent and a romantic attachment to the parent of the opposite sex. Working through these relationships helps the adolescent move on to love relationships outside the family. The teenager vacillates between emulating the same-sex parent and irritably trying to prove how different he or she is. The parent of the opposite sex is at times viewed through rose-colored glasses. Hence mother-son and father-daughter relationships are frequently smoother than those between parents and adolescents of the same sex, and the stage is set for family conflict unless the parents consistently agree on how to respond to their child.

Adolescence is as difficult a time for parents as it is for their teenagers. Parents have historically raised their children the way they were raised. In today's advanced society, that is no longer easy. Adolescents today have access to the vast array of all our society has to offer. They are courted by the media to use their significant purchasing power to buy cosmetics, clothes, records, magazines, cars, etc. Parents want to provide their children with more than they had but are often hard-pressed financially to do so.

Conflicts frequently occur over such issues as curfew, study hours, friends, dress, makeup, and allowance. Teenagers constantly test the limits set by parents, who interpret this to mean that teenagers want no limits placed on their behavior. The opposite is true. They want and need limits as an expression of their parents' love and concern. Adolescents who have no parental rules governing their behavior often are secretly envious of their peers who have curfews or other family rules to follow. Teenagers need to know that their parents have controls on which they can depend. The parent who sets no limits will make adolescence more difficult for all concerned. Consistent discipline strengthens teenagers' security.

A frequent struggle between adolescents and their parents centers on the issue of privileges. Parents usually view privileges as being earned by responsible behavior. Because the behavior of most adolescents vacillates between that of a mature adult and that of a toddler who throws tantrums, it is hard for parents to decide how much responsibility to give them.

Parents who have unresolved conflicts from their own adolescence will have a more difficult time raising a teenager. Parents who were raised in a controlling family may be too lax with their own children, and those raised in an exceedingly permissive environment may be too controlling. Parental expectations are often greater than teenagers can be expected to meet, causing unhappiness and frustration for all. The son who is expected to be a better football player than his father and the daughter who is expected to follow in her mother's footsteps and become a nurse are rarely seen by parents as having the right to make their own life choices. Parental attitudes have a significant effect on adolescent behavior, as Table 13-3 shows.

Adolescents and their parents live best in an atmosphere of mutual trust. Teenagers need to know that they can depend on their parents' love and support. Parents need to be able to trust that their teenagers will use good judgment in making decisions. Perhaps the areas of greatest difficulty are sexuality and drugs. The age of first intercourse continues to be lower, and the incidence of teenage pregnancy rises. Many parents are justifiably concerned that their teenagers will become involved in a sexual relationship before they are able to handle it (see Chap. 25). Likewise, with adolescent drug use rampant and many students attending classes "high," parents are frightened about the use of drugs and their effect. However, parents who have always attempted to keep the line of communication with their children open will have a closer relationship than parents who periodically search their teenagers' possessions for drugs and birth control devices.

By late adolescence, parent-child relationships usually improve markedly; both the teenager and the parents have gained confidence in the young person's increasing ability to manage himself or herself, and the fears and frustrations of both have lessened considerably. Until this time comes, parents need to maintain their own "center," a sense of keeping calm while living in the eye of a hurricane. When parents can maintain their control while adolescents are losing theirs, teenagers will feel more secure in their periods of instability, uncertainty, and regression.

There are four ways in which adolescents achieve their emancipation from parents:*

1. Teenagers may abruptly leave home and subsequently be viewed as adults.
2. Adolescents may gradually move from being dependent children to becoming independent adults without ever having left home. As inflation soars and as rents and the cost of living increase, many young people are continuing to live at home. This gradual role change while remaining in the parents' residence may complicate and extend the separation struggle.
3. Young people may leave home to be independent, and then feel the need for the family unit and move back home. This pattern will be repeated until they are finally able to manage independently away from home.

*This section on the four ways of achieving emancipation was written by Jean I. Clarke.

Table 13-3 Influence of Parents on Adolescent Behavior

Parental attitude or behavior	Adolescent reaction or behavior
1. Overcoercive: rigid, demanding, very high, and controlled standards for children. Perfectionistic, compulsive, often belittling or punitive, or both (child can't possibly satisfy)	1. (*a*) Adoption of same behavior; hypercritical of self, drives self ("workaholic"); *or* (*b*) rebellion or resistance, or both (active or passive): to protect his or her individuality; *or* (*c*) withdrawal or regression or somatic symptoms, or all three: downgrades self, poor self-esteem, depression
2. Overpermissive (indulgent): oversubmission, overindulgence, unable or unwilling to set limits, rarely punish or deny child privileges or gratification	2. Decreased capacity for self-control; increased need for immediate gratification. Bored and not easily impressed. Expects much reward without effort or responsibility. Needs and seeks new thrills and pleasures
3. Overprotective: shielding child from ordinary or imaginary hazards of living. Parent(s) often have phobias; may be narrow or generalized fear. Parent(s) may have guilt and fear of retribution and therefore overprotect	3. (*a*) Fearful person with lowered self-esteem, decreased curiosity, and fear of new experiences; *or* (*b*) anger at having been so restricted; rebellious toward parent(s) who have caused the adolescent's fears and bad feelings about self
4. Rejecting: feelings of not wanting or not loving the child openly or subtly conveyed by parent(s). Ambivalent feelings conveyed or actual neglect or belittling behavior. Child may be scapegoat or "black sheep" or actually unwanted. Distrustful: parent has little faith and tends to assume child has same weaknesses as parent	4. Child feels unwanted or unloved, may retaliate and evoke further rejection. Feeling of worthlessness; poor self-concept. Strangers are perceived as rejecting. Defenses used—aggression, self-aggrandizement, withdrawal, clowning (all these interfere with interpersonal relationships). Child yearns for friendships; has great need for acceptance and approval. May develop strong talents or skill or close relationships. Child tends to fulfill the parents' distrust
5. Symbiotic: abnormally close tie between one parent, usually the mother, and a child. Prevents normal contact with peers and outside world. "You and I against the world" attitude	5. Damaged self-concept: doesn't develop independent personality. Feels inadequate when separated. Social relationships and curiosity are damaged. As adolescent realizes handicap, anger and hostility develop to parent and others
6. Vicarious: the parent lives through the child. Pressure on child to achieve in areas important to parent	6. At first compliance, then anxiety, and finally rebellion or withdrawal. Self-concept suffers since never quite lives up to parent's expectations. Socialization may suffer because of narrowing of activities
7. Inconsistent: opposite of rigidity, rules constantly changing. Parents unpredictable in their response. Often marital disharmony, alcohol, or drug abuse	7. Adolescent may show frustration, anxiety; may withdraw, or may rebel
8. Neglectful: parents who show lack of responsibility or actual emotional or physical abuse of their children	8. Self-esteem damaged, not able to trust or rely on others. Seeks out others (individuals or groups, e.g., "gangs") to substitute for parents. Often angry

Source: G. Comerci, E. Lightner, and R. Hansen, *Adolescent Medicine Case Studies*, Medical Examination Publishing, New York, 1979, pp. 510–511.

4. Adolescents who need a "kick" out of the family nest may be ready to leave but unable to do so. Through repetitions of unacceptable behavior, they force the family to provide the impetus to leave, often in the form of a parental order to pack their belongings and go.

Relationships with peers The peer group plays an essential role for adolescents. It provides security and support as teenagers separate from their families. Peer groups are usually made up of people of the same sex in early adolescence, in midadolescence are composed of one or both sexes, and in late adolescence incorporate couples. Within these groups, conversation revolves around school, clothes, and the opposite sex. The insular safety of the peer group allows adolescents to practice adult roles, social skills, and communication with the opposite sex. Peers provide a group conscience to determine appropriate behaviors and a review board to pass judgment on actions that have already taken place. There are teenagers who "march to their own drummer" and reject or are rejected by the peer group. The lives of most adolescents, however, are centered on the peer group. It dictates how they walk, talk, act, and dress. To behave differently is to risk exclusion from the group, a risk that most adolescents are unwilling to take. Adolescents need others like themselves with whom to share the joys and sorrows experienced in the transition from childhood to adulthood.

The adolescent peer group is a subculture of society. A subculture has distinctly different values, sets of expectations, and approved behaviors that separate it from the mainstream of society. The members of a subculture may have insecure, fragile self-concepts and therefore isolate themselves from threatening outside opinions. They live in protected, closed environments that insulate them from potentially threatening influences. This isolation reinforces their acceptance of only rigidly approved behaviors. Much of the adolescent's seemingly strange behavior can be explained by understanding the characteristics of a subgroup. Every subculture has the following characteristics:

1. There is a distinctive communication system—for example, slang—which reduces communication with outside groups, such as parents.
2. There are distinctive behaviors that isolate members of the subculture and help them identify with their chosen peer groups. This isolation also reinforces their own rigid definitions of acceptable behavior. Earmarks of the adolescent subculture include distinctive dress, dance, hairstyles, body posturing, and other nonverbal behavior.
3. Accepted behaviors change quickly, even every few days.

Identification with, and participation in, the adolescent subculture provides opportunities to try out (and eventually adopt, adapt, or discard) many attitudes and behaviors of other people who are not members of one's family. This experience provides a necessary bridge for emancipating oneself from the overinfluence of parents and finally developing one's own sense of identity, which makes mimicking others unnecessary. In middle adolescence, teenagers readily adopt the peer group's style of dress, language, ideas, and values. Gang activity is seen in some lower economic groups. Gangs are usually made up of young people with a poor or negative sense of identity. (See Chap. 37.) By becoming part of a gang, they achieve a status and recognition they would not have otherwise. Unfortunately, the destructive activities that the gang engages in may hamper the adolescent's chances of becoming a successful, contributing member of society.

Peer activities and dating During early adolescence, boys and girls tend to remain socially separate and to join in group activities (Fig. 13-6). Young teenagers frequently participate in sports and attend athletic events in groups. Each teenager shares his or her most intimate confidences with a best friend. Girls frequently spend hours at the mirror perfecting their hairstyles and makeup. They also spend tremendous amounts of time talking on the telephone—a potential source of family conflict. Teenagers use the telephone to share ideas, judge their clothes according to the peer group's standards of dress, and seek support from peers. Today's trend toward early dating is evidenced in group dating at school dances by the eighth or ninth grade.

During middle adolescence, an automobile or motorcycle is the optimal status symbol among peers. The "wheels" allow increased freedom and independence from parents. Many young people get part-time jobs, which give them an opportunity to earn spending money and to practice adult roles without assuming the responsibilities of an adult breadwinner. For a teenager who is unable to find a job, the lack of money may severely limit group participation. By the tenth grade, couples pair up and go on group dates.

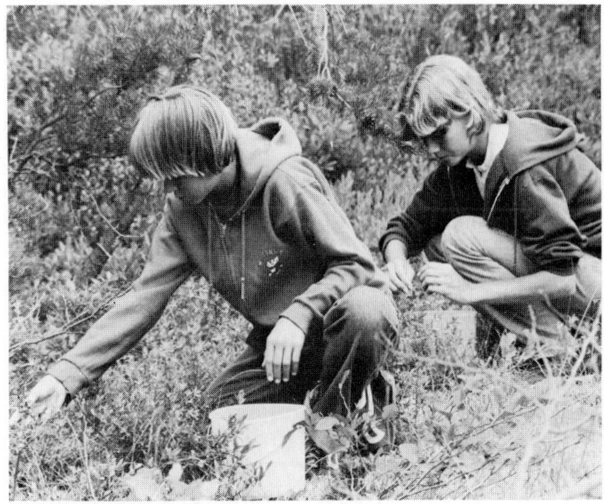

Figure 13-6 Adolescents enjoy activities with peers.

Older adolescents continue to enjoy attending rock concerts, listening to their stereos, reading, and having conversations. Double dating is common in the eleventh grade, and single dating in the twelfth grade.

Throughout adolescence, dating is a means of discovering self-identity through interaction with others. "Going steady" means not having to worry about having a date and gives teenagers a sense of security and belonging. The young person who is sexually promiscuous is often searching for sexual identity but has not yet achieved that goal. A broad range of social and sex role–related skills as well as more specifically sexual attitudes and behaviors are gradually refined by dating, and each refinement brings the young person closer to a sense of identity. Young and middle adolescents use dating primarily as a medium for finding out who they are and how others feel about them. It is generally not until late adolescence that love in the sense of deep concern for the well-being of the other person is possible.

Sexuality and sex role identity The adolescent must achieve a mature sexual identity—an understanding and acceptance of self as a sexual male or a sexual female. Young adolescents often have difficulty accepting their maturing bodies, particularly when they appear to be changing almost daily. Girls, especially those who mature earlier than their friends, often slouch and wear baggy clothing to hide their breasts and hips. The pleasure of becoming an adult male is mixed with displeasure for the young man who experiences ill-timed erections.

Psychosexual development Freud has termed adolescence the *genital stage* of psychosexual development. The Oedipus conflict of the preschool years reemerges; the teenager becomes extremely critical of and rejects the same-sex parent, while loving and subconsciously wanting to possess the opposite-sex parent. The older teenager feels new sexual urges as a result of the secretion of secondary sex hormones and frequently fears loss of control over these urges. The teenager must, then, channel these sexual urges in socially acceptable ways. Today's adolescents do this by finding sexual partners. Many teenagers are sexually active by age 17 but resist using birth control methods regularly. (See Chap. 25.) Teenagers also relieve sexual tension by masturbating. Non-sexually active teenagers masturbate frequently.

Adolescents also normally progress through a homosexual stage that is self-limiting and acts to strengthen sex role identity to prepare them for heterosexual relationships. Close same-sex friendships, manifested in "chum" relationships and hero worship, help reinforce the teenager's ego strength, which is necessary in order to become independent from the parents.

As adolescents progress toward adulthood, they must integrate the biological and psychological aspects of sexuality into their lives. Sexuality is a major theme of adolescence. Sexual self-concept, sex roles, and sexual behavior are affected by each young person's past experiences as a male or female and by his or her ideas about what it means to be a man or a woman.

Society has an impact on adolescent sexuality. Social values and cultural patterns vary according to the adolescent's social subgroup and the times in which he or she lives. Economic and political conditions and laws regulating marriage, contraception, abortion, drinking, and equal rights influence sex roles and sexual behavior. The feminist movement has loosened sex role restrictions for both men and women, and now marriage, child rearing, and careers outside the home are truly options for all. In many segments of society, greater permissiveness has developed in recent years; and marriage is no longer the only setting in which sexual intimacy and long-term love relationships are acceptable. While these social changes give young people a wider range of options, they also can make choosing life-styles and life goals more confusing.

As has been pointed out earlier, adolescents actively involve other people in their search for identity. Sexual self-concept and sex role identity are largely developed in an interpersonal context. By middle adolescence, teenagers want to feel that they are attractive to members of the opposite sex, and many are eager to try out their own sexual capacities. Preoccupation with one's own and others' physical attractiveness intensifies (Fig. 13-7). Crushes and going steady are common ways of experimenting with adult romantic and sexual behavior.

According to Feinstein, adolescents pass through four stages of sexual development:[8]

1. *Sexual awakening* Usually between ages 13 and 15, adolescents are confronted with their body image in comparison with their peers' bodies. They scrutinize and compare breast or penis size, height, weight, and pubic hair

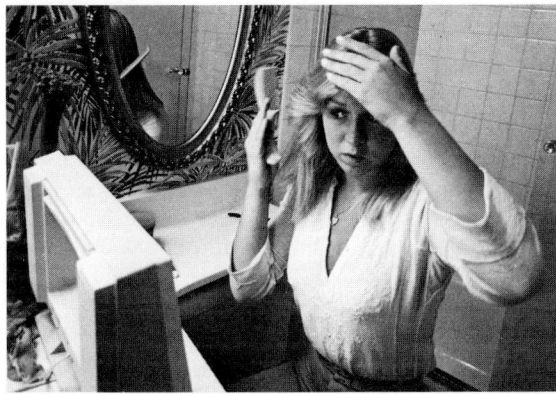

Figure 13-7 Middle adolescents strive for physical perfection.

development. These comparisons can be devastating if the teenager is "out of sync" with the peer group.

2. *Practicing stage* Generally extending from about age 14 to 17, this involves experimenting with and practicing the social skills necessary to form intimate relationships. Often the skills valued by the family and society are not those valued by the peer group, and therefore conflict results for the adolescent.
3. *Acceptance of sexual role* Between the ages of about 16 and 19, the adolescent develops a sense of comfort with the sexual role he or she has chosen. Couple dating replaces some of the activities that earlier involved the larger peer group.
4. *Permanent relationship choice* This stage may take place between ages 18 and 25 or so and is often delayed by prolonged post-high school education. In choosing a life partner, the adolescent must also decide between either a fairly traditional marriage, in which the husband is responsible for family support and finances and the wife is responsible for the home and children and usually does not have a career, or a companionship marriage, in which mutual love and support are considered most important and the responsibilities for financial support and nurturing the family are shared.

Career choice In order to achieve adult status and to acquire the part of identity that has to do with occupation, adolescents must work out an adequate career choice. This choice must be one that is compatible with their sense of who they are, and it must gain them self-sufficiency and recognition from family and friends.

Career choice usually begins to be an issue in middle adolescence, and many teenagers take part-time jobs at that time. Work gives them a sense of responsibility, reduces their financial dependence on parents, and allows them to experience the work role and a particular kind of work. Working also gives teenagers a glimpse of their own adulthood, which is rapidly approaching, without the extensive responsibilities of an adult's career commitment and management of a home.

Independence, which includes financial independence, is an important goal of adolescents. For many young people, the temptation to quit school and take a full-time job is strong. However, most people who go to work without graduating from high school, and often also those who do not acquire post-high school career training, put themselves at a disadvantage in terms of competing in the job market. Hence, many who begin work early instead of going on to school find that they cannot qualify for the kind of work that would give them the degree of financial independence they desire. Those who do choose post-high school education or other career training usually continue to depend on their families for economic support until their career preparation is completed. In this era of high technology and specialization, the length of graduate and postgraduate training programs may prevent the young person from achieving financial independence until his or her middle or late twenties.

Cognitive development

According to Piaget, between approximately 11 and 12 years of age, the final stage of cognitive development takes place. The adolescent enters the stage of *formal operations* and acquires adult cognitive capacities. Formal operations are characterized by abstract thinking. People at this stage now become capable of thinking *hypothetically;* that is, they are no longer limited to thinking only about things they have experienced or observed but can conceptualize beyond the realm of reality to reason about things that are contrary to fact or beyond the range of possibility. They can conceptualize the worlds of historical and future time and geographical and celestial space.[9] The adolescent is able to understand and use the rules of logic for the first time and can think both deductively and inductively.

The person in the stage of formal operations grasps symbolic meanings and hence can appreciate and interpret jokes with double meanings, art forms such as symbolic poetry and abstract paintings, and sayings like "A rolling stone gathers no moss." This person's understanding goes beyond the surface meanings of things, and he or she picks up subtleties and deeper meanings.

The capacity to use abstract thought has a lot to do with the adolescent's general behavior. For example, the formulation of a personal code of ethics or a set of religious beliefs requires the ability to think about hypothetical possibilities beyond the scope of one's own past experience.

In early adolescence and to a lesser degree in middle adolescence, the young person's thinking is characterized by *egocentrism*. Young teenagers are heavily engaged in thinking about themselves in abstract ways that they were not capable of as children: "Am I normal?" "Why am I behaving this way?" "What do I mean to others?" "Who am I, really?" As a consequence of this egocentrism, young people behave much of the time as if they were as central and important in the thoughts of others as they are in their own thoughts. They imagine that they are the center of everyone's attention and interest and that others are impressed by their good points (from character traits to facial features) and critical of their every flaw—whether those good points and flaws are real or only imagined by them. Adolescents frequently experience a "personal fable," in which they truly believe that they are unique among all of humanity and that no one has ever loved, enjoyed, or despaired as deeply as they. Adolescents may see themselves as "saviors" who will be able to solve problems that others have been unable to correct. Teenagers also tend to believe that they are not subject to the laws of probability that affect "ordinary" people and that they can safely engage in drug use, sex, and dangerous activities without suffering any serious consequences.

Moral development

A child's simplistic way of looking at right and wrong is inadequate for the needs of the adolescent, who must build a philosophy of life—a collection of moral values and truths to give meaning, direction, and purposes to life. In gradually establishing their own systems of moral and ethical beliefs, adolescents become greatly interested in moral viewpoints that differ from those of their parents. Adolescents have a keen eye for noticing differences that may exist between their parents' *standards* and their parents' *practices*, that is, between what their parents claim to believe in and what they actually do. Whether their parents live up to their own standards or not, most adolescents go through a stage of questioning, condemning, and rebelling to some degree against the family's beliefs about morality. Teachers and other authoritative adults are also subjected to the critical evaluation of adolescents as they sort through various moral standards in search of those which they will incorporate into their own identity.

Preadolescents and adolescents must be cognitively functioning at the stage of formal operations in order to achieve Kohlberg's stages 3 and 4 of moral development. Adolescents and adults use abstract thinking to make moral judgments. The teenager now analyzes everyone's thinking, anticipates the effect of personal actions on others, finds all solutions to a problem, compares opposing viewpoints, and ponders the ideal answer to moral dilemmas. A recent study found that most 13- to 14-year-olds are at stages 2 and 3 of moral development and that one-half of older adolescents are at stage 3.[10]

Level II: Conventional (moral)

Stage 3: Interpersonal concordance—good-boy–nice-girl orientation The older adolescent strives to conform to the rules and role expectations of parents, teachers, and peers. He or she obeys rules (curfews), does his or her duty (completes household chores), and respects authority (avoids getting demerits and being expelled from school) in order to be thought of as a "good boy" or a "nice girl" and get approval from authority figures. The teenager views an action as desirable and valuable if it supports good, conventional behavior.

The teenager's sense of justice is based on good interpersonal relationships.[11] By being nice, helping those who are weaker, following the golden rule, and showing love, gratitude, respect, and loyalty in relationships, the teenager seeks to maintain fulfilling relationships with others. He or she admires same-sex authority figures with positive qualities. The older child's respect for authority and conformity to rules are apparent in the belief that lying to peers is as bad as lying to adults.[12]

Loyalty to peers and friends becomes increasingly important as the teenager's peer group functions as a conscience. The peer group determines the punishment if cheating or lying occurs within the group. When the peer group values conventional behavior, the adolescent will slowly develop the inner strength to avoid antisocial behavior that could cause ostracism from the group.[13] The teenager thus slowly develops empathy for others and values loving and stable relationships.[14]

Stage 4: Society-maintaining orientation (law and order) Older adolescents and adults continue to conform in terms of the duties, responsibilities, and expectations of their conscience and society. The older teenager defines justice as a system of rules and roles that are shared and maintained by the community in order to prevent the destruction of society.[15] The teenager upholds rules and laws, accepts responsibility, and strives to maintain good relationships with authority figures in the community. The adolescent views authority as a merit to be earned or withdrawn if undeserved.[16]

While the older adolescent may occasionally lie to protect a friend, the urge to preserve self-respect becomes more important than the urge to disobey.[17] The older teenager examines moral values that conflict with his or her own values, but quickly rejects them, and usually associates with persons who have the same values and follow the same rules.

Many adolescents turn to religion to strengthen their identity and to provide a set of clear-cut rules for belief and behavior. Until they have their own well-established, internalized code of behavior and philosophy of life, they find security and control their impulses by adopting external rules of conduct. Religion may take the place of family authority and provide peer acceptance. Adolescents think deeply about religion (see Fig. 13-8). They may view themselves (when they are not despondent, embarrassed, or self-accusing) as pure spirit. Adolescents frequently feel a special link to the mysteries and austerities of religion, the beauties of nature, and poetry or music. These alliances are part of the process of loosening one's ties to one's family and childhood in order to search in broader fields for beliefs and standards that can be used in building one's identity, not only as a member of one's family but also as a member of the human family and the universe.

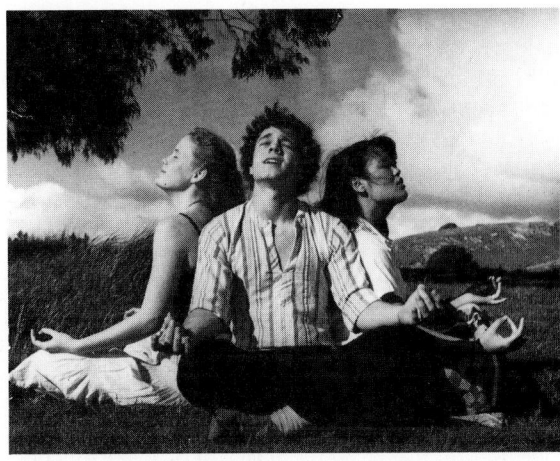

Figure 13-8 Some adolescents turn to religion in order to express their need to establish an identity, both personal and in relation to the universe. (*Photo by Karl Bauer.*)

HEALTH MAINTENANCE

Morbidity and mortality

Adolescents are often considered to be the healthiest segment of the population. It is true that mortality rates are highest for infants under 1 year of age, decline precipitously during childhood, and reach their lowest level during adolescence. 1982 statistics reflect a long-term downward trend in mortality and morbidity rates among adolescents. Fifteen-to-24-year-olds had one of the largest declines in mortality rates.

Accidental injuries remain the leading cause of death among teenagers (51.2 per 100,000) with motor vehicle accidents close behind at 36.9 deaths per 100,000. All other accidents follow with 14.4 deaths per 100,000. Fifteen-to-24-year-olds continue to have a high number of fatalities due to drowning. Most spinal injuries and fatalities due to diving accidents involve teenage and young adult males.

Adolescents die from other forms of violence besides accidents. Homicide is the second leading cause of death in the 15-to-24-year-old group behind accidents (13.7 deaths per 100,000). Suicide is a close third (12.1 deaths per 100,000) in this age group. Suicide among adolescent males is 3 times higher than among females.

Neoplasms, both malignant and benign, and rheumatic fever are the fourth and fifth leading causes of death, with mortality rates approximating 4.6 and 0.2 deaths per 100,000 young people, respectively.

The low incidence of disease among adolescents presents an inaccurate impression of abundant health and reduced health care requirements for this age group. Nurses and teenagers need to be aware that adolescents, who have primary control of their day-to-day health-related behavior, adopt many practices that compromise their health in ways that typically do not show up for several years. Among the common health hazards for young people are poor nutrition, including obesity; cigarette smoking, which involves about one-fourth of adolescents; and use of alcoholic beverages by about one-third. Experimental use or frank abuse of other drugs can of course damage health, as can sexual practices that lead to infection.

Mental health problems are substantial during adolescence, although their exact incidence is unknown. Signs that the nurse should be alert for are drug abuse (see Chap. 39), fatigue, lack of sleep, frequent accidents or visits to health care professionals, poor school attendance or a decline in school performance, "acting-out" behavior, and lack of friends or a peer group. These are indications that a young person is psychologically in trouble and needs intervention by a mental health professional.

Delivery of health care to adolescents

There has been much debate over who should provide health care to the adolescent (see Fig. 13-9). Traditionally, parents took their children to a pediatrician until they rebelled against going to a "baby doctor." At that point, the pediatrician was often replaced by an internist. Over the past few years a new physician specialty, adolescent medicine, has developed; physicians who complete a period of specialized training become skilled in dealing with the medical and psychosocial needs of adolescents. Nurses may obtain postgraduate degrees or certification as adolescent health care nurse practitioners. These physicians and nurses frequently work in adolescent clinics, whose aim is to provide primary care. Many hospitals have adolescent inpatient units with special facilities and a specially trained staff.

Teenagers may also obtain health care at free clinics in many communities. These clinics usually provide a wide range of service—medical and dental care, counseling, and job placement. Free clinics usually are staffed by volunteers and provide service without charge, since cost is a severe problem for adolescents, who generally have limited funds. Clinics associated with high schools have been successful at reducing teenage pregnancy.

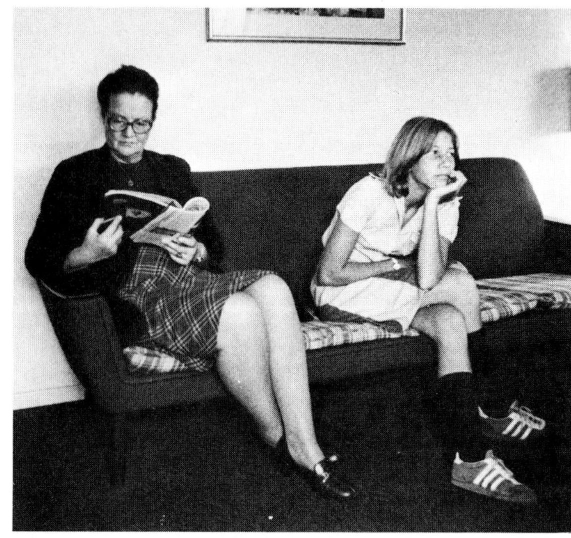

Figure 13-9 Adolescents may be embarrassed to receive care in a pediatrician's office.

Legal issues in health care of adolescents

Until the mid-1960s, minors were legally totally under the control of their parents and had few rights of their own. While laws are changing very rapidly, the right of minors to give legally binding consent for health care varies from state to state. In many states a minor may give consent for routine or emergency medical care, marriage, treatment of venereal disease, contraceptive counseling and supplies, and abortion. Parental consent is not required; in fact, giving parents confidential medical information without the minor's consent subjects the health care provider to prosecution.

In situations in which minors are allowed to give consent for certain health care procedures, the care-giver must first be sure that the adolescent is intelligent and mature enough to understand the treatment and its consequences. A full explanation must be given of the proposed treatment, its risks, and alternatives. *Informed consent* is a patient's agreeing to receive treatment that has been thoroughly explained. Recent Supreme Court decisions have struck down barriers that previously prevented adolescents from obtaining, without their parents' consent, health care related to sexual activity. As laws change, nurses have a responsibility to their adolescent patients to keep informed about the laws in their state. Sources of legal information include:

Regional Planned Parenthood Offices
Regional bar associations
State and county medical associations
State and federal departments of health and social services
State attorney general's office
Counsel for the health provider's malpractice insurance company

Safety

The role of accidents in adolescent mortality and morbidity mandates that accident prevention be a major component of health maintenance for teenagers. Because adolescents are so mobile and independent, it is too late now for the "don't touch" approaches and close adult supervision that were helpful in promoting safety for young children. The focus of accident prevention must be on teaching adolescents how to operate safely in their expanded environment and on helping them to identify hazards and act responsibly to avoid injury to themselves and others.

School-sponsored driver's education courses, provided by law in some states, should be strongly encouraged. The same educational principles—instruction about the hazards involved and supervised teaching about how to proceed safely—need to be applied to other activities besides driving. Adolescents must be taught (and need attractive role models who demonstrate) that certain activities are never to be undertaken without a companion who knows the rules of safety and can provide help in case the need arises. Hunting, wilderness hiking, swimming, and activities involving such hazardous equipment as power saws are examples. Health educators should take advantage of the natural influence of attractive peers or older role models with whom adolescents identify and whom they believe and trust. Particularly in the area of alcohol and other drug use, which is heavily linked to accidents in adolescence, there is probably no preventive or corrective educational approach to equal the effectiveness of peers who "have been there," who can tell what their experience was like, and who can convincingly testify that it was not worth it.

Sex education

Adolescents desperately need information about their sexuality. While an understanding of male and female anatomy and physiology is necessary, they need to understand more than just their "plumbing." Sex education must not focus only on reproduction. Adolescents need to recognize how sexuality can help or harm them and how sexual relationships can enhance or destroy their sense of worth. To learn this, it is imperative that they have adult role models from whom they can learn honest, responsible behavior.

A 1976 study found that 55 percent of young women were sexually active by age 19 and that only 30 percent consistently used birth control methods (see the section "Adolescent Sexuality" in Chap. 25). A number of factors are probably responsible for the low use of contraceptives among adolescents:

1. An inability to accept the fact that they are sexually active.
2. Ignorance about body function and about types of contraceptives and their availability.
3. Embarrassment. Many teenagers find it difficult to purchase tampons or sanitary pads, let alone contraceptive foam or condoms.
4. Adolescent magical thinking and denial: "It can't happen to me."
5. Poor impulse control.
6. The belief that the use of contraceptives will inhibit spontaneity and pleasure.
7. A lack of male teenagers' commitment to the prevention of pregnancy.
8. Fear of the side effects of using contraceptives.
9. A wish to become pregnant.

According to a 1985 survey of teenagers, 37 percent learned about birth control in school, 20 percent from books and the media, 17 percent from friends, 17 percent from parents, 4 percent from a clinic or doctor, and 4 percent from siblings.

Teenagers need answers to their questions about sex. While nurses should have this information and be able to relay it to their teenage patients, this does not mean that they must have all the answers. A nurse who does not have the information should refer the teenager to an appropriate person and emphasize that the teenager is not being put off, but merely referred to another source, such as a health educator or one with training in human sexuality.

Sex education for adolescents should include anatomy and physiology, clarification of value systems, and information about sexually transmitted diseases, pregnancy, contraception, abortion, parenting, communication in marriage, alternative life-styles, and sexual function and dysfunction.

Nutrition

Nutrition is a prime factor in health maintenance during adolescence. Growth is greater during adolescence than at any other time except the fetal period and infancy. The nutritional needs of the adolescent are greatest during the growth spurt (Tanner's stage 1 in girls and stage 2 in boys). During the years of most rapid growth (ages 10 to 14), the adolescent girl's caloric requirements increase to 48 kcal per kilogram of body weight and then decrease to 38 kcal per kilogram of body weight. In contrast, adolescent boys require 60 kcal per kilogram of body weight between the ages of 11 and 14. Their energy needs then decrease to 42 kcal per kilogram of body weight from age 15 to age 18.[18] Nutritional needs are summarized in Appendix C. While these recommended dietary allowances (RDAs) are estimates for age groups and cannot be applied stringently to individuals, they are helpful in evaluating nutrition.

A guide to assessing the nutritional status of adolescents is presented in Table 13-4. A growth chart (see Appendix B) should also be used with every adolescent to plot height and weight in order to assess growth.

The efforts of teenagers to become independent of family and conform to peer group standards and cultural ideals have an effect on their nutritional practices. Young people make their own decisions about what to eat. Adolescents need to be taught that healthful foods have a direct, positive effect on health, appearance, physique, and physical function; this information often positively influences their eating habits.

Nutritional research indicates no evidence of calorie or protein deficiency among American adolescents as a group today. Studies do, however, reveal deficiencies in both vitamins and minerals, particularly calcium, iron, vitamin A, and ascorbic acid (vitamin C). Table 13-5 shows the nutrients most lacking in the diets of adolescents and lists the foods in which they are found. To ensure proper nutritional intake, the teenager should have daily servings of whole-grain breads, cereals, dark-green leafy and yellow vegetables, beans, and fresh fruit.[19] See Appendix C, Table C-5, for the recommended number of servings of foods in the four basic food groups for the teenager.

Table 13-4 Guide to Nutritional Assessment of Adolescents

History

Family: Obesity, diabetes mellitus, or heart disease in close family members? Preventive diet may be indicated

Dietary: Appetite, total daily food intake, special diet, frequency of meals, snacking habits, food preferences and allergies, vitamin supplements

Medications: On oral contraceptive? If so, may need increased vitamin C, pyridoxine, and folic acid

Exercise: Daily exercise pattern. Participation in sports. Which sports? How often? May need increased calories, vitamins C and B complex, water, and salt

Past health problems: Significant weight gain or loss? Obesity, anemia, thyroid imbalance, or diabetes?

Special considerations: Pregnant? Consider needs for increased calories, protein, calcium, iron, B vitamins, and vitamins C and A. Intrauterine device in place? May need increased iron to replace losses during menstrual flow

Review of systems

If the following symptoms are present, consider corresponding mineral and vitamin deficiencies.

Drying and cracking of skin or lips, itching of genital area—*riboflavin*

Nervousness, irritability, insomnia, muscle cramps—*calcium*

Indigestion, constipation, nervousness, irritability, fatigue, mental depression—*thiamine*

Night blindness, roughness of skin, dryness of hair—*vitamin A*

Bleeding of gums, slow wound healing, easy bruising—*vitamin C*

Fatigue, irritability, anorexia, headache, increased menstrual flow—*iron*

Physical assessment

Height and weight: Far below mean on growth chart for age? Consider protein and calorie deprivation. Far above mean? Consider obesity, overweight

Clinical signs: Lethargy; general depression; dry skin or hair; lesions on lips, skin, or genitalia; dental caries, swollen or bleeding gums; tachycardia; and enlarged thyroid may indicate nutritional inadequacies

Laboratory data

Consider iron deficiency anemia if hemoglobin and hematocrit levels are low

Source: C. Torre, "Nutritional Needs of Adolescents," *American Journal of Maternal-Child Nursing* **2**(2):118–127 (March–April 1977).

Table 13-5 Food Sources of Nutrients Commonly Deficient in Adolescents' Diets

Common nutrient deficiencies	Foods high in these nutrients
Vitamin A	Direct sources: liver, fish liver oils, butter, cheese, eggs, and milk Sources of carotene (a substance the body converts to vitamin A): yellow vegetables, green leafy vegetables, tomatoes, yellow fruits
Vitamin C	Citrus fruits, strawberries, broccoli, bell peppers, tomato juice, rose hips
Calcium	Milk, cheese, yogurt, ice cream, soybeans, mustard and turnip greens
Iron	Red meats (especially liver), wheat germ, brewer's yeast, egg yolks, dark-green leafy vegetables, apricots, whole-grain cereals, fish
Riboflavin	Milk, liver, brewer's yeast, whole grains, green leafy vegetables, fish, eggs
Thiamine	Brewer's yeast, wheat germ, rice polish, pork, milk, nuts, whole grains, liver, peas, lentils

Source: C. Torre, "Nutritional Needs of Adolescents," *American Journal of Maternal-Child Nursing* **2**(2):118–127 (March–April 1977).

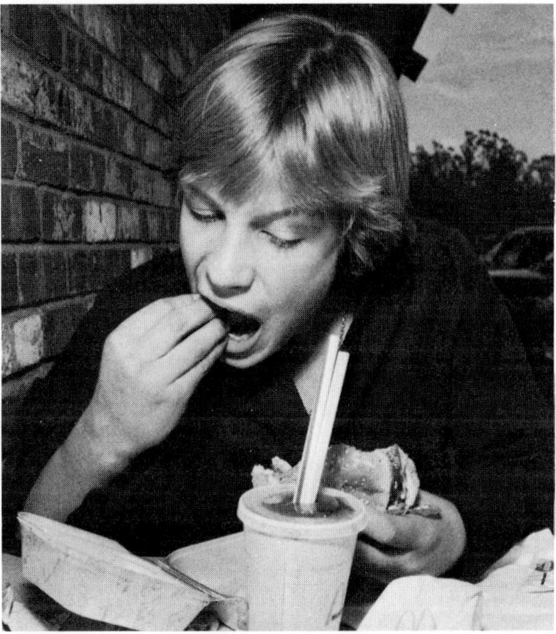

Figure 13-10 Fast foods are a staple of the teenager's diet. (*Photo by Karl Bauer.*)

Fast foods* Adolescents, like others, frequently eat at fast-food restaurants. In the United States, sales of fast food increased by more than 300 percent between 1970 and 1980 (Fig. 13-10). To assess the impact of fast food on an adolescent's diet, the nurse must consider how much fast food the adolescent eats, the nutritional value of the food, and which fast foods the teenager most frequently selects. Each of these topics will be discussed below.

Fast food is simply ordinary food packaged in boxes or wrappers. It is generally high in protein and contains variable amounts of fat and minerals. An analysis of several fast-food menus showed that they all contained items that would provide a meal with 20 to 30 percent of a teenager's recommended daily requirements for thiamine, riboflavin, ascorbic acid, and calcium. The sodium content of some fast-food items is high. Most fast-food menus are deficient in vitamin A, biotin, folacin, pantothenic acid, iron, and copper. These inadequacies result from a lack of fruits and vegetables.

Fast food, then, may be a nutritional triumph rather than a nutritional disaster.[22] The nutritional value of fast food in an adolescent's daily diet depends on his or her making choices. Effective nutrition education programs are needed to teach adolescents and others to choose wisely from fast-food menus and to include the nutrients missed in fast-food meals in the other meals of the day. While the nurse would probably not recommend a diet consisting only of fast food, an adolescent's occasional or daily visit to a fast-food restaurant is not unreasonable.

Although fast food is often classified as "junk food," it is important for the nurse to realize that there are no "good" or "bad" foods. A food is acceptable or unacceptable for a person depending on whether its nutrient content complements the nutrient contents of other foods in the daily or weekly diet. The nurse should provide education about a well-balanced diet for adolescents and family members who frequently eat snacks and prepared meals at fast-food restaurants.

*The next two sections on nutrition were written by Diane M. Huse, M.S., R.D.

Vegetarianism An increasing number of adolescents and young adults are turning to vegetarianism for philosophical, religious, and health reasons. Vegetarianism is not a reason for concern unless it is practiced to an extreme degree. There are three types of vegetarians; they are classified according to the types of animal foods that they include in their diets. The *vegan,* or pure vegetarian, eats only plant foods, such as vegetables, fruits, grains, nuts, and legumes. The *lactovegetarian* consumes milk and dairy products in addition to plant foods. The *lacto-ovovegetarian* eats eggs, milk, and dairy products as well as plant foods. The above classifications are imprecise, however, because vegetarians are also categorized according to their belief systems and life-styles. The Zen macrobiotic diet, for example, consists of plant foods coupled with natural and organic foods. Those who adhere to it advance through 10 stages of progressive dietary restriction and ultimately eat a diet composed only of cereals. Many Seventh Day Adventists are lacto-ovovegetarians who abstain from eating animal foods that they regard as having been obtained by destroying life. Trappist monks are also lacto-ovovegetarians who include natural and organic foods in their diets. They abstain from eating meat because they consider it a luxury that conflicts with their vow of simple living.

Nurses and other health professionals must understand the motivations of people who eat these diets and must be aware of their dietary restrictions. Vegetarian diets can be nutritionally adequate if they are carefully planned to prevent deficiencies. Purely vegetarian diets may be inadequate in terms of providing proteins (including all eight essential amino acids), iron, zinc, calcium, vitamin D, vitamin B_{12}, and riboflavin. These diets are high in bulk because of the amount of vegetables, fruits, and cereals included and are generally low in calories. High-fiber foods create a feeling of fullness even when small amounts are eaten. Adolescents, children, and infants on purely vegetarian diets should drink fortified soy milk. These diets must be carefully planned to meet nutritional needs.

Lactovegetarian and lacto-ovovegetarian diets are usually nutritionally adequate, except for possible deficiencies in iron and zinc. People on these two diets rarely suffer from deficiencies of calcium, vitamin B_{12}, vitamin D, or riboflavin because fortified milk and eggs are good sources of these nutrients.

The adolescent who adopts a vegetarian diet should be counseled by a nurse or nutritionist who is familiar with the particular needs of vegetarians. Some vegetarian diets, such as the Zen macrobiotic diet, increase the risk of dietary deficiencies, malnutrition, and serious disease or death. A vegetarian diet is sometimes mistakenly believed to be a panacea that will prevent or cure all diseases, and therefore believers may not seek necessary medical care. The nurse must therefore assess the diets and belief systems of adolescent vegetarians. The Seventh Day Adventist Church, which advocates vegetarian diets, is an excellent source of information on nutrition and menu planning.[23]

Snacks Adolescents are often ravenous snackers. Snacks are perfectly acceptable and, if well planned, can significantly contribute to a teenager's total daily nutritional intake. Teenagers tend to snack on whatever is available—too often this means that they rely on foods that are high in sugar and starches (which contain too many calories and cause dental caries) but low in calcium and iron. Nutritious snacks, such as milk, eggs, cheese, fruits, nuts, vegetables, and other foods high in calcium and iron, should be offered to the adolescent. There is currently a trend in schools toward replacing soda and candy vending machines with those dispensing juices and fresh fruits. The substitution of nutritionally sound snacks should be promoted and supported by school nurses (see Table 13-6).

Breakfast Adolescents frequently skip breakfast because they fear gaining weight or have little time in the morning. Breakfast is probably the most important meal of the day because the needed amount of ascorbic acid, calcium, and riboflavin may not be adequately provided by other meals. It has been shown that teenagers, particularly girls, who routinely eat breakfast rely less on "junk food" snacks for energy than those who skip breakfast. Eating such "nontraditional" breakfasts as a grilled cheese sandwich is perfectly acceptable.

Athletics and nutrition Adolescents who take part in athletics must meet nutritional needs for growth and energy expenditure (see Table 13-7). Their diets should include sufficient protein, calories, carbohydrates, fat, water, vitamins, and minerals. Caloric intake should range from 2300 to 5000 cal per day for those involved in strenuous exercise. A greater percentage of the additional calories (up to 70 percent) should come from complex carbohydrates (bread and ce-

Table 13-6 Snack Foods Common in Adolescents' Diets

Food	Portion size	Approximate cal
Devil's food cake with chocolate icing	1 (2 × 3 × 2 in)	203
Plain cake donut	1	125
Oreo cookie	1	50
Vanilla wafer	1	15
Plain Jell-O	1 cup	130
With whipped cream	1 tbsp	182
D-Zerta gelatin	1 cup	20
With whipped cream	1 tbsp	72
With Dream Whip topping	1 tbsp	34
Thin pretzel stick	1	1
Potato chip	5	54
Popcorn	1 cup	54
Chocolate milk shake	8 oz	421
Whole milk (white)	8 oz	161
Skim milk	8 oz	81
Coca-Cola	8 oz	104
Tea	8 oz	2
With sugar	1 tsp (level)	18
Ice cream (vanilla)	4 oz	145
Sherbet (orange)	4 oz	134
Ice milk (vanilla)	4 oz	102
Popsicle (twin)	1	95

Source: Derived from H. V. Barnes, "Physical Growth during Puberty," *Medical Clinics of North America* **59:**(6):1305 (November 1975).

reals); these provide a readily available source of energy before an event. Because athletic events may lead to sodium depletion and water loss, the teenage athlete should be instructed to:

1. Avoid dehydration by maintaining an adequate fluid intake before and during a game.
2. Avoid sodium depletion by eating salted foods. Salt tablets are usually not indicated.

Athletes competing for a particular weight class should be counseled to avoid crash dieting to lose weight or binge eating to gain weight. Crash dieting, causing a rapid loss of water, is common among wrestlers. A rapid water loss, representing 5 percent of body weight, decreases the work capacity of the muscles by 20 to 30 percent.

Contraceptives and nutrition Oral contraceptives have no serious effect on nutritional status, although blood levels of some vitamins and minerals are reported to be altered. Folic acid deficiencies have also been reported. Young women who take birth control pills should perhaps be given supplemental folic acid. Those who have IUDs may have increased menstrual bleeding, and their iron intake should be supplemented.

Underweight adolescents The adolescent who is underweight needs nutritional guidance. Teenagers who are too thin are often envied by their obese peers but are often no happier with their body image. A steady weight-gain program should be encouraged, with extra calories obtained from regular, nutritionally balanced meals and frequent, nourishing snacks.

Obesity Obesity among adolescents is a significant problem. Recent evidence suggests that "excessive weight gain during critical periods of development may result in laying down of excessive numbers of fat cells which will remain for the rest of that person's life."[24] Obese infants often become obese children and adults. The odds against an overweight adolescent's becoming an average-weight adult are 28 to 1. Studies have shown that obese young people experience less acceptance from their peers and from significant adults and have greater body-image disturbances and poorer self-concepts than their normal-weight peers. Obese adolescents are also at risk for such physical illnesses as diabetes and cardiovascular problems. (See Chap. 37.)

A normal increase in fat deposition usually occurs in girls between 11 and 13 years of age and in boys between $12\frac{1}{2}$ and $14\frac{1}{2}$ years. By the end of adolescence, as a result of sex differences in hormone secretion and physical activity, males' body composition is 7.9 percent fat, and females' is 22.8 percent fat.

An adolescent is considered overweight if his or her weight falls more than 2 standard deviations from the mean on a growth chart. The diagnosis of obesity also depends on what proportion of the excess weight is fat, measured by use of a skin caliper.

Obese adolescents often find it difficult to lose weight. Often they are more sedentary than their normal-weight peers. A genetic or familial pattern of obesity may exist. Exercise has been shown to be extremely valuable in the treatment of obesity. Overweight teenagers, embarrassed by their weight and poor body image, usually restrict their activity. This further blocks their attempts at weight loss. They become more overweight and restrict their activity even more. This frustrating cycle of events is shown in Fig. 13-11.

The nurse can assist the teenager in treating obesity. Adolescents are more successful at los-

Table 13-7 Energy Expenditures of Various Activities

Activity	Cal/min	Activity	Cal/min
1. Personal necessities		Doing stonemasonry	6.3
Sitting and eating	1.5	Making truck and auto repairs	4.2
Sleeping	1.2	**6. Recreation**	
Washing and dressing	2.6	Playing baseball (not pitcher)	4.7
2. Sedentary activities		Playing basketball	8.6
Listening to a classroom lecture	1.7	Canoeing	
Sitting and reading	1.3	2.5 mi/h	3.0
Sitting and playing cards	2.0	4.0 mi/h	7.0
Standing at ease	1.7	Dancing	
Lying at ease	1.4	Waltz	5.2
Typing 40 words per minute	1.3	Rock	8.5
3. Locomotion		Playing football	10.2
Cycling		Gardening and weeding	4.8
5.5 mi/h	4.5	Golfing	5.0
9.4 mi/h	7.0	Doing gymnastics	
Driving a car	2.8	Balancing	2.5
Walking		Trunk bending	3.5
2 mi/h	3.2	Horseback riding	
4 mi/h	5.8	Walking	3.0
Downstairs	7.1	Trotting	8.0
Upstairs	18.6	Mountain climbing	
4. Domestic work		Light load with slope	10.7
Making a bed	3.5	Heavy load with slope	13.2
Dusting	2.5	Playing ping-pong	4.9
Preparing a meal	2.5	Running cross-country	10.6
Scrubbing floors	4.0	Playing squash	10.2
5. Light industry		Swimming	5.0–11.0
Doing assembly work in a factory	2.3	Skiing, hard snow	
House painting	3.5	Level, moderate speed	10.4
		Sprinting	23.3
		Playing tennis	7.1
		Playing volleyball	3.5

Source: Adapted from J. V. G. A. Durnin and R. Passmore, *Energy, Work & Leisure,* Heinemann, London, 1967, pp. 49, 57, 72, 76; R. Passmore and J. V. G. A. Durnin, "Human Energy Expenditure," *Physiological Reviews* **35:**(4):811–813 (1955); and C. F. Consolazio, R. E. Johnson, and L. J. Pecora, *Physiological Measurements of Metabolic Functions in Man,* McGraw-Hill, New York, 1963, pp. 330–332.

ing weight after age 15.[25] First, however, the nurse should assess the following critical areas in the individual adolescent:

1. Duration and degree of obesity
2. Depression
3. Maturity and independence
4. Motivation
5. Self-esteem
6. Eating and activity patterns
7. Socialization

By reviewing these areas, the nurse can set realistic treatment goals with the adolescent. The depressed, poorly motivated teenager will probably not respond well to a weight-loss program, but would benefit from counseling.

Guidelines to assist nurses who are concerned about management of obese adolescents are found in Table 13-8.

COMMUNICATING WITH ADOLESCENTS

Communicating with teenagers can be easy to do if simple guidelines are followed:

1. *Don't preach* Teenagers often believe that their parents and teachers preach to them; they do not want this from health care providers either.
2. *Listen* Let adolescents know you are inter-

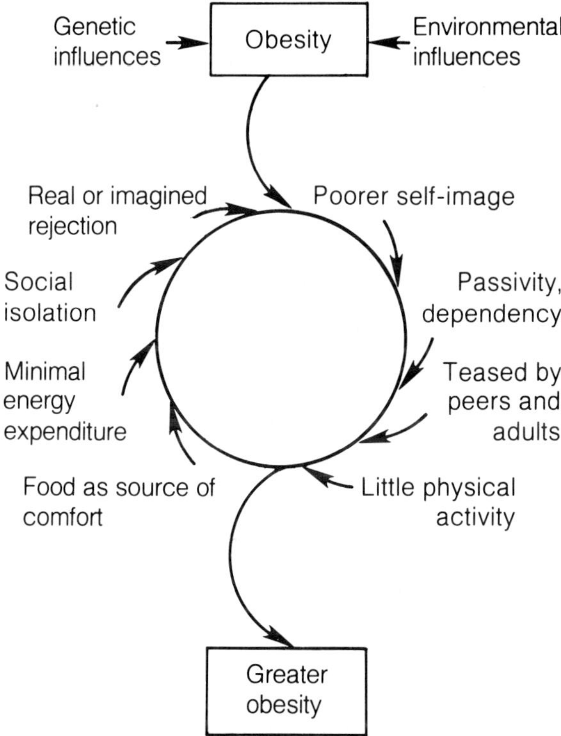

Figure 13-11 Factors that combat obesity.

ested in what they have to say, and then let them say it. Use therapeutic interviewing techniques; do not "jockey" for the floor.

3. *Be aware of nonverbal cues* Often the manner of speaking and posture of people indicate their feelings. Does the adolescent make eye contact with you, sit comfortably in the chair, fidget, or turn away?
4. *Use as few words as possible when asking questions* This encourages a lengthy response.
5. *Ask open-ended questions and avoid "why" questions* Open-ended questions are those which allow for more than a "yes" or "no" answer. "Why" questions require a self-evaluation that promotes defensiveness. For example:

Closed-ended questions	*Open-ended questions*
"Do you like school?" "Do you and your parents get along?"	"What's school like for you this year?" "What do you think about the way you and your parents get along?" "What happened then?"

Table 13-8 Nursing Management of Obese Adolescents

1. Provide supportive counseling
See obese adolescents on a regular basis whether weekly, biweekly, or monthly.

2. Encourage eating regular meals
Eating breakfast will improve performance and may lead to a lowered carbohydrate intake throughout the day.

3. Set realistic goals with the teenager
Encourage a weight loss of no more than 1 to 2 lb per week. Focus on the amount of weight that can be lost in a week or a month, rather than on the total amount, which often sounds unmanageable to an obese teenager.

4. Encourage exercise
Exercise will burn calories (Table 13-7) as well as help teenagers look and feel better.

5. Provide nutrition counseling
Teenagers need nutrition education. Often they are not aware of the calorie content of their favorite foods (Table 13-6).

6. Provide psychosocial support
Often obese adolescents feel different from their peers. Encourage involvement in support groups. Refer the obese teenager to Overeaters Anonymous, Weight Watchers, or a summer camp which offers exercise.

7. Encourage family involvement
Family members responsible for doing the marketing and cooking should be involved and counseled on nutrition. Encourage them to eliminate high-calorie foods and to prepare nutritious, low-calorie meals.

8. Have patience and show patience
Remind the teenager that losing weight takes time, just as gaining weight did. Treatment of a teenager's obesity consists of long-term management.

REFERENCES

1. Bandura, A., "The Stormy Decade: Fact or Fiction?" *Psychology in the School* **1**(3):224–231 (1964).
2. Kenniston, Kenneth, *The Uncommitted: Alienated Youth in American Society,* Harcourt, Brace & World, New York, 1965, p. 7.
3. Nicholson, Sally, "Growth and Development," in J. Howe (ed.), *Nursing Care of the Adolescent,* McGraw-Hill, New York, 1980, p. 3.
4. Berndt, T. J., "The Features and Effects of Friendship in Early Adolescence," *Child Development* **53**:1447–1460 (1982).
5. Tanner, J. M., *Growth at Adolescence,* Blackwell, Oxford, 1962.
6. Erikson, Erik, *Childhood and Society,* 2d ed., Norton, New York, 1964, p. 261.
7. Sorenson, C., *Adolescent Sexuality in Contemporary Society,* World, Tarrytown-on-Hudson, N.Y., 1973.
8. Feinstein, S., and M. Ardon, "Trends in Dating Pat-

terns—Adolescence," *Journal of Youth and Adolescence* **2**(6):157 (June 1973).

9. Elkind, David, "Teenage Thinking: Implications for Health Care," *Pediatric Nursing* **10**(6):383–385 (November–December 1984).
10. Colby, Anne, and Lawrence Kohlberg, "Relationship of Moral Judgment to Age," in "Invariant Sequence and Internal Consistency in Moral Judgment," in William M. Kurtines and Jacob Gerwirtz (eds.), *Moral Behavior and Moral Development,* G. Allen, London, 1984, p. 47.
11. Kohlberg, Lawrence, *Philosophy of Moral Development, Moral Stages and the Idea of Justice,* Harper & Row, New York, 1981, p. 150.
12. Piaget, Jean, *The Moral Development of the Child,* Harcourt, Brace, New York, 1932, p. 308.
13. Ginott, Haim, *Between Parent and Child,* Macmillan, New York, 1971, p. 61.
14. Wilcox, Mary, *Developmental Journey,* Abingdon, Nashville, 1979, p. 105.
15. Kohlberg, loc. cit.
16. Wilcox, op. cit., p. 125.
17. Gruenberg, Sidonie M., *The Parent's Guide to Everyday Problems of Boys and Girls,* Random House, New York, 1958, p. 283.
18. Howard, Rosanne B., and Nancie H. Herbold, *Nutrition in Clinical Care,* McGraw-Hill, New York, 1978, pp. 282–283.
19. Mahan, L., and J. Rees, *Nutrition in Adolescence,* Mosby, St. Louis, 1984.
20. "Fast Food and the American Diet," *Report of the American Council on Science and Health,* April 1983.
21. Wallace, J. U., and B. Raskin, "Who's Afraid of the Long Shadow of Fast Foods?" *Institutions* **76**(4):41, (April 1975).
22. Finberg, L., "Fast Foods for Adolescents: Nutritional Disaster or Triumph of Technology?" *American Journal of Diseases of Children* **130**:362 (1976).
23. Rudy, C., "Vegetarian Diets for Children," *Pediatric Nursing* **9**(5):329–333 (September–October 1984).
24. Pipes, P., and J. Aus, "Special Concerns of Dietary Intake during Infancy–Adolescence," in *Nutrition in Infancy and Childhood,* Mosby, St. Louis, 1977, p. 146.
25. Howard and Herbold, op. cit., p. 280.

14

Barbara Goergen

Children: assessment, maintenance, and promotion of health

Upon completion of this chapter, the student will be able to:

1. List the two goals of child health maintenance.
2. Describe the role of the nurse in child health maintenance.
3. List four common causes of death and injury among children and describe at least one preventive measure for each one.
4. Describe the techniques used in interviewing children.
5. List the information needed for a health history.
6. Explain the four techniques used in making a physical assessment.
7. Describe four common screening tests in terms of the ages at which they are given, their purpose, and method of administration.
8. State the four major factors that contribute to dental health.
9. Describe the major components of a nutritional assessment.
10. List the immunizations for children that are required by law.
11. Define *health promotion*.

Health is defined not only in terms of the absence of disease but also in terms of the person's level of physical, psychological, and social well-being. Both the child and the adults who are responsible for the child must plan care to maintain his or her state of health. The goal of health care is to motivate the child and the family to use their own resources to attain, maintain, or regain optimal health and functioning.[1] Children are the nation's most important resource, and they have truly unique needs and are subjected to unique pressures. Child health maintenance is the management of routine preventive care and includes counseling about growth and development and common health problems.

The family members, as well as the child, must be active participants in implementing the child's health maintenance. The family, as the child's main support system, is responsible for seeing that health maintenance continues during the child's developmental years. Eventually, the child will become responsible for his or her own health maintenance. Active participation by children increases their interest, understanding, and sense of responsibility; it also encourages them to develop their own health-maintenance strategies.

The goals of child health-maintenance programs are twofold:

1. To help the child reach adulthood in the best possible state of health by enhancing the process of physical and emotional development
2. To enable the child—the future adult—to become ultimately responsible for his or her own health maintenance

THE RELATIONSHIP OF NURSING TO CHILD HEALTH MAINTENANCE

State laws regulating nursing practice commonly define professional nursing to include "diagnosing and treating human responses to actual or potential health problems through services such as casefinding, health teaching, health counseling, and the provision of care supportive to or restorative to life and well-being."[2] Thus nursing has a critical role in and can make a significant impact on child health maintenance.

The nurse should be familiar with the signs of health as well as those of illness. Nursing includes assessing the total health status of the child, diagnosing responses to actual or potential health problems, and maintaining the child's normal health status through preventive and promotive health regimens.

The nurse can minimize the child's loss of health by early diagnosis and intervention. Anticipatory planning with the family can assist in developing patterns of living that are conducive to health. Nurses also promote child health by functioning as health teachers and counselors for children, families, and communities. Sometimes nurses must act as advocates for children to ensure that their health-maintenance needs are met.

THE NURSE'S ROLE IN CHILD HEALTH MAINTENANCE

Anticipatory guidance

Anticipating potential child health problems and effectively intervening to avert them are nursing interventions used to promote child health. Many health problems are avoided by early detection and reduction of risk factors. By anticipating problems and assisting families to avoid or minimize them, the nurse promotes health maintenance.

Earlier chapters in this book described normal growth and development from before birth to adolescence. For each age group the developmental steps, psychosocial tasks, and typical health problems were outlined. Using that information, the nurse can make an assessment of the child, the child's family (Chap. 2), and the child's developmental status to provide anticipatory guidance to the family.

A typical health-maintenance guide for a 6-month-old infant is outlined in Table 14-1. The nurse can construct similar guides for the younger and older child.

In addition to a health history, a physical examination, screening tests, and immunizations, consideration is given to counseling and health education regarding nutrition; sleep; play and exercise; safety; physical, emotional, and social development; sexuality; discipline; language skills; and school adjustment. Whether the child is seen on a health-maintenance visit or is hospitalized for an acute illness, the nurse has an obligation to anticipate the educational needs of the child and the family.

For example, since accidents are a leading cause of death and injury among children, parents need to be counseled regarding potential dangers for each age group (Fig. 14-1). Table 14-2 describes safety hazards for each age group and appropriate interventions.

Nurses need to review common safety practices with the parents during the child's health-maintenance visits and in the acute care setting as well. Questions can be asked about the safety hazards common in each age group (Table 14-2). The following are examples of questions to ask:[3]

Does your child play with small objects such as beads or nuts (birth to 9 months)?
Do you ever leave your child alone in the bathtub?
Do you have working fire extinguishers in your home?
Do you have safety plugs on unused outlets?
Do you have gates across entrances to stairways?
Do you keep household products, medicines, and sharp objects in locked cabinets?
Do you keep firearms in your house?

Table 14-1 Health-Maintenance Guide for a 6-Month-Old Child

Assessment	Counseling and health education
Height, weight, and head circumference	Weight should double by 5 months; plot on growth chart.
Physical examination	Complete examination is performed.
Hearing	Infant should localize sound by turning to it.
Vision	Check ability to follow an object and recognize the mother.
Hematocrit	This is the appropriate time to check for anemia, since fetal iron stores are depleted.
Immunizations	DPT no. 3 is given.
Dental screening	Time of first tooth eruption. Discuss use of fluoride. Relate use of sugar to caries. Discourage putting child to bed with bottle.
Nutrition	Begin solids—1 tbsp of rice cereal mixed with formula and fed from a spoon. Can be increased to 2–4 tbsp daily. Add one new food every 4–5 days—first cereal, then 2 weeks later start vegetables, and then fruits. Next begin protein foods (chicken, meat, and eggs). Review label reading and home preparation of baby food. Add finger foods—soft cooked vegetables, crackers, and fruits (counsel regarding choking).
Sleep	Infant should be sleeping all night; total sleep 14–15 h.
Elimination	Observe behavior with wet and soiled diapers; check number of voidings and stools per day.
Play	Infant plays with hands and feet; rolls over into various positions; likes mobiles and swings.
Language	Babbling intensifies. Baby imitates sounds and makes sound "m-m-m" when crying.
Physical development	Baby sits without support; grasp—hand to mouth.
Safety considerations	Electric outlets; discuss syrup of ipecac; falls and accidents.
Responses to people	Infant is beginning period of separation anxiety. Observe how baby acts with the mother and with strangers.
Parenting	How is the primary caregiver getting time away from the baby? Does the family agree on child care procedures and discipline?
Sexuality	Baby has usually found genitals. Discussion of early sexuality is appropriate.

Does your child ride in the car in a safety seat (or with a seat belt on if over age 4)?
Do you leave your child alone in the house?

Written guidelines, appropriate for each age group, are helpful to parents.

The nurse must also be alert to common potential health problems in children. In 1978 the American Nurses' Association appointed a commission to investigate the unmet health needs of children and young people. In its 1979 report[4] the commission listed the following health problems that still must be solved:

1. Teenage pregnancy and venereal disease. The rate of sexual activity among young people is increasing; more than 1 million girls become pregnant each year.
2. Drug abuse. Children are using drugs at an earlier age. (Nevertheless, illicit drug use among high school seniors is continuing its decline, which began in 1980.[5])
3. Child abuse. Most cases go unreported. Possibly 1 million children are abused each year.
4. Sexual exploitation. The incidence of sexual assault, incest, child pornography, and child prostitution is increasing.

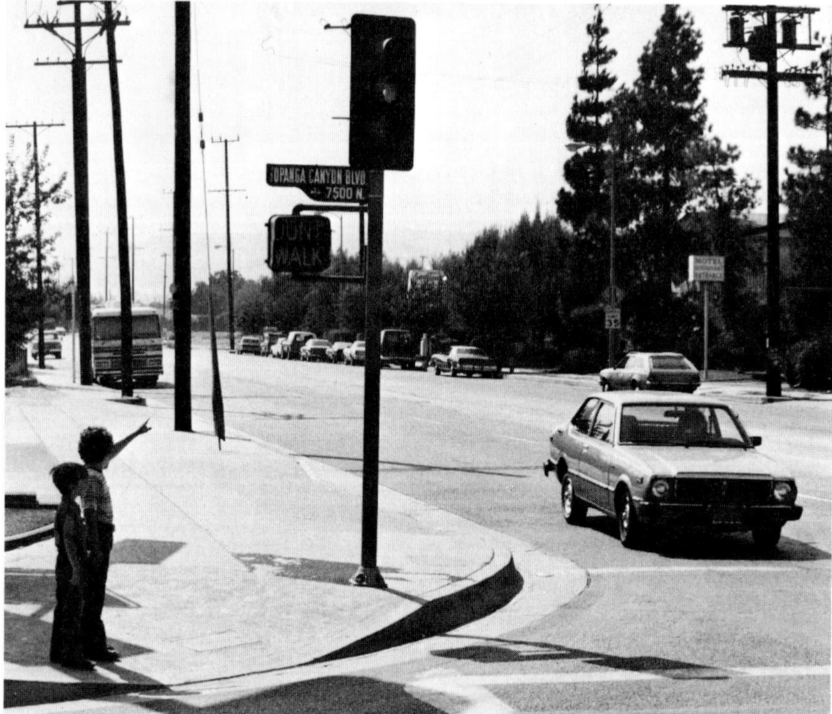

Figure 14-1 Learning to cross the street with "stop" and "go" lights.

5. Suicide. Suicide is the second leading cause of death among young people aged 12 to 24.
6. Accidents, nutritional problems, and dental problems.
7. Developmental disabilities and chronic illness. Estimates suggest that 7 to 10 million children are handicapped.
8. Lack of immunization. It was estimated that in 1977, 20 million out of 52 million children had not been immunized against the most common preventable diseases.

Current literature indicates that these needs have still not been met. These needs must be considered by all health professionals in all health maintenance settings.

Teaching and counseling

Nurses have a social and professional responsibility to promote good health practices by meeting the health learning needs of children and their families. In teaching, an essential component of the nursing process, the nurse transmits knowledge to families and children to ensure continuity of care and long-term health maintenance. When teaching families, the nurse should attempt to elicit feedback from them in order to judge whether information was heard and understood. Even though the nurse may believe that the information was clear and descriptive, if the family does not understand or misinterprets instructions, the teaching has been ineffective. Family members may be embarrassed to admit that they do not understand what the nurse or physician has told them. To confirm that they understand, the nurse may request that family members describe in their own words what the nurse has told them. The nurse should also ask questions that cannot be answered by a simple "yes" or "no." It is the nurse's responsibility to clarify any misconceptions or gaps in his or her teaching. The nurse should be supportive and encourage families' questions about points they do not understand. Effective teaching is planned and measured by the comprehension of learning. Therefore, the nurse must have a thorough understanding of the principles of teaching and learning and must be able to apply them in nursing settings.

Table 14-2 Developmental Safety: Anticipatory Guidance

Age	Developmental characteristics	Hazard	Preventive intervention
6 months–1 year	Creeping	Falls	Do not leave child on high unprotected surface. Close open stairways.
	Exploring	Putting foreign objects in mouth	Pick up buttons, pins, and small objects from the floor. Keep medicines and poisons locked up. Discard broken toys.
		Scalding	Keep hot liquids away from reach.
		Car accidents	Use car safety seats (not parent's lap) fitted according to child's height and weight.
1–3 years	Walking; curious	Running in front of cars; Drowning	Supervise constantly. Enclose yard with fence. Do not let child cross street alone. Set up practice situations so child can learn to cross street. Do not leave child alone in tub or by water.
		Shock from electrical outlets	Cover outlets with plastic plugs.
		Overdosing on medication Poisoning	Keep safety caps on medications. Keep poisons out of reach. Have ipecac at home, and know how and when to use it. (Check with a doctor or poison control center before using.)
		Car accidents	Use car safety seats.
3–6 years	Investigating; wants to play in neighborhood	Car accidents	Give intensive safety instruction. Supervise activities. Use car seats up to 4 years of age and seat belts thereafter.
		Drowning	Do not allow child to swim without responsible adult present. Have child wear life jacket while playing near a lake or pool. Teach child appropriate behavior at lakes and pools.
		Setting a fire	Keep matches locked up. Equip home with fire and smoke alarms.
6–12 years	Tries to be independent in play	Causing fires; using dangerous household equipment; being hit by a car while on a bicycle	Teach safe use of household tools and appliances. Practice fire drills at home. Teach bicycle safety. Use lights. Put reflectors on bike and child.
		Bunk beds	Protect from falls or top bed falling down.
		Car accidents	Use safety belts.
9–18 years	Competes in sports and tournaments	Falls; knee injuries; head injuries	Use appropriate safety equipment (padding, helmets, etc.).
	Uses skateboards		Continue adult supervision.
12–18 years	Wants to drive a car, motorcycle, or three-wheeler.	Moped, motorcycle, three-wheeler, and car accidents; accidents with firearms	Require completion of driver's education classes and use of helmets. Keep firearms out of reach. Teach gun safety if hunting.
	Identifies with peer group Is tempted to experiment with cigarettes, drugs, alcohol, and sex	Long-term effects to lungs, liver, brain cells; teenage pregnancy	Counsel regarding harmful effects of cigarettes, drugs, and alcohol on the body. Continue to monitor activities. Promote peer group support to say "no."

Because of the nurse's expertise, families may request advice from the nurse about their life situations. In counseling, the nurse refrains from making a decision for the family. At the same time, the nurse can listen to the problem, help the family focus on the real issues, and assist family members in making their own decision. The individual nurse, in applying these principles, will make modifications and adaptations to special situations and will continually evaluate the effectiveness of teaching and learning with the child and family.

Advocacy

Since children are not often in a position to advocate effectively for themselves, others must do so for them. Legal measures have been instituted to help ensure child health maintenance. Most states have laws that require nurses to report any suspected incidence of child abuse to official authorities. These rulings are based on the doctrine of *parens patrice,* which gives the state the authority to protect children.[6] Federal regulations requiring child-proof medication caps, flame-retardant nightclothes, and safety standards for car seats are examples of legislation designed to protect the health of children. Many states now require that children aged 4 and under (or weighing 40 lb and under) be placed in federally approved car restraints.

Protection of children's rights Previously, health professionals adopted a paternalistic attitude and included neither the family nor the child in the treatment plan. Increased emphasis on patients' rights and consumer pressure have forced professionals in recent years to include the patient in the decision-making process. More recently, children's rights, an outgrowth of the patients' rights movement, have been clarified.

In 1974 the *Pediatric Bill of Rights* was adopted by the National Association of Children's Hospitals as a proposed legislative model.[7] This bill of rights provides that every person, regardless of age, has the right to seek and consent to treatment involving contraception, venereal disease, pregnancy (including consent for abortion), and psychiatric problems. The bill protects the confidentiality of the patient and prevents the physician from disclosing any information to the child's parents without the child's consent.

Although court cases have not yet arisen, the child may have the right to refuse treatment when the parents want the child to have it. Therefore, the nurse should see that consent is also obtained from any minor aged 14 or over.

Rehabilitation

Through rehabilitation, the health maintenance of the handicapped child is emphasized. Rehabilitation involves retraining the handicapped child to the fullest physical, emotional, social, and vocational usefulness possible. Federal legislation (P.L. 94–142) mandates that handicapped children receive the same education in the same classrooms as normal children. This concept, called *mainstreaming,* is based on the philosophy that integration is necessary for optimal rehabilitation. The nurse promotes positive attitudes toward handicapped children and helps change negative ones.

Referral

Nurses frequently refer children and families to other health care professionals or agencies. Community resources may include physicians, psychologists, social workers, dentists, physical therapists, and nurses. Children with developmental delays can be referred to infant stimulation programs and day activity centers. Handicapped children's services provide care to children with orthopedic problems; fees are based on the family's income. Local health departments are excellent sources of information on immunizations, well-child clinics, treatment for communicable diseases, screening programs, and developmental and psychological testing.

Preparing the child for self-care

The ultimate goal of child health maintenance is self-care. Effective transmission of knowledge and responsibility to the child and the family enables them to be their own advocates. Both continuity of care and lifetime health maintenance are thus ensured. Nurses need to understand children as individuals who are different from adults and as members of their time and their community.

To facilitate health care, both the child and the family should be actively included in the decision-making process for the health-maintenance plan from the beginning. This involvement enables the child to develop problem-solving skills for health maintenance and increases the child's level of compliance. If children as well as adults are included in decision making, they will feel more involved in, and committed to, the resulting plan. For example, it may be appropriate to ask a school-age child whether he or she prefers to receive a penicillin injection or take the penicillin orally.

With effective health-maintenance programs, children and their families can eventually do much of the screening for disease and the preventing of potential health problems themselves. Health habits formed during childhood will continue throughout adulthood. Nurses must be intimately involved in the promotion of healthy adults and potential parents.

HEALTH ASSESSMENT

The health history

A child's health history helps the nurse make an organized assessment of the child's current health. It includes information about the child's development, health practices, health problems, and environment. The history is obtained from the child, the family, or other knowledgeable persons. Personal interviews with the child and the family are the most common way of obtaining a health history.

The interview is the most frequently used tool in understanding and managing the problems, vulnerabilities, and strengths of children and their families. To be effective during an interview, the nurse must have an extensive data base, experience, good judgment, self-assurance, sensitivity, and a deep interest in personal care. The nurse has the ability to see, to hear, to feel, to empathize, and to "read" children and their parents. Communication is both verbal and nonverbal. Nurses should not interrogate. The nurse must be very attentive to the way words and phrases are used and to the way they conceal, reveal, or suggest thoughts and feelings. While most children and parents come to the nurse wishing and expecting to be helped, they may have reservations. They have their own agenda of concerns and their own ideas about what will be helpful. Parents of infants who fail to thrive or who are retarded, psychotic, or handicapped are likely to have feelings of anger, shame, inadequacy, anxiety, despair, and guilt. These feelings influence the interview. A friendly, nonjudgmental, but direct approach will usually help the nurse obtain the necessary information without delay or embarrassment. The nurse should be tactful and courteous and should provide a comfortable and private setting for the interview. The sequence of questioning and the language level used by the nurse are important.

The interview

Children may be initially apprehensive and fearful about the interview. Saying, for example, "I bet you were a little nervous about coming here," may help the child to relax. It is important for the nurse to be perceived as one who likes children. If the nurse is comfortable and friendly, that will usually put the child at ease. The child will usually talk readily and often will respond only to direct questions. The cooperation of older children can be gained by admiring their clothes, conversing with them on their own level, and discussing mutual interests. The nurse may reassure and distract preschool children with interesting objects, such as puppets or dolls. Adolescents should be interviewed without the parents present to ensure confidentiality. If it becomes necessary for the nurse to share information with the parents, it is the nurse's responsibility to tell the adolescent this.

The goals of the history-taking process are:

1. To establish a relationship with the child and the family that will help them trust and confide in the nurse
2. To establish a data base to use in formulating the nursing care plan
3. To help the child and the family, through education or counseling, to learn about development or solve problems

Taking a health history can be facilitated by deciding what information is needed and by using the specific interview technique that is expected to elicit the information. Collecting data in an organized way helps the nurse gain parents' and children's confidence and obtain complete data quickly. Table 14-3 lists guidelines for interviewing a child and his or her family.

The depth and form of the health history vary with its purpose. A complete history is obtained the first time the patient is seen. During subsequent visits, the nurse obtains an interval history relating to the specific problem for which the child is now being seen.

The health history provides both subjective and objective data. A physical examination and laboratory tests furnish objective data used to confirm information obtained in the health his-

Table 14-3 Techniques for Successful Interviews

Set the stage
Provide privacy and comfort.
Introduce yourself and explain your role.
Be interested and concerned about this family—focus on the child.
Young children may need a play activity while parents are being interviewed.

Open-ended questions
Begin interview with such statements as:
"Before I ask any questions, do you have any?"
"How have things been?"
"Tell me why you came today."
"Tell me about your daughter's health."
"Is there anything you want to remind me about?"

Less directive techniques
Listening:
Let the parent or child tell you how it is.
Observe the facial expression, posture, movement. (Adolescents usually do not tolerate silence as well as adults do.)
Facilitation:
Show by your manner, words, or actions that you want to hear more, but don't specify a topic: "Mm-hmm," "Yes," "I understand."
Reflection:
Repeat appropriate words, and watch for cues.
Clarification:
"Tell me what you mean by . . ."

More directive techniques
Confrontation:
Describe something striking about verbal or nonverbal behavior: "You seem to have difficulty talking about that." "You seem worried about ______."
Ask directly about feelings and problems.
Adolescents may ask questions about a "friend's" problem when it is really their own.

Direct questions
Use questions to encourage a chronological account, to fill in gaps, or to go from general information to specific information.
Avoid *leading* questions.
Ask one question at a time.

Miscellaneous
Answer specific questions that parents have as you are able to during the interview.
Avoid asking, "Why did you ______?" Instead say, "Tell me your reasons for ______."
How, who, where, how much, and *how often* are all good words to use to begin questions.

Terminating the interview
Before ending the interview ask:
"Are there any other concerns that you have?"
"Is there anything else bothering you that you'd like to talk about?"
"Is there anything else you think I should know?"

tory. Table 14-4 shows an outline of a pediatric health history. The following is a general discussion of the kind of information that should be obtained under each major heading of the health history.

Identifying data It is important to record not only age, sex, name, nickname, and address, but also the country of origin and primary language of the child. Any serious or chronic illness should also be noted. The parents' names are usually included.

The chief complaint A short, simple statement in the child's or the parent's own words clarifies the primary reason for seeking health care for the present problem—for example, "Fever for 24 h" or "Vomiting and diarrhea for the past 2 to 3 days." The duration of symptoms should be noted.

The historian The reliability of the historian should be noted. It is possible for a parent not to be aware of details relating to a present problem. For example, a divorced father may be spending just a few hours with the child when an earache develops. He may not be aware of a recent upper respiratory infection. Teachers and other care-givers can also be helpful historians.

Sources of health care The names and addresses of other care-givers should be included.

The current problem If the child has come for a health-maintenance visit, the nurse should describe the child's current health status. If the child is ill, the nurse describes, in chronological order, such pertinent factors as the date of onset, the character of the complaint, the course and duration of the illness, the chronological sequence of events, the relation of the illness to other symptoms, anything that aggravates or relieves the symptoms, any treatment and its effects, and exposure to contagious diseases within the past 3 weeks. It is important always to include pertinent negative data. For example, a child may have abdominal pain but not have vomiting or diarrhea.

The birth history The birth history is especially important during the early years. It includes information about the mother's previous pregnancies and/or abortions (spontaneous or induced), obstetrical complications, the mother's health and nutritional status, infections during the pregnancy, medications or drugs taken

Table 14-4 Outline of a Pediatric Health History

Date of interview

Identifying data

Chief complaint

- Location, quality
- Intensity, chronology
- Duration, frequency
- Aggravating or alleviating

Historian (sources)

Sources of health care

Present problem or current health status

Past health

- Birth history
    - Prenatal factors
    - Mother's obstetrical history
    - Child's condition at birth
    - Neonatal period
- Early infancy
- Childhood and adolescent health
    - Common childhood illnesses
    - Serious illnesses
    - Obstetrical, menstrual, and contraceptive history
    - Accidents and injuries
    - Medications, drugs, alcohol
    - Allergies
    - Immunizations
    - Screening procedures

Patient profile

- Current life situation (social history)
    - Household members
    - Physical characteristics of home
    - Primary caregivers at home
    - Cultural beliefs, religious traditions
    - School and educational data
    - Economic situation
    - Agencies involved in care
- Development
    - General description of personality
    - Affect, energy, fears, and feelings about self
    - Child's relationship with family members or caregivers
    - Ages at which milestones were reached
- Habits
- Child-school relationships
- Play
- Language and communication skills
- Motor skills (large and small muscles)
- Adaptive or problem-solving ability
    - School performance
    - Interest in learning
- Social skills
    - Responsibilities
    - Independence
    - Self-control

Family health history

- Family members—age, sex, health status (construct a pedigree)
    - Incidence of heart disease, hypertension, diabetes, kidney disease, stroke, cancer, tuberculosis, arthritis, birth defects, genetic disease, headaches, mental illness

Review of symptoms (subjective data—gathered in response to questions)

- General—fever, vomiting, weight change, fatigue
- Skin, hair, nails—rashes, dryness
- Head—headaches, head injury
- Eyes—vision, cross-eyes, increased tearing
- Ears—earaches, decrease in hearing, infection
- Nose—incidence of colds, drainage, nosebleeds, nasal stuffiness
- Mouth, teeth, gums, and tongue—dental care, tooth eruption, bleeding
- Throat and neck—infections, swallowing, stiffness, lumps
- Respiratory—chest, difficult breathing, pneumonia, infections, wheezing
- Cardiovascular—any history of murmurs, edema
- Gastrointestinal—nausea, vomiting, abdominal pain, stools
- Genitourinary—frequency, pain, menstruation, hernias
- Musculoskeletal—joint pain, muscle soreness, weakness
- Neurological—seizures, head injury, fainting, tremors, weakness
- Endocrine—growth pattern, sweating, thirst
- Mental health—ability to get along with peers and family; fears

Source: Adapted from J. Deborah Ferholt, *Clinical Assessment of Children,* Lippincott, Philadelphia, 1980, pp. 21–22.

during the pregnancy, the length of gestation, the duration of labor, and postpartum procedures or complications. Trauma to the infant and his or her weight, length, and condition at birth should also be noted.

Health in early infancy Information about the child's health, behavior, routines, and family relationships is noted, as well as the type of feeding (breast or bottle), the child's initial eagerness to take food (vs. refusal), the type and amount of formula fed, and any feeding difficulties, such as colic, regurgitation, gas, vomiting, and diarrhea.

Health in childhood and adolescence This section of the health history includes an organized account of the child's past physical and emotional health. The past medical history allows the nurse to determine the adequacy of health maintenance, identify current immunization needs, assess the frequency and types of illnesses or accidents and the presence of allergies, and be alert to patterns that suggest more serious problems.

Current life situation This part of the health history includes the names, ages, and relationships of all household members as well as other primary care givers. Any significant deaths should be recorded. The nurse should also note where the family lives (in a house, apartment, or room); how large the dwelling is; whether anyone lives with the family (grandparents, aunts, uncles, or friends); what the financial situation of the family is; whether the father works; whether the mother works; how they are employed, how they are living if neither one works; whether there is any outside help (baby-sitters, day-care centers, or schools); the general relationship of the family members; and whether the family seems happy, chaotic, sad, depressed, or violent. The nurse must also be aware of any beliefs and practices concerning health and the treatment of illness that are part of the child's culture. Nurses must become sensitive to beliefs and behaviors so that they can anticipate what is culturally acceptable behavior for a particular family. The nurse should ask appropriate questions to determine the meaning that a symptom, illness, or health practice may have to the family. Table 14-5 lists questions and topics that the nurse can use when assessing beliefs about health care practices. When nurses do not understand a family's cultural system, they can make inappropriate value judgments and cause the family to lose confidence in the health care system.

Development The nurse can obtain an impression of the child's past and current developmental status by combining a developmental history with structured and unstructured observations. This is an important way to evaluate brain development. The developmental history should always be age-related. (See Chaps. 8 to 13 for more specific details on developmental tasks.) The nurse should ask whether the child was quicker or slower to learn than siblings; when the child began to sit, stand, roll over, talk, and walk; what kinds of activities the child engages in now; and whether the child has done anything new since the last visit.

Table 14-5 Assessment of Cultural Beliefs and Practices

1. What does this condition or illness mean to the child and/or family?
2. What bodily responses are viewed by the cultural system as life-threatening?
3. What foods, herbs, or objects are viewed as possessing qualities of healing?
4. Are there behaviors of the nurse (or caregiver) that could be threatening to the well-being of the child?
5. Are the family's (or child's) goals compatible with those of nurses or other caregivers?
6. Depending on the age of the child, it may be helpful to determine what beliefs the mother, father, and grandparents have in regard to:
   a. The umbilical cord—wearing a bellyband is very important in some cultures until the cord falls off.
   b. Skin care—some cultures bathe the infant with oil.
   c. Feeding—some Mexican-American women believe that colostrum is filthy. What foods are avoided and why? Some traditional Chinese foods are considered "hot" or "cold."
   d. Outings—a Chinese mother may miss a 2-week checkup because she will not take her baby out for 1 month after birth.
   e. Crying—it may be an indication that evil spirits are lurking around the baby.
   f. Naming—a child may be named after religious figures or family members.
   g. Interactions with others—Filipinos have a great concern for interpersonal relationships and will follow the health professional's advice exactly.
   h. Discipline—Indians quietly tell a child what is expected. Physical punishment and loud reprimands are not used.
   i. Religious practices and healing—Mexican-Americans may believe that *mal ojo,* or "evil eye," can be caused when someone wishes to hold an infant but does not. Touching the child is thought to keep the *mal ojo* away.

The nurse should ask the parent to describe what the child is like, and how he or she responds to other people and to separation. When discussing relationships, the nurse questions the parents about discipline, and when a particular kind of behavior is described, the nurse should ask how the parent feels about it. It is very important to observe the child's behavior during the interview. In assessing play, the nurse should determine what the child likes to do best, both with others and alone. The parents of a younger child should be asked how the child communicates his or her needs. The nurse can evaluate the communication skills of an older child according to the intelligibility and age-appropriateness of the child's language. Often the nurse must respond to parents' concerns about language delays in children. Language disorders are viewed in terms of receptive or expressive disabilities. When speech is unintelligible, the child has articulation difficulties. Table 14-6 lists guidelines for determining whether a child is delayed or has a disorder in the area of either language or articulation.[8]

In assessing motor skills, the nurse observes fine and gross motor development and determines how the child solves a problem such as drawing a circle, completing a puzzle, or naming a color. (See the section "Developmental Screening Tools" later in this chapter.)

Habits It is also important to assess habits, such as eating, sleeping, and toileting. The nurse should ask whether the child's appetite is good, poor, or varied. If the child is on formula, the nurse asks what kind, how it is mixed, how frequently it is given, and how much the child takes in during a 24-h period. It must also be noted what kind of food the child eats, whether the child takes vitamins, and what the child's bowel patterns are—frequency, consistency, color, and discomfort. In the case of a child who is toilet-trained, the nurse should ask whether he or she has accidents, whether they happen during the day or at night, how often they happen, and whether they are frequently associated with emotional upsets. The nurse should also ask when the child goes to bed and wakes up; whether the child awakens during the night, how often, what happens, and what the mother does; whether the child has any nightmares or night terrors; whether the child takes naps; where the child sleeps; and, when the child is awake, whether he or she is alert or seems to need more sleep.

Table 14-6 Guidelines for a Speech-Language Referral Evaluation

Language

1. The child is not talking at all by age 2.
2. The child does not use three-word sentences by age 3 or is using only nouns at age $2\frac{1}{2}$.
3. The child is using excessive, indiscriminate, or irrelevant verbalizing or jargon after age 2.
4. The child's sentence structure is consistently faulty after age 5.
5. The child has unusual difficulty expressing himself or herself after age $2\frac{1}{2}$.
6. The child understands or produces language inconsistently or inaccurately.
7. The child is not labeling things or using language to make requests or comment about things by age 2.
8. The child does not initiate language interactions with the parents.

Articulation

1. The child's speech is unintelligible, or the child omits beginning sounds after age 3.

Source: Robin Goldberg, "Identifying Speech and Language Delay in Children," *Pediatric Nursing* **10**(4):253 (July–August 1984).

The family health history Reviewing the family health history and constructing a pedigree chart (see Fig. 6-18) give the nurse the opportunity to look for hereditary or familial factors that would predispose the child to illness. The child's and the family's reaction to a disability can also be evaluated. Serious infectious diseases should be noted.

The review of symptoms The review of symptoms (ROS) helps establish the data base and helps the nurse assess the effectiveness and pattern of the child's functioning and coping behaviors, which may vary, depending on the child's problem. For example, in the case of a child with a seizure disorder, a complete history of the neurological system is necessary. The ROS is essentially a checklist of recent symptoms related to illnesses in each organ system. (Review Table 14-4.)

The interval history On subsequent visits, after a child's complete history has been recorded, only an interval history is needed. This includes:

1. Symptoms and signs relevant to the present illness
2. New symptoms
3. Developmental achievements and changes in relationships and the environment

The physical assessment

The process of physical assessment begins during the interview as the nurse observes the child's appearance and behavior, using all the senses but relying mainly on sight, touch, and hearing. The physical assessment does not begin with inspection. The nurse must have some background knowledge of anatomy and physiology in order to better understand what is being examined within each section of the body. The inspection consists of observation of the child for physical signs; inspection is the most difficult technique to master, but more diagnoses are made as a result of inspections than by all other methods combined.[9] The technique of applying the hands to the body of the child to evaluate the size, shape, contour, and consistency of organs or tissues is called *palpation*. The technique of listening with a stethoscope is termed *auscultation*. Tapping on the body to produce sounds is called *percussion*. Table 14-7 provides a detailed guide for the physical assessment of a well child.

Table 14-7 Guide for Physical Assessment of Well Children

Sequence of examination	Description of physical examination
Body measurements	**Head circumference** Measure at greatest diameter, occiput to frontal area **Height** Measure recumbent length until age 2; measure standing height after age 2 without shoes **Weight** Measure infants without clothing and older children with light clothing or a gown
Vital signs	**Temperature** Check oral, rectal, or axillary temperature **Pulse** Auscultate in infants **Respiration** Check while child is quiet **Blood pressure** Using accurate cuff size, measure both arms lying and sitting
General health	Assess: Personal appearance, relative to chronological age and appropriateness of clothing Nutritional status Hygiene Responsiveness Affect and facial expression Cooperation State of health

Table 14-7 Guide for Physical Assessment of Well Children (*Continued*)

Sequence of examination	Description of physical examination
Skin and mucous membranes	Check for: Color Rashes Bruises Edema Moisture Texture Lesions Turgor
Nails	Check: Texture Color (apply pressure, release, and observe return of coloring)
Head Hair and scalp Cranium Face	Check fontanels Transilluminate an infant Palpate head for nodes, subcutaneous or subdural swelling, and tenderness Check quantity, distribution, texture, and color of hair Check facial expressions for symmetry, alertness, response to others, and movements Percuss facial sinuses Check CN* V (trigeminal)—pain and light touch intact Check CN VII (facial)—make faces for child to mimic; e.g, smile, frown, or show teeth
Eyes	Check CN II (optic)—visual acuity (Snellen chart) Check visual fields Test for amblyopia with cover test Test for strabismus with light reflex Check movement of eyelids and alignment Inspect conjunctiva, sclera, cornea, iris, anterior chamber, and tears Check extraocular movements: CN III (oculomotor) CN IV (trochlear) CN VI (abducens) Check lacrimal apparatus Check pupils—size, shape, and symmetry

*Cranial nerve

Table 14-7 Guide for Physical Assessment of Well Children (*Continued*)

Sequence of examination	Description of physical examination
	Check PERRLA (pupils equal, round, and react to light and accommodation) Make ophthalmological examination—disk, vessels, retina, and macula
Ears	Inspect auricle and canal Remove wax if obstructing view of tympanic membrane Appraise hearing—CN VIII (acoustic) Administer Rinné and Weber tests Make otoscopic examination—color and presence of landmarks
Nose	Check patency of each nostril Check CN I (olfactory)—identify odor Check for presence of discharge and lubrication of oral mucous membranes
Mouth and throat	Check: Lips Buccal mucosa Gums Teeth Posterior pharynx Tonsils Hard and soft palates Taste CN XII (hypoglossal—movement and strength of tongue) CN IX (glossopharyngeal—phonation) CN X (vagus—gag reflex)
Neck	Check: Full ROM Symmetry Thyroid gland Position of trachea Glands and nodes CN XI (accessory—strength on each side)
Breasts	Inspect nipples and breast tissue for discharge, masses, dimpling, or retraction Palpate axillary, supraclavicular, and infraclavicular nodes
Chest and respiratory system	Check: Shape and symmetry of breasts Shape and symmetry of throat Respiratory movements Retractions Rate and rhythm of breathing Palpate for masses, tenderness, respiratory excursion, and vocal or tracheal fremitus Percuss: note dullness, flatness, resonance, hyperresonance, and tympany Auscultate quality and intensity of breath sounds and adventitious or abnormal sounds
Cardiovascular system	Inspect for bulge and pulsation Palpate apical pulse, thrusts, heaves, and thrills Auscultate rate and rhythm Assess character of S_1 and S_2 and how they compare in aortic area, pulmonic area, Erb's point, bicuspid area, and mitral area Check for heart murmurs Check arterial pulses
Abdomen	Inspect for scars, size, shape, symmetry, muscular development, bulging, and umbilicus Auscultate bowel sounds Palpate masses Check for tenderness Check tone of musculature, liver, spleen, and kidneys Percuss liver and spleen
Extremities	Check for edema Check: Color Temperature Check for lesions, nodules, and pulses Inspect: Palmar creases Nail beds
Musculoskeletal system	Check joints: range of motion and tenderness Assess muscle strength, tone, size, and symmetry Inspect symmetry and structure of back and spine Observe gait

Table 14-7 Guide for Physical Assessment of Well Children (*Continued*)

Sequence of examination	Description of physical examination
Neurological System	Assess: Developmental age and behavior State of consciousness Intellectual performance Memory Coordination Check for: Babinski's sign Romberg's sign Assess: Heel-to-toe walking Sensory acuity Cranial nerves Reflexes
Genitalia Female	Inspect: Labia Urinary meatus Vaginal orifice Pubic hair Check for hernia (inguinal or femoral) Check inguinal nodes
Genitalia Male	Check: Penis Scrotum Urinary meatus Circumcision site Testes Pubic hair Check for: Hernia (inguinal or femoral) Inguinal nodes
Anus	Assess: Patency Rectum Sphincter tone Check for hemorrhoids Check stool for color and presence of occult blood Inspect for masses

Sequence of examination procedures The child's age and health problems influence the sequence and manner in which the physical examination is performed. Newborns must be examined quickly and protected from heat loss. (See Chap. 8 for details about neonatal examinations.) An attempt to elicit a social response from the child should be made before proceeding with the examination (Fig. 14-2). A hurried approach should be avoided; this will alarm the child. Usually the examination is performed while a parent is present. If the child is frightened or clings to the parent, sending the parent out of the room usually serves only to frighten the child more.

Before beginning an examination, nurses should always wash their hands with warm water to cleanse and warm them. In the case of a toddler, the examination should begin with the child on the parent's lap. Eye contact with the child should be maintained as much as possible during the examination. It is best to show the instruments to the child before using them and to tell the child what is going to happen (Fig. 14-3). If the youngster grabs repeatedly at the examining instrument, the nurse can offer the child a toy or a tongue blade.

The physical assessment must be done systematically so that no area is overlooked. The nurse begins at either the head or the feet and

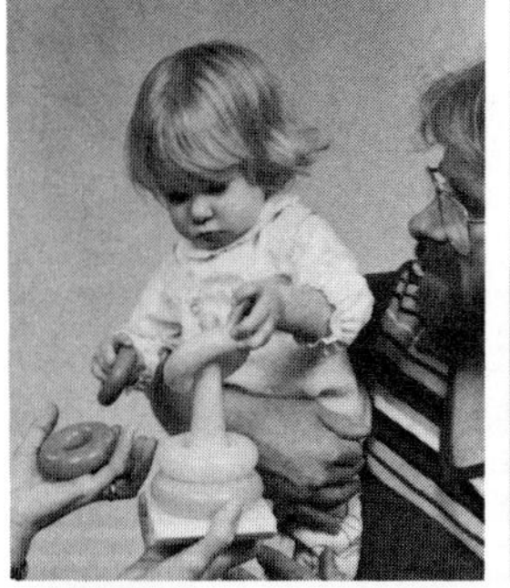

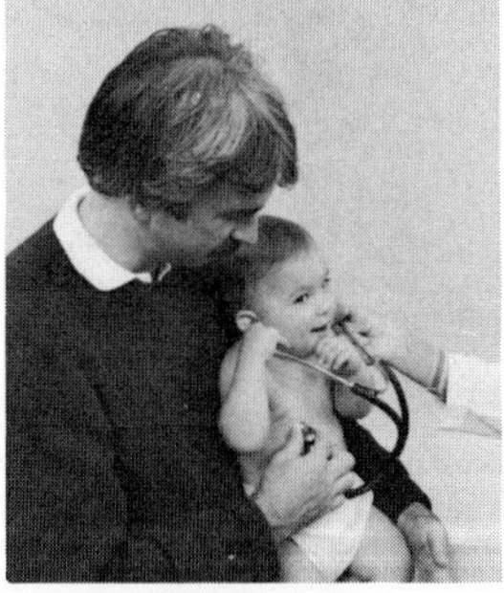

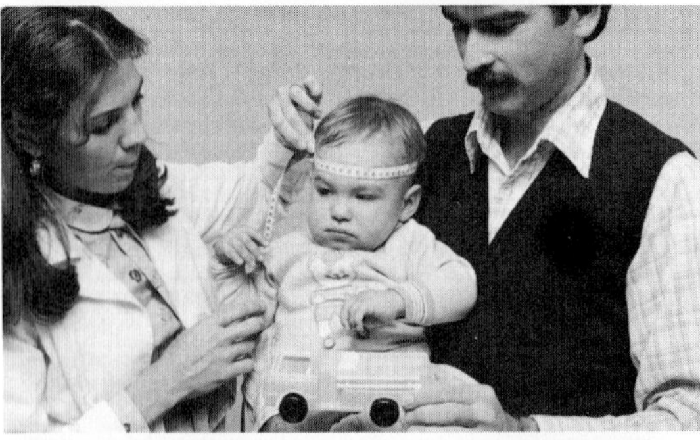

Figure 14-2 Establishing a relationship with the parent and the child before doing a physical examination (*From D. A. Jones, M. K. Lepley, and B. A. Baker, Health Assessment across the Life Span, McGraw-Hill, New York, 1984, p. 445. Used with permission.*)

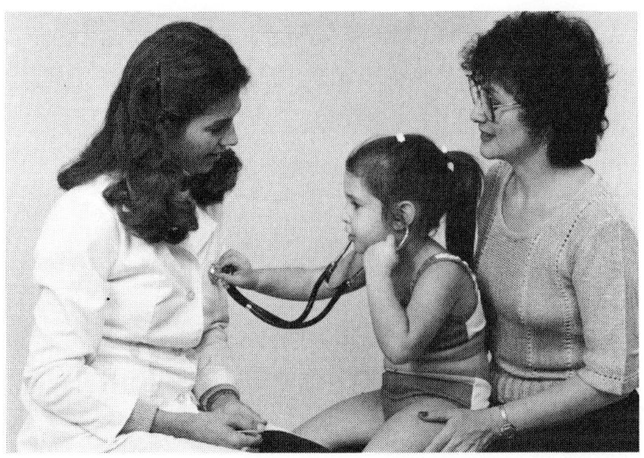

Figure 14-3 The preschooler should be involved in the physical examination. (*From D. A. Jones, M. K. Lepley, and B. A. Baker, Health Assessment across the Life Span, McGraw-Hill, New York, 1984, p. 545. Used with permission.*)

examines all nearby structures before moving upward or downward. The assessment usually begins at the head, although the nurse may begin elsewhere with very young children. Sometimes it is best to undertake auscultation of the chest as the first part of the examination, while the child is still quiet. Allowing the young patient to view the instrument that will be used will often do much to allay the child's fears. For example, the nurse can dangle the stethoscope in front of a baby or show an otoscope to a toddler, saying, "See my little light? I'm going to shine it into your ear. Maybe I'll see some birdies." When examining older children, the nurse should warn them when a procedure will be painful or uncomfortable. Only then will they develop trust in the nurse. Forceful restraint should be used only when absolutely essential; nurses can often enlist the parent's cooperation in restraining a child. For example, a small child's ears can usually be examined best by having the child sit on the mother's lap with the head immobilized against the mother's chest. Restraining the child this way is obviously much less frightening than holding the child's head down on the examining table. The nurse can start the physical examination by observing the hands and feet and then the chest or abdomen; then the nurse can auscultate, percuss, and palpate these areas and follow with the remainder of the examination. The nurse should first do those things which are least upsetting and for which the child's cooperation is needed. The parts of the examination that will most upset the child should be done last. For example, the nurse should not look at the throat first because this is very upsetting to most children, and they will be crying when the time comes to auscultate the heart.

A complete physical assessment requires that the nurse learn new skills of auscultation and percussion; inspection and palpation have long been part of the nurse's responsibility. The physical assessment requires the use of a systematic approach, along with patience, tact, and sensitivity to the needs of the child and the parent.

Although the parts of the examination may be performed in the sequence that best suits the particular child in the specific circumstances, recording the findings of the examination should be done in an orderly, systematic fashion, essentially from head to toe. Orderly recording not only prevents omissions but also, as in the case of the history, facilitates future reviewing of the medical chart. At the very least, the examination of a child should include auscultation of the heart and lungs, inspection of the genitalia, palpation of the abdomen, an examination of the ears with an otoscope, and an examination of the throat.

The nurse constantly makes decisions, both large and small. Does this visit require a complete assessment or only an investigation of the particular symptoms presented? How should the child be positioned for the examination? Is lighting in the room adequate for evaluating jaundice, cyanosis, and pallor? Is the child too tired to continue the examination, and, if so, when should the return visit be scheduled? Is this a normal variant or an abnormal finding? If it is an abnormal finding, what should be done about it? Should the parent be reassured, or is referral to a physician necessary? If a child is unable to perform a particular task, the nurse must decide whether the child understands the question or instructions, has the necessary maturity and motor skills to perform the task, or is simply refusing to cooperate. The ability to make sound decisions and judgments is developed with practice. Feedback from nursing colleagues, from other health care workers, and from children and their families will help the beginning nurse to perfect both decision-making and assessment skills. Nurses whose scope of responsibility includes making regular physical examinations of children are referred to health assessment texts which include complete descriptions of the methods used to perform a thorough physical examination and which provide guidance in performing specific techniques and differentiating between normal and abnormal findings. This text describes the assessment of each body system in the appropriate chapter in Part III.

Temperature Taking temperatures rectally is more reliable than taking them orally in the case of pediatric patients up to 5 years of age. The average rectal temperature usually does not drop below 37.5°C (99°F) until the child reaches the age of 36 months; a variation of 1 to 2°F in 24 h is not unusual. Illness does not always accompany a temperature rise in children. Anxiety, physical activity, and a high environmental temperature may cause body temperature to increase. Infants may have normal or subnormal temperatures with severe infections and also may have temperatures up to 40.6°C (105°F) with only minor illness.[10]

Pulse A child's heart rate is more readily affected by exercise, illness, and emotion than an adult's. An infant's pulse can be taken by palpation at the anterior fontanel or the femoral or carotid artery or by auscultation over the heart. Auscultation is the preferred method if the rate is irregular or very rapid.

A single measurement of pulse, respiratory rate, temperature, and blood pressure is not nearly as useful as a series of measurements of each of these taken over a period of time and under similar conditions. Each child has his or her own normal rate for each vital sign. (For average normal pulse and respiratory rates, see Table 16-19.)

Respirations The nurse must assess the rate, quality, and depth of respirations. Respiratory rate is more variable in children than in adults and is easily influenced by illness, exercise, and anxiety. Because babies and young children use primarily the diaphragm in breathing, there is little chest movement; it is easier to count the respirations by observing abdominal movement. Respiration is predominantly costal by 7 years of age, and so it is easier after that to count respirations by looking at chest movement. The nurse also observes for chest expansion and retraction.

Blood pressure Blood pressure measurement is considered part of routine screening for all children over 3 years of age. Emotion and activity affect the accuracy of blood pressure readings, as does cuff size. Blood pressure should be measured after other vital signs have been checked and before the child becomes excited or upset.[11] Having a variety of cuff sizes enables the nurse to choose the correct size after measuring the arm. (See Table 16-21 for guidelines in selecting sphygmomanometer cuffs.) Percentiles for blood pressure measurements for girls and boys are shown in Fig. 14-4.

Weight and height Periodic assessment of a child's general pattern of growth and development is important in promoting health and progress toward maturity. Measurements of height and weight should be taken at least five times during the first year of life (these usually coincide with well-child visits at 2 weeks and at 2, 4, 6, and 9 months of age) and then yearly throughout childhood and adolescence. The readings are plotted on a graph that shows the child's measurements in relation to percentile norms compiled from data on large groups of children in the same age groups. The chart shows weight, length in the lying position, height in the standing position (stature), and head circumference as they relate to age. Different charts are available for boys and girls. The consistency of a child's measurements over time and the consistency of different measurements at the same time are better indicators of maturation for that child than comparison with the average.[12] It must be kept in mind that the standards are always based on average measurements of a sample population and that individual children can be expected to deviate.

The National Center for Health Statistics (NCHS) growth charts of 1976 were prepared from data obtained in three separate surveys taken from 1962 through 1974. Figure 14-5 shows a sample chart. The complete set of the NCHS growth charts is included in Appendix B. Each chart shows curves at the 5th, 10th, 25th, 50th, 75th, 90th, and 95th percentiles.

A child below the 5th percentile is considered small or underweight. A child above the 95th percentile is considered large or overweight. Family patterns of growth and size must be considered when evaluating children at the extremes of height or weight. Newborns who are in the 50th percentile for height and weight will usually remain in that percentile throughout their lives. Patterns of growth that need further investigation are:

1. A wide disparity between height and weight
2. A failure to show expected increases in height and weight

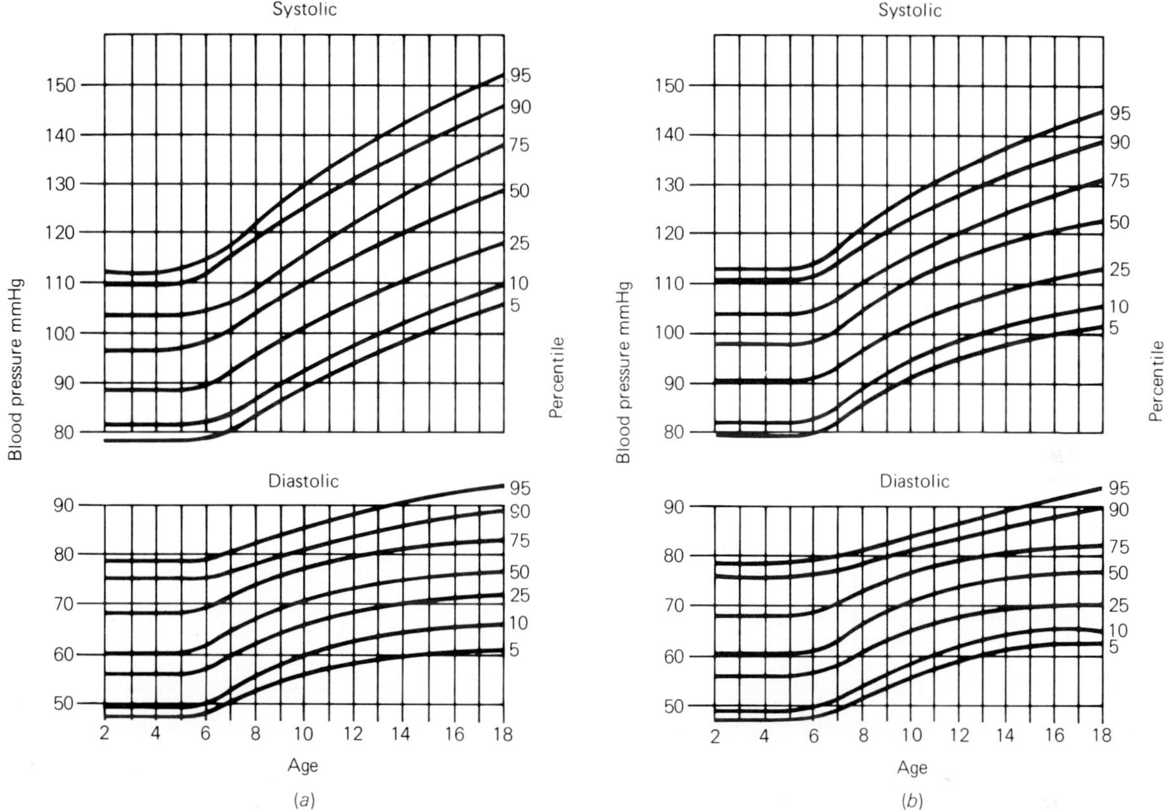

Figure 14-4 Percentiles of blood pressure measurement (done on the right arm when the child is seated). (*A*) Girls. (*B*) Boys, (*From "Report of the Task Force on Blood Pressure Control in Children," Pediatrics,* **59**(suppl):803 [May 1977].)

3. Sudden increases or decreases in height, weight, or head circumference when previous growth was steady
4. Between 2 and 3 (or more than 3) standard deviations below the mean for age[13]

It is important to note that children from the Asian and Pacific countries should not be matched to the standard charts. There are charts available specifically for use with Asian children. In evaluating the growth of a 6-year-old Caucasian boy, his measurements should be compared with those of other 6-year-old Caucasian boys, and with his growth record from birth to age 6.

DEVELOPMENTAL SCREENING TOOLS

Developmental screening tools are available to help nurses assess children's development. Early detection of developmental delays can be vital in determining a child's potential for leading a normal life. A variety of factors influence a child's development. They include neurological, developmental, and environmental factors; the circumstances of the child's birth; family relationships and interpersonal relationships; and outside stimulation. The tests described in this chapter are only a few that are available for assessing children's development. Table 14-8 summarizes a sample of developmental screening tests used with children.

The Denver Developmental Screening Test

The Denver Developmental Screening Test (DDST) is a tool designed to identify developmental delays in babies and children under 6 years of age.[14] The DDST provides a developmental profile of a child in the areas of gross motor, language, personal/social, and fine motor/

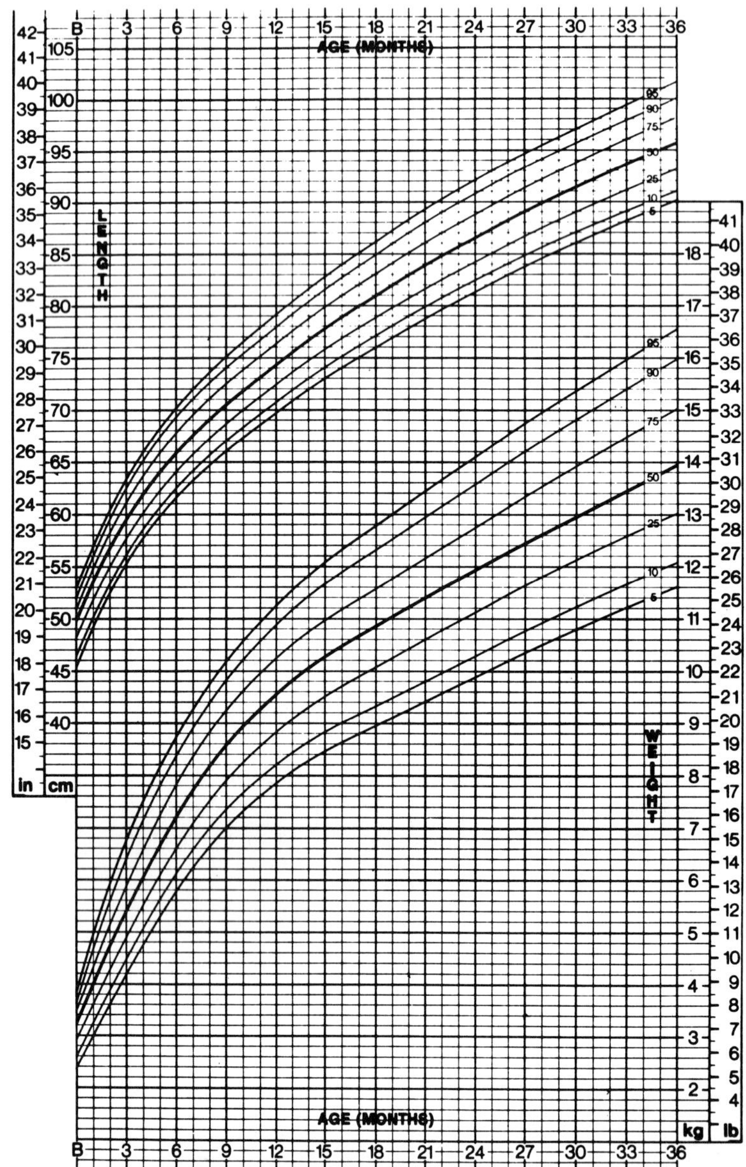

Figure 14-5 Physical growth of girls from birth to 36 months of age. [*Courtesy of Ross Laboratories Columbus, Ohio. Adapted from National Center for Health Statistics, NCHS growth charts, 1976, Monthly Vital Statistics Reports* **25**(*3*) *suppl. (HRA) 76–1120. Health Resources Administration, Rockville, Md., June 1976. Data from the Fels Research Institute, Yellow Springs, Ohio.*]

Table 14-8 Developmental Screening Tests

Screening test and age	Purpose	Administration
Dubowitz Test 1 to 5 days	To determine gestational age of the newborn by assessment of external characteristics and neurological signs	The examiner needs demonstration and practice. An instruction manual and scoring sheets are available. The test takes about 10 min. Observation includes skin, sole creases, lanugo, genital development, and neurological signs.
Neonatal Behavioral Assessment Scale (T. Berry Brazelton) Birth to 4 weeks	To observe and rate the infant's interactive behavior with the environment. Examines state, temperament, and behavior in terms of habituation, orientation, motor maturity, variation, self-quieting abilities, and social behavior	The examiner needs training and evaluation to achieve reliability. The infant is observed in a quiet, somewhat darkened room. Repeated assessments are useful. Responses vary with the state of the infant. The test is useful for teaching parents and takes 20 to 30 min, plus scoring time. A text, films, and a trainer are needed. The test is more sensitive in predicting future development than traditional neurologic evaluation tools.
Neonatal Perception Inventory (Elsie Broussard): Birth to 1 month	To detect potential disturbances in developmental course. Based on the assumption that an infant who is not perceived by the mother as better than average is at much higher risk for development of subsequent emotional difficulty. Can identify newborns at risk for developing an emotional disorder and can identify infants who need watching	The mother completes the Average Baby Inventory and Your Baby Inventory at 2 to 3 days and then these two plus the Degree of Bother Inventory at 1 month. Standard instructions are available for each inventory. The principles of interviewing, guidance, and reassurance are used to counsel a mother who is having difficulty with her infant.
Denver Developmental Screening Test (DDST): birth to 6 years	To detect developmental delays in children in five areas: gross motor, language, fine motor, adaptive, and personal-social skills	The examiner needs training and periodic evaluation and uses a test kit, forms, and manual. A training film is available. The examiner enlists the cooperation of the parents and the child and interprets the results to the parents. The test takes 15 to 30 min.
Denver Prescreening Developmental Questionnaire (PDQ): 3 months to 6 years	To decide whether to test the child with the DDST or to follow the child at well-child visits	A 10-item checklist (yes-no), according to the child's age, is answered by the parent. Immediate referral is indicated if the score is 6 or less; a child who scores 8 or less is retested. Referral is indicated if a child scores less than 8 twice.
Developmental Profile: Questions relate to 6-month period from birth to $3\frac{1}{2}$, then yearly to 12 years	To assess five areas of development: physical, self-help, personal-social, academic, and communication skills	An interview guide is administered to parents or caregiver. Begin with one year level below chronological age. Administration and scoring are easily taught and learned. There are no referral criteria.

Table 14-8 Developmental Screening Tests (*Continued*)

Screening test and age	Purpose	Administration
Carey-McDevitt Infant Temperament Questionnaire: 4–8 months. (Other, similar scales are available for children aged 1–3, 3–7, and 8–12 years.)	To obtain descriptions of the infant's temperament in nine categories: activity, rhythmicity, adaptability, approach, sensory threshold, intensity, mood, distractibility, and persistence. These descriptions should be the basis for discussing the infant's temperament and needs and for helping the mother with the infant	The mother answers 95 questions using six frequency options describing her infant and gives supplementary data. The test takes about 25 min plus 10–15 min to score. Babies are designated as "difficult," "intermediate," or "easy." Areas of questioning cover sleeping, feeding, elimination, diapering, dressing, and bathing.
Home observation for measurement of the environment: birth to 3 years, 3 to 6 years, and 6 to 12 years	To sample the quantity and quality of social, emotional, and cognitive support available to the child in the home from the child's perspective	The observer visits the home when the child is awake, observes the child, and interviews the parent. It takes 60 min and is predictive of scores on the Stanford-Binet at 3 years. It can also be used as a teaching tool for parents. An instruction manual is available.
Vineland Social Maturity Scale: Birth to adolescence	To sample levels of functioning in the areas of self-help, dressing, eating, communication, self-direction, locomotion, and socialization. Provides a scale of normal behaviors and can show mental deficits or emotional disturbances	The examiner asks the parent questions about various activities, starting below the anticipated level. The test takes 20–30 min. Examiners should have formal training or work in pairs to ensure reliability.
Goodenough-Harris Drawing Test: 3–5 years	To assess intellectual development nonverbally	The child's drawings are compared with 12 ranked drawings. Each drawing is scored for 73 items. There are standard scores for both sexes. The test takes 10–15 min.
Self-Esteem Inventory: Grades 4–12	To assess self-esteem through judgment of self-worth	There is a long form (58 questions) and a short form (25 questions). The number of high self-esteem responses is multiplied by 4. Top 25% = high self-esteem, middle 50% = medium self-esteem, and low 25% = low self-esteem.

Sources: Patricia Castiglia and Marcia Petrini, "Selecting a Developmental Screening Tool," *Pediatric Nursing* **11**(1):8–17 (January–February 1985); Suzanne H. Johnson, *High-Risk Parenting: Nursing Assessment and Strategies for the Family at Risk*, Lippincott, Philadelphia, 1979; Marcene Lee Powell, *Assessment and Management of Developmental Changes and Problems in Children*, Mosby, St. Louis, 1981; and Sharon R. Stangler, Cathee Huber, and Donald Routh, *Screening Growth and Development of Preschool Children: A Guide for Test Selection*, McGraw-Hill, New York, 1980.

adaptive abilities (see Figs. 14-6 and 14-7). If a child is scored as questionable or abnormal in any of the four areas of the DDST on two administrations of the test, the child should be referred for further evaluation.[15] Even though the DDST is fairly simple for both professionals and nonprofessionals to administer, score, and interpret, it should not be used without adequate training. An instructional program is available that includes a manual, a workbook, a film, and a practice testing session with proficiency evaluation. Periodic checks of the screening practices of all examiners who use the DDST should be done in order to ensure the accuracy of test results.

The Denver Prescreening Developmental Questionnaire

The Denver Prescreening Developmental Questionnaire (PDQ) is a simplified version of the DDST that can be used to decide whether a child needs to be tested with the DDST. The PDQ is a 10-item questionnaire that is answered by the parent. The questions vary according to the child's age. Like the DDST, the PDQ is suitable for use with children from infancy through the sixth birthday. Immediate testing with the DDST is done when a child has a score of 6 or less; a child who has a score of 8 or less is retested. If the score is still 8 or less, the DDST is administered.[16]

The Developmental Profile

Another questionnaire used with parents is the Developmental Profile. This interview guide relies heavily on verbal answers from a person who knows the child well. It includes five age scales that measure physical, self-help, social, academic, and communication development.[17] It is one of the few tests used to screen children in the middle childhood years.

When developmental screening tests indicate that a child may have a delay, referral to a qualified health provider who regularly administers developmental tests is mandatory. That person may be a psychologist, a nurse practitioner, or a pediatrician.

The Gesell Developmental Test

The Gesell Developmental Test is a somewhat more detailed assessment of development. This test assesses five major areas:

1. *Adaptive behavior,* which is concerned with the organization of stimuli, the perception of relationships, and the dissection of wholes into their component parts and the reintegration of these parts in a meaningful fashion.
2. *Gross motor behavior,* which includes postural reactions, head balance, sitting, standing, creeping, and walking.
3. *Fine motor behavior,* which consists of the use of the hands and fingers in grasping and manipulating objects.
4. *Language behavior,* which assumes distinctive patterns that furnish clues as to the organization of the child's central nervous system. The term *language behavior* is used broadly to include all visible and audible forms of communication, including facial expressions, gestures, postural movements, vocalizations, words, phrases, and sentences. It also includes mimicry and comprehension of the communications of others.
5. *Personal and social behavior,* which includes the child's personal reactions to the social culture in which he or she lives. The child's performance of a variety of tasks is evaluated on a pass-fail basis, and a developmental age is estimated for the child.[18]

The Neonatal Behavioral Assessment Scale

An assessment of behavioral responses should be a part of the examination of every newborn. The Neonatal Behavioral Assessment Scale (NBAS) attempts to measure the complex behavioral responses to social stimuli as the neonate moves from sleeping to alert states of consciousness to crying. The NBAS reflects the infant's capacity for integration of the central and autonomic nervous systems and therefore is a window to the newborn's well-being. The NBAS evaluates a combination of 26 behavioral items and 20 neurological reflexes over a 20- to 30-min period. The six behavioral dimensions are:

1. *Habituation*—the infant's ability to shut out disturbing environmental stimuli
2. *Interaction (orientation)*—the newborn's ability to attend to and process simple and complex environmental events
3. *Motor performance*—the neonate's ability to maintain adequate tone to control motor behavior and to perform integrated motor activities
4. *Range of state*—the intensity and variability of the newborn's state of consciousness during the assessment
5. *State regulation*—the infant's ability to control and modulate the states as he or she attends to social and inanimate stimuli
6. *Autonomic regulation*—the newborn's vulnerability to his or her physiological immaturity as he or she recovers from labor and delivery[19]

Figure 14-6 The Denver Developmental Screening Test form.

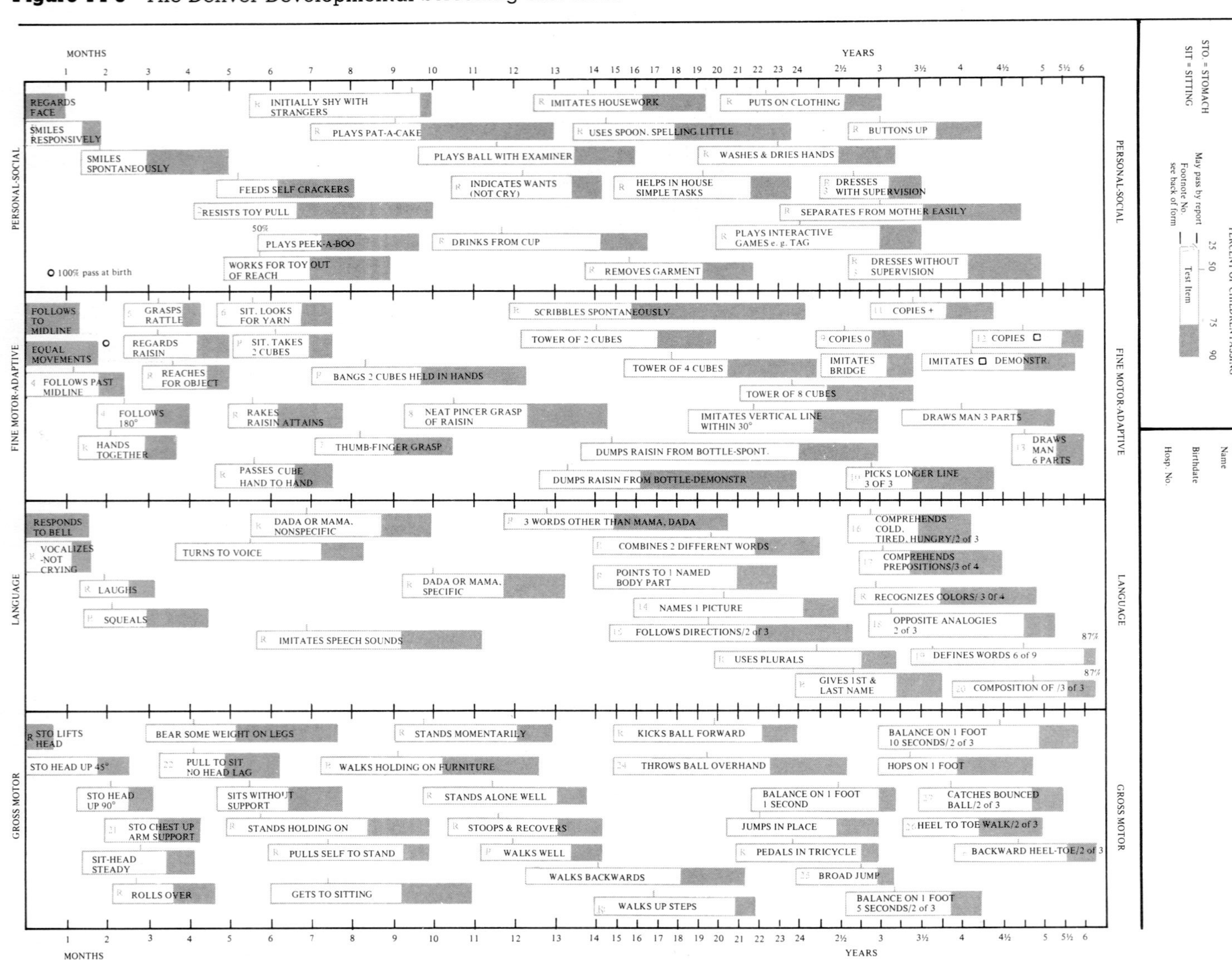

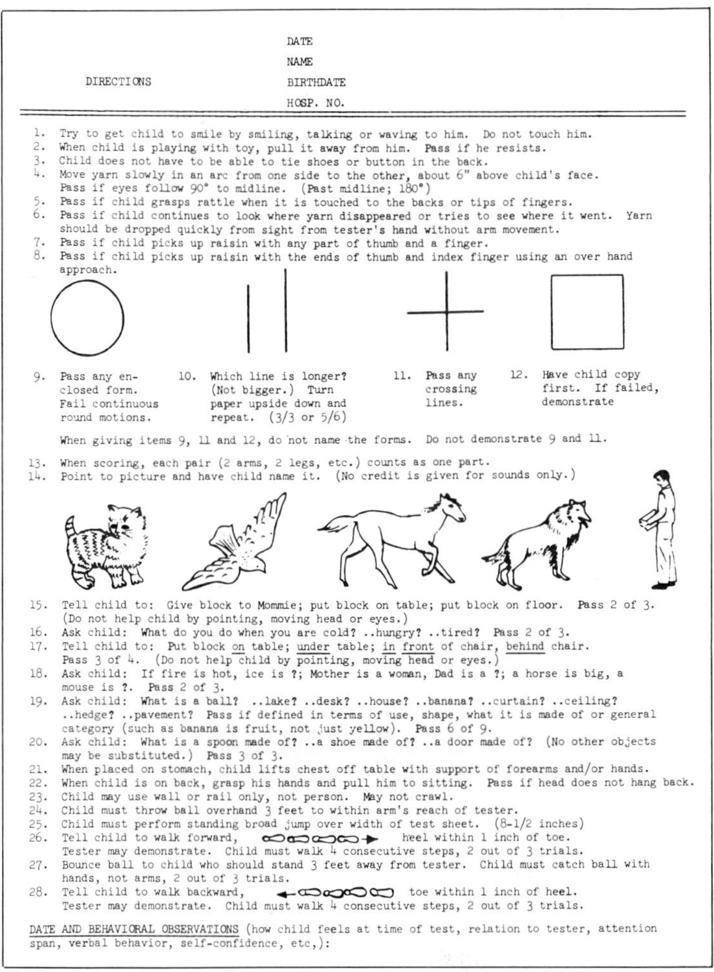

DATE
NAME
DIRECTIONS BIRTHDATE
HOSP. NO.

1. Try to get child to smile by smiling, talking or waving to him. Do not touch him.
2. When child is playing with toy, pull it away from him. Pass if he resists.
3. Child does not have to be able to tie shoes or button in the back.
4. Move yarn slowly in an arc from one side to the other, about 6" above child's face. Pass if eyes follow 90° to midline. (Past midline; 180°)
5. Pass if child grasps rattle when it is touched to the backs or tips of fingers.
6. Pass if child continues to look where yarn disappeared or tries to see where it went. Yarn should be dropped quickly from sight from tester's hand without arm movement.
7. Pass if child picks up raisin with any part of thumb and a finger.
8. Pass if child picks up raisin with the ends of thumb and index finger using an over hand approach.

9. Pass any enclosed form. Fail continuous round motions.
10. Which line is longer? (Not bigger.) Turn paper upside down and repeat. (3/3 or 5/6)
11. Pass any crossing lines.
12. Have child copy first. If failed, demonstrate

When giving items 9, 11 and 12, do not name the forms. Do not demonstrate 9 and 11.

13. When scoring, each pair (2 arms, 2 legs, etc.) counts as one part.
14. Point to picture and have child name it. (No credit is given for sounds only.)
15. Tell child to: Give block to Mommie; put block on table; put block on floor. Pass 2 of 3. (Do not help child by pointing, moving head or eyes.)
16. Ask child: What do you do when you are cold? ..hungry? ..tired? Pass 2 of 3.
17. Tell child to: Put block on table; under table; in front of chair, behind chair. Pass 3 of 4. (Do not help child by pointing, moving head or eyes.)
18. Ask child: If fire is hot, ice is ?; Mother is a woman, Dad is a ?; a horse is big, a mouse is ?. Pass 2 of 3.
19. Ask child: What is a ball? ..lake? ..desk? ..house? ..banana? ..curtain? ..ceiling? ..hedge? ..pavement? Pass if defined in terms of use, shape, what it is made of or general category (such as banana is fruit, not just yellow). Pass 6 of 9.
20. Ask child: What is a spoon made of? ..a shoe made of? ..a door made of? (No other objects may be substituted.) Pass 3 of 3.
21. When placed on stomach, child lifts chest off table with support of forearms and/or hands.
22. When child is on back, grasp his hands and pull him to sitting. Pass if head does not hang back.
23. Child may use wall or rail only, not person. May not crawl.
24. Child must throw ball overhand 3 feet to within arm's reach of tester.
25. Child must perform standing broad jump over width of test sheet. (8-1/2 inches)
26. Tell child to walk forward, heel within 1 inch of toe. Tester may demonstrate. Child must walk 4 consecutive steps, 2 out of 3 trials.
27. Bounce ball to child who should stand 3 feet away from tester. Child must catch ball with hands, not arms, 2 out of 3 trials.
28. Tell child to walk backward, toe within 1 inch of heel. Tester may demonstrate. Child must walk 4 consecutive steps, 2 out of 3 trials.

DATE AND BEHAVIORAL OBSERVATIONS (how child feels at time of test, relation to tester, attention span, verbal behavior, self-confidence, etc,):

Figure 14-7 Instructions for administering some of the items on the Denver Developmental Screening Test. (*Available from LADOCA Project and Publishing Foundation, East 51st Ave. and Lincoln St., Denver, Colorado, 80216.*)

The NBAS guides the examiner in documenting and describing the neonate's performance on each behavioral item but does not yield an overall good or bad score.[20] Because the assessment shows the individuality of the infant, researchers have found it to be a powerful influence in shaping the outcome of his or her relationship with caregivers.[21] It is important to do an NBAS with the parents in attendance so that they can observe all the individual characteristics of their new baby and the tasks that he or she can perform. This often promotes attachment and bonding between the infant and the parents. (See Chap. 8, section on behavioral assessment.)

VISION AND HEARING SCREENING

Vision

Vision defects are among the most common handicapping conditions of childhood. Effective screening is of special importance, since many of these problems are correctable. Vision screening is done to detect conditions that may cause blindness or visual impairment which is less se-

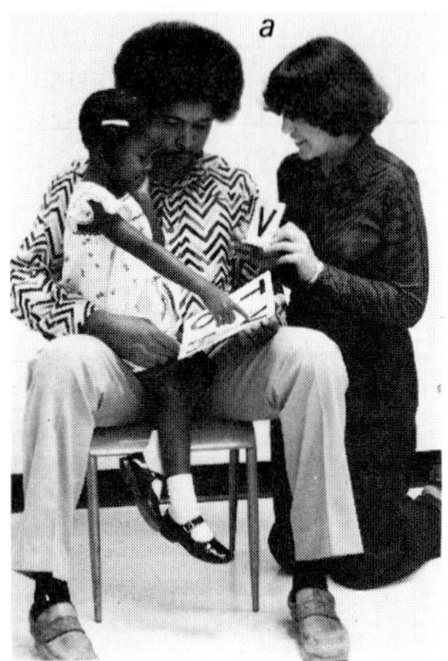

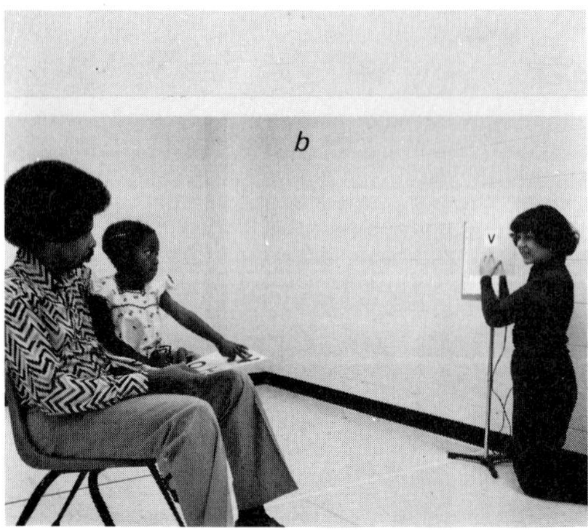

Figure 14-8 (*A*) Teaching a child to take the HOTV test. (*B*) Testing a child with the HOTV test. (*From S. Stangler, C. Huber, D. Roth, Screening Growth and Development of Preschool Children: A Guide for Test Selections, McGraw-Hill, New York, 1980. Used with permission.)*

vere but which is sufficient to delay development or interfere with education. Reduced visual acuity is a common problem with children. *Amblyopia*, or lazy eye, is a major problem and is detectable by screening. Further loss of vision in the unused eye is preventable if amblyopia is detected and treated early (see Chap. 31). A spelling chart with letters of different sizes is used to measure the visual acuity of children who have learned the alphabet. First, both eyes are tested together, and then each eye is tested individually. If vision in either eye is less than 20/30, the child should be referred to an ophthalmologist. For children aged 2 to 5 years, the HOTV test is used. The HOTV test incorporates those four letters; a 10-ft testing distance is used with visual targets of several sizes, and there is a response panel which the child uses to match the letters that he or she sees. Letter shapes are easily learned by children aged 2 and over.[22] A parent can be with the child when the test is given. Figure 14-8 shows a child being tested with the HOTV.

In order to detect strabismus, the nurse should test the corneal light reflex and perform an alternate cover test. The corneal light test is done by shining a light at the bridge of the nose 13 to 15 in before the child's eyes and by observing whether the light reflection falls in the center of both pupils or slightly toward the nasal edge. If one light reflection is out toward the edge of the iris, the test indicates strabismus. To administer the alternate cover test, the nurse has the child look at an object about 12 in before the eyes. Then one eye is covered and the nurse looks for movement of the uncovered eye inward or outward. The other eye is then tested in the same way.[23] The cover must always be kept at the same level. In case of eye movement or suspected latent strabismus, the child should be referred to an ophthalmologist. The Minnesota Department of Health recommends vision screening of all children at birth, at 3 years of age, before entering school, in kindergarten, and in grades 1, 3, 4, 5, 7, and 10. Suspected problems should be verified with repeated screening before a child is referred.

Hearing

Hearing screening is done to detect hearing loss and ear disease, since both are often treatable. Hearing tests are done using mechanical devices that produce either pure tones of different frequencies at different decibels of intensity or the sound of a human voice at different intensities. A child should be referred for hearing testing if he or she:[24]

1. Does not respond to sound or localized sound at any age

2. Responds to people only when they are in visual range
3. Delays for a long time when responding to verbal information at any age
4. Needs to have directions or statements repeated several times

The above may also indicate the need for a speech and language referral evaluation. Finding severe hearing loss is crucial in infants because the development of language skills depends on the child's ability to hear. Severe hearing loss at birth is present in 1 in 2000 infants; by 2 years of age about 1 in 25 children has mild to moderate hearing loss.[25] The incidence of hearing loss is greater in disadvantaged children. Screening is recommended from birth through early childhood by gross hearing testing and assessment of language development. Pure-tone audiometry can be used at 3 to 4 years of age and then repeated every 2 to 3 years. Any child who has otitis media may develop temporary or permanent hearing loss and should be retested. Chapter 31 discusses vision and hearing screening in more detail.

SCOLIOSIS SCREENING

Scoliosis is a lateral curvature of the spine. There are two types: functional and structural. *Functional scoliosis* is often the result of poor posture. *Structural scoliosis* occurs most frequently among children between the ages of 12 and 16 and affects girls more often than boys. The cause of an individual case of structural scoliosis is often not known, but may be due to multiple conditions such as shortening of one leg, muscle spasms secondary to trauma, or structural defects of the spine. Diagnosis is made by means of inspection and x-ray examination. The child is examined from the front, back, and side while standing upright and while bending forward with the hands touching and the arms extended. The nurse looks for abnormalities such as unlevel shoulders, a prominent shoulder blade, unlevel hips, and sideways deviation of the spine. Asymmetry of the chest or rib hump—the classic, most important finding in structural scoliosis—is apparent when the child bends forward. The postural abnormalities of excessive roundback and swayback are visible from the side. All children who are suspected of having scoliosis should be referred to an orthopedic surgeon. The benefits of early detection are twofold. First, most mild progressive curvatures can be arrested, thus preventing the need for surgery. Second, when surgery is required, it will be more successful because the curve can be repaired earlier, when surgery is easier and safer and results in better correction of the problem. Although the heart grows normally in children with structural scoliosis, lung growth is abnormal because of crowding of the organs in the chest cage; these children may develop pulmonary hypertension. Early counseling can help a child cope with the altered body image.[26] Screening for scoliosis is recommended throughout the school-age years. It is usually done by the community or school health nurse (see Chap. 29).

OTHER SCREENING TESTS

Recently, the number of conditions for which screening is recommended and legislated has increased greatly. The following factors are taken into consideration when making decisions about what, whom, when, and how to screen:

1. What is the law?
2. What is the incidence of the condition in the particular area? For example, certain areas have a high incidence of lead toxicity.
3. What is the ethnic background of the population? (Sickle cell disease, for example, is more prevalent among blacks than among Caucasians.)
4. What will be the cost to the patient?
5. Is treatment available at an acceptable cost?

It is important to screen for the following:

1. Conditions that can be diagnosed with certainty
2. Conditions in which early diagnosis and treatment can be beneficial
3. Conditions for which the screening procedures are highly accurate

When considering any screening test, the nurse must be concerned about (1) the adequacy of the descriptive and teaching information available; (2) whether the test is appropriate for the child in terms of his or her age; (3) reliability, i.e., whether a repeat test will produce the same results or whether different testers will get the same results; (4) validity, i.e., whether the test measures what it is supposed to measure; and (5) acceptability in terms of cost, ease of administration, and the reaction of the child and the family.[27]

To justify a screening program it is essential that results on a screening test can be followed up by appropriate evaluation and treatment, and that the benefits of screening tests will be great in terms of the number of affected children identified or the number of disabilities prevented.[28]

Galactosemia affects approximately 1 in 60,000 neonates.[29] Jaundice, poor eating, vomiting, weight loss, and an enlarged liver usually are indications of the disease during the first weeks of life. Untreated infants usually die within 6 weeks, and the few who recover are severely handicapped.[30] Babies should be screened for the disease if symptoms are present or if the family is known to be at risk for the disease. Many physicians screen all newborns. Treatment consists of a lactose-free diet in which milk substitutes are used; infants so treated usually develop normal intelligence.

Phenylketonuria (PKU) occurs in about 1 in 10,000 births and is due to an absence or deficiency of the enzyme necessary to process phenylalanine, an essential amino acid found in natural protein foods.[31] Signs and symptoms (mental retardation, eczema) are not usually apparent until after the child is 4 months old, when some brain damage has already occurred. PKU is treated by restricting the consumption of foods containing phenylalanine: bread, meat, fish, cheese, nuts, and eggs. Even with such treatment, the outcome is sometimes poor, but if the diet is restricted very early in life, mental retardation can be prevented. Planning the diet will be necessary during most of the affected person's life, particularly in the case of girls who must consider the possibility of becoming pregnant.

PKU testing is required by law in some states. Some hospitals screen for PKU before babies are discharged from the nursery, using a Guthrie test on blood from the heel; this ensures that babies are tested at least once. Testing is done again at 3 to 4 days of age, because by that time, a baby who has PKU has ingested enough milk to raise the phenylalanine in the blood to abnormal levels.

Congenital hypothyroidism, or cretinism, results from too little secretion of thyroid hormone and is one of the most common endocrine diseases in children; it affects 1 in 4000 newborns. There is a male/female ratio of approximately 3 to 1.[32] No signs or symptoms are present at birth, but they may appear during the first weeks or months of life (see Chap. 24). Damage to the central nervous system may occur before clinical manifestations are apparent. Testing for hypothyroidism is commonly done by measuring levels of T_4 (thyroxine) during the neonatal period. Treatment consists of replacing thyroid hormone with synthetic levothyroxine.[33] (See Chap. 24.) Even when treatment is successful and is begun early, the child may have some degree of mental retardation. Studies suggest that early treatment leads to a better outcome.[34]

Tuberculosis can affect children of all ages. Children under 3 years of age and adolescents are especially susceptible. When children live for extended periods of time with persons who have tuberculosis, they often develop the disease. It is important to screen a child who lives in the same house with a person who has an active case of tuberculosis, no matter how old he or she is. Routine screening for tuberculosis using the Mantoux test should be done at 12 months of age or at the same time that the 15 mo measles, mumps, and rubella (MMR) vaccine is given. If screening is not done at this time, it is necessary to wait 30 days after the MMR vaccine to avoid the possibility of a false-negative result. The test is given again at 5 and 12 years of age. Children who are regularly exposed to persons with the disease should be tested every 1 to 2 years.

Anemia is a common childhood disorder that can impair health and development and may be indicative of numerous underlying problems. Hemoglobin and hematocrit (see Chap. 23) should be evaluated routinely at birth, at 1 and 5 years of age, and in early adolescence.

Urinary tract infections are also common and require treatment to prevent structural damage to the urinary tract as well as impairment of health and development. Because of their shorter urethras and greater risk of fecal contamination through the urinary meatus, girls have more urinary infections than boys. A urine culture should be done on all toilet-trained girls at 2 to 3 years of age and then again at ages 5 to 6 and 8 to 9. The urine protein of preschoolers and preadolescents of both sexes should be evaluated.

Lead poisoning is also common among children who are at high risk because of their environment or life circumstances. They should be screened at 9 to 12 months of age and at least yearly thereafter until the age of 5. High-risk children are those who live in cities near busy freeways or in houses built before the mid-1940s, when lead paints were used on interior surfaces; those who practice pica, or the ingestion of nonfood substances, which may include paint chips containing lead; and those with previously elevated levels of lead.

Sickle cell hemoglobin should be routinely screened in neonates of African, Mediterranean, or Arab ancestry. If a prenatal diagnosis has not been made, certainly all newborns of parents who are known carriers of the sickle cell disorder should be screened by subjecting hemoglobin from cord blood to electrophoresis.

COMPONENTS OF ROUTINE HEALTH MAINTENANCE

Dental care

Dental health begins with a good prenatal diet, since some of the primary teeth calcify in utero. At approximately 6 months of age, the first of the primary (deciduous) teeth erupt. Formation of the permanent teeth begins soon after birth. The permanent teeth do not erupt until the primary teeth are lost, between 6 and 12 years of age (Fig. 14-9). Two important functions of the primary teeth are to enable the child to chew food and to maintain space in the mandible and the maxilla for the permanent teeth. If a primary tooth is lost early, the child should see a dentist, who will decide whether a space-maintaining device is necessary. Infants and young children do not have the manual dexterity to clean their teeth thoroughly. Their parents must be totally responsible for their oral hygiene. Beginning with the eruption of the first tooth, the parents should perform the daily cleaning process, using a piece of gauze or a washcloth wrapped around a finger. As more teeth erupt, the parents may start to use a soft brush and develop a systematic approach to toothbrushing.[35] Handicapped children, such as those with cerebral palsy, may need special help.

The major factors in dental health are brushing the teeth regularly, eating an adequate diet, applying fluoride or drinking fluoridated water in order to prevent cavities, and preventing or correcting malocclusion. All the surfaces of the teeth should be brushed for 3 min within 10 min after eating (Fig. 14-10). Flossing between the teeth is essential. The diet should be balanced, adequate in amount, and low in foods containing sugars and starches.

Carbohydrates are the main cause of dental caries, but not the only one. Some children are more susceptible than others. The bacteria in dental plaque break down the carbohydrates in the mouth to form organic acids. These acids cause the teeth to demineralize, and decay results. The longer a carbohydrate remains in contact with the teeth, the greater the chance of decay. Sticky foods, such as caramel and dried fruits, are more apt to cause decay than carbonated beverages. Because many medications, such as cough syrups and cough drops, contain over 50 percent sugar, children should brush their teeth after taking them.

Proper nutrition and dental hygiene are important in preventing caries. The nurse should educate parents and children about the importance of consuming adequate amounts of calcium, phosphorus, vitamin D, and fluoride for strong tooth formation (mineralization is completed at approximately 16 years of age).

Children who drink water containing approximately 1 part per million of fluoride throughout the period when their teeth are forming may have approximately 50 to 75 percent fewer caries, and there are strong indications that this effect continues throughout life.[36] Fluoridation of community water supplies is of tremendous value in reducing dental decay.

Periodontal disease is caused by bacterial plaque, genetic susceptibility, diet, or poor oral hygiene. Enzymes and toxic substances are formed by bacteria, causing gingivitis, or inflammation of the gums. Eventually the bone recedes away from the infection. Eighty percent of teenagers have gingivitis, the early form of periodontal disease. Children who wear braces on their teeth must cleanse their teeth very carefully to prevent caries and plaque formation.

Malocclusion is faulty alignment of the teeth; the upper and lower teeth do not come together correctly when the mouth is closed. Common causes of malocclusion are teeth that are too large or too small, one jaw that is too large or too small, thumb-sucking, early loss of the primary teeth, failure of a tooth to form where one should be, and a delayed or distorted pattern of tooth eruption. Malocclusion can interfere with chewing, cause facial deformity, interfere with speech, and cause body-image problems. Parents should be encouraged to obtain regular dental care for their children, beginning at 3 years of age (or earlier), and to seek dental care immediately when injuries to the mouth, gums, or teeth occur. Family patterns of missing teeth, abnormal tooth eruption, or malocclusion are significant factors to note in the health history. When assessing chil-

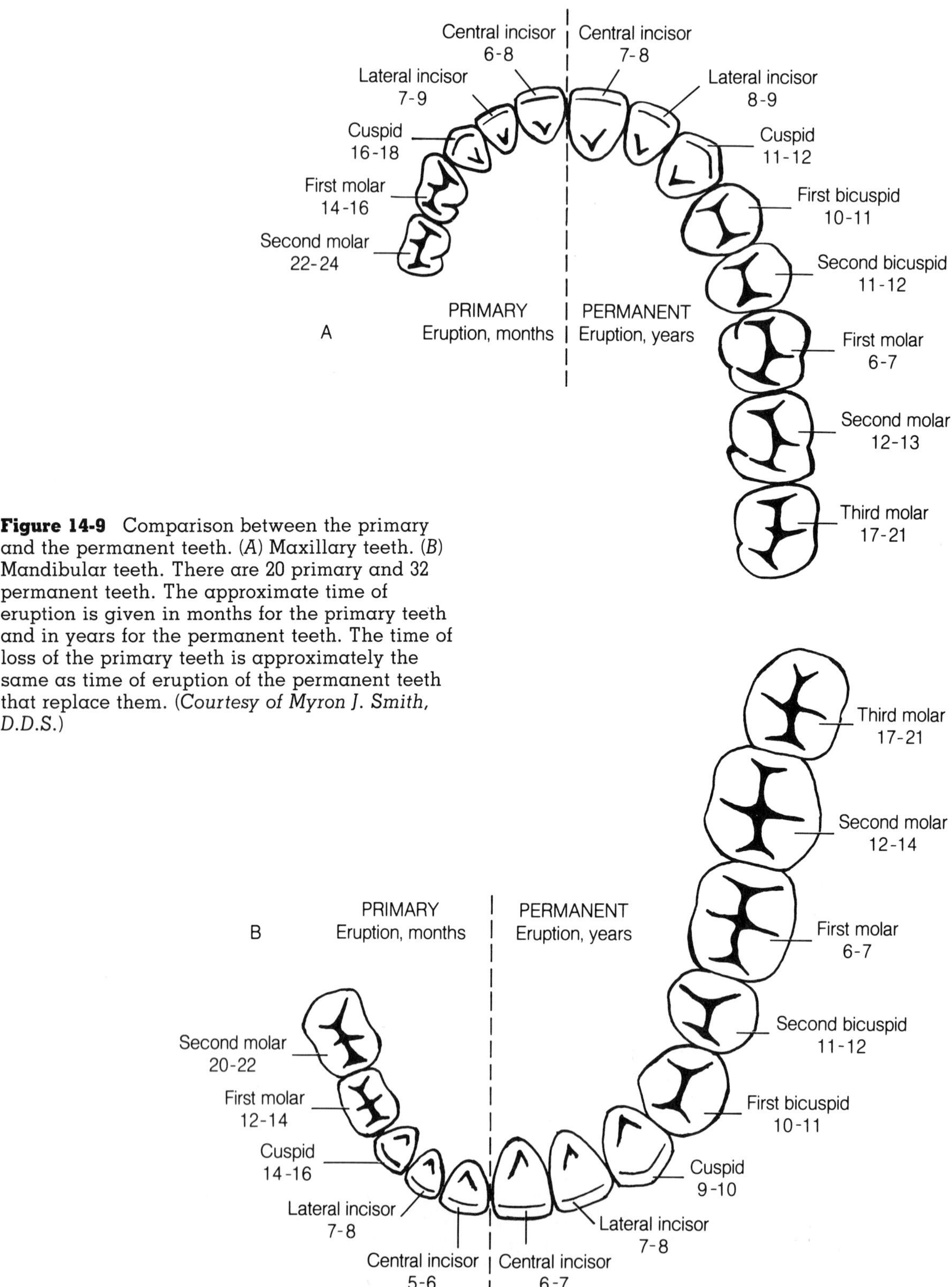

Figure 14-9 Comparison between the primary and the permanent teeth. (*A*) Maxillary teeth. (*B*) Mandibular teeth. There are 20 primary and 32 permanent teeth. The approximate time of eruption is given in months for the primary teeth and in years for the permanent teeth. The time of loss of the primary teeth is approximately the same as time of eruption of the permanent teeth that replace them. (*Courtesy of Myron J. Smith, D.D.S.*)

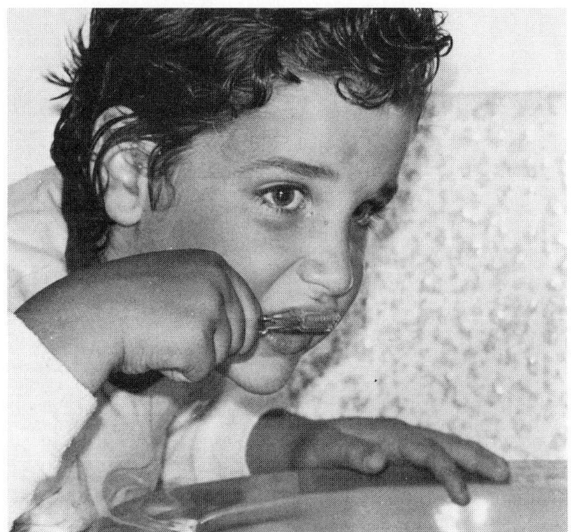

Figure 14-10 Brushing the teeth after meals and before going to bed helps prevent tooth decay.

dren, it is the responsibility of the nurse to recognize and diagnose many common dental problems, including malocclusion. It is important to carefully examine each dental arch and the relationship of each individual tooth to its neighbor. Appropriate referral will help a child have a healthy and attractive smile and good oral health. Comprehensive assessment and education can help reduce the number of caries that the child develops and can help prevent periodontal disease.

THE NUTRITIONAL ASSESSMENT*

The nutritional assessment can be part of a routine health-maintenance visit, or it can be a more specific evaluation in high-risk children. Children who are at risk for nutritional deficiencies include those with feeding problems resulting from either oral motor difficulties or psychosocial factors, those with unusual eating habits, those on special diets, those who are chronically ill, and those from poor, single-parent, or uneducated families. Adolescents are at particular risk for nutritional deficiencies because their nutritional requirements, which are great, may not be met as a result of psychological and cultural factors that influence what adolescents choose to eat.

*This section was prepared by Diane M. Huse, M. S., R. D.

The nutritional assessment is the evaluation of an individual's nutritional status. Inadequate dietary intake results in nutrient deficiencies. Deficiencies develop gradually or rapidly, depending on the severity of the nutrient deprivation, the extent of the body's reserves, and the body's need for nutrients. Both decreased intake and increased utilization of nutrients cause the body to draw on its nutrient reserves. These reserves dwindle, tissues become "desaturated," cells are deprived of essential nutrients, and biochemical disorders appear if the nutrient deficiency persists. Biochemical disorders gradually upset body physiology, resulting in the appearance of clinical lesions denoting malnutrition. The nutritional assessment enables the health care team to identify the type and possible cause of an individual's nutritional problems and forms the basis for developing a comprehensive care plan. The assessment process includes an evaluation of dietary intake, a clinical examination of physical signs, anthropometric measures, and laboratory measurements.

Evaluation of dietary intake

A variety of methods are available for collecting dietary data; they all have limitations and varying degrees of reliability. The methods most often used in the clinical setting are the 24-h recall, the dietary history, and the 3- and 7-day food records. Determining frequency of food intake is important in some situations also.

The interview is the most important aspect of any of the methods used. The validity of the data obtained during the interview, however, depends on the parent's or the child's willingness to discuss diet with the interviewer. To aid in establishing rapport, the interviewer should clearly describe the purpose of the interview and the reasons for asking the questions. Parents may feel threatened by questions about the foods they serve because providing a healthy diet is considered an important part of parenting. If the interviewer takes a nonjudgmental attitude and makes the purpose of the interview clear, the parent and the child will feel more at ease. Beal found that with few exceptions, girls under 12 years of age and boys under 13 to 14 years of age are unlikely to give reliable nutritional histories.[37] If there is considerable disagreement between a preadolescent and a parent about food intake, it may be useful to interview each one individually.

Food	Never	Seldom	Once a Month	Once a Week	Daily
Milk					
Cheese					
Ice Cream					
Pudding, Custard					
Peanut Butter					
Eggs					
Liver					
Beef, Lamb, Pork					
Chicken, Turkey					
Fish					
Dried Beans (Lentils, Navy, Pinto, Kidney)					
Spinach					
Carrots					
Orange, Grapefruit					
Salad					
Squash					
Broccoli					
Cauliflower					
Corn					
Peas					
Green Beans					
Fresh Fruit					
Fruit Cocktail					
Applesauce					
White Bread					
Noodles					
Rice					
Cold Cereal (specify)					
Hot Cereal					
Whole Wheat or Rye Bread					
Potatoes					
Candy					
Soda					
Kool-Aid					
Chewing Gum (specify)					
Cake					
Popcorn					
Pizza					

Figure 14-11 A food-frequency questionnaire

The interviewer should avoid suggesting the correct time to serve meals, the right foods to serve, or the amounts that should be eaten. For example, the question, "What does your child have for a beverage with meals?" is appropriate, whereas the question, "How much milk does your child drink each day?" is inappropriate.

The 24-h recall (see Appendix C-1) is the most common method used for collecting dietary data and is the least burdensome for parents because it is done during the interview and does not require record keeping. The interviewer asks the parent or the child what foods were eaten in the last 24 h, and the amounts. The information given may be incorrect because parents or children cannot remember exactly what was eaten, because they have difficulty establishing portion sizes, or because they lack commitment.[38] The 24-h recall is suitable for use in screening children who are at risk for nutritional deficiencies and in evaluating compliance with a prescribed dietary regimen.

The 3- or 7-day food record is used to identify the current intake and food patterns of a child. The parent is instructed to measure or weigh the portions of all foods offered for meals and snacks and to indicate the amounts not eaten. Careful instructions need to be provided to ensure that such things as jelly, sugar, butter, mayonnaise, and catsup are not omitted from the record. Records covering fewer than 20 consecutive meals or 7 days may not provide valid information.[39] A 3-day record provides an estimate of the general quality of the diet, while a 7-day record provides an estimate of nutrient intake.[40] For parents, the most difficult part of keeping food records is remembering to make an entry each time the child eats.

The diet history is another method of evaluating dietary intake. During an interview, an estimate of the amounts and kinds of foods eaten, usually in the past 1 to 6 months, is made. Food likes, dislikes, preferences, and aversions, as well as meal and snack patterns, are identified. The diet history is usually cross-checked with a food record. This method requires a skilled interviewer; it is time-consuming and should be used only by a dietitian-nutritionist.

A food-frequency questionnaire (Fig. 14-11) is a simple method of detecting unusual dietary patterns. The parent is asked to estimate how often the child currently eats specific foods and the sizes of the portions.

The nurse can identify potential areas of nutritional deficiencies by using the four basic food groups to evaluate the 24-h recall or the 3- or 7-day food record. (See Appendix C-5.) The foods in each group supply similar nutrients. A fifth group, the "extras," consists of such foods as candy and potato chips. The nurse can determine whether the child is eating the recommended number of servings of the foods in each group (see Table 14-9). Occasional or slight deviations are not harmful. When foods in specific groups are consistently missed or are taken in inadequate amounts and/or when meal patterns are erratic or meals are often skipped, there should be further investigation by a dietitian-nutritionist, who will identify specific deficiencies of individual nutrients and provide education about nutrition.

Table 14-9 Evaluation of a Teenager's Diet Using the Four Basic Food Groups (for a 24-h recall)

Food	Amount	Food group
Breakfast		
None		
Lunch		
Hamburger	3 oz	Meat
Roll	1	Bread
French fries	½ cup	Fruit and vegetable—fat
Ketchup		
Cola drink	12 oz	Extra
Apple	1 medium	Fruit and vegetable
Snack:		
Ice-cream cone	½ cup	Milk (⅓ of a full serving)
Chewing gum		Extra
Supper:		
Chicken thigh	2 oz	Meat
Mashed potatoes	½ cup	Fruit and vegetable
Green peas	¼ cup	Fruit and vegetable—½ serving
Lemonade	12 oz	Extra
Yellow cake	1 slice	Extra
Snack:		
Cola drink	16 oz	Extra
Potato chips	¼ bag—2 oz	Extra
Chocolate bar	3 oz	Extra

Clinical examination of physical signs

A physical examination is essential in making a nutritional assessment. Knowing the physical signs and symptoms of malnutrition is valuable in detecting nutritional deficiencies. These may include apathy, irritability, and pallor of the skin, the mucous membranes of the mouth and eyes, the nail beds, or the palm surfaces. More serious signs of advanced protein-calorie malnutrition are changes in hair color and body appearance, such as edema. However, these symptoms may be related to nonnutritional factors, such as poor hygiene or excessive exposure to the sun.

Table 14-10 lists physical signs and their nutrition-related causes. For example, the nurse may note that a child is pale and has pale conjunctivas and brittle, ridged nails. If laboratory

Table 14-10 Physical Signs and Causes of Malnutrition

Body area	Signs associated with malnutrition	Nutrition-related causes
Hair	Lack of natural shine; dull, dry, sparse, straight; color changes (flag sign); easily plucked	Protein-calorie deficiency; often multiple coexistent nutrient deficiencies
Face	Dark skin over cheeks and under eyes (malar and infraorbital pigmentation), scaling of skin around nostrils (nasolabial seborrhea)	Inadequate caloric intake; lack of B-complex vitamins, particularly niacin, riboflavin, pyridoxine
	Edematous (moon face)	Protein deficiency
	Color loss (pallor)	Iron deficiency, general undernutrition
Eyes	Pale conjunctivas	Iron deficiency
	Bitôt's spots, conjunctival and corneal xerosis, soft cornea (keratomalacia)	Vitamin A deficiency
	Redness and fissuring of eyelid corners (angular palpebritis)	Niacin, riboflavin, pyridoxine deficiency
Lips	Redness and swelling of mouth or lips (cheilosis), angular fissure and scars	Niacin or riboflavin deficiency
Tongue	Red, raw and fissured, swollen (glossitis)	Folic acid, niacin, B_{12}, pyridoxine deficiency
	Magenta color	Riboflavin deficiency
	Pale, atrophic	Iron deficiency
	Filiform papillary atrophy	Niacin, folic acid, B_{12}, iron deficiency
	Fungiform papillary hypertrophy	General undernutrition
Teeth	Carious or missing	Excess sugar (and poor dental hygiene)
	Mottled enamel (fluorosis)	Excess fluoride
Gums	Spongy, bleeding; may be receding	Ascorbic acid deficiency
Glands	Thyroid enlargement (goiter)	Iodine deficiency
	Parotid enlargement	General undernutrition, particularly insufficient protein
Skin	Follicular hyperkeratosis, dryness (xerosis) with flaking	Vitamin A deficiency; insufficient unsaturated and essential fatty acids
	Hyperpigmentation	B_{12}, folic acid, niacin deficiency
	Petechiae	Ascorbic acid deficiency
	Pellagrous dermatitis	Niacin or tryptophan deficiency
	Scrotal and vulval dermatosis	Riboflavin deficiency
Nails	Spoon nails (koilonychia); brittle or ridged	Iron deficiency
Muscular and skeletal systems	Muscle wasting	Protein-calorie deficiency
	Frontal and parietal bosselation; epiphyseal swelling; soft, thin infant skull bones (craniotabes), persistently open anterior fontanel; knock-knees or bow-legs	Vitamin D deficiency
	Beading of ribs (rachitic rosary)	Vitamin D and calcium deficiency
Internal systems: gastrointestinal, nervous	Hepatomegaly	Chronic malnutrition
	Mental confusion and irritability	Thiamine, niacin deficiency
	Sensory loss, motor weakness, loss of position sense, loss of vibration, loss of ankle and knee jerks, calf tenderness	Thiamine deficiency
Cardiac	Cardiac enlargement, tachycardia	Thiamine deficiency

Source: Rosanne B. Howard and Nancie H. Herbold, *Nutrition in Clinical Care*, McGraw-Hill, New York, 1978. Used by permission of the publisher.

investigation indicates that hemoglobin and hematocrit are significantly below normal, iron-deficiency anemia is diagnosed. A physical finding suggesting a nutritional abnormality is an indication that further investigation is required.

Physical findings are meaningful primarily in identifying diseases that may interfere with growth and general health. While such disorders (e.g., congenital heart disease and chronic liver disease) may lead to nutritional deficiencies, these deficiencies must be distinguished from those which result from failure to provide a child with adequate amounts of nutritious food.

Anthropometric measurements

Anthropometric measurements provide useful data for analyzing growth and determining body composition. Weight, height (or length), head circumference, skinfold thickness, and arm muscle circumference are the body measurements that are most commonly used in making a nutritional assessment. Measurements of weight and height (length when lying down for children under 2 years of age) and of head circumference should be done periodically to assess growth. These are plotted on a growth chart. A child who is short for his or her age may have a relatively long-term illness or a nutritional deficiency. On the other hand, in the case of a child whose height is above the 10th percentile but whose weight is below the 5th percentile, the nurse might suspect the presence of an acute or subacute nutritional deficiency.[41] Plotting several measurements of height and weight at different ages enables the nurse to visualize how the child's growth is progressing. Growth charts are available for head circumference from birth to 36 months. Sequential measurements plotted on these charts can be used to identify children whose cranial growth is deviating from normal. A rapid increase in rate of growth may indicate hydrocephalus. In cases of malnutrition, the growth of head circumference up to 2 years of age is so closely related to growth in body length that head circumference measurements indicate no more about a child's nutritional status than body length measurements.[42] After 2 years of age, head circumference grows so slowly that it is a good indicator of past malnutrition. The growth chart is the single most useful clinical tool for assessing a child's nutritional status and should be maintained and preserved as part of the child's health record.

Other measurements which can be made in addition to height and weight are skinfold thickness and midarm muscle circumference. Skinfold thickness (Table 14-11) is a good indicator of body-fat reserves, since approximately 50 per-

Table 14-11 Triceps Skinfold Percentiles (Triceps Skinfold Measurements Based on Data Obtained Using Lange Skinfold Calipers on White Subjects Included in the Ten-State Nutrition Survey, 1968–1970)

Age, Yr	Percentiles, mm									
	Males					Females				
	5th	15th	50th	85th	95th	5th	15th	50th	85th	95th
Birth–	4	5	8	12	15	4	5	8	12	13
0.5–	5	7	9	13	15	6	7	9	12	15
1.5–	5	7	10	13	14	6	7	10	13	15
2.5–	6	7	9	12	14	6	7	10	12	14
3.5–	5	6	9	12	14	5	7	10	12	14
4.5–	5	6	8	12	16	6	7	10	13	16
5.5–	5	6	8	11	15	6	7	10	12	15
6.5–	4	6	8	11	14	6	7	10	13	17
7.5–	5	6	8	12	17	6	7	10	15	19
8.5–	5	6	9	14	19	6	7	11	17	24
9.5–	5	6	10	16	22	6	8	12	19	24
10.5–	6	7	10	17	25	7	8	12	20	29
11.5–	5	7	11	19	26	6	9	13	20	25
12.5–	5	6	10	18	25	7	9	14	23	30
13.5–	5	6	10	17	22	8	10	15	22	28
14.5–	4	6	9	19	26	8	11	16	24	27
15.5–	4	5	9	20	27	8	10	15	23	31
16.5–	4	5	8	14	20	9	12	16	26	31
17.5– 24.4–	4	5	10	18	25	9	12	17	25	

Source: A. R. Frisancho, "Triceps Skinfold and Upper Arm Muscle Size Norms for Assessment of Nutritional Status," *American Journal of Clinical Nutrition* **27**:1052–1058 (1974). Table courtesy of Ross Laboratories, Columbus, Ohio.

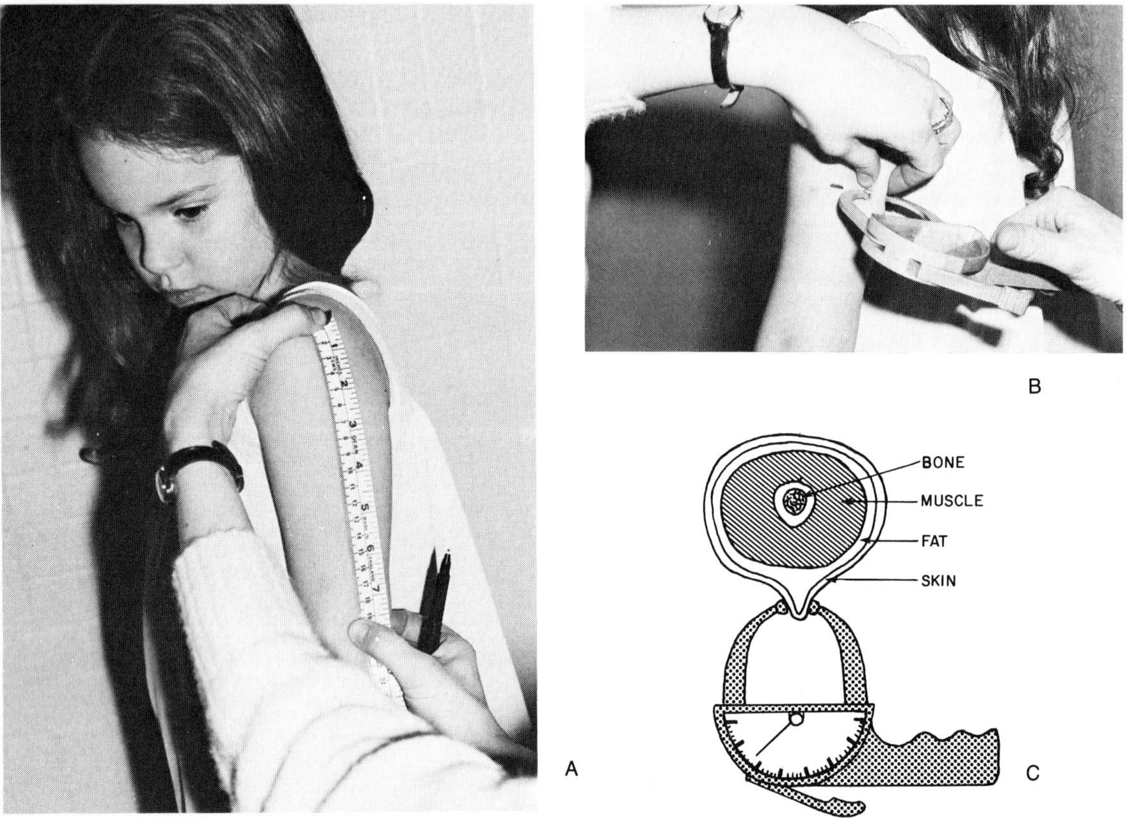

Figure 14-12 Taking skinfold measurements. (*A*) Location of the midpoint of the upper arm. (*B*) Application of the Lange calipers for measurement of the triceps skinfold. (C) Representation of the tissues of the arm (bone, fat, and skin) and measurement of skinfold thickness. (*From Rosanne Howard and Nancie Herbold, Nutrition in Clinical Care. McGraw-Hill, New York, 1978. Used with permission.*)

cent of adipose tissue is located in subcutaneous areas (Fig. 14-12). Midarm muscle circumference reflects both adequacy of caloric intake and muscle mass. However, body height and weight standards are better methods of evaluation for measurement of change; they are readily accessible and do not require extensive training or expensive tools.

Biochemical information

Laboratory evaluation of nutritional status is more objective and precise than dietary or clinical assessments. Biochemical tests are used to measure levels of nutrients in body fluids (blood and urine) or to evaluate certain biological functions that are dependent on an adequate supply of essential nutrients. The primary purpose of laboratory tests is to identify nutritional deficiencies that are indicated by dietary or clinical assessments. Laboratory evaluations often suggest marginal or acute deficiencies even when a child appears clinically normal, since clinical signs usually occur only after prolonged inadequate intake of nutrients. A deficiency in one nutrient can be considered an almost certain indicator of other nutritional deficiencies, which should then be investigated. Laboratory investigation is of little use if it merely confirms a known clinical diagnosis.

A minimal laboratory screening should include a hematocrit and measurements of hemoglobin and serum albumin. A hemoglobin determination is used to detect iron-deficiency anemia. The hematocrit, which measures the percentage of packed red cells in whole blood, is an indicator of nutritional iron deficiency. A low value indicates that there is insufficient hemoglobin formation. For this reason, hemoglobin and hematocrit should be evaluated together.

A measurement of serum albumin indicates visceral protein status. A low level may be caused by malnutrition as well as trauma, sepsis, edema, and blood loss.

More extensive laboratory evaluations can include measurements of serum iron, total iron-binding capacity, and blood urea nitrogen, as well as vitamin and enzyme assays.

Additional information

When evaluating nutritional status, other information should be obtained and recorded. Food allergies or food intolerances will influence daily food intake. A child's food intake will also be modified if he or she is on a vegetarian or weight-control diet. When evaluating such a child, the specific foods or categories of foods that are being either emphasized or avoided in the diet should be noted.

It is useful to identify vitamin, mineral, and food supplements that the child is taking. Medications and dosages should also be noted. These factors can potentially enhance or pose a risk to the child's nutritional and health status. Appendix C-2 gives the recommended daily dietary allowances for children; Appendix C-3 gives the amounts of vitamins and minerals needed, and Appendix C-4 gives mean heights and weights and recommended food intake.

IMMUNIZATIONS

Vaccinations are an inexpensive and effective way to prevent several common childhood diseases. Recent outbreaks of these illnesses indicate that some parents have become apathetic about immunizations. Many states now require up-to-date immunizations for any child who enters public school.

The nurse is often responsible for preparing the vaccines, for discussing the risks and benefits of each vaccine with the parents, and for explaining its purpose, the immunization schedule, and possible reactions. Knowledgeable nurses can safely evaluate a child's immunization status and plan an appropriate immunization schedule. If the schedule is interrupted, final immunity can be achieved as long as the schedule is resumed and completed.

Table 14-12 is a recommended schedule for active immunization of infants and children. Table 14-13 is a schedule for infants and children who

Table 14-12 Recommended Schedule for Active Immunization of Normal Infants and Children

Recommended age	Vaccine or vaccines	Comments
2 mo	DTP[a], OPV[b]	Can be initiated earlier in areas of high endemicity
4 mo	DTP, OPV	2-mo interval desired for OPV to avoid interference
6 mo	DTP (OPV)	OPV optional for areas where polio might be imported (e.g., some areas of southwestern United States)
12 mo	Tuberculin test[c]	May be given simultaneously with MMR at 15 mo
15 mo	Measles, mumps, rubella (MMR)[d]	MMR preferred
18 mo	DTP, OPV	Consider as part of primary series—DTP essential
4–6 yr[e]	DTP, OPV	
14–16 yr	TD[f]	Repeat every 10 yr for lifetime

[a]DTP—Diphtheria and tetanus toxoids with pertussis vaccine.

[b]OPV—Oral, attenuated poliovirus vaccine contains poliovirus types 1, 2, and 3.

[c]Tuberculin test—Mantoux (intradermal PPD) preferred. Frequency of tests depends on local epidemiology. The committee recommends annual or biennial testing unless local circumstances dictate less frequent or no testing.

[d]MMR—Live measles, mumps, and rubella viruses in a combined vaccine.

[e]Up to the seventh birthday.

[f]TD—Adult tetanus toxoid (full dose) and diphtheria toxoid (reduced dose) in combination.

Note: For all products used, consult manufacturer's brochure for instructions for storage, handling, and administration. Biologics prepared by different manufacturers may vary, and those of the same manufacturer may change from time to time. The package insert should be followed for a specific product.

Source: American Academy of Pediatrics, Committee on Infectious Diseases, 1982.

Table 14-13 Recommended Immunization Schedules for Infants and Children Not Initially Immunized at Usual Recommended Times in Early Infancy

	Recommended schedules				
		Alternatives			
Timing	Preferred schedule	No. 1[a]	No. 2[b]	No. 3[c]	Comments
First visit	DTP no. 1[d], OPV no. 1,[e] tuberculin test (PPD)[g]	MMR,[f] PPD	DTP no. 1, OPV no. 1, PPD	DTP no. 1, OPV no. 1, MMR, PPD	MMR should not be given sooner than 15 mo.
1 mo after first visit	MMR	DTP no. 1, OPV no. 1	MMR, DTP no. 2	DTP no. 2	
2 mo after first visit	DTP no. 2, OPV no. 2	—	DTP no. 3, OPV no. 2	DTP no. 3, OPV no. 2	—
3 mo after first visit	(DTP no. 3)	DTP no. 2, OPV no. 2	—	—	In preferred schedule, DTP no. 3 can be given if OPV no. 3 is not to be given until 10–16 mo.
4 mo after first visit	DTP no. 3 (OPV no. 3)	—	(OPV no. 3)	(OPV no. 3)	OPV no. 3 optional for areas where there is likely to be importation of polio (e.g., some southwestern states).
5 mo after first visit	—	DTP no. 3, (OPV no. 3)	—	—	
10–16 mo after last dose	DTP no. 4, OPV no. 3, or OPV no. 4	DTP no. 4, OPV no. 3, or OPV no. 4	DTP no. 4, OPV no. 3, or OPV no. 4	DTP no. 4, OPV no. 3, or OPV no. 4	—
Preschool	DTP no. 5, OPV no. 4, or OPV no. 5	DTP no. 5, OPV no. 4, or OPV no. 5	DTP no. 5, OPV no. 4, or OPV no. 5	DTP no. 5, OPV no. 4, or OPV no. 5	Preschool dose not necessary if DTP no. 4 or no. 5 is given after fourth birthday.
Ages 14 to 16	TD[h]	TD	TD	TD	Repeat every 10 years.

[a]Alternative no. 1 can be used for children more than 15 mo old if measles is occurring in the community.

[b]Alternative no. 2 allows for more rapid DTP immunization.

[c]Alternative no. 3 should be reserved for those whose access to medical care is compromised by poor compliance.

[d]Diphtheria and tetanus toxoids with pertussis vaccine.

[e]Oral, attenuated poliovirus vaccine; contains types 1, 2, and 3.

[f]Live measles, mumps, and rubella viruses in a combined vaccine.

[g]Mantoux (intradermal PPD) preferred. Frequency of tests depends on local epidemiology. The committee recommends annual or biennial testing unless local circumstances dictate less frequent or no testing.

[h]Adult tetanus toxoid (full dose) and diphtheria toxoid (reduced dose) in combination.

Notes: For all products used, consult manufacturer's brochure for instructions for storage, handling, and administration. Biologics prepared by different manufacturers may vary, and those of the same manufacturer may change from time to time. The package insert should be followed for a specific product.

Source: American Academy of Pediatrics, Committee on Infectious Diseases, 1982.

were not immunized at the usual recommended times in infancy.

Diphtheria, pertussis, and tetanus (DPT)

Children can be protected against these three diseases with combined vaccines administered at 2, 4, and 6 months of age. Booster shots should be given at 18 months of age and again at 4 to 6 years of age. Booster shots for pertussis are usually not necessary after the age of 6, since this disease is not as serious after early childhood. Tetanus booster shots are given every 10 years or when a person suffers a deep wound more than 5 years after the last booster shot. A prior severe reaction to pertussis vaccine, such as a temperature greater than 39°C (103°F), screaming, shock, seizures, or other central nervous system manifestations, contraindicates the administration of additional doses of the DPT vaccine in most circumstances.[43] Parents must be assured that routine vaccination of all children is necessary to continue the reduced incidence of diphtheria, pertussis, and tetanus.

Poliomyelitis

Trivalent oral polio vaccine is a live virus vaccine containing three different viruses that can cause the same clinical disease. One dose does not give active immunity for all three types, although multiple doses are given beginning at 2 months of age and again at 4 months and 18 months. A booster dose is needed at 4 to 6 years of age.

Measles

Measles (rubeola, or 10-day measles) is a clinically severe, highly contagious disease. With the naturally occurring form of the disease, there is a 1:1000 incidence of measles encephalopathy.[44] Other complications include bronchopneumonia and middle ear infections. Until about 13 months of age, infants are protected from rubeola with antibodies received from their mothers. Passive immunity from the vaccine can be destroyed by these antibodies if the immunization is given before 13 months of age. During an outbreak of measles, infants 6 months of age and older can be immunized. Reimmunization is necessary at 15 months of age. The measles vaccine is usually administered in combination with the mumps and rubella vaccines (MMR) at 15 months. The most common side effects, a fever and rash occurring 7 to 10 days after the vaccination, should be discussed with the parents.

German measles (rubella)

Immunization against rubella is recommended for all children and is usually given at 15 months of age in combination with the measles and mumps vaccine. Special emphasis should be placed on immunizing all preschool and elementary school children. Children of pregnant women can receive the vaccine, but pregnant women should not be vaccinated because of risk to the fetus.

Mumps

The mumps vaccine can be given at 1 year of age but is usually given at 15 months in combination with the measles and German measles vaccine. Twenty to thirty percent of males who get mumps after puberty develop mumps orchitis. Orchitis (testicular inflammation) can cause sterility in a small percentage of those infected. Other complications of mumps are meningitis, encephalitis, and deafness. The mumps vaccine is recommended for all older children and adolescents who are still susceptible to the disease.

Smallpox

Vaccination for smallpox is not recommended for children living in the United States because the risk of getting the disease is so slight. Because reactions to the vaccine have resulted in death, reactions are considered a greater risk than the chance of getting smallpox at this time.

Hemophilus influenzae Type B

Some state health departments now advocate vaccination of children aged 2 to 5 against a common form of meningitis caused by the bacteria *Hemophilus influenzae* Type B (HIB). Although HIB is more common in children under 2 years of age, the vaccine does not work well in children in that age group. HIB causes meningitis in two-thirds of infected children and can cause severe swelling of the throat, leading to suffocation. If children are vaccinated at 18 months of age, as they may be if they are highly susceptible or are at risk in day-care institutions, they will need a repeat vaccination at 2 years of age to guarantee immunity against HIB.

Contraindications to immunizations

Immunizations are contraindicated for:

1. Children who have an acute febrile illness, a chronic debilitating disease, or an acute neurological disease
2. Children who have cancer or an immunological disease or who are undergoing anticancer therapy
3. Pregnant women (except for the polio vaccine)
4. Children who have had previous allergic reactions to the vaccines
5. Children who have a sibling who had a severe reaction to the DPT vaccine

Parents should be instructed to keep careful records of their children's immunizations and the dates of administration. They should understand the recommended schedule of immunizations. Parents also need to know the common reactions that a child might have to an immunization. The nurse should explain the use of antipyretics and appropriate doses for mild reactions. Table 14-14 lists the common side effects of immunizations.

Table 14-14 Possible Side Effects of Recommended Immunizations

Immunization	Reactions
Diphtheria	Fever within 24 to 48 hours; soreness, swelling, and redness at site of vaccination
Tetanus	Same as reactions to diphtheria immunization plus urticaria and malaise
Pertussis	Same as reactions to diphtheria immunization. Rare reaction includes loss of consciousness, convulsions, thrombocytopenia
OPV	Usually no side effects
Rubeola	Transient rash, anorexia, fever; malaise may occur 7–10 days later
Rubella	Rash, lymphadenopathy, transient pain in peripheral joints
Mumps	Usually no side effects except brief, mild fever

PHYSICAL EXAMINATION SCHEDULES

Well infants are usually examined at birth and at 2 weeks, 2 months, 4 months, 6 months, 9 months, and 15 months of age. Sick infants should be assessed at the time of each illness. If a child has had a recent well-child assessment, then a complete examination need not be done when an illness occurs. The focus should be on the system showing the signs and symptoms. A yearly assessment of a child's physical and developmental status is generally recommended up to the age of 4 years and at any time the parent feels that the child is not progressing normally. After the age of 4, if the child appears well, has no symptoms, and is doing well socially and academically, routine examinations can be done every 2 to 4 years.

EMPHASIS ON HEALTH PROMOTION

Traditionally, health care professionals have focused on an illness model in which a specific illness is diagnosed and treated. Today, this focus is changing, and there is a definite trend toward preventing illness. Health promotion efforts include a consideration of the psychosocial and the physiological aspects of health and illness and how they affect each other. There is a growing awareness on the part of the public, the government, and health care professionals of the logic of utilizing nurses in such new roles as pediatric nurse practitioner and pediatric nurse associate. The demand for accessible health care at a more reasonable cost is another force operating to create these new roles for nurses in the health care system. It is important that nurses think about the services they provide and about how they can be designed to be comprehensive and family-centered in scope, how parents and children can use their services, and what areas of health care should receive priority. It is also important for nurses to examine the families in the community in which they live so that they can determine what changes are desired. Changes in current health care systems point clearly toward changes in health care delivery in the future.

Within the profession of nursing, there is beginning to emerge a renewed sense of direction, identity, and commitment to providing comprehensive health care for children. Nurses who are skilled in making a physical assessment take patient histories and perform physical examinations. From the data collected, they make a judgment regarding whether growth, development, and behavior are progressing in a normal pattern and at a normal rate. Using the interpreted data, they develop nursing diagnoses and evaluations of children's health status. In some settings, nurses assume the responsibility for meeting nearly all the health care needs of children, referring to other health professionals only those children whom they judge to have complex problems. In other settings, nurses see only well children for assessment, and they may be obligated by agency policy to refer to other health professionals any child who has symptoms of illness or whose laboratory and physical findings are abnormal. In most agencies, nurses coordinate health services for children and assist families in setting health care goals.

Care that is extended to parents should support their efforts to meet the needs of their children. By reflecting on the problems of parenthood, nurses become more involved in assuring the optimal development of all children. Increased competence and confidence call for sharing professional knowledge and skills in such a way that parental self-esteem will be enhanced. Health and adjustment in later life have their roots in appropriate health care and experiences in early childhood. Often, extending care to parents is the most challenging and rewarding component of professional practice in the nursing of children. If both nurses and parents make a mutual investment in promoting optimal development and health for all children, the world of tomorrow will be a better place.

REFERENCES

1. Chin, Peggy, *Child Health Maintenance,* 2d ed., Mosby, St. Louis, 1979, p. 1.
2. Numerof, Rita, "Expanded Nursing Role from the Perspective of the New Medicine," *Health Care Management Review* **3**(3):45–51 (Summer 1978).
3. Halperin, Sharon, Joel Bass, and Kishor Menta, "Knowledge of Accident Prevention among Parents of Young Children in Nine Massachusetts Towns," *Public Health Reports* **98**(6):550–551 (November–December 1983).
4. *A Report on the Hearings of the Unmet Health Needs of Children and Youth,* American Nurses' Association, Kansas City, 1979.
5. Johnson, Lloyd, *1984 Nationwide Survey of High School Seniors,* University of Michigan, Press, Ann Arbor, 1985.
6. Halder, Angela R., *Legal Issues in Pediatrics and Adolescent Medicine,* Wiley, New York, 1977, p. 220.
7. Raitt, Emmett G., "The Minor's Right to Consent to Medical Treatment," *Southern California Law Review* **48**:1417 (1975).
8. Goldberg, Robin, "Identifying Speech and Language Delay in Children," *Pediatric Nursing* **10**(4):253 (July–August 1984).
9. DeGowin, Elmer L., and Richard L. DeGowin, *Bedside Diagnostic Examination,* 2d ed., Macmillan, Collier Books, New York, 1969, p. 28.
10. Bates, Barbara, *A Guide to Physical Examination,* Lippincott, Philadelphia, 1979, p. 376.
11. Ibid., p. 377.
12. Valadian, Isabelle, and Dorothy Porter, *Physical Growth and Development,* Little Brown, Boston, 1977, p. 5.
13. Stern, Nancy, and Holly Zaiken, "Assessing the Child with Short Stature," *Pediatric Nursing* **11**(2):107 (March–April 1985).
14. Powell, Marcene L., *Assessment and Management of Developmental Changes and Problems in Children,* Mosby, St. Louis, 1981, p. 183.
15. Castiglia, Patricia, and Marcia Petrini, "Selecting a Developmental Screening Tool," *Pediatric Nursing* **11**(1):10 (January–February 1985).
16. Stangler, Sharon, C. Huber, and D. Routh, *Screening Growth and Development of Preschool Children: A Guide for Test Selection,* McGraw-Hill, New York, 1980, p. 102.
17. Ibid., p. 113.
18. Knoblock, Hilda, Frances Stevens, and Anthony Malone, *Manual of Developmental Diagnosis,* Harper & Row, New York, 1980, pp. 1–4.
19. McCarthy, John, and Berry Brazelton, "Neonatal Behavioral Assessment," *Drug Therapy* **10**(2):103, 107 (February 1980).
20. Brazelton, Berry, *Neonatal Behavioral Assessment Scale,* Lippincott, Philadelphia, 1973, p. 1.
21. Ibid., p. 4.
22. Stangler, op. cit., pp. 148–150.
23. Ibid., p. 229.
24. Goldberg, op. cit., p. 253.
25. Hoekelman, Robert A., et al., *Principles of Pediatrics: Health Care of the Young,* McGraw-Hill, New York, 1978, p. 197.
26. Zarab, P. A., *Scoliosis Proceedings of a Fifth Symposium, September 21 and 22, 1976,* Academic, New York, 1977.
27. Stangler, op. cit., pp. 55–88.
28. Hoekelman, op. cit., p. 182.
29. Hudson, F. P., "Screening for Inborn Errors of Metabolism in Infancy," *Nursing Mirror* (August 28, 1975), p. 64.
30. Ibid., p. 63.
31. Stanbury, J., J. Wyngaarden, D. Fredrickson, J. Goldstein, and M. Brown, *The Metabolic Basis of Inherited Disease,* McGraw-Hill, New York, 1983, p. 270.
32. Coody, Deborah, "Congenital Hypothyroidism," *Pediatric Nursing* **10**(5):342 (September–October 1984).
33. Ibid., p. 344.
34. Ibid., p. 345.
35. Kilman, Carol, and Mark Halpin, "Update on Dentistry for Children," *Pediatric Nursing,* **7**(5):41 (September–October 1981).
36. Ibid., p. 43.
37. Beal, V. A., "The Nutrition History in Longitudinal Research, *Journal of the American Dietetic Association* **51**(5):426 (November 1967).
38. Todd, K. S., M. Hudes, and H. Calloway, "Food Intake Measurements: Problems and Approaches" *American Journal of Clinical Nutrition* **37**(1):139 (January 1983).
39. McHenry, E. W., H. P Ferguson, and J. Gurland, "Sources of Error in Dietary Surveys," *Canadian Journal of Public Health* **36**(9):355 (September 1945).
40. Stuff, J. E., et al., "A Comparison of Dietary Methods," *American Journal of Clinical Nutrition* **37**(2):300 (February 1983).
41. Fomon, S. J., *Nutritional Disorders of Children—Prevention, Screening, and Follow-Up,* U.S. Department of Health Education, and Welfare Publication no. 76–5612, 1976.
42. Malina, R. M., J. P. Habicht, R. Martorell, A. Lechtig, C. Yarbrough, and R. E. Klein, "Head and Chest Circumferences in Rural Guatemalan Latino Children, Birth to Seven Years of Age," *American Journal of Clinical Nutrition* **28**:1061 (1975).
43. Williams, Lucinda, "Childhood Immunizations," *Pediatric Nursing* **8**(1):19 (January–February 1982).
44. Ibid., p. 21.

PART III

Alterations in Child Health: Biophysical Emphasis

15

Nancy Lockwood Ramsey

Effects of hospitalization on the child and the family

Upon completion of this chapter, the student will be able to:

1 List at least two causes of stress in hospitalized children in each age group.
2 Identify at least three factors influencing the child's ability to cope with hospitalization.
3 List at least four functions of play.
4 Describe situational (directive) and free (nondirective) play and ways the nurse can use each to communicate with the child.
5 Identify the child's concept of illness at different ages.
6 Compare the procedures for preoperative preparation of an infant, a toddler, a preschooler, school-age child, and an adolescent.
7 List at least five common feelings of parents of hospitalized children.
8 Describe the reactions to hospitalization of children in each age group and appropriate nursing interventions.

During the past 30 years there has been an increasing emphasis by medical and nursing personnel on meeting the child and the family's psychological needs. In the early twentieth century it sometimes happened that children were given meticulous physical care but died of emotional starvation. Parents were allowed to visit their hospitalized children for only 2 to 3 h per week. Many nurses believed that parents upset their children and excluded the parents from the children's care.

Hospitals have gradually become more family-centered. Nurses have discovered the valuable part that parents play in their children's recovery. The child's sense of security, reaction to the hospital, psychological health, and physical recovery are greatly influenced by the parents. With a knowledge of growth and development, the nurse can create a hospital environment that will prevent psychological trauma and enhance the child's development. Through the nurse's interventions, hospitalization can be a positive, constructive experience for the child and the child's family.

THE CHILD-CENTERED HOSPITAL

Ideally, children's hospital units are homelike and geared to the child's developmental age and size. Small tables and chairs are there for use in family-style dinners (Fig. 15-1). Beds are close to the floor. Rockers and parents' cots are available on each unit. Nurses wear colored uniforms to prevent children from associating white with fear and discomfort. Colorful rooms, play areas, and lofts with toys invite healing play. Children are encouraged to bring favorite toys, "security blankets," and clothes from home whenever possible.

Children's units should welcome visits by parents and siblings. Rooming-in and open visiting hours enable parents to be available during stressful events, for feeding, and at bedtime. Many hospitals have short-admission surgery rooms, where the child is admitted and discharged the same day. Other hospitals have outpatient areas where children can be observed or treated without formal admission. Ill children can be successfully cared for in parent-participation units. Improved admission procedures reduce the child's anxiety; these are discussed in Chap. 16.

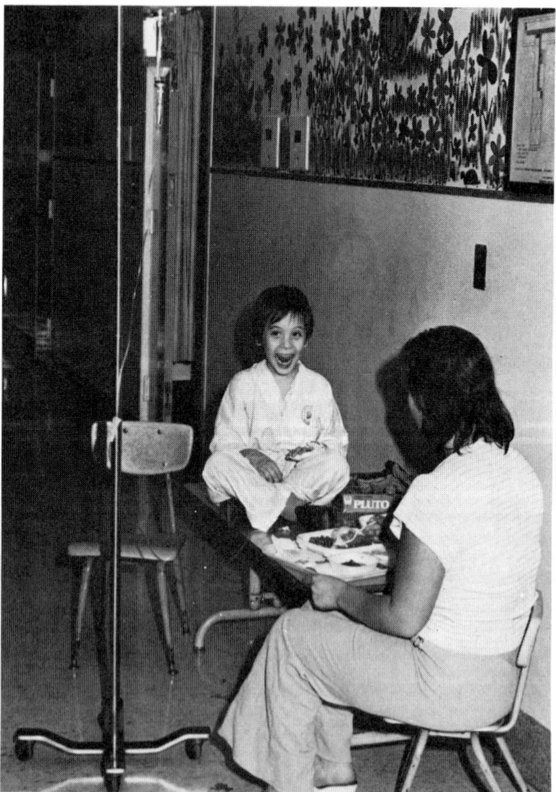

Figure 15-1 Child-sized furniture and unlimited visiting hours make the hospital more homelike. This child eats better at a small table with his mother present. (*Photo by Theresa Friedrich. Courtesy of LAC/USC Medical Center.*)

Many hospitals have preadmission tours that allow children to manipulate hospital equipment, observe the strange environment, and play out or verbalize their concerns about hospitalization. Although hospital tours can help children deal with the stress of hospitalization, the strange sights and stimuli encountered in hospitals can be overwhelming and potentially harmful.[1] Children experience less stress when a nurse or play specialist prepares them for hospitalization in a setting that is familiar to them.[2]

HOSPITALIZATION AND STRESS

Whenever a child is sick or hospitalized, stress is created within the entire family. A child or adult in stress or crisis is at a turning point. When the child or adult cannot solve the problem by using previously developed coping mechanisms, anxiety increases; the child or adult may feel helpless, overwhelmed, and unable to find workable solutions to the problem.

Nursing interventions are crucial to help the child and the family deal with the stresses of hospitalization. By helping the parents and the child meet both psychological and physical needs, the nurse can help them experience success in coping with the hospitalization.

Hospitalization separates children from a familiar and predictable environment and places them in an unfamiliar world dominated by strange people and unknown equipment (Fig. 15-2). They must cope with situations for which they lack preparation. Children fantasize to get the missing information.[3] Lack of control increases their anxiety. Intrusive procedures can threaten children's body image. They may feel dependent, insecure, and vulnerable. A child's ability to cope with hospitalization depends on numerous factors, among which are the following:

1. Age and cognitive development. The older child can more easily understand the reasons for hospitalization. The younger child has an increased tendency to indulge in fantasy and distort reality.

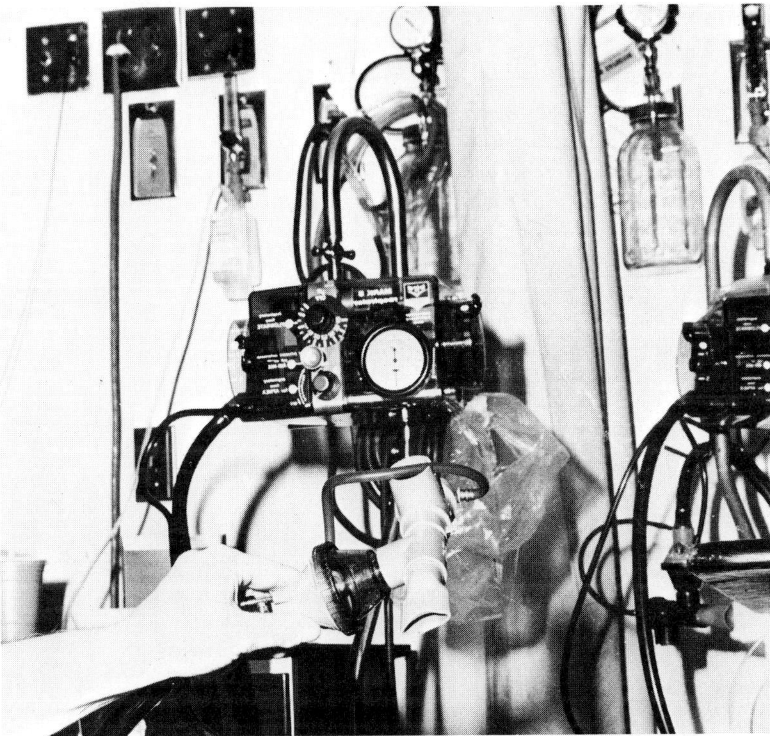

Figure 15-2 Strange, unfamiliar equipment may increase the young child's anxiety level. (*Photo by Theresa Friedrich. Courtesy of LAC/USC Medical Center.*)

2. Previous experience with illness or hospitals. The child's past experience will establish expectations for the present hospitalization.
3. Relationship to parents. The stronger the parent-child relationship, the longer the child trusts the parents to return and protect the child in the hospital.
4. Length and severity of the illness. Stores of psychic energy may be depleted by pain or illness, leaving the child less able to adapt to hospitalization. The acutely ill child needs different nursing interventions during this unstable period from those needed by the child who is not acutely ill.[4]
5. Types and frequency of intrusive procedures. For a preschooler, several needle punctures within a short time may be overwhelming.
6. Anxiety level of the parents. Anxiety in the parents increases anxiety in a child.[5]
7. Preparation. A child's anxiety will be less if he or she knows what to expect and how to act.
8. Prior stresses. If the child has been under stress before hospitalization, he or she will have less energy available to focus on recovery. On the other hand, a child who has learned to cope with stress is likely to deal with hospitalization well.

COMMUNICATING WITH CHILDREN

Children respond not only to words but also to the nurse's "feeling tone." Furthermore, they pick up unspoken attitudes. For this reason, the guidelines listed in Table 15-1 may be helpful in communicating with the young patient.

Television provides an innovative way of communicating with children of all ages. Children delight in seeing their friends' get-well messages flashed on a closed-circuit TV screen and hearing a puppet read the personal greeting. Some-

Table 15-1 Guidelines for Communicating with Children

1. Be gentle in manner and tone.
2. Talk soothingly in a low voice to a distressed or shy child.
3. Talk to preschoolers at their level of understanding:
   a. Use concrete terms: "You'll get well," or "I am busy now giving medicines. When I am finished in 5 minutes, I will play with you."
   b. Give them one direction at a time.
   c. Meet them at their eye level.
4. Praise school-age children for their accomplishments.
5. Be sensitive to teenagers' ambivalent need to approach and withdraw. Join them in their "dance" of moving toward and away from you.
6. Be honest and sincere; teenagers sense dishonesty immediately.
7. Children want to please. They want to know what is expected of them. Emphasize what they *can do*.
8. Give clear, brief directions. Reward them for correct actions. Praise *increases* in learning.
9. Place yourself in the child's position. How would you react and feel?

times a child's favorite stuffed animal is used to give a special message, like "Drink lots of juice and water today, Amy" or "Take your medicine, Jason." Parents and nurses coach the TV director on appropriate messages. Before going to surgery, one boy wanted to see the rocket he had drawn make a safe landing. After surgery he said that seeing his rocket land safely made him feel "good." Children can also participate in these TV productions as they recuperate. Self-esteem is increased, and the child is entertained and even educated.

Play and the hospitalized child

Play is the child's natural means of dealing with new experiences and stress. Play enables the child to express or project anger, aggression, insecurity, fear, fantasy, and conflict. If these emotions are suppressed instead, psychic energy is lost that could have been directed toward physical recovery. Much can be learned by watching a child at play (Table 15-2).

The value of toys No child should be in a hospital bed without a toy. Even in isolation the child should have an age-appropriate toy. Toys that stimulate the imagination and permit manipulation can be made inexpensively in the hospital. The characteristics of safe toys are reviewed in Chap. 16.

By manipulating a small world of easily managed toys, the child gains feelings of control, power, and security. He or she can practice new methods of coping with problems. Furthermore, if play can be combined with procedures (Table 15-3), the child is helped to tolerate and even enjoy some procedures.

Ideally, every pediatric ward has a playroom. Playrooms provide a sanctuary from painful procedures and promote normal growth and development. Here the child can control the environment, make decisions, and be active.

Play for communication The nurse may use two types of play for communicating with the child: *situational,* or *directive,* play and *nondirective,* or *free,* play. In the former the play sit-

Table 15-2 Guidelines for Observing a Child's Play

Observation	Rationale
What toy did the child first select?	The preferred toy is usually the most healing one.
Did the child reject toys that were related to his or her treatment or diagnosis?	Refusal of toys is a method of denying the fear or of maintaining a distance from the fear. For example, a chronically ill child may refuse to play with a hospital model.
Is the child able to play?	Inability to play is a symptom of severe anxiety.
What emotions (affect) were expressed by the child as he or she played? Did the child's facial expression change? How did the child's body move during the play? Did the child express aggression in play? What toys did the child use to express it? What themes did the child communicate in his or her play?	The child expresses inner feelings through play. Observing the young child's body movements and actions is especially revealing if the child cannot talk fluently. Many children have been taught not to express aggression. They may gingerly begin to play aggressively and look at the nurse for approval to continue.
Did the child interact with others during play?	Children play alone and side by side (parallel play) until 4 years of age; then they learn to share (cooperative play).
Did the parents choose the child's toys or allow him or her to play freely?	Many parents need information about the benefits of free play.

Table 15-3 Playing to Ease Procedures

Procedure	Examples of Play
Soaks	Playing with small toys or objects (cups, syringes, soap dishes) in water. Washing dolls. Adding bubbles to bath water.
Range-of-motion exercise	Throwing beanbags at a fixed or movable target. Touching or kicking balloons held or hung in different positions.
Circulation check	Playing "tickle toes"; wiggling them on request.
Deep breathing exercise	Blowing bubbles with a straw (no soap). Blowing on a pinwheel, feathers, a whistle, or a harmonica. Drawing a face on a rubber glove, which will expand when the glove is inflated.
Changing diapers	Nurse sings nursery rhymes or lullabies. Nurse smiles and laughs. Nurse moves child's legs and arms in rhythmical manner. Nurse plays peek-a-boo.
Tuberculin testing	After the injection, nurse or child draws face around site with washable ink.
Examination	Nurse has child "blow out" little flashlight. Nurse lets child listen with stethoscope.
Observing or feeding (when there are many young children in a noninfectious ward)	Nurse places children and toys on floor (covered with sheet) for playtime.
Forcing of fluid	A game of taking sip when turning page of a book. Use small medicine cups. Color water with food coloring. Have a tea party. Pour at a small table.

Source: Adapted from Lucille F. Whaley and Donna L. Wong, *Nursing Care of Children*, Mosby, St. Louis, 1979, pp. 947–950.

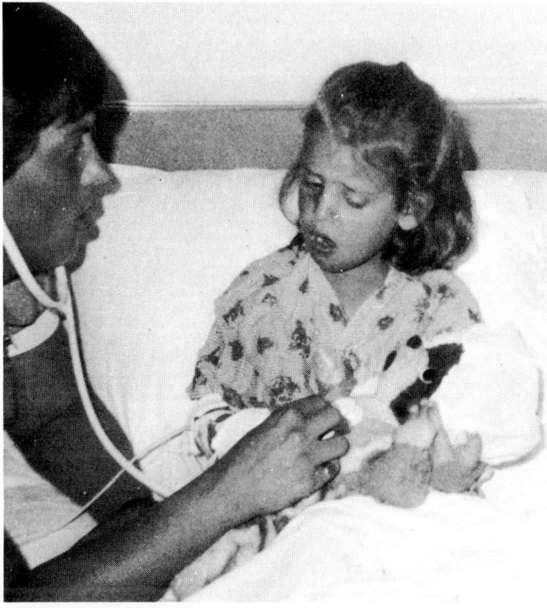

Figure 15-3 This nurse is using play to prepare a child for a procedure. Note the child's anxious facial expression. (*Courtesy of Nancy Conroy. From G. Scipien, M. U. Barnard, M. A. Chard, J. Howe, and P. J. Phillips* [eds.], *Comprehensive Pediatric Nursing, 3d ed., McGraw-Hill, New York, 1986, p. 444. Used with permission.*)

uation is structured around the procedure or other cause of the child's distress: injections, blood pressure cuff, diagnostic test, operation, or separation anxiety (Fig. 15-3). Materials and equipment used in the situation, such as syringes and alcohol sponges, should be gathered together. The nurse should take part in the play, for example, by shouting "ouch" when pretending to give or receive an injection. The child is allowed to handle the objects to make them less frightening and more familiar.

The nurse may use a nurse-doll to teach a child the reasons for a procedure. After a procedure, the child and the nurse play through it to assess the child's fantasies and distortions about the procedure. The nurse-doll can then be used to reteach or clarify the child's misconceptions. The nurse can also gently question the child and provide appropriate information. The nurse's sharing in, and approval of, such play gives the child confidence and strength to master the problem.[6, 7] By the proper use of play, a child can be instructed and persuaded so that it is unnecessary to use force. For example, if a toddler refuses her medicine, a doll can be used as a subject, given medicine, made to tell what it tastes like, and used to instruct the child to accept the medicine. The preschooler will spontaneously give the doll her own name and diagnosis and will project her feelings onto it. The nurse should reflect the child's words back, especially the themes revealed in play.

Nondirective, or free, play is based on the belief that children have the ability to solve their own problems and have a drive toward satisfying, normal behavior.[8] Children therefore instinctively choose comforting, healing toys.

Before the play session begins, the nurse establishes safety limits with the child. The child is then encouraged to choose toys. The child must learn that the nurse accepts the child without evaluation or pressure to change. When trust is established he or she can play freely.

Desensitization

Desensitization is a psychological technique used to lessen a child's anxiety about a stress-producing event. A high anxiety level usually results from a previous encounter with a stress-producing stimulus. To decrease sensitivity, the nurse structures the child's encounter with the stimulus from least to most stressful. It is useful to start with a concrete example (e.g., a syringe) and only later present the abstract concept (sterility).[9] For example, the nurse can show the child the syringe (without a needle) in a basin of bubbly water and in a later session show the child the needle (or a facsimile thereof).

Modeling

Watching other children successfully cope with stressful events helps children master their own fears and model their behavior after others'. Films showing children adapting to hospitalization and surgery have been used to prepare children as young as 3 years old for surgery.[10, 11]

Relaxation techniques

Imagery and neuromuscular relaxation techniques can also be used to lower children's anxiety levels, reduce pain, and promote sleep. Relaxation techniques work well with children as young as 3 years of age. Table 15-4 describes relaxation techniques that the nurse can use with children.

Cognitive rehearsal

Cognitive rehearsal enables the child to mentally rehearse successful coping strategies to deal with the stresses of hospitalization. The child acts out roles of health professionals and patients and manipulates a doll or a piece of equipment. Dur-

Table 15-4 Using Relaxation Techniques with Children

Preparation Phase

1. Provide a calm, restful environment by dimming the lights, reducing the noise level, and planning ahead to prevent interruptions for 10-20 min. Relaxation can be taught before or at any time during hospitalization. The child who is comfortable and familiar with relaxation training will use it more easily during stressful events.
2. Prepare the parents and child for the training. Tell them that the child learns to consciously tighten and then relax each set of muscles throughout the body. Each time the child practices, it becomes easier to relax. This technique was first developed by Dr. Herbert Benson in 1920. Tell them they may stop whenever they wish.
3. Prepare yourself by being as anxiety-free as possible. Plan this time each day to prevent distraction from responsibilities. Talk in a low, soothing, monotone voice. Relax!

Training Phase

1. Instruct the child: "Lie back on your bed [or any comfortable place] and get comfortable. Close your eyes and listen only to me. Try to do what I tell you. If you want to stop, it's okay. Imagine yourself in a happy, quiet place where you are relaxed. You feel wonderful. The sun is warming your body. You can feel it ooze down into your arms, skin, and even hands. Your breathing is slow and relaxed. Let the air breathe for you. Feel your chest moving up and down. It feels lighter and lighter. Now take a deep breath and let it out slowly. Good. Take another deep breath and hold it. Good. Let it out slowly, and as you blow the air out, pretend seeing the worries go out too. Now you are starting to feel relaxed and calm. Make a tight fist with both your hands. Really tight. Feel how tight they are. Let them go, and feel how relaxed they are now (perhaps like a rag doll's)."
2. Tell the child to tense and relax other body parts using the above technique (hands, fingers, arms, shoulders, chest, stomach, buttocks, lower and upper back, neck, face, jaw, legs, feet, and toes). The number of body parts relaxed can be adapted to the child's age, attention span, and physical condition.
3. Have the child practice 1-2 times each day for at least 10 days in a stress-free environment. Only then should the child be coached to prepare for a stressful event such as a dressing change.
4. Praise and encourage the child frequently during the practice sessions and during stressful events. Commercial tapes can be used, or the sessions may be taped by the child's parents or other personnel. The tape can be used whenever the child is threatened by a stressful event.

Sources: Elizabeth Poster, "Stress Immunization: Techniques to Help Children Cope with Hospitalization," *Maternal-Child Nursing Journal* **12:**119–134 (Summer 1983); and Barbara Blattner, *Holistic Nursing*, Prentice-Hall, Englewood Cliffs, N.J., 1981, p. 239.

ing the sessions the child anticipates fears and "plays out" the fears to allow for some mastery over them. When the child knows what will happen, he or she can use cognitive control to decrease anxiety.[12]

PARENTS AND THE HOSPITALIZED CHILD

Reactions of parents

Parents experience a variety of feelings when their child is hospitalized. The majority of parents experience *anxiety,* which directly affects the anxiety level of the hospitalized child.[13] If the child's progress is unknown or recovery is questionable or if the parents' sense of competence is threatened, their anxiety level will be high. In severe anxiety the parents' perceptual field narrows. Their attention focuses on one segment of the environment; what they hear is often distorted, and they cannot learn from, or listen to, others. These parents frequently question nurses repeatedly and appear to test the nurses' competence. Characteristic behaviors of anxiety are rapid talking, a high-pitched voice, agitated hand movements, diaphoresis (sweating), and diarrhea. Anxiety must be recognized and reduced, for it is depleting and highly contagious.

Parents may also experience *fear.* Common causes of parents' fears are inadequate information about test results, treatments, procedures, or prognosis; leaving the child alone; distrust of nursing and medical staff; strange equipment; and the costs of hospitalization. Parents may also worry about other children at home, especially if the child care there is inadequate. An ill or hospitalized child causes reverberations throughout the family constellation; children at home absorb their parents' anxiety. They may become jealous because their parents spend time at the hospital and may become increasingly accident-prone. (See Chap. 34.)

A feeling of powerlessness is a common parental reaction (Fig. 15-4). Before hospitalization, the parents were the experts in control of their child's life. In the hospital, medical and nursing personnel assume control of the child's care. Parents may feel helpless, dependent, uninformed, and powerless. Inadequacy is a common parental feeling. Parents may lack information about their role in the hospital. They do not know how they are expected to act. (One mother confided, "I haven't eaten in two days, but if I finish my daughter's tray, the head nurse will bawl me out!" The nurses had not assessed the mother's needs.)

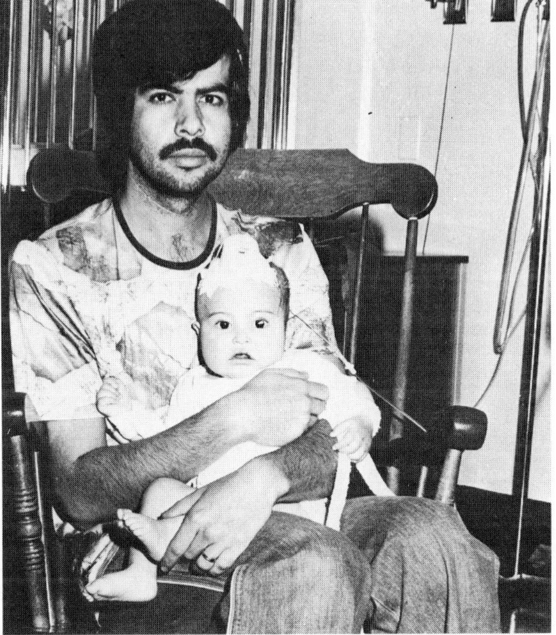

Figure 15-4 Hospitalization increases parents' feelings of anxiety, distrust, and powerlessness. Note this father's protective posture. *(Photo by Theresa Friedrich. Courtesy of LAC/USC Medical Center.)*

Parents frequently feel *guilt,* blaming themselves for their child's illness. (See Chap. 35 for a discussion of grief and the grieving process.) Anger turned inward can result in guilt and depression. Parents express *anger* when they ask, "Why me? Why didn't the doctor diagnose it sooner? Why would God let this happen?" Anger is often directed at nurses or doctors because they are close, convenient targets. It is important for nurses to recognize the parents' anger, acknowledge it, help them express it, and realize that it is not a personal attack. Parents may *deny* (or not consciously acknowledge) their child's illness. They take the child to various doctors and are unable to comprehend or believe the doctors' diagnoses or explanations. They may appear to disbelieve the diagnosis or search for errors. *Jealousy* of nurses occurs because parents feel inadequate, powerless, useless, and unimportant in the child's care. *Physical exhaustion* changes the parents' behavior. Inadequate sleep may reduce their ability to make rational decisions, cope with the stresses of the illness, and maintain a functioning routine at home. Parents who need sleep become irritable and unable to concentrate. Changed behavior toward the child may occur as a result of the child's illness. One parent may become indulgent, while another may become more restrictive.

Parents in the hospital

Parents often have unclear expectations about their role in the hospital.[14] When people in any social encounter perceive their roles in the same way, they are in *role congruency*. If they do not, they may react unacceptably to one another. This is called *role incongruency* and often occurs between parents and nurses. Giving parents role cues or role information helps them learn how they are expected to act in a hospital.[15] Parents who are knowledgeable about the hospitalization and the child's illness feel competent and better able to support their child.[16] Such aid is especially helpful when there is a cultural difference between the nurse and the parents. The four-step method shown in Table 15-5 may help the nurse increase the parents' sense of competence and ease any role incongruency that exists.

In most hospitals, the teaching of role expectations begins before hospitalization. Usually there are booklets available that instruct parents on visiting hours, rooming-in, cafeteria hours, and other policies. Ideally, such guides also welcome them and encourage them to participate in their child's care.

The nurse can offer important help to parents who are in search of an appropriate role. The following are a few guidelines:

1. Parents should be allowed to be with the child during procedures, provided this makes the parents and the child less anxious.
2. Parents should be encouraged to participate in their child's care (Fig. 15-5). According to one study, parents want to do more for their children than nurses realize.[17] They gain a feeling of competence if they actively contribute to their child's recovery. Performing a physical task will also decrease their anxiety level. The nurse who wishes to ensure that parents get to provide care can learn which jobs they prefer to do and establish a contract, written on the Kardex, listing the parents' and the nurse's tasks (Fig. 15-6). Parents should be assured that the nurse will teach them, answer questions, and check the child frequently.
3. Parents should be praised for rearranging schedules in order to be with the child and should be assured that they are making an important contribution to the child's recovery. At the same time, their ability to cope with the illness should be assessed. Can other family members support the parents by caring for children left at home? If appropriate, parents should be referred to sources of financial aid.
4. The nurse should support and help parents when it is time for them to separate from the child and explain that they should honestly tell the child they are going home and that this truthfulness will increase the child's trust. Parents should be educated about separation anxiety and encouraged to leave a personal

Table 15-5 Four-Step Teaching Method

1. *Paying attention* This step validates your nursing diagnosis of the mother's source of anxiety. Directly address her, turn your body toward her, and say, for example, "Mrs. Smith, you look as if you're ready to cry. You seem really reluctant to pick up your child since she's had her IV." The mother then has the opportunity to agree with (and validate) or reject your assessment. You then know whether the observations and nursing diagnosis are correct. Focus your communication and teaching on the mother's main source of increased anxiety.
2. *Information-giving* Give the mother information about her role. Tell the mother that her feelings of fright are acceptable by saying, for example, "Yes, Mrs. Smith, it must be frightening to pick up Jennifer with all those tubes and wires attached to her body. Has anyone told you the reasons for them?" After giving an explanation for the IV, say, "Would you like me to teach you how to pick her up?" Demonstrate the procedure, telling her the essential points in *simple* words.
3. *Participation* Have the mother pick up the child, and stress the important points. Encourage the mother to ask questions.
4. *Evaluation* Evaluate your teaching: Did you consider the mother's main concern? Was your information given in small amounts and simple language during the demonstration? Document the mother's learning. In what areas was she strongest and weakest? What teaching methods appeared most effective? How did the mother's behavior change after the teaching? What were her main concerns? Document these on the chart.

Source: Adapted from Sister Mary Callista Roy, "Role Cues and Mothers of Hospitalized Children," *Nursing Research* **16:**178–182 (Spring 1967).

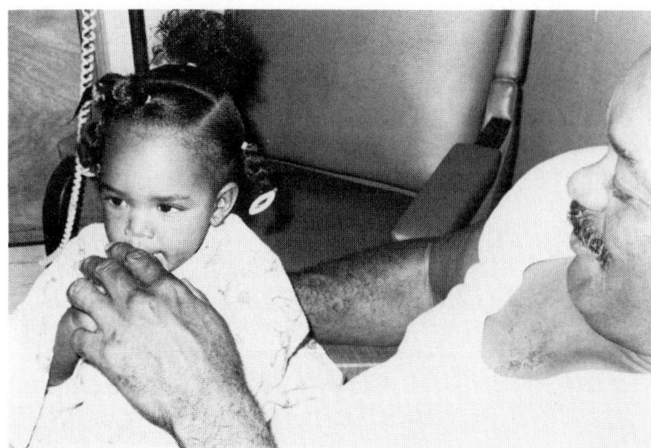

Figure 15-5 Children need their parents. Being given his medicine by his father increases this child's sense of trust.

article (e.g., a sweater, a tie, or keys) with the child and to telephone the child.

In one study, the majority of parents surveyed (52 percent) were concerned about such child and family matters as normal growth and development, parenting skills, language, discipline, safety, and poison prevention. Medical concerns (childhood diseases, emergency care for poisoning, and medications) were expressed by 33 percent. Only 15 percent of the parents were concerned about nutrition. These parents preferred to be taught through newsletters, telephone tapes, discussion groups, personal discussions, and telephone calls.[18]

The nurse should make it a priority to win the parents' trust. They should be asked each day whether they have questions, and these should be answered carefully; following through is important in establishing trust. After a doctor has finished an explanation, the parents should be asked what they understood the physician to mean. In this way the nurse can assess their understanding. Many parents see nurses as less threatening than physicians and as persons who have more time to talk. Finding out how parents interpret what the doctors said gives the nurse an opportunity to teach, clarify, and reinforce the physician's explanations. Simple, everyday words should be employed. If necessary a translator, perhaps another family member, should be used. Medical phrases can be written out on cards in two languages.

It will help communication if the nurse addresses the parents while turned toward them, using direct eye contact, after greeting them courteously by name. (The author once observed two nurses in an intermediate intensive care unit who failed to speak to, or even acknowledge the presence of, five of the six parents who were present over a 6-h period!)

Parent Participation in Hospital Care

What would you like to do for your child during his or her hospitalization as far as physical care is concerned?

Feed child ________
Bathe child ________
Take temperature ________
Give pills or liquid medications ________
Record amount child eats and drinks ________
Record amount of urination or bowel movement ________
Stay with child during doctor's examination ________
Stay with child during painful procedures ________
Take child to bathroom or change diaper ________
Go with child to x-ray department or bathroom ________
Change bed linen ________

Is there anything else you would like to do for your child during this hospitalization? ________

Figure 15-6 A completed nurse-parent contract is placed in the Kardex. (*From Annette Ayer, "Is Partnership with Parents Really Possible?" American Journal of Maternal-Child Nursing 3(2):109* [*March–April 1978*].)

PREPARING THE CHILD FOR PROCEDURES

Nurses who understand how children think and who know how to communicate and play with them are more successful in preparing them for procedures than nurses who lack this understanding and knowledge. The nurse may need guidelines concerning the needs of children in each age group, which naturally differ a great deal. Table 15-6 reviews the preteaching phase. Table 15-7 identifies the concerns and expectations of patients in the age groups from infancy to adolescence and offers suggestions for appropriate teaching and nursing care.

Concepts of illness

One goal in assessing the child's concept of illness is to improve communication between the nurse and the child.[19] Improved communication results in improved compliance with treatment and increased knowledge of health and illness.

Children's beliefs about illness are affected by their cognitive level as well as by their past ex-

Table 15-6 Preparing the Child for Procedures: Preteaching Phase

Preparation for Teaching	Rationale
A nurse who has established trust should teach the child; a relief person should be designated on the Kardex and introduced to the child. Preoperative teaching should start 1 day before surgery at a time when the child is rested.	If the child trusts the nurse-teacher, the child's anxiety will be less, and he or she will be better able to grasp and believe what is said.
Assess the child's cognitive development	Teaching must be adapted to the child's ability to think.
Confer with doctors or nurses in ICU or in surgery regarding special treatments, procedures, etc. Many hospitals use a "roller file" of doctors' special instructions about procedures. Notebooks of teaching plans are also used (e.g., whether anesthesia will be given by mask and whether the child will be on a respirator).	It is important for the nurse to maintain trust by giving the child correct information.
Assess whether the child wants the parents present. Many preschoolers and school-age children do.	The parents' presence increases the child's sense of security.
Assess the child's anxiety level and coping mechanisms.	A highly anxious child cannot learn.
Gather together equipment for teaching: a doll with tubes, IV tubing, etc. Determine whether a school-age child or adolescent is embarrassed by a doll.	The child needs to see equipment. Toddlers and preschoolers think concretely and respond best to dolls.

Table 15-7 Preparing the Child for Procedures: Information-Giving Phase

Characteristics of Cognitive Development	Guidelines for Teaching and Nursing Care
Infant (birth to 1 year)	
Has no understanding of the procedure or the effect.	No preparation needed. Keep the procedure brief. Prepare the parents for the procedure.
Feels pain.	Comfort and hold the infant securely. Talk in a soothing voice during the procedure.
Familiar routines of care establish security and trust in the mother and the nurse.	Have a familiar person hold the infant during the procedure. Give a pacifier if appropriate. Encourage the mother to comfort the infant during the procedure.
Relates to world through touch. Greatest comfort is in sucking.	After the procedure, hold and cuddle the infant. Give a bottle or pacifier.
Toddler (1 to 3 years)	
Fear of separation from parents causes greatest anxiety. Parent provides greatest security, even while the child is experiencing pain.	Urge the parents to stay with and comfort the child during the procedure. Suggest that a parent cuddle the child afterward and provide a security blanket.
Has no vocabulary for explaining fears and anxieties. A toddler has less experience than an older child in dealing with stress. Understands only one concept at a time.	Use simple words. Explain one concept at a time (e.g., "Hold your leg still," not "Hold your leg still and don't cry"). Tell the child how to act (e.g., first say, "Hold your leg still," then later, "You can cry").
Relates to the world by touch, feel, and taste. Uses play to learn about equipment and how to act in a new situation. Mixes up reality and fantasy; misinterprets events.	Use doll play to teach the child about the procedure. Let the child use a syringe (without needle), catheter, etc., and play at giving you or a doll an injection. Tell the child how it will feel. If possible, leave equipment for the child to play with.
Has no concept of passing time	Prepare the child $\frac{1}{2}$ h ahead or just before the procedure.
Preschooler (3 to 5 years)	
Still has no concept of passing time.	Prepare the child $\frac{1}{2}$ h ahead (if surgery is complicated, divide the information in sections). Tell the child when the procedure is completed.
Is egocentric. Thinks he or she is the center of everything and causes everything to happen. Cannot analyze own thinking. Only his or her opinion matters.	Tell the child that he or she did not cause the procedure. Use doll play to discover thoughts. (The doll will "say" what the child thinks.) Have the child play through the procedure. Don't argue about the procedure with the child.

Table 15-7 Preparing the Child for Procedures: Information-Giving Phase (*Continued*)

Characteristics of Cognitive Development	Guidelines for Teaching and Nursing Care
Lives in the present. Is interested only in "how it will feel." Still relates to the world primarily by touch.	Tell the child what will happen now and how it will feel. (He or she has no interest in the cause of the disease.)
May be unable (though willing) to cooperate during a procedure; he or she may not have full control of emotions. Wants to please adults.	Tell the parent what you expect of the child. Allow the child some control by giving him or her a choice (e.g., "Which leg do you want the shot in?"). If the child procrastinates, announce that you are going to give the injection, and proceed.
	Do not punish or get angry. Instead say, "I will help you hold your leg still this time. Maybe you can hold it still next time." Praise the child for something he or she did well (even crying loudly).
May feel anger (without knowing the name for it) because he or she cannot escape the procedure. Has limited coping mechanisms.	Encourage expressions of anger through play (e.g., clay, hammer, or beanbags). Tell the child that he or she is angry and that it is all right.
As part of establishing boundaries of self, fears body intrusion. Fantasies of body mutilation are very vivid.	Stress that only a limited part of the body will be involved. Describe how the body will feel, look, or "work" afterward.
May fear that general anesthesia is like dying.	Stress that "special sleep" keeps pain away and that he or she will wake up.
Thinks that parent (or nurse) is omnipotent and can do anything for him or her.	Support the need for the procedure. Do not say, "I don't want to, but I have to."
School-age child (6 to 12 years)	
Needs to maintain emotional control.	Carry out the procedure in a room away from the child's peers to prevent embarrassment. Tell the child what to do and say during the procedure. Explain the procedure beforehand.
With increase in vocabulary, wants to know cause of the disorder, how the procedure affects body functioning, and how the procedure will feel.	Ask the child to label a body outline or to draw a picture of the affected part. Reinforce his or her correct associations and correct any mistakes about anatomy, and physiology. Explain the cause of the disorder. Draw a picture of the body and part, describing function, the procedure, and the aftermath. Tell the child how the procedure will feel.
Despite larger vocabulary, may not understand meaning of medical words he or she uses.	Ask the child word meanings. Teach the child scientific terms for body parts and procedures.
Tends to blame himself or herself for illness.	Correct this misunderstanding.
Needs to feel proud of accomplishments. May display more self-confidence than he or she actually has. Praise increases self-esteem.	After the procedure, praise the child for what he or she did correctly (no matter how trivial). Encourage the child to visit other well-adjusted children facing similar treatments.
Adolescent (12 to 21 years)	
Wants to be well informed on how procedure may affect body image.	Describe anatomy and physiology. Explain the procedure and its effect on the body; tell the adolescent what clothes or activities will be possible afterward. With a mutilating operation (e.g., a colostomy or amputation) stress how the adolescent's normal activities can be adapted. Have a well-adapted teenager who has experienced the procedure visit.
Needs to have some control and feeling of independence.	Allow the adolescent to wear his or her own clothes. Encourage the adolescent to make health care decisions and to execute them. Give the adolescent privacy when requested. If he or she appears unduly dependent on parents, ask the adolescent necessary questions when he or she is alone.
Fears loss of acceptance by peers.	Encourage visits by friends and other adolescent patients. Encourage the adolescent to eat with friends in the cafeteria. Discuss school and friends with the adolescent.

periences with illness. To make an assessment of the child's knowledge and to plan appropriate interventions, the nurse must understand the developmental changes that occur in children's concept of illness. The assessment requires determination of:

1. The child's conceptual stage (fuzzy, concrete, or abstract)
2. The child's awareness or unawareness of the objective indicators of illness
3. The accuracy or inaccuracy of the child's information

Children's concepts of illness develop through different stages, from global and undifferentiated to concrete and abstract. Their ideas are usually a mixture of facts and imaginative distortions.[20]

Nurses should understand that many young school-age children believe that illness is a punishment for wrongdoing. It is useful to have children describe what is making them sick and why. Children may need permission to express their ideas. Some children may not be ready to learn about their illness. The nurse needs to be able to determine this to avoid increasing the child's anxiety by providing unwanted information. Children with a chronic illness need continuing education to help them develop and revise their understanding of their illness. Table 15-8 describes developmental stages in the child's concepts of illness and suggests appropriate communication techniques for each conceptual level.

Table 15-8 The Child's Concept of Illness: Implications for Nursing

	Concept of Illness	Useful Communication Techniques
Category 0: Incomprehension	The infant cannot understand questions about illness, much less explain it.	Touch, hold, and reassure the child. Keep the parent nearby.
Preoperational thought: 18 months to 6 to 7 years (prelogical)		
Category 1: Phenomenism	Illness is attributed to a concrete phenomenon external to the child. Illness is seen as existing in the present, not the past or the future. "How did you get a cold?" "From the trees."	Focus on the here and now. Use pictures. Use familiar names for body parts. Allow the child to handle equipment and perform procedures on dolls. Assure the child that the parent will return. Point out body cues of illness.
Category 2: Contagion	Illness is attributed to persons or objects in close proximity to the child. The child might say that he or she got a cold from a sibling, but does not know *how* he or she got it.	Provide models of coping responses. Help the child rehearse coping responses to painful, stressful procedures. Help distinguish attainable goals. Reassure the child that he or she did not cause the illness.
Concrete operational thought: 7 to 11 years (logical)		
Category 3: Contamination	The child can separate the illness from its cause. Often the child believes the external cause to be a bad or harmful action or a contaminated article. Children often attribute illness to their own actions.	Give simple explanations, and correct misconceptions. Explain the cause of the illness and contributing factors. Use concrete models, drawings, and diagrams to describe and explain. Ask the child to describe the illness process; make it more clear by adding new steps. Point out the relationship between signs of illness and the illness process (e.g., excessive blood sugar and diabetes).
Category 4: Internalization	The child often links the cause of the illness to something inside his or her body. There is increasing differentiation between external and internal causes as the child matures. "I caught a cold because I got my feet wet."	Help the child sort out the information. (For example, the child may believe that he or she has a fixed quantity of blood that can be permanently depleted.) Avoid using words with two meanings (e.g., *die* vs. *dye* and *take* a sample of blood vs. *draw* blood).

Table 15-8 The Child's Concept of Illness: Implications for Nursing (*Continued*)

	Concept of Illness	Useful Communication Techniques
Formal operational thought: 11 to 12 years to adulthood (formal logical)*		
Category 5: Physiological	The child relates the cause of the illness to malfunction of internal organs. He or she will tell how a cold feels and what it does and may relate it to a virus. The child explains illness in terms of a sequence of events. Children in this age group also believe that everyone around them (imaginary audience) thinks about them and is concerned with them. This leads to the construction of a "personal fable" or a shield of invulnerability. Anything that challenges this fable is very stressful.	Explain the illness in terms of physiological processes and in terms of internal organs and their malfunctions. With children who have a chronic illness, it may be necessary to check for misconceptions. Children may tend to minimize the severity of an illness; therefore, check symptoms carefully. Show that others with a similar illness still carry on. Children in this age group are concerned with how the imaginary audience reacts to them. (Test their personal fable; do not deny it—e.g., that they cannot get pregnant because they are not in love or that they cannot get hurt on a motorcycle.)
Category 6: Psychophysiological	This is the most mature response. The teenager can see the possible psychophysiological cause of an illness, and feels some control over the onset and the cure of the illness. Mature teenagers can think about thinking—and think about what others think about.	Identify future implications of the illness and the treatment; give the adolescent some control in planning schedules and solving problems. Many adolescents want more information about the cause of their illness and the prognosis than the physician gives them.

*Some, but not all, adolescents will be at the stage of formal operations.

Sources: R. Bibace and M. Walsh, "Developmental Concepts of Illness," *Pediatrics* **66**(6):912–917 (1980); L. Dorn, "Children's Concepts of Illness: Clinical Applications," *Pediatric Nursing* **10**(5):327 (1984); D. Elkind, "Teenage Thinking: Implications for Health Care," *Pediatric Nursing* **10**(6):383–385 (1984); and V. Pidgeon, "Children's Concepts of Illness: Implications for Health Teaching," *Maternal-Child Nursing Journal* **14**(1):23–35 (1984).

THE INFANT'S REACTIONS TO HOSPITALIZATION

All infants have similar reactions to hospitalization. Because of their immature body systems, they frequently experience instability in temperature regulation, fluid and electrolyte balance, and absorption of medicine (see Chaps. 8 and 9). Furthermore, the parent-child relationship is likely to be disturbed. The trusting infant perceives the world as safe when experiencing consistency, continuity, and sameness in the daily routine. The inevitable disruptions brought on by hospitalization may promote distrust. The bonding process may be interrupted (see Chap. 8), and the older infant may experience separation anxiety, discussed later in the section "The Toddler's Reactions to Hospitalization."

To offset these reactions, the nurse should attempt to adapt hospital routines to resemble those of the home. It has been found helpful to provide a "primary" nurse for each child and to encourage a family member to be with the child each day.

The remainder of this section will focus on the impact of disturbing a child's daily routines, such as feeding, sucking, sleeping, and crying. It will also examine how a changed sensory environment like the hospital affects a child.

Feeding

A reluctance to eat is very common in sick infants. This makes feeding a very time-consuming and frustrating experience for the nurse and the parents. Feeding suggestions are given in Table 15-9.

Infants need their mothers to hold and feed them whenever possible. Infants are acutely sensitive to the person who feeds them; the environment; the texture, temperature, and taste of food; the type and size of nipple; the bottle;

Table 15-9 Feeding Problems of the Hospitalized Infant

Problem	Nursing Intervention	
Excessive crying, gas, or pain from colic	Burp the infant before feeding and frequently during feeding. Place the infant on his or her abdomen or use a suppository, thermometer, or rectal tube to expel gas. Keep formula cool or at room temperature. Comfort the child to decrease crying. Be sure that diapers are not wet. Offer a pacifier if the infant is unable to take enough formula to appease hunger.	When crying, the infant swallows air, which distends the stomach, increasing pressure and discomfort. Release of air when burping brings food with it. Excessively warm formula increases pressure in the enclosed stomach.
Anxiety and anorexia	A relaxed, secure nurse or preferably a parent should rock and comfort the child before, during, and after feeding. Assess sucking ability. Feed small amounts of food.	A relaxed attitude on the part of the caretaker will be communicated to the infant. Rocking simulates intrauterine movement and increases sense of security.
Frequent regurgitation or vomiting	Burp the infant before feeding and often during feeding. Thicken the formula slightly with rice cereal. Take time in feeding. Allow the child to rest in nurse's arms between feedings. Keep the child in an upright position before, during, and after feeding. Do not feed in infant seat. Perform any scheduled procedures before feeding. Do not overfeed.	Normal newborn children have weak cardiac sphincters, which allows food to ascend easily to the mouth. This may be accentuated in sick infants.
Refusal of solid foods or inability to take in adequate quantities although hungry	Flavor cereal slightly with fruit (apricots, bananas). Thin formula. Serve in a small demitasse spoon. Offer small amounts of food using a gloved, clean finger. Give the child small, frequent feedings, with rest periods between. Reassess hospital routine. Is it homelike and consistent with data from the admission interview?	A critically ill child (e.g., one with cardiac disease) may lack the energy to suck or eat. In premature or brain-damaged infants, the sucking reflex is weak. Sucking requires considerable energy.

Note: Although some of these measures may help the nurse feed the normal newborn, certain others will not. For instance, a pacifier is not to be used to appease a well infant instead of feeding. Furthermore, the nurse should not thicken the feeding of a normal infant to prevent regurgitation.

and the feeding schedule. All these must be considered when feeding the infant, and the experience should be made as homelike as possible. Painful procedures should be scheduled between feedings to avoid upsetting the baby just before or just after eating.

Sucking

Sucking is the infant's main source of emotional satisfaction and brings food and pleasurable feelings to the infant. Sick infants often have difficulty sucking. When the infant's sucking needs are not met through feeding, provide a pacifier, and position the infant to make the pacifier accessible.

Sleeping

Changes in routine and the environment result in disturbances of sleep patterns. Use information obtained in the admission history to simulate the home routine. Pay attention to bedtime, favorite position, nighttime bottle, bedtime rituals, and type and location of bed. Tightly wrapping the infants and placing them against a towel or a diaper roll, to simulate the restricted intrauterine environment and the mother's backbone, prolong sleeping.

Crying

Infants communicate their needs by crying. Cries of pain are high-pitched and shrill; cries of hunger are lower-pitched and increase in loudness to reflect the intensity of hunger. Cries of anger are loud.

Learn to interpret infants' cries. Ask the parents to interpret the cries and suggest successful remedies.

First check the baby's physical comfort: Are the diapers wet? Does the infant have diaper rash? When was the infant last fed? How much was eaten? Does the infant need to be burped? Does the child have appropriate toys? When was the child last taken out of the crib to play? Is the child in pain? Make the necessary corrections, and then comfort the child by rocking or walking, singing and cooing, or offering toys.

Place babies in backpacks while working in noninfectious areas. Hold babies on laps while charting. Utilize others (such as foster grandparents) to consistently feed and care for infants when parents are unable to visit.

Sensory stimulation: Impact of the hospital

Infants and children need stimulation of their senses for normal psychological and neurological development. The newborn is especially alert immediately after birth. Infants move their eyes searching for human faces, which they prefer to other visual stimuli. They also prefer colorful, moving objects to unmoving, colorless forms.[21]

Auditory stimuli, like visual ones, can be highly significant. Hospitalized infants are soothed almost immediately when recordings of intrauterine sounds are placed close by. It is probably no accident that a mother naturally cradles her child over her heart. The heartbeat may simulate intrauterine sounds. Infants also move in synchronous rhythm with the sounds of the parent's speech.[22] All such auditory stimuli are believed to promote a feeling of security and the process of bonding.

Sensory stimulation of certain kinds also appears to foster physical development. Infants who are stimulated with rocking and tape recordings of a woman's voice and heartbeat have been shown to grow better than infants who do not receive the stimulation[23] In another study, infants who were exposed to auditory, visual, tactile, and motor stimulation matured faster than children who were not exposed to this stimulation.[24] Several studies have found that premature infants are especially vulnerable to developmental delays if the hospital environment provides inadequate stimulation and does not encourage the mother's presence.

For these reasons the modern-day pediatric unit is a far different place from the one of years past, when infants were placed in white rooms, enclosed in bassinets with white-sheeted sides, and viewed by parents through a window. Infants were handled and rocked minimally. The practices of such institutions may have unintentionally contributed to developmental delays and inadequate parent–child bonding.

Sensory deprivation The importance of sensory stimulation appears to derive from the need of the cerebrum for a certain level of input from the environment by way of the nervous system. The level is believed to be preset in each individual by hereditary and learned means. A prolonged drop below this level brings about *sensory deprivation*. Premature infants, chronically ill children, isolated children, and institutionalized children are at risk for sensory deprivation.

If a child's crying brings no response from an adult, the child cries less and learns not to expect adults to meet his or her needs. Infants who rarely see adults will not learn to imitate the facial expressions, body movements, or speech of adults. The faces of these infants have stonelike or bland expressions. Speech development is delayed. Their speed of response is below normal, as is the number of words they learn to speak. Severely deprived infants fail to develop stranger anxiety (a behavior indicative of bonding) and to learn to mold to the caretaker's arms.

Older sensory-deprived children may exhibit self-stimulatory behavior such as body-rocking, head-banging, and repetitious rubbing or picking of the sheets. Such children are more likely than others to experience hallucinations, which are a self-stimulatory behavior.[25]

Sensory overload Excessive sensory stimulation may lead to *sensory overload*. Infants and children in critical care units are especially vulnerable, given the constant beeping of cardiac monitors, the sound of respirators, and the continuous, monotonous lighting. The behaviors of sensory overload are similar to those of sensory deprivation. The infant has difficulty perceiving and selecting new stimuli among the inflow of others. He or she needs a general reduction in stimuli and an individualized, age-appropriate plan for sensory stimulation.

Nursing management Using appropriate stimuli, the nurse is the critical person to design the plan for enrichment of the infant's environment. The nurse should assess the child for symptoms of sensory deprivation or overload and identify environmental sources if either condition exists.

Chosen stimuli should have maximal meaning for the child. A recording of the mother's heartbeat or voice may be right for an infant but less effective for an older child. The stimuli should relate to the child's greatest need. If the child screams for the mother, for example, the nurse should fetch her or provide a substitute. The intensity of the stimulus should be varied. Television should not be the source for an extended period. The visual and auditory stimuli, especially in the daytime, when there are continuous game shows, may become monotonous and hence ineffective. Because of infants' short attention span, stimuli for infants should be varied frequently.

Stimuli selected by the nurse for an infant should be age-appropriate and engage the infant's main ways of experiencing the world: touch, movement, vision, and hearing. Suggestions are given in Table 15-10.

Table 15-10 Suggestions for Sensory Stimulation

Tactile
Fuzzy blankets
Toys of different colors and textures to touch and hold
Holding and cuddling during feedings and whenever possible
Diaper rolls to place behind the infant's back (to simulate the mother's backbone)
Pacifiers to bring pleasurable feelings and satisfaction
Movement
Rocking chairs to simulate intrauterine movement
Cradle gyms to pull self up
Toys to bounce, crunch, and squeeze
Minimal restraint on the child, with toy in reach
Visual
Mirrors in crib or incubator
Pictures of parents and pets
Brightly colored mobiles placed in the child's line of vision, not at foot of bed
Auditory
Singing lullabies
Recordings of mother's heartbeat
Recording of parent's voice
Music boxes and records

THE TODDLER'S REACTIONS TO HOSPITALIZATION

Toddlers usually react to hospitalization with three main behaviors: (1) separation anxiety (which begins in infancy but peaks in the toddler years), (2) regression, and (3) disturbances in daily routines. Each of these behavioral disturbances will be discussed in this section.

Separation anxiety

This is essentially a grief reaction and is characterized by stages of (1) protest, (2) despair, and (3) denial or detachment. Children from 7 months to 3 years of age are most vulnerable to separation anxiety. The toddler's response to separation is greatly influenced by the existence of a strong parental bond, the severity of the illness, and previous experiences with separation.

Stage 1: Protest After the mother has gone, the toddler angrily protests (Fig. 15-7). The toddler refuses to eat, tries frantically to climb over the siderail, keeps watching for her return, and cries loudly and angrily until dropping from exhaustion. The toddler immediately goes to the mother when she returns. The toddler depends on the mother. Her absence increases feelings of vulnerability. The hospitalized child needs the mother as much as food. The environment is strange. The toddler may feel punished or abandoned by the mother. This lowers self-esteem and increases feelings of shame and doubt. Behavior is thus focused on regaining the mother. This is psychologically healthy behavior because the toddler still trusts that the mother will return and outwardly expresses his or her anger.

Nursing management The goal during protest is to preserve the child's trust in the parents. Do not feel rejected if the child stiffens when comforted; the child simply prefers the mother. Nurses instinctively say, "Shh, don't cry." In-

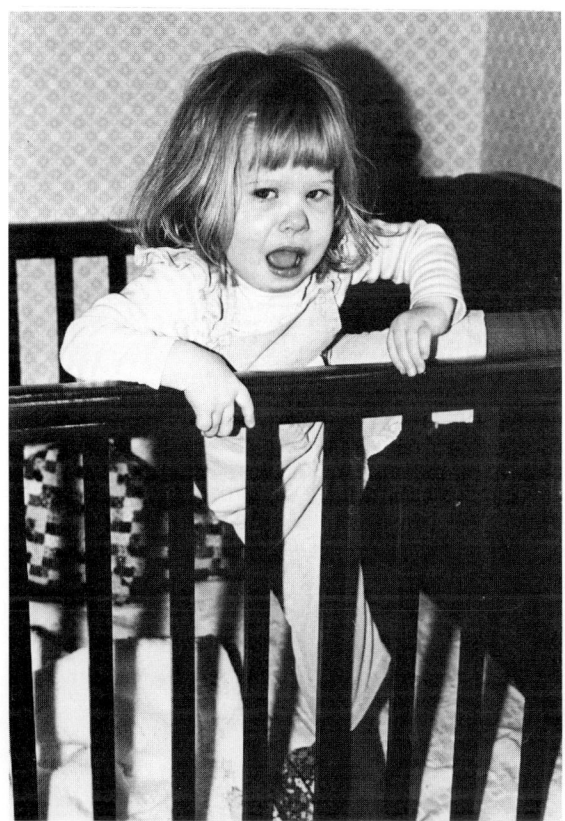

Figure 15-7 This toddler is in the protest stage of separation anxiety. She angrily protests her mother's departure.

stead, encourage the child to cry and express anger by saying, "Go ahead, cry! I know you want your mommy." Expressing, instead of suppressing, anger is psychologically healthy for the child. Encourage and accept expression of aggression in play: pounding boards or clay, throwing beanbags, or hitting balloons hung from the bed. Tell children that you will stay with them. Help toddlers remember their parents by talking about them and their activities together at home. Toddlers think in the present: "My parents are gone and may not return." Because their security is associated with objects, they believe that the parents will return for an object. The parents should leave a personal object from home: a tie, purse, or scarf, for example.

Favorite toys, pajamas, dishes, or security blankets bridge the transition from home and bring hours of comfort. New toys and clothes brought by the parents are not the same. Pictures of family members and pets can be taped to the crib to connect the child to home. If the mother cannot come in, her voice can be tape-recorded telling a story or singing a bedtime lullaby. Foster grandparents can also help the child when parents cannot be present. Allowing the parents to *room-in* is ideal for promoting the toddler's security.

Stage 2: Despair In this stage the child's depression deepens, and anger is turned inward (Fig. 15-8). The child begins to wonder whether the parents will ever return, and his or her trust in the parents wavers. The child becomes sad, withdrawn, subdued, and less angry. He or she submits to intrusive procedures with little resistance, picks at food, and sits quietly and forlornly in the crib. The child's cry is whining, listless, and pitiful. Behavior regresses. When the parents return, the child may not go to them immediately, but stands back as if to say, "You

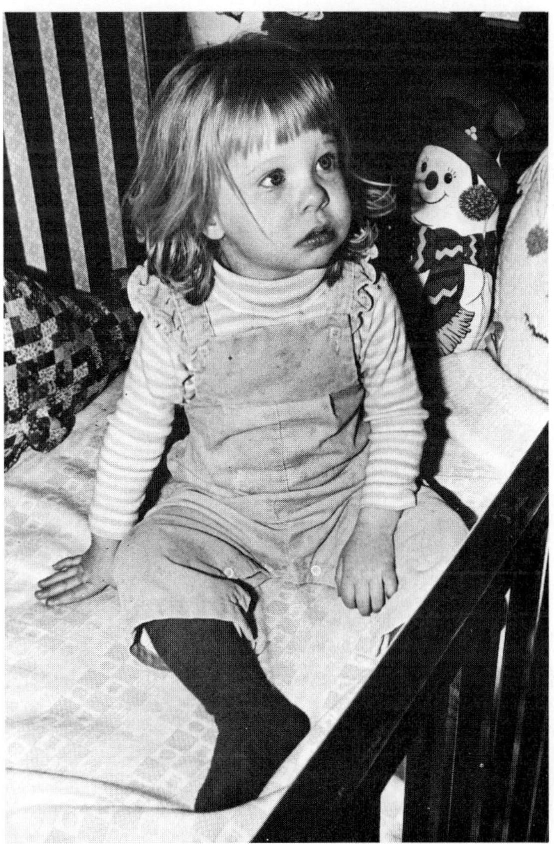

Figure 15-8 This toddler is in the despair stage of separation anxiety. Her depression deepens; she sits listlessly in the crib.

have caused me so much pain that I really don't know if I want to be closely involved with you again." When the child does approach them, he or she may cry, show anger, or frantically cling to them. The child occasionally runs away from the mother as if to punish and reject her, but soon clings tightly to her again.

Nursing management The nurse's goal with a child in despair is to increase the child's trust in the parents and to facilitate the expression of anger. If rooming-in is not possible, have the same nurses care for the child so that he or she will develop trust in consistent caregivers. Encourage the child to talk about the parents. Use the interventions described in the section "Stage 1: Protest" to promote the child's trust in the parents. Encourage the parents or a familiar person to consistently visit and feed the child. When nurses do not actively intervene with a child in despair, the child's depression will deepen and progress to distrust of the parents.

Stage 3: Denial or detachment In past years nurses erroneously thought that settling-in, or an outward denial of parents, was a positive change in the child's behavior. Certainly a compliant child is easier to care for than a screaming protester. If the nurse does not strengthen a child's trust in the parents and if the child's hospitalization is traumatic and prolonged, the child may lose trust in the parents.

The child in the denial stage eats, plays with toys, begins to resist intrusive procedures again, and makes "overtures" to all nurses on the unit. He or she appears to have sad eyes, brimming with tears, and a permanent, fake smile. The child rejects the parents and their presents when they return and deliberately expresses affection for the nurses. The child denies the need for the parents' love and suppresses longing and hostility toward them. Instead he or she relates to others on a superficial level and is no longer willing to risk intimate, trusting involvement with the parents. If the health team does not actively promote the child's trust, he or she may no longer be able to maintain in-depth, intimate relationships with adults.

Nursing management Encourage the child to express fears and perceptions (doll play is the ideal medium for toddlers' self-expression, where one can show them that the parents will return and take them home). Promote the consistent presence of the mother or other caregiver, and continue to use all the nursing interventions described earlier.

Regression

While all children and adults regress to some degree when ill or when faced with a stressful situation, regression is an especially common coping mechanism during the toddler and preschool years. The child usually drops the most recently learned behavior and returns to an earlier, more firmly established and satisfying behavior.[26]

Toddlers may revert to the bottle, refuse to drink from a cup, and wet their pants. Regression enables the child to withdraw, conserve energy, and eventually develop new methods of problem solving. This healthy, beneficial, "time-out" behavior is an attempt to regain control. The amount of regression is directly related to the degree of frustration and stress experienced by the child.

Nursing management Accept the child's behavior. Many nurses respond to regression in a cold, disapproving manner and label it as bad or obstructive.[27] This increases the child's stress. Therefore, let the child play "baby" or drink from a bottle. Hold, rock, and cuddle the child. Help the parents understand the healthy psychological benefits of regression. Relate regression to their own need for hot chicken soup and tender, loving care when ill. Explain that regression reduces the child's anxiety level, helps him or her regain control, and facilitates the child's physical recovery. The toddler's readiness to stop regressing can be assessed by noting his or her willingness to share and play with the nurse.[28]

Disturbance of daily routines and behavior

Toilet training Make a Kardex note about stage of training, specific words, and usual time of elimination. Instead of automatically placing toddlers in diapers, establish a routine for placing them on the potty-chair (see Chap. 10).

Sleeping Continue the child's bedtime ritual in the hospital with a story, lullaby, favorite animal, or security blanket (see Chap. 10).

Eating behavior The toddler's eating patterns are erratic and ritualistic. The child is very sensitive to changes in the environment, type of food, and the person doing the feeding. Provide small portions of foods that can be easily handled and eaten by the child without help (see Chap. 10).

Negativism The toddler often says "No!" to everything from a cookie to a nap. This is the toddler's method of proving that he or she is an individual with needs that are separate from the mother's.

Avoid asking questions that invite a "No!" answer, such as, "Do you want to take a nap now?" Help the child respond by holding his or her hand and leading the child to the bed. Emphasize what to *do*, rather than what *not to do*. If the child is immersed in a forbidden activity, say "No" and divert the child's attention to another toy. Give the toddler a choice between two acceptable alternatives: "Do you want the red or the green medicine first?" (see Chap. 10).

Temper tantrums Temper tantrums provide a safety valve for releasing pent-up, explosive emotions. Toddlers have limited control over their feelings. Ignore tantrums, rather than punishing children for having them. Some children respond well to being held firmly while regaining control. Hold the child and say, "I will help you hold still. The way you feel is called 'mad.' " If a toddler is biting a child or behaving in some other unacceptable manner, move his or her head away from the other child, get on the child's eye level, and say, "Stop biting him now. That hurts." Avoid saying "You're a bad girl," since this may diminish the child's self-esteem.

Ritualistic behavior Toddlers depend on familiar routines and objects for security (Fig. 15-9). They cannot reason, have a short attention span, and live in the present; toddlers have less ability than older children to control and understand their environment. They seek to gain control and security by ritualistically controlling objects. Provide homelike routines to meet basic needs and a safe environment that is appropriate for toddlers' size.

Dawdling Toddlers dawdle when caught in an ambivalent situation and should be helped to perform a necessary activity (see Chap. 10).

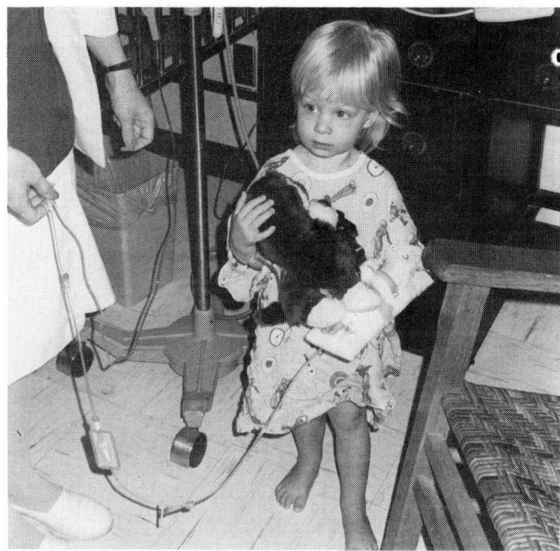

Figure 15-9 This child's transitional object provides security.

Reactions at home after hospitalization

Help parents anticipate possible changes in their child's behavior when he or she returns home. After a prolonged or traumatic hospitalization, the child may show any or all of the following behaviors: aggression, regression, nightmares, fear of falling asleep or of the dark, eating disturbances (food refusal, overeating, or rituals), overdependence, and unwillingness to let the mother out of his or her sight.[29] The child is afraid that if the parent disappears, he or she will again be left alone. One mother said this about her daughter Sara:

> She follows me everywhere! I can't even go to the bathroom alone. She wakes up screaming five or six times at night, shaking and crying, "The nurses are giving me shots! I can't run away! They're tying me down." She's regressed, and when I approach her, she backs away and shakes like a hurt puppy!

Before her hospitalization, Sara had gone to nursery school, fed herself, and was toilet-trained. After hospitalization, which included 22 injections in 2 days, she regressed. The nurse reviewed the child's illness and history with the parents to analyze their effects on Sara's behavior. Together they planned methods of handling her fears that would neither punish nor reward the behavior. For example, the nurse advised the mother to use the interventions described earlier for dealing with protest behavior: stay with Sara, help her return to meaningful activity, allow her to regress, and use needle play. She gleefully "shot" everything in the house—walls, pillows, the couch, and her father—and within a few weeks her behavior returned to normal.

THE PRESCHOOLER'S REACTIONS TO HOSPITALIZATION

Preschoolers have the following reactions to hospitalization: (1) they fear bodily mutilation, (2) they misinterpret hospital events, (3) they exhibit withdrawn behavior, (4) they exhibit aggressive behavior, (5) they have sleep disturbances, (6) they engage in masturbation, and (7) they experience separation anxiety. Each of these reactions will be discussed in this section.

Fears of mutilation

The main fear of preschoolers is loss of body integrity. They have violent fantasies about mutilation (Fig. 15-10). Preschoolers are just defining their bodies' outer boundaries, are unsure about their completeness, and are acutely sensitive to physical sensations and threats of attack. When asked to open his mouth and say "Ah," one preschooler refused and clutched his penis as if to reassure himself of its intactness. Preschoolers are acutely interested in physical deviations among people. Preschoolers suppose that such deviations are the results of violence and egocentrically assume that bodily intrusions or mutilation may also happen to them.

Preschoolers have only general ideas about body functions. For example, they picture a whole hamburger or cola drink inside the body and are unable to visualize the digestion and elimination of food. Preschoolers may know that they have a heart, but lack information about its function

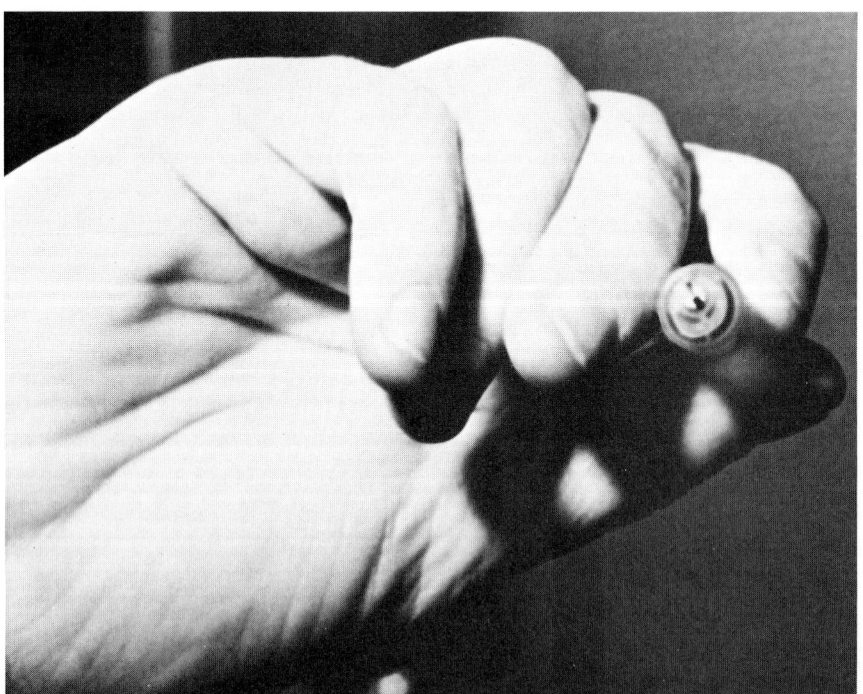

Figure 15-10 An injection seen through a child's eyes. Preschoolers fear body invasion and mutilation. (*Photo by Theresa Friedrich. Courtesy of LAC/USC Medical Center.*)

and location. They have minimal knowledge of other body organs and fantasize the information they lack.[30] Selected nursing interventions to promote body integrity are described in Table 15-11.

Misinterpretation of events

Preschoolers commonly misinterpret hospital events. Thinking at this age is magical and concrete, and these children readily create fantasy explanations for events that they do not understand. They do not clearly differentiate their fantasies, which are very real to them, from facts, which they poorly comprehend. They believe that thoughts and actions have equal power and that angry thoughts can make bad things happen. For example, if a child is angry with the mother and then the mother leaves, the child will think that he or she caused her to go away.

Children's thinking is egocentric; hence they are unable to understand or accept the points of view of others. They "know what they know," and arguing does not change their opinions. (See the section "Cognitive Development" in Chap. 11.)

Preschoolers focus on one aspect of an event while overlooking its other features. This characteristic causes them, for example, to attend only to the anticipated pain of an injection and to be unconsoled by promises that it will hurt only for a moment.

Table 15-11 Nursing Interventions to Reduce a Preschooler's Fears about Medical Procedures

Source of fear	Intervention
Bleeding, even a tiny amount	Use adhesive bandages liberally, including after every injection and finger-stick and for small abrasions. Tell the child the bandage will plug the hole. Explain that when the blood comes out, it gets "gluey" and "fixes" the hole and that the body makes new blood all the time.
Surgery	In preparation for surgery, explain that the doctor stops the bleeding and fixes the skin with needle and thread. Explain that surgery does not hurt because the child is in a special sleep. Have the child sew a doll's skin and apply a bandage. Avoid words like *cut* and *knife*; use words like *take away, sew up,* and *fix*. Describe postoperative body function, e.g., "You will go to the bathroom just like before."
Casts and cast removal	Have the child apply and remove a cast from a doll. Explain that the body part is protected inside the cast and remains attached to the body and that body parts do not "break off" from people, as the child may have seen happen to toys and dolls or in cartoons. Demonstrate a cast remover; use on your own skin or the parent's to show that it doesn't cut.
Disfigurements observed in others, especially other patients	Explain how the observed person's condition differs from the child's and reassure the child (realistically) that whatever happened to the other person (amputation, burn, birthmark, etc.) will not happen to the child. Emphasize restoration of body intactness; for example, "The doctors and nurses give her medicine and a new bandage every day, and her arm is getting better so that she will be able to play again."
Teasing, "jokes," and other threatening remarks about body damage	*Never* joke or threaten about accidental or intentional body injury. Young children interpret such remarks literally.
Equipment (sphygmomanometer, thermometer, traction, oxygen tents, respirators, etc.)	Emphasize the therapeutic purpose of equipment; for example, "That machine helps the boy breathe until he gets better and can breathe by himself." Arrange doll play and manipulation of the sphygmomanometer, thermometer, and other equipment used in the child's care. Demonstrate use and explain what the child will experience; for example, take a doll's or a parent's blood pressure and say, "It doesn't hurt. It feels tight like a belt. Now it's getting looser and I will take it off." When using a rectal thermometer say, "See, it isn't sharp. It only goes in this far. It tells me how hot you are, and then I take it out again." Allow the mother to insert the thermometer.
Injections	See Chap. 16.

They also are very present-oriented and cannot spontaneously anticipate that the current situation will improve (for example, that a procedure will soon be completed or that the mother will return and eventually take the child home).

The thinking of young children is animistic; that is, they think that everything that makes noise or has moving parts or blinking lights is alive. Consequently, preschoolers are commonly frightened of respirators, elevators, monitors, and other unfamiliar and noisy equipment.

Preschoolers also think that adults are omnipotent and that adults' motivations for causing or allowing unpleasant things to happen to children must be malevolent, since they imagine that adults have the power to exercise control over such events.

A forthright, honest, sympathetic, firm approach does much to support young children during hospitalization, even though they are still developmentally limited in their ability to understand what they are experiencing. Help children separate fact from fantasy; tell them, for example, that they have to take medicine because it helps them get well faster so that they can go home, not because they are naughty, and that the mother leaves the hospital because it is time for her to go to work, not because they are misbehaving. Use play to discover children's perceptions and imaginings, and use play, story telling, and simple explanations to correct misperceptions and reduce fears. Prepare children in advance of procedures by demonstrating and explaining what will be done and by providing opportunities to examine and manipulate equipment. When a child is too upset about an injection or other treatment to tolerate explanations about it, it is usually best to provide external controls (restraints) and proceed as quickly and kindly as possible; preschoolers often are more amenable to teaching and reassurance after a procedure than before. Do not argue or coax. Offer choices only if a choice truly exists; otherwise, explain what will be done and do it. Tell the child when the procedure is over. Provide simple explanations about equipment that do not support fearful fantasies. Adults' motives can be explained without making the child feel powerless. For example, in the case of a venipuncture, say, "The doctor needs to see a little of your blood so that we can tell how to make your stomachache go away. We are sorry the needle will hurt for a few minutes," rather than, "We don't want to do this, but we have to."

Withdrawn behavior

Some preschoolers withdraw from threatening stimuli. They often appear passive, immobile, and apathetic when faced with threatening procedures or separation from parents. Accept such behavior. Help them to recognize and accept their emotions, to learn new methods of coping with stress, and to express themselves in play. The nurse must be consistent in order to maintain the child's trust.

Aggressive behavior

Aggressive behavior is common among preschoolers. Many children want to, but are unable to, control their impulsive behavior. Preschoolers are less socialized than older children and have not yet learned to hide their true feelings. Label the child's emotion, saying, "The way you feel is called 'anger.' It is *okay* to be angry. I understand that you want your mommy, not me. Let's talk about what else you can do besides kicking me when you feel angry. You can. . . ." Restrain the child so that he or she will not hurt others. Explain the reasons for holding the child. "I am holding you until you stop biting. You cannot bite Andy again. Chew on this biscuit or bite the rubber duck. I will help you stop biting. It hurts." Accept the child's feelings of anger, and provide an outlet for his or her aggression, such as letting the child hit a punching bag or pound clay.

Sleep disturbances

Fear of "monsters" at bedtime peaks at $2\frac{1}{2}$ to 4 years of age (Fig. 15-11). The boundary between dreams and reality is shadowy. Preschoolers cling to bedtime rituals to increase control over their lives. Repeat the home bedtime ritual. If a child is afraid of monsters, comfort the child and emphatically tell the child that monsters are *not* real. Pretending to search for monsters is a questionable approach, since it may reinforce belief in their possible existence.

Masturbation

Preschoolers are establishing sexual identity. They learn that masturbation is pleasurable and tension-releasing. Instead of shaming them, which communicates that sexual organs are bad, tell them to rub themselves in their room instead of in the hall, or divert their attention (see Chap. 11).

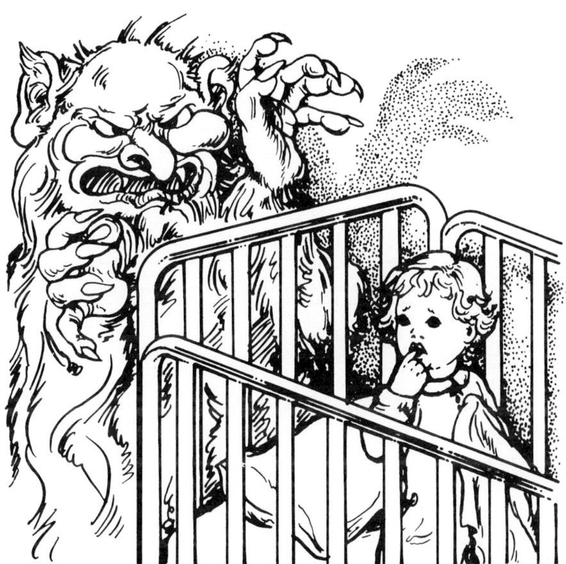

Figure 15-11 Fear of nighttime "monsters" peaks during the preschool years.

Separation anxiety

The separation anxiety of preschoolers is less intense than that of toddlers. Preschoolers have learned to handle their parents' absence, and they may previously have been away from home overnight. Their security is still closely bound to their parents, however, and during times of stress they need their parents nearby. The reactions to separation described in the section "The Toddler's Reactions to Hospitalization" may also be seen in the preschooler, and the nursing interventions are the same.

THE SCHOOL-AGE CHILD'S REACTIONS TO HOSPITALIZATION

School-age children frequently react to hospitalization with (1) fear of pain and bodily injury, (2) the perception of illness as punishment, (3) fear of loss of control, and (4) distress over separation from friends, school, and family. Each of these topics will be discussed in this section.

Fear of pain and bodily injury

These are important concerns of school-age children. Furthermore, they fear that bodily changes will make them different and result in rejection by their friends. They no longer focus on how the illness will feel, but are interested in learning about the causes and *results* or outcomes of the disease or surgery.

School-age children's understanding of things is likely to be incomplete. They use words correctly but fantasize to fill the gaps in their knowledge. School-age children have a basic understanding of body organs and functions but do not understand the terms used for them.[31] A nursing student reported:

> My patient, a 10-year-old hemophiliac, seemed to know everything about his disease. When I asked him what happened when he bled, he said, "Oh, well, there's a hemophiliac bug eating his way in and out of my blood vessels, and that's what makes me bleed." And when asked what caused his disease, he answered, "Well, it's 'cause I ate too much candy after my mom told me not to."

Carefully question children to reveal and clarify their fantasies. Guidelines for teaching the school-age child are given in Table 15-7.

Use a projective technique for older school-age children who are reluctant to discuss their fears. Encourage them to draw a picture of the hospital and describe it or to make up a story about a child in the hospital. Use one of the prepared and validated tests, such as The Hospital Picture Test (developed by Dr. Pauline Barton at the University of Florida).[32]

As children unconsciously project their feelings in pictures or stories, the nurse learns about their level of growth and development, their perceptions of the hospital, and their relationships with others.[33] In one study, children drew pictures of the hospital. After discussing the pictures with the nurse, they had a greater sense of confidence, a better focus on reality, and a decrease in fear of the unknown.[34]

Perception of illness as a punishment

Children have a very rigid, moralistic code of behavior. Because they are learning new roles, they scrutinize their own behavior and compare it with their parents' expectations. By acting "good" and following rules, they can win approval and increase their self-esteem. Since they associate pain and hospitalization with unpleasant, negative feelings, they assume that they are being punished for breaking a rule. Assess their beliefs about their illness, and reassure them about the cause of their condition and the motivations behind the therapy.

Fear of losing emotional control

All children want to be courageous and successfully cope with a frightening event; this bravery enhances their self-image. They mobilize their resources to control their emotions and want to receive praise for remaining in emotional control. Help them discuss their feelings and methods of handling emotions. Never demand total submission.[35] Plan play activities to allow expression of aggression (see Table 15-12). Encourage activities based on their individual interests and hobbies.

Immobilized children feel powerless and vulnerable. School-age children have endless energy to explore and gain information about their environment. Being able to move quickly is associated with being in control and with being able to express aggression and protect themselves. Immobilized children have fewer opportunities to express aggression and feel less able to protect themselves from intrusive procedures.

Separation anxiety

Younger school-age children may occasionally experience separation anxiety during traumatic procedures, but their reaction is shorter and less intense than that of preschoolers. Older children may miss their friends and activities more than they do their parents. They often have difficulty finding stimulating activities and become bored, frustrated, and lonely.

Table 15-12 Activities that Allow Teenagers to Express Aggression

1. Using boxing gloves or punching bags. (At one hospital the teenagers demolished one every 3 to 4 months!)
2. Writing on "graffiti boards." This encourages anonymous expression of feelings (both washable walls and large, wall-size sheets of paper work well).
3. Playing darts (with suction cups for safety).
4. Hammering and sawing.
5. Having pillow fights.

Note: Always establish safety limits and rules before beginning these games, like "No throwing above the head. If a pillow hits someone's head or an IV, the game is over."

Nursing management of the school-age child

Promoting self-esteem The security of school-age children is directly related to living in an organized, predictable, and scheduled world. Children who know the rules of expected behavior will know how to react and gain approval. Tell them what to expect and how to act. Promote self-esteem by affirming their success in coping with hospitalization.

Increase children's sense of power or control over their hospital environment by allowing them to make decisions about daily routines and giving them appropriate mobility (Fig. 15-12). School-age children can help make beds, straighten rooms, pass out food, answer lights,

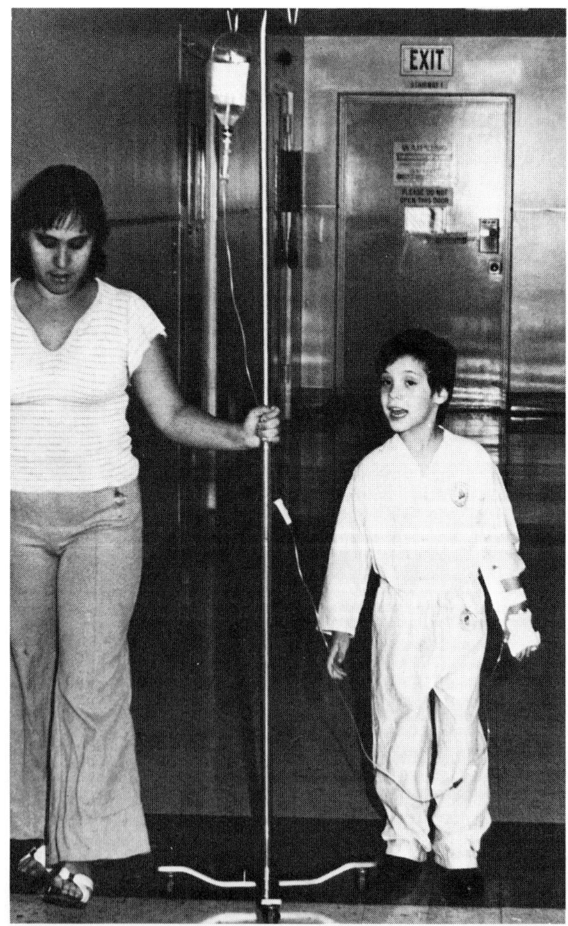

Figure 15-12 This school-age child's increased mobility enhances his feelings of self-control and power. (*Photo by Theresa Friedrich. Courtesy of LAC/USC Medical Center.*)

put charts together, and orient new children to the unit.

Dealing with rigid, moralistic behavior School-age children may have rigid, moralistic behavior because they are learning precisely how to act in a new role. They want to "play by the rules," and to them things are either right or wrong. They cannot yet think abstractly to learn the principle underlying social expectations. Therefore, they must still rely on actions, and if they gain approval from their parents or other authority figures, their self-confidence will be bolstered.

Compulsive, ritualistic behavior pervades all aspects of the lives of school-age children. They may increase their feelings of control over procedures by "ordering" nurses' actions in a certain way.

> Johnny, aged 10, was crying and extremely upset during his dressing change. He said, "I want Judy to do it! She changes my bandage different!" Later during the dressing change, Johnny whined, "You're doing it all wrong! Why don't you put on the tape this way? No! It's not put on that way! Your tape is too long!" The nurse recognized his distrust, slowed her pace, and explained her upcoming actions. She knew this was one of his only ways left of maintaining control; therefore, she didn't scold him or tell him to be quiet. Instead, she let him tell her exactly how he wanted it done and followed his directions. To promote trust, she also wrote down his directions on the Kardex. Because she knew he was interested in the reasons for her actions, she explained them to him. Johnny's behavior the next day was vastly different; he greeted her with a smile. She suggested he help, play nurse, and wear sterile gloves. He glowed with satisfaction and maintained sterile technique; during the procedure the nurse asked him questions to assess his views of the procedure.

Communicate acceptance of children's ritualistic behavior by discussing it in an honest, open manner. Explore the causes of their fear and discuss the "rules" of their behavior. Other team members can follow the same routine when it is reported verbally and recorded in the Kardex.

Preserving communication with school, friends, and home Since most of the school-age child's day is spent in school, it is logical for the hospital day to include educational activities. Observe the child's attitude toward homework, give help when needed, schedule time for homework, assess areas of difficulty, and communicate observations to the teacher. Before discharge, contact the school nurse, and plan for home teachers if they will be required.

Preserving communication with friends at home is difficult for school-age children. They are dependent on parents to form car pools and bring friends and siblings to the hospital. Call the school requesting the class to send letters. School-age children love to collect cards from their friends and tape them on the wall. Help children write letters or make tape recordings about hospital life to send to friends. List their favorite toys and games on the Kardex. The toys should allow children to complete a task successfully (e.g., crossword puzzles, erector sets, and embroidery sets), promote their motor coordination (e.g., Ping-Pong, jumping rope, and painting), and teach them to follow rules (e.g., card games and hide-and-seek).

Provide opportunities for school-age children to interact with members of the same sex. Place children together in rooms with others of the same age and sex. Encourage volunteers to form clubs built around crafts, interests, or activities. For chronically ill children, arrange visits from local celebrities, rock stars, puppet groups, dramatic groups, or zoo personnel.

THE ADOLESCENT'S REACTIONS TO HOSPITALIZATION

Adolescents who become hospitalized are concerned chiefly about (1) the loss of their independence and identity, (2) the possibility of changes in body image, (3) peer rejection, and (4) loss of emotional control.

Feelings of loss of independence and identity

Major threats to the hospitalized adolescent are loss of independence and identity. The enforced dependency caused by illness and hospitalization occurs just when the adolescent is trying to establish independence and identity at home. Illness may prevent the teenager from driving a car, from participating in peer group activities, or even from going to the bathroom alone. These feelings of powerlessness, or lack of control over the environment, cause anger, frustration, and withdrawal (Fig. 15-13).

Nursing management Plan nursing care *with* teenagers. Too often, decisions are made about treatments, medicines, and daily routines without asking the patient. Joint planning will increase feelings of power, independence, cooperativeness, and control: "Adolescents are . . . best equipped to know which actions will fit most comfortably into their own life-styles. They know their home routines and school days better than anyone else and they need to help determine what actions are reasonable and workable for them in their own lives and settings."[36]

Adolescents thrive on demonstrating feelings of responsibility and independence. Encourage them to take care of a younger child, answer lights, or take snack orders to maintain their recently established identity in the hospital. Allow them to order preferred foods (within dietary guidelines), order double portions, prepare food in a kitchen on the unit, wear their own clothes, and visit and eat in friends' rooms. Adolescents successfully orient new patients, help prepare each other for tests, and publish unit newsletters.

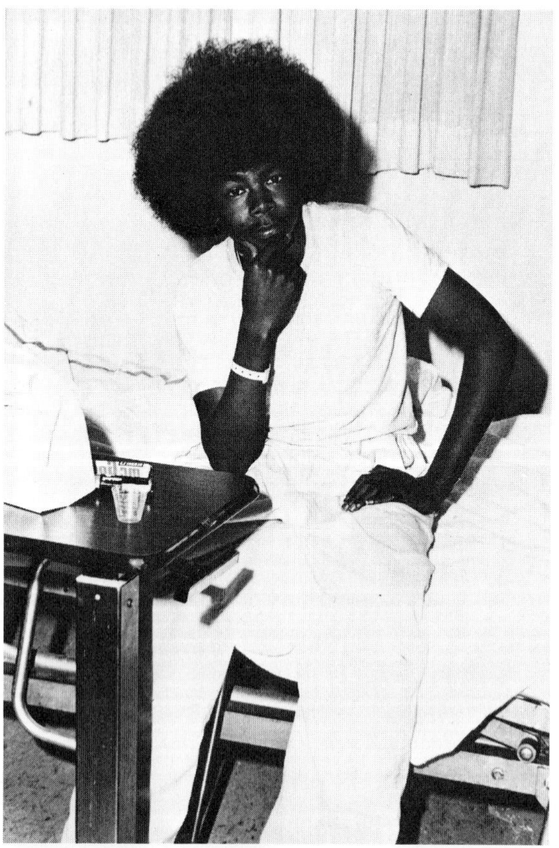

Figure 15-13 This teenager has lost his independence and identity and is bored. He stated, "There ain't no action here!" (*Photo by Theresa Friedrich. Courtesy of LAC/USC Medical Center.*)

Families and friends remain an important base in their security system. Visiting hours should be liberal, allowing parents, friends, and siblings to visit freely. Place adolescents in their own section or ward. Imagine an adolescent's chagrin and embarrassment at being assigned to a room with a baby!

Continuation of schoolwork in the hospital provides relief from boredom. Tutoring allows the adolescent to maintain academic progress on a par with that of peers. Obtain a school referral. Assess the teenager's motivation for doing homework, his or her favorite classes, and areas needing improvement. Communicating this information to the teacher will ensure an individually designed school program.

Discuss with the teacher the teenager's physical limitations, upcoming stresses, and their effect on the child's ability to learn. After eye surgery, for example, the adolescent may be able to tolerate only 1 h of studying at a time. The seriously ill child may not be able to manage the entire school program.

Fear of body-image changes

A second cause of the hospitalized teenager's anxiety is the fear of body-image changes (Fig. 15-14). This anxiety increases in direct proportion to the severity of the threat to the body image. Body image is defined as a changing or evolving mental picture of one's own body. Teenagers believe that their bodies are the main criterion by which others will accept or reject them. The normal adolescent experiences rapid physical growth and changes in body shape. When these normal changes are coupled with any threat to body image from surgery or illness, the adolescent's feelings of vulnerability increase. The threat of more body changes makes the adolescent feel more insecure, less in control, and incapable of succeeding.

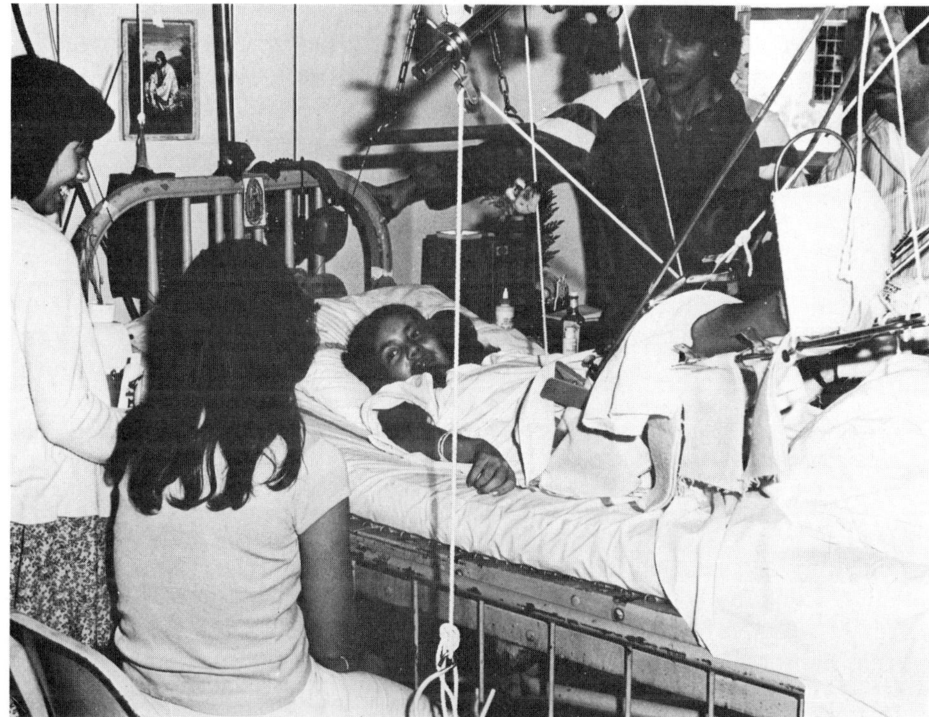

Figure 15-14 Teenagers fear body-image changes and rejection by peers. This girl is being visited by family and friends. (*Photo by Theresa Friedrich. Courtesy of LAC/USC Medical Center.*)

Nursing management For a teenager with a body-image change:

1. Assess the importance of the teenager's body image.
2. If surgery has been performed, assess the teenager's understanding of what went on during the operation.
3. Assure the teenager that his or her body has been "resewn" and is still intact.
4. Discuss and provide opportunities for the teenager to see the bodily changes, but do not force this.
5. Assess talents which can be used to compensate for lost body functions.
6. Help the teenager value his or her positive attributes.
7. Have another adolescent who has successfully adjusted after the same procedure or body alteration visit the teenager.

Help adolescents feel successful in using their bodies. This will promote a more positive self-image. Postsurgical adolescents can join a group meeting and discuss common adjustment problems, such as, "How do I go to a dance in a wheelchair?" "What can I wear around these body casts?" Group members are very tolerant about practicing social behavior on one another. One 14-year-old boy stated, "It's easier for me if I talk about what's happening to me, and it's better to talk to a group my own age—I feel less uncomfortable with teenagers than adults."[37]

Meetings of teenagers were begun at the University of Minnesota hospitals to encourage adolescents to share their feelings, to increase awareness of adolescent conflicts, to help them support one another during the stresses of hospitalization and the transition to home, and to convey the nurses' caring and concerned attitudes toward them. The teenagers who had become disfigured were able to be accepted within the group.[38] For meetings like these to succeed, a high level of commitment is necessary from the group leaders and nursing staff. Treatments and doctors' appointments must be scheduled around group meeting times.[39]

Provide privacy. Hospitalized teenagers' need for privacy is often overlooked. Body-image changes make them especially sensitive to being displayed in front of medical personnel or strangers. All shared information must be kept confidential. Members should have mutual respect and are free to leave the group at any time.[40]

Fear of rejection

Normal adolescents are acutely aware of their bodily defects. Physical perfection is idealized by our culture. Any physical imperfection may exclude them from the peer group. The peer group's acceptance of behavior is rigidly controlled, is centered on physical perfection, and changes very quickly. Adolescents' fear of peer rejection is, therefore, very real.

Nursing management During the hospitalization, assess teenagers' interactions with peers of both sexes. Do they initiate conversation (and with what sex), or do they withdraw? Do they enter other teenagers' rooms? What are the behavioral reactions and common interests of their chosen friends? How are they treated by their roommates? Are they acknowledged as worthwhile people, or are they ignored by other patients? Are they likely to go to the activity room? Certainly, young people who refuse to interact with other adolescents, who keep the curtains drawn and the door closed, and who stay alone need nursing interventions designed to increase social interaction. Encourage peer interaction through parties, games, visits from friends, and flexible visiting hours. If an adolescent is consistently withdrawn, arrange a team meeting with a mental health nurse to assess behavior and plan an appropriate, consistent 24-h plan of care.

Fear of losing emotional control

Teenagers are famous for rapid mood changes. They are also afraid of losing control of their emotions and may be reluctant to express their frustration, anger, and aggression. Teenagers may lose control or overextend themselves. Their emotions may be released in temper tantrums or crying. This leads to anxiety and fear. They then retreat to reassess their actions and plan more mature coping behavior. Their withdrawal and regression make them feel guilty, since teenagers are not supposed to act like babies.

Nursing management Accept teenagers' regressed, dependent behavior. When they experience approval, their self-esteem soars. Regression allows them to recharge their psychological energy and then forge on ahead, independently.

Refrain from immediately reacting to their outbursts. Wait a few moments, and their behavior will usually change to a more easily tolerated, more balanced, and more mature level.

Respect teenagers' need to be alone. Observe "Keep out" signs, and accept their behavior by saying, "You look really sad today," or "I will leave you alone. But call me if you need me. I will help you." Avoid saying, or implying, "Don't act like a baby!" Plan activities to encourage the expression of aggression (Table 15-12).

Success in communicating with teenagers depends on understanding their needs, growth, and development and on gaining genuine satisfaction from working with them. Help them to achieve self-esteem and to learn self-reliance. When the nurse shows flexibility, openness, acceptance, and tolerance, teenagers respond. Adolescents talk with a vengeance. As Eileen Tiedt has written:

> The nurse must consider it equally important to listen. As a listener she must allow the patient to tell about his plans, his successes, and failures. Those nurses who "cannot take the time," and those who have been "trained" to feel most useful when they're active, will find it hard to listen to them. The patient feels much more comfortable when a nurse is willing to sit and listen. And no other person is so insistent on attention as the adolescent. He is susceptible to the advances of anyone who shows genuine interest in him, but he is equally quick to reject anyone who tries to impose his will or ideas on him, whose interest is feigned, or who seems to have little regard for what the adolescent is, does, thinks, or says. The nurse, therefore, must pay as much attention to him as she does to his symptoms.[41]

REFERENCES

1. Azarnoff, Pat, "Preparing Well Children for Possible Hospitalization," *Pediatric Nursing* **11**(1):53–56 (January–February 1985).
2. Ibid.
3. Kunzman, Lucy, "Some Factors Influencing a Young Child's Mastery of Hospitalization." *Nursing Clinics of North America* **7**:13–26 (March 1972).

4. Birchfield, Marilyn E., "Nursing Care for Hospitalized Children Based on Different Stages of Illness." *American Journal of Maternal-Child Nursing* **6**(1):46–52 (January–February 1981).
5. Hunsberger, Mabel, et al., "A Review of Current Approaches Used to Help Children and Parents Cope with Health Care Procedures," *Maternal-Child Nursing Journal* **13**(3):145–164 (Fall 1984).
6. Hott, Jacqueline, "Play PRN in Pediatric Nursing," *Nursing Forum* **9**(3):288–309 (1970).
7. Betz, Cicely L., "After the Operation—Postprocedural Sessions to Allay Anxiety," *American Journal of Maternal-Child Nursing* **7**(4):260–263 (July–August 1982).
8. Axline, Virgina, *Play Therapy,* Random House, New York, 1947, p. 10.
9. Poster, Elizabeth, "Stress-Immunization: Techniques to Help the Child Cope with Hospitalization," *Maternal-Child Nursing Journal* **12**(2):119–134 (Summer 1983).
10. Hunsberger et al., op. cit., pp. 146–147.
11. Poster, op. cit., p. 129.
12. Ibid., p. 127.
13. Hunsberger et al., op. cit., p. 153.
14. Roy, Sister Mary Callista, "Role Cues and Mothers of Hospitalized Children," *Nursing Research* **16**:178–182 (Spring 1967).
15. Ibid.
16. Poster, op. cit., p. 128.
17. Merrow, Dorothy, and Betty S. Johnson, "Perceptions of the Mother's Role with Her Hospitalized Child," *Nursing Research* **17**(2):155–156 (March–April 1968).
18. Ryberg, J. W., and E. B. Merrifield, "A Questionnaire for Assessment of Parent's Needs in a Child Health Clinic," *Pediatric Nursing* **8**:318–319, 322 (1982).
19. Dorn, Lorah D., "Children's Concepts of Illness: Clinical Applications," *Pediatric Nursing* **10**(5):325–327 (September–October 1984).
20. Pidgeon, Virginia, "Children's Concepts of Illness: Implications for Health Teaching," *Maternal-Child Nursing Journal* **14**(2):23–31 (Spring 1985).
21. Lipsitt, L. P., "The Study of Sensory and Learning Processes of the Newborn," *Clinics in Perinatology* **4**:163–186 (March 1977).
22. Condon, W., and L. Sander, "Neonate Movement Is Synchronized with Adult Speech: Interactional Participation and Language Acquisition," *Science* **18**(1):99–101 (January 1974).
23. Kramer, L., and M. Pierpont, "Rocking Waterbeds and Auditory Stimuli to Enhance Growth of Preterm Infants," *Journal of Pediatrics* **88**(2):297–299 (February 1976).
24. Katz, V., "Auditory Stimulation and Developmental Behavior of Preterm Infants," *Nursing Research* **20**(3): 196–201 (May–June 1972).
25. Kagan, Jerome, "Personality Development," in Nathan Talbot, Jerome Kagan, and Leon Eisenberg (eds.), *Behavioral Science in Pediatric Medicine,* W. B. Saunders, Philadelphia, 1971, pp. 282–349.
26. Audette, Marjorie S., "The Significance of Regressive Behavior in the Hospitalized Child," *American Journal of Maternal-Child Nursing* **3**(2):44–48 (Spring 1974).
27. Ibid., p. 33.
28. Ibid., p. 34.
29. Wilkinson, Anne L., "Behavioral Disturbances Following Short-Term Hospitalization," *Issues in Comprehensive Pediatric Nursing* **3**:12–18 (July 1978).
30. Gellert, Elizabeth, "What Do I Have inside Me? How Children View Their Bodies," in *Psychological Aspects of Pediatric Care,* Grune & Stratton, New York, 1978, p. 22.
31. Denehy, Janice, "What Do School-Age Children Know about Their Bodies?" *Pediatric Nursing* **10**(4):290–292 (July–August 1984).
32. Barton, Pauline H., "The Relationship between Fantasy and Overt Stress Reactions of Children to Hospitalization," unpublished Ed.D. dissertation, University of Florida, Gainesville, 1964.
33. Allen, Jeanine M., "Influencing School-Age Children's Concepts of Hospitalization," *Pediatric Nursing* **4**(6): 26–28 (November–December 1978).
34. Gelhard, Helen L., "Drawing and Development," *Pediatric Nursing* **4**(6):23–25 (November–December 1978).
35. Lamb, Jacqueline M., and Denise R. Rodgers, "Assisting the Hostile Hospitalized Child," *American Journal of Maternal-Child Nursing* **8**(5):336–339 (September–October 1983).
36. Denyes, Mary Jean, and Anne Altschuler, "Illness: The Adolescent," in G. Scipien, M. U. Barnard, M. A. Chard, J. Howe, and P. J. Phillips (eds.), *Comprehensive Pediatric Nursing,* 2d ed., McGraw-Hill, New York, 1979, p. 478.
37. Altschuler, Anne, and Ann H. Seidl, "Teen Meetings: A Way to Help Adolescents Cope with Hospitalization," *American Journal of Maternal-Child Nursing* **2**(6): 348–353 (November–December 1977).
38. Ibid.
39. Ibid., p. 349.
40. Pazola, Kathryn J., and Ann K. Gerberg, "Teen Group: A Forum for the Hospitalized Adolescent," *American Journal of Maternal-Child Nursing* **10**(4):265–269 (July–August 1985).
41. Tiedt, Eileen, "The Adolescent in the Hospital: An Identity-Resolution Approach." *Nursing Forum* **1**(2):126–140 (1972).

16

Linda W. Olivet

Basic care of the hospitalized child

Upon completion of this chapter, the student will be able to:

1. Describe the role of the nurse in preparing and admitting a child and the child's family for hospitalization.
2. Describe nursing approaches to the common procedures to be performed during admission.
3. Explain how to use various restraints.
4. Describe feeding techniques and methods for motivating children to eat.
5. Compare dehydration and volume overload.
6. Describe the role of the nurse in starting and maintaining intravenous therapy in children.
7. Describe methods for administering and monitoring moist oxygen.
8. Demonstrate emergency procedures for choking and cardiopulmonary resuscitation in children.
9. Explain how to measure temperature, pulse rate, respiratory rate, and blood pressure in children.
10. Name potential problems and appropriate nursing intervention in the assessment of vital signs.
11. Describe hygiene for the hospitalized child.
12. List manifestations of pain in children.
13. Describe the nurse's role in the care of the child with fever, pain, and nausea and vomiting.
14. Determine the dosage for a common pediatric drug using body surface area (BSA).
15. Describe approaches to administering oral medications to children.
16. Compare the various sites for intramuscular injection in children.
17. List safety measures to be taken when administering any medications to children.
18. Discuss the role of the nurse in dismissal planning for the hospitalized child.

In recent years the number of children being hospitalized has decreased. This is due partially to improved health education and outpatient services and to an emphasis on cost-effectiveness. Nevertheless, there are some occasions when a child must enter a hospital for health care.

When a child becomes a hospital patient, whatever the medical diagnosis, there are many areas of need that make the nursing care special. The fact that a hospitalized child is usually accompanied by a parent or concerned loved one makes pediatric nursing family-centered as well as patient-centered. Hospitalization has the potential for being an enriching experience for the family and the child; it can also be difficult, emotionally draining, and even devastating. Appropriate intervention by caring, knowledgeable nurses can make the difference.

ADMISSION TO THE HOSPITAL

Preparation for admission

A child must be prepared in advance for hospitalization whenever possible. Preparation lessens anxiety and fear because the "unknown" becomes somewhat familiar. The child may work through uncomfortable feelings and determine some methods of coping with the anticipated experience. Even if a child has multiple hospitalizations, adequate preparation is essential to identify misconceptions and fears. Preparation also helps parents examine their own fears, expectations, and feelings and prepares them to cope in the hospital setting (see Chap. 15).

Role of the hospital Over the years, hospital personnel have identified specific activities that prepare children for hospitalization. Some programs are offered in cooperation with the local schools. Children learn about hospital activities and the roles of health professionals. This approach increases their awareness of certain "helpers" in the community and may decrease their fears of hospitals.

Another type of program is set up specifically for children who are soon to be admitted. A puppet show, preadmission party, tour, or similar activity is held at the hospital. Children can see the hospital setting, meet other children who may be with them as patients in the hospital, and prepare for a specific experience. These sessions may include time for the children to handle equipment and play "doctor" or "nurse" with dolls. They may also try on masks, gowns, and gloves like those worn by hospital personnel in surgery (Fig. 16-1). Some programs include films or slides that show many aspects of hospital life.

In addition to specific admission orientation programs, the hospital provides the environment that affects the child as a patient. An awareness of the needs of children and parents and a desire to provide for them is reflected in the facilities available. Brightly colored walls and curtains, playrooms and toys, sleeping provisions for parents, age-appropriate furniture, child-proof nurses' stations, and personnel wearing colorful uniforms—these are a few of the ways a hospital says, "We want to make your time as a patient in our institution as easy and pleasant as possible."

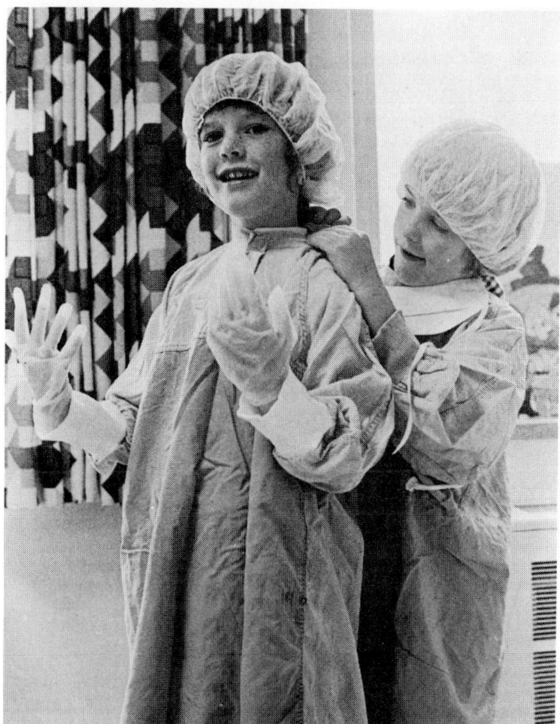

Figure 16-1 Children dressing up in masks and gowns during a "come-and-see" hospital orientation program. (*Photo by Beverly K. Bisek.*)

Role of the parents

Children reflect the attitudes of parents. If parents are anxious and worried, the child will react in a similar manner. A calm, informed parent encourages the child's confidence and trust in the caregivers.

Parents need to be encouraged to ask questions and express concerns to the doctor and nurse in the outpatient setting. This increases their understanding and allows them to be more effective as a resource and support to their child. Because each person faces a new experience in light of the past, an assessment of the parents' previous hospital experiences and present concerns provides the nurse with vital information in preparing both the parents and the child.

Specific preparation should begin a few days prior to admission. There are many ways in which parents can prepare the child at home. Reading appropriate books can answer many questions (see Table 16-1).

Children may also act out being in a hospital by role-playing various procedures. Informal discussions among the family members and simu-

Table 16-1 Books about Hospitalization

1. Bettina Clark and Lester Coleman, *Pop-Up Book: Going to the Hospital,* Random House, New York, 1971.
2. F. H. Erickson, *Play Interviews for Four-Year-Old Hospitalized Children,* Kraus Reprint, Millwood, N.Y. 1958.
3. Harold Geist, Manson Geist, and P. Morse, *Children Going to the Hospital,* Manson Western Corporation, Los Angeles, 1965.
4. Harold D. Love et al., *Your Child Goes to the Hospital: A Book for Parents,* Charles C Thomas, Springfield, Ill., 1972.
5. H. A. Rey, *Curious George Goes to the Hospital,* Houghton Mifflin, Boston, 1966.
6. Florence Whitman Rowland, *Let's Go to the Hospital,* Putnam, New York, 1968.
7. Arthur Shay, *What Happens when You Go to the Hospital,* Contemporary Books, Chicago, 1969.
8. Sara Bonnet Stein, *A Hospital Story,* Walker, New York, 1974.

lated situation storytelling ("If this happened, what would you do?") are also helpful. Siblings should be included in the preparatory activities to decrease their unspoken fears.

Some children enjoy making scrapbooks about hospitals. This kind of activity increases their involvement in preparation. The child may select toys, pajamas, and a "security blanket" and can help with the packing. Special "homecoming" activities to be enjoyed when hospitalization ends may also be planned with the child.

Throughout this preparatory period, parents should be encouraged to answer the child's questions simply, directly, and honestly. If questions arise that they cannot answer, they may call the hospital for clarification.

Role of the outpatient clinic nurse

Many of the ideas mentioned in the section "Role of the Parents" are alternatives that the outpatient or clinic nurse may suggest to the parents. The parents will determine the methods that seem most appropriate for their circumstances, but the outpatient nurse has the responsibility for encouraging them to prepare the child.

The outpatient nurse also acts as a resource person and may be asked questions about hospitalization by both the child and the child's family. By visiting the hospital periodically, the nurse can become familiar with hospital staff routines. If the child or the family has special needs, the nurse should call before admission and share these with the hospital staff. Ideally, a written nursing care plan should be forwarded for the hospital nurse to use as a resource.

Teaching, explaining, and preparing—all are functions of the outpatient nurse. An accurate assessment of the child's and the family's present knowledge can make the approaching hospitalization much easier for them.

The admission process

During admission to the hospital the child and the parents develop their first impressions. It is very important that they be greeted warmly and welcomed to the nursing unit as guests. Hospitality can be expressed in any hospital setting if the nursing staff values such an approach. Being welcomed, called by name, and accompanied to the appropriate room can help the child and the family feel important and reassured.

Orientation to the environment Upon arriving in the room, the child and the family should receive an orientation to the surroundings. The extent of the orientation may vary depending on the time available to the nurse at that moment and whether the child has been hospitalized there previously. Explain where the bathroom is and how to call the nurse, turn on the TV, and operate the buttons or cranks on the bed. Make the child and the parents as comfortable as possible, and tell them when the admission procedures will begin and what they can do in the meantime. Explain about visiting hours and facilities that are available for parents—cafeteria, sleeping facilities, and so forth.

As soon as possible, preferably before any procedures are done, take the child and the family on a brief tour of the nursing unit. This allows time for the child to see the surroundings and for the nurse to begin an informal assessment. Introductions of the child to the staff convey that the unit is friendly, pleasant, and nonthreatening. During the tour the child may walk or be carried in the parent's arms. Give the child a chance to see the playroom or, if no playroom is available, a chance to observe other pleasant activities which are provided for young patients. Wait until later in the admission to undress the child or begin procedures.

A tour is not meant to mislead a child into thinking that all is "fun and games," but it is one way to develop rapport. Children will respond in a variety of ways according to their level of growth and development, their previous experiences with hospitalization, and their illness.

If a child is acutely ill or is anticipating major surgery, decide whether a tour is appropriate. The anxiety level of the child, the parents, or both may be so great that the admission procedure must begin another way. Sit down and talk with them to plan the admission together. Establish a climate of reassurance and understanding.

Whatever the initial activity, the nurse begins assessment of the child's and the family's needs at the time of the first encounter. The nurse may then determine well-chosen interventions on the basis of that assessment.

In the immediate environment, items and equipment that are routine and normal to the nurse may be very strange and frightening to the child. Determine the unspoken concerns through attention to nonverbal cues. Brief, honest explanations of equipment or of what another nurse is doing can alleviate fears.

Admission procedures Many hospitals provide admission packets containing helpful information about services available, routines, visiting hours, facilities for families, patients' rights and responsibilities, and similar items. Encourage use of the material by mentioning it in conversation and using it when questions arise.

During initial conversations the child and the family may comprehend only part of the information. Give general information at first; prior to each activity give a more detailed explanation.

Table 16-2 provides an outline of admission activities and information to be given.

The admission history The Kardex nursing history card (Fig. 16-2) contains items of information that should be obtained during the admission interview. If a child is to be in the hospital for a very brief stay, the Kardex history may be adequate. It is the most practical approach if a child is admitted and then whisked off for surgery or diagnostic tests.

The American Academy of Pediatrics has developed information guidelines for use with children in various age groups (see Appendix D). These are useful for obtaining more detailed information about the child and are essential for longer stays.

It is important that parents be available for the admission interviews by the nurse and the physician. Advise them to remain until these are completed. Direct appropriate questions to the child so that he or she will feel included. If the parent or the child is exhausted, delay a long interview.

The Kardex and American Academy of Pediatrics forms can be used as a guide for setting up personal information forms for pediatric patients of various ages and can be adjusted to fit the needs of particular hospital units.

Table 16-2 Admission Activities

1. Tour of the unit
2. Orientation to the room and equipment
3. Identification
4. Admission history
5. Vital signs
6. Height and weight
7. Give information about:
   a. Clothing in the hospital
   b. Mealtimes and snack times
   c. Rules about bringing food from home
   d. Daily activities—bath, naptime, and bedtime
   e. Visiting hours
   f. Facilities for parents
   g. Physician's examination and visits
   h. Laboratory tests

Identification and checking vital signs Identification (ID) of the child during admission and throughout the hospital stay is a necessary safety precaution. The ID band contains information such as the child's name, hospital number, room number, age, address, and date of admission. It is attached to the wrist with approximately the space of a finger between the band and the arm to prevent constriction.[1] A preschooler or early school-age child will not usually object to the band if told that it is a bracelet that tells who he or she is. An infant or toddler may need to have the ID band placed on an ankle rather than a wrist if it is irritating or slips off easily. If the child's skin is sensitive to the plastic or tape, the band can be pinned to the child's clothing. The child should wear an ID band at all times throughout the hospital stay.

Vital signs include temperature, pulse rate, respiratory rate, and blood pressure. Procedures for checking vital signs are described later in this chapter. Taking a rectal temperature is an intrusive procedure for a young child and may cause crying. Perform this toward the end of the physical assessment. The assistance of parents in holding the thermometer in place or in remaining beside the child may help alleviate fears. Use dolls or puppets, if appropriate, to show how procedures are to be done.

Determining height and weight Height and weight determinations are very important and must be obtained soon after admission. The phy-

Name .... Date .... By ....

Nickname .... Age .... Religion ....

DIET: Food Allergies .... NURSING Food Dislikes ....

Formula, Kind .... HISTORY Amount ....

Bottle .... Breast .... Cup .... Warm .... Cold ....

Types of foods: Strained .... Junior .... Regular ....

SLEEPING: Usual Bedtime .... Does he climb out of crib ....

What, if anything, does he take to bed with him ....

Any problem with sleeping .... If so, what helps ....

ELIMINATION: Any problems bowel .... Urine .... If so, what helps ....

Toilet trained .... Taken to B.R. at regular times .... at noc ....

Term used bowel movement .... Urination ....

PLAYING: Favorite toy with him ....

Hospitalized before .... Why .... Unpleasant experiences ....

Exposed to any communicable diseases within the past 2 weeks ....

Has he been on any drugs at home ....

What is your understanding of your hospitalization ....

FAMILY - INTERESTS - HOBBIES ....

ORIENTATION	Pt. Unit	Telemike	Visiting Hrs.	Pamphlet to Parents	Pre-Op Teaching Post-Op Teaching	Chaplain

Figure 16-2 An example of Kardex information to be obtained during admission of a young child to the hospital. (*Courtesy of Rochester Methodist Hospital, Rochester, Minn.*)

sician calculates fluid and drug amounts using these data. Upright scales for weight may be used by any child who can stand alone. Young children may be frightened of the scales and refuse to cooperate. Stand on the scale first or ask a parent to do so, demonstrating that being weighed is painless. If this is ineffective, a parent can hold the child and both can be weighed. The parent is then weighed alone, and the weight is subtracted from the total. Ideally, weighing should be done when the child is wearing only underwear. It may be done in the room while the child is changing from street clothes to pajamas in order to avoid embarrassment.

Since weight is one of the critical indicators of fluid balance in children, weight measurements must be correct. Many hospitals number the scales on which children are weighed, and a child is weighed on the same scale each time. The scale number is recorded next to the weight. Any discrepancy from one weighing to the next indicates the need to recheck the weight and report the difference to the physician if appropriate. Ideally, the child should wear the same clothes every time he or she is weighed.

Height determinations are made pleasant through the use of decorative tape measures on the wall. A demonstration by the nurse or parent of how to stand against the wall may be adequate preparation for the child. Comments about how tall the child is can reward the child for cooperative behavior.

Infants' height and weight must be determined in a different manner. Infant scales allow the child to be weighed lying down or sitting. Weigh when the infant is wearing as little clothing as possible—preferably none. The younger the child, the more significant a few ounces will be in weight determination. The child's length can be determined by placing him or her on a measuring board (Fig. 16-3). Measure from the crown of the head to the stretched-out heel. Recording height and weight on a growth chart is a good method of determining general health status (see Appendix B).

The use of a bed scale may be necessary when weighing an acutely ill child. More than one person will be required to gently move the child from the bed to the scale and back again. A metal tape measure which remains straight will give a rough estimate of height, or the parents or the child may know the child's height.

Personal belongings The child may bring various personal belongings to the hospital. Store them in the area provided in the room. Write the child's name and room number on toys, stuffed animals, security blankets, and other personal equipment which might be confused with hospital items or other children's toys.

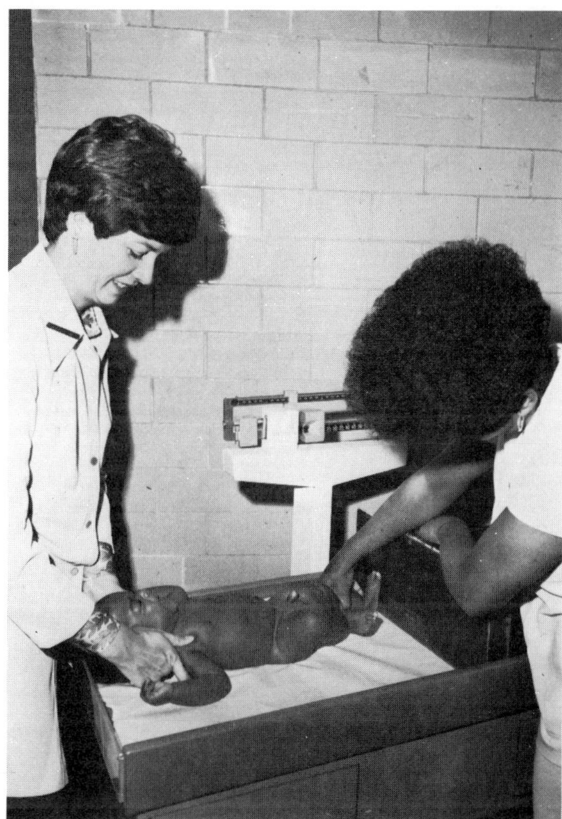

Figure 16-3 Using a measuring board to determine the length of an infant. (*From G. Scipien, M. U. Barnard, M. A. Chard, J. Howe, and P. J. Phillips* [eds.], *Comprehensive Pediatric Nursing, 3d ed., McGraw-Hill, New York, 1986, p. 367. Used with permission.*)

Clothing The child may wear his or her own clothes and pajamas or hospital clothing. Some children need and want the security of their own clothes. Honoring this desire as much as possible is another way to make hospitalization easier. A surgical patient must wear a hospital gown to the operating room. Gowns are easier than pajamas to change when intravenous lines and other equipment are in use, but the emotional needs of the child should have priority in influencing what will be worn upon return to the hospital room.

Obtaining specimens Routine laboratory tests during admission include blood work and a urinalysis. A stool specimen, an x-ray, and various cultures may also be necessary. Each of these tests is brief, and explanations are most effective and least frightening if given just prior to the test.

Blood work A heel stick in an infant or a finger stick in an older child or adolescent is used to obtain capillary blood. Certain tests require venipuncture with a needle and syringe.

Blood work can be painful, and the child may need restraining in order to lie still. Give a brief explanation just as the procedure begins, describing how it will feel.[2] Have the child squeeze your hand, count to 10, or hold the siderail of the bed when it hurts. Tell the child that you will help him or her hold still during the procedure so that it will be over faster.

The nurse can be a patient-advocate in this situation by suggesting appropriate sites for venipuncture. If the child is right-handed, suggest that the left arm be used. Though the laboratory technician may not find adequate veins at the suggested site, such an effort reassures the child. When blood is drawn from the antecubital fossa, restrain the arm at the joints above and below the elbow—the shoulder and wrist. Placing your hand under the child's elbow also helps facilitate the procedure.

Urine specimens Routine urinalysis is done on admission to identify the presence of infection in the urinary tract or changes in the end products of metabolism. It is nonintrusive and less threatening than some tests. When obtaining a urine specimen, do not try to encourage voiding by forcing the child to drink fluids. This dilutes the urine and may produce false results.[3]

Urinalysis is done on a clean specimen of urine. Assist the child to clean gently around the meatus with a warm, moist cloth, or use betadine and rinse with sterile water. Explain how to hold the container without touching the inside. A child of either sex can obtain the urine by voiding directly into the container. If this is difficult for a girl, place a clean bedpan or collecting pan in the toilet, replace the seat, and have her void normally. Transfer the urine from the pan to the specimen bottle.

Although obtaining a urine specimen is one of the simpler diagnostic procedures, it can be embarrassing to children. The school-age child wants privacy and can usually collect the specimen alone. Preschoolers and toddlers will need adult assistance, preferably from a parent.

Obtaining specimens from infants and toddlers in diapers requires the use of plastic urine bags—unless one happens to catch a specimen during a diaper change (keep the specimen bottle nearby at this time). Figure 16-4 illustrates the use of the U-bag pediatric urine collector for boys and girls. The procedure requires three steps: (1) cleaning, (2) applying the collector, and (3) removing and folding the bag.

1. The child is placed on his or her back on a clean towel folded in quarters. The entire area between the legs is washed with a soapy washcloth and rinsed.
   a. With a boy, first the testicles and then the penis are washed. The rectal area is washed last with a different corner of the washcloth. A cup of lukewarm water is used to rinse the area. The area is gently dried with a towel or dry washcloth.
   b. With a girl, each skinfold is washed with a different corner of the soapy washcloth. A top-to-bottom motion is used, and care is taken not to touch the rectum. The rectum is cleaned with a fourth corner of the washcloth. The area is rinsed with a cup of lukewarm water. Next, with the left thumb and index finger, the nurse separates the skinfolds and repeats the entire cleaning procedure with a second soapy washcloth. After another rinse, the area is dried gently and thoroughly with a towel or dry washcloth.
2. The protective paper is removed from the bottom of the collector bag. The bag is fitted over the boy's penis and testicles; a girl's skinfolds are separated to expose the urethra, and the bag is placed over it. Be sure that the bag

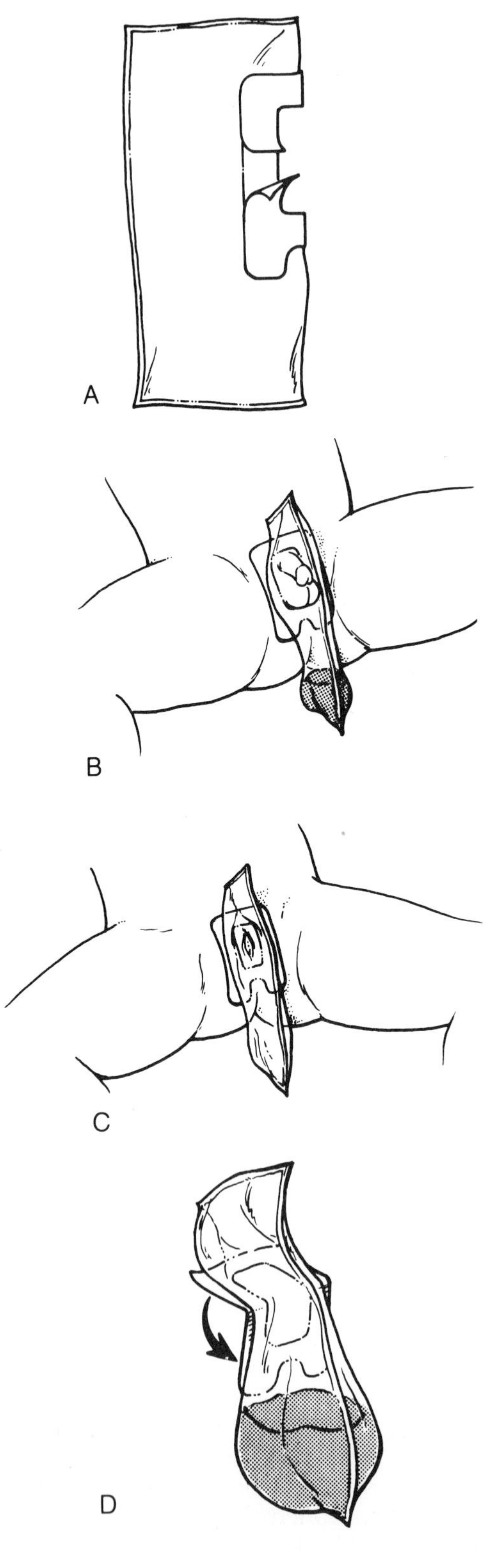

Figure 16-4 Collection of a urine specimen by means of a U-bag. (*Courtesy of Hollister, Inc.*) The perineum is first carefully washed and dried. (*A*) The collector is opened by removing the protective paper from the bottom section first. (*B*) The bag is placed over the penis and testicles, flaps pressed firmly to the area between the anus and testicles. The remaining protective paper is removed, and adhesive is pressed to the skin. (*C*) After the skinfolds are separated, the bag is placed over the vagina. Adhesive is pressed firmly against the bridge of skin separating the rectum from the vagina. The remaining protective paper is removed, and the adhesive surface is pressed against the skin. (*D*) When the specimen is obtained, the bag is removed and closed by folding the sticky, adhesive sides together. It may be placed into a cup for transportation.

adheres securely, especially to the perineum (most leaks occur there). A diaper may be reapplied to help secure the bag in place.
3. When the specimen is obtained, the bag is removed and closed by folding the sticky, adhesive sides together.

Stool specimens With infants and toddlers the stool specimen may be obtained from the diaper. It should be a fresh specimen and uncontaminated by urine. Older children may use a clean bedpan or potty-chair. Explain to the child that the stool specimen must be obtained before he or she voids into it. The stool is transferred to a cardboard container with a tight-fitting lid and is sent to the laboratory immediately.

This can be an embarrassing procedure and is best handled matter-of-factly. Terminology used for explanations should include words for bodily functions which the child understands.

School-age children and adolescents may not have a daily bowel movement. A child who has been told that a stool specimen is needed may, out of embarrassment or lack of understanding, try to avoid having a stool or may go to the bathroom without telling the nurse. Use tact and good observation to intervene appropriately.

Other procedures Common procedures with which the nurse assists are x-rays, enemas, and throat and nasopharyngeal cultures.

X-rays If a child needs a chest film on admission, explain that it is like having a picture made of the inside of the body and that it is important to hold still "just like when Mommy or Daddy takes your picture at home." Practice taking a deep breath with the child. Encourage the parent to accompany the child to the x-ray department, but explain that the parent will remain in the waiting area during the procedure.

Enemas Discuss with the physician the purpose and type of solution to be used before proceeding with an enema. Pediatric disposable enemas are available and easy to use. Normal saline is also a safe solution for a cleansing enema. Do not use tap water on a child suspected of having megacolon.[4] Some of the enema solution might be retained, and if tap water is absorbed in large quantities, the child might suffer water intoxication. Only isotonic solutions should be used with these children.[5]

Table 16-3 describes the steps in giving an enema to a child and the amounts of solution used for children in different age groups.

Table 16-3 Enema Procedure for Children

Recommended Amounts of Solution
Infant: 150 to 250 ml
18 months to 10 years: 250 to 500 ml
10 to 14 years: 250 to 750 ml

Position for infant or toddler
1. Place pillow under head and back.
2. Pad infant bedpan and place under buttocks.

Position for older child
1. Turn to left side.
2. Pad bed well with towel and/or bath blanket.
3. Instruct the child to hold enema solution after instillation. Use the bedpan or assist the child to the bathroom for expulsion.

Procedure
1. Use a no. 10 or 12 French catheter inserted 2 to 4 in into the rectum. Lubricate tip with a small amount of water-soluble lubricant. (Commercially prepared enemas are prelubricated and may be inserted without additional lubrication.)
2. Use an enema can or a 50-ml syringe barrel for solution. Warm to no greater than 40.6°C (105°F).
3. Instill by gravity with solution no higher than 18 in above the level of the hips.
4. For the infant or toddler, the solution and the stool will be expelled simultaneously during the procedure. If a retention enema is necessary, hold the buttocks together for a short time.†
5. Be gentle and do not exhaust the child. If results are inadequate, allow a rest time and repeat the procedure.
6. Clean the buttocks, bed, and equipment after the procedure.
7. Chart the amount and type of solution, the results of the enema, and the condition of the child after the procedure.

Source: *Leifer [6], †Whaley and Wong [7].

Throat cultures When a throat culture is ordered, the nurse is usually responsible for obtaining it. Throat Culturettes are self-contained (Fig. 16-5), and the only additional equipment needed is a tongue blade. (It may be necessary to have an assistant help complete the procedure.) Ask the child to open his or her mouth; an infant needs help in opening the mouth. Stabilize the tongue with the tongue blade. Use the swab from the Culturette to sweep down the right tonsil; cross the posterior pharyngeal wall, touching the tissue with the swab; and then sweep up the left tonsil.[8] Avoid touching the uvula. Going down, across, and up facilitates getting a sufficient specimen. Return the swab to the Culturette without contaminating it, crush the culture medium in the lower portion of the tube to saturate the swab, and send the specimen to the laboratory immediately.

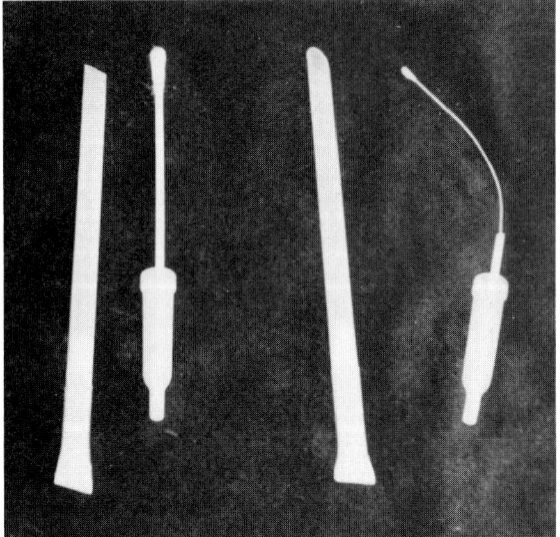

Figure 16-5 Equipment for obtaining throat and nasopharyngeal cultures. The throat Culturette is made of stiff material; the nasopharyngeal culture swab is made of wire and is very flexible, allowing for easy insertion through the nasal passage.

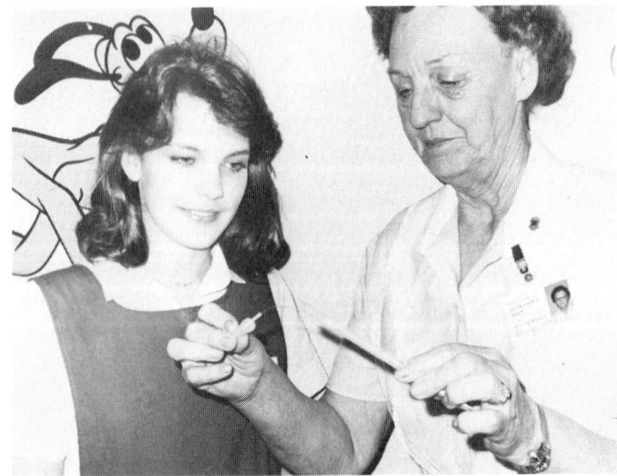

Figure 16-6 This staff nurse is showing a student how to bend the nasopharyngeal culture swab when removing it from the tube, while maintaining sterile technique.

Nasopharyngeal cultures The nasopharyngeal culture is obtained by inserting a sterile swab (Fig. 16-5) through the child's nostril into the nasopharynx. The swab is made of wire and curves gently as it is removed from the culture tube (Fig. 16-6). Touch only the handle when removing the swab from the tube. When the culture is obtained, the swab is returned to the tube and is handled like a throat culture.

Preoperative preparation When a child is admitted for a surgical procedure, preoperative preparation is a vital part of the admission routines. Good preoperative teaching lessens anxiety, postoperative pain, and other complications.

The admission assessment allows the nurse to determine what the child and parents already know. The nurse must also determine the child's level of development and select approaches that are most effective for the age of the child.

Children under 3 years of age have difficulty conceptualizing and have no awareness of time. Pictures and explanations may be of no value to them but can be helpful to their parents. Using equipment and dolls to show what will happen may be of some help to young children. Preoperative preparation is further discussed in Chap. 15.

The presence of parents is most important to children in the hospital. Throughout the preparation, references to where the parents will be during surgery can provide continuing reassurance.

The following are content areas to be covered in preparing the child for surgery:

1. Nothing by mouth (NPO)—"So that your tummy will be empty and you won't throw up during your operation."
2. Surgical cart—"A bed on wheels to carry you to the operating room."
3. Preoperative medications—Explain to the child receiving medicine that it will make him or her sleepy before leaving the room to go to surgery. If an injection is to be used, explain it just prior to administration rather than the evening before. Nevertheless, if the child asks, "Will I have a shot?" be honest but brief in discussing it. Say that it will "pinch" or "sting" but will be over very quickly.[9] Describe things to do to make it easier—count to 10 or squeeze the bedrail or the nurse's hand. (See the section "Intramuscular Medication" later in this chapter.)
4. Anesthesia—"A special sleep so that you won't feel the operation." Children may be very fearful of mask anesthesia. In order to decrease anxiety, some institutions allow a parent to hold the young child during induction by mask anesthesia. Intravenous medications are an alternative for older children. Com-

municate with the anesthesiologist preoperatively if the child is extremely anxious.

5. Descriptions of, visits to, and pictures of various areas of the hospital, the preoperative area, the surgical suite, and the recovery room are helpful to the child and the parents.
6. How the child may feel—"You may be dizzy and sleepy when you wake up. A nurse will be with you until you are brought back to your room with your parents." It is most helpful to the child to describe the sensations he or she will feel.
7. Location of parents during the procedure.
8. Postoperative nursing care—Vital signs will be checked frequently. Describe intravenous fluid, O_2 therapy, emesis basin, coughing and deep breathing, and other routines and equipment. Allow the child to see and touch equipment. Use terms that are appropriate for his or her level of understanding, and describe activities according to how the child will feel.

SUPPORT OF THE FAMILY

A great deal of emphasis is being placed on family-centered nursing care. *Family-centered* means that there is an awareness that the family is important, has the right to be involved in what happens to the child, and can be therapeutic in the child's recovery from illness. Giving the family support and encouragement may assist the child as much as, or more than, working directly with the child! When the family members have their emotional needs met, they are much more able to support the child.

Parental anxiety

It is very important to identify the causes of parents' anxiety in order to effectively intervene. Table 16-4 lists some possible causes of parental anxiety.

Anxiety is manifested in various behaviors. For instance, a mother who is afraid may avoid touching her child or helping with care. She may be fearful of doing the wrong thing and causing harm to her child. If the nurse takes time to determine the reasons for her lack of involvement in care, teaching can be done to decrease the mother's insecurity. The nurse is a helper, not a substitute parent. The nurse's role is to help parents meet their child's needs, since they are the most significant people to the child. (See Chap. 15 for a further discussion of parents of the hospitalized child.)[10]

Table 16-4 Causes of Parents' Anxiety During a Child's Hospitalization

1. Concern for the child's recovery
2. The hospital environment—strange, frightening equipment with which they are unfamiliar
3. Feelings of loss of control
4. Feelings of being subordinate to the nurse
5. Sense of guilt or self-condemnation because of the child's illness
6. Concern about other family members at home
7. Financial concerns

Source: Compiled from G. Scipien, M. V. Barnard, M. A. Chard, J. Howe, and P. J. Phillips (eds.). *Comprehensive Pediatric Nursing,* 2d ed., McGraw-Hill, New York, 1979, pp. 417–418.

Rooming-in

Some hospitals provide facilities for sleeping, personal hygiene, and cooking so that a parent may remain with a child overnight (see Chap. 15).

When rooming-in is possible, one parent may tend to remain at the hospital constantly. This can be very tiring and can decrease that parent's effectiveness as a support person. It also divides the family and deprives those at home of parental attention. Encourage a system of taking turns so that some other familiar person is with the child at times. Show interest in what is happening at home: "How are your other children being cared for while Billy is in the hospital?" Arrange for the parent to take breaks and leave the room. Assure the parent that it is all right to leave. Arrange for open visiting hours for siblings to encourage family solidarity and increase the family's understanding of what is happening in the hospital.

Parents' rights

In order to decrease the parents' anxiety and increase effective support for the child, the nurse must be aware of parents' rights. Following are the parents' rights identified by Hilt[11] and the nursing approaches designed to ensure them:

1. Right to be with their child
   Nursing approaches
   a. Provide rooming-in facilities.
   b. Encourage their involvement in care.
   c. Talk with them while giving care.

2. Right to understand the diagnosis and treatment

   Nursing approaches
   a. Accompany the physician on rounds.
   b. Spend time with the parents after rounds to clarify what they have been told.
   c. Explain each treatment and medication before administration.
   d. Use pamphlets and books to increase their understanding.
3. Right to question anything they do not understand or feel may be detrimental to their child

   Nursing approaches
   a. Listen carefully to the parents' concerns.
   b. Encourage questions by maintaining an open attitude.
   c. Intervene with the physician or other health team members and explain the parents' concerns.
4. Right to participate in decisions on their child's behalf

   Nursing approaches
   a. Confer with the parents about all planned activities. Keep their phone number handy, and call them if they are away when a new treatment is to begin.
   b. Include them in setting goals for the child.
   c. Ask their opinion about what is best for their child.

Cultural differences

The nurse should identify and record specific cultural needs and determine nursing interventions at admission. The child's and the parents' anxiety can be greatly decreased when cultural needs are recognized.

For example, an Orthodox Jewish boy was admitted to a pediatric unit for 2 weeks of treatment for a skin problem. The admitting nurse learned that he always wore a skullcap, said prayers twice a day for 30 min, and needed kosher food to meet religious requirements. This information was recorded on the Kardex. His treatment schedule was arranged so that he could have his prayer times undisturbed. A sign was placed on his door to prevent interruptions. The nurse discussed the schedule with the physician so that rounds could be planned accordingly. The nurse also conferred immediately with the dietitian so that the boy's first meal in the hospital met the requirements. This took extra time during admission but made the hospital experience very positive for the child.

Language differences may indicate the need for an interpreter. Use word charts showing common hospital terms in the child's language and the corresponding English word. Learn to pronounce the words in the foreign language. Use pictures to communicate with the child who cannot read. Label toys and equipment with the appropriate word in the child's language.

Identify ethnic food preferences, and obtain the preferred foods through the kitchen if possible. Allow parents to bring food from home to ensure adequate nutrition.

According to Farris, culturally different people generally intend to retain their respective identities. "Becoming aware of cultural differences and similarities is the first priority in becoming an effective health care provider."[12] The nurse's role is to be sensitive to the differences, understand reticence in accepting new and strange ideas, and move slowly and patiently if changes are necessary for improved health.[13]

BEHAVIOR AND DISCIPLINE

Discipline can be considered guiding behavior. In the past it was equated with punishment. As efforts have been made to encourage effective parenting, the concept of discipline has been broadened to include a more positive approach.

Care of pediatric patients involves their activities both as individuals and in groups. Many pediatric units have written guidelines for children's activities. These should be explained to the child and the parents during admission. Most children will follow the rules if they understand them. Use a kind but firm approach when setting limits.

Rewards

Rewards may be used as positive reinforcements of acceptable behavior. School-age children respond favorably to "star charts" or schedules. Star charts can include any activities the child resists that are a necessary part of nursing care. The child receives a star upon successful completion of an activity.

Schedules provide time limits for unpleasant activities and encourage doing homework, resting, and playing during the day. The child will respond to the schedule more cooperatively if he or she helps develop it. The schedule can be combined with a star chart and posted near the child's bed so that it can easily be seen (Fig. 16-7).

It may seem unrealistic to encourage the busy nurse to use these methods. They can, however, significantly increase children's cooperation, decrease inappropriate behavior, and ultimately save time.

Television

When children are hospitalized, they can easily spend many hours watching television. In a study by McCain and Bies, it was reported that hospitalized children watched an average of $8\frac{1}{2}$ h of television a day. Television viewing was most likely to occur when there were no planned activities on the hospital unit.[14]

Ill children are more vulnerable to fears of separation, mutilation, and death—frequent themes of TV programs. These fears may be increased by long hours of watching TV. Small children vent feelings and fears through creative play. TV viewing does not encourage this kind of expression. In addition, parents and visitors may become absorbed in TV programs and ignore the needs of the sick child.[15] Encourage appropriate TV viewing in the following ways:

1. Assist the child and the parents in choosing programs appropriate for the age of the child.
2. Encourage parental participation in viewing.
3. Plan treatments and care so that the child is free to watch a selected program.
4. Provide play activities, crafts, music, and games that are interesting, stimulating alternatives.
5. Help the child select times when the TV is to be turned off.
6. Make the TV an ally in health teaching by developing closed-circuit TV systems and videotapes appropriate for children (see Chap. 15).

PROVIDING FOR SAFETY DURING HOSPITALIZATION

Safety during activities and procedures

Identification of the child During the admission procedure the child receives an ID band and must wear it at all times. A card on the bed is used as a double check of the child's identity. It should include the same information that is on the ID band and should be securely attached to the bed or the wall above the bed.

On occasion, children will find it amusing to swap beds or try to exchange identity with another child. Difficulties may occur also if siblings are hospitalized in the same room. Check the ID band and bed card carefully to ensure that the right child receives the right care.

	Sun.	*Mon.*	*Tue.*	*Wed.*	*Thur.*	*Fri.*	*Sat.*
BATH (8:30–9:00 A.M.)	★	★					
SHAMPOO (9:15–9:30 A.M.)		★					
DRESSING CHANGE		★					
HOMEWORK (11:00 A.M. to noon, 2:00–3:00 P.M.)	★ ★	★					
MEDICINE (9:00 A.M., 1:00 P.M., 5:00 P.M.)	★★ ★	★★ ★					

Figure 16-7 A schedule of daily activities. Stars are used to indicate successful completion of tasks. (*Courtesy of Teresa Atkinson.*)

Siderails Siderails are available on cribs, youth beds, and adult beds to prevent falls. Cribs are available in two lengths—one for infants and one for toddlers. They are generally used for children under 3 years. Youth beds may be used up to age 10. Practice raising and lowering siderails so that care may be given without disturbing a sleeping child.

When caring for an infant in a crib, lower the siderail only halfway. When alone, have only one side down at a time. When leaving an infant in bed—even in restraints—be sure that the siderails are *up all the way*. Everyone on the nursing unit should check siderails frequently. (When a child is in a mist tent, the plastic sides tucked under the mattress may give a false sense of protection. Make sure that siderails are not accidentally left down.)

A youth bed looks like a high twin bed with siderails. Because the bed is higher than the child's bed at home, the siderails act as a reminder to the child to seek assistance before getting out of bed. A stool or the supportive arms of an adult are adequate to assist the child when the rails are down. These siderails can be raised 1 ft above the mattress. Although rails can prevent a young patient from falling out of bed when lying down, they cannot prevent the child from *climbing out*. The nurse must choose the appropriate bed according to the child's age and ability to call for assistance. Restraints other than siderails may be necessary.

Teach parents how to use the siderails. Stress the importance of raising them when leaving the child alone in bed.

Restraints The use of restraints as a safety measure may be a necessary, but unpleasant, part of caring for hospitalized children. The nurse must assess the need for restraints and select the appropriate kind. Restraints should be used sparingly. Dowd, Novak, and Ray, in a study of 29 children, found that none of the children attempted to remove or disturb their tubes and suture lines when restraints were removed.[16] Restraints are not essential for every child with a tube or line attached. Simply covering the area with a cloth or dressing may adequately prevent disturbance.

If a child must remain in a certain position, or if he or she is tampering with equipment and interfering with necessary treatments, some way of decreasing mobility must be employed. Restraints are necessary if no other means (e.g., a parent who will hold the child) are available. Carefully explain restraints to the child and the parents to lessen fears and increase cooperation. Use a kind, gentle approach when applying them.

Various kinds of restraints are available or can be improvised. The following are discussed below:

1. Bubble tops and crib nets
2. Elbow restraints
3. Mittens
4. Clove-hitch restraints
5. Mummy restraints
6. Jacket restraints

Bubble tops and crib nets Full siderails will usually prevent infants and small children from falling out of cribs. However, a toddler may be able to climb over the rail. If a child is too young to be moved to a youth bed, a bubble top (Fig. 16-8) or net can provide further protection.

A clear, heavy plastic bubble top can be secured on a track attached to the top of the endrails. When care is being given, the top can be made to slide to the side by releasing a catch at each end. A bubble top allows the child to stand in the crib and see out through the clear top.

An alternative to the bubble top is a crib net placed snugly over the top of the crib and attached securely to each corner of the bedsprings. It will stretch to allow the child to stand, but activity is more restricted than with the bubble top.

Elbow restraints Elbow restraints (Fig. 16-9) are most often used when children have had head or neck surgery or a scalp-vein infusion. Elbow restraints keep the arms extended. The child is unable to bend the elbow or touch his or her head. The restraint consists of a rectangular heavy-duty cloth divided into compartments. Tongue blades are placed into each compartment. If presewn restraints are not available, tape tongue blades close together across a washcloth or use a cardboard cylinder. Wrap the restraint around the child's arm so that it extends about halfway up between the elbow and shoulder and down to the wrist. Secure with gauze ties or pins. To prevent slipping, extend the child's gown or pajama sleeve below the restraint, turn it up, and pin it to the restraint. Apply the restraint loosely enough to allow insertion of a finger underneath it. Check the circulation of the arm frequently.

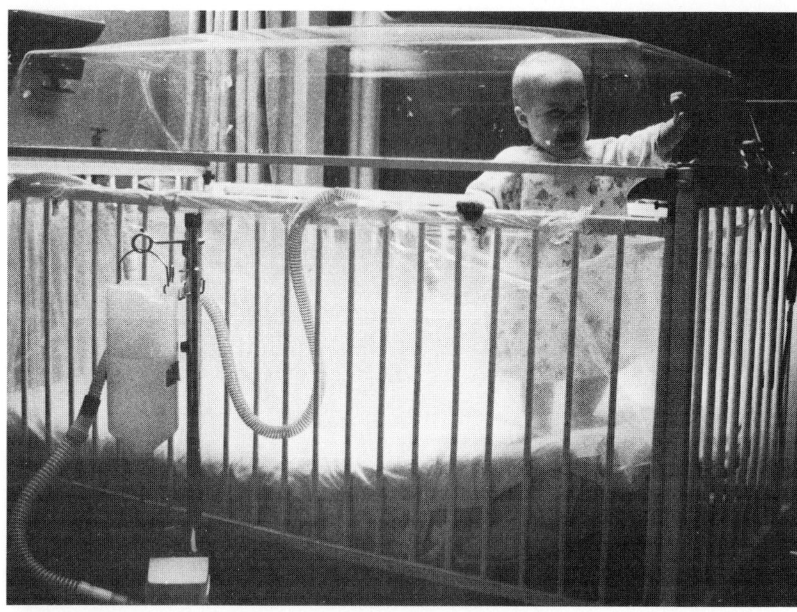

Figure 16-8 The bubble top attached to the crib prevents the toddler from climbing out and provides visibility of surroundings. The ultrasonic nebulizer attached to the crib provides a high-humidity environment for the child with respiratory problems. (*Photo by Pearl Sheps.*)

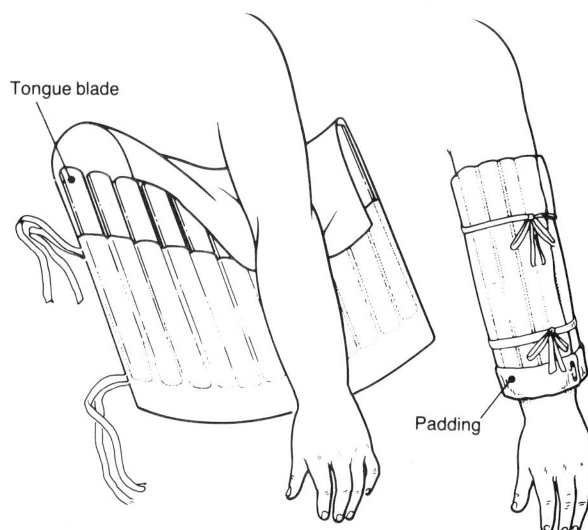

Figure 16-9 An elbow restraint (*From G. Scipien, M. U. Barnard, M. A. Chard, J. Howe, and P. H. Phillips* [*eds.*], *Comprehensive Pediatric Nursing, 3d. ed., McGraw-Hill, New York, 1986, p. 1406. Used with permission.*)

Mittens These can be used to prevent the child's fingers from manipulating tubes or to prevent scratching in dermatologic disorders. Use snug socks over the hands, and pin the socks to the sleeves of the gown.

Clove-hitch restraints This restraint secures the extremities but cannot tighten to decrease circulation. Place a gauze pad over the wrist or ankle before the restraint is applied. Use a long piece of gauze or heavy-duty cloth, and loop it around the limb as illustrated in Fig. 16-10. Secure the restraint to the mattress spring, not to the siderail.

Somewhat similar to the clove-hitch restraint is a commercially manufactured cuff restraint padded with sheepskin or foam. This may be adequate for older children, but active toddlers and infants can slip their small fists out of them.

Mummy restraints This is useful when a small child must be positioned for a jugular venipuncture, a scalp-vein infusion, or a subdural tap. (See Fig. 16-11 for steps in applying a

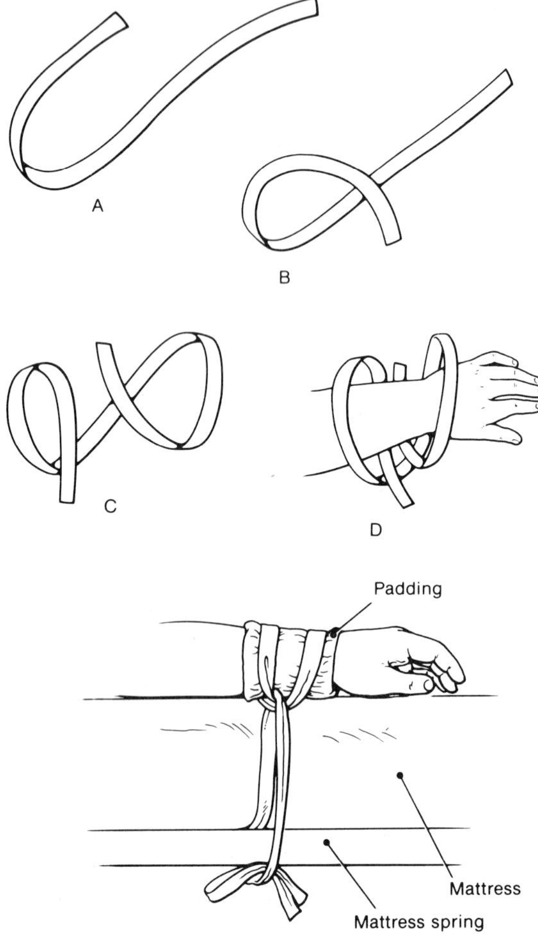

Figure 16-10 A clove-hitch restraint. A figure eight is formed with gauze and then placed over padding on an extremity and tied by a slip knot to a stationary part of the crib. (*From G. Scipien, M. U. Barnard, M. A. Chard, J. Howe, and P. J. Phillips* [eds.], *Comprehensive Pediatric Nursing, 3d ed., McGraw-Hill, New York, 1986, p. 1406. Used with permission.*)

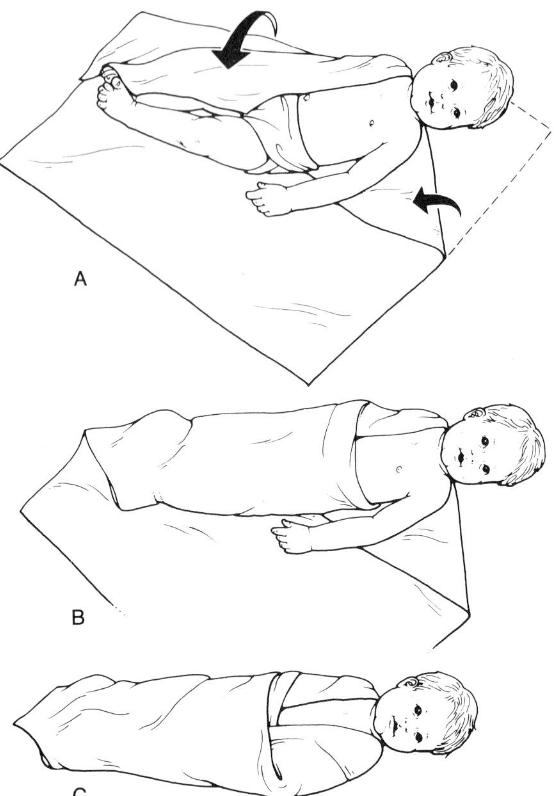

Figure 16-11 A mummy restraint. (*A*) and (*B*) Material is first folded over the right arm, and then the corner is tucked under the left side. (*C*) The opposite corner is then folded over the infant's left arm and tucked under the right side to secure it. (*From G. Scipien, M. U. Barnard, M. A. Chard, J. Howe, and P. J. Phillips* [eds.], *Comprehensive Pediatric Nursing, 3d ed., McGraw-Hill, New York, 1986, p. 1405. Used with permission.*)

mummy restraint.) When applying a mummy restraint, use tape to secure it on the outside and to prevent the child from wiggling out of it. Leave the bottom of the mummy restraint open when feasible to allow the child to express anger by kicking. Continue to hold the upper part of the body.

Jacket restraints Jacket restraints are available in various sizes and are applied with ties at the back. Long tapes extending from the sides of the jacket are tied to a chair. In the past the jacket was used as a bed restraint to allow some mobility, but this proved unsafe because children frequently became entangled in the long tapes. It is best to use the jacket only when positioning a child in a high chair, feeding table, wheelchair, or stroller. Secure the tapes snugly.

Nursing management of the restrained child Table 16-5 presents some nursing approaches to be used with any child who is restrained. Remember that the patient is a child and that the restraints may seem like punishment. Give the child attention frequently. Hold and cuddle often and provide distractions. Change the child's position and check circulation fre-

Table 16-5 Intervention Regimen for Children in Restraints

Nursing action	Rationale
Explain to the child why his or her body part is restrained. This may be done through the use of a doll, puppet, or story for a toddler or preschooler.	It is important that the child understand why he or she is not allowed to use mobility at this time to meet his or her needs.
While remaining with the child, remove the restraints for 10 min every 2 h and allow random movement.	Removing the restraints will allow the child to have some means of self-expression, to maintain contact with the environment, and to preserve his or her physiological integrity.
Change the child's position in relation to gravity as much as possible while he or she is unrestrained.	Position change is necessary to increase respiratory volume, to maintain autonomic control of the heart and peripheral circulation, and to provide the proprioceptive stimulation which is necessary for neuromuscular function.
Talk soothingly to the child while he or she is unrestrained; use touch and body contact and provide play as appropriate.	Interaction with the child increases sensory input, encourages self-expression, and decreases boredom and feelings of loneliness and helplessness.
Before reapplying necessary restraints, change the child's position and talk soothingly. Restrain as little and as loosely as possible to maintain safety while allowing enough freedom so that the child can touch some part of the body.	Position change helps prevent skin ischemia and breakdown, provides comfort, and allows for a variety of stimulation. The emotional attitude of the restraining person plays a role in the child's response*. The degree of restriction influences the effect of restraints on the child†. The infant and toddler develop a knowledge of their bodies and distinguish their bodies from other objects through motor sensations.
Provide stimulation for the child while he or she is restrained.	Restricting the child's mobility has deprived the child of most of his or her important means of learning about and mastering the environment. Compensatory stimulation will facilitate the child's development.

Source: From E. L. Dowd, J. Novak, and E. Ray, "Releasing the Hospitalized Child from Restraints," *American Journal of Maternal-Child Nursing* **372** (November–December 1977). Used with permission.
**Source:* Bernabeau [17].
†Source: O'Grady [18].

quently. Take special care not to restrain the child supine in a spread-eagle fashion. Leave at least one extremity free. If a child is restrained on the back, elevate the head of the bed at least 15° to prevent aspiration in case of vomiting. Give the child stroller or wagon rides to increase mobility.

Positioning for procedures Proper positioning of a child is essential for the child's safety and the successful completion of a procedure. Provide a good explanation and a comfort measure (e.g., a pacifier, stuffed animal, blanket, or parent). When holding the child, use a minimum number of personnel. Imagine what it is like for a 4-year-old in a strange, new place to be approached by several strangers who restrain the child for a painful procedure! With advance planning, two people can usually provide restraint while the third performs the procedure.

Find ways in which the child can help during the procedure, such as holding some of the equipment. Plan something pleasant to anticipate following the procedure. Praise the child frequently for helping. Encouraging children's cooperation and allowing them to make some decisions will increase their feeling of control over what is happening.

When positioning the child, be sure that adequate light is available and that those restraining the child do not obstruct the light source. Position the child as comfortably as possible while maintaining adequate restraint.

Positions for injections Common sites for intramuscular injections are the thigh and hip. When the thigh is used, position the child on his or her back in bed. Maintain the knees in an extended position, since the tendency is to flex the knees when the needle penetrates the skin. Restrain the hands by asking the child to squeeze your hands, or place the hands on the chest and restrain the hands and chest simultaneously. The latter prevents the child from sitting up during the injection.

Vary the location of the procedure so that the child does not associate the bed with shots and refuse to sleep. One alternative is for the nurse or parent to hold the young child on the lap; the adult can hold the child's hands with one hand and restrain the knees with the other. The child's lower legs can also be restrained between the thighs of the adult.

When the site for the injection is the hip, position the child on the abdomen. Extend the child's hands over the head so that he or she can grip the head of the bed or the mattress. Have the child turn the toes inward to enhance relaxation of the hip muscles. Ask the child to concentrate on something (e.g., count to 10 or take slow, deep breaths). Maintain the knees in an extended position, and restrain the child's trunk to prevent flexion of the hip.

When giving an injection to an infant, turn toward the child's feet (Fig. 16-12) and secure the buttocks between your elbow and hip. Use the appropriate sites in the thigh. (See Fig. 16-48 for intramuscular sites.)

An experienced nurse can administer injections safely and also restrain the child. For example, the nurse can extend an arm across the child's knees and still have a hand free to hold the syringe. Avoid becoming overconfdent, however, because children's movements can be quick and unexpected. An inexperienced nurse must concentrate on the injection itself and have adequate assistance in positioning the child so that there is no need to worry about sudden movement.

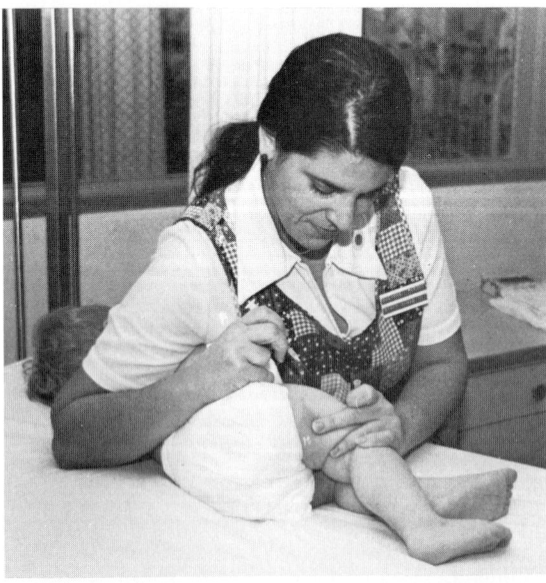

Figure 16-12 A small child is being restrained for an intramuscular injection. (*From L. Whaley and D. Wong, Nursing Care of Infants and Children, Mosby, St. Louis, 1979, p. 940. Used with permission.*)

Positions for venipuncture Careful selection of a potential site for venipuncture must be done before the child is held down. This lessens the restraint time and may also allow the child to participate in the procedure.

When the site is determined, ask for the child's cooperation so that the procedure can be completed quickly. Tell the child that you will help him or her, if necessary, to stay in position. Restrain the child's hands or joints near the site. Remind the child that after the needle is in place, it will not hurt or "stick."

Use a mummy restraint (Fig. 16-11) for a venipuncture of the jugular vein. Turn the child's head to the side and extend it slightly over the edge of the bed (Fig. 16-13*A*). This hyperextends the neck so that the jugular vein is more accessible. (*Note:* After puncture of the jugular vein, apply pressure for at least 10 min to prevent hematoma formation.)

For a scalp-vein infusion, use a mummy restraint, and position the child flat in bed. Hold the child's head firmly to one side. Avoid obstructing the nose and mouth.

Femoral sticks may be necessary for infants when no other veins are available or when arterial blood tests are needed. Place the infant's legs in a frog-leg position, with the knees flexed and the hips abducted (Fig. 16-13*B*). Place a diaper over the genitalia to prevent contamination of the site. (Infants commonly void during this kind of procedure.) Restrain the infant by holding the knees from above. The person performing the procedure works from below.

Positions for lumbar puncture Position the child on the side with the knees and head flexed toward the abdomen (Fig. 16-13*C*). Position the child at the edge of the treatment table. As the physician begins cleansing the skin, hold the child, but do not flex the neck and knees until the physician is ready to insert the needle (Fig. 16-14*A* and *B*). Place one arm behind the knees and one behind the neck to maintain the flexion. This produces separation of the spinous processes

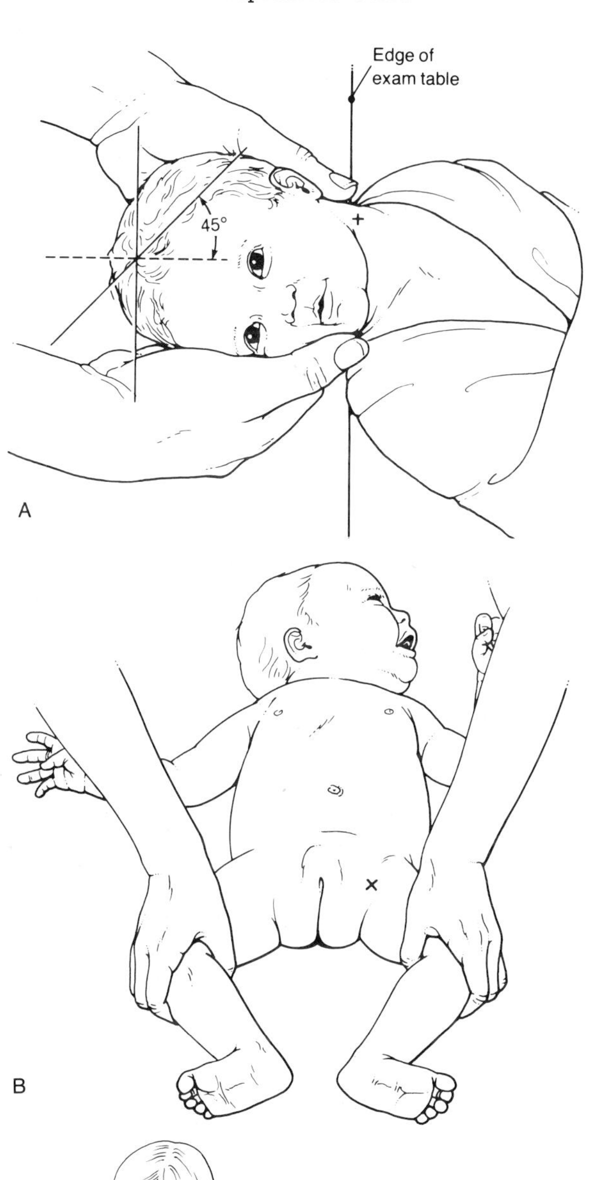

Figure 16-13 Positions for venipuncture. (*A*) Position for jugular venipuncture. The puncture site is indicated by X. The mummy restraint shown in Fig. 16-11 is being used. (*B*) Position for femoral venipuncture. The X indicates the puncture site. (C) (Left) Position for lumbar venipuncture with the back at or over a table edge. The X indicates the puncture site. (Right) View of lumbar puncture restraint from above. (*From G. Scipien, M. U. Barnard, M. A. Chard, J. Howe, and P. J. Phillips* [*eds.*], *Comprehensive Pediatric Nursing, 3d ed., McGraw-Hill, New York, 1986, pp. 1406–1407. Used with permission.*)

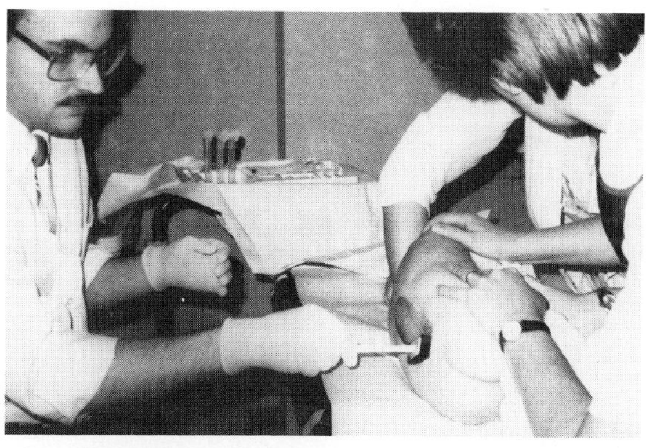

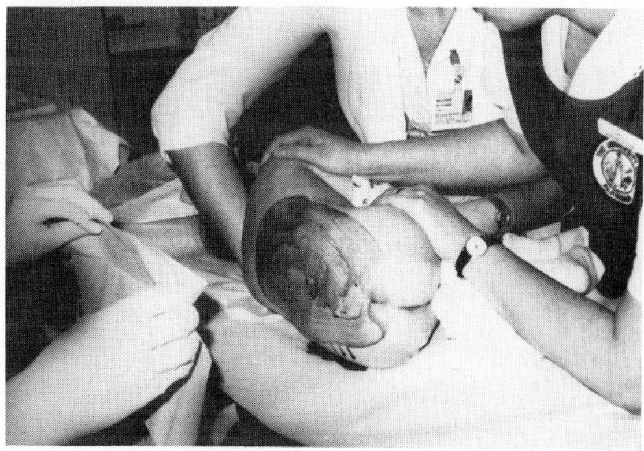

Figure 16-14 (*A*) The nurses are restraining the child gently while the physician cleanses the skin for the lumbar puncture. (*B*) When the physician is ready for the needle insertion, the child's back is rounded, the drape is placed, and she is held securely until the procedure is completed.

and assists the physician in inserting the spinal needle properly. Keep the child's back parallel to the edge of the bed or treatment table, and maintain the flexion throughout the procedure. Remember to talk to the child. Observe his or her appearance and check respirations as you hold the child.

The sitting position for a lumbar puncture may be used with premature infants who have a low spinal-fluid pressure.[19] Infants are supported sitting and leaning forward so that the spine is rounded.

Positions for physical examination of the head To position a small child's head securely, place the child in a supine position, extend the arms up beside the head, restrain the elbows, and hold the head simultaneously. This facilitates eye, ear, nose, and throat examinations.

Reassurance following procedures During any procedure remember that you are holding a frightened child who is uncomfortable. He or she may also be very ill. Observe the child closely. Check vital signs and appearance during and after any stressful procedure. As soon as it is over, give comfort and reassurance. Though other nursing responsibilities are necessary (getting specimens to the lab, cleaning trays and equipment, etc.), the comfort and well-being of the child have top priority. Encourage parents to hold the child. Provide a play activity or a treat as a pleasant change.

Role of parents in restraining for procedure There are a variety of opinions about whether parents should hold their children during painful procedures. Some authors feel that children do not understand why the parents will allow them to feel pain. Their presence may cause the child to distrust them. Others believe that when parents assist, children know that the procedure, though painful, is necessary for getting well. This enhances their acceptance of the procedure and increases feelings of security. Each situation must be assessed individually. Remember that some parents cannot tolerate seeing their child in pain and prefer to leave the room. A child may become anxious if he or she senses the parents' anxiety. Maintain open communication between the parents, the child, the physician, and the nurses to determine what role the parents should play.

Toy safety Most of a child's waking hours are filled with play activities. Toys of all kinds are usually available on a pediatric unit, and each child will find some object to play with—whether it is a "real" toy or not. Be aware of the safety hazards of all toys and equipment within the child's reach. A set of tiny building blocks appropriate for a 7-year-old can be lethal to a 14-month-old who puts everything in his or her mouth. Be aware of the developmental needs at various ages in order to determine what is appropriate and safe for each child.

In general, toys for children through age 5 should have the following safety characteristics: they should have no sharp edges, be nonallergenic, have no small removable parts, and be unbreakable, washable, and lead-free.[20] With older children it is difficult to restrict toys to those which meet these requirements.

Explain to both children and parents that toys must be put away when no longer in use. Have all children keep their own toys at their bedsides or on a nearby shelf that is inaccessible to other children. Make sure that each child has age-appropriate, safe, and varied toys so that he or she will be less likely to look for unsafe toys.

Carrying and holding infants Being held gently but firmly increases an infant's feelings of security and comfort. Safe methods for holding and carrying infants are as follows:

1. *Cradling the child* Hold the infant in your arm with the head above your elbow. Hold the thigh with your hand in order to keep the infant securely in place (Fig. 16-15).
2. *Using the football hold* Support the infant's head with your hand, and with the back on your forearm, press the infant's buttocks between your elbow and hip (Fig. 16-16). This leaves one hand free for changing bed linen, shampooing the hair, etc.
3. *Holding the child upright* Support the infant's buttocks on one forearm, and rest the head against your shoulder. Keep the other hand on the back to catch the unexpected backward movement that can easily occur. This hold is modified for the toddler, as shown in Fig. 16-17.

The movements of small children are unpredictable. While carrying a young child, always remain alert to the possibility of sudden move-

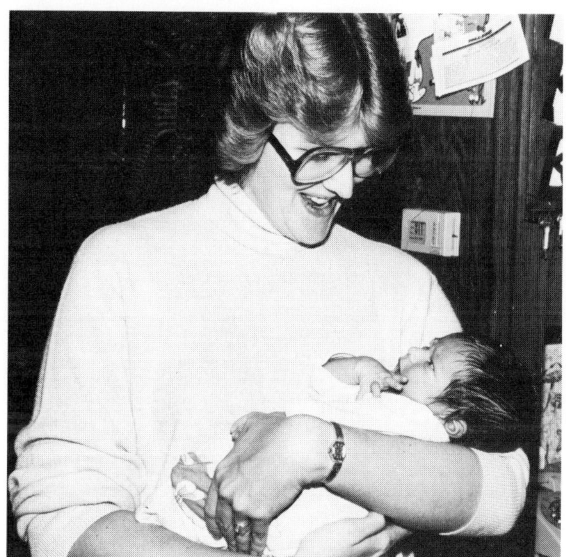

Figure 16-15 An infant being cradled in the caregiver's arms. Note the eye-to-eye contact between the adult and the child.

ment, and be able to compensate for it immediately.

Supervising children's activities Maintaining safety when caring for children involves looking at the hospital unit with a critical eye and constantly identifying safety hazards.[21] Written guidelines developed by the nursing staff should be shared with children and parents. These must be supported and reinforced by all the staff—nurses, physicians, nursing assistants, housekeeping personnel, and other hospital workers.

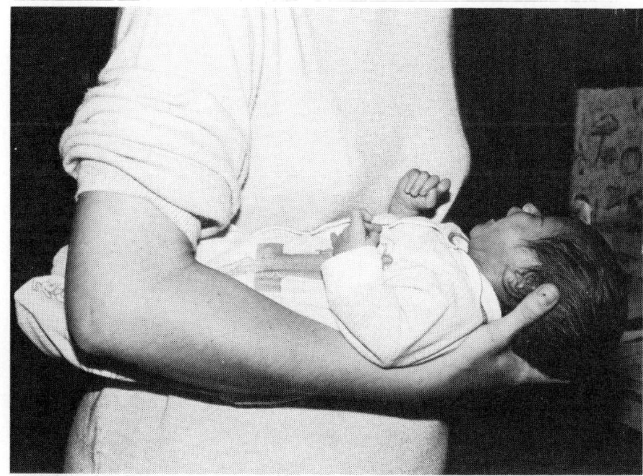

Figure 16-16 The football hold.

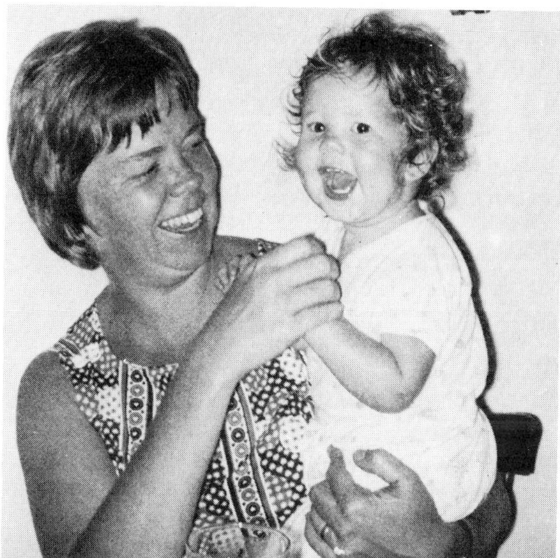

Figure 16-17 Holding a small child in an upright position. The caregiver holds the child's arm to prevent her from falling backward. (*From G. Scipien, M. U. Barnard, M. A. Chard, J. Howe, and P. J. Phillips* [eds.], *Comprehensive Pediatric Nursing, 2d ed., McGraw-Hill, New York, 1979, p. 220. Used with permission.*)

When parents are well informed about the guidelines, they can help their own child and other patients as well. See Table 16-6.

To provide a safe means of expanding the young child's environment and decreasing boredom, place the child in a playpen at the door of

Table 16-6 A Sample of Nursing Unit Guidelines for Children's Activities

The following guidelines have been developed for the safety of all the children who are patients in the unit. Please try to follow them. If you have questions, contact one of the nurses. Thank you!

1. Do not run on the nursing unit.
2. Please remain outside the medication area at all times.
3. Return toys to the playroom shelves after use.
4. Feel free to use playroom toys in your room, unless you are in isolation. In that case, talk with a nurse before taking toys into the room.
5. Daily quiet time: 12:30 P.M. to 2:00 P.M.
6. Playroom hours: 7:30 A.M. to 8:30 P.M.
7. Please be in your own room by 8:30 P.M.
8. Talk with the nurse before bringing in food from outside.
9. Small children must be accompanied by an adult when out of bed.

the room or at the nurses' station. Use strollers, wagons, or wheelchairs to give the child rides around the unit or to transport the child to other departments. Use restraints to ensure the child's safety, and do not leave a child alone in the movable equipment unless the child is old enough to safely get in and out and operate the vehicle (e.g., a 12-year-old can easily move a wheelchair alone).

Infection control

Medical asepsis The word *asepsis* means "germ-free," and the purpose of medical asepsis is to eliminate all *disease-producing* organisms from the environment.[22] A clean noninfectious item or area becomes contaminated if it comes in contact with anything infected.

Hand-washing Hand-washing is the *single most important factor in infection control* on a nursing unit. Good, thorough, and frequent hand-washing prevents the accumulation of bacteria. Soap mixes with and loosens dirt and oils on the hands, while friction—good rubbing—actually removes the germs. Hands should be washed after each patient contact and after handling contaminated materials (e.g., elimination products). Table 16-7 describes proper hand-washing techniques.

Maintaining a clean environment One aspect of the nurse's role in infection control is to help maintain a clean environment. Housekeeping personnel are responsible for *daily* cleaning of floors, furniture, and equipment. Maintain close communication with the housekeeping department, and notify them when an area needs additional cleaning.

If children eat together in the playroom, it is important that the floors be cleaned immediately afterward. Food is a potential source of bacterial growth. Periodically check the bedside or overbed tables for snacks or leftover food, which may be a source of bacteria. Children may hide sweets or snack foods in bedside tables or closets. These attract ants, cockroaches, and even mice. Check these areas frequently also.

Provide a mat, sheet, or rug for play on the floor. This allows children to play without sitting directly on the floor; the covering can be cleaned after each use.

Playroom toys are used by many different children and should be cleaned regularly—especially those used by young children, who will put them in their mouths. Develop a plan for effectively accomplishing this task, perhaps by including it in the daily assignments for the nursing assistants.

Toys used by children in their rooms should be cleaned before being returned to the playroom. Send the equipment to a central cleaning department for terminal sterilization, or wash it with an antibacterial solution. Consult the hospital's infection control policies for specific guidelines.

Preparing food Nurses commonly prepare snacks, food, and formula for infants on the nursing unit. A kitchenette with a sink and refrigerator for patients' foods should be available. No medications or staff lunches should be kept in the same refrigerator. Careful hand-washing before preparing any food is essential.

Presterilized formula and disposable bottles for juice or milk are often used for infants in the hospital. Parents may ask that a child's own bottle be used. The nurse must decide whether the facilities permit proper cleaning without cross-contamination. On a busy nursing unit, the safest way is to use only hospital equipment.

Keep a good supply of prepared cereal and baby food on the unit. Infants do not conform to routine food service hours.

When preparing food, use a clean cup and spoon for each child. Close dry cereal boxes securely after use so that the contents remain clean and dry. When a jar of baby food is opened, re-

Table 16-7 Hand-Washing Techniques

With the Newborn

1. Keep nails short and carefully trimmed.
2. Remove all jewelry, including watch.
3. Perform a 2- to 5-min scrub upon entering the nursery:
   a. Moisten hands, apply soap, and, using friction, wash palms, backs, and sides of hands and between fingers. Use a brush for most effective scrubbing. Clean nails.
   b. Rinse hands.
   c. Moisten arms and apply soap, scrubbing to the elbows.
   d. Rinse hands and arms.
4. Dry carefully with disposable towels.
5. Wash hands for at least 30 s between infants.

With Older Children

1. Keep nails short and carefully trimmed.
2. A watch and plain ring may be worn.
3. Perform initial scrub of 1 min on the hands (as above).
4. Wash hands for 30 s between patients.

move the amount needed, close the jar tightly, and label it with the date and time opened. Store it in the refrigerator no longer than 24 h. Do not feed an infant directly from a jar of food. The saliva that adheres to the spoon contaminates the food in the jar and provides a medium for bacterial growth. Discard a partially used bottle of milk or juice and *use a fresh bottle for each feeding*.

Making room assignments The nurse has the primary responsibility for selecting appropriate rooms and beds for patients. When possible, group patients by age and similarity of diagnosis. Be alert to signs that isolation may be necessary, and report these to the physician. (See Table 16-8 for some signs of possible infection.) If in doubt about the need for isolation, place the child in a private room until diagnostic tests are done to determine the presence of a communicable disease. If the child has had recent exposure to a communicable disease, note this on the Kardex, and be alert for symptoms during the child's hospitalization.

Cleaning equipment Various items such as stethoscopes and blood pressure cuffs are kept in the nurses' station for use in physical assessment. Wipe the bell, ear pieces, and tubing of the stethoscope with alcohol and allow it to dry before use. Blood pressure cuffs should be cleaned periodically by terminal sterilization. When feasible, wipe all equipment with an antiseptic solution before and after use. If a child is isolated, frequently used equipment should remain in the room throughout his or her stay and should be sterilized after dismissal.

Isolation procedures Table 16-9 lists a variety of communicable diseases and the type of isolation precautions necessary.

Preparing the child and the parents Explain carefully why isolation is needed. Sometimes a child does not fully understand the reason for isolation and believes it is punishment for wrongdoing. It may help to use play techniques—providing dolls with masks and gowns and drawing pictures—to explore the child's feelings. Meehan's *Isolation Coloring Book* may be a helpful resource.[23]

Instruct not only the child but also the parents in hand-washing and gown procedures. The involvement of the parents in care should be encouraged by teaching them proper isolation techniques. However, the nurse should continue working with them rather than leaving them alone once they are trained. Use color-coded cards on doors to indicate the type of isolation.

Disposition of equipment Check daily for adequate supplies, and reorder from central supply (Fig. 16-18). Room facilities should include:[24]

1. A table or cart outside the door for gowns, masks, gloves, and plastic bags
2. Facilities for hand-washing
3. Separately covered containers for soiled linen and diapers
4. Individual equipment for the child's care
5. Paper towels

Organize activities and gather necessary equipment and medications before entering the room.

If a piece of equipment is needed one time only (e.g., an otoscope), place it on a paper-towel barrier on the bedside table. Wash it off with an antiseptic solution and return it to the unit.

Provide toys which can be easily sterilized after isolation is terminated.

Use disposable trays and dishes for mealtimes and snacks.

Personal hygiene Practice good hand-washing before and after each patient contact. Remove your rings and watch before scrubbing and during care. Wear long hair pinned up off the shoulders. Wear a fresh disposable gown when entering the room. When a mask is necessary, cover both your nose and mouth. Wear a mask for only 30 min, and then replace it.

Do not touch your hair, face, neck, uniform, or other "clean" item with contaminated hands. Wash your hands before removing the gown (i.e., do not handle the neck of the gown with contaminated hands).

Do not assign a staff member who is pregnant, has skin lesions, or has an upper respira-

Table 16-8 Signs of Possible Infection

1. Nasal discharge	7. Stiff neck
2. Cough	8. Malaise
3. Skin rash	9. Enlarged lymph nodes
4. Fever	10. Vomiting
5. Draining wound	11. Diarrhea
6. Headache	

Table 16-9 Infectious Diseases Grouped According to Degree of Recommended Isolation

Private Room	Mask	Gown	Gloves	Excreta and Excreta-Soiled Articles	Blood	Secreta and Secreta-Soiled Articles	Diseases
Strict Isolation							
R*	R	R	R			R	Anthrax, inhalation; eczema vaccinatum; melioidosis, pulmonary, or extrapulmonary with draining sinus or sinuses; plague, pulmonary or bubonic; smallpox; vaccinia, generalized and progressive
R	C†	C	C			R	Burns, extensive (when infected with *Staphylococcus aureus* or Group A streptococcus)
R	R	C	C			R	Staphylococcal enterocolitis; staphylococcal or streptococcal pneumonia
R	R	C				R	Diphtheria
R		C		R	R	R	Neonatal vesicular disease (herpes simplex); rubella, congenital syndrome
R			C			R	Rabies
Respiratory Isolation							
R	R					R	Tuberculosis, pulmonary—sputum-positive (or suspect); Venezuelan equine encephalitis
R	R						Meningitis, meningococcal; meningococcemia
R	S‡					R	Chickenpox; herpes zoster; measles (rubeola); mumps; rubella (German measles); pertussis (whooping cough)
Enteric Precautions							
D§		C	C	R			Cholera; *Escherichia coli* gastroenteritis; salmonellosis, including typhoid fever; shigellosis
D				R	R		Hepatitis, infectious or serum
Wound and Skin Precautions							
D						R	Gas gangrene
D	C	C	C			R	Staphylococcal skin or wound disease
D		C	C			R	Impetigo; streptococcal skin infection; wound infections, extensive—other than staphylococcal; burns, extensive—infected other than with *Staphylococcus aureus* or Group A streptococcus

Table 16-9 Infectious Diseases Grouped According to Degree of Recommended Isolation (*Continued*)

Discharge Precautions		
Special handling of excreta and excreta-soiled articles is recommended for the following diseases:		
Herpangina	Pleurodynia	Viral diseases, enteric (if not covered elsewhere)
Leptospirosis	Poliomyelitis	
Meningitis, aseptic	Taeniasis, pork	
Special handling of secreta and secreta-soiled articles is recommended for the following diseases:		
Actinomycosis with draining lesions	Gonococcal ophthalmia neonatorum	Scarlet fever
Anthrax, cutaneous	Gonorrhea	Staphylococcal food poisoning
Brucellosis with draining lesions	Granuloma inguinale	Streptococcal pharyngitis
Burns and wounds, minor (infected)	Herpes simplex	Syphilis, mucocutaneous
Clostridium perfringens food poisoning	Keratoconjunctivitis, infectious	Trachoma, acute
Coccidioidomycosis with draining wounds	Listeriosis	Tuberculosis, extrapulmonary with open lesions
Conjunctivitis, acute bacterial (including gonócoccal)	Lymphogranuloma venereum	Tularemia, cutaneous
Cryptococcosis	Pneumonia, bacterial (if not covered elsewhere)	Viral diseases, respiratory (if not covered elsewhere)
	Psittacosis	Wound infections, not extensive (other than staphylococcal)
	Q fever	
Blood Precautions		
Special handling of secreta and secreta-soiled articles is recommended for the following diseases:		
Arthropod-borne viral fever (dengue and so forth)	Anthropod-borne viral hemorrhagic fever	Hepatitis, infectious or serum
		Malaria

*Recommended.

†With direct contact.

‡For susceptible children.

§Desirable but optional.

Source: Hospital Care of Children and Youth, American Academy of Pediatrics, Committee on Hospital Care, Evanston, Ill., 1978, p. 94–96. Used with permission.

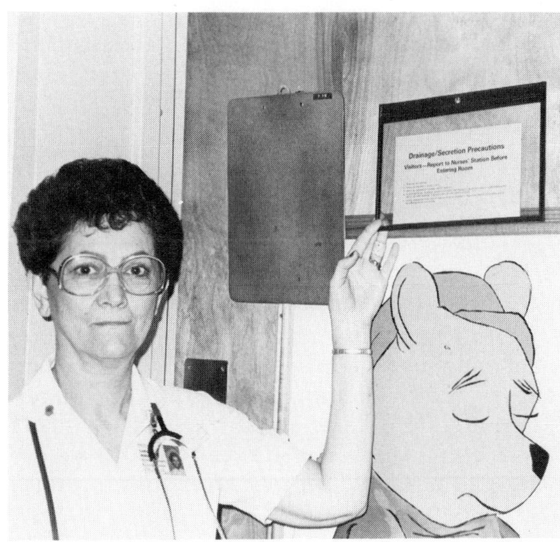

Figure 16-18 Equipment for maintaining isolation on the hospital unit.

tory infection to care for a child with a communicable disease. A nurse who is caring for a child in isolation should not concurrently be assigned to another patient with a fresh surgical incision or lowered resistance to infection.

Disposal of contaminated items Dispose of diapers, contaminated dressings, and linen in covered containers kept in the room. Make certain that the child cannot get into these containers.

At the end of each shift, clean the room and remove all trash and linen. This requires two staff members dressed in isolation attire. One works inside the room, while the other remains at the door and holds a clean bag. A soiled bag from the room is placed into the clean bag at the door. The outside person secures the bag and disposes of it properly. *No contaminated articles should be carried outside the room unless double-bagged.*

Reverse isolation This technique is used to protect a child who has a reduced resistance to disease (e.g., a severely burned child or one with a reduced white blood cell count). A mask, a gown, and gloves are required for direct care. Staff members with any sign of infection must not care for these patients.

Surgical asepsis Surgical asepsis is an extension of medical asepsis. It includes good handwashing, maintenance of a clean environment, and use of sterile technique in the care of surgical wounds. It is more rigorous because open wounds are more vulnerable to infections than normal, intact tissues.[25]

Sterile dressings are applied to surgical wounds in the operating room. The initial dressing may be large and bulky in order to provide pressure to minimize bleeding. It is usually removed after the first day and replaced by either a smaller dressing or none at all.

Soiled, wet dressings act as a wick and allow bacteria to soak through to the site of the incision. In order to prevent this, the dressing can be changed or reinforced (added to) with additional sterile dressings. The physician must be notified if drainage is excessive; the physician's instructions regarding dressing care should be followed.

The physician may prefer to do the first postoperative dressing change, but the nurse may be asked to perform subsequent ones. Steps in performing dressing changes are as follows:

1. Explain the dressing change to the child and the parents. Demonstrate dressing application and removal on a doll. Encourage the child to do the same.
2. Gather dressing supplies, masks, two pairs of sterile gloves, and a plastic bag.
3. Have the parent or another nurse assist in restraining the child or handling equipment.
4. Open all dressings and gloves on the table at the bedside.
5. If masks are necessary (determined according to the type of incision or wound, the doctor's recommendation, and hospital policy), each attendant and the child must wear one. A crying child may be unable to tolerate a mask, in which case turn the child's head away when the wound is exposed.
6. Remove old tape gently by pulling the skin and the tape away from each other. This may be the most painful part of the procedure for the child. Encourage the child to help with the tape removal.
7. Put on gloves.
8. Remove all old dressings and discard them in plastic bag.
9. Note the condition of the incision or wound, the type of drainage, and the surrounding skin.
10. Remove gloves and discard them in the bag. Put on a sterile pair.
11. Replace the dressings and secure them well with gauze and tape. Prevent future discomfort of tape removal by using paper tape rather than adhesive tape, or wrap the area securely with gauze and apply tape to the gauze rather than the skin.
12. Remove gloves and discard them in the bag.
13. Discard the bag in a closed container that is inaccessible to the child.
14. Comfort the child.
15. Chart the dressing change and the condition of the incision.

Documentation to promote safety

Safety requires that complete charting be done *as soon as possible after care is given*. A young patient cannot and will not always tell the nurse, "Oh, I've already had that medicine." As a result, omissions in charting can cause errors in care.

Nursing care of children under 10 should be documented on a flow sheet at least every hour. Observe the child's activities frequently when not giving direct care. With infants or seriously ill children, charting may be more frequent. Write a thorough nurses' note at least once a day to document needs and progress. Observe the child for problems or needs related to the medical diagnosis, emotional status, growth and development, or parental concerns.

Keep accurate records of fluid intake and output throughout the hospitalization. Record all intake in milliliters and the number of voidings. When a child is receiving intravenous fluids or has a condition affecting renal function, the urinary output should be measured and recorded. The parents and the child may assist in documenting intake and output by keeping a record at the bedside.

NUTRITION OF HOSPITALIZED CHILDREN

Requirements for different nutrients vary according to the growth rate of various body tissues and the child's sex, stage of maturation, physical activity, and body build. The child's general health and conformity to percentiles of growth in height and weight are the best indications of nutritional state. Sample growth charts for males and females are presented in Appendix B.

Caloric needs

The total caloric needs of children increase with age and with gains in height and weight. Appetite is a good indication of a child's caloric needs. During the period of early infancy, when growth occurs at a fast pace, the appetite is good and the caloric intake tends to increase accordingly. At the beginning of the second year there is a decrease in the rate of weight gain, as the child becomes more mobile and growth slows. Throughout childhood there are times when growth speeds up and the caloric needs increase, such as in adolescence.

Segar has developed a simple method of determining caloric needs according to body weight (Table 16-10).

Assessing nutritional patterns

On admission, determine the child's weight and height, and plot these on a growth chart to show how the child compares with others of the same age. Discuss with the parents and the child the child's eating habits and food preferences, and share this information with the dietitian. If a detailed nutritional history is needed, have the mother recall and write down a typical day's intake at home. Since a child's eating habits may be altered significantly by hospitalization and illness, the child's "normal" nutrition cannot be determined only by what is eaten in the hospital.

Calorie counts When a child is not eating properly in the hospital, it may be necessary to determine the child's daily caloric intake. Adequate caloric intake for the ill child is based on replacing the calories normally expended plus extra calories used in recuperating from the disease or in healing after surgery. To estimate the child's caloric intake, observe and record exactly how much he or she eats. The child and the family can be taught to help keep this record so that nothing will be overlooked. The dietitian will know exactly what amount was served and can help calculate the calorie count. Be sure that everything the child eats during a period of "calorie count" is served from the diet kitchen. Obtain daily weights on any child whose nutritional status is questionable.

Table 16-10 Caloric Expenditures of Children

Body Weight in Kilograms*	Caloric Expenditure Per Day
3 to 10 kg	100 kcal/kg
11 to 20 kg	1000 kcal plus 50 kcal/kg for each kg over 10
Above 20 kg	1500 kcal plus 20 kcal/kg for each kg over 20

*1 kg = 2.2 lb.

Source: V. C. Vaughan and J. R. McKay, *Nelson Textbook of Pediatrics,* 10th ed., Saunders, Philadelphia, 1975, p. 252. Used with permission.

Feeding techniques

In order to encourage good nutritional intake in the hospitalized child, the nurse must use creativity, initiative, and intuition. A child who is away from home and family, is feeling ill, is in a strange environment, and has an intravenous line in one arm and a cast on the other cannot be expected to eat enthusiastically when served a tray of food in bed.

Positioning Assist a bedridden child to assume a natural position at mealtime. If the child can sit with the legs over the side of the bed and the feet on the floor, he or she will eat more easily. Free a hand for the child to use at mealtime if at all possible. If the child must remain in bed, support the child in an upright position to facilitate eating. Use an over-bed table for an older child or a bed tray in a youth bed or crib. (A bed tray allows siderails to be left up during mealtime.) Remove equipment like oxygen masks or mist tents during the meal.

Feeding infants Infant feedings of baby food and formula are usually prepared on the nursing unit rather than in the diet kitchen. (Review the discussion of cleanliness when preparing infant foods in the section "Infection Control.") The food and formula may be served warm or cold according to the infant's routine at home. Dilute dry cereal with the formula to a liquid consistency. Prepared baby foods require no dilution. Have food and formula available on the nursing unit before needed. Babies won't wait! Table 16-11 lists methods for feeding infants.

Although an infant usually requires only formula or breast milk until the age of 6 months, the physician may choose to start the child on solid foods earlier. Do not overfeed the infant. Stop feeding when the infant begins to spit food back or lose interest.

An infant who can sit alone should be secured in a high chair with a strap or jacket restraint. Never leave an infant alone in a chair. Falls from high chairs are a major cause of injury in young children.

An older infant can be encouraged to participate in the meal by holding a piece of dry toast and "gumming" it. Offer the infant a cup with a small amount of liquid at about 6 months to prepare the child for weaning later on. Toward the end of the first year, children can begin to feed themselves as the diet progresses to include chopped table foods.

Even though an infant is old enough to have a meal in a high chair, hold the baby for the bottle-feeding. Some infants are accustomed to taking a bottle to bed during naps or at bedtime. If the child demands a bottle in bed, remove it as soon as it is empty or the child falls asleep. It is unwise to try to break this habit in the hospital. It is far better to talk with the parents about how this can be done at home. Explain that going to sleep with a bottle of milk or sweet liquid increases the chance of dental caries and ear infections.

Table 16-11 Feeding the Infant

1. Put a bib on the infant and have a cloth handy.
2. Position the infant in your lap or in an infant seat or high chair for solid foods.
3. If the infant is very hungry and crying vigorously, offer a few sips from the bottle before feeding solids.
4. Using an infant spoon, put a small amount of the food on the end of the spoon and place it on the center of the infant's tongue, not on the tip.
5. Burp the newborn after every ounce. Set him or her upright and support the head and chest by placing the fingers over the mandible (the lower jaw) and upper chest. (See Fig. 16-19.) The older infant can be burped after every 2 to 3 oz. Pat the infant's back gently to obtain a burp.
6. When solids are completed, cradle the infant in your arms for the bottle feeding.

Source: G. Leifer [26].

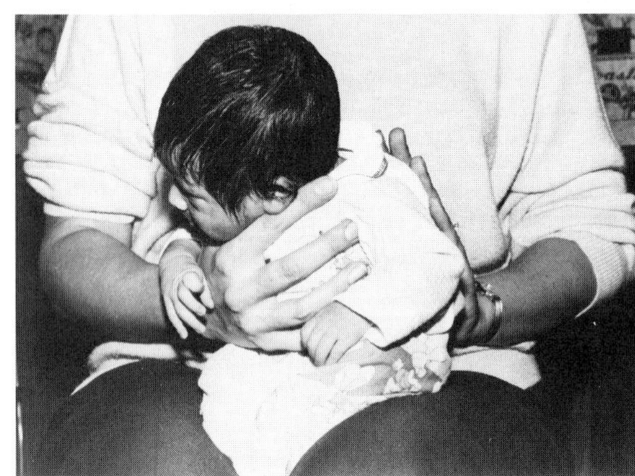

Figure 16-19 A method of holding an infant when burping. The mandible is supported to hold the head upright.

Exclude sweetened foods such as desserts, pastries, candy, and soft drinks from the infant's diet. If clear liquids are necessary, use plain water, sugar water, and clear juices, such as apple juice, rather than soft drinks or prepared drink mixes. When an infant is teething or needs a snack, offer hard toast, a cracker, or pieces of a bagel served with fruit juice. Ice chips may also be given to a teething infant.

Feeding toddlers and preschoolers Use a feeding table or high chair for toddlers. Allow toddlers to help feed themselves (Fig. 16-20). Preschoolers can use a bed tray or sit at a small table in the hospital room or in the playroom. These children are at an age when the time between one meal and the next may be too long. Provide a carefully planned midmorning and midafternoon snack; this creates a pleasant change of pace and decreases irritability and crying due to hunger or thirst. A drink of water or juice after naptime also helps the child wake up and be in a more pleasant mood.

Gavage feeding When an infant or child is too ill to eat normally or when oral feedings are contraindicated, gavage feeding may be the method of choice. A nasogastric tube is passed into the stomach for a single feeding and re-

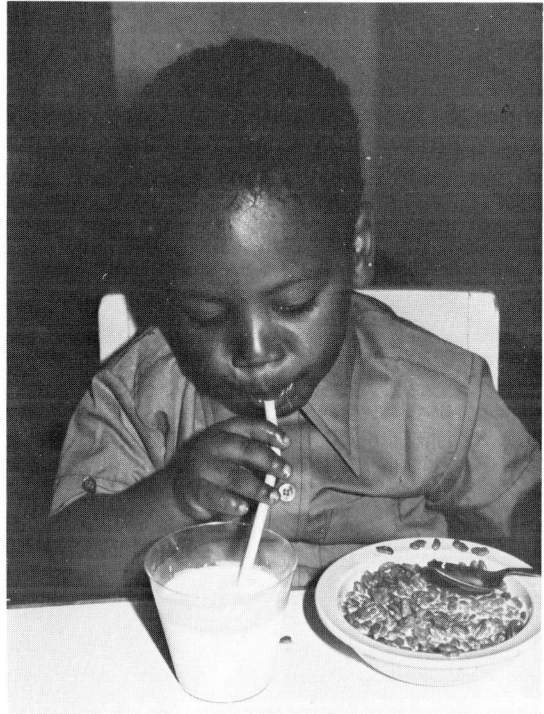

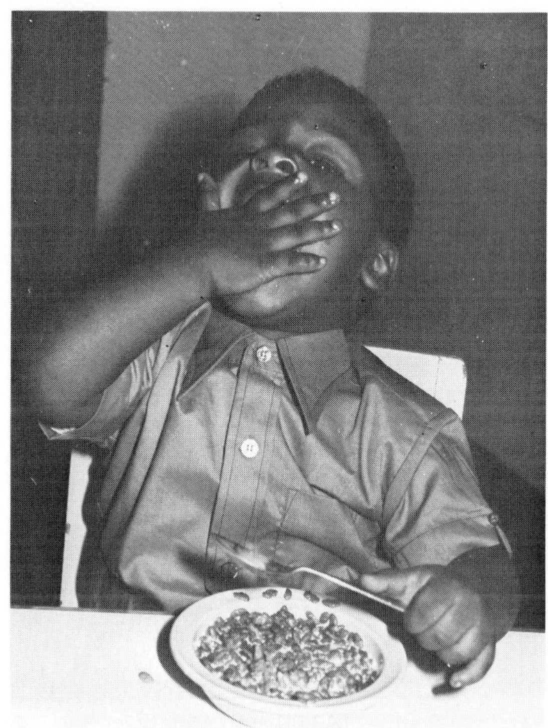

Figure 16-20 Toddlers like to feed themselves. (*From R. B. Howard and N. H. Herbold, Nutrition in Clinical Care, McGraw-Hill, New York, 1978, p. 233. Used with permission.*)

moved, or it may be left in place for 2 to 3 days before replacement is needed. The equipment required for gavage feeding is listed in Table 16-12. The steps in tube insertion and gavage feeding are described below. The technique outlined is for infant gavage feedings, but the principles are the same for older children. Modifications in the size of the tube and the type of feeding are necessary to accommodate the older child's nutritional needs.

Inserting the tube Using the nasogastric tube, measure from the tip of the infant's nose to the ear to a point midway between the xiphoid process and the umbilicus.[27] Using a small piece of tape, mark the tube to show how far it should be inserted.

Place the infant on his or her back. While restraining the head with one hand, quickly insert the tube through one nostril to the tape marker. (Use a mummy restraint to position the child if necessary.) Lubricate the tube with normal saline if mucous membranes are dry and the tube does not pass easily. If the infant begins to cough or choke or becomes cyanotic, remove the tube and reinsert it.

Check placement of the tube as follows:

1. Hold or tape the tube in place. Inject 1 ml of air while listening with a stethoscope over the stomach. A "pop" indicates correct placement. Gently withdraw the injected air.
2. Aspirate gently for gastric contents.

Table 16-12 Equipment Needed for Gavage Feeding

1. No. 5 to 8 French catheter 15 in long (nasogastric tube)
2. Nonallergenic tape
3. 3-ml syringe
4. Cup of sterile water
5. Stethoscope
6. Bulb suction
7. 30-ml syringe
8. Formula as ordered by the physician (warmed to room temperature)

3. Stimulate the infant to cry.
4. Invert the tube in a cup of sterile water while the child exhales. If bubbles appear, the tube may be in the lungs and should be removed immediately. Test only during exhalation to avoid the possibility that, if the tube is in the respiratory tract, the child might pull water from the cup into the lungs during inhalation.
5. Ask an older child to hum. If the tube is malpositioned and is between the vocal cords, the child will not be able to hum.

Once correct placement is confirmed, secure the tube by wrapping one strip of tape around it, and attach the free end above the upper lip. Place a second strip of tape over the tube. Secure the tube to the cheek by means of a third short strip of tape. Take care not to obstruct the nose.[28] Avoid taping the tube in any position that could cause pressure necrosis of the nasal cartilages. For example, this might happen if the tube were bent upward in order to tape it to the forehead.

The position of the tube should be checked every hour in infants and immediately prior to any feeding, using the preceding steps.

Feeding procedure Check the physician's order for the type, amount, and frequency of feeding. Draw up the formula in a 30-ml syringe. Position the infant on the right side, with the back supported by a blanket roll.[29] Elevate the head of the bed 15 to 30°.

Attach a syringe of formula to the tube, and infuse the contents by gravity at the rate of 3 ml/min. If the infant coughs, gags, or vomits, stop the feeding until this passes. (If respiratory distress occurs, stop the feeding, suction the infant, and recheck the tube's position.)[30]

To add formula, pinch the tube just before the syringe becomes empty. Refill the syringe and reattach it to the tube. Unclamp the tube so that flow resumes.

At the conclusion of the feeding, clear the tubing with 1 to 2 ml of sterile water, and either clamp the tube or leave it unclamped, according to the physician's orders. If vomiting is a problem, it may be necessary to leave it unclamped so that aspiration does not occur. The infant should be left undisturbed on his or her right side for 30 to 45 min, with the bed elevated 15 to 30°.

To remove the tube, first remove the tape at the nose, clamp the tube so that formula does not drip into the pharynx, and remove the tube quickly.[31,32]

Prior to each feeding, gastric contents should be aspirated. If residual fluid measures more than 2 ml, refeed it, and subtract the amount from that ordered for the next feeding. Report to the physician any abdominal distention and excessive amounts of formula remaining in the stomach at the time of the next feeding. Amounts fed may need to be reduced temporarily until the infant's tolerance increases.

Chart the time and location of gastric-tube insertion. Record the time, type, and amount of each feeding and the amount of the residual measured prior to the feeding.

Give oral care every 3 h while the tube is in place by wiping the infant's mouth with wet sterile gauze. Check for irritation of the nostril.

During the feeding, talk to the infant and stroke the back gently to increase relaxation and comfort. Provide a pacifier so that the infant can associate the feeling of fullness with sucking. If intermittent oral feedings are given, it is preferable to remove the nasogastric tube. This should be discussed with the physician. Hold and cuddle the infant during all oral feedings.

Snacks

Children need additional fluids and nutrients between meals. Confer with the physician (and dietitian) about the child's specific needs so that snacks—as well as meals—can be planned wisely.[33] Plan a snack time in the midmorning, midafternoon, and evening. This may be an excellent time to increase the caloric intake of a child who is recuperating from surgery (by giving a milk shake or other high-calorie food), but the snack must be planned so that it will not interfere with the appetite at mealtime. Snacks should not be given 1 to $1\frac{1}{2}$ h before mealtime. Some hospitals use a "five-meal-a-day" plan so that the diet is divided into five small meals rather than three large ones. This may be a good alternative for a child who is not eating well and cannot tolerate a large meal all at once.

The problem eater

Motivation Hospitalization and illness may decrease appetite and increase dependence. This is especially noticeable in young children who are accustomed to feeding themselves and then refuse to do so in the hospital. During the acute phase of an illness, it is appropriate to feed children. Each meal can be a time to encourage their involvement. As they improve, help them assume a normal position for eating at a table. Use small servings and remind them that they are improving and can now do more for themselves.

School-age children may be motivated by recording their own intake and output. Provide an easily accessible chart at the bedside so that they can write down what they eat and drink. A star chart or similar poster can also be a good motivational tool.

Give praise liberally for all evidence of improvement in eating habits. Include the doctor in the efforts to encourage a child to eat. The doctor's praise may be very significant to the child.

Improving the appearance of food Institutional food prepared in large amounts may not look very appetizing to a young child. Work with the dietitian to make the food trays look more attractive. Request small servings for young children. Tray favors and placemats made by volunteers or other patients can brighten up the serving trays.

Offer children the opportunity to request foods which they would like to eat or which are special favorites. Hamburgers, pizza, peanut butter and jelly sandwiches, milk shakes, and foods specific to a particular ethnic group can be highly nutritious. If the diet kitchen cannot provide them, encourage the parents to do so when appropriate.

Socialization at mealtime An area with child-sized tables and chairs is a pleasant eating environment. Sometimes children who are not eating well will be encouraged by seeing others eating. The distraction provided by the conversation of others may also help children forget about their discomforts and fears for a while and encourage them to eat.

When a child cannot leave his or her room to eat in the playroom, the parents may help by eating with the child in the room. Provide guest trays or allow them to bring in their own meals.

FLUIDS FOR HOSPITALIZED CHILDREN

Fluid requirements

A child's metabolic rate is much faster than that of an adult. As a consequence, a child needs more fluid in proportion to body weight than an adult. This is especially true of the younger child, whose fastest-growing tissues are the ones most active metabolically. It has been pointed out that, because the younger child weighs so much less than an adult, "there's a greater chance of overhydration through improper intravenous therapy."[34]

Determining fluid needs

The Segar table (Table 16-10) gives guidelines for determining caloric expenditures per kilogram of body weight. Since water needs (in milliliters) are approximately equal to caloric needs (in calories), the Segar guide can also be used to determine fluid needs. Fluid needs for infants weighing less than 3 kg must be determined by a more specific guide for neonates (see Chap. 8) and low-birth-weight infants (see Chap. 17). For example, to determine how much fluid a 30-lb child needs per day, convert pounds to kilograms:

30 lb ÷ 2.2 lb/kg = 13.6 kg

Then find weight excess over 10 kg:

13.6 − 10 = 3.6 kg

From the Segar formula:

100 kcal/kg for first 10 kg
= 100 × 10 = 1000 kcal

50 kcal/kg for each kilogram over 10 kg
= 50 × 3.6 = 180 kcal

Total caloric requirement = total fluid requirement = 1000 + 180 = 1180 kcal, or ml per day

This child requires maintenance fluids of 1180 ml per day.

The Segar formula provides minimal requirements. Additional fluids may be required to make up deficits. Infants and children who fail to grow need at least $1\frac{1}{2}$ times their normal requirement to gain weight.

Dehydration results from inadequate fluid intake in relation to normal or excessive fluid losses. When the body is unable to eliminate fluids adequately, fluid retention occurs. Signs of dehydration and fluid retention are listed in Table 16-13.

A child may receive an excessive amount of fluid and tolerate it well as long as electrolyte balance and renal function are normal. Such a situation would be accompanied by passage of a

Table 16-13 Signs of Dehydration and Fluid Retention

Dehydration	Fluid Retention
1. Dry skin and mucous membranes	1. Edema—puffy eyes, face, and ankles
2. Depressed fontanel	2. Dyspnea
3. Poor skin turgor	3. Abdominal distention
4. Sunken eyeballs	4. Weight gain
5. Thirst	5. Scanty urine output
6. Elevated temperature or, in severe cases, lowered temperature	6. Elevated blood pressure
7. Increased pulse rate	7. Decreased hematocrit
8. Weight loss	8. Distended neck veins
9. Dark or concentrated urine, increased specific gravity	
10. Decreased urine output	
11. Exhaustion and collapse	
12. Increased hematocrit	
13. Decrease or absence of tears	

large volume of dilute urine. Treatment involves decreasing the intravenous rate or oral intake.

The physician is responsible for calculating and ordering the fluids needed by the child, but the nurse should double-check the orders for accuracy and appropriateness according to the child's size. Fluids for maintaining adequate balance are made up of water plus electrolytes and such nonelectrolytes as dextrose and proteins. (Chapter 18 describes fluid and electrolyte balance in children.) The amount and type of fluids required are influenced by diagnosis, general condition, blood chemistry, and intake and output. Consideration must be given not only to maintenance fluid requirements but also to existing fluid deficits and abnormal, ongoing fluid losses.

Fluid intake and output

Measuring fluid intake The nurse must accurately measure the fluid intake of every pediatric patient. The child and the parents can help by keeping a daily record at the bedside. Transfer this information to the chart and make a cumulative total every 24 h. Fluid intake includes the following:

1. Fluids taken orally, including ice cream, popsicles, gelatin desserts, and so forth
2. Fluids given intravenously
3. Medications in liquid form taken orally
4. Medications given intravenously
5. Irrigating fluids

The child can also absorb fluids from a high-humidity environment (a mist tent or oxygen hood) or may lose excessive fluid during phototherapy (e.g., for hyperbilirubinemia). Discuss these factors with the physician when fluid needs are being determined.

It is helpful to have a standard list of the amount of fluid contained in cups and containers of various sizes, as shown in Fig. 16-21. Any nurse who removes a tray or soiled cup from a child's room is responsible for reporting or charting the amount taken.

Maintaining "nothing by mouth" It is challenging to care for the child whose fluid intake is restricted. Children may get water from the sink when thirsty. Roommates sometimes share their drinks. Carefully explain the rationale for fluid restriction to the child, the parents, and roommates and their families. Place signs on the door, on the bed, and on the child as reminders (Figs. 16-22 and 16-23).

Measuring fluid output Urine output in a child is monitored in a general way by placing a checkmark on the chart each time the child voids. Keeping accurate measurements of urine is essential when fluid balance is questionable. It is far better to measure urine when it is unnecessary than to overlook a measurement. When uncertain—measure! Have the child void in a bedpan, urinal, or potty-chair, or place a collecting device in the toilet.

Coffee mug	240 ml	Creamer	15 ml
Fruit juice cup	120 ml	Isolation bowl	270 ml
Soup bowl	240 ml	All soft drinks (12-oz can)	360 ml
Styrofoam cup	240 ml	Milk shake (7 oz)	210 ml
Disposable cup	120 ml	Sherbet-ice cream (Dixie cup)	65 ml
Milk: 8 oz.	240 ml	Gelatin	200 ml
Milk: 4 oz.	120 ml	Popsicle	120 ml
Isolation cup	210 ml		

Figure 16-21 A chart of the fluid volume of various containers appears on the flow sheet of each chart at Rochester Methodist Hospital to facilitate recording fluid intake. (*Courtesy of Rochester Methodist Hospital, Rochester, Minn.*)

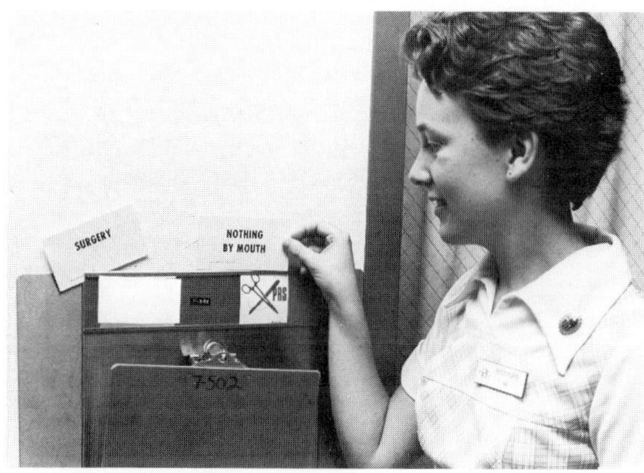

Figure 16-22 A nurse placing an NPO sign on a child's door. (*Photo by Brian Kaihoi.*)

Measure and record each voiding and calculate 24-h cumulative totals on any child who:

1. Is receiving intravenous fluids
2. Is receiving medication which requires urinary output for excretion (to be sure that the child will not be overdosed by an accumulation of medication) or which affects renal function
3. Is dehydrated, is retaining fluids, or is in acid-base disequilibrium
4. Has a known or suspected impairment of renal function
5. Has had surgery performed within the last 24 h or more, if necessary

All types of fluid output must be measured to give an accurate picture of fluid needs. Measure fluid from drains, chest tubes, nasogastric tubes, liquid stools, and emesis.

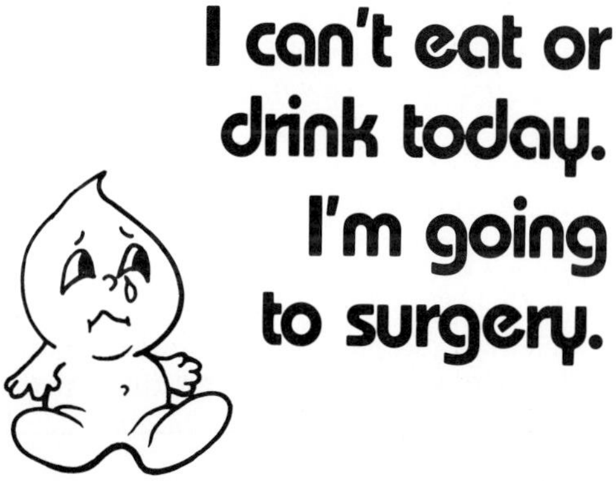

I can't eat or drink today. I'm going to surgery.

Figure 16-23 An NPO sign to be placed on a child's bed or back as a reminder that nothing is to be taken by mouth. (*Courtesy of Teresa Atkinson.*)

Weighing diapers Diapers are weighed to determine an infant's output. Use a metric scale (Fig. 16-24) and weigh the diaper immediately; do not let it dry out. Subtract the weight of a dry diaper from that of the wet one. Diapers can be weighed before using, and the weight written on the diaper. The difference (in grams) is approximately equal to the amount of urine (in milliliters) in the wet diaper; 1 ml weighs approximately 1 g. Record the amount of urine on the chart and indicate that it was obtained by weighing the diaper.

Measuring body weight Body weight is an indicator of fluid needs and should be measured daily before breakfast for any child on accurate intake and output. Weight is always obtained on admission. Closer monitoring is required, however, if a child receives intravenous fluids or begins retaining fluids.

Methods of encouraging fluid intake Pain or drug therapy which causes drowsiness or irritability may adversely affect the child's ability to cooperate and willingness to drink. A thorough assessment of all the reasons why the child's intake is diminished must be done before appropriate intervention can be initiated.

Encourage the child to take fluids orally by offering choices. Popsicles, ice cream, milk shakes, slushes, and juices provide variety. Use small cups—even medicine cups—rather than large containers. Give pain medication judi-

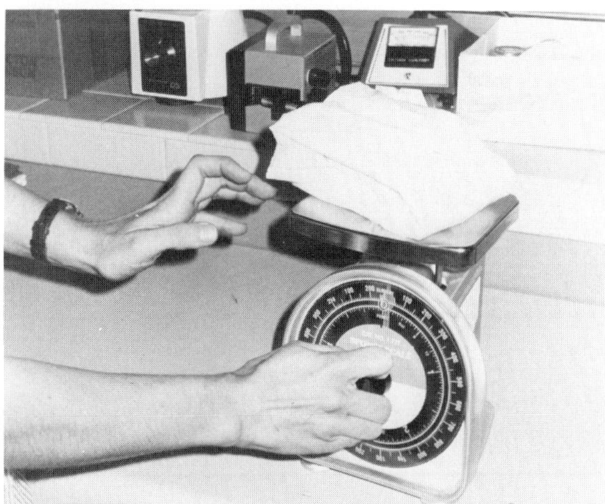

Figure 16-24 The gram scale is calibrated with a dry diaper. The wet diaper is then placed on the scale in order to measure urine output; 1 g equals 1 ml.

ciously to increase comfort before encouraging intake. Star charts, "cup" posters (the child makes paper symbols and pastes one on the poster for each cup of liquid he or she drinks), and tea parties in the playroom are other possibilities. Effective approaches should be documented on the Kardex nursing care plan. It is well worth spending time to get a child to drink if intravenous therapy can be avoided.

Intravenous fluid therapy

Intravenous (IV) fluid therapy is used to:

1. Provide adequate fluids to the child who cannot take them orally
2. Provide a means for the safe and effective administration of parenteral medications
3. Correct electrolyte imbalance

Initiating intravenous therapy Because children have smaller veins than adults, different sites for intravenous infusions may be used. Scalp veins are often used in infants. Superficial veins of the arms, hands, and lower legs may be used in a child of any age.

Of special concern to the nurse is prevention of circulatory overload and subsequent heart failure. To ensure the child's safety, the nurse must provide the correct equipment, monitor the infusion closely, and maintain the patency of the infusion.

Intravenous fluids are usually available in plastic bags or glass bottles in sizes of 250 ml, 500 ml, and 1000 ml. A volume control chamber (Soluset or Buretrol), attached to the intravenous fluid container, allows only small amounts (100 to 150 ml maximum) to be available for infusion at a given time (Fig. 16-25). A stopcock between the chamber and the IV bag allows the nurse to control the flow to the chamber and is a safety feature in preventing fluid overload. Intravenous infusion sets have either the standard drip chamber (15 gtt/ml) or the "minidrip" chamber (60gtt/ml). Minidrip sets are preferable for use with children because the flow can be regulated to a very slow rate. Various intravenous pumps are also available. (Refer to the section "Intravenous Therapy Monitors" later in this chapter.)

Intravenous tubing is available in various lengths and with Y connections to allow IV medications to be attached and infused as needed. Needles used include scalp-vein needles, short

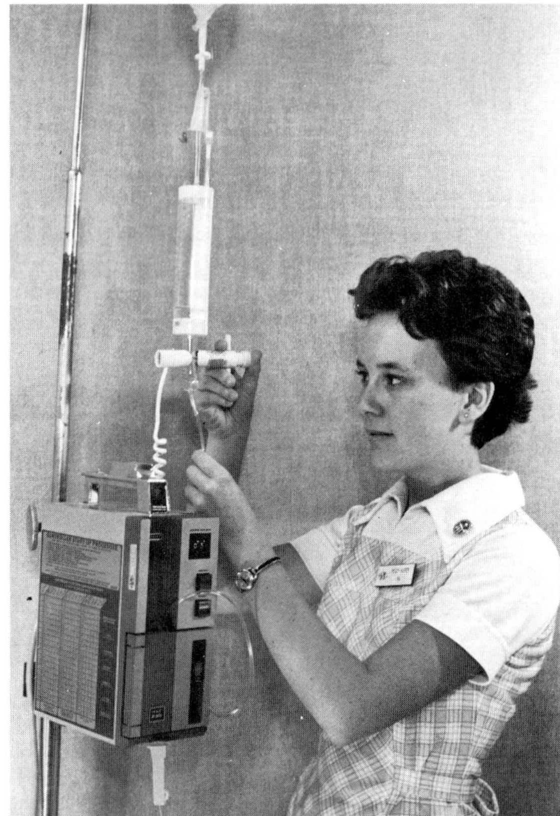

Figure 16-25 This nurse is preparing intravenous fluid. The clear plastic chamber (volume control chamber) and the pump are safety features to control rate and volume. (*Photo by Brian Kaihoi.*)

plastic needles for standard infusions, and intravenous catheters for infusion into a cutdown site (Fig. 16-26).

The nurse's role in starting IV therapy is described below.[35] It is assumed that the physician or specially prepared nurse will perform the venipuncture.

1. Prepare the child and the parents for the procedure. Describe how it will feel and the child's expected activity level during the infusion. Remind the child that the needle will not hurt after the initial venipuncture. Show the child the equipment. Begin the procedure soon after preparation is completed.
2. Wash hands well.
3. Gather and prepare equipment (Table 16-14).
4. Bring the child to a treatment room away from other patients.

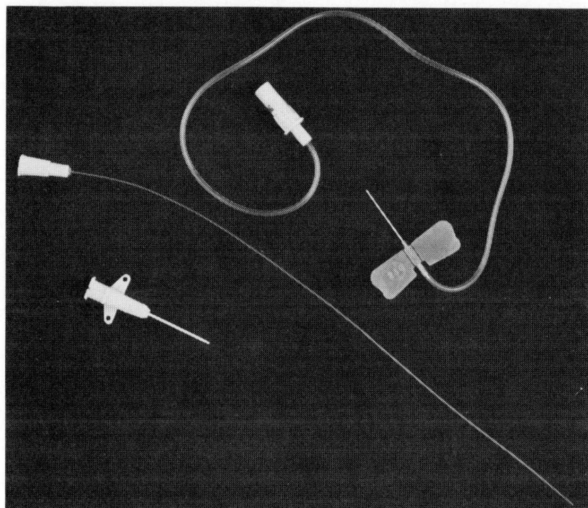

Figure 16-26 Various needles used in intravenous therapy.

Table 16-14 Equipment Needed for Intravenous Therapy

IV fluid. (Check type and amount. Make sure it is clear and free of foreign material.)
Tubing with minidrip chamber, needles, and scalp-vein sets. (Have a variety of sizes available.)
T connector
5-ml syringe
Bottle of parenteral normal saline
Volume control chamber
IV filter
Tourniquet or rubber band (used as a tourniquet for scalp-vein influsions)
Safety razor
Tape
Padded arm board
Gauze roll or stockinette
Betadine and alcohol (for cleansing site)
Antibiotic or iodine ointment for application to site after insertion
Half of a medicine cup padded with tape for site protection (see Fig. 16-28).
3- by 3-in gauze pads and cotton balls
Infusion pump
Intravenous pole
Light source

Source: Modified from D. A. Millam, "How to Insert an IV," *American Journal of Nursing* **79** (7):1268 (July 1979).

5. Get adequate assistance: one nurse to help restrain the child, one to handle equipment, and the physician or intravenous nurse to perform the venipuncture. It is generally best to have the parents wait outside and comfort the child afterward, unless they or the child insists on their presence.[36]
6. Prepare a syringe of sterile saline in case it will be needed to check the site.
7. Connect the tubing and volume chamber to the IV fluid and hang them on the pole. Fill the volume chamber and clear the tubing of air.
8. Mount the pump on the pole and check the alarm and battery. Plug the pump in, but leave the switch off until needed.
9. Help with site determination so that the dominant hand may be free for play, thumb-sucking, or eating. Millam advises: "If infusion time is to be long-term and successive starts are anticipated over a number of days, beginning with the superficial vessels in the hand will permit progressively upward selection of later sites."[37]
10. Position the child and talk to the child gently during site selection. Do not restrain the child until absolutely necessary for needle insertion. Tell the child that it is okay to cry but that he or she can help by being very still during the procedure.
11. If an extremity is used, assist in securing it to an arm board. Place gauze pads under tape to decrease discomfort and prevent skin abrasion. Check circulation to make sure that the tape is not too tight. A scalp site must be shaved, and the head positioned securely for needle insertion.
12. The site is cleansed, and the needle inserted (Fig. 16-27*A*). Apply small strips of tape to secure the needle. Use clear tape over the site to increase visibility. Figure 16-27*A* and *B* shows two methods of taping the needle at the site.
13. Cover the site with half a medicine cup and tape the cup in place (Fig. 16-28), or wrap the site and board with gauze or stockinette to cover the site and prevent the need for a restraint. The site must be checked every hour for signs of infiltration or phlebitis, and so it must be accessible as well as protected.
14. Tape connections throughout the tubing, and place the tape on the tubing and the bag, which should be labeled with the date and the time the intravenous therapy was started.
15. Attach the intravenous line to the pump, set the rate, and switch the pump on.
16. Comfort the child and have the parents come in to be with the child.

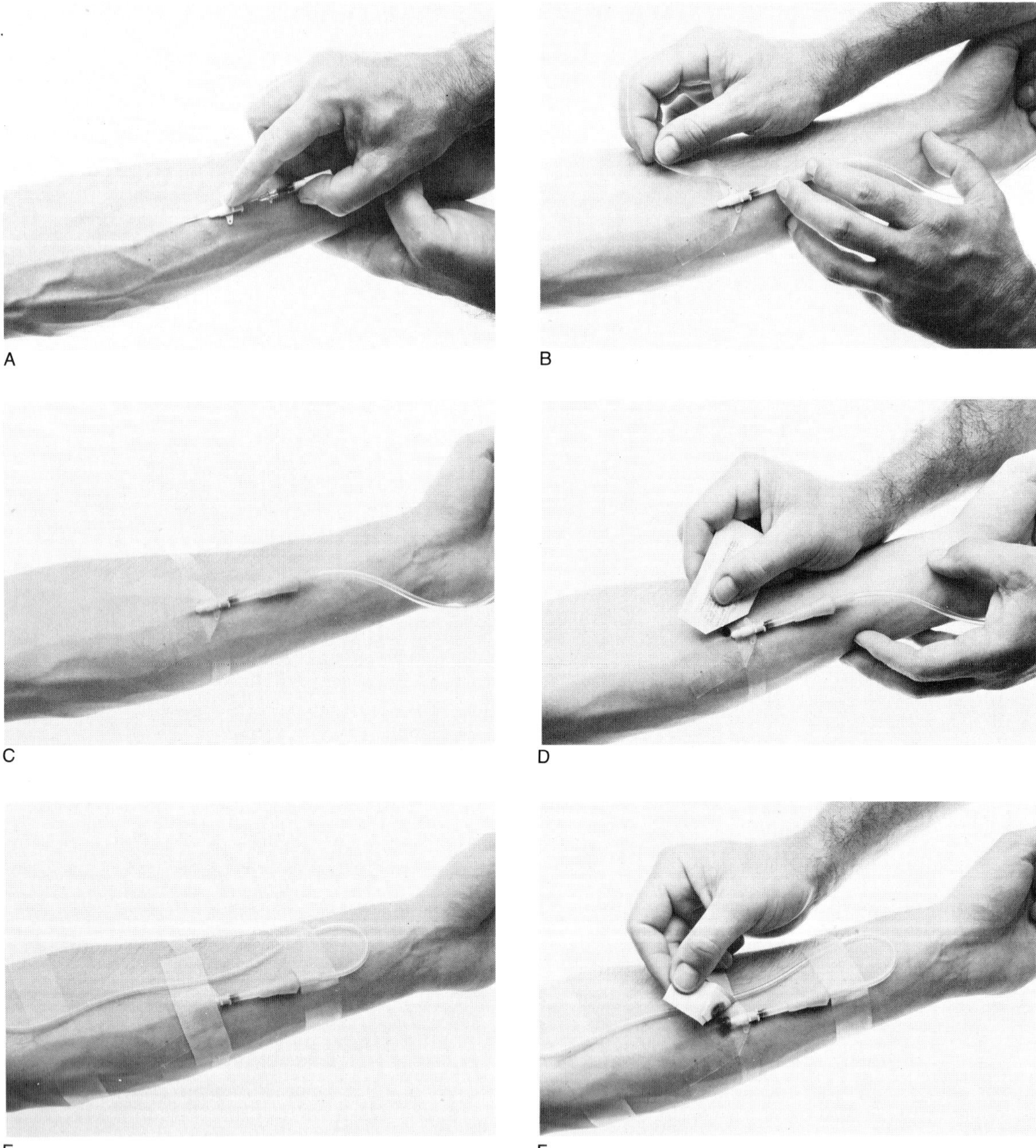

Figure 16-27 A method of securing an intravenous needle for infusion. (*A*) The intravenous catheter is inserted into the vein. (*B*) To secure the catheter properly, a piece of tape 5 in long and $\frac{1}{2}$ in wide is placed under the wings of the catheter, adhesive side up. (*C*) Each end is folded forward in the direction of the catheter insertion, forming a V configuration. A second piece of tape should be placed over the catheter hub. The tape is not placed over or near the skin puncture site. (*D*) Topical ointment can be applied after the catheter is securely taped to the patient. (*E*) The skin puncture site should be covered with a sterile dressing. (*F*) The dressing can be removed easily for site inspection and maintenance without risk of disturbing or cutting the tape securing the catheter hub. (*Courtesy of Vicra Division, Travenol Laboratories, Inc.*)

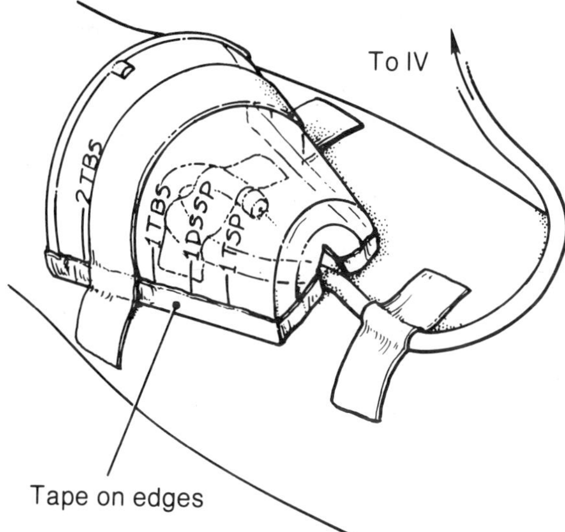

Figure 16-28 Half a medicine cup to be used for protecting an intravenous site. The edges should be padded for comfort.

17. Check the pump rate by counting the drops infused per minute.
18. Return the child to his or her room and provide a pleasant activity.
19. Clean and replace the equipment used.

Maintaining the IV site A major part of the nurse's role is that of maintaining the site after intravenous therapy is initiated. The younger and more active the child is, the more difficult it is to maintain the site. Being aware of the possible problems is essential.

Infiltration is the accumulation of intravenous fluid in extravascular tissue. It is the most common complication of an infusion and occurs when the venipuncture device penetrates the vein and the wall beyond or becomes dislodged during normal insertion.[38]

Phlebitis is an inflammation of a vein. Some factors that contribute to the development of phlebitis include:

1. Chemical irritation by the intravenous solution
2. Mechanical irritation by the intravenous device
3. An allergic reaction to the intravenous device
4. Trauma during venipuncture
5. Infection via a skin defect or contamination of the intravenous apparatus[39]

Although the signs of phlebitis and infiltration are similar, there are a few differences, which are important to note (Table 16-15).

In maintaining the intravenous site, the nurse must maintain the correct flow rate, prevent infection, and keep the needle in place. Specifically, the nurse must take the following steps:

1. Check and record the intravenous rate every 30 to 60 min.
2. Watch for kinks in the tubing and position the child so that he or she is not lying on the tubing. Assist the parent who wishes to hold the child and keep the tubing free of obstruction.
3. If the flow rate is affected by normal movement:
   a. Use sandbags to prevent an infant's head from resting on the scalp-vein site.
   b. Use a short, padded, lightweight arm board. Secure it to the skin with adhesive padded with gauze.[40]
   c. Secure the arm board to the bed with a pin or tape if necessary.
4. Observe the site at least every hour for signs of infiltration. Stop the intravenous flow and call the physician or venipuncture nurse if infiltration occurs. Since certain drugs and electrolytes are extremely irritating and can cause tissue damage, infiltration should be the signal to stop infusion.
5. Perform site care according to the hospital's infection control policies. This usually means changing the tape, cleansing with antiseptic, and applying an iodine or antibiotic ointment at the site every 24 to 48 h.
6. Secure the needle well at the site. If the flow seems to be obstructed, the bevel of the needle may be against the vein wall; a small piece

Table 16-15 Signs of Infiltration vs. Phlebitis

Infiltration	Phlebitis
Blanching	Redness
Cold skin	Hot skin
Pain	Palpable, cordlike vein
Sensation of heaviness	Pain
Swelling	Sensation of heaviness
Tenderness	Swelling
	Tenderness

Source: Adapted from "Fundamentals of IV Maintenance," programmed instruction, *American Journal of Nursing* 1275, (July 1979).

of cotton placed under the hub of the needle may position it properly.

7. Restrain the child's other extremity (i.e., the opposite leg or arm) if it interferes with the intravenous infusion.

Cutdown At times it is impossible to find an appropriate venipuncture site on a small child, and a cutdown (incision into a vein) becomes necessary. This is a sterile procedure which can be performed in the nursing unit. In addition to standard IV fluid equipment, a cutdown tray, sterile gloves, masks, and an intravenous catheter are needed. The physician incises the skin, dissects a vein free, inserts the sterile catheter, sutures it in place, and attaches the intravenous tubing. The ankle is a common site for a cutdown on an infant. Check the specific hospital procedure for information about site care. Observe the site and the skin above it frequently for signs of phlebitis, since the catheter may extend several inches into the vein. The physician is responsible for discontinuing a cutdown.

Discontinuing an intravenous infusion Explain what is going to be done and reassure the child that taking the needle out does not hurt, as inserting it did. Allow the child to assist in tape removal.

To discontinue the infusion, turn off the IV pump, clamp off the tubing, loosen and remove the tape. Hold sterile gauze—alcohol stings and has an anticoagulant property—over the site and withdraw the needle. Elevate the extremity and apply pressure with a gauze pad over the site of skin puncture and over the site of entry into the vein, which may be 1 to 2 cm higher in the extremity. Maintain pressure for 1 to 2 min. Place an adhesive bandage over the site. If a large-gauge needle (no. 19 or larger) was used for the infusion, a pressure dressing (a gauze pad secured tightly with gauze bandage) may be necessary for 10 to 15 min to stop the bleeding.[41]

Safety during intravenous therapy There are a number of areas of concern during intravenous therapy with children. The following are important:

1. Use a volume control chamber with all pediatric patients except when the child is receiving more fluid per hour than the chamber will hold.
2. Do not put more than a 2-h supply of fluid into the volume chamber at any time.
3. Change the fluid and the tubing every 24 h and label the bag with the date, the time changed, and your initials.
4. The physician's order should include the type of fluid and a specific rate—not KVO (keep vein open).[42]
5. Frequently check the restraints and the tape to make sure that they are effective and are allowing adequate circulation. Release the restraints every 2 h and do range-of-motion exercises, unless contraindicated by the intravenous site.
6. Frequently check the extremities and scalp for signs of pressure sores.
7. Tape connections and the rate control clamp to prevent tampering by a curious child.[43]
8. Supervise a child who has an intravenous infusion at all times when he or she is out of bed.
9. Do not develop a false sense of security when the intravenous pump is used. Double-check the pumping rate by your watch. Use an *air-eliminating filter with infusion tubing when a pump is to be used.* Some pumps will pump air as well as fluid.[44] Know the pump's limitations and check it frequently.
10. Throughout intravenous therapy remember that you are caring for a child and not an intravenous bag. Observe the child's general condition, vital signs, and emotional response to the infusion. Provide comfort and diversional activities; remember that a child can sit up in a chair or ride in a wagon and have a change of scenery, even with an intravenous infusion.
11. *Document* the following carefully: date, time, and type and amount of fluid hung; rate and volume infused every hour; site care and condition of the site; accurate intake and output; and daily weight.

Heparin lock The heparin lock is an ideal temporary measure for maintaining an infusion site for intermittent use. There is less chance of fluid overload and phlebitis, and the child is more mobile and comfortable.[45]

Heparin sodium is an anticoagulant available in a heparin lock flush solution (Wyeth). A heparin lock infusion set (a needle and a short catheter with an injection cap) is inserted into a vein, usually in the arm, and taped securely. Dilute heparin sodium is injected via the injection hub in a quantity sufficient to fill the set to the needle tip. The dilute heparin must be reinstilled after each use (e.g., after an intravenous medication is infused or blood is drawn).[46] For children, a heparin solution of 10 units per milliliter should be adequate to keep the lock open.[47] If a drug to be administered is incompatible with heparin, the entire heparin lock set should be flushed with sterile water or normal saline before and after the medication is administered; following the second flush the dilute heparin may be reinstilled into the heparin lock set.[48]

Contraindications to a heparin lock include an allergy to heparin and the presence of any type of bleeding disorder.

To maintain a heparin lock, the nurse must check the site frequently, give site care, and protect the site by wrapping, using a medicine cup, or both.

Intravenous therapy monitors A variety of intravenous therapy monitors are available to facilitate maintenance of safe IV flow rates, vein patency, and controlled administration of medications. Most pumps also contain a battery unit so that they will function when unplugged for a short time (e.g., during tub baths, walks, or trips for tests).

Peristaltic pumps, such as the IVAC monitor shown in Fig. 16-25, move fluid by compressing the IV tubing with either a rotary or a linear device. Rotary devices use a disk that alternately squeezes and releases a section of the tubing. Linear devices use a series of fingerlike projections to propel the fluid through the tubing.[49]

The IMED pump (Fig. 16-29) is a cassette-piston pump that applies pressure to the fluid rather than the tubing. The sterile cassette is connected to the IV tubing and then is attached to the pump itself.[50]

Another type of pump is the small-volume infusion system, which consists of a spring-loaded infuser, flow-regulating tubing, and a syringe. Flow controllers are available to administer rates of 0.5, 1.0, 10, and 30 ml per hour. In a research study by Bosso, the infusion system was used to instill medications through heparin locks intermittently and to deliver very small amounts of fluid at very slow infusion rates. In the latter use, the small-volume pump was especially effective in maintaining venous and arterial lines in premature infants because of the even, consistent pressure and flow provided. This type of pump is also small and easily portable, making it very useful when working with pediatric patients[51] of all ages.

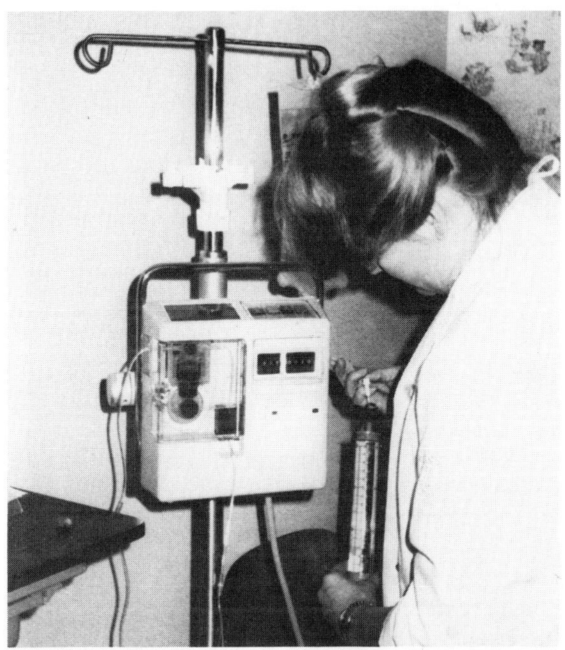

Figure 16-29 The IMED intravenous pump uses a cassette and positive pressure on the IV fluid to produce movement into the vein.

Central venous catheters (right atrial catheters) Central venous catheters may be inserted into the right atrium of the heart to provide a semipermanent means of administering drugs (as in cancer chemotherapy and bone marrow transplantation), total parenteral nutrition (TPN), and blood products and to access blood samples for diagnostic tests. When the catheter is not in use, it may be "heparin-locked" to ensure patency and allow the child freedom of activity. Port-a-Cath is an implantable catheter system that consists of a self-sealing injection port placed under the skin, where it is connected to the central arterial or venous catheter.[52] The system can be repeatedly accessed through the skin for blood sampling, drug delivery, or TPN (see Fig. 16-30).

There are several commonly used right atrial catheters. The Hickman and Broviac are two types. These can be combined in one sleeve. Double lumen atrial catheters permit delivery of

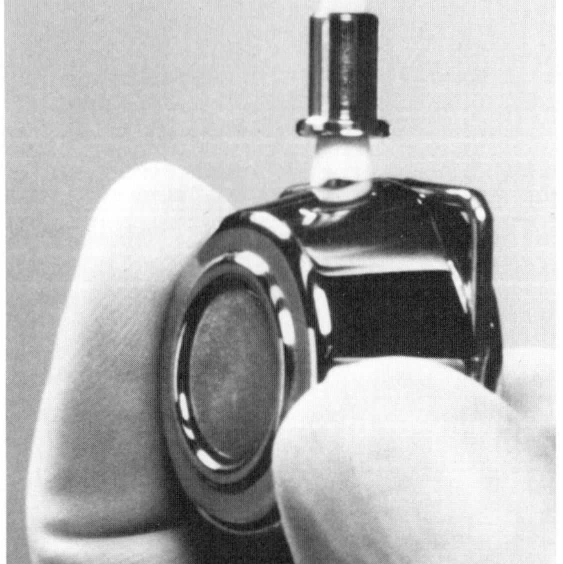

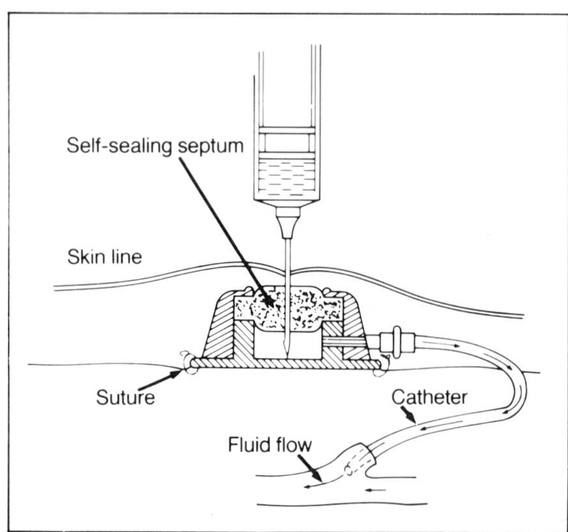

Figure 16-30 (*A*) The Port-a-Cath, which is placed under the skin. (*B*) The port is located by palpation; the needle is inserted perpendicular to the septum through the skin until it hits the bottom of the portal chamber. (*Photo courtesy of Pharmacia Inc.*)

blood products and antibiotics in the larger line and use of the smaller line for TPN.[53]

The central catheter is inserted during a surgical procedure through either the external jugular vein or the cephalic vein. After the vein is identified through a surgical incision, a subcutaneous tunnel is formed, exiting at a site between the sternum and the nipple. The catheter is pulled through the tunnel into the vein and is positioned at the entrance to the right atrium in the lower superior vena cava. A Dacron cuff attached to the catheter is positioned in the subcutaneous tunnel; it acts as a barrier to infection and also prevents removal of the catheter.[54] To prevent tunnel infection, dressing changes at the exit site are done twice daily with sterile technique using hydrogen peroxide, betadine swabs, and ointment. These lines also must be flushed with heparinized solutions to maintain patency. The parents (and the child, if old enough) are taught about the care and maintenance of these lines before discharge.

Detailed instructions for the care of central venous catheters are not included here, since they may vary from hospital to hospital as well as from product to product. Doran's review of the specific differences between care of the catheter in adults and care of the catheter in children is a helpful reference.[55] A further discussion of nursing management of the child who is receiving total parenteral nutrition appears in Chap. 19.

OXYGENATION

Methods of providing moist oxygen

When a respiratory problem is identified, one important treatment may be the provision of oxygen with moisture. Increased oxygen in the inspired air facilitates the transfer of oxygen to the blood in the lungs. Added moisture prevents drying of mucous membranes and may help in decreasing inflammatory processes in the airway.

Oxygen hoods Oxygen hoods are effective for administering high levels of oxygen to an infant. The cylindrical plastic hood fits over the infant's neck and surrounds the head. Checks of vital signs and other care can be given without affecting the oxygen concentration. The hood allows administration of oxygen in concentrations of up to 100 percent. Since it covers the head, nursing responsibilities include maintaining a warm environment and monitoring the infant's temperature so that oxygen requirements are not unduly increased by efforts to stay warm. The moist oxygen should be warmed (31 to 34°C [87.8 to 93.2°F]) to prevent cold stress. An oxygen hood (Fig. 21-7) has an attached thermometer which constantly registers the temperature of the hood air.

Oxygen masks and face tents Moist oxygen can also be administered through masks or face tents. They are convenient for use with older children, but the child's and the family's cooperation is essential. Although the percentage of oxygen delivered is variable, masks are usually adequate for the administration of moist oxygen during the immediate postoperative period. A face tent (Fig. 16-31) is better tolerated by most children than a face mask because it fits loosely and does not resemble the anesthesia mask, which is frightening to some children. The face tent is held near the child's face while the child sits with a parent or is placed near the child in bed. As the child moves in his or her sleep, the family member in attendance helps by moving the tent with the child. Although straps are available to secure the tent to the child's face, they usually are not tolerated well.

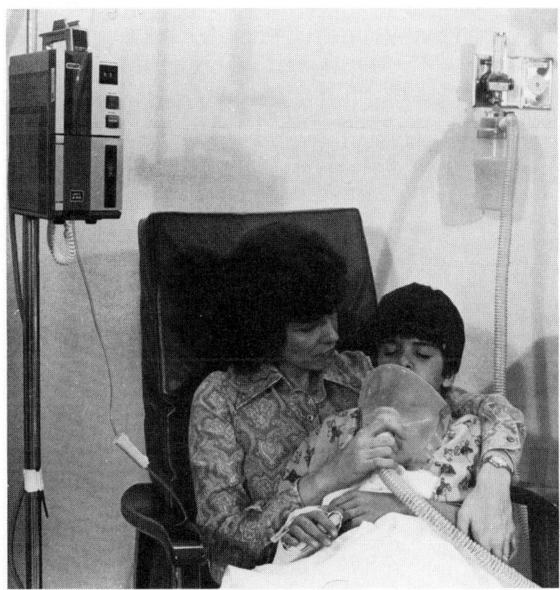

Figure 16-31 An oxygen face tent on a child. The child can be held by the mother despite the presence of the equipment. (*Photo by Brian Kaihoi.*)

Nasal cannulas and catheters Nasal cannulas and catheters are important tools used in oxygen therapy. Nasal cannulas are useful when transporting oxygen-dependent infants and children for diagnostic tests or other procedures. Humidity should be maintained during oxygen administration to prevent drying and irritation of mucous membranes.

Nasal catheters have been used effectively with infants requiring long-term oxygen therapy. In a study by Guilfoile and Dabe,[56] the nasal catheter provided oxygen concentrations comparable to those provided by the oxygen tent and head hood during sleeping, waking, and crying states. The nasal catheter provided better oxygenation than the conventional method of holding an oxygen line to the infant's face during feeding. Nasal catheters allow increased mobility of the infant, provide more consistent oxygen concentrations, and allow more sensory stimulation. A nasal catheter is inserted just out of sight, with the tip in the oropharynx behind the uvula. This position seems to be well tolerated. Complications such as excessive nasal discharge, inflammation of the nasal mucosa, and frequent catheter dislodgement may occur, but the use of nasal catheters in certain infants can be very appropriate and effective.[57]

Mist tents A mist tent is a large plastic canopy that can be used for a child of any age. It provides high-humidity oxygen and allows the child freedom of movement. Its small counterpart, the croupette, can be used with infants and children under 3.

Mist tents are available with a nebulizer for the water and may have an open-topped canopy or closed canopy with an air-conditioning unit (Fig. 16-32). In the first type, the top is open to allow circulation of the air and escape of the carbon dioxide. Since oxygen is heavier than room air, it settles to the lower part of the tent. Do not place a towel or blanket over the open top to keep the mist from escaping. Though such a covering does not totally prevent the escape of carbon dioxide, it creates a "stuffy" atmosphere. If a greater mist concentration is needed, an ultrasonic nebulizer may be attached through the zippered opening or the top of the canopy. Some tents have ice troughs, which may be used to

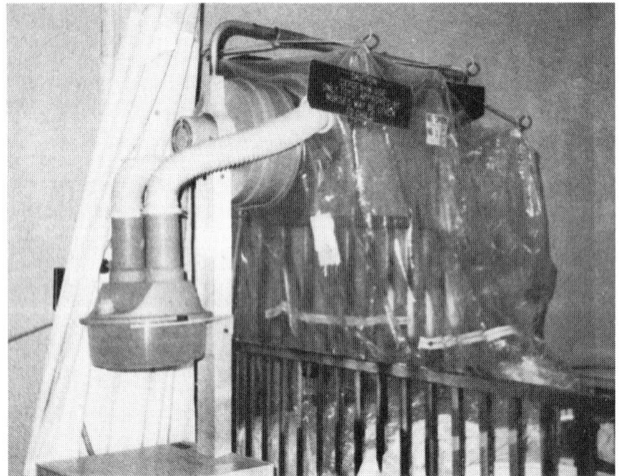

Figure 16-32 An oxygen mist tent over the crib of a child with a respiratory infection.

decrease the tent temperature and cool a feverish child. Some mist tents use compressed air.

Nursing care activities for a child in a mist tent are as follows:

1. Prepare the child and the parents by age-appropriate means:
   a. Set the tent up. Let the child feel the mist and hear the sound inside.
   b. Place a safe toy inside.
   c. Have a parent extend his or her head inside.
   d. Explain how, why, and when the mist tent will be used.
2. Before placing the child inside, turn on the oxygen flow for 10 to 15 min so that it is mist-filled and cool.
3. Place the child inside with a safe toy. (See the section "Fire Prevention" later in this chapter.)
4. Tuck the top and sides of the tent under the edge of the mattress. Secure the bottom edge by folding a blanket over the end and securing it under the mattress on each side.
5. Check the oxygen concentration periodically—every 4 to 24 h, according to the respiratory therapy policy of the hospital—and record it on the chart.
6. Check the nebulizer or water reservoir and refill with sterile distilled water every 8 h or more often as needed.
7. Change the child's clothing and bed linen when it is damp. Use a bath blanket on top of the bottom sheet. (A blanket is more comfortable and warm in the tent because it absorbs some of the moisture.)
8. Organize nursing care to decrease the number of times the tent is opened.
9. Set times for the child to be out—e.g., during meals, and every 2 h to be held—according to the child's needs and tolerance for room air. Return the child to the tent if signs of respiratory distress develop. (See Chap. 21 for signs of respiratory distress.)
10. Keep the tent oxygen on if the child is out for a brief period. For longer periods, turn it off and then flush with oxygen 15 min before the child returns to it.
11. When transporting a child in bed with the tent, raise the sides of the tent to prevent hypoxia when the oxygen is turned off.
12. Monitor the child's physical response, color, rate and type of respirations, and other vital signs frequently, and chart this information on the nurses' notes or flow sheet.
13. Give the child attention and diversion. Play with the child even though he or she is in the tent.
14. Change the tent and equipment according to hospital policy. Mist tents readily become contaminated with bacteria.

Ultrasonic nebulizers Ultrasonic nebulizers provide high humidity in very fine droplets which are easily absorbed and helpful in resolving inflammation of the airway (Fig. 16-8). Because the ultrasonic nebulizer provides large amounts of easily absorbed moisture, some authors recommend that it not be used for small children because it may alter fluid balance. If an infant receives treatment with an ultrasonic nebulizer, monitor the infant's weight and vital signs frequently.

Vaporizers Vaporizers, which increase the humidity in room air, are available in a variety of types. Figure 16-33 shows two different kinds used in hospitals. The cold vaporizer is used 24 h a day after the child's respiratory illness no longer indicates the need for a mist tent. Parents are encouraged to use cold vaporizers for home care of children with respiratory illnesses. (Hot vaporizers can cause burns.)

Safety factors in oxygen therapy

Maintaining oxygen saturation Room air contains approximately 20 percent oxygen; 40 percent oxygen is generally considered therapeutic, though physicians may order higher con-

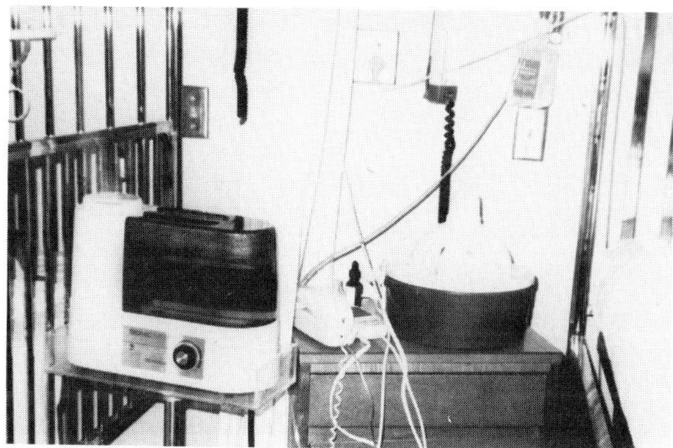

Figure 16-33 Two types of cold vaporizers or humidifiers for use at the bedside.

centrations in certain situations. In order to maintain a saturation of approximately 40 percent, the following flow meter rates are recommended:

2 to 4 liters per minute—infant incubator
5 to 8 liters per minute—croupette
10 to 12 liters per minute—larger tents[58]

Monitoring oxygenation When a child is receiving oxygen therapy, the oxygen concentration must be monitored with an oxygen analyzer at least every 8 h. Oxygen for the newborn must be monitored continuously. For older children, periodic analysis is usually sufficient.

To accurately determine the oxygen content of the child's environment, place the analyzer tube near the child's face—not just inside the top of a mist tent or isolette. The analysis should be done when the tent or isolette has been closed for at least 15 min.

Since various types of oxygen monitors are available, check the instructions for use printed on the side of the monitor. To ensure accuracy, each monitor must be calibrated (i.e., checked for the accuracy of its reading) periodically according to the manufacturer's instructions.

Chart the results of oxygen analysis on the child's medical record and indicate calibration of the monitor as necessary.

Checking for oxygen toxicity Prolonged exposure to high oxygen tensions can be damaging to some body tissues and functions.[59] Use of oxygen for a long period or high concentrations of oxygen (70 to 80 percent) for a short time may result in pulmonary changes.[60] There is evidence to indicate that damage to lung capillaries can occur, causing diffuse microhemorrhagic changes, diminished mucus flow, and inactivation of surfactant. Ventilation is gradually impaired as these changes occur.[61]

The premature infant treated with high concentrations of oxygen can develop *retrolental fibroplasia*. In this condition of the eyes, vasoconstriction of the blood vessels of the retina progresses to endothelial damage, obliteration of the vessels, and eventual blindness.[62]

The nurse who cares for a child receiving long-term or high concentrations of oxygen must be alert to signs of oxygen toxicity: depressed respirations, somnolence, and coma. Check vital signs and oxygen concentration every 1 to 4 h (or continuously in the newborn and premature infant). Periodic blood gas determinations are made to monitor arterial oxygen levels.[63]

Infection control during oxygen therapy The high-humidity environment used in oxygen administration provides a good medium for bacterial growth.[64] The following steps are helpful in maintaining cleanliness of the equipment:

1. Change all equipment every 5 to 7 days.
2. When needed, add sterile distilled water to the water reservoir or nebulizer in the following manner:
   a. Discard any remaining water first.
   b. Rinse the nebulizer and tubing before adding sterile distilled water.

   Distilled water is used in respiratory equipment because the minerals and salts in tap water or saline are damaging.
3. Take periodic cultures of the equipment according to the recommendations of the infection control committee.

Accumulation of moisture With the mask, hood, or ultrasonic nebulizer, there may be accumulation of moisture in the tubing connecting the oxygen source to the equipment. This interferes with oxygen flow, makes a disturbing "bubbling" noise, and can soak the child thoroughly if the tubing is moved. Watch the tubing for moisture accumulation, and drain the water into a basin rather than returning it to the nebulizer.

Fire prevention Because oxygen supports combustion, several safety principles must be adhered to during its use:

1. *Do not* use electric equipment in an oxygen tent.

2. Use all-cotton clothing and bed linens to prevent production of static electricity.
3. Do not use alcohol or oil products on a child or infant during oxygen therapy.
4. Choose toys carefully so that they meet the above guidelines (e.g., no toys which produce sparks).
5. Check room electrical cords for frayed wires.
6. Do not allow smoking by visitors.
7. Place signs in the room, on the bed, and on the door of the room indicating that oxygen is in use and that necessary safety precautions must be taken.

Techniques to improve oxygenation

Positioning Elevate the head of the bed to facilitate an open airway and chest expansion. This may be accomplished for an infant by elevating the mattress with a blanket or pillow or positioning the child in an infant seat. Do not use a pillow under the head of an infant or young child. A pillow may push the head forward and obstruct the trachea. Elevating the mattress provides a more physiologically normal position. If an infant seat is used, secure it with a sandbag and strap the infant in place to prevent falling.

Suctioning Keep a bulb suction in the crib of an infant for aspiration of mucus and emesis from the child's mouth and nose. Turn the infant to the side to suction so that obstructing fluids are more accessible. Rinse the bulb with water after each use. Replace with a clean one daily.

If congestion is severe, use a mechanical suction machine with a catheter small enough to pass easily though the nose and into the child's throat. Table 16-16 lists the steps in suctioning a child.

Table 16-16 Steps in Suctioning a Child

1. Use normal saline for lubrication.
2. Clamp the catheter during insertion. Pass the catheter through the nose to the back of the throat.
3. Unclamp and suction during catheter removal.
4. Suction quickly (5 to 10 s maximum in the airway) and allow the child to catch his or her breath before reinserting the catheter.
5. Rinse the catheter in saline and reinsert.
6. Suction only in the back of the throat. Do not perform deep tracheal suction. There is a danger of laryngospasm and apnea, especially in young infants.
7. Suction the mouth as needed.

Chest physiotherapy Chest physiotherapy is used to prevent or treat conditions in which there is excessive mucus in the bronchi that is not being removed by normal coughing or ciliary action.[65] Techniques used include deep breathing, coughing, postural drainage, percussion, vibration, and suctioning when necessary.

Deep breathing Have the child take several deep breaths. Ask the child to blow up a balloon, or use "blow bottles" or an incentive spirometer (Tri-Flow R) to stimulate deep breathing.[66] Make a game of blowing objects across the bedside table.

Coughing Encourage periodic coughing during deep breathing as well as during other components of chest physiotherapy. Have the child sit up. Encircle the child's chest with your hands and compress the rib cage as he or she tries to cough. Splint any abdominal or chest incisions with a folded bath blanket or towel to decrease discomfort during coughing.

Postural drainage Position the infant over a pillow, or elevate the foot of the bed 15 to 25°, to encourage removal of secretions by gravity. Position the older child over the elevated knee rest of the bed.

Postural drainage is especially helpful with the infant who cannot cough or breathe deeply on command. The following nursing actions are needed:

1. Raise the end of the mattress by using a towel or blanket roll.
2. Position the infant on the abdomen with the head down for 10 to 15 min. Support the head with a pillow or blanket roll to prevent slipping.
3. Suction the nose and mouth as drainage accumulates and at the end of the procedure.
4. Repeat every 4 h or as needed.
5. Chart (*a*) time, (*b*) length of procedure, (*c*) type and amount of mucus, (*d*) suctioning done, and (*e*) the child's response.

Percussion Percussion (or clapping) involves cupping the hands or using an object to trap air over portions of the chest wall to loosen secretions during postural drainage. See Fig. 16-34 for positions and areas to percuss to achieve drainage of specific portions of the lungs. The physician will determine which areas need percussion. Vibration may be done in conjunction with percussion.

Figure 16-34 Positions for postural drainage and percussion. (*A*) Cupped hand position for percussion. Percussion is done in all positions for 1 ½ to 2 min. (*B*) Hand position for vibration. Vibration is done two to three times in positions 1 to 9. (*Demonstrator: Surina Geoffroy, R.P.T., California Medical Center, Los Angeles. Photo by Theresa Friedrich.*)

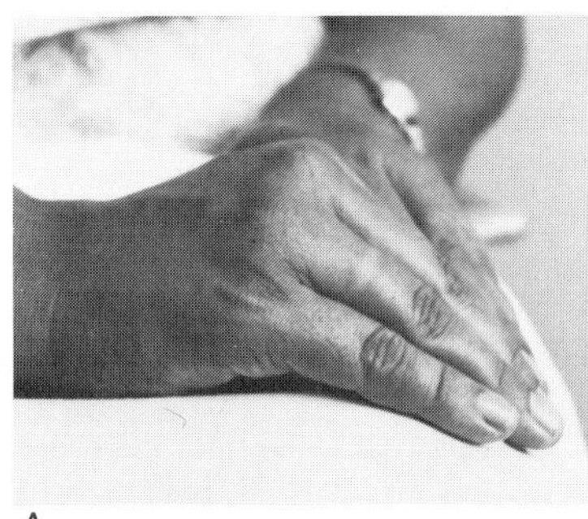

A

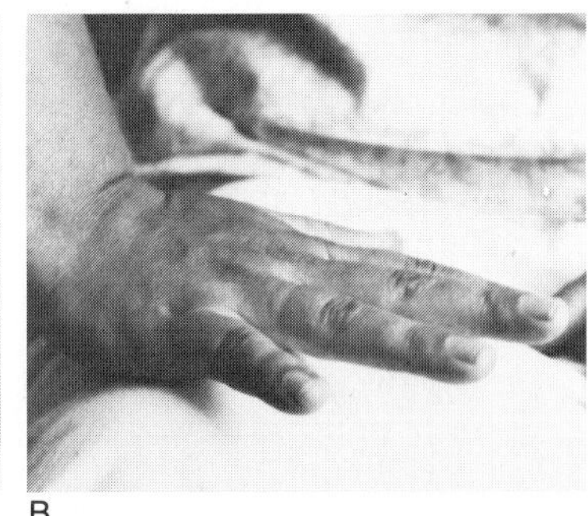

B

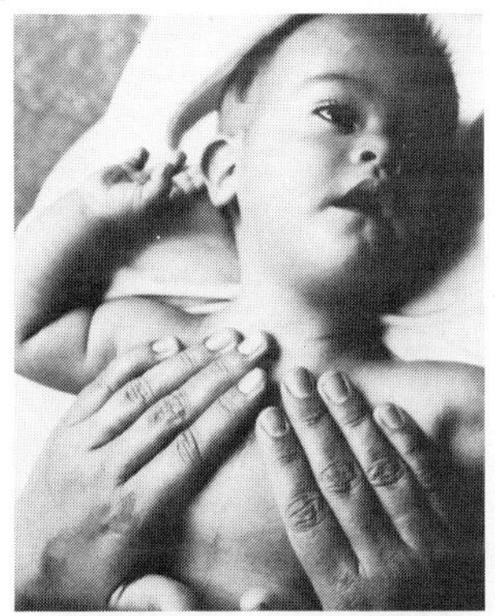

(*1*) Anterior upper lobes. Patient is supine.

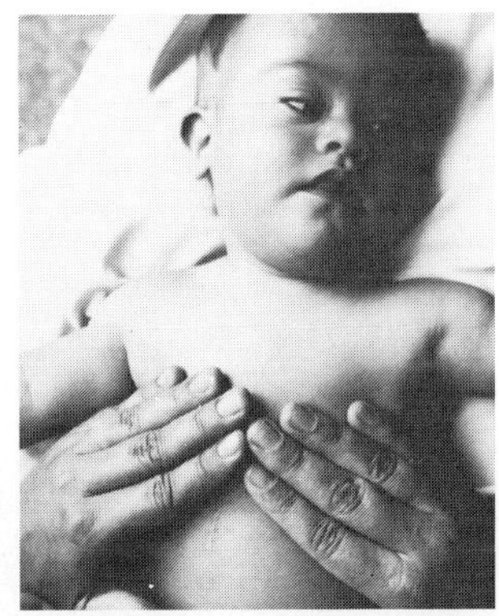

(*2*) Anterior lower lobes. Patient is supine with head lowered 45°.

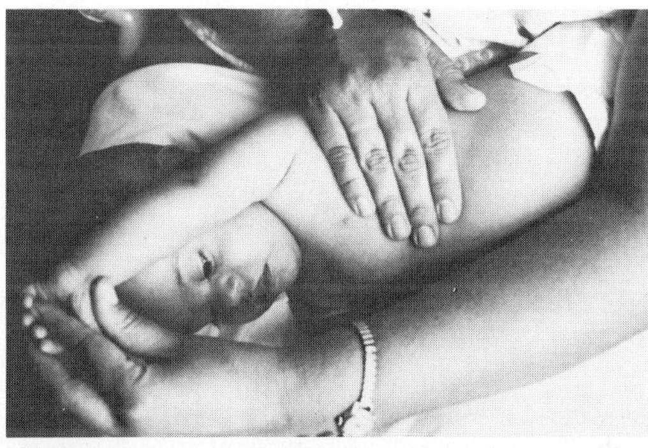

(*3*) Left lateral lobes. Patient is placed lying on the right side with left arm overhead. Head is lowered 45°.

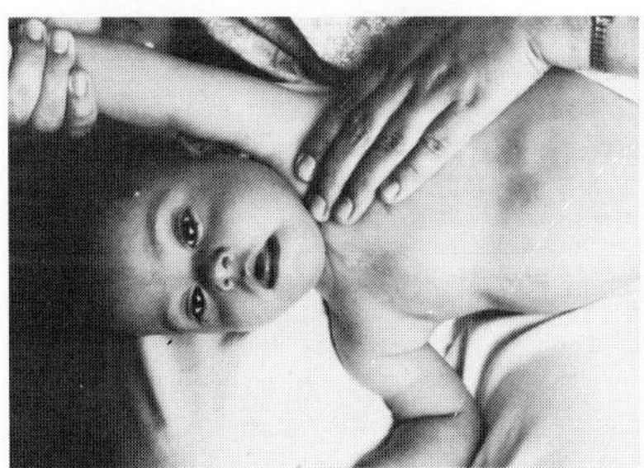

(*4*) Left lingual lobe. Patient is placed with half side lying on right with left arm over head. Head is lowered 45°.

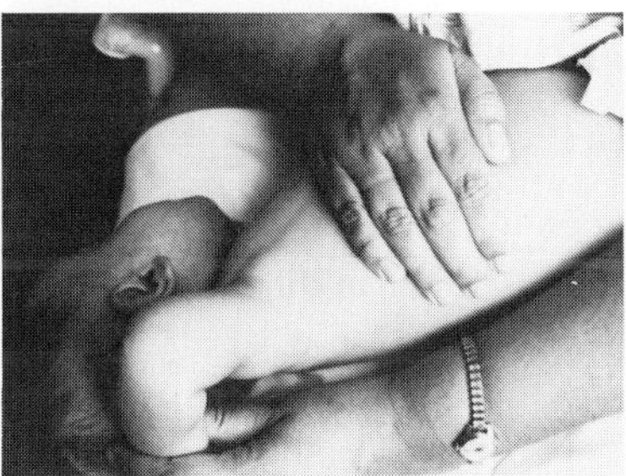

(*5*) Right lateral lobe. Patient is placed lying on right side with left arm over head. Head is lowered 45°.

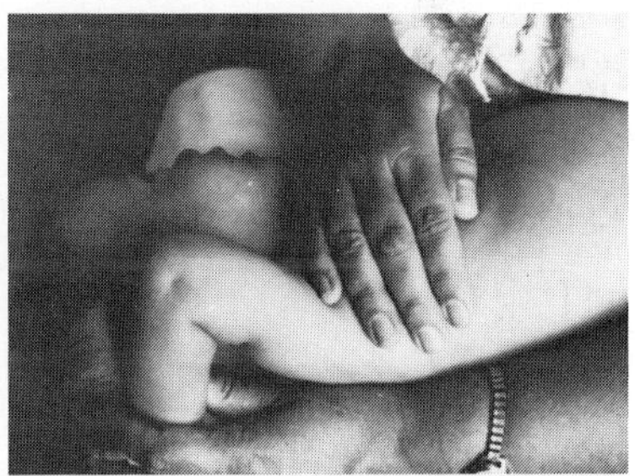

(*6*) Right middle lobe. Patient is placed with half side lying on left with right arm over head. Head is lowered 15°.

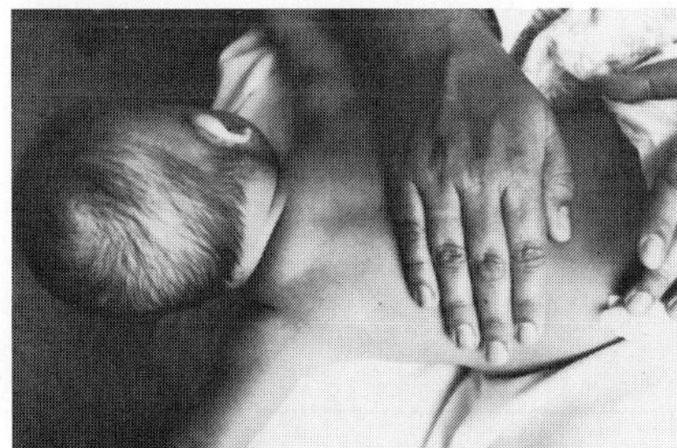

(*7*) Posterior lower lobes. Patient in prone position with head down 45°.

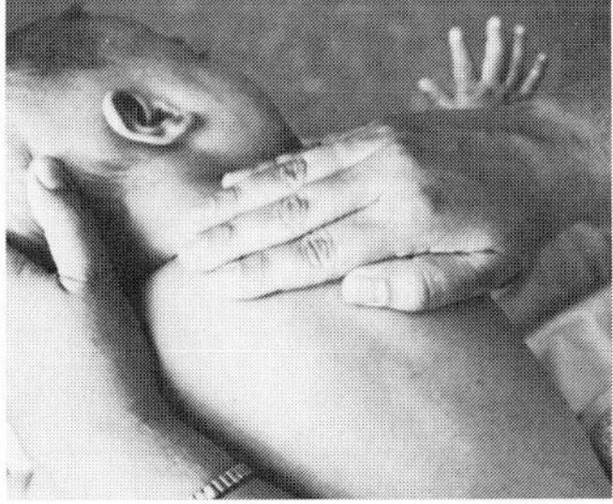

(*8*) Right posterior upper lobe. Patient prone with left shoulder elevated 30°.

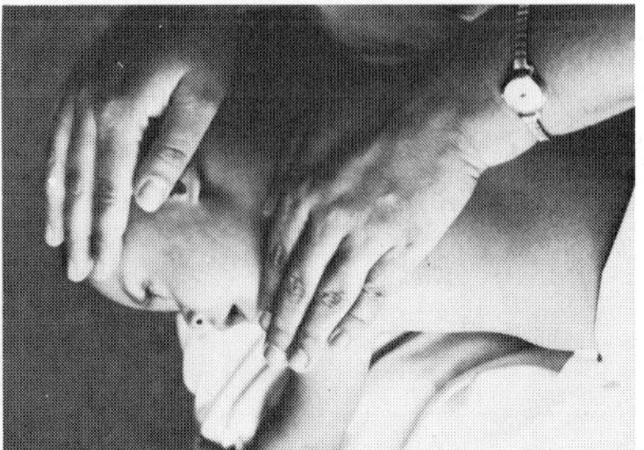

(*9*) Left posterior upper lobe. Patient prone with left shoulder elevated 45°.

Special precautions Chest physiotherapy requires the following precautions:

1. It should be performed 1 h before meals to improve nutritional intake. If procedures must be done after meals, delay at least 1 h to avoid vomiting.
2. Modify the length of treatment and positions for drainage according to the child's tolerance and physical limitations.
3. Do not percuss over the kidneys, lower back, or clavicle.[67]
4. Use cupped hands—do not slap—conforming to the contour of the chest, and percuss over the rib cage. A rubber bottle stopper, small anesthesia mask, padded stethoscope head, or two to three fingers tented together should be used for the infant.[68]
5. If postoperative pain interferes with chest physiotherapy, give pain medication approximately 30 min before the procedure.

CARDIOPULMONARY RESUSCITATION

Cardiopulmonary resuscitation for infants and children is patterned after that for adults, with a few modifications to accommodate size differences.

If you are the rescuer

In an emotionally charged situation like a respiratory or cardiac arrest, speed is essential, but accuracy of diagnosis is equally important. The first step is to make sure that resuscitation is needed.

1. Shake the child, shout, and call his or her name. Slap the feet of an infant. To determine whether there has been respiratory arrest, place the child in a horizontal position and listen at the nose and mouth to hear or feel whether air is being exhaled. This allows you to focus on actual ventilation rather than chest movements, which may not be achieving ventilation.
2. Open the airway by extending the neck slightly. Shout for help simultaneously. Note the time. Avoid hyperextending the neck of infants and small children. The tissues of the trachea are very soft and pliable; if hyperextended, they may obstruct the airway.
3. Carry out rescue breathing (mouth to mouth) and ventilate four times. Use:
   a. Puffs of air from cheeks for infants
   b. Small breaths for young children
   c. Normal breaths for children over 8 years of age

   With a young child, cover the mouth and nose to ventilate; release to allow exhalation. Forward traction on the mandible keeps the root of the tongue from obstructing the airway in the hypopharyngeal area. Use enough air to cause the chest to rise and fall.
4. Palpate the carotid or femoral artery for pulse.
5. If there is no pulse, begin cardiac massage (see Table 16-17).
6. Continue cardiopulmonary resuscitation until the child begins breathing or until you are relieved by another rescuer.

If you are the helper

Your job is to mobilize the resources of the hospital and to supplement the actions of the rescuer:

1. Get additional help by following hospital protocol.
2. Bring emergency equipment to the bedside—suctioning equipment, oxygen, and medications.
3. Connect the manual resuscitation bag (e.g., Ambu) and mask and ventilate the child.
   a. Stand at the child's head.
   b. Pull forward on the angles of the lower jaw to keep the tongue from obstructing the airway.

Table 16-17 Cardiac Massage of Children

1. Ventilate after every five compressions (watch the chest rise to determine adequacy of ventilation).
2. **Chest Compression:**
   a. *In the infant:* Draw an imaginary line between the nipples; place the index finger just under this line where it crosses the sternum. The area of compression is one finger-breadth *below* this line. With a hand or solid surface under the back, use 2 or 3 fingers to compress the sternum, 0.5 to 1 in, 100 times per min.
   b. *In the child:* Locate the lower margin of the child's rib cage. Follow it with the index and middle fingers to the notch where the ribs and sternum meet. With the middle finger on the notch, place the index finger on the sternum. Then place the heel of the other hand next to the index finger, parallel to the sternum. Compress the sternum 1 to 1½ in, 80–100 times per min. Keep fingers off the ribs. If the child is large or older than 8 yr, use the two-hand method for adults.
3. Remember that the purpose of compression is to produce blood flow to vital organs by compression of the heart and the spinal column. Adequate compression is indicated by the presence of femoral, carotid, or temporal pulse.

Source: Standards for CPR and ECC, *Journal of the American Medical Association,* June 6, 1986, 225(21):2958.

c. Hold the mask securely with the thumb over the mask at the bridge of the nose, the forefinger over the mask at the chin, and three fingers under the jaw to keep it forward.
d. Gently inflate the bag and watch for the rise of the chest to check adequacy.
e. Release the bag quickly.
f. Use caution to prevent overinflation of the lungs. (Ventilation with a bag and mask should be assumed by specially trained personnel as soon as possible.)

4. Check the femoral or temporal pulse for adequate compression. Check the pupils for reaction to light.
5. When relieved, set up intravenous infusion equipment and other items as needed. (See Chap. 33 for information on advanced cardiac life-support and emergency drugs.)
6. Document all activities. Be very aware of time and length of resuscitation effort.

Throughout any resuscitation effort, the child must be checked frequently to see whether he or she is breathing and whether the heart is beating on its own.

During cardiopulmonary resuscitation, an infant's stomach can easily become distended with air. Compress the stomach periodically during the procedure, but not simultaneously with chest compression. If decompression is not effective, consider passing a nasogastric tube.

Locate all emergency equipment (Fig. 16-35) soon after arriving on any nursing unit, and be familiar with the steps in cardiopulmonary resuscitation. Be prepared to act quickly.

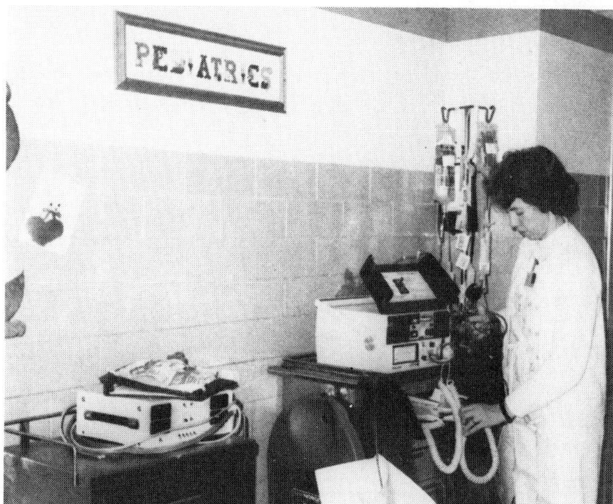

Figure 16-35 This head nurse is checking the emergency cart to ensure that all necessary equipment is available and in working order in case of a cardiac arrest.

CHOKING AND FOREIGN-BODY ASPIRATION

Airway obstruction with secondary cardiac arrest is much more common among infants and children than cardiac arrest followed by airway obstruction. It is imperative that a nurse be able to institute emergency measures to relieve or remove the obstruction quickly and safely. Obstruction of the airway can be caused by a foreign body (such as food or a toy), an accident, or an infectious process. When an infection causes the obstruction, the child should be attended by a physician as quickly as possible so that medications and artificial airways can be started.

The most important rule in managing an aspirated foreign body is: *Never start emergency treatment if the airway is partially open and the child is moving air adequately.*

The common signs of true choking are:[70]

1. Grabbing at the throat
2. Inability to cry or speak
3. Turning blue
4. Collapsing

Place the infant in a position with the face and head down to facilitate expulsion of the object. For an older child, let the child assume the position that is most comfortable for breathing. If the airway is completely obstructed, emergency measures are needed. If you see the object, use your fingers to sweep the mouth and pharynx, approaching from the side to prevent pushing the object further down the airway.

The 1986 guidelines from the American Heart Association for dealing with an obstructed airway are summarized below.

For the *conscious* infant:

1. Determine airway obstruction and observe for breathing difficulties.
2. Support head with one hand, keeping the head lower than the trunk, and place the infant face down so he or she straddles your forearm or thigh. Deliver *4 back blows* between the shoulder blades with the heel of the hand.
3. Continue to support the head, sandwich the infant between your hands, and turn the infant on its back keeping the head lower than

the trunk. Deliver *4 chest thrusts* to the midsternal region in the same manner as external chest compressions but at a slower rate.
4. Repeat steps 2 and 3 until either the foreign body is expelled or the infant loses consciousness.

For the *unconscious* infant:

1. Call for help.
2. Assess airway. Do head tilt/chin lift maneuver to neutral position. (Head tilt: Place thumb in mouth over tongue; lift tongue and jaw forward with fingers wrapped around lower jaw.) Look, listen, and feel for breathing. Seal mouth and nose; attempt to ventilate (1–1.5 s/ventilation).
3. Do steps 2 and 3 as described above for the conscious child.
4. Check mouth and remove foreign body if visualized.
5. Reattempt ventilation. Repeat steps 3, 4, and 5 until successful.

For the *conscious* child:

1. Determine whether there is complete airway obstruction (in the infant, look for blue lips; in the older child, look for the inability to speak).
2. Stand or kneel behind the child. Wrap arms around the child's waist. Place one fist, thumb side in, against the child's abdomen well below the tip of the ziphoid and slightly above the navel. Grasp this fist with the other hand.
3. Apply 6–10 quick upward thrusts; each thrust should be distinct and delivered with the intent of relieving the airway (see Fig. 16-36). (Do not slap the child's back, give fluids, hold the child upside down, or turn the head to the side during the maneuver.)
4. Repeat thrusts until the foreign body is expelled or the victim becomes unconscious.

For the *unconscious* child:

1. Turn on back, place face up, arms at side; call for help.
2. Open the airway with tongue-jaw lift. Remove foreign body *only if* visualized. Attempt ventilation (1–1.5 s/ventilation).
   a. Activate the emergency code system if someone responded to call for help.
3. Perform abdominal thrusts.
   a. Kneel at victim's feet if on floor or stand by feet if victim is on table.
   b. Place the heel of one hand against the abdomen slightly above the navel and well below the tip of the ziphoid.
   c. Put second hand on top of first hand.
   d. Press into abdomen with *6–10 quick upward thrusts*.
4. Open the mouth; if the foreign body is visible, remove it with a finger sweep or forceps.
5. Reposition the head, open the airway and attempt to ventilate. If the child cannot be ventilated repeat steps 2 and 3.

Once the object is removed, check for spontaneous breathing. If present, monitor breathing and pulse closely. If breathing is absent, perform rescue breathing 20 times/min for the infant or 15 times/min for the child.

It is far better to prevent choking if at all possible. The guidelines listed below are for general use but can also be applied in the hospital setting.

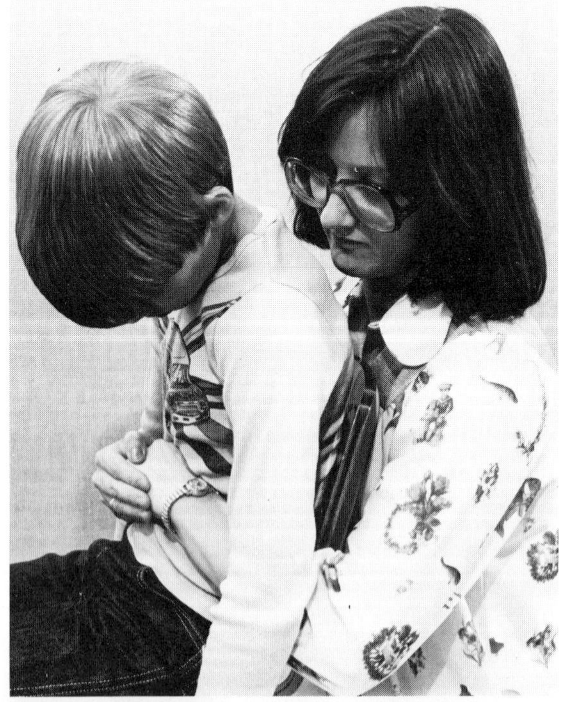

Figure 16-36 Abdominal thrust with the child sitting. The fist is placed with the thumb next to the sternum. The other hand is used to push on the fist and extend it in an inward and upward thrust. (*Photo by Brian Kaihoi.*)

To prevent choking:[72]

1. Introduce solid foods to infants only when they have teeth for proper chewing.
2. Do not give children under $2\frac{1}{2}$ years of age such foods as peanuts, popcorn, whole-kernel corn, potato chips, and pieces of apple.
3. Do not let children eat while lying down or when overly active—running or playing—since a bolus of food can become lodged in the larynx at such times.
4. Remove small objects from the reach of young children. When changing diapers, close safety pins and remove them from the infant's reach.
5. Teach by example—do not hold objects such as tacks, pins, and pencils between your lips or in your mouth.

VITAL SIGNS

Temperature

Average normal temperatures for children are shown in Table 16-18. Variations of a degree or more can occur after activity, crying, or periods of excitement. There are also slight differences in temperature according to age. Since the body temperature reflects metabolic rate, heat production steadily declines as the child grows. During the first year, for example, the average normal temperature is 37.5°C (99.5°F). This decreases to 37.2°C (99.0°F) at 3 years. Body temperature also fluctuates with room temperature.

Taking the temperature Ideally, a child should rest in bed 5 min or more before the temperature is taken. However, this is not always possible. The nurse should stay with the child throughout the procedure. If a standard thermometer is used, be sure the child's thermometer holder is labeled with his or her name, room, and bed number, as well as the type of temperature taken. Wash the thermometer with soap under cold running water after each use, and store it safely out of children's reach. Change the thermometer weekly or more often according to infection control procedures at the hospital. When charting temperatures, note "R" or "A" if rectal or axillary temperatures have been taken rather than oral temperatures.

Electronic thermometers (Fig. 16-37) are used frequently in the hospital setting. Thermometers should be designated for oral, axillary, or rectal use. Temperatures can be obtained quickly with an electronic thermometer, and it also makes the procedure less unpleasant. Barrus found that the axillary temperatures of 50 hospitalized preschoolers were 0.4°C lower than their rectal temperatures when measured electronically. In 20 percent of her sample, however, axillary temperatures were higher than rectal temperatures.[74]

Rectal method Take a rectal temperature if a child is under 6 years of age. However, there are several exceptions. The rectal method should be avoided if the child is facing rectal surgery, has diarrhea, or suffers from other rectal problems.

An oral or axillary temperature may be taken if the child has grown accustomed to either method or finds the rectal method unduly frightening.

Finally, another exception is the newborn. The first temperature should be rectal so that the nurse can check for imperforate anus. Subsequent temperatures for a neonate should be axillary.

Every method starts with shaking the mercury in the thermometer down below 35.6°C

Table 16-18 Average Normal Temperatures and Normal Temperature Ranges for Children

	°C	°F
Rectal	37.6 (37.2 to 37.8)	99.6 (99 to 100)
Oral	37 (36.7 to 37.2)	98.6 (98 to 99)
Axillary	36.3 (36.1 to 36.7)	97.4 (97 to 98)

Source: S. M. Tucker et al. [73].

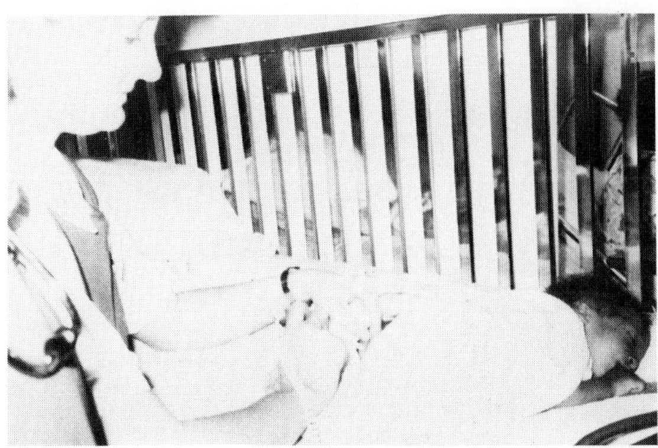

Figure 16-37 An electronic thermometer is quick and easy to use and may allow the nurse to take an infant's temperature without disturbing the child.

(96°F). After that, the rectal procedure is as follows:

1. Lubricate the thermometer with a water-soluble lubricant.
2. Position the child on the abdomen or side. The infant may be placed on the back, side, or abdomen (Fig. 16-38).
3. Look at the anus and insert the thermometer the length of the bulb.
4. Hold the thermometer in place for 3 to 5 min, or until the mercury stops rising or the electronic device indicates completion.
5. Keep a diaper over the infant's genitalia because the child may be stimulated to void.
6. Withdraw the thermometer, read the temperature, and wipe the child's rectal area with a tissue to remove the lubricant.

Oral method An oral thermometer is used for children 6 years of age and older. The procedure is as follows:

1. After shaking it down, insert the thermometer under the child's tongue. Tell the child to keep the lips closed during the procedure and not to bite the thermometer. (Be certain that the child has not just had a meal, snack, or cold drink!)
2. Do not let the child move around the room with a thermometer in his or her mouth. It is best to keep the child seated or lying down. *Stay with the child.*
3. After about 3 to 5 min, or when the electronic device indicates, remove the thermometer and record the reading.

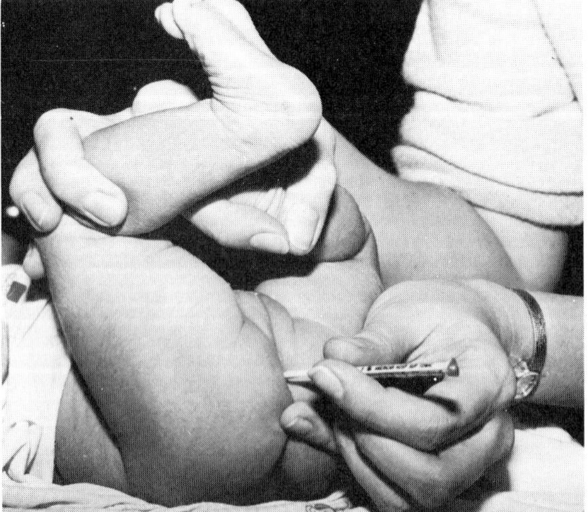

Figure 16-38 Taking an infant's rectal temperature. The thermometer is steadied by the little finger and the fingers holding it, while the other hand restrains the feet and legs.

Axillary method A clean oral or rectal thermometer should be used. The procedure is as follows:

1. After shaking down the thermometer, insert it under the child's arm in the axilla and hold it in place, with the child's arm at his side. Do not allow movement.
2. After 5 to 8 min, when the mercury has stopped rising, remove the thermometer and record the reading.

Kresch found that axillary temperatures are poor indicators of fever, have a low predictive value, and take 8 min or more to record when a glass thermometer is used.[75]

Temperature variations If a child has a $\frac{1}{2}$°C increase or decrease in temperature, a recheck is required. If it is confirmed, the variation should be reported to the physician (either at once or on the next medical rounds). A certain percentage of glass thermometers lose accuracy after some months of use.[76] It is wise for a nurse to question the accuracy of any temperature reading which does not fit the child's signs and symptoms. A second thermometer should be used for the recheck. Temperature variations are significant in children.

Oral temperature rises from 36.1°C (97°F) during the morning to a peak of 37.2°C (99°F) or higher between 6 P.M. and 10 P.M., before it drops to its lowest point between 2 A.M. and 4 A.M.[77] Alertness, character of the cry, spontaneous activity, visual movements, motor behavior, and interest in eating are more important in the febrile child than the pattern of temperature elevation.[78] In the newborn, hypothermia may indicate sepsis, just as an elevated temperature (hyperthermia) indicates possible infection in an older child. A continuous low-grade fever (37.8 to 38.3°C [100 to 101°F] rectally) may indicate that tests need to be done to determine the source of the fever.

When the temperature exceeds 40°C (104°F) rectally, a young child may have seizures. Efforts must be made to reduce a temperature approaching the high range. (See the section "Discomfort" later in this chapter.)

Antipyretics—aspirin (acetylsalicylic acid) and acetaminophen (Tempra, Tylenol, Datril, and other trade names)—should be reserved for temperatures over 38.9°C (102°F) rectally. Otherwise, they may mask the course of the fever and prevent accurate diagnosis by the physician. Antipyretics are most useful for reducing fevers caused by an infectious disease. They work by lowering the body's set point (which is elevated by the infection) and preventing shivering during temperature lowering.[79]

Pulse

The heart rate is very rapid at birth and slows down with age, as shown in Table 16-19. Factors that influence pulse rate are (1) age; (2) sex of the child; (3) fever, which increases the rate; (4) drugs (including anesthetics), which may increase or decrease pulse rate or cause arrhythmias; (5) emotions (excitement and anxiety); (6) activity; and (7) environmental temperature—pulse rate increases as metabolic rate increases to provide warmth.

If the child is under 10, the nurse should take an apical pulse while the child is sitting or lying quietly (Fig. 16-39). Warm the bell of the stethoscope by holding it in your hand for a short time, or carry it in a pocket close to your body. Check the rate for a full minute. A radial pulse is accurate in a child over 10, but should also be checked for a full minute.

Respirations

Respirations are counted for a full minute by observation or with a stethoscope. The latter is more accurate for children under age 10, and can be done along with an apical pulse. This also provides an opportunity to assess respiratory sounds. Normal respiratory rates by age are given in Table 16-19.

Table 16-19 Normal Pulse and Respiratory Rates for Children of Specific Ages*

Age	Pulse	Respirations
Newborn	110 to 160	30 to 60
2 years	100 to 140	28 to 32
4 years	90 to 96	24 to 28
6 years	80 to 90	24 to 26
8 years	80 to 84	22 to 24
10 years	80 to 84	22 to 24
12 years	78 to 80	18 to 20

*These are averages only and vary with the sex of the child.

Source: G. Scipien, M. U. Barnard, M. A. Chard, J. Howe, and P. J. Phillips (eds.), *Comprehensive Pediatric Nursing*, 2d ed., McGraw-Hill, New York, 1979, p. 28. Used with permission.

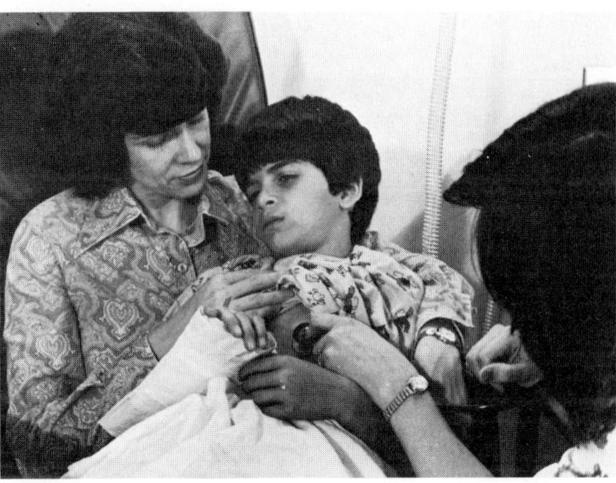

Figure 16-39 Apical pulse rate being determined while the child sits with the mother. (*Photo by Brian Kaihoi.*)

Count respirations when the child is quiet. If the child cries, defer the count until a later time. Otherwise, indicate C for *crying* when recording the respiratory rate.

Blood pressure

Blood pressure determination should be a routine part of taking vital signs in children 3 years and over because of the possibility of hypertension.[80] Detection is essential because:[81]

1. Hypertension in children and adolescents is usually secondary to a primary disease and may be cured by treating the underlying cause.
2. Unrecognized and uncontrolled high blood pressure may interfere with normal growth and development during the critical childhood years.
3. Hypertension can cause irreversible damage to major organs.

Blood pressure measurement is also necessary to identify hypotension (e.g., postoperatively), although in infants the blood pressure may drop suddenly rather than decrease gradually, as in adults.

Normal blood pressure readings at different ages are listed in Table 16-20. It is important to realize that one reading is unreliable because the

Table 16-20 **Average Normal Blood Pressure Values by Age***

Age	Systolic / Diastolic
Neonate (birth to 1 month)	80 ± 16* / 46 ± 16
Infant (1 to 12 months)	96 ± 30 / 65 ± 25
Preschooler (2 to 6 years)	60 to 110 / 40 to 75
School-age child (8 to 10 years)	105 ± 15 / 60 ± 10
Adolescent (11 to 16 years)	85 to 130 / 45 to 85
Adult	90 to 140 / 60 to 90

*The student should interpret a range presented in this way as follows: the average extends from 64 (80 − 16) to 96 (80 + 16).

Source: S. M. Tucker et al., *Patient Care Standards*, Mosby, St. Louis, 1975, p. 350–353. Used with permission.

Table 16-21 **Guidelines for Selection of Standard Blood Pressure Cuffs (*Dimensions of approximate size cuff*)***

	Range of Dimensions of Bladder	
Cuff Name	Width, cm	Length, cm
Newborn	2.5 to 4.0	5.0 to 10.0
Infant	6.0 to 8.0	12.0 to 13.5
Child	9.0 to 10.0	17.0 to 22.5
Adult	12.0 to 13.0	22.0 to 23.5
Large adult arm	15.5	30.0
Adult thigh	18.0	36.0

*Selection of proper size is dependent on the size of the extremity, not cuff name.

Source: "Report of the Task Force on Blood Pressure Control in Children," *Pediatrics* **59**(5):801 (May 1977). Used with permission.

normal range is wide. The most useful blood pressure readings in children are serial readings, which show an upward or downward trend.

Cuff size Appropriate cuff size is essential for accurate blood pressure measurement. A cuff that is too small causes an incorrectly high reading, and a cuff that is too large causes an erroneously low reading. The cuff width should be no less than one-half and no more than two-thirds of the width of the upper arm, or it should be 20 percent wider than the limb on which it is used. Guidelines for selecting blood pressure cuffs are given in Table 16-21.

Standard blood pressure The standard procedure for taking a blood pressure measurement on the arm is as follows:

1. Prepare the child by explaining how the blood pressure cuff will feel ("It will feel tight") and letting the child handle the equipment.
2. Help the child assume a relaxed position on the bed or in the mother's lap. (Place the infant supine in bed.) Measure the blood pressure after the child has been quiet for a few minutes to ensure greater accuracy.
3. Apply the cuff snugly. (Do not apply the cuff over clothing. Remove the clothing or raise the sleeve.)
4. Place the aneroid gauge so that it can be seen directly, not at an angle. If a mercury manometer is used, make sure that the meniscus of the mercury is at zero and can be viewed at eye level.
5. Palpate the radial pulse and inflate the bag 20 to 30 mmHg past the point at which the pulse disappears.
6. Place the stethoscope over the brachial artery. (The stethoscope must not be applied under the edge of the cuff. The cuff's inflatable bag can cause uneven pressure and distort the reading.)[82]
7. Release the cuff at a rate of 2 to 3 mmHg per second.
8. Repeat the reading once if in doubt. If still uncertain, have a coworker check it, or delay another reading for 15 to 20 min.

Under normal circumstances two pressure readings are noted: (1) systolic pressure, or the highest reading at which two consecutive sounds are heard, and (2) diastolic pressure, or the reading when the sound becomes muffled. The two consecutive sounds are known as *Korotkoff sounds*. If they cannot be heard with the stethoscope, the brachial or radial artery should be palpated with two fingers. The cuff should be inflated and released. Where the pulse can be felt is the systolic reading. The diastolic reading cannot be determined by palpation.

If the child is suspected of having hypertension,[83] three numbers are recorded: (1) systolic pressure, (2) diastolic pressure, and (3) where the sound ceases.

Thigh blood pressure Blood pressure readings may also be obtained in the lower extremity. The cuff must be 20 percent wider than the diameter of the thigh. Place the child on his or her abdomen or back. Apply the cuff over the midthigh, with the compression bag (the part that fills with air) over the *back* of the thigh. Place the stethoscope over the popliteal space behind the knee. (If the child is on his or her back, flex the knee slightly to place the stethoscope.) Note whether the right or left thigh was used when recording blood pressure.

In children under 1 year of age, the thigh blood pressure is the same as the arm blood pressure. In children over 1 year of age, the thigh systolic pressure is 20 mmHg higher, but the diastolic pressure remains the same.[84]

Flush blood pressure Flush blood pressure is an indirect method used in children under 1 year of age when a standard blood pressure reading is not obtainable (see Fig. 16-40). The procedure is as follows:

1. Select an appropriate infant cuff.
2. Place the cuff on the infant's wrist or ankle.
3. Elevate the extremity.
4. Compress the extremity distal to the cuff by wrapping it firmly with an elastic bandage.[85]
6. Remove the bandage. The extremity should appear blanched.
7. Gradually lower the manometer at a rate of 2 to 3 mmHg per second.
8. Take a reading at the moment the extremity appears flushed.

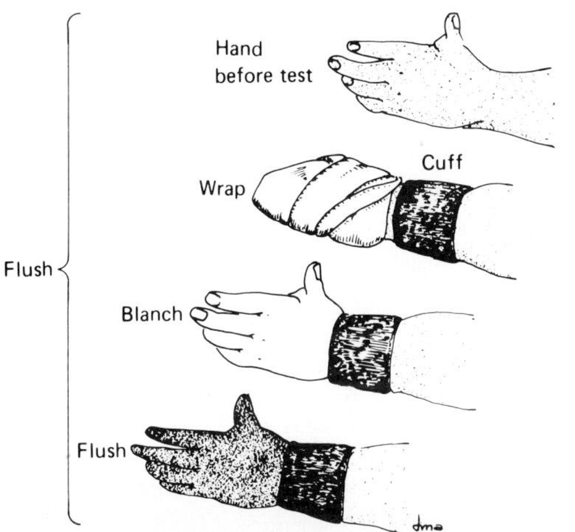

Figure 16-40 Flush blood pressure. (*From G. Scipien, M. U. Barnard, M. A. Chard, J. Howe, and P. J. Phillips* [eds.], *Comprehensive Pediatric Nursing, 3d ed., McGraw-Hill, New York, 1986, p. 168. Used with permission.*)

It is wise to have two people present: one to watch the manometer and one to signify when the flush occurs. Be sure that the room is well lighted. If alone, place the manometer so that it can be seen simultaneously with the extremity.

The pressure determined by the flush method is the mean blood pressure—a point between the systolic and the diastolic. A range of 30 to 60 mmHg is considered normal for an infant over 2500 g (5.5 lb).[86]

The Doppler method The use of *oscillometry*, or instrument measurement of pulsation, for determining blood pressure is popular in intensive care areas. An instrument using the Doppler effect is especially useful in neonates. It translates changes in sound frequency caused by blood motion to audible sound. It can also measure both systolic and diastolic pressures.[87] (See Fig. 16-41.)

A sphygmomanometer cuff is wrapped snugly around the child's limb. The transducer is applied with connecting gel over the brachial or popliteal artery. The cuff is then inflated 20 to 30 mmHg above the systolic sound and then slowly deflated. The systolic reading is the first sound heard, and the diastolic pressure is the point at which the sound changes from loud and sharp to soft and muffled.[88]

COMFORT

Daily care

Bathing A daily bath can be pleasant and relaxing for a sick, anxious child. Allow flexibility in scheduling bath time so that it is as much like bath time at home as possible. For instance, if a parent is able to assist, a child who is embarrassed at being bathed by a "stranger" will feel more at ease. Furthermore, for the younger child, toys should be provided. Young children enjoy having toys at bath time—even for a bed bath from a small basin. Rubber water toys, cups, bubbles, and washcloth mittens may be welcome.

An individual bath basin, infant tub, or regular tub can be used for the infant. The older child can bathe in a tub or shower. (Check to make sure that the child bathes the genitalia and

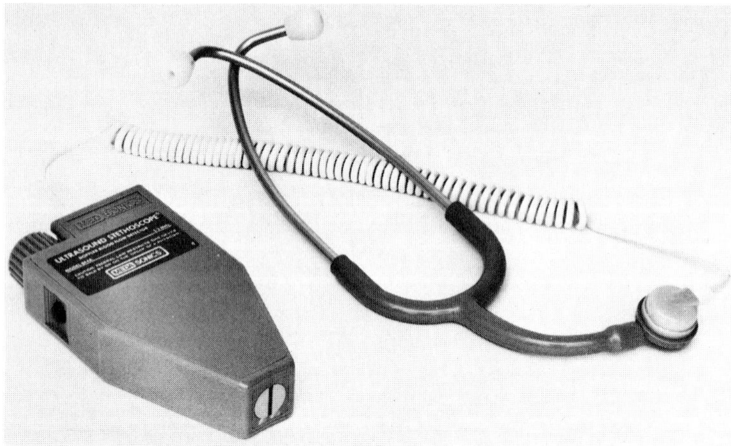

Figure 16-41 An ultrasound stethoscope, an instrument for the detection of blood flow using the Doppler effect. (*Courtesy of MedaSonics, Inc., Mountain View, Calif.*)

anal area. A tub bath allows better cleansing of these areas for the child who bathes reluctantly.)

The following safety precautions should be observed:

1. A water thermometer should be used to check the temperature just before placing the child into the water. The water should be tepid or slightly warmer (31.1 to 34.4°C [88 to 94°F]). Young children are especially sensitive to extremes in temperature; bath water that seems too cold to an adult may be just right for a child. Prepare the bath for the child. The water controls may be different from those in the child's home. Do not let the child play with the water controls during the bath.
2. *Stay with an infant or young child at all times when he or she is in a tub or basin.* Check frequently on an older child or adolescent. Show the child the nurse's call light in the bathroom and tell the child to call for assistance if needed.
3. When children have been bedridden, accompany them to their first tub bath or shower. Remain there or outside the door.
4. While bathing an infant, support the infant behind the shoulders and hold the opposite arm firmly.

The bath routine will be carried out more efficiently if the nurse increases the temperature in the room 15 to 30 min prior to bath time and gathers equipment before the child is undressed or the water is prepared. At the end of the bath, the tub or basin should be cleaned with a disinfectant solution.

Routine skin care Good skin care includes cleansing as well as preventing dryness and itching. Skin dryness is a result of lack of moisture in the skin and can be remedied by the appropriate use of bath oils, lubricants, and proper bathing and drying techniques.

Use a nonirritating, unscented, and inexpensive bath oil (e.g., Robathol) in the basin or tub or on the skin for a shower. (Oil should not be used for newborns and teenagers with acne.) Unscented bath oil is soothing and prevents dryness; the use of soap is unnecessary unless desired for the groin or axillary area. After the bath, gently pat the skin dry. Do not rub vigorously. Use additional lubrication, such as a water-in-oil emulsion (e.g., Eucerin), to hold moisture in the skin.[89]

Shampoos A shampoo is very beneficial in helping a child, and especially a teenager, feel that he or she is returning to normalcy. The nurse must be familiar with hospital policy regarding the need for a doctor's order. When in doubt, discuss the plan for the shampoo with the physician. Suggestions for giving shampoos are listed in Table 16-22. Figure 16-42 shows a good position for giving an infant a shampoo.

Nail care It is easy to overlook care of the nails because the child will not remind you about it.

Table 16-22 Steps in Giving a Child a Shampoo

1. Prepare for the shampoo. Various shampoos are available, and each hospital has its stock supply of recommended products. Do not use bar soap for shampooing because it is drying and difficult to apply and rinse off. A nonallergenic shampoo which can be used for all patients is desirable.
2. Moisten the hair, apply the shampoo, lather, massage the scalp gently, and rinse well. Repeat the procedure. (A second shampoo is usually unnecessary in infants.)
3. Keep the temperature of the water warm, but not hot.
4. Young children:
   a. Give an infant a shampoo during the bath, but avoid getting soap and water in the infant's eyes.
   b. Use the football hold while holding the child's head over a basin or sink (see Fig. 16-41).
   c. Sing and/or talk pleasantly to the infant to make the procedure more tolerable.
   d. Ask a toddler to help by holding a cloth over the eyes or rubbing his or her scalp.
5. Older children:
   a. Allow capable older children to give themselves shampoos in the tub or shower.
   b. Use bed shampoo equipment when necessary.
   c. An older child may be placed on a cart and moved to the sink. Extend the child's head over the end of the cart and support it during the procedure.
6. After the shampoo assist the child to towel dry his or her hair. Use a hair dryer for an older child if towel drying is inadequate.

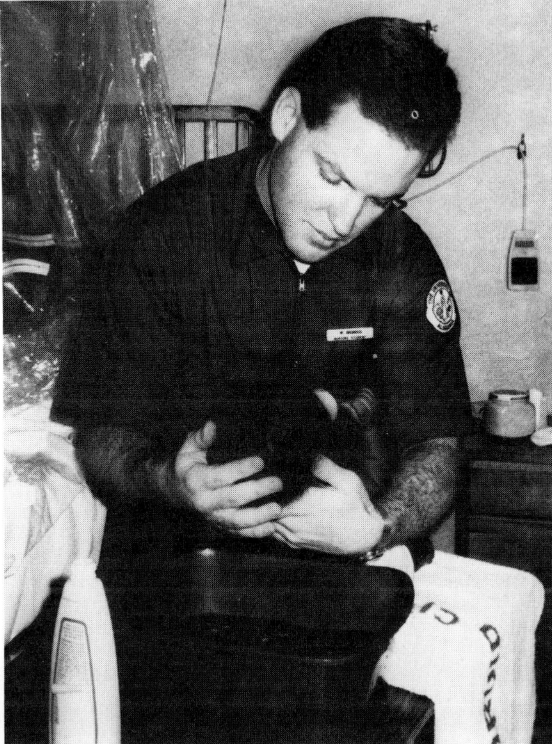

Figure 16-42 This student nurse is holding an infant in a football hold and has one hand free to give the shampoo.

Safety clippers or nail scissors should be available on every unit. Wipe them with alcohol before and after each use. A doctor's order is necessary for nail care in some hospitals.

Young children's nails should be clipped straight across, and care should be taken not to leave sharp edges. Trim hangnails carefully. Nail care can sometimes be done for infants and toddlers when they are sleeping. When a young child is awake, he or she can hold a toy or be distracted by someone else while the nails are being clipped.

Oral hygiene As soon as a child has teeth and shows an interest in brushing (around 12 to 18 months), parents can begin brushing the child's teeth. Even before that, the teeth should be wiped with a clean cloth or gauze sponge after meals. Regular toothbrushing habits should be established by age 3, but children should be *supervised* until age 8. Morning and evening routines in the hospital should include brushing and flossing the teeth.

Toothbrushing techniques Most dentists recommend a brush with (1) soft bristles, (2) a straight handle, (3) a flat brushing surface, and (4) a head small enough to reach every tooth. When the bristles become bent and the brush does not clean well, the child should have a new brush.[90]

The following brushing procedure was modified from *Care of Children's Teeth,* published by the American Dental Association in 1978:

1. Place the head of the toothbrush alongside the teeth.
2. Angle the bristle tips against the gum line.
3. Gently "scrub" the brush back and forth with short, quick strokes.
4. Brush the inner, outer, and biting surfaces of each tooth, both top and bottom.
5. Use the front of the brush to clean the inside area of the front teeth.
6. Gently brush the tongue.
7. Rinse the mouth with water.
8. Floss carefully between the teeth.

Teaching the technique requires spending time with the child and using the same procedure consistently. Older children who have already developed toothbrushing habits will probably prefer to continue to brush as usual, but a tactful discussion of appropriate methods may be well received. Bedridden children will need to be taught to use a cup and basin for brushing.

When children are seriously ill and unable to brush their own teeth, the nurse or parent must assist them. Use a toothbrush or sponge stick with toothpaste, followed by a mouthwash. When oral surgery has been done or the gums are susceptible to bleeding, an oral irrigating device is helpful. Discuss this with the physician.

Nursing bottle mouth As soon as a child's teeth appear, they are susceptible to decay. If the child is allowed to go to bed with a bottle of sugary liquid, the teeth can be badly damaged. The liquid pools around the teeth, and bacteria in the mouth change the sugar into decay-causing acids. Milk, fruit juices, formula, and other drinks can also be harmful under these circumstances.[91]

To prevent "nursing bottle mouth":

1. Clean the infant's mouth after each feeding with a clean washcloth or gauze pad.
2. Do not give the child a bottle of sugary liquid at bedtime. Use water if he or she must take a bottle to bed.[92] Remove the bottle as soon as the child is asleep.

Dressing Dressing young children can be made easier by allowing them to wear their own clothes if possible, encouraging their help, and learning their idiosyncrasies. When putting on a T-shirt, gather the excess fabric up to the neck opening so that the child's face is covered only briefly. Gather up a sleeve or pant leg and pull the child's extremity through it. Use a loose-fitting gown or shirt which opens up the front or back for a seriously ill child.

Do not allow children to walk barefooted in the hospital. Provide slippers with nonskid soles in a variety of sizes, or ask the parents to bring slippers from home. Slippers can be made by taping washcloths around the child's feet.

Diapering The nurse who is inexperienced in caring for infants may have difficulty applying diapers snugly. The following suggestions may be helpful:

1. Use disposable diapers or cloth diapers if the child is sensitive to plastic. (Figure 16-43 shows how to fold cloth diapers.)
2. Place the diaper underneath the child—provide extra thickness at the back for girls and at the front for boys.
3. Secure the diaper with self-adhesive tabs or pins. To pin the diaper, place the fingers of one hand between the diaper and the child's skin to guide the pin through the cloth and prevent the infant from being stuck. Pin the

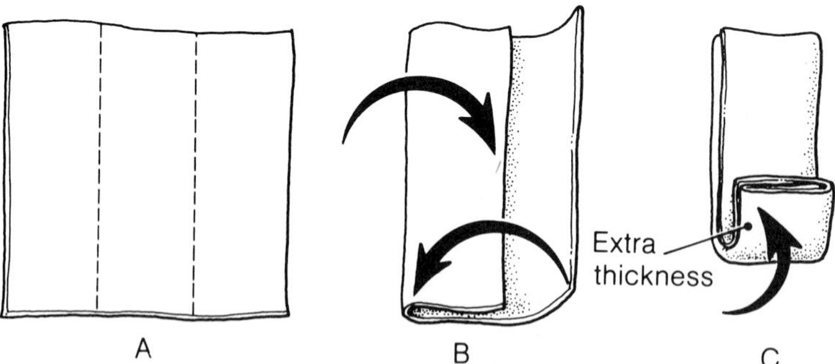

Figure 16-43 Folding the diaper to provide extra thickness. (*A*) Place the diaper on a flat surface. (*B*) Fold it into thirds. (*C*) Place the thickest part under the buttocks for a girl and over the penis for a boy. (*From G. Leifer, Principles and Techniques in Pediatric Nursing, Saunders, Philadelphia, 1977, p. 48. Used with permission.*)

back over the front to fit body contours. Direct both pins horizontally and posteriorly in case a pin should accidentally open.

4. Change the diaper frequently. As an infant walks, the diaper will stretch and loosen. Voiding will compound the problem.
5. For an older infant, apply two diapers at naptime or bedtime. Use plastic pants or a waterproof flannel pad on the bed.

Diaper rash is often caused by skin irritation from urine. See Chap. 9 for care of diaper rash.

Sleep Adequate rest and sleep are essential for normal growth and development in children as well as for recovery from illness (Fig. 16-44). When they are sick, children need more sleep than usual. Table 16-23 shows the average sleep needs of children at different ages.

Determine the child's sleep pattern at home. Some small children want or need both morning and afternoon naps. Others take one long nap. Children use various comfort measures to help them go to sleep—a blanket, a stuffed animal, or thumb-sucking. Many parents will hold and rock a child to sleep when he or she is in the hospital simply because the child needs the extra love and security during this time. As a child's condition improves, the parents may prefer to break this habit and try to help the child regain the ability to go to sleep without being rocked.

Provide a quiet rest time each day. Turn the lights down, close the doors of rooms, and turn off TVs to enhance the rest time. Even older children and adolescents may welcome a time to read, be alone, or take a nap as they recuperate. On an adolescent unit it is important to post rest and "lights out" times.

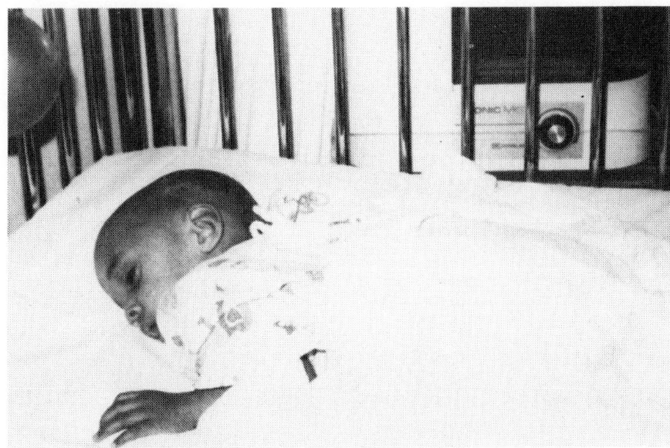

Figure 16-44 Nursing activities should be planned to allow the sick child to get as much rest and sleep as possible.

Table 16-23 Sleep Needs

Age	Hours per Day	Naps
Infant	16 to 18	Morning and afternoon
Child aged 1 to 3 years	13	2 h in the afternoon
Child aged 3 to 6 years	11 to 13	2 h in the afternoon
Child aged 6 to 12 years	8 to 10	Rest time
Adolescent	8	

Source: S. M. Tucker et al., *Patient Care Standards*, Mosby, St. Louis, 1975, p. 407.

Parents may want to "sneak away" while a child is asleep so that they will not have to see the child cry when they leave. This should be discouraged because children may resist sleep if they think that their parents will leave each time they try to rest. Honest, open communication with children about when parents are leaving is the best approach. Refer to Chap. 15 for ways of dealing more effectively with separation anxiety.

Rest and nursing care Plan vital sign checks, dressing changes, medications, and other activities so that the child does not have to be awakened from a nap or a night's rest. When it is necessary to awaken the child, maintain a quiet atmosphere and use a flashlight rather than the room light. When possible, take vital sign measurements while the child is still sleeping. If the child *must* be awakened, rub his or her back or sing lullabies to encourage the child to fall asleep again.

Sometimes children are awakened by nursing care given to other children in the same room. Plan room assignments to allow children with similar care schedules to be in the same room.

DISCOMFORT

Pain

When a child is in pain, it may be difficult to assess. This is especially true of preschoolers and toddlers, who may be unable to verbalize effectively. (See Chap. 34 for additional information on pain assessment.)

Identifying pain In a study of pain in children aged 2 to 7 years, Smith[93] identified some ways in which pain may be expressed:

1. Aggressive behavior
2. Dependency
3. Some verbalization
4. Physiological response (adrenal and sympathetic stimulation)
   a. Vasoconstriction of vessels to the internal organs (except the heart, lungs, and brain), causing hypomotility of the gastrointestinal tract
   b. An increase in circulating blood glucose with an increased amount of energy available
   c. Vasodilatation of peripheral vessels, increasing oxygen content and glucose in the muscles.
5. Observable manifestations
   a. Flushing of the skin
   b. Vomiting
   c. Elevated pulse and respiratory rate
   d. Restlessness (whole body movement)
   e. Dilatation of the pupils

If pain is identified and treated early, the child is more comfortable, more cooperative, and more tolerant of hospitalization. The nurse must observe the child carefully and be alert to behaviors indicative of pain.

Pain management Pain management does not necessarily mean use of medications. In fact, narcotics for pain relief are generally unnecessary for children because relief can be obtained with safer analgesics and nursing measures. Ways to help a child become more comfortable include providing a change of position, loosening tight dressings, wrapping the child comfortably in a blanket, rocking the child, singing, and providing a favorite drink or play activity.

If comfort measures are inadequate, confer with the physician about medications. For some children the thought of a shot is worse than tolerating pain. The nurse must be alert to all the signs of pain to determine whether medication is needed—especially if the child is denying pain because of fear of an injection. Explain that the pain of the medication is very brief and will make his or her body feel better. Consider the possibility of oral or rectal medications as alternatives to injections. Give medications as often as needed to control the discomfort.

Persistent pain that is not relieved by mild analgesics and comfort measures should be reported to the physician. There may be complications occurring which will require additional medical intervention.

Irritability and crying

Irritability and aggressive behavior may be the result of conditions other than pain. Crying may occur simply because a child is hungry or tired. Try a cracker, some juice, or a nap as a means of helping the child.

Children also cry because of the presence of strangers, separation from parents, fear of the environment or procedures, uncertainty about what is happening, and boredom. Talk with the parents and spend time with the child to assess the causes of the irritability and to determine relief measures.

Some anesthetics cause irritability and irrational behavior. Reassure the parents and use comfort measures—rocking, singing, and giving back rubs—so that the child can "sleep off" the side effects of the anesthetic.

Fever

Fever can cause irritability, crying, and lethargy. It is the most frequent cause of seizures in young children and may be a sign of infection. An elevated body temperature requires attention when:[94]

1. The temperature is above 39.4°C (103°F)
2. The child is under 6 months of age
3. The child has a disease
4. The fever lasts longer than 8 days
5. No localizing signs are present

Report a fever to the physician and discuss the control measures needed.

Antipyretics may be ordered by the physician. The most common drugs for temperature control are aspirin (acetylsalicylic acid) and acetaminophen (Tylenol, etc.). For a high fever it has been recommended that half doses of aspirin and acetaminophen be used together. The combination works better than either antipyretic used alone, and the effect is prolonged.[95] Aspirin should not be given to a child with a viral illness because it increases the risk of Reye syndrome.

Additional nursing measures are as follows:

1. Dress the child lightly. Remove the bedclothes to promote heat loss.
2. Encourage taking fluids to replace those lost because of fever and to overcome any mild dehydration, which can raise the temperature.
3. Give a sponge bath (see Table 16-24).

Nausea and vomiting

Nausea and vomiting occur as symptoms of gastrointestinal disease or as side effects of medications, pain, surgery, and anxiety.

If a child is in the immediate postoperative period, the nurse must be familiar with the side effects of the preoperative medications and the anesthesia which the child received. The side effects will be relieved when the drugs have been metabolized and eliminated. Blood and mucus swallowed during surgery may cause postoperative vomiting, which is relieved when the stomach empties itself.

Young children cannot verbalize the feeling of nausea. They may become restless, perspire, look flushed or pale, and begin to cough, gag, or hold the stomach or throat. They may say "my throat hurts!" Nursing measures for care of the child who is vomiting include the following:

1. Keep an emesis basin, tissues, and a washcloth at the bedside at all times. Provide these when preparing *all* postoperative beds.
2. Tell the child and the parents why the basin is available and to call a nurse if any vomiting occurs.
3. Have a child who is vomiting sit up and lean over the basin. Support the head and wipe the child's mouth as needed. If sitting is contraindicated, turn the child to the side.
4. Position the child on the abdomen or the right side or with the head of the bed elevated at least 15° while resting.
5. Place a cool cloth on the child's throat or head.
6. Provide a quiet environment and use a soft speaking voice.
7. Measure and record the amount of emesis; then rinse the basin quickly and return it to the bedside.
8. Remove soiled clothing and linen and use an air deodorizer to freshen the room.
9. Provide a mouthwash or water with which the child can rinse his or her mouth. Tell the child not to swallow it.
10. Confer with the physician about restricting the oral intake to avoid stimulating the gastrointestinal tract. Discuss the use of antiemetics. (Great care must be taken when using phenothiazines in children.)
11. Resume the consumption of fluids and food by slowly progressing from ice chips or sips of carbonated beverages and popsicles, to full servings of liquids, and then to a regular diet.

Table 16-24 **Sponge-Bath Technique for a Child with a Fever**

1. Fill a tub with 1 to $1\frac{1}{2}$ in of lukewarm water.
2. Place the child in the tub, and sponge him or her for 30 to 45 min.
3. Do not use alcohol or ice to enhance the cooling effect. This may cause chills and shivering, which tend to raise body temperature. There is also a danger of alcohol intoxication.
4. If the child cannot be moved from bed, use a basin of water at the bedside. Sponge the extremities, trunk, axilla, and groin with light, gentle strokes. Chilling can be prevented by keeping half the body covered while sponging the other part.
5. If the child feels chilled or begins to shiver, stop the sponging and resume it later if necessary.
6. Check the child's temperature occasionally during bathing and at $\frac{1}{2}$-h intervals afterward until it is down or at least has stopped rising.

MEDICATIONS

Dosages

Pediatric dosages are calculated according to body weight (for instance, 10 mg/kg per 24 h) or body surface area (BSA). BSA is considered to be a more accurate means of determining dosage than body weight alone.

Determination of BSA with the West nomogram (Fig. 16-45) is made using the child's height and weight. The dose is then determined as follows:

$$\text{BSA in m}^2 \times \text{recommended dose/m}^2 = \text{approximate child's dose}$$

For example, assume that you want to determine the appropriate dose of Benadryl for a child who weighs 30 lb and is 30 in tall. The recom-

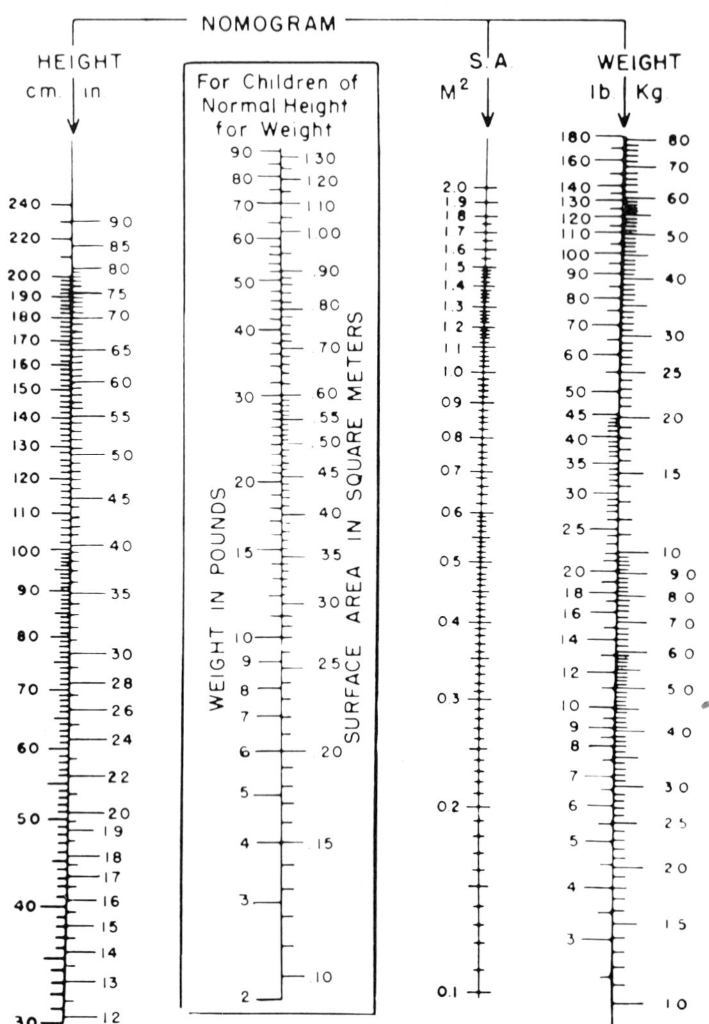

Figure 16-45 The West nomogram (for estimation of surface areas). The surface area is indicated where a straight line connecting the height and weight intersects the surface area (SA) column or, if the patient is roughly of normal proportion, from the weight alone (enclosed area). *(Nomogram modified from data of E. Boyd by C. D West, from H. C. Shirkey in V. C. Vaughan and R. J. McKay* [eds.], *Nelson Textbook of Pediatrics, 10th ed., Saunders, Philadelphia, 1975, p. 1713. Used with permission.)*

mended dosage is 150 mg/m² per 24 h. To find the answer using the West nomogram, draw a straight line between 30 lb and 30 in; the BSA is 0.56 m². Therefore:

$$0.56 \text{ m}^2 \times 150 \text{ mg} = 84 \text{ mg per day}$$

This amount is then divided into four evenly spaced doses.

BSA determinations can be made through the entire life-span *except* with premature and full-term neonates. Because their excretory function is immature, neonates must receive special care in all drug administration; BSA determinations are not appropriate.[96]

Factors affecting dosage are listed in Table 16-25.

Table 16-25 Factors that Affect Drug Dosage in Neonates and Older Children

Factors Related to Drug Absorption

The reduced intestinal motility typical of the neonate slows passing of drugs taken orally.

The delay in intestinal enzyme development of the newborn impairs the ability of intestine lining cells to process the drug for absorption.

Reduced acidity within the neonate's intestinal tract lowers drug uptake by lining cells.

Factors Related to Drug Distribution

Continual changes in relative tissue mass and fat content during growth and development make predictions as to drug delivery and tissue uptake unreliable.

The greater volume of body water in the neonate relative to total weight requires adjustment of dosage calculations for certain drugs if the desired serum concentration is to be achieved; adult water-vs.-tissue proportions are achieved in the teenage years.

Factors Related to Drug Metabolism

The normal slow maturing of hepatic enzymes during the first 2 to 3 weeks postnatally, if unrecognized, may lead to unmetabolized drugs accumulating to toxic levels.

From about the fourth week, the fully functioning liver can process larger quantities of drugs than BSA calculations would indicate because the liver is proportionately larger in the child than in the adult.

Factors Related to Drug Excretion

The expected decreased glomerular filtration rate (GFR) during the first 3 weeks must be recognized to avoid drug accumulation to toxic levels. Full renal function at adult levels is reached by 5 to 7 months.

The neonate's decreased renal tubular function poses the same danger as decreased GFR.

Source: Adapted from G. Udkow, in R. Hoekelman et al. (eds.), *Principles of Pediatrics*, McGraw-Hill, New York, 1978, pp. 235–245.

Understanding medications

The nurse is responsible for knowing or learning about each drug to be given. Specific resources usually available are the *Hospital Formulary*, *Physician's Desk Reference*, a pediatric source such as Shirkey's *Handbook of Pediatric Dosages*, and the hospital pharmacist. Some hospital units have a drug dosage file with commonly used drugs and dosages on individual cards. A list of drugs used for emergencies is usually kept with the resuscitation equipment.

In checking physicians' orders, note any aspect of an order which may be inappropriate, and discuss it with the physician before the drug is administered (Fig. 16-46). Dosages for drugs are based on the average amount of medication needed to achieve therapeutic effects without causing signs of overdose. The physician may have a specific reason for giving more or less than the average. However, the nurse must communicate *specific concerns* so that dosages can be determined with all aspects of correct therapy in mind.

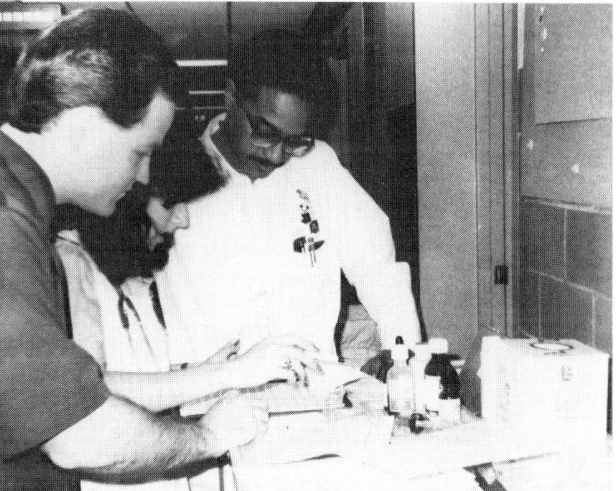

Figure 16-46 This staff nurse and student nurse are conferring with the physician about a medication dosage.

Administering medications

Before giving any medication, explain to the child and the parents what the medication is and why it is given. Use terms that the child understands—how it will feel, taste, and look—but make the explanation brief, and then give the medication. It is best to have the medication prepared when the explanation is given so that a long period of time will not elapse between explanation and administration. (See Chap. 15 for more details about preparation for procedures and use of therapeutic play.) In some instances the parent may be more effective than the nurse in obtaining the child's cooperation.

When administering medications, the nurse must choose the appropriate route (enteric vs. parenteral) as well as the appropriate interval between doses to maintain the desired serum drug level. The child's response is influenced by fever (increased metabolic rate), the disease process itself, other drugs being taken, and the time of administration (with meals or between meals).

Time of administration The nurse should be aware of which drugs are to be given with or without food. Clarify orders for medications to be given three times a day or four times a day. Every 6 h or every 8 h may be more appropriate for maintaining therapeutic blood levels.

Oral medications These include tablets, capsules, liquids, and, occasionally, powders. Equipment for oral administration includes a medicine cup, spoon, plastic dropper, and plastic syringe.

Ormond and Caulfield have developed a helpful guide for administering oral medications to children aged 1 month through 6 years based on developmental tasks and behaviors (Table 16-26). The authors note that the charts are presented as "guides for normal behavior, but 'normal' is not an absolute and there is plenty of room for variation.[97]

Some additional suggestions are given below.

Tablets Chewable tablets are generally taken easily by young children as long as a "chaser" such as water or a soft drink is provided. If it is

Table 16-26 Pediatric Medication Guidelines

Developmental Tasks and Behaviors	Nursing Implications
1 to 3 Months	
Motor	
Reaches randomly toward mouth; shows strong palmar grasp reflex.	The infant's hands should be monitored or controlled to prevent spilling of medications.
Head drops or exhibits bobbing control.	The head must be well supported.
Feeding	
Sucks reflexively in response to tactile stimulation.	Medication should be administered using this natural behavior: medication should be given via nipple.
The corners of the mouth may not seal effectively, and the tongue may be reflexively forced against the palate.	Correct position of the nipple, if used, must be assured for adequate sucking.
Tongue movement may project food out of the mouth.	A syringe or dropper, if used, should be placed in the center back portion of the mouth. If placed along the gums, it must be toward the back of the mouth.
Sucking strength increases (3 months)	The amount of medication presented must be controlled. Infants may choke or drool because they can take in more medication than they can handle.
Stops taking fluids when full; sucking reflex begins to fade (3 months).	Medication more easily given in small volumes and when the infant is hungry.
Interactive: Stage: Basic trust vs. mistrust	
Becomes socially responsive.	Medication administration requires feeding behavior which establishes an easy, comfortable situation. This is part of the child's learning to form a trust relationship.
3 to 12 Months	
Motor	
Advances from sitting well with support (3 to 4 months) to crawling (10 months).	Safety precautions regarding where medications are placed and kept become extremely important.
Begins to develop fine motor hand control.	
Advances from lying as placed (3 months) to standing with support (12 months).	A child who does not want to cooperate has the ability to resist with his or her whole body.
Feeding	
Starting at 12-month-old level:	
Smacks and pouts lips in act of shifting food in mouth and in swallowing. Lower lip is active in eating.	Children may spit out food and medicine they do not want.
Tongue may protrude during swallowing.	Eating is inefficient, and so medications may need to be retrieved and refed.
Learns to drink from cup. Generally has poor approximation of corners of the mouth when drinking.	A small medicine cup may be more effective than a nipple or syringe because the cup can catch parts of the medicine the baby spits out.
Learns to finger-feed self.	
Feeding behaviors become individualized.	Feeding patterns and routines at home need to be considered.

Table 16-26 Pediatric Medication Guidelines (*Continued*)

Developmental Tasks and Behaviors	Nursing Implications
3 to 12 Months	
Interactive: Stages: Basic trust vs. mistrust and oral sensory	
Communication skills develop from random social responses (3 months) to making simple requests by gesturing (12 months).	Be alert to children's indicating their own needs (12 months).
Is sensitive and responsive to tactile stimulation. Begins developing responsiveness to other stimuli.	Physical comforting will be most effective. Verbal comforting is secondary.
Recognizes immediate family and, very importantly, may exhibit intense separation anxiety.	The child exhibits early memory and may recall negative experiences, precipitating negative response in another, similar situation.
12 to 18 Months	
Motor	
Advances from standing with support to independent walking.	Have children choose a position for taking medication or hold them to provide control and comfort. Forcing children to take medicine when they are lying down takes away their sense of independence and will frequently result in very resistive behavior.
Feeding	
Begins independent self-feeding but is still messy.	Home feeding habits should be considered.
Develops voluntary tongue and lip control.	The child spits out something that tastes disagreeable. Disguise crushed tablets and contents of capsules in a small amount of a familiar solid food. Be prepared to refeed.
Spits deliberately.	
Interactive: Stage: Autonomy vs. shame and doubt	
Indicates needs and wants by pointing.	
Speaks four to six words. Uses individual jargon.	Find out what words children use for drinking and swallowing and how oral medicines have been given at home.
Responds to familiar commands.	
Responds to, and participates in, the routines of daily living.	Let children explore an empty medication cup. They will probably be more cooperative if familiar terms are used.
	When possible, involve the parents. They are familiar and trusted persons, which is an important factor during an unfamiliar experience.
	Tell the parents and staff the approach used for medication. Report its effictiveness.
Exhibits notable independence, resistance, self-assertiveness, and ambivalence. Begins to have temper tantrums.	Allow children as much freedom as possible.
	Allow children to assert themselves by choosing a drink to wash down the medicine.
	Use games to gain cooperation.
	Tell children what you expect and then follow through. A consistent, firm approach is essential.
18 to 30 Months	
Motor	
Walks and climbs into chair (18 months).	The child is able to run away and kick.
Advances to running without falling (24 months)	
Advances to obtaining and throwing small objects.	Children may throw materials placed within their reach. Never leave medications sitting on the bedside stand.
Feeding	
Generally feeds self. Advances to proficiency with minimal spilling.	Allow children to drink liquids from a medicine cup by themselves.
Second molars have erupted (20 to 30 months).	Give children more opportunities to choose forms of medication.
Exhibits increased rotary chewing; manages solid food particles.	
Controls mouth and jaw proficiently.	The child can spit out unwanted medications and can shut the mouth tightly in resistance.

Table 16-26 Pediatric Medication Guidelines (*Continued*)

Developmental Tasks and Behaviors	Nursing Implications
18 to 30 Months (*Continued*)	
Interactive: Stage: Autonomy vs. shame and doubt	
Has some sense of time, but no words for time (18 months). Then responds to "just a minute" (21 months). Advances to understanding, "Play after you drink this" (24 months).	Tell the child who is getting medicine that any bad taste will last only "a minute." Find out the child's level of time awareness from the nursing history.
Carries out two to three directions given one at a time.	Give simplified directions: "Open your mouth, drink, and then swallow."
Shows ability to respond to, and participate in, the routines of daily living. Helps put things away; carries breakable objects.	Include the child in establishing a medicine-taking routine.
Exhibits independence, resistance, self-assertiveness, and ambivalence. Has temper tantrums frequently.	Use a firm, consistent approach. Resistive behaviors are at a peak.
Shows pride in accomplished skills. Does not know right from wrong.	Give immediate, positive tactile and verbal response to cooperative taking of medicine. Ignore resistive behavior.
Shows conflict between holding on and letting go.	Give choices when possible: "Do you want to sit in the chair or on my lap to take your medicine?"
$2\frac{1}{2}$ to $3\frac{1}{2}$ Years	
Motor	
Continues to develop proficiency. Basic skills have all been initiated.	The child may be quite adept at showing resistive behavior.
Feeding	
Is becoming more proficient in skills. Eating likes and dislikes are definite but changeable.	The taste of medications can be disguised with variable effectiveness.
May be influenced by others' reactions in responding to new food experiences.	A calm, positive approach is needed to gain a cooperative response from the child; a quick, tense approach is likely to produce similar behavior in the child.
Interactive: Stage: Initiative vs. guilt	
Gives full name.	Begin to ask children to state their names before giving medications.
Is ritualistic.	Communicate administration methods.
Has little understanding of past, present, or future.	Use concrete and immediate rewards.
Shows concrete thinking and egocentricity.	The child tolerates frustration poorly. His or her initial response to reason appears positive, but without consistent effect. Prolonged bargaining is frustrating and frightening to the child because no one is in control of the situation.
Exhibits early aggressiveness and coercive, manipulative behavior.	Give a choice when possible. Do not give a choice if the child does not have one.
Has many fantasies.	Begin giving simple, honest explanations of why a medication is given.
May be frightened by his or her "power."	The child's sense of security is dependent on the nurses' consistent expectations of his or her behavior.
$3\frac{1}{2}$ to 6 Years	
Motor	
Develops proficiency of coordination. Can identify the parts of a complete movement or task.	The child can attempt and master pill taking.
Feeding	
Exhibits olfactory, gustatory, and kinesthetic refinement.	Disguising tastes is generally less effective than with younger children. The child can distinguish medicine tastes and smells.
Begins to lose temporary teeth (5 years).	Loose teeth may need to be considered when selecting a form of medication.

Table 16-26 Pediatric Medication Guidelines (*Continued*)

Developmental Tasks and Behaviors	Nursing Implications
Interactive: Stage: Initiative vs. guilt	
Makes decisions.	Children should be active in making decisions which affect them.
Sense of time allows enjoyment of delayed gratification. Is able to tolerate frustration. Seeks companionship. Shows pride in accomplishments.	Rewards which are not immediately received and social interaction can be used as effective motivators. The child is able to understand the purpose of medications in simple terms.
Has ability to follow directions and remember several instructions for a period of minutes to hours.	Teaching can have long-term benefits.
Exhibits developing conscience. Needs limits set to help control frightening sense of "power."	Prolonged reasoning or arguing may frighten the child; a simple command by a trusted adult may be more effective.
Exhibits interest in genitals and has general fears of mutilation.	Explain the relationship between cause, illness, and treatment. Use simple terms.
Often sees illness as punishment.	Give control when possible—the child needs to make choices.
Shows changeable response to parents.	The child may be more cooperative about taking medicine with the nurse than with the parent.

Source: E. A. R. Ormond and C. Caulfield, "A Practical Guide to Giving Oral Medications to Young Children," *Journal of Maternal-Child Nursing* 320–325 (September–October 1976). Used with permission.

necessary to crush a tablet in order to give only part of it, ask the pharmacist to crush it for greater accuracy in dosage. If this must be done on the unit, crush the tablet between two spoons.

Crushed medications may be mixed with a *small* amount of syrup, jelly, or applesauce to facilitate administration. Do not mix the medication with food (e.g., eggs, milk, or formula) because the child may not eat the food later. Mix the medication and the camouflage thoroughly on a small spoon and administer it in one or two bites. Have a drink of the child's choice immediately available.

For the child on extremely limited fluid intake, offer the medications in baby food, thus saving the fluids for later.

Capsules Capsules should not be opened to facilitate administration without conferring with the pharmacist. If a child refuses a capsule, another form of the drug or another drug with similar actions may need to be substituted by the physician.

Liquids Because the stomach is not primarily an organ for absorption, oral medication must pass into the small intestine. Liquids pass more quickly and easily than tablets. Hence a liquid is the preferred form of oral drug for infants and small children. Measure the dose in a syringe to ensure accuracy. Do not depend on a medication cup for any amounts smaller than 5 ml. Use a tuberculin syringe if the amount is smaller than 1 ml.

Giving liquid medications to infants To prevent aspiration, always hold the infant in an upright position or with the head and shoulders elevated when giving liquid medications. Use a soft plastic dropper or small plastic syringe for administration. Insert it into the side of the mouth between the cheek and the gums. Slowly release the medicine so that it passes around the gums and into the esophagus. The sucking reflex may be used, as indicated in Table 16-26, by placing the dropper or syringe directly on the tongue.

Very young infants may take medications easily if they are given through a nipple. Dilute the medication in a little water or juice and administer when the infant is hungry. Use only a small amount of diluent so that the infant will be more likely to take the whole amount.

When a child is crying vigorously, do not give the medication. Help the child settle down and then try again. Never hold the child's nose to forcefully give medicine. The child will associate the medicine with the feeling of suffocation and will fight harder the next time. Forcing also creates a risk of aspiration.

Giving liquid medications to toddlers Older toddlers should be given a good explanation before receiving medications. If the child resists the medication, give choices between using the medicine cup, a paper cup, a straw, or a syringe. If this does not help, the child should be held firmly on the parent's or nurse's lap (see Fig. 16-47). Explain kindly, but firmly, that the medication must be taken now. Open the child's mouth by pressing on the chin, and put the medication in. If the child spits it out, give it again so that the child understands that the medicine is essential. Remind the child that as soon as the medicine is taken, he or she can play.

If a child regurgitates the medication immediately after receiving it, give the total amount again. If vomiting occurs within 30 min after taking the medication, contact the physician so that new orders about readministering the drug can be given.

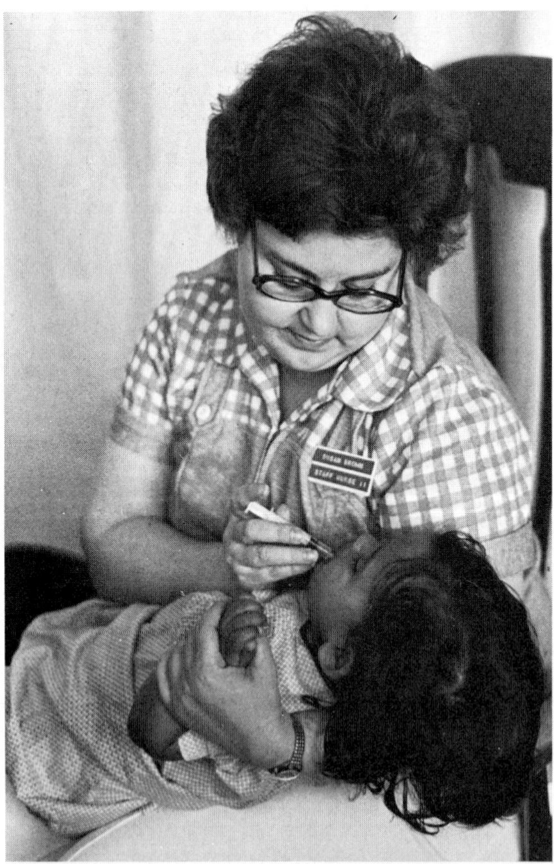

Figure 16-47 A small child being restrained while being given oral medication from a syringe. *(From L. Whaley and D. Wong, Nursing Care of Infants and Children, Mosby, St. Louis, 1979, pp. 937. Used with permission.)*

Rectal medications The advantages of rectal medications are that there is no chance of aspiration; they may be given without concern about excessive oral fluid intake; the chid cannot spit them out; they can be used when oral intake is contraindicated, as in the presence of nausea and vomiting; and insertion is brief and painless, when compared with injections. Though medications given rectally may not be absorbed as readily as those given orally, there are times when they are the best alternative available.

Prior to administration, use a finger cot to check the child's rectum for the presence of stool. A suppository administered into a bolus of stool is *totally* ineffective. Lubricate the suppository *as directed*. Most are prelubricated, but moistening with a small amount of warm water may be helpful. Insert the suppository past the anal sphincter. Remain with a young child for a few minutes, and hold the buttocks together in order to prevent expulsion of the medication. While waiting, talk, sing, and play with the child as a distraction. Fifteen to thirty min after the suppository is administered, check the child's diaper or underwear for expulsion.

Most suppositories cannot be divided because the manufacturer does not guarantee that the drug is evenly dispersed throughout the suppository.[98] Talk with the pharmacist before attempting to divide a suppository.

Intramuscular medications Because an injection is a very brief procedure, it is best to prepare the child just before giving it so that the child does not have a long time to build up unnecessary anxieties.

Sites In children the appropriate sites for intramuscular injections are as follows:

1. Vastus lateralis (used in newborns) or anterolateral thigh (Fig. 16-48*A* and *B*). These sites are recommended in children under age 2 in order to avoid the gluteal site. The gluteal muscle is not well developed until the child is walking.
2. Posterolateral gluteal (Fig. 16-48*C*). In children over 2, the upper outer quadrant of the gluteal may be used.
3. Ventrogluteal (Fig. 16-48*D*). This is an excellent site because there are no important nerves or blood vessels in the area.

4. Deltoid (Fig. 16-48*E*). The deltoid should not be used for intramuscular injections in small children but can be used in school-age children and adolescents for small dosages (e.g., immunizations). Thick, long-acting antibiotics should always be administered in the large muscles of the leg or hip.

The deltoid has a faster absorption rate than the larger muscles, and so it is appropriate when faster absorption is desired.

Needle size The needle chosen should be long enough to ensure that it will insert the medication in the muscle without hitting the bone and large enough for the medication to pass through easily with minimal tissue trauma.

Suggested sizes are as follows:

Infants and toddlers $\frac{5}{8}$ in (very small infants) to 1 in (most infants)
Older children 1 to $1\frac{1}{2}$ in, depending on the size of the child and the injection site
Thin liquid medications 23 to 25 gauge
Thick antibiotics 21 to 22 gauge

Tubex syringes are available for many pediatric injections. Because these are sometimes frightening to children, the plastic disposable syringes and needles may be preferred.

Administration Table 16-27 lists the steps in administering an intramuscular injection to a child.

Intravenous medications When administering an intravenous medication, the nurse must be thoroughly familiar with the drug and its side effects, the correct dosage, the length of time necessary for administration, and the compatibility of the drug with the other intravenous medications and fluids being given. The effect of intravenous drugs is immediate, and errors which may be well tolerated by an adult can be fatal in a small child.

Intravenous medications may be given:

1. Directly into the IV line through a medication inlet
2. Via the intravenous volume control chamber (Fig. 16-49)
3. Via a separate intravenous medication bag or bottle.

When medication is given through the volume control chamber, it is added through the medication inlet on top of the chamber. The volume of intravenous fluid added to the chamber for medication administration is determined by the amount needed to prevent pain and irritation to the child's vein and the length of infusion time desired.

Use of a separate medication bag or bottle is the safest means of intravenous medication administration. The pharmacist prepares the medication and carefully determines the appropriate amount of diluent. The medication is administered through secondary intravenous tubing attached to the primary tubing through a Y inlet (Fig. 16-50).

Several important precautions to consider when administering intravenous medication are listed in Table 16-28.

Ear drops Warm ear drops to body temperature prior to administration. An infant may be held on the mother's lap, but an older child should be positioned on the bed so that he or she can remain in bed for a few minutes after the drops are inserted. To accommodate for anatomic differences at different ages, use the following guidelines.[99]

Children under 3. Hold the pinna of the ear *down* and back.
Children over 3. Hold the pinna of the ear *up* and back.

Turn the child's head to the opposite side, insert the ear drops, and keep the head turned for 2 to 3 min. It may be more comfortable to the child to have a cotton wick inserted loosely into the ear upon completion of the procedure to prevent the drops from rolling out during activities.

Eye drops Restrain the child as necessary. The hand which holds the dropper should rest on the child's head.[100] Pull down the lower lid and insert the drops in the center of the pocket formed by the lid (Fig. 16-51). The child should remain flat on his or her back for several minutes after the drops are inserted so that the medication can reach the entire cornea. Provide a tissue to absorb tears, but restrain the child from rubbing the eyes.

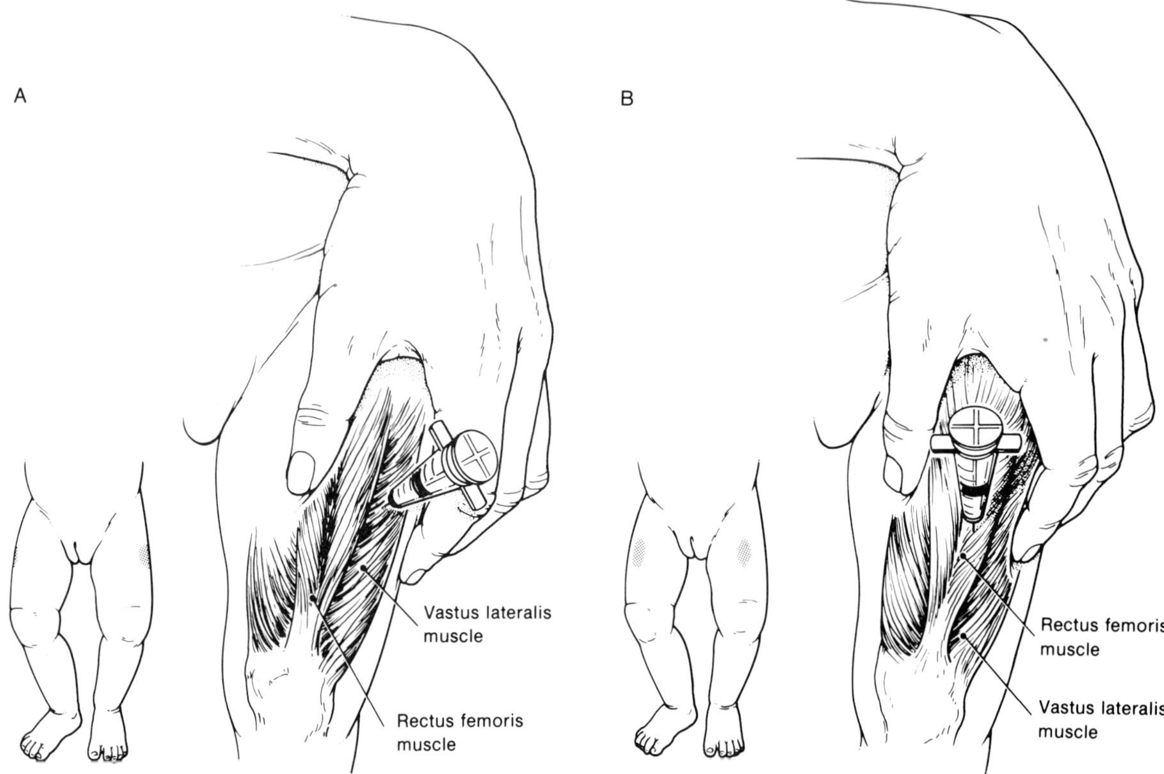

Figure 16-48 Sites for intramuscular injections in children. (*A*) The vastus lateralis. The vastus lateralis is the primary site for intramuscular injections in the thigh. The needle penetrates on a front-to-back course of the midlateral anterior thigh. Grasp the thigh as shown to stabilize the extremity and concentrate the muscle mass. (*B*) The anterolateral thigh. An alternate site for intramuscular injections in the thigh is the anterolateral surface. The needle is directed distally into the rectus femoris muscle at a 45° angle to the horizontal and long axes of the leg. Compress the thigh as suggested in (*A*). (*C*) The posterolateral gluteal. The posterolateral aspect of the gluteal area is located by palpating the posterior superior iliac spine and the head of the greater trochanter. An imaginary line is drawn, and the needle is inserted on a straight back-to-front course as shown. (*D*) The ventrogluteal area. The ventrogluteal area provides good muscle density and is free from major nerves and vessels. If the injection is to be given on the child's left side, use the right hand in determining landmarks, and vice versa. Place the palm on the greater trochanter, the index finger on the anterior iliac spine, and the middle finger on the posterior edge of the iliac crest. The intramuscular injection is given in the center of the V or triangle formed by the hand, with the needle directed upward toward the iliac crest. (*E*) The deltoid. The injection site is determined by the acromion and the axilla as shown. Because muscle mass is limited in the middeltoid area, repeated injections and large quantities of medication are not recommended. Compress the muscle mass prior to inserting the needle. (*From G. Scipien, M. U. Barnard, M. A. Chard, J. Howe, and P. J. Phillips* [eds.], *Comprehensive Pediatric Nursing, 3d ed., McGraw-Hill, New York, 1986, pp. 1403–1404. Used with permission.*)

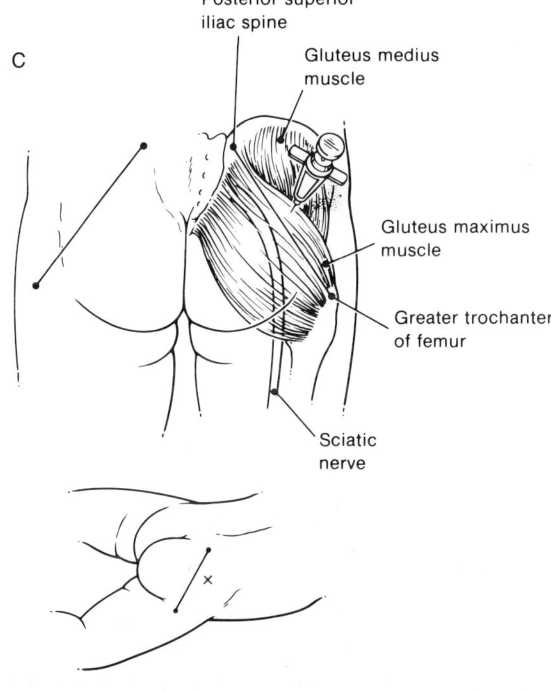

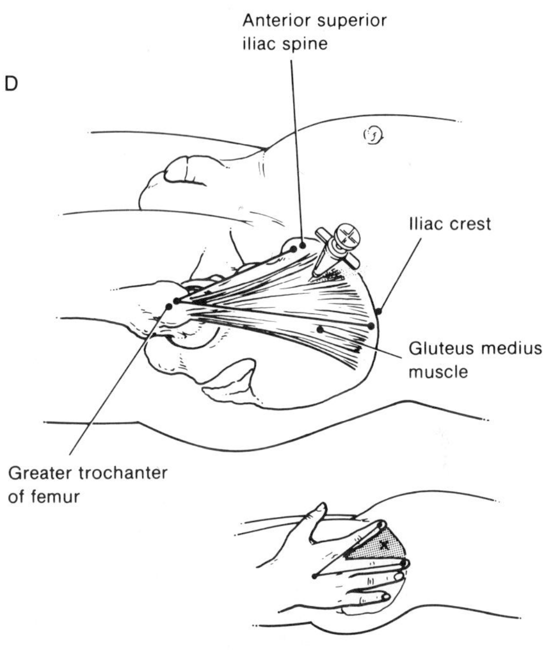

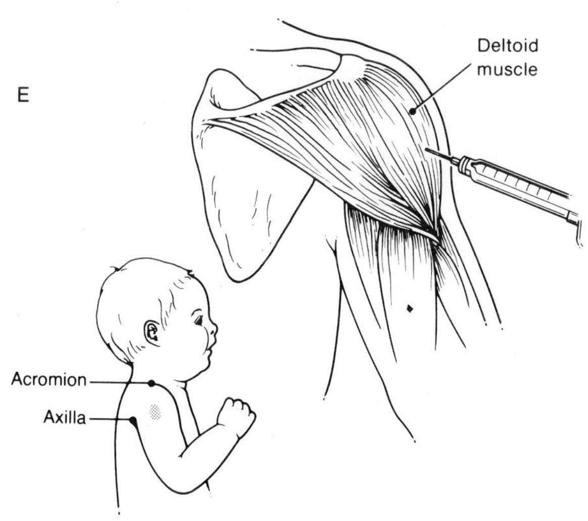

Nose drops Nose drops should be given before meals to open the nasal passages and make eating easier. This is especially necessary for infants who are still nursing because it is very difficult for them to suck when they cannot breathe through the nose.

Position the child's head by placing a towel roll under the neck or extending the head over the edge of the mattress. Keep the head back for 2 to 3 min after the drops are inserted.

Table 16-27 Steps in Administering an Intramuscular Injection

1. Prepare the medication out of the child's sight. Bring it in inconspicuously on a tray.
2. Explain briefly that the medicine is needed to help the child get well or prepare him or her for surgery. It will stick or sting and be over quickly. (See the earlier section "Restraints.")
3. Position the child as needed for the appropriate site. Ask the child to help by turning toes in, squeezing the side-rail, counting, and remaining as still as possible.
4. Cleanse the skin with an alcohol sponge and keep the sponge on hand to cleanse the site afterward.
5. Pinch up the skin and muscle for a thigh injection on a small child, but release when injecting the medication.
6. Insert the needle with wrist positioned as if throwing a dart. If the injection must be given at a 45° angle, as in the anterior thigh, turn the bevel up to aid smooth insertion.
7. Aspirate the syringe and slowly inject the medication.
8. Maintain firm restraint of the child throughout the injection. The pain of the medication entering the tissue may be more uncomfortable than the needle, and the child may try to move away.
9. Remove the needle and apply the alcohol sponge to the site. If bleeding occurs, apply pressure with a dry cotton ball for a few seconds.
10. Let the child help with the application of a Band-Aid or similar dressing.
11. Explain that the injection is over and change the child's position to increase comfort. Distract the child with a pleasant activity. Apply ice to the site if the child continues to complain.

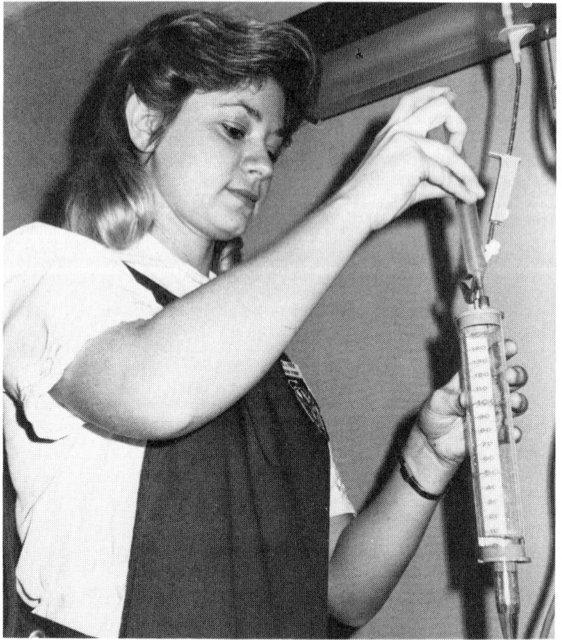

Figure 16-49 Intravenous medication can be infused through the volume control chamber on the IV.

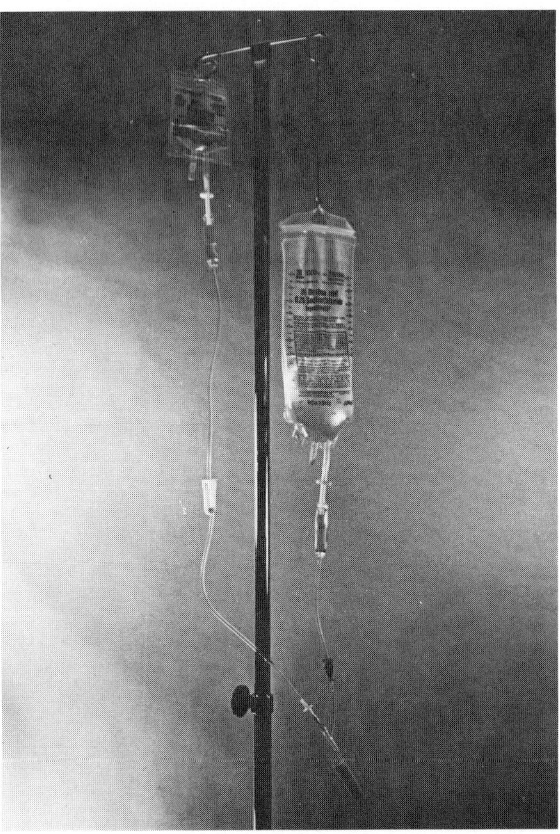

Figure 16-50 Intravenous medication being infused through a Y inlet in the main tubing. Note that the medication bag must be raised above the regular intravenous bag during medication administration.

After frequent use, certain kinds of nose drops create a chemical congestion in the nose and are no longer useful. It is best to use them only 2 to 3 days at a time.

Comfort measures after giving medications

The child may be very frightened or uncomfortable after a medication has been administered. Spend time with the child, and provide comfort and distraction through a pleasant play activity. Help the child realize that the medication was not given as a punishment and that he or she is still loved. This may be a good time for the child to try "giving medicine" to a doll or toy animal. Encourage the parents to provide comfort measures and distraction, because parents are the most significant "comforters."

Record on the nursing care plan specific approaches and comfort measures that are helpful to individual children.

Safety factors in giving medications

The following *"five rights"* of medication administration are vital in giving drugs safely to children:

1. Right medication.
2. Right dosage.
3. Right route.
4. Right time.
5. Right child.

Because small amounts of medication are involved, incorrect measurement or loss of some of the medication is a proportionately greater error when giving medications to children than when giving them to adults.

Be aware of the side effects of medications on children, which may be different from those on adults.

Be cautious and never leave medications at the child's bedside. After an injection, remove the equipment from the room immediately. Even such seemingly harmless items as topical creams and lotions should never be left near a young child, who may decide to apply them or eat them.

Table 16-28 Precautions in Administering Intravenous Medications

1. Check the intravenous site for patency before beginning the medication infusion.
2. Label the medication bag or volume control chamber with the drug name, date, time hung, time of expiration, and your initials or name.
3. Administer the drug as soon as possible after it is prepared, and complete the infusion before the expiration time to ensure drug potency.
4. Clear the secondary set tubing of all medication solution before discontinuing. Not all the medication is infused unless the line is cleared.
5. Use an intravenous pump to regulate the flow rate accurately.
6. Observe for signs of phlebitis or infiltration.
7. If there is local irritation of the vein only during infusion of the medication, the following alternatives may be helpful:
   a. Talk with the pharmacist about increasing the dilution of the medication. Confer with the physician about limits on fluid intake.
   b. Slow down the rate of infusion.
   c. Apply warm packs to the site (e.g., a warm washcloth changed frequently).
8. Flush the medication out of the tubing before another drug is infused. If a secondary set is used, as in Fig. 16-50, use different secondary tubing for each drug to prevent drug incompatibility.
9. Include the amount of fluid used for intravenous medications in the child's total daily fluid intake.

Document medication administration immediately. Chart the name, time, dosage, and route. Indicate effective approaches on the nursing care plan.

DISMISSAL PLANNING

According to Scipien,[101] the general objectives of dismissal planning are:

1. To ensure that there will be no interruption in the care required by the child and the family
2. To provide the family with adequate information and instructions to care for the child
3. To involve other appropriate agencies as needed and provide them with the necessary information to ensure continuity of care

Dismissal planning begins during the initial nursing assessment of the child and the family (Fig. 16-52). Assess the home situation and the level of understanding of the illness. Confer with the physician about the probable length of the child's hospitalization, and discuss the anticipated care needed at home. Continue to assess learning needs throughout the hospitalization.

Involve the child and the family in setting goals and planning for the return home. They need to

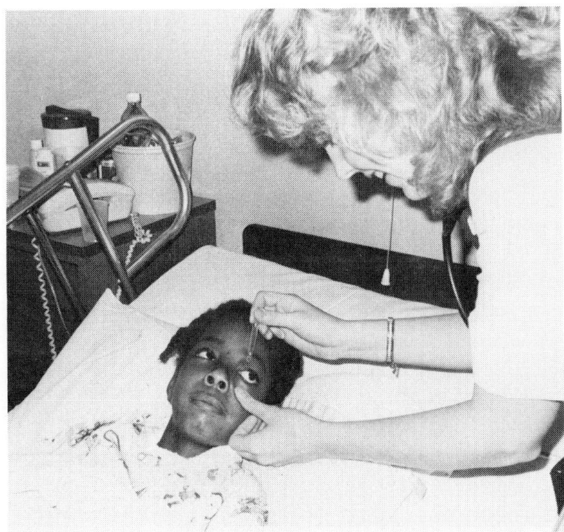

Figure 16-51 Eye drops being inserted into the sac formed by the lower lid. The child is asked to lie flat for several minutes after the insertion.

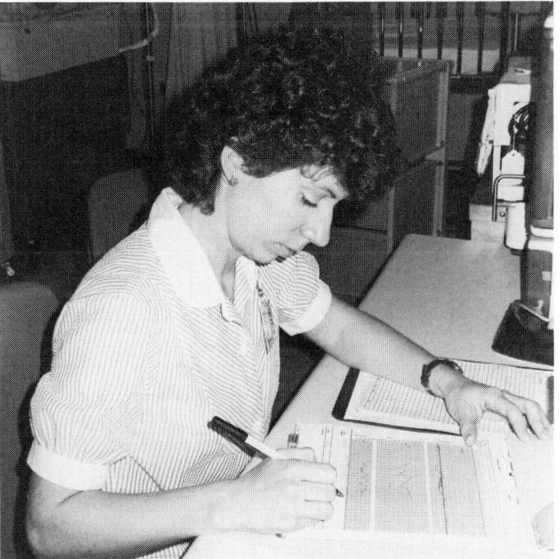

Figure 16-52 This nurse is reviewing a child's chart in order to make appropriate plans for dismissal.

know what is to be accomplished before dismissal and to anticipate home care needs in order to make arrangements in advance. Prepare a written plan on the Kardex containing goals for the child and the family and specific instructions needed to carry out the plan. Provide the child and the family with a copy.

Preparing the child and the family

Use the following principles of teaching and learning in preparing the child and the family for dismissal:

1. Determine readiness to learn. Teach when the parents and the child are receptive and motivated to learn.
2. Determine reading and comprehension level. Do not assume that printed instructions can be understood.
3. Repeat information. When the parents and the child are anxious, they may remember only portions of what they hear. Be prepared to repeat information patiently. Remind them, in the physician's presence, of those questions they "needed to ask the doctor but forgot."
4. Build on present knowledge. Be sure that there is *real* understanding of simple information before moving to more complex information.
5. Use teaching aids—pamphlets, books, and films—as appropriate.
6. If medications are to be continued at home, be sure that the parents (and the child) have a clear understanding of the dosage, the frequency and length of administration, and the possible side effects of the drugs involved. Be aware of what equipment will be used at home, and teach with that in mind.
7. Provide time for questions, discussion, demonstration, and practice in giving care.
8. Evaluate teaching effectiveness through quizzes and repeat demonstrations.[102]

Community resources

Community resources include public health nursing agencies, school nurses, support groups for patients with specific illnesses and their families, clergy, educational facilities, friends, relatives, and others. Determine those which are appropriate for the child and the family. Talk with a representative of any community agency needed, and arrange a meeting in the hospital before dismissal.

A written referral may be necessary to ensure adequate follow-up. Consult the child and the family and obtain their permission. Complete a written nursing referral including:

The child's diagnosis
Treatments during hospitalization
Medications and treatments to be administered at home
Reasons for the referral
Special needs of the child and the family
Teaching done in the hospital
Goals for the child
Planned follow-up activities
A hospital resource person who may be contacted

Documentation

1. Chart all teaching on the nursing care plan and in the nurses' progress notes to ensure continuity of care from one shift to the next. Indicate the receptiveness of the child and the family and an evaluation of learning.
2. Record plans for a nursing referral in the nursing care plan (or attach a copy to the chart).
3. Obtain the parents' and the child's permission for referral to a community agency, and chart this in the nurses' notes.
4. Give written instructions to the child and the family about medications and treatments.
5. Complete a written referral at dismissal time.
6. Chart the dismissal procedure; include medications and equipment taken home and the child's physical and emotional state.

The dismissal procedure

When dismissal is ordered, the nurse must confer with the physician about all medications and treatments to be administered at home. Obtain medications and review the schedule of administration with the child and the family. Review all previous teaching and written instructions. Help the child get dressed and gather his or her belongings. Encourage the parents to go to the hospital business office to complete dismissal details before they take the child from the room. Give the child an opportunity to say good-bye to staff members and other children who are patients. Some pediatric units provide a dismissal gift (such as a stuffed animal or a coloring book) as a memento of the hospitalization.

It is important to accompany the child and the family to the entrance of the hospital to help carry belongings and to ensure that they are safely dismissed. Encourage them to call the nursing unit or the physician if questions arise.

A follow-up telephone call by the child's primary nurse a few days later may be welcomed by the family. Any questions can be answered, and the current conditions at home can be assessed.

REFERENCES

1. Leifer, G., *Principles and Techniques in Pediatric Nursing,* Saunders, Philadelphia, 1982, p. 19.
2. Johnson, J., K. T. Kirchoff, and P. M. Endress, "Easing Children's Fright during Health Care Procedures," *American Journal of Maternal-Child Nursing* **1**(4):206 (July–August 1976).
3. Scipien, G., M. U. Barnard, M. A. Chard, J. Howe, and P. J. Phillips (eds.), *Comprehensive Pediatric Nursing,* 2d ed., McGraw-Hill, New York, 1979, p. 837.
4. Leifer, op. cit., p. 88.
5. Marlow, D., *Textbook of Pediatric Nursing,* Saunders, Philadelphia, 1977, p. 456.
6. Leifer, op. cit., p. 89.
7. Whaley, L., and D. Wong, *Nursing Care of Infants and Children,* Mosby, St. Louis, 1983, p. 929.
8. Erb, B. D., and G. R. Wilson, "Rheumatic Heart Disease," *Cardiovascular Nursing* **4**(1):4 (January–February 1968).
9. Johnson, Kirchoff, and Endress, loc. cit.
10. Scipien, Barnard, Chard, Howe, and Phillips, op. cit., p. 418.
11. Hilt, N., "Pride, Prejudice, and Parents," *Pediatric Nursing* **2**(3):34 (May–June 1976).
12. Farris, L. S., "Approaches to Caring for the American-Indian Maternity Patient," *American Journal of Maternal-Child Nursing* **1**(2):82 (March–April 1976).
13. Ibid., pp. 80–87.
14. McCain, G. W., and D. C. Bies, "Television Viewing and the Hospitalized Child," *Pediatric Nursing* **9**(1):33 (January–February 1983).
15. McCown, D., "TV: Its Effects on Children," *Pediatric Nursing* **5**(2):19 (March–April 1979).
16. Dowd, E. L., J. C. Novak, and E. J. Ray, "Releasing the Hospitalized Child from Restraints," *American Journal of Maternal-Child Nursing* **2**(6):373 (November–December 1977).
17. Bernabeu, E. P., "The Effects of Severe Crippling on the Development of a Group of Children," *Psychiatry* **21**:169–194 (May 1958).
18. O'Grady, R. S., "Restraint and the Hospitalized Child," in B. S. Bergerson et al. (eds.), *Current Concepts in Clinical Nursing,* vol. 2, Mosby, St. Louis, 1969, pp. 192–202.
19. Leifer, op. cit., p. 81.
20. Ibid., p. 39.
21. Scipien, Barnard, Chard, Howe, and Phillips, op. cit., p. 501.
22. Seedor, M. M., *Introduction to Asepsis,* 2d rev. ed., Teachers College, New York, 1979.
23. Meehan, R. M., "Isolation—To Be or Not to Be Afraid," *American Journal of Maternal-Child Nursing* **5**(4):257 (July–August 1980).
24. Leifer, op. cit., p. 93.
25. Seedor, op. cit.
26. Leifer, op. cit., p. 104.
27. Zeimer, M., and J. S. Carroll, "Infant Gavage Reconsidered," *American Journal of Nursing* **78**(9):1543 (September 1978).
28. Ibid.
29. Ibid.
30. Ibid.
31. Leifer, op. cit., p. 120.
32. Marlow, op. cit., p. 198.
33. Leifer, op. cit., p. 60.
34. Guhlow, L. J., and J. Kolb, "Pediatric IVs: Special Measures You Must Take," *RN* **42**(3):40 (March 1979).
35. Millam, D. A., "How to Insert an IV," *American Journal of Nursing* **79**(7):1268 (July 1979).
36. Guhlow and Kolb, op. cit., p. 47.
37. Millam, op. cit., p. 1270.
38. "Fundamentals of IV Maintenance," programmed instruction, *American Journal of Nursing* **79**(7):1275 (July 1979).
39. Ibid.
40. Millam, op. cit., p. 1269.
41. Millam, op. cit., p. 1270.
42. Guhlow and Kolb, op. cit., p. 50.
43. "Pediatric IVs: Nursing Implications at a Glance," tear-out guide, *RN* **42**(3) (March 1979).
44. Guhlow and Kolb, op. cit., p. 47.
45. Guhlow and Kolb, op. cit., p. 50.
46. *Wyeth R Heparin Lock Flush Solution,* USP, Wyeth Laboratories, Philadelphia, 1978.
47. Guhlow and Kolb, loc. cit.
48. *Wyeth R Heparin Lock Flush Solution.*
49. Bosso, J. A., "Experience with a New Small-Volume Infusion System in Pediatric Patients," *Hospital Formulary* **17**(2):214 (February 1982).
50. Ibid.
51. Ibid., pp. 214–222.
52. Joyner, S., and S. Peristein, *Nursing Protocol for Port-a-Cath System,* Pharmacia, 1983.
53. Anderson, M., S. Aker, and R. Hickman, "The Double Lumen Hickman Catheter," *American Journal of Nursing* **82**(2):272–273 (February 1982).
54. Doran, E. M., "Care of the Hickman Catheter in Children," *Nursing Clinics of North America* **18**(3):579–580 (September 1983).
55. Ibid., pp. 579–583.
56. Guilfoile, T., and K. Dabe, "Nasal Oxygen Therapy for Infants," *Respiratory Care* **26**(1):35 (January 1981).
57. Ibid.
58. Shirkey, H. C. (ed.), *Pediatric Therapy,* 5th ed., Mosby, St. Louis, 1975, p. 306.
59. Whaley and Wong, op. cit., p. 1166.

60. Scipien, Barnard, Chard, Howe, and Phillips, op. cit., p. 590.
61. Ibid.
62. Whaley and Wong, loc. cit.
63. Ibid.
64. Ibid., p. 1312.
65. Ibid., p. 1166.
66. Tecklin, Jan S., "Positioning, Percussing, and Vibrating the Patient for Effective Bronchial Drainage," *Nursing* **79**9(3):68 (March 1979).
67. Ibid., p. 69.
68. Ibid., p. 68.
69. *A Study Guide to Basic Cardiac Life Support,* West Alabama Emergency Medical Services, Aug. 20, 1980.
70. Block, C. R., and C. E. Block, "Help, My Child Is Choking," *Pediatric Nursing* **2**(5):48 (September–October 1976).
71. "Standards for CPR and ECC," *JAMA,* June 6, 1986, vol. 255, no. 21, pp. 2955–2960.
72. Block and Block, loc. cit.
73. Tucker, S. M., et al., *Patient Care Standards,* Mosby, St. Louis, 1975, pp. 350–353, 407.
74. Barrus, D. H., "A Comparison of Rectal and Axillary Temperatures by Electronic Thermometer Measurement in Preschool Children," *Pediatric Nursing* **11**(6):425 (November–December 1983).
75. Kresch, M. J., "Axillary Temperature as a Screening Test for Fever in Children," *Journal of Pediatrics* **104**(4):598 (April 1984).
76. Abbey, J., et al., "How Long Is That Thermometer Accurate:" *American Journal of Nursing* **78**(8):1375–1376 (August 1978).
77. Younger, J. B., and B. S. Brown, "Fever Management: Rational or Ritual?," *Pediatric Nursing* **11**(1):26–29 (1985).
78. Ibid.
79. Ibid.
80. Botwin, E. D., "Should Children Be Screened for Hypertension?" *Journal of Maternal-Child Nursing* **1**(3):152 (May–June 1976).
81. Greenfield, D., R. Grant, and E. Lieberman, "Children Can Have High Blood Pressure Too," *American Journal of Nursing* **76**(5):771 (May 1976).
82. Lancour, J., "How to Avoid Pitfalls in Measuring Blood Pressure," *American Journal of Nursing* **76**(5):774 (May 1976).
83. Ibid., p. 775.
84. Whaley and Wong, op. cit., p. 178.
85. Ibid.
86. Ibid.
87. Greenfield, Grant, and Lieberman, loc. cit.
88. Hernandez, A., D. A. Meyer, and D. Goldring, "Blood Pressure in Neonates," *Contemporary OB/GYN* **5** (March 1975).
89. Daniels, J., "Winter Skin Care: Change Your Skin's Personality," *Rochester Methodist Hospital News,* Rochester, Minn., Winter 1977, pp. 10–11.
90. *Care of Children's Teeth,* American Dental Association, 1976, p. 15.
91. *Your Child's Teeth,* American Dental Association, 1976, p. 4.
92. Ibid.
93. Smith, M. E., "The Preschooler and Pain," in P. A. Brandt, P. L. Chinn, and M. E. Smith (eds.), *Current Practice in Pediatric Nursing,* Mosby, St. Louis, 1976, p. 206.
94. Younger and Brown, loc. cit.
95. Dube, S. K. and S. H. Pierog, *Immediate Care of the Sick and Injured Child,* Mosby, St. Louis, 1978, p. 14.
96. Shirkey, op. cit., p. 22.
97. Ormond, E. and C. Caulfield, "A Practical Guide to Giving Oral Medications to Young Children," *American Journal of Maternal-Child Nursing* **1**(5):325 (September–October 1976).
98. Whaley and Wong, op. cit., p. 924.
99. Ibid.
100. Ibid.
101. Scipien, Barnard, Chard, Howe, and Phillips, op. cit., p. 506.
102. Ibid., p. 508.

17

Julie A. Goodman

Nursing care of the high-risk infant

Upon completion of this chapter, the student will be able to:

1. Relate the mother's preconceptional health to the health of the fetus and the newborn.
2. Describe the use of prenatal assessment tools to predict fetal well-being.
3. Use the gestational age assessment tool to evaluate gestational age.
4. Identify the role of transport and the neonatal intensive care unit in the care of the high-risk infant.
5. Identify the immediate care needs of the depressed newborn.
6. Describe the problems specific to an infant whose growth is inappropriate for gestational age.
7. Identify the common problems of postmature infants.
8. Relate the physiological immaturity of a preterm infant to the physiological handicaps of that infant.
9. Contrast the methods of feeding the high-risk infant.
10. Describe the alterations caused by faulty oxygenation of the high-risk newborn.
11. Contrast physiological and pathological jaundice.
12. Compare the disease processes of, and the supportive care for, ABO and Rh hemolytic disease.
13. Describe the effects of maternal diabetes on the infant.
14. Identify the signs of fetal alcohol syndrome in an affected newborn.
15. Describe the signs of drug addiction in a newborn.
16. Discuss the commonalities underlying birth trauma.
17. Discuss the ways in which the steps in parenting are affected by the birth of a high-risk infant.

High-risk is a comprehensive term applied to a wide range of infants, from the minimally ill to the critically ill. Whatever the cause or severity of the problem, a high-risk newborn needs special medical and nursing assistance to maintain the bodily functions that normal newborns are capable of maintaining independently. A special report by the Robert Wood Johnson Foundation states that one out of every seven births has some element of high risk.[1]

IDENTIFICATION OF THE HIGH-RISK INFANT

Preconceptional factors

The fetus is totally dependent on its mother for a healthy environment; therefore, preparation for pregnancy needs to begin long before conception occurs. Ideally, this preparation begins by maintaining a high level of wellness between puberty and the childbearing years. The initial opportunity to evaluate a woman's health often arises at the time she comes to a clinic for information about birth control or for a premarital physical examination. The history and physical examination will reveal any physical problems present and the visit can be used to educate the woman about preventing future childbearing risks. Some of the most important topics that should be covered during counseling for preconceptional health and the prevention of diseases that threaten maternal and fetal health follow below.

Timing of pregnancy Ages 20–35 are optimal ages for childbearing. Women 16 and under and those over 35 are at a higher risk. At least a 2-year interval between pregnancies is recommended.

Nutrition An effort should be made to ensure a well-balanced diet and appropriate weight control. Women who begin pregnancy 10 percent or more under their normal weight are at a greater risk for perinatal complications, even though they have an adequate weight gain during pregnancy. The incidence of low-birth-weight babies among underweight women is twice that among women of normal weight.[2] Obesity presents the hazards of soft tissue dystocia (fatty tissue impairs the baby's movement through the pelvis) and an increased incidence of hypertension and diabetes.

Prenatal care The need to have a prepregnancy physical examination to correct or control health problems should be emphasized. The nurse should discuss the need for beginning prenatal care when the woman first knows that she is pregnant.

Drugs Women should avoid taking all nonprescription drugs and should consult a doctor regarding prescribed medications both while trying to become pregnant and during the first trimester of pregnancy. There is uncertainty about the absolute safety of many drugs when taken during pregnancy, but many are known to pass the placental barrier. For example, tetracycline prescribed for acne can cause discoloration of the fetal tooth buds. Aspirin has been linked to increased intracranial bleeding at birth. Sulfonamides are toxic to the fetal liver when taken during the last trimester. The effects of street drugs and pot are not completely known, but these should be avoided because fetal addiction to some drugs is known to occur.

Alcohol It is best not to drink during pregnancy, especially during the first trimester. At the most, no more than one drink (2 oz of liquor) a day should be consumed. Fetal alcohol syndrome is discussed later in this chapter.

Genetic counseling Premarital genetic counseling should be considered if a close relative has a disorder that is considered to be inherited. Indications for genetic counseling are listed in Table 6-1.

Smoking Smoking retards fetal growth and should be discontinued before pregnancy. Women should be told that reducing cigarette smoking and stopping entirely even late in pregnancy is of some benefit. Recent research has shown that women who cut their smoking in half, even in their eighth month of pregnancy, still had babies who were 92 g heavier and 0.6 cm longer than the babies of women in a matched control group.[3]

Diseases that can be transmitted and cause disease in the fetus Additional information regarding these diseases is given in Chap. 28.

Rubella (German measles) Rubella causes cataracts, hearing defects, and heart defects in the fetus during the first 3 months of pregnancy and may cause chromosomal damage, with slower cell division and shorter cell life span, causing mental retardation and motor impairment that will be apparent at a later time.

Five to fifteen percent of women of childbearing age are susceptible to rubella. In the United States, newly immigrated Asian women constitute one of the largest groups of women at risk. In addition, a small number of previously immunized women have low antibody titers and need to be revaccinated. A rubella titer to check immunity should be done on all women of childbearing age. A titer greater than 1:10 indicates immunity. In 1982, the Immunization Practices Advisory Committee made the following recommendations: (1) Pregnancy should be considered a contraindication to rubella vaccination because of the small risk of congenital rubella, (2) vaccination should take place at least 3 months prior to conception, and (3) accidental vaccination of a pregnant woman should not be considered to necessitate an abortion, since the risk of the fetus's contracting congenital rubella from vaccination is so small as to be negligible.[4]

Toxoplasmosis The protozoan causing toxoplasmosis has as its primary host the cat. When infected the cat sheds oocysts during the days 7–20 following the infection. The human becomes infected by coming in contact with the cat feces. Infection is also caused by handling or eating undercooked red meat, drinking unpasteurized milk, eating raw eggs, and receiving blood transfusions. After the initial human infection, the second stage of the life of the protozoan begins with the formation of tissue cysts that persist throughout the person's life. The cysts rupture continuously, and the body maintains a continuous antibody production. Eighty percent of those infected have no symptoms during the initial infection; the rest have only flulike symptoms. The fetus is affected only at the time of the primary infection; the disease is most severe during the first trimester and is only mild or asymptomatic during the second and third trimesters. Maternal infection acquired during pregnancy is transmitted only about 50 percent of the time. For those fetuses that are affected hydrocephalus, mental retardation, seizures, intracranial calcifications, and impaired vision (chorioretinitis) may result. Children with a subclinical infection (seropositive only) show a propensity toward subnormal IQs and late-developing chorioretinitis.[5]

Gonorrhea Early treatment of gonorrhea will prevent infertility due to obstruction related to tubal adhesions. Pregnant women who have gonorrhea must be treated prior to vaginal delivery, since blindness in the newborn can result from contact with a birth canal that is infected with gonorrhea.

Syphilis A premarital blood test for syphilis is required in most states. If the disease is present, it is treated with penicillin.

Herpes simplex: Type I (oral) and Type II (genital) Both types of herpes can cause genital infections in the susceptible woman and can be transmitted to the fetus and the newborn if the disease is active at birth. Primary genital herpes that is transmitted to the fetus is associated with an increased incidence of spontaneous abortions and premature births. Thirty to fifty percent of infants delivered through a birth canal that is contaminated with herpes are infected, regardless of whether the mother is symptomatic.[6] Fetal infection carries the danger of massive fetal encephalitis and dissemination to the liver, the adrenal glands, and the central nervous system. A cesarean section is indicated when blisters or lesions are present, when there has been a positive culture in the 2 weeks preceding the anticipated birth, and when membranes are intact or have been ruptured for less than 6 h.

Cytomegalovirus Cytomegalovirus (CMV) is a very common infectious agent; it is related to the herpes virus and is usually present in adults in a subclinical state. It causes disease in persons who are immunosuppressed or in conjunction with another disease. In the pregnant woman, it is transmitted to the fetus with the primary infection 50 percent of the time and can also be transmitted from an infection prior to pregnancy. Twelve to twenty percent of infected fetuses are born with systemic cytomegalovirus inclusion disease. Sequelae are not related to gestational age at the time of the infection. The child is at risk for lower IQ, deafness, motor defects, and learning disabilities. Early treatment of infected infants with antimetabolites or antiviral agents may prevent central nervous system destruction. Immunization with CMV strains is still experimental.[7]

Hepatitis B virus Infants born to asymptomatic women who are positive for hepatitis B surface antigen develop the disease. Pregnant women should be screened, and immunoprophylaxis should be given to all newborns of women who are surface-antigen-seropositive. The long latency period of 4 months complicates the disease. Hepatitis B immunoglobulin plus hepatitis B vaccine is expensive, but can be used for infants born to seropositive mothers. Some of these infants will become chronic carriers, and others will show symptoms that range from mild disease to cirrhosis, chronic hepatitis, and fulminating hepatitis B, leading to death.[8]

AIDS The fetus can contract acquired immune deficiency syndrome (AIDS) transplacentally from an infected mother or from infected transfusions. Some sources also indicate that the AIDS virus is present in the breast milk of affected women. See Chaps. 26 and 28 for additional information.

Prenatal factors

Prenatal factors that have proved to be important predictors of the newborn's health are quality of prenatal care, the parents' levels of education and socioeconomic status, the father's occupation, the mother's nutritional status, genetic factors, and race.

The pregnant woman who lives in poverty is often poorly educated and has little access to nutritious food; prenatal care is a luxury that she cannot afford. She is also more frequently a member of a minority population. A recent survey of 45 cities in the United States showed that the gap in survival rates between black and white infants is widening. Low birth weight, the factor most predictive of infant death, rose to 13.08 percent in the black population in 1981, while in the white population it remained at 6.8 percent.[9]

There is no mystery concerning what must be done to increase birth weight and reduce infant mortality. For many years, the most positive influence on the health of newborns has been early, comprehensive prenatal care. The outlook for improving prenatal care is not good. A 1981 survey showed that the number of both black and white women who receive prenatal care during the first trimester has declined and that the number of women who receive no prenatal care has risen.[10]

The United States ranks first in the world in terms of the outcome for a very low birth weight baby who is admitted into a center that provides tertiary care; but it ranks tenth in overall infant death rates. The attempts to break the high-risk cycle prenatally by providing federal or state funding for free or low-cost neighborhood health clinics, nutrition counseling, and supplemental food programs for pregnant women and infants have been poorly funded. An increased financial commitment to maternal and child health is desperately needed and would prove to be cost-effective, since it would lower, at least to some extent, the huge cost of caring for sick newborns.

Tools for assessing fetal well-being There are many assessment tools for evaluating risks to the mother and the fetus during the prenatal and perinatal periods. It is important to have information about the mother's health before conception and about diseases she has that can affect the fetus. Scoring Form for the Serial Identification of the High-risk Fetus (Table 17-1) and Factors That Place the Fetus at Risk (Table 17-2) give an overview of the risk factors that are responsible for most of the alterations of the high-risk infant discussed in this chapter. The value of assessing prenatal health risks lies in using the assessment as a health-maintenance and evaluation tool. When risks are recognized and treated prenatally, they become the basis of preventive care during the perinatal period.

Advances in fetal medicine have made it possible to study the fetus in utero. Biochemical samples are obtained to determine the fetus's sex, condition, and level of maturity and to determine whether congenital anomalies or genetic diseases are present. Tests are also used to diagnose chronic fetal distress and to make decisions regarding safe delivery dates and routes. Fetal monitoring is used to diagnose acute fetal distress during labor and to closely observe the status of an infant known to be previously distressed. Table 17-3 summarizes some of the tests that are frequently used to evaluate the high-risk fetus. More detailed information regarding fetal medicine can be found in any current obstetrics textbook.

NEONATAL CARE OF THE HIGH-RISK INFANT

Neonatal intensive care

Since the development of the neonatal intensive care unit (NICU) in the 1960s, there has been a rapid increase in the use of intensive care for newborns. This trend has greatly decreased the neonatal mortality rate. At first, no guidelines for establishing a neonatal intensive care unit existed, and units proliferated without specified standards of care.

In 1971, the American Medical Association formally recognized the need to centralize and organize newborn care facilities to ensure quality of care. The association issued a statement supporting the regionalization of care by geographic area and recommending levels of caregiving. The National Foundation–March of Dimes financed a committee on perinatal health, which studied the issue and recommended three levels of care. Level 1 care, or primary care, is the least complex and can be given in the community hospital that handles uncomplicated deliveries of full-term infants; level 2 care, or secondary care, is provided at a large obstetric unit which is equipped to care for moderately ill newborns and which has an organized transport system; and

Table 17-1 Scoring Form for Serial Identification of the High-Risk Fetus

Check off all risk factors present (even if the maximum score is reached), and tabulate the fetal risk score and gestational age at each visit.

Part A: Score 0, 1, 2, or 3 to a maximum of 3	A
Part B: Score 0, 1, 2, or 3 to a maximum of 3	B
Part C: Score 0, 1, 2, 3, or 4 to a maximum of 4	+C

A. Baseline Data

Factor	Score	
Age less than 15	2	☐
35+	1	☐
40+	3	☐
Para 0	1	☐
6+	2	☐
Interval less than 2 years	1	☐
Weight less than 100 lb	1	☐
Obesity (200 lb+)	1	☐
Diabetes		
Class A	1	☐
Class B, C, or D	2	☐
Class F, R	3	☐
Chronic renal disease	1	☐
With diminished renal function	3	☐
Preexisting hypertension		
140+/90+	1	☐
160+/110+	2	☐
Interpregnancy cardiac failure	3	☐
Previous Obstetrical History		
Abortion		☐
Stillbirth		☐
Neonatal death		☐
Surviving premature infant		☐
Antepartum hemorrhage		☐
Toxemia		☐
Mid-forceps delivery		☐
Cesarean section		☐
Major congenital anomaly		☐
Baby 10 lb+		☐
Cervical incompetence		☐
One instance of above	1	☐
Two or more instances of above	2	☐
Rh isoimmunized mother with homozygous husband	2	☐
Also history of erythroblastosis (affected infant)	3	☐

B. Present Pregnancy

Factor	Score	
Bleeding, before 20 weeks		
Alone	1	☐
With pain	2	☐
Bleeding, after 20 weeks		
Ceased	1	☐
Continues	2	☐
With pain	3	☐
With hypotension	3	☐
Spontaneous premature rupture of membranes	1	☐
Latent period 24 h+	2	☐
Anemia 8 to 10 g	1	☐
Less than 8 g	2	☐
No prenatal care	2	☐
One to three prenatal visits	1	☐
Toxemia (mild to moderate)	1	☐
Eclampsia	3	☐
Hydramnios (single fetus)	3	☐
Multiple pregnancy	2	☐
Gestational diabetes, diagnosis before 36 weeks	1	☐
Diagnosis after 36 weeks	2	☐
Decreasing insulin requirement	3	☐
Maternal diabetic acidosis	3	☐
Maternal pyrexia	1	☐
Pyrexia and FHR greater than 160	2	☐
Rh-negative—rising antibody titer	2	☐
Heart disease, classes III–IV	2	☐

C. Gestational Age (at Time of Scoring)

Factor	Score	
28 weeks or under	4	☐
29 to 32 weeks	3	☐
33 to 35 weeks	2	☐
36 to 37 weeks	1	☐
38 to 41 weeks	0	☐
42 weeks	1	☐
43 weeks or more	2	☐

Source: Adapted from J. Goodwin, J. Dunne, and B. Thomas, "Antepartum Identification of the Fetus at Risk," *Canadian Medical Association Journal* **101**(458):57–65 (October 1969).

level 3 care, or tertiary care, involves the highest degree of medical specialists and an NICU with a highly sophisticated transport system (Fig. 17-1).

Transport of the high-risk mother and infant

Referral involves moving a high-risk pregnant woman (maternal transport) or a high-risk baby after birth (neonatal transport) from a smaller community hospital to a larger medical center or hospital that provides secondary or tertiary care. *Transport* is accomplished through the use of a van or ambulance equipped with special life-support systems. Some NICUs also have the capability for airplane or helicopter transport. Specially trained perinatal nurses and a pediatrician are members of the transport team for a critically ill newborn. Recent experience has shown that the infant's outcome is equally good if the transport team consists only of experienced NICU nurses.[11]

Table 17-2 Factors That Place the Fetus and the Newborn at Risk

Decreased Oxygenation in the Fetus
Placenta previa or abruptio placentae
Placental insufficiency
Uterine rupture with hemorrhage
Maternal hypertension, diabetes, heart disease, toxemia, renal disease, or Rh sensitization
Anemia
Sickle cell disease
Effects of anesthetic, analgesics, or drugs
Cord prolapse or knot in cord
Trauma to the Baby During the Birth Process
Prolonged labor
Arrest of labor
Cephalopelvic dysproportion
Dystocia related to large baby, twins, breech birth, or face presentation
Difficult delivery (mid forceps)
Precipitous delivery
Dysmaturity and Alteration in the Health of the Baby
Prematurity
Postmaturity
Low birth weight
Congenital anomalies
Respiratory distress syndrome
Respiratory distress related to cesarean section
Aspiration of meconium, blood, or mucus
Sepsis:
Prolonged rupture of membranes
Bacterial or viral disease

Since the uterus is the ideal incubator, it is best for the high-risk woman to be transported *before* delivery. This significantly decreases the severity of illness in the newborn, subsequent complications, and fetal mortality. If transport occurs after delivery, the neonate must be stabilized before being moved to the NICU.

Factors related to transport that increase the stress to the family and the health care personnel involved are:

1. Separation of the mother and the infant from the family
2. Separation of the infant from the mother when the baby is put in the NICU
3. The increased costs of intensive care, transport, and lengthy hospitalization
4. Problems with the actual transport (e.g., a poorly supervised or disorganized transport)
5. Poor communication between referral centers (which may make the physician reluctant to refer patients)
6. Lack of education on the part of personnel in referring communities
7. Failure to recognize the perinatal risks and the need to refer a mother and her infant[12]

Stabilizing the infant after birth

Stabilization of the sick newborn begins in the delivery room. Premature labor, a maternal his-

Table 17-3 Fetal Assessment Procedures

Test	Method	Purpose
1. Amniocentesis a. Analysis of fetal cells	Amniotic fluid is withdrawn from the amniotic cavity through a needle, often in conjunction with ultrasound to determine where the placenta, cord, and fetus are located.	At about 16 weeks of gestation, the test can determine sex and many genetic defects. See also Chap. 8.
b. Analysis of bilirubin in the amniotic fluid	Done for isoimmunization after 26 weeks of gestation.	Bilirubin usually disappears from the amniotic fluid by 36 weeks of gestation. Increased levels after 30 weeks indicate destruction of red blood cells. The test is done to evaluate Rh incompatibility.
c. Analysis of creatinine in the amniotic fluid		A value of 2 mg per 100 ml at 36 weeks of gestation indicates maturity of the kidneys.
d. Analysis of the color of the amniotic fluid (normally is straw-colored)		Meconium will color the fluid brown or green. Bilirubin will color the fluid yellow-brown.
e. Analysis of phospholipids level		L/S (lecithin-sphingomyelin) ratio of 2:1 indicates fetal lung maturity. Sphingomyelin is present all during pregnancy and decreases at term. Lecithin increases with gestational age.

Table 17-3 Fetal Assessment Procedures (*Continued*)

Test	Method	Purpose
f. Analysis of alpha fetoprotein		A possible neural tube defect is indicated by the presence of alpha fetoprotein due to leakage of spinal fluid into the amniotic fluid.
2. Serial estriols	Twenty-four-h urine specimens are collected several times to obtain a baseline. Can also be done using blood.	The test measures the hormonal function of the placenta. The estriol content of urine and blood during pregnancy rises from 28 weeks of gestation to delivery. Urine values of 12 mg or above indicate adequate placental and fetal adrenal function; values of 4 to 12 mg usually indicate fetal death. A sudden drop of 25% is a warning that the fetus is in danger.
3. Shake test	Amniotic fluid is collected (or, in a newborn, gastric aspirant) and is shaken with alcohol.	A positive result indicates the presence of lecithin and stability of surfactant. There is a 95% chance that the infant will not have respiratory distress syndrome if enough bubbles form to make a ring around the fluid in the test tube. Few or no bubbles constitute a negative result.
4. Ultrasound	A scan using ultrasound waves is used. The patient must have a full bladder.	The test detects some abnormalities of the fetus (e.g., hydrocephalus, anencephaly, and hydatidiform mole), intrauterine growth retardation, and twins.
a. Measurement of the biparietal diameter (BPD) of the fetal head		The test assesses fetal gestational age and growth rates; 8.9 to 10.1 cm is the normal range of a full-term BPD. The average is about 9.4 cm.
5. Oxytocin challenge test (OCT), or stress test	An external fetal monitor is used to check fetal heart tones and contractions. Then Pitocin is given to produce three contractions in 10 min. Contractions can also be produced by nipple stimulation.	The test establishes the baseline fetal heart rate. A delay in return of fetal heart tones to normal after a contraction indicates uteroplacental insufficiency (late deceleration). The baby may tolerate the stress of labor poorly. A cesarean section must be considered. There are both false-negative and false-positive results, and the test should be used as only one of many evaluation tools.
6. Nonstress test (NST); sometimes called *fetal acceleration determination* (FAD)	An external fetal heart monitor is attached. Mild, normally present (Braxton Hicks) contractions or fetal activity is used, and each movement is marked.	The fetal heart should accelerate with fetal movement or contractions. Lack of fluctuations (5 to 20 per minute), a straight baseline (poor variability), or a decrease in heart rate predicts a poor reaction to the stress of labor. This is called a *nonreactive test*.

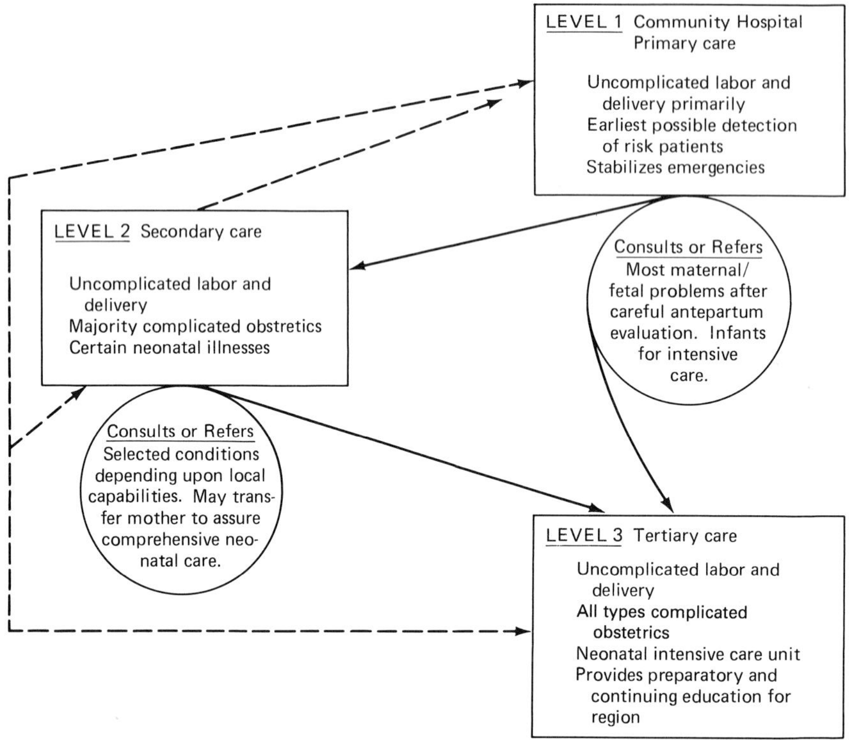

Figure 17-1 A schematic representation of regionalized perinatal care. Note the equal responsibility and reciprocal interaction between the levels. (*From R. Hoekelman et al.* [eds.], *Principles of Pediatrics: Health Care of the Young, McGraw-Hill, New York, 1978. Used with permission.*)

tory of disease, and fetal distress alert the nurse to prepare for a compromised newborn. The nurse is often responsible for calling the transport team, coordinating the care, and ensuring that a pediatrician or a neonatal nurse who is skilled in resuscitation will be available when the infant is born. It is important to have one person in the delivery room whose sole responsibility is the well-being of the depressed baby.

The major goals of care immediately after birth are to:

1. Establish ventilation
2. Maintain temperature
3. Provide fluids and electrolytes
4. Prevent infection
5. Maintain vital signs

Assessing the high-risk newborn

Physical assessment The components of the routine physical assessment of a newborn's body systems and of the minor and major abnormalities that can cause potential problems are listed in Table 8-2. Chapter 8 also describes the routines for admitting a newborn to the nursery; obtaining a health history of the mother and the newborn; checking the newborn's temperature, heart rate, and blood pressure; and administering medications routinely given at birth. Because it is not appropriate to exhaust a sick newborn by giving a detailed physical examination, these general assessment guidelines can be modified and used as a basis for assessing the status of a high-risk infant.

Statistics Statistics show that the risk of neonatal death is greatest during the first hour of life and then during the next 24 h, after which the risk decreases significantly. In reporting statistics, the following terms are used. A *fetal death* is the death of a viable fetus. A *viable fetus* is legally defined as a fetus between 20 weeks of gestational age and birth. A *neonatal death* is the death of a newborn during the first 28 days of life. A *perinatal death* is the death of a fetus or a newborn from 20 weeks of gestational age through the first 28 days of life expressed in deaths per 1000 live births.

Gestational-age assessment

Most mortality (death) and morbidity (illness) is related to low birth weight and prematurity. In the past, the word *premature* was sometimes used to refer to any infant weighing 2500 g or less ($5\frac{1}{2}$ lb), regardless of gestational age. The American Academy of Pediatrics has defined birth weight and gestational age as follows:

1. *Low birth weight* Less than 2500 g
2. *Gestational age* Preterm or premature—less than 37 full weeks of gestation, regardless of weight; full-term—38 to 42 weeks of gestation; and postterm—more than 42 weeks of gestation

Lubchenco's newborn classification (Fig. 17-2) is a tool for assessing the appropriateness of intrauterine growth for gestational age. Using this chart, it is possible to determine whether an infant is appropriate for gestational age (AGA), falling between the 10th and the 90th percentiles in growth; is small for gestational age (SGA), falling below the 10th percentile in growth; or is

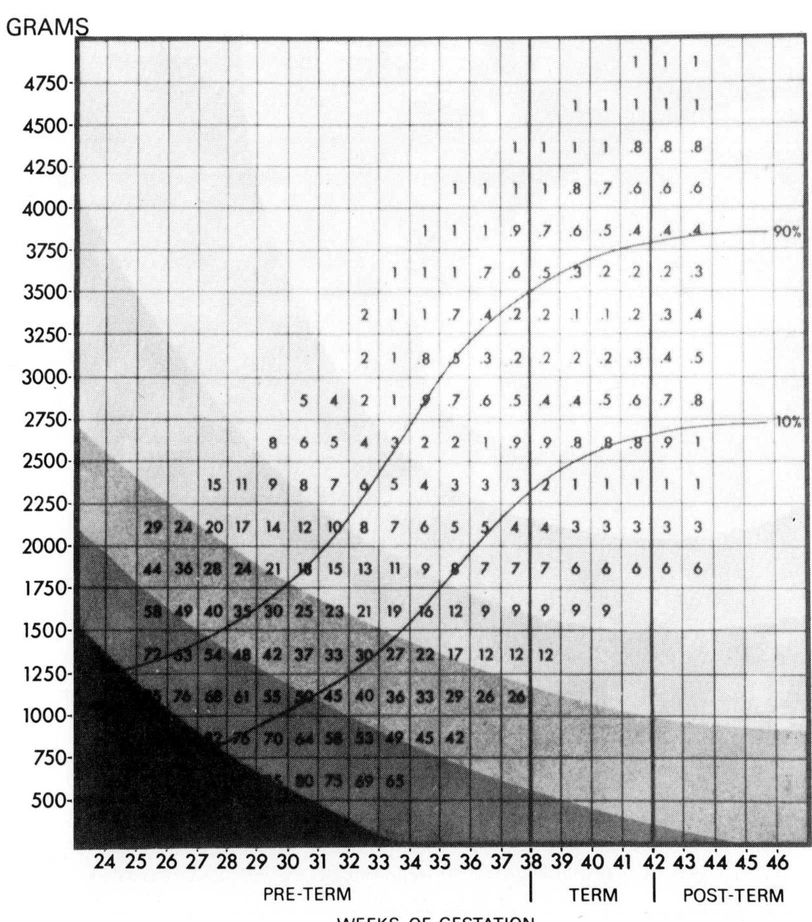

Figure 17-2 Classifications of newborns and neonatal mortality risk by birth weight and gestational age. (*From L. O. Lubchenco, D. T. Searls, and J. N. Brazie, Journal of Pediatrics 81:814–822* [1972].)

large for gestational age (LGA), falling above the 90th percentile in growth. For example, using Fig. 17-2, the nurse can estimate that a 1500-g fetus at 28 weeks of gestation is AGA and that a 34-week newborn weighing 1500 g is SGA. Mortality rates among premature infants have declined significantly since 1972, when this growth chart was printed, and while it is no longer accurate in this regard, it is a good tool for assessing appropriateness of growth.

Gestational-age assessment, using the traditional criteria of estimated date of confinement, uterine size, quickening, and time when the first fetal heart tones are heard, is sometimes unreliable. Using ultrasound to measure biparietal head diameter is a more accurate way of monitoring intrauterine fetal growth and of estimating gestational age. However, after the baby is born, gestational age can be assessed quite accurately. Dubowitz has proposed 10 neurological criteria (Fig. 17-3 and Table 17-4) and 11 physical criteria (Table 17-5) that can be used to assess the status of a newborn in less than 10 min. Table 17-6 is the maturity score sheet for esti-

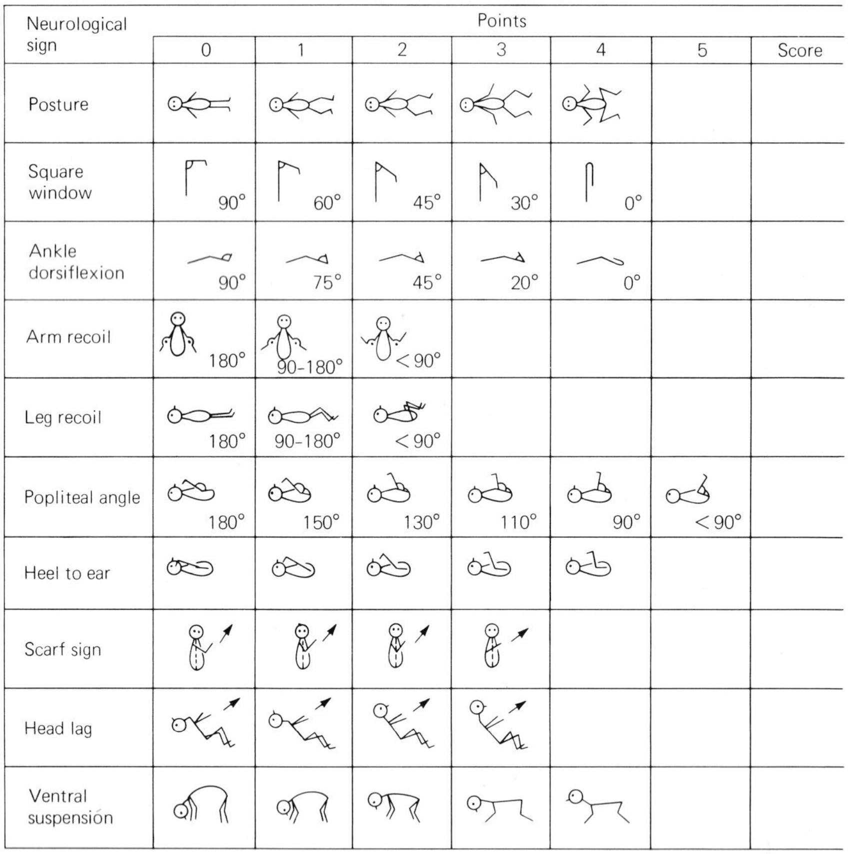

Neurological sign	Points						
	0	1	2	3	4	5	Score
Posture							
Square window	90°	60°	45°	30°	0°		
Ankle dorsiflexion	90°	75°	45°	20°	0°		
Arm recoil	180°	90–180°	< 90°				
Leg recoil	180°	90–180°	< 90°				
Popliteal angle	180°	150°	130°	110°	90°	< 90°	
Heel to ear							
Scarf sign							
Head lag							
Ventral suspension							

Neurological Total: ________

External Total: ________

TOTAL SCORE: ________

Gestation Age: (in weeks) ________

Figure 17-3 A score sheet for rating neurological characteristics of the neonate. Instructions for using this chart are presented in Table 17-4, and the infant's gestational age can then be determined using Table 17-5. (*From L. M. S. Dubowitz, Victor Dubowitz, and Cissie Goldberg, "Clinical Assessment of Gestational Age in the Newborn Infant," Journal of Pediatrics 77:1–10* [*1970*].)

Table 17-4 Instructions for Scoring the Neurological Assessment of the Newborn*

Posture

With the infant supine and quiet, score as follows:

The arms and legs extended	= 0
Slight or moderate flexion of the hips and knees	= 1
Moderate to strong flexion of the hips and knees	= 2
The legs flexed and abducted; the arms slightly flexed	= 3
Full flexion of the arms and legs	= 4

Square Window

Flex the hand at the wrist. Exert pressure sufficient to get as much flexion as possible. The angle between the hypothenar eminence and the anterior aspect of the forearm is measured and scored according to Fig. 17-3. Do not rotate the wrist.

Ankle Dorsiflection

Flex the foot at the ankle with sufficient pressure to get maximum change. The angle between the dorsum of the foot and the anterior aspect of the leg is measured and scored as in Fig. 17-3.

Arm Recoil

With the infant supine, fully flex the forearms for 5 s; then fully extend by pulling the hands and release. Score the reaction according to whether:

The forearms remain extended or make random movements	= 0
There is incomplete or partial flexion	= 1
There is a brisk return to full flexion	= 2

Leg Recoil

With the infant supine, fully flex the hips and knees for 5 s; then extend them by traction on the feet and release. Score the reaction according to whether:

There is no response or slight flexion	= 0
There is partial flexion	= 1
There is full flexion (less than 90° at the knees and hips)	= 2

Popliteal Angle

With the infant supine and the pelvis flat on the examining surface, flex the leg on the thigh, and fully flex the thigh with one hand. With the other hand extend the leg; then score the angle attained as in Fig. 17-3.

Heel-to-Ear Maneuver

With the infant supine, hold the infant's foot with one hand and move it as near to the head as possible without forcing it. Keep the pelvis flat on the examining surface. Score as in Fig. 17-3.

Scarf Sign

With the infant supine, take the infant's hand and draw it across the neck and as far across the opposite shoulder as possible. Assistance to the elbow is permissible by lifting it across the body. Score according to the location of the elbow:

The elbow reaches the opposite anterior axillary line	= 0
The elbow reaches between the opposite anterior axillary line and the midline of the thorax	= 1
The elbow reaches the midline of the thorax	= 2
The elbow does not reach the midline of the thorax	= 3

Head Lag

With the infant supine, grasp each forearm just proximal to the wrist, and pull gently so as to bring the infant to a sitting position. Score according to the relationship of the head to the trunk during the maneuver:

No evidence of head support	= 0
Some evidence of head support	= 1
The infant maintains the head in the same anteroposterior plane as the body	= 2
The infant tends to hold the head forward	= 3

Ventral Suspension

With the infant prone and the chest resting on the examiner's palm, lift the infant off the examining surface and score according to the posture shown in Fig. 17-3.

*The score obtained from this table is added to the score obtained from Table 17-5, and the infant's estimated gestational age is determined using Table 17-6. See also Fig. 17-3.

Source: L. M. S. Dubowitz, Victor Dubowitz, and Cissie Goldberg, "Clinical Assessment of Gestational Age in the Newborn Infant," *Journal of Pediatrics* **77**: 1–10 (1970).

mating gestational age. If gestational-age assessment is done within the first 24 h after birth, it is usually accurate to within 1 to 2 weeks. The neurological examination is the most difficult and should be done on an alert, quiet newborn. Some parts of the neurological examination may produce inaccurate results when performed on a depressed newborn or may be too exhausting to perform safely on a sick baby. Ballard's modified gestational-age assessment is a shorter version using fewer criteria; it can be used more easily with a sick baby in an NICU and is quite accurate (see Fig. 17-4).

Large-for-gestational-age babies Ninety percent of LGA babies weigh 4000 g (9 lb), and 10 percent weigh 4500 g (10 lb) or more. Large size is associated most frequently with two factors: heredity and a diabetic mother. The large size makes it difficult for the head and shoulders to pass through the birth canal, contributing to the frequent problem of traumatic injury during labor and delivery. The injuries to the infant are the result of pulling and stretching during the birth process. The best choice of delivery for a baby that is too large for the mother's pelvic size is a cesarean section. The diabetic infant and

Table 17-5 Score Sheet for External Physical Characteristics of the Newborn, for Use in Estimating Gestational Age*

External Sign	Points					
	0	1	2	3	4	Score
Edema	Obvious edema of hands and feet; pitting over tibia	No obvious edema of hands and feet; pitting over tibia	No edema			______
Skin texture	Very thin and gelatinous	Thin and smooth	Smooth; medium thickness; rash or superficial peeling	Slight thickening and peeling, especially of hands and feet	Thick and parchment-like; superficial or deep cracking	______
Skin color	Dark red	Uniformly pink	Pale pink; variable over body	Pale; pink only over ears, lips, palms, or soles		______
Skin opacity (trunk)	Numerous veins and venules clearly visible, especially over abdomen	Veins and tributaries visible	A few large vessels clearly visible over abdomen	A few large vessels visible indistinctly over abdomen	No blood vessels visible	______
Lanugo (over back)	No lanugo	Abundant; long and thick over whole back	Hair thinning, especially over lower back	Small amount of lanugo and bald areas	At least one-half of back devoid of lanugo	______
Plantar creases	No skin creases	Faint red marks over anterior half of sole	Definite red marks over > anterior one-half; indentations over < one-third	Indentations over > anterior one-third	Definite deep indentations over > anterior one-third	______

Nipple formation	Nipple barely visible; no areola	Nipple well defined; areola smooth and flat; diameter < 0.75 cm	Areola stippled; edge not raised; diameter < 0.75 cm	Areola stippled; edge raised; diameter > 0.75 cm	_____
Breast size	No breast tissue palpable	Breast tissue on one or both sides; diameter < 0.5 cm	Breast tissue on both sides; one or both 0.5 to 1.0 cm	Breast tissue on both sides; one or both >1 cm	_____
Ear form	Pinna flat and shapeless; little or no incurving of edge	Incurving of part of edge of pinna	Partial incurving of whole upper pinna	Well-defined incurving of whole upper pinna	_____
Ear firmness	Pinna soft and easily folded; no recoil	Pinna soft and easily folded; slow recoil	Cartilage to edge of pinna, but soft in places; ready recoil	Pinna firm; cartilage to edge; instant recoil	_____
Genitals:					
Male	Neither testis in scrotum	At least one testis high in scrotum	At least one testis down		
Female (with hips one-half abducted)	Labia majora widely separated; labia minora protruding	Labia majora almost cover labia minora	Labia majora completely cover labia minora		_____
				External total:	_____

*The score obtained from this table is combined with the score obtained from Table 17-4, and then Table 17-6 is consulted for gestational-age determination.

Source: L. S. M. Dubowitz, Victor Dubowitz, and Cissie Goldberg, "Clinical Assessment of Gestational Age in the Newborn Infant," *Journal of Pediatrics* **77**:*1–10 (1970)*.

Table 17-6 Maturity Score Sheet for Estimating Gestational Age of a Newborn*

Total Score	Gestational Age, Weeks
5	26
10	27
15	29
20	30
25	31
30	33
35	34
40	35
45	36
50	38
55	39
60	40
65	42
70	43
75	44

*For estimating gestational age after scores have been obtained on the basis of neurological characteristics (see Fig. 17-3 and Table 17-4) and external physical characteristics (see Table 17-5).

Source: L. M. S. Dubowitz, Victor Dubowitz, and Cissie Goldberg, "Clinical Assessment of Gestational Age in the Newborn Infant," *Journal of Pediatrics* **77**:1–10 (1970).

birth-related trauma will be discussed later in this chapter.

The postmature newborn

Incidence Twelve percent of all newborns are postmature, i.e., delivered after 42 weeks of gestation. The mortality rate among these infants is 2 to 3 times higher than that among full-term infants.

Manifestations Many postmature infants exhibit signs of inadequate intrauterine nutrition. Intrauterine weight loss is common and is thought to result from placental aging, leading to decreased intrauterine blood flow. When transplacental nutrients decrease, the fetus begins to use its own body stores as sources of energy, including the subcutaneous fat. Because the subcutaneous fat is absent at birth, the skin of postmature infants looks loose and baggy. The loss of this insulating layer also makes it difficult for these babies to maintain their body temperature.

Decreased placental blood flow also causes hypoxia and stimulates the fetus to pass meconium. Meconium aspiration is a common problem, and the skin is stained yellow-green as a result of contact with the meconium. No vernix is present to protect the skin; it is dry and parchment-like and frequently peels off in scales (desquamates) after birth. In addition, little lanugo is present on the skin, the hair is long, and the nails are long and ragged and extend beyond the fingertips. The newborn appears to be 1 or 2 weeks old, is wide-eyed and alert, and suffers from problems similar to those of the SGA baby. Hypoxia, hypoglycemia, hypothermia, polycythemia, and respiratory distress are common problems of the postmature infant (see Fig. 17-5).

Treatment Confirming postmaturity by determining exact gestational age is sometimes a difficult process. Prior to inducing labor, ultrasound, amniocentesis, tests of serial estriol levels, and stress and nonstress tests are used to determine the fetus's maturity and response to stress. Seventy-five to eighty percent of fetal deaths among postmature infants occur during labor and delivery. Fetal mortality is significantly decreased by accurately determining fetal gestational age and delivering the baby within 2 weeks of term. When a firm diagnosis of postmaturity is made, the method of delivery—induction of labor or a cesarean section—is determined. A cesarean section will be chosen when tests have indicated a poor fetal response to being stressed: late decelerations on the stress test, poor heart rate variability on the nonstress test, and declining serial estriol levels.

Meconium aspiration A wide variety of mild to severe respiratory problems result from meconium aspiration. Meconium aspiration, although it occurs in other babies who experience intrauterine distress, is most common in postterm babies.[13]

Etiology Meconium is passed when fetal circulation responds to an episode of decreased oxygenation with a mechanism that conserves blood flow to vital organs, such as the brain and the heart, and restricts blood flow to less vital areas, such as the intestines. The intestines' response to lack of oxygen is hyperperistalsis and rectal sphincter relaxation. Thus meconium is moved through the stimulated intestines and passes unobstructed through the rectum into the amniotic fluid.

Meconium mixes with the amniotic fluid and can be aspirated by the baby before, during, or after birth. Intrauterine hypoxia causes a temporary increase in the fetus's breathing efforts, resulting in strong reflex gasps. This causes the meconium to be aspirated when the baby

NEWBORN MATURITY RATING
and
CLASSIFICATION

ESTIMATION OF GESTATIONAL AGE BY MATURITY RATING

Side 1

Symbols: X - 1st Exam O - 2nd Exam

Scoring system: Ballard JL, *et al:* A Simplified Assessment of Gestational Age, Pediatr Res 11:374, 1977. Figures adapted from "Classification of the Low-Birth-Weight Infant" by AY Sweet in Care of the High-Risk Infant by MH Klaus and AA Fanaroff, WB Saunders Co, Philadelphia, 1977, p. 47.

NEUROMUSCULAR MATURITY

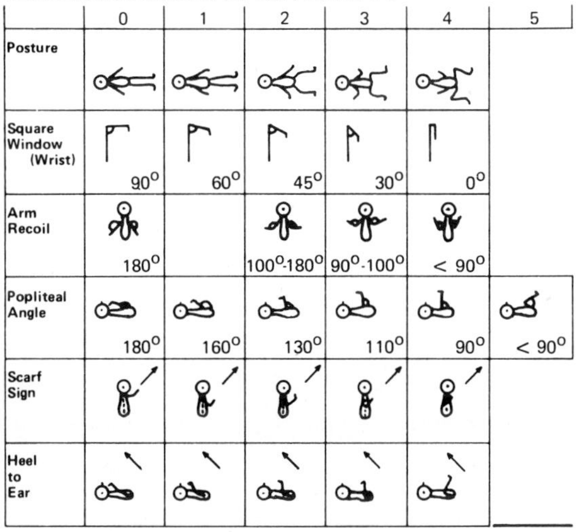

	0	1	2	3	4	5
Posture						
Square Window (Wrist)	90°	60°	45°	30°	0°	
Arm Recoil	180°		100°-180°	90°-100°	< 90°	
Popliteal Angle	180°	160°	130°	110°	90°	< 90°
Scarf Sign						
Heel to Ear						

PHYSICAL MATURITY

	0	1	2	3	4	5
SKIN	gelatinous red, trans-parent	smooth pink, visible veins	superficial peeling &/or rash, few veins	cracking pale area, rare veins	parchment, deep cracking, no vessels	leathery, cracked, wrinkled
LANUGO	none	abundant	thinning	bald areas	mostly bald	
PLANTAR CREASES	no crease	faint red marks	anterior transverse crease only	creases ant. 2/3	creases cover entire sole	
BREAST	barely percept.	flat areola, no bud	stippled areola, 1–2 mm bud	raised areola, 3–4 mm bud	full areola, 5–10 mm bud	
EAR	pinna flat, stays folded	sl. curved pinna, soft with slow recoil	well-curv. pinna, soft but ready recoil	formed & firm with instant recoil	thick cartilage, ear stiff	
GENITALS Male	scrotum empty, no rugae		testes descend-ing, few rugae	testes down, good rugae	testes pendulous, deep rugae	
GENITALS Female	prominent clitoris & labia minora		majora & minora equally prominent	majora large, minora small	clitoris & minora completely covered	

Gestation by Dates __________ wks

Birth Date __________ Hour __________ am pm

APGAR __________ 1 min __________ 5 min

MATURITY RATING

Score	Wks
5	26
10	28
15	30
20	32
25	34
30	36
35	38
40	40
45	42
50	44

SCORING SECTION

	1st Exam=X	2nd Exam=O
Estimating Gest Age by Maturity Rating	_____ Weeks	_____ Weeks
Time of Exam	Date _____ Hour _____ am pm	Date _____ Hour _____ am pm
Age at Exam	_____ Hours	_____ Hours
Signature of Examiner	_____ M.D.	_____ M.D.

Figure 17-4 Newborn maturity rating and classification (scoring system). (*From J. L. Ballard et al., "A Simplified Assessment of Gestational Age," Pediatric Research 11:374* [1977]. *Used with permission.*)

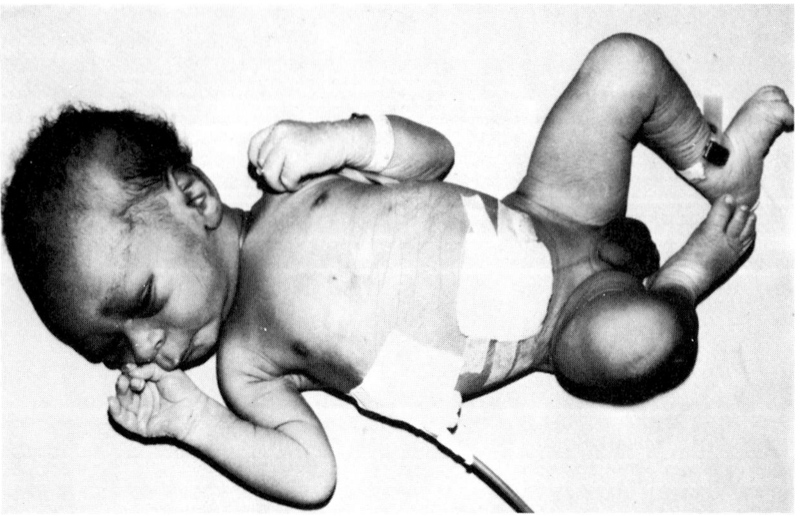

Figure 17-5 A postmature 2-day-old black male born at 43 weeks of gestation and weighing 2840 g (6 lb 4 oz). Note the diminished subcutaneous fat, the cracking skin, and the long nails, which are typical of a postmature infant. The chest tube was inserted for treatment of pneumothorax after meconium aspiration. (*From G. Scipien, M. U. Barnard, M. A. Chard, J. Howe, and P. J. Phillips [eds.] Comprehensive Pediatric Nursing, 3d ed., McGraw-Hill, New York, 1986. Used with permission.*)

breathes. The severity of respiratory distress depends on the amount of meconium aspirated, how deeply it has spread into the lungs, and how much airway obstruction occurs.

Management When meconium is present in the amniotic fluid, aggressive suctioning will significantly reduce complications. Respiratory complications can be reduced from 25 percent in nonsuctioned infants to 1 percent in suctioned infants.

To prevent the newborn from aspirating meconium-stained fluid with the first breath, the oral and nasopharyngeal airways are suctioned before the chest is born. After birth, the respiratory passages and stomach are suctioned. The stomach is suctioned because amniotic fluid is swallowed and can be regurgitated and aspirated into the lungs. The vocal cords are inspected for the presence of meconium using an endotracheal tube, and if meconium is present, gentle and repeated suctioning is done. Mouth suction on the endotracheal tube is maintained while the tube is being withdrawn. This holds meconium at the base of the tube, removing it from the airway. The process of inserting and removing the endotracheal tube is repeated until the meconium is cleared. When resuscitation is needed, suctioning must be completed before beginning positive pressure ventilation, since this process will spread meconium throughout the lungs, causing severe meconium aspiration pneumonia.

The newborn who has aspirated meconium is transferred to an NICU and receives the same respiratory care as other high-risk infants with respiratory distress. Most newborns recover rapidly from meconium aspiration if they have been adequately suctioned and have received good respiratory care. Mild symptoms usually subside in 1 to 2 days. In the case of infants who are inadequately treated or who have aspirated meconium deeply into the lungs, the symptoms become gradually more severe. Resolution is slow, and death or permanent damage may result.

Complications Meconium aspiration can cause the complete blockage of portions of the lungs; as a result, some parts of the lungs are uninflated (atelectasis). Because the airways expand on inspiration and become smaller on expiration, meconium can be inspired, but expiration is obstructed. Air is trapped, overdistending the lungs and leading to a rupture of the alveoli.

If air escapes from the lungs into the chest or mediastinum, it will result in pneumothorax or pneumomediastinum with signs of severe respiratory distress. Pneumothorax causes a shift in the position of the chest contents (a mediastinal shift), and displaced heart sounds are heard on the affected side. To expand the lungs, the air must be removed from the chest. This is done by using needle aspiration and chest tubes and by maintaining chest suction until the air leak is sealed.

Small-for-gestational-age babies

Incidence SGA babies weigh less than 2500 g ($5\frac{1}{2}$ lb) and may be preterm, full-term, or postterm infants. However, the majority of these babies are born near term. There are two distinct subgroups of SGA newborns: those who are proportionally small without appearing wasted and those who are dysmature and appear thin and wasted, although their length is normal and they have a normal head circumference.

Intrauterine growth retardation is related to inadequate maternal nutrition, especially late in the pregnancy; placental insufficiency; maternal disease, smoking, or excessive alcohol intake; and/or intrauterine infections. Dysmature SGA babies with normal head circumference appear to have been growing too slowly for a long period of time and tend to have more anomalies.[14] Some problems seen more frequently in SGA babies are rubella syndrome, trisomies, congenital heart anomalies, and gastrointestinal and genitourinary anomalies.

When intrauterine growth is not progressing normally, the doctor will investigate by checking biparietal diameter by using ultrasound, checking estriol levels, by doing an amniocentesis, and, near term, by doing nonstress and stress tests. If the intrauterine environment is very poor and if tests demonstrate sufficient lung maturity to survive, poor response to stress, and/or falling estriol levels, the baby may be delivered early by cesarean section or induction of labor.

At birth, the SGA infant appears long, thin, and wasted and has poor muscle development, especially over the buttocks and cheeks. Loss of subcutaneous fat, which was used as an energy source before birth, gives the skin a loose, baggy appearance. Loss of body fat also reduces body insulation and makes the baby vulnerable to chilling. The skin is dry and parchment-like, and the hair is sparse. The nails, skin, and umbilical cord are often stained yellow as a result of contact with meconium-stained amniotic fluid. Chronic low levels of oxygen trigger the fetus to pass meconium in the uterus. Polycythemia, an increase in red blood cells with a resulting high hematocrit, also may occur as a response to prolonged hypoxia (see Fig. 17-6).

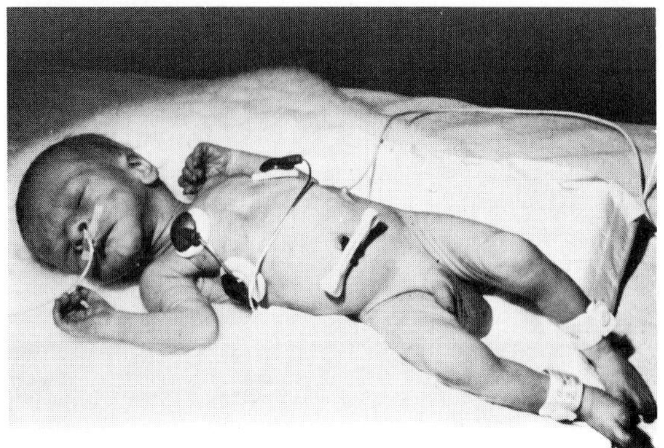

Figure 17-6 This infant has the typical appearance of an intrauterine-growth-retarded baby. The infant appears long, thin, and wasted.

Management At birth, the SGA baby frequently suffers from hypoxia, hypothermia, and hypoglycemia. Resuscitation and thorough suctioning are needed to remove as much meconium as possible. The baby had depleted its glucose stores prenatally and will need to have oral and/or intravenous glucose. These babies are usually very active and have a strong sucking reflex; they act starved, suck on their hands and clothing, and appear wide-eyed, alert, and almost birdlike. A pacifier helps satisfy the strong sucking urge and also helps prevent overfeeding. These babies need a calming, soothing environment because they are often irritable and difficult to comfort.

The preterm infant Mortality rates among preterm infants are directly related to maturity of the body systems (gestational age), birth weight, and availability of intensive care. An AGA baby of 35 to 37 weeks of gestational age has only a slightly higher risk of mortality than a full-term infant, whereas the mortality rate of infants between 26 and 29 weeks of gestational age is over 60 percent, by most estimates. Table 17-7 lists the percentages of preterm infants who survive as related to weight.

Physical characteristics The typical physical attributes of the preterm infant are given in

Table 17-7 Percent of Survival of Preterm Infants Related to Weight

Weight	Survival
1501 to 2500 g	95 to 100%
1251 to 1500 g	87%
1001 to 1250 g	72 to 79%
751 to 1000 g	57%
500 to 750 g	Less than 10%

Table 17-5 and Fig. 17-3, which list the physical and neurological characteristics of infants used for gestational-age assessment. The common characteristics of infants of various gestational ages are shown in Fig. 17-7*A*, *B*, *C*, and *D*.

Weight Preterm infants weigh less than 2500 g.

Length Preterm infants are less than 47 cm (18 in) in length.

Head Circumference The head circumference of preterm infants is about 33 cm (13 in), which is large in proportion to body size—about one-third. The bones of the skull are incompletely calcified, soft, and spongy, and the hair is fine and sticks out from the head in clumps. The eyes appear large.

Ears The cartilage in the ears of preterm infants is soft. The ears fold easily and stay bent; there is little incurving of the outer edge.

Body The body of the preterm infant is long, with a protruding abdomen. Lanugo is increasingly abundant, covering the forehead, the tops of the ears, the shoulder, the body, and the thighs. Thick, white, cheeselike vernix covers the body. The amounts of lanugo and vernix begin to decrease at about 36 weeks. The nipples are not palpable, but at 32 weeks the nipples and areolae are visible.

Extremities The peripheral circulation of preterm infants is poor, and the legs become mottled when chilled. The nails are soft and extend to the ends of the nail beds of the fingers and toes. Sole creases are beginning on the anterior part of the foot and will spread until the entire foot is covered at term.

Skin The skin of preterm infants is thin and delicate; that of Caucasian babies is reddish pink and almost gelatinous in appearance. The lack of subcutaneous fat makes the skin look loose or wrinkled. Blood vessels are easily seen through the skin and are very obvious on the abdomen. Because subcutaneous fat is deposited during the last trimester, the skin of the full-term infant is less red and is generally more durable.

Genitalia The scrotum of a preterm male infant is small, with few rugae (folds), and the testicles can be palpated at the external inguinal ring after 30 weeks. The testicles generally descend into the scrotal sac by 36 weeks. At 32 weeks the labia majora of the preterm female infant are small and widely separated, and the labia minora and clitoris are prominent. Hymenal tags are much more common in preterm than in full-term newborns.

Physiological handicaps

Temperature Regulation The preterm infant's labile temperature is related to an immature brainstem temperature regulatory mechanism, limited subcutaneous fat and body activity, and a large body surface area. The brainstem regulatory center is completely formed, but does not yet effectively control temperature in response to internal or external stimuli. Heat conservation through vasoconstriction and heat loss through vasodilatation are poor. The normal heat production through muscle contraction is limited. The preterm infant typically lies with the extremities extended or in a froglike position; the arms and legs are hypotonic, with little flexion or active movement. The proportion of body surface to body weight is very high, which increases heat loss substantially. Since body fat and glycogen in the liver are stored during the last trimester, little subcutaneous fat and glucose are available as energy sources. Capillary blood flow dissipates heat rapidly through the infant's thin skin layer, since little insulation is present to conserve heat. Brown fat, another concentrated source of calories in the newborn, is available in small amounts or not at all.

Circulation Congenital heart disease and a continuation of fetal circulation patterns, accompanied by failure of the patent ductus arteriosus (PDA) to close, are especially prevalent in premature infants. Failure of the PDA to close is related to failure of the newborn's lungs to expand and to the presence of a reduced pulmonary vascular pressure below that of the aorta; it is most often discovered at 5 to 10 days of age, when the ventilator-supported infant is beginning to be weaned. Respiratory distress syndrome and decreased lung perfusion can cause enough back pressure to precipitate eventual congestive heart failure and left-to-right shunting of the blood through the PDA. Severe gen-

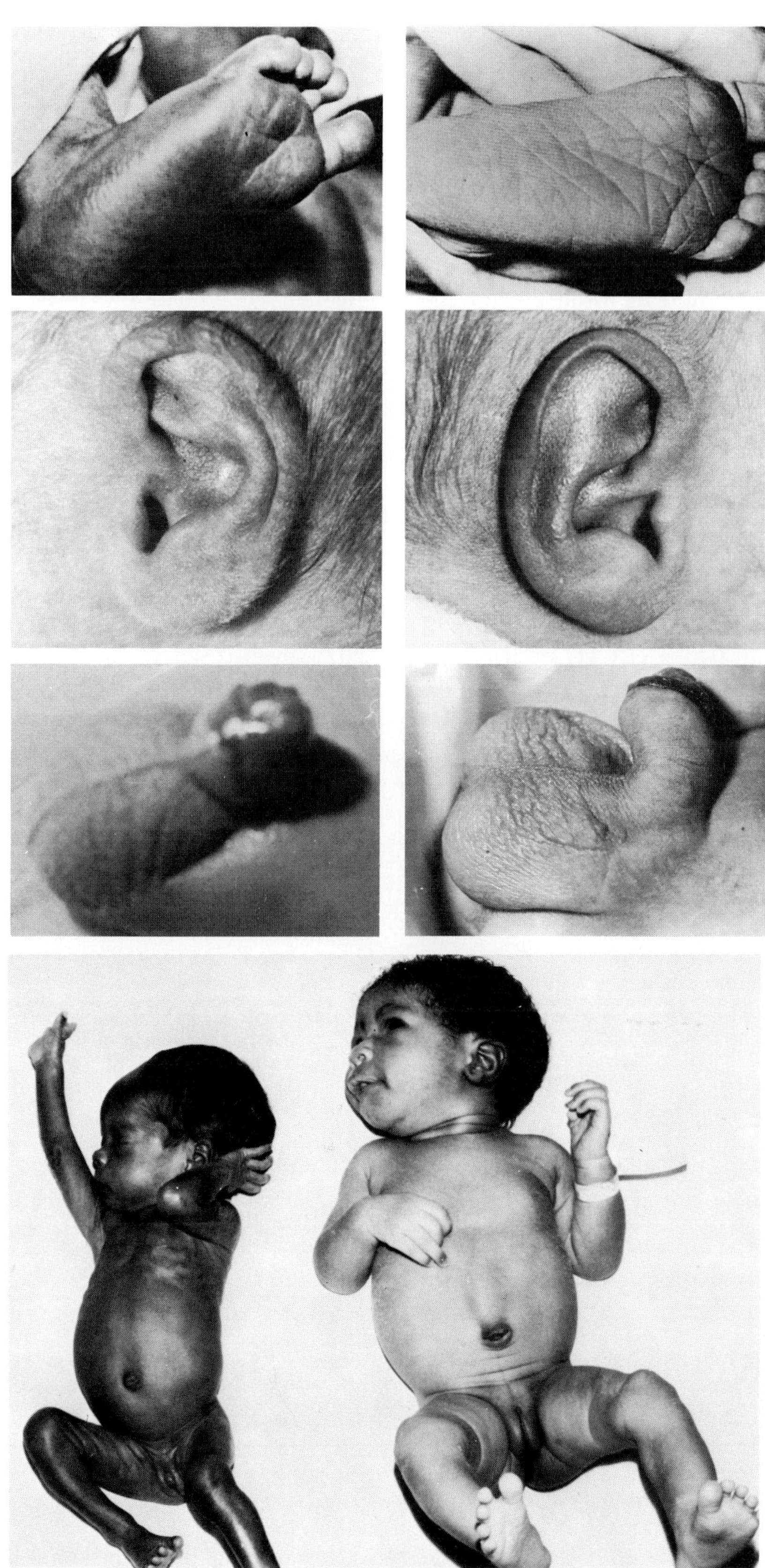

Figure 17-7 (*A*) A comparison of the sole creases of a full-term infant and a preterm infant. Creases cover the entire sole of the full-term infant's foot. The preterm infant's is smooth and shiny, with only a few creases in the anterior part. (*B*) A comparison of the ears of a full-term infant and a preterm infant. The full-term infant's ear is well formed, with much incurving on the pinna and good, firm cartilage. The preterm infant's ear has much lanugo on it, is much softer, and has less shape and incurving. (*C*) A comparison of a full-term male infant's genitalia and a preterm male infant's genitalia. The full-term scrotum is full and pendulous, and the testes have descended. The preterm infant's scrotum is small with few rugae, and the testes are undescended. (*D*) A 38-day-old preterm black female infant weighing 1415 g (3 lb $1\frac{1}{2}$ oz). Her birth weight was 1300 g at an estimated gestational age of 32 weeks. Note the thinness of the skin. The absence of subcutaneous fat is especially noticeable in the thigh folds, in the labia majora, and over the ribs. The open hands and extended position show the diminished muscle tone of the preterm infant. The 2-day-old black female infant, weighing 3140 g (6 lb 14 oz) at a gestational age of 40 weeks, shows the full-term infant's greater muscle tone, curlier hair, and more abundant subcutaneous fat, especially in the genital area where the labia majora cover the clitoris. The open, mature eyes contrast with those of the preterm infant, whose eyelids are birdlike. *(From G. Scipien, M. U. Barnard, M. A. Chard, J. Howe, and P. J. Phillips [eds.], Comprehensive Pediatric Nursing, 3d ed., McGraw-Hill, New York, 1986. Used with permission.)*

eralized cyanosis, which responds poorly to the usual oxygen and respiratory therapy, is related to the decreased systemic blood oxygen levels. A murmur, bounding pulses, and a heaving pericardial impulse (a sign of the working of the overloaded left ventricle) are present.[15] If pulmonary edema is advanced, crepitant rales will be heard. Surgical ligation and treatment with indomethacin are discussed in Chap 22.

The capillaries of preterm infants are profuse and fragile, and the vessel walls are poorly supported by connective tissue. Birth trauma produces an increased incidence and severity of hemorrhage and the subsequent complications of anemia, jaundice, and neurological damage from intracranial hemorrhage. Each of these complications is discussed in detail later in this chapter.

Immunity The usual defenses against infection—the skin barrier, antibodies, and phagocytosis (the ability to localize infections)—are all less effective in the preterm infant. Antibodies against specific bacteria and diseases from the mother cross the placenta in small numbers after the first 3 months of pregnancy and in the largest numbers during the third trimester. Most full-term newborns manufacture their own antibodies by 3 months of age. Preterm infants do not receive a full complement of maternal antibodies, and their own immune response is delayed. The decreased number of white blood cells reduces their ability to localize infections. Even a mild infection can cause systemic sepsis with pneumonia or meningitis in the preterm infant.

Digestive Function and Nutrition A high metabolic rate and large caloric and fluid requirements, which increases per kilogram of body weight as size decreases, make providing adequate nutrition to the preterm infant complicated. Adequate nutrition is needed so that the infant can continue the rapid rate of intrauterine growth that was interrupted by the early birth. The immature gastrointestinal tract is limited in its ability to hold and absorb the needed nutrients. The stomach is very small; in a 1200-g baby it may hold 2 ml, while in a 2000-g baby it may hold 15 ml ($\frac{1}{2}$ oz). Over a period of time the size of the stomach increases, until at 40 weeks the stomach is able to hold from 1 to 3 oz. Overdistention of the stomach, with pressure on the diaphragm and subsequent regurgitation is a common, frequent cause of respiratory distress in the preterm infant. The hypotonic cardiac sphincter may also cause reflux from the stomach and regurgitation, with possible aspiration. The poor sucking ability of preterm infants may make it impossible to feed them by nipple, since feeding may be so tiring that it uses an inordinate number of calories. Typically, the feeding reflexes—rooting, sucking, swallowing, and gagging and coughing—are weak and uncoordinated. This combination of immature reflexes, a small stomach, and an immature cardiac sphincter makes sucking and swallowing difficult, and the weak gag and cough reflex prevents the infant from clearing aspirated milk from his or her air passages. The acidity of the digestive juices is low, and although carbohydrate metabolism is normal, the digestive tract fails to absorb 20 to 40 percent of the fat in milk feedings.[16]

Respiratory Function The lungs of the premature infant are not ready for birth. Fetal lung development is discussed in Chap. 21. The poor alveolar development and the decreased amount of surfactant lead to severe respiratory problems, which increase with shorter gestational age and lower birth weight. Respiratory distress syndrome, apnea, and the complications of oxygen toxicity, which are frequent problems in preterm infants, are discussed later in this chapter.

STABILIZING AND MAINTAINING VENTILATION

Establishing ventilation

The Apgar score, which is determined at 1 and 5 min after birth, is a good indicator of the infant's overall respiratory, cardiac, muscle, and reflex response at birth. Low-birth-weight infants frequently have a score below 3 at 1 min, whereas this score is uncommon among infants with a higher birth weight. The 5-min Apgar score is generally more predictive of neonatal mortality and of abnormalities that will appear during the first year than the 1-min Apgar score.

Most newborns breathe spontaneously in less than 30 s after birth. If spontaneous respirations do not begin, resuscitation is required to establish respirations within 1 min of birth. For all infants, the head is held downward and is gently suctioned with a bulb or DeLee suction. The infant is kept warm by being dried and put under a radiant warmer. If the 1-min Apgar score is 7 to 10, no resuscitation is necessary. The nurse listens to the chest to make certain that the heart rate and respirations are within the normal ranges

(120 to 160 and 35 to 50, respectively). If the 5-min Apgar is stable or rising, no additional action is taken.

When spontaneous respirations are not effectively established within 1 min, steps must be taken to resuscitate the infant. There can be many different causes of asphyxia in the newborn. If depression is due to narcotics given to the mother during labor, the narcotic antagonist naloxone (Narcan) is administered intramuscularly in a dosage of 0.01 ml per kilogram of body weight. Narcan is the drug of choice because it does not have the respiratory-depressant effects of nalorphine (Nalline) and levallorphan (Lorfan) if the agent causing the depression is not an opiate derivative. The peak effect of Narcan occurs at 1 to 2 min after injection; the effect lasts for 2 to 3 h. The dose may be repeated after 15 min.[17]

The *moderately depressed infant* (with an Apgar score of 4 to 6) looks cyanotic or pale and appears limp. The cry is weak, and respirations are irregular and shallow, but the heart rate is above 100. During the first minute, management is the same as for the normal infant, but, in addition, oxygen by mask is given after suctioning. If effective spontaneous respirations are not established, a laryngoscope is inserted, allowing direct visualization of the larynx, and any foreign material, blood, mucus, or meconium is removed. The infant receives 100% oxygen with a tight-fitting face mask and bag. An assistant listens for breath sounds as the chest rises. If color and respirations are not improved after 1 min and the heart rate is below 100 or is dropping, endotracheal intubation is indicated. Usually, normal respirations begin and color and muscle tone improve rapidly with ventilation.

The *severely depressed infant* (with an Apgar score of 0 to 3) looks pale, blue, and limp and has few spontaneous respirations, no cry, and a heart rate below 100. This infant needs immediate resuscitation. The laryngoscope is inserted, the airway is suctioned, and oxygen therapy with the bag ventilator is begun immediately. Dramatic improvement is usually evident with oxygenation. If the heart rate drops to 60, it is a sign of imminent cardiac arrest, which can result when oxygen does not reach the cardiac muscle. If cardiac arrest occurs, external cardiac massage is started after 3 to 4 breaths are given.

Acidosis is usually present in the depressed, hypoxic newborn. Oxygen alone will not correct this state, and half-strength sodium bicarbonate (2 to 4 mEq) is given by direct infusion through the umbilical catheter. Continued doses will be needed until resuscitation is completed. Hypoglycemia may also result. An infusion of 10% glucose is started to replace the glycogen stores lost as a result of hypoxia and chilling and to prevent further acidosis.

Blood gas measurements Blood gas measurements of oxygen (P_{O2}), carbon dioxide (P_{CO2}), and pH are done frequently on the infant with respiratory distress. Measurement of arterial oxygen level is repeated every 5 to 15 min during resuscitation and then is continued at least every 4 h for sick infants. Normal ranges of blood gas values are listed in Table 17-8. The P_{O2} in the blood should be maintained above 50 mmHg, although cyanosis is not visible until it drops to 40 mmHg. Many NICUs regulate the arterial oxygen (Pa_{O2}) at 60 to 80 mmHg. Blood oxygen levels are measured using arterial blood, usually from an arterial umbilical catheter.

The *arterial catheter* is inserted into the umbilical artery soon after birth. Although the complications of blood clots, infection, and reflex arterial spasms may occasionally occur, arterial catheterization is the most frequently used method of obtaining repeated arterial blood samples. Without catheterization, repeated venipunctures would have to be made in the temporal, radial, or brachial artery. Capillary blood from heel or finger sticks is usually not adequate for arterial blood oxygen readings. If capillary blood is used, the values will be much lower than if blood from an arterial source is used. Blood drawn for blood gas measurements should never be left at room temperature because the pH drops

Table 17-8 Normal and Abnormal Blood Gas Values for the Newborn

Blood Component	Normal Range	Range in Respiratory Depression
P_{O_2}	80 to 100 mmHg	Below 50 mmHg (hypoxia)
P_{CO_2}	35 to 45 mmHg	Above 65 mmHg (hypercapnia)
pH	7.35 to 7.45	Below 7.20 (acidosis)

and the P_{CO2} rises. The nurse should put the blood on ice or refrigerate it immediately and not use it if there has been a 10-min time lapse.

A *transcutaneous oxygen tension* (tcP_{O2}) monitor is used to continuously monitor the oxygen and carbon dioxide levels in the capillaries of the skin surface. The monitor uses a skin contact plate or sensor that warms the skin to produce vasodilatation in the capillary bed and gives a fairly accurate Pa_{O2} reading. The skin is cleansed with alcohol, and a contact gel or distilled water is put under the electrode. Flat surfaces permit a more airtight seal, but the face should never be used because of the risk of a burn. Abrasions occur frequently when the adhesive plate is removed from the preterm infant's delicate skin. Erythema and skin craters can be caused by the electrode; reducing the temperature of the probe and changing the site every 2 h will help prevent these skin problems.[18] The values fluctuate widely with nursing care, especially suctioning, feeding, and routines such as bathing. In addition wide deviations are seen with crying and positioning. The nurse can use the transcutaneous blood oxygen measures as a valuable guide to how the infant is tolerating the care and can adjust the care given accordingly. Transcutaneous P_{O2} readings have recently been categorized into reactive and nonreactive patterns. The nurse can use these categories as a guide in determining whether the baby's hypoxia is caused by pulmonary disease or some other problem resulting in circulatory shunting. (See Table 17-8 for normal and low blood gas levels.)

Maintaining oxygenation The infant's oxygen needs after respirations are stabilized can be met in a number of different ways. If the baby is breathing spontaneously, environmental oxygen may be provided in an Isolette or a hood. Respiratory distress syndrome, low blood oxygen or high blood carbon dioxide, or the inability of the infant to maintain respirations may indicate the need to use an endotracheal tube, a mechanical ventilator, and continuous positive airway pressure (CPAP). The decision about which method of oxygen administration to use depends on the disease process, the amount of oxygen needed to maintain P_{O2} above 50 percent, and the infant's physical condition. It is important to keep the oxygen adjusted to a level that is therapeutic and yet does not damage the infant's developing eyes and lungs.

A *mask* and a *nasal cannula* are not usually used for high-risk newborns. An *incubator* or *Isolette* is often used, but it is very difficult to raise the oxygen concentration above 40% in an incubator or Isolette. The lid and portholes permit oxygen loss. An *oxygen hood* can increase oxygen concentration and can be used either in an incubator or under an open radiant warmer (see Fig. 17-8). The hood is a small plastic bubble placed over the infant's face; it can remain in place during most care-giving procedures. The oxygen concentration can be raised to almost 100%. It is essential that the oxygen be warmed to prevent chilling, since it blows directly over the sensitive thermal sensors on the infant's face. Continuous positive airway pressure (CPAP) provides constant distending pressure in the lungs to keep the alveoli partly inflated. The distending pressure in the lungs is maintained by adjusting the outflow setting to keep the lungs pressurized between 2 and 13 mmHg. This is gradually decreased as the respiratory condition improves. Continuous positive airway pressure can be given through an endotracheal tube or, less effectively, nasally through a tight-fitting adapter. Positive end expiratory pressure (PEEP) is another way of maintaining a higher level of constant airway pressure. Both CPAP and PEEP are used when the lungs are not compliant, as in an infant with hyaline membrane disease or apnea. Maintaining a constant airway pressure is thought to make the work of breathing less difficult by keeping the lungs partially inflated and therefore decreasing the level of inspired oxygen needed.

Severely depressed infants, infants with high levels of carbon dioxide (P_{CO2} over 70 percent), and infants who are using too much energy and

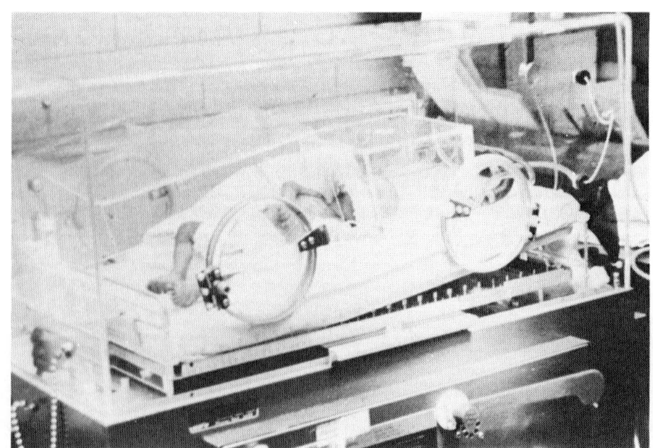

Figure 17-8 A preterm infant in an incubabtor with an oxygen hood in place.

exhausting themselves breathing require mechanical ventilation (see Fig. 17-9). An infant on a ventilator must be maintained with an endotracheal tube. The respirator must be checked for appropriate functioning and settings. Since secretions accumulate in the endotracheal tube, observing the endotracheal tube for patency and suctioning when needed are essential. Suctioning can cause a significant drop in oxygen levels, which can be seen on the transcutaneous oxygen monitor or determined through blood gas measurements. Hypoxemia and bradycardia due to suctioning can be reduced significantly if supplemental oxygen is given for 15 s after suctioning. Suctioning and techniques to maintain oxygenation during suctioning are discussed in Chap. 21.

High-frequency ventilation (HFV) is being used on a trial basis around the country. As many as 120 respirations per minute are delivered by a ventilator. It is hoped that HFV will reduce the pressure of inspired oxygen, since high pressure seems to be related to increased incidence of bronchopulmonary dysplasia. It is too soon to predict how successful this technique will be; at present the outcomes in infants are questionable, and there are great variations in reported success when judged by improved ventilation in the infant.[19]

Signs of respiratory distress

Respiratory distress in infants follows a pattern that includes the following symptoms (going from the least to the most severe): tachypnea, grunting, nasal flaring, retractions, and cyanosis.

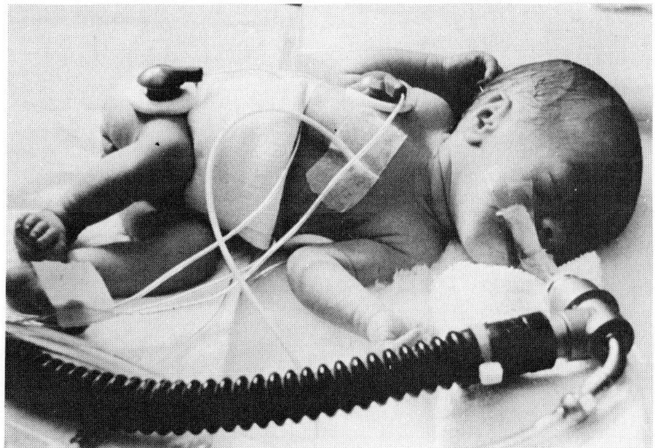

Figure 17-9 An intubated preterm infant attached to a ventilator with an endotracheal tube. A heat sensor and cardiac leads are in place.

Tachypnea, a respiratory rate above 60 breaths per minute, is often the first sign of distress; the rate may rise as high as 80 to 100 breaths per minute. Breathing faster is the infant's first response when he or she tries to increase blood oxygen levels. As the infant expends energy to increase respirations, further signs of progressive respiratory distress may occur.

Expiratory *grunting,* or *sighing,* is the sound made when the infant closes the glottis to temporarily stop exhalation. It is an effort to increase back pressure in the lungs to keep the alveoli partially expanded. The epiglottis is held so that the glottis closes; when it is suddenly released, a grunting sound is made as the air passes over the vocal cords. Grunting may improve the baby's respiratory status temporarily but cannot be continued for long because the infant becomes exhausted. Intubation eliminates grunting, because it does not permit closure of the glottis, but it may be needed along with artificial ventilation to maintain respiratory status. An artificial means of keeping the alveoli partially expanded, such as PEEP or CPAP, can be used; such methods provide constant distending lung pressure and are frequently used as an adjunct to a ventilator.

Nasal flaring, a primitive reflex, is frequently seen in response to respiratory distress. It is a widening of the external nostrils and seems to be a way of reducing the resistance of the narrow nasal passages to respirations.

Retractions are the visible effects of incomplete lung expansion created by the negative pressure between the lungs and the chest wall. They are an effort to aid respirations by using the auxiliary muscles to expand the chest. In infants with respiratory distress syndrome, retractions are increased because the lungs are very stiff and do not easily fill the chest cavity and the bones and cartilage of the premature infant's flexible chest wall, diaphragm, and accessory muscles are soft. Retractions are much more common in preterm infants with respiratory distress syndrome. The different types of retractions are named for the specific locations in which they occur: *intercostal* (the chest wall is pulled in between the ribs), *suprasternal* (above the sternum), *substernal* (below the sternum), *supraclavicular* (above the clavicle), *subclavicular* (below the clavicle), and *xiphoid retractions.* Retractions may actually decrease the volume of lung expansion. If the inflation of the lungs is greatly decreased, the chest appears flattened and the abdomen bulges. This is called *see-saw* or *paradoxical* respirations. The only effective muscle left in this case is the diaphragm, which still ventilates the lower part of the lungs.

The Silverman-Anderson index (see Fig. 17-10) can be used to assess degree of respiratory distress. The higher the score, the more serious the respiratory distress. The maximum score is 10.

Cyanosis in room air is a late, major sign of respiratory distress. Central cyanosis, or blueness of the body and head, is a serious sign of oxygen deprivation. Cyanosis around the mouth—circumoral cyanosis—often precedes central cyanosis. Peripheral cyanosis—acrocyanosis—is not a significant sign of respiratory distress and is commonly present in newborns. Cyanosis is not apparent until the arterial blood oxygen is about 40 mmHg, even though respiratory distress may be present earlier.

Management The nurse carefully monitors the condition of the infant who is receiving oxygen, observing and charting the course of the disease and the infant's response to treatment and watching for indications of complications.

Whatever the method of administration, oxygen is warmed to 31 to 34°C and is humidified between 40 and 60 percent. An oxygen analyzer is used to measure the oxygen content of the air in incubators. A continuous analyzer can be used, or oxygen is monitored every hour and each time blood gases are drawn. Chapter 16 discusses oxygen analysis. Blood gas measurements are used to adjust the oxygen level for high-risk newborns who are receiving oxygen by other methods. Pulmonary care includes suctioning, postural drainage, chest physiotherapy, and position changes every 2 h. Pulmonary care is discussed in Chap. 16. Recent research has shown that pulmonary care must be performed cautiously to prevent dangerously stressing the sick infant, and at times procedures such as chest physiotherapy need to be abbreviated. Listening to the chest for air flow into the lungs and respiratory rales is done to determine the necessary pulmonary care. The respiratory rate, the heart rate, and blood pressure are indicators of the infant's response to oxygenation. A respiratory rate of 60 or above, a heart rate below 100 or above 180, and a drop or elevation in blood pressure may indicate problems with ventilation.

Removing the infant from oxygen Oxygen is adjusted by using blood oxygen level concentrations and by observing for cyanosis. The infant is gradually weaned off the oxygen. The oxygen concentration is lowered by no more than 10 percent at a time about every 3 to 4 h. If the infant becomes slightly cyanotic, the level may have to be increased. It is important to keep the

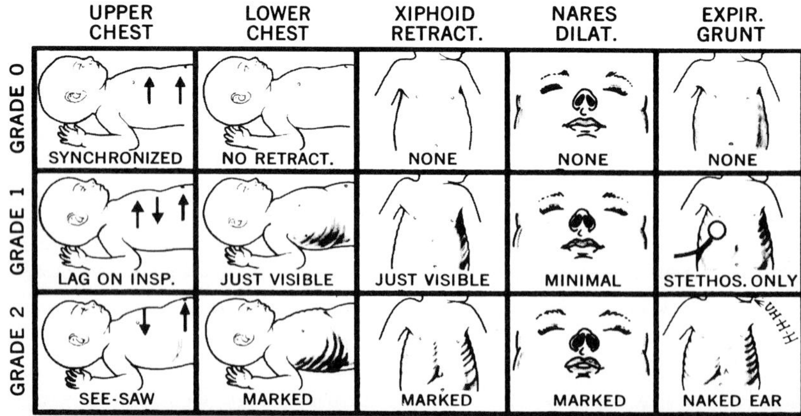

Figure 17-10 The Silverman-Anderson index for evaluation of respiratory status. Five criteria are used to arrive at a retraction score. The values of 0, 1, and 2 are assigned to each factor, and the total score indicates the degree of distress, from 0 (none) to 10 (severe). (*After W. A. Silverman and D. H. Anderson, Pediatrics **17(1)** [1956]. Used with permission.*)

oxygen adjusted to a therapeutic level and yet at the lowest possible level to prevent oxygen toxicity. High concentrations of oxygen can cause damage to the developing eyes (retrolental fibroplasia) and lungs.

ALTERATIONS ASSOCIATED WITH OXYGENATION

Respiratory distress syndrome

Respiratory distress syndrome (RDS), also known as hyaline membrane disease and idiopathic respiratory distress syndrome, is the largest cause of respiratory disease in the newborn infant. It is responsible for thousands of deaths annually in the United States.[20]

Incidence RDS is primarily a disease of the premature infant. The incidence is 65 percent in babies weighing less than 1000 g, 57 percent in infants weighing between 1000 and 1500 g, and 10 to 20 percent in infants weighing 2000 to 2500 g.[21] There is also a higher incidence of RDS in babies of women who have diabetes, or in babies of women who have experienced placental bleeding, and in babies delivered by cesarean section. In each of these cases, it is the baby's immaturity that precipitates the RDS. For example, there is a high rate of RDS among immature infants delivered by emergency cesarean section, while RDS is less common in mature infants delivered by elective cesarean section. Another major cause of RDS is fetal asphyxia, which can cause pulmonary vasoconstriction and inhibit surfactant production, initiating RDS even in mature babies. Among the variety of other causes of RDS are birth trauma, cold stress, and hypoglycemia.

Pathology The lungs of a normal newborn are salmon pink, spongy, and air-filled. The lungs of an infant with RDS are livery red and solid. The terminal bronchioles and alveolar ducts are filled with products of cellular necrosis, bloody exudate, and fibrin. The so-called hyaline membrane is found only in previously aerated portions of the lungs and therefore is the result, not the cause, of RDS. X-rays of severely affected infants' lungs show atelectasis (collapse of the alveoli) as dark, comma-shaped areas of density; blocked, air-filled bronchi (air bronchograms) are shown as dark streaks. The lungs also have a clouded appearance, with the grainy look of ground glass (reticulogranular pattern), which can be seen on an x-ray.

Etiology Understanding fetal lung development and surfactant production is essential to understanding RDS. The alveoli of the fetal lungs multiply rapidly during the third trimester and continue vigorous, active growth, as demonstrated by a threefold increase in the number of alveoli during the first 3 months of life.

Prior to 28 weeks of gestation, the fetal lungs have thick-walled alveoli and a scanty capillary blood supply. After 28 weeks, the alveoli gradually increase in number and mature. As this happens, the alveolar walls become thinner and more closely approximated to the capillary membranes, facilitating oxygen–carbon dioxide exchange. There is a large amount of connective tissue in the preterm infant's lungs, and it is this condition that makes the lungs stiff (low lung compliance) and promotes edema through fluid accumulation in the spongy connective tissue.

Surfactant The fetal lungs secrete a fluid, surfactant, that is found in the lungs at birth. It contains approximately 10 different phospholipids, of which sphingomyelin and lecithin are predominant. Sphingomyelin is present early in fetal life and decreases in amount toward term, while the amount of lecithin increases as the fetal lungs mature. The fetus breathes amniotic fluid, contaminating it with phospholipids from the lungs. Therefore, testing amniotic fluid using the lecithin/sphingomyelin (L/S) ratio will reflect the phospholipid levels and the fetal lung maturity. A ratio of 2 parts lecithin to 1 part sphingomyelin (L/S = 2:1) in the amniotic fluid indicates mature fetal lungs. The lungs are usually mature at 32 to 35 weeks of gestation. Another test of lung maturity is the Shake test. This can be done using amniotic fluid or secretions from the newborn's respiratory passages or stomach; it is described in Table 17-3. A detailed discussion of embryology and assessment of the newborn's lungs appears in Chap. 21.

A baby born with immature lungs and low surfactant production will develop RDS. Surfactant, which is composed largely of lecithin, is secreted by the fetal alveoli in two cycles. Type II cells producing surfactant appear in the alveolar walls at about 24 weeks of gestation. At first, only a small amount is produced and is easily inhibited by fetal asphyxia and the stressful events commonly associated with premature birth.

The second and larger surge of surfactant production occurs at 32 to 35 weeks of gestation; at this time, the amount secreted increases until birth, and its production becomes more stable.

The purpose of surfactant is to make respiration less difficult by decreasing surface tension in the alveoli. Surfactant exerts the strongest influence on relaxed lungs, where it coats the alveoli with a thick layer and can counteract surface tension most effectively. As the alveoli expand with inspiration, the layer of surfactant thins. Its effect decreases, reducing resistance to the recoil of the lungs and allowing expiration to occur. The presence of adequate surfactant keeps the alveoli partially distended after the first breath and makes subsequent breaths easier. Various sources estimate that the *functional residual capacity,* which is the continuous amount of expansion of the lungs maintained by surfactant, remains at 25 to 50 percent.

A factor recently associated with increased surfactant production is fetal stress. Fetal stress is believed to stimulate the fetal adrenals to produce glucocorticoids (steroids) that speed production of surfactant and increase lung maturity. To replicate this stress effect, corticosteroids—betamethasone or dexamethasone—are given to the pregnant woman to stimulate surfactant production. They are given 24 h to 7 days before delivery when a premature birth is imminent. This treatment, when administered before 32 weeks of gestation, has demonstrated increased lung maturity by a 21 percent decrease in the incidence of RDS. Betamethasone was proved ineffective when administered after 32 weeks of gestation, and there was no positive effect when hydrocortisone was given to premature newborns.

Manifestations The infant with decreased surfactant accommodates effective breathing for a short time. When surfactant is used up, a normal functional residual capacity is not maintained, and the alveoli that were inflated on inspiration collapse again on expiration. The work of breathing is increased, since lung compliance (elasticity of the lungs) is greatly reduced; the infant becomes exhausted and has difficulty continuing the effort of breathing.

The alveolar collapse causes widespread atelectasis and results in increased pressure in the lungs and reduced pulmonary blood flow. Eventually these changes cause the cardiopulmonary circulation to revert to the fetal circulation pattern, largely bypassing the lungs. These factors cause reduced oxygen in the blood (hypoxemia) and increased carbon dioxide levels (hypercapnia), as well as a low blood pH, which results in metabolic and respiratory acidosis. The potassium level is elevated because potassium is released from damaged alveolar cells.

The infant may show signs of RDS immediately requiring resuscitation, or may seem stable and develop signs of distress within 2 to 3 h after birth. The course of the disease ordinarily runs 3 to 5 days; death is much less likely after the infant has survived the first 72 h. When prolonged ventilator-controlled breathing is needed, the prognosis is poor.

Management There is no definitive treatment for RDS. Treatment is supportive in nature and centers on providing effective ventilation, correcting acid-base imbalance, providing optimal temperatures, and maintaining fluid balance and normal hematocrit and blood pressure.

The nurse performs all the general assessments and supportive functions discussed previously in this chapter. All vital functions, respirations, heart rate, blood pressure, temperature, and intravenous intake and output are carefully monitored. The baby will frequently require oxygen and may need an endotracheal tube to maintain ventilation. An arterial umbilical catheter is usually inserted and is used to draw the blood needed for the frequent laboratory tests and for measurements of arterial blood gases. Good skin care is necessary to avoid breakdown, and respiratory care—including gentle suctioning, chest physiotherapy when indicated by decreased lung sounds, and observation for signs of deterioration—is also required. Signs indicative of sepsis, intraventricular hemorrhage, and pneumothorax must be carefully monitored and reported.

Complications Intraventricular hemorrhage is a leading cause of death among babies on a ventilator and is also a complication of endotracheal intubation and suctioning. Neurological defects are primarily hydrocephalus or cerebral palsy, presumably as a result of intracranial hemorrhage. Pulmonary complications include significant apnea, increased infections, and bronchopulmonary dysplasia.

Periodic breathing and apnea

Periodic breathing Periodic breathing is a common finding in full-term infants and is even more common in preterm infants; it is probably caused by immature central nervous system respiratory control. Respirations are characterized by cessation of breathing for up to 10 s without bradycardia (a heart rate below 100) or cyanosis; this is rare during the first 24 h of life. Respirations resume spontaneously, and there are no ill effects.

Apnea Apnea should not be confused with periodic breathing. In apnea, spontaneous respirations cease for periods of 15 to 20 s or more; it is accompanied by functional changes, such as bradycardia, visible cyanosis, and hypotonia, and is indicated in the blood by acidosis. Episodes of apnea can cause brain damage and are related to increased mortality; they can progress in severity if left untreated.

Etiology Apnea is found in about one-third of preterm infants with a gestational age of 32 weeks and more frequently in preterm infants under 30 weeks of gestational age. Apnea decreases spontaneously with increasing age and the resolution of any underlying disorder. Research has shown an interaction between pulmonary function and central nervous system immaturity in apnea in preterm infants. Measures of pulmonary function of apneic infants with a mean gestational age of 30 weeks showed a decrease in tidal volume and alveolar ventilation and an elevated arterial P_{CO2}. Medullary respiratory center immaturity with decreased carbon dioxide response appears to be a major mechanism for idiopathic apnea in preterm infants.[22] Irregular respirations associated with repeated episodes of apnea are often secondary to depressed central nervous system functioning caused by severe hypoxia or intracranial hemorrhage. Apnea can have many different underlying causes. These are listed in Table 17-9.

Treatment For almost a decade, therapy has included theophylline, continuous positive airway pressure (CPAP), mechanical stimulation, and rocking water beds. Only the first two are in common use. Theophylline has been tested in research, and early use in cases of "mild" apnea has resulted in a more positive outcome in terms of both a lowered requirement for mechanical ventilation and decreased mortality.[23] Continuous positive airway pressure has been demonstrated to improve oxygenation, but it may increase the work of breathing and diminish minute ventilation. If theophylline is unsuccessful, doxapram (a respiratory stimulant) can be used in cases of unresponsive apnea (four or five severe spells) and has been shown to reduce the frequency of the episodes.[24]

Nursing management includes accurate monitoring of respirations and heart rate and close observation of the infant for signs that might indicate underlying disorders. Routine infant stimulation for 5 out of every 15 min is done for babies who are at risk for apnea. Position the infant with a small head roll placed at the base of the head to slightly extend the neck to prevent airway obstruction from the tongue. An alternating pressure mattress or a rocking water bed can also be used to stimulate breathing. When a baby has frequent episodes of apnea, a mechanical apnea monitor, set to sound an alarm when breathing stops for 10 to 15 s, is used to alert nurses. These alarms are very sensitive and if the alarm goes off the nurse should quickly assess the color and respirations and then investigate the possible causes of a false alarm. If the infant is observed to be apneic, he or she is stimulated by light rubbing of the body and face.

Table 17-9 Underlying Causes of Apnea

1. Respiratory	Airway obstruction; alveolar collapse; pulmonary pathology; exhaustion due to the effort of overcoming airway resistance in respiratory distress syndrome
2. Central nervous system	Intracranial bleeding; apnea may precede a seizure; drug depression
3. Infection	Sepsis; meningitis; necrotizing enterocolitis
4. Gastrointestinal	Increased vagal tone caused by overdistended abdomen and pressure on the diaphragm;
5. Vascular	Dehydration; cardiac anomaly; hypotension; hypertension; anemia
6. Electrolyte imbalances	Decreased calcium and sodium levels; hypoglycemia

This will usually initiate breathing. If it does not, suctioning of the airway to remove any obstruction and suctioning of the stomach to relieve overdistention may initiate breathing. If these measures are unsuccessful and bradycardia persists, oxygen and ventilation with an Ambu-bag and mask are used until a mechanical ventilator can be started. Medications (usually theophylline) and sometimes CPAP are ordered by the physician. Apnea usually improves gradually and disappears with increased maturity and physical status; it is not usually seen after about 11 days.

Home apnea monitoring A few infants continue to have spells of apnea and are sent home on apnea monitors. Most spells cease by 1 year of age. The parents need to be given detailed instructions about use of the equipment and must be taught to deal with false alarms. They need to be given accurate descriptions of spells of apnea and should be taught cardiopulmonary resuscitation and be allowed to practice on a "resusci-baby" and to ask questions. Dimaggio and Shutz studied the changes in families with an infant on an apnea monitor and asked the parents to rank their concerns. Parents listed the following: (1) emotional stress as a result of being on call 24 h a day, with the accompanying changes in life-style; (2) a need to feel confident about their ability to do cardiopulmonary resuscitation, to understand the equipment, and to make adaptations in the home; and (3) concerns about whether the infant was growing properly, about feeding, and about traveling with the infant.[25] A study that included home follow-up showed that in a period of $2\frac{1}{2}$ years, nine parents resuscitated their infants, eight of whom are alive and well today; one died after cardiac surgery.[26]

Oxygen toxicity

The improved efficiency of oxygen administration equipment has made it possible to give high-concentration oxygen and to monitor oxygen levels more precisely. Technology has improved the equipment and advances in nursing practice have improved the nursing care of preterm infants. Despite these lifesaving advances, incidents in which oxygen has toxic effects on the eyes and lungs of very premature infants still occur, though less frequently than in the past. It is the new population of very low-birth-weight infants, who are surviving as a result of today's improved care, who are most likely to become ventilator-dependent and to suffer from the destructive effects of oxygen.

Retrolental fibroplasia

Etiology Blindness in preterm infants—*retrolental fibroplasia* (RLF) or *retinopathy of prematurity*—was first reported in 1942. About 10 years later, oxygen was discovered to be the cause. The lower the infant's gestational age, the higher the risk of RLF. The eyes of preterm infants are susceptible to damage because the retinal capillary development is incomplete and the blood vessels are extremely fragile. High blood levels of oxygen cause vasoconstriction and spasm of the retinal blood vessels.

Manifestation Retrolental fibroplasia progresses in two stages. The first stage involves retinal arterial constriction that persists as long as the high levels of blood oxygen are present. At this point the process may be reversible if exposure to oxygen is of short duration.

The second stage, or the proliferative stage, usually begins within 1 to 2 months after the oxygen therapy has been terminated. There is retinal edema and dilation of the capillaries and vascular overgrowth in the retrolental space (the area behind the lens). When the disease has progressed to the point of hemorrhage, scarring, and retinal detachment, the damage is permanent and the outcome is blindness. Approximately 25 percent of infants who experience retinal vasospasm during early oxygen treatment will become blind. (See Chap. 31 for a further discussion of RLF.)

Management The effect of oxygen on the eyes depends on the maturity of the infant, the level of oxygen in the blood, and the length of oxygen exposure. It is impossible to set an exact level as safe. Good nursing practice indicates that oxygen concentration should be maintained at the lowest possible therapeutic setting, reduced as the infant's condition permits, and used for the shortest time possible. A low level of vitamin E, commonly found in the preterm infant, can be related to hemolysis and anemia and has some relationship to RLF. Vitamin E has been used in conjunction with other measures to reduce the severity of RLF with some reported success, and it continues to be studied to determine its exact action.[27]

Controlling only the oxygen flow rate, monitoring the oxygen level in the environment, and keeping it at 40% concentration, as has often been suggested in the past, does not guarantee safety for the preterm infant's eyes. Carefully monitoring blood gases and keeping the level of oxygen in the blood between 50 and 70 mmHg is most effective in preventing eye damage. At present, it is the consensus that a Pa_{O2} of 100 mmHg increases the likelihood of eye injury and is not of value in treating hypoxia. It is also important that preterm infants routinely have eye examinations, both while in intensive care and during routine health care visits after discharge in order to detect developing retinal vasospasm.

Bronchopulmonary dysplasia

Etiology For almost 20 years, oxygen toxicity has been identified as the cause of *bronchopulmonary dysplasia* (BPD), a chronic pulmonary disease found predominantly in infants with RDS but occasionally also in infants who have received mechanical ventilation. There is a correlation between high oxygen concentration of inspired air (Fi_{O2}), mechanical ventilation through an endotracheal tube, and incidence of chronic lung disease. The flow of high-concentration oxygen into the lungs causes thickening of the basement membranes and the epithelial lining of the alveoli, impairing gas exchange. In addition, the presence of the endotracheal tube during mechanical ventilation impairs ciliary action and prevents mucus and debris from being cleared from the lungs. Surfactant production is inhibited by a combination of these stressors, and hyperventilation of obstructed bronchioles may lead to atelectasis and cystlike areas in the lungs.

Incidence In one study that covered a 12-year period, it was reported that about 21 percent of 299 infants with RDS who required mechanical ventilation with oxygen for at least 24 h developed BPD.[28] The incidence of moderate to severe cases of BPD has been decreased by about one-half since CPAP (continuous positive airway pressure) has been used.

Manifestations Early warning signs of BPD are increased oxygen and ventilator pressure requirements in infants with RDS at about 5 to 10 days, when they should be in the process of recovering. The nurse will also note increased signs of respiratory distress such as retractions, crepitant rales, and decreased breath sounds. Diffuse lung changes seen on early x-ray are replaced by signs of atelectasis due to obstruction of the small bronchioles and progressive air cysts that indicate developing emphysema. As emphysema progresses, barrel chest becomes obvious, respiratory acidosis is present, and right heart failure caused by increased pulmonary hypertension develops. Right heart failure is the leading cause of death.

The recovery process is extremely slow, requiring lengthy, gradual weaning from oxygen and the respirator. With improved ventilation techniques, the chances for survival have improved in recent years. Most infants recover by 1 year of age, and survival beyond 7 to 8 months is generally associated with normal cardiopulmonary function by 5 to 6 years of age. Some children develop a chronic lung condition and continue to suffer from recurrent pulmonary infections and wheezing. A few have bouts of acute pulmonary edema and respirator dependence.

Treatment Prevention of BPD centers on reducing trauma to the lungs from ventilation. New techniques that allow for lower oxygen pressures, such as high-frequency ventilation, are being introduced in an effort to prevent lung damage. The usual careful respiratory care and meticulous attention to hydration and cardiac function are the basis of nursing management. Treatment of right heart failure by using digitalis and diuretics and by very slowly and carefully weaning these infants from oxygen is the key to their survival.[29]

Bronchodilators such as Isuprel (isoproterenol) may be used to decrease airway resistance, and research is being conducted on an enzyme, superoxide dismutase (SOD), which may prevent or lessen the adverse effects of oxygen.[30] Parents will need support services to assist them in caring for a child with chronic lung disease at home. (See Chap. 34 for a discussion of the care of chronically ill children.)

Pulmonary dysmaturity

Pulmonary dysmaturity (Wilson-Mikity syndrome) is difficult to distinguish from BPD and may be a continuum of the same disease or a separate entity. Its onset, symptoms, and treatment are very similar to BPD. The chief manifestation is the appearance of multiple cystlike bubbles visible in the lungs on x-ray. Symptoms become severe in 4 to 8 weeks and take 6 months to 2 years to resolve.

REGULATION OF BODY TEMPERATURE

Temperature maintenance

One of the nurse's most important tasks in caring for a high-risk newborn is to keep the baby warm. Because of immaturity, asphyxia, or hypoxia, the baby cannot maintain his or her body temperature. A wet newborn in a cold environment can become chilled very quickly. The simple measures of drying and warming the newborn are essential for survival.

The full-term infant loses heat much more rapidly than an adult because the body surface area of the newborn represents 15 percent of the adult's body surface whereas the newborn's weight is only 5 percent that of the adult's. Heat loss in low-birth-weight newborns is an even greater problem because the proportion of body surface area to weight is even larger. The lack of subcutaneous fat, which is usually stored during the third trimester of pregnancy, can be a special problem for the preterm or intrauterine-growth-retarded infant. When the insulation of the subcutaneous fat is not present, capillaries are very close to the surface and release heat to the cool outside environment quickly.

An adult responds to cold by shivering and using muscle activity to produce heat. This is called *shivering thermogenesis*. An infant is unable to shiver and is capable of little muscle flexion or activity to produce heat. The sick or low-birth-weight newborn is hypotonic, and movement is infrequent. The infant responds to cold stress by nonshivering thermogenesis and raises body heat by metabolism. Norepinephrine is released in response to chilling. This stimulates metabolism, using oxygen and glucose to raise body heat. This is a very inefficient response and burns many times the normal number of calories.

Chilling initiates a cycle leading to hypoxia. After available glucose and oxygen are depleted, glycogen is converted without oxygen. Lactic acid is a by-product of this conversion and builds up in the body, leading to metabolic acidosis. Increased intrapulmonary vasoconstriction causes the circulation to return to the fetal circulatory pathways. As blood flow and gas exchange decrease, respiratory acidosis is the outcome.

In the mature newborn, brown fat is an excellent source of calories. It is found at the nape of the neck, between the scapulae, in the mediastinum, and around the kidneys. It is used for heat production during the first few weeks of life and then atrophies. In the preterm infant, brown fat may never have been formed; in the stressed fetus, it may be used up prior to birth; and in the cold-stressed infant, it is depleted rapidly.

In addition to causing impaired pulmonary function, cold stress decreases the amount of glucose available to other organs, particularly the muscles, the liver, and the brain. Cold stress depletes organ stores of glucose, particularly in the liver, and produces hypoglycemia. Because the brain requires a constant source of glucose, prolonged glucose deprivation can cause subsequent mental retardation.

Management Measures taken by hospital personnel to prevent cold stress to the infant can be lifesaving. Simple measures taken at delivery, such as drying the infant, wrapping the infant in a warm blanket, and putting the dry infant under a radiant warmer, can reduce heat loss by 65 percent.[31] Being alert to such things as cold coming from windows or walls and using commonsense measures can prevent cold stress and help the infant maintain body temperature.

The axillary or rectal temperature is measured every hour until it is stable and then is measured every 2 to 4 h. Rectal temperatures reflect the internal body temperature more accurately and take longer to drop in the face of cold stress than axillary temperatures. However, axillary temperatures are safer and are preferred because there is no risk of perforating the bowel with the thermometer. Most high-risk nurseries have automatically controlled heat regulators called *Infant Servo-controls*. They respond to a skin temperature sensor that is put on the abdomen over the area of the liver, the point of maximum body skin temperature. To prevent an inaccurate reading, the temperature sensor is protected from outside sources of heat by a foam-backed aluminum shield. When the infant is turned, the temperature sensor is moved to the flank to maintain an accurate reading.

Critically ill infants are especially vulnerable to cold stress because they are left naked for easier observation and frequently are under an open radiant heater (see Fig. 17-11). Four factors control the infant's thermal environment: the temperature of the surrounding air, the temperature of the radiant surfaces, the air flow, and the relative humidity. The smaller the infant, the

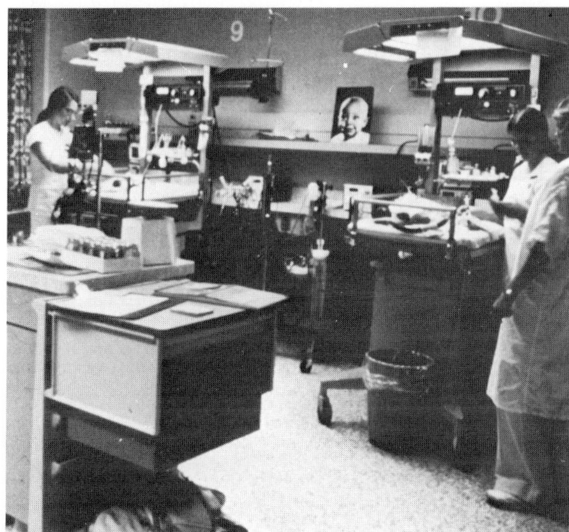

Figure 17-11 A neonatal intensive care unit with a nurse/patient ratio of about 1:2. Note the radiant warmers, which are typically used with the source of heat from the overhead lights.

more strict the temperature control must be. In the nursery an attempt is made to provide a *neutral thermal environment* to maintain the infant's skin temperature at 36.6 to 36.8°C (97.8 to 98.2°F). The core body temperature should be about 37°C (98.6°F). This temperature range does not require either great heat loss to cool the body or heat production to raise the body temperature.

Environmental heat is usually raised by placing the baby in an incubator or under a radiant warmer. Incubators lose heat by radiation through the single-walled construction and when portholes and lids are opened. Radiant heat loss can be decreased by surrounding the infant with a plastic heat shield that acts as a "minishelter" and by keeping the infant away from exterior sources of cold. A humidity level of 40 to 60 percent is optimum for maintaining body temperature because this level of humidity decreases evaporation loss. However, stagnant water is a good source of bacteria, and except in the case of very small infants, incubators are used without humidity. If water is used, sterile distilled water, changed every 8 h, is preferable.

An open radiant-heated bed is an even more serious problem in terms of heat loss. Air currents in the nursery may make it difficult to keep the baby warm, and the direct radiant heat on the heat sensor may cause the warmer to reduce the output of heat. Insensible water loss is higher when open radiant warmers are used; water loss and heat loss can be counteracted by the use of a plastic heat shield. Some hospitals use plastic cling wrap, attached from one side of the radiant-heated bed to the other, instead of a plastic heat shield because plastic wrap is convenient, cheap, and disposable. It is also important to remember that the baby's face has heat sensors and that even if the body is warm, a baby can be cold-stressed if cold oxygen is blowing on his or her face. Be sure to heat and humidify oxygen as discussed earlier in this chapter.

Whenever an infant is under an artificial source of heat, it is important to monitor both the baby's temperature and the temperature of the warmer. It is easy to overlook a drop in body temperature when it is automatically compensated for by a rise in the warmer's temperature. A drop in body temperature may signify an important change, such as hypoglycemia or infection.

Changing levels of heat

Etiology Some sources suggest that severely chilled infants should be warmed gradually with a heat source that is a degree above the body temperature. Too rapid warming, as well as too rapid chilling, can cause apnea. Overheating occurs when the core body temperature reaches 37.5°C (99.6°F) and should be avoided, since the newborn does not easily lower body temperature. Signs of hyperthermia are flushed skin, tachycardia, labored respirations, and seizures; severe hyperthermia can be fatal.

External temperatures should also be reduced gradually, a degree or less at a time. The infant's temperature should be closely monitored to make sure that it remains stable. When the nurse transfers infants from an incubator to an open crib, they can be kept warm by dressing them in a shirt, diapers, booties, and a stocking cap and wrapping them snugly in blankets. The head accounts for 25 to 33 percent of the infant's body surface, and the brain is a major heat-producing organ; thus the head of an infant who has temperature control problems should be covered.

CONTROL AND PREVENTION OF INFECTION

The trauma and stress of resuscitation experienced by the high-risk infant increase the danger of infection. Preterm babies face the additional risk posed by immature body defenses and reduced immunity, since immunity is usually transferred from the mother during the last trimester of pregnancy. A diverse group of infections are seen in the perinatal period and are produced by organisms that are not associated with disease in older children.

The birth canal is a source of infection when organisms ascend from the vagina through a ruptured amniotic sac to the fetus. Passage through the birth canal may result in infections, and postnatal infections from parents, nursery personnel, and contaminated equipment are also possible.

While many different organisms are responsible for infections in newborns, there are three major infectious diseases: pneumonia, septicemia, and meningitis.[32] *Listeria monocytogenes* from the mother is the most common cause of septicemia and meningitis today, but this is always subject to change. Group B streptococci and *Escherichia coli* cause many of the infections that originate in the birth canal. Postnatal infections are more likely to be nosocomial infections caused by "water bugs" such as *Pseudomonas* and *Serratia,* which thrive in any source of standing water such as soap dishes and respiratory equipment. While staphylococcal disease has never again reached the epidemic proportions of the early 1960s, hospitals are still indicated as sources of contamination when it occurs. Thirteen viruses are known to cross the placenta and cause fetal disease. These viruses are discussed in Table 28-9. Transmission from the mother can cause chronic intrauterine infections and postnatal infections. The symptoms of these diseases in infants are not the same as the symptoms of the same diseases in older children and adults.

Management

When infection is suspected in a newborn, appropriate cultures are taken 1 to 2 h after birth. In the delivery room, cultures of the stomach aspirate, the placenta, membranes, and the amniotic fluid may be diagnostic. The infant's external ear, nares, throat, axillae, inguinal folds, cord, and rectum are also cultured. A complete sepsis workup will be done if the infant shows signs of infection, but it is done with caution because it is traumatic. A complete workup includes urine, blood, and spinal fluid cultures. Infections can at first appear deceptively mild with few symptoms in the newborn and then become overwhelming and fatal, even with vigorous treatment.

Vague, nonspecific symptoms that mimic the symptoms of other illnesses are the rule in sepsis. The nurse notices that the baby does not "act right" or "looks funny." Fever is not a good indicator of infection, since the newborn frequently does not respond with a fever. The following signs may indicate sepsis:

1. Lethargy or hyperirritability.
2. Changes in color, activity, or muscle tone (hypotonia).
3. Changes in temperature. Hypothermia is more frequently a response than fever.
4. Feeding problems, spitting up, a poor sucking reflex, a distended abdomen, slowed digestion, vomiting, and diarrhea.
5. Rapid respirations, cyanosis, and/or apnea, especially in a preterm infant.
6. A drop in blood pressure, which may be related to septic shock.
7. Jaundice.
8. Hypoglycemia.
9. Signs of increased intracranial irritation.

If the organism cannot be specifically identified, broad-spectrum antibiotics—often kanamycin or gentamicin plus ampicillin—are given immediately. Care is used when administering antibiotics because they predispose the infant to infection from an opportunistic fungus or yeast, particularly *Candida*. The prognosis for outcome after sepsis is grave. The mortality rate is high, and infants may be left with residual central nervous system deficits. Supportive therapy includes giving blood transfusions, oxygen, and intravenous fluids and paying careful attention to temperature control.

Infections that are acquired postnatally can be greatly reduced through careful attention to nursery procedures. The following are some simple infection prevention measures that nursery personnel must take:

1. Wash hands carefully when entering the nursery, before and after handling a baby, and before going into central supply areas.
2. Maintain strict sterile techniques when invasive procedures are performed and when medications are administered.
3. Observe umbilical artery catheters, total parenteral nutrition lines, and intravenous sites carefully for signs of infection.
4. Although caps, masks, and hairnets are no longer advised, wear a scrub suit or gown that

can be changed before handling different babies.

5. Isolate infants who have a known infection, and provide protective isolation (in an Isolette) for infants who are extremely susceptible to infection.
6. Routinely culture equipment and sinks in the nursery as a preventive measure.
7. Avoid having stagnant water in equipment, and do not use Zephiran chloride. It will grow *Pseudomonas* and should not be used in the nursery.

ALTERATIONS ASSOCIATED WITH INFECTION

Necrotizing enterocolitis

Etiology *Necrotizing enterocolitis* (NEC) is an infectious process which leads to ulceration and at times perforation of the intestines. The mortality rate is high. It occurs in 2 to 15 percent of low-birth-weight (1250 g or less), sick, or preterm infants, and the incidence varies greatly among intensive care units. There are many theories, but the cause of this disease is unclear. It has been said to be related to an ischemic insult to the bowel, tube feedings, sepsis, an exchange transfusion, the use of umbilical catheters, and hypertonic formulas.

Manifestations Decreased blood supply to the bowel causes large numbers of mucus-producing cells to be damaged. These cells stop secreting the mucus barrier that protects the bowel wall. Without this barrier, the normally present acids erode the bowel wall, allowing bacteria to invade. As the bacteria infiltrate the submucosa and subserosa, gas is released. This results in the distinguishing sign of NEC, *pneumatosis intestinalis*—free gas in the intestinal wall or the peritoneum.

Signs of NEC may develop insidiously. The first signs may be those of sepsis: poorly controlled temperature, poor feeding, vomiting, lethargy, gastric distention, reduced or absent bowel sounds, blood in the stools, and jaundice. Eventually, apnea, shock, and circulatory collapse will occur.

Management The infant who is receiving gastric tube feedings should have abdominal girth measured to assess abdominal distention. The nurse should also observe for signs of infection, large residuals left in the stomach from the previous feeding, and blood in the stools.

Animal studies also indicate a relationship between NEC and hypertonic feedings.[33] Breast milk, which has a human-specific composition and contains immune substances and macrophages that combine to inhibit bacterial action in the bowel, is used by some pediatricians for babies at risk for NEC. Another often overlooked source of hyptertonic feedings is oral medications. White suggests that drugs given to high-risk infants should be diluted, that companies should develop lower concentrations of oral medications, and that intravenous administration should be preferred for some drugs.[34]

If signs of NEC are observed, intravenous feedings are started, and oral feedings are stopped. A nasogastric tube is inserted, and suction is begun to decompress the stomach. Broad-spectrum antibiotics are given systemically and by nasogastric tube. X-rays are done to confirm the presence of free abdominal air. Surgery is indicated when there is perforation or when the disease is severe. Often an intestinal resection and a colostomy or ileostomy are done. The course of recovery is prolonged, and the prognosis is poor.

NUTRITIONAL NEEDS OF THE HIGH-RISK INFANT

Most high-risk newborns have some fluid and electrolyte imbalances at birth that are related to their physical condition and stress they have endured. The method of correcting these deficiencies depends on the infant's condition. For most, an intravenous line is started for fluids, and an umbilical artery catheter is used for monitoring blood gas levels and giving medications. After the infant has stabilized, other types of feedings may be used if the infant's condition permits. The sick or low-birth-weight baby may not have the strength or maturity to suck, and the stomach may be too small to hold the amount of food needed to gain weight. The infant may have intravenous and gavage feedings or receive part of the feedings from a bottle. The goal is to ensure an adequate intake of calories and fluids so that the infant will gain weight and maintain hydration in the least stressful way.

The nutritional needs of the high-risk newborn vary with gestational age, weight, and condition. Caloric and fluid requirements are usually calculated on the basis of weight. The caloric, fluid, electrolyte, mineral, and vitamin requirements of low-birth-weight infants vary because they depend on the body stores and on the infant's absorption, rate of utilization, expenditure, and excretion of the substances.

Table 17-10 gives general estimates of the daily nutritional requirements of low-birth-weight infants. It is impossible, however, to present a single guideline for use with all infants. Many preterm infants have deficiencies of sodium, potassium, chloride, phosphorus, magnesium, and vitamins A, B, C, D, and E. Iron and calcium, which are usually stored during the third trimester of pregnancy, are also deficient. The fluid requirements of low-birth-weight infants are high because the body composition is 80 to 90 percent water and because the immature kidneys are unable to conserve water and electrolytes. Artificial heat and phototherapy lights also increase fluid losses through the skin by about 10 percent.

Methods of feeding

Intravenous feeding Most low-birth-weight infants will require intravenous feedings until adequate nourishment can be provided in another way. All infants who are under 32 weeks of gestational age and who weigh less than 1500 g will need intravenous feedings for at least the first 24 to 48 h, and usually longer. A 10 percent glucose solution is given at a rate of 80 to 100 ml/kg of body weight per 24 h for the first day, and then the amount is increased to about 150 ml per kilogram of body weight per 24 hours. This is an extremely small flow rate—4 to 6 ml per kilogram of body weight per hour—and must be monitored carefully to prevent error. Volume overload and cardiac failure can result if the intravenous feeding is infused too rapidly, and dehydration may result if it is administered at too low a rate. An intravenous pump is used to deliver these small amounts at a steady, controlled speed.

The intravenous site that is most frequently used is the umbilical artery; the second most frequently used site is the scalp vein or a cutdown into the saphenous vein of the leg. The veins are fragile and small, and the nurse must carefully protect and observe the site for infiltration. Intravenous therapy is discussed in Chap. 16.

Table 17-10 Daily Nutritional Requirements for Low-Birth-Weight Infants

Nutrients	Amount per Kilogram of Infant's Weight
Calories	110 to 150 (120 average)
Water	130 to 200 ml
Protein	3 to 4 g (10 to 15% of diet)
Carbohydrates	12 to 15 g (45 to 55% of diet)
Fat	5 to 8 g (30 to 45% of diet)

Total parenteral nutrition Adequate nutrition to maintain the body organs and promote growth is difficult to provide with intravenous feedings over a long period. Total parenteral nutrition (TPN) is used with infants who continue to be too ill to take food through the gastrointestinal tract for a long period of time. Total parenteral nutrition solutions are highly concentrated solutions of protein, glucose, and other nutrients and are injected into a large blood vessel using a constant-infusion pump; meticulous nursing care is required in order to prevent infection. Total parenteral nutrition is discussed in Chap. 19.

Oral and gavage feedings Before beginning feedings that require the gastrointestinal tract to function, the nurse must be sure that the infant can tolerate them. The following conditions must be met before feedings are begun:

1. There must be normal respirations (fewer than 60) with no signs of respiratory distress.
2. There must be no abdominal distention.
3. Bowel sounds must be audible.
4. The infant's color, tone, and cry must be normal.
5. There must be a strong sucking and swallowing reflex.

The first oral feeding is usually sterile water because if it is aspirated, it will be less irritating then either 5 percent glucose or milk. Formulas may be diluted for early feedings and gradually brought to full strength. Concentrated, high-calorie lipid solutions are used to provide additional calories; formulas for preterm infants contain 24 cal per ounce, instead of the usual 20 per ounce.

Recently pediatricians have expressed concern about high concentrations of solutes in formulas. The immature kidneys of the preterm baby may be damaged by excreting this additional load of solutes. Some centers use breast milk because it is more dilute and more compatible with the needs of a sick infant.

Gavage feedings are used when the infant can digest the feeding but cannot take a bottle. A feeding tube is inserted through the nose or mouth. The disadvantages of nasogastric insertion include the danger of blocking the nostrils, since babies are nose breathers; bleeding and irritation of the nares caused by the tube can lead to infection and obstruction. Oral gastric insertion gives the nurse an opportunity to watch the infant's sucking response and is the preferred method. Tube placement and the feeding technique are described in Chap. 16.

Continuous feeding cycles, which involve placing the feeding tube in the jejunum or duodenum, are usually reserved for very small infants who need long-term tube feedings. The advantages of this type of feeding include less fatigue, less gastric distention and irritation, and no reflux from the stomach into the esophagus and therefore less danger of aspiration.

Feedings usually begin with a few milliliters and are increased 2 to 3 ml at a time every 1 to 2 h. The stomach is aspirated before each feeding to determine whether the milk has been digested. When two ml or more from the previous feeding is present, the stomach aspirate is replaced, and the current feeding is reduced by that amount. Large amounts of residual formula are a sign of inadequate digestion and may signify a worsening physical condition.

It is important to protect the infant from abdominal distention caused by overfeeding. A distended abdomen puts pressure on the diaphragm, with resulting respiratory distress and apnea. Respiratory distress may indicate a need to stop oral feedings. Other signs of overfeeding are vomiting and "spitting up" formula. The stomach can also be overdistended with air. Leaving the feeding tube in place and open after feeding is a way to decompress the stomach. Complications that sometimes accompany gavage feedings include intestinal perforation, changes in intestinal flora, and more frequent occurrence of necrotizing enterocolitis.

Bottle feedings The nurse watches for signs that indicate readiness for bottle feedings. The baby will begin to suck on the tube during feedings and to be awake before feedings and will root when the cheek is touched. Encouraging the infant who is being fed through a gastric tube to suck on a pacifier stimulates and strengthens the infant's sucking reflex and facilitates bottle-feeding. At first, bottle feedings are given once a day, and then the number is increased gradually. Gavage feedings and bottle feedings are often alternated. The nurse watches the baby carefully to make sure that the amount of energy used in eating is not so great that weight gain is sacrificed.

Most well infants over 32 weeks of gestational age can coordinate sucking and swallowing. Preterm infants suck in short, rapid bursts and then rest. It is important to let them follow this natural pattern. Many nurses become frustrated because the high-risk infant is lethargic and sucks poorly. It is helpful to use a soft nipple, sit the baby upright, and burp the infant frequently. Patience is needed, but the feeding time is usually limited to 20 to 30 min to prevent exhausting the baby. Inability to feed for that length of time or respiratory distress usually signifies a need to return to gavage feedings.

Breast-feeding Breast milk contains more easily digestible protein and fat and more carbohydrates than cow's milk. It also contains antibodies and macrophages that can help prevent infection. At present, there is much controversy among pediatricians regarding the benefits of feeding breast milk to sick babies. Donor breast milk is not used as frequently as in the past because research suggests that the mother's antibodies are beneficial only to her own baby. Breast milk is no longer frozen; it is used fresh, refrigerated, and discarded when it is 12 h old. Some of the formula companies are now producing formulas intended to simulate breast milk.

Sick or low-birth-weight infants do not have sufficient energy to suck from a breast. The mother who wants to breast-feed should be encouraged to use a breast pump every 3 to 4 h to build up her supply of milk. Lemons's has described a protocol that has been used successfully to breast-feed preterm infants. Both the mother and the infant must be ready for breast-feeding. The mother must express the amount of milk that is needed to support the infant's growth—about 110 to 130 cal per kilogram of body weight per day (20 cal per ounce). The low caloric content of breast milk and the large caloric requirements of the low-birth-weight infant may make this difficult. The mother should also be available to the infant through rooming-in on a 24-h-a-day basis. In Lemon's study, rooming-in was provided for 2 days prior to discharge of the infant. Success was judged according to whether the infant gained weight, continued to breast-feed, wet six to eight diapers a day, and slept between feedings.[35]

Management The nurse monitors the baby's response to intravenous feedings and watches for signs indicating that gavage or oral feedings can be given. The baby is handled gently after feedings to prevent regurgitation of milk through the weak cardiac stomach sphincter. The nurse positions the baby on the right side so that air can leave the stomach more easily and places the baby with the head up or on the abdomen after feeding.

The nurse watches the infant's response to feeding carefully and observes for abdominal distention, vomiting, or respiratory distress. All feedings, amounts taken, and any observations concerning how the feedings were tolerated are charted. Dextrostix or Chemstrips are used to determine blood glucose levels. Intake and output are carefully monitored; diapers are weighed, and color, amount, and consistency of the stools are charted. The baby is weighed several times a day, since weight is the most accurate indicator of hydration. A weight loss between 5 and 10 percent in the first week is acceptable, but after this, the baby should gain 10 to 30 g a day.

Nurses who are responsible for feeding preterm babies (weighing over 1800 g) should consider the findings of a research study showing that infants who were fed on demand did better than infants on scheduled feedings. Infants who were allowed to sleep until they woke up and who were fed when alert required fewer tube feedings, compared with infants on scheduled feedings. In addition, bottle feedings were taken in much less time, and although the initial weight gain was slightly less, the babies who were fed on demand were discharged an average of 6 days earlier.[36]

SPECIFIC PROBLEMS OF THE HIGH-RISK INFANT

Hypoglycemia

Etiology *Hypoglycemia* is found most frequently in four broad categories of newborns: small-for-gestational-age babies, preterm infants (weighing not more than 1250 g), infants of diabetic mothers and erythroblastotic infants, and infants with rare genetic disorders (e.g., galactosemia).[37] In addition, hypoglycemic effects will occur in infants suffering from hypoxia, cold stress, respiratory distress, or sepsis.

The fetus receives its supply of glucose from the mother. At birth, the newborn's blood glucose drops from cord blood levels of 70 or 80 to about 50 mg per 100 ml in 2 h. Further decline is prevented by release of glycogen from the liver. After this source is depleted, the neonate begins to break down fat stores to use as fuel. Ultimately, external sources of glucose are needed to maintain energy levels. When neither glycogen nor fat has been stored, because of prenatal stress or because of birth prior to the third trimester when storage normally takes place, hypoglycemia is very severe unless glucose is replaced through oral or intravenous feedings.

Manifestations Hypoglycemia usually develops in 1 to 4 h after birth, but it may develop 1 or 2 days later or as long as a week later. Few signs of hypoglycemia are specific, and it can easily be confused with hypocalcemia or central nervous system trauma. The most frequently seen signs are refusal to feed, a weak cry, lethargy, rapid and irregular breathing, apnea, dyspnea, cyanosis, tremors, rolling of the eyes upward, convulsions, and coma.

A blood glucose level less than 30 mg per 100 ml in the full-term infant and less than 20 mg per 100 ml in the preterm infant during the first 3 days of life, and less than 40 mg per 100 ml thereafter, is regarded as indicating hypoglycemia. Glucose levels should be monitored during the first 1 to 2 h for all babies. Two consecutive low glucose levels are considered diagnostic of hypoglycemia. If blood levels are low, glucose is given, and blood glucose levels are monitored for 1 to 2 days until they stabilize. Infants with questionable symptoms can be treated with glucose. The symptoms will disappear after about 5 min if the problem is due to hypoglycemia. An infant on normal feedings will have a gradual increase to blood glucose levels of at least 45 mg per 100 ml as registered on a Dextrostix.

While blood sugar levels are more accurate for diagnosing hypoglycemia, Chemstrips or Dextrostix are often used for screening. A heel prick is used to obtain the blood sample. Warm the heel for 5 min to dilate the capillaries, and prick the heel less than 2 mm deep; and never use the bony back of the heel. Use the lateral heel and good antiseptic technique to prevent bone necrosis and future problems with heel pain. A level less than 45 percent on a Dextrostix is considered diagnostic of hypoglycemia.

Management Giving oral glucose and normal feedings will prevent or treat hypoglycemia in the infant who feeds well and has no contraindication to oral feedings. If the infant is unable to feed orally, glucose is given intravenously. The following regimen is often used:

1. Twenty-five percent glucose (2 to 4 ml per kilogram of body weight) given intravenously immediately to treat symptoms
2. Fifteen percent glucose (65 to 75 ml per kilogram of body weight) given intravenously for 24 h until the infant is stable
3. Ten percent glucose given intravenously for 12 h and then 5 percent glucose given intravenously for the next 12 h

Intravenous infusions of glucose are gradually tapered to prevent a severe rebound hypoglycemic reaction. Untreated hypoglycemia has serious consequences and can lead to brain deprivation of glucose with retardation or even death.

The infant of a diabetic mother

More effective control of diabetes and improved techniques for maternal and fetal assessment have decreased the maternal mortality rate among diabetic women to a rate close to that among other pregnant women. Despite improved prenatal care, the incidence of stillbirths, perinatal deaths, and congenital anomalies remains significantly higher among infants of diabetic mothers.[38] Estimates of perinatal mortality range from 10 percent in centers that specialize in high-risk infants to 20 to 30 percent in less specialized centers.[39]

Experience with an increasing number of pregnancies in diabetic women has led to an awareness of the need for close supervision of prenatal care and care of the newborn and of the need to time the birth precisely. Women in White's classes D through F have the poorest fetal outcomes. These are women with diabetes of early onset (prior to 10 years of age) and of long standing (20 years) and women with vascular changes. Women with vascular changes (class C and below) may give birth to intrauterine-growth-retarded babies, whereas class A and class B women characteristically give birth to large babies.

Carefully controlling maternal blood glucose to keep it within a normal range, through close medical supervision and home self-monitoring of blood glucose, has improved the fetal and maternal outcomes. The timing of the delivery is also critical; most physicians prefer to deliver the infant at 36 to 37 weeks of gestation. It is at about this time that placental dysfunction begins to take place. The risk of prematurity is balanced against the risk of stillbirth. The physician's past experience and tests performed to determine the fetus's size, level of maturity, and intrauterine conditions and the placental function all play a part in determining the exact time to deliver the baby. Table 17-3 describes the prenatal tests that are done to determine fetal condition and placental function. Tests of estriol levels are begun at 32 to 34 weeks and are done at least several times a week to establish a baseline of placental function. Ultrasound helps determine fetal growth and normality of parts and gestational age on the basis of the biparietal head diameter. Amniocentesis is used to assess fetal lung and renal maturity. The nonstress test evaluates the fetus's condition, and the stress test helps determine whether the infant can tolerate a normal vaginal delivery or needs to be delivered as quickly as possible by cesarean section.

The decision about when to deliver and whether the delivery should be vaginal or by cesarean section is made on the basis of the above tests and the size of the mother's pelvis in relation to the size of the baby. Babies of diabetic mothers are typically large, and a pelvis that is too small can cause severe trauma to both the mother and the baby. Frequently a cesarean section is the safest choice; about 70 percent of infants of diabetic women are delivered by cesarean section.

Manifestations The typical infant of a diabetic mother is very large, weighing over 4500 g (10 lb), and has fat cheeks, a red face, and a flushed, edematous appearance (see Fig. 17-12). The muscles are often hypotonic, but a slight stimulus will cause a tremulous, hyperirritable response. Babies of diabetic mothers frequently suck poorly and are not interested in eating. They are usually premature, and their physiological characteristics reflect their gestational age, despite their large size. A small intrauterine-growth-retarded infant may be born to a diabetic woman with severe vascular involvement.

Many of the problems of the infant of a dia-

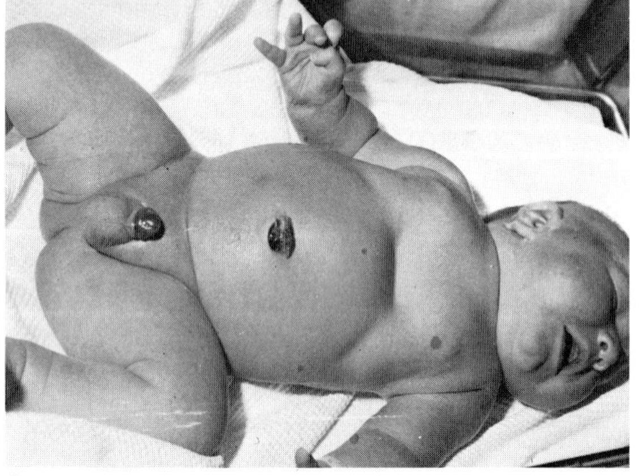

A

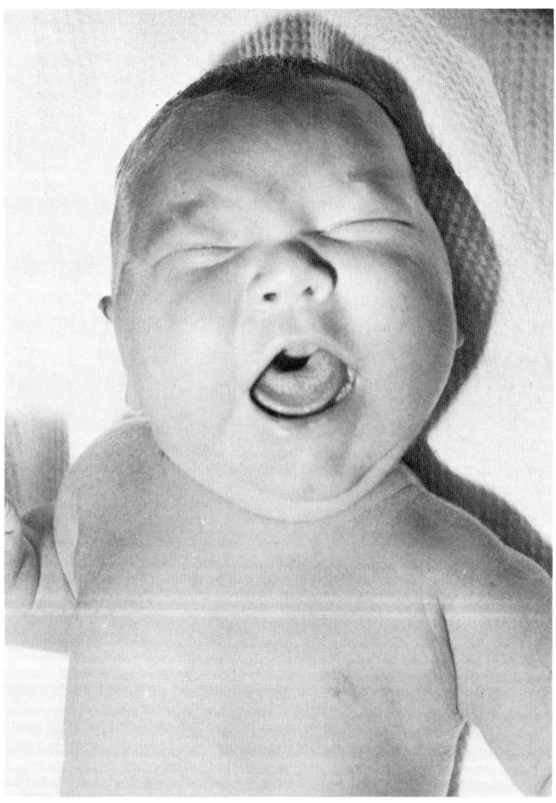

B

Figure 17-12 A 4500 g infant of a diabetic mother at 36 weeks of gestational age. Note the typical round face and fat, edematous body.

betic mother are based on the response of the fetus to a hyperglycemic environment. The large size, the deposits of subcutaneous fat, and the frequent occurrence of hypoglycemia are the result of this intrauterine environment. Maternal insulin does not pass through the placenta; maternal glucose does, however, and the fetus's blood glucose level is generally 80 percent that of the mother. If maternal hyperglycemia exists, it is reflected in the blood glucose level of the fetus. The fetus responds by increasing insulin production to an amount sufficient to metabolize the glucose. By the time of birth, the part of the pancreas responsible for producing insulin—the islets of Langerhans—has hypertrophied. Although glucose is no longer received from the mother, the newborn's insulin production continues, and the lack of a new source of glucose creates an imbalance that results in hypoglycemia.

Complications Infants of diabetic mothers have frequent complications. Some of the most common are hypoglycemia, hypocalcemia, respiratory distress syndrome, prematurity, hyperbilirubinemia, congenital anomalies, polycythemia, and renal vein thrombosis (quite rare).

The newborn continues to produce excessive amounts of insulin for the first few days after birth. The degree of hypoglycemia is affected by the prenatal control of blood glucose levels and the severity of the mother's diabetes. If the mother's blood is very hyperglycemic during labor and delivery, the resulting hypoglycemic reaction of the newborn will be severe. If the mother's blood sugar has been maintained at relatively normal levels, the newborn's hypoglycemic response will be much less severe. It is important to expect a sharp drop in blood glucose levels to 20 to 30 mg per 100 ml within 1 to 4 h after birth. Closely observing blood glucose levels with Chemstrips or monitoring blood glucose levels every 1 to 2 h for the first 8 h and then every 4 h for the next 24 h is required. Refer to the discussion earlier in this chapter of the manifestations and treatment of hypoglycemia.

Infants of diabetic mothers frequently develop hyberbilirubinemia related to polycythemia, preterm vascular fragility, and extravascular bleeding if the delivery was traumatic. Polycythemia can also be related to renal vein thrombosis, which is a rare complication. A calcium level below 7 mg per 100 ml (4 to 5 mEq per liter) is another common problem in these infants. Hypocalcemia is likely to occur either 24 to 48 h after birth or 5 to 10 days later. The early signs of hypocalcemia may be similar to those of hypoglycemia. Chapter 18 discusses the signs of hypocalcemia and its treatment.

Birth trauma is associated with vaginal delivery of a large baby. Common birth injuries are fractures of the clavicle, facial nerve paralysis, and brachial nerve plexus damage.

Major congenital anomalies are 2 to 3 times more common in infants of diabetic mothers than in other infants. The most common anomalies are congenital heart defects, spinal defects, tracheoesophageal fistulas, and malformations of the lower extremities. In a recent study by Fuhrman, 0.8 percent of newborns of diabetic women who were under strict control prior to conception had anomalies, compared with 7.5 percent of infants of a group of diabetic women who were under strict metabolic control after 8 weeks of gestation.[40] The implications of these research findings in terms of prenatal care are obvious.

Management Information that is essential in planning nursing care includes the newborn's history and the results of physical examinations, the mother's diabetic classification, the infant's gestational age, the type of delivery and any complications, and the newborn's Apgar score, blood glucose levels, calcium levels, and respiratory status. The infant of a diabetic mother may have a multitude of problems and needs the close observation available in an intensive care nursery. Details of nursing management are given in the discusions of each complication in other sections of this chapter.

Injuries related to birth trauma

The process of being born is traumatic to some degree to all babies. Minor soft tissue injuries include petechiae, conjunctival hemorrhage, and subperiosteal hemorrhage (cephalohematoma). These heal spontaneously, and recovery is usually complete.

The more serious injuries are those to the skeletal system and the central nervous system. These are related to the serious trauma associated with large fetal size and small pelvic size, breech deliveries, and complicated deliveries that exert excessive force on the infant's body parts. Central nervous system injuries have four main causes: hypoxia, birth trauma, hemorrhage, and infection.

Fractures Fractures most commonly involve the clavicle, but the spine, the skull, and the long bones of the extremities (the femur and the humerus) are also sometimes broken. Fractures of the clavicle occur as a result of shoulder dystocia (the shoulders are too large for the pelvis), and the clavicle breaks during delivery. A swelling is seen, or a snapping sensation is felt in the area. The break will heal spontaneously without any specific treatment. The arm on the affected side is supported and immobilized by pinning the long sleeve of the shirt to the body of the shirt. Skull fractures are usually caused by pressure of the head against the contracted pelvis, particularly the sacral promontory. Mid forceps or high forceps can also produce fractures, which are usually linear rather than depressed. Linear fractures (cracks) are not treated; depressed fractures are treated by elevating or removing the depressed bone. Fractures of the extremities are treated with immobilization, and if casts are applied, they must be observed carefully for tightness and must be changed frequently to allow for rapid growth. Care of fractures and casts is discussed in Chap. 29.

Peripheral nerve trauma Damage to the peripheral nerves is most often related to hemorrhage, excessive twisting of the neck and spine, and excessive manipulations during a traumatic delivery. *Brachial nerve plexus palsy* affects the arm and shoulder, causing paralysis of the upper extremity on the injured side. Paralysis is usually partial and disappears when the swelling of the nerves resolves.

Erb-Duchenne paralysis Erb-Duchenne paralysis, or Erb palsy, involves the fifth and sixth cervical spinal nerves. The newborn's arm is flaccid, with the elbow extended and the fist clenched. The arm is adducted and internally rotated. The condition is obvious because the usual flexion of the injured arm is absent. There is muscle weakness on the affected side, and there is little or no movement. The disorder involves primarily the shoulder and the arm muscles, not the hand muscles. The Moro reflex on the affected side is absent, but the grasp reflex is intact.

Klumpke paralysis Klumpke paralysis is due to an injury of the seventh and eighth cervical spinal nerves and the first thoracic nerve, which supply the brachial plexus. The principal involvement is in the lower arm. The wrist and hand are flaccid, and the grasp reflex is absent. Lower plexus injuries are usually more severe; children with these injuries have a poorer chance of recovery than those with Erb-Duchenne paralysis.

Management The affected arm and shoulder are protected from further injury by gentle handling and support with a figure-eight bandage. Care is taken to avoid trauma to the shoulder joint, since the lack of muscular support makes it susceptible to being dislocated. Gentle range of motion to the shoulder, elbow, wrist, and hand is required. Recovery is spontaneous, and there are minimal residual effects in over three-fourths of infants with this injury.[41] If the nerve has been disrupted rather than just traumatized, the return of function will be determined by the degree of regeneration. After about 6 months it is possible to determine the degree of recovery.

Facial paralysis Facial paralysis results from damage to the VIIth cranial nerve. Pressure on the face just posterior to the lower earlobe during pregnancy or delivery is the most frequent cause. This can happen during normal deliveries; a comparison of forceps deliveries and normal deliveries showed no increase in facial palsy as a result of the use of forceps.[42]

Central nervous system trauma Intracranial hemorrhage in the newborn is most often related to asphyxia or mechanical trauma. It can be classified according to the areas of the brain that are affected by the hemorrhage.

Subdural hemorrhage Subdural hemorrhage is caused by stretching and tearing of the large veins in the dural membrane (the tentorium cerebelli) that separates the cerebral hemispheres from the cerebellum. Abrupt compression of the skull, such as during a precipitate delivery, can cause bleeding in the full-term as well as the preterm infant. The same kind of pressure can also be exerted by high forceps or mid forceps. The prognosis for newborns with subdural hemorrhage is very poor, and death occurs frequently.

Subarachnoid hemorrhage Subarachnoid hemorrhage may be mild or severe and occurs in full-term and preterm infants as a result of hypoxia or birth trauma. Large amounts of blood in the subarachnoid space may interfere with cerebrospinal fluid absorption and lead to hydrocephalus.

Intraventricular hemorrhage Intraventricular hemorrhage is a major cause of death in preterm infants. CAT scans have shown intraventricular hemorrhage in 43 percent of infants weighing less than 1500 g. Hemorrhage into the ventricular wall frequently ruptures into the cerebrospinal fluid and blood circulates within the ventricular system. The flow of cerebral spinal fluid can be blocked, and as a result the ventricles dilate. Hydrocephalus results from dilatation and blockage of the ventricles. CAT scans have shown hydrocephalus in 44 percent of infants with intraventricular hemorrhage.[43]

Preterm infants are more susceptible to intraventricular hemorrhage because a very early vascular developmental structure of the brain, the germinal matrix, is present. The fragile capillaries in the germinal matrix lack support and are easily ruptured.

Three-quarters of the intraventricular hemorrhages are found within 30 h after birth; they are related to hypoxia and trauma and are complicated by hypoglycemia. Intraventricular hemorrhages occur more frequently in infants who have other complications that require resuscitation and stressful suctioning at birth and mechanical ventilation with an endotracheal tube. Extreme respiratory difficulty not improved by mechanical ventilation may indicate increasingly severe intraventricular hemorrhage. Drops in blood pressure and temperature, lethargy, hypotonia, apnea, hypercapnia, hypoxemia, and signs of increased intracranial pressure, such as a bulging anterior fontanel and seizures, are indications of intraventricular hemorrhage. With progressive intraventricular hemorrhage, the hematocrit drops, and the spinal fluid becomes bloody. A CAT scan shows ventricular dilatation, and finally hydrocephalus occurs.

The care of a child with neurological impairment requires close observation of neurological function. Chapter 30 discusses in detail the care of a child with neurological impairment and increased intracranial pressure.

Fetal alcohol syndrome

Since 1973 studies have described the pattern of fetal alcohol syndrome (FAS) in babies of chronically alcoholic women. Research has shown that maternal blood alcohol levels determine the effects on the fetus. "Binge drinkers," or women who drink large amounts periodically, are also at risk for having babies with FAS. Even social drinkers may be causing damage to their offspring.

Harmful effects of alcohol can be seen in children who do not have fetal alcohol syndrome. Alcohol intake has been related to decreased birth weight, head size, and length and to a greater risk of congenital anomalies. Since a large number of young women known to be alcoholics are reaching childbearing age, the problem will reach greater proportions in the future. Prenatal injury cannot be reversed; only prevention works.

Manifestations Not all children of chronic alcoholic women are affected. Smith estimates that the risk of FAS in the offspring of alcoholic women is about 33 percent and that the risk of mental deficiency is about 50 percent.[44] The fetus seems to be affected during the first 11 weeks of gestation. The defects result from a decreased number of cells, or hypoplasia, which causes an uneven rate of body growth. In affected children, a small head with undersized eyes and a small midface are typical. Diagnostic criteria suggested by the FAS Study Group of the Research Society on Alcoholism are delayed psychomotor development, mental retardation, microcephaly, midfacial hypoplasia, prenatal and postnatal growth retardation, and small palpebral fissures/microophthalmia. Other associated problems are cardiac septal defects, genitourinary anomalies (renal hypoplasia, hypospadias, and septate vagina), hemangiomas, hyperactivity, low Apgar scores, neonatal irritability, eye problems, and skeletal defects (club feet and congenital hip dislocation).[45] See Fig. 36.2.

Management Diagnosis is made on the basis of the mother's history and the appearance and symptoms of the child. Pregnant women should be told to abstain from drinking alcohol or to limit the alcohol intake to no more than one drink (2 oz) of alcohol a day. Health professionals must actively educate pregnant women regarding the dangers of alcohol and must take accurate histories concerning alcoholism. The advantages of using birth control should be discussed with the known alcoholic.

The infant of a drug-addicted mother

Heroin, methadone, and barbiturates are the drugs most commonly abused by pregnant women. Drug abuse affects the quality of the woman's pregnancy and motherhood. The typical pregnant drug abuser is in her early twenties, and the pregnancy was unplanned. Poor prenatal care, malnutrition, and diseases often related to drug abuse—such as hepatitis, septicemia, preeclampsia, and sexually transmitted diseases—are common.

Manifestations The addicted fetus may show signs of hyperactivity, such as kicking a lot, at the times the mother is due to take drugs. As many as 50 percent of these newborns have a low birth weight. Forty percent are small-for-gestational-age babies, and 60 percent are appropriate-for-gestational-age preterm infants. The small size of these infants relates to hypoplasia, or a reduced number of organ cells. It is known to occur independently of poor nutrition in heroin and morphine addicts.

Severe addiction in early pregnancy may lead to abortion and stillbirth. Two-thirds of the newborns of addicted mothers are affected and show visible signs of addiction. Problems of hypoxia, hypoglycemia, and hypothermia frequently complicate the birth.

Symptoms usually appear 24 to 96 h after birth, with occasional delays up to a week or more. The newborn shows such signs of central nervous system stimulation as hyperactivity, hypertonicity, irritability, tremors, high-pitched crying, and, infrequently, convulsions. Gastrointestinal symptoms include vomiting, diarrhea, poor feeding, and a constant sucking need. The newborn may also sweat, sneeze, yawn, and have excessive mucus.

A complete maternal history concerning addictive drugs is essential. Observing newborns for the symptoms listed above will help the nurse detect addicted infants. A urinalysis done within 12 h after birth will show traces of morphine and quinine, a substance often used to dilute morphine.

Medical and nursing management Withdrawal symptoms are controlled by administering chlorpromazine or phenobarbital to relieve central nervous system symptoms and by giving paregoric to control diarrhea. Intravenous therapy prevents dehydration. These babies are extremely irritable, tense, and difficult to comfort. A pacifier relieves their tension and satisfies their sucking needs. These babies need a calm, quiet environment and soothing activities such as swaddling and very gentle rocking. The nurse must anticipate that the mother may experience long-term difficulty caring for the infant. Referral to a community health nurse and follow-up by a counselor or social worker are essential. Symptoms of hyperirritability and learning disabilities persist as the infant grows up. The chances that the baby will fail to grow, will be abused or neglected, or will die of sudden infant death syndrome are all increased.

HYPERBILIRUBINEMIA IN THE NEWBORN

Hyperbilirubinemia, or an elevated blood bilirubin level that produces jaundice, is frequently seen in the newborn. Most jaundice is physiological, and its course is benign and self-limiting; however, physiological jaundice must be differentiated from pathological jaundice, which is more serious and may require aggressive treatment.

The basic process of bilirubin production is the same in pathological and physiological jaundice. Red blood cell breakdown, with the release of hemoglobin, produces 80 to 85 percent of bilirubin. When the red blood cells become aged or damaged, the fragile cell membranes rupture, releasing their contents. The hemoglobin portion divides into *globin,* a protein that is reused in the body, and *heme,* the iron-containing portion, which is converted to bilirubin after the iron is salvaged.

The major portion of red blood cell destruction takes place in the liver and spleen; macrophages, found in other parts of the reticuloendothelial system, also reduce hemoglobin to bilirubin by phagocytosis. Through the action of enzymes, these macrophages produce *unconjugated* (fat-soluble, or indirect) bilirubin, which will attach to other molecules in the body. In the blood, it attaches to the protein albumin and is carried to the liver. The liver separates bilirubin from the blood albumin through the action of the enzyme *glucuronyl transferase* and converts it to *conjugated* (water-soluble, or direct) bilirubin. Water-soluble bilirubin cannot diffuse through the cell membranes and is carried as a part of bile, through the bile ducts, to the duodenum. In the intestines it interacts with bacteria to produce urobilinogen and stercobilin. The stercobilin is excreted in the stool, giving it a dark-brown color. Urobilinogen is absorbed and is excreted in the urine, which will be brown when the level is elevated.

Jaundice

The yellow color of the skin, or *jaundice,* is seen when the albumin binding sites in the blood are filled and the unconjugated bilirubin attaches to molecules elsewhere in the body. Bilirubin commonly deposits in the subcutaneous fat, the eyes, and under the nails, and eventually, in an unexplained process, it crosses the blood-brain barrier and deposits in the brain cells.

Normal bilirubin levels are higher in newborns than in adults—0.2 to 1.4 mg per 100 ml of blood. Levels must exceed 5 mg per 100 ml of blood before jaundice in the newborn becomes visible. Levels of 12 mg per 100 ml of blood are usually treated. Jaundice progresses in a cephalocaudal direction, beginning in the head and gradually moving down the body to the legs and feet. Pathological levels are generally not present until it has spread below the upper part of the body.

Physiological jaundice Physiological jaundice is the most common cause of elevation of bilirubin levels in healthy, asymptomatic newborns. The levels reach about 12 mg/dl; the jaundice peaks at about the fourth day of life, and the levels fall by the end of the first week. Healthy preterm infants, who have less mature liver function than full-term infants, have physiological jaundice that peaks at levels of 15 mg/dl, and the levels take about 10 days to fall.

A number of factors contribute to jaundice in the newborn: fetal hemoglobin levels of 18 to 22 g, 5 to 6 million red blood cells at birth, a 90-day average life span of fetal red blood cells (the life span of adult red blood cells is 120 days), low blood albumin levels, immature liver function, and delayed meconium passage. The number of red blood cells is reduced to 4 to 5 million in about a week, as the newborn adjusts to higher extrauterine oxygen levels and thus does not need the additional oxygen-carrying power of high hemoglobin. The rapid breakdown of red blood cells and the impaired ability to excrete bilirubin during the first few days of life raise the newborn's bilirubin levels. Additionally, meconium can be reabsorbed through the intestines if its passage is not stimulated by early feeding. Also, the liver has a deficiency of glucuronyl transferase and cannot respond to an increased load from all these sources. Intestinal bacteria necessary for breaking down conjugated bilirubin for excretion are not present at birth, and a fetal enzyme—beta glucuronidase—is still present in the newborn and converts bilirubin back to the unconjugated form. As much as 1 mg of bilirubin per gram of meconium can be reabsorbed into the bloodstream.

Breast-feeding jaundice The management of jaundice in breast-fed babies has been a controversial subject for many years. It has been suggested that two substances found in breast milk—pregnandiol and a free fatty acid—inhibit the activity of glucuronyl transferase in the newborn's liver. From the fourth or fifth day of life, when physiological jaundice recedes, a small number of breast-fed babies continue to be jaundiced for 3 or more weeks. According to a recent study, serum bilirubin peaks at 13 mg per 100 ml, with jaundice still present on the twenty-first day but with no ill effects apparent in the infants.[46] Other sources suggest that the bilirubin can peak between 10 and 27 mg per 100 ml and that when breast-feeding is discontinued for several days, bilirubin declines to normal levels. Once the diagnosis is confirmed, breast-feeding can be resumed.

Pathological jaundice Pathological jaundice is an increase in the bilirubin level that poses a threat to the baby's health. It begins early, and the bilirubin level may become very high or remain high for a prolonged period. Hyperbilirubinemia may be the first indication of the presence of an undiagnosed disease or of a complication of an existing disorder. Table 17-11 lists conditions related to hyperbilirubinemia. A distinction between physiological and pathological jaundice can be made on the basis of the time of onset, the course of the jaundice, the bilirubin level, and the infant's general maturity and condition. Table 17-12 compares these two types of jaundice.

Kernicterus

Kernicterus (bilirubin encephalopathy) is the most serious complication of hyperbilirubinemia. Bilirubin passes the blood-brain barrier, attaching to the cells and causing disruption in function or even death. This usually occurs at levels above 15 mg per 100 ml in a preterm baby and at levels above 20 mg per 100 ml in a full-term infant. It is possible to have brain damage in dehydrated, sick, or very low birth weight infants at lower levels. In infants with low levels of albumin in the blood, bilirubin will bind to other sites, in-

Table 17-11 Conditions Related to Hyperbilirubinemia

Classification	Examples and Further Information
1. Hemolytic disorders	Rh and ABO incompatibilities; genetic red blood cell abnormalities
2. Extravascular blood	Intraventricular hemorrhage; cephalohematoma; swallowed blood
3. Polycythemia	Excessive numbers of red blood cells
4. Drug reactions	Sulfonamides and aspirin taken by the mother
5. Infections	Prenatal or neonatal infections (see Table 17-1)
6. Delayed meconium passage	Meconium ileus; bowel obstruction; delayed feeding
7. Metabolic factors	Infants of diabetic mothers; hypothyroidism; breast milk jaundice
8. Prematurity	Low albumin; fragile blood vessels; immature body systems
9. Impaired liver function	Biliary atresia or obstruction; immaturity
10. Hypoglycemia	Delayed oral intake; prematurity; cold stress; hypoxia; infants of diabetic mothers
11. Hypoxemia	Asphyxia; respiratory or cardiac disease

Table 17-12 Comparison of Physiological and Pathological Jaundice

Physiological Jaundice	Pathological Jaundice
Onset	
After 24 h—full-term infants After 48 h—preterm infants	Before 24 h
Course	
Full-term infants—disappears in 1 week Preterm infants—disappears in 9 to 10 days	Full-term infants—lasts more than 1 week Preterm infants—lasts more than 2 weeks
Level	
Less than 12 mg per 100 ml	20 mg per 100 ml in full-term infants 15 mg per 100 ml in preterm infants
Peak	
Full-term infants—3 to 4 days Preterm infants—5 to 6 days	
Rate of Elevation	
Less than 5 mg per 100 ml daily	More than 5 mg per 100 ml daily
General condition	
Infant is well	Infant is sick: anemia; hepatosplenomegaly; Coombs—positive

Table 17-13 Central Nervous System Signs of Kernicterus

CNS Depression	CNS Excitation
Lethargy	Tremors
Poor feeding; decreased sucking and rooting	Twitching
Decreased reflexes; absent Moro reflex	Seizures
Decreased muscle tone (hypotonia)	High-pitched cry
	Opisthotonus (hyperextension of the back)

cluding the brain. Cold stress, acidosis, hypoglycemia, and drugs that compete for binding sites (sulfonamides and salicylates) reduce the binding power of albumin.

Kernicterus often begins with central nervous system depression and progresses to central nervous system excitation (see Table 17-13). The damage to the infant may range from mild developmental delays to permanent damage or death. Mental retardation, sensorineural hearing loss, and delayed or abnormal motor function may be found in babies who survive.

ISOIMMUNE HEMOLYTIC DISEASE IN THE NEWBORN

Most *isoimmune hemolytic disease* in the newborn is the result of ABO and Rh incompatibilities. Rh incompatibility has been greatly reduced since the advent of anti-Rh gamma globulin, and most isoimmunizations are at present due to ABO incompatibility. When an isoimmune reaction takes place, antibodies are produced by the mother against red blood cells from her baby, endangering the infant's survival.

If the parents have different blood types (A, B, AB, or O), the baby can inherit a blood type that is incompatible with that of the mother. The Rh and ABO blood group systems are the most significant. Although thousands of other red blood cell antigens are present, they are rarely involved in maternal-fetal blood incompatibilities.

ABO incompatibility

ABO incompatibility most commonly involves a mother with type O blood and an infant in the A or B group. Type B infants of type A mothers are occasionally affected, and type O infants are never affected (see Table 17-14).

The infant's reaction may vary from mild to severe disease. The natural anti-A and anti-B antibodies that exist in the type O mother's blood may pass to the fetus without previous sensitization of the mother as the result of leaking of fetal blood to the maternal circulation. Therefore, the first infant may be mildly or severely involved. The presence or severity of the disease in future pregnancies is not related to the disease in the first infant.

The severe complications of stillbirth, hydrops fetalis, and significant anemia are rare. Varying degrees of jaundice are commonly present, and enlargement of the liver and spleen may sometimes occur. After birth, a *direct Coombs test,* which measures antibodies attached to the infant's red blood cells, may be negative or weakly positive. An *indirect Coombs* test on the baby's serum may be strongly positive. Spherocytes—red blood cells that are smaller in diameter and thicker than mature red blood cells—will be found in increased numbers and confirm the diagnosis of ABO incompatibility. Treatment consists of phototherapy and exchange transfusion with type O blood, never the baby's own type, if the bilirubin level becomes very elevated. Phototherapy and exchange transfusions are discussed later in this chapter.

Table 17-14 ABO System of Antigens and Antibodies for Determining Blood Compatibility

			Compatibility	
Blood Group	Antigen	Antibody	Can Be Donor to Person With	Can Receive Transfusion from Person With
A	A	Anti-B	Type A or AB	Type A or O
B	B	Anti-A	Type B or AB	Type B or O
AB	A and B	No antibodies	Type AB	Type A, B, AB, or O
O	No antigen	Anti-A and anti-B	Type A, B, AB, or O	Type O

Source: Adapted from G. Scipien, M. U. Barnard, M. A. Chard, J. Howe, and P. J. Phillips (eds.), *Comprehensive Pediatric Nursing,* 2d ed., McGraw-Hill, New York, 1979.

Rh incompatibility

The Rh factor was named for the rhesus monkey, in which it was discovered in 1940. Six major factors are present in the Rh system—C, c, D, d, E, and e—but it is the capital D that is responsible for 95 percent of the incompatibilities. The term *Rh-positive* means that the Rh antigen is present on the outer membrane of the red blood cell; *Rh-negative* means that it is absent. The Caucasian population is 85 percent Rh-positive and 15 percent Rh-negative. Other racial groups, such as blacks and American Indians, have fewer Rh-negative members.

When the mother is Rh-negative, her chances of having an Rh-positive baby depend on whether the father is heterozygous or homozygous for Rh-positive. If he is homozygous, all the babies will be Rh-positive because he carries only the dominant Rh-positive genes. If he is heterozygous, there is a 50 percent chance of passing either Rh-positive or Rh-negative genes because he carries both.

Rh incompatibility occurs when the mother is Rh-negative and the fetus she carries is Rh-positive. The placenta usually acts as an effective barrier to the mixing of maternal and fetal blood; however, sometimes fetal red blood cells enter the maternal circulation. A small amount of fetal blood (0.1 to 0.2 ml) may pass during pregnancy but is not normally enough to sensitize a mother during her first pregnancy. It is not until the events of labor and delivery cause placental tears and disruption that the larger dose of fetal blood, about 0.5 ml, passes to the mother and stimulates a primary immune response.

This response is also known as *sensitization*. In addition to pregnancy or miscarriage, it is also possible to be sensitized by a blood transfusion. A primary response takes about 72 h to be stimulated, and from 6 weeks to 6 months is required for a full complement of antibodies to be produced. Future exposures to Rh-positive red blood cells will stimulate a secondary "memory" response and more rapid, higher-level antibody formation. See the section "Immune Response" in Chap. 26 for a full explanation of this process.

Once the mother has been sensitized, her body will produce antibodies against Rh-positive fetal red blood cells (antigen) that enter her body, and these antibodies will pass through the placenta into the fetal circulation, where they will attach to and destroy the fetal red blood cells. The degree of red blood cell hemolysis depends on the degree of sensitization of the mother, but it becomes worse with each pregnancy that is not treated with RhoGAM (see Fig. 17-13).

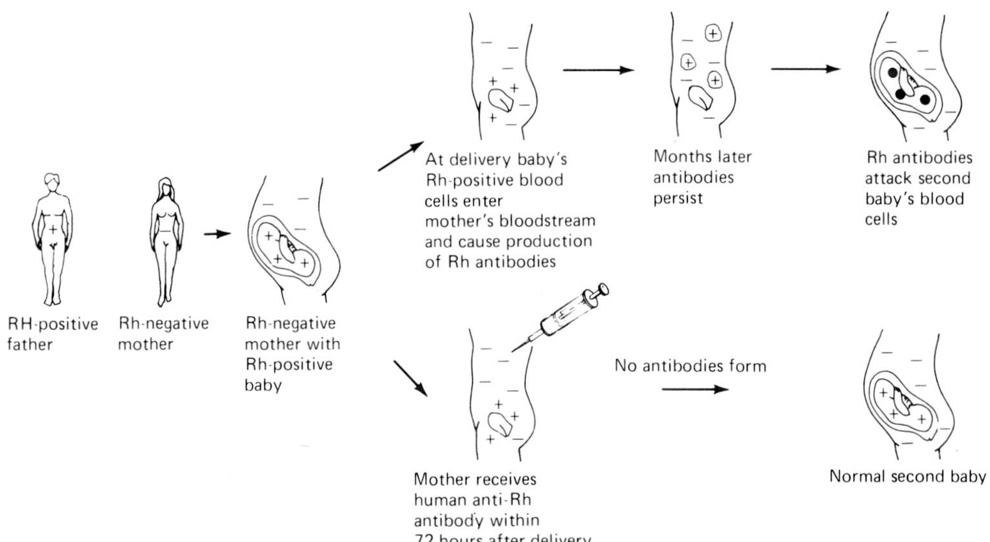

Figure 17-13 Maternal Rh sensitization and prevention using RhoGAM, or Rh_o(D) immune globulin (human). (*From S. H. Pierog and A. Ferrara, Medical Care of the Sick Newborn, 2d ed., Mosby, St. Louis, 1976, p. 188. Used with permission.*)

RhoGAM *RhoGAM*, or $Rh_0(D)$ immune globulin (human), gives the mother artificial antibodies that destroy the Rh-positive fetal red blood cells that have passed through the placenta into her circulation. These antibodies remain in her circulation for about 4 to 6 weeks and then are destroyed. Since the mother's own immune system was never activated in a primary response, it will have no "memory" of this antibody reaction. Without RhoGAM, the body actively produces antibodies during the first pregnancy, and in each pregnancy that follows there is a stronger, secondary antibody response, since the body "remembers" the first reaction. RhoGAM should be given within 72 h after a miscarriage or the birth of an Rh-positive baby to an Rh-negative mother. New research indicates that the number of sensitized women can be further reduced if RhoGAM is used prenatally at 28 weeks to clear the maternal circulation of any Rh-positive cells and prevent isoimmunization.[47]

Hemolytic disease of the newborn

Hemolytic disease of the newborn (erythroblastosis fetalis) is generally a result of ABO or Rh incompatibility. The severity of the hemolytic reaction depends on the strength of the antibody response in the mother and the length of time the fetus is exposed to the antibodies. Anemia is the primary sign in the fetus, and severe anemia causes the liver and spleen to enlarge and leads to edema as a result of low blood protein. Massive total body edema of the fetus is known as *hydrops fetalis* and may result in pulmonary edema and heart failure. Jaundice is rarely present in the fetus because the placenta continues to clear bilirubin. The severity of the hemolytic response is measured by several prenatal tests. A red blood count will demonstrate that immature red blood cells (erythroblasts) are present and are trying to replace the red blood cells that are being destroyed. An indirect Coombs test is done on Rh-negative women to measure anti-D antibody levels in the serum. Initially this test is done at 16 to 20 weeks of gestation; if the results are positive, it is repeated at frequent intervals during the pregnancy. A direct Coombs test will show the presence of anti-D antibody attached to the fetus's red blood cells.

Amniocentesis is performed if the maternal indirect Coombs test shows rising antibody titers. Bilirubin levels in the unaffected fetus peak between 16 and 30 weeks of gestation and bilirubin disappears by 36 weeks. A rising or very high level of bilirubin in the amniotic fluid indicates progressive red blood cell destruction and may indicate the need for an intrauterine transfusion or delivery of the fetus.

Intrauterine transfusions

An intrauterine transfusion can be given to a severely anemic fetus that is too immature to survive and is suffering from such severe hemolytic disease that its life is in danger. In a procedure much like an amniocentesis, radiopaque dye is put into the amniotic fluid. When the fetus swallows the amniotic fluid containing the dye, the peritoneal cavity is outlined and can be seen with a fluoroscope. Type O Rh-negative blood—about 75 to 100 ml of packed red blood cells—is injected into the peritoneal cavity of the fetus. The red blood cells are absorbed and alleviate the anemia. The intrauterine transfusion may need to be repeated. There is a risk of injuring the infant through inadvertent needle puncture. The nurse checks the fetal heart tones and observes for amniotic fluid leakage and the onset of labor.

Exchange transfusions

Giving exchange transfusions to newborns is the most effective way to treat severe anemia and stop the rise of bilirubin levels before the anemia progresses to kernicterus. An exchange transfusion will replace the infant's sensitized red blood cells, remove circulating maternal antibodies, lower the bilirubin levels, and increase the hematocrit. Fresh Rh-negative blood is best—either the infant's own type or, in the case of ABO incompatibility, type O. Blood that is more than 48 h old has high potassium levels, and acidosis has to be corrected if it is used. If heparinized blood is used, protamine sulfate must be given at the completion of the transfusion to prevent bleeding. Blood preserved with sodium citrate combines with the infant's serum calcium and depletes it. Infusions of calcium gluconate are given after each 100-ml transfusion of citrated blood to prevent hypocalcemia. Giving albumin intravenously, before an exchange transfusion, in amounts of 1 g per kilogram of body weight will increase the binding sites in the blood; this procedure is called *priming*. It increases the amount of bilirubin removed during an exchange transfusion.

In a continuous-volume exchange, 5 to 20 ml of the newborn's blood is withdrawn from the umbilical artery catheter, and an equal volume of exchange blood is replaced into the umbilical vein catheter. This is continued until double the infant's volume has been given (170 ml per kilogram of body weight).[48] This replaces about 85 percent of the infant's blood. The procedure takes about an hour. Serum bilirubin is decreased by about 50 percent, but rises as bilirubin is drawn out of the tissues. The infant may need several repeat transfusions and may continue to show a progressive decrease in hemoglobin as long as maternal antibodies are present, which is about 6 weeks (see Table 17-15).

Management The nurse warms the blood to body temperature, accurately determines the blood type and Rh, and verifies the infant's name. The baby is kept warm during the procedure, and cardiopulmonary status is carefully monitored. Sterile technique is scrupulously maintained, and detailed records of the amount of blood transfused and of cardiac and respiratory status are kept.

Phototherapy

Phototherapy is the use of a light source to stabilize the level of bilirubin in the newborn and prevent further increases. Many sources suggest using phototherapy when the level reaches 12 to 15 mg per 100 ml, but other researchers have found that waiting until the level reaches 20 in an otherwise healthy baby does no harm.[49] Phototherapy should not be used as a substitute for exchange transfusions, and the physician should attempt to find the cause of elevated serum bilirubin levels. The laboratory tests discussed earlier should be done, and less obvious causes such as sepsis and biliary atresia should be considered. Even with this careful examination, a cause of the jaundice will be discovered in only about one-half of the cases.

Whatever type of light is used for phototherapy, a Plexiglas shield is used to prevent undesirable ultraviolet rays from reaching the baby and causing a burn. Usually a bank of four to eight incandescent lights is used, and the hours of use are accurately recorded, since some lights lose their effectiveness after 200 h of use. An accurate way of judging a light's effectiveness is to use a light meter that monitors energy output, although this is not commonly done. The nurse should observe for harmful effects of the lights on both the baby and the nursing personnel. When nurses are working with blue lights, wearing sunglasses and a hair covering may reduce nausea and dizziness.

The naked baby is placed under the light source, with the eyes shielded and a paper mask covering the gonads. Before the eyes are covered, make sure that they are shut, and secure the mask so that it does not obstruct breathing. The mask is removed every 4 h, and the eyes are cleansed and checked for corneal abrasion. The nurse should encourage the parents to interact with the baby while the eyes are uncovered and should reassure them that nothing is wrong with the baby's eyes. The baby is turned about every 2 h to increase exposure of all skin surfaces to the light. Infants under lights can have difficulty controlling their temperature, and the insensible water loss can be increased twofold to threefold. The skin turgor and the fontanels (depressed) are observed for signs of dehydration. The infant is weighed every 8 to 12 h, since weight loss is an accurate sign of dehydration. Fluid intake should be large enough to compensate for the losses. Fluids are also lost through the stools, and loose green stools are to be expected. Careful attention should be given to care of the skin in the diaper area. The body temperature is controlled by putting the baby in a radiant warmer or an Isolette with a properly shielded constant temperature probe. The temperature is checked every 4 h. Care should be taken to maintain skin integrity (see Fig. 17-14).

A maculopapular skin rash is common and disappears spontaneously. A severe gray-brown discoloration of the skin, called *bronze baby syndrome,* occurs in infants with liver disease who are treated with phototherapy. The discoloration clears up about 3 weeks after therapy is discontinued.

Table 17-15 Indications for Exchange Transfusion

Cord blood bilirubin over 4 mg per 100 ml at birth
Bilirubin—rising more than 0.5 to 1 mg per 100 ml in 1 h:
15 mg per 100 ml in a preterm infant
20 mg per 100 ml in a full-term infant
Hemoglobin:
Under 14 g in a preterm infant
Under 12 g in a full-term infant

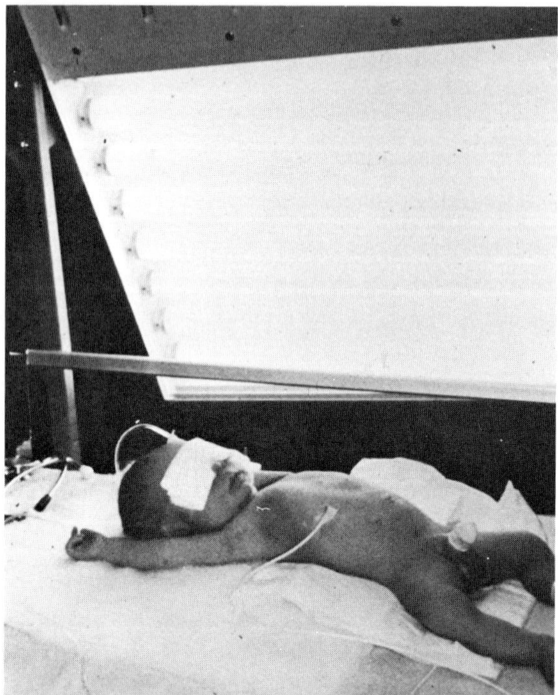

Figure 17-14 An infant with the eyes and gonads covered and a heat sensor in place under a bank of eight fluorescent lights; the baby is being given phototherapy. Note that all the skin surface is exposed.

Parenting is easily disrupted at this early stage, and the nurse should reassure the parents that the jaundice is not related to neglect on their part or to any factors under their control. The parents should be allowed in the nursery to hold the baby for feedings with the eye patches off and to touch and stroke the baby between feedings. The sensory deprivation of an infant under lights can be severe, and relief from the isolation of the environment is an absolute necessity.

THE NICU: A HIGH-RISK ENVIRONMENT

Sensory overload

Infants who are cared for in an NICU often receive inappropriate sensory stimulation. Overstimulation can be the result of excessive environmental noise levels, excessive exposure to light, and painful stimuli from treatments. A decrease in transcutaneous blood oxygen readings and an increase in intracranial pressure have been observed when noise levels rise. In animal studies, ototoxic drugs that are often given to sick newborns, such as kanamycin, neomycin, and gentamicin, have been shown to magnify the effect of noise one-hundred-fold.[50] Light deprivation due to eye patches, the phototherapy lights, and failure to establish diurnal (night and day) rhythms are other examples of inappropriate sensory stimulation.

Nurses should be alert to ways of providing appropriate stimulation. Research on loving and stroking care has shown that infants receive this kind of stimulation least frequently and that some infants receive none.[51] Most care involves a technical procedure. Nurses should try to feed infants when they become alert so that they can establish their own waking-sleeping cycles. The lights should be turned down at night to establish the diurnal cycle. Nurses should stroke and talk to infants during and after care, handle them gently, and avoid sudden changes in position.

Both nurses and parents should learn to recognize the cues that indicate readiness to respond or that indicate overstimulation. Signs of overstimulation include facial grimaces, increased jerky and startled movements, labile color changes, decreased muscle tone, instability of respiration and heart rates, hiccuping, and turning the head away from the source of stimulation. Because overstimulation is painful to the newborn, these are responses to pain. The infant responds to pain with generalized body movements because the motor pathways are too immature to permit specific responses.

In a study using foster grandmothers to provide stimulation in a nursery for preterm infants, muscle tone and alertness were shown to improve, especially around the time of the stimulation, when the babies were rocked, talked to, and shown bright objects. This was done twice a day for 2 weeks. The foster grandmothers in this study also became advocates for the babies.[52]

Alterations in parenting of high-risk infants

Parents of high-risk infants have special parenting and attachment needs as a result of the disruption of the usual process of attachment and the birth of a "less than perfect" baby. How the parents respond to these crises is influenced by their past experiences with pregnancies; their own parenting; the planning, course, and events of the pregnancy; relationships with their spouse and other family members; their cultural and socioeconomic background; and their level of maturity.

Pregnancy, labor, and birth The usual tasks of midpregnancy include bonding to the fetus and preparing physically and emotionally for the baby's arrival (nesting). The final task of pregnancy—separation—establishes the baby as an entity, apart from the mother. Separation is mastered in part through fantasy. The baby is imagined as having certain characteristics—blue eyes "like mine" or black hair like the father's, for example. The baby is thought of as either a boy or a girl, and always as "normal." Producing a perfect baby is an extension of the mother's body image and self-esteem. The pregnant woman mentally readies herself for motherhood.

A premature birth interrupts the normal psychological development of mothering. While this is not an insurmountable obstacle to normal mothering, it is a disruptive and traumatic event for the woman and the entire family. Labor is usually a happily anticipated event; premature labor is often a disastrous emergency situation. The joy and calmness associated with normal birth are not present. Feelings of guilt are common and may be expressed by the parents.

The delivery is an anxious time for the father, who may be separated from the mother and anxiously waiting for information. Fathers are not usually allowed in the delivery room when the birth is "complicated." The delivery room is often crowded with medical experts, but there may be no one there to support the mother. The nurse should be sure to spend time close to the mother's head, telling her what is happening and holding her hand. After the birth, it is very important that the mother be given a quick summary of the infant's condition and be allowed to look briefly at the infant. Seeing the baby dispels the mother's fear that the baby has died and no one is telling her.

Sick infants are usually stabilized by the pediatric team before being moved to an NICU. A baby who is being taken to another hospital can be brought in the transporter to visit the mother. Seeing the baby and, if possible, touching the baby will begin the attachment process. The father often follows the transport team and is the one who relays information to the mother. It is important to explain the purpose of all the tubes and equipment and to give the father a truthful report on the baby's condition.

Meeting the needs of the parents of a high-risk infant Caplan has identified four major tasks that the mother needs to complete after the birth of a high-risk infant.[53]

1. She must realize that she may lose the baby, and she may do some anticipatory grieving; she still hopes for survival, but she prepares for death. Interventions include talking with the parents about the baby and giving them realistic, correct information. Klaus and Fanaroff suggest stressing the positive aspects and being optimistic, since the outlook for high-risk infants is now greatly improved. Once a parent believes that a baby will die, mourning takes place, which makes it more difficult to attach to the infant.[54] A woman who has held and cared for her baby is very distressed if the baby dies, but there is no evidence of a dangerous increase in grief among women who have no emotional health problems. When NICU nurses take pictures of the baby and make telephone calls to the parents, this is reassuring to the parents and helps make the baby a reality. Doctors' visits are also essential. As soon as possible, the parents should visit the NICU. Nurses should tell the parents about the equipment, tubes, and monitors and tell them what to expect the baby to look like. The policies of the unit should also be discussed. Nurses should arrange for transportation, if necessary, and should go with the parents to visit the baby if they can. The first visit may be extremely overwhelming and may have to be broken up into short intervals. The nurse should stay with the parents the first time, but during later visits it is important to give them some privacy.

2. She must acknowledge her failure to deliver a full-term baby. Interventions include encouraging the mother to retell her experience—how labor began, her account of the delivery, and how the baby appears to her. Allow parents to grieve, and accept their crying and even their anger. Help them in their grief work by describing reality. At times, being in a private room may help the mother express herself and work out her feelings. While parents may direct their anger toward the people around them, it is a response to deep fear and hurt. Remember that withdrawal can also be a protective mechanism; when parents are overloaded, or have heard as much as they can bear, they may mentally shut down.

Depression, loneliness, isolation, and a deep sense of loss are common feelings, especially during the first few days, when a mother may not see her baby. The father may be busy serving as a messenger between the maternity ward and the intensive care unit; he may feel exhausted and torn between spending time with the mother and the baby and meeting the needs of other family members. It is also very difficult to explain to other children in the family why the baby has not come home. The other children may also feel neglected. Showing them pictures of the baby and letting them visit the hospital to see their mother and the baby help them understand what is happening (see Fig. 17-15).

3. If the baby improves, she must respond with hope and anticipation. After the separation from the infant, due to a prolonged hospital stay, she must resume her interrupted relationship with the baby in preparation for the infant's homecoming. Once the mother feels physically able to visit the baby, she gradually resumes her acquaintance process with the infant. This involves asking herself three questions: "What are you really like?" "What do you think of me?" and "What do I think of you?" The mother answers these questions through interaction with the baby. She can touch and stroke the newborn, and many times it is possible for her to hold the baby. According to Rubin's classic description, touching progresses from poking and handling the extremities to stroking and whole-hand touching and then from holding the baby away from the mother's body to holding it close. Establishing eye-to-eye contact is very important. A sign of progressing attachment is presented in Fig. 17-16, which shows the mother lining her face up with the baby's face in the *en face* position. When the baby opens his or her eyes and looks at the mother, she will often say, "He knows me" or "She knows I'm her mother."

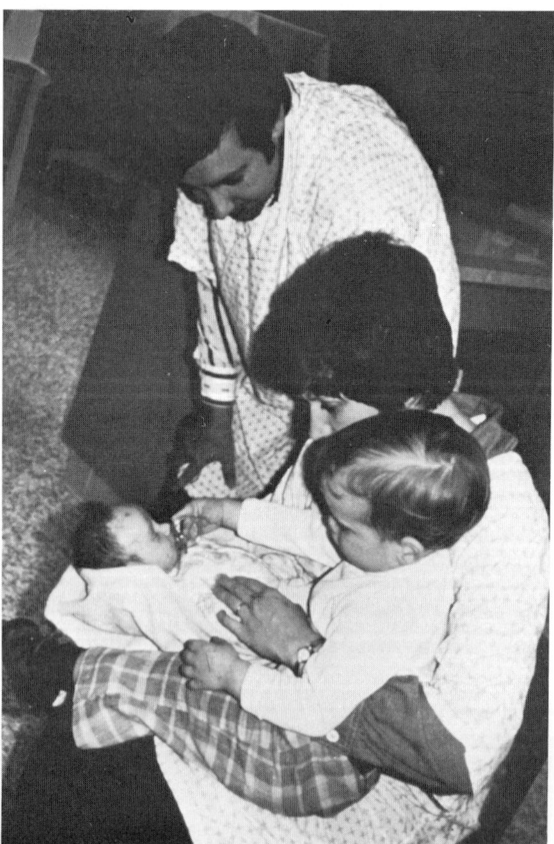

Figure 17-15 This family is getting acquainted with the newborn in the intensive care area. Notice the brother's attention to the pacifier.

The critical period for attachment is during the first few hours and then during the first 10 to 14 days. If the parents are not permitted contact during this time, their interest wanes, and visiting decreases. In the early 1900s, Dr. Martin Cooney treated more than 5000 premature infants in incubators. He prohibited parents from having contact with their babies. After the babies were well, Dr. Cooney had extreme difficulty persuading some parents to take their infants home.[55]

Fortunately, NICU policies now permit early visiting, touching, and caretaking by parents and siblings. Visiting hours are unrestricted, and many units have areas for overnight stays. The staff members orient the parents to the area and implement a systematic teaching and discharge plan.

4. She must prepare herself for the job of caring for the baby through understanding the baby's special needs and growth patterns, while still recognizing that the baby will eventually develop normal growth patterns. The amount of caretaking progresses with the parents' readiness and the improvement in the baby's condition. The nurse is an ally, not a competitor. It is important to praise the mother's care and give her a job that will make her feel competent. Encourage her to touch, stroke, and talk to the baby. Help her feel good about what she is doing by pointing out things like the way the

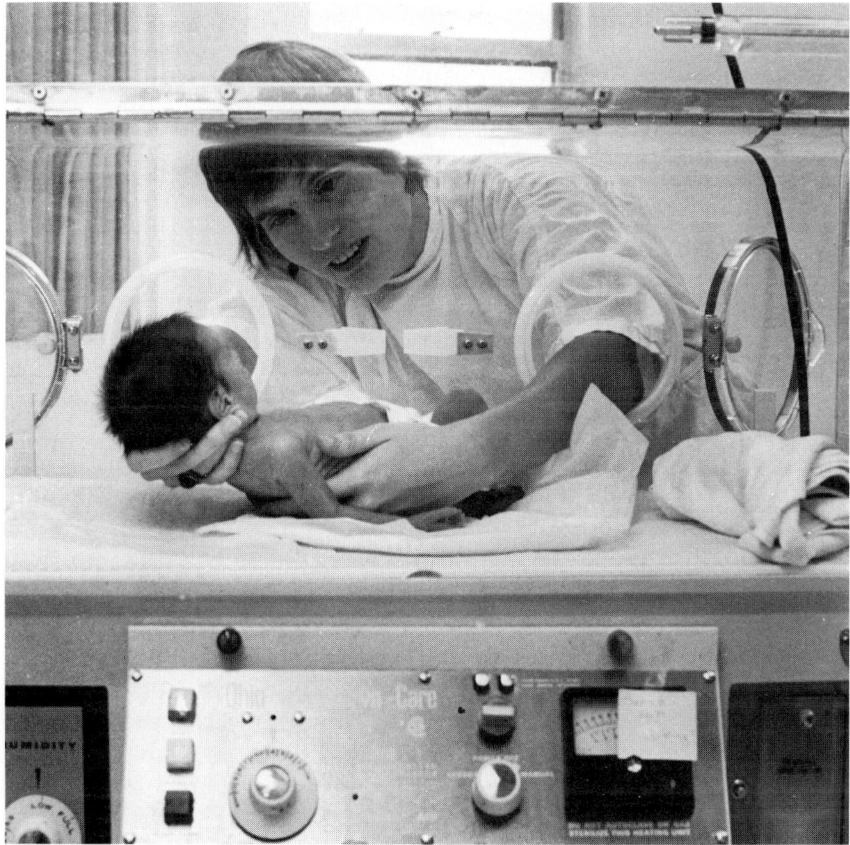

Figure 17-16 This mother is getting acquainted with her premature baby. Notice the *en face* position. (*From G. Scipien, M. U. Barnard, M. A. Chard, J. Howe, and P. J. Phillips* [eds.], *Comprehensive Pediatric Nursing, 2d ed., McGraw-Hill, New York, 1979. Used with permission.*)

baby responds by holding on to her finger. Have the mother bring in special toys or clothing, such as a soft stocking cap for the baby. Leave notes on the crib for her, saying things like, "Hi, Mom. I'm glad you came to feed me." Mother the parents so that they in turn will be able to care for the baby.

The nurse can help the parents have realistic expectations for the baby by using the preterm infant's expected date of birth rather than the actual date of birth when making comparisons of size, weight, and food intake. It is normal for preterm infants to be behind their age group by at least the amount they are premature. As preterm infants grow older, the parents have problems setting normal limits and tend to be more restrictive and to be more unduly concerned about minor illnesses and body functions than the parents of full-term, normal babies. Preterm infants are more likely to fail to thrive and to be abused than full-term, normal babies. This reflects the mother's inability to complete Caplan's fourth task: seeing the baby as normal.

Preparing for discharge Criteria for discharge are not as rigid as they were in the past, when preterm infants had to weigh 5 lb in order to be discharged. Usually, a preterm infant is discharged when:

1. The baby's condition is stable.
2. Body temperature is maintained.
3. The baby is gaining weight and feeds easily.
4. The mother is willing and able to care for the infant.
5. The home environment is free of infection.

When the parents are spontaneously interacting with the baby and when the baby's condition is stable, the nurses can focus on discharge. It is very helpful throughout the infant's stay to have continuity of caregivers. Parents need to feel that their baby is in the hands of competent nurses who know what the baby needs so they will feel comfortable about accepting the teaching offered by the nurses and will also take time to rest and recuperate before the baby comes home. Teaching is a continuous process that begins when the baby comes to the NICU. It is helpful to have a formal teaching tool to make sure all of the information given will be complete. Table 17-16 is a sample discharge planning tool. The nurse should also note the number of times the parents phoned the hospital or visited the baby and the length of the visits, since these are indications of how parenting is progressing. After the parents have gained some proficiency in comforting and caring for the infant, they are ready to take the baby home.

The tension associated with taking the baby home is reduced if rooming-in for a night or two at the hospital is possible. The fears of having the baby home alone are frequently recounted by parents of normal, let alone high-risk, infants. The parents may continue to be fearful after the baby comes home. This fear is gradually reduced as the baby grows and remains healthy.

Death of an infant The grieving process of the parents of a child who dies is discussed in detail in Chap. 35. There are some nursing interventions that are specific to the death of an infant in an NICU. The University of Colorado and Children's Hospital have instituted a concept of hospice care for babies that are critically ill and not responding to care that is designed to help the family members and the staff cope with a less active form of therapy for the infant. Three aspects of hospice care that have been instituted are: joint decision making regarding the level of care; a family room that is fully equipped to support the critically ill neonate but provides a homelike, private atmosphere where families can hold and interact with the baby (average time spent by families is 2 to 3 hours); and a trained

Table 17-16 Discharge Planning Tool

Infant's name ____________ Birth date ____________ Discharge date ____________
Parents' names ____________ Address ____________ Telephone ____________
Physician ____________ Primary nurse ____________
Summary of birth events: Reason for admission ____________
Gestational age ______ Weight ______ Height ______ Head circumference ______ Eye examination ____________

The parent:	Yes	No	Comments
1. Bathes the baby			
2. Feeds the baby			
3. Diapers the baby			
4. Cares for the cord			
5. Takes the rectal and/or axillary temperature			
6. Cares for the circumcision site			
7. Knows how to prepare formula			
8. Is comfortable with breast-feeding, and milk supply is established; identifies a support source			
9. Gives additional treatment: ____________			
10. Gives medications; knows actions, side effects, and correct schedule.			
11. Has prepared for the baby at home and has planned for integrating the baby into the family.			
12. Has correct expectations for development and knowledge of techniques for appropriate stimulation			
13. Demonstrates bonding (calls, visits, and cares for the infant—include behaviors)			

Follow-up: Referral: Public health nurse ____________
Social worker ____________ Parent support group ____________
Appointment: Dr. ____________ Clinic ____________
Date ____________ Time ____________

NICU staff that visit and call families after the death of an infant.[56]

In all settings it is important for parents to have an opportunity to touch and hold their dying baby, take pictures of the baby before and after death, and discuss funeral arrangements. Expressing grief is appropriate, and being with the baby even after death, with a time alone to hold, rock, caress, and even bathe the baby, facilitates grieving. Mothers demonstrate the same attachment behavior toward a dead infant as they do toward a live infant: poking, touching, and finally embracing. Denial is eliminated, and the infant's death becomes a reality.

Parent support groups can also be a source of comfort and provide an opportunity for valuable interaction. The nurses who cared for the baby should contact the parents 2 to 3 weeks after the death. Since many parents never receive a report about the autopsy findings, it is appropriate to review the autopsy findings and communicate these to the parents. The parents should be contacted again 2 to 3 months later, when they will usually be feeling depressed, angry, and isolated. Depression indicates acceptance of the reality of the infant's death. Inappropriate responses include total denial of loss, inappropriate hostility or cheerfulness, severe depression, psychosomatic disorders, and inability to cope. The parents should be referred for psychiatric counseling if they need assistance working through their grief.

Nursing Care Plan: Premature Infant

Patient: Boy Peterson | *Age*: 2 hours | Date of Admission: 9/3

ASSESSMENT

Male infant with diagnosis of RDS arrived from the referring hospital accompanied by a neonatal transport nurse and a registered respiratory therapist. He is 2 h old and presents with moderate subcostal retractions, prominent expiratory grunting, and nasal flaring. Air entry in the lungs is decreased bilaterally. The coloring of the mucous membranes is pink when the infant is ventilated with 68% oxygen, although acrocyanosis and half-nail-bed cyanosis continue. Generalized hypotonia is present.

Physical examination
Length: 44 cm. Weight: 2020 g. Occipitofrontal circumference: 32.5 cm. Dubowitz score: 32 points, 33 weeks gestation. Temperature: 37°C (98.6°F), axillary. Pulse: 158. Dextrostix: 45 mg%. Hematocrit: 56%. Respiratory rate: 68. Blood pressure: 50/20 (arterial); 34 mean, 40 flush.

Skin
Generalized pink coloring when in oxygen. Acrocyanosis is present. Vernix covers half the skin surface. The skin is smooth. Lanugo covers the entire body, except the face.

Head
The anterior and posterior fontanels are present. The hair is fine.

Eyes and ears
Normal positioning. The ears are flat and shapeless with scant cartilage.

Nose
A catheter passes easily through both nares.

Mouth
Negative.

Chest
Intercostal retractions. There is no palpable breast tissue. The areola and nipple are visible.

Abdomen
No masses are palpable. There are three cord vessels.

Genitalia
Normal in appearance, with undescended testes. The testes are palpable in the inguinal canal. The scrotum has few rugae.

Extremities
Symmetrical movement. Two anterior sole creases are present.

Hips
Negative.

Spine
Negative.

Reflexes
The Moro reflex and the sucking reflex are present.

Heart
A soft systolic murmur is present.

Elimination
Has voided 10 ml of urine and has passed a small amount of meconium. The anus is patent.

Psychosocial history
The parents have been married for 8 years. There is a 6-year-old female sibling. This is the second-born child; the pregnancy was planned. The families of the parents live in close proximity. The parents carry insurance through the husband's business.

Maternal history
The mother is gravida 2, para I, a 30-year-old white female with blood type A, Positive. Prenatal care was sought prior to conception for infertility problems. EDC: 11/4. No medications were taken during the pregnancy other than

multiple vitamins and iron. The mother is a nonsmoker and is a light social drinker (two or three glasses of wine per month). Weight gain during the pregnancy was 25 lb. Vital signs remained within normal limits during the course of the pregnancy. The pregnancy was uncomplicated until the event of premature labor and delivery. Spontaneous rupture of membranes occurred 12 h prior to delivery. The amniotic fluid was clear and odorless. Betamethasone was given 16 h prior to delivery. The fetal heart tones remained stable during labor and delivery. The delivery was vaginal.

Neonatal history

The infant's Apgar score was 6 at 1 min (points off for heart rate, color, respiratory effort, and muscle tone) and 8 at 5 min (points off for color and respiratory effort). An umbilical arterial catheter was put in place. The infant was intubated and placed on a ventilator with pressures of 20/5 at a rate of 20. Initial blood gases were Pa_{o2} = 52, Pa_{co2} = 62, and pH = 7.20 on 68% oxygen. When stabilization measures were completed, the infant was transported to the regional neonatal referral center, which was located in the same city.

Nursing Diagnosis	Outcome Criteria	Nursing Interventions	Evaluation and Modifications
1. Impaired gas exchange associated with inefficient ventilation of the alveoli and immaturity of the lungs	☐ The infant's mucous membranes and skin will be pink. ☐ The infant's respiratory rate will be 30 to 50 per minute without retractions. ☐ The infant's circulatory flow will be maintained at the level needed for adequate oxygenation and perfusion.	☐ Wean from the ventilator to CPAP as ordered, assess blood gases and respiratory status, and maintain transcutaneous oxygen readings of 60 to 80.	☐ 9/6 Is tolerating CPAP trials. ☐ 9/7 Was placed in 28% humidified hood oxygen. Respirations are easy; lungs are clear.
		☐ Administer warm, humidified oxygen as ordered according to blood gas determinations and assessment of respiratory status and color.	☐ 9/13 Was placed in room air. Pa_{O_2} maintained above 70 mmHg; presently is 88.
		☐ Observe for signs of respiratory distress, degree and location of retractions, grunting, nasal flaring, tachypnea, character of breath sounds, and rate of respirations. Record and report.	☐ 9/13 Respiratory rate is 38 to 50. Respirations are easy, without retractions. Breath sounds are clear.
		☐ Assess the rate, rhythm, and quality of heart sounds. Record and report.	☐ 9/11 Heart rate is 120 to 146 and regular. A soft systolic murmur is present. ☐ 9/14 No murmur is present.
		☐ Administer chest physiotherapy (percussion, vibration, and postural drainage) q1h to q2h, as indicated by the quality of breath sounds and secretions. Maintain a patent airway by suctioning.	☐ 9/7 Minimal secretions. Chest physiotherapy is now q2h to q3h. ☐ 9/14 Chest physiotherapy was discontinued. Breath sounds are clear.
		☐ Change position frequently, at least q2h. Assess positioning in reference to color and respiratory status.	☐ 9/6 Color improves when the infant is on the abdomen or the right side.

Nursing Diagnosis	Outcome Criteria	Nursing Interventions	Evaluation and Modifications
			☐ 9/13 Color remains pink when the infant is on either the side or the abdomen.
		☐ Assess perfusion of the extremities by observing quality of pulses, color of the skin, capillary filling, and warmth.	☐ 9/6 Pulses are equal. Extremities are warm and pink. The skin, when blanched, quickly returns to normal.
		☐ Record the arterial blood pressure, noting the systolic and diastolic components, the mean, and pulse pressure.	☐ 9/7 Arterial blood pressure is 62/36; mean remains 40 to 50. ☐ 9/9 Umbilical arterial catheter was removed. Flush blood pressure is 50.
2. Potential for hypoglycemia related to increased intake and decreased energy stores of brown fat and glycogen	☐ The infant's blood glucose level will consistently remain above 45 mg per 100 ml.	☐ Administer constant infusion of intravenous glucose as ordered. Record accurately.	☐ 9/8 10% glucose with 0.2% sodium chloride infusing; rate was decreased from 8 ml per hour to 3 ml per hour. Nasogastric feedings were started.
		☐ Observe, record, and report signs and symptoms such as jitteriness, lethargy, seizures, change in color, heart rate, and respiratory effort.	☐ 9/4 No symptoms noted. ☐ 9/8 No symptoms noted.
		☐ Monitor Dextrostix values. Report if below 45 mg per 100 ml or above 130 to 170 mg per 100 ml.	☐ 9/4 Dextrostix values are 45 to 90. ☐ 9/8 Values are as stated above.
		☐ Assess the potential for hypoglycemia by determining gestational age, weight, and length and plotting these values on an intrauterine growth curve. Determine whether the infant is the appropriate size for his gestational age.	☐ 9/3 Weight, 50th percentile; is AGA. Length, 50th percentile.
		☐ Feed as early as can be done with safety. Advance to oral gastric feedings cautiously; gradually increase amounts. Advance to oral feedings as indicated by the infant's clinical course.	☐ 9/8 Nasogastric feedings of 5 ml of breast milk per hour were initiated. ☐ 9/12 Nasogastric feedings were increased to 15 ml per hour. ☐ 9/16 First oral feeding (15 ml) was given.
3. Instability of body temperature associated with prematurity, decreased layer of subcutaneous tissue, and immature neuromuscular control	☐ The infant's temperature will remain between 36.5 and 37°C (97.7 and 98.6°F) (axillary) or between 37 and 37.5°C (98.6 and 99.5°F) (rectal).	☐ Prevent heat loss due to evaporation, radiation, conduction, and convection. Keep the baby dry and out of drafts. Avoid chilling.	☐ 9/3 Environment was adjusted to prevent heat loss.

Nursing Diagnosis	Outcome Criteria	Nursing Interventions	Evaluation and Modifications
		☐ Assist maintenance of temperature with use of a radiant warmer or incubator. Apply a shielded servo-control probe to the exposed skin area. Set the control to maintain skin temperature at 36.5°C.	☐ 9/9 Temperature remains 36.5 to 37°C (97.7 to 98.6°F) (axillary). ☐ 9/10 Was moved from warmer to incubator.
		☐ Have the infant wear a cap as necessary to maintain body temperature.	
		☐ Record the axillary temperture q1h initially. When the temperature has stabilized, record it q2h.	☐ 9/4 Temperature remains within normal limits.
		☐ Monitor the temperature q1h when weaning from the incubator begins.	☐ 9/20 Was weaned from incubator. Temperature is 36.7°C (98°F) (axillary) and above.
		☐ Double-wrap the baby and put on a cap when he is out of the warmer or incubator.	☐ 9/10 Is double-wrapped in blankets when being held. The mother brought in a baby cap.
4. Potential for fluid and electrolyte imbalances related to immature regulatory mechanisms and inadequate intake	☐ The major body electrolytes will remain within normal limits. ☐ Hydration will remain within normal limits.	☐ Administer calcium and potassium as ordered.	☐ 9/8 While on IV fluid, 200 mg/kg of calcium gluconate and 10 mEq per liter of potassium chloride is given per day.
		☐ Observe for signs and symptoms of electrolyte imbalance. Record and report: **a.** Hypocalcemia—twitching, tremors, and jitters **b.** Potassium imbalance—cardiac irregularities **c.** Sodium imbalance—neurological changes, feeding intolerance, and edema	☐ 9/8 No symptoms noted. Serum values: sodium, 136 mEq per liter; potassium, 4.0 mEq per liter; calcium, 8.8 mg per 100 ml.
		☐ Observe for any change in alertness, pattern of activity, or movement.	☐ 9/10 No changes noted.
		☐ Observe and report skin turgor.	☐ 9/12 Elasticity of skin is present. No "tenting."
		☐ Accurately record output (nasogastric, blood loss, urine, and stools). Weigh diapers.	☐ 9/8 Intake is approximating output. Urine output is adequate.
		☐ Measure specific gravity q8h.	☐ 9/8 Specific gravity averages 1.010. Frequency of testing changed to once per day.
		☐ Weigh daily.	☐ 9/5 Weight is 100 g below birth weight. ☐ 9/10 Has regained birth weight.
		☐ Administer Lasix as ordered.	☐ 9/20 Is gaining an average of 10 to 15 g per day.

Nursing Diagnosis	Outcome Criteria	Nursing Interventions	Evaluation and Modifications
5. Alteration in nutrition: less than body requirements related to gastrointestinal immaturity and an immature sucking reflex	☐ The infant will be feeding orally and gaining weight at the time of discharge.	☐ Encourage the mother to breast-feed, if this was her initial intention. Discuss breast care, milk expression, and how she can keep her supply of breast milk while the infant is not nursing. Identify a source of support for her.	☐ 9/3 The mother wishes to breast-feed. Obstetric nurses are giving the mother information. Someone from the LaLeche League will be contacting the mother.
		☐ Invite the mother to an infant nutrition class taught by the hospital dietitian.	☐ 9/14 The parents attended an infant nutrition class.
		☐ Gavage feedings may be indicated initially. Follow the procedure for insertion of the gastric tube. Allow the feedings to flow in over the time it would take for normal oral feedings. Check gastric residuals prior to each feeding. Measure abdominal girth prior to each feeding. Increase the amount of feedings gradually.	☐ 9/8 Nasogastric feedings were started at 5 ml of breast milk per hour. ☐ 9/12 Nasogastric feedings were increased to 15 ml per hour. ☐ 9/10 Gastric residuals are consistently less than 20% of total feeding. Abdominal girth is 28 cm.
		☐ Provide pacifier practice q3h while the baby is on gavage feedings in order to develop the sucking reflex.	☐ 9/12 Sucking movements are weak.
		☐ Gradually switch from gavage feedings to oral feedings, depending on the infant's tolerance of activity and ability to take adequate amounts, until all feedings are oral.	☐ 9/14 Sucking is improving; coordination with swallowing is present. Feeding cycles are one oral and two gavage. ☐ 9/16 Sucks strongly on a soft nipple. Alternating gavage and oral feedings. ☐ 9/18 All feedings are oral.
		☐ Use a premature (soft) nipple when feeding orally.	
		☐ Allow the infant to sleep or rest 1 h before feeding. Allow for cuddling and rocking before and after feeding.	☐ 9/20 Takes feedings with increased vigor if allowed to rest.
6. Potential for hyperbilirubinemia associated with liver immaturity	☐ The infant's bilirubin will remain below 15 mg per 100 ml (indirect).	☐ Maintain fluid intake as specified according to protocol for the infant's age. Anticipate increased insensible fluid loss with phototherapy.	☐ 9/6 Appears well hydrated—skin is elastic. ☐ 9/10 Urine output is adequate.
		☐ Record intake and output accurately. Note stool pattern, frequency, type, and consistency of stools.	☐ 9/6 Meconium stools five times per day. ☐ 9/9 Transitional stools.

Nursing Diagnosis	Outcome Criteria	Nursing Interventions	Evaluation and Modifications
		☐ Initiate phototherapy as ordered if indicated by the bilirubin level. Place protective shields over the eyes. Remove the shields q4h to cleanse and note the condition of the eyes.	☐ 9/7 Indirect bilirubin reached level of 13 mg per 100 ml and then decreased. ☐ 9/9 Bilirubin lights are not indicated.
		☐ Provide time for parental interaction during the period of phototherapy. Allow the parents to hold and touch their infant. If the parents do not visit frequently, nurses should provide for stimulation.	☐ 9/9 Not applicable.
7. Delayed parent-infant bonding related to the separation of the parents and the infant and parental anxiety	☐ The parents will demonstrate appropriate bonding behaviors. ☐ The baby will give positive feedback (eye-to-eye contact and quieting) to the parents when touched.	☐ Allow the parents to see and touch their infant prior to transport.	☐ 9/3 The parents touched the baby prior to transport.
		☐ Encourge the father to come to the referral hospital as soon as possible. Have him take pictures of the infant back to the mother.	☐ 9/3 The father followed the ambulance to the hospital. He brought pictures of the infant to the mother.
		☐ Encourage early initial contact. Provide for 24-h visiting and phoning.	☐ 9/4 The mother came to visit the infant while on pass from the hospital.
		☐ Provide information to the parents about their infant's problems. Repeat concepts as necessary. Emphasize the normal as well as the abnormal.	☐ 9/3 Basic information was provided. A unit handbook was given to the parents. ☐ 9/4 The parents received a more in-depth explanation of the infant's problems.
		☐ Encourage the parents to touch, hold, caress, and talk to their baby. Comment on their baby's individuality and things he can do.	☐ 9/5 The parents verbalized what their baby's major problem is. ☐ 9/5 The parents held the baby for the first time.
		☐ Call the mother frequently while she is hospitalized to update her on the infant's condition. Encourage her to call at any time. Arrange a schedule of the most convenient times for phone calls and visits.	☐ 9/5 The mother called five times yesterday. She was dismissed from the hospital. ☐ 9/6 The parents wish to call at their convenience. We will call if there are any significant changes.
		☐ Contact health care personnel from the referral hospital daily while the mother is hospitalized and weekly until the infant is discharged.	☐ 9/6 Nurses at the referral hospital say the mother is coping well; her spirits improved after seeing the infant yesterday.

Nursing Diagnosis	Outcome Criteria	Nursing Interventions	Evaluation and Modifications
		☐ Provide continuity of care through primary nursing.	☐ 9/4 A primary nurse was identified; a core group of consistent nurses were assigned.
		☐ Record on the parent interaction sheet (to permit easy evaluation of phone calls, visits, types of interaction, and caretaking skills).	☐ 9/3 An interaction sheet was started.
		☐ Encourage the grandparents to visit the infant so that they will begin to feel attached and will provide support to the parents.	☐ 9/4 All the grandparents visited. ☐ 9/13 The grandparents visit every other day with the parents.
		☐ Encourage the parents to visit frequently and give care to the infant. Have them spend time alone with the infant, if possible. Try to coincide their visits with the baby's alert states. Help the parents interpret the baby's behavior.	☐ 9/6 The parents changed the infant's diapers. The mother gave him a bath. ☐ 9/16 First time the parents were completely alone with the baby.
		☐ Plan a patient care conference every week with the unit staff to evaluate the family's progress and reassess attachment behavior. Record.	☐ 9/4 Weekly conferences will be held on Monday mornings. See nurse's notes for comments.
8. Parental anxiety and grieving related to the premature infant's illness and the loss of the anticipated perfect baby	☐ The parents will be able to verbalize their feelings regarding their baby's illness and hospitalization.	☐ Assess the parents in the following areas: **a.** Their reaction to the illness **b.** Their perception of the infant's condition	☐ 9/6 The mother states, "We didn't expect any problems. It really overwhelmed us. We feel everything will turn out fine, but how does anyone ever know?"
		c. Their behaviors in relation to the baby	☐ 9/7 The parents continue to touch and talk to their infant.
		d. Their coping mechanisms (what support systems are available to them, how have they handled stress before, and what their religious ties are)	☐ 9/5 The parents have had their minister visit every day with them. The parents talk to and touch each other during visits.
		e. Their relationships with each other **f.** Family support and reaction	☐ 9/7 The grandparents came with the parents to visit.
		☐ Involve the social service representative.	☐ 9/5 Ms. Johnson met with the parents.

Nursing Diagnosis	Outcome Criteria	Nursing Interventions	Evaluation and Modifications
		☐ Be aware of the grieving process that the parents are going through (the loss of the normal child they anticipated during the pregnancy and the realization that the baby is less than perfect initiate a grief reaction).	☐ 9/8 The mother has cried quite often today. She stated, "This is not what we expected. We had been so happy with the thought of the baby. Everything was going so perfectly."
		☐ Encourage the parents to express their feelings. Reflective statements may help.	
9. Altered parenting and nurturance related to limited parent-child interactions and a lack of privacy	☐ Upon discharge, the baby will: **a.** Participate actively in his environment through visual perception **b.** Socialize with his caretakers **c.** Become alert and quiet with tactile stimulation ☐ The parents will verbalize their expectations for the infant's development and will plan for appropriate stimulation. ☐ The parents will assume the primary role as their infant's advocate. ☐ The parents will verbalize their concerns and will plan ways to deal with sibling rivalry and to integrate the infant into the family unit. ☐ The parents will be able to verbalize ways to involve the sibling in activities with the infant.	☐ Encourage the parents to participate in the infant's care, Emphasize that this is one area in which they can really be of assistance.	☐ 9/13 The parents usually do physical chores, such as bathing and diapering, when visiting. They stroke and hold him as much as possible.
		☐ Provide tactile and sensory stimulation in the following ways: **a.** Frequently change the infant's position (turning, using an infant seat, rocking, and cuddling). **b.** Provide appropriate toys, such as a brightly colored rattle, a brightly colored mobile attached to the crib or warmer, a music box, cuddly toys, bells, and brightly colored pictures placed within 9 in of the infant's face. **c.** Play classical music and tapes of the parents' voices.	☐ 9/10 The parents brought a music box, a mobile, and a cuddly toy for the baby. ☐ 9/20 The infant quiets when talked and sung to. His movements have become calmer and slower. ☐ 9/20 The parents continue to bring appropriate toys. They verbalize the rationale behind the activities.
		☐ Provide the baby with brightly colored blankets, clothing, and crib materials, when his condition is stable. Encourage the parents to bring these for the baby.	☐ 9/15 The mother brought in sleepers and knitted caps.
		☐ Have the sister visit the unit as much as possible.	
		☐ Send the family members postcards from the infant.	
		☐ Encourage the parents to record hospitalization events in a baby book.	

Nursing Diagnosis	Outcome Criteria	Nursing Interventions	Evaluation and Modifications
		□ Encourage the parents to room in prior to discharge.	□ 10/5 Parents roomed in and managed all tasks with confidence.
10. Knowledge deficit related to the special care needs of a premature infant		□ Provide a darkened atmosphere to establish the infant's sleep pattern and maintain a day-night cycle.	□ 9/15 The lights continue to be dimmed at night.
		□ Provide the parents with information so that they can continue the stimulation program at home.	□ 9/20 The parents have been instructed about the infant stimulation program for their baby.
	□ The parents will exhibit confidence in their ability to care for their infant at the time of discharge. They will: **a.** Demonstrate their ability to bathe the baby, take the baby's axillary or rectal temperature, use a bulb syringe for suctioning secretions, and feed the baby by breast or bottle **b.** Demonstrate a knowledge of the actions and side effects of prescribed medications, administer medications, and verbalize the schedules **c.** Verbalize the time and place for follow-up care of the infant **d.** Verbalize situations in which the physician should be called on for advice	□ Assess the parents' readiness to perform care activities. Observe the parents for signs of stress. Initiate caregiving activities early, and gradually increase the amount of care that the parents give. Reinforce the parents' positive interactions with their infant. □ Demonstrate bathing, temperature taking, feeding, and using a bulb syringe, and have the parents do a demonstration. □ Discuss medications, side effects, and the schedule for administration. Have the parents administer the medications at least twice prior to discharge.	□ 9/13 The mother is consistently giving the baby his bath each day. The father changes the diapers. The parents stay at the baby's bedside for long periods. □ 9/20 The mother is spending the entire afternoon with the infant. □ 9/27 Demonstrations were given to the parents by the primary nurse. □ 9/28 A demonstration of care activities was done by the mother. □ 10/5 The parents were instructed by the nurse and the pharmacist about the administration of vitamins. The parents verbalized reasons why their child was on the preparations and how to administer them.
		□ Inform the parents of the premature infant's special needs: temperature regulation, development of the sucking reflex, the need for touch and stimulation, and nutritional needs.	□ 9/23 The parents attended a scheduled class for the parents of premature infants.
		□ Explain what types of signs and symptoms the parents should be alert for and concerned about regarding their baby's actions and behaviors, and tell them when they should call their physician.	□ 10/5 The parents verbalized to the primary nurse the symptoms they should be alert for that may signify that their baby is in need of medical care.

Nursing Diagnosis	Outcome Criteria	Nursing Interventions	Evaluation and Modifications
		☐ Provide for follow-up care when the child is discharged (a public health nurse, a social service worker, a physician, a follow-up clinic, and follow-up calls).	☐ 9/14 The county public health nurse was notified of the baby's admission to a high-risk nursery. ☐ 10/6 The parents were informed of a scheduled follow-up clinic visit on 10/24. ☐ 10/6 The primary nurse will call the family on 10/9, 10/24, and 11/9.

*Prepared by LiAnne M. Kitchen, RN, MS.

References

1. Robert Wood Johnson Foundation, "Special Report—Perinatal," abstracted in *Perinatal Press* **3**(1):9 (January 1979).
2. Leonard, Linda, "Underweight and Pregnant," *Maternal-Child Nursing* **9**(5):332 (September–October 1984).
3. Sexton, M., and J. R. Hebel "A Clinical Trial of Change in Maternal Smoking and Its Effect on Birth Weight," *Journal of the American Medical Association* **251**(7):911–915 (February 17, 1984).
4. Sever, John L., "Rubella Vaccine Given during Pregnancy," *Perinatal Newsletter* **8**(1):3 (1984).
5. Sand, Pat, "Congenital Toxoplasmosis," *Perinatal Newsletter* **8**(8):119 (1984).
6. DeVore, N., et al., "Torch Infections," *American Journal of Nursing* **83**(12):1660–1665 (December 1983).
7. Ibid, p. 1664.
8. Delaplane, D., et al., "Fatal Hepatitis in Infancy," *Pediatrics* **72**(2):176 (August 1983).
9. "Infant Death Gap Widening: Black vs. White Babies," *NAACOG Newsletter* **10**(8):1 (September 1983).
10. Ibid.
11. Reedy N. J., et al., "Maternal-Fetal Transport: A Nurse Team," *Journal of Obstetric and Gynecological Nursing* **13**:(91):94 (1984).
12. Harris, T. L., et al., "Maternal Transport at Work," *Obstetrics and Gynecology* **52**(3):295 (September 1978).
13. Bacsik, Robert D., "Meconium Aspiration Syndrome," *Pediatric Clinics of North America* **24**(3):463 (August 1979).
14. Gross S. J. et al., "Head Growth and Developmental Outcome in Very Low Birth Weight Infants," *Pediatrics* **71**:70 (1983).
15. Korones, Sheldon B., *High-Risk Newborn Infants,* 3d ed., Mosby, St. Louis, 1981, p. 235.
16. Ibid., p. 133.
17. Wiener, M. B., et al., *Clinical Pharmacology and Therapeutics in Nursing,* 2d ed., McGraw-Hill, New York, 1985, p. 1029.
18. Kuller, J., et al., "Improved Skin Care for Premature Infants," *Maternal Child Nursing* **8**(3):210 (May–June 1983).
19. Boros, S. J., "Using Regular Ventilators at Unconventional Rates," *Pediatrics* **74**(4):487 (October 1984).
20. Korones, op. cit., p. 205.
21. Ibid.
22. Gerhardt, T., et al., "Pathophysiology of the Apnea of Prematurity," *Pediatrics* **74**(1):58 (July 1984).
23. Jones, R. A. K., "Theophyllin vs. CPAP: Early vs. Late Treatment," *Archives of Diseases of Childhood* **57**(10):761 (October 1982).
24. Alpan, G., et al., "Treating Unresponsive Apnea," *Journal of Pediatrics* **104**(4):634 (April 1984).
25. Dimaggio, G. T., and A. H. Shutz, "Concerns of Mothers Caring for an Infant on an Apnea Monitor," *Maternal-Child Nursing* **8**(4):294 (July–August 1983).
26. Rehm, R. S., "Teaching Cardiopulmonary Resuscitation to Parents," *Maternal-Child Nursing* **8**:411 (1983).
27. Hittner, H. M., et al., "Retrolental Fibroplasia: Further Clinical Evidence and Ultrasturctural Support for Efficacy of Vitamin E in the Preterm Infant," *Pediatrics* **71**:423 (1983).
28. Korones, op. cit., p. 222.
29. Klaus, M. H., and A. A. Fanaroff, *Care of the High-Risk Neonate,* 2d ed., Saunders, Philadelphia, 1979, p. 195.
30. Rosenfeld, F. W., et al., "Preventing BPD with SOD," *Pediatrics* **105**(5):781 (November 1984).
31. Korones, op. cit., p. 93.
32. Ibid., p. 317.
33. White, K. C., and K. L. Harkavy, "Hypertonic Formula Resulting from Added Oral Medications," *American Journal of Diseases of Children* **136**:931–933 (1984).
34. Ibid., p. 932.
35. Lemons, P. H., "Breast-Feeding the Premature," *Perinatal Newsletter* **7**(6):83 (1983).
36. Collings, J., et al., "Demand versus Scheduled Feedings

in Premature Infants," *Journal of Obstetric and Gynecological Nursing* **11**:362 (1982).
37. Korones, op. cit., p. 304.
38. Klaus and Fanaroff, op. cit., p. 8.
39. Ibid., p. 9.
40. Fuhrman, K., et al., "Diabetic Care," *Pediatrics* **6**(3):219 (May–June 1983).
41. Schaffer, A., et al., *Diseases of the Newborn*, 4th ed., Saunders, Philadelphia, 1977, p. 701.
42. Ibid., p. 698.
43. Korones, op. cit., p. 347.
44. Smith, K., and F. Jones, "The Fetal Alcohol Syndrome," *Teratology* **12**:1–10 (1975).
45. Danis, R. P., et al., "Pregnancy and Alcohol: A Difficult Mix," *Ortho Forum* **3**(4):9 (November–December 1983).
46. Kivlahan, C., et al., "Neonatal Jaundice: Long-Term Natural History," *Pediatrics* **74**(3):364 (September 1984).
47. Hammer, Rita M., et al., "The Prenatal Use of RHo (D) Immune Globulin," *Maternal-Child Nursing* **9**(1):29–31 (January–February 1984).
48. Korones, op. cit., p. 271.
49. Cashore, W. F., et al., "Neonatal Jaundice: Exchange Transfusion, Phototherapy, or Observation?" *Consultant* **23**(12):57 (December 1983).
50. Hansen, H., "Nursing Care in the Neonatal Intensive Care Unit," *Journal of Obstetric and Gynecological Nursing* **11**(1):17–20 (January–February 1982).
51. Blackburn, S., "The Neonatal ICU: A High-Risk Environment," *American Journal of Nursing* **82**(1):1708–1712 (November 1982).
52. LaRossa, M. M., and J. V. Brown, "Foster Grandmothers in the Premature Nursery," *American Journal of Nursing* **82**(1):1834–1835 (November 1982).
53. Caplan, G., E. Mason, and D. Kaplan, "Four Studies of Crisis in Parents of Prematures," *Community Mental Health Journal* **1**(2):149–160 (Summer 1965).
54. Klaus and Fanaroff, op. cit., p. 159.
55. Ibid., p. 98.
56. Whitfield, J. M., et al., "The Application of Hospice Concepts to Neonatal Care," *American Journal of Diseases of Children* **136**:421–424 (1982).

18

Pauline C. Beecroft

Fluid and electrolyte balance

Upon completion of this chapter, the student will be able to:

1 List five reasons why fluid balance is more critical in children than in adults.
2 List the major solutes of the extracellular, intracellular, and intrastitial fluid compartments.
3 Compare the percentage of total water weight of the neonate, infant, toddler, preschooler, school-age child, adolescent, and adult.
4 Identify the composition and functions of body water and the physiological mechanisms for movement of body water.
5 Define osmosis, diffusion, filtration, active transport, and pinocytosis.
6 List the three mechanisms that regulate body water balance.
7 Calculate maintenance fluid requirements for children using either body weight or body surface area.
8 Compare the changes that occur as a result of isotonic, hypotonic, and hypertonic fluid deficit and excess and relate these changes to the signs and symptoms seen in the child.
9 Identify the function, regulation, and dietary sources of sodium, potassium, calcium, phosphorus, and magnesium.
10 Contrast the etiology, pathophysiology, symptoms, and treatment of hyponatremia, hypernatremia, hypocalcemia, hypercalcemia, hypomagnesemia, and hypermagnesemia.
11 State the normal range for blood pH and identify states of metabolic and respiratory acidosis and alkalosis.
12 Describe the differences between volatile and nonvolatile acids.
13 List the three pathophysiological regulatory mechanisms that interact to maintain pH within normal limits.
14 Describe the effects of potassium and chloride on pH.
15 List the assessment parameters and nursing interventions for a child with potential or actual fluid and electrolyte disturbances.

The special fluid and electrolyte requirements of the young patient demand that the nurses understand the different needs of pediatric patients for the management of their fluid and electrolyte balance.

WHY CHILDREN ARE DIFFERENT

1. In the newborn, total body water (TBW) as a percentage of body weight is *80 percent;* this is *20 percent* greater than in the adult. By the

time the child is about 2 years of age, TBW has declined to approximately 60 percent, which is the adult percentage.

2. Extracellular fluid (ECF) in the infant may be almost double that in the adult.[1]

	ECF
Infant	28 to 57% of body weight
Child	21 to 30% of body weight
Adult	18 to 26% of body weight

Extracellular fluid is more accessible for loss than intracellular fluid (ICF). Therefore, the infant and the young child show the effects of fluid imbalance twice as fast as the adult. For example, daily fluid output can constitute more than one-third of the young child's ECF, in comparison with that of the adult, whose daily output is less than one-sixth of his or her ECF.[2]

3. The metabolic rate of the child is 2 to 3 times that of the adult. The greater the metabolic rate, the more fluid is required to remove waste products. For every 100 cal expended, approximately 100 cc of water is needed. The number of calories expended per kilogram of body weight decreases as body weight increases.[3] For example, 1 to 10 kg of body weight equals 100 cal per kilogram, 10 to 20 kg of body weight equals 50 cal per kilogram, and more than 20 kg of body weight equals 20 cal per kilogram. Therefore, the increased energy expenditure of infants and children requires a greater water intake to make up for normal ongoing losses.
4. The body surface area of children per unit of body weight is greater than that of adults, and therefore there is a larger surface area over which evaporative losses occur.
5. The infant's and the child's kidneys are less mature than the adult's and do not concentrate urine, excrete fluid, or conserve fluid as effectively.
6. The child's buffer systems are less mature, predisposing the child to rapid development of acid-base problems.

WATER AS A BODY CONSTITUENT

Distribution of body water

Body water is divided into two main compartments: the intracellular and the extracellular compartments. *Intracellular fluid* is the water content of all body cells, including blood cells. *Extracellular fluid* is all other body water. It is subdivided into *intravascular fluid* (plasma within the vascular system), *interstitital fluid* (the fluid that bathes the tissue cells), and *transcellular fluid,* which includes fluid located in the eyes (ocular fluid), in the joints (synovial fluid), in the cerebrospinal system (cerebrospinal fluid), around the heart (pericardial fluid), in the abdominal cavity (peritoneal fluid), and sometimes in the gastrointestinal and urinary tracts.[4]

Table 18-1 Body Water as a Percentage of Body Weight*

Age	Extracellular Fluid	Intracellular Fluid	Total Body Water
Infant	28 to 57%	25 to 40%	80%
Child	21 to 30%	40 to 45%	65%
Adult	18 to 26%	40 to 50%	60%

*Variations reflect individual differences, such as amount of body fat.

Volume of body water

The amount of total body water as a percentage of body weight varies not only with age but also with the amount of body fat (see Table 18-1).

As the amount of body fat increases, the amount of body water decreases. There is 10 percent water in fat cells, 75 to 80 percent water in other body cells.[5] The young person with more adipose (fatty) tissue has less water weight. This is also true of girls, who tend to have more adipose tissue than boys.

Composition of body water

The body fluid is composed of water and dissolved substances, or solutes. There are two kinds of solutes: electrolytes and nonelectrolytes.

Electrolytes are substances which carry an electric charge when in solution. In solution, electrolytes dissociate into positive and negative ions. Chloride, bicarbonate, and phosphate are negatively charged ions, or *anions*. Sodium, potassium, calcium, and magnesium are positively charged ions, or *cations*. They are present in both the intracellular and the extracellular compartments, but their concentrations in each are significantly different (see Table 18-2). Sodium,

Table 18-2 Approximate Concentrations of Ions in the Two Fluid Compartments of the Body

Ion	Extracellular concentration, mEq per liter	Intracellular concentration, mEq per liter
Sodium	140	10
Potassium	5	150
Calcium	5	<1
Magnesium	2	40
	152	200
Chloride	101	2
Bicarbonate	25	12
HPO_4	1	110
SO_4	9	16
Protein	16	60
	152	200

chloride, and bicarbonate are the dominant electrolytes of the extracellular compartment; potassium and phosphate dominate the intracellular compartment. The number of positive charges equals the number of negative charges in each of the compartments, resulting in electrical neutrality.

Nonelectrolytes are substances that do not ionize or dissociate in solution and do not carry an electrical charge. Glucose is an example of a nonelectrolyte.

Functions of body water

In addition to being a solvent for body electrolytes and proteins, water has several other important functions: (1) It is a transport medium for the blood cells and substances traveling through blood vessels and it carries enzymes, nutrients, and hormones to tissue cells and carries waste products from these cells; (2) within the cells, water provides the environment for the chemical reactions that fuel the body and maintain homeostasis; (3) in the interstitial compartment, water is a lubricant for the tissues, such as in the joints and the pleural spaces; and (4) water regulates body temperature. Through diaphoresis (sweating), water is released to the skin surface. As it evaporates, body heat is lost, and the skin surface is cooled. Furthermore, blood carries heat from internal organs to blood vessels near the body surface, where some of it leaves the body by radiation. Body heat carried by the blood also leaves with air expelled during expiration.

Movement of body water

Along with the electrolytes found in body fluids, there are other substances that have a role in the maintenance of fluid balance. Nonelectrolytes—such as urea, glucose, creatinine, and plasma proteins dissolved in body water—exert forces that affect water movement. These forces cause the constant movement of water (body fluids) back and forth across the semipermeable membranes of the body compartments.

Diffusion is the movement of solute through a solution down its concentration gradient, from an area of higher concentration to an area of lower concentration. Diffusion results from the natural random movements of particles, which lead them to spread evenly through a solution. Even a membrane, as long as it is permeable to the solutes, will not interrupt diffusion (see Fig. 18-1). Movement down a concentration gradient is characteristic of *passive transport*. Water and many metabolites that enter and leave the cells move by passive transport, and many substances are capable of moving up a concentration gradient from areas of low concentration to areas of high concentration. This kind of movement, termed *active transport*, requires assistance and energy expenditure. The active transport mechanism of a given substance is known as a *pump*. For example, nerve cells maintain sodium in high concentration outside the membrane but in low concentration inside the cell, despite the tendency of sodium to enter by diffusion. The sodium pump of the membrane is so efficient that in the resting nerve cell, there is approximately 14 times the concentration of sodium outside the cell as inside it.

Osmosis is the movement of water through a semipermeable barrier in response to a concentration gradient of solute, i.e., a difference in solute concentration from one side of the barrier to the other. The *water* moves from the side where the solutes are in low concentration to the side where the concentration of solutes is higher. In doing so, the water equalizes the concentration of solutes on the two sides of the barrier (see Fig. 18-2).

Any solution is said to exert *osmotic pressure* if it contains osmotically active particles. Proteins exert strong osmotic pressure. Osmotic pressure due to proteins is called *colloid osmotic pressure* or *oncotic pressure*.

The osmotic pressure of a solution can be stated in terms of its osmolarity. *Osmolarity* is the con-

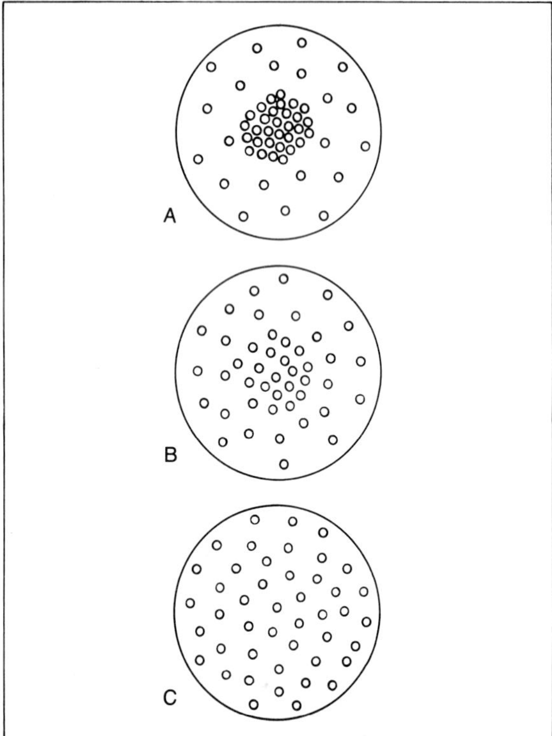

Figure 18-1 Diffusion. (*A*) As molecules randomly move, they bounce off one another, and the concentration is unequal. (*B*) The concentration becomes progressively more equal. (C) The molecules are equalized. (*From Dorothy Jones, Claire Ford Dunbar, and Mary Marmoll Jirovec* [*eds.*], *Medical-Surgical Nursing: A Conceptual Approach, McGraw-Hill, New York, 1978. Used with permission.*)

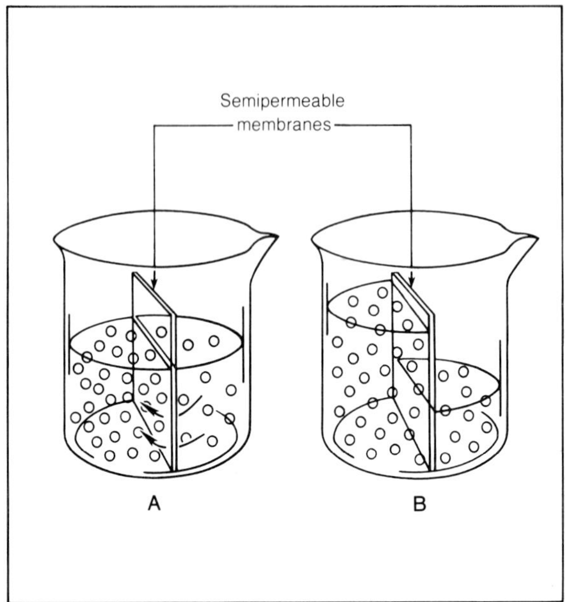

Figure 18-2 Osmosis. (*A*) A concentration gradient exists between the two sides of the semipermeable membrane. (*B*) The concentration gradient causes the water to move to the more concentrated side. (*From Dorothy Jones, Claire Ford Dunbar, and Mary Marmoll Jirovec* [*eds.*], *Medical-Surgical Nursing: A Conceptual Approach, McGraw-Hill, New York, 1978. Used with permission.*)

centration of osmotically active particles in a solution. Solutions can also be classified in terms of their tonicity. An *isotonic* solution has the same solute concentration as one used for reference—plasma, for example. Adding an isotonic solution to plasma does not change the osmotic balance between the plasma and the cells carried in it. A *hypertonic solution* is one with a greater solute concentration. Adding a hypertonic solution to plasma would cause blood cells to shrink, as fluid crossed the cell membrane and entered the plasma. The opposite effect would follow the addition of a *hypotonic solution*. Cells would swell as water from the plasma entered, seeking to equalize the solute concentration.

Filtration is the transfer of water and solutes down a concentration gradient. The force behind filtration is hydrostatic pressure. In the vascular system, this pressure is created by the outward thrust of blood against the vessel walls that confine it. The driving force is the pumping action of the heart.

Regulation of body water balance

The thirst mechanism Osmoreceptors in the hypothalamus are stimulated by increased plasma osmolarity and decreased blood volume. The thirst sensation occurs and urges the person to obtain water. Comatose or mentally retarded children do not always have an appropriate response to thirst and are dependent on others to fulfill their water intake needs. They can rapidly develop dehydration unless an early assessment is made and intervention occurs.

Hormonal control

Antidiuretic hormone Thirst works to control water intake, while antidiuretic hormone (ADH) functions to control water output. ADH

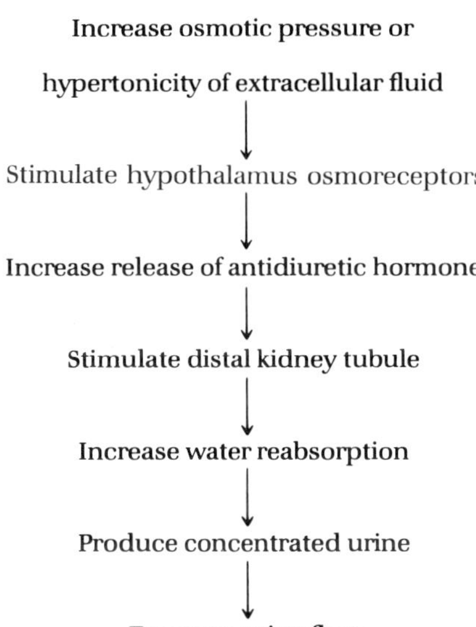

Figure 18-3 Antidiuretic hormone and water reabsorption. Interactions between the release of antidiuretic hormone by the hypothalamus and water reabsorption by the kidneys serve to stabilize the osmotic pressure of the body fluids. *(From Rosanne B. Howard and Nancie H. Herbold, Nutrition in Clinical Care, McGraw-Hill, New York, 1978. Used with permission.)*

is released by the posterior pituitary gland in response to decreased blood volume or increased plasma osmolarity. ADH decreases urine output and causes the body to retain water through its action on the collecting ducts of the kidneys. Because ADH causes water reabsorption, the ECF osmolarity is decreased, and blood volume is increased (see Fig. 18-3).

In Syndrome of Inappropriate ADH (SIADH), other factors besides plasma osmolarity and blood volume have been found to stimulate the release of ADH. The most common form is acute and usually self-limited in children. Head injury with rupture of the pituitary stalk, meningitis, encephalitis, brain abscess, subarachnoid hemorrhage, and Guillain-Barré syndrome have been reported to produce SIADH.[6] In addition, certain medications (e.g., morphine), anesthesia, trauma (including surgery), pain, and emotional stress may stimulate an increase in ADH. In SIADH, the water retention contributes to a fall in the serum sodium level (dilutional), an increase in weight, and a decrease in urine output.

Diabetes insipidus is a condition that occurs when ADH secretion is significantly *decreased* from normal. (See Chap. 24 for a further discussion of diabetes insipidus.) Decreased ADH secretion causes massive urine excretion and results in hypovolemia unless there is adequate fluid replacement.

Both SIADH and diabetes insipidus require the nurse to pay close attention to urine output, urine specific gravity, and unusual weight changes, since these are warnings of possible fluid imbalance.

Aldosterone *Aldosterone* is a mineralocorticoid that is secreted from the adrenal cortex. It has two important regulatory functions. The first is regulation of ECF volume. Aldosterone production is stimulated by hypovolemia, by decreased amounts of sodium in the bloodstream, and, indirectly, by release of renin from the kidneys. Renin is converted to angiotensin I and angiotensin II. Both renin and angiotensin increase blood pressure through vasoconstriction and direct stimulation of aldosterone production. Aldosterone promotes sodium and water retention, thereby increasing blood volume.

The second important activity of aldosterone is regulation of potassium metabolism. Under normal conditions, aldosterone favors urinary excretion of potassium. Aldosterone acts at the level of the distal convoluted tubules of the kidneys, where sodium is saved from tubular urine and is exchanged for either a hydrogen ion or a potassium ion. Thus, sodium reabsorption and urinary excretion of potassium and hydrogen ions occur. This is an obligatory excretion of potassium and must be matched by dietary or parenteral intake of potassium.

The kidneys The kidneys have both an excretory and a regulatory function. They participate in the adjustment of the composition of extracellular body fluids by determining both the volume of fluid and the amounts and kinds of electrolytes to be excreted or retained.

The *nephron* is the major functioning unit of the kidneys; it regulates composition and volume of body fluid. There are about 1 million nephrons in each kidney; each nephron is composed of an afferent arteriole, a glomerulus encased in Bowman's capsule, an efferent arteriole, the proximal convoluted tubule, collecting tubules, and peritubular capillaries. Each part of the nephron plays a specific role in water and electrolyte balance (see Fig. 18-4). The kidneys' ability to accomplish water and electrolyte bal-

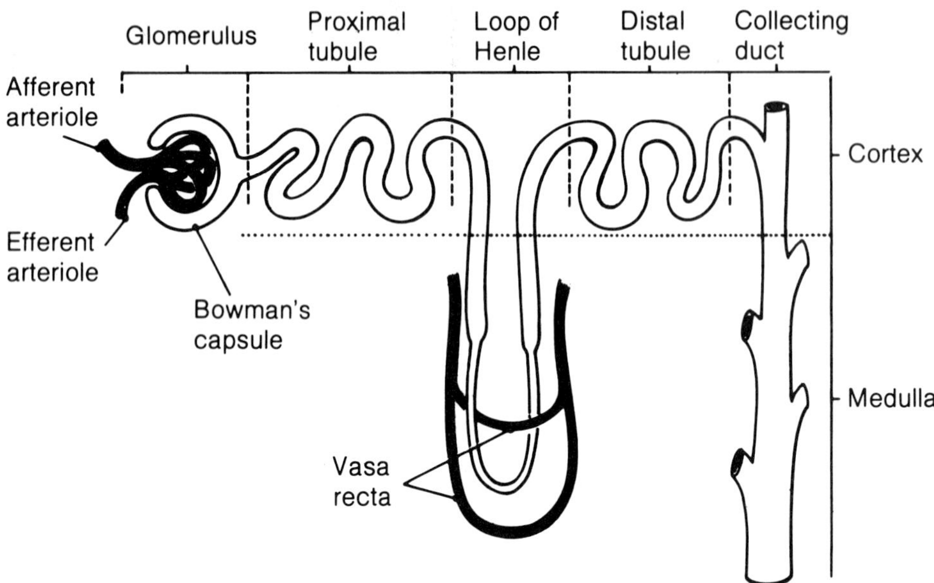

Figure 18-4 A schematic view of a nephron, with its functional units identified. (*From Rosanne B. Howard and Nancie H. Herbold, Nutrition in Clinical Care, McGraw-Hill, New York, 1978. Used with permission.*)

ance depends in part on the hormones aldosterone and ADH, as mentioned previously. Other important mechanisms that influence water regulation and sodium balance are glomerular filtration, tubular reabsorption, and tubular secretion.

Glomerular filtration Filtration is the result of pressures that force fluids and solutes through a membrane. *Glomerular filtration* occurs between the capillaries of the glomerulus and Bowman's capsule. The *colloidal osmotic pressure* created by blood proteins is the force that holds fluid within the glomerulus. Under normal circumstances, almost all substances with a molecular size less than that of the plasma proteins will be filtered out into Bowman's capsule.

Although glomerular hydrostatic pressures remain relatively constant with variations in blood pressure, a significant decrease in arterial blood pressure will affect glomerular hydrostatic pressure and, consequently, filtration rate. Conditions such as idiopathic nephrotic syndrome cause changes in the glomerular membrane, resulting in protein loss into the filtrate (and the urine) and thus changing colloidal osmotic pressures. (See Chap. 20 for a discussion of nephrotic syndrome.)

Tubular reabsorption *Tubular reabsorption* is the movement of substances from the tubular fluid into the blood. Reabsorption of water and solutes in the glomerular filtrate takes place as a result of both active and passive transport in all parts of the renal tubules. Reabsorption of water is influenced by the osmotic pressure (pull) from the movement of solutes, such as sodium, and by the amount of ADH present.

Tubular secretion *Tubular secretion* is the movement of substances from the blood into the tubular fluid. This can occur by either active or passive transport from the tubular cells into the tubular fluid.

Insensible losses While the kidneys play a significant role in regulating the volume and composition of body fluids, insensible losses via the skin, lungs, and stool also contribute to maintaining body fluid balance. The lungs utilize 15 ml of fluid per 100 cal metabolized and release this in exhaled air at the rate of 0.5 ml/kg per hour.

The normal skin expenditure is 30 ml per 100 cal and does not include diaphoresis. Sweating usually begins after the environmental temperature reaches 30°C (86°F).[7] Fluid loss increases by 30 ml per 100 cal for each 1°C rise in the environmental temperature. Children are much more susceptible than adults to increased insensible fluid loss during increases in both body temperature and the environmental temperature because of their larger body surface area. Roughly 5 ml/kg per day (5 ml per 100 cal metabolized) is excreted in the feces of chidren, compared with the adult's output of 2.5 ml/kg per day.[8]

FLUID AND ELECTROLYTE REQUIREMENTS

Metabolic rate, body weight, and body surface area must be considered when determining electrolyte and fluid expenditure and requirements. It has already been mentioned that the child's metabolic rate is twice that of the adult per unit of body weight. The body surface area of an infant is 3 times that of an adult per unit of weight, creating an opportunity for a greater loss of heat and fluid.

Fluid and electrolytes required to replace *normal* ongoing losses through the skin, lungs, stool, and kidneys are calculated in terms of body surface area or body weight in kilograms.

Body surface area

To calculate maintenance requirements, first calculate the child's body surface area (BSA) in square meters (m^2) (see Fig. 18-5 for a nomogram).

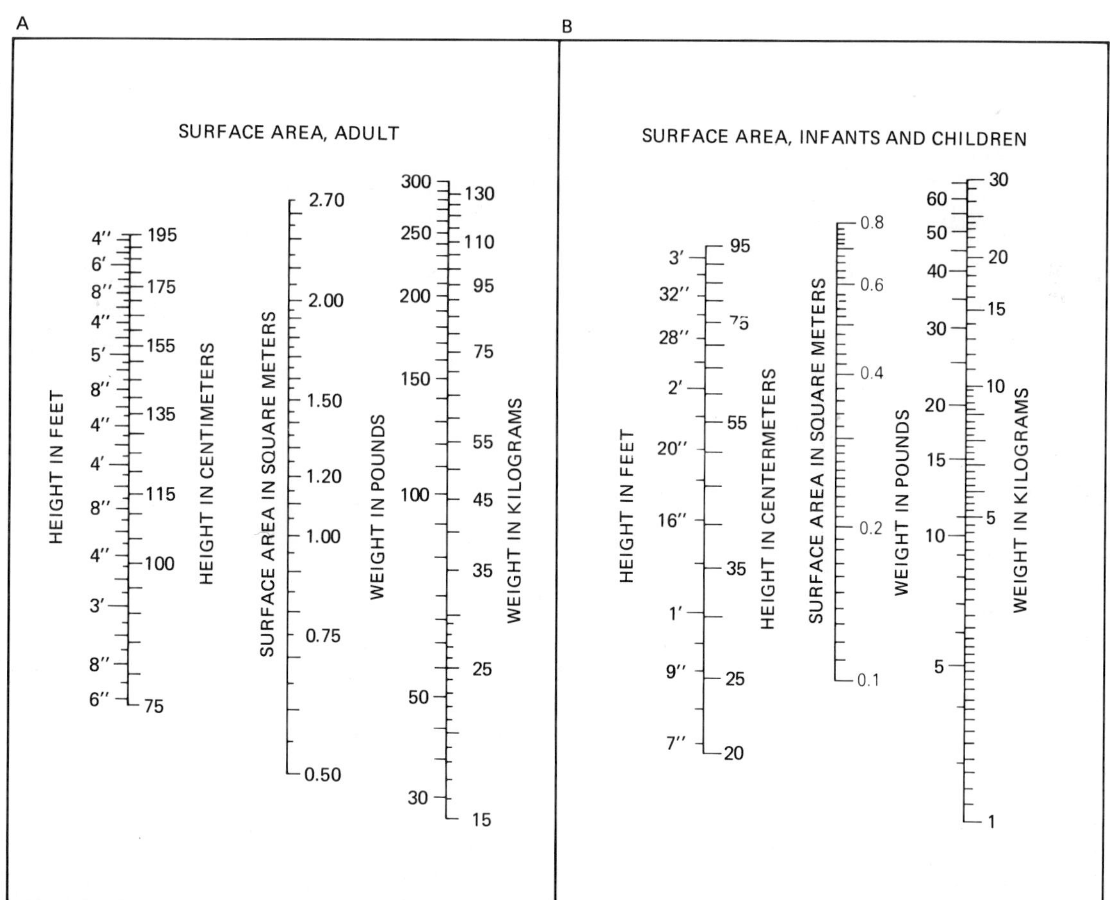

Figure 18-5 (*A*) A nomogram for body surface area (adults). (*B*) A nomogram for body surface area (infants and children). (*From C. E. Hollerman, Pediatric Nephrology, Medical Examination Publication, Garden City, N.Y., 1979, pp. 84–85. Used with permission.*)

Table 18-3 Calculations of Daily Fluid and Electrolyte Requirements by Body Surface Area*

1. From the nomogram, BSA is calculated as $0.4m^2$.
2. Water maintenance requirement is calculated as 1500 cc/m^2 per 24 h × 0.4 m^2 = 600 cc per 24 h.
3. Sodium maintenance requirement is calculated as 35 mEq/m^2 per 24 h × $0.4m^2$ = 14 mEq per 24 h.
4. Potassium maintenance requirement is calculated as 30 mEq/m^2 per 24 h × $0.4m^2$ = 12 mEq per 24 h.

*For a 2-year-old child who weighs 7 kg and is 85 cm in height.

Then, for fluid requirements, multiply the BSA by 1500 to 2000 cc per m^2 per 24 h. For electrolyte requirements, multiply the BSA by 35 to 50 mEq of sodium per m^2 per 24 h, and multiply the BSA by 30 to 40 mEq of potassium per m^2 per 24 h (see Table 18-3).[9]

Maintenance requirements should not exceed 1500 cc per square meter per 24 h if the child is not dehydrated. Use 2000 cc per m^2 per 24 h if the child is dehydrated.

For the newborn on the first day of life, fluid and electrolytes are calculated at one-half maintenance of 750 cc per m^2 per 24 h, 20 mEq of sodium per m^2 per 24 h, and 15 mEq of potassium per m^2 per 24 h. Maintenance requirements are gradually increased during the first week of life.[10]

Body weight

To calculate maintenance fluid requirements, multiply the body weight in kilograms by (1) 100 cc per kilogram per 24 h for the *first 10 kg,* (2) 50 cc per kilogram per 24 h for the *second 10 kg,* and (3) 20 cc per kilogram per 24 h for *each kilogram over 20 kg* (see Table 18-4).[11]

Table 18-4 Calculations of Daily Fluid Requirements by Body Weight

For a 4-month-old infant weighing 4 kg
4 kg × 100 cc per kilogram of body weight per 24 h = 400 cc per 24 h

For a 5-year-old child weighing 17 kg
For the first 10 kg of body weight, 1000 cc + 7 kg × 50 cc per kilogram of body weight per 24 h = 350 cc = 1350 cc per 24 h

For a 9-year-old child weighing 30 kg
For the first 20 kg of body weight, 1500 cc plus 10 kg × 20 cc per kilogram of body weight per 24 h = 200 cc = 1700 cc per 24 h

Table 18-5 Calculations of Electrolyte Requirements by Body Weight

For a 4-month-old infant weighing 4 Kg
4 kg × 4 mEq of sodium per kilogram of body weight per 24 h = 16 mEq of sodium per 24 h
4 kg × 2 mEq of potassium per kilogram of body weight per 24 h = 8 mEq of potassium per 24 h

For a 5-year-old child weighing 17 Kg
17 kg × 4 mEq of sodium per kilogram of body weight per 24 h = 68 mEq of sodium per 24 h
17 kg × 2 mEq of potassium per kilogram of body weight per 24 h = 34 mEq of potassium per 24 h

For a 9-year-old child weighing 30 Kg
30 kg × 4 mEq of sodium per kilogram of body weight per 24 h = 120 mEq of sodium per 24 h
30 kg × 2 mEq of potassium per kilogram of body weight per 24 h = 60 mEq of potassium per 24 h

To calculate maintenance electrolyte requirements, multiply the body weight in kilograms by 4 mEq of sodium per kilogram per 24 h and 2 mEq of potassium per kilogram per 24 h (see Table 18-5).[12]

ALTERATIONS IN BODY WATER

Disturbances in fluid volume—either too much or too little—are among the most common and potentially life-threatening problems in the nursing care of children (see Table 18-6).

Isotonic disturbances

Extracellular volume depletion

Pathophysiology Extracellular volume depletion is an isotonic water deficit that results when sodium and water are lost in the same proportions in which they occur in the ECF. Extracellular fluid osmolarity remains unchanged, and there is no shift of water between the intracellular and the extracellular fluid compartments (see Fig. 18-6).

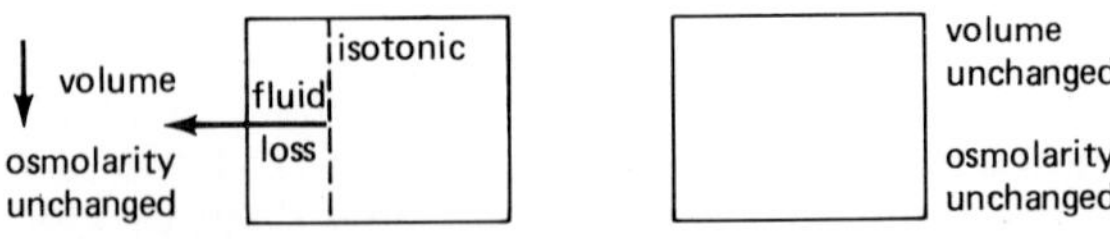

Figure 18-6 Isotonic disturbance due to extracellular depletion.

Table 18-6 Pathogenesis and Fluid Effects of Volume Expansion and Contraction

Disorder	Example	Changes in volume		Changes in ECF[a] concentration			
		ECF[a]	ICF[b]	Na$^+$	Protein	Osm	Hct[c]
1. *Isosmotic contraction* Loss of isosmotic fluid from plasma. ISF[d] moves into plasma. The result is contraction of the entire ECF volume. No shift of fluid from intravascular spaces occurs. Plasma circulatory compromise sets in early.	Diarrhea with concurrent loss of electrolytes in urine	↓	—*[e]	—	↑	—	↑
2. *Hyperosmotic contraction* Water is lost in excess of solute. Water is lost first from plasma. ISF flows in to replace water lost from plasma, and intracellular water flows into the interstitium. The volume of all major compartments is reduced. Symptoms of contraction are less severe than with isotonic contraction because the ECF volume is protected by ICF shift into ECF.	Dehydration, insensible water loss, or fever	↓	↓	↑	↑	↑	—
3. *Hyposmotic contraction* Loss of solute in excess of water relative to normal plasma. NaCl is lost from ECF, and so osmolality decreases. Fluid shifts from ECF into cells.	Dehydration	↓	↑	↓	↑	↓	↑
4. *Isosmotic expansion* A positive balance of an isosmotic solution (NaCl). Selective expansion of ECF due to solute retention here (edema).	Edema	↑	—	—	↓	—	↓
5. *Hyperosmotic expansion* A positive balance of ECF solute in excess of water causes a shift of water from the ICF into the ECF space until osmotic equilibrium is reached.	NaCl poisoning	↑	↓	↑	↓	↑	↓
6. *Hyposmotic expansion* A positive balance of water. Both ECF and ICF spaces expand.	SIADH[f]	↑	↑	↓	↓	↓	—

[a]Extracellular fluid.

[b]Intracellular fluid.

[c]Hematocrit

[d]Interstitial fluid.

[e]No change.

[f]Syndrome of inappropriate antidiuretic hormone.

Source: Janis B. Smith (ed), *Pediatric Critical Care*, Wiley, New York, 1983.

Etiology Extracellular fluid volume losses are commonly caused by vomiting, gastric suction, hemorrhage, or diarrhea. Diarrhea in young children produces large losses of water and sodium, causing ECF depletion in varying degrees (see Table 18-7). It is important to consider that small losses in children may be critical, when compared with their total blood volume (approximately 80 ml per kilogram of body weight). The decreased ability of the kidneys to concentrate urine during the first 1 to 2 years of life predisposes the child to the rapid development and progression of dehydration.

Prevention is aimed at rectifying the cause of

Table 18-7 Degrees of Dehydration

	Degree		
	Mild	**Moderate**	**Severe**
Weight loss:			
Infants	5%	10%	15%
Older children	3%	6%	9%
Skin turgor	Mild decrease	"Tenting"	Severe decrease
Mucous membranes	Dry	Dry	Parched
Tears	Normal	Absent	Absent
Fontanels	Flat	Sunken	Sunken
Eyeballs	Normal	Sunken	Sunken
Pulse	Rapid	Rapid	Rapid and weak
Blood pressure	Normal	Normal to low	Low

Source: C. E. Hollerman, *Pediatric Nephrology*, Medical Examination Publication, Garden City, N.Y., 1979. Used with permission.

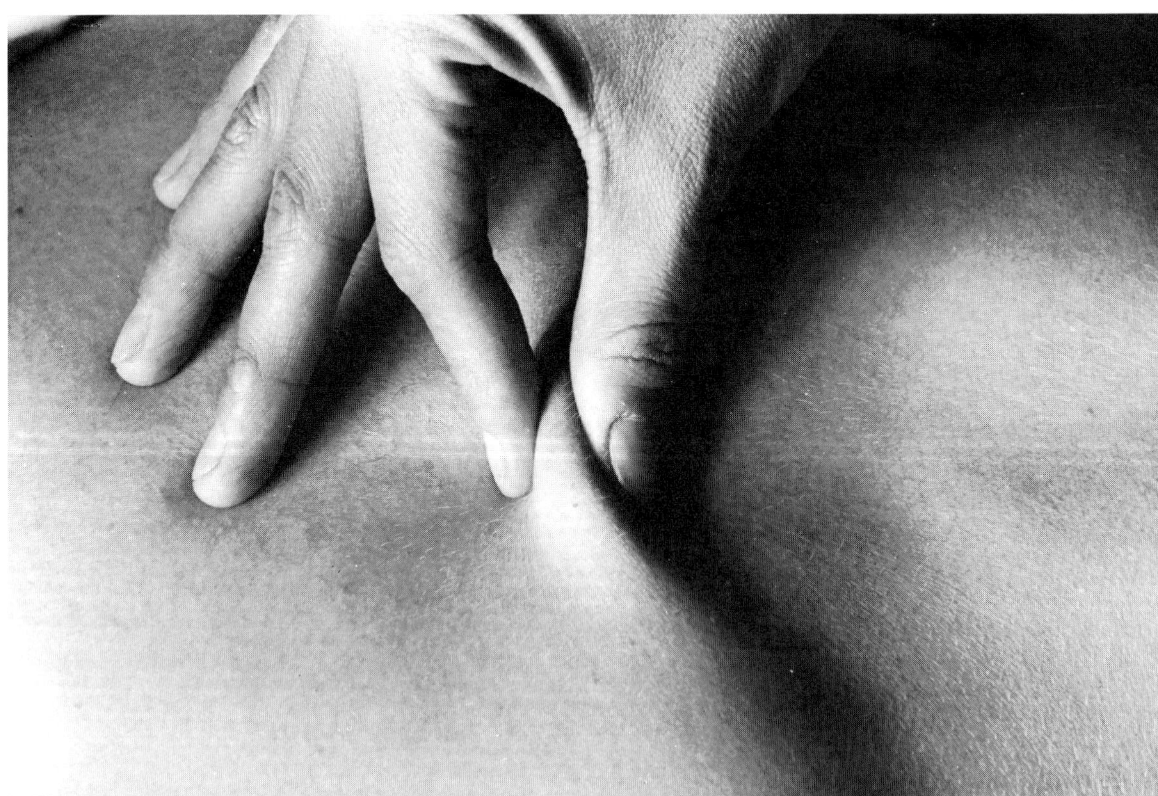

Figure 18-7 The technique for determining skin turgor. A fold of skin over the sternum is lifted with the thumb and index finger and is then released. In a young child, the abdomen near the umbilicus is used. In an older child, the inner thigh may also be used. (*From Dorothy Jones, Claire Ford Dunbar, and Mary Marmoll Jirovec* [eds.], *Medical-Surgical Nursing: A Conceptual Approach, McGraw-Hill, New York, 1978. Used with permission.*)

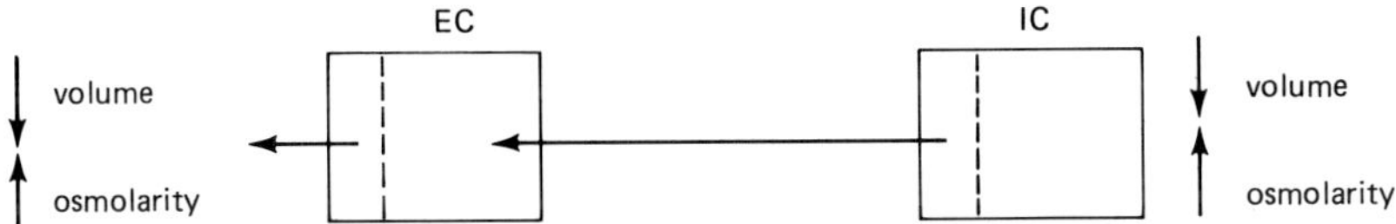

Figure 18-8 Hyperosmolar imbalance related to water deficit.

the ECF volume losses. In the young child with diarrhea, the nurse would teach the parents to observe for dehydration (see Fig. 18-7), to intervene by increasing appropriate fluid intake, and to seek further medical advice if dehydration continues.

Extracellular volume excess

Pathophysiology Fluid remains in the extracellular compartment (vascular and interstitial) when isotonic fluid is added to the extracellular compartment. An extracellular volume excess may be caused by the administration of excessive amounts of isotonic fluids at a rate that exceeds renal capacity for excretion. This is a risk for children with immature or impaired kidney function. Children who have renal disease and a limited ability to excrete sodium and water are at risk for extracellular volume excess. Conditions which impair circulation of the kidneys, such as congestive heart failure, or which cause an increase in sodium and water reabsorption, such as cortisone administration, will contribute to extracellular volume excess.

Parents and their children will need to be taught about fluid limits in renal and cardiac disorders. Children on steroids must be carefully monitored for signs of fluid overload (see Table 18-8). Although the physician is responsible for ordering intravenous fluids, the nurse should always evaluate the amount ordered to be sure that it is correct. Intravenous fluids should be monitored and recorded by the nurse at least every hour. Delivery of intravenous fluids should be controlled by a pump to prevent overadministration or underadministration (see Chap. 16). The laboratory results, clinical manifestations, treatment, and nursing management of fluid and electrolyte imbalances are listed in Table 18-8.

Osmolarity disturbances

Hyperosmolar imbalance

Pathophysiology A water deficit or a solute (sodium) excess causes *hyperosmolarity*. A water deficit due to water loss or decreased intake leads to an increase in the concentration of sodium per liter of water. As a result, water moves from the intracellular space to the extracellular space (see Fig. 18-8). A sodium excess due to increased intake or inadequate output of sodium causes loss of fluid from the intracellular space and expansion of the extracellular space (see Fig. 18-9).

Etiology Decreased water intake may be due to several factors: (1) inability of the infant, the young child, or the comatose patient to feed himself or herself, (2) a dislike of available liquids, (3) a sore throat, (4) extreme fatigue, (5) impaired response to thirst (e.g., due to a cerebral injury), and (6) unavailability of water.

Increased water output may be due to (1) fever, (2) diaphoresis, (3) watery diarrhea, (4) diabetes insipidus, and (5) diabetic acidosis. The condition of sodium excess will be discussed later in the section "Hypernatremia."

Because of the etiology of *hyperosmolar imbalance*, there is a need for careful nursing care based on a knowledge of the fluid requirements of children. The nurse must carefully assess the signs and symptoms of fluid imbalance (see Table 18-9).

Hypoosmolar imbalance

Pathophysiology A water excess or a solute deficit can cause *hypoosmolar imbalance*. The addition of electrolyte-free water to the extracellular space or a solute loss causes dilution of

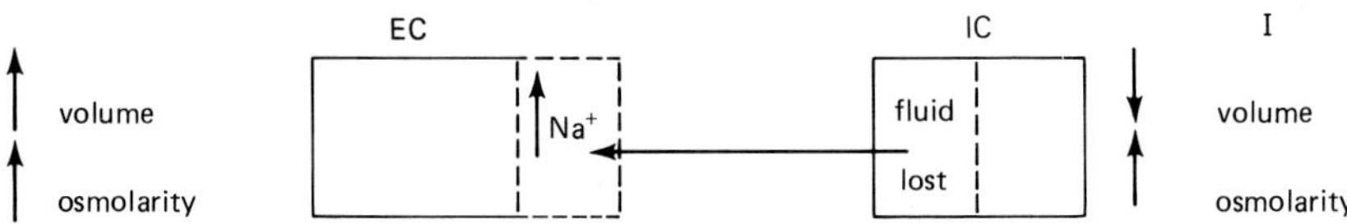

Figure 18-9 Hyperosmolar imbalance related to sodium excess.

Table 18-8 Fluid and Electrolyte Imbalances: Clinical Manifestations and Nursing Management

Imbalance	Laboratory results	Clinical manifestations	Nursing management
Hyponatremia	Serum sodium is less than 130 mEq per liter. Mild: 120 to 130 mEq per liter; moderate: 114 to 120 mEq per liter; severe: below 114 mEq per liter. Urine sodium is decreased. Urine specific gravity is decreased.	Mild: anorexia, nausea and vomiting, apprehension, anxiety, weakness, twitching, and sense of impending doom. Severe: headache, lethargy, confusion, convulsions, vasomotor collapse (decreased blood pressure and rapid, thready pulse), and fingerprinting of sternum	Prevent by always irrigating nasogastric tubes with normal saline and monitoring serum sodium levels of children at risk for developing a solute deficit. Infuse an isotonic or occasionally a hypertonic saline solution intravenously. Restrict fluids (because of intracellular fluid excess). Monitor fluid intake and output balance (to prevent fluid volume deficit). Weigh daily. Frequently reassure the confused child. Take precautions against seizures. Encourage intake of foods that are high in sodium.
Hypernatremia	Serum sodium level is increased above 150 mEq per liter. Urine specific gravity is elevated.	Neurological symptoms, including lethargy and dullness; irritability when disturbed; tremors and convulsions; nuchal rigidity; muscle rigidity; dry, sticky mucous membranes; flushed skin; immense thirst; increased extracellular fluid volume; edema ("doughlike" feel to the skin); oliguria or anuria	Prevent by providing adequate fluid intake with high-protein feedings, and always dilute sodium bicarbonate by one-half for infants under 1 month of age. Increase fluid intake orally, or infuse 5% dextrose solution intravenously. Observe for changes in blood pressure. Evaluate intake and output for fluid volume changes. Weigh the child daily. Assess urine specific gravity and volume. Observe for signs of congestive heart failure. Offer fluids frequently. Give meticulous skin and mouth care. Take precautions against seizures.
Hypokalemia	Serum potassium is decreased to less than 3.5 mEq per liter. pH is increased if the child has metabolic alkalosis. Plasma bicarbonate is increased above 29 mEq per liter if the child has metabolic alkalosis. Plasma chloride may be decreased below 98 mEq per liter.	Cardiac arrhythmias; muscle weakness (especially in the legs); diminished reflexes; flaccid paralysis; abdominal cramps; nausea; anorexia; paralytic ileus; abdominal distension; hypotension; weak, shallow respirations; weak, irregular pulse	Administer potassium orally or intravenously. Monitor the IV rate with potassium closely (less than 20 mEq per hour). Place on a cardiac monitor. Assess serum potassium levels. Review drugs to determine which drug is causing potassium loss (e.g., steroids). Assess urine output (never give potas-

Table 18-8 Fluid and Electrolyte Imbalances: Clinical Manifestations and Nursing Management (*Continued*)

Imbalance	Laboratory results	Clinical manifestations	Nursing management
			sium until renal functioning is assured). Assess vital signs for changes in pulse, respirations, and blood pressure. Administer potassium supplements (if given orally, observe for gastrointestinal bleeding; if given intravenously, observe the IV site for pain and irritation). Encourage intake of foods high in potassium. Plan nursing care to conserve the child's energy and lessen weakness and fatigue.
Hyperkalemia	Serum potassium is elevated above 5.5 mEq per liter. Serum sodium is decreased. Renal tests may be impaired.	Muscle cramping; weak, flaccid muscles; irritability; paresthesias (numbness and tingling of the face, arms, hands, and legs); hyporeflexia; cardiac arrhythmias; diarrhea; nausea	Administer glucose intravenously with insulin and/or sodium bicarbonate (to move potassium into the cells as emergency treatment). Administer Kayexalate resin via a nasogastric tube or enema (to exchange nitrogen for potassium). Administer fresh blood transfusions (fresh blood contains less potassium than banked blood). Decrease oral or IV potassium intake. Monitor serum potassium levels. Administer calcium gluconate in an emergency (to decrease cardiac muscle irritability). Give diuretics or place the child on dialysis if appropriate (peritoneal dialysis or hemodialysis). Monitor ECG for arrhythmias and possible cardiac arrest. Restrict intake of foods high in potassium. Increase carbohydrates in diet (to prevent further catabolism and potassium loss). Decrease environmental stimuli.
Hypocalcemia	Serum calcium level is decreased below 8 mg per 100 ml. Serum phos-	Numbness and tingling in the ends of the fingers and the circumoral re-	Administer 10% calcium gluconate intravenously. Educate the par-

Table 18-8 Fluid and Electrolyte Imbalances: Clinical Manifestations and Nursing Management (*Continued*)

Imbalance	Laboratory results	Clinical manifestations	Nursing management
	phate level is increased in renal failure.	gion; muscle cramps; carpopedal spasm; tetany and convulsions; positive Chovstek's sign (the face twitches when the facial nerve is tapped); laryngeal spasm; rickets; memory lapse; irritability; seizures; hallucinations; cardiac arrhythmias	ents about a diet high in calcium and vitamin D. Assess tingling in the ends of the fingers or muscle spasm (for early detection). Monitor ECG for arrhythmias and bradycardia during IV calcium infusion. Assess serum calcium levels. Assess vital signs.
Hypercalcemia	Serum calcium level is increased above 12 mEq per 100 ml. Serum phosphate level is decreased. Blood urea nitrogen is increased (because of calculi damage to the kidneys).	Lethargy; depression; confusion; stupor; coma; weakness; fatigue; hypotonia; hyporeflexia or absent reflexes; anorexia; nausea; vomiting; abdominal pain; constipation; paralytic ileus; cardiac arrhythmias; bone pain and possible bone fractures; polyuria; kidney stones	Infuse isotonic saline intravenously (to increase urinary excretion). Administer oral phosphates or steroids (to decrease interstitial absorption). Evaluate digitalis dosage (calcium potentiates the action). Place the child on dialysis if ordered. Assess the child for signs of acute hypercalcemic crisis: nausea and vomiting, dehydration, stupor, delirium, hallucinations, coma, and/or cardiac arrest. Assess for kidney stones. Provide rest, a quiet environment, and diversional activities.
Hypophosphatemia	Serum phosphate level is decreased below 3 mg per 100 ml. Hemoglobin and hematocrit are decreased (because of red blood cell hemolysis).	Bleeding (nosebleeds, gastrointestinal bleeding, and ecchymosis due to platelet dysfunction); weakness; tremors; malaise; ataxia; memory loss; confusion; coma; pathological fractures; anorexia; nausea; vomiting; acute respiratory failure	Add maintenance requirements of phosphate to the TPN solution. Administer phosphate salt replacements (especially for a child with diabetic ketoacidosis). Administer oral phosphate supplements. Assess the child for hazards associated with IV administration of phosphate: hyperphosphatemia, hypotension, hyperkalemia (if the phosphate supplement is given as potassium phosphate), dehydration, and hypernatremia (due to the osmotic diuretic effect of filtered phosphate). Increase the intake of dairy products.

Table 18-8 **Fluid and Electrolyte Imbalances: Clinical Manifestations and Nursing Management (*Continued*)**

Imbalance	Laboratory results	Clinical manifestations	Nursing management
Hyperphosphatemia	Serum phosphate level is increased above 5.0 mg per 100 ml.	Crystal deposits in soft tissues and vital organs (even when calcium levels are normal)	Administer phosphate binders (e.g., aluminum hydroxide) with meals. Assess serum calcium and phosphate levels. Dialysis may be ordered.
Hypomagnesemia	Serum magnesium level is below 1.5 mEq per liter. Serum calcium and serum potassium levels are decreased.	Changes in mental status (insomnia, hallucinations, confusion, and depression); muscle twitches or cramps; convulsions; hyperactive reflexes; carpopedal spasm; positive Chvostek's sign; nausea; vomiting; anorexia; diarrhea; abdominal distension; tachycardia; arrhythmias; hypotension	Administer magnesium supplements orally (e.g., Mylanta, Maalox, or Gelusil) or intravenously (magnesium sulfate). Monitor blood pressure during IV magnesium sulfate supplementation. Encourage the intake of foods high in magnesium. Reassure and reorient the confused child. Take precautions against seizures.
Hypermagnesemia	Serum magnesium level is elevated above 2 mEq per liter.	Neuromuscular depression (drowsiness, apnea, and possible coma); hyporeflexia; muscle paralysis; muscle flaccidity; hypotension; diaphoresis and sensation of heat; bradycardia; cardiac arrhythmias; possible cardiac arrest	Dialysis may be ordered (to reduce high magnesium level). Stop all magnesium supplements. Give antacids that do not contain magnesium. Monitor cardiac and respiratory status. Assess neurological signs. Assess level of consciousness and neuromuscular depression. Monitor serum magnesium levels.
Extracellular fluid volume depletion	Hemoglobin and hematocrit are increased (are decreased if there is blood loss). Blood urea nitrogen is increased. Urine specific gravity is over 1.030. Potassium level is decreased (if diaphoresis, stools, or gastric suction is excessive).	Decreased blood pressure; increased pulse rate; decreased pulse pressure; increased body temperature; decreased skin turgor (see Fig. 18-7); dry skin and mucous membranes; sunken fontanels; absence of tears; weakness; lethargy; confusion; sunken, soft eyeballs; oliguria or anuria; thirst	Infuse isotonic solutions intravenously. Infuse colloids if lost from vascular bed. Monitor central venous pressure if volume depletion is severe. Monitor vital signs for signs of hypovolemic shock and/or elevated temperature. Measure intake and output strictly. (With adequate intake, output should be 0.5 to 1.0 ml per kilogram of body weight per hour. A slightly reduced urine volume can indicate a significant change in renal perfusion or function.) Monitor urine specific gravity (a spe-

Table 18-8 Fluid and Electrolyte Imbalances: Clinical Manifestations and Nursing Management (*Continued*)

Imbalance	Laboratory results	Clinical manifestations	Nursing management
			cific gravity above 1.030 indicates dehydration). Weigh the child daily (weigh small children more frequently). Measure abnormal fluid output (diarrheal stools, gastrointestinal losses, pleural drainage, and wound drainage). Assess for signs of fluid overload (especially when colloidal or plasma albumin solutions are being administered, since these can cause rapid fluid shifts). Assess the IV fluid rate and the IV site for infiltration. Encourage fluid and electrolyte intake (usually by giving Infalyte or a similar product). Turn the child frequently, and massage bony prominences (tissues are more susceptible to breakdown). Provide skin and mouth care (especially if dry).
Extracellular volume excess	Hemoglobin and hematocrit are decreased.	Elevated blood pressure; full to bounding pulse; neck vein distention; elevated central venous pressure; increased abdominal girth; periorbital edema; sudden or abnormal weight gain; pulmonary edema with dyspnea, cough, and crackles; fluid intake greater than output; bulging fontanels	Give diuretics (to increase water excretion). Reduce the IV fluid rate, and limit oral intake. Limit sodium intake. Assess vital signs for signs of fluid overload (especially respiratory effort). Monitor intake and output (checking especially for decreased output). Weigh the child daily. Measure abdominal girth. Assess breath sounds (especially crackles). Assess edema (especially sacral and periorbital edema in infants and young children). Elevate the head of the bed (for a child with pulmonary edema). Inspect edematous areas of the skin for circulation and potential breakdown. Prevent dry skin.

Table 18-8 Fluid and Electrolyte Imbalances: Clinical Manifestations and Nursing Management (*Continued*)

Imbalance	Laboratory results	Clinical manifestations	Nursing management
Hyperosmolar fluid imbalance	Hemoglobin and hematocrit are increased. Sodium level is increased above 150 mEq per liter.	Decreased skin turgor, or "tenting" (see Fig. 18-7); sunken or soft eyeballs; feelings of apprehension; mental changes; possible convulsions	Over a period of 48 to 72 h, infuse IV fluids containing some solute (sodium) to prevent too rapid osmotic changes where shrunken brain cells may swell as a result of too rapid rehydration. Monitor serum sodium levels. Assess for symptoms of extracellular fluid volume depletion (include condition of the eyeballs). Assess mental status.
Hypoosmolar fluid imbalance	Serum sodium level is less than 135 mEq per liter. Hemoglobin and hematocrit are decreased.	Increased urine output; decreased urine specific gravity (below 1.001); signs and symptoms of congestive heart failure; signs and symptoms of extracellular volume excess; neuromuscular signs and symptoms (confusion, stupor, coma, and seizures due to swollen brain cells); muscle weakness	Restrict fluids given intravenously and orally (to decrease total body water). Possibly restrict sodium in the diet, and give diuretics. Possibly infuse 5% hypertonic saline for children who have seizures. Assess for symptoms of extracellular fluid volume excess. Monitor serum sodium level. Assess neuromuscular signs. Protect the child from falls (due to muscular weakness). Take precautions against seizures.

Table 18-9 Signs and Symptoms Related to Isotonic, Hypotonic, or Hypertonic Disturbances

	State		
	Isotonic	Hypotonic	Hypertonic
Skin turgor	Poor	Quite poor	Fair
Mucous membranes	Dry	Perhaps moist	Parched
Mental status	Lethargic	Coma (if severe)	Hyperirritable
Pulse	Rapid	Rapid	Moderately rapid
Blood pressure	Low	Quite low	Low
Serum sodium (mEq per liter)	135 to 150	Below 135	Above 150
Serum osmolality (mOsmol per liter)	280 to 310	Below 280	Above 310

Source: C. E. Hollerman, *Pediatric Nephrology*, Medical Examination Publication, Garden City, N.Y., 1979. Used with permission.

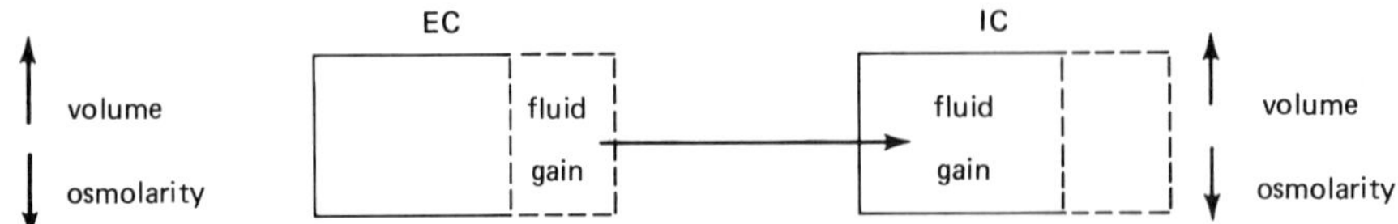

Figure 18-10 Hypoosmolar imbalance related to water excess.

solutes and a shift of water to the intracellular space (see Figs. 18-10 and 18-11).

Etiology Excessive ADH secretion by the posterior pituitary can cause a decreased serum osmolarity through retention of electrolyte-free water by the kidneys. Increased ADH secretion is discussed in the "Hormonal control" subsection of "Regulation of body water balance."

Tap-water enemas given to children can cause water absorption through the bowel. The inability of the kidneys to excrete the increased amounts of water may contribute to water excess and hypoosmolar imbalance. The condition of sodium deficit is discussed later in the section "Sodium Deficit (Hyponatremia)" and in Table 18-8.

ALTERATIONS IN ELECTROLYTE BALANCE

Sodium balance

Sodium is the major cation of the extracellular fluid, including interstitial and intravascular fluid (see Table 18-2). The normal sodium concentration in plasma is 135 to 145 mEq per liter (see Table 18-10).

The major function of sodium is to maintain the osmotic pressure of the extracellular fluid and thus regulate extracellular fluid volume. The sodium level is regulated by the kidneys. Sodium is reabsorbed by the kidneys and influences water reabsorption. When the concentration of sodium falls, aldosterone secretion promotes sodium reabsorption. As the kidneys retain sodium, they also retain water. A deficit in body fluid volume causes a decrease in the glomerular filtration rate and enhances sodium retention. The body retains sodium so effectively that a person can remain on a low-sodium diet for a long time without experiencing sodium depletion.

In contrast, when the sodium concentration in the extracellular fluid rises, ADH release causes the kidneys to retain water. The retained fluid dilutes the sodium to more normal concentrations. Sodium is excreted in the urine, feces, and sweat when the level exceeds normal.

Sodium has two additional functions. First, it is one of the ions responsible for the cell membrane's potential, essential for nerve impulse conduction and muscle contraction. Second, sodium participates in maintaining the acid-base balance as a component of the buffer, sodium bicarbonate. Commercially prepared foods contain high levels of sodium. Examples include pickles, catsup, canned soups, processed meats, ham, and bacon. Other high-sodium foods that children like include potato chips, french fries, hot dogs, and cheese. The recommended intake of sodium is 2.5 mEq per 100 cal metabolized.

Sodium imbalances

Sodium deficit (hyponatremia) *Hyponatremia* can occur in association with a water excess, dilutional hyponatremia, or an actual solute deficit. Dilutional hyponatremia was discussed earlier.

Etiology Hyponatremia (serum sodium deficit) is uncommon because of the body's excellent ability to conserve sodium. When it does occur, hyponatremia is likely to be caused by decreased salt intake, gastroenteritis, renal salt-losing states, a potent diuretic, irrigation of naso-

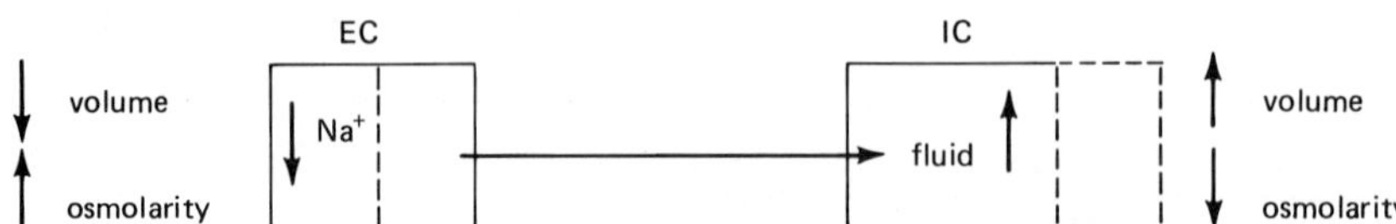

Figure 18-11 Hypoosmolar imbalance related to solute deficit.

Table 18-10 Laboratory Test Values and Clinical Implications

Test	Normal value	Some causes of excess	Some causes of deficit
Sodium	135 to 145 mEq per liter	High-protein formula, diabetes insipidus, hydrocephalus, hypertonic dehydration	Gastroenteritis, hypotonic dehydration, inappropriate ADH secretion, fluid overload
Potassium	3.5 to 5.0 mEq per liter	Renal failure, exchange transfusion, crushing injury	Diarrhea, vomiting, diuretics, adrenocorticoid steroids
Calcium	9.0 to 11.0 mg/dl	Idiopathic hypercalcemia, vitamin D metabolism defects, multiple fractures, bone tumors	Renal failure, inadequate dietary intake, diarrhea, hypothyroidism
Magnesium	1.5 to 1.9 mg/dl	Renal disease, newborn of mother treated with magnesium sulfate	Hypoparathyroidism (familial), high-calcium dietary intake, malnutrition
Chloride	94 to 104 mEq per liter		Vomiting, diarrhea, diuretics
Protein	6.2 to 8.0 g per 100 ml		Malnutrition, starvation
Glucose	80 to 120 mg per 100 ml	Diabetes mellitus, acute injury, brain lesions	Hyperinsulinism, liver disease, malnutrition
BUN (blood urea nitrogen)	5 to 15 mg per 100 ml (children aged 1 to 2 years) and then 10 to 20 mg/dl	Renal disease, increased protein catabolism	
pH	7.35 to 7.45	Metabolic or respiratory alkalosis	Metabolic or respiratory acidosis
O_2 saturation	95% arterial 70 to 75% venous		High altitude, polycythemia
P_{O_2}	80 to 100 mmHg arterial 35 to 40 mmHg venous	Hyperventilation, high O_2 atmosphere	Hypoventilation
Total CO_2	20 to 26 mEq per liter (infants) 24 to 30 mEq per liter (older children)	Hypoventilation, respiratory acidosis	Hyperventilation, respiratory alkalosis
P_{CO_2}	35 to 45 mmHg arterial 41 to 51 mmHg venous	Hypoventilation, respiratory acidosis	Hyperventilation, respiratory alkalosis
Phosphate	Up to 6 mg/dl (infants) 3.0 to 4.5 mg/dl (children over 1 year)	Acute and chronic renal failure, urate nephropathy associated with leukemia	Malabsorption, small bowel disease, starvation, TPN without phosphates, thiazine diuretics
CO_2 (as bicarbonate)	20 to 26 mEq per liter, infants 24 to 30 mEq per liter (older children)	Metabolic alkalosis	Metabolic acidosis
Hematocrit	Newborn—46 to 68% Child—35 to 38% Adolescent—38 to 40% Adult male—42 to 52% Adult female—37 to 47%	Hemoconcentration, isotonic dehydration	Physiological anemia, blood loss, fluid overload
Urine:			
Electrolytes	Varies with diet		
Sulkowitch test	Positive	Heavy positive—hypercalcemia	Hypocalcemia
Protein	Negative	Renal disease, anabolic state, glomerular nephritis	
Glucose	Negative	Diabetes mellitus	
Ketones	Negative	High-protein diet, diabetes mellitus	
Creatinine clearance (24 h)	60 to 80 ml/min/m^2	Renal failure, decreased glomerular filtration rate	
pH	4.6 to 8.0	Alkalosis	Acidosis
Specific gravity	1.010 to 1.030	Fluid volume excess, high fluid intake, diabetes insipidus	Fluid volume deficit
Osmolality	50 to 1200 mOsmol per kilogram	Fluid volume excess, high fluid intake, diabetes insipidus	Fluid volume deficit
Volume	Varies with age	Fluid volume excess	Fluid volume deficit

Sources: Sarko M. Tilkian, Mary Boudreau Conover, and Ara G. Tilkian, *Clinical Implications of Laboratory Tests,* Mosby, St. Louis, 1979; and *Children's Hospital of Los Angeles Resident Manual,* Section XIX, "Normal Laboratory Values and Nomograms," Children's Hospital, Los Angeles, pp. 1–15.

gastric tubes with plain water, and replacement of sodium and water losses with only water. The laboratory results, symptoms, treatment, and nursing care are described in Table 18-8. The neurological symptoms result from swelling of the brain cells with water as fluid shifts from the extracellular to the intracellular compartment.

Sodium excess (hypernatremia) *Hypernatremia* occurs in association with a water deficit or a solute (sodium) excess. Hyperosmolar imbalance related to a water deficit was discussed earlier in this chapter. This section focuses on hypernatremia related to solute excess.

Etiology Hypernatremia can be caused by high protein feedings with minimal fluid intake, saltwater drowning, and accidental addition of salt instead of sugar to formula. Infants who are given sodium bicarbonate during cardiopulmonary arrest may become severely hypernatremic, which causes cerebral bleeding, pulmonary edema, and systemic hypertension. Additional symptoms, laboratory results, treatment, and nursing management are described in Table 18-8.

Potassium balance

Potassium is the major cation of the intracellular fluid. Values of intracellular potassium are inaccessible and are therefore approximated by the serum level. The normal serum potassium level is 3.5 to 5.0 mEq per liter (see Table 18-10).

Potassium helps maintain the normal fluid and electrolyte distribution of the intracellular compartment. As a component of a buffer pair, potassium guards the acid-base equilibrium of the intracellular fluid. The potassium ion, like sodium, establishes the membrane potential necessary for nerve impulse conduction and muscle action. Abnormal potassium levels are immediately reflected in disturbed functioning of nerves or muscles.

In the kidneys, potassium is completely filtered out of the blood at the glomerulus and is entirely reabsorbed in the proximal convoluted tubules. In the distal convoluted tubules, potassium is often excreted in exchange for sodium. Absorption is fairly complete in the upper gastrointestinal tract, but potassium may be exchanged for sodium in the lower gastrointestinal tract.

Daily dietary intake of potassium is required because it is lost daily in the feces and urine. The recommended potassium intake is 2.5 mEq per 100 cal metabolized. Bananas, oranges, potatoes, carrots, celery, peaches, and salt substitutes are excellent sources of potassium.

Potassium deficit (hypokalemia) *Hypokalemia*, or loss of potassium, occurs rapidly and frequently in sick children. Potassium must be ingested daily to maintain a normal level. Diarrhea may cause a child to lose one-fourth of the total body potassium in 1 day. Any child who has taken nothing by mouth for 24 h should be assessed carefully and routinely for potassium deficit.

Etiology Diuretics are another main cause of hypokalemia. Other causes include decreased dietary intake (in patients who have anorexia or who can take nothing by mouth), wound drainage, gastric suctioning, steroid therapy, therapy with carbenicillin or amphotericin B, diabetic ketoacidosis, and massive trauma. Metabolic alkalosis causes a temporary serum hypokalemia as potassium enters the cell when sodium and hydrogen leave the cell; it rectifies itself when the alkalosis is corrected.

Symptoms of hypokalemia are related to impaired nerve conduction in cardiac, skeletal, and smooth muscle. The laboratory results, symptoms, treatment, and nursing management are described in Table 18-8.

Potassium excess (hyperkalemia)

Etiology *Hyperkalemia*, or excess serum potassium, may result from renal failure, hemolysis, excessive or too rapid infusion of potassium supplements or banked blood, and severe burns or crushing injuries. Metabolic acidosis may temporarily cause a rise in serum potassium, but this is usually reduced as the acidosis is corrected.

Symptoms of potassium excess, laboratory results, clinical manifestations, and nursing management are presented in Table 18-8.

Calcium and phosphate balance

Both *calcium* and *phosphate* are found primarily in the bones; 99 percent of the body's calcium is in the teeth and bones. The remaining 1 percent is in the plasma and cells. The normal value for serum calcium is 9.0 to 11.0 mg per 100 ml. About 85 percent of phosphate is in the skeleton; the remaining 15 percent is in soft tissues. Phosphate is critical for cellular metabolism, especially metabolism of red blood cells. In addition, it is part of the energy storage system (adenosine triphosphate). In children, the normal serum value of phosphate varies between 3.0 and 4.5 mg per 100 ml.

Calcium is a component of cell cement, which determines the thickness, strength, and permeability of cell membranes. Furthermore, calcium is essential for contraction of muscles. Calcium abnormalities cause cardiac irregularities and skeletal muscle problems, such as leg cramps.

Calcium is required to metabolize and absorb vitamin B_{12}, to activate enzymes for chemical reactions, and to convert prothrombin to thrombin in the clotting mechanism.

Vitamin D promotes calcium absorption from the intestines, while increasing renal excretion of phosphate. *Parathormone*, a parathyroid hormone, regulates the plasma phosphorus and calcium levels. Parathormone enhances calcium absorption from the intestines and the kidneys to raise the serum calcium level. It also increases osteoclastic (bone-destroying) activity, which releases calcium into the bloodstream to raise the serum concentration. This results in the release of calcium from the bones and occurs in rickets (soft, porous bones). *Calcitonin*, a thyroid hormone, facilitates calcium excretion by the kidneys as the serum calcium level increases.

Dairy products are sources of both calcium and phosphate. Green, leafy vegetables are high in calcium. Children who refuse milk can be given cheese, ice cream, yogurt, puddings, and custards. Instant milk can also be camouflaged in baked goods.

Calcium imbalances

Calcium deficit (hypocalcemia)

Etiology *Hypocalcemia*, or calcium deficit, occurs when the serum calcium level falls below 8 mg per 100 ml. It results from prolonged inadequate dietary intake. Inadequate vitamin D intake and decreased absorption due to altered metabolism, diarrhea, or copious wound exudate may cause hypocalcemia. Exchange transfusions with citrated blood, hypoparathyroidism, and increased excretion due to renal failure may also contribute to hypocalcemia. Mothers with diabetes mellitus or hyperparathyroidism may deliver a newborn with transient hypoparathyroidism. Because the parathyroid gland controls the calcium level, this results in a temporary low serum calcium level.

With inadequate calcium, the body's nerves become increasingly excitable and fire spontaneously. This causes contraction of muscles and paresthesias. Laboratory results, symptoms, and nursing management are described in Table 18-8.

Calcium excess (hypercalcemia)

Etiology *Hypercalcemia*, or excessive calcium, is present when the serum calcium level exceeds 12 mg per 100 ml. It is caused by vitamin D metabolism deficit or vitamin D intoxication during pregnancy or childhood, excessive milk ingestion, hyperparathyroidism, and bone tumors. Metabolic acidosis and idiopathic (cause unknown) hypercalcemia can also occur.

Calcium enhances the movement of sodium into the cell, causing depolarization. Excess calcium inhibits proper functioning of the sodium pump and sedates nerve transmission.

Phosphate imbalance

Phosphate deficit (hypophosphatemia)

Etiology *Hypophosphatemia* occurs when serum levels fall below 3.0 mg per 100 ml. It is caused by decreased intake or absorption in conditions such as malabsorption, small bowel disease, and starvation and when total parenteral nutrition solutions without phosphate are given. Phosphate losses via the kidneys can occur as a result of taking thiazide diuretics and with hyperparathyroidism and diabetic ketoacidosis.

The signs and symptoms result from the decreased production of adenosine triphosphate and from alterations in all cellular functions. Laboratory results, other clinical manifestations, and nursing management are described in Table 18-8.

Phosphate excess (hyperphosphatemia) *Hyperphosphatemia* is almost always present in cases of acute and chronic renal failure. It may be severe in the urate nephropathy associated with leukemia and rhabdomyolysis. Hyperphosphatemia occurs at levels of more than 5.0 mg per 100 ml. Clinical manifestations are listed in Table 18-8.

Magnesium balance

Magnesium is found in the bone cells (50 percent); specialized cells of the heart, liver, and skeletal muscles (49 percent); and the extracellular fluid (1 percent). The normal serum magnesium level is 1.5 to 1.9 mEq per liter.

The functions of magnesium are similar to those of calcium. Magnesium has been used successfully to treat cardiac arrhythmias and to reduce hyperactive muscle response in toxemia of pregnancy. This leads to the belief that magnesium has a role in nerve impulse transmission and muscle function. Magnesium is also used as a supplement to antihypertensive agents.

Recently, it has been found that magnesium activates enzymatic reactions related to vitamin B functions and the body's use of potassium, calcium, and protein. Like calcium, it inhibits muscle contraction.

Magnesium, like calcium, is regulated by the parathyroid gland. Magnesium and calcium compete for absorption, and as the absorption rate of one increases, the absorption rate of the other decreases. Magnesium is also regulated by the renal system. As the magnesium level of the blood drops, the renal excretion of magnesium slows.

Magnesium imbalances

Magnesium deficit (hypomagnesemia)

Etiology *Hypomagnesemia* (a serum magnesium level of less than 1.5 mEq per liter) is related to decreased intake (as in malnutrition or starvation), to decreased absorption (as in malabsorption syndromes), to small bowel resections, or to increased dietary intake of calcium. In the newborn, it may occur as a result of a familial condition, hypoparathyroidism, or renal damage.

Since magnesium stabilizes nerve impulse transmission, inadequate magnesium causes increased nerve irritability and other symptoms listed in Table 18-8.

Magnesium excess (hypermagnesemia)

Etiology *Hypermagnesemia* (a serum magnesium level elevated above 2 mEq per liter) is more rare than hypomagnesemia. Renal disease, decreasing magnesium excretion, uncontrolled diabetic acidosis, and excessive administration may cause this electrolyte abnormality. When a pregnant woman has received magnesium sulfate or has taken magnesium-containing antacids or magnesium salt cathartics excessively, the residuals may be found in the newborn.

Excess magnesium has a sedative effect on the nerves. Other symptoms are presented in Table 18-8.

ACID-BASE BALANCE

The *acidity* of a solution is usually expressed as *pH;* pH can be translated as "power of hydrogen" and is a means of expressing hydrogen concentration.

The pH of the blood is held within a very narrow range, about 7.35 to 7.45, with a mean value of 7.40. Extremes of 6.70 (low) and 7.70 (high) can be tolerated only for short periods of time. Body cells cannot live in an environment with too little or too great a concentration of hydrogen; therefore, the acidity (hydrogen concentration) of body fluids is of great importance. Several physiological regulatory mechanisms interact to maintain pH within normal limits.

Normal acid production

On a daily basis, the processes of cellular metabolism produce an excess of acid. This excess must be neutralized or eliminated from the body in order to maintain normal pH. Acids formed are of two types: volatile and nonvolatile.

Volatile acids are so named because they dissociate into carbon dioxide (CO_2) gas, which easily diffuses across the alveolocapillary membrane and is removed during ventilation. Most of the acid produced daily is carbonic acid, which is formed when the carbon in foods is oxidized to yield carbon dioxide. The carbon dioxide combines with water (H_2) to form carbonic acid (H_2CO_3) as follows:

$$CO_2 + H_2O \rightleftharpoons H_2CO_3 \rightleftharpoons HCO_3^- + H^+$$

However, carbonic acid is a weak acid and can be dissociated into bicarbonate (HCO_3^-) and hydrogen (H^+). As indicated by the arrows, though, these reactions are reversible to carbon dioxide and water.

Nonvolatile acids are excreted by the kidneys, not the lungs. Sulfuric acid and phosphoric acid are examples. They are produced in the metabolism of proteins, carbohydrates, and fats.

Control of pH

There are three physiological regulatory mechanisms that interact to maintain pH within normal levels: (1) buffers, (2) ventilation via the lungs, and (3) excretion through the kidneys. Buffers tend to make their corrections within seconds; the lungs, within minutes; and the kidneys, within hours to days.

Buffers *Buffers* are compounds that enable body fluids to correct changes in pH when acidic or alkaline substances are added. Most buffers of the body consist of a pair of compounds and hence are called *buffer systems*. The three main ones are (1) the bicarbonate buffer system, (2) the phosphate buffer system, and (3) the protein buffer system.

The bicarbonate buffer system is the primary buffer system of the plasma and interstitial fluid. It consists of bicarbonate and carbonic acid. When hydrogen is added to a solution containing this buffer system, some of it immediately combines with bicarbonate molecules to form carbonic acid. The carbonic acid and bicarbonate ions are normally maintained at a ratio of 1 to 20 (see Fig. 18-12). The pH remains stable as long as this ratio is maintained.

$$H^+ + HCO_3^- \rightleftharpoons H_2CO_3$$

As a result, the increase in hydrogen in the solution is much reduced. The carbonic acid ties up much of the added hydrogen and holds the solution close to its original pH. The opposite would follow a decrease in hydrogen below normal levels. The reactions would shift to the right, with a breakup of carbonic acid and an increase in hydrogen and bicarbonate.

$$H_2CO_3 \rightleftharpoons H^+ + HCO_3^-$$

The phosphate and protein buffer systems predominate in the intracellular fluid. The phosphate buffer is filtered at the glomerulus and is poorly reabsorbed. Alkaline phosphate (HPO_4^-) picks up excess hydrogen from the renal tubular cells to become phosphoric acid (H_2PO_4). The acid is then excreted in the urine. To offset the loss of a positive (hydrogen) ion, a sodium (Na^+) ion is reabsorbed, increasing sodium bicarbonate ($NaHCO_3$) in the ECF.

The protein buffer system is found in the intravascular fluid in the form of plasma proteins. Some proteins have extra acid radicals (^-COOH), and others have extra base radicals ($^-NH_2$). Proteins can therefore donate or accept hydrogen ions as needed to maintain the normal pH of intravascular fluids.

Hemoglobin is an example of a protein buffer which functions to attach carbon dioxide directly or indirectly. Buffering occurs when carbon dioxide diffuses into the red blood cells and forms carbonic acid. The carbonic acid then dissociates into hydrogen and bicarbonate. The hydrogen attaches to the hemoglobin molecule, and bicarbonate is available for buffering in the plasma.

Respiratory mechanisms The lungs are able to excrete or retain carbon dioxide by altering ventilation. Changes in hydrogen and carbon dioxide affect the respiratory center in the cerebral medulla in such a way as to increase or decrease the rate and depth of ventilation. *Hypoventilation* causes an increase in carbon dioxide and therefore increases the acidity of the blood. *Hyperventilation*, on the other hand, causes a decrease in carbon dioxide, and, therefore, the blood becomes alkalotic. Respiratory adjustment begins within minutes of a change in pH. Res-

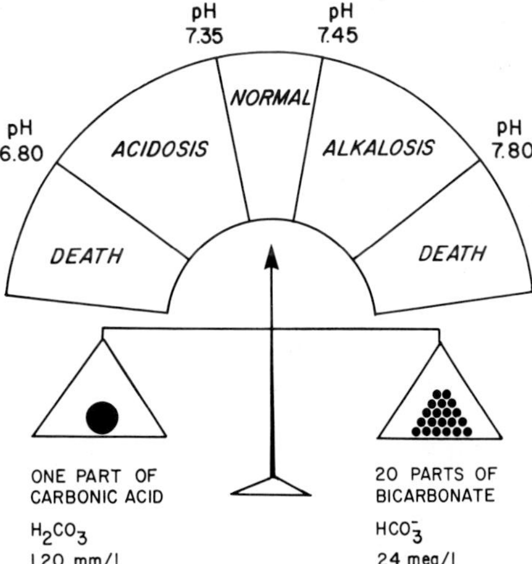

Figure 18-12 The bicarbonate buffer system. The body maintains a ratio of 1 part carbonic acid to 20 parts bicarbonate. An alkaline deficit or an acid excess will bring a shift to the left. An alkaline excess or an acid deficit will bring a shift to the right. (*Adapted from Abbott Laboratories, "Fluid and Electrolytes: Some Practical Guides to Clinical Use," in Rosanne B. Howard and Nancie H. Herbold, Nutrition in Clinical Care, McGraw-Hill, New York, 1978. Used with permission.*)

piratory ability to normalize pH, however, is limited.

Renal mechanisms For a buffer system to work, the buffer compounds have to be available in the right amounts. Maintaining the proportion of about 1 carbonic acid molecule for every 20 bicarbonate molecules is the job of the kidneys.

The kidneys return pH to normal through three mechanisms: (1) bicarbonate reabsorption, (2) formation of a titratable acid, and (3) the ammonium mechanism.

Bicarbonate reabsorption involves the reabsorption of sodium and bicarbonate ions in exchange for hydrogen ions. The rate at which this occurs depends on the pH of the blood. The formation of phosphoric acid has already been described in the discussion of the phosphate buffer system.

The ammonium mechanism functions to eliminate excess hydrogen ions. Ammonia (NH_3), which is formed by the renal tubules, is changed into ammonium (NH_4). The ammonium combines with a negative ion, such as a chloride ion, and releases a sodium ion, which is reabsorbed and adds sodium bicarbonate to the blood. Renal tubular synthesis of ammonia is controlled by the amount of hydrogen ion secreted.

Acid production in children is normally 2 to 3 mEq per kilogram of body weight per day. This acid is buffered by bicarbonate ions that form carbon dioxide. In addition, sodium sulfate and sodium phosphate are excreted by the kidneys as ammonium and phosphate ions. Sodium and bicarbonate then return to the ECF via the kidneys.

Alterations in acid-base balance

A change in the concentration of hydrogen ion or bicarbonate ion will produce a state of acidosis or alkalosis.

Acidosis refers to an elevation of the hydrogen ion concentration above normal or to a decrease in the bicarbonate ion concentration below normal. This situation results in a pH of body fluids below 7.35. Either respiratory (volatile) or metabolic (nonvolatile) changes can cause acidosis.

In *alkalosis,* there is a decrease in the hydrogen ion concentration or an elevation in the bicarbonate ion concentration. The pH of body fluids will be above 7.45. The cause of depleted hydrogen ion may be respiratory, with hyperventilation eliminating carbon dioxide (acid), or metabolic, with primary base bicarbonate excess.

Effects of potassium on pH Potassium and hydrogen are cations that can be exchanged between the intracellular and extracellular compartments. Potassium or hydrogen is secreted into the tubular fluid of the kidneys as sodium is reabsorbed. Thus, in hypokalemia there is a decrease in the number of potassium ions available for secretion, which allows for an increase in hydrogen ion secretion into the urine. Since hydrogen is lost, alkalosis results. The opposite situation—acidosis—can occur with hyperkalemia. In this case, hydrogen moves into the cells, and potassium moves out. Consequently, serum potassium levels increase approximately 0.6 mEq per liter for every 0.1 decrease in pH. Alkalosis has the opposite effect on serum potassium levels: hydrogen moves out of the cells, and potassium moves in to take its place and maintain a balance.

Effects of chloride on pH When there is a need for an ion exchange, chloride and bicarbonate can replace each other. There is a reciprocal relationship between serum chloride and serum bicarbonate levels. Thus, when chloride levels increase, the bicarbonate concentration decreases. *Hyperchloremic acidosis* occurs when excess levels of chloride are present, and *hypochloremic alkalosis* occurs when an increase in pH results from decreased serum chloride levels.

Metabolic acidosis

Etiology *Metabolic acidosis* is a decrease in plasma pH below 7.35, resulting from an accumulation of acids or a primary bicarbonate deficit. Newborns and young children are at risk of becoming acidotic because their buffer systems are immature. Furthermore, the young child's high metabolic rate increases the formation of acids and the potential for acidosis. Metabolic acidosis appears most often in children with diabetic or starvation ketoacidosis, diarrhea, vomiting, salicylate intoxication, and renal disease. Babies who are fed cow's milk also have a greater tendency to develop metabolic acidosis because of the high phosphate and sulfate content of cow's milk. Any gastrointestinal losses (e.g., from diarrhea or vomiting) from below the pyloric sphincter cause acidosis because the excreted fluid contains large amounts of bicarbonate. The normal newborn may be acidotic at birth, but this acidosis is resolved by the second day of life. Excessive addition of chloride to the body—for example, by administering drugs such as ammonium chloride—can also contribute to acidosis.

To compensate for metabolic acidosis, the kidneys excrete hydrogen ions or conserve bicarbonate ions. In addition, the respiratory system responds with hyperventilation as a means of excreting excess carbon dioxide. Primary metabolic acidosis usually results in pallor, tachypnea, and lethargy. See Table 18-11 for further signs of acid-base imbalance.

Metabolic alkalosis

Etiology *Metabolic alkalosis* (primary bicarbonate excess) occurs when a metabolic malfunction brings about an increased amount of a base or a decreased amount of an acid. Four of the most common causes are (1) administration or ingestion of excess sodium bicarbonate, (2) loss of chloride as hydrochloric acid during vomiting or gastric suctioning, (3) excessive excretion of acid in the urine, and (4) decreased serum potassium, due to the movement of hydrogen ions out of the cells and into the serum and to the movement of potassium ions into the cells. The clinical manifestations of metabolic alkalosis are listed in Table 18-11.

Respiratory acidosis

Etiology *Respiratory acidosis* (carbon dioxide excess) in infants and children may be caused by obstructive pulmonary problems such as cystic fibrosis, asthma, croup, respiratory distress syndrome, and foreign-body aspiration; it can also be caused by neuromuscular disorders such as muscular dystrophy or Guillain-Barré syndrome. These diseases generally reduce pulmonary ventilation, causing retention of carbon dioxide (increased carbon dioxide) and an increase in the serum carbonic acid level. This results in respiratory acidosis.

Table 18-11 Acid-Base Imbalances: Clinical Manifestations and Nursing Management

Imbalance	Laboratory results	Clinical manifestations	Nursing management
Metabolic acidosis	Normal or decreased pH (see Table 18-10); decreased bicarbonate; normal to decreased P_{CO_2}; negative base excess; increased potassium (or decreased ketoacidosis); decreased CO_2 combining power; urine pH less than 6 (see Table 18-10)	Weakness; lethargy; nausea and vomiting; hyperventilation; Kussmaul respirations; abdominal pain; acetone breath; stupor and coma; pallor; tachypnea	Infuse glucose, insulin, and potassium intravenously for diabetic ketoacidosis. Infuse sodium bicarbonate intravenously. Infuse IV fluids (to replace vomiting and diarrheal losses). Possibly place the child on dialysis for renal failure. Assess symptoms of metabolic acidosis. Monitor intake and output strictly. Monitor serum electrolytes. Monitor vital signs (to check for symptoms of fluid volume deficit). Assess neurological status: level of consciousness and pupillary response. Take precautions against seizures (if indicated). Monitor serum glucose level and glucose in urine (if the child has diabetic ketoacidosis). Monitor urine pH and specific gravity.

Table 18-11 Acid-Base Imbalances: Clinical Manifestations and Nursing Management (*Continued*)

Imbalance	Laboratory results	Clinical manifestations	Nursing management
Metabolic alkalosis	Increased pH; increased bicarbonate; slightly increased P_{CO_2}; decreased serum potassium; possibly decreased serum chloride (in children with hypochloremic alkalosis); increased CO_2 combining power; urine pH elevated over 7	Hypoventilation (to increase P_{CO_2} and conserve carbonic acid); hypertonicity of muscles with tetany, tremors, and convulsions; irritability; confusion; vertigo; numbness and tingling	Infuse fluids intravenously (to replace lost fluids). Infuse electrolytes intravenously, especially potassium and chloride. Possibly infuse acidifying drugs (ammonium chloride as a temporary treatment). Monitor intake and output. Monitor signs of hypokalemia: vital signs, arrhythmias, and muscle weakness. Monitor serum potassium level. Assess respiratory depression. Take precautions against seizures. Assess and care for vomiting. Monitor dosages of sedative drugs (to avoid further respiratory depression).
Respiratory acidosis	Decreased pH; normal to increased bicarbonate; increased P_{CO_2}; increased serum potassium; urine pH below 6	Weakness and listlessness; disorientation, somnolence, stupor, and coma (with high P_{CO_2}); diaphoresis; rapid, irregular pulse; decreased respirations; dyspnea and breathlessness; possible arrhythmias	Administer sodium bicarbonate intravenously or orally. Use mechanical ventilation (if indicated). Perform postural drainage, suctioning, and oxygen prn. Assess respiratory function. Turn the child, and have the child cough and deep-breathe. Assess pulse changes. Assess level of consciousness. Monitor hydration status. Carefully use pain medications and sedatives.
Respiratory alkalosis	Increased pH above 7.45; normal P_{O_2}; normal bicarbonate; decreased P_{CO_2}	Headache; vertigo; tetany, tremors, convulsions, and coma; numbness and tingling of the hands and face; deep, rapid respirations; confusion; irritability	Infuse chloride intravenously (to neutralize bicarbonate). Use rebreathing bag (to increase P_{CO_2} level). Administer sedatives. Assess respiratory rate and status. Monitor serum potassium level (it may decrease with renal compensation). Observe for vertigo. Encourage the child to breathe more slowly.

Respiratory alkalosis

Etiology *Respiratory alkalosis* (primary carbonic acid deficit) occurs in children as a result of hyperventilation, hysteria, meningeal irritation, brain tumors, or salicylate ingestion. The increased respirations cause an excessive loss of carbon dioxide, resulting in a carbonic acid deficit. The clinical manifestations, treatment, and nursing management are listed in Table 18-11.

ASSESSING FLUID AND ELECTROLYTE DISTURBANCES

All hospitalized children are at risk for developing fluid and electrolyte imbalances. The nurse is responsible for thoroughly assessing changes in the child's fluid and electrolyte status.

The history

During the admission interview the nurse should obtain a complete history from the parents and review what is already known about the child. The nurse should determine whether the disease process, liquid feedings, or medication could result in a fluid and electrolyte loss or gain. For example, pyloric stenosis causes vomiting of hydrochloric acid, diuretics such as Lasix may cause potassium depletion, and liquid feedings may increase serum sodium levels.

Information about the child's normal and current intake and output should be obtained. If the child has had diarrhea or vomiting, it is important to obtain information about (1) the frequency, duration, and character of the stools; (2) the volume of lost fluid; and (3) whether the diarrhea or vomiting is related to any changes in the child's diet. Past colds or fevers, recent immunizations given or antibiotics taken, and trauma may be significant factors in the illness.

General appearance and behavior

Observe the child's general appearance, and then confirm your conclusions with the parents. Parents are usually very alert to even the most subtle changes in their child's behavior. Watch for tremors, lack of coordination, or purposeless movements. Also observe the child for lethargy, irritability, or inappropriate responses to stimulation.

The physical examination

As part of the physical examination, the nurse should observe the following:

1. *Skin color and turgor* The *color* of the child's skin is important in assessing hydration. Mild fluid loss will change the normal color to a pasty, pale color. Moderate to severe dehydration will change the skin color to a grayish, mottled hue as a result of decreased peripheral circulation. Skin or tissue *turgor* refers to the elasticity of the skin. It is evaluated by pinching up a section of tissue and then observing it as it falls back into place. The skin turgor can be assessed on the abdomen near the umbilicus in a young child or on the inner thigh in an older child. The well-hydrated child's skin returns quickly to a normal state when released. The skin of a child with a fluid volume deficit remains in a tented (raised) position for several seconds after release (see Fig. 18-7).

   Normal skin turgor begins to be lost after a 5 percent fluid volume loss. Malnutrition may also decrease skin turgor because not enough protein is being ingested to firm the cells. Sodium deficit and fluid loss cause a shift of fluid from the extracellular to the intracellular compartment, causing the tissues to have a characteristic fingerprinting. Hypernatremia will cause the tissue to take on a thick consistency.
2. *Signs of edema* Edema occurs in cases of fluid overload and hypernatremia. Often periorbital edema may be one of the first indications of fluid overload in infants and young children. In addition, dependent edema of the extremities or sacrum may occur.
3. *Mucous membranes* The mucous membranes should be observed for any signs of decreased salivation. Be sure to observe for mouth breathing, since this will also cause dry mucous membranes.
4. *Vein filling* Distended or flat neck veins may give valuable information about fluid volume overload or deficit. The neck veins should be observed with the child at a 45° angle. Venous filling is not easy to assess in infants because their necks are short and often chubby.
5. *Fontanels and suture lines* In the infant, the fontanels become depressed, and the skull suture lines are more prominent, when a fluid deficit exists.

6. *Eyes* The absence of tearing indicates a fluid deficit and occurs in cases of moderate dehydration (10 percent). Moderate to severe dehydration will cause a decrease in the extracellular fluid around the eyes, causing them to appear sunken.

Age and body surface area

A vital part of any assessment of a child includes an evaluation of fluid intake based on calculated requirements. This requires using the child's body surface area or body weight to compute daily requirements.

Output

To assess for fluid balance or imbalance, estimate total output. Both sensible and insensible fluid losses must be considered. Sensible fluid losses are the obvious fluid losses, such as fluid lost in the urine and stool. Insensible fluid losses are less apparent, such as fluid lost through skin evaporation and respiration.

Normal urine output should be more than 1 ml per kilogram of body weight per hour.[13] When fluid balance is critical for the very ill child, output should be *accurately recorded*. This may be done by using a 24-h urine collection bag or by weighing diapers on a gram scale before and after voiding; 1 g equals 1 ml (see Chap. 16).

Abnormal losses, such as fluid lost in diarrhea stools, vomiting, wound drainage, and gastric drainage, must be carefully measured and recorded, and total output must be calculated. Infants and young children show the effects of fluid imbalance much more rapidly than older children and adults because a greater percentage of their fluid volume remains in the extracellular compartment (see Table 18-1).

Other factors influence insensible fluid loss. Fever increases insensible fluid losses via evaporation through the skin; there is about a 12 percent increase for each degree of fever above a rectal temperature of 37.8°C. Infants who are receiving bilirubin phototherapy or who are placed in radiant warmers lose from 10 to 20 percent more fluid through evaporation via the skin.[14]

Weight

The child's weight is a very sensitive indicator of fluid loss or gain. Compare the present weight with the past weight. This provides a baseline for fluid and electrolyte replacement and for assessment of fluid gains or losses. The child should be weighed at the same time each day, before eating, and on the same scale to ensure accuracy. Record the time, the clothing worn (preferably none) and intravenous lines or dressings that are in place, and the scale used. Small changes in daily weight may be significant. A weight gain or loss of 50 g per day in an infant, 200 per day in a child, and 500 per day in an adolescent should be brought to the attention of the physician.[15]

Vital signs

Temperature Fluid shifts in dehydration may initially cause an elevated temperature, but as energy production decreases, the temperature may decrease. Severe fluid volume loss causes the skin to become cool; this is especially noticeable in the extremities. The young child's peripheral blood vessels have poor perfusion, which is further decreased as blood is shunted to the vital organs.

Respirations The rate, depth, regularity, and character of the child's respirations must be assessed. *Hyperpnea* increases insensible water loss from the lungs. *Kussmaul breathing* is an attempt to reduce metabolic acidosis by blowing off carbon dioxide. Respirations should be counted for a full minute, and any abnormalities in depth or rhythm should be noted.

Pulse The pulse rate increases as the fluid volume and blood pressure decrease. The increased pulse rate is a compensatory mechanism whereby the heart pumps faster to provide adequate nutrients within a smaller amount of fluid to the cells. Irregularities in the heart rhythm may result from electrolyte imbalances, such as hypokalemia. The pulse should be taken apically for a full minute to detect abnormalities.

Blood pressure Blood pressure may not be the most reliable indicator of fluid volume deficit in children. The increased elasticity of children's arteries causes them to close around a diminishing blood volume in order to keep blood pressure stable.

Laboratory test results Laboratory test results provide additional information about the child's status (see Table 18-10). The hematocrit, serum electrolytes, blood urea nitrogen, and carbon dioxide are often tested every 4 to 8 h to assess the degree of fluid volume deficit. An elevated hematocrit, elevated levels of blood urea nitrogen and hemoglobin, and an elevated urine specific gravity reflect hemoconcentration due to fluid volume deficit. When the values are below normal, hemodilution due to fluid volume excess may be indicated. The serum sodium level indicates the type of dehydration present. In cases of hypertonic fluid deficit, the sodium level is elevated; in cases of hypotonic fluid deficit, the sodium level is lowered; and in cases of isotonic fluid deficit, the serum sodium level is normal.

Table 18-12 Composition of Common Hydrating Solutions

Solution	Sodium (mEq per liter)	Osmolality (mOsmol per liter)
Dextrose in water, 5%	—	250
Dextrose in water, 10%	—	505
Dextrose in saline, 5% in 0.2%	34	320
Dextrose in saline, 5% in 0.45%	77	405

Source: R. M. Perkin and D. L. Levin, *Pediatric Clinics of North America*, **27**:567–586 (1980).

MANAGEMENT OF FLUID AND ELECTROLYTE DISTURBANCES

Fluid and electrolyte replacement

There are four main classes of parenteral solutions: protein, plasma-expanding, hydrating, and replacement solutions.

Protein solutions contain amino acids and may be given in the form of total parenteral nutrition to supply protein, calories (dextrose is added), and fluid. They may also be given as 5 percent albumin solutions to control third spacing (fluid accumulation in areas that normally have minimal or no fluid, e.g., ascites, edema from burns) of fluid in postsurgical patients or to increase plasma protein levels in conditions such as nephrotic syndrome (see Chap. 20).

Plasma-expanding solutions are colloidal solutions that pull fluid into the vascular space, thereby expanding the intravascular (plasma) volume. Protein solutions such as 5 percent albumin are also colloids and are commonly given to children who are in early shock to correct hypovolemia.

Hydrating solutions include dextrose—either 5 or 10 percent—with sodium chloride of varying amounts (see Table 18-12). These solutions are used for daily maintenance of body fluids. A 5 percent dextrose solution is used for older infants and children. Young infants, because they have immature livers and deplete their glucose stores much more rapidly when under stress, may require a 10 percent dextrose solution. The sodium chloride amounts will vary, depending on the daily requirements of the individual child; 0.2 percent is commonly used.

Replacement solutions are designed to replace lost fluids and electrolytes; 5 percent dextrose and 0.45 percent sodium chloride with 20 mEq of potassium chloride per liter of solution is commonly used to replace lost gastric fluids in children.

The osmolarity of body fluids, 280 to 290 milliosmols per liter, is used as a reference to describe parenteral fluids. Therefore, parenteral fluids may also be described in terms of their tonicity or osmolarity, i.e., described as hypertonic, hypotonic, or isotonic. Very hypotonic solutions will cause red blood cells to swell and burst. Water is an example of a very hypotonic solution and must never be used without the addition of a solute, such as dextrose. A 5 percent dextrose solution contains 280 milliosmols per liter, which is isotonic with body fluids. When 0.45 percent sodium chloride or 0.2 percent sodium chloride to 5 percent dextrose is added, the solution becomes slightly hypertonic (see Table 18-12).

Intravenous therapy

See Chap. 16 for a discussion of the initiation and maintenance of intravenous therapy in children.

APPLICATION TO THE CHILD WITH DIARRHEA

Etiology

Diarrhea is an increase in the number of stools or a decreased firm consistency of the stools. It is classified as either acute or chronic. *Acute diarrhea* is a sudden change in the frequency or consistency of the stools. It is usually self-limiting, whereas chronic diarrhea may persist for 2 weeks or more. Acute diarrhea is related to infection (viral or bacterial), ingestion of a toxic substance (e.g., arsenic, lead, or iron), administration of antibiotics (e.g., ampicillin), overfeeding, changes in diet (e.g., new foods, excessive carbohydrates, or unripe fruits), emotional stress, fatigue, and other infections (e.g., otitis media and urinary tract infections).

Chronic diarrhea is often associated with malabsorption disorders (e.g., cystic fibrosis and celiac disease), nutritional deficiencies (e.g., kwashiorkor and marasmus), allergies (e.g., to milk), inflammatory disorders (e.g., ulcerative colitis), and anatomic defects (e.g., intermittent or incomplete small bowel obstructions).

Pathophysiology

The intestinal contents are propelled along so rapidly that there is inadequate time for absorption of digested foods, water, and electrolytes. The resultant stool contains undigested fats, carbohydrates, and, to a lesser extent, protein. It is green, watery, mucus-streaked, possibly blood-tinged, and expelled with force. Water losses in the stool may be increased to 250 to 500 ml per 24 h. This is 10 to 15 times the normal rate. Electrolytes—specifically sodium, chloride, bicarbonate, and potassium—are also lost in amounts 10 times greater than normal. Altered fluid and electrolyte balance is the primary pathophysiological consequence of diarrhea. The child presents with symptoms of dehydration and metabolic acidosis.

Clinical manifestations

The signs and symptoms observed are directly related to the severity of the diarrhea, which determines the percent of dehydration and acid-base imbalance. Diarrhea is generally classified according to the percent of dehydration present. Table 18-7 lists the physical changes that occur according to the percent of dehydration.

Treatment

Hospitalization is necessary to reverse the symptoms of fluid and electrolyte imbalance in cases of moderate and severe dehydration. Medical treatment focuses on prescribing intravenous fluids to meet the child's normal fluid requirements and to replace fluid lost through diarrhea. In addition to maintenance fluid requirements, an estimated 50 ml per kilogram of body weight is needed to replace fluid lost in cases of mild diarrhea (5 percent dehydration), 100 ml per kilogram of body weight to replace fluid lost in cases of moderate diarrhea (10 percent dehydration), and 125 ml per kilogram of body weight to replace fluid lost in cases of severe diarrhea (10 to 15 percent dehydration). This additional fluid is administered over 8 to 16 h to prevent fluid volume excess. The intravenous solution contains glucose for calories and normal saline.

Potassium is added only after adequate kidney function has been documented, since without sufficient kidney function, potassium is retained, and hyperkalemia results.

Nursing management

The nurse should carefully assess the child who is at risk for developing fluid and electrolyte imbalances. Precisely determine the child's hydration status by observing:

1. The child's skin turgor and mucous membranes, fontanels, and neurological function.
2. The child's weight, to determine whether there has been a weight loss.
3. The child's stool, to check for color, odor, consistency, amount, pH, and the presence of pus, blood, and sugar (reducing substances).
4. The child's urine, to check for amount, color, concentration, and specific gravity.
5. The child's vital signs, to check for changes that indicate fluid volume deficit. The axillary temperature must be taken, not the rectal temperature, because rectal stimulation may provoke intestinal motility and increase stooling.
6. The rate at which intravenous fluid is being infused and the site.
7. The skin in the diaper area, to check for redness, rash, or excoriation.

Children need frequent attention to oral hygiene during the period when they can take nothing by mouth. They also need meticulous diaper care to prevent diaper rash. Infants and young children who are unable to eat may receive emotional satisfaction from sucking on a

Table 18-13 Composition of Fluids Given Orally

Fluid	Sodium	Potassium (mEq)	Chloride	Solute (mOsmol per liter)	Calories (kilocalories per liter)
Water 0	0	0	0	0	0
Sugar water (56%)*	0	0	0	0	200
Lytren	25	25	30	135	280
Pedialyte	30	20	30	115	280
Coca-Cola	0.5	13	0	27	435
Pepsi Cola	7	1	0	15	480
Ginger ale	3	1	1	10	380
Seven-Up	7.5	0.5	0	15	420
Orange juice	2	48	2	100	410
Gatorade	0.23	2.5	—	50	167
Boiled skimmed milk†	27	43	31	350	410
One-half boiled skimmed milk‡	13	21	15	175	205

Note: This table presents the electrolyte, solute, and caloric content of fluids commonly given to infants who are unable to take their usual diet.

*Prepared at home by using 3 tbsp per quart of water.

†Assuming no evaporation. In practice, boiling creates an evaporative loss, producing higher values than those shown.

‡Equal amounts of water and skimmed milk.

Source: W. Weil, *Fluid and Electrolyte Metabolism in Infants and Children,* Grune & Stratton, New York, 1977, p. 111. Reprinted with permission.

pacifier. The child who cries often needs frequent bubbling to expel swallowed air. Enteric isolation should be scrupulously maintained.

When the child is ready to resume eating, begin with clear liquids. Ice chips, weak tea, diluted grape or apple juice, diluted liquid gelatin desserts, Gatorade, and "flat" carbonated beverages are appropriate choices (see Table 18-13). When the child can tolerate the clear fluid, he or she is progressed to a bland diet. Offer white toast, plain crackers, cooked rice or puffed rice cereals, ripe bananas, and unsweetened applesauce. Milk should be avoided at this stage because the milk sugar is thought to increase stooling.

The child can resume a regular diet when he or she can tolerate the bland diet without an increase in stooling or abdominal cramping. The stools should remain free of pus, blood, and other reducing substances. The child can progress from half-strength skim milk to full-strength skim milk over a period of 2 to 3 days. The child can also be given antidiarrheal medications.

Nursing Care Plan: Fluid Volume Deficit

Patient: Karen White *Age:* 9 months *Date of Admission:* 3/18

ASSESSMENT

Karen White, a 9-month-old infant, was admitted to the pediatric nursery at 9 A.M. with a tentative diagnosis of viral gastroenteritis and 5 percent dehydration. The following information was given by her mother during the admission interview.

Two days ago, Karen began vomiting and passing frequent watery stools, approximately 10 per day. She usually has three soft, formed stools per day. Karen's 3-year-old brother and 5-year-old sister had vomiting and diarrhea for the last 3 days.

Mrs. White called her doctor and followed his instructions to limit Karen's oral intake to clear liquids, but the vomiting and diarrhea have continued. Over the past 24 h, Karen has been sleeping more and, when awake, is very irritable. Karen's axillary temperature has ranged from 37.8 to 38.3°C (100° to 101°F).

Her mother seems exhausted and very concerned. She commented, "I am so tired, with all three children sick. The other two children seem to be getting better. They, at least, have stopped vomiting and are keeping down sips of soda. But I'm really worried about Karen. She's not even keeping soda down and is still having diarrhea. She hasn't had a wet diaper since eight o'clock last evening."

Physical examination

Weight: 8.1 kg. Prior to illness at the last well-child checkup 2 weeks ago, weight was 8.5 kg (19 lb). Temperature: 38°C. Pulse: 108. Respiratory rate: 28. Blood pressure: stable at 104/64.

Behavior

Is lethargic at present. Dozes when left alone, passively submits to all procedures, and is very irritable when aroused. Has a weak, whining cry. Hesitates to go to her mother, and then clings to her mother.

Hydration

Skin turgor is decreased; a slight delay in return to normal. Mucous membranes dry along the cheek and gum line.

Eyes

No tearing is evident; the eyeballs are sunken and soft.

Fontanel

Slightly depressed.

Intake

Has sipped only water in the last 24 h; has vomited all intake within 10 min after each sip.

Output

Wet last diaper at 8 P.M. yesterday, 13 h ago. The mother states that the urine was bright yellow.

Abdomen

Is tense when palpated; hyperactive bowel sounds.

Extremities

Are pale and cool to the touch.

PHYSICIAN'S ORDERS

1. Private room, enteric isolation.
2. Strict record of intake and output.

3. Check urine specific gravity with each voiding.
4. Laboratory work: hematocrit, blood urea nitrogen, sodium, chloride, potassium, bicarbonate, stool specimens for ova and parasites, occult blood, sugar, and pH.
5. NPO.
6. IV of D5/0.2 NaCl to run at 63 ml per hour. After child voids, add 20 mEq of KCl per liter to D5/0.2 NaCl; then run at 38 ml per hour (810 ml per 24 h is maintenance fluid; 405 ml per 24 h is replacement fluid).
7. Vital signs q 4 h.
8. Weigh daily.
9. Record and describe all stools and emesis, including color, consistency, amount, pH, and presence of sugar or blood.

Nursing Diagnosis	Outcome Criteria	Nursing Interventions	Evaluation and Modifications
1. Fluid volume deficit and altered electrolyte status related to abnormal fluid loss from vomiting and diarrhea	☐ Karen will attain normal fluid and electrolyte balance, as evidenced by: **a.** Skin turgor—rapid recoil **b.** Moist mucous membranes **c.** Tearing, and eyeballs no longer sunken **d.** Fontanel no longer depressed **e.** Urine output of at least 8 ml per hour with a specific gravity less than 1.020 **f.** Vital signs within normal for age **g.** Serum electrolytes within normal limits	☐ Maintain IV fluids as ordered: **a.** Monitor IV rate closely. **b.** Check IV site frequently for infiltration: edema, coolness, or pain. **c.** Stabilize extremity on an arm board (tie to bed frame for additional security, if necessary). **d.** Monitor circulation of IV extremity. **e.** Add potassium chloride to IV solution after Karen voids. ☐ Monitor serum electrolytes and report abnormal values to the physician. ☐ Monitor hydration status: **a.** Vital signs **b.** Skin turgor **c.** Fontanel **d.** Tearing **e.** Urine output and specific gravity ☐ Measure intake and output: **a.** Use a medicine cup to measure oral intake. **b.** Apply a 24-h urine collection bag to collect and measure urine accurately.	☐ IV solution is infusing at the desired rate without signs of infiltration or phlebitis. ☐ IV is maintained adequately on the IV board without the need for additional security. ☐ Serum electrolytes are within normal limits. ☐ Hydration status: **a.** Vital signs are within normal limits. **b.** Skin turgor—rapid recoil. **c.** Tearing was evident when Karen cried after her mother's arrival. ☐ Urine output for the last 4 h was 70 cc; urine specific gravity was 1.018.
2. Alterations in bowel elimination: diarrhea	☐ Karen will have a return of normal bowel function, as evidenced by: **a.** Three soft, formed stools per day **b.** Normoactive bowel sounds	☐ Observe and record amount, color, consistency, presence of blood, and pH of stool. ☐ Take the axillary temperature. ☐ Observe for abdominal cramps. ☐ Monitor frequency of bowel sounds.	☐ During the last 8 h, Karen has had 100 cc of liquid green stool; this is a decrease from 150 cc in the previous 8 h. ☐ Bowel sounds continue to be hyperactive.

Nursing Diagnosis	Outcome Criteria	Nursing Interventions	Evaluation and Modifications
		☐ Give mouth care when Karen is NPO. ☐ Tell the mother the reasons for NPO. ☐ Maintain enteric isolation, and instruct the parents in the correct technique for isolation.	
3. Impaired skin integrity related to interaction of bacteria and digestive juices on the skin	☐ Karen will attain normal skin integrity, as evidenced by no redness, irritation, or excoriation.	☐ Change diapers after each voiding and stooling. ☐ Cleanse the perianal area after each voiding or stooling with warm water and soap. Dry carefully. ☐ Apply Desitin or A&D ointment to the perianal area. ☐ As the diarrhea becomes less frequent, place Karen prone and expose the buttocks to air; apply lights 18 in away from buttocks for 20 min QID. ☐ Assess the mother's knowledge of diaper rash care; instruct her as needed.	☐ The diaper area continues to be red and excoriated. ☐ Start leaving the buttocks exposed to air, and apply lights.
4. Potential alteration in nutrition: less than body requirements related to vomiting, diarrhea, and current NPO status	☐ Karen will not suffer nutritional impairment, as evidenced by return of weight to 8.5 kg within 1 week.	☐ Introduce clear liquids as ordered. Offer small amounts—30 cc at a time—and progress as tolerated, i.e., when there is no vomiting or diarrhea ☐ Introduce solid food as ordered: bananas (raw), rice cereal, and toast (white). ☐ Advance to a regular diet as tolerated per the physician's orders.	☐ Karen remains NPO.
5. Potential anxiety related to separation from primary caretaker and hospitalization	☐ Karen will not exhibit signs of advanced separation anxiety, as evidenced by protest phase of separation anxiety.	☐ Encourage the mother to stay with Karen while she is in the hospital. ☐ If the mother cannot stay, encourage frequent visits, pictures from home, and security objects from home (such as blanket or favorite toy). ☐ Explain Karen's behavior to the mother whenever she leaves or visits. ☐ Schedule consistent nurses.	☐ The mother will stay at the hospital during the day and go home at night; the grandmother cares for the siblings during the day. ☐ Karen cried when she saw her mother this morning.

Nursing Diagnosis	Outcome Criteria	Nursing Interventions	Evaluation and Modifications
6. Knowledge deficit (mother): related to medical procedures and terminology	☐ Karen's mother will be knowledgeable regarding Karen's illness.	☐ Explain to Karen's mother the reasons for: **a.** IV therapy **b.** Use of restraints **c.** Isolation **d.** Collection of stool **e.** Specimens **f.** NPO status ☐ Assess the mother's understanding of the above explanations.	☐ The mother was able to explain the reason for treatments listed this morning after being instructed last night.

References

1. Kemp, C., H. Silver, and D. O'Brien, *Current Pediatric Diagnosis and Treatment,* 6th ed., Lange, Los Altos, Calif., 1980.
2. Weil, William B., and Michael B. Baille, *Fluid and Electrolyte Metabolism in Infants and Children: A Unified Approach,* Grune & Stratton, New York, 1977, p. 91.
3. Winters, Robert W. (ed.), *The Body Fluids in Pediatrics,* Little, Brown, Boston, 1973, p. 118.
4. Hoekelman, Robert A., et al. (eds.), *Principles of Pediatrics: Health Care of the Young,* McGraw-Hill, New York, 1978, p. 248.
5. Levin, Daniel L., Francis C. Morriss, and Gerald C. Moore (eds.), *A Practical Guide to Pediatric Intensive Care,* Mosby, St. Louis, 1984, p. 306.
6. Ibid., p. 311.
7. Winters, op. cit., p. 120.
8. Weil and Baille, op. cit., p. 49.
9. Jacobs, Robert A. (ed.), *Children's Hospital of Los Angeles, Resident Manual,* 4th ed. Children's Hospital, Los Angeles, January 1975, p. V-3.
10. Ibid., p. V-4.
11. Levin, Morriss, and Moore, op. cit., p. 94.
12. Ibid.
13. Hazinski, Mary Fran, *Nursing Care of the Critically Ill Child,* Mosby, St. Louis, 1984, p. 4.
14. Levin, Morriss, and Moore, loc. cit.
15. Hazinski, loc. cit.

19

Cindy Smith Greenberg

Gastrointestinal function

Upon completion of this chapter, the student will be able to:

1 Describe the embryological development of a patent gastrointestinal tract.
2 Identify the major functions of each organ in the gastrointestinal tract.
3 Identify the deficiency diseases associated with a lack of selected nutrients.
4 Identify vitamins which are toxic if taken in excessive amounts.
5 Describe the correct procedure for administering enteral nutritional supplements.
6 List two methods of delivering total parenteral nutrition and the rationale for using a particular method.
7 Describe the nursing care of a child who is receiving total parenteral nutrition through a central catheter.
8 Identify appropriate nursing interventions for psychological problems associated with total parenteral nutrition.
9 List nursing assessment components for the child with gastrointestinal tract alterations.
10 Compare the care of a colostomy patient and an ileostomy patient.
11 Describe the preoperative and postoperative nursing care of a child who is having gastrointestinal surgery.
12 Contrast the preoperative and postoperative nursing care given to an infant with cleft lip and an infant with cleft palate.
13 List the signs that indicate the presence of an esophageal anomaly.
14 Discuss the postoperative nursing care of a child with a tracheoesophageal fistula.
15 Describe dehydration in the infant with pyloric stenosis.
16 Describe the anatomic defect present in omphalocele and contrast it with the defect found in gastroschisis.
17 Compare the immediate care of a newborn with the postoperative care of an infant who has an omphalocele or gastroschisis.
18 Describe the nursing care of an infant with a diaphragmatic hernia.
19 Describe the nursing care of children with ulcers.
20 Compare ulcerative colitis and Crohn's disease.
21 Describe the possible courses of therapy for ulcerative colitis.
22 Identify the bowel anomalies related to defects in fetal development.
23 Differentiate between inguinal and umbilical hernias.
24 Describe the signs that might be seen in a child with appendicitis.
25 List the foods that must be eliminated from the diet of a child with celiac disease.
26 Compare the repair of high and low defect in imperforate anus.
27 List the functions of the liver.
28 Write an appropriate nursing care plan for a child with biliary atresia.

EMBRYOLOGY OF THE GASTROINTESTINAL TRACT

The digestive tube is formed from the part of the yolk sac contained within the embryo. The developing digestive system is divided into the foregut, midgut, and hindgut.

The *esophagus* begins as a short tube that develops from the foregut. It rapidly increases in length, and the lining proliferates, almost completely obstructing the lumen.

The *stomach* begins as a dilation of the foregut during the fifth week of gestation. The dorsal border grows to become the greater curvature of the stomach. The lesser curvature is formed from the anterior border.

The *duodenum* is formed from the end of the foregut and the first portion of the midgut. As with most of the esophagus, the cells lining the duodenum completely obstruct the lumen. Later, these cells degenerate, and recanalization occurs. The *liver* and *pancreas* develop from buds on the duodenum.

The *jejunum, ileum, cecum, appendix, ascending colon,* and *proximal two-thirds of the tranverse colon* develop from the midgut. At 6 weeks of gestation the midgut elongates rapidly. The small abdominal cavity is occupied by the relatively large liver and kidneys. The growing gut loops out into the umbilical cord as a normal stage of development. The tip of the loop attaches to the vitelline duct (yolk stalk), which gradually degenerates. A small pouch appears at the caudal end of the loop and evolves into the cecum and the appendix. The midgut returns to the abdominal cavity at about 10 weeks and rotates, thus positioning the cecum and the appendix on the right side of the abdomen.

The *descending colon, pelvic colon, rectum,* and *upper half of the anal canal* evolve from the hindgut. This ends in a dilated blind pouch called the *entodermal cloaca*. A portion of the hindgut forms a structure called the *allantois*, which branches off and passes into the umbilical cord. The allantois and hindgut are separated by a wedge that forms gradually and penetrates the entodermal cloaca. This wedge, the *urorectal septum*, eventually divides the cloacal membrane into the urogenital membrane and the anal membrane. The anterior structure becomes the primitive bladder, and the posterior part forms the anorectal canal. The anal membrane breaks down when the protodeum (from the anus) invaginates at the end of the eighth week, establishing a connection between the upper and lower anal canals.

PHYSIOLOGY OF THE GASTROINTESTINAL TRACT

The transformation of edible substances into chemical energy utilized by the body involves the processes of ingestion, digestion, absorption, and elimination. *Ingestion* is the intake of food and is controlled by both physiological and psychological factors. *Mastication* (chewing) of food occurs in the mouth, and *deglutition* (swallowing) propels the bolus of food into the esophagus. This completes ingestion.

Digestion is the process that converts food into an absorbable form. This function begins in the mouth and is continued in the stomach and small intestine. Digestion is both mechanical and chemical. *Mechanical digestion* involves the changing of foodstuffs into minute particles and their movement through the gastrointestinal tract. *Chemical digestion* is the hydrolysis (breakdown) of proteins, carbohydrates, and fats into absorbable units.

In the *mouth*, ptyalin is secreted and initiates starch digestion. Peristaltic waves of the esophagus move the bolus of food to the stomach. The cardiac sphincter at the base of the esophagus prevents the reflux of stomach contents into the esophagus.

The *stomach* acts as a reservoir for food and mixes it with solution. This mass is called *chyme*. Hydrochloric acid and pepsin are secreted by the stomach and aid in the digestion of proteins. Mucus forms a protective covering over the gastric epithelial cells and buffers strong acids. The gastric mucosa cells secrete gastrin, which is absorbed into the circulation, increasing gastric motility and acid secretion. The intrinsic factor, responsible for vitamin B_{12} absorption, is also secreted by the stomach. Small amounts of chyme are slowly moved into the duodenum.

The *small intestine* is the final site of digestion. Table 19-1 lists the many secretions that act in the small intestine.

The *pancreas* releases into the small intestine proteolytic enzymes that convert protein molecules into smaller amino acids. Fat metabolism is carried out by pancreatic lipase. Pancreatic amylase breaks down polysaccharides. The beta cells of the pancreas secrete insulin, while the

Table 19-1 Digestive Secretions Acting in the Small Intestine

Secretion	Action
Maltase, sucrase, and lactase	Convert disaccharides to monosaccharides
Amylase	Breaks down polysaccharides to disaccharides
Protease	Breaks down proteins to peptides and amino acids
Peptidase	Breaks down proteins to amino acids
Lipase	Changes neutral fats to fatty acids and glycerol
Enterokinase	Activates pancreatic trypsin
Enterogastrone	Released by stimulus of fat in the small intestines to decrease gastric activity
Bile	Emulsifies fat

alpha cells secrete glucagon. Both are important factors in carbohydrate metabolism.

The liver secretes bile, which is either stored in the gallbladder or released into the small intestine. Cholecystokinin-pancreozymin (CCK-PZ) is secreted by the small intestine in the presence of fat. This hormone stimulates the gallbladder to contract, which releases bile into the small intestine. Bile is responsible for fat emulsification. CCK-PZ also causes the secretion of pancreatic juice with a high enzyme content.

The liver is responsible for glycogenesis (production of glycogen), glycogenolysis (freeing glucose from glycogen in the liver), and gluconeogenesis (formation of glucose from noncarbohydrate sources), which are essential components of carbohydrate metabolism. The liver also synthesizes serum proteins, such as prothrombin, fibrinogen, and albumin, and plays a role in fat metabolism through the synthesis and release of bile.

Absorption occurs mainly in the small intestine through diffusion, filtration, osmosis, and active transport. Limited absorption of glucose, water, and alcohol takes place in the stomach. The most absorptive areas are the lower part of the duodenum and the first segment of the jejunum. Villi cover the mucosa of the small intestine, greatly increasing the surface area and therefore its absorptive abilities. The large intestine absorbs water and electrolytes.

The large intestine is responsible mainly for *elimination*. It secretes mucus that causes the waste material, or feces, to adhere as peristaltic waves move it through the large intestine. The waste products accumulate in the rectum, causing the descending colon to contract. The act of defecation is the release of fecal contents from the rectum. It occurs as a result of voluntary and reflex actions.

ANATOMY OF THE GASTROINTESTINAL TRACT

The location of the gastrointestinal viscera in infants and young children is similar to that in adults, but there are some age-related differences. In newborns the liver edge can often be palpated 2 to 3 cm below the right costal margin. It is normal to be able to palpate the liver 1 cm below the costal margin throughout childhood.

Infants and young children have relatively shorter omentums than adults, and so they do not localize infections as well. They also have small abdominal cavities; thus the organs are in closer proximity to one another. Both these factors increase the chance that an infection will spread and develop into generalized peritonitis.

Young children have a higher costal arch than adults, and the pelvic portion of the body cavity is small; therefore, the abdominal organs are not as well protected by the bony skeleton. Because of these factors, the young child is at greater risk for abdominal injury if trauma does occur.

NUTRITION

Alterations in vitamin and mineral intake

Vitamins and minerals are nutrients with specific functions needed by the body in small amounts. Although they interact with one another, they cannot substitute for one another. Vitamins are essential for a wide range of metabolic reactions. When inadequate amounts are consumed, signs and symptoms of deficiency develop (see Table 19-2).

Vitamins A, D, E, and K are fat-soluble. The body stores rather than excretes excessive amounts, and so toxic levels may build up. The B vitamins and vitamin C are water-soluble. They are not stored in the body in appreciable amounts. Thus, if intake is inadequate, deficiencies will occur in a fairly short period of time. Megadoses of water-soluble vitamins are less likely to have toxic effects than megadoses of fat-soluble vitamins, but toxic effects are not unknown.

Table 19-2 Physical Signs and Causes of Malnutrition

Body Area	Signs Associated with Malnutrition	Nutrition-Related Causes
Hair	Lack of natural shine; dull, dry, sparse, straight; color changes (flag sign); easily plucked	Protein-calorie deficiency; often multiple coexistent nutrient deficiencies
Face	Dark skin over cheeks and under eyes (malar and infraorbital pigmentation); scaling of skin around nostrils (nasolabial seborrhea)	Inadequate caloric intake; lack of B-complex vitamins, particularly niacin, riboflavin, pyridoxine
	Edematous (moon face)	Protein deficiency
	Color loss (pallor)	Iron deficiency, general undernutrition
Eyes	Pale conjunctivae	Iron deficiency
	Bitôt's spots, conjunctival and corneal xerosis, soft cornea (keratomalacia)	Vitamin A deficiency
	Redness and fissuring of eyelid corners (angular palpebritis)	Niacin, riboflavin, pyridoxine deficiency
Lips	Redness and swelling of mouth or lips (cheilosis), angular fissure and scars	Niacin or riboflavin deficiency
Tongue	Red, raw and fissured, swollen (glossitis)	Folic acid, niacin, B_{12}, pyridoxine deficiency
	Magenta color	Riboflavin deficiency
	Pale, atrophic	Iron deficiency
	Filiform papillary atrophy	Niacin, folic acid, B_{12}, iron deficiency
	Fungiform papillary hypertrophy	General undernutrition
Teeth	Carious or missing	Excess sugar (and poor dental hygiene)
	Mottled enamel (fluorosis)	Excess fluoride
Gums	Spongy, bleeding; may be receding	Ascorbic acid deficiency
Glands	Thyroid enlargement (goiter)	Iodine deficiency
	Parotid enlargement	General undernutrition, particularly insufficient protein
Skin	Follicular hyperkeratosis, dryness (xerosis) with flaking	Vitamin A deficiency; insufficient unsaturated and essential fatty acids
	Hyperpigmentation	B_{12}, folic acid, niacin deficiency
	Petechiae	Ascorbic acid deficiency
	Pellagrous dermatitis	Niacin or tryptophan deficiency
	Scrotal and vulval dermatosis	Riboflavin deficiency
Nails	Spoon nails (koilonychia); brittle or ridged	Iron deficiency
Muscular and skeletal systems	Muscle wasting	Protein-calorie deficiency
	Frontal and parietal bosselation; epiphyseal swelling; soft, thin infant skull bones (craniotabes), persistently open anterior fontanel; knock-knees or bow-legs	Vitamin D deficiency
	Beading of ribs (rachitic rosary)	Vitamin D and calcium deficiency
Internal systems: gastrointestinal and nervous	Hepatomegaly	Chronic malnutrition
	Mental confusion and irritability	Thiamine, niacin deficiency
	Sensory loss, motor weakness, loss of position sense, loss of vibration, loss of ankle and knee jerks, calf tenderness	Thiamine deficiency
Cardiac	Cardiac enlargement, tachycardia	Thiamine deficiency

Source: Rosanne B. Howard and Nancie H. Herbold, *Nutrition in Clinical Care*, McGraw-Hill, New York, 1978. Used with permission.

Reports of vitamin intoxication outnumber reports of vitamin deficiency, suggesting a need for a reappraisal of current vitamin use.* In preschool children of lower socioeconomic status, the most prevalent nutritional problem is simply an insufficiency of food. Other preschool children show little evidence of vitamin deficiencies. Therefore, there is little evidence to support giving vitamin supplements routinely to normal children.

The use of large doses of certain vitamins, characteristically more than 10 times the recommended dietary allowance to maintain health,

*The section on alterations in vitamins was written by Diane Huus, R.D., M.S.

is popular. The term *megavitamin therapy* was originally coined for the use of extremely large doses of nicotinamide in the treatment of schizophrenia. The American Psychiatric Association has, however, concluded that megavitamin therapy is useless for the treatment of schizophrenia. In some rare inborn errors of metabolism, the metabolic defect may be partially or completely corrected by large doses of a specific vitamin. Vitamin supplements in excess of normal requirements are also needed by children with intestinal malabsorption.

There is no scientific basis for the consumption of vitamins in amounts far in excess of the recommended dietary allowance by people who are generally healthy. Indeed, reports of harmful consequences from excessive use of vitamins are increasing.

Vitamin A Vitamin A (retinol) aids in vision, growth, epithelial tissue health, tooth and bone development, and reproduction. Inadequate intake can lead to night blindness due to interferences with the chemistry of the retina. The cornea becomes dry, and eventually Bitôt's spots form. If this is unchecked, severe visual damage and eventual blindness will result. Scaliness (keratinization) will also occur throughout all epithelial tissue, such as the skin, oral cavity, and respiratory tract. When the epithelial cells become dry, hair is lost and the body is more open to invasion by infectious organisms. In children, vitamin A deficiency can also cause growth retardation.

Since vitamin A is fat-soluble, it is stored in the body. Consequently the development of a deficiency is generally slow. A diet which contains organ meats, whole milk, eggs, and butter will supply preformed vitamin A. Provitamin A (a precursor) is found in deep-green leafy or yellow vegetables (squash, spinach, pumpkin, and carrots) and is readily used by the body. These items should be consumed every other day.[1] If a deficiency does develop, administration of vitamin A will correct the problem—unless irreversible damage has been done.

Since vitamin A is stored in the body, it can be toxic if taken in large doses over a period of time. Early signs of overdose in children are anorexia, growth failure, headache, and pruritus. Other symptoms of toxicity include nausea, irritability, flaky skin, rashes, liver and spleen enlargement, and bone fragility. Infants are more susceptible to toxicity than adults. The nurse should educate parents and children in the correct administration and dosage of vitamin supplements. Some vitamin A is good, but too much can be harmful.

Vitamin D Vitamin D aids in calcium absorption from the intestinal tract, bone mineralization, and regulation of serum calcium and phosphorus levels. In children, the deficiency of vitamin D is known as *rickets*. The mineralization of long bones is inadequate, resulting in bowlegs and knock-knees. Since teeth contain calcium, they generally are poorly calcified and erupt late in children with rickets. Treatment consists of daily administration of vitamin D supplements until the bone ends have calcified.

Rickets can be prevented with an adequate daily intake of vitamin D. The most important sources of this vitamin are fish liver oil and fortified milk. Milk is fortified with 400 IU of vitamin D per quart. Exposure to sunlight is also a good source of the vitamin. This causes ultraviolet light to change 7-dehydrocholesterol into cholecalciferol, a form of vitamin D. Since few young children drink 1 qt of milk each day, it is important that the nurse encourage parents to expose children to sunlight. Playing or walking outdoors when the weather is nice is generally sufficient. Since breast milk is a poor source of vitamin D, nursing infants should be given a supplement of this vitamin until they are 1 year of age. Care should be taken to prevent excess supplementation. This vitamin is stored, and so toxic levels can accumulate and cause elevated levels of serum calcium. Symptoms of acute toxicity include anorexia, nausea, diarrhea, weight loss, and headache. Chronic hypervitaminosis may result in calcification of soft tissues and kidney stones, with kidney failure.

Vitamin E Vitamin E (tocopherol) has received much publicity in recent years. It has been associated with sexual functioning, heart disease, and aging. Its exact function in the human body is unknown. It does function as an antioxidant, helping to stabilize unsaturated fats, vitamin A, and certain enzymes and cell components. Deficiencies have been recorded in premature infants and individuals with fat malabsorption problems (e.g., cystic fibrosis and biliary atresia). Vitamin E levels are low in the newborn and are especially limited in the premature infant. The mother's vitamin E levels do not increase until late in pregnancy, and so the premature infant does not benefit from maternal supplies. Hemolytic anemia has been noted in premature infants and in infants who receive iron supplements or fortified formulas and whose serum levels of tocopherol are low. Iron (which acts as an oxidant) and high concentrations of oxygen (red blood cell membranes contain large amounts of polyunsaturated fatty acids, which need protection from oxidation when exposed to oxygen) increase the need for vitamin E. A deficiency suppresses the immune system. Other symptoms of vitamin E deficiency include irritability and edema. Water-miscible preparations of vitamin E should be given to those at risk for deficiency, particularly premature infants and individuals with fat absorption problems.

Vitamin E is widespread in the diet. Fats and oils, especially unsaturated fats, are the major food sources. Liver, egg yolks, cereal grains, and green leafy vegetables are minor sources of this vitamin. An excessive intake does not appear to have toxic effects.[2]

Vitamin K Vitamin K is one nutrient that is essential but does not need to be consumed regularly. The main source is bacterial synthesis in the intestinal tract. This vitamin may also be obtained from liver, eggs, spinach, kale, lettuce, broccoli, cabbage, cauliflower, and other leafy vegetables. A deficiency of vitamin K manifests itself as a disorder of the blood-clotting mechanism. Vitamin K aids in the formation of prothrombin, which is necessary for blood clotting. Deficiency is rare under normal conditions. Use of anticoagulants (coumadin) and salicylates is antagonistic to the action of vitamin K. Newborns have a very low storage level of vitamin K. This does not increase rapidly, since the gut flora are absent at birth and take time to be established. Newborns are given 1 mg of vitamin K intramuscularly at birth. Another pediatric population at risk is adolescents on prolonged antibiotic therapy (e.g., tetracycline) for acne. Such drugs diminish the bacterial flora, therefore decreasing the vitamin K supply to the body. Supplements need not be taken, especially since an excess is toxic. The nurse should encourage patients on antibiotic therapy to consume cultured milk products, such as buttermilk and yogurt, to maintain the gastrointestinal flora and prevent possible problems.

Thiamine Thiamine is a B-complex vitamin needed by the body primarily for carbohydrate metabolism. Its deficiency disease is known as *beriberi*. This affects the gastrointestinal tract, causing anorexia, indigestion, severe constipation, and vomiting; the nervous system, causing apathy, fatigue, and eventual damage of the myelin sheaths; and the cardiovascular system, causing cardiac muscle fatigue and peripheral dilation leading to edema (wet beriberi). Foods high in thiamine include pork, beef liver, whole or enriched grains, and legumes. These foods should be consumed daily by all children and adolescents to prevent the adult form of beriberi.

Daily needs for thiamine depend on the caloric level of the diet and range from 0.3 mg for infants to 1.4 mg for adolescent males. Surplus thiamine is excreted in the urine, and so excesses should not build up in the body.

Riboflavin Riboflavin is another B-complex vitamin. It functions as a coenzyme in protein and energy metabolism. A deficiency is most likely to occur as a result of alcohol abuse; during stress, such as that which results from rapid growth, severe burns, surgery, or trauma; and when there is impaired absorption and utilization. Ultraviolet rays and fluorescent lights destroy riboflavin, and so milk should be stored in opaque containers.[3] Phototherapy for neonates with jaundice may also cause a deficiency.[4] Clinical symptoms include cheilosis (lesions of the lips), seborrheic dermatitis, glossitis, and eye irritations. Riboflavin deficiency often occurs along with other B-vitamin deficiencies. Treatment includes supplements of the vitamin and a diet rich in riboflavin. The main dietary sources of riboflavin are milk and other dairy products, organ meats, eggs, and green leafy vegetables. Enriched cereals contain small amounts of riboflavin but do contribute significantly to the total daily intake. No toxic side effects are associated with megadoses of this vitamin, but its excretion may cause the urine to turn bright yellow.

Niacin Niacin, another B-complex vitamin, functions as a coenzyme to help obtain energy from glucose. *Pellagra,* a disease due to a deficiency of niacin, is characterized by the 3 D's—dermatitis, dementia, and diarrhea. Death occurs if pellagra is untreated. Treatment is similar to that of the other B-vitamin deficiencies. Supplements of nicotinamide (a form of niacin) are given. Often other B vitamins are also given, since their respective deficiencies may also be evident. A diet containing meat, enriched grains, and peanuts should be eaten. Since tryptophan can be converted to niacin in the body, foods (meat, fish, and poultry) containing this amino acid should also be eaten.

Niacin has been found to have toxic effects. When large doses of nicotinic acid (a form of niacin) are taken, vasodilation may occur. The person will become flushed and feel a tingling sensation. Liver toxicity, skin rashes, elevated serum levels of glucose and uric acid, and peptic ulcers are other possible complications associated with long-term megadoses of niacin.[5]

Pyridoxine Pyridoxine, vitamin B_6, plays a role in cellular reactions involving carbohydrates, protein, and fat. It is also necessary for the formation of the heme molecule and for the conversion of tryptophan into niacin. Pyridoxine deficiency is rare. Symptoms of this deficiency are irritability, convulsive seizures, and a greasy skin disorder. It may also impair the immune response. Children who are receiving isonicotinic acid hydrozide are at risk for developing pyridoxine deficiency. Oral supplements are usually used in conjunction with isonicotinic acid hydrozide therapy. Dosages are determined on an individual basis. Normal daily needs range from 0.3 mg for infants to 2 mg for adolescent males. These levels are easily obtained from a diet which includes meat, liver, poultry, fish, wheat, and corn. Large doses of pyridoxine have been shown to inhibit lactation and cause permanent nerve damage.

Folic acid Folic acid is associated with blood cell production. Megaloblastic anemia is the disease associated with a deficiency of this vitamin. Other signs and symptoms of folate deficiency include diarrhea, glossitis, and growth retardation. Megaloblastic anemia may be seen in infants whose diets are low in ascorbic acid (ascorbic acid aids in the conversion of folic acid to the coenzyme form) and in children who are receiving anticonvulsant drugs (DPH, primidone, or barbiturates) or who suffer from malabsorption problems. In infant megaloblastic anemia, 5 mg of folic acid daily will reverse the condition in a few days.[6] Children who are receiving anticonvulsant medications should take 1 mg of folate daily.[7] Large doses of folic acid can mask signs of vitamin B_{12} deficiency. For this reason, over-the-counter preparations cannot contain more than 0.1 mg of folic acid.[8] When larger doses of folic acid are prescribed, vitamin B_{12} is often given also to prevent this problem. Food sources of folic acid include liver, meat, green leafy vegetables, asparagus, kidney beans, and whole grains.

Vitamin B_{12} Vitamin B_{12}, cobalamin, is needed for blood cell production. Unlike other water-soluble vitamins, B_{12} is stored in the liver. Healthy individuals have approximately a 3- to 5-year store of this vitamin. Growing children do not have as extensive stores. Deficiency signs and symptoms include pernicious anemia and neurological disturbances. Children who regularly consume meat, milk, eggs, and other foods from animal sources usually get adequate amounts of vitamin B_{12}. (This vitamin is not found in plant foods.) Malabsorption disorders may lead to a deficiency. Vitamin B_{12} (the extrinsic factor) must combine with the intrinsic factor in the stomach for absorption to occur. Parenteral doses of vitamin B_{12} are indicated in malabsorption. The child or parent can be taught how to give these injections.

One area of concern is the child on a vegan (strict vegetarian) diet. Without animal foods, the diet lacks vitamin B_{12}. A diet which includes eggs and dairy products is therefore recommended for children and adolescents who are vegetarians. (This also assures adequate amounts of complete protein needed for growth.) Oral supplements of vitamin B_{12} or soybean milk fortified with vitamin B_{12} can be used as a source of the vitamin also. Excessive intakes of vitamin B_{12} have not been proven harmful and are generally excreted in urine.

Vitamin C Vitamin C (ascorbic acid) is required for collagen formation and therefore forms a base for all connective tissue. Thus, there are high concentrations in active tissue during growth and healing. Vitamin C is involved in the metabolism of some amino acids, facilitates the gastrointestinal absorption of iron, and is involved in the release of epinephrine and norepinephrine during times of stress. Studies have failed to prove that megadoses of vitamin C can prevent or cure the common cold or cancer.[9] More research is needed on these controversial topics.

The ascorbic acid deficiency disease, *scurvy*, results in impaired bone formation and wound healing. The vascular network appears to be very sensitive to decreased vitamin C stores. Petechial hemorrhage and bruising are noted with scurvy. Other symptoms include anorexia; weakness; tender joints, bones, and muscles; swollen and bleeding gums; and loose teeth. Most infants who are receiving commercial formula have an adequate vitamin C intake. Breast-fed infants also generally have an adequate intake unless the mother's intake is very poor. Cow's milk is a poor source of vitamin C because pasteurization destroys the small amount of ascorbic acid in this food. Therefore, infants who are receiving cow's milk or a home-prepared modified cow's milk formula should be given a vitamin C supplement. Liquid drops are generally used. Orange juice and grapefruit juice, once they have been introduced into the diet, will meet the child's daily vitamin C needs. Other foods which supply vitamin C are broccoli, strawberries, and cantaloupe. Raw cabbage, tomatoes, green peppers, and potatoes are fair sources of this vitamin. Children and their parents should be instructed by the nurse not to leave these foods exposed to air (especially after cutting) or to cook them for long periods of time. Such preparation methods destroy the vitamin C in the food.

Although vitamin C is water-soluble, some toxic reactions have been observed as a result of megadose intakes. Kidney stones, false-positive urine glucose test results, and impaired white blood cell function, nausea, diarrhea, abdominal cramps, and elevated vitamin requirements in newborns whose mothers took large doses during pregnancy are among the possibilities.[10]

Minerals Iron is a mineral needed by the body in relatively small amounts daily. Iron is stored in the liver, bone marrow, and spleen. In red blood cells, iron acts to transport oxygen to all body cells for respiration and metabolism. Iron deficiency is observed as anemia and may result from various causes. Nutritional anemia is due to an inadequate intake of iron; hemorrhagic anemia results from excessive blood loss; and malabsorption of iron and increased iron requirements also result in iron-deficiency anemia. The anemic individual experiences weakness and fatigue and appears pale. Tests of hemoglobin levels and of the hematocrit are used to confirm a diagnosis of anemia. When a diagnosis of iron-deficiency anemia is made, supplements of ferrous gluconate or ferrous sulfate are prescribed. Care should be taken to avoid excessive iron intake, since this may lead to hemosiderosis. Foods such as organ meats, egg yolks, red meats, green leafy vegetables, dried fruits, fortified cereals, and legumes should also be eaten. (Chapter 23 discusses anemia in detail.)

In the pediatric population, several groups are at risk of developing iron-deficiency anemia. Infants are born with a 3- to 6-month supply of iron. At approximately 4 months of age, iron supplementation should be started to prevent anemia. Generally, cereals are introduced at this age. Since infant cereals are fortified with iron, they can be used as the source of iron supplementation. If the introduction of cereals is delayed, iron-fortified formula or iron drops can be used. Supplementation must be done, since cow's milk is a poor source of iron. If, during the first year, a child continues to take more than 1 qt (32 oz) of formula or milk a day, the chances of anemia increase. This excessive quantity of milk generally satiates the child and prevents adding iron-containing foods to the diet. A good diet history will identify such an occurrence. The nurse should instruct the parent to introduce solid foods, especially those rich in iron; to have the older infant use a cup (especially at meals); and to discontinue extra between-meal bottles. By assisting the parent with weaning, infant nutritional anemia may be prevented.

Some iron-deficient children may develop pica. Pica is an abnormal desire to eat nonnutritious substances such as ice, starch, clay, and paint. Anemia may also result from pica when the substances ingested cause lead poisoning. Nursing care should include giving information about foods that contain iron.

This same information should be given to girls when menstruation begins. At this point, daily iron requirements nearly double, to 18 mg. This amount is very hard to consume without overeating. For this reason, a small dosage (30 to 60 mg) of an iron supplement may be recommended.

When oral iron administration is prescribed, certain procedures should be followed. If liquid supplements are used, caution should be taken to put the liquid far back in the mouth to avoid staining the teeth. Water or juice should be given afterward to rinse the teeth. For maximum iron absorption, the supplement should be taken on an empty stomach with orange juice (iron is absorbed in an acid medium). This method may cause gastrointestinal irritation. If the iron is taken approximately 10 to 15 min before meals, less irritation may occur. When iron is taken after meals, the absorption is decreased, and larger doses may be needed to correct the problem. Small, frequent doses will also help prevent gastric problems. The iron should be started slowly and gradually increased to full dosages. Iron therapy should be continued for 6 to 12 months to ensure that iron stores are replenished.

Calcium is essential for skeletal and dental development, influences cell membrane permeability, is required for muscle contractility, and plays a role in blood clotting. Calcium deficiency causes rickets, and was previously discussed in the section "Vitamin D." Hypocalcemia will cause tetany. Milk and milk products are the main sources of calcium. Other foods, such as green leafy vegetables, egg yolks, legumes, shellfish, canned fish with bones (salmon and sardines), and nuts, supply some calcium. For children who refuse milk, such foods as puddings, ice cream, soups made with milk, yogurt, and cheese can be substituted. Dry milk solids can be added to sauces, ground-meat dishes, and casseroles to increase milk consumption. Some mothers have even blended powdered milk into peanut butter. If the child is unable to consume milk because of allergies or lactose intolerance, other foods containing calcium and calcium supplements should be given. Soybean-based infant formulas used for babies with lactose intolerance will supply adequate calcium.

Zinc, which is receiving increased attention, functions in growth and maintenance of body tissues, digestion, cellular respiration, and glucose oxidation. Symptoms of zinc deficiency may include growth retardation, alterations in taste acuity, impaired wound healing, sexual immaturity, and immune incompetence. Good food sources of zinc are seafood, meat, egg yolks, whole grains, and legumes. Oral supplements of zinc can be administered to correct deficiency states.

Fluoride is important for children. This mineral helps prevent dental caries and possibly strengthens bone structure. For most people, fluoridated drinking water is the major source of this nutrient. In areas where the drinking water is not fluoridated or where well water is used, children should be given fluoride tablets or multiple vitamins containing fluoride. *Fluorosis,* or excessive fluoride intake, can cause the teeth to become discolored (gray or brown) and pitted (mottled). Fluorosis can also cause opaque spots on the teeth. For these reasons, the nurse should be sure that parents know how to administer fluoride supplements accurately.

Enteral nutrition

The body's need for nutrients changes during periods of physical stress such as fever, burns, infection, and malignancies. These conditions require an increase in calories because of an increased metabolic rate. Protein requirements are also increased in the latter three conditions to promote healing and prevent physical deterioration. Three meals and three snacks daily generally provide the needed calories and protein, without requiring the ingestion of excessive quantities at one time. Such items as milk shakes, eggnogs, and sandwiches can be eaten. If necessary, special concentrated products, such as Meritine, Vivonex, Sustacal, and Ensure, can be given. Total parenteral nutrition may be necessary if the gastrointestinal tract is unable to handle food.

When special enteral feedings are given, it is important that proper administration techniques be used. Such supplements as Meritine, Sustacal, and Ensure (lactose-free) can be given in the same way as a milk drink. Small amounts should be given initially so that the nurse can check for any signs of intolerance. These products come in several flavors to encourage acceptance by the child.

Elemental or low-residue supplements such as Vivonex or Precision may need to be given more carefully. These products often have a disagreeable taste. If these liquids are flavored and given ice-cold, they may be more palatable. When giving elemental products, such as Vivonex, which are hypertonic, encourage the child to sip them slowly. This will aid absorption and decrease the chances of osmotic diarrhea. Often these products are given through a nasogastric tube. When given properly, enteral supplements can supply the needed calories, protein, and other nutrients to aid healing and prevent nutritional deterioration.

Total parenteral nutrition

Generally, if the gastrointestinal tract is functioning, it should be used to nourish the child. In the case of many congenital anomalies of the gastrointestinal tract, short bowel syndrome, intractable diarrhea, inflammatory bowel disease, extensive burns, and other disorders, it is not possible to use the gastrointestinal tract to maintain nutritional status. In these situations, total parenteral nutrition (TPN) may be a lifesaving therapy. It supplies the needed protein, carbohydrates, vitamins, minerals, trace elements (except iron), and water in usable form directly into the circulatory system. Fat emulsions (Intralipid or Liposyn) are frequently administered in conjunction with TPN solutions to prevent essential fatty acid deficiencies and to provide calories.

TPN solutions are very concentrated and therefore require infusion through a large central vein, such as the superior vena cava. Central venous catheter insertion is a surgical procedure. A Silastic catheter is first tunneled under the skin and then is inserted into the desired vein. Catheter placement is checked by x-ray. Tunneling the catheter helps stabilize its position and makes it more difficult for microorganisms to invade the central system. Potential complications of TPN infusion are listed in Table 19-3.

Peripheral veins may be used for TPN infusion if the child does not require long-term therapy or an excessive amount of calories. The maximum glucose concentration of peripheral infusions cannot exceed 12.5 percent.[11] Skin sloughing from tissue damage due to infiltration may be severe enough to require skin grafting and plastic surgery. When peripheral veins are used, fat emulsions often provide the major source of calories (1.1 cal per cc). They also decrease the incidence of thrombophlebitis by lowering the osmolarity of the infusate.[12]

TPN solutions are high in nutrients and therefore provide an excellent medium for bacterial growth. To prevent contamination, solutions should be mixed by qualified personnel under laminar flow. Solutions should not be mixed more than 24 h prior to use and should be kept under refrigeration. Once a bottle is in use, it should not hang for more than 24 h. The entire tubing system should be changed at least every 24 h. A millipore filter should be placed in the tubing system to filter out potential contaminants and to help trap air. The central catheter dressing should be changed every 24 to 72 h using aseptic technique. The insertion site and the catheter are usually scrubbed with alcohol and povidone-iodine (Betadine), an antibacterial ointment applied, and the site covered with an occlusive dressing (see Fig. 19-1).

Catheter-associated infection is one of the most common complications of TPN therapy. Most infections are bacterial, caused by common skin flora (staphylococcus and streptococcus). *Candida* causes the most common fungal infection. The nurse must check daily for redness or swelling near the catheter site. The child's temperature must be monitored closely. Blood cultures for septicemia should be done when infection is suspected.

When TPN is initiated, it is done gradually so the child can accommodate the glucose load. TPN solutions should be administered via infusion

Table 19-3 Potential Complications of TPN Infusion

Central Catheter	Infusate
Malpositioning and dislodgment	Metabolic complications:
Air embolism	Hyperglycemia
Central vessel perforation	Hypoglycemia
Cardiac arrhythmias	Electrolyte imbalance
Pneumothorax	Acid-base disturbance
Hemothorax	Vitamin and mineral disorders
Infection	Fluid overload
	Hyperosmotic dehydration
	Hepatic dysfunction
Peripheral Catheter	**Fat Emulsion**
Vessel thrombosis	Hyperlipemia
Vessel sclerosis	Decreased pulmonary diffusion
Phlebitis	Eosinophilia
Tissue damage due to infiltration	Bilirubin displacement from albumin

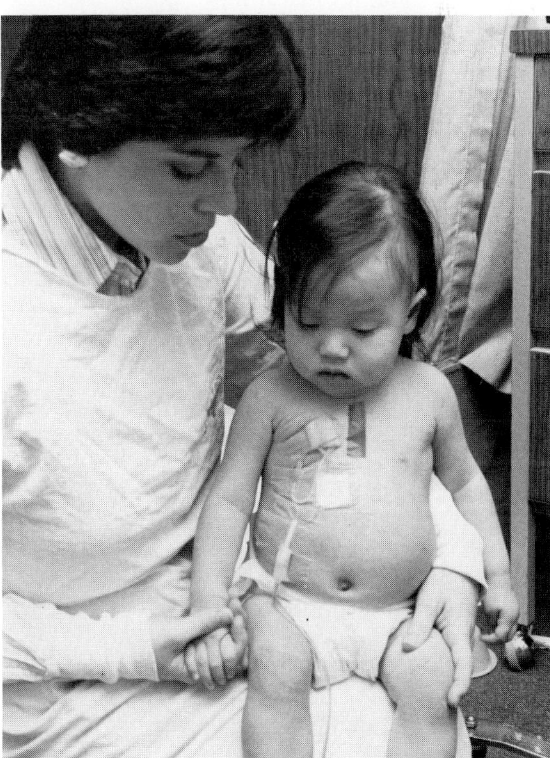

Figure 19-1 A child with a central line infusion. (*Photo by Al Jones.*)

pumps to maintain a constant flow rate. Rates should not be increased or decreased, since this may cause hyperglycemia or hypoglycemia. When TPN is to be discontinued, the rate should be gradually decreased so the body can adapt to the decreased glucose load.

Protein in TPN solution is usually supplied as crystalline amino acids. The vitamin and mineral content of a child's TPN solution is higher per unit of body weight than that of an adult's TPN solution. This is due to the increased need for growth. Vitamins A, D, E, K, and C, the B-complex vitamins, and folic acid are generally added.[13] If some vitamins are not included, they will need to be given in another appropriate route (e.g., intramuscularly or orally). Iron is not in the TPN solution. It is given when needed.

Fat is not contained in the primary TPN infusate, and so fat emulsions may be administered. These provide a more concentrated form of calories and therefore may decrease fluid intake. They are also a source of essential fatty acids. Some manifestations of essential fatty acid deficiency are eczema, diminished growth,[14] sparse hair, and thrombocytopenia. When administering fat emulsions, make sure that the solution is stable. It has a milky appearance and does not need shaking. Fat emulsions are administered via a separate infusion pump and tubing setup and "piggybacked" into the TPN infusion tubing as close to the patient as possible. Once the infusion is started, monitor vital signs and watch for signs of an adverse reaction (e.g., fever, headache, nausea, dyspnea, chest and back pain, and respiratory distress). Lipid binds with albumin and therefore displaces bilirubin. Infants with hyperbilirubinemia may be at risk for developing kernicterus,[15] and so fat emulsion infusions are contraindicated.

The nurse has many responsibilities in caring for a child who is receiving TPN. The contents of the solution are double-checked against the doctor's order to ensure that the correct solution is given. Vital signs are obtained every 4 h, or as the child's condition warrants. Growth parameters must be monitored, usually by weighing the child daily and by measuring head circumference (in infants) and height weekly. Accurate records of intake and output are kept. Urine should be tested for specific gravity, glucose, and ketones at least every shift as an indicator of how the body is handling the glucose load. Blood is drawn weekly (or more often if indicated) to monitor serum glucose, electrolytes, minerals, albumin, triglycerides, liver function (SGOT, SGPT, and alkaline phosphates), and kidney function (blood urea nitrogen and creatinine). A complete blood count, including a differential, is also obtained. Abnormal values should be reported to the physician.

Children who are receiving TPN should be watched closely to prevent dislodgment of the catheter and kinks in the line. Toddlers and older children should be monitored so that they do not step on the line or place objects on the tubing that could cause the line to kink or break. If the tubing is gently coiled near the entry site and under the dressing, less pressure will be exerted on the catheter as the child moves about.

Psychological and developmental complications can occur. Since there is no oral intake, infants receiving TPN lack needed sucking. The use of a pacifier may stimulate this important reflex and prepare the child for eventual resumption of oral feedings. When permitted, hard sour candies or chewing gum can be given to older children. Older children are deprived of the social interaction associated with meals. Some other activity may be planned for these children during mealtimes.

When food is reintroduced, it should be done slowly. The gastrointestinal tract is unaccustomed to food after a prolonged rest. Food is better tolerated if small, frequent meals are given. This also eliminates the chance of overwhelming the child with too much food. Many children who receive TPN for long periods of time do not have much appetite. The sight of a large meal may therefore discourage them. They should be encouraged to eat what is tolerable. They also need reassurance that physical hunger and appetite will increase as the IV solution is slowly decreased.

The family is included in the care of the child who is receiving hyperalimentation. The procedure is thoroughly explained so parents can feel at ease working with their child. Hygienic or mouth care can easily be given without disturbing the IV setup. It is important that the child receive this care and attention from the family often. Generally, the child receiving TPN in the hospital is there for a long period of time. This may fragment the family unit if total family involvement is not encouraged by the nurse.

Home hyperalimentation has been developed to try to avoid some of the family and social problems which arise from prolonged hospital stays. The time required (approximately 10 to 14 h) to administer the solution can be scheduled so that

Table 19-4 Nursing Care Responsibilities for the Child Receiving TPN

1. Monitor for signs of infection:
   a. Inspect the infusion site.
   b. Monitor vital signs (particularly the temperature) qid.
2. Maintain aseptic technique:
   a. Apply central line dressings.
   b. Scrub the site with alcohol and Betadine.
   c. Apply an antibacterial ointment.
   d. Apply an occlusive dressing.
3. Maintain infusion:
   a. Change the bottle and tubing every 24 h.
   b. Maintain a constant infusion rate.
   c. Increase the rate gradually when beginning TPN.
   d. Decrease the rate gradually when discontinuing TPN.
4. Monitor for nutritional deficiencies:
   a. Check caloric intake.
   b. Check vitamin intake.
   c. Check intake of essential fatty acids.
   d. Obtain daily weight.
   e. Obtain weekly height and head circumference.
5. Monitor for biochemical imbalance:
   a. Measure intake and output.
   b. Test the urine q4h for specific gravity, glucose, and ketones.
   c. Make sure that required blood tests are done.
   d. Check and report the results of blood tests.
6. Give psychological support.
7. Educate the parents and the child appropriately.

the child may still participate in school or other activities. Another benefit is that the hospital costs are eliminated.

When home TPN is used, the nurse needs to provide in-depth patient and family education. The proper techniques for tube changes, solution storage, and administration must be taught to all family members who will be working with the child. Needed reinforcement can be given by a visiting nurse or during subsequent visits to the doctor, clinic, or hospital (see Table 19-4).

ASSESSMENT OF COMMON GASTROINTESTINAL TRACT ALTERATIONS

Gastrointestinal signs and symptoms can be the result of either systemic diseases or gastrointestinal alterations. It is essential to obtain baseline data of the child's usual state of health before the significance of alterations can be established.

An accurate nursing history is beneficial to both health professionals and the child-family unit. The child's usual appetite, diet, meal schedule, food preferences, dislikes, and intolerances should be noted. Toileting habits, elimination patterns, and stool characteristics are also included in the nursing history. Medication intake (including over-the-counter drugs) should also be noted in the nursing history.

Observation of the child's general appearance and nutritional state are important components of the assessment process. This can be beneficial in discriminating between an acute and a chronic illness. The child's weight and height are measured and recorded on growth charts. These parameters can then be compared with previous measurements. The onset and duration of symptoms are discussed after baseline data have been obtained.

Physical assessment begins with examination of the oral cavity. The mouth is inspected for any condition that can interfere with sucking or chewing. In the older child, inspection of the gums for bleeding or ulcers is necessary. The condition of the teeth is important to note. Dental caries can seriously hinder chewing and, consequently, nutrition.

The child or parents can be asked about swallowing problems *(dysphagia)*. Difficulty with only solid foods probably indicates a mechanical obstruction such as a foreign body or a cyst. A neurological problem is indicated when swallowing difficulties extend to include liquids. A distinction must be made between dysphagia and a sore throat.

The abdomen is divided into four quadrants for the purposes of physical assessment. An imaginary line is drawn from the middle of the sternum through the umbilicus to the symphysis pubis. A horizontal line intersects at the umbilicus. This separates the abdomen into the right upper, the right lower, the left upper, and the left lower quadrants. Table 19-5 lists the organs located in each quadrant.

The color of the abdomen is inspected, and any distention is noted. In children, distention must be differentiated from a normal "potbelly." The abdomen is also inspected for visible peristalsis and any masses. The abdominal girth is measured in children with suspected gastrointestinal alterations. Tissue turgor can be assessed by gently pinching a fold of skin and then quickly releasing it. Normally, the tissue immediately assumes its regular contour. If it remains creased, the dehydration is present.

The location of pain must be determined. Children have trouble verbalizing the source of

Table 19-5 Organs Located in Each of the Four Quadrants of the Abdomen

Right Upper Quadrant	Left Upper Quadrant
Liver and gallbladder	Left lobe of liver
Pylorus	Spleen
Duodenum	Stomach
Head of pancreas	Body of pancreas
Right adrenal gland	Left adrenal gland
Portion of right kidney	Portion of left kidney
Hepatic flexure of colon	Splenic flexure of colon
Portions of ascending and transverse colon	Portions of transverse and descending colon
Loops of small bowel	Loops of small bowel
Right Lower Quadrant	**Left Lower Quadrant**
Lower pole of right kidney	Lower pole of left kidney
Cecum and appendix	Sigmoid colon
Portion of ascending colon	Portion of descending colon
Bladder	Bladder
Ovary and salpinx	Ovary and salpinx
Uterus (if enlarged)	Uterus (if enlarged)
Right spermatic cord	Left spermatic cord
Right ureter	Left ureter
Loops of small bowel	Loops of small bowel

pain. Hence, the nurse must observe the child's facial expression while gently palpating the abdomen to determine the locus of pain. Auscultation of the abdomen reveals the presence or absence of peristalsis. The gurgling sound heard is caused by air and fluid in the intestine. Gastrointestinal alterations can result in absent or diminished bowel sounds.

Sucking and feeding difficulties

Sucking and feeding difficulties in the neonate are sometimes due to congenital anomalies such as cleft lip, cleft palate, or tracheoesophageal atresia or fistula. These defects require adaptive devices or alternative methods of feeding. They are discussed in detail later in this chapter. Infants with large, protruding tongues (as in Down syndrome) may also have difficulty sucking.

Swallowing foreign bodies

Children under the age of 5 are the most likely to swallow foreign bodies. Safety pins, buttons, coins, and any number of objects have been retrieved from the alimentary tracts of pediatric patients. Foreign bodies that lodge at the junction of the upper and middle third of the esophagus are removed by esophagoscopy with forceps extraction.

After esophagoscopy, humidity is provided by a mist tent or face mask, depending on the child's age. Diet restrictions are unnecessary. Observation is required for a 24-h period, after which the child is discharged.

Objects that reach the stomach will generally move through the gastrointestinal tract without difficulty. It may take 3 weeks for some to be eliminated in the stool. Surgery is necessary if the object remains in the alimentary tract or obstructs the pylorus or ileocecal valve. Periodic x-rays are utilized to follow the progression of the foreign body.

Parents of children who swallow things frequently feel guilty and responsible for the child's predicament. The nurse should reassure the parents that no one is at fault.

Nausea and vomiting

Vomiting can indicate a host of problems, both inside and outside the gastrointestinal tract. Nausea may or may not precede vomiting. Bile-stained vomitus usually indicates an obstruction below the ampulla of Vater, as in duodenal atresia or stenosis. Reflux of bile from the duodenum into the stomach can account for bile-stained vomitus without gastrointestinal obstruction in older children with persistent vomiting. Nausea and vomiting are symptoms of some underlying pathology. The definitive cause must be determined and treated.

It is the nurse's responsibility to record the color, consistency, and amount of vomitus and any relationship between vomiting and other events, such as meals or stressful situations. Vomiting in children can easily result in dehydration and fluid and electrolyte imbalance. Intravenous fluids with added electrolytes may be necessary to prevent or treat imbalances. The nursing care of a child with vomiting is discussed later in this chapter.

Diarrhea

Diarrhea is the passage of loose or liquid stools, usually with increased frequency. It may have an acute onset or become a chronic condition. The cause of diarrhea may be bacterial, viral, food- or drug-related, the result of a disease process (either a gastrointestinal disease or another disease, such as an upper respiratory infection), or unknown. In some instances, fever is present, increasing water losses.

Many intestinal and other disorders have diarrhea as one of the symptoms. Diarrhea causes rapid passage of nutrients from the body. This decreases digestion time and the availability of nutrients for absorption. Initially, food is withheld, and intravenous fluid and electrolytes are administered to correct imbalances. Once oral feedings are permitted, the diet progression is similar to that for gastroenteritis. The addition of banana flakes, pieces of apple, or pectin agar will help decrease diarrhea. Infants may be given diluted formula, which is slowly increased to full strength. A lactose-free formula may be used initially to prevent any problems due to temporary decreased lactose tolerance. When fat absorption is impaired, medium chain triglyceride (MCT) oil may be given. This is more readily absorbed and will aid in absorption of fat-soluble vitamins. The treatment and nursing management of a child with diarrhea are discussed in Chap. 18.

Constipation

Constipation is the passage of hard, dry stools or stools of insufficient quantity. The feces eliminated vary from a large mass to small, hard pellets. An anal fissure may cause the stool to be blood-streaked.

Constipation in infancy is usually due to insufficient fluid intake or to an incorrect formula composition. Formulas with a high renal solute load draw water from the bowel contents to provide enough water for urine solute clearance.[16] Older children may withhold bowel movements for a variety of reasons, resulting in constipation. Emotional stress also contributes to constipation. Diets that are low in bulk or contain excessive protein can also contribute to the problem.

Increasing the fluid intake or adding carbohydrates to the formula can remedy the infant's constipation. The addition of fiber and fluids to the older child's diet can be beneficial. Instruct parents to include fruits, vegetables, and whole-grain cereals that are moderately high in fiber in the child's diet. A stool softener or mild laxative may be employed on a temporary basis but should not be used for long-term management. If an anal fissure has resulted from dry, hard stools, the area must be kept clean and dry. Healing is usually spontaneous.

Gastrointestinal bleeding

Gastrointestinal bleeding is caused by various disorders. *Hematemesis*, vomiting of blood, usually indicates bleeding in the upper gastrointestinal tract. However, swallowed blood, as from epistaxis (nosebleed) or dental extractions, may also produce hematemesis. "Coffee-ground" emesis usually indicates bleeding in the esophagus, stomach, or duodenum.

Anal fissures or polyps are responsible for blood-streaked stools. Massive upper gastrointestinal bleeding may stimulate hyperperistalsis, with the result that unaltered blood appears in the stools.[17] "Currant-jelly" stools are associated with intussusception. An infectious process produces acute bloody diarrhea, while chronic diarrhea with bleeding is more often associated with ulcerative colitis.

Tarry stools (melena) result from upper gastrointestinal bleeding. The darker the blood in the stool, the higher it originates in the alimentary tract. The underlying cause of the bleeding must be determined and treated.

The color, amount, and characteristics of the bleeding are noted by the nurse. Hematest tablets, Hemoccult slides, or guaiac reagents may be used to test stool and vomitus for the presence and amount of bleeding. Labstix should not be used to test for blood. They are designed for noting microscopic blood in urine, not for stool and vomitus testing. A nasogastric tube may be inserted if hematemesis is continuous or of significant amounts. Transfusion of whole blood or packed red blood cells may be necessary if the child's hemoglobin is not stabilized. Frequent checks of vital signs are essential to monitor the child's systemic response to blood loss.

Bleeding is very anxiety-provoking for both the child and the parents. Even small amounts may appear great to them. It is the nurse's responsibility to provide support, reassurance, and an explanation of treatments and nursing measures.

Gastrointestinal obstruction

Obstruction in the gastrointestinal system produces vomiting, abdominal pain, and distention. Bile-stained vomitus indicates that the obstruction is in the small intestine below the ampulla of Vater. Bile-stained vomiting occurs in obstructions such as duodenal atresia, duodenal stenosis, and meconium ileus.

Colonic obstruction causes vomiting of fecal material. Hyperperistalsis results from the bowel's attempt to move the contents past the obstruction. Bowel movements are absent.

Signs and symptoms of obstruction also occur with *paralytic* or *adynamic ileus*. In this condition, the nerve impulses that trigger peristalsis are absent or greatly decreased. Thus, bowel sounds are absent or diminished. Abdominal pain, distention, and vomiting are present. Foreign bodies may also cause obstruction. However, the clinical manifestations differ according to the size and location of the object.

Obstruction can progress to perforation and peritonitis. Fluid and electrolyte imbalances as well as dehydration are a result of vomiting, bowel edema, and the accumulation of secretions within the intestine. The obstruction must be identified and corrected.

Gastrointestinal pain

Abdominal pain in children is a fairly common complaint and has numerous causes. It is essential to inquire about the acuteness or chronicity of the pain. The location, duration, and characteristics of the pain must also be assessed. The child frequently is unable to provide this information, and so parents' observations are very helpful. Associated problems such as fever, vomiting, and nausea are important. Any modification in the child's activity, particularly if self-imposed, is noted in the assessment.

Palpation of the abdomen helps determine the pain locus. Most children tend to guard their abdomens, and so it is important to help the child relax. Generalized abdominal pain with rigidity may indicate peritonitis. *Rebound tenderness* (an increase in pain following the release of pressure applied to the abdomen) frequently occurs with appendicitis.

Pain is only a symptom. Efforts must be made to determine the etiology. In some children, the cause is never identified but is attributed to "school phobia" or other psychogenic factors. Such labels should not be used without a thorough evaluation of the child.

Astute observation of the child validates the information obtained from the parents. Any change in pain must be noted and reported to the physician. Heat should never be applied to the abdomen in the presence of undiagnosed pain. Perforation can result from such action. Cathartics and laxatives are also withheld for the same reason.

Types of stools

The newborn's stool cycle is discussed in Chap. 8. Stools similar to adults' are seen by the time the child reaches 2 years of age.

Stools vary greatly in appearance. Small amounts of mucus in stools are of no significance. Large amounts occur in inflammatory bowel disease. In starvation, stools are mucoid with a brownish tint.

Green stools result from the oxidation of bilirubin to biliverdin. Diarrhea stools are commonly green and watery. However, a green stool is not always abnormal. Swallowed blood, upper gastrointestinal tract bleeding, and iron cause the stools to turn black.

Protein stools are brownish yellow or green-black and malodorous. These are found in children who either consume large amounts of protein or are unable to digest it completely. Children with malabsorption syndromes, such as celiac disease or cystic fibrosis, have fatty stools. These are gray, greasy, and bulky and have a foul odor.

Clinitest and guaiac tests are routinely done on stools of children who have elimination or digestive alterations. Guaiac testing reveals the presence of blood, while Clinitest tablets monitor sugar content. Litmus paper may be used to measure stool pH.

Fluids and electrolytes

The stomach contains large amounts of hydrochloric acid. High concentrations of sodium are present in the gastric mucus. Fluid from the small intestine contains bicarbonate and sodium, with lesser amounts of chloride and potassium. The large intestine absorbs water and electrolytes. Diarrhea, vomiting, gastric and intestinal suction, and other gastrointestinal alterations all contribute to electrolyte loss. Hypovolemic shock, electrolyte imbalances, and acid-base disturbances are potential complications of both alterations and treatments. The clinical manifestations and nursing management of these problems are discussed fully in Chap. 18.

MEDICAL ASSESSMENT AND TREATMENTS

Diagnostic tests

Barium studies Alterations occur in all areas of the gastrointestinal tract. Many problems produce similar clinical manifestations. Diagnostic tests are used to determine the location and severity of the alteration.

Barium is a contrast material that outlines organ systems on x-ray examination. Barium is used for both upper and lower gastrointestinal x-ray studies. The child consumes barium prepared as either a liquid or a pudding. Fluoroscopy follows the progress of the contrast agent down the esophagus, into the stomach, and through the small intestine. Pictures are taken and examined in greater detail later. Barium is given by rectum to outline the lower gastrointestinal tract.

Food and fluids are withheld for 8 h prior to the barium swallow. Only clear liquids are allowed for 8 h prior to the barium enema. Mineral oil and cleansing enemas are given to empty the intestinal tract the night before the lower gastrointestinal study. After both procedures, all the barium must be eliminated to prevent impaction. Laxatives or enemas may be necessary to expel the barium. Check the stool for barium, which is white. A normal diet is resumed after the completion of the studies, provided that there are no contraindications.

Endoscopy *Endoscopy* is a broad term that refers to the visualization of an internal body cavity. It is possible to use a fiber-optic instrument (with an internal light source) to examine many parts of the gastrointestinal tract.

Esophagoscopy is utilized to (1) retrieve foreign bodies in the esophagus, (2) determine the presence and extent of stenosis, (3) determine the extent of esophageal varices, (4) assist in dilatation procedures, and (5) perform a biopsy. Esophagoscopy is usually done after administration of intravenous sedatives. Nothing is given by mouth for 8 h prior to the procedure (possibly less time in the case of younger children). Normal activities and a regular diet are resumed when the child is fully alert.

Proctoscopy, sigmoidoscopy, and colonoscopy are used to diagnose intestinal conditions such as Hirschsprung's disease, ulcerative colitis, regional enteritis, and rectal polyps. The flexible fiberscopes (such as the colonoscope) allow the examiner to see the entire colon. Biopsies can also be performed at the time of examination.

Proctoscopy, sigmoidoscopy, and colonoscopy can be done without anesthesia or sedation. Bowel preparation (enemas and laxatives) is frequently deferred because it could cause mucosal changes that would distort the examination. The nurse is responsible for explaining the procedure to the child and enlisting his or her cooperation. The child is placed in either a knee-to-chest or left lateral position. The nurse should stay with the child to provide support and to help maintain the proper position. No restrictions are necessary after the procedure. The child should be observed for signs and symptoms of perforation and bleeding.

Biopsies A *rectal biopsy* is performed under anesthesia. After the specimen is obtained, the small surgical wound is closed with sutures. *Nothing* is inserted into the rectum for several days postoperatively.

A *liver biopsy* can be performed on the unit. Premedication with sedatives, narcotics, or tranquilizers promotes comfort. The child must be immobilized during the procedure. A small incision is made between the eighth and ninth ribs, and a Menghini or Jamshidi needle is used to obtain the tissue specimen. Baseline vital signs are taken before the biopsy and frequently thereafter. Hemorrhage is a dangerous potential complication. Pressure is applied to the site for 10 min after the biopsy. The child remains in bed for 24 h and is positioned on the right side for splinting purposes.

Enemas

Enemas are not diagnostic tools but may be used prior to lower gastrointestinal studies or surgery to ensure adequate visualization of the bowel. They must be used judiciously to prevent electrolyte imbalances. Many commercial enema preparations are available for bowel preparation, and the specific directions for their use in children should be followed (see Table 16-13).

Colonic lavage, or irrigation, differs from enema administration. In this procedure, small amounts of solution are inserted and then aspirated back. It is most often used for children with Hirschsprung's disease and, occasionally, for those with encopresis.

The rubber catheter is lubricated and inserted into the rectum, using a gentle rotating motion, until resistance is felt (this is the initial point of aganglionic bowel, the underlying lesion in Hirschsprung's disease). Thirty ml of solution is instilled through the catheter, using a large syringe. This is then aspirated back. The process is repeated until the aspirate is free of fecal particles.

The entire length of the catheter is then inserted, using the same rotating motion. Force should not be used because of the danger of bowel perforation. The procedure is continued, with small amounts of solution instilled and aspirated back until the returns are clear. The catheter is withdrawn 1 in, and the process is repeated until the catheter is completely out.

Finally, the catheter is reinserted for its entire length to check for missed areas, and the lavage is repeated if necessary. All the solution instilled must be returned to prevent absorption into the circulatory system through the intestinal wall.

Gastric intubation

Gastric intubation is the insertion of a nasogastric tube for the purposes of preoperative and postoperative decompression, removing gastric contents, obtaining specimens for diagnostic tests, or giving feedings and medications. The catheters vary in size and have either single or double lumens (see Chap. 16). The older child is placed in an upright position for tube insertion. The child is encouraged to swallow as the catheter is inserted. Drinking water, if not contraindicated, may be helpful in this process.

Preoperatively, gastric intubation may be necessary to relieve distention and prevent vomiting. Manipulation of the bowel during surgery results in paralytic (adynamic) ileus. Decompression and drainage of gastric and intestinal secretions are necessary until peristalsis returns. The tube may be attached to suction to facilitate drainage. The maximum suction force that can be used without causing mucosal damage is 25 mmHg.[18] Intermittent suction, set at "low," must be used with single-lumen (Levin) tubes. The "high" setting is used with Salem sumps, which have double lumens. The vent lumen of the Salem sump keeps the suction pressure below 25 mmHg. Because of the air vent, the Salem sump tubes may also be connected to continuous suction at 30 to 40 mmHg without adverse effects.[19] This vent must never be occluded, or pressure will exceed the maximum and cause gastric mucosal injury.

It is a nursing responsibility to ensure patency of the nasogastric tube. Irrigations are performed with normal saline at specified intervals. The amount instilled is recorded as intake, and the aspirate as output. The color and amount of the aspirate are noted, as well as any changes in its characteristics. Difficulty in irrigating or withdrawing solution, nausea, vomiting, distention, or discomfort must be reported to the physician. Nasogastric tubes are never clamped without a physician's order. When peristalsis returns, they are removed.

Gavage feedings are used for children whose physical condition is such that oral feedings place an extreme burden on them (see Table 16-3). The formula is given slowly and at room temperature or slightly warmer. Feeding pumps and constant-flow drips are other methods used for gavage feedings. The nurse must routinely check these to ensure that the correct volume is infusing.

When the nurse is giving an infant a gavage feeding, a pacifier should be used to stimulate sucking. The infant can then associate the action of sucking with a feeling of fullness. Studies have shown that nonnutritive sucking during feeding may accelerate weight gain and make the transition to oral feedings easier.[20]

Ostomies

An *ostomy* is a surgically created opening between an internal cavity and the body surface. After procedures such as ileostomies and colostomies, a *stoma* (opening) is present on the external surface.

An *ileostomy* may be performed for ulcerative colitis or temporarily for meconium ileus. The terminal ileum opens onto the right side of the abdomen. The drainage from an ileostomy is liquid and continuous and cannot be regulated. In a continent ileostomy, an intraabdominal reservoir, or *Kock pouch,* is made from the terminal ileum; the pouch stores fecal contents until the patient drains it with a catheter. Just distal to the pouch the terminal ileum is telescoped upon itself (similar to intussusception) to form a valve that prevents leaking. The stoma is almost flush with the skin. The purpose of the reservoir is to eliminate the need for an external appliance. This procedure may be more acceptable for patients, particularly adolescents, who are concerned with their body image. One disadvantage of the Kock pouch is that if for some reason the pouch needs to be taken down, the patient loses that portion of the ileum. This is an important factor when considering absorptive surface.

There are several types of *colostomies*. The sigmoid colostomy is the most common. A transverse colostomy is performed for some types of imperforate anus and for Hirschsprung's disease. It is the most common type of temporary colostomy. A transverse colostomy is created either by the loop method or with surgically severed proximal and distal stomas (double barrel). The stool is eliminated from the proximal stoma. The fecal discharge from a transverse colostomy is more formed than that from an ileostomy because the stool contains less water.

Children with either an ileostomy or a colostomy require meticulous nursing care. The peristomal area is vulnerable to skin breakdown (excoriation), particularly with an ileostomy. Digestive enzymes are present in the waste material and are harmful to skin integrity. The area must be protected from leakage and kept clean and dry (see Table 19-6).

The ostomy appliance (bag) must fit securely around the stoma to prevent spillage. Skin barriers such as zinc oxide or karaya powder can be used for infants. Stomahesive or karaya rings are better for older children.[21] Both these protectors adhere directly to the peristomal area. The appliance is then fixed to either the Stomahesive or the ring. The appliance should be drainable so that it can be left in place for several days. Careful attention to skin care and appliance fixation minimizes the possibility of leakage and subsequent excoriation (skin breakdown). Odors from ostomies can be controlled with a variety of agents. Some experimentation may be necessary to find one that works optimally for the individual child.

It is a nursing responsibility to teach the parents ileostomy or colostomy care. Initially the parents may be frightened or overwhelmed by the surgery. They need support, guidance, and encouragement to participate in their child's care. The parents begin with small tasks in the care of the ostomy and gradually are able to assume total care. Teaching should take place over a period of time so that the parents can perform the tasks several times in a nurse's presence. The child who is old enough can also be responsible for some aspects of ostomy care.

Table 19-6 Nursing Care Responsibilities for the Child with an Ostomy

1. Change the appliance regularly:
   a. Gather equipment (consider the type of appliance).
   b. Empty the old appliance.
   c. Remove the old appliance gently (use water or solvent if necessary).
   d. Hold gauze over the stoma to absorb leakage.
2. Cleanse the area (use mild soap, rinse with water, and dry completely).
3. Assess the stoma (color, bleeding, edema, retraction).
4. Assess the condition of the peristomal skin:
   a. Apply a skin barrier.
   b. Consider the age of the child and the type of appliance. Prepare the skin, using a karaya product and stomahesive.
5. Prepare the appliance:
   a. Temporary: measure and cut the opening.
   b. Permanent: apply adhesive.
6. Apply the appliance (smooth out bubbles).
7. Monitor intake and output (quantity and quality).
8. Answer questions and give instructions during the process.
9. Provide psychosocial support for the child and the family.

It is important to observe the type and amount of drainage. If the child has diarrhea, large amounts of sodium and water can be lost rapidly with an ileostomy. Dehydration can occur in a short period of time with either a colostomy or an ileostomy. Parents need to be provided with this information.

Body image and body integrity are important concerns for both the child and the parents. It is imperative that nurses recognize these issues and allow time for discussion. Peer relationships are major concerns of school-age children and adolescents, and anxieties can surface in regard to these relationships and the ostomy. The nurse must answer any questions the child has and provide reassurance that the child's social life need not be adversely affected.

A *cervical esophagostomy* is performed for esophageal atresia that ends in a proximal blind pouch. A stoma is created from the end of the pouch and opens onto the base of the neck, usually on the left side. A plastic or rubber catheter is inserted and remains in place for several days postoperatively. Nasal and oral secretions drain from the stoma.

Cervical esophagostomy does not cause skin breakdown because there are no proteolytic enzymes in saliva. A mild ointment will suffice to protect the skin from irritation due to constant wetness. The area needs to be wiped frequently with tissues and washed two to three times daily. A small dressing can be taped over the site and changed every 1 to 2 h, or an absorbent "bib" can be used.

To provide nutrition for the child with a cervical esophagostomy, a *gastrostomy* is also performed. The child with a gastrostomy and an esophagostomy may be given "sham" feedings.[22] Fluid is given orally, and a towel or cup is used to catch the fluid as it comes from the esophagostomy. This promotes essential learning of sucking, swallowing, and eating and avoids the difficulties of teaching the infant how to eat after the atresia is surgically corrected.

A *gastrostomy* (Fig. 19-2) is created by inserting a mushroom or Foley catheter through a

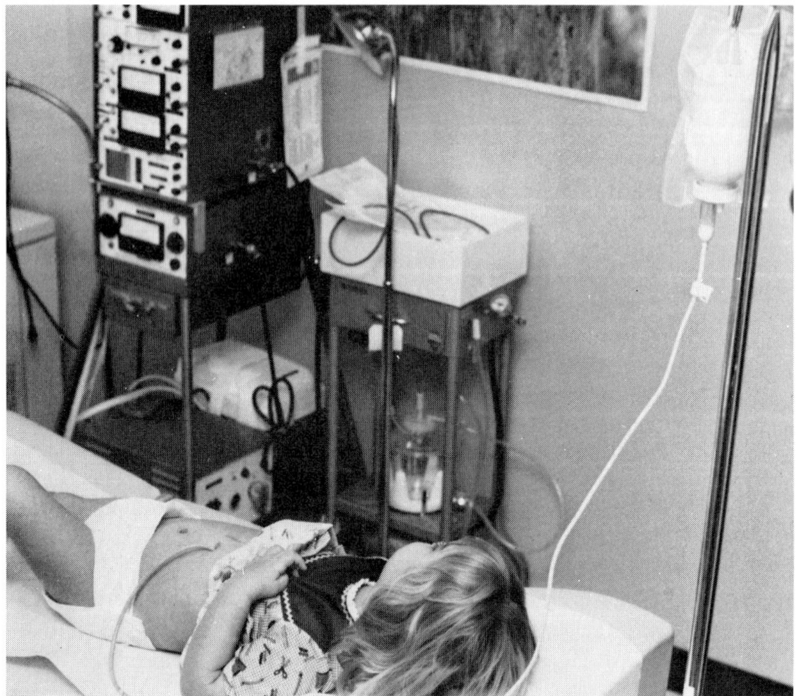

Figure 19-2 A child receiving a gastrostomy tube feeding. (*From L. Shortridge and E. J. Lee, Introductory Skills for Nursing Practice, McGraw-Hill, New York, 1980. Used with permission.*)

small incision in the abdomen into the stomach. The anterior stomach wall is sutured to the anterior peritoneum to prevent seepage of gastric material into the peritoneal cavity. The gastrostomy tube is secured to the abdominal surface by a purse-string suture.

Another technique of insertion, which is still being tested for use with pediatric patients, involves inserting the catheter percutaneously while the child is undergoing an esophagoscopy. In addition to the sedation used for the esophagoscopy, a local anesthetic is used at the insertion site. This procedure eliminates the risks of general anesthesia and is much less expensive.

Tension on the gastrostomy tube should be avoided. It can widen the opening, causing leaking. The area is inspected for redness, excoriation, and leakage of gastric secretions. The skin can be protected by the use of a karaya paste, zinc oxide, or other products.

Feedings initially consist of clear liquids and are advanced to full-strength formula according to the individual child's tolerance. Infants with long-term gastrostomy feedings should have diets that progress as a normal infant's would. Cereal and strained baby foods can be mixed with the formula at the normal developmental times. The tube should be flushed with a small amount of water after feedings to maintain patency. The gastrostomy tube is elevated and left unclamped to allow for the reflux of air and formula. The tube is clamped between feedings after the child demonstrates tolerance for the amount and type of formula used.

Dilatations

Esophageal dilatation is done to relieve strictures or prevent scar tissue formation such as may follow tracheoesophageal fistula repair or lye ingestion. Tucker or mercury dilators are the instruments used for esophageal dilatation. The procedure itself varies with the dilator used, but the principles are the same. Rubber tubes of various sizes are threaded into the esophagus. Dilatations are performed on a regular basis until the larger tubes pass easily. Anesthesia is usually required because of the child's difficulty in swallowing the dilators.

Anal dilatation is performed using Hager dilators. These are cone-shaped metal instruments of different sizes which are inserted into the anus. Dilatation may be required after pull-through surgery for Hirschsprung's disease or imperforate anus. The dilator is inserted and held in place for several minutes. It should be warmed and lubricated before insertion.

PRINCIPLES OF NURSING CARE FOR THE CHILD WHO UNDERGOES GASTROINTESTINAL SURGERY

Preoperative nursing management

Preoperatively, teaching is an essential component of nursing management for the child and the family (see Chaps. 15 and 16).

The child is shown where the incision and dressing will be. If an ostomy procedure is to be done, the child must be told about it and prepared for the alteration.

Postoperative nursing management

When the child returns to the unit, he or she is positioned on the side to prevent aspiration and promote drainage of oral secretions. The child is encouraged to cough and deep-breathe frequently to prevent atelectasis. Infants and small children may require oral or nasotracheal suctioning of secretions. The patency of both the intravenous line and the nasogastric tube must be maintained. The dressing is inspected for drainage, and the color, odor, and amount are recorded.

It is important to observe for abdominal distention because this raises the diaphragm and exerts pressure on the abdominal cavity and the incision. Distention also compromises respiratory function, particularly in children under the age of 7, who are primarily abdominal breathers. Measuring abdominal girth once a shift, or more frequently, is a means of detecting distention.

Accurate intake and output are necessary, as well as urine specific gravity. Fluid and electrolyte balance can be precarious in children with gastrointestinal alterations, and it is essential to account for all gains and losses. The nurse must also be alert to any clinical manifestations of electrolyte imbalances.

Mouth care is given frequently for the child's comfort and to moisten the mouth and lips. Nothing is given by mouth until peristalsis resumes. This is indicated by the passage of flatus or stool and the presence of bowel sounds.

The incision should be inspected for signs of infection such as redness, warmth, and drainage. A culture should be taken of any wound exudate. Wound *dehiscence* is the separation of the edges of the incision. *Evisceration* is the protrusion of abdominal contents (usually bowel) through the separated incision. These two complications are not common in pediatric patients but may occur in debilitated children. The physician must be notified immediately. The wound edges are brought together and held in place with either a dressing or Steri-strips for dehiscence. If evisceration occurs, the abdominal contents are covered with a sterile towel which has been wet with normal saline. Vital signs should be monitored frequently, since shock is associated with evisceration.

ALTERATIONS OF THE MOUTH

Cleft lip

Cleft lip is a facial malformation involving a congenital fissure or fissures of the upper lip. Cleft lip with or without cleft palate occurs in about 1 in 1000 births, with about three-quarters of the cases involving a unilateral (one-sided) cleft. Of the unilateral clefts, 70 percent are on the left side, and 30 percent are on the right side.[23] Cleft lip occurs twice as frequently in males as in females and is more common in the relatives of affected persons. The defect is believed to be either an autosomal recessive or a conditioned dominant inheritance.[24]

Etiology The etiology of cleft lip is not conclusively known. Heredity is one possible factor; approximately 15 to 20 percent of children with clefts of the lip or palate have another family member with the condition. Recent research indicates that the etiology is a combination of genetic and environmental factors. Possible environmental factors include nutritional deficiencies, radiation, maternal infection, and a deficiency in the embryonic mesoderm.

Cleft lip may result from the failure of the facial processes to fuse between the fifth and eighth weeks of embryonic life. An alternative hypothesis is that it is due to a rupture that occurs after the fusion process is completed.[25]

The defect is visible and is diagnosed imme-

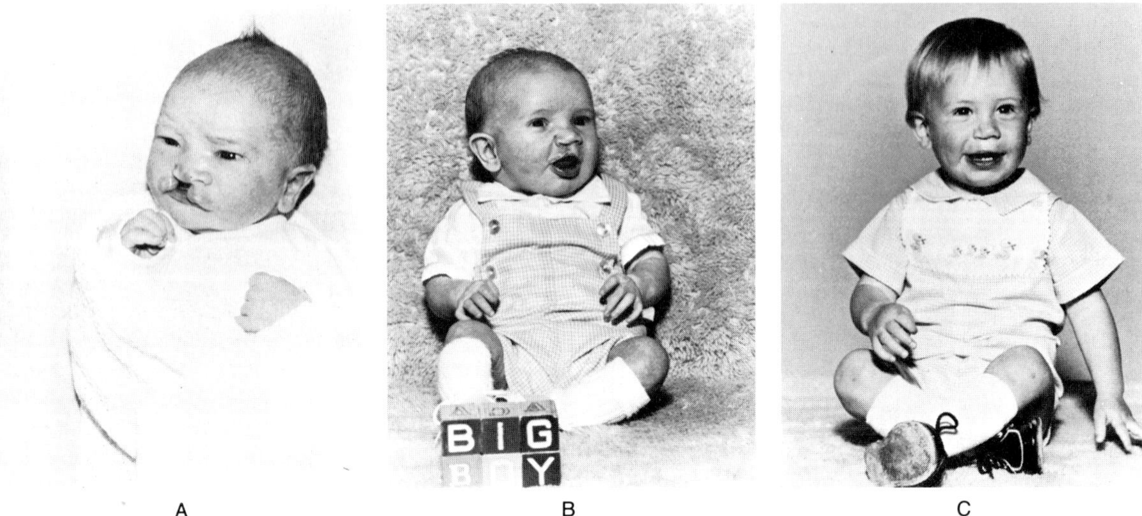

A B C

Figure 19-3 (*A*) A 3.6-kg newborn with a cleft lip and a cleft palate, which cannot be seen in this picture. (*B*) The same infant after repair of the cleft lip at about 8 weeks of age (and weighing 4.5 kg). (*C*) The same child at the age of about 11 months. Note the lower teeth. The upper teeth are in good position, except for the one that is missing. The cleft palate has not yet been repaired.

diately at birth (see Fig. 19-3*A*). Cleft lip varies in severity from an incomplete cleft lip, which can be simply a notch in the vermilion (red) border of the lip, to a complete separation of the lip extending into the nostril and floor of the nose. The affected nostril is wider than normal, and there is a high incidence of poorly positioned, missing, or supernumerary (extra) teeth in the line of the cleft.

In a bilateral cleft lip, the middle portion of the lip, the *prolabium,* is isolated in the midline and remains attached to the *premaxilla* and the *columella* (nasal septum). The nostrils are stretched and wide.

Medical management The treatment is surgical closure of the cleft. Some surgeons do this in the first week of life. However, most prefer to wait until 2 to 3 months of age, when the child has demonstrated a satisfactory weight gain and is completely free of oral, respiratory, and systemic infection. The rule of 10 may be utilized: The infant should be 10 weeks of age, weigh 10 lb, and have a hemoglobin of 10 (see Fig. 19-3*B* and *C*). The time delay also allows for the development of normal maternal-infant bonding and gives the parents time to adjust to the defect and accept the child. Cleft lip may be accompanied by other congenital anomalies. The child needs thorough evaluation to detect the presence of any anomalies.

Surgical correction The surgical objective is to unite the cleft edges and produce a lip that is both functional and cosmetically attractive. The surgery, *cheilorrhaphy,* involves a Z-plasty technique, which employs a staggered, Z-shaped suture line. Notching of the lip from retraction, which usually occurs with healing, and scar formation are reduced using this incision. To protect the lip and to relieve tension on the suture line, the *Logan bar,* a wire bow, is attached to the infant's cheeks with tape (see Fig. 19-4), or a butterfly adhesive strip is placed over the suture line.

The defects that may remain after corrective surgery are a widened nostril and flattened tip of the nose on the side of the repair, a thinner area on the bottom of the upper lip, a lumpy or irregularly shaped vermilion lip margin, and a fine-line surgical scar. The lip may need one or more revisions. Additional nasal corrective surgery is often done in later childhood or early adolescence. The success of surgery depends on the severity of the cleft and the freedom from postoperative infection.

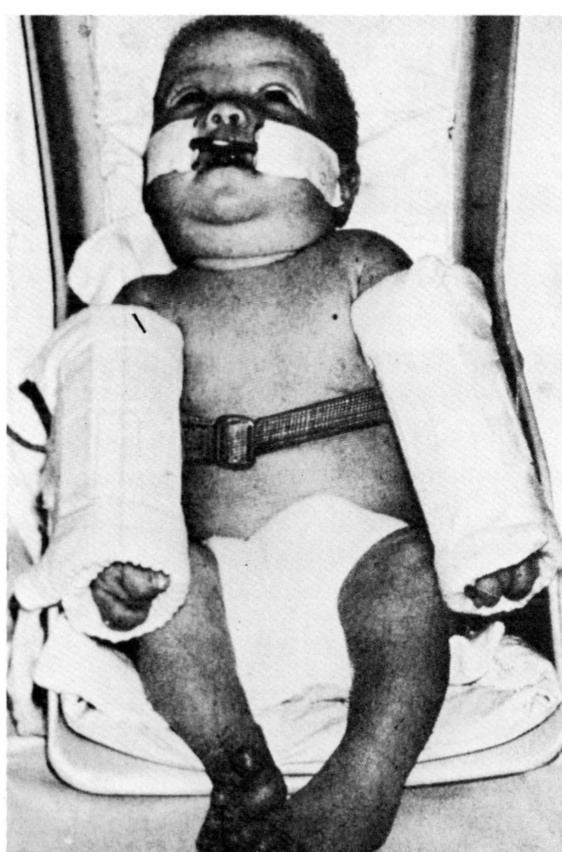

Figure 19-4 An infant in elbow restraints and with a Logan bow in place to prevent tension on the suture line following cleft lip repair. (*From A. J. Ingalls and M. C. Salerno, Maternal and Child Health Nursing, 4th ed., Mosby, St. Louis, 1979. Used with permission.*)

Preoperative nursing management Preoperatively, the role of the nurse focuses on providing support for the parents, ensuring adequate nutrition, and preventing aspiration and infection. Feeding an infant with a cleft lip takes longer than normal and may be frustrating. Each child is individual and has different needs, depending on the characteristics of the cleft. There are a variety of feeding methods available. The nurse should support the parents in finding the method that works best for their child. An infant with a cleft lip may be able to breast-feed. In addition to its nutritional value, breast milk contains immunoglobulins that help prevent upper respiratory infections and otitis media, which occur frequently in these children. To breast-feed, the mother should manually extend the nipple and place it in the child's mouth. Milk is released through the pressure of the baby's jaws, gums, and tongue on the areola, even if the cleft makes sucking ineffective. The attitude of the mother is very important. The nurse and family members should give her extra support. The local chapter of the LaLeche League can provide additional guidance and printed material for the mothers of babies with cleft lip. Careful growth records must be kept to ensure that the infant is obtaining enough milk. If the mother does not opt to breast-feed or is unable to, the nurse should suggest other feeding techniques.

Soft, regular cross-cut nipples or nipples for premature babies, in which the hole is slightly enlarged, are often used successfully. A Nuk nipple turned upside down; a cleft lip–cleft palate nurser (Mead Johnson), which has a long nipple with a broad base (see Fig. 19-5*A* and *B*); or a long, thin rubber nipple (Ross Laboratories) (see Fig. 19-5*C*) may also be used. Breast-feeding and nipple-feeding encourage the use of the facial and sucking muscles, leading to proper facial growth and development[26] and later speech development. When nipple-feeding, be sure that the nipple is placed in a normal feeding position, not in the cleft. Encourage the infant to suck by moving the jaw or stroking the cheek. Placing the thumb or index finger over the cleft lip may help the infant create suction. A soft bottle enables the person giving the feeding to apply gentle pressure, thus maintaining milk flow when the infant's suck is ineffective. Another technique involves the use of a large rubber-tipped syringe, sometimes referred to as a *Breck feeder*, which is similar but not the same (see Fig. 19-5*D*). A Lamb's nipple (which is very soft and long and requires little sucking for milk flow) may occasionally be used. Using a medicine dropper or a spoon is tedious, time-consuming, and fatiguing for both the infant and the mother, but should be considered if other feeding methods are unsatisfactory. On occasion, gavage feedings may have to be given.

The infant should be held in an upright position, fed slowly, and burped frequently. Infants with a cleft lip swallow large amounts of air before and during feedings and are at increased risk for vomiting and aspiration. Choking is a frequent feeding problem. Some milk may come out of the nose. Warn the parents that because of incomplete suction, the feedings may be noisy but should not be continually interrupted. This frustrates the baby, increases crying, and adds

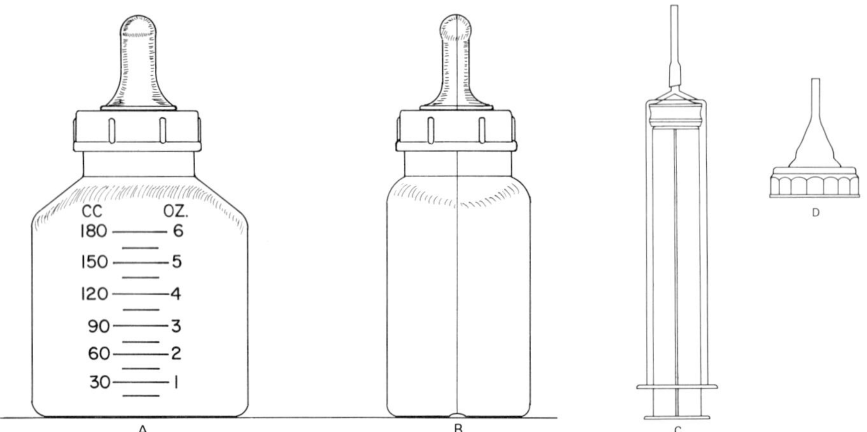

Figure 19-5 Methods of feeding infants with cleft lip and/or palate. (*A*) A cleft lip–palate nurser, front view. (*B*) Side view, showing the broad part of the nipple positioned against the tongue and the cleft. (*C*) A rubber-tipped syringe. (*D*) A cleft palate assembly; a long nipple bypasses the cleft.

to the problem. When a feeding is completed, the mouth should be rinsed with water. After feeding, position the child in an infant seat or on the side to prevent vomiting and aspiration. It is best not to get the baby accustomed to sleeping on the abdomen, since this position is contraindicated after surgery.

A few days before surgery, the infant should be taught the feeding techniques to be used after surgery. It is also wise to introduce the restraints so that the baby will become accustomed to restricted positioning and decreased mobility. The restraints used should immobilize the arms so that the infant cannot rub or disturb the suture line or turn over onto the abdomen. Jackets with pockets in the arms for tongue blades or arm restraints that do not allow bending of the elbows are needed.

Postoperative nursing management Postoperatively, the role of the nurse is to prevent trauma and infection of the suture line and maintain nutrition. The restraints should be sent with the infant to the operating room and applied in the recovery room. They also need to be pinned to the infant's clothing or diapers to prevent the infant from rubbing the mouth against the shoulder. The infant wears the restraints until the lip is completely healed. They should be removed one at a time at least every 4 h to allow range of motion and inspection of the skin condition. Discharge instructions should stress the correct use of restraints, precautions that must be taken, and the necessity for using the restraints (see Chap. 16).

Postoperative feeding will be by rubber-tipped syringe for about 3 weeks because a nipple would cause suture line pressure. The rubber tip should be directed toward the side of the mouth to avoid the suture line and prevent sucking motions. The feeding principles previously discussed should be utilized. After feeding, the mouth is rinsed with water to cleanse the oral cavity and prevent infection. Suture care of both the inner and outer lip is done to prevent crusting, infection, and subsequent scarring of the incision. Care consists of cleansing, not rubbing, the site gently with sterile swabs and a solution of water and hydrogen peroxide and then rinsing with sterile water or saline. Once the lip is cleansed, a thin layer of antibiotic ointment, such as bacitracin, may be applied to promote a supple suture line and prevent infection. The Logan bar or butterfly adhesive is not disturbed; any bleeding or separation of the suture line should be reported immediately to the surgeon. Crying stresses the suture line, increasing the chance of scarring. It is important to anticipate the infant's needs in order to prevent crying. Holding may be needed to keep the baby content.

Positioning of the infant postoperatively is very important. The infant may be positioned in an infant seat or on the back, but never on the abdomen. The side-lying position can be used, taking care to prevent the infant from rolling over and rubbing the face on the mattress.

Increased mucus production and laryngeal edema due to endotracheal intubation may cause airway problems. The nursing goal is to prevent aspiration and respiratory complications. The infant must be observed closely and constantly; humidifying the air may help reduce edema and make breathing easier. If suctioning is needed, it is done with care to avoid damaging the lip. A very soft catheter and low suction are employed. Avoiding the suture line is mandatory. If the infant develops acute respiratory distress, these precautions must be modified because preservation of life is primary. Positioning with the infant's head elevated—for example, in an infant seat—will make breathing easier. The side-lying position prevents aspiration.

The nurse's role as teacher and counselor is extremely important. After the initial diagnosis of the defect, the parents will have to be taught to care for the child. They will need to know why the child cannot suck efficiently and learn the appropriate feeding techniques. The parents should begin caring for and feeding the infant early so that they will gain confidence before the infant's discharge. If the mother and the baby are at different hospitals, the mother visits the baby when she is physically able to. Initially, learning to feed the infant can be a frustrating and time-consuming experience. The parents will need constant support and praise from the nursing staff. The parents should be told of future surgeries, as well as the other problems that can occur, such as increased numbers of upper respiratory and ear infections. After surgery, discharge instructions need to cover feeding techniques, restraints, positioning, and lip care.

When the parents are told of the defect initially, they will go through a grieving process for the loss of the normal, perfect child they had anticipated for 9 months and now do not have. With the resolution of this grieving process, the parents will begin to accept the child. The nurse can support the parents by listening to their concerns, encouraging them to care for the infant, praising their care-giving achievements, and encouraging them to make realistic plans. A positive aspect of this type of defect is that it can be surgically repaired.

A major determinant of the parents' reaction to a cleft lip is its location. The face is the main means of communication in most cultures. Such a visible facial defect is one of the most difficult congenital defects to accept. The nurse is a role model for the family in showing acceptance for the baby as an individual. The nurse should point out positive things about the child (e.g., turning toward a parent's voice or having beautiful eyes). The parents should be encouraged to cuddle, hold, and talk to the child, particularly emphasizing eye-to-eye contact. These interactions are needed for the development of normal parent-child relationships and for the normal emotional and social development of the infant.

A Nursing Care Plan for a child who has undergone surgery for a cleft lip is presented at the end of this chapter.

Cleft palate

Etiology *Cleft palate* is thought to be inherited as a simple dominant trait; it has an incidence of about 1 in 2500 live births.[27] Cleft palate is frequently associated with other congenital anomalies, especially those involving intellectual impairment. It is also found with many syndromes involving chromosomal abnormalities. The cleft palate results from the failure of the maxillary processes to fuse completely. The formation of the hard and soft palates takes place from the seventh to the twelfth weeks of intrauterine life. The lateral palatal processes of the maxilla grow upward and arch over the tongue. During the eighth week, the fusion of these processes begins anteriorly and extends posteriorly. This fusion is completed at the uvula during the twelfth week. Due to this directional developmental process of growth, from front to back, it is impossible to have a cleft of the hard palate without a cleft of the soft palate (see Fig. 19-6).

The extent of a unilateral cleft palate may range from an incomplete submucous cleft in the soft palate to separation through the entire soft and hard palates. With a bilateral complete cleft palate, the clefts extend through the hard and soft palates and the alveolus (dental ridge) on each side of the premaxilla. As a result, there is a direct connection between both nasal chambers and the oral cavity. Feeding problems are similar to those of the infant with a cleft lip. The child cannot suck properly, and food is regurgitated through the nose.

Medical management Cleft palate, unlike cleft lip, may go undetected for a period of time. It can be detected in the newborn by exploring the palate with a finger. Some overt signs of cleft palate that might be noted by the nurse who is

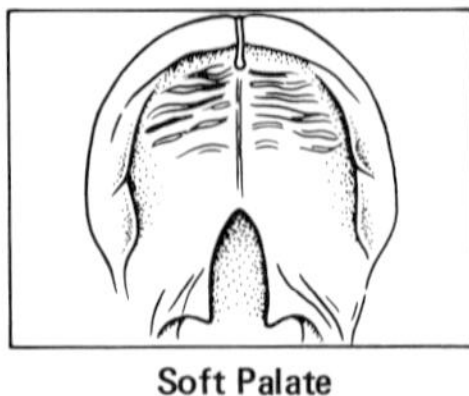
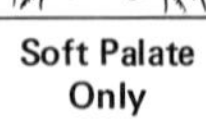

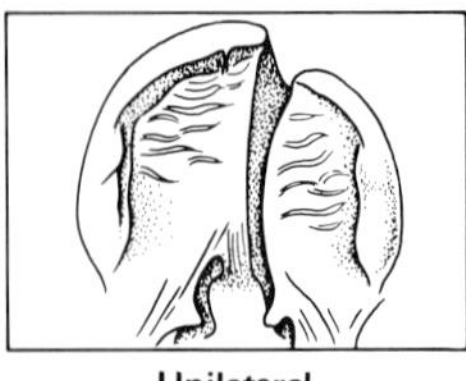

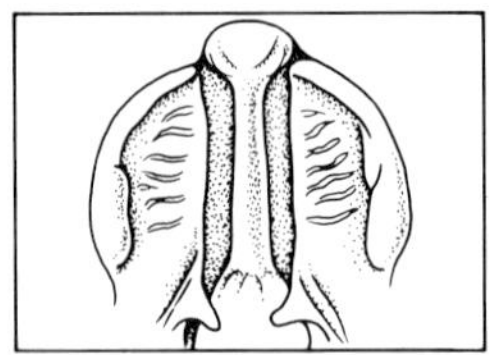

Figure 19-6 Three variations of a cleft palate defect. The palate fuses from the front, hard palate to the back, soft palate, with the more severe defect signifying an origin earlier in fetal life. (*From Ross Laboratories, Clinical Education Aid No. 11, Columbus, Ohio, February 1979. Reprinted with permission.*)

feeding the newborn include the inability of the infant to suck properly, regurgitation of fluids through the nose, and difficulty in swallowing or breathing.

The primary objective of medical treatment is union of the cleft segments and achievement of intelligible and pleasant speech. Surgery can be done at any time after 3 months of age.[28, 29] Surgical correction at 3 months is controversial, and some surgeons prefer to wait until the child is older (1 to 2 years). Some surgeons believe that making the repair too early may damage the developing tooth buds. Others believe that if the teeth are in line with the cleft, they will be malformed or malpositioned anyway. If the cleft is severe, repair may have to be done later to take advantage of changes in the palate occurring with growth. Consonant-vowel sounds begin between 6 and 9 months of age,[30] and so articulation defects may be minimized by early repair. The best speech outcome correlates with early correction. If surgery is to be delayed beyond 3 years, a palatal appliance may be used to allow speech development to take place. If repair is not technically feasible or is medically contraindicated, a prosthodontic obturator (a plastic device that covers the palate defect) may be used to create an artificial palate.

Preoperative nursing management Preoperatively, the goals are the same as those for the infant with a cleft lip: adequate nutrition and prevention of infections. Similar feeding principles and techniques are used. Prior to surgery, the child needs to be fed by the technique to be employed postoperatively. The infant can become accustomed to the method, thus facilitating fluid intake in the postsurgical period. A cup or the side of a spoon can be used; a nipple would disturb the surgical line. The mouth should be rinsed after feeding to prevent the collection of milk as a medium for bacterial growth.

Postoperative nursing management In the postoperative period, the nurse wants to prevent both trauma to the repair and infection. Respiratory problems can occur in the immediate postoperative period. Laryngeal edema due to intubation and learning to breathe through the smaller nasal passages may lead to respiratory difficulties; a croupette with mist will help alleviate these problems. Suctioning should not be done routinely, but only as needed, because the catheter may injure the palate repair. Close observation of respiratory status and color is mandatory. Clots have been known to fall off the repair and block the airway.

Restraints are used to prevent the child from injuring the suture line by placing fingers or objects in the mouth. Positioning on the abdomen can be done; this will facilitate drainage of secretions and help prevent aspirations. An upright position in an infant seat is also useful.

Feeding should be done using the method selected preoperatively. A paper cup or the side of a plastic spoon is best. Metal utensils, straws, or any device that could harm the suture line must be avoided. The child will be fed only fluids for 3 to 4 weeks, until healing is complete; a normal diet can then be resumed.

On discharge, the parents should be aware of the need to keep hands and toys away from the child's mouth. Sucking, laughing, and blowing all cause strain and should be avoided. Feeding techniques and restraints also need to be discussed. Parents should be aware that further surgery may be needed to close any small residual fistulas of the palate, for scar revisions, and for correction of nasal deformities. The eustachian tube may also be partially blocked or abnormally positioned in the pharnyx. Thus it may not drain properly, causing a high frequency of otitis media. Myringotomy (insertion of polyethylene drainage tubes into the eardrum) to treat chronic serous otitis media may need to be done.

The problems of the child with a cleft palate are multiple and require the coordinated efforts of the entire health team. Recurrent ear infections can lead to permanent hearing loss. Dental decay and malpositioned teeth require extensive dental and orthodontic work. Speech defects may remain, even after closure of the palate, and speech therapy is required. The child's speech will have a hypernasal quality when he or she makes certain sounds—*p, b, d, t, s, h,* and *g*—due to the inadequacies remaining in the function of the palatal and pharyngeal muscles.[31]

The palate team is an interdisciplinary team of pediatric specialists who repair the defect and deal with dental, hearing, speech, social, and emotional problems. The child's physical problems can lead to social problems due to the speech impediment. Problems with self-image and peer relationships are common. The whole habilitative effort is team-centered. Well-established cleft palate clinics have these wide-ranging facilities available for the child and family. The nurse plays an important role in coordinating care and dealing with the child on a long-term basis.

ALTERATIONS OF THE ESOPHAGUS

Esophageal atresia and tracheoesophageal fistula

Embryology The esophagus develops from the primitive foregut. Between the third and sixth intrauterine weeks, it lengthens and separates from the trachea, which lies in front of it. Figure 21-1 shows the lung bud branching off the esophagus. At one point in development, the esophagus is a solid tube that later hollows out.

Etiology The embryological failure of the esophagus to develop as a continuous, intact passageway results in the defects of *esophageal atresia* and *tracheoesophageal* (TE) *fistula.* Figure 19-7 lists six types of esophageal defects and the frequency of the defects. Complete esophageal atresia occurs when the esophagus ends in two blind, separate pouches with no connection between the mouth and stomach (Type I). The most common (87 percent) atresia and TE fistula is Type III.[32] In this defect, the proximal (upper) esophagus ends in a blind pouch, while the lower esophageal segment has a fistula (opening) into the trachea or primary bronchus. The connection from the stomach to the trachea allows reflux of gastric contents into the lungs.

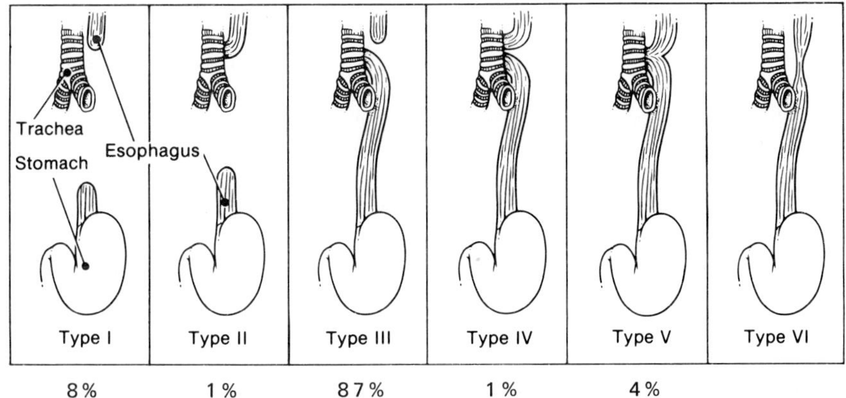

Figure 19-7 Types of esophageal atresia. Type I: esophageal atresia with no fistula and blind pouches. Type II: lower esophageal atresia with a fistula from the upper pouch. Type III: esophageal atresia with a blind upper pouch and a fistula from the lower pouch. Type IV: esophageal atresia with fistulas from both pouches. Type V: no esophageal atresia, with a connecting fistula present. Type VI: esophageal stenosis—not a true atresia. (*From G. Scipien, M. U. Barnard, M. A. Chard, J. Howe, and P. J. Phillips* [*eds.*], *Comprehensive Pediatric Nursing, 3d ed., McGraw-Hill, New York, 1986, p. 1055. Used with permission.*)

Passage of air from the lungs through the TE fistula progressively distends the stomach.

The etiology of the anomaly is unknown. The incidence is from 1 in 3000 to 1 in 4500 live births, and one-third of these infants are premature.[33] The anomaly occurs equally in both sexes, and there is often a history of maternal hydramnios (excessive amniotic fluid). The normal fetus swallows amniotic fluid that is absorbed through the intestine. If the fetus cannot swallow or if the gastrointestinal tract is blocked, maternal hydramnios results.

In over 40 percent of infants with esophageal anomalies, other congenital defects are present.[34] The major associated defects are cardiac, anorectal, genitourinary, and vertebral.

Manifestations Detection of this life-threatening defect immediately after birth is imperative. The usual symptoms are excessive oral and pharyngeal mucus, often flowing from the nostrils and bubbling from the mouth. Drooling, choking, and coughing are characteristic. Symptoms may not appear until the infant is fed for the first time; the baby may take a few swallows, but immediately chokes and becomes cyanotic due to laryngospasm. Overflow of fluid from the blind esophageal pouch is aspirated into the trachea and bronchi. Suctioning temporarily relieves the respiratory distress, but it will recur. Death may result from aspiration or aspiration pneumonia following feeding. (Since sterile water causes less irritation than glucose or milk, it is often used for a neonate's first feeding.) In animal studies, pathological changes and decreased P_{O2} values have been shown to occur if gastric contents are aspirated.[35]

Diagnosis This problem is diagnosed by passing a radiopaque nasogastric catheter into the esophagus. Passing of a nasogastric tube and aspiration of stomach contents are done routinely in some delivery rooms to rule out TE fistula and atresia. Failure to aspirate gastric contents, obtaining mucus and saliva instead, and a catheter that is visualized by x-ray coiled in the upper esophageal pouch are diagnostic of atresia. Radiopaque contrast material is not recommended unless absolutely necessary for diagnosis of TE fistula because it can be aspirated into the lungs.

Medical management The medical management of the infant is directed toward treatment and prevention of pneumonia, which causes 75 percent of the deaths, and repair of the defect. Depending on the type of defect, the surgery may be done in one stage or several. With a Type III defect, if the infant is a good surgical risk, the repair is done in one stage through a thoracotomy, with ligation of the fistula and an end-to-end anastomosis of the two segments of the esophagus. A gastrostomy may be done for decompression of the stomach and feeding. Occasionally the surgery is done in stages (repeated operations separated by a period of time so that growth can occur). A premature or very sick infant with extensive pneumonia, other anomalies, or very short esophageal segments often has the surgery done in stages. In such cases, the fistula will be ligated, and a gastrostomy done for gastric decompression and feeding. Primary fistula repair and esophageal anastomosis are done later.

The esophageal segments may be too short to allow for primary anastomosis. If so, the method of repair will depend on the individual situation and the surgeon's preference. One method involves preoperatively lengthening the proximal segment by repeatedly stretching it with a bougie. After a period of time, surgery is done to join the two segments. Multiple circular myotomies (which involve cutting the muscle) may be done during surgery to further lengthen the segments.[36] Where muscle is cut, there is no peristalsis, and so there may be problems with food propulsion postoperatively. In another type of surgery, a colon interposition, a portion of colon is used to connect the esophageal segments. The surgery is usually delayed until the child is 6 to 24 months of age. To allow the child to survive until reparative surgery is done, the fistula, if present, is ligated, and a gastrostomy is performed for feedings.

A *cervical esophagostomy* may be done to prevent aspiration by allowing drainage of the oral secretions. At the time of transplant or esophageal surgery, the cervical esophagostomy is closed, and the gastrostomy removed. A cervical esophagostomy and its care were discussed earlier in this chapter.

Complications following reconstruction of the esophagus include leakage at the anastomosis site, recurrence of the fistula, and stricture of the anastomosis due to the scar formation that accompanies healing. Many surgeons routinely do *esophageal dilatation* to eliminate strictures following surgery and repeat it as often as monthly after discharge and at periods when growth occurs. Stenosis (narrowing) of the esophagus can occur at any time after surgery. The parents should be aware of signs indicating this condition: dysphagia (difficulty in swallowing), increased coughing and choking, increased pharyngeal secretions, and decreased nutritional intake with weight loss. After surgery, the swallowing mechanism is not entirely normal, and gastroesophageal reflux (the backing up of gastric contents into the esophagus), with its attendant *peptic esophagitis,* is common. The child experiences heartburn and has bad breath, and vomiting may increase. The child is more susceptible to respiratory infections. A harsh, brassy cough may be present for as long as a year after surgery.

Preoperative nursing management The essential components of nursing care are removal of the secretions and promotion of adequate air exchange. Until surgery, oral secretions must be removed from the blind upper pouch to prevent overflow to the trachea. One method of accomplishing this is nasopharyngeal and oral suctioning as frequently as every 10 to 15 min. Another technique is to place an indwelling nasal catheter into the blind pouch and apply low, intermittent suction. The catheter is easily obstructed and needs to be changed daily.

Other nursing care to promote air exchange includes the provision of humidified oxygen, usually by Isolette. Positioning is important. A head-down position can be used to facilitate mucus drainage if there is no fistula to the stomach. With the presence of fistulas, the supine position, with the head elevated from 20 to 30°, will decrease gastric reflux. If the child is turned from side to side, more time should be spent on the right side than on the left.

Intravenous fluids are needed to maintain fluid and electrolyte balance; total parenteral nutrition may be instituted if there is prolonged nutritional deprivation. Broad-spectrum antibiotics, such as penicillin and kanamycin, are used to combat respiratory infection. The infant is given nothing by mouth, and mouth care is essential. A pacifier should not be offered at this point. It will increase secretions in an infant unable to handle them adequately.

A gastrostomy is used to decompress the stomach and to prevent gastric aspiration. The gastrostomy tube drains by gravity; preoperatively, feedings and fluid irrigations are contraindicated. If the tube needs to be irrigated, air should be used.

When surgery is delayed, a gastrostomy provides the means of giving nutrition. The gastrostomy tube is placed immediately after diagnosis. Feedings are initiated usually within 24 h if no TE fistula is present. The feeding techniques and care are similar to those for children with regular gavage tubes. Gavage feeding was discussed in Chap. 17.

Postoperative nursing management Many of the principles employed preoperatively also apply postoperatively. Once healing of the anastomosis has progressed sufficiently, oral feedings are begun. If a gastrostomy tube is present, it will be left open and positioned above the level of the stomach to promote gastric decompression and prevent gastroesophageal reflux, which could irritate the anastomosis and contribute to breakdown of the site. Suctioning, monitoring of intravenous fluids, positioning, and careful observations are essential. When suctioning, care must be taken not to disrupt the integrity of the suture line.

The interval between surgery and the initiation of feedings depends on the child's individual condition and the extent of the surgery performed. Postoperative feedings are often started after the first week via the gastrostomy or after approximately 2 weeks orally. Oral feedings are started slowly and cautiously. The initial feeding is a few milliliters of glucose water. Feedings are given every 2 h by medicine dropper. The volume and type of fluid are advanced slowly until the infant is taking normal formula from a nipple every 2 to 3 h. This may take as long as 2 to 3 weeks to accomplish. The nurse must be careful when feeding the infant and must use methods that minimize coughing, choking, and swallowing of excessive air. A slightly elevated position is best for feeding. The baby should be allowed to rest frequently during feedings and should be burped thoroughly. The care plan should include the feeding schedule and the reactions to feeding so that normal feeding behavior and experiences can be promoted. The feedings may be supplemented via gastrostomy until the infant's nutritional needs can be met by oral feedings. When the infant is taking adequate amounts and gaining weight, the gastrostomy tube is removed, and the child is ready for discharge.

Parental discharge teaching includes effective feeding techniques, observations indicating increasing respiratory distress, the need to prevent swallowing of foreign objects, respiratory infections, and the possible need for further dilatation. If the child has esophageal atresia and has had palliative surgery, the parents need to know how to do gastrostomy feedings, suctioning, and esophagostomy care. They also need guidance concerning normal development and stimulation, and they must understand the need for later surgeries.

Gastroesophageal reflux

Etiology *Gastroesophageal reflux* (GER) occurs when the lower esophageal sphincter is relaxed or is incompetent, allowing stomach contents to reflux up into the esophagus. Some degree of reflux is normal in the newborn. GER is abnormal when it is excessive and causes problems. The etiology is unknown, but it may be due to a motility disorder of the intestines[37] or to a delay in the maturation of lower esophageal neuromuscular function.[38] It occurs more frequently in children with cerebral palsy, mental retardation, or Down syndrome and after TE fistula or esophageal atresia repair.

Manifestations The signs and symptoms of GER are related to the exposure of the esophagus to acid stomach contents. Vomiting is frequently noted and may be in amounts large enough to cause weight loss or failure to thrive. Refluxed material may easily be aspirated into the lungs, causing pneumonia, bronchitis, and respiratory symptoms. Apnea is rare, but may occur in infants. The acidity of gastric contents within the esophagus may lead to esophagitis. There may be iron-deficiency anemia from chronic blood loss or, less commonly, hematemesis.[39] Older children may complain of heartburn. Infants cannot verbalize this, but they may be very irritable, particularly after eating. Esophagitis may lead to stricture formation.

Diagnosis A good history and physical examination are important in diagnosing GER. Height, weight, and head circumference (in infants) are plotted on growth curves. A barium esophagram will be done but may not show reflux, since it occurs intermittently. A pH test will be done by inserting a probe into the esophagus and monitoring the pH for a period of time. An esophagoscopy may be done to check for esophagitis. Other tests include esophageal manometry and gastroesophageal scintiscan, which detects reflux after a radioisotope feeding.

Treatment The treatment of GER depends on the severity. It may include giving small, frequent (every 2 to 3 h) feedings; thickening formula with cereal; or positioning the child prone at a 30° angle.[40] Older, more active children may sit upright, and as the symptoms improve, they may crawl around just prior to meals. Antacids may be given if esophagitis is present.

If, after 6 weeks, the child does not respond to intensive medical therapy, surgery is indicated. The procedure most commonly performed is the Nissen fundoplication in which the fundus of the stomach is wrapped around the distal esophagus. Operative mortality is low, and the procedure is usually successful with cessation of vomiting immediately after the operation and weight gain shortly thereafter.

Nursing management Preoperatively, nursing care is aimed at supporting the family in maintaining a schedule of small, frequent feedings and at teaching proper positioning. The child should be handled gently and burped frequently. Creative techniques are used to keep the child upright and yet support normal growth and development. Growth parameters and respiratory status must be monitored.

Postoperative care is similar to that for any child who undergoes gastrointestinal surgery. Respiratory status is monitored closely, since pneumothorax is a potential complication from surgery done so close to the pleural cavity. If a nasogastric tube is in, be sure that it is placed securely. Do not reposition it, since this may disrupt the integrity of the suture line. A nasogastric tube helps prevent "gas-bloat syndrome." After surgery, the child may be unable to burp; gas then accumulates and causes abdominal distention. This may lead to tachycardia and dyspnea. The clinical status of the child determines when oral feedings are begun. The parents need to be supported during all aspects of care, especially when beginning oral feedings. Preoperatively, feeding was likely to have been a frustrating, anxiety-producing procedure. Negative feeding behaviors may have developed. Encouragement by the nurse and the absence of vomiting by the child often reverse these patterns and make feeding a positive experience.

ALTERATIONS OF THE STOMACH AND DUODENUM

Pyloric stenosis

Pyloric stenosis is an obstruction at the outlet of the stomach as a result of progressive hypertrophy of the circular muscle of the pyloric sphincter. It is the most common entity, after inguinal hernia, requiring surgery in the first few months of life. Pyloric stenosis is 5 times more common in males than in females[41] and is more likely to occur in full-term infants. Black and Oriental infants are rarely affected. The incidence is 1 in 500,[42] and tends to be familial. If the parents (especially the mother) or siblings are affected, the child has a greater tendency to develop pyloric stenosis.

Etiology The cause of the pyloric enlargement is unknown. One theory suggests that the circular, smooth fibers of the pyloric sphincter hypertrophy due to spasm of the sphincter or possibly due to peptic ulcer disease.[43] The circular muscle of the pylorus is thickened and elongated. The pyloric canal leading from the stomach to the duodenum becomes narrow and progressively obstructed. Diffuse hypertrophy and hyperplasia of the smooth muscle of the antrum of the stomach are present.[44] As peristalsis attempts to push food through the pylorus (Fig. 19-8), the stomach's musculature becomes thickened. Pyloric obstruction leads to prolonged stasis of gastric secretions and may cause gastritis and bleeding.[45]

Manifestations Vomiting is the cardinal symptom and usually begins between the third and fourth weeks after birth, but it may occur from the first week of life to as late as the fourth month. Initially, the history reveals that the infant does well after birth, with occasional vomiting or regurgitation, and may even have gained weight. During the second to fourth weeks, the infant begins vomiting more frequently and forcefully shortly after being fed. As the obstruction becomes more complete, the vomiting becomes more projectile, shooting out as far as 30 to 120 cm, and begins to occur after every feeding. The emesis is partially digested or undigested food without bile, although it may be brownish-tinged periodically, secondary to the bleeding from gastritis.

Hunger is ever-present, and the child refeeds eagerly. Progressive weight loss occurs. Varying degrees of dehydration may be present. The infant demonstrates the signs of dehydration: poor skin turgor, depressed fontanel, decreased urinary output, dry mucous membranes, and lethargy. With the inability to retain nutrients, severe nutritional depletion results, and the infant appears malnourished. The infant's stools and voidings decrease in number, quantity, and frequency, depending on the amount of food and fluid reaching the intestinal tract.

Acute abdominal pain does not accompany pyloric stenosis, but the infant does seem uncomfortable. The upper abdomen is distended, and the enlarged pylorus is palpated as a hard, mobile, nontender, olive-shaped tumor in the right epigastrium. It is felt more easily right after eating or vomiting. After feedings, peristaltic waves may be seen as the stomach works against the hypertrophied, closed sphincter. These waves move from left to right across the epigastrium.

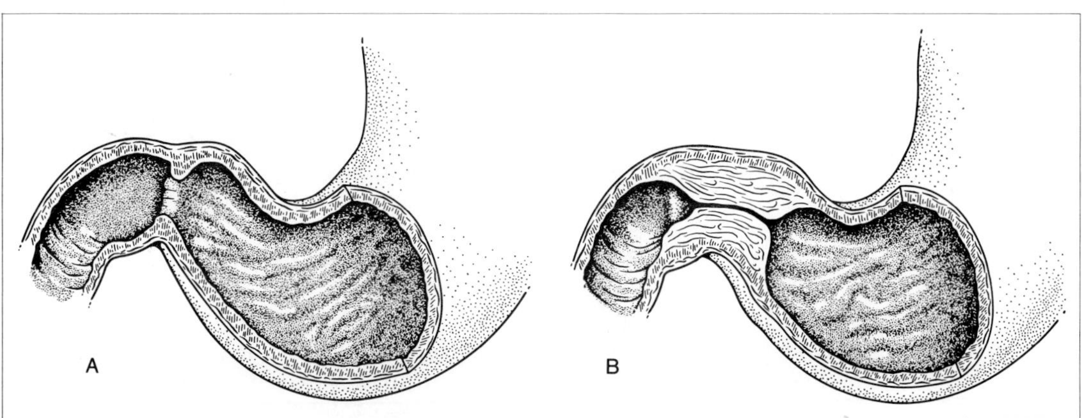

Figure 19-8 (*A*) A normal pylorus. (*B*) Pyloric stenosis. Notice the hypertrophied muscle mass and the narrowed lumen. (*From M. Armstrong et al. [eds.], McGraw-Hill Handbook of Clinical Nursing, McGraw-Hill, New York, 1979. Used with permission.*)

Diagnosis Once the tumor is palpated, upper gastrointestinal barium x-rays are usually not needed. Clinical symptoms and the history confirm the diagnosis. In some cases, a barium x-ray will demonstrate delayed gastric emptying and the "string" sign, showing the threadlike, elongated pyloric canal. X-rays may be used to rule out other possible diagnoses.

Jaundice is found in a small number of infants with pyloric stenosis. It disappears soon after surgery and is thought to be related to increased circulatory bilirubin, poor nutrition, and impaired liver enzyme function.[46]

Prolonged, frequent vomiting produces severe fluid and electrolyte disturbances that are revealed by laboratory tests. Loss of acid gastric juice containing chloride, sodium, and potassium causes hypochloremic metabolic alkalosis. With the alkalosis, bicarbonate and pH are elevated. The hematocrit and hemoglobin are increased secondary to the hemoconcentration of dehydration.

Medical management The preferred method of treatment is surgical—the *Fredet-Ramstedt pyloromyotomy.* The mortality rate is only 1 percent. A right-upper-quadrant incision is made, and a longitudinal incision through the muscular fibers down to the submucosa of the pylorus is accomplished. This procedure is safe and has a very high success rate, and reoperation is rarely necessary.

Nonsurgical treatment is seldom used, except in a baby who would be a poor surgical risk. With this treatment, there is a higher mortality rate, and improvement is very slow, taking up to 8 months. The long hospitalization can have deleterious effects on the emotional development of the infant. The conservative treatment consists basically of giving thickened (with cereal), frequent, small feedings. The infant is fed in a semiupright position, is burped frequently, and is placed upright in an infant seat for 1 h after feeding. If the infant vomits, he or she is immediately refed an amount equal to that vomited. Drug therapy includes sedation and cholinergic blocking agents, such as methylscopolamine nitrate, given 15 to 20 min prior to feeding to relax the sphincter. Intravenous fluids may be used to restore and maintain normal fluid and electrolyte balance. When gastric distention is present, a nasogastric tube used prior to feeding decreases the possibility of emesis with feeding.

Preoperative nursing management The surgical repair of pyloric stenosis is not an emergency. The nursing goal is to help restore the fluid and electrolyte balance so that the child will be a good surgical risk. The infant who is well hydrated and demonstrates no evidence of electrolyte imbalance will go to the operating room immediately. If severe fluid and electrolyte depletions are present, surgery will be delayed until the deficits are corrected, usually 24 to 48 h. Severe nutritional depletions of fat and protein may require a longer restorative period.

The infant is given nothing by mouth, and a nasogastric tube is put in place to prevent further vomiting and possible aspiration and to empty the stomach for surgery. Intravenous fluids with replacement of potassium and fluid deficits are maintained and are closely monitored for signs of water intoxication and circulatory overload. Vital signs and other indications of the infant's hydration are checked frequently. Intake and output, urinary specific gravity, daily weights, and skin turgor are evaluated. Restraints will be needed to prevent disruption of the intravenous and nasogastric tubes. Emesis and stools are noted for frequency and amount. Mouth care is very important, since the child is dehydrated, can take nothing by mouth, and has a nasogastric tube in place. The infant needs to be protected from possible sources of infection because of particular susceptibility due to a poor nutritional status. Sensory stimulation should be provided, and a pacifier may meet some sucking needs.

The parents are usually apprehensive. The mother especially is often anxious and may even feel guilty, believing that in some way her skill as a mother and her feeding techniques have been a failure. It is important to help allay these very normal concerns and to prepare the parents for the various diagnostic procedures and the surgery.

Postoperative nursing management The nursing goal postoperatively is to return the infant to a normal feeding pattern and diet. A nasogastric tube is often left in place until feedings are begun in order to provide gastric decompression and prevent vomiting, which would strain the pylorus. The infant may have occasional postoperative vomiting. If vomiting persists for 3 to 5 days, it may indicate an incomplete division of the hypertrophied pyloric muscle, and reoperation is necessary. Intravenous fluids are continued until the child is taking adequate amounts of formula. Checking vital signs, recording intake and output, and other preoperative nursing interventions are continued.

Feeding is initiated when the infant is alert and has bowel sounds and when the nasogastric tube is out, from 4 to 24 h after surgery, usually in the first 6 h. Small amounts of glucose water are started; then feedings progress slowly from half-strength to full-strength formula. An example of a feeding regimen would be 3 to 5 ml for the first feeding, repeated hourly. If no emesis occurs, the infant progresses a few milliliters more with each feeding until 2-h feedings have been achieved. Normal feeding amounts and timing should be accomplished within 2 days. If vomiting occurs at any time, the baby is given nothing by mouth for 4 h, and the regimen is started again from the beginning.

The infant is held in a sitting position, fed slowly, burped frequently, and handled gently. Feeding techniques used preoperatively are continued. Turning the infant on the right side with the head elevated after feedings will aid emptying of the stomach. Intravenous fluids can be discontinued when daily weights indicate satisfactory oral intake.

With the breast-fed infant, two approaches can be taken. The mother can express her milk into a bottle and then feed it to the infant, or she may breast-feed the baby. For the first feeding, it is desirable to allow the baby only 1 min at each breast and then lengthen the time as the baby tolerates it.

The incision should be checked for inflammation and infection. Postoperative complications may include apnea, pneumonia, and hypoglycemia due to the preoperative glycogen depletion.

The parents should be included in the care and taught to feed the infant. A pacifier may be used to satisfy additional sucking needs, and sensory stimulation such as cuddling and holding is very important. The mother particularly may be apprehensive and hesitant after her prior feeding experiences, but should be encouraged to participate in the child's feeding and care.

The infant will be ready for discharge by the third or fourth postoperative day. The parents need to learn about feeding techniques, positioning, and care of the incision, and they must know the signs of incisional infection and signs that might indicate pyloric or bowel obstruction.

Omphalocele

Etiology *Omphalocele* is an anomaly in which abdominal contents protrude into the umbilical cord (see Fig. 19-9). The size of the defect depends on its contents, which may vary from a small amount of intestine to most of the intestines and the liver. The sac can rupture easily, with resulting peritonitis, sepsis, and death. The cause of omphalocele is unknown, but it seems to result from failure of the intestines to return to the abdomen during the tenth week of fetal life. Since the abdominal contents remain externalized, an associated defect is an underdeveloped abdominal cavity. The incidence is 1 in 3000 to 1 in 9000 births.[47] Omphalocele is associated with other gastrointestinal problems, such as malrotation and small bowel atresia, because the bowel normally rotates as it returns to the abdominal cavity. Cardiovascular and genitourinary anomalies are also commonly found with omphalocele.[48]

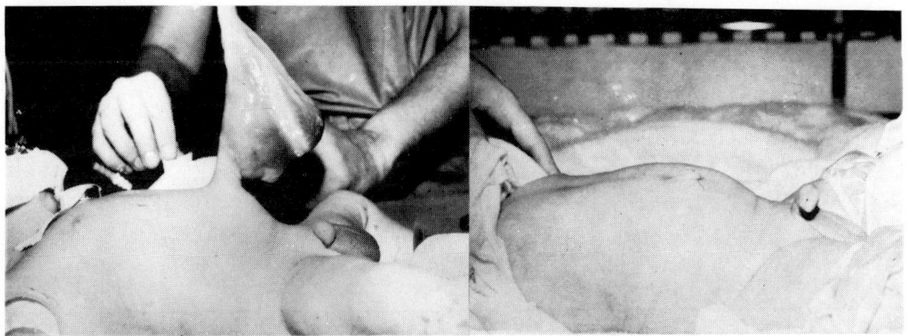

Figure 19-9 An omphalocele before and after surgery. (*From G. Scipien, M. U. Barnard, M. A. Chard, J. Howe, and P. J. Phillips* [*eds.*], *3d ed., McGraw-Hill, New York, 1986, p. 1062. Used with permission.*)

Medical management The defect constitutes a medical emergency. Immediately after birth, the goals of care are to minimize heat and fluid loss, prevent trauma and rupture of the sac, and prevent infection. The treatment is surgery. With a small defect, complete closure of the muscular wall, with the return of the bowel to the abdominal cavity, is done.

Returning the contents of a large defect to a small abdominal cavity will cause elevation of the diaphragm, resulting in respiratory distress, and may compress the inferior vena cava or compromise intestinal integrity. Thus, a large defect may necessitate several stages of repair accomplished over days or weeks. A gastrostomy tube is put in place for gastric decompression. A staged repair involves covering the sac with a prosthetic material (Dacron, Silastic, Teflon mesh, or Op-Site).[49] This material creates a silo, which is sutured around the edges of the abdominal opening. The silo is suspended perpendicular to the infant and is attached to the top of the Isolette with a rubber band. The sac is wrapped in gauze soaked in a solution such as Betadine, and parenteral antibiotics are started. Progressive shortening of the silo and consequent stretching of the abdominal cavity may require a number of surgical procedures over a period of days. This eventually permits removal of the silo and complete repair. The risk of mortality increases if the silo is left in place for more than 10 days.[50]

Preoperative nursing management Preoperatively, the nurse's major role is to provide care that prevents sac rupture and infection. Immediately after the birth, the infant is placed in a warmed, humidified Isolette. The exposed bowel is covered with sterile gauze soaked in warmed normal saline and covered with dry sterile towels to maintain the sterility of the inner dressings. *All* dressings are done with sterile technique. The intestine is not pushed into the abdominal cavity in any manner because respiratory distress, trauma, and shock may result. Prevention of tension on the area is mandatory. Extreme care should be taken positioning, turning, and using restraints with the infant. Moving the infant for procedures such as x-rays may take two people.

Intravenous fluid therapy is essential to promote perfusion of the major organs, to replace fluid lost through the bowel, and to prevent shock. The amount of fluid required varies with the size of the infant, the extent of the omphalocele, and the subsequent amount of bowel exposed. Shock is an ever-present problem, and the nurse must be constantly observant for the indications of fluid and protein losses. They occur continuously at varying rates until the abdomen is closed and healed. A volume expander, albumin, may be used to deal with this problem. A gastrostomy tube or nasogastric tube with low, intermittent suctioning keeps the stomach empty. Respiratory distress is often evident. The infant will need suctioning and humidified oxygen, either by hood or through the Isolette. Cyanosis of the lower extremities is caused by the increased pressure on the descending aorta and its femoral branches. It is dangerous to try to move the bowel to correct this impaired circulation. Surgery should correct the problem.

Postoperative nursing management The major postoperative nursing goal is to promote healing and prevent trauma and infection. Respiratory assistance with oxygen provided by a hood or a ventilator may be required. Shock remains a major concern because of the possible fluid shift from the intestine to the silo and because of the surgical manipulation of the intestine. Close observation for the signs of shock—tachypnea, tachycardia, decreased urinary output and increased specific gravity, and hypotension—is mandatory. If the lower extremities remain mottled or dusky, the surgeon may shift the silo or increase its tension; the nurse does not do this. The infant may remain NPO for up to several weeks and will be maintained on total parenteral nutrition.

Positioning and moving the infant are done with extreme caution to prevent trauma and tension to the wound. Sterile technique is used whenever the nurse is dealing with the wound, and parenteral antibiotics will be continued.

Complications after the repair include intermittent episodes of gastroenteritis, vomiting, abdominal distention, and malabsorption. Bowel obstruction and adhesions are not uncommon.

Maternal bonding may be delayed because of prolonged hospitalization of the infant immediately after birth, the shocking appearance of the defect, and difficulty in handling the infant with the omphalocele. The parents should be encouraged to visit and care for the infant.

Gastroschisis

Etiology *Gastroschisis* is the herniation of intestine through an abdominal wall defect, usually to the right of the umbilicus. There is a normal umbilical cord. Gastroschisis is a different entity from omphalocele, although the presentation and problems are similar. The incidence of gastroschisis is 1 in 6300 to 1 in 50,000 births.[51] Seventy-five percent of these infants are premature.[52] The cause of the defect is controversial, but it is postulated that failure of the abdominal wall's lateral folds to fuse may cause it. As with omphalocele, the size of the defect may vary. Since the intestines are not protected by a covering, they are edematous, and peritonitis is usually present. Twenty-five percent of infants with gastroschisis have associated malrotation, intestinal atresia, or stenosis.[53] Medical management and preoperative and postoperative nursing care are very similar to the management and care of an infant with an omphalocele.

Diaphragmatic hernia

Diaphragmatic hernia is the protrusion of varying amounts of abdominal contents through a defect in the diaphragm into the chest cavity. This congenital defect is an acute emergency in the newborn; the mortality rate is 30 to 60 percent.[54] The incidence is 1 in 5000 to 1 in 2200 births.[55] It results from failure of the *pleuroperitoneal canal* (the opening between the chest and the abdomen) to close completely during fetal development and/or from the early return of the intestines to the abdominal cavity (see Fig. 19-10). Usually the herniation is on the left side; bilateral hernias are rare.

Small hernias produce few symptoms and may not be discovered until later in infancy when the child is seen for increased respiratory infections. Severe cases of herniation may include upward displacement of the stomach, the small intestine, the spleen, the left lobe of the liver, the left kidney, and even the large intestine. These organs enter the thorax, displacing the heart and lungs. The left lung is usually *hypoplastic* (underdeveloped) and may be collapsed as a result of the pressure of the other organs.

Manifestations Respiratory status is complicated by atelectasis, and the movement of the diaphragm is impaired as the herniated intestine and stomach fill with air and distend from the swallowing of air. Clinical signs include mild to severe respiratory distress usually within a few hours of birth. Chest sounds are dull to percussion, and breath sounds are decreased or absent on the left side; bowel sounds may be heard instead. The chest appears barrel-like, especially on the left side. In contrast to the normal newborn's protruding abdomen, the abdomen will appear small and *scaphoid* (sunken) because of the absence of the abdominal contents. Heart sounds are shifted to the opposite side as the pressure in the left thorax increases.

Diagnosis Diagnosis is made by anterior-posterior chest x-ray, which differentiates this defect from other problems such as lung cysts and paralysis of the diaphragm due to phrenic nerve involvement. A definitive diagnostic sign is *dextrocardia* (a shift of the heart to the right), with spasmodic attacks of cyanosis and difficulty in

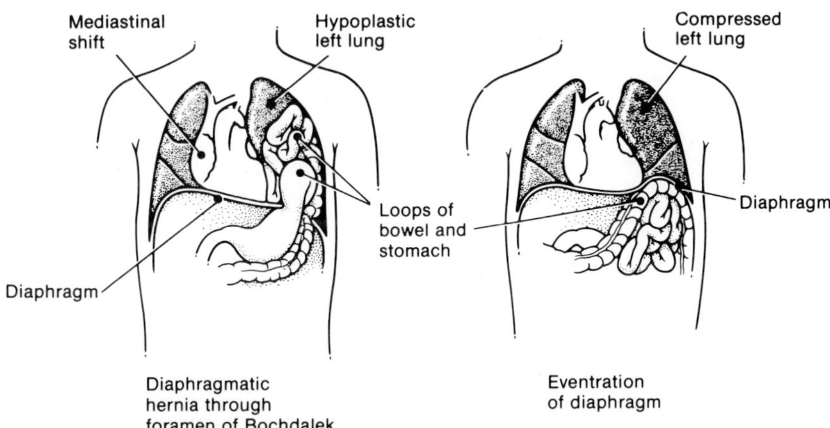

Figure 19-10 A comparison of the pathological anatomies of diaphragmatic malformations. (*From G. Scipien, M. U. Barnard, M. A. Chard, J. Howe, and P. J. Phillips* [eds.], *Comprehensive Pediatric Nursing, 3d ed., McGraw-Hill, New York, 1986, p. 1054. Used with permission.*)

feeding; gas-filled bowel loops are seen in the chest on x-ray. Signs of intestinal obstruction will also eventually occur.

Medical management The treatment is immediate surgery. A laparotomy is done to put the displaced abdominal contents back into the abdominal cavity and to close the defect. The abdominal approach permits exploring for other defects and stretching the abdominal cavity. The abdominal cavity may be small, since the intestines develop outside the cavity. If the abdominal cavity is too small to accommodate the intestines, only the skin may be closed over the defect. After the child grows, the muscle will be closed for complete repair. The prognosis depends on the size of the defect, the degree of hypoplasia of the left lung, and the respiratory status of the right lung. Complications after surgery include spontaneous pneumothorax, pulmonary infection, pulmonary hypertension, and circulatory problems. Pharmacological treatment of pulmonary hypertension is being investigated, but there has been little success as yet.[56]

Preoperative nursing management Prior to surgery, the infant's respiratory status is stabilized, and the respiratory and metabolic acidosis is corrected. If oxygen is administered, it must be by endotracheal intubation to prevent further inflation of the intestine and stomach. Place the infant in the semi-Fowler's position to allow expansion of the thorax and prevent pressure on the lungs, diaphragm, and viscera. The baby is turned on the affected side to allow the unaffected lung to expand. Nasopharyngeal suctioning of secretions is needed to preserve airway patency. A nasogastric tube is essential for gastric decompression and will improve lung expansion. The child will take nothing by mouth, and intravenous fluids containing prophylactic antibiotics will be infused.

Close observation of respiratory effort and status to facilitate respiratory functions is essential. The infant should also be kept from crying to prevent an increase in intrathoracic pressure and the swallowing of air.

Postoperative nursing management The infant's respiratory status continues to be of primary concern. Oxygen therapy is continued, and often the infant is placed on a positive-pressure ventilator. Suctioning and chest physiotherapy will help prevent atelectasis and other respiratory complications. Positioning is similar to that done preoperatively. The thoracotomy tube is removed in 2 to 3 days when the left lung has expanded and air has been removed from the chest. Intravenous fluids are continued, and a nasogastric tube remains in position.

Feedings are initiated slowly and cautiously. The infant often seems apathetic and fatigued, and gags and vomits easily. The feedings should be small and frequent, with a maximum amount set for any one feeding. The infant should be fed in a semiupright position and bubbled frequently. The infant is prone to abdominal obstruction. Vomiting, decreased number and frequency of stools, and abdominal distention should be noted and reported immediately. Before discharge, the parents should be taught appropriate feeding techniques, should be cautioned particularly to avoid overfeeding, and should know the signs of respiratory distress, respiratory infection, and bowel obstruction.

Peptic ulcer

Etiology and pathology The incidence of *peptic (gastric* and *duodenal) ulcers* in children is not precisely known. A family history of ulcers is often present. Acute peptic ulcers occur most frequently in children between 12 and 18 years of age. Boys are affected more frequently than girls.[57] In children under the age of 6, ulcers are related to an underlying condition (a malignancy, trauma, burns, sepsis, or bronchopneumonia) or to a toxic substance and are referred to as *stress ulcers*. Ulcers in children this age develop in the stomach and the duodenum with equal frequency. In children over 6 years of age, ulcers are usually primary (not related to another condition). In children between 6 and 18 years of age, ulcers occur mainly in the duodenum.[58]

It has been postulated that acute peptic ulcers, which are the result of erosion of the mucosal wall of the stomach, pylorus, or duodenum, have two causes. One is the increased rate of gastric juice production. The other involves interference with the normal protective mechanisms of the mucosal lining. As a result, there is a loss of normal mucosal barriers, and gastric acids digest the lining of the stomach and duodenum. Progressive edema, hemorrhage, and erosion of the mucosal lining occur. Drugs implicated in the development of ulcers in children include aspirin and steroids. The evidence linking the development of ulcers with the administration of steroids is weak, if children with chronic renal disease or a history of peptic ulcers are excluded.[59] Emotional stress is frequently a factor in older children.

In neonates, the ulcer formation is associated with birth hypoxia, a difficult labor and delivery, sepsis, dehydration, allergic disease, hypoglycemia, and tube feeding. Perforation and hemorrhage can occur very rapidly in the neonate. The baby needs to be observed for the signs of perforation—shock, rectal bleeding, distention, and absent bowel sounds. Emergency surgery may be necessary, with ligation of the bleeding points.

Manifestations The clinical symptoms may be few or may include vomiting, poor eating, *hematemesis* (bloody emesis), melena, abdominal distention, crying after feeding, and anemia. Children up to the age of 10 may not consistently exhibit vomiting and abdominal pain before or after meals. They often have chronic anemia and a family history of peptic ulcers. The child over 10 follows the adult pattern of symptomatology. Complications of peptic ulcers are hemorrhage, perforation, pyloric obstruction, and intractable ulcers (those which do not respond to treatment).

Diagnosis Diagnostic assessment includes the history, with specific attention to the family history of ulcers, and an explicit description of the presence and pattern of pain. Tests may include an upper gastrointestinal barium swallow; endoscopy (visualization of the gastric wall), which can be done as early as 1 month of age; and selective celiac and mesenteric arteriography studies. Blood studies reveal anemia subsequent to chronic blood loss. Gastric acid measurements (to look for hypersecretion) may also be done. The stools are tested for occult blood. Studies are also done to rule out the possibility of other problems, such as functional abdominal pain or gallbladder or pancreatic disease.

Treatment The goals of treatment are to relieve pain, promote healing, and prevent recurrences and complications. Aspirin should be avoided; acetaminophen (Tylenol) is an acceptable substitute. Antacids are used to increase the pH of the gastric secretions. H_2-receptor antagonists, such as cimetidine, act to inhibit acid secretion. These may be used to help heal ulcers, although rebound acid hypersecretion may occur after discontinuing treatment.[60] The use of anticholinergic agents is controversial and not recommended.[61]

Nursing management Management of peptic ulcers is aimed primarily at reducing acid production and protecting the mucosal tissues. Prolonged fasting and giving foods that cause the child discomfort should be avoided. A bland diet that does not include substances that increase gastric secretion and irritation is given. Substances to be avoided are tea, coffee, spices, fried foods, citrus, carbonated beverages, alcohol, and colas. Milk, given hourly, between meals, and at bedtime has been shown to stimulate acid secretion because of its calcium and protein content. For this reason, milk is no longer suggested.[62] Cigarette smoking increases the incidence of duodenal ulcers, and therefore adolescents who smoke should be advised to stop.[63]

Antacid dosage is adjusted to the age and size of the child. It is recommended that antacids be given 1 and 3 h after meals and at bedtime. Many antacids contain magnesia, a cathartic, while others cause constipation. An alternating schedule of the two types may be appropriate. Liquid antacids are more effective than tablets. As the child improves, the frequency of administration of antacids should decrease; when a child has been symptom-free for 3 months, some physicians discontinue them completely.

Nursing care involves close observation for bleeding and signs of shock. Vital signs are taken frequently; emesis and stools are examined for the presence of blood. "Coffee grounds" or frank, bright-red blood may be seen in the vomitus. Stools can be tarry; the presence of bright-red blood in the stool indicates rectal rather than gastric bleeding. The amount, color, and site of any bleeding are recorded. Dyspnea and cyanosis indicate perforation. If active bleeding is occurring, the abdominal girth is measured hourly, and blood replacement is done. During these acute episodes, the child takes nothing by mouth, and a nasogastric tube is inserted to decompress the stomach and to allow iced saline lavages to be done to provide local hemostasis.

Other therapy may include psychotherapy to help the child identify and deal with environmental stresses that have contributed to the ulcer formation.

Recurrent ulcers may lead to perforation of the ulcer and surgery. The surgery is a gastric resection, often involving the removal of 70 to

80 percent of the stomach, or a vagotomy with pyloroplasty. The aim is to reduce the amount of gastric acid. The child and the family need support and teaching. Acute bleeding episodes are frightening, and the child and the parents require ongoing information concerning tests, treatment, and possible surgery.

Upon discharge, the child and the family should be knowledgeable about prescribed drugs and antacids, dietary restrictions, and general health maintenance measures. After a gastric resection, the possibility of dumping syndrome and its treatment should be discussed.

Table 19-7 Food Sources of Lactose

Milk: fluid, evaporated, condensed, dry, and flavored	Candies, chocolate, caramels, and toffee
Commercial baked products	Luncheon meats
Instant cereals	Monosodium glutamate
Ice cream, ice milk, and sherbet	Spice blends
Custard and pudding	Breaded meats and vegetables
Cream: sour and sweet	
Butter and margarine	
Creamed meats, vegetables, and soup	

ALTERATIONS OF THE LOWER GASTROINTESTINAL TRACT

Lactose intolerance

Etiology and pathology *Lactose intolerance* is a congenital or acquired disorder in which the enzyme lactase is lacking. Without lactase, a person is unable to digest lactose to form galactose and glucose. Lactose then ferments, causing severe cramping, increased flatulence, intestinal distention, and diarrhea. Failure to thrive and muscle wasting in children will result because of decreased nutrient absorption. Lactase levels are highest during the first 3 years of life and decrease after that. Therefore, lactose intolerance (other than that caused by disease processes, such as diarrhea) is more commonly seen in older children and adults. The incidence is higher among blacks and Orientals than among Caucasians.

Diagnosis A lactose tolerance test may be used to confirm a possible diagnosis of lactose intolerance. An oral test load of lactose (2 g per kilogram of body weight, up to 50 g per dose) is given. The H_2-breath test is the procedure of choice for children. For about 3 h after the lactose load is administered, periodic breath samples are obtained. Results of over 20 parts per million are diagnostic of malabsorption. Other disaccharide intolerances may be tested for in the same manner, using the suspected agent for the test load. Another, less desirable method of testing is to obtain periodic blood samples after the test load is administered. A lactose level of 20 mg or less confirms the diagnosis.

Treatment Treatment consists of eliminating lactose from the diet. Lactose, also known as *milk sugar,* is present in milk. Therefore, all milk and milk products are eliminated from the diet. For infants, this generally means the use of soybean-based formulas, such as Isomil and ProSobee. The parents (and the child, when old enough) should be instructed to read all food labels carefully. Table 19-7 lists some foods that contain lactose. Many infants with lactose intolerance also have a soybean intolerance. If this is the case, a lactose- and soybean-free formula, such as Pregestimil or Nutramigen, should be given.

Other disaccharides (e.g., galactose and sucrose) may also not be tolerated. These intolerances occur less frequently than lactose intolerance. Treatment consists of eliminating the particular disaccharide from the diet.

Intestinal atresia and intestinal stenosis

Etiology *Intestinal atresia* is an interruption in the continuity of the bowel, resulting in total obstruction. *Intestinal stenosis* is a narrowing or constriction of the bowel, causing incomplete obstruction. Single or multiple areas of atresia or stenosis involving varying lengths of bowel may exist.

Intestinal atresia and intestinal stenosis are due to the failure of the embryological gut to recanalize. Duodenal obstruction usually occurs in the area where the common bile duct and the pancreatic duct enter. Atresia or stenosis below the duodenum is thought to be caused by ischemic injury to the bowel during intrauterine life.[64] The incidence is estimated to be 1 in 20,000 births.[65]

Manifestations *Duodenal atresia* is the most frequently encountered form of intestinal atre-

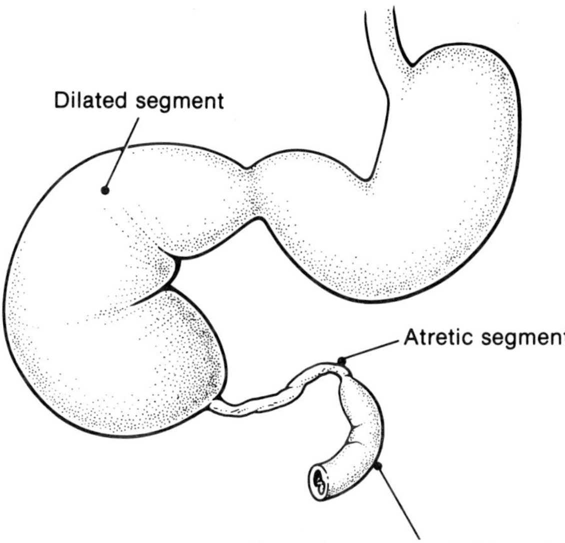

Figure 19-11 The "double-bubble" effect is seen in jejunal atresia as a result of the relationship of distended bowel to the atretic and normal nonexpanded bowel. (*From G. Scipien, M. U. Barnard, M. A. Chard, J. Howe, and P. J. Phillips [eds.], Comprehensive Pediatric Nursing, 3d ed., McGraw-Hill, New York, 1986, p. 1059. Used with permission.*)

sia. This defect produces symptoms in the newborn within a very few hours after birth. Polyhydramnios is usually present during pregnancy. Bile-stained vomiting occurs within the first 24 h of life. Abdominal distention is present intermittently, since the vomiting decompresses the bowel. The neonate fails to continue to pass meconium. Dehydration and weight loss occur rapidly. A flat plate x-ray of the abdomen reveals a "double-bubble" pattern due to the distended duodenum (see Fig. 19-11). A significant number of children with Down syndrome have duodenal atresia.

Duodenal stenosis has clinical manifestations similar to those of duodenal atresia. However, symptoms may appear later and may be less severe and more intermittent, depending on the degree of stenosis. An upper gastrointestinal barium study may be required to establish a definitive diagnosis.

In *jejunal atresia* and *ileal atresia* there is a more gradual onset of symptoms. Vomiting is less frequent, but larger amounts are lost. Abdominal distention is present and persistent. X-rays show dilated loops of bowel that relate to the length of intestine above the obstruction. A barium enema is performed to determine the presence or absence of large intestine atresia.

Medical management Surgery involves resection and anastomosis of the affected intestinal segment. One procedure performed for duodenal atresia, a duodenoduodenostomy, surgically joins the proximal and distal segments of the duodenum. Another corrective procedure, a duodenojejunostomy, involves a side-to-side anastomosis between the duodenum and the proximal jejunum. Surgical management of jejunal or ileal atresia includes resection and end-to-end anastomosis. The type of surgery performed depends on the segment of bowel affected. A gastrostomy is also done in conjunction with these procedures. Total parenteral nutrition is given until enteral feedings can be resumed.

Nursing management Preoperatively, gastric decompression and fluid and electrolyte balance are of primary importance. The danger of aspiration is always present for a neonate who vomits persistently. The nurse must position the infant on the abdomen or side to avoid aspiration and observe for signs of this complication. Once the nasogastric tube is inserted, patency must be maintained. Observations for distention include measurement of the infant's abdominal girth. Intravenous fluids to correct imbalances and maintain hydration are initiated. Thermoregulation of neonates is essential, and some may require humidified oxygen if respiratory compromise is evident.

Postoperatively, gastric decompression and parenteral fluids are continued. Oral feedings begin when gastric drainage decreases, bowel sounds are present, and stools are passed. These feedings are initially small amounts of clear liquids. They are advanced slowly to full-strength formula according to the neonate's tolerance.

The nurse should be alert to vomiting, poor intake, diarrhea, and abdominal distention and should notify the physician if these symptoms occur. These signs may indicate leakage of the anastomosis, obstruction, formula intolerance, or short bowel syndrome. If formula intolerance is present, other formulas may need to be tried. Once feedings begin, the nurse must observe the stools and note changes related to feedings. Testing the stools for blood, sugar, and pH is done routinely.

Total parenteral nutrition may be utilized for premature neonates, for newborns with malabsorption problems or paralytic ileus, or at the discretion of the physician. Nursing management of the child who is receiving total parenteral nutrition was discussed earlier in this chapter.

Meconium ileus

Etiology *Meconium ileus*, or obstruction of the neonate's bowel caused by very thick, sticky meconium, is usually indicative of cystic fibrosis. While this complication occurs in only 15 percent of children who have cystic fibrosis,[66] almost 90 percent of infants with meconium ileus have cystic fibrosis. The meconium is thick and tarry due to the deficiency of pancreatic enzymes and mucus from intestinal secretory glands. The meconium obstructs the distal ileum. Antenatal perforation can occur, and at birth, the infant manifests meconium peritonitis.

Manifestations Although the prognosis has improved, neonates with meconium ileus are critically ill. They appear toxic, vomit bile-stained material, and display uneven abdominal distention. Palpation reveals a firm, puttylike consistency to the intestinal contents. These newborns fail to pass meconium.

Diagnosis The diagnosis is difficult to confirm as the findings mimic those of other intestinal obstructions. A family history of cystic fibrosis may be instrumental in the final determination. X-rays show air bubbles interspersed within the meconium, resulting in a "ground-glass" appearance. A barium enema shows a small, unused colon.

Medical management Gastrografin enemas are used to dislodge the impacted meconium. This solution is hypertonic and causes fluid to shift to the bowel and loosen the stool. Intravenous fluids must be administered at the same time to prevent hypovolemia. Electrolyte status must be monitored. If the first enema is unsuccessful and the patient is stable, a second enema may be administered. This technique cannot be utilized if bowel perforation is evident. Surgery is indicated if perforation has occurred or if the Gastrografin enemas fail to relieve the obstruction.

There are several surgical procedures that can be used. In some instances, an abdominal incision is made, the meconium is manually extracted, the remaining portion of the bowel is irrigated with warm normal saline, and the abdomen is surgically closed. Often a temporary ileostomy is necessary. A Mikulicz, or "stovepipe," ileostomy allows for the irrigation of the intestine postoperatively to dislodge the meconium.

Postoperative nursing management Postoperatively, these neonates require close observation and expert nursing care. Respiratory complications can be prevented through the use of humidification and suctioning of secretions. Chest physiotherapy helps loosen thick pulmonary secretions. Hypothermia is prevented by placing the neonate in an incubator or on a warming table.

The ileostomy may require irrigation if impacted meconium is still evident. Various solutions are used for this purpose. It is important to observe the color and amount of return from the irrigations. The stoma and the peristomal area must be inspected for excoriation and breakdown. The skin must be kept clean and dry.

Feedings are initiated when peristalsis has resumed and the ileostomy is functioning adequately. Total parenteral nutrition may be used postoperatively until oral intake is sufficient.

Malrotation and volvulus

Etiology The cecum normally rotates into the lower right quadrant during the tenth week of gestation. At the same time, the mesentery of the ascending colon attaches to the posterior abdominal wall. Failure of the cecum to assume its normal anatomic position results in *malrotation* and failure of fixation of the mesentery. Peritoneal bands may form from the cecum and compress the duodenum, causing partial or complete obstruction. The mesentery remains unattached or is only loosely connected and allows the small intestine to twist around it. The twisted loop of intestine *(volvulus)* causes bowel strangulation and obstruction (see Fig. 19-12).

Malrotation and volvulus are found primarily in newborns. Most patients present in the first month of life; however, there are several reports of adolescents and adults with malrotation and volvulus.[67]

Manifestations The clinical manifestations are bile-stained emesis, pain, and diminished or absent stools. The symptoms are proportional to the degree of obstruction. Bowel strangulation may cause mucus and blood to ooze from the

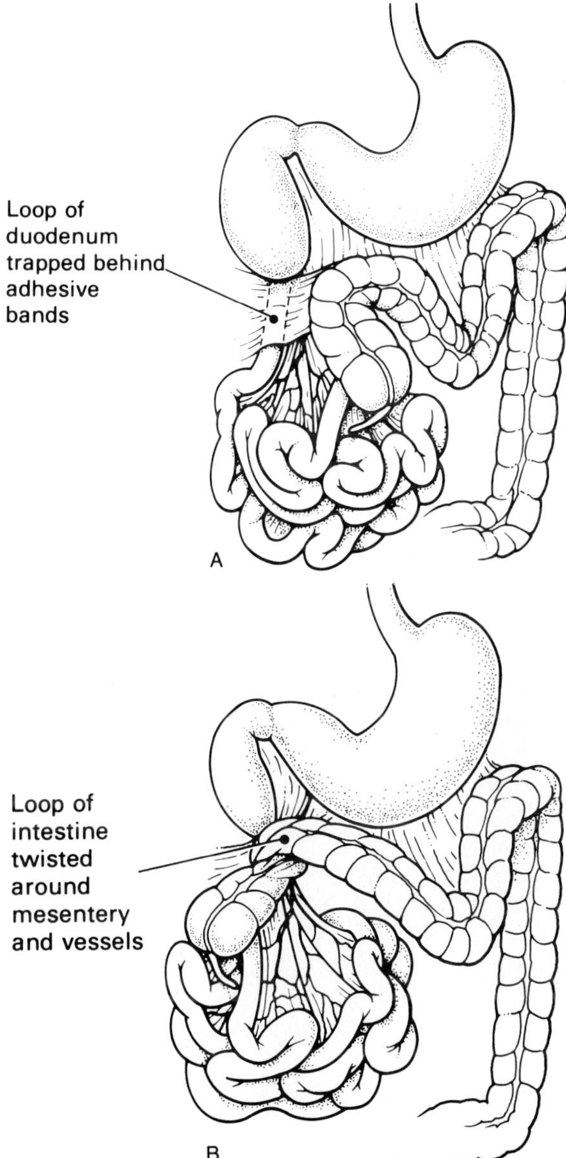

Figure 19-12 Malrotation and volvulus—causes of obstruction. (*A*) Loops of intestine trapped behind the mesentery of the descending colon. (*B*) A loop of intestine wrapped around the mesentery. (*From G. Scipien, M. U. Barnard, M. A. Chard, J. Howe, and P. J. Phillips* [eds.], *Comprehensive Pediatric Nursing, 3d ed., McGraw-Hill, New York, 1986, p. 1072. Used with permission.*)

rectum. The infant may appear toxic or demonstrate signs of shock. The diagnosis is established by upper gastrointestinal series and a barium enema.

Medical management The surgical procedure involves correcting the volvulus, releasing the constricting bands across the duodenum, and freeing the cecum. If the bowel is gangrenous, the affected segment is resected. If the resection is extensive, it may compromise oral nutrition or make it an impossibility, and so total parenteral nutrition may be used to maintain the child's nutritional status.

Nursing management Both preoperatively and postoperatively, intravenous fluids and gastric decompression are utilized. Nursing management is essentially the same as previously discussed under postoperative care for children who have undergone intestinal surgery.

Meckel's diverticulum

Etiology and pathology This anomaly is due to the persistence of the embryological vitelline duct. It remains as a small outpouching on the terminal ileum (see Fig. 19-13). The diverticulum can become infected, produce obstruction, and cause intussusception or perforation. It may also remain asymptomatic. It is present in 1.5 percent of the population.[68]

A previously healthy child may suddenly pass a bloody stool. Bleeding is of large volume and is initially dark, but rapidly becomes bright red with clots. There is no evidence of pain. Rectosigmoidoscopy and an abdominal scan using sodium pertechnetate may aid in the diagnosis. However, a negative scan does not rule out Meckel's diverticulum. Screening tests for bleeding disorders should also be done. Treatment is resection of the diverticulum and anastomosis.

Nursing management The child's massive bleeding can easily result in shock. Nursing responsibilities include frequent monitoring of vital signs along with blood pressure measurements. The child may have tachycardia and pallor due to blood loss. Transfusions may be necessary. Stool characteristics are also noted, particularly the amount of blood present.

Postoperatively, nursing care is similar to that for children who have undergone other intestinal procedures. Recovery is usually uneventful.

Intussusception

Etiology *Intussusception* is the telescoping of one portion of intestine in another, often causing

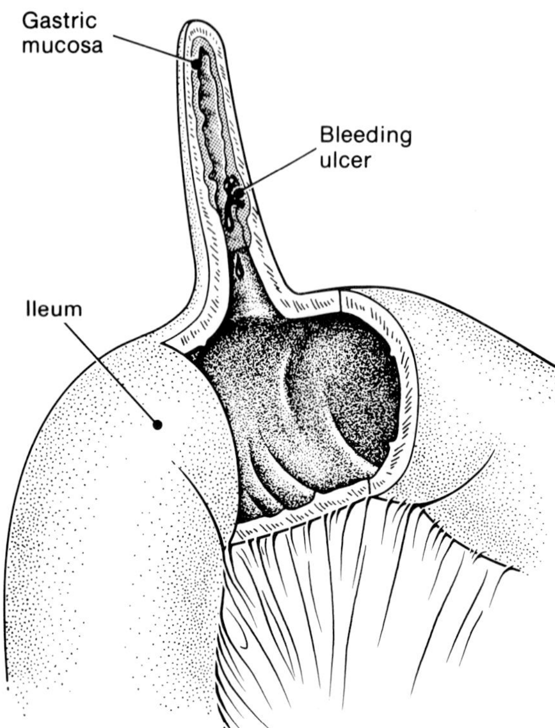

Figure 19-13 This outpouching is an example of the type of abnormality present in Meckel's diverticulum. (*From G. Scipien, M. U. Barnard, M. A. Chard, J. Howe, and P. J. Phillips* [eds.], *Comprehensive Pediatric Nursing, 3d ed., McGraw-Hill, New York, 1986, p. 1079. Used with permission.*)

intestinal obstruction (see Fig. 19-14). The terminal ileum and ascending colon are the segments most commonly involved. This problem occurs most frequently in healthy, well-nourished male children at approximately 6 months of age; 80 percent of affected children develop the disorder by age 2.[69]

Manifestations The child experiences extreme episodic abdominal pain, appears sweaty and pale, vomits reflexively, and tends to draw the legs up toward the abdomen. The pain episodes last 5 to 10 min, after which the child has some temporary relief.

The temporary relief is due to the initially incomplete bowel obstruction. As complete obstruction occurs, vomiting and "currant-jelly" stools (blood and mucus) occur, along with abdominal distention. Between attacks of pain, an upper transverse tubular abdominal mass can be palpated.

In the first 1 to 2 days, a barium enema may correct the invagination. The pressure created by the flow of barium pushes out the telescoped bowel. This cannot be used if (1) evidence of complete mechanical small bowel obstruction is present or (2) peritonitis, sepsis, or shock has occurred. Surgery involves manual reduction of the telescoped bowel. Resection is done only if manual reduction fails or if the intestine is severely damaged.

Nursing management After barium enema reduction, the child is observed for signs and symptoms of recurrence. Intravenous fluids are administered during this time. If clinical mani-

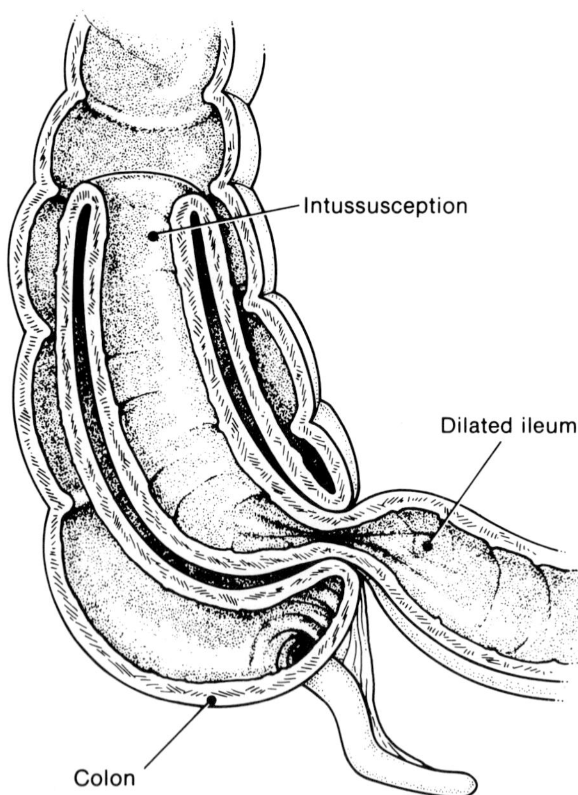

Figure 19-14 The presence of telescoped bowel produces the clinical symptoms in intussusception. (*From G. Scipien, M. U. Barnard, M. A. Chard, J. Howe, and P. J. Phillips* [eds.], *Comprehensive Pediatric Nursing, 3d ed., McGraw-Hill, New York, 1986, p. 1071. Used with permission.*)

festations are absent, oral feedings are resumed within 24 h. The child is discharged shortly thereafter. If surgery is necessary, the usual postoperative care is given. Recovery is usually rapid and uncomplicated.

Ulcerative colitis

Etiology and pathology *Ulcerative colitis* and Crohn's disease are both referred to as *inflammatory bowel disease*. Ulcerative colitis is an inflammatory process that involves the colon mucosa, eventually extending to the submucosa. The rectum is first involved, and the disease progresses proximally. A *crypt* (a glandular cavity in the intestines) abscess is the most typical lesion of ulcerative colitis. Ulceration occurs when these lesions become necrotic. The more extensive the mucosal damage, the less absorptive surface is available (see Table 19-8).

Ulcerative colitis affects people in all age groups, but the incidence is greatest among those between the ages of 10 and 28.[70] It is more severe in children and adolescents, who may need surgery earlier than people who are older. The etiology is unknown, but there is a familial pattern. Males and females are equally affected.[71] It is more frequent in the Jewish population.[72] Emotional and psychogenic factors may play a role in exacerbations after the disease occurs,[73] but patients with ulcerative colitis do not seem to have a higher incidence of emotional problems than others with chronic illnesses.[74] One suggested cause of ulcerative colitis is that a bacterial or viral invasion produces inflammation; another is that an autoimmune response takes place.[75]

Manifestations Ulcerative colitis is characterized by exacerbations and remissions. The course of the disease is variable. Two patterns of the disease have been observed. The first, and most common, is remitting colitis. The disease produces episodic acute attacks, but between the attacks the child is relatively free of symptoms. There is usually a good response to medical treatment. With time, the disease either terminates or becomes chronic. The second pattern is chronic, continuous colitis, in which there are never any complete remissions. This form of the disease tends to be milder but is always present. Chronic anemia and malnutrition occur. The response to medical treatment is usually poor, and complications are frequent.[76]

The most common clinical manifestations are diarrhea with tenesmus, rectal bleeding, and abdominal pain. *Tenesmus* is the continued feeling of a need to defecate. Pain is usually but not always located in the left lower quadrant. Stools may contain pus, mucus, and blood. Other signs and symptoms include weight loss, nausea, vomiting, fever, and weakness.

Diagnosis Diagnosis begins with a family history. An upper gastrointestinal series with small bowel follow-through is performed, and a barium enema is given. Ulcerations of the colon may be outlined by these studies. A rectal examination is done to rule out other diseases. Sigmoidoscopy and colonoscopy are also done to determine the

Table 19-8 Comparison of Ulcerative Colitis and Crohn's Disease

Feature	Ulcerative Colitis	Crohn's Disease
Onset	Gradual (may be acute)	Insidious (may be acute)
Manifestations:		
Pain	Less frequent and colicky	Frequent and crampy; triggered by food
Stools	Often severe diarrhea with blood, mucus, or pus	Absent to moderate diarrhea, occasionally bloody
Growth retardation	Present, usually mild	Frequently severe
Area involved	Rectosigmoid	Primarily terminal ileum (rectal sparing)
	Continuous segments	Discontinuous segments
	Mucosal lesions	Transmural lesions
Response to medications	Fair to good	Poor to fair
Total parenteral nutrition	Helps in cases of malnutrition, but rarely induces remissions	Helps in cases of malnutrition and can aid healing and induce remission
Surgery	Curative	Palliative
Cancer risk	High risk; increases with duration of the disease	Some risk; less than with ulcerative colitis

extent of bowel involvement. A rectal biopsy for the presence of lesions and inflammation aids in the diagnosis.

Medical management Children with *mild attacks* of ulcerative colitis require rest and dietary management. A low-residue, high-calorie, high-protein diet is necessary. Roughage is restricted during active periods of the disease. Sulfasalazine is one of the major therapeutic agents employed in the treatment of ulcerative colitis. It relieves diarrhea and the associated symptoms and decreases the number of relapses. Sulfasalazine is introduced gradually because of its gastrointestinal side effects. Anticholinergics are used to relieve muscle spasm, and antidiarrheals may also be prescribed to decrease the frequency of stools. The nurse should be aware of the side effects of such medications and note the child's response to them.

Children with more *severe attacks* require intravenous fluid therapy to correct dehydration and electrolyte imbalance. Albumin, plasma, or blood transfusions may be necessary if severe anemia or hypoalbuminemia exists. Corticosteroids are administered parenterally to control the inflammatory process. Vitamins and iron are given as the child's symptoms subside and solid foods are tolerated. Sulfasalazine is added to the regimen after steroids are discontinued. Electrolyte imbalance can occur rapidly. Potassium and bicarbonate losses are high because of hyperperistalsis and decreased intestinal absorption. Metabolic acidosis can result from these losses.

The child with severe or prolonged symptoms is given nothing by mouth. Nasogastric intubation and parenteral fluids are initiated. Total parenteral nutrition is given when weight and protein losses are severe. Antibiotics may be added to the treatment protocol to control inflammation and prevent peritonitis.

Toxic megacolon is another indication for the use of antibiotics. This rare complication causes complete bowel obstruction and can produce perforation and peritonitis. Ampicillin, chloramphenicol, and clindamycin are usually given, although other antibiotics may also be used. Arthritis is the most common systemic complication of ulcerative colitis; it occurs in 20 percent of affected children.[77]

If conservative measures do not control the inflammatory process or if toxic megacolon, peritonitis, profuse hemorrhage, malignancy, or chronic growth failure occurs, surgery is indicated. A total proctocolectomy with an ileostomy may be done. Other options include a continent (Kock pouch) ileostomy and an endorectal ileoproctostomy (in which the diseased rectal mucosa is stripped from the muscle and the ileum is sutured to the remaining rectum or anus). The latter procedure usually permits continence but does result in frequent, loose stools, which may be controlled by giving Lomotil or Imodium.[78] Immediately after the surgery, 10 to 15 stools a day may be normal. The number usually decreases to fewer than 10 per day as the remaining lower bowel dilates. The procedures discussed above are usually considered curative for ulcerative colitis.

Nursing management Nursing responsibilities include accurately measuring intake and output, administering medications and recording their effects, maintaining fluid balance, and providing for physical and emotional rest. It is essential that the nurse record the frequency and characteristics of the stool. The child's environment should be as free of stress as possible. Odor control is also important to the child's sense of well-being. Skin care is important, as excoriation easily occurs. The anal area should be washed gently after each bowel movement, and ointment applied.

Because of the child's debilitated condition, infection is always a potential hazard. Vital signs are monitored frequently to detect temperature elevation. Abdominal girth measurements are taken to check for distention. The nurse should also be alert for signs and symptoms of obstruction, which may indicate a worsening of the child's condition.

Psychosocial support is very important for these children and their families, since they are dealing with a chronic, debilitating disease. The consequent growth failure and delayed sexual maturation may be particularly distressing to adolescents.

Preoperative nursing management Preoperatively, every attempt is made to stabilize the child's condition. Electrolyte and blood values must be corrected to normal limits if the child is to withstand the stress of major surgery. The bowel is prepared through the use of neomycin or another agent which affects bacterial flora. Cleansing enemas are not given because of the risk of inducing an acute exacerbation, bleeding, or toxic megacolon.[79]

Preparation also includes teaching the child and the parents about the particular surgery to be performed, including ileostomy care if applicable. The nurse must expect to deal with concerns and questions expressed by the child and the family. Alterations in body image and in elimination are the major issues that need to be explored. The nurse should reassure the child and the parents that a normal life can be resumed with minimal, if any, restrictions. If the child will have a stoma, the stoma site that is best in terms of the child's activities is selected preoperatively. The child should be shown the appliance that will be used postoperatively and should be allowed to wear it. If the child is very ill or has had drastic changes in life-style because of the illness, surgery may be regarded positively and as giving the child a chance to lead a more normal life.

Postoperative nursing management Fluid and electrolyte balance continues as a primary need postoperatively. Since the portion of bowel that is responsible for absorption of fluids has been removed, the stools (or ileostomy drainage) are initially very liquid. Sodium losses from an ileostomy are great. The losses in a child who has a Kock pouch or who has undergone an endorectal ileoproctostomy are not as great, since stool stays in the intestine longer, facilitating sodium reabsorption. The nurse must note any signs of hyponatremia and be aware of the child's possibly low serum sodium level. The absorption of fat-soluble vitamins may also be impaired, and supplements may be necessary.

A nasogastric tube is used for decompression, and patency must be maintained. Drainage from this tube is noted, and the amount is recorded. This loss is included in the calculation of the child's fluid requirement. The nasogastric tube is removed when peristalsis resumes.

The nurse is responsible for ascertaining the condition of the stoma, the integrity of the peristomal and perianal areas, and the type and amount of drainage. Ileostomy contents will never resemble formed stool, but will gradually become thicker once the child begins to eat a more normal diet.

After peristalsis resumes, the child is allowed to drink clear liquids and, gradually, to eat solids. The feedings are small to give the intestine a period of adjustment. The initial diet is high in protein and carbohydrates and low in residue. However, the child is allowed and even encouraged to consume a liberal diet after the postoperative period. Most children will avoid foods that cause discomfort or diarrhea. If an ileostomy is present, its care must be taught to the child and the parents (see the section "Ostomies"). The nurse should take into account the child's concerns regarding body image and loss and should expect periods of depression and rebellion as the child adapts to the ileostomy. The parents must also be prepared for their child's mood swings.

Ulcerative colitis is considered a premalignant disease. There is an increased risk of colon cancer in individuals in whom the disease has been present for over 10 years.[80]

Children who do not undergo surgery for ulcerative colitis should have biennial examinations, including a sigmoidoscopy. These measures are essential for the early detection of malignant changes.

Crohn's disease

Etiology and pathology *Crohn's disease* is also known as *regional enteritis* and differs significantly from ulcerative colitis (see Table 19-8). The cause is unknown, but infectious agents and an autoimmune process have been suggested. It occurs more frequently among blacks and those of Jewish descent. It affects males and females equally.

Inflammatory changes occur in all layers of the bowel wall. Inflammation and edema lead to ulcerations, which often form fistulas.[81] Granuloma formation is common. The most commonly affected area is the terminal ileum. Edema leads to thickening of the bowel wall, which may lead to obstruction.

Diagnosis Unlike ulcerative colitis, which affects a continuous bowel segment, Crohn's disease affects several parts of the intestines simultaneously. The involved segments are separated by bowel that does not appear diseased. Therefore, the bowel has "cobblestone" markings, which are seen on barium swallow. A sigmoidoscopy shows rectal sparing, as opposed to ulcerative colitis, which involves the rectosigmoid area. A rectal biopsy is done as a component of the diagnostic process.

Manifestations The onset of Crohn's disease is usually insidious but may be acute. Systemic signs such as arthritis, arthralgia, growth failure, and anemia may precede gastrointestinal manifestations by several years. Abdominal pain and diarrhea are the predominating symptoms. Pain is initially described as crampy and intermittent; when the disease is advanced, it becomes a constant aching. Rectal bleeding may be present. Surgery is not indicated unless severe complications such as perforation, obstruction, or fistulas are present. Recurrences after surgery can be expected.

Nursing management The nursing management of children with Crohn's disease is similar to that for children with ulcerative colitis. The child may require hospitalization both for evaluation and for hydration. Total parenteral nutrition may be required for severe attacks. A diet high in protein and carbohydrates and low in fat is used to control the diarrhea. If malabsorption is present concurrently, an individualized diet for the child is necessary. Raw fruits and vegetables are eliminated, as well as high-residue foods.

Vitamins, iron, and folic acid are prescribed for deficiencies and anemia. Sulfasalazine is also used in the treatment of Crohn's disease. However, it may not be as effective as in the treatment of ulcerative colitis. The risk of bowel cancer is increased, but less than in children with ulcerative colitis.

Gluten-sensitive enteropathy

Etiology *Gluten-sensitive enteropathy* (GSE), also known as *celiac disease* and *nontropical sprue*, is second only to cystic fibrosis as a cause of malabsorption in children. The average age of onset is between 8 and 24 months.[82] Symptoms are usually noted 3 to 6 months after the introduction of gluten into the diet.[83] The incidence ranges from 1 in 300 in western Ireland to 1 in 3000 in the United States.[84] Males and females are affected equally,[85] and there seems to be a familial pattern. Two theories have been proposed to explain the cause of GSE. One suggests that an enzyme that digests gluten is lacking, which results in an accumulation of material that is toxic to the mucosa. The other theory suggests that the cause is an immunologic dysfunction of the intestinal mucosa.[86] GSE is characterized by an inability to digest and absorb gluten, a protein found in wheat, oats, rye, and barley.

Manifestations Anorexia, irritability, chronic diarrhea, severe abdominal distention, muscle wasting, and failure to thrive are the clinical manifestations. Stools are bulky and foul-smelling and contain large amounts of fat (steatorrhea) due to incomplete digestion and absorption. Abdominal pain and vomiting are present in some children.

Anemia is common due to iron, folate, or vitamin B_{12} malabsorption. Serum albumin and globulin studies reveal a protein-losing enteropathy. Hypokalemia is common, and hypocalcemia can lead to tetany in severe cases. Stool analysis shows a high fat composition.

Diagnosis A barium x-ray reveals dilatation of the small intestine lumen and segmentation due to hypersecretion of intestinal fluid. Biopsy of the small intestine shows mucosal changes in the jejunum that confirm the diagnosis of celiac disease.

Nursing management The child with GSE frequently has osmotic diarrhea. The nurse must be alert to symptoms of fluid and electrolyte imbalance. A gluten-free diet is the treatment for GSE. The mucosal changes are reversible if the diet is followed. Vitamins and iron are prescribed to correct deficiencies. The anorexic and irritable child is a nursing challenge. Patience and persistence are required to get the child to accept a diet high in calories and protein. Small, frequent feedings are better tolerated than a few large ones. Lactose, which is found in milk products, may also be eliminated for 4 to 6 weeks to allow the mucosa to heal.

A dietitian should be consulted to help with meal planning. The parents and the child must be taught dietary management to avoid foods containing gluten (wheat, rye, barley, and oats). Generally, gluten is found in bakery products, cereals, pastas, and soups containing barley. All ingredient labels must be read carefully. Hydrolyzed vegetable products containing grains are used often as food additives.[87] Rice, corn, and potato flours[88] can be substituted for grain products that contain gluten. Recipes using these grains are available from community health departments, hospital dietitians, and allergy associations. Wheat starch (from which all protein has been removed) is also available, and manufacturers can provide recipes in which it is used. Some health and specialty stores carry baked products made with rice, soybean, and corn flours. The parents and the child must understand the necessity of dietary controls. The nurse must provide periodic reinforcement and support, since it is difficult to stay on the strict diet when the child appears healthy. The child will begin to gain weight and to grow taller once the diet is implemented. The child must continue the gluten-free diet for the rest of his or her life.

Appendicitis

Etiology and pathology *Appendicitis* is the inflammation of the vermiform appendix and is a common surgical problem of school-age children and adolescents. It is rare in infants. The appendix is located on the cecum and serves no discernible purpose. When the lumen becomes obstructed, the walls of the appendix become inflamed. Infection develops as a result of fecal stasis within the appendix. Perforation and peritonitis can result.

Because the omentum is larger in older children, peritonitis can remain localized in the right lower quadrant or lower abdomen. In young children, generalized peritonitis often results from perforation.

Manifestations The earliest sign of appendicitis is colicky, periumbilical pain. Vomiting may follow but is less common in older children than in younger children. An infant is usually irritable and tends to lie quietly with the hips flexed. In the older child, the pain shifts to McBurney's point, in the right lower quadrant, after a few hours. As the pain progresses, the child guards the abdomen, and there is rebound tenderness. The temperature may be slightly elevated if the appendix has not ruptured. The white blood cell count is usually elevated but is unlikely to be higher than 15,000 in an older child and 20,000 in an infant.

Management An appendectomy is the surgical treatment. Preoperatively, the nurse helps in establishing the diagnosis. A good nursing history and behavioral assessment are important. Postoperatively, the child receives intravenous fluids and is given nothing by mouth. A nasogastric tube may be used for gastric decompression. The child must be observed for signs and symptoms of abscess formation, such as prolonged postoperative pain and irritability.

The operative site is examined for inflammation, pain, and drainage. The recovery period for an uncomplicated appendectomy is generally short.

Peritonitis

Perforation may occur within a few hours of the onset of symptoms. Immediately after perforation, the child may appear improved, since the pain is relieved. This is short-lived, and as peritonitis occurs, pain recurs. The child appears severely ill. The temperature is elevated to 38.3 to 40°C (101 to 104°F), and tachycardia is present. The child lies quietly, breathing shallowly and rapidly. The right leg may be drawn up in an attempt to relieve the pain. Vomiting is more frequent after perforation, and the vomitus may contain small bowel contents. A small amount of mucoid diarrhea may be passed. Eventually, bowel motility decreases, resulting in diminished or absent bowel sounds. Peritoneal inflammation leads to plasma loss within the abdominal cavity (third spacing), and the child becomes dehydrated.

Management An appendectomy is required immediately. Preoperatively and postoperatively, the child receives intravenous fluids, and gastric decompression is done. Broad-spectrum antibiotics, such as ampicillin, gentamycin, and clindamycin, are given parenterally preoperatively and for 10 days postoperatively to prevent abscess formation. A Penrose drain is inserted at the time of surgery to drain exudate.

The child may be positioned on the right side or in a semi-Fowler's position to facilitate drainage from the lower abdomen through the Penrose drain. The nurse must change the dressing as often as necessary. The characteristics of the exudate, such as color, odor, and amount, must be noted. The drain is advanced, by the physician, over a 1- to 2-week period and is finally removed. Continued observation of the operative site is necessary to detect abscess re-formation.

Accurate measurement of intake and output are important nursing responsibilities. Albumin may be necessary to maintain intravascular fluid volume, since plasma loss within the abdominal cavity is high. Patency of the nasogastric tube and the intravenous line must be preserved by the nurse. These measures are necessary for a longer period of time than in the case of a simple appendectomy. The child is given nothing by mouth until the peritoneal inflammation subsides and stooling resumes.

The recovery period for the child with peritonitis is prolonged. The bed-rest restriction limits interactions with other patients. The nurse should spend time with the child, engaging in quiet activities. The child needs reassurance that the condition will improve and that normal activities can be resumed.

Hirschsprung's disease

Etiology and pathology *Hirschsprung's disease* is characterized by constipation and megacolon. It is caused by the congenital absence of parasympathetic nerve ganglion cells. The aganglionic segment extends from the internal anal sphincter through varying lengths of the rectum and colon (see Fig. 19-15). The rectosigmoid area is the site most frequently affected. There is a 4:1 ratio of boys to girls. It is not uncommon for two or three siblings to have Hirschsprung's disease.

The diseased bowel segment lacks peristalsis and is unable to propel fecal material through the colon. The normal bowel proximal to it becomes greatly dilated (megacolon) in an attempt to move the accumulated fecal mass. Hyperperistalsis develops in the dilated bowel because of the functional obstruction of the affected segment.

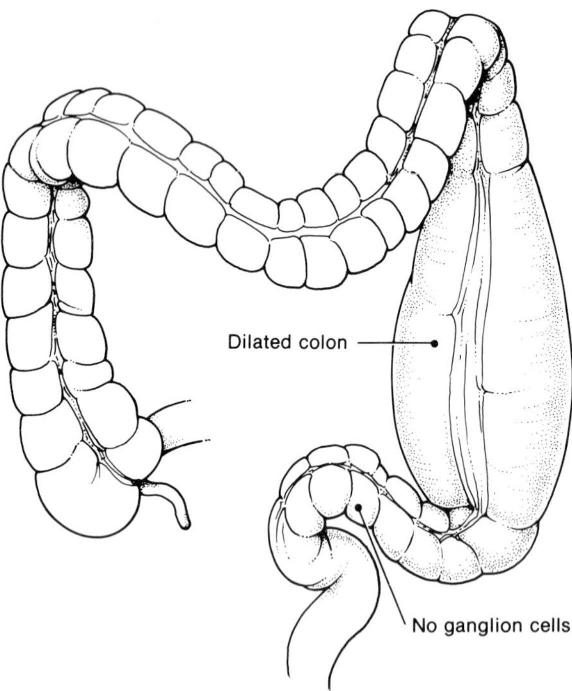

Figure 19-15 Notice the portion of the intestine without ganglia distal to the dilated colon, which is typical of Hirschsprung's disease. (*From G. Scipien, M. U. Barnard, M. A. Chard, J. Howe, and P. J. Phillips* [*eds.*], *Comprehensive Pediatric Nursing, 3d ed., McGraw-Hill, New York, 1986, p. 1069. Used with permission.*)

Manifestations In the neonate, manifestations range from complete intestinal obstruction to intermittent episodes of distention, feeding difficulties, and various degrees of constipation. Failure or delay in passing meconium, abdominal distention, and bile-stained vomitus are suspicious signs. Digital rectal examination results in immediate evacuation of meconium with or without the meconium plug. Infants with complete obstruction require immediate surgery. The diagnosis in newborns with intermittent problems may not be made until intestinal obstruction or severe, persistent constipation occurs later in infancy.

The older child displays failure to thrive, a protuberant abdomen, chronic constipation, and megacolon. Anorexia and muscle wasting are related to poor dietary intake and protein loss. Diarrhea may occur in both infants and older children because of the seeping of liquid stool around the fecal impaction. However, significant diarrhea may indicate the onset of enterocolitis. This complication can occur at any time and is the major cause of death in untreated infants. Sudden abdominal distention, fever, dehydration, and shock are the manifestations of enterocolitis.

Diagnosis Abdominal x-rays show a distended colon that ends in an unexpanded rectum. A barium enema aids in the diagnosis by outlining the dilated bowel segment. The usual bowel preparation before the enema is omitted, since it would alter the radiological picture. Manometric studies are done by inserting a balloon into the rectum and inflating it. Normally, rectal distention will cause the internal sphincter to relax and the external sphincter to contract. In individuals with Hirschsprung's disease, distention causes both sphincters to contract.[89] A rectal biopsy confirms the absence of ganglionic nerve cells.

Medical management Medical management of Hirschsprung's disease involves the use of colonic irrigations and anal dilatations, discussed earlier in this chapter. These procedures are used until a colostomy can be done on children who are in poor condition. Fluid and electrolyte balance must be closely monitored. A temporary colostomy is created as soon as possible after diagnosis because of the risk of enterocolitis. The definitive treatment is surgical removal of the aganglionic portion of the bowel. This is done sometime after the child is 6 months of age. In cases diagnosed in older children, the colostomy should remain for at least 3 months.[90] The temporary colostomy may be closed at the time the definitive repair is done or a few months later in a separate procedure. A number of surgical procedures can be used for final repair.

Swenson's abdominoperineal pull-through involves pulling the aganglionic bowel through the anus and anastomosing normal bowel to the anal canal.

The *Duhamel procedure* involves resecting the aganglionic segment and bringing normal bowel down to a surgically created retrorectal space. This segment is pulled through the posterior rectal wall. Using a surgical stapler, normal colon is anastomosed to the retained lower aganglionic rectum.[91] This creates a new rectum with aganglionic rectum anteriorly and ganglionic colon posteriorly, which is sufficient to propel feces through the intact external sphincter.

The *Soave procedure* involves resection of the aganglionic bowel with separation of the mucosal layer of the rectum. This layer is then excised, and a rectal cuff remains. The normal bowel is brought down through this conduit and is allowed to protrude. A spontaneous or autoanastomosis forms in 15 to 20 days. After this time, the protruding bowel is excised, and the anastomosis is sutured. A rectal tube is in place from the time of surgery.

A *modified Soave procedure* involves the same procedures, except that the normal bowel is sutured to the rectal cuff at the time of surgery, and the protruding bowel is also excised.

Nursing management Preoperatively, bowel preparation is essential. Colonic irrigations are continued, with neomycin or kanamycin added to the solution. These drugs may also be given orally to suppress intestinal flora. A clear liquid diet is given for 24 to 48 h prior to surgery.

Postoperatively, intravenous fluids are required for several days. Gastric decompression is managed by insertion of a nasogastric tube. Perineal care is important for the child's comfort. Small amounts of bloody drainage or dark mucus are usually expelled from the anus. This area must be kept clean and dry. If a Soave procedure has been performed, the rectal tube must not be disturbed.

Stooling resumes approximately 4 days postoperatively and is usually liquid. The number and characteristics of the stools are observed and recorded. Large volumes of fluid and electrolytes can be lost, and it is important to have accurate measurements. Assessment of stool characteristics aids in establishing whether intestinal functioning is progressing toward normal or is compromised. Stools are routinely tested for occult blood and sugar.

The child needs to be observed during the postoperative period for signs and symptoms of anastomosis breakdown or leakage. Sudden abdominal distention, fever, and irritability may signal the presence of this complication. Some children have intermittent periods of abdominal distention because of an inability to evacuate. Gentle insertion of a rectal tube will alleviate the problem. The diet initially consists of clear liquids and is gradually advanced to normal. If any foods contribute to diarrhea, they are avoided temporarily.

The success of surgery cannot be determined until the child reaches the toilet-training stage. Parents should receive support from the nurse during toilet training, as it may be very stressful for them. Long-range problems include delays in toilet training, staining, constipation, and intermittent incontinence with diarrhea. The overwhelming majority of children experience satisfactory surgical results. However, perfect bowel function is not always attained.

Encopresis

Encopresis is a psychogenic dysfunction in which the child displays chronic constipation and persistent soiling. A functional megacolon develops as the result of stool retention. However, there are significant differences between the child with encopresis and the child with Hirschsprung's disease. Table 19-9 compares encopresis and Hirschsprung's disease. There is disagreement over treatment modalities for this problem. However, the fecal impaction must be evacuated before any therapy can be instituted.

Emotional disturbances in the child and/or in the family are sometimes encountered in cases of encopresis but are not necessarily its cause. Parents are involved in the training program once

Table 19-9 Comparison of Encopresis and Hirschsprung's Disease

Encopresis	Hirschsprung's Disease
Cause is psychogenic.	Cause is absence of colon ganglion cells.
Onset is at approximately 2 years of age.	Onset is during the neonatal period.
Stools are large and formed; there is incontinence and soiling.	Stools are small ribbons or liquid; there is no soiling or incontinence.
General state is healthy.	General state is characterized by anorexia, muscle wasting, anemia, growth retardation.

the initial bowel cleansing has been done. To prevent reimpaction, a regimen of cathartics and a high-fiber diet, along with specified toileting times, is instituted. Gradually, medications are eliminated from the program. Several months are required for the bowel training to be successful.

Nursing management Both the parents and the child require nursing support to deal with this difficult problem. The child should be praised for using the toilet appropriately. Incontinence is handled tactfully. Criticizing or punishing the child for soiling is not effective. One approach is to have children with encopresis rinse out their clothes and clean themselves after soiling.

Consistent adherence to the regimen is essential for success. The nurse should emphasize the necessity of this to the parents and should praise both the child and the family for their efforts.

Imperforate anus

Etiology *Imperforate anus* is the result of imperfect fusion of the entodermal cloaca with the proctodeum. (Refer to the section "Embryology of the Gastrointestinal Tract" for a further discussion.) Imperforate anus manifests itself in several ways, but is commonly categorized according to whether the rectum passes through the puborectalis muscle or not (Fig. 19-16 shows the types and the frequency of occurrence). High and low agenesis, type III, are by far the most common. Fistulas to the vagina and rectum may coexist with imperforate anus. The incidence is between 1 in 5000 and 1 in 15,000.[92]

Manifestations The manifestations of imperforate anus depend on the type of defect present. Failure to pass meconium or difficulty in doing so and the development of symptoms of intestinal obstruction, if there is no associated fistula, are present in all types. Anal stenosis may cause the infant to pass dots of meconium or ribbonlike stools. Straining during defecation is usually present. An imperforate anal membrane will present with a bulging, greenish membrane at the anus. The anal dimple is present in low types of agenesis but not in high types. If a fistula is present, stool may come from the perineum, the vagina, or the urethra.

Diagnosis An abdominal x-ray may be taken with the infant held upside down and with a marker placed in the anal dimple. This position allows gas in the colon to rise and outline the blind rectal pouch and its distance from the anal opening. This technique is not diagnostic and has many disadvantages. The infant must be at least 24 h old for air to have passed through the intestines, meconium may block air passage and give false results, or the marker may be misplaced. Ultrasound scanning may help in differentiating the lesions. An intravenous pyelogram, urography, and cystography will be done preoperatively and postoperatively.

Medical management The low anomalies may be treated surgically by removing the anal membrane, anoplasty, and anal dilatation. The high anomalies require more extensive surgery over many years. The degree of surgical difficulty is directly proportional to the space between the anus and the rectal pouch. A colostomy is performed in the neonate until definitive treatment can be undertaken. When the infant is 6 to 10 months of age[93] or older, a pull-through procedure, such as those discussed in connection with Hirschsprung's disease, can be performed. Studies which evaluate the innervation status of the pelvic muscles should be done prior to the pull-through procedure. Bowel continence is dependent on the levator ani muscle sling. If nerve impulses are weak or lacking, continence will not be achieved, and a permanent colostomy would be preferable.

Nursing management Frequently, the nurse discovers that the neonate has an imperforate anus when attempting to insert a rectal thermometer. Newborns may also develop signs of

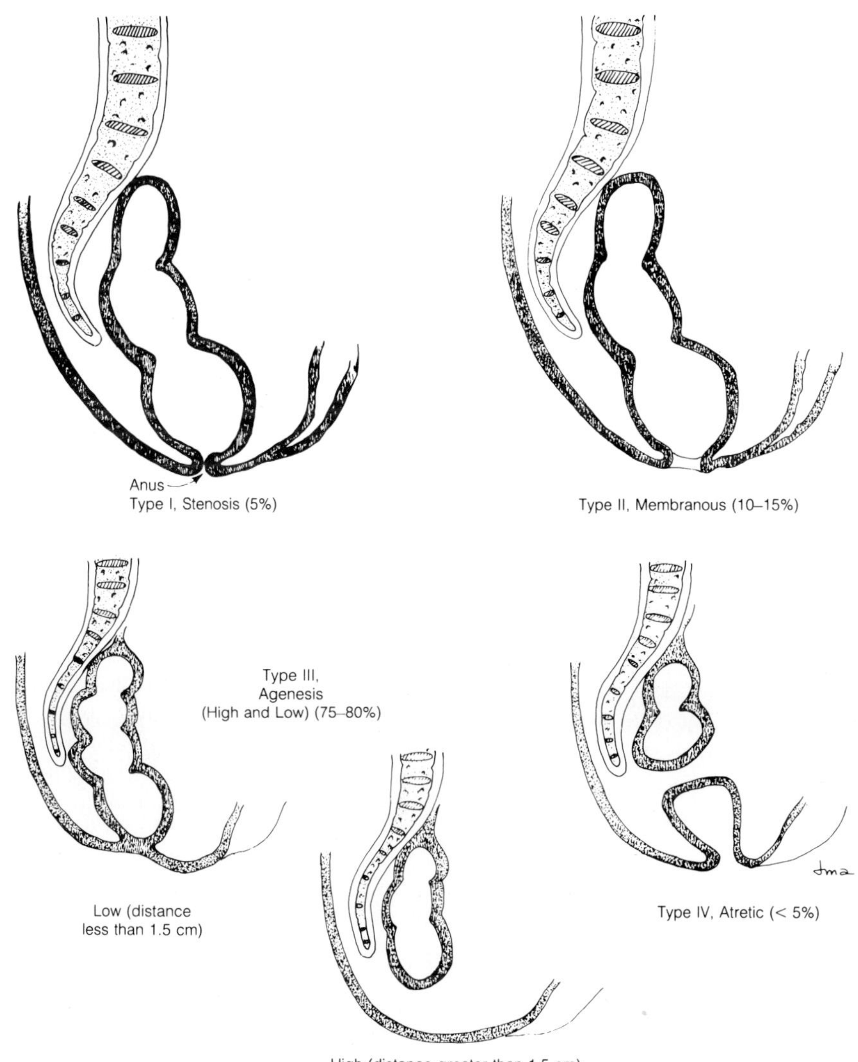

Figure 19-16 The different types of imperforate anus. (*From G. Scipien, M. U. Barnard, M. A. Chard, J. Howe, and P. J. Phillips* [eds.], *Comprehensive Pediatric Nursing, 3d ed., McGraw-Hill, New York, 1986, p. 1058. Used with permission.*)

obstruction such as vomiting and abdominal distention. Postoperatively, the infant who has an anoplasty is positioned on the side to prevent tension on the suture line. The diaper is left off, and the area must be kept clean and dry. Ointments are not used, and nothing should be inserted into the rectum. Dilatation is initiated once healing has begun and is continued at home. The parents must be taught this procedure.

If a colostomy has been done, the infant will have a nasogastric tube and an intravenous line. These are continued until peristalsis resumes. The parents need to be taught colostomy care prior to the infant's discharge. To allay their anxieties, they also should receive an explanation of why definitive surgery has been postponed.

Nursing care of the child after the pull-through procedure is similar to that of the child with Hirschsprung's disease. Continence cannot be assessed until the child is older. A second procedure may be necessary to replace the colon in the puborectalis sling if bowel continence has not been completely achieved. Anal dilatations are necessary after the pull-through procedure and are continued at home. The parents need support during the toilet-training period, since they have many concerns in regard to the child's ability to master this task. These children and their parents should receive long-term follow-up by nursing personnel.

Hernias

Inguinal hernia *Etiology and manifestations* *Inguinal hernia* is the prolapse of a portion of the intestine through the inguinal ring. The prolapse occurs as a result of a congenital weakness or an incomplete closure of the inguinal ring. During fetal development, at about the eighth month, the testes descend with a portion of the peritoneum down the inguinal canal. This tract, called the *processus vaginalis,* closes and atrophies, except for the peritoneum enclosing the testes in the scrotum. Incomplete closure can allow intestine or fluid to enter the scrotum. Inguinal hernias occur infrequently in females; 90 percent occur in males.[94] There is a high incidence among premature infants, frequently associated with hydroceles and undescended testicles. The processus vaginalis in girls extends from the external inguinal ring to the labia minora. Usually hernias produce few symptoms. When a child cries vigorously or strains, a bulging mass can be felt, or the hernia becomes larger.

Management Hernias can become incarcerated or strangulated. An incarcerated or strangulated hernia becomes tightly bound in the inguinal ring. The blood supply to the bound intestine may be cut off, and bowel necrosis can occur. To prevent bowel damage, the hernia must be reduced (moved back out of the inguinal ring). Sedation may be necessary because the pain can become intense. The surgeon will apply pressure to the site for several minutes in an attempt to reduce the hernia. If this is unsuccessful, the child is placed in the Trendelenburg position, and ice is applied to the scrotum. The hernia is usually manually reduced, but surgery will be done when the edema subsides, usually in about 48 h. When symptoms persist or worsen (increased crying, vomiting, abdominal distention, and bloody stools), surgery is done on an emergency basis.

When hernias are diagnosed at birth, reparative surgery is usually done as soon as the infant's condition permits. Inguinal hernia repair is not a complicated surgical procedure and in some settings is done on an outpatient basis.

Postoperative nursing management Postoperatively, the child is allowed to ambulate freely. The biggest nursing challenge is keeping the operative site clean and dry. Frequent diaper changes and careful attention to hygiene are necessary.

Umbilical hernia *Etiology* *Umbilical hernia* is the bulging of the intestine at the umbilicus. The umbilical ring that allowed the umbilical cord to penetrate the abdominal wall usually closes soon after birth.

Management When an umbilical hernia is present, the umbilical ring remains as an opening of varying size. Strangulation is rare with umbilical hernias. Most of these begin to regress and gradually close as crawling and walking strengthen the abdominal muscles. Umbilical hernias are more common among premature and black infants. The home remedies once commonly used are of no benefit. Assure parents that taping the umbilicus and using bellybands will not prevent or cure an umbilical hernia. Surgery is indicated if the defect persists past the age of 5 years.

Postoperatively, the child will have a large pressure dressing over the abdomen. This is left in place for a week to 10 days. The hospital stay is 2 or 3 days.

ALTERATIONS OF THE LIVER

Normal liver function

The liver is essential for health and accomplishes multiple functions in the healthy child. Table 19-10 lists liver functions and some of the effects of impairment.

Liver dysfunction

Disease or obstruction of the liver can result in cell death, fibrosis, scarring, and decreased efficiency.

Table 19-10 Summary of Liver Functions and the Results of Impaired Function

Liver Function	Results of Impairment
Synthesis of fibrinogen, prothrombin, and clotting factors V, VII, IX, X	Clotting times and prothrombin and partial thromboplastin times are prolonged; the patient bleeds and bruises easily; possible hemorrhage and melena.
Synthesis of albumin	Decreased albumin levels; edema and ascites result.
Production of enzymes (SGOT, SGPT, LDH, and alkaline phosphatase)	Elevated enzymes are released from damaged liver cells.
Metabolism and conjugation of bilirubin	Increased bilirubin levels. Indirect indicates damage to the cells, and direct indicates a problem in the ducts. Jaundice; itching.
Deamination of amino acids to ammonia to urea	Increased levels of ammonia; confusion; toxic encephalopathy; hepatic coma.
Drug metabolism and detoxification	Increased toxic levels of drugs; smaller dosages than normal are needed.
Production of bile (pigments)	Stools are white or clay-colored; there is reduced bile to the intestines and impaired fat digestion.
Storage of glycogen	Hypoglycemia.
Metabolism of fats, proteins, and carbohydrates	Decreased metabolism and utilization of foods; reduced glycogen.
Storage of vitamins and iron	Avitaminosis.
Bile for absorption of fat-soluble vitamins (A, D, E, and K)	Anemia: D—possible rickets; K—not absorbed in intestines, influencing clotting factors that require vitamin K for formation.
Filtration, detoxification, and excretion of corticosteroids (ADH and aldosterone)	Poor detoxification causes accumulation in the body; there is sodium retention and potassium loss.

The liver is a very vascular organ, supplied with blood from two main sources: the portal vein and the hepatic arteries. Blood from the digestive tract normally passes through the portal veins to the portal circulation of the liver and then to the inferior vena cava and back to the heart. Obstruction of the portal blood flow, whether due to disease inside *(intrahepatic)* or outside the liver *(extrahepatic)*, leads to the development of increased portal pressure *(portal hypertension)*.

The blood flowing through the portal veins is impeded by this pressure and is forced to use an alternative route in its return to the vena cava. This results in the development of *collateral circulation*. The blood uses the collateral circulation provided by veins at the cardia of the stomach and lower esophagus, umbilicus, anus, and retroperitoneum.

As the pressure within the venous portal system increases because of obstruction or disease of the liver, it results in a large, tense liver; esophageal and gastric varices; hemorrhoids; distended umbilical veins; and ascites. The major danger is rupture of the varices and hemorrhage, resulting in shock and death.

Diagnostic tests The laboratory tests that are usually done to diagnose liver disease are tests of:

1. Clotting function.
2. Albumin levels.
3. Bilirubin levels.
4. Blood ammonia (NH_3) level and blood urea nitrogen.
5. Blood glucose.
6. Serum enzyme levels:
   a. SGOT (serum glutamic oxaloacetic transaminase) is an enzyme found in the liver and heart. Acute cell destruction will cause an increase after about 8 h, with a peak in 24 to 36 h and a decrease in 4 to 6 days.
   b. SGPT (serum glutamic pyruvic transaminase) is an enzyme found only in the liver, but this test is not as sensitive an indicator as the test for SGOT.
   c. Serum alkaline phosphatase is an enzyme produced in the liver and bone and excreted in the bile. Its level in the blood is increased if the biliary pathways are obstructed.

A liver biopsy and liver and spleen scans are commonly done. Nuclear scanning tests using technetium 99m isotopes are done to establish patency of the bile ducts. I^{131} rose bengal tests may be done.

Medical management *Conservative management* of liver dysfunction includes providing good nutrition and rest, protecting against infection and trauma, and taking measures to increase comfort. The diet is adjusted according to the specific problem. Carbohydrates are generally increased because of their protein-sparing effect. High-quality protein is given in moderation to promote the healing process in cases of acute hepatic illness. Excessive amounts of fats are avoided. Additional fat-soluble vitamins, iron preparations, and intramuscular vitamin K will be needed. If the child is admitted to the hospital with bleeding, transfusions may be required.

Clinical symptoms seen in the child are jaundice; edema; ascites; portal hypertension; esophageal varices; dry, itching skin; splenomegaly; and color changes in the stool (clay-colored) and urine (dark). In children with portal hypertension, massive hemorrhage with symptoms of vomiting of blood and melena may be seen. Control of bleeding from esophageal varices is essentially the same as for adults. The major method of control is gastric compression using a Sengstaken-Blakemore tube. Esophageal varices may be treated by sclerotherapy, but this is controversial.[95]

Surgery is usually done in children with severe hemorrhaging from esophageal varices. The surgical objective is to divert the blood through another pathway, around the liver, and thereby to relieve the pressure on the gastrointestinal tract. The *portocaval shunt* has the highest success rate and is done in children over 5 years old with intrahepatic obstruction. The portal vein is anastomosed to the inferior vena cava, thus bypassing the liver. The *splenorenal shunt* joins the splenic vein to the renal vein. It is used with extrahepatic obstruction. The splenic vein is too small to be used in children under 10 years of age.

Biliary atresia

Etiology The cause of *biliary atresia* is uncertain; it may be due to an insult (infectious, chemical, or vascular) in utero that progresses in postnatal life.[96] Obstruction of the ducts, inside or outside the liver, is present, and as a result, bile builds up in the liver. It cannot be absorbed and causes jaundice, itching, and other symptoms of liver impairment. The incidence is 1 in 8000 to 1 in 20,000.[97]

Manifestations The primary symptom is persistent jaundice continuing in the newborn after 2 weeks of age. The direct bilirubin level is elevated, and the stools are white or clay-colored and puttylike in consistency. The urine is dark. Hepatomegaly and abdominal distention are common. Laboratory studies reveal anemia, elevation of the serum alkaline phosphatase level, and increased clotting times. Later (a few months to a year), if surgery is not done, fibrotic changes occur within the liver. This leads to cirrhosis and the development of portal hypertension. An enlarged spleen, esophageal varices, and ascites appear. As the child grows older, the skin color becomes more greenish gray or bronze, and itching becomes intense due to the buildup of bile salts. Growth is impaired, with malnutrition (especially hypoproteinemia) and wasting due to nutritional deficits. Hyperammonemia can result in hepatic coma and eventually death. If surgery is not done, the child usually dies between the ages of 18 and 36 months.[98]

Diagnosis No single laboratory test is diagnostic of biliary atresia. Technetium 99m scanning tests and a liver biopsy will be done. An exploratory laparotomy and operative cholangiography are often done to make a definitive diagnosis.

Medical management The surgical procedure performed depends on the location of the atresia. If it is in the common bile duct, the patent proximal duct and the duodenum can be connected by means of an anastomosis or conduit.

If the intrahepatic ducts are patent but there is extrahepatic atresia, a modification of the *Kasai procedure* (portoenterostomy) is done. This involves using a segment of jejunum to connect the liver to a double-barreled stoma. Bile drains out the proximal stoma into a collection bag and then may be refed into the intestine via the distal stoma. Surgery must be done early (at 2 to 3 months of age). Postoperative complications include infection (cholangitis), portal hypertension, and cirrhosis. Surgical failures have the same outcome as inoperable cases—death in 8 to 15 months. When bile flow is sustained, there is a 10-year survival rate of 38 percent.[99] With advancing techniques, the quality of life and survival rates of children with biliary atresia are improving.

If the atretic segment includes intrahepatic ducts as well as extrahepatic ducts, the prognosis is poor. A liver transplant may be an option.

Nursing management Nursing care is directed toward providing good nutrition and comfort for the child, appropriate for his or her age. Intravenous fluids may be used until the infant has stabilized after the diagnostic workup. Formulas that contain medium chain triglycerides and do not need bile to digest the fats, such as Pregestimil and Portagen, are given. Water-miscible forms of vitamins A, D, E, and K are administered. The child may be deficient in vitamin K, which is needed for the synthesis of prothrombin. Any signs of bleeding are noted, and gentle handling is necessary to prevent trauma and bruising.

Phenobarbital may be ordered to enhance bile drainage. The infant may have respiratory distress due to ascites and abdominal distention. Frequent measurements of abdominal girth may be required to monitor this. A semi-Fowler's position is usually most comfortable.

The skin is edematous, and the increase in bile salts causes intense pruritus, resulting in a fussy, irritable infant. Cholestyramine and antihistamines (Benadryl) may be used to decrease discomfort. Giving frequent cool or tepid baths, applying lotions, carefully cutting the fingernails, and placing mittens on the hands will prevent scratching and subsequent skin infections. The infant may seem so uncomfortable that the parents need extra encouragement to hold and cuddle the child.

If surgery has been performed, routine postoperative care is given. Bile drainage is very irritating, and so meticulous skin and ostomy care (discussed earlier in this chapter) are essential. Bile must be measured, and its characteristics noted. The nurse should be alert for, and teach the parents about, the symptoms of cholangitis. These include decreasing bile output, increasing bilirubin levels, fever, and lethargy. Cholangitis is treated with broad-spectrum antibiotics. The parents need much support, as do the parents of any child with a chronic, and potentially fatal, illness.

Nursing Care Plan: Cleft Lip Surgery

Patient: James Martin **Age:** 3 months, 3 days **Date of Admission:** 7/1

ASSESSMENT

James Martin, age 3 months, 3 days, was admitted to the pediatric unit on 7/1. The reason for hospitalization was primary repair of a unilateral cleft lip, which was performed on 7/2. The infant has no history of hospitalization. He has no known allergies. His parents are married, and there are no siblings.

General Appearance
Is a healthy, well-nourished active infant. Is alert and responsive to people.

Health History
Was diagnosed at birth as having a unilateral cleft lip and cleft palate. He is the first child of young (22-year-old) parents; there is a paternal family history of cleft lip. He has had two colds and one episode of otitis media. Both parents seem to be dealing well with the baby, holding, cuddling, playing with, and feeding the child. Immunizations have not been started.

Diet and Elimination
Takes 112 to 208 ml of Enfamil with iron 4 to 5 times per day. A soft, cross-cut regular nipple has been used, but he has been fed with a rubber-tipped syringe for the last week. It takes him about 30 to 35 min to eat. Both parents are comfortable feeding the child. Voids 8 to 10 times a day and stools once per day—soft, brown, and formed.

Sleep
Usually sleeps through the night, but may wake once during the night. His mother gives him formula, and he readily falls asleep.

Physical Examination
Weight: 4.5 kg 84g. (Birth weight 3.15 kg 280g). Height: 57.5 cm. Temperature: 37.5°C (99.4°F). Pulse: 126. Respiratory rate: 30. Blood pressure not obtained.

Skin
Is intact, pink, and warm. Cleft of lip on left side is complete and extends into nostril. Buttocks—pinpoint maculopapular rash on inner thighs and buttocks.

Respiratory Function
Lungs are clear to auscultation. Respirations are regular and easy.

Neurological Function
Has normal reflexes for an infant his age.

Growth and Development
Smiles socially; is beginning to roll over by himself, babbles; sucks left fingers.

Family History
The father was recently laid off from work. Blue Cross/Blue Shield is in force temporarily. They live in an apartment—the baby has his own room.

Laboratory Data
Hbg 12g; Hct 36%; WBC 4500. Urine clear and without WBC. Chest x-ray clear.

PHYSICIAN'S ORDERS

Surgery 7/2. Postoperative orders include:

1. Provide a mist tent for 24 h.
2. NPO until alert and then start clear liquids via a rubber-tipped syringe; advance diet as tolerated.
3. IV fluids: 5% dextrose and 0.2% NS to run at 15 ml per hour. Discontinue when taking fluids well.
4. Use arm restraints at all times.
5. Cleanse incision with hydrogen peroxide and normal saline and then apply bacitracin tid and prn.

Nursing Diagnosis	Outcome Criteria	Nursing Interventions	Evaluation and Modifications
1. Potential for respiratory complications related to anesthesia, cleft palate, and poor immune system of infancy	☐ The infant's lungs will remain clear to auscultation, with normal temperature, no cough, normal respiratory rate, and a clear chest x-ray.	☐ Note respiratory rate, color, and breath sounds every hour until stable; then q2h. ☐ Turn from side to side q2h. ☐ Check mist tent for misting q2h; check linens for dampness. ☐ Take the rectal temperature q4h. ☐ Suction only if absolutely necessary.	☐ 7/2—11 P.M.: Temperature increased to 38.3°C (101°F). Ice placed in croupette. Temperature was 38.3°C at 1 A.M. Lungs are clear; respiratory rate is 32. No cough or excess secretions. ☐ 7/3—12 noon: Respirations are stable, and there is no stridor or dyspnea. Temperature was 37.8°C (100°F) at 11 A.M. Mist tent discontinued.
2. Potential fluid volume deficit related to hemorrhage from surgery	☐ The infant's pulse and respiratory rate will remain within normal limits. The infant's hematocrit and hemoglobin will remain within normal preoperative limits.	☐ Check the apical pulse and respiratory rate every hour until stable; then q2h. ☐ Note any bleeding from the wound. ☐ Note color, skin temperature, and urinary output frequently.	☐ 7/3: Pulse and respirations are stable; vital signs now q4h. No visible bleeding. Color is pink, and has good urinary output. Hct 36.
3. Potential for infection of wound	☐ The surgical site will remain intact and have normal wound healing without signs of infection or bleeding.	☐ Use arm restraints at all times. Remove q4h to check skin and circulation. Logan bar in place. ☐ Place on side or back—*not* abdomen. ☐ Cleanse lip with hydrogen peroxide and normal saline after feeding and apply bacitracin—sterile technique. ☐ Check for signs of infection—temperature, erythema, and purulent drainage. ☐ Try to prevent crying and fussing.	☐ 7/3: No signs of bleeding, and incision is intact. Incision is being cleansed and appears clean and supple.
4. Decreased hydration related to decreased fluids with surgery	☐ The infant will have adequate hydration, as indicated by good urinary output, good skin turgor, moist mucous membranes, and normal pulse.	☐ IV fluids—D_5/0.2 NS to run at 15 ml per hour. Check rate hourly. Note signs of circulatory overload. ☐ When alert, and bowel sounds present, start feeding with glucose water via a rubber-tipped syringe. If retained, continue feedings and work up to normal formula, feeding q4h. ☐ Disconnect IV when taking fluids well.	☐ 7/3: Is taking clear liquids well; tolerated one feeding of half-strength Enfamil with iron. IV has been discontinued. Has good urinary output, good skin turgor, and moist mucous membranes.

Nursing Diagnosis	Outcome Criteria	Nursing Interventions	Evaluation and Modifications
		☐ Check urinary output, skin turgor, and mucous membranes.	
5. Disruption of skin integrity on buttocks, related to diaper rash	☐ The infant's skin will be intact, pink, and healthy.	☐ Cleanse buttocks well after every voiding. Check diapers frequently and change. ☐ Air-dry buttocks 20 min, tid. ☐ Apply A and D ointment at each diaper change.	☐ 7/3: Diaper rash is decreasing.
6. Increased parental anxiety related to surgery and financial worries	☐ The parents will have decreased anxiety, as evidenced by fewer questions and fewer verbal and nonverbal expressions of anxiety.	☐ Explain the surgery to the parents and keep them informed of all procedures and tests. Answer all questions as fully as possible. ☐ Encourage visiting and caring for the child. ☐ Explore any concerns they may have, i.e., finances.	☐ 7/3: The parents remained concerned, but less than immediately after the surgery. They did express worry about finances; a social services referral has been initiated.
7. Knowledge deficit related to care of the child's lip repair and health maintenance	☐ The parents will demonstrate knowledge of health maintenance and discharge teaching.	☐ Review immunizations—need and schedule. ☐ Discuss growth and development—play, safety, and normal milestones. ☐ Give discharge instructions regarding feeding, restraints, lip care, signs of infection, and diaper rash.	☐ 7/3: Plan to do this 2 days prior to discharge. Need to discuss future plans also—work with cleft lip–cleft palate team and future surgeries for lip and palate.
8. Health maintenance, potential alteration in, related to maturational factors.	☐ The infant will exhibit normal growth and development, as evidenced by achieving the normal motor and social milestones.	☐ Have mobiles in crib. No toys which could injure the mouth. ☐ Sing, talk to, hold, and cuddle with feedings and when awake. ☐ Encourage the parents to visit frequently and care for and play with the child. ☐ Keep crib rails up at all times. ☐ Discuss normal growth and development with the parents after assessing their level of knowledge and their needs.	☐ 7/3: The child seems happy and smiles in response to the parents. The parents are visiting frequently.

References

1. Hamilton, Eva May, Eleanor Noss Whitney, and Frances Sizer, *Nutrition: Concepts and Controversies*, 3d ed., West, St. Paul, Minn., 1985, p. 227.
2. Pipes, Peggy L., *Nutrition in Infancy and Childhood*, 2d ed., Mosby, St. Louis, 1981, p. 54.
3. Hamilton, Whitney, and Sizer, op. cit., p. 237.
4. Pipes, op. cit., p. 59.
5. Hamilton, Whitney, and Sizer, op. cit., p. 240.
6. Hui, Y. H., *Human Nutrition and Diet Therapy*, Wadsworth Health Services Division, Monterey, Calif., 1983, p. 121.
7. Taylor, Keith B., and Luean E. Anthony, *Clinical Nutrition*, McGraw-Hill, New York, 1983, p. 319.
8. Hamilton, Whitney, and Sizer, op. cit., p. 244.
9. Ibid., pp. 250–251.
10. Ibid.
11. Kanarek, Keith S., Paul R. Williams, and John S. Curran, "Total Parenteral Nutrition in Infants and Children," *Advances in Pediatrics* **29**:151–181 (1982).
12. Gryboski, Joyce, and W. Allan Walker, *Gastrointestinal Problems in the Infant*, 2d ed., Saunders, Philadelphia, 1983, p. 881.
13. Kanarek, Williams, and Curran, op. cit., pp. 165–167.
14. Ibid., p. 163.
15. Ibid.
16. Ling, Lyllis, and Sarah P. McCamman, "Dietary Treatment of Diarrhea and Constipation in Infants and Children," *Issues in Comprehensive Pediatric Nursing* **3**:20–28 (October 1978).
17. Raffensperger, John G., and Susan R. Luck, "Gastrointestinal Bleeding in Children," *Surgical Clinics of North America* **56**:413 (1976).
18. McConnell, Edwina A., "Ensuring Safer Stomach Suctioning with the Salem Sump Tube," *Nursing '77* **7**:54 (September 1977).
19. Ibid., p. 56.
20. Bernbaum, Judy C., Gilbert R. Pereira, John B. Watkins, and George J. Peckham, "Nonnutritive Sucking during Gavage Feeding in Premature Infants," *Pediatrics* **71**:41–45 (January 1983).
21. Watt, Rosemary C., "Ostomies: Why, How, and Where," *Nursing Clinics of North America* **11**:396 (September 1976).
22. Martin, Lester W., Alice Gilmore, Judith Peckham, and Jean Baumer, "Nursing Care of Infants with Esophageal Anomalies," *American Journal of Nursing* **66**:2462–2468 (November 1966).
23. Gryboski and Walker, op. cit., p. 16.
24. Ibid.
25. Whaley, Lucille F., and Donna L. Wong, *Nursing Care of Infants and Children*, 2d ed., Mosby, St. Louis, 1983, p. 378.
26. Styker, Grace Witmer, and Kathy Freeh, "Feeding Infants with Cleft Lip and/or Palate," *Journal of Obstetric, Gynecologic, and Neonatal Nursing* **10**:329–332 (September–October 1981).
27. Behrman, Richard E., and Victor C. Vaughan, *Nelson Textbook of Pediatrics*, 12th ed., Saunders, Philadelphia, 1983, p. 881.
28. Kaplan, I., M. Ben-Bassat, E. Taube, J. Dresner, and A. Nachmani, "Ten Year Follow-up of Simultaneous Repair of Cleft Lip and Palate in Infancy," *Annals of Plastic Surgery* **8**(3):227–228 (March 1982).
29. Kaplan, E. N., "Cleft Palate Repair at Three Months?" *Annals of Plastic Surgery* **7**(3):170–190 (September 1981).
30. Dorf, Debra S., and John W. Curtin, "Early Cleft Palate Repair and Speech Outcome," *Plastic and Reconstructive Surgery* **70**(1):74–81 (July 1982).
31. Behrman and Vaughan, op. cit., p. 882.
32. Ibid., p. 893.
33. Ibid.
34. Silverman, Arnold, and Claude C. Roy, *Pediatric Clinical Gastroenterology*, 3d ed., Mosby, St. Louis, 1983, p. 51.
35. Jose, James H., D. Wade Clapp, William C. Kirby, and Richard L. Schreiner, "Perinatal Aspiration Syndrome: Current Concepts," *Respiratory Therapy* **15**(15):18–25 (January–February 1985).
36. Holder, Thomas M., and Keith W. Ashcraft, "Developments in the Care of Patients with Esophageal Atresia and Tracheoesophageal Fistula," *Surgical Clinics of North America* **61**(5):1051–1061 (October 1981).
37. Herbst, John J., "Diagnosis and Treatment of Gastroesophageal Reflux in Children," *Pediatrics in Review* **5**(3):75–79 (September 1983).
38. Whaley and Wong, op. cit., p. 1254.
39. Herbst, op. cit., p. 75.
40. Ibid.
41. Silverman and Roy, op. cit., p. 162.
42. Ibid.
43. Gryboski and Walker, op. cit., p. 226.
44. Behrman and Vaughan, op. cit., p. 904.
45. Ibid.
46. Ibid., p. 905.
47. Gryboski and Walker, op. cit., p. 287.
48. Ibid.
49. Silverman and Roy, op. cit., p. 132.
50. Schwaltzberg, Steven D., William J. Pokorny, Charles W. McGill, and Franklin J. Harberg, "Gastroschisis and Omphalocele," *The American Journal of Surgery* **144**:650–654 (December 1982).
51. Gryboski and Walker, op. cit., p. 284.
52. Ibid., p. 285.
53. Ibid.
54. Silverman and Roy, op. cit., p. 100.
55. Harrison Michael R., and Alfred A. deLorimier, "Congenital Diaphragmatic Hernia," *Surgical Clinics of North America* **61**(5):1023–1035 (October 1981).
56. Ibid.
57. Silverman and Roy, op. cit., p. 165.
58. Ibid.

59. Rudolph, Abraham M., *Pediatrics,* 17th ed., Appleton Century Crofts, New York, 1982, p. 973.
60. Silverman and Roy, op. cit., p. 176.
61. Behrman and Vaughan, op. cit., p. 903.
62. Silverman and Roy, loc. cit.
63. Ibid.
64. Rudolph, op. cit. p. 955.
65. Gryboski and Walker, op. cit., p. 439.
66. Ibid., p. 127.
67. Rudolph, op. cit., p. 957.
68. Silverman and Roy, op. cit., p. 134.
69. Sabiston, David C. (ed.), *Davis-Christopher Textbook of Surgery: The Biological Basis of Modern Surgical Practice,* 12th ed., Saunders, Philadelphia, 1981, p. 1380.
70. Hoekelman, Robert A., Saul Blatman, Philip A. Brunell, Stanford B. Friedman, and Henry M. Seidel, *Principles of Pediatrics: Health Care of the Young,* McGraw-Hill, New York, 1978, p. 832.
71. Silverman and Roy, op. cit., p. 353.
72. Gryboski and Walker, op. cit., p. 517.
73. Rudolph, op. cit., p. 982.
74. Silverman and Roy, op. cit., p. 351.
75. Ibid., pp. 349–350.
76. Rudolph, op. cit., pp. 982–983.
77. Ibid.
78. Fonkalsrud, Eric W., "Inflammatory Bowel Disease in Childhood," *Surgical Clinics of North America* **61**(5):1125–1135 (October 1981).
79. Ibid.
80. Gryboski and Walker, op. cit., p. 523.
81. Hughes, James G., *Synopsis of Pediatrics,* 5th ed., Mosby, St. Louis, 1980, p. 302.
82. Silverman and Roy, op. cit., p. 267.
83. Shah, Praful C., and Emanuel Lebenthal, "Gluten Sensitive Enteropathy (GSE): A Practical Approach," *Pediatric Basics* **34**:4–8 (December 1982).
84. Gryboski and Walker, op. cit., p. 602.
85. Ibid.
86. Silverman and Roy, op. cit., p. 266.
87. *Pediatric Nutrition Handbook,* American Academy of Pediatrics, Evanston, Ill. 1979, p. 193.
88. Ibid.
89. Gryboski and Walker, op. cit., p. 504.
90. Silverman and Roy, op. cit., p. 410.
91. Lavery, Ian C., "The Surgery of Hirschsprung's Disease," *Surgical Clinics of North America* **63**(1):161–174 (February 1983).
92. Gryboski and Walker, op. cit., p. 492.
93. Silverman and Roy, op. cit., p. 74.
94. Behrman and Vaughan, op. cit., p. 949.
95. Atkinson, James B., and Morton M. Woolley, "Treatment of Esophageal Varices by Sclerotherapy in Children," *The American Journal of Surgery* **146**:103–106 (July 1983).
96. Silverman and Roy, op. cit., p. 539.
97. Gryboski and Walker, op. cit., p. 304.
98. Kempe, C. Henry, Henry K. Silver, and Donough O'Brien, *Current Pediatric Diagnosis and Treatment,* 7th ed., Lange, Los Altos, Calif., 1982, p. 476.
99. Silverman and Roy, op. cit., p. 548.

20

Lois L. Lux
Karen E. Roper

Renal function

Upon completion of this chapter, the student will be able to:

1 Relate urinary system congenital anomalies to embryological development.
2 Explain the method and purposes of selected renal diagnostic tests.
3 Describe the methods of collecting serum or urine specimens for renal diagnostic tests.
4 Interpret the results of urine culture and sensitivity tests.
5 Describe three radiological examinations used in the diagnosis of urinary system disorders.
6 Identify three measures employed after a closed renal biopsy to detect or minimize internal renal hemorrhage.
7 Differentiate the signs of lower and upper urinary tract infections.
8 List the common organisms responsible for urinary tract infections.
9 Formulate a plan of care for a child with a urinary tract infection.
10 Describe the anatomy and physiology present with vesicoureteral reflux.
11 Explain the treatment modalities for obstructions of the urinary tract.
12 Describe the physical appearance of a child with exstrophy and epispadias.
13 Prepare a preoperative teaching session for the parents of an infant with hypospadias.
14 Describe the treatment modalities for children with neuropathic bladders.
15 Describe three symptoms of acute glomerulonephritis and the nursing measures for each.
16 Compare the drug therapies generally utilized for acute and chronic glomerulonephritis.
17 Describe four nursing care measures used for a child with severe active nephrotic syndrome.
18 Compare the advantages of peritoneal dialysis vs. hemodialysis in children.
19 Compare the advantages of an internal and an external shunt for hemodialysis.

EMBRYOLOGY

Although the renal and reproductive systems are intimately related embryologically, they are discussed independently in this text to facilitate comprehension.

The kidneys begin to function at approximately the eighth week of development after passing through three stages. The first stage is marked by the development of the *pronephros*, or forekidney, which is a primitive, transitory, nonfunctional unit that appears early in the fourth week. Later in the fourth week, during the second stage, it gives rise to the *mesonephros*, or midkidney. The mesonephros may function as a temporary renal unit for a few weeks until the *metanephros*, or hind kidney, is formed during the third stage. The mesonephros gradually disintegrates after the eighth week except for the mesonephric duct (which buds to form the ureters, renal pelvis, calyces, and collecting tubules) and a few tubules which later form part of the male reproductive system. The metanephros, or permanent kidney, begins to develop in the fifth week and is producing urine in the eighth week, signifiying completion of the third stage of development.

The nephrons, the basic functioning units of the kidneys, are derived from the metanephric mass of the mesoderm. The number of nephrons does not increase after birth except in premature infants. As a child matures, the increase in renal size results from a growth in nephron size, not from an increase in the number of nephrons.

Initially, the permanent kidneys are located in the pelvis, but their ascent to an abdominal position begins by the seventh to the ninth weeks of gestation. As they ascend, they rotate 90° and are supplied by successively higher arteries. At birth, one renal artery and one renal vein supply each kidney. Infrequently, the kidneys do not ascend, resulting in ectopic kidneys. Fusion may also occur during ascent, producing a horseshoe (U-shaped) kidney.

By the seventh week, the *cloaca* (the chamber to the hindgut and the urogenital sinus) is divided by the urorectal septum into the rectum and the urogenital sinus (the bladder, urethra, and lower vagina in the female). The mesonephric duct and the ureteric bud have separate openings into the urogenital sinus. In the male, the mesonephric duct eventually becomes the ejaculatory duct, whereas in the female, it simply degenerates. The ureteric bud, derived earlier from the mesonephric duct, becomes the ureter.

In the male, the urethra, except for the glandular portion of the penile urethra, develops from the urogenital sinus. The glandular portion of the urethra is formed by tubularization of a cord of cells that enter the glans by way of the tip. Various degrees of hypospadias occur if the urethra does not form correctly. In the female, the entire urethra is formed from the urogenital sinus (Fig. 20-1).

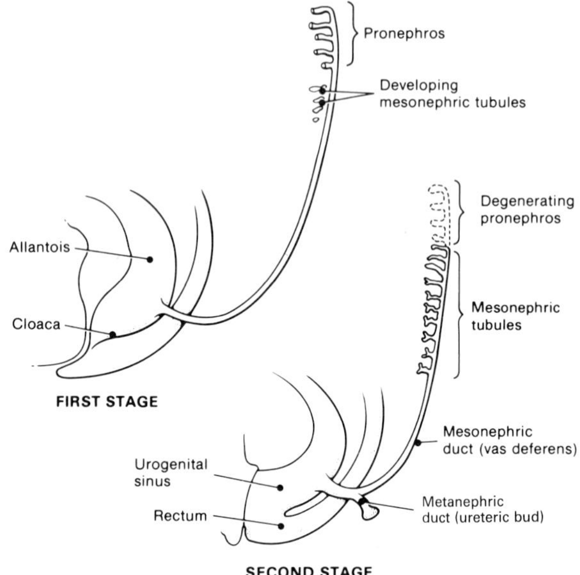

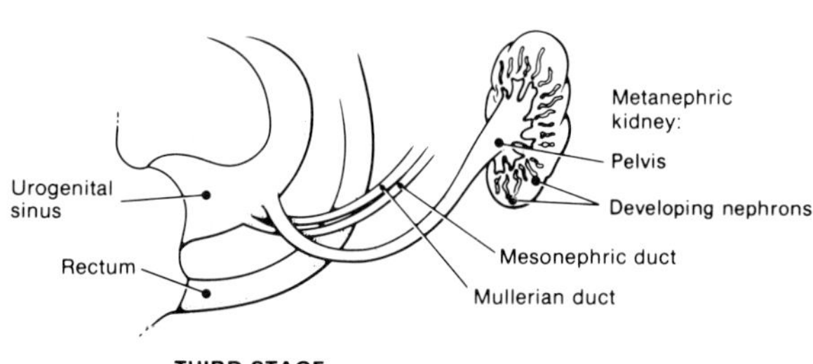

Figure 20-1 The three stages of development of the embryonic kidneys in the human fetus and the embryonic development of the collecting system. (*From G. Scipien, M. U. Barnard, M. A. Chard, J. Howe, and P. J. Phillips* [eds.], *Comprehensive Pediatric Nursing, 3d ed., McGraw-Hill, New York, 1986. Used with permission.*)

ANATOMY AND PHYSIOLOGY

The urinary tract is composed of an upper tract (the kidneys and ureters) and a lower tract (the bladder and urethra). The kidneys are located in the retroperitoneal space, on the dorsal aspect of the abdominal cavity on either side of the vertebral column. Because of the location of the liver, the right kidney is usually lower than the left kidney. They are not rigidly attached to the abdominal wall, but are supported by the renal fascia, renal arteries and veins, and perirenal fat. The kidneys of a newborn infant are proportionally about 3 times larger than those of an adult, when general body mass is taken into consideration.

The kidneys participate in the regulation of fluids and electrolytes, body pH, and excretion of the end products of metabolism. Each kidney has approximately 1 million nephrons that serve as its functioning units. A nephron is composed of a glomerulus (a tuft of capillary loops) surrounded by Bowman's capsule and the renal tubule system (Fig. 20-2). The glomerulus is the center for filtration of water and solutes from the

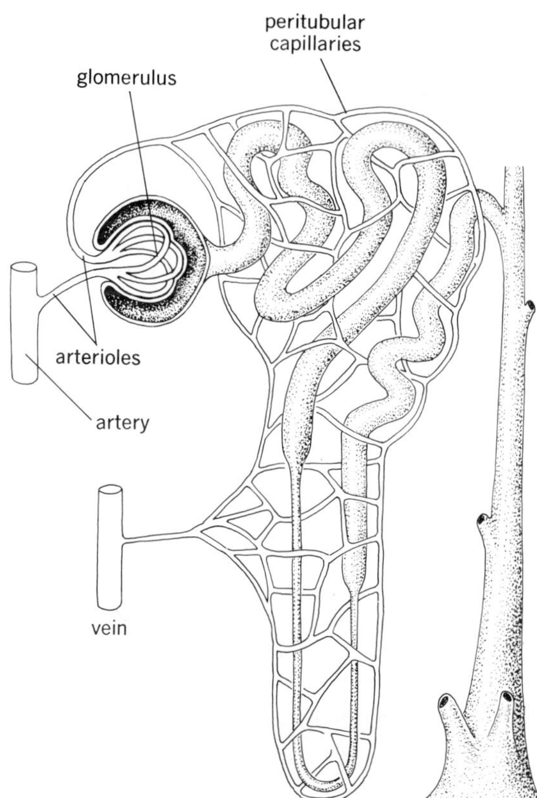

Figure 20-2 The basic structure of a nephron and the relationship between the blood supply and the renal tubular system. (*From A. Vander et al., Human Physiology: The Mechanisms of Body Function, 3d ed., McGraw-Hill, New York, 1980. Used with permission.*)

blood. The renal tubules are responsible for reabsorbing essential substances as well as for allowing waste products to remain in the filtrate and to be passed into the collecting tubules. The collecting tubules join to form central tubes, called *the ducts of Bellini*. The contents of these tubes pass through the calyces into the renal pelvis. Urine is then transported into the bladder by way of the ureters. (For additional information on the role of the kidneys in fluid and electrolyte management, refer to Chap. 18.)

The bladder is a hollow muscular organ that functions as a reservoir for urine. The internal urethral orifice, located at the upper border of the symphysis in a neonate, gradually sinks until it is at the level of the lower border of the symphysis in the adult. For this reason, the bladder of a child is truly an abdominal rather than a pelvic organ. It is therefore more accessible for suprapubic aspiration of urine or suprapubic surgery.

ASSESSMENT OF THE CHILD WITH ALTERATION OF THE URINARY TRACT

Interview and history

The interview, history, and physical examination should be conducted in a manner conducive to health teaching. Participation by the child, appropriate for his or her age, should be elicited during the assessment. Standard questionnaires designed to identify specific patterns of disease (such as urinary tract infections and enuresis) may be beneficial in establishing a data base and in planning for comprehensive care. They can also be important in providing continuity of care in a clinical setting.

A family history should be obtained, as should the physical and emotional history of the child. Any familial predispositions to renal disease, hypertension, urinary tract infections, and syndromes associated with urinary tract abnormalities are important to note. Specific questions to be asked include those pertaining to unexplained fever, flank or abdominal pain, changes in voiding habits (urgency, dysuria, enuresis, or change in stream), and changes in the character of the urine (color and odor). Medications the child is taking should be noted, and the nurse should pay particular attention to those that are potentially nephrotoxic or that may affect bladder function.

One must remember that some chronic renal conditions progress slowly and may not be associated with pain; in contrast, acute pyelonephritis causes a sudden onset of renal edema and will usually be accompanied by flank pain. Discomfort from the renal and ureteral areas may also be referred to the bladder, scrotum, and testicle in the male and to the bladder and vulva in the female.

Observation and the physical examination

The general condition of the child is observed throughout the initial assessment. General malaise and failure to thrive may be associated with chronic urinary tract conditions. General skin condition and the presence or absence of periorbital, facial, or generalized edema should be noted.

The physical examination should include palpation of the kidneys and bladder (if partially distended) and inspection of the genitalia. Accurate measurements of height and weight should be plotted on a standard growth chart. Blood pressure should be taken, especially in children with reflux or renal disease. Follow-up physical examinations may not need to be as extensive, depending on the past history and the presenting symptoms.

Diagnostic tests

The nurse should discuss with the family the rationale for performing any diagnostic test, remembering to include an age-appropriate explanation for the child. If a urine specimen must be obtained, the method of collection should also be discussed and explained. Children (and parents) tend to be more cooperative when they understand the procedure as well as their role.

Urine tests A voided sample usually is easily obtained, although catheterization of the bladder, catheterization of a urinary stoma, or suprapubic aspiration may occasionally be necessary. A voided specimen may be obtained with a clean-catch, midstream collection or with a U-bag (refer to Chap. 16).

The procedure for catheterizing children is essentially the same as that for catheterizing adults. The use of a no. 5 or 8 French infant feeding tube is appropriate when catheterizing an infant or small child. The child should be told that the procedure will probably not be painful but will be uncomfortable. If a urine specimen is needed for culture and sensitivity testing in a child with a *urostomy* (a nephrostomy, ileal conduit, or other urinary stoma), it will be necessary to obtain a catheterized specimen because of the high incidence of contamination associated with "bagged" or clean-catch specimens in these children. The procedure for stomal catheterization is essentially the same as for sterile urethral catheterization.

Suprapubic aspiration is performed by a physician or pediatric nurse practitioner and should be attempted only in a child with a full bladder (i.e., not immediately following voiding). The bladder is situated just beneath the skin and can be easily palpated in an infant or small child. The skin should be prepared with Betadine solution. A needle of an appropriate size is used to puncture the bladder about 1 cm above the symphysis, and the specimen is aspirated using a syringe (Fig. 20-3). Suprapubic aspiration of the male newborn is recommended to avoid the significant risk of iatrogenic injury to the urethra during catheterization.

Routine urinalysis When a routine urinalysis is ordered, instructions may include obtaining a fresh morning specimen. At this time, the urine will be more concentrated. Drinking large quantities of water to facilitate voiding is not advised because it may change the concentration.

Urine obtained for urinalysis should be kept at room temperature, since refrigeration can cause precipitation of phosphates or urates, which could interfere with the microscopic examination. It must not, however, be kept at room temperature for more than 1 to 2 h before examination. If it is allowed to stand at room temperature for a longer period of time, red cells may break up, casts may disintegrate, and bacteria may multiply, thereby affecting the accuracy of the test.

Color Urine is normally pale yellow or amber. A change in color may be due to food ingestion (dyes from beets or other vegetables), medications such as phenazopyridine (Pyridium) and Urised, red blood cells, or hemoglobin. It can also be very pale as a result of a low specific gravity or an osmotic diuresis (e.g., in diabetes mellitus).

Odor An acetone odor is present with keton-

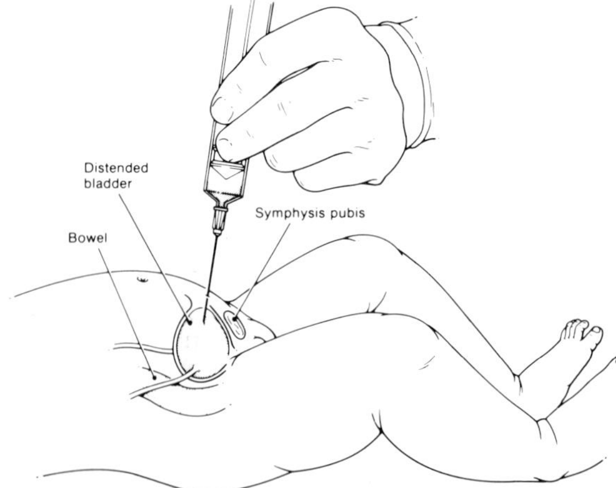

Figure 20-3 Suprapubic bladder aspiration is frequently the preferred method of obtaining a sterile urine specimen in infants. (*From G. Scipien, M. U. Barnard, M. A. Chard, J. Howe, and P. J. Phillips* [eds.], *Comprehensive Pediatric Nursing, 3d ed., McGraw-Hill, New York, 1986, p. 1151. Used with permission.*)

uria, and a strong ammonia-like or fecal odor may be present with bacterial growth.

Specific Gravity The normal range for children is approximately 1.000 to 1.030. Infants do not concentrate urine as well as older children, and normally their urine specific gravity will not exceed 1.020. If fluids are restricted, the child's urine should become more concentrated, and the specific gravity should reach the upper limits of normal. The specific gravity may be elevated if glucose, protein, or radiographic contrast material is present. Specific gravity can be measured easily on a nursing unit with a hydrometer or a refractometer; the latter requires only one drop of urine.

pH Normal kidneys participate in the control of total body pH by excreting urine in pH ranges of 4.5 to 7.5. Levels greater than 7.5 indicate that urea-splitting organisms are present (usually *Proteus*). These organisms make the urine very alkaline by releasing ammonia. Acid or alkaline food or medication may also affect the pH.

Other Urine Assessments A dipstick screening test for protein, blood, ketone, and glucose is performed. Normally, these elements are not present in the urine. A microscopic examination is done to determine the presence or absence of red blood cells, white blood cells, epithelial cells, casts, crystals, bacteria, and yeasts.

One must consider the entire urinalysis when evaluating the results. For example, hematuria in the presence of bacteria and white blood cells would probably indicate a bladder infection. Hematuria with proteinuria and tubular casts would probably be the result of a glomerular disorder.

Urine culture and sensitivity Urine that has been collected for culture and sensitivity testing should be sent to the laboratory immediately, since the number of bacteria doubles approximately every 30 min. An alternative to this practice is to use a dip-slide. This is a commercially prepared slide with culture media on both sides that can be dipped into the fresh specimen immediately and placed back in its plastic container. If dip-slides are not available, the urine may be placed in the refrigerator prior to transportation to the laboratory. A urinary tract infection is diagnosed if more than 100,000 colonies of a single strain of bacteria are present in a voided specimen. Recent evidence shows that bacterial count should not vary significantly whether the specimen is obtained by voiding, catheterization, or suprapubic aspiration if the urine specimen is collected and handled properly. Antibiotic sensitivity testing should then be done so that appropriate antibiotic therapy can be initiated. A positive urine culture obtained on a specimen collected by U-bag is not reliable, since contamination from the skin or from possible reflux of the urine into the vagina of female patients may occur. Suprapubic aspiration or catheterization is indicated when positive results are obtained with U-bag specimens.

The importance of collecting a urine specimen correctly cannot be overemphasized. The risk of contamination is significant. A positive culture obtained from a single, clean, voided specimen has a validity of only 80 percent. If two consecutive cultures are done correctly and they demonstrate the same organism and a high colony count, the validity rate increases to 95 percent.[1]

Timed urine collections When a 12- or 24-h urine collection is required for an outpatient, written instructions are helpful. The child should be instructed to void before the test starts, discarding the urine. *All* the urine that is voided from the time the test is initiated to the time it is completed should be saved. Timed collections begin and end with an empty bladder. The nurse should inform the family whether a preservative (Formalin) or refrigeration is necessary.

Creatinine Clearance This is a timed urine collection performed in conjunction with a serum creatinine test. (Refer to the section "Blood Tests".)

Proteinuria A patient with persistent proteinuria may undergo a timed test for total protein excretion. It is important to remember that transient proteinuria may occur with *orthostatic proteinuria* (caused by standing or exercising for long periods) or acute febrile illnesses or may follow a blood transfusion, exercise, or extensive burns. Therefore, it is not necessarily indicative of a severe renal disorder. Persistent, massive proteinuria generally accompanies glomerular disease and nephrosis. Mild proteinuria may be present or absent in many other renal conditions.

Osmolality The ability to concentrate urine is decreased in such renal conditions as chronic renal failure and obstructive uropathy with hydronephrosis. In general, children over 2 months old should be able to concentrate urine to 900 mOsmol per liter after a 12-h period of fluid restriction.

Renal function tests

Blood tests Renal function may be studied by blood tests and radiological examinations. The most common blood studies are of blood urea nitrogen (BUN), creatinine clearance, and urea clearance.

Urea and creatinine are the major nitrogenous waste products normally cleared from the circulation by the kidneys. Their concentration in the blood increases as kidney function decreases. These tests are considered only gross indicators of renal function since their values do not change until renal function is markedly impaired. The BUN and creatinine levels are elevated only after approximately 60 percent of kidney function is impaired.

Clearance tests report the milliliters of plasma that are completely cleared of a test substance each minute. Clearance values may relate primarily to glomerular function or to both glomerular and tubular function, depending on the test substance being measured. The creatinine clearance test is generally considered more valuable than the urea clearance test because creatinine clearance values are not affected by diet, fluid intake, or rate of urine flow. Normal values for the creatinine clearance test are approximately 100 ml/min. Normal urea clearance is approximately 70 ml/min.

Estimation of glomerular filtration rate is another important measure of kidney function. The glomerular filtration rate is measured by the clearance (removal from the bloodstream into the urine) of certain test substances. A normal glomerular filtration rate is 70 ml/min in children over 1 year of age.

Radiological tests The most common radiological test of renal function is the *intravenous pyelogram* (IVP). This is a study of the upper urinary tract. An iodinized dye is given to the child through an intravenous line. The kidneys concentrate and excrete the iodine compound, so that the kidneys, ureters, and bladder can be visualized on x-rays. Some patients are allergic to the dye compound, and so a small test dose is usually given prior to the examination. IV diphenhydramine (Benadryl) should be available in case of reactions. Patients are sometimes given a cleansing enema the evening before the examination so that bowel contents will not obscure the IVP films. Fluids are usually restricted for some hours before the examination.

A voiding cystourethrogram (VCUG) may be performed to study the lower urinary tract. This examination consists of introducing contrast media into the bladder via a catheter. The bladder is filled, and the child is asked to void. The child should be warned about this and told that it is part of the test. Films of the bladder, bladder neck, and urethra are taken during voiding. This test is not done in the presence of an acute urinary tract infection, since filling the bladder via a catheter may force infected urine up into the kidneys by reflux, causing upper urinary tract infection. (See Fig. 20-4*A* and *B*.)

Aortography and *renal angiography* may be performed for the diagnosis of problems such as tumors, cysts, aneurysms, and trauma. An arteriogram provides detailed visualization of the large and small renal arteries. A cutdown is performed, and a catheter is passed via the femoral artery into the abdominal aorta. Contrast media can be injected into the aorta, thereby filling both renal arteries. The catheter can be directed into one of the renal arteries if only one kidney needs to be visualized. Digital subtraction angiography is now possible using the venous system.[2]

Ultrasonography utilizes very high frequency sound waves transmitted through fluids and tissues. With this examination, the kidneys can be localized and measured. A mass can be identified as cystic, solid, or a mixture of both. This method is noninvasive and painless.

Radioisotope scanning is used to obtain detailed pictures of the pattern of blood flow and the excretory functioning of each kidney. A radioactive isotope is injected into the bloodstream. Films are taken as the kidneys concentrate and excrete the isotope. The test can define nonfunctional areas of the renal cortex and is of particular value in studying unilateral renal diseases and anomalies.

Computed tomography is a reconstruction by a computer of an image depicting a tomographic plane (slice) through the body. It is used selectively as a complementary imaging technique for diagnosing urinary system abnormalities.

Magnetic resonance imaging is still in its developmental stages but is expected to become one of the most significant advances in diagnostic body imaging. There is no ionizing radiation, and contrast medium is unnecessary.[3]

Cystoscopy

Cystoscopy is a means of visualizing the lower urinary tract directly. In children, this procedure is usually performed under general anesthesia.

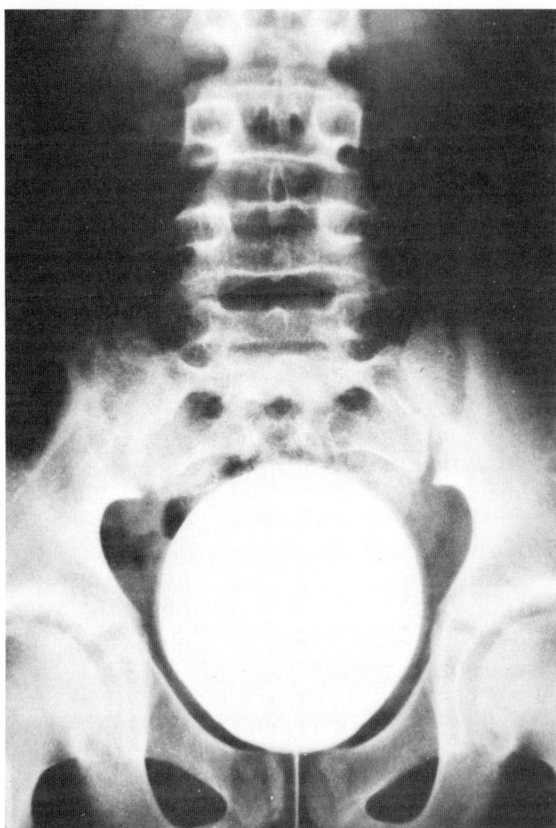

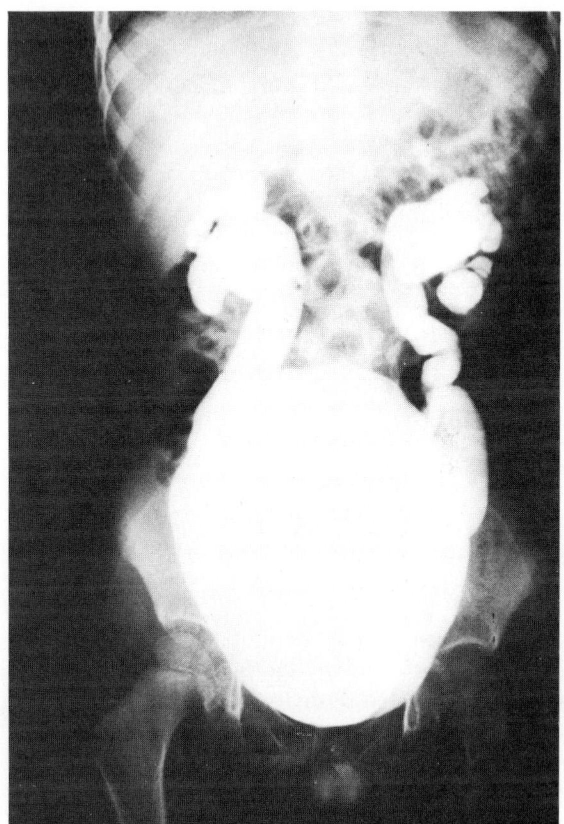

Figure 20-4 (*A*) A radiographic study demonstrating a normal voiding cystourethrogram. (*B*) A voiding cystourethrogram showing gross reflux. (*Courtesy of J. W. Duckett, M. D., Director of the Division of Urology, Children's Hospital of Philadelphia.*)

The surgeon inserts the tubular cystoscope through the urethra into the bladder so that the bladder wall and the ureteral openings can be visualized. In addition to cystoscopy, the surgeon may perform *retrograde pyelography.* This involves visualizing the ureteral openings with the cystoscope and injecting contrast material into the openings through a catheter. The contrast material will ascend to the ureters, and the appearance of the kidneys and the ureters may then be filmed.

Renal biopsy

At times, it may be necessary for the physician to examine a small piece (the diameter of a pencil lead) of kidney tissue to accurately diagnose a renal disorder and decide on appropriate treatment. A renal biopsy may also be done to determine the progression of a chronic kidney disease or to evaluate the status of a transplanted kidney.

An "open" renal biopsy is a surgical procedure that exposes the kidney. It is done under general anesthesia. The preoperative and postoperative nursing care is similar to that of most pediatric surgical patients. A "closed" renal biopsy is performed under local anesthesia, using a long needle to enter the kidney tissue. The procedure may be conducted using fluoroscopy or ultrasonography to assist in the placement of the needle. The child is premedicated to promote relaxation and is positioned on the stomach. The biopsy should not be painful, although the child will feel the pressure of the needle.

To assure maximum cooperation, the child should be told ahead of time what to expect during and after the procedure. The most common complication of renal biopsy is internal renal hemorrhage. Postoperative care is designed to minimize hemorrhage and to detect it as early as possible. Strict bed rest is maintained for 24 h after a renal biopsy. The pressure dressing over the biopsy site should be checked frequently for bleeding. Vital signs, including blood pressure, should be taken every $\frac{1}{2}$ h for 4 h and then every hour for 4 h. Drinking fluids must be encouraged in order to maintain a good urine flow. Urine should be saved in separate containers, with the date and time noted. Any profuse or persistent hematuria should be reported to the physician. Severe loin pain or abdominal pain should also be reported.

STRUCTURAL AND POSITIONAL ALTERATIONS OF THE URINARY TRACT

Urinary tract infections

Urinary tract infections are very common in children. Girls, except as neonates, have a much higher incidence of urinary tract infections than boys, with a ratio of approximately 9 to 1.[4] At any given time, 1.2 percent of all school-age girls (through high school) have bacteriuria.[5] Many of them are asymptomatic. Five percent of all school-aged girls have had a urinary tract infection by the time they graduate.[6] Generally, bacterial invasions that cause urinary tract infections occur by a hematogenous (blood-borne) route in newborns (more commonly males) and a urethral route in older children (predominantly females).

Escherichia coli infections account for approximately 80 percent of all urinary tract infections. The next most common organisms are *Klebsiella*, enterococci, *Proteus*, *Pseudomonas*, and *Enterobacter*. Antibiotic treatment is usually instituted after sensitivity tests are done, taking into consideration the child's age, renal function, past allergies, and history of urinary tract infections (including response to treatment) as well as normal expected serum and urine concentrations of the antibiotic. Follow-up urinalyses are done at appropriate intervals to monitor the child's status.

Not all children with bacteria in their urine will develop an infection. Other factors are significant. The frequency of bladder emptying plays an important role. Overdistention will cause stagnant urine to remain in contact with bladder mucosa for prolonged periods. This may occur in a child who has a neuropathic bladder or in one with a functional disorder who holds large amounts of urine in the bladder before voiding. Obstruction, renal calculi, foreign bodies, and reflux may also interfere with the child's resistance. The characteristically short urethra in the female may be one of the reasons for the increased incidence of infection in girls. The body does, however, have natural defenses. For example, *Escherichia coli* does not colonize at pH levels of less than 5.5 or more than 7.5.[7] Some people advocate drinking alkaline juices (e.g., cranberry juice) that produce an acid ash to maintain or create an acid urine. If this is to be part of the treatment plan, the pH of the urine should be checked routinely because the amount of cranberry juice necessary to acidify the urine varies with the individual and, unfortunately, is usually large. This type of preventive care would probably be beneficial for a child who is prone to infections and who drinks large quantities of acidic juices (citrus juices). The family could then substitute cranberry juice for some of the citrus-juice intake, thus reducing the chances for an alkaline urine. It is also thought that the bladder mucosa itself may have an intrinsic factor that repels colonization.

Symptoms of a urinary tract infection depend on the child's age and whether the upper or lower urinary tract is involved. An *infant* may present with anorexia, lethargy, irritability, abdominal pain, temperature change, or failure to thrive. Because of the wide range of symptoms in this age group, almost any unexplained illness could be a urinary tract infection, and it is wise to obtain urine for culture. *Older children* with upper urinary tract infections may have the same symptoms as adults: elevated temperature, flank or back pain, and general malaise. Those with lower urinary tract infections urinate frequently and urgently with a burning sensation and have urethral or lower abdominal pain after voiding or enuresis. Symptoms of a lower urinary tract infection, in conjunction with a negative culture, may indicate a local urethral irritation. This may be secondary to taking a bubble bath, being infected with pinworms, or sexual activity.

Management A child with a urinary tract infection may have less pain if he or she increases oral fluid intake. Many children with lower urinary tract infections who complain of burning on urination are naturally reluctant to void. The nurse may suggest placing the child in a warm tub to stimulate voiding.

Children who are prone to urinary tract infections should be encouraged to empty their bladders frequently to prevent overdistention and should be told to avoid bubble baths. Girls should be taught to wipe from front to back after bowel movements to prevent fecal contamination of the urethra.

Vesicoureteral reflux

After a child has recuperated sufficiently (3 to 5 weeks) from the first urinary infection and a sterile urine is documented, a voiding cystourethrogram and an intravenous pyelogram should be obtained to rule out urinary tract abnormalities. According to King, 45 percent of his female patients under 2 years of age and 20 percent of older girls who presented with a urinary tract infection demonstrated reflux.[8] Approximately 40 to 60 percent of all boys who have urinary tract infections will have a renal abnormality, most commonly reflux, demonstrated radiographically.[9] Because of this high degree of occurrence, radiography is a necessary diagnostic tool.

Vesicoureteral reflux occurs when urine backs up (refluxes) from the bladder into the ureters and possibly into the kidneys. Reflux may vary in severity and may occur only at the time of voiding. After voiding, refluxed urine returns to the bladder, creating a good medium for infection. In a normal system, the ureters enter the bladder at an oblique angle. The intravesical sections of the ureters, which are located in the submucosal tunnels, clamp off when the bladder contracts during voiding. In children who reflux, the ureter or ureters tend to enter the bladder laterally. The configuration of the ureteral orifices, the position of the ureters in the bladder, and the length of the submucosal tunnels may be abnormal (Fig. 20-5). Diagnosis of reflux is confirmed by a voiding cystourethrogram, and its degree of severity is graded. If there is a small degree of reflux, the child may outgrow it and may be able to be managed conservatively. Medical treatment consists of low-dose antibiotic suppressive therapy and periodic urine cultures and radiographic examinations. The importance of continuous suppressive therapy must be emphasized to the parents because infections associated with reflux may cause permanent renal damage and arrested renal growth.

Ureteral reimplantation is performed when the child has a high degree of reflux, abnormal renal growth as evidenced on comparative x-ray films, breakthrough infections while on suppressive therapy, noncompliance with drug treatment, or all of the above. The operative procedure consists of reimplanting the ureter or ureters obliquely into the bladder, simultaneously fashioning the submucosal tunnels. Postoperative care is generally the same as for all children who have undergone abdominal surgery. The child will have a catheter in the bladder for 4 to 5 days. The catheter will drain bloody urine because the bladder is a vascular organ. The catheter may cause bladder spasms, which may be treated with propantheline (Pro-Banthine) tablets or Banthine bromide and opium (B&O) suppositories.

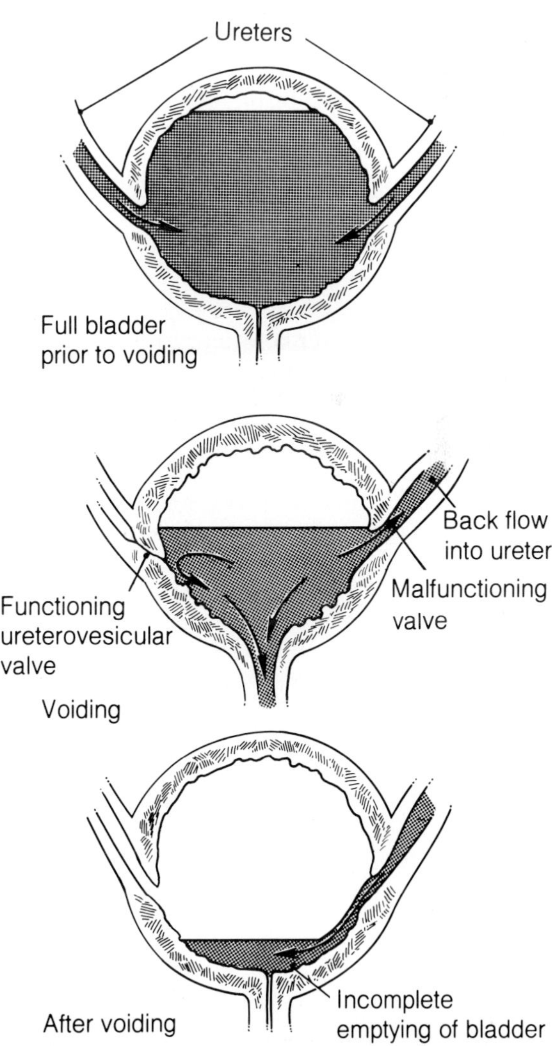

Figure 20-5 Vesicoureteral reflux occurs if there is a malfunctioning ureterovesicular valve that permits urine to flow back into the ureter when the bladder becomes full. After voiding, when pressure within the bladder is lower, the refluxed urine reenters the bladder.

Ureteral *stents* (tubes) may be used, depending on the preference of the surgeon. If the anastamosis has been difficult (because of the size of the ureters or the thickness of the bladder), stents will maintain patency by preventing edema from obstructing the flow of urine. It is important to measure all drainage from the catheter and stents separately so that it will be easy to detect obstruction of a tube. Kinking of these small stents does occur, and the nurse should be alert to this.

Ureteral reimplantation has a very high degree of success in children with nonneuropathic bladders. The absence of reflux postoperatively should be verified by a voiding cystourethrogram. This is routinely obtained a few months after surgery. The child may continue to have bladder infections, but infected urine will not be refluxing up to the ureters. For this reason, it is important to emphasize to the family that the primary reason for reimplantation is kidney preservation, not the prevention of future bladder infections.

Upper urinary tract obstruction

Obstruction of the urinary tract creates an increased pressure above the point of obstruction. The degree of dilatation in the ureters and kidneys depends on the severity and location of the obstruction. If the obstruction and backflow of urine raise the intrapelvic pressures to equal the glomerulus capillary pressure, filtration will cease. Early diagnosis and treatment of an obstruction are essential to prevent permanent renal structure damage and dilatation of the upper urinary tract, which may result in hydronephrosis.

Obstruction of the ureteropelvic junction (hydronephrosis) The ureteropelvic junction (UPJ) is the most common site for obstruction in the kidneys and upper ureters. In most cases it is considered to be a congenital defect caused by mechanical (narrowing or kinking of the ureter) or functional (no definitive etiology known) obstruction.

UPJ obstruction causing hydronephrosis is the most common renal mass that occurs in children under 1 year of age.[10] A palpable kidney mass and failure to thrive are the most common presenting symptoms in this age group. An older child will usually have vague gastrointestinal symptoms or recurrent attacks of colicky flank pain. Because of the vague symptoms, the correct diagnosis may not be made at the initial examination.

Surgical intervention in the form of pyeloplasty is required or, rarely, nephrectomy may be indicated for a nonfunctioning kidney. The choice of treatment depends on the severity of the obstruction and the resultant damage to the collecting system.

Occasionally, a temporary nephrostomy tube may be placed in the renal pelvis following a complicated pyeloplasty or preoperatively to decompress the system. One of the major advantages of the nephrostomy tube, its ease of reversibility, is also a disadvantage. If the tube should accidentally be dislodged, the tract can close off in just 2 to 3 h, making replacement of the tube difficult. Nephrostomy tubes are usually sutured to the skin and taped in place to avoid this complication.

Lower urinary tract obstructions

Meatal stenosis The premise that meatal stenosis is the cause of most recurrent urinary tract infections and reflux is not accepted by many pediatric urologists. Meatal stenosis may, however, be the cause of abnormal voiding symptoms (narrowing and deflection of the stream), and dilatation may occasionally be required.[11] In the male, the primary indications for a meatotomy are extreme narrowing of the urinary stream and prolonged voiding times. In both males and females, diagnosis is made by examining the urethra and observing the child while voiding.

Urethral strictures Basically, four types of strictures can be identified: congenital, inflammatory, traumatic, and iatrogenic. *Congenital strictures,* if they exist at all, are rare and occur mainly in boys. *Inflammatory strictures* are also rare in children and may be a sequela of gonorrhea. *Traumatic strictures* may occur following urethral trauma secondary to straddle or penetrating injuries. *Iatrogenic strictures* can be caused by the use of instruments and catheters of inappropriate size.

Diagnosis in all but the traumatic strictures is difficult because the symptoms vary. Strictures may become symptomatic because of a decrease in caliber or strength of the urinary stream or incomplete emptying of the bladder from outflow obstruction. A retrograde urethrogram may be necessary to establish a diagnosis. Depending on the severity of the stricture, urethral dilatation, urethrotomy, or urethroplasty may be performed.

Congenital posterior urethral valves Posterior urethral valves are membranous diaphragms found within the prostatic urethra that partially obstruct the flow of urine. The size of the opening in the valve determines the severity of the obstruction. Chronic bladder distention in utero may lead to a thickened bladder wall, ureterovesical junction obstruction, and, eventually, hydronephrosis. Reflux, if present, may cause further renal damage.

In newborn male infants, bilateral or unilateral smooth flank masses and a distended bladder would be suggestive of congenital posterior urethral valves. A dribbling stream is likely; however, significant valve obstruction has been observed in infants with a good stream. Many children with obstructive uropathy do not concentrate urine effectively. This becomes significant when the child has severe diarrhea or vomiting, as it can result in rapid dehydration.[12] If the diagnosis is not established during the newborn period, subsequent chronic urinary tract infections and failure to thrive may be diagnostic. In older boys, the symptoms may not be as definitive. The diagnosis should be confirmed by radiographic studies.

The treatment of choice is surgery, which may be performed transurethrally or by perineal urethrostomy. Surgical treatment may have to be postponed in infants until their general condition has stabilized. They may need fluids to correct dehydration and azotemia (elevated BUN), electrolytes to correct imbalances, and adequate urinary drainage to relieve hydronephrosis. Drainage may be provided by a temporary vesicostomy or placement of a nephrostomy tube.

Genital, bladder, and abdominal wall anomalies

External defects of the genitourinary tract are usually found during the physical examination at birth. Some may be mild, requiring little treatment. Severe defects, such as exstrophy of the bladder, require costly, time-consuming surgical repairs. Even minor defects may have a significant emotional impact on the parents because the genitourinary system is involved.

Patent urachus *Patent urachus* occurs when the epithelialized tube (the urachus) that connects the bladder with the umbilicus prior to birth fails to close. When the urachus remains patent, urine leaks onto the abdomen, and a persistently moist umbilicus may be noted. This anomaly may be seen alone or in conjunction with prune-belly syndrome or obstruction of the urinary tract. If the urachus does not close during the newborn period, surgical intervention will be necessary.

Exstrophy of the bladder *Exstrophy of the bladder* results from failure of the anterior wall of the abdomen and bladder to fuse, leaving the bladder open and exposed on the abdomen (Fig.20-6). Exstrophy occurs in approximately 1 in 30,000 births.[13] It is seen more often in males than in females.

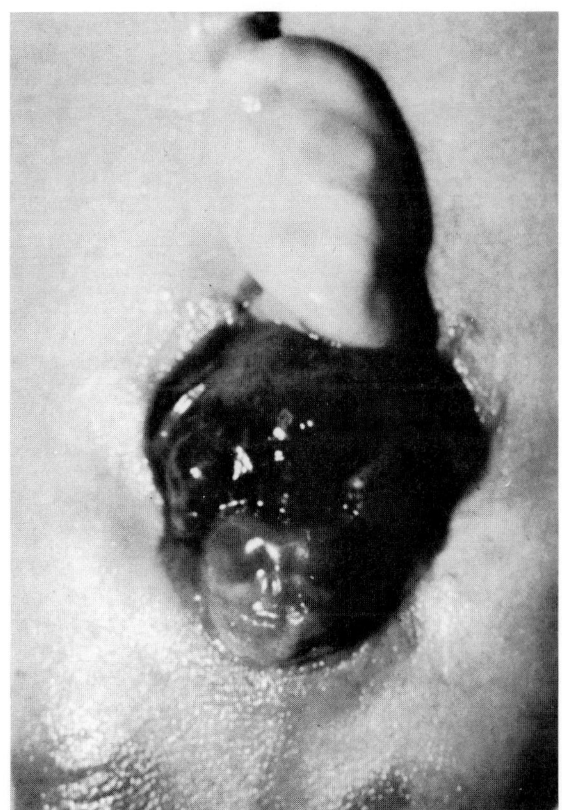

Figure 20-6 A newborn with exstrophy of the bladder. The pubic bones are widely separated. *(Courtesy of J. W. Duckett, M. D., Director of the Division of Urology, Children's Hospital of Philadelphia.)*

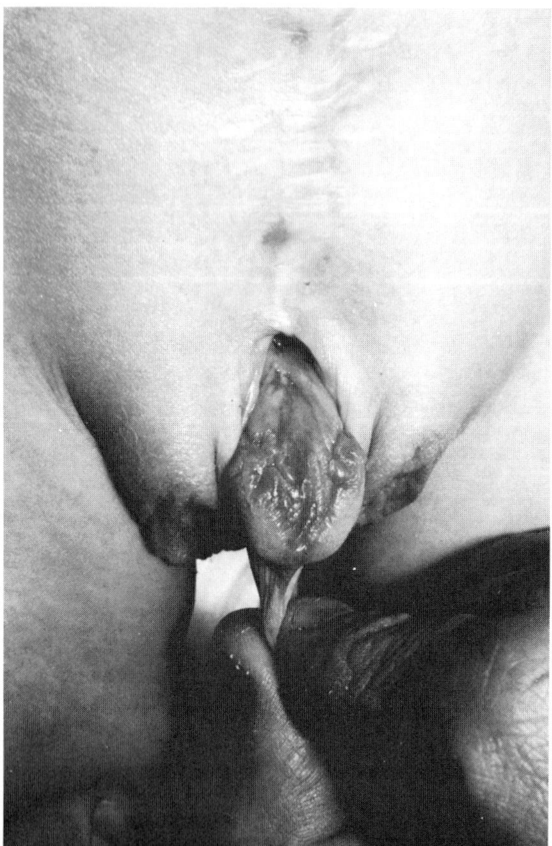

Figure 20-7 Surgical correction of bladder exstrophy in a male. Notice the splayed, open penis with uncorrected subsymphysial epispadias. (*Courtesy of J. W. Duckett, M. D., Director of the Division of Urology, Children's Hospital of Philadelphia.*)

The most common form of the condition is bladder exstrophy with complete epispadias. In this form, the bladder is turned out, and the ureteral orifices are visible and are draining urine (Fig. 20-7). In the male, the urethra is splayed open with a dorsal groove, and the testicles, although lying in the canal, are frequently undescended. In the female, there is an epispadiac urethra, a bifid clitoris, and widely separated anterior labia. The pubic bones are widely separated, and the femoral heads are externally rotated. The child's gait will appear broad-based, but there is no associated permanent orthopedic disability. The separated pelvis often does not provide good suspensory support for the rectum, and rectal prolapse may result. This tends to correct itself as the child grows older.

Many pediatric urologists operate on children with exstrophy within 48 h after birth. The rationale for this practice is that the pelvic structures move more freely during this period, allowing reconstruction without the aid of iliac osteotomies. This increased pliability is thought to be secondary to the same factors that allow the molding of the fetal skeleton during delivery.[14, 15]

During this first surgical procedure, the bladder is closed. The defect is thus partially corrected, leaving the child with an epispadiac urethra. Often a penis-lengthening procedure is necessary to ensure adequate sexual function in the male. This may be done at the time of the initial surgery, or it may be postponed.

Future surgical procedures may include repair of the epispadias, bladder neck surgery for incontinence if the bladder is of adequate size, or a urinary diversion if it is not.

Some urologists prefer to delay the initial surgery until the child is older. In this case, the nurse will teach the parents how to protect the bladder mucosa and the surrounding skin against infection and irritation.

Management Family support is especially difficult initially because the mother may still be hospitalized when the baby is transferred to a tertiary pediatric center. The father is then faced with the task of trying to spend time at both hospitals.

Often, the nurse serves as the liaison who coordinates care, education, and communication between the family and all the involved disciplines. The nurse must foster positive feelings about the eventual outcome, while helping the family realize that long-term medical supervision and multiple surgical procedures will be necessitated by this anomaly.

When the initial surgery is postponed, a fine-mesh petroleum gauze is placed over the bladder mucosa, and a protective ointment is placed on the surrounding skin to prevent irritation. Frequent diaper changes and immediate cleansing after bowel movements are essential.

After the initial surgery, the baby is hospitalized for a few weeks, depending on the general condition. For 6 weeks postoperatively, the infant's legs may be flexed and wrapped in Kling or Ace bandages so that the femoral heads are internally rotated. The flexed knees keep additional pressure off the abdominal wall and the site of skin closure, facilitating healing. The wrapped legs maintain the hips in an internally rotated position and reduce tension on the sutures holding the pelvis together. Diapers must be applied in the same manner as a wraparound skirt in order to maintain correct alignment during this period. As an alternative to this method of immobilization, a cast or orthopedic traction may be used.

If a urinary diversion is required, either an *ileal conduit* or a *ureterosigmoidostomy* is usually performed. The major advantage of a ureterosigmoidostomy is that there is no abdominal stoma. There are also disadvantages that make this type of diversion controversial. In this procedure, the ureters are taken out of the bladder wall and implanted into the sigmoid colon using an antireflux technique. The colon then becomes a reservoir for both stool and urine. Only children with normal kidneys and ureters and with good rectal tone (no history of rectal prolapse) are selected for this procedure. The parents should be made aware of the care and long-term follow-up required. The parents and the child should receive continual support, since it will take time for the child to develop fecal and urinary continence and for the parents to feel confident of their ability to manage all aspects of the child's care. Some children develop full continence, whereas others are plagued with leakage.

Epispadias *Epispadias* is a rare congenital condition, found more frequently in males than in females, in which a dorsal cleft of the urethra is present. In females, there is an associated bifid clitoris, and the urethral cleft extends to and involves the bladder neck. In males, the cleft may involve only the glans (balanic epispadia), the glans and the penile shaft (penile epispadia), or the entire penis and the bladder neck (subsymphysial epispadia). If it involves the bladder neck, the child is incontinent (Fig. 20-7).

The primary objectives of treatment are to (1) reconstruct the urethra, (2) straighten the penis (or bring the bifid clitoris together), (3) produce a penis (or female genitalia) that is cosmetically acceptable and functional, and (4) restore continence.[16] All these goals are accomplished through surgical intervention. Achieving bladder continence continues to be the major problem.[17, 18, 19]

Hypospadias *Hypospadias*, or the congenital occurrence of an abnormally placed urethra on the ventral surface of the penis or the perineum, has a high incidence (5 of 1000 male births).[20] There is no known single cause of this condition, although there is a familial tendency.

In hypospadias, the ventral foreskin is absent, a dimple or groove is often present at the tip of the penis, and the glans is usually spade-shaped. *Chordee*, a cobra-head-like bending of the penis, is often present and is corrected at the time of the hypospadias repair. Chordee may be noticeable only with erections (Fig. 20-8). Significant associated upper urinary tract anomalies are unusual. When the testes are undescended or nonpalpable, sexual determination may be difficult. Buccal smears and a karyotype may be necessary to determine gender.

Hypospadias in girls is uncommon and rarely causes problems. Occasionally, incontinence is present if the urethra is extremely short.

Surgery is usually performed after the child's penis is of sufficient size to facilitate the procedure (18 months to 2 years of age) and before the child starts school so that he will be able to void like his male peers. Depending on the severity of the defect and the preference of the urologist, the repair may be done in one or two stages. Neonates with hypospadias must not be circumcised. The foreskin is needed to repair the urethra.

During the neonatal period, the parents have to be reassured of the child's future normal sexual development. Often, they do not believe that the penis will be normal after surgery, and they may have difficulty verbalizing their fears.

A parent should be encouraged to stay in the hospital with the child. Children this age do not

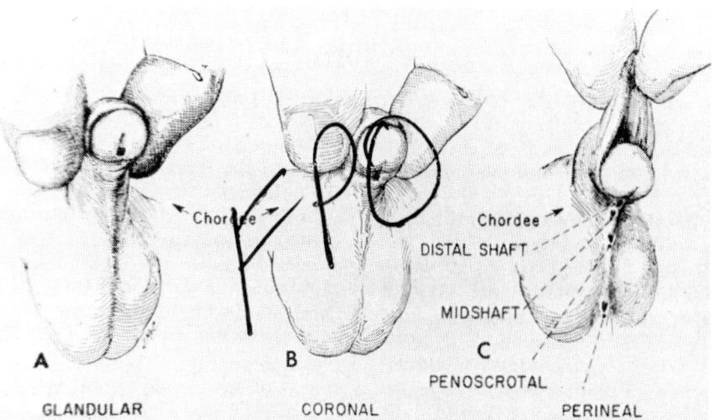

Figure 20-8 Classification of hypospadias based on anatomic location of the urinary meatus. Associated chordee is best described in terms of its severity: mild, moderate, or severe. (*From P. Kalalis and C. King, Clinical Pediatric Urology, Saunders, Philadelphia, 1976. Used with permission.*)

tolerate separation from their parents well and are very concerned about their genitalia.

Preoperative instructions, including an explanation of dressings, catheter placement, and probable bladder spasms secondary to the presence of the catheter, are imperative. Propantheline (Pro-Banthine) tablets or Banthine bromide and opium (B&O) suppositories may be prescribed to relieve these spasms. A "well-bandaged" penis and a Foley catheter or suprapubic tube that is adequately taped down will make it possible to leave the child's hands unrestrained. These children are usually out of bed the day following surgery and are in the playroom soon thereafter. They are not allowed to straddle toys or other objects, but because children usually limit themselves appropriately, they are otherwise unrestricted. Most hypospadias repairs are done on an outpatient basis. Written directions like those listed in Table 20-1 should be provided.

Table 20-1 Information for Parents: Home Management for a Child with Hypospadias Repair

We have designed this information sheet to help you with the care that your son will require at home after his surgery.

1. Your son may play as he wishes except that he may not straddle a bicycle, rocking horse, or any other toy until your urologist says he can. This is to prevent him from damaging the operative area.
2. He will have a tube (catheter) in for approximately 10 days to 2 weeks after surgery. You will be furnished with a leg bag for daytime use and a larger drainage bag for overnight use. Most children do not like the feeling of the plastic bag against their leg. Before going home, please obtain a piece or two of stockinette from your nurse or the urology office on the third floor. This may be worn as a thigh-high sock so that the plastic will not bother him. If either of the bags develops urine crystals on the inside, you may rinse it with a solution of one-half plain white vinegar and one-half water.
3. As long as the tube (catheter) is in, your son may have bladder spasms. These cramping pains can be treated with B&O suppositories or Pro-Banthine tablets. Please follow the directions on the label. You may want to fill the prescription for B&O suppositories at the hospital pharmacy, because most outside pharmacies do not carry them.
4. Your son should take tub baths twice a day for 20 to 30 min when he goes home. He may get completely wet, even the tube.
5. It is important to keep the tip of the penis from crusting over. You will be receiving a tube of Lacrilube to use to keep the opening at the end of the penis free of crusts. This is to be done while your son has a suprapubic tube in his bladder. Obviously, if he has a Foley catheter (tube) going into the opening of his penis (meatus), this will be done after the tube is removed.
6. Try to avoid constipation. Good oral fluid intake will help.

Please do not worry if:

1. There is bloody urine in the tubing or bag, especially when your son has bladder spasms.
2. There is mucus or sediment (whitish particles) in the urine.
3. Your son voids (passes water) in small amounts through his penis (if he has a suprapubic catheter in his bladder).
4. There is some swelling (edema) of his penis. Call us if it increases significantly.
5. The sutures on his penis start to come out. (They are dissolvable and will gradually fall out over the next several weeks.)

Please call us if there are any problems or questions.

Prune-belly syndrome A child with this rare congenital syndrome is identified by a wrinkled, prunelike abdomen. This condition is actually composed of a triad of symptoms: abdominal muscle deficiency, cryptorchidism, and urinary tract anomalies. These anomalies usually consist of varying degrees of dysplastic kidneys; tortuous and redundant ureters; a large, thick-walled bladder; and an abnormal urethra (Fig. 20-9). Some children do not meet all three criteria, and their condition is therefore known as *pseudo-prune-belly syndrome*. Only a few girls have been

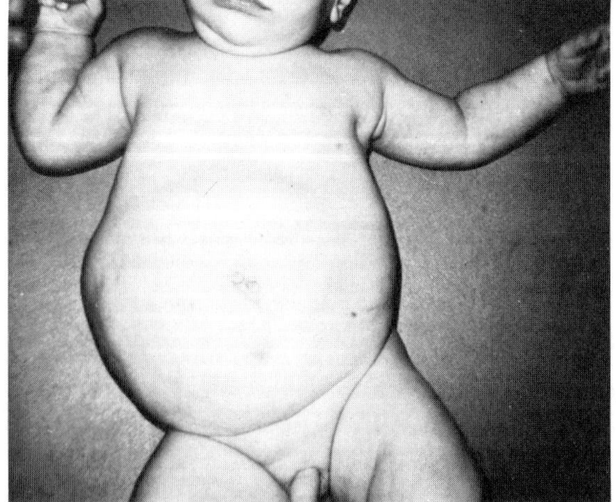

Figure 20-9 This male infant has the large, distended abdomen of prune-belly syndrome. A vesicostomy is present approximately midway between the umbilicus and the symphysis pubis. *(Courtesy of J. W. Duckett, M. D., Director of the Division of Urology, Children's Hospital of Philadelphia.)*

known to have pseudo-prune-belly syndrome, and obviously no girls have been diagnosed as having true prune-belly syndrome, since they have no testes.

The prognosis for these children seems to depend on the degree of renal dysplasia rather than on the severity of the abdominal wall defect.

Because of the large bladder and refluxing ureters (70 percent of the cases), stasis of urine leading to urinary tract infections is a primary problem. A cutaneous vesicostomy (see the section "Neuropathic Bladder") may be necessary to alleviate the situation. Because of the lack of abdominal musculature, these children have difficulty coughing and are prone to upper respiratory tract problems. Support of the abdomen when coughing is generally beneficial.

Neuropathic bladder A *neuropathic* or *neurogenic bladder* is one that fails to function normally as a result of a neuromuscular defect. Children with neuropathic bladders may be divided into three groups. The first and most common group is composed of children with congenital sacral agenesis or myelomeningocele. The children in the second group have acquired lesions as a result of traumatic injuries to the spinal cord, tumors of the spinal cord, sacrococcygeal teratomas, and surgical trauma associated with the repair of imperforate anus or extensive bladder dissections. The third group, which is composed of children who have occult neuropathic bladders, is not well defined. This discussion will be limited to neuropathic bladders in children with myelomeningocele.

Neuropathic bladders may be classified as either functional or neurological disorders. Further division into those that involve a failure to empty and those that involve a failure to store facilitates an understanding of treatment modalities.

Failure to empty An infant with a myelomeningocele should be initially evaluated with an intravenous pyelogram and a voiding cystourethrogram. If an infant fails to empty the bladder completely on voiding and does not demonstrate reflux, the parents may be taught to use the Credé method (manual bladder pressure) to express the residual urine from the child's bladder at specified intervals. This may be continued by the child in conjunction with the Valsalva maneuver (holding a deep breath while contracting the abdominal muscles and straining) when the child is mature enough to be responsible and physically able to do it effectively.

If a child with this type of neuropathic bladder has reflux, the Credé method should not be used because the high pressure obtained during this mechanical decompression of the bladder will force urine up the ureters into the kidneys. Routine urine cultures and radiographic monitoring of renal growth and function are essential.

The objectives of treatment are to decompress the system in order to preserve renal function, to keep the child as free of infection as possible, and to promote the child's social acceptance. These goals may be achieved by temporary urinary diversion (usually a vesicostomy), clean intermittent catheterization, or a permanent diversion such as an ileal or colon conduit. Permanent urinary diversion is rarely indicated.

In a newborn infant or young child, a *cutaneous vesicostomy* (an opening into the bladder) is probably the most desirable solution (Fig. 20-10). This technique is advocated because of its ease of reversibility as well as its ease of management for the parents.[21] The dome of the bladder is brought to the skin surface, forming a 1- to 1.5-cm stoma that is situated between the umbilicus and the pubic symphysis. It allows urine to flow freely, decompressing the upper tracts. These children usually drain urine into diapers, since urostomy appliances do not seem to adhere well in this area. Many ingenious parents have devised their own methods for keeping their children dry. One child may wear an elasticized band over a section of disposable diaper that covers the vesicostomy, allowing the child to wear panties rather than diapers. Another parent may have found that taping an undershirt over the diaper helps keep the diaper over the vesicostomy.

Clean intermittent self-catheterization (CIC) is initiated when these children reach an "age of concern," defined as the age when they become tired of being wet, be it at 5 years or 25 years. This clean, nonsterile method of emptying the bladder was introduced in this country in 1970. Patients who were on a regimen of self-catheterization demonstrated improvement, including continence and a decreased incidence of urinary tract infections.[22]

Teaching the child and the family clean intermittent catheterization before the vesicostomy is closed and without emphasizing a projected date of competency takes the pressure

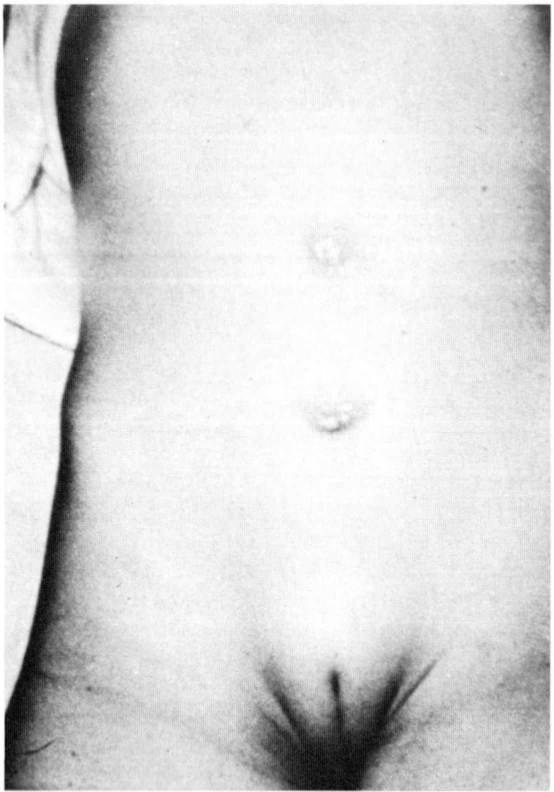

Figure 20-10 A cutaneous vesicostomy (an opening into the bladder). The stoma is about 1 to 1.5 cm and is situated between the umbilicus and the symphysis pubis.

off everyone. In this way, the family is not faced with a closed vesicostomy and the absolute necessity of learning clean intermittent catheterization before discharge from the hospital. The parents may be taught the procedure if the child is very young. Sometimes clean intermittent catheterization, rather than a vesicostomy, is undertaken in neonates, and the responsibility is then transferred from the parents to the child when the child is old enough.

It is important to evaluate the child's understanding and acceptance of the procedure and his or her mental or physical ability to perform the task. The parents' attitudes and willingness to comply play an important role and must also be assessed. A knowledgeable, relaxed, and perceptive nurse-teacher is definitely an asset. Changes in body image and individual feelings regarding the genital area are a few of the major concerns that must be dealt with effectively.

A review of basic anatomy and physiology, using diagrams and pictures, will provide a sound basis for instruction. Boys, because they can see their meatus, are generally easier to teach than girls. Girls may be taught by learning to locate their urinary meatus by touch or by using a mirror. For specific information regarding types of catheters, lubricants, care of equipment, teaching methods, and follow-up, refer to selected readings on clean intermittent self-catheterization.[23, 24] It is essential to remember that the school nurse and the public health nurse are integral members of the health team and should be advised of treatment and consulted for assistance and follow-up when appropriate.

Failure to store Approximately one-third of children with myelomeningocele and neuropathic bladders fail to store urine. These children are constantly wet and may require a permanent urinary diversion for social reasons alone if all other treatment modalities fail. This failure to store may be due to uninhibited bladder contractions or hypertonicity of the bladder itself. Medication such as propantheline (Pro-Banthine), imipramine (Tofranil), and oxybutynin chloride (Ditropan) is often given in an attempt to block uninhibited contractions and to decrease the hypertonicity of the bladder. The goal is to convert the problem with the child's bladder to one of "failure to empty," which can then be managed by the Credé method or clean intermittent self-catheterization.

An artificial sphincter was devised in 1973 and has been successful in selected children. This is an implantable Silastic prosthesis composed of a cuff which surrounds the bladder neck, a small reservoir for fluid used to inflate the cuff, and a bulb that moves the fluid from the cuff to the reservoir by releasing the pressure on the bladder neck and urethra each time the child voids. The bulb is located in the scrotum or in the labial folds and is activated by manual squeezing. The major problems associated with this device have been infection and erosion.[25]

Ileal conduits Candidates for ileal conduit diversion may include children with exstrophy of the bladder, unresolved urinary incontinence, or unremitting urinary tract infection with renal deterioration. When describing this surgery to the patient, it will be necessary to have diagrams or to draw pictures to illustrate the various steps. A small segment of ileum is excised, and one end is sutured shut and is used to form the conduit. The remaining ileum is then rejoined, leaving a normally functioning intestinal tract. The ureters are disconnected from the bladder and inserted into one end of the conduit. The other end is then brought out onto the skin surface at a previously determined site, turned back, and fastened to the abdominal wall, creating a stoma. This ileal segment is not meant to function as a substitute bladder; rather, it is a tube through which urine flows and should not store more than 5 to 10 ml of urine. Normal peristaltic movement of the ileal segment will assist urine flow (Fig. 20-11). The child will have to wear an external appliance to collect urine. Obviously, these children and their families will have to deal with feelings regarding an altered body image. A sound preoperative understanding of the surgery, the types of appliances available, skin care products, and general daily care will alleviate some of their fears (Fig. 20-11*B*). Children will develop an understanding of the way an appliance functions and how it feels if they are enocuraged to wear one that contains water for a day or two prior to surgery. This practice also aids in the selection of the stomal site.

The child will come back from the operating room with an appliance in place; this will be hooked up to a bedside drainage bag. Once the child is ambulatory, the use of the bedside drainage bag will be necessary only at night. Teaching is individualized, and participation in care is encouraged as the child and the family indicate their readiness.

Families should be made aware of the available community resources, such as public health nurses, visiting nurses, ostomy groups, and enterostomal therapists. An enterostomal therapist is a nurse or technician who has received specialized training in ostomy management and who is certified by the International Association of Enterostomal Therapists. The United Ostomy Association, with headquarters in Los Angeles, publishes comprehensive educational material for children and adults. A list of publications and the locations of United Ostomy chapters in the area may be obtained by writing to the association.

Emphasis should be placed on the positive aspects of diversion. The child will ultimately wear an appliance that will maintain continence and will allow the resumption of a normal life-style, while providing protection against renal deterioration.

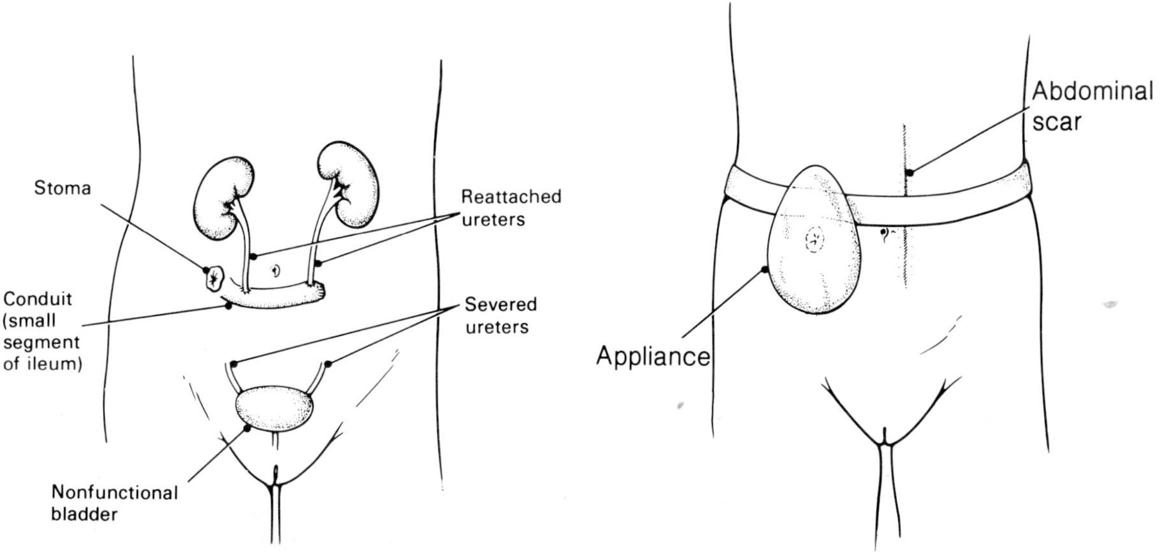

Figure 20-11 (*A*) An anatomic drawing of an ileal conduit. (*B*) The position of the permanent drainage appliance after the ileal conduit procedure has been done. (*Adapted from G. Scipien, M. U. Barnard, M. A. Chard, J. Howe, and P. J. Phillips* [*eds.*], *Comprehensive Pediatric Nursing, 2d ed., McGraw-Hill, New York, 1986, p. 1178. Used with permission.*)

STRUCTURAL AND POSITIONAL ALTERATIONS OF THE KIDNEYS

Renal agenesis

Renal agenesis is the congenital absence of one or both kidneys. Unilateral agenesis is more common than bilateral agenesis and occurs more frequently in males. Renal agenesis is caused by degeneration of the ureteric bud during early fetal development.[26] Unilateral renal agenesis is usually associated with the absence of the ureter on the affected side. The opposite kidney is usually hypertrophied but otherwise normal. The single kidney may be in the pelvis.

Children with one missing kidney may be asymptomatic unless the existing kidney is abnormal. On physical examination, the child with bilateral renal agenesis has no palpable renal masses, and intravenous pyelograms will show no renal visualization. Since bilateral agenesis is incompatible with life, these children die during the neonatal period.

Renal hypoplasia

Renal hypoplasia may involve one or both kidneys. In a true primary renal hypoplasia, the kidneys are much smaller than usual, but the anatomic structures present are normal. Normal kidneys have 10 or more calyces, while a hypoplastic kidney contains five or fewer.

Most hypoplastic kidneys also function poorly. The severity of the kidney disease will depend on whether one or both kidneys are affected and on the amount of functional tissue present. Unilateral renal hypoplasia is usually asymptomatic and is not treated. If the disease is bilateral, varying degrees of renal insufficiency will be present. As the child grows older and as greater demands are placed on the renal structures, problems can develop. These children are treated for chronic renal failure, as discussed later in this chapter.

Renal dysplasia

The term *renal dysplasia* refers to a kidney that contains poorly functioning or nonfunctioning tissue. Renal structures are disorganized, and some are abnormally developed.[27] Renal dysplasia may be bilateral, unilateral, or segmental within the kidney. The renal pelvis is usually absent, and the ureter on the affected side is almost always abnormal. The involved kidney is often hypoplastic and may contain cystic formations.

Children with dysplastic kidneys often have anomalies of other organ systems. Congenital obstruction of the lower urinary tract is frequently associated with renal dysplasia.[28] Unilateral renal dysplasia may be asymptomatic, or the child may have a mild degree of hypertension. Bilateral dysplasia generally leads to chronic renal failure.

Polycystic kidney disease

There are several types of *polycystic kidney disease*, each causing clinical symptoms at a different age. The prognosis depends on the severity of interference with kidney function.

The infantile form of the disease is bilateral and is genetically transmitted as an autosomal recessive. The male/female ratio is 2 to 7. The kidneys are enlarged and filled with minute cysts. The anatomic structures of the kidneys may be present but are distorted, and there is little functioning renal tissue. There are often associated cystic malformations of the liver. It is believed that the main cause of cystic disease in the kidneys is abnormal embryological development of the collecting tubules.[29]

The large kidneys produce abdominal distention, and the infant may exhibit respiratory distress as a result. Because there is little functioning kidney tissue, progressive renal failure develops. Urinary tract infections may complicate the course of the disease, and severe hypertension may be present early in the disease.

Treatment is directed toward preventing chronic renal failure. Death generally occurs early. Dialysis and eventual transplantation must be considered if the child is to survive. Genetic counseling should be offered to parents.

HEREDITARY RENAL DISEASE

Inherited nephritis

Inherited nephritis, or *familial nephritis*, is transmitted as an autosomal dominant trait. The renal manifestations of the disease are similar to those of chronic glomerulonephritis. The most common type of inherited nephritis is known as *Alport syndrome*.

Alport syndrome is often initially diagnosed as acute glomerulonephritis until similar findings are discovered in other family members. It is more severe and progressive in males than in females. Remissions are common, and exacerbations may be associated with acute infections. The syndrome may include progressive nerve deafness, abnormality of the optic lens, and neurological dysfunction. Alport syndrome is treated symptomatically and supportively with the therapy used for chronic glomerulonephritis. Steroids and cytotoxic drugs do not appear to alter the disease course. Genetic counseling should be made available to the family.

ACQUIRED RENAL ALTERATIONS

Acute nephritic syndrome

Acute nephritic syndrome is a clinical condition, a collection of signs and symptoms, that indicates a disease affecting the glomeruli of the kidney. There are several varieties of acute nephritic syndrome, the most important being acute glomerulonephritis itself. There are other variants of the syndrome, such as recurrent hematuria and proteinuria. Acute nephritic syndrome may be seen occasionally as part of a generalized disease affecting small blood vessels, such as Henoch-Schönlein purpura.[30] The treatment depends on the cause of the syndrome.

Acute glomerulonephritis

Broadly defined, *acute glomerulonephritis* may be considered an inflammation of the glomeruli. The cause is uncertain but is probably an antigen-antibody reaction stimulated by an infection somewhere else in the body. Any infection caused by group A beta hemolytic streptococcus may lead to acute glomerulonephritis. The infection is generally an upper respiratory tract infection but may also be scarlet fever, impetigo, or infected eczema.

Etiology The actual glomerular injury is caused by the antigen-antibody complexes trapped in the glomerulus. Endothelial cellular swelling and proliferation obstruct the glomerular capillaries, decreasing the amount of glomerular filtrate. All the glomeruli in the kidney are involved, although the amount of proliferation varies among them. With the decreased glomerular filtration, the amount of sodium and water that is passed to the tubules for reabsorption is reduced, and the end result is fluid retention with increased plasma volume and edema.

Manifestations Acute glomerulonephritis tends to occur in males between the ages of 3 and 7 years. The onset of symptoms generally occurs 1 to 3 weeks after the streptococcal infection. The symptoms vary from child to child and may be mild enough to be ignored or rapid and severe. There may be some or all of the following symptoms:

1. *Hematuria* Hematuria is the usual presenting symptom. The urine will be grossly bloody, but not bright red. After a few days, the urine becomes a smoky-brown color. This is caused by hemolysis and the release of hemoglobin, which is converted to brown hematin by the urine acidity.
2. *Edema* Edema is also commonly seen in children with acute glomerulonephritis. Periorbital edema is most common, but the edema may become generalized. It usually does not proceed beyond a moderate degree.
3. *Mild hypertension* This is also a common symptom. The diastolic pressure may rise as high as 100 to 120 mmHg. Hypertensive encephalopathy may then occur, with headaches, vomiting, blurred vision, disorientation, and/or convulsions.
4. *Oliguria or anuria* Oliguria or anuria may occur in some cases. It is accompanied by a high urine specific gravity. The urine contains protein, red blood cells, white blood cells, and casts.
5. *Transient anemia* This symptom may develop because of the expanded plasma volume. As a result, these children are pale, tire easily, and have poor appetites.
6. *Abnormal laboratory values* The blood urea nitrogen and creatinine may be mildly elevated. The erythrocyte sedimentation rate (ESR), which is a nonspecific indication of acute inflammation, will usually be elevated. Serologic tests for streptococcal infection (ASO titers) are often elevated.
7. *Severe circulatory congestion* This may occur in the seriously ill child because of the greatly expanded plasma volume. Cardiac enlargement and pulmonary vascular congestion may ensue.

Treatment There is no specific treatment for acute glomerulonephritis. Medical management is largely supportive and symptomatic, and many children can be cared for by their parents in the home. Since the course of the disease is variable, the child should be initially assessed in the hospital.

Many children will limit their own activity, and so strict bed rest is not usually necessary. Some ambulation and mild activity are generally acceptable to the child. If the child is hypertensive or at risk for cardiac failure, bed rest or hospitalization may be necessary. Most children will be able to resume their normal activities after 2 to 3 weeks.

During the acute phase of the disease, fluid intake should be limited to the amount of the previous 8-h output plus the calculated insensible water loss. Intake need not be limited when the child's output again reaches normal levels. Salt intake is usually not restricted unless the child is hypertensive or edematous. Potassium-free foods and fluids may be necessary if the child has a decreased urine output. Lowering dietary protein is usually not necessary unless blood urea nitrogen levels are grossly elevated. Dietary restrictions are usually moderated when diuresis ensues.

Drug therapy varies with the symptoms. Penicillin may be given if the child's infection was previously untreated. Penicillin, however, will not prevent acute glomerulonephritis from developing if the child has been exposed. It will not cure or reduce the severity of acute glomerulonephritis once it has developed. Antihypertensive drugs are given if the diastolic blood pressure is greater than 100 mmHg or if symptoms of encephalopathy develop. Hydralazine and reserpine are used initially for mild hypertension. Digitalization and diuretics may be prescribed if the child develops severe circulatory congestion. If the child develops acute renal failure, dialysis may be necessary during the crisis phase.

Acute glomerulonephritis is a relatively brief disease. Improvement usually begins within 1 to 2 weeks. At that time, the grossly visible blood in the urine will disappear. The prognosis for acute glomerulonephritis is generally good although somewhat unpredictable. Reoccurrences are unusual, and death is very rare.

Management The nursing management of a child with acute glomerulonephritis is based on an accurate assessment of the child and the family (see the Nursing Care Plan at the end of this chapter). Initial observations are important for establishing baseline data about the child's condition. Vital signs (including blood pressure) should be frequently checked. In children who show signs of encephalopathy, blood pressure should be checked at least every 2 h. Any elevated reading should be reported to the physician, along with the symptoms of encephalopathy that the child is exhibiting. Symptoms include headache, vomiting, blurred vision, and convulsions.

In the acute phase, the child should be weighed daily, and a careful record of intake and output kept. Urine must be carefully observed for amount and color. Testing for blood and protein is done as ordered. If the child is edematous, meticulous skin care should be part of the nursing care. Folds in the skin should be bathed and powdered frequently, and the child's position changed as needed.

The activity level allowed the child will depend on the acuteness of the illness. Quiet, ambulatory activities will enable the child to maintain relationships with peers. If bed rest must be maintained, it is helpful if the child can be positioned to see out a window or into the hallway. Games, puzzles, and books will help relieve the boredom of enforced bed rest.

Prevention of any further infection is an important part of the nursing care. The child should always be kept warm and dry and away from anyone with an active infection. Family members may need cultures for streptococcal infections. Children who are returning to an infected environment may be placed on prophylactic penicillin for a few months. Discharge planning for the hospitalized child should include information from the nurse, physician, and dietitian. The social worker may also be involved if needed. The child can usually return home on a regular diet with no fluid restrictions and generally can return to school 2 weeks after discharge from the hospital, if no further hypertension or hematuria occurs. Competitive sports and other strenuous activities should be avoided until the urine is free of red blood cells.[31]

Chronic glomerulonephritis

Chronic glomerulonephritis is a term that can be used to refer to any idiopathic, progressive form of renal disease. The clinical picture of proteinuria, hematuria, and hypertension indicates major involvement of the glomeruli.[32] There are several forms of chronic glomerulonephritis. The disease may be a late manifestation of nephrotic syndrome, result from hereditary nephritis, or occur as a complication of other diseases.

Etiology Chronic glomerulonephritis reduces kidney size. Many of the renal tubules are atrophic or have totally disappeared. The tubules that remain are enlarged, although there is a reduction in the total number of glomeruli. The arterioles in the kidneys are narrowed, thereby reducing the blood supply. This probably contributes to the increasing renal destruction.

Manifestations The progression of this disease is highly individualized. Symptoms vary from no obvious symptoms to those associated with severe renal failure and hypertension. Proteinuria is constant, although variable in amount. Creatinine and other urinary clearance tests and tests of blood urea nitrogen indicate a gradual but progressive loss of function. The specific gravity is low and fixed, indicating the kidneys' inability to concentrate urine. Hematuria is usually present, although it may be seen only microscopically. Anemia is present and progressive. The child is pale, tires easily, and has a poor appetite.

Periorbital edema is generally present. The edema may be limited to the eye region and to the ankles, or it may be severe and generalized. Hypertension is usual in chronic glomerulonephritis, and the child may suffer from episodes of encephalopathy and cardiac failure.

As the final stages of the disease are reached, the child may have muscular cramps, diarrhea and vomiting, headaches, anorexia, and convulsions. Overt uremia is not uncommon.

Treatment There is no known cure for chronic glomerulonephritis. The disease may be rapidly progressive or interrupted by intervals of freedom from symptoms. Each exacerbation may result in progressive functional deterioration of the kidneys. With recent advances in dialysis and transplantation, there is some hope for these chronically ill children.

The treatment of chronic glomerulonephritis is symptomatic and supportive. The child may restrict his or her activities somewhat. During periods of exacerbation, the child may need to be kept in bed, depending on the amount of edema and degree of hypertension.

Adequate caloric intake is important in meeting the nutritional needs of the chronically ill child. A large body of research has accumulated suggesting that malnutrition, primarily caloric malnutrition, is a cause of growth failure in children with renal disease.[33] Salt is restricted only in the presence of edema or severe hypertension. Protein intake may be reduced if the blood urea nitrogen levels exceed 50 or 60. Supplemental vitamins and minerals are usually prescribed.

Varying drug therapies are ordered, depending on the child's symptoms. *Antihypertensives*, such as reserpine and Apresoline, are useful if the diastolic blood pressure rises over 100 mmHg. If the child develops heart failure, digitalization may be attempted. *Antibiotics* are utilized for infection. *Steroids and cytotoxic* drugs have been utilized in chronic glomerulonephritis, but the results to date have been unsatisfactory in most children.[34] All drugs excreted primarily by the kidneys should be given in reduced amounts, since an overdose due to poor renal function is possible. A *blood transfusion* for anemia may be given when the child's hemoglobin is low.

Peritoneal dialysis or *hemodialysis* is utilized for those children who may later be candidates for renal transplantation. Without dialysis, transplantation, or both, the life expectancy of children with chronic glomerulonephritis is generally 5 to 10 years after diagnosis.

Management The nursing management of the child with chronic glomerulonephritis presents many problems. The problem of dealing with a chronic disease may be devastating to both the child and the family. It is difficult for the child to accept frequent bouts of illness while friends and siblings are actively pursuing their interests at home and at school. The stunting of growth may make the child and the family embarrassed about the child's physical appearance. The nurse should play an active role in helping the family cope with chronic disease and the disruptions it causes. The parents must be helped so that the ill child is not treated like an invalid at the expense of other family members. Feelings of parental guilt often arise when siblings are neglected so that the ill child can receive most of the parents' attention. The parents must be taught about the disease and treatment so that they feel they have gained some control over the situation. Drug and dietary therapies must be carefully taught so that the treatment plan will be followed when the child is at home.

When the child with chronic glomerulonephritis is hospitalized with an acute exacerbation, the nursing management is similar to that for the child with acute glomerulonephritis. Frequent checks of vital signs, emotional support, observation of symptoms, and monitoring drug therapy are all important. Discharge planning should always be done by the renal team.

Nephrotic syndrome (nephrosis)

The term *nephrotic syndrome* may be used to refer to several clinical entities that have common symptoms and varied pathological manifestations, prognoses, and responses to therapeutic agents.[35] The cause of nephrotic syndrome is uncertain. Recurrences and exacerbations may sometimes be associated with acute respiratory infections.

Etiology Children with nephrotic syndrome have increased glomerular membrane permeability to large molecules, specifically proteins. The exact pathological lesion in the kidneys varies with the type of nephrosis. In all types, large losses of protein from the blood into the urine occur. Albumin is lost in the largest quantities, and the body is unable to replace it as fast as it is lost. The resulting low levels of blood protein decrease capillary osmotic pressure and result in a fluid leak from the capillaries. This causes a decrease in circulating blood volume, which stimulates the kidneys to retain sodium and water. The end result of the process is edema.

Several forms of nephrotic syndrome are recognized. The three most common are *minimal-change glomerular disease, focal glomerulosclerosis,* and *chronic proliferative glomerulonephritis*. The differentiation is important since the various types differ in terms of clinical course, response to drugs, and prognosis.[36]

Manifestations More males are affected than females. Each type of nephrosis is characterized early by edema, heavy proteinuria, hypoalbuminemia, and hypercholesterolemia.

The symptoms of minimal-change nephrotic syndrome usually appear between the ages of $1\frac{1}{2}$ and 4 years. Edema is the usual presenting symptom (Fig. 20-12*A* and *B*). Initially it occurs around the eyes and in the ankles and may then progress to the rest of the body. The child may develop ascites, which can cause respiratory distress. The genitalia, especially the scrotum, tend to become very swollen.

Proteinuria is probably the most important laboratory finding. The protein in the urine is mostly albumin. The urine specific gravity is elevated. Hyaline, granular, and cellular casts are also found in large numbers in the urine, and the urine appears foamy or frothy. Gross hematuria is not present.

The urinary output is decreased in relation to the amount of edema. Hypertension may occur, although the blood pressure is usually normal. Children with nephrotic syndrome exhibit pallor, poor appetite, lassitude, and irritability. Malnutrition may become severe since protein is lost in the urine and is not replaced. These children are unusually susceptible to infection.

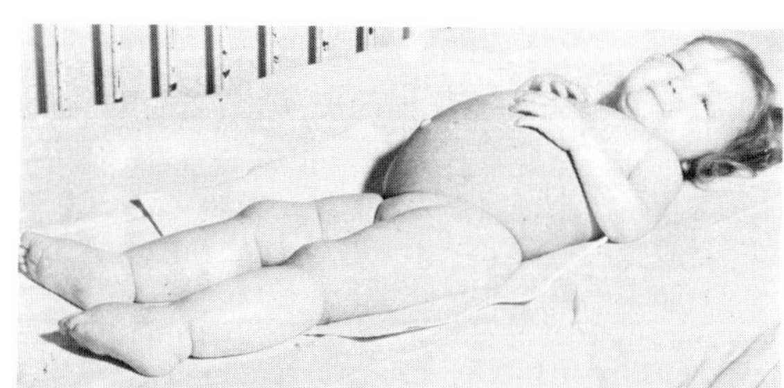

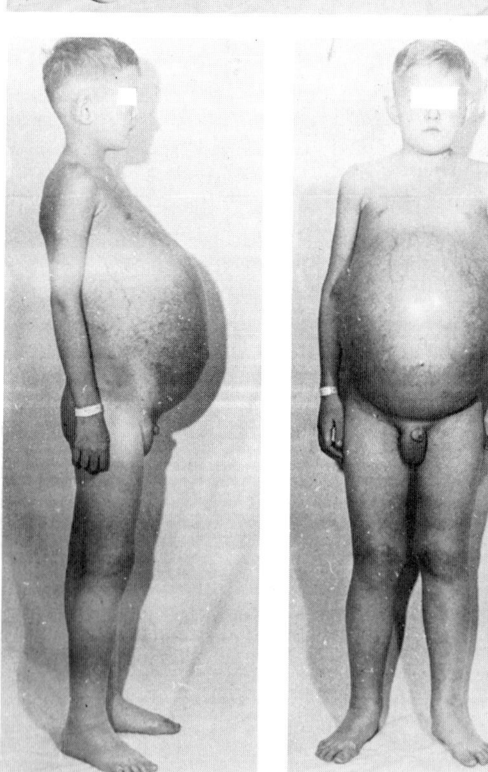

Figure 20-12 (*A*) A girl with active nephrosis. Note the severe generalized body edema and the periorbital edema, which almost closes the eyes. (*B*) A boy with massive ascites associated with nephrosis. Note the scrotal edema.

Treatment Nephrotic syndrome is a chronic disease. The course is one of recurrent accumulations of edema after partial or complete remissions. The duration and severity of nephrotic syndrome are variable.

Minimal-change glomerular disease is the most common form of nephrosis. More than 90 percent of children with this form of nephrosis will have remissions, and most have a good prognosis for eventual preservation of normal kidney function. The prognosis of children with chronic proliferative glomerulonephritis is not as good, because there is no known effective treatment. Children with focal glomerulosclerosis progress inexorably to renal failure.[37]

The treatment of nephrotic syndrome is aimed at prevention and control of acute infections, establishment of good nutrition, control of edema, and control of the progression of the renal lesion. During acute infections and when undergoing diuresis, the child may need to be in bed with only limited ambulation. Adequate rest is always important so that the child does not become fatigued. Generally, these children set their own activity limits.

Prevention of infection is important since edema fluid is an excellent culture medium. The edematous skin must be protected from injury, since it is stretched thin and easily breaks down.

Since malnutrition is common in nephrotic children, dietary therapy is important. Sodium may be restricted to 1 to 2 g per day, or the child may simply be placed on a "no added salt" diet, depending on the degree of edema. Potassium is generally added to the diet. Water is usually restricted only during extreme edema. At those times, the child is generally allowed an intake equal to the previous day's output plus the calculated insensible water loss. There are varying opinions about the amount of protein that should be allowed. A high-protein diet is usually advocated since the child loses so much protein in the urine. Protein is necessary to help offset the growth failure and muscle wasting often seen in these children.

Drug therapy is usually effective with minimal-change glomerular disease. Corticosteroids are given, with the goal of relieving edema. Diuresis usually occurs between days 8 and 14, after which the child's appetite and activity should improve. Prednisone is the steroid of choice because it has less tendency to cause sodium retention and potassium loss. The steroids may be given only every other day in an attempt to minimize side effects. Steroids are given for as short a time as possible because of their side effects, which include obesity, growth failure, hypertension, gastric ulcer, bone demineralization, and hypercoagulability. Nephrosis associated with focal glomerulosclerosis and chronic proliferative glomerulonephritis does not usually respond well to corticosteroids.[38]

Cyclophosphamide (Cytoxan) is an immunosuppressant given to children who are steroid-resistant. It is given with prednisone. Immunosuppressants are used to attempt to prolong remissions. Serious side effects of Cytoxan include leukopenia, hair loss, cystitis, gastric ulceration, and sterility.

Diuretics are given to help control the edema. Thiazide diuretics are usually used. Spironolactone may also be given to enhance the effectiveness of the thiazides. Intravenous salt-poor albumin is given on occasion and helps reverse hypovolemia and replace plasma proteins.[39]

Paracentesis may be necessary to relieve fluid pressure in the abdomen and to ease the respiratory effort. Hypertension, if it occurs, is treated with antihypertensive drugs and bedrest. Infections are vigorously treated with antibiotics.

Management The nursing care of a child with active nephrotic syndrome is complex and challenging. Meticulous skin care is necessary to prevent breakdown, since the tissues have poor tone owing to stretching by the interstitial fluid and since skin infections from abrasions can be very serious. Frequent position changes are necessary, although few positions may be truly comfortable. The head of the bed may need to be elevated to prevent respiratory embarrassment from ascites. Special localized care may be necessary for edematous areas such as the male genitalia. Frequent bathing, careful drying, and powdering should be done. Scrotal support may make the child more comfortable. Watch for hydrocele and rectal prolapse. Diarrhea may occur as a result of intestinal malabsorption secondary to edema of the bowel wall. This may further compromise an already stressed area of the skin. The child should be kept as clean and dry as possible.

Vital signs (including blood pressure) should be checked frequently. Respiratory efforts should be observed, since some respiratory distress is likely to develop. The child's temperature should be watched because nephrotic children are susceptible to infection. Edematous tissue is an excellent culture medium, and steroids often mask infection. The child should be kept away from crowds and infected persons. Weighing the child daily and accurately measuring intake and output help in monitoring the success of treatment.

The side effects and complications of the drugs should be understood by the nurse and carefully watched for. Tests will be performed to monitor the development of complications, such as leukopenia and diabetes.

The child should be encouraged to eat as much of the prescribed diet as is possible. Since muscle wasting often occurs, a balanced program of rest and activities should be planned.

The child's mental status may be difficult for both the nurse and the family to deal with. The nurse can anticipate that the child will suffer some loss of self-esteem with the changes in body image and appearance. The parents and the child will need assistance in dealing with the restrictions associated with chronic illness.

Parental teaching is an important part of discharge planning. The parents need to know about the disease, diet, side effects of drugs, skin care, and urine testing in order to follow the regimen of care at home.

Acute renal failure

Renal failure may be divided into two classifications: acute and chronic. Both types can have devastating implications for the child and family.

Acute renal failure, *acute renal insufficiency*, and *acute uremia* refer to a varied clinical picture of sudden and severely decreased kidney function that impairs homeostasis.

The symptoms and types of acute renal failure vary with the cause. Acute renal failure can be divided into three subclasses: (1) renal, (2) prerenal, and (3) postrenal. It is vitally important to ascertain the type of failure because prompt, appropriate treatment can prevent irreversible kidney damage and return renal function to within normal limits in relatively short periods of time. A complete examination of the child should be done, since injuries or illnesses unrelated to the kidneys can result in acute renal failure.

Renal failure This type of acute renal failure is relatively uncommon in children. Its causes are still uncertain, but are often external to the kidneys, such as drugs, poisons, gastroenteritis, surgery, and, most frequently, hemolytic-uremic syndrome.

Prerenal failure Prerenal failure results from decreased perfusion of blood to the kidneys. If blood flow and blood pressure are decreased below normal for a period of time, the body responds by trying to increase the blood volume to remedy the situation. This is accomplished by increasing reabsorption of sodium and decreasing the urine volume. The blood flow to the kidneys themselves is also decreased, and they become progressively less efficient. If the decreased circulation is short-lived, no symptoms or problems other than decreased urine sodium with a subsequent drop in urine volume will occur. If the impaired circulation is prolonged and is accompanied by an increase in waste products to be excreted, acute renal failure and permanent kidney damage may result. This situation is called *prerenal* because the conditions causing it arise elsewhere in the body.

The most common cause of prerenal failure in children is dehydration. This frequently is the aftermath of severe diarrhea, gastroenteritis, persistent vomiting, or, less commonly, bodily trauma, hemorrhaging, and burns. Prerenal failure can be easily reversed, and urine flow restored, by appropriate fluid replacement therapy and prompt treatment of the causative condition.

Postrenal failure Postrenal failure is due to obstruction of urine from the kidneys or the lower urinary tract. Obstructive causes of acute renal failure in children are relatively rare. Some cases are seen in the newborn and postoperatively. Sudden and complete obstruction of the outflow of urine from both kidneys will result in anuria and acute renal failure. It must be remembered that as long as one kidney continues to function and eliminate urine from the body, renal failure will not occur. Obstructions may occur anywhere in the system as a result of calculi, blood clots, sloughed tissue, or external pressure with compression of the ureters or the urethra by tumors or retroperitoneal fibrosis. Complete recovery is possible with removal of the obstruction but is considered unlikely when total obstruction has lasted for more than 3 weeks.[40]

Manifestations of acute renal failure In most cases the child with acute renal failure is already very ill. A thorough history must be obtained to ascertain exposure to harmful drugs and chemicals as well as to evaluate symptoms of glomerulonephritis.

The most blatant symptom (probably the only

true symptom) is *oliguria*. Although urine output may be only 40 to 60 ml per 24 h, anuria is relatively rare. Other symptoms, such as nausea, vomiting, and drowsiness, are usually due to the buildup of waste materials in the blood.

Laboratory values are usually abnormal and easily attributed to the lack of cleansing of the blood by the kidneys. *Azotemia*, with rapid rises in serum creatinine and blood urea nitrogen, is always seen. *Metabolic acidosis* occurs more slowly but can be life-threatening. *Hyponatremia* results from lack of urine output, and fluid requirements must be calculated frequently to prevent overhydration. *Hyperkalemia* is seen because of the normal release of potassium from the cells when the body is stressed. In renal failure, the potassium cannot be excreted, and blood levels increase. Many other blood values will change due to the failure itself and as a result of the treatment.

Treatment and management Nurses play a major role in the prevention of acute renal failure. The nurse must be aware of potential situations that will result in renal failure. By observing trends and communicating changes to the physician, acute failure can sometimes be prevented. For example, children undergoing treatment for burns or dehydration or receiving nephrotoxic drugs should be adequately hydrated, and fluid output should be closely monitored.

The role of the physician in acute renal failure is supportive. Initially, the blood and fluid deficits and the electrolyte imbalances must be corrected. Causative factors must be treated. Body fluid homeostasis must be maintained within limits that the body can handle until the failure is reversed or until more drastic measures, such as dialysis, are initiated.

Nursing care of children with acute renal failure involves close observation and monitoring as well as crisis intervention. These children are acutely and often critically ill and are very uncomfortable and irritable. Their families are understandably overwhelmed. The nurse needs to establish a rapport with the family and help them cope with the illness, hospitalization, and possible guilt feelings. Honesty and the sharing of factual data are vital. People can cope more effectively when they know what to expect. A team approach is usually quite helpful.

The child who is already in acute renal failure must have fluid intake and output monitored closely. Intravenous therapy rates must be maintained as ordered, with no "catching up." These children are often anorexic and yet require a nutritious diet. The diet in acute renal failure is usually restricted in fluids, potassium, and protein. Urinary output may require catheters or collection bags. Nurses must be prepared to deal with this equipment and maintain accurate records.

Hyperkalemia can constitute a major emergency for the child and may quickly result in cardiac arrhythmias and cardiac arrest. Laboratory values must be monitored, and changes communicated to the physician quickly. Many children are placed on cardiac monitors. Nurses must observe for elevation of the T wave and for widening of the QRS complex of the electrocardiogram. Both oral and intravenous potassium are severely restricted in patients with hyperkalemia. Dialysis may be needed to relieve the symptoms and prevent permanent kidney damage.

Recovery from acute renal failure varies from complete recovery to permanent kidney damage requiring chronic dialysis or transplantation. The extent of recovery depends partially on the promptness of treatment, but more importantly on the causative agent.

Chronic renal failure

Chronic renal failure leading to end-stage renal disease and finally uremic syndrome may be defined as irreversible changes in the kidneys that result in reduced function to the extent that the kidneys no longer maintain normal body fluid homeostasis. The kidneys are able to maintain normal homeostasis until greater than 50 percent of the functioning renal tissue is destroyed. The signs of beginning chronic failure are more chemical than clinical, and the child's symptoms and degree of illness will vary.

Manifestations The clinical manifestations of kidney failure may be predicted by considering the major kidney functions. The kidneys regulate both the volume and concentration of body fluids, play a role in acid-base balance, and maintain various solutes at optimal levels. They remove waste products of normal metabolism as well as toxic substances that may have been ingested. Their role in blood production revolves around production of *erythropoietin* (a substance stimulating red blood cell production). Another major function centers on blood pressure regulation. All these vital functions suffer when the kidneys no longer function adequately. Although chronic renal failure is defined as irreversible damage to the kidneys, obtaining a thorough history to attempt to find possible causative conditions is necessary. Sometimes treatment may increase renal function. When it is too late for improvement, the knowledge gained from the history may be helpful in preventing failure in siblings or in preventing further damage to the child's kidneys.

As kidney failure progresses, the serum levels of creatinine, urea, and uric acid slowly but steadily increase. The kidneys attempt to compensate through hypertrophy of the functioning nephrons and through increased activity within the tubules. If the failure is treated, the kidneys can usually maintain some capacity to eliminate wastes unless they are overloaded.

Unless stressed, the kidneys can maintain a normal sodium-water balance even with minimally functioning nephrons. Changes occur within the nephrons themselves to increase filtration rates and decrease sodium reabsorption rates. It is only in the final stages of renal failure or when the body is unduly stressed that signs of edema and sodium retention are observed.

While hyperkalemia can be a major problem in acute renal failure, it usually occurs only in the latter stages of chronic renal failure. Potassium secretion by the tubules can be maintained as long as conditions remain within normal limits. If the potassium intake is increased, the kidney in failure may not be able to handle it. If salt intake is decreased, the normal exchange of sodium and potassium will be decreased, and this can lead to hyperkalemia.

In reality, the kidneys will continue to excrete hydrogen ions to maintain acid-base balance but will be less efficient. Thus metabolic acidosis will result from a buildup of acids. A child with renal failure may have a pH of 7.2 to 7.3 and tolerate it well.

Central nervous system changes occur late in chronic renal failure. These may include a dulling of the senses, muscle twitching, weakness and cramping, convulsions, lethargy, restlessness, and irritability. Some children experience a loss of vision. Others may hallucinate, usually because of hypertension and decreased cranial blood flow.

The anemia of chronic renal failure is normocytic and normochromic. The cause of this anemia is a complex interplay of a number of factors. Impaired production and a shortened life span of red blood cells and an increased bleeding tendency with blood loss from the gastrointestinal tract are present. The negative effect on blood cell production is due to decreased erythropoietin production. Bleeding is related to platelet changes. The count is normal, but the platelets themselves lack adhesiveness.

One of the most distinctive and possibly most frustrating complications of chronic renal failure in children is their growth failure. It may be due partially to poor dietary intake. These children experience severe anorexia, refuse most foods, and thus have low caloric intake.

Another major factor in growth retardation is the change in calcium and phosphate metabolism due to the renal failure. Low serum calcium levels and high serum phosphate levels produce bone pain and deformities (rickets and renal osteodystrophy). The inability to excrete phosphates and metabolize vitamin D increases loss of calcium from the bones. With decreased serum calcium, parathyroid hormone is released, resulting in further demineralization of the bones. All these changes result in severe bone disease and an obvious lack of growth.

With all these problems, what picture does this child present? The history states that this usually active child now prefers to sit and watch television or sleep. There may be a history of growth slowing. The blood urea nitrogen and creatinine levels are elevated. The blood pressure may be elevated but could be normal, and anemia may be present. The child eats poorly, is pale and listless, and is apathetic about school and play. Adolescent girls may experience amenorrhea. Even minor illnesses such as colds or gastroenteritis can precipitate major changes in renal function. While these symptoms alone do not mean renal failure, seen in combination they usually are good indicators.

Because of health professionals' increasing knowledge and awareness of the symptoms of chronic renal failure, it is less common to see the end result of untreated failure; however, it can still occur. The clinical manifestations reflect continuation of the symptoms and changes of chronic renal failure already mentioned. These children have anorexia, vomiting, and inflammation or sores of the mouth and lips, and many have bloody stools due to intestinal ulceration. They complain of unrelieved itching and may accumulate urates on the skin, or "uremic frost." The level of consciousness can decrease and progress to coma and death. Hypertension, congestive heart failure, and pulmonary edema are not uncommon findings.

Management Medical management of chronic renal failure often provides only temporary relief of symptoms, and more drastic treatment, such as dialysis or transplantation, is ultimately required.

The goals of medical management of chronic renal failure are few, but vital. These include promotion of renal function (whatever amount is possible), maintenance of body fluid homeostasis, treatment of symptoms, and maintenance of as normal and active a life as possible. Unfortunately, sometimes the treatment of one complication creates other complications, and so the medical regimen is one of constant change.

The team approach is vital in caring for these children. The team includes not only the physicians and nurses but also dietitians, pharmacists, play therapists, radiologists, social workers, psychologists, and psychiatrists. The parents are a vital part of the team and also need to be consulted.

The child with chronic renal failure must be allowed to resume normal activities at his or her own pace. This fosters growth and independence and ultimately ensures the cooperation of the child and the parents (see Chap. 34).

In dealing with these children, the diet involves a great deal of time, energy, and frustration. Adults with renal failure are on very restricted diets. With children, considerations other than just the kidney failure must be taken into account. Children need enough protein and calories to grow, but not enough to cause needless overload to the kidneys. Sodium should not be drastically reduced unless edema or hypertension appears. Potassium can still be excreted, but should be monitored. Care should be taken to avoid overloading the child with such high-potassium foods as orange juice and bananas. The diet is not a regular diet; some foods are avoided. Using salt makes what can be eaten a little more palatable. The nurse must be patient and caring and a good negotiator when helping the child eat. Sometimes it is wise to settle for a meal one-third eaten rather than argue, with the result that the child does not eat at all or becomes so agitated that emesis occurs. If you find a method that works, *write it in the care plan*.

While bone disease is not apparent at first, it is inevitable. Hypocalcemia must be corrected to prevent further release of calcium from the bones. Vitamin D is given, but levels must be increased slowly to prevent toxicity. Parathyroidectomies are done in severe cases to control release of calcium from the bones. The most common and effective treatment is to bind the phosphates with aluminum hydroxide gels and give calcium. This eliminates the exchange of phosphates for calcium in the bones and tissue. Although phosphates are reduced in the diet, they cannot be completely eliminated because high-phosphate foods, such as milk, are also, unfortunately, often high in calcium.

Care must be taken to avoid the central nervous system symptoms of aluminum toxicity. The gels will need to be discontinued or decreased if these occur. Nursing care includes watching for any bone changes, monitoring bone pain, observing for difficulty in walking, and administering the medications.

Children with chronic renal failure are always anemic. They appear pale and bruise easily. They can function quite well on very low hemoglobin, less than 10 g per deciliter, and most centers will not transfuse them until hemoglobin reaches 4 to 5 g per deciliter. Transfusing before this only creates the chance of transfusion reactions and a very temporary rise in blood values. Packed red blood cells are used for transfusion. Iron and folic acid supplements are given, since the dietary intake is not a dependable source. The nurse's role is to monitor the blood values and help the family accept the appearance of their child. Many parents become quite perceptive and can tell when their child has reached the state of having critically low hemoglobin by changes in his or her behavior and color (changes that are imperceptible to most medical personnel).

Cardiovascular involvement, with hypertension as a symptom, is the rule rather than the exception for children with renal failure. Treatment does not begin until the blood pressure is moderately high (higher than normal high values for the child's age), since overtreatment can create as many problems as undertreatment.

Fluid and sodium restriction and diuretics are usually used in management of the hypertension. Antihypertensive drugs may be used to combat elevated blood pressure related to excessive activity of the renin-angiotensin system. Blood pressure needs to be monitored carefully for both hypertension and hypotension. Hypotension may be seen as a result of antihypertensive drugs. Intake and output are closely monitored. Sodium depletion should be avoided since it may increase the severity of the renal failure.

The nurse must know the child and be able to recognize behavior changes, complaints, and changes in attitude that could mean increased blood pressure, pericarditis, or congestive failure. Early detection of these can mean more prompt treatment, shortened duration of treatment, and fewer residual effects.

Children with chronic renal failure tend to be more susceptible to infections, especially of the urinary and upper respiratory tracts. Treatment must be prompt and *specific*, and results of cultures and sensitivities must be obtained before treatment is begun. Remember that most of the drugs available are excreted by the kidneys. Dosages must usually be reduced, and blood values monitored, since the drugs will remain in the bloodstream longer.

Ideally, these children will spend most of their time at home. Follow-up in the community is necessary because many are treated in medical centers far from their homes. Public health nurses, local physicians, the school nurse, and the local hospitals are good sources of follow-up and should be sent a discharge summary. Children with chronic renal failure are pale, have abnormal blood values, are on medications, and have kidney failure. Both the parents and the child should be ready to explain the child's condition—pallor, abnormal blood values, and kidney failure—whenever medical attention is required.

Medical management of chronic renal failure is used for as long as the child's physical condition permits. Unfortunately, it cannot maintain the child forever. Eventually these children require peritoneal dialysis or hemodialysis, and some receive renal transplants.

Hemolytic-uremic syndrome

Hemolytic-uremic syndrome is a combination of acute renal failure, severe hemolytic anemia, thrombocytopenia, and changes in the shape of red blood cells. It is a disease that occurs primarily in the first 3 or 4 years of life and is of unknown etiology.

The onset of hemolytic-uremic syndrome follows an earlier illness, usually gastroenteritis or an upper respiratory tract infection. The child is pale, restless, and prostrate. Severe oliguria or anuria develops rapidly, and the child may become stuporous and have convulsions. Pinpoint cutaneous hemorrhages may be present. The symptoms of severe acute renal failure are evident within a few days. The renal failure may be a result of clot formation in the small renal blood vessels.

Treatment There is no definitive treatment for hemolytic-uremic syndrome. Treatment is symptomatic and includes therapies for acute renal failure. Dialysis may become necessary. Transfusions of packed red blood cells and platelets may be given. Transfusions of fresh frozen plasma may be beneficial. Anticoagulant drugs, corticosteroids, and immunosuppressive agents are not of benefit. Many cases will resolve without permanent renal damage, although some children may progress to chronic renal failure. The prognosis is poor in familial cases.

Management The nursing management is the same as that for children with acute renal failure. Close observation for bleeding is important. So much of the child's clotting factors may be used up that he or she begins to actively bleed.

PERITONEAL DIALYSIS

In peritoneal dialysis, the peritoneum acts as a semipermeable membrane, allowing water and small-molecular-size solutes to pass back and forth, depending on their concentrations. The dialysis works on the basis of osmosis and diffusion. Hypertonic solutions are introduced into the peritoneal cavity, time is allowed for equilibration, and the hypertonic solution is then removed.

Peritoneal dialysis is used most widely with children to treat not only chronic renal failure but also acute renal failure, poisonings, severe metabolic problems, congestive heart failure, and at times hepatic coma and Reye syndrome.

Although acute catheters in pediatric sizes are available, many centers use a permanent Silastic catheter, even for acute dialysis. From a nursing standpoint, the acute catheters are more difficult to stabilize, tend to occlude faster, and are more difficult to maintain. Permanent catheters may be inserted under local anesthesia on the patient unit or in the operating room. The family and child must be told what will happen and what to expect afterward. They may see dialysis as proof that the disease is worse or that the child is closer to death. They must be assured that although the child is indeed very ill, dialysis is another more involved treatment, not a last-ditch effort.

Once the catheter is in place, dialysis is begun. The returned fluid is initially bloody because of the catheter insertion, but it slowly clears. The fluid of chronic dialysis patients is clear and straw-colored, similar to urine, at the beginning of each dialysis and is clear and colorless at the end of the dialysis session. Changes in color or odor, or pain or inflammation at the insertion or exit sites, can be signs of infection.

Children require 30 to 40 h of peritoneal dialysis a week either in the hospital or at home. Many children are dialyzed every other day during the night while they sleep to avoid interrupting their daily routine.

While a child is being dialyzed in the hospital setting, the nurse has the major responsibility for maintaining the dialysis and monitoring the child's progress. Tasks that are usually performed are blood pressure monitoring, weighing at regular intervals, measuring intake and output, and encouraging food intake.

Nurses monitor for and initiate some interventions for complications arising from peritoneal dialysis. A common complication is obstruction to the fluid flow. Failure of the dialysis to flow in or out freely may be due to kinking, blockage, or displacement of the catheter. Repositioning or replacement of the tube and treatment of constipation may be needed. Additional fluid is not infused until the problem is corrected because distention, pain, and, in severe cases, rupture of the peritoneal membrane can occur. While abdominal pain often is present during the first month of dialysis, recurring pain after long periods without pain may indicate peritonitis. Shoulder pain is usually due to air in the abdomen and diaphragmatic irritation. This is treated with a mild analgesic.

Peritonitis may be caused by a bacterial or aseptic infection as well as by a systemic infection. The symptoms may include abdominal pain, cloudy fluid that does not clear, rebound tenderness, and, at times, fever. Cultures of the fluid will usually be positive. Treatment includes adding antibiotics to the dialysate and giving systemic antibiotics.

Other complications include dialysis which is too efficient at removal of fluids or which causes an imbalance of potassium. Giving extra fluids, closely monitoring the weight loss and serum potassium levels, and adding potassium to the dialysate can prevent this.

Long-term or chronic complications are few and are due to the renal failure rather than the dialysis. Peritoneal dialysis is a safe method of maintaining a child who has chronic or acute renal failure, but it is less efficient than hemodialysis. While children can be maintained for lengthy periods on peritoneal dialysis and while some refuse any further treatment, transplantation is usually the next step.

The emotional responses to dialysis differ; some children may shut the world out by sleeping the whole time (usually with their heads covered), by staring out the window, or by watching TV. The nurse must be aware of these behaviors and allow the child *some* time to be alone, but should also make sure that the child interacts with others. Children with end-stage renal disease (chronic renal failure) tend to become depressed because of mental changes caused by the disease itself, the chronicity of their illness, and feelings of abandonment, being "different," and isolation. Dialysis units can be busy, and a quiet child hiding under the covers can be easily ignored. Some units employ a buddy system; two children with possibly opposite temperaments are paired. Especially in the case of adolescents, they provide peer evaluation, support, and companionship to each other.

HEMODIALYSIS

Hemodialysis in children was not successful until approximately 10 years after its clinical use in adults. Much of this delay can be attributed to lack of trained personnel, technical difficulties in adapting adult equipment to pediatric use, and the variability of children in different age groups. Hemodialysis tends to retard or at least does not encourage growth and physical maturation of children. Thus some physicians do not recommend it for long-term chronic use and suggest that it be considered only once transplantation is assured.[41] However, more children are going on chronic hemodialysis programs since Medicare now covers all chronic dialysis and transplantation expenses. There is a tendency to transplant earlier, which may eliminate some problems of long-term hemodialysis. Use of hemodialysis as an acute treatment in children is also limited because peritoneal dialysis is quicker and safer and works sufficiently well in children.

Hemodialysis requires a direct blood access. This is accomplished in two ways: an external shunt and an internal fistula.

An *external shunt* (see Fig. 20-13*A*) consists of two cannulas—one to an artery and one to a vein. During dialysis the cannula to the artery is connected to the dialyzer and carries the patient's blood to the machine. The blood is returned to the patient via the cannula attached to the vein. The largest cannula that will fit into the vessel without harming it is used. In older children, the radial artery and a vein in the forearm are used; in younger children, the brachial artery and the cephalic vein are used; and in small children and infants, the femoral artery and the saphenous vein are used.[42] These shunts are external to the skin and are in areas that require some immobilization for safety. Children

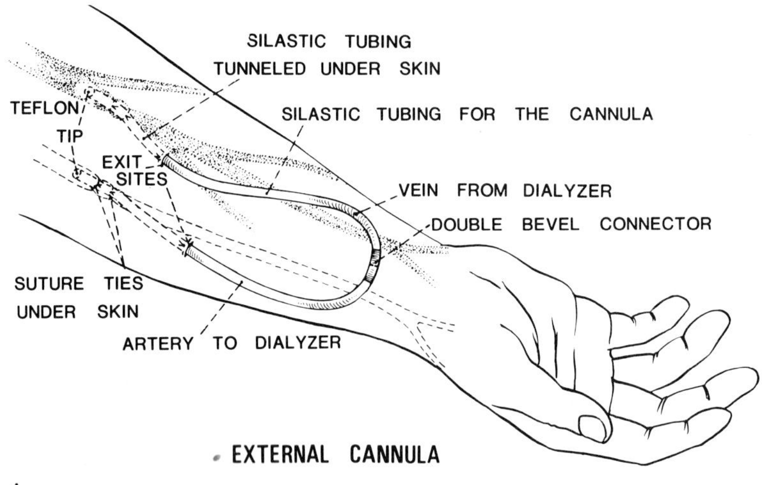

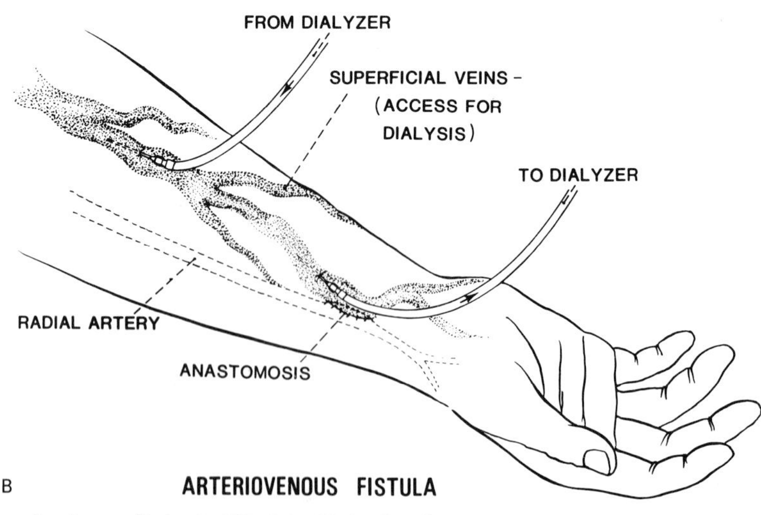

Figure 20-13 (*A*) An external shunt for hemodialysis. During dialysis, the cannula to the artery is connected to the dialyzer and carries the patient's blood to the machine. The blood is returned to the patient via the venous cannula. (*B*) An internal fistula for hemodialysis. The internal arteriovenous fistula is made by connecting the radial artery and the cephalic vein at the wrist. As blood shunts from the artery to the vein, the vein enlarges and can be used for easy venipuncture access.

may respond negatively to this restriction. A shunt also requires dressings that may be hard to maintain and much teaching to prevent infection. The incidence of shunt infections and clotting problems tends to be higher among children, requiring more frequent revisions.

An *internal fistula* is a connection made between an artery and a vein by a surgical procedure (see Fig. 20-13*B*). Since the vessels are quite small in children, grafts from the saphenous vein or bovine grafts are used to accomplish the anastomosis. After anastomosis, the vein will enlarge, become easily visible, and pulsate. During dialysis, two large-bore needles are inserted into the vein and attached to the dialyzer. Since the access is internal, the chance of infection between sessions is minimal. No dressings are required, and movement is not greatly restricted. The major disadvantage is that it requires repeated venipuncture, which can be painful, frightening, and difficult as the skin and venous wall toughen. Many centers prefer this method because of its longer effectiveness.

While connected to the dialyzer, the child is monitored for blood pressure, weight, intake and output, and clotting factors. Children on hemodialysis require dialysis usually two to three times a week for 4 to 6 h at a time. Dietary limitations are necessary and involve sodium, potassium, phosphorus, and fluid restrictions. Usually the child is allowed one meal that is less limited during the dialysis. Medications are still required and must be even more carefully monitored, since many can be removed during dialysis. Children generally respond well clinically to hemodialysis and receive temporary relief of symptoms.

Because home dialysis is costly and requires a great deal of teaching and because the pediatric patient is more difficult to manage clinically, hospital-based outpatient hemodialysis is more commonly used for children. While the families and the child are encouraged to assist in the care, the burden of initiation, maintenance, and discontinuation falls on the nurses and technicians.

The major complications to observe for include the disequilibrium syndrome and hepatitis. The disequilibrium syndrome occurs with a too rapid and efficient dialysis, which causes a rapid shift of water, pH, and osmolarity between the cerebrospinal fluid and the blood. Cerebral edema results, as evidenced by restlessness, confusion, nausea, and vomiting. Usually this is treated with intravenous saline. As with any treatment that involves the blood, hepatitis is always a possibility. The incidence is relatively small, but the precaution of routinely screening patients and staff should always be taken.

RENAL TRANSPLANT

Most children with chronic renal failure ultimately require a kidney transplant. The criteria for accepting children into transplant programs are very liberal. Few children are permanently rejected. Age is not a real factor, since successful transplants have been done on small children (doing transplants on children under the age of 12 months is still debatable). Children with chronic conditions or with controlled malignancies have had successful transplants. Some children will have a reoccurrence of their original disease in the transplanted kidney, but there is no predictable incidence with most diseases. The possibility of full renal function outweighs the chance of reoccurrence. The child should be consulted and involved in the decision concerning transplantation if he or she is old enough.

The nursing assessment of the child and the family must begin once transplantation as a treatment is accepted. The time before hospitalization for the transplant itself is devoted to testing for *histocompatibility* (tissue compatibility), treating any medical problems, and telling the child and the family what is going to happen and what to expect afterward. The prehospitalization time may be quite short or long. The waiting time depends on the type of transplant the child is going to receive, that is, from a related donor or a cadaver. Related-donor (a parent, a sibling, or, best of all, an identical twin) transplants are more successful and require a shorter waiting period. Cadaver transplants require being on a waiting list and being available when a suitable kidney is found.

On admission, the nursing care becomes more intense. The teaching continues, but on admission the child and family often become more tense, anxious, and excited. To combat the risk of overwhelming them, nurses often become coordinators of care and of visits by other team members.

The surgery itself varies little from adult transplantation. Younger, smaller children may have the new kidney placed in a different anatomic position. Some children have nephrectomies either before or at the same time as the transplant; others retain their own kidneys.

Immunosuppression is begun preoperatively and continued postoperatively, sometimes for a year or more. At the present time immunosuppression is general and thus decreases the child's ability to fight infection. Research is being done to find ways to do specific immunosuppression. Teaching about these drugs must be specific and detailed. Many children and their families see a transplant as a cure and expect all to be fine postoperatively. They must be helped to understand that this is the goal but that medical care will still be very much required.

Rejection is still the major problem. It can occur immediately or even 6 months later. The child needs to be monitored for the usual postoperative problems (pneumonia, dehydration, etc.) as well as for decreased urine output (once output is established), abdominal pain, changes in blood pressure, changes in blood urea nitrogen and other blood values, and changes in consciousness, all of which could mean rejection. If rejection occurs, it means returning to dialysis to wait for another kidney.

Any complication can mean a major setback both physically and emotionally for the child and the family. They need added support and teaching. They are frightened and need someone to care and to listen. The nurse is in an optimal position to help.

Nursing care continues long after transplantation and discharge. These children are followed both by the outpatient departments and by the public health department. The team continues to evaluate and reevaluate the child and family for years afterward.

Nursing Care Plan: Acute Glomerulonephritis

Patient: Martin Wilson **Age:** 6 years old **Date of Admission:** 1/6, 2 P.M.

ASSESSMENT

Martin Wilson, a 6-year-old male, was admitted to the pediatric unit with a tentative diagnosis of acute glomerulonephritis. The following information was given by his mother during the admission interview.

Mrs. Wilson had noticed that Martin's eyes were somewhat puffy 2 days prior to admission. The day before admission, Martin looked pale and did not appear to have any energy. Mrs. Wilson called her doctor on the morning of admission when she noticed that Martin was going to the bathroom less frequently, his urine was red-colored, and his other symptoms had not improved. The physician immediately arranged for Martin to be admitted to the hospital. On the way to the hospital, Martin vomited twice.

When questioned, Mrs. Wilson recalled that Martin and his brother had had sore throats about 3 weeks earlier. They had been treated with penicillin for 10 days and recovered without any problems. Mrs. Wilson appeared anxious about her son's illness. She repeatedly questioned the nurse about what was wrong with Martin and asked whether his brother was also going to get sick. Mrs. Wilson stated that Martin had always been healthy and that the doctor said he was growing normally. There have been no previous hospitalizations. She decided to stay with Martin while he was in the hospital, since his brother could stay with his grandparents. Mr. Wilson, a plumber, can also help with child care and visit Martin in the evenings. Mrs. Wilson stated that she was upset with herself for not calling the doctor earlier.

Physical examination

Weight: 21.9 kg (48.3 lb)—50th percentile. Height: 117.5 cm (46.3 in)—50th percentile. Temperature: 37°C. Pulse: 100. Respiratory rate: 23. Blood pressure: 138/98.

General appearance

Is lethargic, does not appear interested in his environment, and vomited on the way to the hospital. When questioned, he denies having a headache or blurred vision. A moderate amount of periorbital edema is present. His color is pale, and the urine is smoky brown.

PHYSICIAN'S ORDERS

1. Bedrest with bathroom privileges.
2. Strict record of intake and output.
3. Complete blood count, BUN, and creatinine.
4. Urinalysis—save urine samples from each voiding to compare color; check urine specific gravity.
5. Regular diet with no added salt.
6. Vital signs q2h, including blood pressure.
7. Notify the physician of diastolic blood pressure greater than 100 mmHg.
8. Administer a chest x-ray.
9. Weigh bid.

Nursing Diagnosis	Outcome Criteria	Nursing Interventions	Evaluation and Modifications
1. Potential for neurological complications related to impaired glomerular filtration	☐ Intact neurological status—no encephalopathy. Diastolic blood pressure is less than 90 mmHg.	☐ Record vital signs including blood pressure q2h. ☐ Notify the physician if diastolic blood pressure is 100 mmHg. ☐ Maintain bedrest with bathroom privileges. ☐ Observe the child for signs of encephalopathy, i.e., headache, vomiting, blurred vision, dizziness, and seizures. ☐ Record intake and output.	☐ Blood pressure ranging from 130/90 to 136/94. ☐ No evidence of encephalopathy. ☐ Maintain bedrest.
2. Potential alteration in fluid volume related to reduced glomerular filtration	☐ Urine output will be 650 to 1000 ml per 24 h.	☐ Maintain accurate intake and output records. ☐ Obtain information from the mother regarding the child's normal voiding patterns. ☐ Report urine output of less than 100 ml per shift to the physician.	☐ Urine output for this 24-h period is 400 ml.
	☐ Urine color will be umber to light yellow.	☐ Observe and record color or urine—save a sample from each voiding to compare color (tape to bathroom wall).	☐ Urine continues to be smoky brown.
	☐ Urine specific gravity will be 1.000 to 1.030.	☐ Check and record urine specific gravity with each voiding.	☐ Specific gravity is 1.020.
	☐ Urine protein will become negative.	☐ Record urine proteins by using Albustix to test each voiding.	☐ Urine is showing 3+ proteins at present time.
	☐ Periorbital edema will gradually disappear.	☐ Record weight twice daily (at same time each day). ☐ Monitor and record degree of edema when taking vital signs.	☐ Periorbital edema is resolving. ☐ Weight loss of 0.5 kg. ☐ Weight is slowly returning to normal.
	☐ There will be improved renal function, as evidenced by normal circulatory blood volume.	☐ Observe for and record any signs of cardiac involvement, i.e., cardiomegaly, tachycardia, diaphoresis, or dyspnea.	☐ No evidence of cardiac involvement at present.
3. Potential for altered body image (self-concept) related to periorbital edema	☐ The child will understand that the changes in appearance are temporary and usually resolve within 5 to 10 days.	☐ Allow the child to express feelings regarding puffy eyes. ☐ Inform the child that the puffiness will disappear as he begins to feel better.	☐ Martin says "I'm looking better."

Nursing Diagnosis	Outcome Criteria	Nursing Interventions	Evaluation and Modifications
4. Potential for skin irritation and excoriation related to edema and immobility	☐ The skin will remain pink, smooth, and intact.	☐ Observe and record skin condition every shift. ☐ Reposition the child q2h. ☐ Bathe and powder skinfold areas bid and prn. ☐ Cleanse eyelids with warm saline qid and prn.	☐ Skin is intact at present time. Continue to assess at every shift.
5. Potential for impaired nutrition related to anorexia and change in diet	☐ The child's appetite will improve as the symptoms subside.	☐ Provide regular diet for age with no added salt. ☐ Obtain information from the mother and the child regarding food likes and dislikes, to aid in planning daily menus. ☐ Provide afternoon and bedtime snacks.	☐ Appetite is only fair, and the child does enjoy snacks.
6. Diversional activity deficit related to continuing lethargy of disease and restricted activity level	☐ Martin will resume his normal activity level; activities of daily living and participation in scheduled unit play activities alternated with rest periods.	☐ Maintain bedrest with bathroom privileges. ☐ Provide age-appropriate toys and games that maintain bedrest. ☐ As the symptoms subside, allow the child to resume activities at his own pace. ☐ When activity increases, encourage interaction with peers.	☐ From his bed, Martin played Star Wars with his mother.
7. Alteration in family processes related to illness and hospitalization of the child	☐ The mother will verbalize her feelings about Martin's illness.	☐ Provide time and a quiet area where the mother can relax and talk with the nurse. ☐ Allow the mother to participate in Martin's care to the extent to which she is able. ☐ Teach the mother about Martin's illness and its treatment so that she will be able to accept what is happening to him. ☐ Tell the mother what the signs of complications are. ☐ Refer the family to appropriate agencies for follow-up after discharge.	☐ The mother talked to the nurse about her understanding of Martin's illness.

References

1. Colodny, Arnold H., "Urinary Tract Infections: Pediatric Urology," *Urology Times* **3** (March 1978).
2. Criss, Elizabeth, "Digital Subtraction Angiography," *American Journal of Nursing* **82**:1707 (November 1982).
3. Williams, Richard, and Hedvig Hricak, "Magnetic Resonance Imaging in Urology," *Journal of Urology* **132**:614 (October 1984).
4. Kleeman, C. R., et al., "Pyelonephritis," *Medicine* **39**:12 (February 1960).
5. Kunin, C. M., et al., "Urinary Tract Infection in School

Children: Epidemiologic, Clinical and Laboratory Study." *Medicine* **127**: (March 1964).
6. Kunin et al., op. cit., p. 122.
7. Woodward, John R., "Urinary Tract Infections," in P. O. Kelalis and L. W. King (eds.), *Clinical Pediatric Urology,* Saunders, Philadelphia, 1976, p. 185.
8. Ibid., p. 347.
9. Colodny, loc. cit.
10. Duckett, John W., "Urologic Considerations," in H. C. Filston (ed.), *Surgical Problems in Children: Recognition and Referral,* Mosby, St. Louis, 1983.
11. Ibid.
12. Gonzales, Edmond, Jr., "Posterior Urethral Valves and Bladder Neck Obstruction," in R. Jeffs (ed.), *The Urologic Clinics of North America,* vol. 5, Saunders, Philadelphia, 1978, p. 64.
13. Sorrentino, R., and P. Leonetti, "Terapia della estrofia vesicale," ESI (1958).
14. Chishol, Tague C., and Felix A. McParland, "Exstrophy of the Urinary Bladder," in M. Ravitch (ed.), *Pediatric Surgery,* 3d ed., Year Book, Chicago, 1979, pp. 1239–1253.
15. Ansell, Julian, "Vesical Exstrophy," in J. F. Glenn (ed.), *Urologic Surgery,* 2d ed., Harper & Row, New York, 1975, p. 316.
16. Duckett, John W., "Epispadias," in Jeffs, op. cit., p. 428.
17. Bredon, H. C., and E. C. Muecke, "Surgical Correction of Male Epispadias with Total Incontinence," *Journal of Urology,* **908** (May 1978).
18. Culp, O. S., "Treatment of Epispadias with and without Urinary Incontinence: Experience with 46 Patients," *Journal of Urology,* **125** (January 1983).
19. Gross, R. E., and S. L. Cresson, "Treatment of Epispadias: A Report of 18 Cases," *Journal of Urology,* **477** (April 1952).
20. Belman, A. Barry, "Urethra," in P. P. Kelalis and L. W. King (eds.), *Clinical Pediatric Urology,* Saunders, Philadelphia, 1976, p. 576.
21. Duckett, John W, and D. M. Raezer, "Neuromuscular Dysfunction of the Lower Urinary Tract," in Kelalis and King, op. cit., p. 416.
22. Lapides, Jack, et al., "Follow-up on Unsterile Intermittent Self-Catheterization," *The Journal of Urology* **187** (February 1974).
23. Altschuler, Anne, et al., "Even Children Can Learn to Do Clean Self-Catheterization," *American Journal of Nursing,* **98** (January 1977).
24. Devlin, K., and D. Rheinheimer, "Clean Intermittent Catheterization in Children," *Pediatric Nursing,* **29** (July–August 1976).
25. Duckett and Raezer, op. cit., p. 413.
26. Langman, Jan, *Medical Embryology,* 4th ed., Williams & Wilkins, Baltimore, 1981, p. 239.
27. Gauthier, Bernard, Chester Edelmann, and Henry Barnett, *Nephrology and Urology for the Pediatrician,* Little, Brown, Boston, 1982, p. 152.
28. Ibid., p. 153.
29. Langman, loc. cit.
30. Gauthier, Edelmann, and Barnett, op. cit., p. 132.
31. James, John A., *Renal Disease in Childhood,* 3d ed., Mosby, St. Louis, 1976, p. 210.
32. Brenner, Barry, and Floyd Rector (eds.), *The Kidney,* 2d ed., Saunders, Philadelphia, 1981, p. 1395.
33. Potter, Donald, and Ira Greifer, "Statural Growth of Children with Renal Disease," *Kidney International* **14**:337 (1978).
34. Brenner and Rector, op. cit., p. 1397.
35. Behrman, R., V. Vaughan, and W. Nelson (eds.), *Nelson Textbook of Pediatrics,* 12th ed., Saunders, Philadelphia, 1983, p. 1322.
36. Gauthier, Edelmann, and Barnett, op. cit., p. 142.
37. Brenner and Rector, op. cit., p. 1435.
38. Garlin, Edwardo, William Donnelly, Dennis Geary, and George Richard, "Nephrotic Syndrome and Diffuse Mesangial Proliferative Glomerulonephritis in Children," *American Journal of Diseases of Children,* **137**:113 (February 1983).
39. Behrman, Vaughan, and Nelson, op. cit., p. 1326.
40. James, op. cit., p. 260.
41. Ibid., p. 261.
42. Ibid., p. 268.

21

Nancy A. Eppich, Elizabeth L'Estrange Simone, and Mary Jo McCracken

Respiratory function

Upon completion of this chapter, the student will be able to:

1 Describe the embryological development of the respiratory system.
2 Describe the structure and functions of the upper and lower airways.
3 Describe the accessory structures of the respiratory system.
4 List eight important nursing assessments for a child experiencing alterations in respiratory function.
5 Discuss the purpose of five methods used to improve respiratory function.
6 List six ways in which a child's respiratory system differs from that of an adult.
7 Describe the pathophysiology, signs, and symptoms of foreign-body aspiration.
8 Describe the nursing responsibilities in suctioning a child with an artificial airway.
9 Describe the nursing management of a child with an upper respiratory infection.
10 Contrast the etiology and treatment of acute otitis media with the etiology and treatment of serous otitis media.
11 List four signs of respiratory failure in chidren.
12 Contrast the nursing care priorities for a child who has epiglottitis with those for a child who has croup.
13 Describe the nursing management of a child with a lower respiratory infection.
14 Compare the clinical signs and symptoms of mild, moderate, and severe asthma.
15 Describe the physiological changes that cystic fibrosis causes in the respiratory, gastrointestinal, and reproductive systems.
16 List six components of the therapeutic regimen used by children with cystic fibrosis.
17 Describe the psychosocial impact of cystic fibrosis on the child and his or her family.

The main function of the respiratory system is to supply oxygen to, and remove carbon dioxide from, the body cells. Accomplishing this task requires normal anatomy and physiology of the respiratory system as well as proper functioning of the cardiovascular, musculoskeletal, and nervous systems.

EMBRYOLOGY OF THE RESPIRATORY SYSTEM

A knowledge of the prenatal and postnatal development and growth of the respiratory system serves as a basis for understanding congenital defects as well as pulmonary function in healthy persons and those with a disease.

The oral and nasal cavities

During the fourth week of development, the beginnings of the nose, the *olfactory pits*, appear on either side of the head end of the embryo as widely separated thickenings of depressed ectoderm (Fig. 21-1). These pits are surrounded by horseshoe-shaped elevations that gradually merge during the sixth week to form the nose and upper lip. Failure of these medionasal processes to merge results in a cleft lip.

Also located on the ventral portion of the head

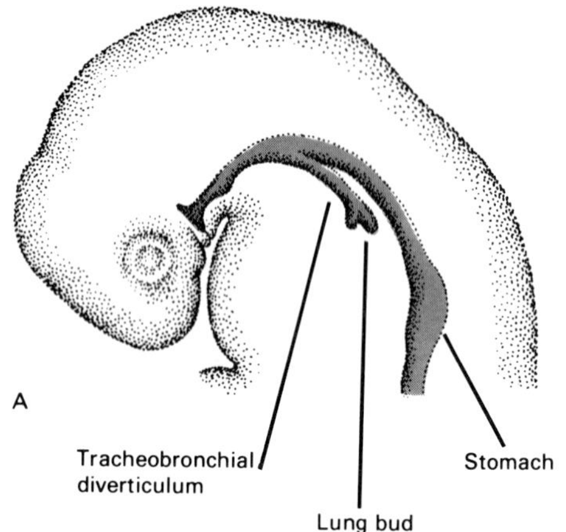

Figure 21-1 Embryonic development of the respiratory system (*From L. L. Langley et al., Dynamic Anatomy and Physiology, McGraw-Hill, New York, 1980.*)

is the *stomodeum,* or mouth, which opens into the primitive pharynx and foregut. At around 6 weeks, the thin membrane separating the stomodeum and nasal cavity disintegrates, creating a large *oronasal cavity.*

At about 7 to 8 weeks, a vertical plate grows down from the roof of the nasal cavity and forms the nasal septum. A horizontal plate grows toward the midline during the tenth to the twelfth weeks, forming the secondary palate. A cleft palate results when the horizontal plate fails to fuse.

The larynx and trachea

The rest of the respiratory system arises from the *laryngotracheal groove,* which appears in the floor of the pharynx at about 26 days. As the groove deepens and grows caudally, a tubular outpouching of endodermal cells is formed. This tube becomes separated from the esophagus by the tracheoesophageal septum. The laryngotracheal tube, along with the splanchnic mesenchyme, develops into the larynx, trachea, bronchi, and lungs (Fig. 21-1). A defect in the development of the tracheoesophageal septum results in a tracheoesophageal fistula (Fig. 21-2).

The bronchi and lungs

Lung development begins at about the 24th day of embryonic life and continues throughout the period of body growth. A lung bud develops at the caudal end of the laryngotracheal tube at 4 weeks and rapidly divides into two. During the 5th week, the lung buds grow laterally. By the 17th week, the bronchial tree is formed. By 24 weeks, the bronchioles have developed (Fig. 21-3).

Lung development takes place in four stages. During the *pseudoglandular period* (4 to 17 weeks), the lungs resemble glands. All major structures, except those involved with gas exchange, are formed. During the *canalicular period* (13 to 25 weeks), the lumina of the bronchi and bronchioles enlarge, and lung tissue increases in vascularity. Primitive alveoli (type 1 alveolar cells) develop, making gas exchange possible.

The *terminal sac period* (24 weeks to term) is marked by the development and thinning of the epithelium of the terminal sacs. At 25 to 28 weeks, the terminal sacs have sufficient vascularity and alveolar surface to support survival. At 23 to 24 weeks, the type 2 alveolar cells begin to secrete surfactant. Surfactant prevents alveolar collapse during expiration by decreasing surface tension.

The *alveolar period* (the late fetal period to about 8 years) is characterized by the development of mature alveoli. The alveoli increase in number until 8 years and in size until the thorax reaches adult size. The alveoli increase in number from about 25 million at birth to several hundred million at full growth.[1]

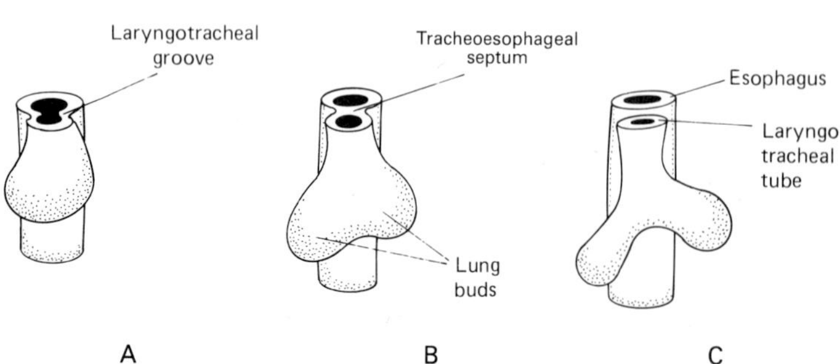

Figure 21-2 Embryonic development of the larynx and trachea. (*A*) The esophageal ridges. (*B*) The esophageal ridges fuse to form the tracheoesophageal septum. (*C*) The tracheoesophageal septum divides the esophagus from the trachea and lung buds. (*From Jan Langman, Medical Embryology, Williams & Wilkins, Baltimore, 1981, p. 204. Used with permission.*)

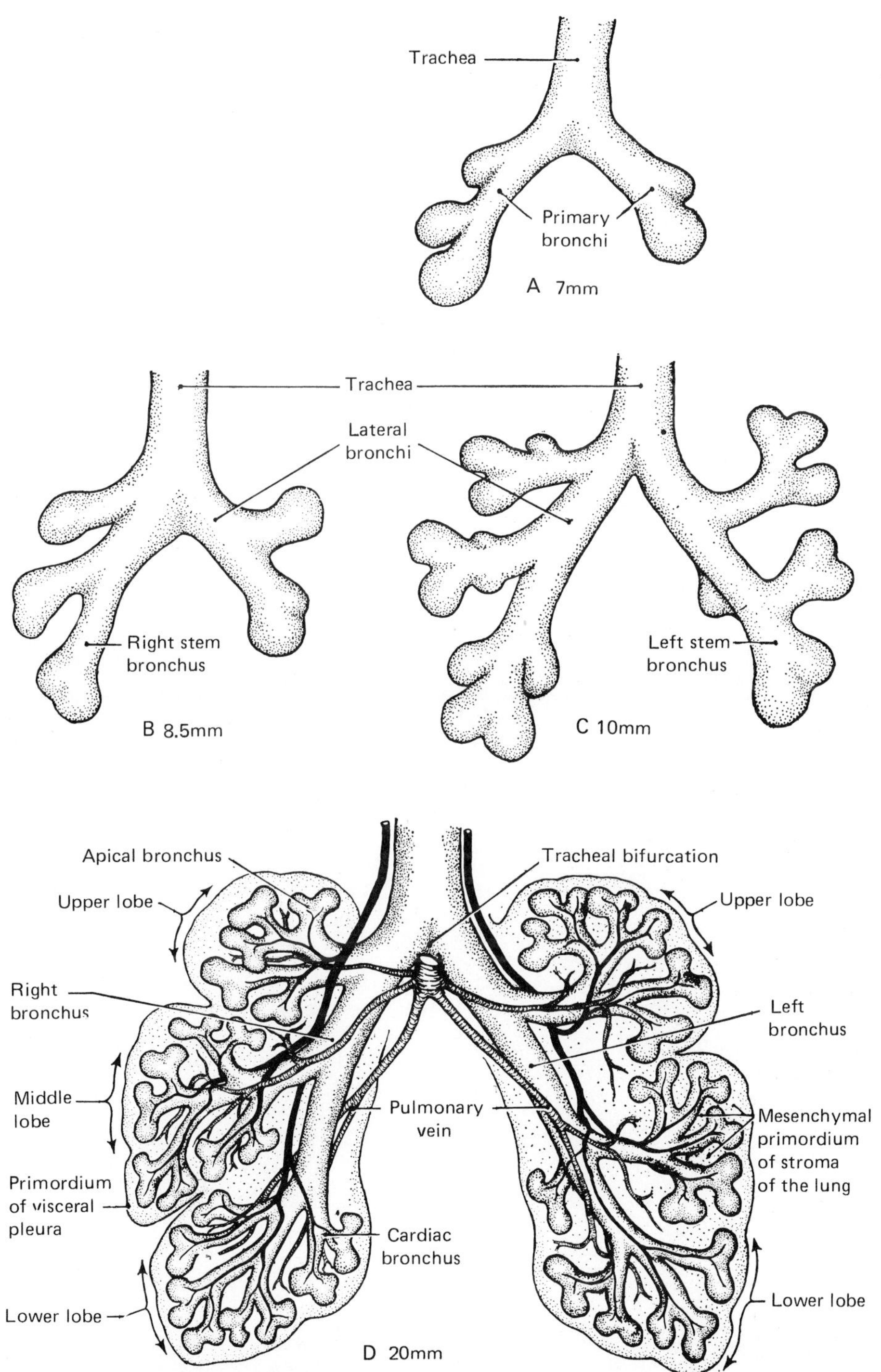

Figure 21-3 Development of the major bronchi and lungs. (*From Patten and Carlson, Foundations of Embryology, McGraw-Hill, New York, 1974, p. 299. Used with permission.*)

STRUCTURE AND FUNCTION OF THE RESPIRATORY SYSTEM

The respiratory system is made up of a series of conducting passages and the functional respiratory apparatus where oxygen–carbon dioxide exchange occurs. The *upper airway* is composed of the nose, nasopharynx, oropharynx, oral cavity, laryngopharynx, and larynx (the transition to the lower airway). The *lower airway* is composed of the tracheobronchial tree (trachea, bronchi, and bronchioles) and lung parenchyma (respiratory bronchioles, alveolar ducts, and alveolar sacs) (Fig. 21-4).

The upper airway

The nasal passages The *nasal passages* serve two important functions, the first of which is to cleanse inspired air. They are the first line of defense against inhaled particles. Long hairs at the nares act as filters. Mucous secretions of the nasal membranes trap particles, and cilia propel them toward the mouth for expectoration.

The second function of the nasal passages is to warm and humidify inspired air. Warmth is supplied by the highly vascular nasal turbinates. Moisture is provided by the mucosa. Inspired air is normally warmed almost to body temperature and is saturated with moisture by the time it reaches the carina of the trachea. In children who are mouth breathers or who have artificial airways, lack of humidification can cause secretions to become dry and crusted.

An additional defense mechanism is the *sneeze reflex*. Irritation of the nasal sensory receptors of the trigeminal nerves by foreign particles results in a deep inspiration followed by a strong expiratory blast, discharging the foreign particles through the nose.

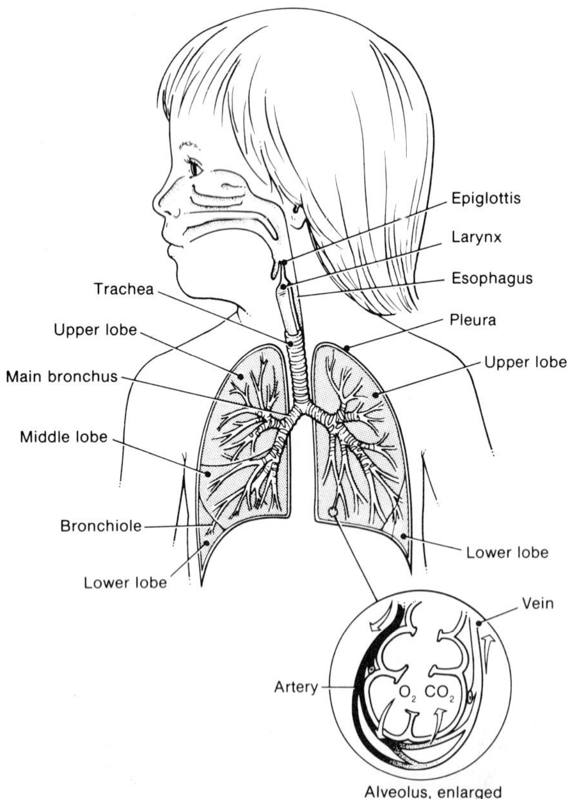

Figure 21-4 Structure of the respiratory system. *(From G. Scipien, M. U. Barnard, M. A. Chard, J. Howe, and P. J. Phillips [eds.], Comprehensive Pediatric Nursing, 3d ed., McGraw-Hill, New York, 1986, p. 843. Used with permission.)*

The pharynx The *pharynx* is common to both the respiratory and the digestive systems. Its primary function is to aid in swallowing. It is composed of three parts:

1. The *nasopharynx,* or the portion lying above the soft palate
2. The *oropharynx,* or the portion between the soft palate and the base of the tongue
3. The *laryngopharynx,* or the portion below the base of the tongue at the opening of the esophagus

The *pharyngeal tonsils* (adenoids) are located on the upper posterior wall of the nasopharynx. When these tonsils become enlarged, they can block either the internal nares or the eustachian tubes. The eustachian tubes are channels connecting the nasopharynx to the middle ear. The eustachian tubes regulate air pressure in the middle ear and drain fluid from it.

The oropharynx receives air from the mouth and nasopharynx and food from the mouth. It contains the *faucial tonsils,* or tonsils.

The laryngopharynx contains the epiglottis, which is a leaflike lid that lies over the glottis and protects it during swallowing.

The larynx The *larynx* connects the upper and lower respiratory systems. It lies higher in the neck of the child than in the adult. Its shape is established by the thyroid, arytenoid, and cricoid cartilages and by the epiglottis, muscles, and ligaments. In the infant and small child, the cricoid cartilage is the narrowest part of the airway. Within the larynx lie the true and false vocal folds. The larynx not only conducts air to the lower airway but also protects it from foreign objects and aids in coughing and speaking.

The lower airway

The lower airway consists of two parts: (1) the tracheobronchial system and (2) the terminal respiratory unit.

The tracheobronchial tree The function of the *tracheobronchial tree* is to conduct, humidify, and heat inspired air. Gas exchange occurs in the lung parenchyma. At birth, the bifurcation of the trachea is at the level of the third thoracic vertebra, and by 12 years it is at the sixth thoracic vertebra. Its diameter is about 6 mm at birth, increasing to 12 mm by age 6 and to 18 mm by adulthood. Because of the small diameter in the young child, infection or inflammation takes on greater significance.

The trachea is a muscular tube in which 16 to 29 C-shaped cartilages are embedded. The area where it branches into two main stem bronchi is called the *carina*. The trachea lies in front of the esophagus.

The right main stem bronchus divides into three secondary bronchi (lobar branches) serving the three lobes of the right lung. The left bronchus divides into two secondary bronchi. Secondary bronchi further divide into segmental bronchi and smaller subsegmental bronchi. As the bronchi divide, their diameters become smaller and smaller. They are composed of (1) an epithelial lining of ciliated, mucus-secreting glands; (2) a loose fibrous tissue layer containing blood vessels, lymphatic vessels, and elastic fibers; and (3) an outer layer of cartilage. The many goblet cells in the tracheobronchial tree secrete a mucous blanket that is designed to trap dust and foreign particles. The cilia continually move this mucous blanket from the respiratory bronchioles toward the larynx, at a rate of 2 cm per minute, creating a self-cleansing mechanism in the normal lung. The cartilage ensures a relatively rigid open tube for air passage.

The bronchi further branch into bronchioles and terminal bronchioles. Bronchioles have diameters of less than 1 mm and lack cartilage. Terminal bronchioles have a diameter of less than 0.5 mm. Both mucus and surfactant are found in these terminal bronchioles, although mucous glands and cilia are absent. The bronchi and bronchioles dilate and contract passively in response to lung inflation and actively in response to chemical and immunologic factors. An understanding of these responses is important to an understanding of many respiratory diseases.

The terminal respiratory unit The *terminal respiratory unit* consists of structures distal to the terminal bronchioles: (1) respiratory bronchioles, (2) alveolar ducts, and (3) alveolar sacs. Although gas exchange takes place in each of these structures, alveolarization increases from the bronchioles to the sacs. The alveolar sacs exist in clusters of 15 to 20 and have common walls between them. The thin alveolar epithelium, which lines all the lung parenchyma, allows for diffusion of oxygen and carbon dioxide. Thirty-five percent of alveolar gas exchange occurs in the ducts, while sixty-five percent occurs in the sacs. The alveolar epithelium is lined with fluid containing type 3 alveolar cells, or *macrophages,* which are an important part of the body's defense mechanism.

Accessory structures of the respiratory system

The thorax The *thorax* is sufficiently rigid to provide protection for the delicate organs it contains and, at the same time, is sufficiently pliable to allow the chest to expand and contract in the respiratory cycle.

Each lung is enclosed in a double-walled serous membrane called the *pleura*. The inner *visceral* layer covers the lung surface. It folds back on itself at the *hilum* (where the bronchi enter the lungs) and becomes the parietal layer, which is attached to the chest wall. The pleural cavity—a serous, fluid-filled "potential" space—acts to decrease friction between the two layers of pleura. The pleura adheres to the chest wall, pulling the lung out with it on inspiration.

The two lungs are separated by the *mediastinum,* which lies in the midline and contains the heart, great vessels, trachea, esophagus, and thymus gland. The *thoracic cage* is composed of the sternum, ribs, and thoracic vertebrae. The thorax has a cylindrical configuration at birth but gradually changes with growth, until the anterior-posterior diameter is less than the transverse diameter.

Muscles of respiration The expansion of the chest during inspiration takes place in three directions: longitudinally, transversely, and anteroposteriorly. Four major groups of muscles function in respiration: (1) the scalene muscles, (2) the intercostal muscles, (3) the diaphragm, and (4) the accessory muscles of respiration.

The first three groups of muscles are used in normal respiration. The accessory muscles are used in times of physical exertion or dyspnea.

The *scalene muscles* elevate the anterior end of the first rib during inspiration in order to increase the anteroposterior diameter of the chest and assist the external *intercostal muscles* in elevating the remaining ribs.

The *diaphragm* is the main inspiratory muscle. Contraction of the diaphragm increases the longitudinal dimension of the thoracic cage. During childhood, ventilation is much more dependent on the diaphragm than it is later in life.

Normal respiration is a passive act, due to gravity and the elasticity of the lungs. Forced expiration is accomplished in two ways: (1) forcing the diaphragm further up with the abdominal muscles and (2) depressing the ribs with the internal intercostal muscles.

The respiratory muscles work continuously without becoming fatigued as long as they receive an adequate supply of oxygen and as long as the amount of mechanical work required to overcome resistance to breathing is normal. However, if the muscles are oxygen-depleted, are weak because of poor nutrition, or are required to overcome increasing impedance over a long period of time, they will become fatigued, and respiratory failure can result.

Nerve supply of the lungs The lungs are innervated by branches of the vagus nerve and the thoracic sympathetic ganglia. The intercostal muscles are innervated by thoracic segments of the spinal cord, whereas the diaphragm responds to the phrenic nerve.

Neurochemical control of respirations

Because respirations are dependent on the action of muscles, they must be controlled within the central nervous system.

Central chemoreceptors The respiratory center in the medulla transmits signals to the muscles of inspiration. When inspiratory neurons fire, inspiration occurs. When they are inhibited from firing, expiration occurs by elastic recoil. The central chemoreceptor cells stimulate inspiration when there is an increase in hydrogen ions (a drop in pH) in the cerebrospinal fluid, signaling an increase in arterial P_{co2}. First the depth of respirations increases, and then the rate. However, if hypoxia and hypercapnia (increased P_{co2}) exist for a long time, the respiratory center becomes depressed.

Peripheral chemoreceptors Chemoreceptors in the aortic arch and carotid bodies are very sensitive to a drop in oxygen supply. They stimulate the respiratory center when there is decreased blood flow, decreased hemoglobin amount or saturation, or increased P_{co2}. Stimulation of these receptors causes increased minute ventilation and cardiac output.

PHYSIOLOGY OF THE RESPIRATORY SYSTEM

The term *respiration* actually encompasses all the processes that are essential for cellular metabolism, not just ventilation. A continuous supply of oxygen and continuous removal of carbon dioxide are vital.

External respiration occurs in the lungs when gas is exchanged between the external environment and the blood. Through *diffusion*, oxygen and carbon dioxide pass across the alveolar epithelium to and from the pulmonary capillaries. Gases are then transported by the blood and body fluids to and from the body cells. Gas exchange that occurs at the cellular level, involving systemic capillaries, is known as *internal respiration*. Thus, there are two different capillary beds where gas exchange takes place: pulmonary and systemic.

Mechanics of ventilation

The process of gas movement in and out of the pulmonary system is termed *ventilation*. Inspiration causes the thorax to enlarge and the diaphragm to descend. The pleural layers, which are held together by pleural fluid, expand the lungs as the thorax volume increases. The pressure inside the lungs decreases, becoming less than the atmospheric pressure, and air flows inward until the pressures inside and outside equalize. With the end of inspiration, the muscles relax, and the elastic forces of the lungs and chest predominate, causing the capacity of the thorax to decrease. The pressure inside the lungs increases above the atmospheric pressure, and gas flows outward.

The term *compliance* is used to describe the elastic forces of the lungs and thorax that must be overcome to expand the lungs. When a lung has high compliance, little force is needed to expand it. When a lung has low compliance, the elastic forces are such that it can be expanded only with great difficulty.

The flow of gas in and out of the lungs is measured by resistance. Any increase in secretions or any narrowing of the airways increases resistance. Normally, the upper airway accounts for 45 percent of total airway resistance.

Pulmonary gas exchange

Gas exchange between the pulmonary capillaries and the atmosphere should equal that of the systemic capillaries. To ensure adequate perfusion across the alveolar epithelium, alveolar inflation (ventilation) and capillary blood flow (perfusion) should match. This means that ideally all alveoli are inflated with air and are surrounded by blood-filled pulmonary capillaries.

This is not the case, however. Air in the upper airways cannot participate in gas exchange and is part of the *anatomic dead space*. It usually equals 1 ml per pound of body weight. *Alveolar dead space* is the portion of ventilation that contacts the alveolar epithelium where there is no blood flow. Together, these two dead spaces make up the *physiological dead space*.

Physiological shunt refers to the part of cardiac output that does not exchange with alveolar gas. Blood passes by an unfilled alveolus and is shunted around a filled alveolus. Atelectasis leads to intrapulmonary capillary shunting and produces a *venous admixture*, the return of unoxygenated blood to the left heart. This condition occurs in pulmonary edema and obstructive pulmonary disease and when there are retained secretions.

DIFFERENCES BETWEEN A CHILD'S RESPIRATORY SYSTEM AND AN ADULT'S

A child's respiratory system differs from an adult's in several important ways. A knowledge of these differences is important to an understanding of the etiology and treatment of respiratory disorders in children.

The upper airway

Smaller upper airway passages and a loose attachment of the mucous membrane lining make the possibility of obstruction edema more likely in a child than in an adult. The soft and more cartilaginous larynx of the infant increases the likelihood of airway obstruction if the infant's neck is flexed or hyperextended. Supporting a supine infant's neck with a small roll helps prevent this problem.

Because the infant's larynx is two to three cervical vertebrae higher than the adult's, the risk of aspiration and possible obstruction is increased.[2] A sitting position, especially during feeding, is helpful for the infant, particularly one with respiratory distress.

An infant is an obligatory nose breather for the first 4 weeks of life. Any condition that interferes with the patency of the nares will cause the infant distress.

The lower airway

Because the respiratory tract of the child is much shorter than that of the adult, bacteria in the upper airway have easier access to the lower portion of the airway. This increases the risk of infection.[3]

Like the upper airway passages, the lower airway passages are narrower, and the mucous membrane lining is loosely attached, providing the same susceptibility to obstruction. Since airflow resistance is inversely proportional to airway radius, a small amount of airway swelling can quickly lead to high resistance, respiratory distress, increased respiratory effort, and respiratory failure.

The smaller bronchioles require increased time for the filling and emptying of air sacs. If a prolonged expiratory phase is not possible owing to a rapid rate of breathing, the alveoli will become overextended and may possibly rupture, causing pneumothorax.[4] Because the child has fewer alveoli, congestion can quickly lead to loss of oxygenation and respiratory compromise.

Accessory structures

The child's chest wall is softer than the adult's because of the greater amount of cartilage in the sternum and ribs. The infant's ribs are attached to the sternum and vertebrae in such a way that the chest wall actually moves in during difficult respiratory effort. This inward movement, or *retraction*, is an important indicator of respiratory distress in a child.[5]

The child is also more dependent on the diaphragm because the accessory muscles of respiration are poorly developed and contribute little to chest wall movement during inspiration. A distended abdomen due to overfeeding, an abdominal mass, or an adbominal incision will impede the diaphragm and limit respiratory effort.

ASSESSMENT OF RESPIRATORY FUNCTION

Assessment of a child with a problem related to the respiratory system involves the collection of both subjective data (the parents' or child's input) and objective data (the nurse's and physician's clinical evaluation). An accurate and complete assessment enables the nurse to effectively plan the care that the child will need. A thorough assessment includes the interview and history, observation, palpation, percussion, and auscultation. As with all procedures and interactions with the child and the family, a gentle, reassuring voice and manner are necessary.

The history

If the nurse is seeing a child for the first time, the history should include details of the current complaint or illness as well as all other components of the nursing history (see Chap. 14). The nurse will want to ask the following questions:

1. Has the child experienced similar problems before? If so, what treatment was carried out and was it effective? Does the child follow any particular treatment plan at home?
2. Has the child had a fever?
3. What have the parents done for, or given to, the child because of this illness?
4. Has there been a change in the child's eating habits?
5. Has the child experienced anorexia, nausea, vomiting, diarrhea, or abdominal pain?
6. Does the child appear frightened or restless?
7. Has the child been worried, fatigued, or irritable?
8. Has the child been exposed to others who were ill?
9. Does the child attend a day-care center or have a baby-sitter?
10. Are the child's immunizations up to date?
11. Are there any pets in the home?

Specific information about respiratory status can be obtained by asking the following:

1. Has the child complained of difficulty in breathing? If so, when?
2. In the case of an infant, does the baby have to pause while sucking at the breast or bottle? Does the baby vomit after eating or appear to choke?
3. Has the child's activity level changed?
4. Are there any abnormal sounds during breathing? If so, describe.
5. Does the child complain of or appear to have pain?
6. Has there been a recent choking episode during play or at a meal?
7. Does the child cough? If so, how frequently and when? What causes the cough, and how does the cough sound? Is the cough productive? If so, what are the color and consistency of the sputum?

Observation

It is extremely important to look closely at a child. Whenever possible, observe the child when he or she is resting, is engaged in a quiet activity, and is distressed in order to make comparisons. Note the child's size and physical characteristics, state of alertness, posture, speech or cry, skin color, respiratory rate, and degree of respiratory effort. Often the child refuses to eat. Young children and infants are not able to tell the nurse how they feel. Therefore, observation must be particularly astute for these age groups.

An orderly observation of general appearance begins with noting the child's size in relation to his or her age and weight. Determining whether percentiles for height and weight are appropriate may give the first clue about a child's health problems. The nurse must note the child's general state of alertness. Sleepiness, fatigue, restlessness, or irritability may all be signs of respiratory dysfunction. The position the child assumes must also be observed. A child who prefers to sit up may be having respiratory difficulties. An infant demonstrates increased respiratory effort by hyperextending the head backward, reaching an almost C-shaped position (opisthotonis). In observing the general shape and size of the chest, the nurse should note whether the child has:

1. A funnel chest (pectus excavatum), characterized by sternal depression.
2. A pigeon chest (pectus carinatum), characterized by a protruding sternum.
3. A barrel-shaped chest, in which the ribs form concentric circles. Infants characteristically have a barrel-shaped chest, but in older children this is a sign of chronic respiratory disease.

The child's speech or cry can alert the nurse to problems associated with respiration. Hoarseness or no voice at all (aphonia) may be a sign of obstruction (an infection or a foreign body) or of a congenital problem (e.g., vocal cord paralysis). A weak cry may be due to fatigue or respiratory distress. A verbal child who must pause frequently while speaking and seems unable to finish a sentence in one breath may be doing so due to shortness of breath. Infants may also be short of breath, as evidenced by frequent pausing to breathe during feeding.

When observing color, look for pallor of the lips, mucous membranes, skin, and nail beds. Cyanosis is a late sign of hypoxia and may indicate the presence of cardiopulmonary disease due to hypoventilation or right-to-left shunting of blood. The fingers and toes are examined for clubbing, which is characterized by hypertrophy of soft tissues at the nail base. The skin over the nail bed becomes stretched and shiny and the terminal phalanges enlarge, becoming puffy and blunt (Fig. 26-3). Clubbing does not appear until 1 year of age, and its intensity can be correlated to the severity of the underlying disease.[6] Clubbing is characteristic of chronic lung disease and cardiac disease.

The rate, depth, quality, and pattern of respirations provide important assessment data (Table 21-1). In infants, it is helpful to count the rise and fall of the central abdomen just below the xiphoid process. The transition from abdominal (diaphragmatic) to costal (thoracic) respirations is gradual and is completed by 7 years of age. Average respiratory rates for children are given in Table 16-19. Ordinarily, there are approximately four pulse beats to every respiration. As body temperature increases, so does the respiratory rate.

The respiratory rate should be monitored often in the newborn; 2 h after birth, a resting rate of more than 45 in a full-term infant and 60 in a preterm infant should be considered abnormal and reported to the physician.[7] Abnormal breathing is often the outstanding feature of cardiac problems in infants with congenital heart disease.[8]

In observing the degree of respiratory effort, the nurse must remember that dyspnea is a subjective complaint of difficulty in breathing. Not all children will be able to communicate this problem to the nurse. Therefore, look for flaring of the nostrils on inspiration, use of the accessory muscles in the neck and abdomen, and retraction of the intercostal muscles. Look for head-bobbing, and listen for grunting and stridor. Also note whether there is bilateral chest expansion or paradoxical (seesaw) movement of the rib cage. (Silverman's index for evaluation of an infant's respiratory status is presented in Fig. 17-10.) Determine the position of the trachea; normally, it is at the midline of the neck, but it may be deflected toward the unaffected side if pneumothorax is present.

With increased respiratory effort there will be an increase in the negative intrathoracic pressure in the chest. A retraction, or a pulling in of the skin and muscles, may be seen over the bony landmarks of the chest (the ribs and sternum). Retractions are seen at the neck (sternocleidomastoid retractions), the suprasternal notch and above the clavicles (suprasternal and clavicular retractions), below the xiphoid process (substernal retractions), between the ribs (intercostal retractions), and below the costal margins (subcostal retractions) (Fig. 21-5).

In addition to making a careful assessment of respirations, the nurse should describe the child's cough. Usually, an infant's or young child's cough is nonproductive. The cough, which is a basic defense mechanism, is an attempt to maintain adequate pulmonary hygiene when there is a problem with the mucous blanket. Coughing is the major defense against retained secretions.[9] The ability to cough is present at birth.

An expiratory paroxysmal cough followed by an inspiratory "whoop" is characteristic of pertussis. A loose, productive cough accompanies bronchitis, cystic fibrosis, and a postnasal drip due to an upper respiratory infection. A sharp, brassy, nonproductive, barking cough is heard with foreign-body aspiration, croup, and tuberculosis. The cough heard with pneumonia is tight

Table 21-1 Classification of Respiratory Patterns

Type	Rate	Rhythm	Depth	Respiratory Cycle
Eupnea (normal)	Infant: 30 to 60; child: 15 to 25	Smooth and even	Variable	Active inspiration; passive expiration
Tachypnea	Increased	Regular or irregular	Within normal range or decreased	Active inspiration; passive expiration
Bradypnea	Decreased	Regular or irregular	Normal to increased	Active inspiration; passive expiration
Apnea	Variable	Irregular	Variable	Active inspiration; temporary cessation in the resting expiratory phase
Hyperpnea	Normal or increased	Regular	Increased	Active inspiration; usually prolonged and deep; passive expiration
Hypopnea	Normal or increased	Regular	Shallow	Shallow, active inspiration; passive expiration
Apneusis	Decreased	Regular or irregular	Variable	Active inspiration; cessation during inspiration; passive expiration
Cheyne-Stokes respiration	Variable	Regular increases and decreases in rate	Sequential changes from increased to decreased	Active inspiration; passive expiration with recurring periods of apnea lasting 10 to 15 s
Kussmaul's respiration	Variable	Regular or irregular	Increased	Active inspiration; passive expiration
Biot's respiration	Variable	Irregular	Shallow	Shallow breathing followed by apnea

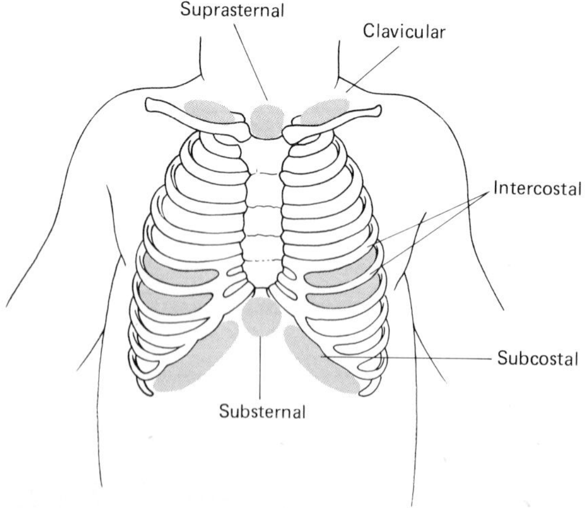

Figure 21-5 Location of retractions in a child. *(From L. Whaley and D. Wong, Nursing Care of Infants and Children, Mosby, St. Louis, 1983. Used with permission.)*

and nonproductive. A dry, irritating, persistent cough is characteristic of measles and laryngitis.

Palpation

When doing *palpation*, the nurse places his or her hands over the sides of the chest wall to feel the degree of movement with each inspiration. The bony landmarks of the chest can be palpated, which will give clues as to the location of the underlying lobes of the lungs (Fig. 21-6). Vibrations caused by the voice (vocal fremitus) are most easily felt over the trachea and bronchi; their absence can mean an obstruction or consolidation. Sometimes vibrations can be felt that are due to secretions or fluid. The grating sensation of a pleural friction rub and the coarse, crackling sensation of crepitation (air) can also be felt by palpation.

The symmetry of chest expansion is best felt by palpation. Palpation of the chest wall will also pinpoint areas of tenderness.

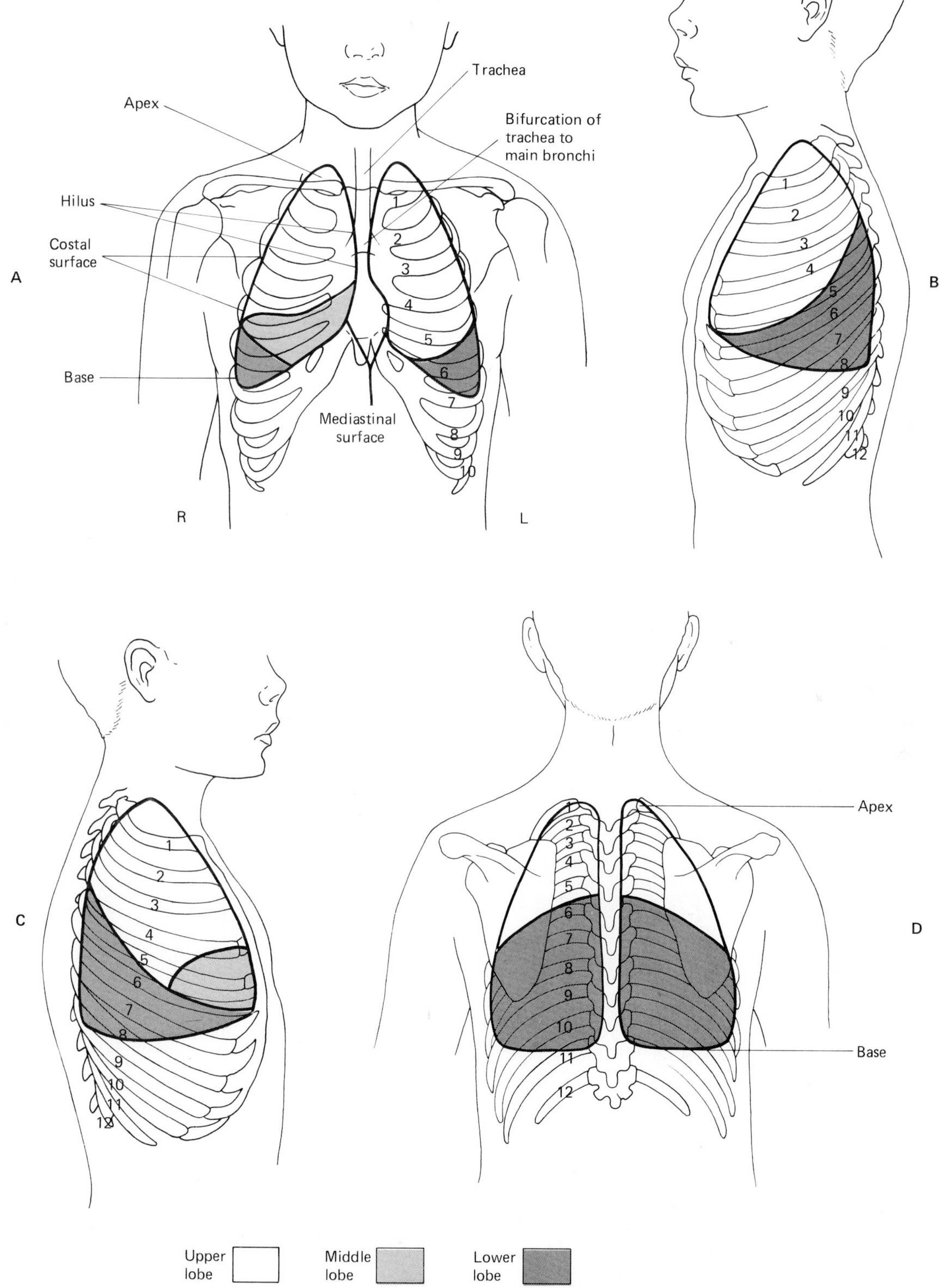

Figure 21-6 Location of the lobes of the lung within the thoracic cavity. (*A*) Anterior view. (*B*) Left lateral view. (C) Right lateral view. (*D*) Posterior view. (*From L. Whaley and D. Wong, Nursing Care of Infants and Children, Mosby, St. Louis, 1983. Used with permission.*)

Percussion

Percussion is an assessment technique that helps identify underlying tissues and whether they are air-filled, fluid-filled, or solid. The left hand is placed on the chest (with the fingers spread), and the middle finger of the right hand is used to strike the middle finger of the left hand with quick, sharp strokes. Percussion penetrates to a depth of 5 to 7 cm, producing vibrations and sounds which differ according to the underlying structures. Percussion over the lungs yields resonance, because the lungs are air-filled. Percussion over the solid diaphragm elicits a dullness. When fluid fills the lungs, resonance can change to dullness.

Auscultation

Auscultation is used to interpret the quality and quantity of breath sounds as air flows through the tracheobronchial tree and to detect the presence of fluid, mucus, or an obstruction of the air passages. Because the chest wall of the child is thin, breath sounds are louder and harsher than they are in the adult.

It is wise for the nurse to listen often to chest sounds in many different children. When a condition is described by a physician, the nurse should listen and learn. Only by doing this will the nurse be able to distinguish the variety of sounds possible and become familiar with the normal ones. The nurse should listen to a complete breath cycle, systematically comparing each position with the same one on the opposite side of the thorax. Auscultation of breath sounds is important in evaluating the effectiveness of suctioning and chest physiotherapy. Auscultation in infants and small children is very difficult because of their inability to cooperate. Offering infants a pacifier or having small children sit in the mother's lap is a great help in obtaining accurate auscultatory findings.

Normal breath sounds *Vesicular breath sounds* are those of normal inspiration. They are heard all over the chest, except over the manubrium and interscapular areas, and are characterized by a louder, longer, higher-pitched inspiration with a shorter, softer, lower-pitched expiration.

Bronchial breath sounds are those heard as air rushes through the large airways. They are normal only over the trachea. Elsewhere they indicate consolidation. They are characterized by a shorter inspiratory phase and a longer expiratory phase and sound like air blowing through a tube.

Bronchovesicular sounds are a combination of vesicular and bronchial sounds commonly heard at the manubrium of the sternum and the upper intrascapular areas. Inspiration and expiration are equal in quality, pitch, intensity, and duration.

Abnormal breath sounds *Adventitious breath sounds* are abnormal sounds, not alterations of normal sounds. There are many, varied descriptions of adventitious sounds. Until the nurse has a vast amount of experience in listening for these sounds, it may be better to describe exactly what is heard rather than trying to apply a label to it.

Rales (French for "rattle") are the most common and indicate the presence of fluid in the small airways and alveoli. They are heard on inspiration. Fine rales sound like the noise made when a lock of hair is rubbed between the thumb and forefinger in front of the ear. Medium rales originate in the bronchioles and sound like the fizz of a carbonated drink. Coarse rales are loud and bubbly. They originate in the trachea or bronchi and are also known as the *death rattle*.

Rhonchi are loud, gurgling noises produced as air passes through airways narrowed by secretions, inflammation, or spasm. They are usually more prominent during expiration. *Sibilant rhonchi* are high-pitched or squeaky and are produced in the smaller bronchi. *Sonorous rhonchi* are lower-pitched and sound like snoring. They are often labeled *coarse rales*. Since rhonchi suggest accumulated or retained secretions (or both), efforts should be made to mobilize the secretions, and an evaluation should be made as to whether they disappear or change.

Rales and rhonchi can be difficult to distinguish from each other. To do this, listen with the bell of the stethoscope to the sounds of breathing produced through the mouth. Compare these with the sounds heard on the chest. Rhonchi can be heard transorally; rales cannot.[10]

Wheezes sound more musical than rales and rhonchi. The sound is produced by high-velocity airflow through a restricted air passage. Wheezes often accompany asthma and bronchoconstriction. Audible wheezes may be heard with aspiration of foreign bodies. Wheezes may be inspiratory or expiratory.

Pleural friction rubs are caused when inflamed pleura rub against one another. If one hand is cupped over the ear and a finger of the other hand is rubbed over the cupped hand, a pleural friction rub can be simulated.[11]

Stridor is produced by the flow of air through an obstructed upper airway. It can be loud or soft, high- or low-pitched, and musical or harsh, depending on the type and extent of obstruction. Inspiratory stridor usually means obstruction at or above the larynx. Expiratory stridor usually indicates obstruction below the larynx. *Grunting* on expiration is a typical sign of severe respiratory distress in the infant (see Chap. 17).

"*Snoring*" while awake is associated with enlarged tonsils or other tissue obstruction of the upper airway.

Measurement of blood gases

One of the most important tools for assessing respiratory status today is the measurement of arterial blood gases and pH (Table 21-2). These values provide information about acid-base balance, alveolar ventilation, and oxygenation. They can be used to determine the degree of respiratory disturbance, to select treatment, and to evaluate the child's progress. The more severely ill the child is, the more important the blood gas measurements become.

The measurement of the partial pressure of carbon dioxide in the arterial blood (Pa_{co2}) is a direct reflection of the adequacy of alveolar ventilation.[12] The normal Pa_{co2} range is 35 to 45 mmHg. When the Pa_{co2} rises (*hypercapnia*), respiratory acidosis results. When it falls (*hypocapnia*), respiratory alkalosis is present.

The measurement of dissolved oxygen gas tension in arterial blood (Pa_{o2}) is closely related to the amount of oxygen carried by hemoglobin, that is, the saturation (Sa_{o2}). The normal Pa_{o2} is 80 to 100 mmHg; the normal Sa_{o2} is 95 to 100 percent. Together, these measurements indicate the oxygen content of arterial blood.

The Sa_{o2} is reflected in the oxygen-hemoglobin dissociation curve. When the curve shifts to the right, as can occur with hyperthermia, chronic hypoxemia, hypercapnia, and acidosis, hemoglobin has less affinity for oxygen, and more can be released to the tissues. When the curve shifts to the left, as in hypothermia, hypocapnia, and alkalosis, less oxygen is released.

The arterial pH measurement—the amount of free hydrogen ion concentration in arterial blood—reflects the acid-base balance in the body. The normal arterial pH is 7.35 to 7.4. A value lower than 7.35 indicates acidosis; a value higher than 7.4 indicates alkalosis. Values less than 7 or more than 7.8 are incompatible with life. The three mechanisms for maintaining the acid-base balance are (1) the buffers in the bloodstream (hemoglobin, protein, and bicarbonate); (2) kidney regulation of bicarbonate; and (3) ventilatory regulation of carbon dioxide.

A decrease in arterial pH will stimulate an increase in the depth and rate of respiration. The Pa_{co2} than falls, and the pH rises. An increase in pH suppresses alveolar ventilation, thereby increasing the Pa_{co2} and lowering the pH. Thus the pH and Pa_{co2} provide a physiological reflection of the ventilatory and acid-base status.

Table 21-2 Normal Arterial Blood Gas Values

	Normal	
pH	7.35 to 7.45	Acidity or alkalinity of blood in terms of hydrogen ion concentration
Pa_{CO2}	35 to 45 mmHg	Partial pressure of carbon dioxide in arterial blood
Pa_{O2}	80 to 100 mmHg; 40 to 60 mmHg in newborns	Partial pressure of oxygen in arterial blood
Sa_{O2}	95 to 100%	Saturation of oxygen—plotted on an oxyhemoglobin dissociation curve—affected by pH, P_{CO2}, and temperature
HCO_3	22 to 26 mEq per liter	Bicarbonate ion, the basis of the buffer system
H_2CO_3	1.05 to 1.35 mEq per liter	Carbonic acid, formed by carbon dioxide and water, is 3% of P_{O2} (the ratio of hydrogen ion to carbonic acid is usually 20 to 1)

Pulmonary-function testing

Perfusion, gas exchange, and ventilation can be measured by pulmonary-function tests. Normal values depend on the height, weight, sex, and age of the child. Normal values are then "predicted" on the basis of these factors. The child's values are expressed as a percentage of the predicted values (100 percent indicates good pulmonary function). Pulmonary-function testing is useful in:

1. Differentiating between *restrictive* and *obstructive* lung disease. Lung expansion is limited with restrictive lung disease (e.g., spinal cord injury or pneumonia). There is an impairment of air movement through the airways with obstructive lung disease (e.g., asthma or bronchitis).
2. Evaluating a particular treatment plan. The effectiveness of a bronchodilator can be assessed by pulmonary-function tests performed before and after treatment.
3. Evaluating the severity and progression of pulmonary disease as well as in making a prognosis.

The cooperation of the child is necessary if accurate values are to be obtained. Therefore, children 5 years and up are better candidates for pulmonary-function testing than younger ones. Lung volumes and flow rates are typically measured. The primary lung volumes are:

1. *Tidal volume* The volume of air inhaled and exhaled with each breath
2. *Residual volume* The volume of air remaining in the lungs after a maximal expiration
3. *Expiratory reserve volume* The extra air that can be exhaled after a normal respiration
4. *Inspiratory reserve volume* The extra air that can be inhaled after a normal inspiration

Lung capacities usually include one or more of the volumes. The common capacities include:

1. *Vital capacity* The total of tidal volume, inspiratory reserve volume, and expiratory reserve volume
2. *Functional residual capacity* The amount of air remaining in the lungs after a maximal expiration
3. *Total lung capacity* The total amount of air that the lungs can hold when at rest.

Pulmonary-function testing is done in a pulmonary-function laboratory. The patient requires sedation beforehand and no special care afterward. Young children (3 to 6 years old) who cannot cooperate and those who are in pain (which may restrict breathing) are not good candidates for pulmonary-function testing.

Diagnostic procedures

Chest x-rays are used to diagnose such clinical conditions as atelectasis, pneumonia, pneumothorax, and mediastinal shift. They are also valuable in validating the correct placement of artificial airways. Anterior, posterior, and lateral views are commonly taken. Lateral neck films may be taken of children with suspected upper airway obstruction, such as would be caused by foreign-body aspiration or epiglottitis.

Bronchoscopy allows the direct visualization of the larynx, trachea, bronchi, and alveoli for diagnostic or therapeutic purposes. Biopsies, aspiration of sputum and cells, as well as removal of foreign bodies may be done using bronchoscopy.

There are many diagnostic tools and procedures available to the medical community to aid in identifying problems associated with the respiratory system. A knowledge of these will help the nurse prepare the child and the family for a procedure, answer questions, and allay concerns.

METHODS OF IMPROVING RESPIRATORY FUNCTION

Respiratory care of a child (or adult) is multidisciplinary. The nurse will share the responsibility for caring for the child with the pediatrician, anesthesiologist, respiratory therapist, and even the physical therapist. Although these other health professionals may have primary responsibility for certain treatment modalities, the nurse becomes involved in all treatment aspects through day-to-day care, as well as in teaching the child and the family.

Oxygen–carbon dioxide exchange can be improved by (1) increasing the amount of oxygen available during the inspiratory phase of respiration or (2) decreasing the work of breathing by making the respiratory effort more effective. Increasing the effectiveness of the respiratory effort can be achieved by improving the patency of the passages of both the upper and the lower airways; this is done by eliminating secretions or relieving an obstruction.

The techniques described below can be used in both a supportive, therapeutic mode and a preventive mode. In most cases, the techniques are used to augment the body's own mechanisms for maintaining respiratory function.

Oxygen therapy

Oxygen therapy is used to treat hypoxemia and increase alveolar oxygen tension as well as to decrease the work of breathing and the work of the heart.[13] Increased oxygen in the inspired air facilitates transfer of oxygen to the lungs for use in external respiration. The amount of oxygen delivered to an infant or child can be increased by giving supplemental oxygen through high-flow systems (PEEP [positive end expiratory pressure] and CPAP [continuous positive airway pressure]) or low-flow systems (cannulas, hoods, masks, and tents) (Fig. 21-7). The choice of the system will depend on the physiological need for flow and the age of the child. For a complete discussion of oxygen therapy and the methods of administering it, see Chaps. 16 and 17.

Whenever oxygen is used, it should be considered a medication. Flow rate and concentrations must be checked frequently and documented on the child's chart. Frequency of checking varies from hourly for the very small infant to every 2 to 4 h for the older child, who is more stable. The nurse must observe the child's response to oxygen therapy: color, vital signs, and respiratory effort. Blood is drawn for blood gas measurements according to a schedule based on the concentration of the oxygen being administered and the response of the child to therapy.

Oxygen toxicity is possible when oxygen is given for too long and at too high a concentration. Lung toxicity, bronchopulmonary dysplasia, and retrolental fibroplasia can result (see Chap. 17 for a discussion of these problems). Children with chronic lung disease, in whom chronic hypoxia triggers the respiratory centers, can rapidly lose consciousness as a result of hypoventilation if they are given too much oxygen.

Whenever oxygen therapy is instituted, it is the responsibility of the nurse to make certain that the oxygen is both humidified and warmed prior to inspiration in order to prevent further irritation or damage to the tracheobronchial tree. This is even more important when oxygen is being delivered through an artificial airway.

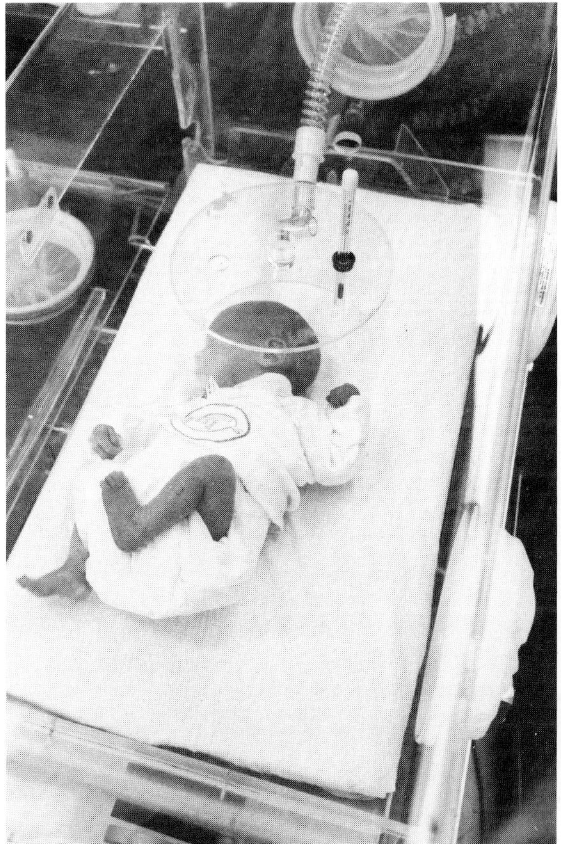

Figure 21-7 An infant receiving oxygen via an oxygen hood. (*Photo courtesy of Olympic Medical Corp., Seattle.*)

Humidification of room air

Normally, air is 100 percent humidified by the upper airway when it reaches the alveoli, thus maintaining the hydration of the mucous blanket. If disease causes drying of the mucous membranes, the following will occur:

1. Ciliary activity will be impaired.
2. Mucus will be thickened, and its movement will be impaired.
3. Secretions will be retained.
4. Inflammation will result.

As a result of the above complications, infection, atelectasis, and pneumonia may follow.

Humidifying inspired room air is an important treatment for the tracheobronchial tree under these conditions. Aerosol machines—ultrasonic or jet nebulizers—break down a liquid (usually water) and suspend it in a gas. The gas and liquid are then deposited in the tracheobronchial tree to aid in bronchial hygiene. The liquid may be water or a medication. The gas is usually room air, but oxygen in varying concentrations may also be used.

In some occasions, intermittent positive-pressure breathing (IPPB) therapy is used to increase airway pressure, mechanically dilate the tracheobronchial tree, decrease the work of breathing, and increase the tidal volume. It is used to deliver medication, but, more important, it is also used to stimulate the child to cough and mobilize retained secretions. IPPB is difficult to use with small children because it is frightening. Clear instructions, patience, and understanding are needed to teach an older child how to use IPPB.

Drug therapy

Medications are used frequently in the treatment of respiratory disease for any of the following reasons: dilatation of the air passages, decongestion, thinning of secretions, reduction of inflammation, and suppression of the cough reflex. The medications used can be given orally or intravenously or by inhalation. Although medications given by inhalation may have a topical effect, they are rapidly absorbed systemically because of the thin alveolar membrane and the generous capillary blood flow through the lungs. The nurse must understand and watch for systemic responses to inhaled medications. Table 21-3 outlines the various types of medications used in the treatment of respiratory disease.

In addition to the medications listed in Table 21-3, numerous antibiotics are used to treat infections that occur in the respiratory system. Since pulmonary infections in children usually present with a temperature elevation, aspirin and acetaminophen are frequently used to lower the fever.

Chest physiotherapy

Chest physiotherapy is used to prevent pulmonary complications in some children (for example, children who have surgical procedures) and to improve function in acute and chronic respiratory disease. It includes postural drainage, chest percussion, chest vibration, coughing, and exercise. Chest physiotherapy may be combined with aerosol or IPPB therapy, especially when an acute illness is superimposed on a chronic illness, such as cystic fibrosis or bronchiectasis. Percussion and vibration mobilize and loosen secretions, which are then moved by gravity as the various postural drainage positions are assumed. (These positions and techniques are explained in more detail in Fig. 16-33.)

In order to help the child breathe properly, the nurse must understand normal respiration. With normal respiration, the abdomen rises as the diaphragm descends, the ribs flare, and there is a slight rise in the upper chest. During expiration, the diaphragm moves up and the abdomen falls.

The nurses must be able to tell a child how to breathe more effectively as well as how to cough. Incentive spirometers, balloons, laughing, and crying may all aid in improving ventilation. To help the child cough properly, have the child take several breaths and then take one large one, hold it, and forcefully contract the abdominal muscles and expel the air by opening the glottis. Incisions will need splinting with hands or pillows.

Nasopharyngeal or oropharyngeal suctioning is useful for removing secretions in infants and children who are unable to clear their own secretions. Suctioning is often done to remove mucus prior to feeding an infant and after a postural drainage treatment. Suctioning also stimulates the cough reflex to help the infant expel secretions.

Positioning the child to maintain a patent airway is important. An infant's or a young child's larynx can be kept open by putting a roll underneath the neck to prevent flexion or hyperextension. An unconscious child should be positioned to allow for full expansion of the chest to prevent atelectasis. Frequent position changes prevent pooling of secretions in the lungs.

A child in respiratory distress may be made more comfortable by being placed in the semi-Fowler's or Fowler's position with the upper body and legs adequately supported. This position aids the contraction of the diaphragm by relieving abdominal pressure.

Artificial airways

When respiratory failure occurs or when there is obstruction of the upper respiratory tract, an artificial airway may be lifesaving. Endotracheal tubes (Fig. 21-8) and tracheostomy tubes (Fig. 21-9) are designed to:[14]

1. *Relieve airway obstruction* due to soft tissue obstruction, edema, or laryngeal obstruction

Table 21-3 Drugs Used in Respiratory Disease

Type	Function
Noninhalation Pulmonary Agents	
1. Bronchospasmolytics	
a. Active bronchodilators	Promote relaxation of smooth muscle fibers and cardiac stimulation
(1) Catecholamines (epinephrine, ephedrine)	Sympathomimetic agents; alpha and beta effects
(2) Methylxanthines (theophylline, aminophylline)	Provide central nervous system stimulation and relax smooth muscle
(3) Corticosteroids (hydrocortisone, methylprednisolone)	Relieve bronchospasm and inhibit mediator release from mast cells
2. Decongestants	Relieve swelling of mucosa and increase capillary blood flow in nasal and pulmonary tree
a. Alpha-adrenergic drugs	Constrict arterioles, thereby decreasing blood flow
(1) Phenylephrine (Neosynephrine)	Most useful as a nasal decongestant
b. Allergic decongestants	Increase and thicken glandular secretions
(1) Antihistamines (Benadryl, Chlor-trimeton)	Decrease histaminelike irritation to tissues and decrease cause of increased blood flow.
3. Mucokinetic agents (expectorants)	Improve removal of sputum
a. Water	Thins mucus and decreases viscosity
b. Vagal stimulants	Stimulate gastric mucosa and cause vagal activation of bronchial glands producing secretions
c. Direct bronchial gland stimulants (supersaturated potassium iodide)	Increase secretions
4. Anti-inflammatory agents	
a. Corticosteroids	Decrease acute and chronic inflammation
5. Antiallergic agents (allergy shots)	Reduce sensitivity to allergen (cause)
6. Antimicrobials	Given when pulmonary infection present
7. Antitussives	Suppress coughs
a. Codeine	
b. Dextromethorphan	
Inhalation Pulmonary Agents	Topical application of drugs to the pulmonary tree through aerosol treatment
1. Bronchodilators	Cause vasodilation of pulmonary mucosal vessels. Side effects: tachycardia, palpitation, flushing
a. Adrenergics	
(1) Epinephrine (Bronkaid, Primatene)	
b. Beta adrenergics (Beta$_1$ and beta$_2$ effects)	
(1) Isoproterenol (Isuprel)	Bronchodilatation; short duration (1 to 2 h)
(2) Isotharine (Bronkosol)	Bronchodilatation; short duration (1 to 2 h)
(3) Metaproterenol (Alupent)	Bronchodilatation; short duration (1 to 2 h)
c. Beta$_2$	
(1) Albuterol (Proventil)	Duration 4 to 8 h No direct cardiac stimulation
(2) Terbutaline (Brethine)	
(3) Fenterol, Carbuterol	
2. Antihistamines	
a. Cromolyn sodium	Stabilize sensitive mast cells; used prophylactically
3. Corticosteroids	Inhibit mediator release from mast cells; enhance bronchodilators; maintenance therapy without systemic effects
a. Beclomethasone (Beclovent)	
b. Triamcinolone, dexamethasone $NaPO_4$	
4. Decongestants	
a. Racemic epinephrine (Micronefrin, Vaponefrin)	Topical vasoconstrictor Aerosol decongestant Mild systemic bronchodilator
b. Phenylephrine	
5. Mucokinetic agents	
a. Hypoviscosity agents	Decrease viscosity of mucus
(1) Water	
(2) Weak electrolyte solutions (sodium bicarbonate)	
b. Mucolytic agents	Liquefy purulent sputum by digesting DNA
(1) Pancreatic agents (Dornavac)	Used only in cystic fibrosis: reduce tenacity of secretions; expectorant
(2) N-acetylcysteine (Mucomyst)	Decrease mucus viscosity and help mobilize secretions

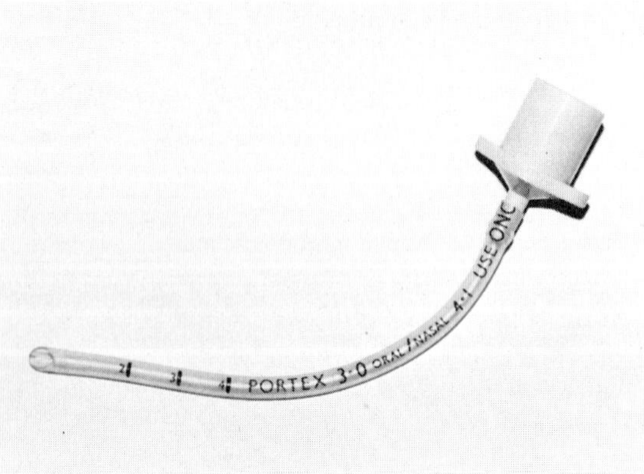

Figure 21-8 An endotracheal tube suitable for a small child. (*Photo by M. Smith.*)

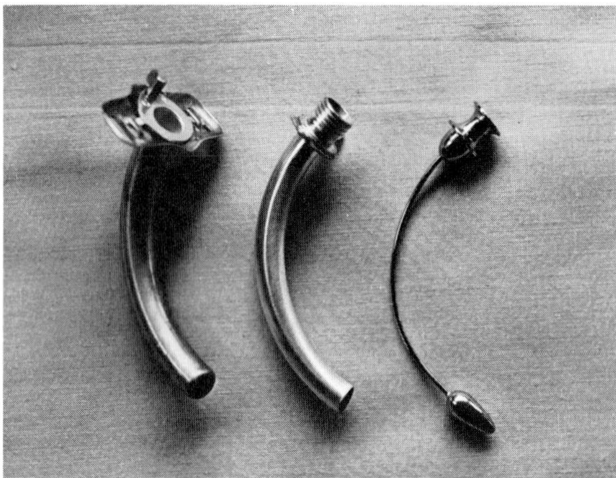

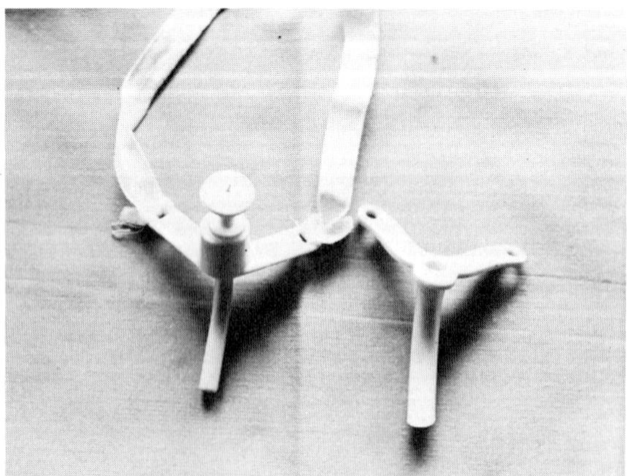

Figure 21-9 Tracheostomy tubes. (*A*) A metal tracheostomy tube. From left to right: (1) outer cannula, (2) inner cannula, and (3) obturator. (*B*) Silastic tracheostomy tubes. From left to right: (1) a tube with ties and obturator in place and (2) a wing-tipped tube. (*Photo by M. Smith.*)

2. *Protect the airway* when the normal protective reflexes (gag, swallowing, and cough) are absent because of anesthesia, drugs, or disease
3. *Facilitate suctioning* and pulmonary physiotherapy
4. *Support ventilation* when it is needed for prolonged periods

Endotracheal intubation involves passing a polyvinyl chloride tube through the nares or mouth and down into the larynx and lungs. Because the tube is passed through the vocal cords, they are unable to vibrate, which prevents speaking or crying. Endotracheal intubation is performed by a physician or nurse who has received special training in this technique. It may be done in an emergency room, an intensive care unit, or any pediatric unit if necessary and if the proper equipment and personnel are available.

Endotracheal tubes come in a variety of sizes and may or may not have a cuff. In general, if the endotracheal tube passes through the nares, it is of an appropriate size to pass also through the larynx and vocal cords. (See Table 33-4 for guidelines for selecting endotracheal tubes and suction catheters of the correct size.) Cuffed tubes are seldom used with children under 10 years of age because the cricoid ring, which is the smallest part of the airway, allows for a secure fit without a cuff. Cuffed tubes are used when there are large amounts of secretions (mucus or blood) in the upper airway, in order to prevent their spread to the lungs, and also when very high pressures are needed for mechanical ventilation.

A tracheostomy involves the insertion of a tube into a surgically created opening in the trachea. The tube is inserted at a point below the glottis and vocal cords, thus making speech or crying impossible and also altering the effectiveness of the coughing mechanism. Tracheostomies are performed by a surgeon in the operating room. Tracheostomy tubes come in a variety of sizes and may or may not be cuffed or have inner cannulas. The smallest tubes, used for infants, are available in two different lengths to accommodate the shorter airway of the newborn. Table 21-4 compares endotracheal intubation and tracheostomy.

Cricothyroid puncture is an alternative to intubation when a temporary airway is needed. This procedure is performed in an emergency room and is done to ventilate a child whose breathing is obstructed. It allows air exchange until a

Table 21-4 Comparison of Endotracheal Intubation and Tracheostomy in Children

Intubation	Tracheostomy
Advantages	**Advantages**
1. Simple procedure	1. Lower incidence of acquired subglottic stenosis
2. Can be done quickly	2. Larger tube, making obstruction less likely
3. No surgery: no scar or bleeding	3. Less discomfort: less sedation needed
4. Simple extubation in most cases	4. Care relatively simple
5. Simpler reintubation after accidental extubation	
Disadvantages	**Disadvantages**
1. Greater risk of acquired subglottic stenosis	1. More difficult procedure
2. Nasal excoriations	2. Surgery: increased chance of infection, bleeding, scar; more frightening
3. More postextubation stridor	3. Removal of tracheostomy more difficult: granulation tissue, edema, dependence
4. Accidental extubation easier	4. Accidental extubation more dangerous
5. Smaller tube: obstruction more likely	5. Intensive care needed initially
6. More discomfort: sedation or restraint more necessary	
7. Intensive care needed	

Source: Adapted from Aubrey Maze and Edward Bloch, "Stridor in Pediatric Patients," *Anesthesiology* **50**:132–145 (1979).

tracheostomy can be performed in the operating suite under better conditions. A large-bore needle is inserted through the avascular membrane between the thyroid cartilage and the cricoid cartilage. Textbooks on pediatric emergencies provide more detailed explanations of this procedure.

Psychologically, the insertion of an artificial airway is frightening, uncomfortable, and traumatic to the child and the family. Research shows that schoolchildren are able to recall at least some of their experiences during intubation, including suctioning, coughing, being unable to talk, and having the tube removed.[15] Communicating with the child and his or her family is of great importance. Gentle handling and a reassuring manner are helpful for the child who is intubated.

Whenever the upper airway is bypassed, its normal function of humidifying and warming inspired air is lost. Children with artificial airways will either be placed in a mist tent or be connected to a special "collar" or "T tube" that delivers humidified and warmed air (Fig. 21-10). When air is properly humidified and the child is properly hydrated, crusting of secretions is unlikely.

If mechanical ventilation is necessary, the child will usually be unable to handle secretions, making suctioning necessary. The child is suctioned only when necessary, or every 2 h, to maintain a patent airway. With suctioning catecholamines are released, causing an increase in heart rate that can lead to arrhythmias. Hypoxia, tracheal irritation, hypotension, and lung collapse are other potential complications of suctioning. Suction pressure limits must be strictly adhered to. For infants, the suction pressure should be 60 to 80 mmHg; for older children, it should not exceed 120 mmHg.

Giving constant reassurance and using the correct techniques are essential in order to make the procedure as nontraumatic for the child as possible. (Guidelines for suctioning a child without an artificial airway are presented in Table 16-16.) Table 21-5 describes a basic suctioning procedure in detail.

If a tracheostomy was done, the child needs to be observed initially for hemorrhage. The tube must be kept securely in place, and removal must be prevented. It will be approximately 7 to 10 days before a patent "tract" through the skin and trachea is formed. After this time, the tube may be changed every week as a precaution against infection. The skin around the stoma should be cared for whenever necessary, but at least once a day. The ties, which hold the tracheostomy tube in place, are changed whenever they become soiled, and the skin under them must be watched carefully. Redness and irritation indicate the need for more frequent changing of the ties and closer attention to skin care. If an inner cannula is present, it must be removed and cleaned daily to prevent accumulation and buildup of secretions. It can be soaked in sterile normal saline.

Although bacterial contamination of the lower airway is inevitable when the upper airway is

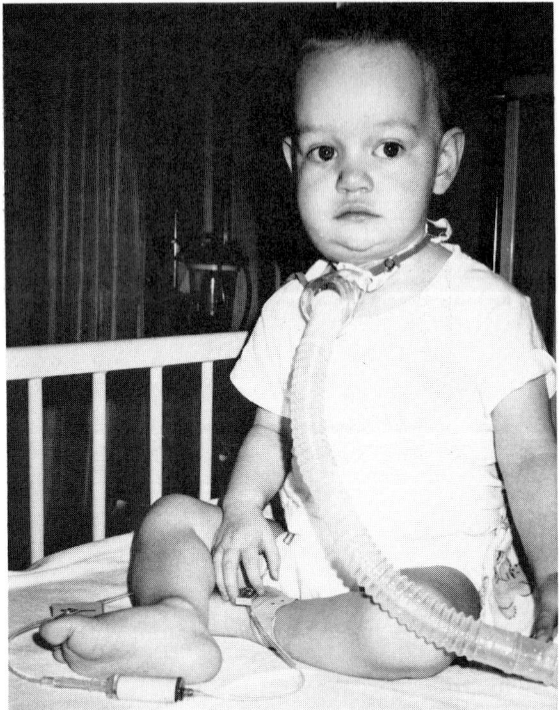

Figure 21-10 A child with a tracheostomy receiving warmed and humidified air. (*Photo courtesy of Elizabeth E. Simone.*)

bypassed, infection must be minimized by using careful aseptic technique during suctioning and tracheostomy site care.

All humidifying equipment should be changed often in the hospital. Endotracheal and tracheostomy tubes are changed according to hospital routine.

Complications of intubation Whenever a foreign body is placed inside the trachea, there is a risk of infection, tissue change, or alteration in the cardiorespiratory function. Placement of the endotracheal tube may precipitate bradycardia or cardiac arrest as a result of vagal nerve stimulation. If the intubation was traumatic, blood may be present in the secretions suctioned from the tube. Once an endotracheal tube is in place, its patency must be constantly monitored. Asphyxia can result if secretions obstruct the tube. Whether the child is nasally or orally intubated, there is a possibility of tissue breakdown and ulceration from the pressure of the tube. This is also possible in the larynx.

Edema of the glottis is caused by trauma during intubation, maintenance care, or an allergic response. One of the first signs of glottal edema is *inspiratory stridor.* The swelling progresses for about 24 h after removal of the tube. The sooner it appears, the more serious it is. Usually reassurance, careful observation, and aerosol treatment are helpful. Racemic epinephrine may be ordered for administration by a hand-held nebulizer. Steroids may also be given by inhalation or intravenously. Usually this treatment will avoid the necessity of reintubation. Subglottal edema is even more serious and often requires the reestablishment of an artificial airway.

After the endotracheal tube is removed, the child will experience a sore throat and hoarse voice for a short peroid of time. Laryngospasm is more common in infants and children than in adults after extubation. It usually lasts 30 s or so and can be relieved by the administration of high oxygen concentrations.

Other complications that can develop from intubation include vocal cord granulomas, vocal cord paralysis, a laryngotracheal web (which develops from several days to weeks after extubation and should be suctioned out), and tracheal stenosis due to scarring.

Home care of a tracheostomy As more and more children with congenital and acquired defects of the trachea and related structures survive with long-term tracheostomies, nurses must be prepared to teach families how to manage their care at home. Aradine has listed the following initial concerns of parents about home care of a tracheostomy:[16]

1. Obtaining the needed equipment and keeping it in working order
2. Hearing the child at night
3. Being unable to provide the proper care in case of complications, such as infection

Once the child is home, the parents find that providing care can be extremely demanding. Their life-styles change, and they may feel isolated and confined to the home. The parents worry about the child's development in relation to language and school.

Parents can be helped to cope with home care of a child with a tracheostomy when the nurse:

1. Includes the family in setting goals for the teaching-learning process
2. Carefully assesses the child's and the family's perceptions, needs, readiness, and resources
3. Includes the parents in the child's care from the very beginning

Table 21-5 Two-Nurse Procedure for Suctioning an Endotracheal or Tracheostomy Tube*

First Nurse

1. Obtains needed equipment:
   a. Disposable suction kit: one sterile glove, aspirating catheter (ratio of catheter size to lumen should be 1 to 3 or 1 to 2), and container for sterile water.
   b. Sterile normal saline (if needed as a lavage to loosen secretions).
   c. Sterile gauze 4- by 4-in gauze pads (no filler).
   d. Sterile deionized water (to rinse catheter and lubricate tip).
   e. Ventilating bag connected to oxygen supply with flow meter.
2. Opens sterile suction kit:
   a. Adds sterile deionized water to container.
   b. Puts on sterile glove (dominant hand).
   c. Using gloved hand, picks up sterile catheter and connects it to suction tubing, held by ungloved hand.
3. Tests suction by occluding side hole and placing tip in sterile deionized water.

Second nurse

4. Stabilizes endotracheal or tracheostomy tube and disconnects it from ventilating machine or tracheostomy tube that delivers humidified air.
5. *Carefully hyperventilates* child with a hand-operated ventilator bag that is connected to oxygen source 10% higher than the child's oxygen.
6. May order sterile normal saline (0.5 to 2 ml) as a lavage to loosen secretions *before* hyperventilating.

First nurse

7. Introduces catheter gently, to end of tube.
8. Intermittently *suctions* (60 to 100 mmHg) while withdrawing catheter. Catheter may be rotated if it has only one opening. Suctioning should take no longer than 10 s. Nurse may estimate time tube should be occluded by holding breath.
9. Rinses catheter in sterile deionized water and wipes clean with the sterile 4- by 4-in gauze pads if necessary after each suctioning.

Second nurse

10. Repeats step 5. This reinflates alveoli that were collapsed by suctioning.

First nurse

11. Repeats suctioning as necessary *after* second nurse has repeated step 5. Hyperventilation must be done before suctioning, between suctions, and at the end of the procedure before the child is reconnected to a ventilator or humidifier.
12. Suctions the oropharynx last if necessary. Glove is turned inside out over used catheter, and both are discarded.
13. Auscultates the child's chest, listening for retained secretions and noting respiratory status. Records the procedure, the child's response, and the amount, consistency, and characteristics of secretions.

*This procedure helps maintain patency of the airway and prevents stasis of secretions. It must take place in sterile conditions, and the nurses must listen to breath sounds before beginning.

Source: Adapted from the nursing procedures of St. Mary's Hospital, Rochester, Minn., and Rainbow Babies' and Children's Hospital, Cleveland, Ohio.

4. Provides consistency in teaching and continuity in teachers and caregivers
5. Begins with simple tasks and progresses to more difficult ones, as the family demonstrates mastery
6. Encourages the siblings to be involved at a level appropriate for their development
7. Encourages self-responsibility in the child and the other family members
8. Includes another caregiver (e.g., a grandparent or a baby-sitter) and the community health nurse in the demonstration of home care techniques
9. Has the child and the family followed by an interdisciplinary tracheostomy clinic, if available, where their teaching can be reinforced and there is a possibility of membership in a parent and/or peer group, in which they can discuss their thoughts and feelings concerning the tracheostomy
10. Investigates all possible resources in the community that may help the family with teaching, baby-sitting, finances, and supplies*

*A helpful resource for the nurse and the parents is *Parents' Guide to Home Tracheostomy Care,* available for $5.00 from the Respiratory Therapy Department, Minneapolis Children's Medical Center, 2525 Chicago Ave. South, Minneapolis, Minn. 55404.

EPISTAXIS

Episodes of *epistaxis* (nosebleed) that are isolated and mild are common in children. The nose is a highly vascular structure and, as such, is highly sensitive to mild trauma to the anterior nasal septum; irritation from foreign bodies, nose picking or rubbing; vigorous nose blowing, and mucosal inflammation due to rhinitis. The manifestations, treatment, and nursing management of epistaxis are discussed in Chap. 33.

OBSTRUCTION OF THE RESPIRATORY TRACT

Foreign-body aspiration

Anything that an infant or child puts into his or her mouth has the potential to be aspirated. By far, pieces of food are the most commonly aspirated objects.[17] Foreign-body aspiration occurs most frequently in children between the ages of 6 months and 3 years. Aspiration of a foreign body into the airway can be very serious and even fatal. With accurate assessment and appropriate intervention, however, the prognosis is very good.

Pathophysiology With normal respirations, the airway expands on inspiration and becomes larger, while on expiration it contracts. This fact is useful in explaining the degree of obstruction which may be seen with foreign-body aspiration. Partial obstruction occurs when the aspirated object is small enough so that airflow around it is still possible during inspiration and expiration. A wheeze is heard. When the aspirated object is somewhat larger, airflow around it may be possible during inspiration, but obstruction occurs when the airway contracts during expiration. This results in air trapping distal to the obstruction. There is total obstruction when the object is large enough to block the airway completely during inspiration and expiration. Air distal to the obstruction is absorbed, and atelectasis results.

A foreign body may lodge anywhere within the tracheobronchial tree. Many objects are small enough to pass through the trachea and larynx and lodge in the main stem bronchi. The right main stem is the more common site because it is shorter and has a straight angle, which makes it easier to enter than the left.

Manifestations Initially, the symptoms are coughing, choking, or gagging. The child may then be symptom-free for a period of days to months. The clinical symptoms that follow depend on the type of foreign body, its location within the tracheobronchial tree, and the degree of obstruction. Sharp, penetrating, or large objects will cause clinical symptoms in a relatively short period of time. Cyanosis and other signs of respiratory distress will be apparent. An object that lodges in the larynx will produce hoarseness, cough, and a crouplike inspiratory stridor. Foreign bodies lodged in the trachea characteristically produce an asthmalike wheeze. An audible slap is heard, as air becomes trapped below the glottis. Objects which lodge in the bronchi may produce symptoms similar to those of pneumonia, and, in fact, repeated episodes of pneumonia may have occurred. Breath sounds may be decreased. Tracheal shift can be seen with significant air trapping. Respiratory distress can be quite marked as a result of atelectasis. Table 21-6 lists the locations of an aspirated foreign body and the accompanying symptoms.

Treatment Many aspirated foreign bodies do not show up on x-ray. Chest x-rays taken on full inspiration may appear normal, but with forced expiration they will show hyperventilation and air trapping distal to the object. If it has been several weeks since the object was aspirated, the chest x-ray may show atelectasis distal to the obstruction. The treatment of choice is removal of the foreign body by bronchoscopy. Antibiotics are given to treat infection. Chest physiotherapy may also be necessary.

Nursing management A complete and accurate history provides the first clue to the possibility of foreign-body aspiration. In one study, more than half the children who were subsequently diagnosed as having aspirated a foreign body had a positive history for choking or gagging while eating or playing.[18] Often the nurse is the first person who interviews the child and the parents while obtaining the admission history. It is also necessary to note the signs of respiratory dis-

Table 21-6 Location of an Aspirated Foreign Body and Accompanying Symptoms

Location	Symptoms
Larynx	Hoarseness, cough, dyspnea, stridor
Trachea	Wheeze, dyspnea, bilateral chest findings
Bronchus	Wheeze, emphysema, atelectasis

tress, the quality of the cough, and the presence and severity of wheezing and stridor. The abdominal thrust (the Heimlich maneuver) and the immediate management of a choking child are discussed in Chap. 16.

Prevention Children under 3 years of age are most prone to foreign-body aspiration and therefore must be watched carefully to prevent its occurrence. Parental education is essential. Small objects such as buttons, coins, and beads must be kept out of children's reach. Balloons also pose a risk. Children's toys should not have removable small parts. Food should be mashed or ground whenever appropriate. Uncut hot dogs or grapes are common hazards. Popcorn, nuts, beans, and hard candies are best avoided. Small children should be cautioned not to run when they have something in their mouths. It is extremely important to educate parents about the possibility of foreign-body aspiration, especially the parents of younger children.

CONGENITAL ALTERATIONS OF THE RESPIRATORY SYSTEM

Congenital alterations of the airway are uncommon. Most abnormalities produce stridor.

Choanal atresia

Choanal atresia is a congenital obstruction of one or both posterior nares at the entrance to the nasopharynx. The obstruction is usually membranous but may be due to bony growth. It occurs once in every 8000 births.[19]

If the obstruction is bilateral, the baby must breathe through the mouth. Because mouth breathing is difficult for the newborn, signs of respiratory distress are likely. The nasal obstruction also prevents the nasal discharge from draining posteriorly. Therefore, unilateral or bilateral rhinorrhea is a significant sign of this anomaly.

The diagnosis is suspected when a soft rubber catheter passed up the nose meets resistance. Contrast x-ray studies are usually done to confirm the diagnosis. An oral airway may be used initially to aid mouth breathing. The atresia plate is then pierced or removed by surgery.

Nursing management The infant must be closely observed for signs of respiratory distress. Feeding is done slowly, with several rest periods. These infants typically have trouble coordinating sucking and swallowing because of nasal obstruction. Usually they become adept at mouth breathing by 3 weeks.

Laryngeal abnormalities

Laryngomalacia is the most common (70 percent) congenital problem of the larynx. The larynx is unusually flaccid, causing collapse of the supraglottic structures. There is a high-pitched "crowing" on inspiration as the baby draws air through the narrow opening in the larynx. Crying, feeding, and a supine position usually make the stridor worse. The etiology is unknown. This condition will normally improve as the larynx grows, and it usually disappears by 1 to 2 years of age.

Nursing management The infant should be placed in a prone position when sleeping and resting; this allows the soft supraglottic structures to fall away from the airway.

The noisy respirations can be very frightening to the baby's parents. They will need continued support and reassurance as they learn to feed and care for their baby. Feeding should be done slowly. Special handling, positioning, and nipples may be necessary. In extreme cases, a tracheostomy or intubation may be required.

Tracheal abnormalities

Tracheomalacia is an uncommon lesion; the tracheal rings have an abnormal shape or are absent. It is usually associated with other congenital abnormalities. The condition resolves spontaneously over time. Severe cases may require a tracheostomy for support of respiratory status.

Tracheoesophageal fistulas are abnormal connections between the trachea and the esophagus. They are recognized at birth by the presence of feeding difficulties and cyanosis. Further details are given in Chap. 19.

Nursing management The infant requires frequent observations to ensure a patent airway. Keeping the airway clear of secretions is a priority. Nurses and parents must be keenly alert to color changes in the infant and must be able to assess respiratory difficulties accurately.

Other congenital alterations causing stridor

Other congenital conditions presenting with stridor include:

Vocal cord paralysis This is the second most common congenital laryngeal anomaly (10 percent).[20] It may be unilateral or bilateral, and intermittent cyanosis and aspiration occur during feedings. The symptoms are generally worse with bilateral paralysis. Pathology of other systems is often present (the cardiac, pulmonary, and central nervous systems). Spontaneous recovery does occur, but in severe cases a tracheostomy is necessary. The prognosis may depend on other, associated anomalies.

Congenital subglottic stenosis This defect consists of soft tissue thickening without inflammatory reaction. The point of greatest obstruction is seen 2 to 3 cm below the level of the true cords. Airway support is indicated in severe cases. Congenital subglottic stenosis can be associated with other congenital defects and syndromes.

Laryngeal webs These account for a small percentage of laryngeal anomalies and may be found above, at, or below the glottis. The majority are at the glottal level. The web can be a thin membrane, which is easily ruptured, or a thick, fibrous band of tissue. Complete absence of the larynx is incompatible with life if not recognized and treated immediately. Overall treatment depends on the thickness of the web. A tracheostomy may be necessary.

Subglottic hemangiomas The subglottic region is the most common site for these hemangiomas. Skin hemangiomas are present in about half the cases. Infants may have a hoarse cry in addition to stridor. There is a girl/boy ratio of 2 to 1. Hemangiomas in the airway usually decrease in size with age and disappear between the ages of 1 and 2 years. A tracheostomy and surgical intervention are necessary in severely obstructed infants.

ALTERATIONS IN RESPIRATORY FUNCTION DUE TO INFECTION

Infants and children are more susceptible than adults to infections of the respiratory tract because of their immunologic immaturity and because of their frequent contact with other immunologically incompetent children. The more contacts a child has, the more likely he or she is to develop a respiratory infection. Anatomic factors, described earlier in this chapter, prevent children from handling respiratory infections as well as adults do.

Infections of the respiratory tract can be classified according to the anatomic portion of the airway that is affected. They include (1) upper airway infections: nasopharyngitis and pharyngitis; (2) lower airway infections: croup syndromes, bronchitis, and bronchiolitis; and (3) lung infections: pneumonia and tuberculosis.

Upper respiratory infections

Upper respiratory infections (URIs) include (1) nasopharyngitis, or the common cold, and (2) pharyngitis or pharyngotonsillitis. Complications of upper respiratory infections include (1) otitis media, (2) retropharyngeal abscess, (3) cervical adenitis, and (4) chronic tonsillitis and adenoiditis. Upper respiratory infections are the most common acute infections in children and are caused by viruses, bacteria, fungi, or *Mycoplasma pneumoniae*. Age, allergies, chronic disease, number of exposures, environment, and the season all affect the incidence and the severity of the child's response to the infection.

Nasopharyngitis Acute viral *nasopharyngitis* (acute viral rhinitis), or the common cold, is the most frequent infectious disease of humans; the highest incidence is among children. Fifteen to thirty percent of all colds are due to the rhinovirus, with peak incidence occurring in the spring and fall. Children 1 to 5 years old are the most susceptible to colds, experiencing 10 to 12 per year. School-age children may have up to 6 colds a year. Younger children are also more apt to develop such complications as otitis media, bronchitis, and pneumonia because viral invasion of the nasopharynx damages the epithelium and makes it more vulnerable to a superimposed bacterial infection.

The symptoms of a cold result from inflammation due to *viral* invasion of the epithelium. Hyperemia and edema cause *rhinorrhea*, the clear, profuse, watery nasal discharge that characterizes the beginning of a cold. Nasal obstruction, sneezing, a mild sore throat and cough, and a low-grade fever often accompany the rhinorrhea. The younger the child is, the higher the fever. After 2 to 3 days, the nasal secretions become yellow and thickened.

The typical cold lasts 4 to 7 days, after an incubation period of 1 to 4 days.

Pharyngitis Infection and inflammation of the pharynx, tonsils, and cervical lymph nodes are characteristics of *pharyngitis*. The child is mildly to moderately ill, with a sore throat, swollen glands, headache, malaise, anorexia, and a fever. Sixty percent of pharyngitis cases occur in children between the ages of 2 and 8 years. Viruses account for the majority of cases. Group A beta hemolytic streptococcus (GABHS) is responsible for about 10 to 15 percent. The incidence peaks in children between 6 to 8 and 12 to 14 years.

Viral pharyngitis typically has a more gradual onset than bacterial pharyngitis. Its symptoms more closely resemble those of a viral upper respiratory infection.

Bacterial pharyngitis ("strep" throat) often presents more suddenly with a temperature increase up to 40°C (104°F), headache, severe sore throat, abdominal pain, and localized tender cervical nodes. A white exudate is typically seen on the reddened, enlarged tonsils.

Untreated children with pharyngitis due to GABHS can develop (1) acute rheumatic fever, (2) acute glomerulonephritis, or (3) abscesses, pneumonia, or osteomyelitis. Therefore, throat cultures are routinely done on all children with pharyngitis. Those with a history of rheumatic fever or other chronic illness may be treated immediately with benzathine penicillin intramuscularly, oral penicillin, or erythromycin. Treatment for those with positive cultures is begun once the results of the culture are obtained. A 48-h delay in starting treatment does not increase the incidence of rheumatic fever or glomerulonephritis and is beneficial in that it gives the child time to develop an antibody response. A new, 10-min test for strep throat is currently being tested. Oral antibiotics must be taken for 10 days to be effective. Since drug compliance decreases rapidly after treatment is begun, many physicians (and parents) prefer one injection of penicillin. Pharyngitis may also be the presenting symptom in diphtheria, gonococcal infection of the throat, or retropharyngeal abscess.

Flu or grippe This third category of upper airway infection is more commonly known as *flu* or *grippe*. The child becomes moderately ill without focal symptoms. There is muscle soreness, malaise, an elevated temperature (37.8 to 41°C [100 to 106°F]), headache, a dry cough, and sometimes mild nausea and diarrhea. The bronchial epithelium is affected, and pneumonia is an infrequent complication.

Nursing management Most children with an upper respiratory infection are treated at home. Therefore, the nurse becomes involved in educating and guiding the parents in giving effective care.

Symptomatic care includes rest, control of fever, hydration, good nutrition, and comfort measures. The child should rest at home, separated from other children. Stories, quiet games, television, and naps as needed help the child relax.

Ingestion of fluids must be encouraged in order to keep the child well hydrated and keep secretions liquefied. Often the child has a favorite, such as a certain soft drink or apple juice. Gelatin desserts, popsicles, pudding, and ice cream are often pleasing. When anorexia or nausea is present, clear fluids may be all that the child will tolerate. When there is diarrhea, dehydration may be likely. The parents should be taught to observe for signs of dehydration (see Chap. 16) and monitor the child's voiding pattern.

When the child has a fever acetaminophen can be given in age-appropriate doses every 4 to 6 h. Tepid sponge baths help reduce a high fever.

A cool mist vaporizer soothes inflamed mucous membranes and liquefies secretions. A warm saline gargle (2 tsp of salt per liter of water) is often soothing for the child who is old enough to manage the technique. If the cough is persistent, increasing hydration and giving lozenges, lollipops, or hard candy may help. Cough suppressants are seldom used, and then only at night. Nose drops are given with caution. There is rebound engorgement of the nasal mucosa if they are used for more than 3 days. For the very young infant, giving saline nose drops before feeding and sleeping may liquefy mucus, facilitating its removal. It is wise to clear the infant's nasal passages with a rubber bulb syringe before feeding. Petrolatum or a mild protective cream may be applied to the nostrils and upper lip to prevent excoriation from nasal secretions.

It is important for parents and children to understand that upper respiratory infections are very contagious. The severity of the infection, the amount of virus shed, and the length of contact all contribute to the possibility of spreading the infection. Careful hand-washing, covering the mouth and nose with a tissue when coughing or sneezing, using paper cups and individual towels in the bathroom and kitchen, and washing dishes in a dishwasher all help reduce the spread of disease. Children should be taught to blow the nose gently, one nostril at a time, to prevent ear infections.

As stated earlier, antibiotics, although ineffective for viral infections, are very important in treating streptococcal pharyngitis. Teaching should emphasize the difference between viral and bacterial infections. Parents should be instructed to seek professional help for their child when (1) the symptoms persist longer than 7 days; (2) the symptoms localize in the ears, throat, or neck; (3) there is localization of the symptoms in the lower chest, with purulent or bloody sputum; or (4) gastrointestinal symptoms or fever is prolonged.[21]

Acute otitis media

Pathophysiology *Acute otitis media* is an infection of the middle ear which occurs frequently following an upper respiratory infection in young children because of the anatomy of the eustachian tube. In infants, the eustachian tube is wider, shorter, and placed more horizontally than in older children. The supine position of the infant also favors the introduction of bacteria from the pharynx through the eustachian tube and into the middle ear. Older children often have enlarged lymphoid tissue, which obstructs the eustachian tube; they also have more frequent upper respiratory infections, predisposing them to otitis media. The most common causative organisms are *Hemophilus influenzae,* streptococci, and pneumococci.

An infant may have vague symptoms, such as irritability, prolonged crying, or fever, vomiting, and diarrhea following a cold. The child may pull at the involved ear. In the older child, infection also follows a cold, and the child complains of earache in addition to having a fever. Pain is due to the distention of the tympanic membrane. On examination, the tympanic membrane may appear red and bulging, with the light reflex muddled. Mobility of the tympanic membrane may be decreased.

Treatment Treatment is usually carried out at home unless an infant becomes dehydrated. Oral ampicillin is usually prescribed for 10 days; decongestants or antihistamines may also be given, although their value has not been substantiated. The physician may reevaluate the child in several days. A *myringotomy,* which is a small incision in the tympanic membrane, may be performed to relieve the pressure and permit drainage from the middle ear. Two weeks after the infection, the ears should be examined again, and the child checked for hearing loss.

Complications of acute otitis media include the development of a chronic form of otitis, mastoiditis, or meningitis. The child with chronic otitis media has recurring episodes of middle ear infection, which can lead to mastoiditis or to hearing loss due to immobilization of the ossicles and damage to the cochlea.

Nursing management Teaching parents how to care for a child with otitis media includes instructions in administering ampicillin and providing comfort measures. Ampicillin is absorbed best when given 1 h before meals. The medication should be given on time to maintain its blood level and continued for the full 10 days. It is tempting to discontinue the medication after the symptoms are relieved, especially if giving it involves a struggle. Occasionally, administration of ampicillin results in the appearance of a maculopapular rash or diarrhea. The physician should be notified; in most instances the medication will be continued.

For relief of pain, aspirin or acetaminophen can be given. Occasionally the child will require codeine. Suggest to the parents that they place the child with the head turned to the affected side and that they put a heating pad on a low setting underneath the ear. When using heating pads with small children, constant supervision is necessary to prevent burns. If pain persists or increases, if the temperature rises, or if the child becomes lethargic and appears to have a stiff neck, the physician should be notified. Tell the parents the importance of returning to the physician for evaluation after the infection has subsided.

Serous otitis media

Pathophysiology *Serous otitis media* is the most common cause of hearing loss among school-age children and is usually the result of eustachian tube dysfunction or adenoid hypertrophy. The eustachian tube serves multiple functions, including drainage of the middle ear secretions into the nasopharynx and ventilation of the middle ear to keep the air pressure in the middle ear equal to the air pressure in the outer ear. Serous otitis media results if any of these functions are compromised by one of the following factors: (1) obstruction of the tube by enlarged adenoids, mucosal edema, or allergic rhinitis; (2) residual purulent otitis media; (3) altitude changes; and (4) secretions by the middle ear mucosa in an allergic child.[22]

The most common symptoms of serous otitis media are a fluctuating hearing loss reported by the teacher or the parents, mild intermittent pain, and a feeling of fullness in the ear. Blockage of the eustachian tube results in a negative middle ear pressure, which leads to increased mucoid secretion and increased permeability of the middle ear capillaries. On ear examination, the tympanic membrane will appear retracted, making the landmarks more visible, and will look dull or blue; a fluid level or air bubbles may be seen behind the drum. A *tympanogram* is a graph which indicates the mobility of the tympanic membrane by measuring the air pressure on either side of it; in serous otitis media, the tympanic membrane is immobile.

Treatment Medical treatment usually consists of administering antibiotics, antihistamines, and decongestants. The child is taught exercises such as blowing balloons to reopen the eustachian tube. If treatment is not successful within 4 weeks, a small Teflon tube, resembling a small dumbbell, may be inserted into the tympanic membrane. The tube acts as a substitute eustachian tube by providing aeration into the middle ear. The tube works itself out into the external ear canal within 6 months. It may need to be reinserted if the condition has not resolved by then. An adenoidectomy may be performed at the time the tube is inserted. A possible complication of tube insertion is a permanent perforation of the tympanic membrane.

Nursing management Insertion of ventilating tubes into the tympanic membrane may be performed in an emergency outpatient department. The child is discharged several hours after the procedure when he or she is taking fluids orally and has voided. The child may be admitted to the pediatric unit if he or she lives some distance from the hospital or if an adenoidectomy is to be performed.

When the child is admitted, ask the parents whether the child has decreased hearing, and if so, note this on the Kardex. Postoperatively, the child returns to the unit awake and alert. Slight serous or mucoid drainage may be noted in the operative ear; the discharge can be wiped away, but cotton balls should not be inserted into the ear.

The nurse's role in preparing the child and the parents for discharge includes demonstrating the procedure for instilling ear drops and teaching the special precautions necessary as long as the tube is in place. Steroid ear drops may be prescribed to reduce inflammation. The medication should be discontinued if the child complains of pain. The parents will note an improvement in hearing when the drainage from the ear subsides.

Since the ventilating tube provides an open pathway into the middle ear, no water should be allowed in the ear. For bathing or shampooing, cotton balls coated with petroleum jelly can be inserted into the ear. Showering should be avoided until the tube is out. Swimming may be permitted if the child has well-fitting earplugs. Diving is contraindicated; without an intact tympanic membrane, the change in pressure that occurs during diving may rupture the oval or round window, leading to permanent deafness. A new type of ventilating tube, which is semipermeable and does not allow water into the middle ear, is now being used with some children.[23]

The parents should contact the doctor if hearing again decreases or if drainage increases. The child will be rechecked about 2 weeks after tube insertion and every 3 or 4 months until the tube is removed.

Retropharyngeal abscess

A *retropharyngeal abscess* results from the bacterial infection of lymph nodes that drain the adenoids or nasopharynx. It occurs almost exclusively in children under 3 years of age. Symptoms include fever, hyperextension of the neck, and painful swallowing, often evidenced by an open mouth and drooling. Examination of the pharynx reveals a bulge on one side of the posterior portion. Soft tissue neck films help confirm the diagnosis.

Surgical drainage of the abscess is done with the child in the head-down position to prevent aspiration of the purulent material. Intravenous hydration and antibiotic therapy are begun prior to surgical drainage.

Cervical adenitis Acute *cervical adenitis* results from secondary bacterial infection of a lymph node that drains the nose or throat. This complication of an upper respiratory infection is most common in preschoolers. The child has a unilateral swollen neck mass and a sustained high fever. An elevated white blood count and a positive throat culture help confirm the diagnosis.

Prompt treatment with antibiotics may prevent suppuration and abscess formation. If the abscess localizes, however, surgical incision and drainage are necessary.

Tonsillitis and adenoiditis *Tonsillitis,* or inflammation of the ring of lymphoid tissue around the entrance to the pharynx, can occur after pharyngitis. Inflammation and swelling of the faucial tonsils cause the child to have difficulty swallowing and breathing. *Adenoiditis,* or inflammation of the pharyngeal tonsils (adenoids), blocks the posterior nasal passages and causes the child to mouth-breathe.

Repeated bouts of pharyngitis and upper respiratory infections lead to chronic tonsillitis and airway interference. At one time, removal of the tonsillar tissue was routine in almost all children. Most physicians currently believe that this surgery is undesirable as a routine procedure because of the great surgical risk and that it is also detrimental because valuable protective lymphoid tissue is removed. Currently, a tonsillectomy, an adenoidectomy, or both are reserved for use in children who have one or more of the following:

1. Persistent nasal obstruction and mouth breathing, resulting in snoring and hyponasal speech
2. Persistent oral obstruction and dysphagia
3. Recurrent peritonsillar abscess
4. Sleep apnea
5. Recurrent aspiration pneumonia

Usually this surgery is performed when the child is around 4 to 6 years of age. Preoperative teaching is extremely important to reduce the trauma of hospitalization. Bleeding and clotting times are checked preoperatively because hemorrhage is the most common surgical complication. Preoperative care is similar to that for children who have undergone other surgical procedures. Postoperative care is summarized in Table 21-7.

Lower respiratory infections

Because the larynx can be considered the transitional area between the upper and lower airways, infections that compromise its function are considered with those of the lower airway. Infections of the larynx are somewhat more likely to extend to the trachea and bronchi than are upper respiratory infections.

When caring for children with any kind of respiratory disease, the nurse must be constantly on the alert for the following signs of respiratory failure and must report them immediately:

1. Decreased or absent inspiratory breath sounds
2. Severe inspiratory retractions and use of the accessory muscles
3. A depressed level of consciousness and a diminished response to pain

Table 21-7 Summary of Postoperative Care for a Child Who Has Had a Tonsillectomy and/or an Adenoidectomy

1. The child is placed on the abdomen or side to facilitate drainage from the mouth until fully alert.
2. The child is constantly observed for signs of hemorrhage such as:
   a. Frequent swallowing (count number per minute)
   b. Tachycardia (more than 120 beats per minute)
   c. Pallor
   d. Vomiting of bright-red blood
3. Suction equipment should be available for airway obstruction. Suctioning must be done extremely cautiously to avoid trauma to the surgical site.
4. Comfort measures are taken to ease sore throat, including:
   a. Ice collar
   b. Analgesics
   c. Mild sedation
5. Once the child is fully awake and alert, give clear fluids—e.g., cool water, Jell-O, apple juice—and then sherbet, soup, ice cream, and pudding. Soft, nonirritating foods are continued for several days.
6. Alert the parents to signs of complications after discharge.
   a. Hemorrhage 5 to 10 days postoperatively due to tissue sloughing during healing
   b. Persistent cough or earache

4. Poor skeletal muscle tone
5. Cyanosis in 40 percent ambient oxygen
6. A Pa_{CO2} equal to, or more than, 75 mmHg or a Pa_{O2} of less than 100 mmHg in 100 percent oxygen
7. Tachypnea and tachycardia

Croup syndromes A variety of respiratory inflammations characterized by inspiratory stridor and hoarse cough, usually of rapid onset, constitute the *croup syndrome*. Acute laryngotracheobronchitis (viral croup) is the most common form, whereas epiglottitis (bacterial croup) is the most serious. Table 21-8 compares three types of croup.

Acute laryngotracheobronchitis The word *croup* is derived from the old Scottish word *croup*, meaning "to cry out in a hoarse voice." *Acute laryngotracheobronchitis* (viral croup) is usually caused by parainfluenza or influenza A viruses. Children between 6 months and 3 years are most commonly affected, with the peak incidence occurring in the second year of life. Viral croup is a much more common cause of stridor in children than bacterial croup. Some children have repeated episodes of viral croup, known as *acute spasmodic laryngitis*.

Pathophysiology The vocal cords, subglottic tissue, trachea, bronchi, and bronchioles are all involved in the inflammatory exudative process. Edema of the subglottic area, however, causes the characteristic inspiratory stridor and makes the greatest contribution to obstruction of the airway.

Typically, the child has what at first appears to be a mild upper respiratory infection. As the disease progresses, the child develops a characteristic barking or brassy cough and a hoarse voice. Often the child goes to sleep in fairly good condition and awakens later at night with inspiratory stridor.

Because air is sucked in through the narrowed subglottic area, the negative pressure on inspiration tends to narrow further the already compromised airway (like sucking on a plugged

Table 21-8 Comparison of Three Types of Croup

	Type of Croup		
	Bacterial Croup (Epiglottitis)	**Viral Croup (Laryngotracheobronchitis)**	**Spasmodic Croup (Spasmodic Laryngitis or "Midnight Croup")**
Location of obstruction	Supraglottal, at the epiglottis	Subglottal, below the vocal cords	Glottal, at the vocal cords
Age at onset	3 to 7 years	1 to 3 years	3 months to 3 years
Etiology	Usually *Hemophilus influenzae* type B pneumococci	Viral, often parainfluenza virus	Unknown—mild virus, allergy, or emotional component suspected
Onset	Rapid, 4 to 12 hours	Gradual, often during the course of an upper respiratory infection	Sudden, usually at night
Clinical manifestations	High fever; inspiratory stridor; severe sore throat with pain on swallowing; drooling; secretions; muffled voice	Slight temperature elevation; inspiratory stridor; brassy cough; retractions; a high pulse	Stridor on inspiration; cough; retractions; high pulse
Diagnosis	By lateral neck films; white blood count 15,000 to 25,000; observation of inflamed epiglottis	By clinical manifestations and absence of inflamed epiglottis	By clinical manifestations
Treatment	IV ampicillin; observation for increasing respiratory distress; cool mist; IV hydration; fever control; intubation and mechanical support of respirations	Cool mist; observation for increasing respiratory distress; IV hydration; racemic epinephrine aerosols; tracheostomy for severe obstruction	Cool mist, usually managed at home

straw). Respiratory effort is increased. The child appears distressed, frightened, and anxious. Suprasternal, supraclavicular, and substernal retractions are common. The respiratory rate increases to 50 or more per minute. Coarse rales may be heard on auscultation.

As the obstruction increases, so does hypoxemia. Cyanosis may develop when the Pa_{o2} falls below 60 mmHg. Decreased perfusion and decreased ventilation can combine to produce respiratory failure in severe cases, making artificial ventilation necessary.

Treatment When arterial blood gases indicate hypoxemia, the child is given humidified oxygen to raise the Pa_{o2}. Humidification is usually given by ultrasonic nebulizer to thin secretions (Fig. 2-11). Fluids are administered parenterally to improve hydration. Antibiotics are not useful in treating this viral infection unless a bacterial infection is superimposed on it.

If the child is particularly fatigued and is experiencing respiratory distress, racemic epinephrine by IPPB may aid in decreasing stridor and retractions. Mechanical ventilation becomes necessary when (1) the Pa_{co2} rises progressively (above 45 mmHg), (2) oxygen therapy does not improve hypoxemia, and (3) the child has copious secretions that cannot be mobilized by coughing or increasing hydration.

Nursing Management Although most children with viral croup can be managed at home with increased humidity, fluids, antipyretics, and measures to decrease anxiety, some need hospitalization. The child and the parents will be frightened and anxious and will need calm reassurance.

Assessment of the child's respiratory status must be made frequently by monitoring color, cyanosis, arterial blood gases, respiratory pattern and difficulty, and vital signs. Often the mist tent or croup tent prevents soothing of the child by the parents, thus adding to the discomfort. The child also needs to be kept dry and prevented from being chilled in the moist environment.

The nurse must observe the child's responses to humidity and oxygen. An increase in heart rate, restlessness, retractions and cyanosis, along with a decrease in respiratory rate, indicate the need for an artificial airway and mechanical respiratory support.

Some very young children will continue to have periodic bouts of viral croup that always occur at night. The child does not have a fever but may have been exposed to excessive cold or may have a history of allergies. The parents learn to cope with stridor and respiratory distress by providing cool or warm humidity at night. They need to know that they can provide quick relief by sitting with the child near a hot shower for 15-20 min that is producing steam in a closed bathroom. This procedure may prevent a trip to the emergency room. Table 21-9 summarizes the nursing care for a child with viral croup.

Epiglottitis *Epiglottitis* (bacterial croup) is a life-threatening disease that can occur at any age. Without prompt treatment, it can progress rapidly to death by closing off the airway.

Pathophysiology This acute bacterial infection is usually due to *Hemophilus influenzae*. Its onset is rapid—less than a day. The symptoms

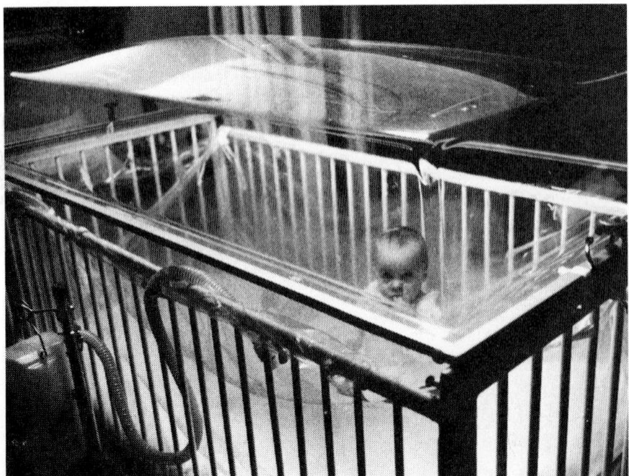

Figure 21-11 A 14-month-old child with croup. Note the ultrasonic nebulizer at the left. (*Photo by P. Sheps.*)

Table 21-9 Summary of Nursing Care for a Child with Viral Croup (Laryngotracheobronchitis)

1. Administer cool mist with humidified oxygen to relieve swelling and liquefy secretions.
2. Assess respiratory status continually:
   a. Assess rate and quality of respirations.
   b. Monitor blood gas values.
   c. Assess skin color and perfusion of extremities.
3. Maintain adequate level of hydration by oral fluid intake or IV supplements.
4. Provide a quiet environment to encourage restfulness. Arrange nursing care to allow for periods of uninterrupted rest.
5. Support the parents' involvement in the child's care in order to reassure the child and the parents.

are a sore throat, a high fever, a muffled voice, and quickly developing signs of respiratory obstruction: inspiratory stridor, retractions, restlessness, inability to swallow, drooling of secretions, and respiratory distress. The child assumes an upright position, leaning forward and drooling, with the mouth open and the tongue protruding. The child appears pale, "shocky," and frightened.[23]

Treatment A definitive diagnosis of epiglottitis is made on the basis of clinical signs and symptoms, laboratory findings that include an elevated white blood count (above 15,000), and lateral neck films suggesting swelling at the epiglottis. Direct visualization of the swollen epiglottis confirms the diagnosis. The examination should be made in an area where intubation can be done quickly, since visualization and manipulation often lead to airway spasm with complete obstruction.

Once elective intubation has been done, the child will be cared for in an intensive care unit. Mechanical ventilation or PEEP is used, along with oxygen therapy and humidification of the airway. The antibiotic of choice is chloramphenicol given intravenously. The endotracheal tube can be removed when the swelling has decreased and the child's temperature has returned to normal, usually in about 48 to 72 h.

Nursing Management Since epiglottitis is an emergency, the nurse must make an immediate assessment of the child's respiratory status and notify the physician. The parents and the child will be extremely frightened. A calm, knowledgeable nurse is essential. The nurse's initial responsibilities include assisting the physician with airway placement, oxygen therapy and humidification, intravenous fluids and antibiotics, measurement of arterial blood gases, and cultures. Once these emergency measures are instituted, the child will need rest and reassurance, endotracheal tube care, careful observation and frequent assessment of respiratory status, management of secretions, and care directed toward meeting his or her basic human needs.

Bronchitis *Bronchitis* refers to a condition in which the child has a chronic or acute nonproductive cough. The cough may be due to an infection or to chemical or mechanical irritation of the bronchial epithelium. In children, bronchitis usually follows croup, pneumonia, or an upper respiratory infection. Increasing humidity at night, lozenges and cough drops, postural drainage, and expectorants may be helpful.

Bronchiectasis Whenever a child develops a chronic cough that produces sputum, *bronchiectasis* may be present. It can follow repeated cases of pneumonia or measles or aspiration of a foreign body. It is also a complication of cystic fibrosis.

In bronchiectasis, saccular deformities of the bronchi and bronchioles develop, and secretions accumulate within them. The sputum is grayish white. Usually the diagnosis is made by bronchoscopy. A child who has a positive throat culture should be treated with an appropriate antibiotic. Mist and postural drainage are helpful. If the disease continues to progress, surgery to remove the diseased area of the lung may be indicated.

Bronchiolitis *Bronchiolitis* is an infection of the lower respiratory tract caused by the respiratory syncytial virus. It is seen most commonly during the winter in infants under 1 to 2 years, especially those aged 2 to 6 months.

Pathophysiology Initially the infant may appear to have an upper respiratory infection with a watery nasal discharge. The infection of the bronchiolar mucosa soon causes inflammation, edema, and the production of mucosal exudates that lead to obstruction of the small and medium airways.

Air passes into the air sacs but becomes trapped, eventually causing overinflation. This condition leads to obstructive emphysema and patchy areas of atelectasis. Because of the increase in airway resistance, the infant has prolonged and difficult expirations.

The heart rate increases up to 200/min. Respiratory rates may go as high as 80 per minute. Wheezing and rhonchi are heard on auscultation. The baby may have a troublesome, distressing cough. The chest takes on a barrel shape, and retractions are common. The infant appears anxious and restless and is often unable to eat. Bronchiolitis will often get worse before it gets better, lasting 7 to 14 days.

Nursing management Basic supportive care is essential for an infant with bronchiolitis. Usually, humidified oxygen is necessary to increase the Pa_{O2}. Elevating the head of the bed 30° or placing the baby in a padded seat makes the work of breathing easier. Aerosol therapy may also be used occasionally. Sedation is avoided because of the danger of depressing respiration.

During the acute phase, intravenous fluids are necessary to maintain hydration. Arterial blood gases and pH are measured, and respiratory status is monitored frequently.

Because bronchiolitis epidemics can occur in hospitals, especially among chronically ill children, it is imperative to isolate these infants from others and to use proper hand-washing techniques. Any respiratory equipment used must be thoroughly cleaned before being used with another child.

Lung infections

Pneumonia *Pneumonia* is an inflammation of the alveoli and pulmonary interstitium. It results from a number of factors, including (1) continuous spread of infection from other portions of the lower respiratory tract, (2) aspiration of infectious agents from the upper respiratory tract, (3) a secondary invasion by pathogenic organisms in a compromised lung, and (4) aspiration of a foreign body or substance.

Incidence Because acute respiratory infections are so prevalent in young children, the infrequent complication of these infections, pneumonia, becomes a relatively common pediatric diagnosis. The incidence of pneumonia is approximately 40 per 1000 in preschool-age children and drops gradually to 9 per 1000 in 15-year-olds.[24]

Pathophysiology *Pneumonia* is a generalized inflammation and infection of the lung parenchyma. It may be disseminated throughout the lungs (bronchopneumonia) or confined to a specific area (lobular pneumonia). An elevation in the white blood cell count, a characteristic infiltration that shows on x-rays, and cultures of organisms from the trachea or blood all help in the diagnostic process.

A logical way to classify pneumonias is by causative agent. The most common causative agents are viruses, bacteria, *Mycoplasma pneumoniae,* and foreign substances. See Table 21-10.

Viral pneumonia is seen in children of all ages. It has a gradual onset, often after an upper respiratory infection.The child develops a dry, hacking, nonproductive cough; has a slight increase in respiratory rate; and appears mildly ill. Abdominal distention is often present as a result of air swallowing and paralytic ileus. The child's temperature ranges from 37.8 to 40°C (100 to 104°F). On auscultation, inspiratory crepitant rales and expiratory rhonchi may be heard. X-rays reveal infiltration. Treatment of viral pneumonia is symptomatic.

During winter and early spring, the respiratory syncytial virus is the most frequent cause of lower respiratory disease in infants under 6 months of age as well as of upper respiratory disease in older children. This virus spreads easily in families and hospitals. The most effective prophylactic measure is careful hand-washing. Pneumonia caused by this virus produces severe distress in infants because of the plugging of smaller airways with necrotic cells, fibrin, and mononuclear cells. This mechanical obstruction results in areas of hyperaeration and atelectasis.[25] Supportive treatment for very young and debilitated infants with this infection frequently involves mechanical ventilation.

Bacterial pneumonia, in contrast to viral pneumonia, usually has a sudden onset. The child appears very ill with a high fever, respiratory distress, and sometimes chest pain. The child may be restless and apprehensive. Circumoral cyanosis, retractions, tachypnea, and tachycardia indicate the seriousness of the illness. See Table 21-11.

In *pneumococcal pneumonia,* the alveoli become edematous and filled with inflammatory cells. Then, during the stage of *red hepatization,* serum and red blood cells enter the alveoli, thereby interfering with gas exchange. The stage of *gray hepatization* follows when leukocytes and fibrin fill the alveoli. Resolution occurs when the inflammatory reaction is over.

Most bacterial pneumonias are caused by pneumococci, but *Staphylococcus, Streptococcus group A,* and *Hemophilus influenzae* are also culprits.

Ten to twenty percent of hospital admissions for pneumonia involve the *M. pneumoniae* organism, which causes atypical primary pneumonia. Usually school-age children are affected. Signs and symptoms include fever, chills, malaise, myalgia, anorexia, sore throat, and a dry, hacking cough that later becomes mucopurulent.

Pneumonia also occurs after aspiration of hydrocarbons and lipids. Hydrocarbon pneumonia results from aspiration following coughing and vomiting after ingestion of gasoline, kerosene, or solvents. Respiratory symptoms develop within the first few hours and may be severe because of the pneumonitis and atelectasis that ensue. Treatment is similar to that for any lower respiratory tract inflammation and consists of humidification, oxygen therapy, hydration, ventilatory support, and treatment of any secondary infec-

Table 21-10 Comparison of Four Major Types of Pneumonia

	Viral Pneumonia	Bacterial Pneumonia	Mycoplasma Pneumonia	Pneumonia Due to a Foreign Substance
Epidemiology	Any age; may be seasonal. Common agents include respiratory syncytial virus, adenovirus, and influenza virus	Any age, but occurs most frequently in infants. Most common in winter and early spring	Most common cause of lower respiratory tract infections in children over 5 years of age; follows an upper respiratory infection	All ages. May be chronic or emergent. Incidence related to a specific substance, e.g., meconium aspiration in newborns, gastric acid in children with reduced consciousness or an incompetent cardioesophageal sphincter, and complications of ingestion of a foreign substance
Pathophysiology	Usually involves both airways and alveoli. Interstitial pneumonitis; inflammation of mucosa of the bronchi and bronchioles	Varies according to specific agent (see Table 21-11)	Infectious agent *Mycoplasma pneumoniae*	Clinical pneumonitis
Clinical manifestations	Mildly elevated temperature (below 39°C); tachypnea, cough, sore throat, conjunctivitis; diffuse bilateral rales and retractions	History of abrupt onset of mild upper respiratory infection with high temperature (above 39°C) and shaking chills; productive cough, chest pain, rhonchi, wheezing	Mildly elevated temperature (below 39°C); gradually worsening upper respiratory infection; rash; conjunctivitis, pharyngitis, diarrhea, nonproductive cough, bilateral wheezing	Cough, cyanosis, tachypnea, rales, wheezing
Laboratory and x-ray findings	Interstitial infiltrate in diffuse distribution; white blood count above 15,000; lymphocytes predominate	Alveolar infiltrate; patchy or consolidated distribution; white blood count above 15,000; granulocytes predominate	Alveolar-interstitial patchy infiltrates in single or contiguous lobes; white blood count normal or slightly elevated	Depends on substance; white blood count within normal limits
Therapy	Humidified oxygen; vigorous pulmonary physiotherapy; tracheal intubation and mechanical ventilation if necessary; antibiotics only for secondary infections	Antibiotics specific for agent (see Table 21-11)	Erythromycin and tetracycline for 7 to 10 days	Supportive care; humidified oxygen; pulmonary physiotherapy; antibiotics only for secondary infections
Complications	Atelectasis, bronchiectasis, fibrosis; may lead to respiratory failure in very young infants and compromised patients	Septicemia, septic shock, lung abscess, pleural effusion, emphysema, pneumothorax, respiratory failure	Very rare	Respiratory failure

Table 21-11 Bacterial Pneumonias

Organism	Children Affected	Signs and Symptoms	Laboratory Reports	Treatment
Staphylococcus	Infant, under 1 year of age	History of furunculosis, recent hospitalization, or maternal breast abscess. Respiratory infection, upper or lower, for several days to 1 week followed by abrupt change—fever, cough, respiratory distress, tachypnea, grunting respirations, sternal and subcostal retractions, cyanosis, anxiety. Lethargic if undisturbed and irritable if roused. Pyopneumothorax, pneumatoceles, and empyema as the clinical course progresses	White blood count within normal range in young infants, 20,000 per cubic millimeter, with predominant polymorphonuclear leukocytes in older infants. Tracheal aspiration and/or pleural tap culture positive. X-ray: patchy infiltration or dense (bronchopneumonia or lobar pneumonia)	Symptomatic and supportive. Oxygen, semi-Fowler's position, parenteral fluids during acute phase, methicillin or penicillin G for 3 weeks IV or IM, thoracentesis, closed-chest drainage with extensive involvement for 5 to 7 days, hospitalization for 6 to 10 weeks
Streptococcus group A	Children 3 to 5 years of age	Mild prodromal symptoms followed by sudden onset of high fever, chills, respiratory distress. Clinical course similar to that of staphylococcal infections. Complications: empyema and bacterial foci in bones and joints	White blood count elevated with polymorphonuclear leukocytes predominating. ASO titer elevated, positive culture. X-ray: disseminated infiltration	Symptomatic and supportive. Penicillin G, thoracentesis, closed-chest drainage
Hemophilus influenzae	Infants and young children	Mild or severe. Insidious onset. Clinical course subacute and prolonged, of several weeks' duration. Signs and symptoms similar to those of pneumococcal infections. Signs and symptoms in young infants associated with bacteremia and emphysema. Complications: bacteremia, pericarditis, cellulitis, empyema, meningitis, pyarthrosis	Bacteremia, positive cultures, moderate leukocytosis with lymphopenia. X-ray: lobar consolidation	Symptomatic and supportive. Ampicillin.
Pneumococcus	Children 1 to 4 years of age	Sudden onset preceded by upper respiratory infection. High fever and chills in older children. Tachypnea, productive cough, chest pain, depressed breath sounds, abdominal pain, anorexia	White blood count elevated, 18,000 to 40,000 per cubic millimeter, with polymorphonuclear leukocytes. X-ray: patchy infiltrates. Positive sputum culture	Supportive and symptomatic. Penicillin G

Source: Adapted from G. Scipien, M. V. Barnard, M. A. Chard, J. Howe, and P. J. Phillips (eds.), *Comprehensive Pediatric Nursing*, 3d ed., McGraw-Hill, New York, 1986, pp. 874–5. Used with permission.

tions with antibiotics. Death after hydrocarbon ingestion is usually due to hepatic failure rather than to respiratory complications.[26] (See the section, "Hydrocarbons" in Chap. 33.)

Lipid pneumonia results from the aspiration of oily substances such as medications suspended in oil or formula and the accumulation of these substances in the alveoli. Children especially at risk for this type of pneumonia are those with cleft palates, those debilitated by poor gag reflexes, and those who are force-fed. Supportive treatment includes humidification, postural drainage, and treatment of secondary infections. Nursing care involves not only supportive measures but also preventive measures when feeding or administering medications to children at risk.

Treatment Children usually recover from viral pneumonias with supportive care at home. Bacterial pneumonias were a serious threat to a child's life before antibiotic therapy was developed.

Antibiotics, fluids, antipyretics, and rest are the principal elements of care for children with pneumonia. For very young children, hospitalization may be more appropriate because of the availability of oxygen and intravenous therapy and because of variability in illness.

Because pneumonia is treated thoroughly and early, the complications of pneumothorax and empyema (accumulation of pus) do not occur as often as they once did. Nevertheless, a thoracentesis may be necessary to remove fluid or pus from the pleural cavity. If purulent fluid is obtained, continuous closed-chest drainage is begun (see Figs. 22-18 to 22-20 for care of a child with chest suction).

Signs of *pneumothorax*, the accumulation of air between the parietal and visceral layers of the pleura, include chest pain, difficulty in breathing, and cyanosis. Breath sounds are absent over the affected lung. With large amounts of air or fluid, there can be *mediastinal shift*—displacement of the heart, trachea, esophagus, vena cava, and aorta to the unaffected side. Arterial blood gases reveal a decreased Pa_{o2}. Pulmonary-function studies indicate a decrease in forced expiratory volume, vital capacity, and compliance. A thoracentesis must be done, a chest tube inserted, and a connection made to a closed-chest drainage system to allow reexpansion of the lung.

Nursing management Nursing management of the child with pneumonia is directed toward supporting vital functions and meeting basic needs as well as carrying out the medical treatment plan. Oxygen therapy using cool, humidified mist helps improve alveolar gas exchange.

Airway patency is helped by proper positioning, postural drainage of secretions, humidification, and suctioning if necessary.

Supporting the child in a semierect position alleviates pressure on the diaphragm from the abdominal contents. When the pneumonia is unilateral, lying on the affected side may reduce discomfort from pleural rubbing by splinting of the chest.

Fever should be treated with antipyretics as ordered. Although the cool environment of the mist tent may also be helpful in reducing fever, tents are seldom used. Frequent changes of clothing and bed linen will prevent chilling in the moist environment of the tent.

The child with pneumonia must be monitored for signs of dehydration leading to electrolyte imbalance. If the child is in severe respiratory distress, he or she will be given nothing by mouth in order to prevent aspiration and will need intravenous fluids for maintenance. If the child is well enough to drink, cool, high-calorie fluids are given slowly and in small amounts to prevent aspiration and abdominal distention.

Rest and conservation of energy are important. Parental presence is very reassuring to the young child and can be very important in keeping the child calm. Nursing care should be organized so as to provide undisturbed periods of rest for both the child and the parents.

Perhaps the most important intervention in the nursing care of the child with pneumonia is frequent assessment of the child's respiratory status to determine response to medical and nursing treatment as well as to quickly identify any complications. The frequency of assessment is determined by the condition of the child and may vary from continuous monitoring by an individual or a cardiopulmonary monitor to periodic observations every 1 to 4 h.

The nurse's judgment is crucial in recognizing the signs and symptoms of serious complications, such as pneumothorax or impending respiratory failure. The signs of respiratory failure include cyanosis, nasal flaring, increased retractions, wheezing, prolonged expirations, headache, and restlessness. The more immediate signs of respiratory failure include increasing restlessness, tachypnea or apnea, and diaphoresis. Prompt initiation of mechanical ventilatory support can be a lifesaving measure.

Tuberculosis *Tuberculosis* is no longer a major cause of morbidity and mortality in the United States because of the introduction of chemotherapeutic agents in the 1940s and improvements in public health standards.[27] Despite the eradication of epidemic tuberculosis, it still occurs in some parts of the United States, such as metropolitan ghettos, Indian reservations, and areas with high concentrations of immigrants.

Because the dormant tubercle bacilli can remain alive in the host for years, complete extinction of the disease is unlikely. The decrease in the incidence of tuberculosis has resulted in an increased number of susceptible individuals. Children with multiple drug resistance, although few in number, also remain a problem.[28]

Individuals who are more susceptible to infection from the tubercle bacilli include nonwhites, the very young and very old, pregnant women, and people in certain occupations, such as nurses, chefs, and truck drivers.[29]

Screening Screening for tuberculosis is now recommended only when there is a high risk that a group of people will develop the disease or when a sporadic case would represent a significant hazard. Screening is directed toward those who have not been identified as having the disease. Current guidelines suggest that screening be done when:[30]

1. A group of people have a high rate of tuberculosis (e.g., Mexican immigrant workers and American Indians)
2. A group of people have a high rate of tuberculosis and are at risk for developing the disease (e.g., persons over 50 years and Asian-American immigrants)
3. People are in an environment in which they are at high risk for becoming infected (e.g., health care and correctional institutions)
4. People, although at low risk for getting tuberculosis, have the potential of infecting young children or others with a suppressed immune response if they develop the disease (e.g., teachers in schools, day-care centers, and resident facilities for young people and workers in acute or long-term health care facilities and correctional institutions)

Primary tuberculosis *Primary tuberculosis* is the initial infection with *Mycobacterium tuberculosis*. After the primary infection occurs in the lung, any one of the following can happen:

1. The infection can heal. This happens in more than 90 percent of those infected. Hypersensitivity to the tuberculin organism then occurs, causing a positive tuberculin skin test. A fraction of 1 percent of children entering school, but more than 50 percent of persons over 60 years, show evidence of infection (a positive tuberculin skin test).
2. The primary infection can develop into active disease. Active disease is usually discovered through a positive skin test or because of a history of exposure to a person with tuberculosis.
3. The primary infection heals, but months or years later becomes reactivated. Factors that predispose a person to reactivation tuberculosis include the menarche, poor nutrition, a debilitating disease, diabetes, pregnancy, cancer, and steroid or immunosuppressive therapy.[31] About 30,000 people in the United States develop active or reactivation tuberculosis each year.[32]

Pathophysiology The tubercle bacillus is carried on an airborne droplet nucleus produced when an infected person coughs, sneezes, sings, talks, or laughs. Because these droplets are so small, they can be kept airborne by normal room air currents. These droplet nuclei then enter the body through the respiratory tract in almost all cases. Rarely, *M. tuberculosis* enters through the gastrointestinal tract or through a break in the skin or a mucous membrane.

When tubercle bacilli reach the lungs in a susceptible host, they lodge in a respiratory bronchiole or alveolus. During the incubation period of 3 to 5 weeks, the bacilli multiply. They spread through the lymph channels to the lymph nodes and into the circulation. Systemic reticuloendothelial tissues usually destroy the disseminated organisms. The alveolar macrophages are the body's first line of defense and may be able to decrease the concentration of *M. tuberculosis* in the alveoli.

Locally there is an inflammatory reaction resembling pneumonia. Edema, fluid, and white blood cells surround the bacilli. Within 2 to 10 weeks the T lymphocyte system is activated, producing cellular immunity.

Once the infected person acquires active immunity, further multiplication of the organism is limited unless primary pulmonary tuberculosis develops after the incubation period. Children, especially those under 2 years, are at higher risk for development of active disease. In most people, however, the lesion is walled off and healed by calcification. The individual then has a positive skin test and may have a positive x-ray showing a calcified, healed lesion and regional lymph node involvement—the *primary complex* or *Ghon complex*.

Diagnosis

Tuberculin Skin Test The best way to diagnose tuberculosis in children is with a skin test. When the antigen (culture extracts of tuberculin) is injected intradermally, an area of induration results in sensitized persons. The test is done using a tuberculin solution made from old tuberculin or from purified protein derivative stabilized with Tween 80. Table 21-12 describes the interpretation of skin test reactions. A positive skin test in a child under 1 year indicates active disease and in a 1- to 3-year-old is highly suggestive of active disease.

Chest X-ray X-rays are generally used only in tuberculin-positive children to look for the presence of a primary complex. The x-ray is often diagnostic in reactivation tuberculosis. Signs indicating disease include infiltration, fibrosis, calcification, cavity formation, and pleural thickening.

Demonstration of the Tubercle Bacillus Diagnosis of tuberculosis is confirmed by culturing the tubercle bacillus from sputum or other body fluids. Since the culture grows slowly, as many as 8 weeks may be required before a culture is considered negative.

Children, because they are poor coughers, generally swallow their secretions, making sputum specimens difficult to get. Often gastric or bronchial washings are needed. It is important to get at least three specimens prior to beginning treatment. In older children, sputum may also be obtained by aerosol induction using hypertonic saline. Because mycobacterial disease can locate in any part of the body, urine, cerebrospinal fluid, pleural fluid, pus, or bone marrow biopsy specimens may be collected.

Once specimens are obtained, a smear is stained to look for acid-fast bacilli. If it is positive, the number of organisms present is significant. The smear is not diagnostic, however, because there are acid-fast bacilli other than *M. tuberculosis*. The culture allows precise identification of the organism and drug susceptibility testing.

Manifestations Usually primary tuberculosis in children is discovered because the child has been in close contact with an affected adult. The clinical picture is variable. The child may be asymptomatic or may show any or all of the following: fatigue, anorexia, low-grade fever, irregular menses, night sweats (older children), and weight loss. Pulmonary signs and symptoms include an increasingly severe cough, upper respiratory infection, production of sputum, and a dull aching or tightness in the chest.

Extension of tuberculosis into other body systems causes a variety of symptoms. In *miliary tuberculosis* the organisms erode the blood vessels in the lungs, giving them a "snowstorm" appearance on the x-ray. Miliary tuberculosis is associated with osteomyelitis, arthritis, menin-

Table 21-12 Interpretation of Skin Test Reactions

Test	Positive Reaction	Doubtful Reaction	Negative Reaction
Intracutaneous Mantoux Test			
0.1 ml (5 tuberculin units [TU]) PPD tuberculin or jet injection tests (read 48 to 72 h after injection)	10 mm or more induration	5 to 9 mm of induration	0 to 4 mm of induration
Multiple Puncture Test			
Tine test read in 48–72 h; Heaf (qun) read in 3–7 d.	Vesiculation	2 mm or more of induration	Less than 2 mm of induration

Source: Diagnostic Standards and Classification of Tuberculosis and Other Mycobacterial Diseases, American Lung Association, New York, 1974, pp. 17–19.

gitis, and infection in the brain, kidneys, and gastrointestinal tract. *Tuberculous meningitis* is characterized by headache, vomiting, and other signs of increasing intracranial pressure. These serious complications of tuberculosis are fatal in children if untreated. These children are very sick and require hospitalization and intensive treatment.

In *glandular tuberculosis* there is extension into regional lymph nodes, often the cervical nodes or tonsils. The nodes become tender and immobile and may drain externally.

Treatment All children under 6 years who are exposed to someone in their home with tuberculosis should receive primary prophylaxis with isoniazid for 3 months. If active tuberculosis exists, the child is treated with a *minimum of two first-line drugs* to which the organism is *sensitive*. First-line drugs (Table 21-13) are effective, easy to administer, and less toxic and usually less expensive than second-line drugs. Second-line drugs are more likely to be used with drug-resistant strains of *M. tuberculosis*. Children receiving them must be watched much more closely for side effects. Occasionally three drugs will be used initially, especially in drug-resistant or systemic tuberculosis.

Chemotherapy reduces the number of infectious droplet nuclei very quickly. Within 2 weeks after treatment begins, children are usually noninfectious. In addition, drug therapy reduces sputum production and coughing. Since children are such poor coughers, they are unlikely to be very contagious unless they have advanced disease.

Oral medications are given on an empty stomach. Normally, drugs are taken once a day, but some treatment regimens with twice-weekly dosages are successful.

Because the single most important cause of unsuccessful treatment is failure to take medications regularly, a shortened period of daily doses or twice-weekly doses may be helpful. In the case of unreliable children or families, the nurse may have to visit to administer the drug. Taking medications irregularly encourages the development of resistant organisms. Education of the child and the family is extremely important in promoting compliance with the treatment and follow-up plan.

Nursing management Isolation of the child with tuberculosis is necessary only if he or she has a productive cough that cannot be made safe for others. The child should be taught to cover the mouth and nose with tissues when coughing. These tissues should be flushed down the toilet or placed in a paper bag and then burned. These protective measures should be used with any tuberculosis patient with a productive cough. The effectiveness of masks is questionable.

Ideally, room air is ventilated outside and is not recirculated. Ultraviolet lights in the ceiling will kill bacilli in circulating droplets and are often used in sputum-collecting areas.

Unless the child is severely ill, hospitalization is rarely necessary. If the child has draining fistulas or cavitating tuberculosis, appropriate isolation techniques become necessary (Chap. 16).

Because motivation is such an important factor in continuing chemotherapy for the prescribed time, enthusiastic and encouraging nursing care is a key factor. It is imperative that parents and children understand and accept the importance of continuing treatment. Nurses must understand tuberculosis if they are to teach the family about its prevention and treatment ramifications.

The nurse must provide continuing support throughout the diagnostic and treatment program. It is helpful to family members if they can develop their own system of reminders to take the drug daily. Obstacles to visiting the clinic or to obtaining drug refills should be removed. The family should be monitored through home visits and clinic visits and by telephone calls to follow up treatment and to observe for adverse effects of drugs. Families need to know what side effects to watch for and must be interviewed monthly.

The need for adequate rest, a nutritious diet, and general health promotion measures should be stressed. Cigarette smoking should be discouraged.

Any case of tuberculosis must be reported to the local health department by the physician. Although the private physician may manage the child's and the family's treatment, the public health department is responsible for follow-up investigation of all contacts. In addition, the public health department is responsible for (1) education, (2) community screening programs, and (3) clinics for diagnosis, treatment, follow-up, and preventive treatment.

The community health nurse becomes involved with (1) contact investigation and follow-up and (2) case follow-up. Case follow-up includes teaching the child and the family about

Table 21-13 Treatment of Mycobacterial Disease in Adults and Children

Drug*	Daily Dosage	Most Common Side Effects	Monitoring Tests for Side Effects	Remarks
Isoniazid (the drug of choice in primary prophylaxis)	5 to 10 mg/kg for children; up to 300 mg PO or IM. Younger children need 20 mg/kg per day or 30 mg/kg per day with tuberculous meningitis. Can be combined with another first-line drug and given twice a week. Treat for 12 months	Peripheral neuritis, hepatitis, hypersensitivity	SGOT and SGPT	Bacteriocidal. Pyridoxine (vitamin B_6) is given to prevent and/or treat peripheral neuritis. Monitor monthly for symptoms of hepatitis. Contraindications: in previous untoward reaction; patient taking diphenylhydantoin; daily use of alcohol; pregnancy.
Ethambutol (used with isoniazid—most commonly for 18 months)	15 to 25 mg/kg PO. Treat for 12 months	Optic neuritis, skin rash	Visual acuity and red-green color discrimination	Use with caution in children younger than 13 yr when eye testing is not feasible. Optic neuritis is reversible with discontinuance of drug—very rare at 15 mg/kg. Rash, GI upset, malaise. Do not give aminosalicylic acid within 8 h of administering drug.
Rifampin (used with isoniazid)	10 to 20 mg/kg up to 600 mg PO. Treat for 6 to 9 months	Hepatitis, febrile reaction, purpura (rare)	SGOT and SGPT	Bacteriocidal. Orange urine color. Negates effect of birth control pills.
Streptomycin	15 to 20 mg/kg up to 1 g IM. Treat for 2 to 3 months	Eighth-nerve damage, nephrotoxicity	Audiogram, vestibular function, blood urea nitrogen, creatinine	Use with caution in older patients and in patients with renal disease.
Ethionamide	15 to 30 mg/kg up to 1 g PO. Treat for 12 months	GI disturbance, hepatotoxicity, depression	SGOT and SGPT	Divided dose may help GI side effects.
Para-aminosalicylic acid	150 mg/kg up to 2 g PO	GI disturbance, hypersensitivity (fever, rash, etc.), sodium load, hepatotoxicity; may be used with isoniazid in very young children	SGOT and SGPT	GI side effects very frequent, making cooperation difficult.

*Isoniazid, ethambutol, nifampin, and streptomycin are first-line drugs. Ethionamide and para-aminosalicylic acid are second-line drugs (more toxic than first-line drugs). Other second-line drugs include viomycin, pyrazinamide, capreomycin, kanamycin, and cycloserine.

Source: Adapted from American Thoracic Society, "Treatment of Mycobacterial Disease," *American Review of Respiratory Diseases* **115**(1) (1977).

the transmission and treatment of tuberculosis, helping with the chemotherapy program, and providing support and counseling.

Prevention The best way to prevent tuberculosis is to identify people with the infection and then treat them. Those living in close proximity to an infected person should be tested and treated if appropriate. A circle of contacts is then tested; once all tests are negative, contact follow-up ceases.

The reduced incidence of tuberculosis and the current low risk of infection have made routine screening of the general population unjustifiable. As the incidence of tuberculosis decreases, however, the tuberculin test becomes more valuable as a screening test. Chest x-rays are also used to screen people over 50 because so many people in this age group have positive skin test results.

Bacillus Calmette-Guérin (BCG) vaccination, which contains antigens, confers definite but only partial protection by preventing extension of the original infection to active disease. It is recommended for children who have negative tuberculin tests but who are known to be exposed to adults with active disease.[33]

ASTHMA

Asthma is an episodic, wheezy breathlessness produced by a narrowing of the tiny airways (bronchioles) leading to the alveoli where gases are exchanged. The narrowing is due to bronchospasm, edematous swelling of the bronchioles, and an increased amount and viscosity of mucus in the airways. It is the *most common chronic disease of childhood* and the major cause of school absenteeism, physical disability, and hospitalization. It affects twice as many boys as girls before puberty, with some reversal of that ratio later.

There are two main types of asthma: *allergic asthma* (also known as *atopic asthma* and *extrinsic asthma*) and *nonallergic asthma* (also known as *intrinsic asthma, infective asthma,* and *idiopathic asthma*). Allergic asthma usually has its onset in childhood (before the age of 2), while nonallergic asthma usually begins after the age of 35. Children with allergic asthma have a positive family history of allergy, probably had infantile eczema, and have a heightened reactivity of the tracheobronchial tree to a variety of stimuli.

Table 21-14 Common Precipitating Factors in Asthma

Allergens
House dust, pollens, weeds, grasses, trees, feathers, animal dander, mold spores, dust mites, wool articles
Specific Irritants
Odors and chemical fumes (paint and gasoline), tobacco smoke, perfumes, cold air, air pollution, sulfiting preservatives
Infections
Colds or other viral infections, sinusitis, bronchiolitis
Foods
Nuts, seafood, fish, eggs, milk, chocolate, tomatoes, strawberries
Nonspecific Irritants
Exercise, emotions (stress, anxiety, and fatigue), nasal polyps

There may also be a history of repeated episodes of bronchiolitis, causing wheezing and respiratory distress. See Tables 26-7 and 26-8 for history and physical assessment guides for a child with an allergic problem.

An acute asthma attack can be precipitated by known allergens or by an unknown cause. Table 21-14 lists several common causes of asthma and bronchospasm. The most common allergens are inhalants; foods are the next most common allergens, followed by substances that come in contact with the mucous membranes. Nonallergic asthma may be precipitated by an upper respiratory infection.

In asthma, the hypersensitive immune response to the allergen is mediated by immunoglobulin E. Antigen-antibody complexes are formed that cause the release of histamine. Histamine causes bronchospasm, capillary dilatation, and increased mucus production. (See Chap. 26 for a further discussion of the immune response.)

Manifestations

Regardless of the type of asthma, hyperirritability of the airway is a common feature. The reason for this hyperirritability is not always understood. The child becomes short of breath and distressed because of smooth muscle constriction and increased secretion of mucus into the edematous airway. Within a relatively short time the child's respirations become rapid and shallow. Noisy respirations, which produce little air movement, are heard on auscultation. The characteristic wheeze is noted at the end of each expiration, as the last bit of air is squeezed through the bronchioles. Some air is trapped in the alveoli. The child pulls his or her shoulders up and uses the abdominal muscles to help pull more air into the lungs. The child experiences shortness of breath and difficulty doing any exercise. Only a few words may be spoken before a breath is needed. Sometimes there is so much frothy mucus that the child seems to be drowning.

Treatment

With treatment, most acute asthma attacks can be reversed in minutes. Some are reversed immediately, especially when the child and the allergen are separated. Trips to the emergency room for epinephrine, however, are common occurrences for asthmatic children.

Until emergency medical treatment is obtained or until the prescribed medication begins to take effect, the child should experience minimal exertion, be encouraged to breathe slowly, be reassured that the treatment will work, and be kept as occupied and distracted as possible. Rocking small children or rhythmically stroking the back of an older child to encourage relaxation may be helpful. Many children will be relieved of excessive mucus by spontaneously vomiting. Asthmatic children will not lie down during attacks. They are most comfortable sitting with their legs under them and leaning forward on their hands.

A child who is having an acute asthma attack needs immediate attention. Bronchodilators (theophylline), beta adrenergics (epinephrine), and corticosteroids (methyl prednisolone) are the mainstay of treatment. The standard emergency treatment has been epinephrine (0.01 mg/kg) given subcutaneously at 20-min intervals for 3 doses. Epinephrine antagonizes the effects of histamine produced by the allergen and dilates the airways. Airway resistance is then decreased, and air exchange is improved. Epinephrine also increases the heart rate and blood pressure dramatically. Recently, isoetharine (Bronkosol), metaproterenol (Alupent), and albuterol (Proventil or Ventilin) have been used. These inhalants have more beta specificity and therefore are less stimulating to the central nervous and cardiovascular systems. Table 21-3 gives brief descriptions of drugs used in the immediate and long-term management of asthma.

Intravenous aminophylline (5 mg/kg) is infused slowly via an infusion pump over a period of 20 min if there is no response to adrenergics. Aminophylline is a potent bronchodilator that produces gastrointestinal, neurological, and cardiovascular side effects. It is always given very slowly over at least a 15-min interval. Side effects indicating that the dose is being given too fast or that the dosage is too high are nausea and vomiting, nervousness, and diarrhea. An overdose can result in convulsions, coma, cardiac irregularities, and death. The nurse must respect the dangers inherent in administering drugs intravenously and must pay special attention to the therapy.

Children who have asthma that is difficult to control may be given corticosteroids to decrease inflammation in the lungs and to potentiate the effects of the other asthma medications. These may be given intravenously initially and then orally or by inhalation. Because exogenous steroids can rapidly suppress the child's own adrenal function, steroid drugs that are to be discontinued must be tapered off rather than stopped abruptly. There is a potential for adrenal insufficiency in children when the drug is being reduced or shortly after discontinuation. Hypothalamic-pituitary adrenal function may be suppressed for several months. Children may need to resume steroids in the event of trauma, surgery, stress, or severe asthma attacks.[34]

Status asthmaticus

Status asthmaticus is lack of improvement after an asthma attack has been treated by giving three doses of subcutaneous epinephrine. Hospitalization, usually in an intensive care unit, is necessary. Intravenous fluids are begun, intake and output are monitored, and respiratory status is checked frequently by auscultation and by observation of the ratio of inspiration to expiration, dyspnea, and retractions. Cardiovascular status and blood gases are monitored. The Pa_{o2} should be kept above 50 mmHg. The child should be in a semi-Fowler's position. In very severe cases, ventilation may be needed.

For children with chronic asthma, around-the-clock treatment with medication is essential. The treatment must be matched to the severity of the disease (Table 21-15). Cromolyn sodium has been successful in preventing asthma attacks. It decreases the hyperresponsiveness of the airways by coating the mast cells in the lungs, thus pre-

Table 21-15 Comparison of Clinical Signs and Treatment Modalities for Children with Mild, Moderate, and Severe Asthma

Mild Asthma	Moderate Asthma	Severe Asthma
Acute attacks less than once a week	Coughing and wheezing episodes once a week	Frequent attacks; may be cyanotic
No signs of asthma between attacks	Coughing or wheezing between attacks	Almost daily wheezing
Good exercise tolerance	Diminished exercise tolerance	Poor exercise tolerance
Good school attendance	School attendance affected	Poor school attendance—frequent absences
Normal chest x-ray	Hyperinflation on x-ray	Barrel chest deformity apparent due to hyperinflation
Medication needed only during acute attacks	Substantial improvement seen in condition with around-the-clock treatment with medication	Requires around-the-clock treatment with medication and possibly steroids on alternate days

Source: Adapted from Elliot Ellis and Elliot Middleton, "Asthma in Children," in Lichenstein, L. and A. S. Fauci (eds), *Current Therapy in Allergy and Immunology,* C. V. Mosby, St. Louis, 1983–84.

venting them from releasing histamine and SRS-A (slow-reacting substance of anaphylaxis). There are no known serious side effects, although bronchospasm and pharyngeal irritation sometimes occur. These can be made less severe by using an inhaled bronchodilator prior to using cromolyn sodium and following the powder with a glass of water.

Nursing management

Along with careful attention to the administration of drugs to the asthmatic child, the nurse has a major role in the management of hydration, oxygenation, and maintenance of a clear airway. Hydration, to maintain body fluid volume and to liquefy secretions, may be done intravenously, orally, or both. Even oxygen, when ordered, must be humidified to avoid drying secretions. Maintaining a clear airway is difficult in the asthmatic child. While coughing is a frequent accompaniment to the onset of an attack, once the airways are narrowed, the forced expiration necessary for coughing is difficult or impossible. Coughing can further diminish airways by inducing bronchospasm. The removal of secretions must be aided by hydration; mucolytic expectorant drugs; deep, slow breathing; chest percussion; frequent turning; and postural drainage (see Fig. 16-34).

Excessive movement increases the child's need for oxygen. Shortness of breath produces anxiety and agitation in the child. It is essential in caring for the asthmatic child *not* to increase his or her anxiety and apprehension. The child should be talked to, not about. Short, direct statements will aid understanding. When medication is to be administered, it should be given with minimal hesitation and maximum efficiency. The child can be told that the epinephrine injection is not painful but will burn or sting for a few seconds.

Most asthmatics require continuous, seasonal, or episodic treatment with bronchodilators, drugs that open up airways by reducing bronchospasm. A frequently used bronchodilator, theophylline (related to aminophylline), comes in liquid and chewable form for young children.

Bronchodilators are often administered via hand-held inhalers (nebulizers), metered dose inhalers, or compressors. Children younger than 5 years may have some difficulty with the technique involved in inhalation therapy. Instructions to the parents concerning the use of inhaled medications should include the following:

1. Be sure that the child's mouth is clear of food, gum, and all particulate matter before inhalation; rinsing the mouth with water is a good idea (this will prevent aspiration of matter into the lungs).
2. Have the airway extended; the chin should be pointing toward the ceiling to facilitate clear passage of the medication into the bronchial tree.
3. Have the child practice exhaling forcibly to empty the lungs of as much air as possible before inhaling the medication.
4. Be sure to shake the aerosol before using it.
5. After exhalation, have the child place the mouthpiece between the lips and actuate the

drug delivery system, while at the same time inhaling slowly to total lung capacity. Tell the child to hold his or her breath for 6 to 10 s and then exhale slowly through pursed lips.

6. Have the child wait at least 1 min before the next inhalation. If cromolyn sodium or steroid preparations are used, they should *follow* the bronchodilator by 5 to 15 min so that maximum bronchodilatation can take place.
7. If steroids are inhaled, have the child rinse his or her mouth carefully after the treatment to avoid *Candida albicans* infection.

Children often have difficulty coordinating exhalation and inhalation with actuation of the aerosol. Improper timing of inhalation and actuation can cause most of the drug to be deposited in the mouth and pharynx instead of the lungs. Placing a tube spacer between the valve of the aerosol and the child's mouth helps overcome this problem.

As with other medications, children and their parents must be taught the proper name, dose, administration methods, and frequency of their medication. This is very important in asthma, since therapy is continuous and the child becomes dependent on the drug. Children must be assured that their asthma medication is nearby and supervised in its administration, especially at night. Otherwise, they may wake up, require medication, take it, fall asleep, wake up later, and take it again. An overdose of many of the drugs used for asthma can be fatal.

Etiology and prevention

Most allergists, pediatricians, and psychiatrists now accept a multiple etiology for asthma. They generally agree that heredity, allergy, infection, and psychology each play a role. Many early theories that asthma is due to emotional maladjustments have not proved accurate. Children with chronic disorders of any type show a higher prevalence of adjustment problems than healthy children.[35] Emotional problems in the asthmatic child must be assessed to determine whether they are primary or secondary to the asthma. Emotions alone may not be able to cause asthma, but it is suspected that in the asthmatic child, emotional stress can precipitate an attack.

As with all allergies, the key to management is *prevention*. Identification of the allergen through skin testing or environmental manipulation is essential. Hyposensitization is the next step if the allergen is known and cannot be removed from the environment. (See Tables 26-9 and 26-10 for guidelines to the assessment, environmental management, and identification of the allergen.)

CYSTIC FIBROSIS

Cystic fibrosis (CF) is a genetically transmitted disorder characterized by widespread dysfunction of the exocrine (the mucous, salivary, and sweat-producing) glands. Chronic pulmonary disease, gastrointestinal disease accompanied by pancreatic enzyme deficiency, and abnormally high sweat electrolytes are manifestations of the disease. In the past, children with CF had little hope of surviving adolescence. Today, with improved treatment modalities, the mean age of survival is over 20 years, with many individuals living productive adult lives.

Incidence

CF is the most common, lethal genetic disease of children. Although it is seen predominantly in Caucasians, especially in central and western European countries and in areas populated by emigrants from these countries, it has been sporadically reported in all ethnic and racial groups. One out of every fifteen to twenty Caucasian individuals (males and females) carries the autosomal recessive gene for CF. In the United States, the incidence of marriage between two carriers is estimated to be 1:400. This carrier rate results in a CF occurrence rate of 1 out of every 1000–1600 live births. This high incidence has sparked speculation that carriers may have an advantage in terms of increased fertility or resistance to disease. The basic genetic defect in CF remains unknown, and therefore carriers of the disease cannot yet be accurately identified. There have been numerous attempts, many of them promising, to produce a reliable carrier test or method for in utero diagnosis, but none have been successful. Genetic counseling cannot offer much more than the explanation that CF is inherited from both carrier parents and what their chances are of having an affected child. With each pregnancy the chance of producing a child with CF is 25 percent, or 1 in 4. The risk of producing a carrier is 50 percent (2 in 4), and the probability of producing an unaffected child is 25 percent.

Pathophysiology

The exocrine abnormality in CF results in an accumulation of, and obstruction by, mucous secretions in nearly all the body organs, particularly those in the respiratory and gastrointestinal systems. Elevated sweat electrolyte concentrations (sodium and chloride) are present at birth and continue throughout life. The clinical manifestations are related to increased mucous secretions, obstruction of organ passageways, and electrolyte losses from sweat. The disease can be present in varying degrees, depending on the severity of organ involvement. Recent research has identified epithelial abnormalities in active sodium absorption and chloride permeability as well as an increased intracellular calcium content in children with CF.[36] Researchers hope that these findings will provide the basis for identification of the CF genetic defect and an ultimate cure.

The majority of children with CF appear normal at birth. Exceptions include newborns with the complication meconium ileus, in which the tenacious meconium blocks the intestinal tract and causes acute bowel obstruction. More commonly, the infant with CF thrives initially but gradually develops deficiencies in growth (weight and height) as a result of maldigestion and malabsorption of nutrients. Excessive oral intake, coupled with frequent, loose, often fatty stools, accompanies the failure to grow. Pulmonary changes often develop gradually, and abnormal bronchial secretions and obstruction cause infection and lung destruction. Early diagnosis and appropriate treatment are essential in controlling complications and lowering morbidity and mortality rates among CF victims.

Diagnosis

The most reliable diagnostic test for CF is the "sweat test" (a quantitative analysis of sodium and chloride concentrations in the sweat). The sweat test, in which either the Gibson Cooke titration or the Orion method is used, stimulates sweat glands on the arm and leg with electrodes and pilocarpine. The sweat produced is collected and analyzed for sodium and chloride concentrations; sodium and chloride concentrations are typically 2 to 5 times above the norm in children with CF. This abnormal sweat electrolyte concentration results in massive salt depletion and heat prostration if dehydration is left untreated.

In addition to a positive sweat test, the diagnosis of CF is established on the basis of objective evidence of pulmonary involvement or pancreatic involvement or a positive family history. The signs and symptoms of CF include:

1. Failure to thrive (poor weight gain despite good intake)
2. Production of a large amount of frothy, foul-smelling, fatty-appearing stool (a result of malabsorption)
3. Rectal prolapse
4. Frequent cough, bronchitis, or pneumonia
5. A salty taste to the skin (a mother may notice this when she kisses her infant)
6. Meconium ileus in the newborn

Because of these symptoms, CF is often confused with allergies, chronic respiratory infection, celiac disease, or failure to thrive.

The respiratory system Progressive respiratory changes occur with age. Mucus accumulation and obstruction in the sinuses may result in chronic sinusitis and edematous, swollen nasal tissues with nasal polyp formation. Obstruction of the eustachian tube can lead to acute and chronic ear infections, particularly in the infant and toddler. Allergies are common and complicate the clinical course of affected children.

Chronic obstructive, infective pulmonary disease of the lower respiratory system is the major cause of disability and death in children with CF. Progressive, irreversible pulmonary involvement is inevitable. It develops from the accumulation and retention of mucus in the airways. Mucus plugs lead to areas of overinflation and atelectasis in the lungs, impairing airflow.

Infection inevitably follows mucus obstruction. A vicious cycle results: infection causes increased mucus production, which leads to inflammation; inflammation in turn causes bronchospasm, which results in further obstruction. Clearance of the airways is significantly limited.

Most infections are caused by *Staphylococcus aureus, Hemophilus influenzae,* and *Pseudomonas aeruginosa*. Infection with the mucoid strain of *Pseudomonas* is occurring more frequently in younger children and is almost impossible to eradicate with current antibiotic therapy. Infections due to *Pseudomonas cepacia* and *Aspirigillus* are becoming more frequent and are associated with a poorer prognosis.

Hyperinflation of the lungs results in chronic emphysema, with bleb or bullae formation. These areas of coalesced, distended alveoli, especially in the upper lobes, are prone to rupture and associated pneumothorax. The presence of bronchiectasis is a universal finding throughout the lungs of a child who has CF. These abnormal airways further complicate the treatment of airway obstruction due to mucus and chronic infection. Areas of abscess result. Bronchiectasis is usually accompanied by bronchial artery hypertrophy and subsequent hemoptysis.

Eventually, a loss of gas exchange surface area leads to pulmonary insufficiency and respiratory failure. With severe pulmonary disease, pulmonary vascular resistance increases. The right side of the heart must work harder to pump blood through the lungs, leading to cardiac hypertrophy or failure (cor pulmonale).

Signs of pulmonary involvement include (1) a chronic cough, (2) purulent sputum production, (3) an increased respiratory rate, (4) use of the accessory muscles of respiration, (5) excessive caloric requirements due to the increased work of breathing, (6) adventitious sounds heard on auscultation (crackles, wheeze, and absent to decreased breath sounds), (7) enlargement of the thoracic cage (barrel chest), (8) clubbing of the ends of the fingers and toes, and (9) cyanosis.

The pancreas Mucus obstruction of the pancreatic ducts inhibits the flow of trypsin, lipase, and amylase (the digestive enzymes) to the duodenum. Maldigestion and malabsorption of food lead to poor weight gain and delays in growth and development. Stools are frequent, bulky, and foul-smelling and contain large amounts of fat (*steatorrhea*) and protein. The fat-soluble vitamins (A, D, E, and K) are poorly absorbed. Because of malabsorption, the child with CF often presents with a protruding belly, thin extremities, and poor muscle mass. With adequate treatment and improved nutrition, these signs should resolve.

Intermittent glucose intolerance is common and progresses to diabetes in approximately 10 percent of the persons with CF. The etiology of glucose intolerance remains unclear, but pancreatic destruction due to mucus obstruction is thought to be a major contributor. Diabetes usually develops in the adolescent and adult years and is managed with insulin injections and diet. The absence of ketoacidosis in diabetics with CF makes diabetes in these individuals different from other types of diabetes.

The liver Focal biliary cirrhosis in the liver can result from mucus obstruction of the bile ducts. A small percentage of patients with CF demonstrate abnormal liver function and clinical evidence of liver disease. Extensive liver involvement, although unusual, can result in portal hypertension, esophageal varices, gastrointestinal hemorrhage, and ascites.

The intestines Meconium ileus (meconium obstruction of the bowel) is the earliest complication and occurs in approximately 10 percent of babies with CF. Surgical correction is frequently required. (See Chap. 19.)

Hypersecretion of intestinal mucus occurs and contributes to the malabsorption seen in CF. Obstruction of the bowel due to the accumulation of dehydrated mucus, stool, and undigested food is a common problem for all affected. This complication, known as *meconium ileus equivalent,* as well as intussusception, can be managed without surgery.

Abdominal pain is a common complaint of children with CF. It is frequently caused by (1) undigested food, which results from failure to take pancreatic digestive enzymes; (2) intussusception of the small and large bowel; (3) partial obstruction by feces and mucus; (4) muscular soreness from coughing; (5) gallstones (10 percent of patients with CF over age 5 develop gallstones); and (6) subacute or chronic pancreatitis.

Rectal prolapse is often the initial symptom of CF in undiagnosed children. It results from excessive stool output due to maldigestion and malabsorption. The problem resolves with appropriate treatment and control of malabsorptive stools. Surgical correction may sometimes be necessary.

The reproductive system Generally, males and females with CF experience delayed development of secondary sex characteristics due to malnutrition and pulmonary complications.

Lack of sperm causes sterility in 97 percent of all males with CF. This defect is believed to occur in utero as a result of mucus obstruction of the vas deferens. Although sterile, males have normal sexual function. Since a growing number of children with CF now live into adulthood and experience normal sexual relationships, sex education should not be neglected.

Females with CF are less fertile because of thick cervical secretions. Menstrual irregularities and failure to ovulate due to malnutrition and chronic pulmonary infection further decrease fertility. Many females with CF are capable of reproduction, however, and a growing number achieve healthy pregnancies and motherhood.

Sweat The sweat of individuals with CF is abnormally high in electrolytes. Excessive losses of electrolytes can lead to hyponatremia. Adequate salt replacement during periods of increased sweating, such as in hot weather, during febrile episodes, or when exercising, prevents problems.

Treatment

A specific treatment for CF is not possible since the basic biochemical defect remains unknown. At the present time no cure exists, but medical advances, especially in the areas of antibiotic therapy and nutritional support, have greatly increased the life expectancy for patients with CF. Since patients are ill from complications, treatment is aimed at controlling and preventing the complications. Control of the pulmonary obstructive process, pulmonary infection, and pancreatic and nutritional deficiencies are the primary objectives of treatment.

Pulmonary therapy Since pulmonary complications account for the majority of disability and death in CF, successful treatment must focus on the maintenance of good pulmonary hygiene. Conventional pulmonary therapy includes the use of (1) a mist tent, (2) aerosol inhalation, (3) postural drainage, (4) antibiotics, and (5) physical exercise. Controversy exists regarding these different aspects of therapy. Research is aimed at discovering more effective and less time-consuming methods of clearing the airways of obstructive mucus.

Mist tents The mist tent is designed to increase humidification of inspired air and to help thin mucous secretions by depositing water particles in the respiratory tract. Patients who use a mist tent usually sleep in it every night. Overnights with friends and vacations are common exceptions. To be effective, the mist cloud should be so dense that the child is barely visible. The usual mist tent solution for home use is a combination of propylene glycol and distilled water. Because of the risk of mold and bacterial growth, the use of a mist tent is controversial. Proper care and daily cleaning of the equipment are imperative if the mist tent is to be used safely and effectively. Many physicians feel there is no clinical evidence that mist tents are beneficial and no longer prescribe them.

Aerosol inhalation Aerosol therapy is designed to thin and liquefy the thick bronchial secretions, thereby improving ventilation of the lungs and oxygenation of arterial blood. Medications used include bronchodilators, mucolytic agents, and antibiotics (see Table 21-3). Aerosol therapy is used both prophylactically and therapeutically on a daily basis prior to postural drainage. If necessary, it may be used as frequently as every 4 h. Children 5 years old and under receive aerosol therapy via a face mask. Usually children over the age of 5 are able to mouth-breathe totally and can receive the treatment via a mouthpiece.

A face mask should replace the mouthpiece apparatus, however, when sinusitis and nasal polyps are present. The ventilatory pattern should be slow, with moderately deep breathing and breath-holding at the end of inspiration to ensure deposition and retention of the aerosol. The use of daily aerosol therapy is also controversial. Some physicians prescribe it only during acute phases of the illness.

Percussion and postural drainage Percussion and postural drainage (P & PD) is an essential part of pulmonary therapy in CF. Its purpose is to (1) increase sputum expectoration and thereby reopen clogged airways and (2) improve ventilation by decreasing bronchial obstruction. This is accomplished through the use of physical maneuvers (percussion and vibration) and gravity, which stimulate the movement of the thick bronchial secretions toward the large airways. The patient is then able to cough up and expectorate the thick mucus. The frequency of postural drainage depends on the extent of pulmonary involvement. It is usually done once or twice daily at home and as often as every 4 h during hospitalization. P & PD should be done at least 1 h after eating to avoid nausea and vomiting. Recent research has clearly established P & PD as one of the most important clinical aspects of CF care. Much effort is currently being put forth by clinical researchers to develop more effective and time-efficient methods to replace P & PD. A promising tool may be the "PEP mask" (a positive expiratory pressure breathing device), currently used in Europe.

Older children with CF are usually able to perform the majority of P & PD therapy independently using a lightweight mechanical percussor-vibrator. It is vital that this self-care activity be initiated during the preadolescent or early adolescent years in order to promote independence. Mechanical percussors-vibrators, combined with forced expiratory breathing techniques, have proved effective in helping children with CF carry out good pulmonary hygiene independently. By midadolescence, teenagers should be responsible for the majority of their own care. Family support with self-care activities is essential for success. Assistance from family members and friends with care activities is needed during periods of decreased energy levels, acute illness, and unusual time constraints.

Antibiotics Antibiotics are used both prophylactically and therapeutically for treatment and control of pulmonary infection in CF. Many patients are routinely placed on prophylactic antibiotics (usually sulfa drugs) to decrease the incidence of pulmonary infection. All patients are placed on antibiotic therapy for treatment of specific organisms cultured out of their sputum.

Hospitalization, with extensive high doses of intravenous antibiotics, is needed during periods of serious disease exacerbation. Aminoglycosides (e.g., tobromycin and gentamicin) are used to treat *Pseudomonas* infections. Many drugs, including aminoglycosides, are rapidly metabolized by the person with CF, and unusually high doses are required for effective treatment. The aerosolization and inhalation of other antibiotics may be used in treating particularly difficult pulmonary infections.

Physical exercise The value of physical exercise cannot be overemphasized. The patient with CF should be encouraged to be as physically active as possible. Exercise loosens mucus and helps remove it from the lungs, strengthens the respiratory muscles, improves pulmonary function, and decreases pulmonary artery pressure. Some form of aerobic exercise, which will increase the pulse and respiratory rates, should be done daily or a minimum of three times a week.

Breathing exercises help establish normal patterns of breathing, strengthen the respiratory muscles, and remove mucus from the lungs. The use of forced expiratory breathing has proved extremely beneficial in avoiding mucus retention and obstruction (see Table 21-16). This breathing technique should be done in conjunction with postural drainage as well as practiced several times a day.

A few words need to be said about coughing. The cough is the CF patient's best friend, for without coughing, mucus is not expectorated and remains in the lungs, where it obstructs airways and causes infection. The patient with CF needs to be encouraged to cough effectively throughout the day.

The child with CF learns early to adopt a shallow breathing pattern to control airflow and help suppress coughing. Cough suppression is widespread in individuals with CF and results in retention of infected, thick pulmonary secretions. The general public fosters cough suppression by expressing annoyance with a person who coughs. The child with CF needs to understand that coughing is a natural mechanism that works to keep him or her healthy. It should not be a source of embarrassment.

Health professionals must desensitize themselves to the child's sputum. Nurses need to assess sputum for quantity, color, and consistency. It is disturbing to the child if nurses and physicians appear uneasy when looking at expectorated sputum. Nurses need to help children with CF value coughing and sputum expectoration as a part of health maintenance.

Nutritional therapy Nutrition is of extreme importance in CF. A well-nourished child will cope better physically with pulmonary disease. A major objective for the child, therefore, is the achievement of an optimal nutritional state. A well-balanced diet with increased caloric intake is needed to offset malabsorptive losses due to the disease process. Dietary intake must be balanced with pancreatic enzyme supplementation to achieve adequate absorption and digestion of food. Nutritional therapy for the patient with CF

Table 21-16 Forced Expiratory Breathing Technique*

Instruct the child to:

1. Take in an average breath.
2. Using *force,* breathe out *all* the air in the lungs.
3. Squeeze the sides of the chest with the arms while breathing out.
4. Do relaxed diaphragmatic breathing. (The child will need to cough to expectorate the mucus produced.)

*The purpose of this procedure is to force mucus out of the small airways. It should be used only one or two times per sitting, as it can be very tiring. It is used with postural drainage and three to four times during the day.

consists of (1) pancreatic digestive enzyme supplements, (2) vitamin supplements, and (3) a high-calorie, high-protein diet.

Pancreatic digestive enzyme supplementation Because CF causes obstruction of the pancreatic ducts, the flow of digestive enzymes is inhibited. Replacement of these absent enzymes is necessary in order for food to be adequately digested and then absorbed. The amount of supplementation taken depends on stool frequency, amount, and consistency. The patient is placed on a dosage that will control steatorrhea and limit stool frequency to once or twice a day.

The commonly used brands of pancreatic digestive enzyme supplements are Viokase (the mildest form), Cotazyme (a medium-strength preparation), and Pancrease Cotazyme S (enteric coated preparations which act in the duodenum). Pancreatic digestive enzyme supplements must be taken with all meals and snacks. To be most effective, the total amount given should be equally divided into three doses and administered at the beginning, middle, and end of the meal. This will ensure proper mixing of foods and enzymes. Bile salts may be added to facilitate fat digestion, and an alkalizing agent (cimetidine or Tagamet) used to improve pancreatic digestive enzyme activity. The parents and child should be responsible for adjusting the dosage of the pancreatic digestive enzyme supplement as needed. Signs and symptoms of inadequate pancreatic digestive enzyme replacement are (1) abdominal cramping and distention; (2) frequent, fatty stools; (3) poor weight gain, despite good intake; and (4) rectal prolapse.

Pancreatic digestive enzyme supplements are usually mixed in applesauce (a good vehicle, which is not easily liquefied by the enzymes) before being administered to infants and toddlers. It is important to protect the skin surrounding the mouth with petroleum jelly if pancreatic digestive enzyme supplements without an enteric coating are administered. Without this coating, tissue is easily irritated, and skin breakdown occurs. School-age children often avoid taking their pancreatic digestive enzyme supplements while eating with friends, in an attempt to be like them. Many schools require children to get their enzyme supplements from the school nurse or principal, which obviously makes it difficult for them to take the supplements at the correct times. This practice fosters noncompliance and may also serve to further isolate children with CF from their peers. A method must be worked out whereby children can manage their own medications in an appropriate and convenient manner. In general, children with CF should be instructed to carry their enzyme supplements with them (in a pants pocket or a purse, for example) at all times, since they often eat away from home.

Fats should not be limited for children with CF because they are a good source of the calories needed for growth, health maintenance, and the work of breathing. Pancreatic digestive enzyme supplementation should be increased with fatty food intake in order to facilitate appropriate digestion.

Vitamin supplementation Supplementation of fat-soluble vitamins (A, E, K, and at times D) in a water-soluble form is prescribed to prevent and correct deficiencies due to malabsorption. High doses of vitamin C may be used in an attempt to increase white blood cell activity against chronic pulmonary infections, especially those caused by *Pseudomonas*.

Nutrition A child with CF should eat a high-calorie, high-protein, well-balanced diet. In general, a 50 to 100 percent increase in calories and a protein intake that is 2 to $2\frac{1}{2}$ times greater than the normal requirement are recommended. Dietary consultation is needed to determine the appropriate caloric intake for each child. Between-meal snacks are usually necessary to meet the above-normal caloric intake requirements.

Infants who are not breast-fed are placed on a predigested formula, such as Pregestimil. Some infants may require formulas with 24 to 28 cal per ounce to ensure adequate growth. Although pancreatic digestive enzyme supplements must be given with all formulas, predigested formulas usually require less enzyme supplementation. Once solids are begun, high-protein foods should be favored, and the amount of enzyme supplementation needed will increase. Cereals should be given in reduced amounts because they provide a less desirable source of calories than high-protein foods.

Overall, it is important to make foods attractive and mealtimes pleasant. The development of good dietary habits is essential for the well-being of the child with CF.

Providing adequate caloric intake is often a major challenge in the presence of such factors as increased work of breathing, pulmonary infection, oxygen desaturation, and malabsorption. Nutritional supplements such as Vivonex, Ensure, Magnacal, and Vitacal often are taken by children with CF. Innovative methods are being tried for children with CF who cannot get adequate nutrition and gain enough weight. Supplemental nighttime nasogastric feedings are often successful. Some children have difficulty, however, with frequent coughing associated with vomiting. Long-term hyperalimentation is becoming increasingly popular for a limited number of children with CF who are plagued by severe malnutrition and excessive caloric requirements.

Central venous catheters, such as Port-a-Cath, have made prolonged parenteral nutrition possible for children with CF. The implantable catheter decreases infection and minimally affects the child's already altered body image.

A small silicone port is surgically implanted beneath the subcutaneous tissue and is securely sutured against a thoracic rib. A catheter is attached to the port and threaded into the subclavian vein (see Fig. 16-30). A straight 90°-angle needle (Huber needle) is used to access the port. The 90° angle allows the needle to lie flat against the skin, making it more comfortable and less of a problem in terms of appearance. The straight needle is used to heparinize the port after each infusion or every 2 to 4 weeks if the catheter is not in use.

Implantable infusion devices make frequent therapy and home intravenous therapy more feasible and safe. With proper education, the child and the family can manage catheter care. Only qualified nurses should perform port access and care and educate the child and the family.

Psychosocial aspects

Like any other chronic illness, CF has a significant psychosocial impact on the child and the family. The stresses of daily therapy, life-style changes, the cost of medical care, and the constant threat of a limited life span can prove overwhelming.

The diagnosis of CF in a child produces feelings of shock, despair, and guilt in the parents. They must cope with the reality that their child has a serious, life-threatening, chronic disease. Parents feel guilty because the disease is genetic. Reassurance is needed that both parents carry the abnormal gene for CF and that mass screening for detecting carriers is not currently feasible.

Caring for the child with CF will make significant changes in the parents' life-style. They must share the burden of prescribed daily therapy. Feelings of anger and hostility may develop when one parent becomes the primary caregiver. A breakdown in communication can result, which can have a profound, long-range effect on the marriage. The parents should be encouraged to be open and honest in talking with each other about CF and its effect on them and their life-style.

A common problem for the parents is the difficulty of getting occasional relief from the daily care routines and regimen that CF imposes. Training baby-sitters, extended family members, or friends in chest physiotherapy and utilizing community resources for assistance can give the parents needed relief and time away from home. Many insurance companies and state medical assistance programs now provide coverage for some of the costs of home health care, home health aids, and respiratory therapy. This has proved beneficial and cost-effective, since it decreases the frequency and length of hospitalization and contributes to improvements in the child's health status and psychosocial function.

Parent support groups provide an opportunity to share experiences and exchange ideas. Contact with another parent at the time of the diagnosis is also beneficial. Knowing that there are other parents who are successfully coping with CF in their lives and that their children are doing well proves supportive and facilitates acceptance.

CF imposes a great financial burden on the family. The cost of home equipment, medications, clinic appointments, and hospitalizations is astronomical. Being able to provide the necessary medical care for the child can be a continued stress for the parents. Often the family goes without other things in order to pay medical bills. This may cause feelings of guilt in the child with CF, who realizes the hardship that the disease has placed on the family. Resources such as state government services for handicapped children can assist qualifying families with medical expenses.

The ongoing, lifelong stress of chronic illness has the potential to result in psychosocial difficulties. The demands of daily home care, clinic visits, hospitalizations, and the cost of health care result in higher than normal stress. Alterations in body image from CF complications — causing chronic, productive cough, barrel chest, clubbed fingers and toes, and small stature—make children with CF feel different from their peers. Concern with body image increases during adolescence.

Absences from school due to illness, frequent hospitalizations, and poor exercise tolerance can separate children with CF from their peer group. A sense of isolation develops. As children attempt to gain some form of control in their lives, they may refuse chest physiotherapy and medications. This becomes a real frustration for the parent, who is trapped between the need for providing prescribed therapy and the need for discipline and limit setting and provision for a quality life.

As the child reaches adolescence, the risk of psychosocial problems increases. Attempting to work through the normal tasks of adolescence while coping with the limitations imposed by CF can prove stressful and depressing. Delays in puberty coupled with an altered physical appearance contribute to a poor body image. Many adolescents with CF are dissatisfied with their bodies and find their obvious physical differences a source of great stress and embarrassment. While the normal adolescent is attempting to develop a positive self-image, the adolescent with CF finds this almost impossible to do. A poor self-image develops, leading to feelings of inadequacy and insecurity.

Gaining peer group acceptance is often difficult for adolescents with CF because of body-image problems, physical limitations, and frequent illness. Adolescents with CF often allow their body-image perception to affect the way other adolescents react to them. Fearing rejection, the adolescent with CF may develop few interpersonal relationships. The idea of dating and marriage produces anxiety, especially for boys, who experience feelings of sexual inadequacy because of sterility. Poor peer group acceptance and the dependency on others for assistance with daily chest physiotherapy inhibit the development of independence, a major task of adolescence.

Awareness of the prognosis for people with CF leads to anxiety and a preoccupation with death and dying. Making career decisions is difficult when adolescents question their ability ever to be physically and financially independent of their parents. The use of denial and avoidance in dealing with these issues leads to rebellion and poor compliance with treatment.

The young adult with CF faces the problems of achieving and maintaining independence from the family unit. Finding a suitable occupation that will provide financial security and not be physically detrimental is often difficult. For the married adult with CF, the need for daily therapy and the financial burden of medical expenses, plus physical limitations and frequent illness, place great stress on the marriage. Family planning decisions are difficult. Many females with CF decide not to have children because of the physical risks involved and the fact that all the children will be carriers. Attempts at adoption are hindered because of the chronicity of the illness and the prognosis.

Artificial insemination may be used by a male with CF and his spouse who decide to have children. Counseling regarding the stresses of parenthood and chronic illness is a necessary part of the care for individuals with CF who are planning a family. Making a marriage succeed when one partner has a chronic illness is a difficult task. With CF, the threat of a serious illness and death from complications is always present.

Nursing management

An essential component of nursing management is providing for the physical, psychological, and social needs of the patient. However, before a nursing care plan can be established, the nurse must make an accurate assessment of the patient's needs. Data obtained from this assessment will provide guidelines for all areas of nursing management. Table 21-17 lists areas of assessment for the child with CF and his or her family.

Once the assessment is complete, the nurse is ready to incorporate the data into a care plan that will establish goals for the nursing staff, the child, and hospitalization. Since pulmonary hygiene is a major component of care in CF, the care plan should reflect this priority. Aggressive chest physiotherapy should be initiated, a sputum sample obtained and sent for culture and sensitivity testing, and appropriate antibiotic therapy begun. Oxygen therapy may be indicated. All equipment should be functioning properly and used safely. The child's exercise tolerance should be evaluated, and an exercise program begun. Continuous assessment of respiratory status is essential, and interventions must be changed accordingly.

Nutrition is another priority of care, and weight gain is a usual goal of therapy. The daily caloric

Table 21-17 Nursing Assessment of a Child with CF

Respiratory Status	Gastrointestinal Status	Psychosocial Status
General appearance:	Height and weight:	Family support system
Discomfort	Growth pattern	Financial status
AP diameter of chest	Usual intake:	Understanding of CF and treatment program
Vital signs:	Number of calories	Compliance with treatment program
Temperature	Type of foods eaten	Other family stressors
Pulse	Use of enzymes—type, frequency, dosage	School adjustment: Peer relationships
Blood pressure	Stools:	Community resources
Respirations:	Quality	CF clinic follow-up
Rate	Quantity	Problem-solving strategies
Quality	Odor	Current limitations
Use of accessory muscles	Abdominal pain or discomfort	
Retractions	Supplements (vitamin supplements, caloric supplements, etc.)	
Breath sounds		
Color, cyanosis		
Clubbing of digits		
Cough		
Usual pulmonary care practiced at home		
Schedule		
Equipment—type and care		
Exercise program		
Medications		

intake should be recorded. High-calorie, high-protein foods should be included in meals and between-meal snacks made readily available. Determining the daily caloric intake necessary for weight gain is important in setting realistic goals for the child. Children must eventually be able to estimate their own caloric intake to know whether it is enough to ensure weight gain. Nutritional supplements may be indicated if weight gain is not achieved.

The nurse is responsible for coordinating all aspects of the child's care effectively and efficiently. Scheduling meals, chest physiotherapy, medications, and exercise time can be a complicated task, but it is necessary for an optimal outcome.

The nurse must also communicate nursing goals to the child, the family, and involved health team members. When it is time to plan for discharge, the nurse must often contact health professionals outside the hospital and clinic. Referrals to community health nurses may be vital to continuity of care.

Sometimes the stress of coping with this demanding illness causes a breakdown in communication or a disruption among family members. Parents and siblings may have difficulty expressing their feelings about how CF affects their relationships and life-style. The nurse should facilitate the development of healthy communication between family members when it does not exist and reinforce it when it does.

Educating the child and the family

When the diagnosis of CF is made, the parents, and even the child or adolescent, are asked to absorb a great deal of information regarding the disease process, its treatment, and home care. The nurse, along with the physician and other health team members, is responsible for implementing a teaching program. Education is an ongoing process for the child and the family, since only so much information can be assimilated at one time. As the child grows older, pulmonary therapy techniques change, medications change, and the disease process may progress, creating new learning needs in the child with CF and his or her family. Techniques of chest physiotherapy require periodic evaluation, whether they change or not. The Cystic Fibrosis Foundation* and state chapter affiliates provide educational materials and services to families and health professionals.

*Cystic Fibrosis Foundation, 6000 Executive Boulevard, Suite 309, Rockville, Md. 20852.

Principles of self-care should be taught as appropriate, often by age 10. CF, with its demanding home therapy, can foster dependency. The child should eventually assume responsibility for home equipment, medications, and chest physiotherapy.

The parents need to understand that their child will experience normal growth and development, even though some steps may be delayed, such as puberty. Discipline, limit setting, and promotion of independence are important topics to explore.

Adolescents who are experiencing their illness with feelings of rejection and rebellion may be helped by support groups of others with CF. Group teaching situations may increase receptiveness and eventual compliance with treatment regimens. Psychologists who specialize in adolescence and CF are a vital component of the care and health promotion of teenagers with this disease.

Health maintenance

Children with CF should be regularly evaluated at a recognized regional CF care center. A CF care center usually provides evaluation and management of complications of CF and then coordinates care with local health professionals. This approach to care greatly increases the survival rates of individuals with CF.

Chest x-rays, pulmonary-function tests, blood gas measurements, sputum cultures, and various other tests are done to monitor status.

Very often the nurse acts as the coordinator of the child's care. The nurse can facilitate referral to genetic and vocational counselors, social workers, respiratory therapists, nutritionists, and community and school health nurses. Providing comprehensive care to the child (or adult) with CF is a demanding, time-consuming job that no one person can accomplish alone.

Nursing Care Plan: Laryngotracheobronchitis*

Patient: Billy Dow Age: 12 months, 7 days Date of Admission: 1/13 at 2:30 A.M.

ASSESSMENT

The child was brought first to the emergency room accompanied by his parents and 3-year-old brother, his only sibling. The mother stated that he "couldn't breathe." He has not been hospitalized before. He has no history of allergies. The medical diagnosis is laryngotracheobronchitis.

General Appearance

The child has circumoral cyanosis; a pale color; substernal, intercostal, and suprasternal retractions; nasal flaring; and prominent inspiratory stridor. He is very anxious and frightened and has a hoarse, "seal-like" cough made worse by crying.

Physical Examination

Weight: 13 kg. Temperature: 38.8°C (101.8°F), rectal. Respiratory rate: 60 to 70. Pulse: 140.

History

One week ago, Billy had an upper respiratory infection for which he was treated with 60 mg of Tylenol q4h to q6h; his rectal temperature was 38.9°C (102°F). On the evening before admission, the mother noticed that he seemed congested and hoarse when she put him to bed at 8 P.M. At midnight she was awakened by the child's severe, brassy coughing and crying. Billy was standing in his crib, coughing; his hair was wet from perspiration. When she changed his diapers, Mrs. Dow noted that his chest seemed to "move in and out funny" with each breath. He made a high, shrill noise on inspiration. His rectal temperature was 38.3°C (101°F). Billy was restless, refused a bottle, and would not settle down, even when his mother rocked him or walked with him. The pediatrician was called, and he told the parents to take Billy to the emergency room, where he would meet them.

In the emergency room the primary pediatrician took chest and lateral neck x-rays. These showed some subglottal narrowing below the vocal cords and edema of the vocal cords. Two trial doses of racemic epinephrine via IPPB were administered by a respiratory therapist, with no improvement in the chest retractions, color, or stridor. Billy was admitted to the pediatric unit at 2:30 A.M.

PHYSICIAN'S ORDERS

1. Chest x-ray.
2. Lateral neck x-ray.
3. Throat culture.
4. Nothing by mouth.
5. Cool mist tent.
6. D5 and 0.2 NS IV or D4mRL to run at a maintenance rate: 100 ml/kg for the first 10 kg per 24 h, 50 ml/kg for the next 10 kg per 24 h, and 2 mEq KCl added per 100 ml of IV fluid when the child is urinating.
7. Vital signs: respirations and pulse q1h, temperature q2h if fever is present, BP on admission and q4h.
8. Provide rest and keep external stimuli to a minimum.
9. Tylenol 60 mg per rectum for rectal temperature above 39°C (102.5°F).
10. Emergency tracheostomy (intubation) equipment at the bedside.
11. Notify the physician if respiratory rate is above 60, heart rate is above 160, temperature is above 38.9°C (102°F), skin color becomes ashen gray, or restlessness or retractions increase.

Nursing Diagnosis	Outcome Criteria	Nursing Interventions	Evaluation and Modifications
1. Ineffective airway clearance related to inability of air to pass the glottis, inflammation, and probable infection	☐ Effective airway clearance, as evidenced by: **a.** Absence of stridor and circumoral, buccal, and nail-bed cyanosis **b.** Absence of retractions **c.** Decreased restlessness, dyspnea, and respiratory rate	☐ Place the child in a cool mist tent with humidified oxygen as ordered, according to blood gas determinations and assessment of respiratory rate, pattern, and skin color.	☐ 1/13: The child was placed in a cool mist tent with 40% oxygen. Pa_{O_2}, 90%; Pa_{CO_2}, 52%; pH, 7.30.
		☐ Assess blood gases (Pa_{O_2}, Pa_{CO_2}, and pH).	☐ 1/14: Pa_{O_2}, 96%; Pa_{CO_2}, 43%; pH, 7.36. Fi_{O_2} reduced to 21% in the mist tent.
		☐ Assess and document: **a.** Respirations—rate, depth, character, and pattern **b.** Breath sounds, noting diminished breath sounds, rales, and rhonchi **c.** Inspiratory/expiratory ratio and equal chest expansion	☐ 1/13: Four h after admission, respiratory rate was 54, and retractions lessened, but were mild to moderate during rest. Skin color remains pale; no cyanosis was noted. Breath sounds were heard bilaterally. Coarse rales were heard in the left lower lobe; the inspiratory phase is prolonged, and equal chest expansion was noted.
		d. Signs of increasing respiratory distress: restlessness, degree and location of retractions, nasal flaring, inspiratory stridor, or expiratory grunting	☐ No signs of increasing respiratory distress were observed. Billy is less restless. ☐ 1/13: Billy had moderate substernal and suprasternal retractions. ☐ 1/14: The retractions lessened to mild substernal retractions during rest. ☐ 1/14: Circumoral cyanosis was present only when the child was crying and agitated.
		☐ Take vital signs q1h and rectal temperature q2h initially.	☐ 1/14: Vital signs were stable: respiratory rate, 48; pulse, 130; temperature, 37.9°C (100.2°F).
	d. The absence of inspiratory stridor and brassy cough	☐ Provide a quiet environment, and group nursing actions together to give longer periods of uninterrupted rest. Limit all nursing care to essentials. Encourage the mother to comfort and hold the child when he is not in the mist tent. Place his favorite toys inside the tent.	☐ 1/13: Billy was transferred to a private room as per the parents' request. The mother said that Billy is a stomach sleeper, and so he was positioned on the stomach and slept better.

Nursing Diagnosis	Outcome Criteria	Nursing Interventions	Evaluation and Modifications
	e. Nonretention of secretions, as evidenced by a loose, productive cough	☐ Check the fluid level in the mist tent hourly and fill with distilled water when appropriate. Change the equipment qod. ☐ Explain to the parents how much oral fluid Billy can have, and schedule 120 ml during the 7 A.M. to 3 P.M. shift, 90 ml during the 3 P.M. to 11 P.M. shift, and 60 ml during the 11 P.M. to 7 A.M. shift. Leave 1-oz paper measuring cups in the room. Teach the parents how to record intake and output and how to remove Billy from the tent and place him back into it. Record the amount and characteristics of secretions.	☐ 1/14: Clear liquids were begun; Billy's favorite is popsicles. ☐ 1/14: The mist tent required filling q6h to maintain mist at the desired concentration. The tent is large enough to cover the entire mattress. Billy has a loose, productive cough now. ☐ 1/15: Billy is allowed to have broth, Jell-O water, and 7-Up to drink, but total oral and IV fluid is not to exceed 1200 ml per 24 h. He is tolerating oral fluids well. ☐ 1/15: Respiratory rate is 34 to 40, with mild retractions intercostally and mild stridor on inspiration. The cough is lessened, but is still productive. ☐ 1/16: IV fluids were discontinued, and a clear liquid diet was maintained; oral intake was 600 ml during the 7 A.M. to 3 P.M. shift and 450 ml during the 3 P.M. to 11 P.M. shift.
	f. Adequate oxygen perfusion to the tissues	☐ Elevate the head of the bed 30°. Permit Billy to assume a comfortable position without compromising the IV line. ☐ Assess perfusion of the extremities by assessing and documenting pedal pulses, capillary filling, and warmth.	☐ 1/14: Oral mucosa are pink when the child is sleeping; circumoral cyanosis returns when he is agitated and crying. ☐ 1/16: Color remains pink when the child is out of the mist tent. No cyanosis was noted. ☐ 1/14: Perfusion was monitored q1h, keeping in mind that the mist tent is cool. Billy was covered with bath blankets to keep the extremities warm and prevent vasoconstriction. The blankets were changed frequently. Pedal pulses strong, equal to the apical pulse. There is prompt capillary filling in the toes of both feet.

Nursing Diagnosis	Outcome Criteria	Nursing Interventions	Evaluation and Modifications
2. Potential fluid volume deficit and electrolyte imbalance related to inability to take oral fluids, tachypnea, and age	☐ Fluids and electrolytes will be maintained within normal limits for a 13-kg infant, as evidenced by: **a.** A fluid intake of 46 ml per hour **b.** Voiding sufficient quantities of straw-colored urine at least four to five times per 24 h **c.** Normal urine specific gravity **d.** Firm skin turgor and moist oral mucous membranes **e.** Weight within 60 g of admission weight	☐ Maintain patency of the IV line and administer fluids at the rate ordered. Secure the left hand to the sheet and place a medicine cup over the insertion site. Check the IV line hourly. ☐ Record intake and output. Weigh diapers. ☐ Check urine specific gravity at each voiding. ☐ Assess skin turgor. ☐ Maintain NPO status for the first 24 h; then progress to clear liquids. ☐ Weigh the child daily before breakfast.	☐ 1/13: IV of D5 0.2 NS with 2 mEq of NCl per 100 ml was started to run at 50 ml per hour. A no. 22 catheter was placed in the dorsum of Billy's left hand and secured to a padded arm board. Serum electrolytes: sodium, 137; chloride, 96; potassium, 3.9. ☐ 1/13: The skin remains elastic; there is no tenting. ☐ 1/14: Urine output is 10 to 15 ml/kg per 24 h; specific gravity is normal. The IV line is patent; there is no edema or erythema at the site. Weight is stable at 13 kg.
3. Parental anxiety, guilt, and feelings of powerlessness related to their son's illness and hospitalization	☐ The parents will experience decreased anxiety, guilt, and feelings of powerlessness, as evidenced by: **a.** Increased satisfaction with their role performance **b.** Decreased self-blame	☐ Assess the parents' anxiety level. Complete nursing admission information sheet during the first 24 h; assign a primary nurse. ☐ Assess and identify: **a.** The parents' feelings and reactions to the child's illness **b.** The parents' knowledge of the child's condition; clarify and reinforce physician's teaching. **c.** The parents' relationship with each other (their support systems) **d.** The parents' coping mechanisms **e.** Family support and reaction	☐ 1/13: A primary nurse and an associate nurse were assigned. ☐ The mother feels guilty and stated, "It was only a cold, and he seemed okay when I put him to bed. What did I do wrong?" ☐ 9 A.M.: The pediatrician told the parents that the child's condition is common at his age, gets worse at night, and occurs in fall and winter. He reinforced the parents' positive actions and praised their ability to assess the need for medical intervention and notification of the pediatrician. ☐ 1/13: The parents appear close; they touch and support each other verbally and ask questions about their son's condition and how to prevent a reoccurrence. ☐ 1/13: The father asked the maternal grandmother to take the 3-year-old brother so that he can stay with his wife at the hospital.

Nursing Diagnosis	Outcome Criteria	Nursing Interventions	Evaluation and Modifications
			☐ 1/13-16: The grandparents, the minister, and neighbors visited and stayed with Billy so that the mother could go home and rest for several hours and be with Billy's brother.
	c. Increased involvement in Billy's care	☐ Encourage the parents to change Billy's diapers, but save the diapers so that they can be weighed. ☐ Allow the parents to take the rectal temperature. Make a chart of the tasks the parents wish to perform and put this in the Kardex. Teach the parents the reasons for the procedure, and answer their questions.	☐ 1/13, 4:30 P.M.: The mother and father seem less frightened and expressed the wish to assist in care. The nurse explained the reason for the mist tent and how to tuck it under the mattress. The mother or father changes Billy's diapers and takes the rectal temperature if Billy becomes anxious when the nurse does it. The nurse instructed the parents to sit with the child next to a hot shower in a closed bathroom for 20 min during the next episode.
		☐ Encourage the mother to feed, rock, touch, and talk to Billy. ☐ Praise the mother for correct actions.	☐ 1/15: The mother enjoys holding Billy and giving him his bottle for short periods when he is out of the mist tent.
4. Irritability and restlessness of the child related to the illness, the strange environment, and separation anxiety	☐ Billy will adjust to the strange environment, as evidenced by decreased restlessness and irritability and resting and napping two or three times per day.	☐ Ask the parents to bring in a familiar blanket or toy from home. ☐ Place pictures of family members on the crib; discuss the parents' activities while caring for the child. ☐ Place mobiles on the crib, or provide soft, squeezable toys and animals; a mirror; or stacking disks. ☐ Encourage the parents to visit and care for Billy as much as they can. Have a cot available if a parent or other family member wishes to stay overnight.	☐ 1/13: The father brought a blanket from Billy's crib. ☐ Billy enjoys seeing mother's picture prior to her arrival and hearing a tape-recorded story or message. ☐ 1/13: Since the grandparents are caring for the 3-year-old sibling, the mother can stay with Billy all day.

*Prepared by Nancy Horvath, B.S.N., and Nancy L. Ramsey, R.N., M.S.N.

References

1. Murry, John, *The Normal Lung: The Basis for Diagnosis and Treatment of Pulmonary Disease,* Saunders, Philadelphia, 1976, p. 46.
2. *Nursing Photobook: Nursing Pediatric Patients,* Nursing 82 Books, Intermed Communications, Springhouse, Pa., 1982, p. 88.
3. Ibid.
4. Hazinski, Mary, *Nursing Care of the Critically Ill Child,* Mosby, St. Louis, 1984, p. 8.
5. Ibid., p. 7.
6. Whaley, Lucille F., and Donna L. Wong, *Nursing Care of Infants and Children, Mosby, St. Louis, 1983, p. 1160.*
7. Weinberg, Arim, Charles Christiansen, and Doreen Wise, "Respiratory Rate: Forgotten Clue in Early Detection of Congenital Heart Disease," *Pediatric Nursing,* **3**(3):40 (May 1977).
8. Ibid.
9. Shapiro, Barry, Ronald Harrison, and Caroll Trout, *Clinical Application of Respiratory Care,* Year Book, Philadelphia, Chicago, 1975.
10. Bates, Barbara, *A Guide to Physical Examination,* Lippincott, Philadelphia, 1983.
11. Whaley and Wong, op. cit., p. 208.
12. Shapiro, Harrison, and Trout, op. cit., p. 106.
13. Ibid., p. 127.
14. Ibid., pp. 231–233.
15. Corbo, Beverly H., and Huda Abu-Huda, "Children's Experience with Endotracheal Intubation," *Dimension of Critical Care Nursing* **3**(3):184 (May–June 1984).
16. Aradine, Carolyn E., "Home Care for Young Children with Long-Term Tracheostomies," *American Journal of Maternal-Child Nursing* **5**:121–125 (1980).
17. Blazer, Shraga, Yehezkel Naveh, and Abraham Friedman, "Foreign Body in the Airway: A Review of 200 Cases," *American Journal of Diseases of Children* **134**:68 (1980).
18. Ibid.
19. Richardson, Mark, and Robin Cotton, "Anatomic Abnormalities of the Pediatric Airway: A Review of 200 Cases," *American Journal of Diseases of Children* **134**:68 (1980).
20. Ibid.
21. Champous, Susan, "Upper Respiratory Tract Infection," *Nurse Practioner* **2**(6):31–35 (July–August 1977).
22. Hoekelman, R. S. Blatman, P. Brunell, S. Friedman, and H. Seidel, *Principles of Pediatrics,* McGraw-Hill, New York, 1978, p. 1468.
23. Maze, Aubrey, and Edward Bloch, "Stridor in Pediatric Patients," *Anesthesiology* **50**:138 (1979).
24. Long, Sarah S., "Treatment of Acute Pneumonia in Infants and Children," *Pediatric Clinics of North America* **30**(2):297–312 (April 1983).
25. Murphy, Shirley, and Alfred Florman, "Lung Defenses against Infection: A Clinical Correlation," *Pediatrics* **72**(7):1–15 (July 1983).
26. Kempe, H., H. Silver, and D. O'Brien (eds.), *Current Pediatric Diagnosis and Treatment,* Lange, Los Altos, Calif., 1984, p. 319.
27. Karus, Celinda, "Tuberculosis: An Overview of Pathogenesis and Prevention," *Nurse Practitioner* **8**(2):21–25 (February 1983).
28. Lorin, Martin, et al., "Treatment of Tuberculosis in Children," *Pediatric Clinics of North America* **30**(2):333–343 (April 1983).
29. Karus, op. cit.
30. American Thoracic Society, "Screening for Pulmonary Tuberculosis in Institutions," *American Review of Respiratory Disease* **115**(5):1 (1977).
31. Hoekelman, Blatman, Brunell, Friedman, and Seidel, op. cit., p. 1207.
32. Fahrer, Lawrence, "Tuberculosis in the United States Today," *American Lung Association Bulletin* **65**(3):2 (1979).
33. Hoekelman, Blatman, Brunell, Friedman, and Seidel, op. cit., p. 1208.
34. Fischer, R., "Pediatric Drug Information (Aerosols Used in Asthma)," *Pediatric Nursing* **11**(1):51 (January–February 1985).
35. Mattson, Ake, "Psychologic Aspects of Childhood Asthma," *Pediatric Clinics of North America* **22**(1):77–78 (January–February 1975).
36. Taussig, Lynn, *Cystic Fibrosis,* Thieme-Stratton, New York, 1981.

22

Sandra Sonnessa Griffiths
Nancy Kosiba Koster

Cardiovascular function

Upon completion of this chapter, the student will be able to:

1. Describe the growth and development of the fetal heart during gestation.
2. Name the components of fetal circulation that differ from those of postnatal circulation.
3. Describe the changes in the heart and circulation that occur at or soon after birth.
4. List alterations in cardiovascular status that may be present if the child has congenital heart disease.
5. Identify the signs and symptoms of congestive heart failure.
6. Discuss the nursing care of a child with congestive heart failure.
7. Describe the hemodynamic components that differentiate acyanotic heart disease from cyanotic heart disease.
8. Suggest two reasons why either medical or surgical treatment may be appropriate for a child with congenital heart disease.
9. Describe selected examples of acyanotic heart defects and cyanotic heart defects.
10. State the nursing management involved in caring for a child after heart surgery.
11. Identify areas of health teaching for children (and their parents) who have atherosclerosis, hypertension, or Kawasaki syndrome.
12. Discuss the etiology and nursing management of acute rheumatic fever.
13. Identify the purpose of drugs commonly used for children with heart disease.
14. Discuss areas of teaching appropriate for the child and the family when the child has congenital heart disease.

Ever since living organisms evolved beyond the size of a few cells, a circulatory system that moves essential substances from the environment to each cell has been a necessity for all but the tiniest creatures. Similarly, as soon as cell division gets well under way in the human embryo, a primitive circulatory system is required, which is then transformed progressively in the developing embryo, ultimately acquiring its fully developed characteristics. The pumping structure of the developed circulatory system provides the force needed to circulate life-sustaining oxygen and nutrients. Any alterations in the normal heart structure affect the transportation of these vital materials.

A malformation in heart structure, or a *congenital heart defect*, occurs during early fetal development. The incidence of congenital heart defects is estimated to be from approximately 10 to 20 per 1000 live births.[1] The exact etiology of a congenital heart defect is often unknown, but theories center on a combination of genetic and environmental influences. It is known that the more genetic defects present in a child, the greater the chances of a coexisting heart defect. Approximately 40 percent of children with Down syndrome have cardiac defects; one-third have endocardial cushion defects; and the rest have a patent ductus arteriosus, atrial septal defects, or tetralogy of Fallot.[2] Thirty-five percent of individuals with Turner syndrome have a defect; the most common is coarctation of the aorta.[3] Prematurity has also been associated with a higher incidence of congenital heart disease in newborns.

FETAL HEART DEVELOPMENT

From the time of fertilization until the third week of gestation, the developing embryo's nutritional needs are supplied by diffusion, since the embryo is merely a few cell layers thick. The heart and vascular system develop rapidly from the third to the eighth weeks of gestation. A primitive hollow, curved tube gradually develops into four highly specialized chambers of the heart. Simultaneously, the cell layers of the *pericardium* (the outer layer of the heart), the *myocardium* (muscle wall), and the *endocardium* (inner lining) develop. During the first 3 weeks, there is no separation of chambers. The blood flows freely into the right and left atria and to the right and left ventricles and leaves the heart in an undivided flow. By the end of the sixth week, the primitive tubular heart is differentiated into a parallel double-pump circulatory system and is a recognizable four-chambered structure similar to that present at birth.

Fetal circulation*

The fetal heart and vascular system develop in a way that will support the fetus in utero and permit rapid transition to extrauterine life at birth. *Arteries* are vessels that take blood away from the heart; *veins* bring blood back to the heart. In adult circulation, all arteries except the pulmonary artery carry blood enriched with oxygen in the lungs from the heart to the body tissues. The pulmonary artery transports oxygen-depleted blood from the heart to the lungs. The oxygenated blood then returns from the lungs via the pulmonary veins to the heart, where it is pumped out of the left ventricle to the systemic circulation. During gestation, the placenta is the site of carbon dioxide–oxygen exchange and nutrient absorption. The lungs do not develop sufficiently to support extrauterine life until 26 to 28 weeks of gestation.

The fetal circulatory system utilizes three blood-diverting mechanisms, called *shunts*, to direct oxygenated blood flow away from the liver and lungs. The three shunt systems are the *ductus venosus*, the *foramen ovale*, and the *ductus arteriosus* (Fig. 22-1).† Closure of these shunts after birth is necessary if a normal extrauterine pattern of blood flow is to exist.

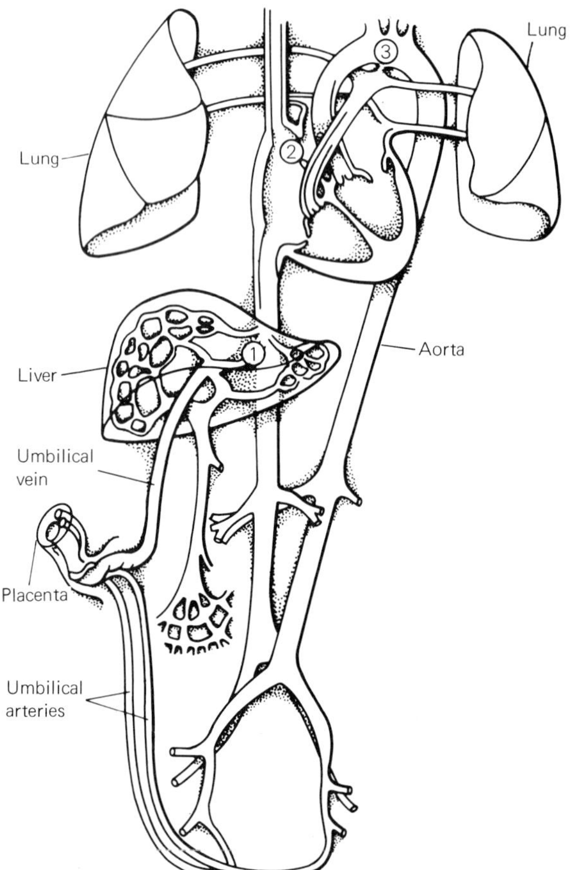

Figure 22-1 Fetal circulation. (1) The ductus venosus. (2) The foramen ovale. (3) The ductus arteriosus (under label).

Oxygenated blood flows from the placenta through the umbilical vein to the liver. Here, some blood is directed into the hepatic circulation, while the rest is shunted directly through the ductus venosus to the inferior vena cava. The blood circulating through the liver returns to the inferior vena cava through the hepatic veins. Blood from the lower extremities and the alimentary canal returns to the heart through the inferior vena cava. Blood entering the heart is a mixture of well-oxygenated blood received from the ductus

*The authors gratefully acknowledge the assistance of Barbara Macpherson, B.S.N., and Sarah Sacksteder, B.S.N., of Fresno Valley Hospital, in the preparation of this section and in the presentation of specific congenital heart defects.

†The authors wish to thank Kathleen A. Nyberg for the sketches on which the anatomic drawings in this chapter are based.

venosus and blood with a lower oxygen saturation received from the gastrointestinal system and the lower extremities.

Upon entering the right atrium, most of the blood from the inferior vena cava is directed through the foramen ovale (an opening between the atria) into the left atrium, bypassing the right ventricle and the lungs. The foramen ovale allows blood to flow unidirectionally from the right atrium to the left atrium. Only small amounts of blood enter the left atrium from the pulmonary veins. Blood entering the left atrium flows into the left ventricle and out through the ascending aorta.

Upper extremity and cerebral blood returns to the heart through the superior vena cava. This blood, low in oxygen content, and some blood from the inferior vena cava, flows from the right atrium into the right ventricle and then into the pulmonary artery. The ductus arteriosus directs most of this blood away from the immature lungs directly into the aorta. The pulmonary vascular resistance (the resistance to blood flow through the lungs) in the fetus is normally high, partly because of the vasoconstriction caused by the hypoxia effect in the lungs of the fetus. A portion of right ventricular output still flows through the pulmonary circulation; this blood returns from the lungs to the left atrium through the pulmonary veins. Blood from the descending aorta is distributed to the alimentary tract and the lower extremities and returns to the placenta through the umbilical arteries. The left ventricle does not meet high resistance when pumping blood into the systemic circulation because the placenta is a low-resistance system.

Before birth, the right atrium receives and accommodates more blood volume than the other chambers of the heart. This causes the right side of the heart, especially the ventricle, to be slightly larger than the left. This normal right heart hypertrophy gradually diminishes after birth as the left ventricle begins to receive blood from the lungs. The left ventricle then enlarges to accommodate the increased blood volume and to overcome the increased systemic vascular resistance that occurs when the placenta is no longer part of the systemic circulation.

Circulatory changes at birth

At birth, the function of the three fetal circulation shunt structures—the ductus arteriosus, foramen ovale, and ductus venosus—changes drastically. The lungs assume the function of oxygen–carbon dioxide exchange. With initiation of respiration, the alveoli expand and blood flow through the lungs increases. Pulmonary vessel resistance decreases as the blood vessels dilate and vessel wall tension is lowered. The increased oxygen concentration is believed to be one of the primary stimuli for closure of the ductus arteriosus. Separation from the placenta causes increased resistance in the arterial system. Left atrial pressures exceed right atrial pressures and the foramen ovale, anatomically structured to permit flow only from right to left, closes. The heart now acts as a functioning unit rather than two parallel pumps. The ductus venosus eventually becomes a nonfunctional ligament.

CIRCULATION IN THE HEART AFTER BIRTH

The heart is a muscular pumping organ designed to circulate oxygen-depleted blood through the pulmonary system and oxygen-enriched blood through the body. The right atrium and ventricle and the left atrium and ventricle serve as two circulatory systems alternately contracting and relaxing in series. Venous blood returning from the systemic circulation enters the right atrium by way of the superior vena cava and inferior vena cava (Fig. 22-2). The oxygen-depleted, dark-red blood is propelled through the tricuspid valve into the right ventricle. The right ventricle pumps blood through the pulmonary artery to the lungs, where carbon dioxide–oxygen gas exchange takes place. Blood returning from the lungs is oxygen-enriched and bright red. It enters the left atrium through the pulmonary veins and is propelled through the mitral valve into the left ventricle. Thus the *oxygen saturation* values (the amount of oxygen combined with hemoglobin) vary between the right and left heart chambers (Fig. 22-3).

The pressure within each chamber differs (Fig. 22-3) and has a characteristic waveform corresponding to a numerical value (Fig. 22-2). Because blood always flows from areas of higher pressure to areas of lower pressure, an increase in pressure in the chambers, lungs, or systemic circulation causes the part of the heart pumping blood into that area to work harder. For example, when the right atrium contracts, its pressure is higher than that of the right ventricle during

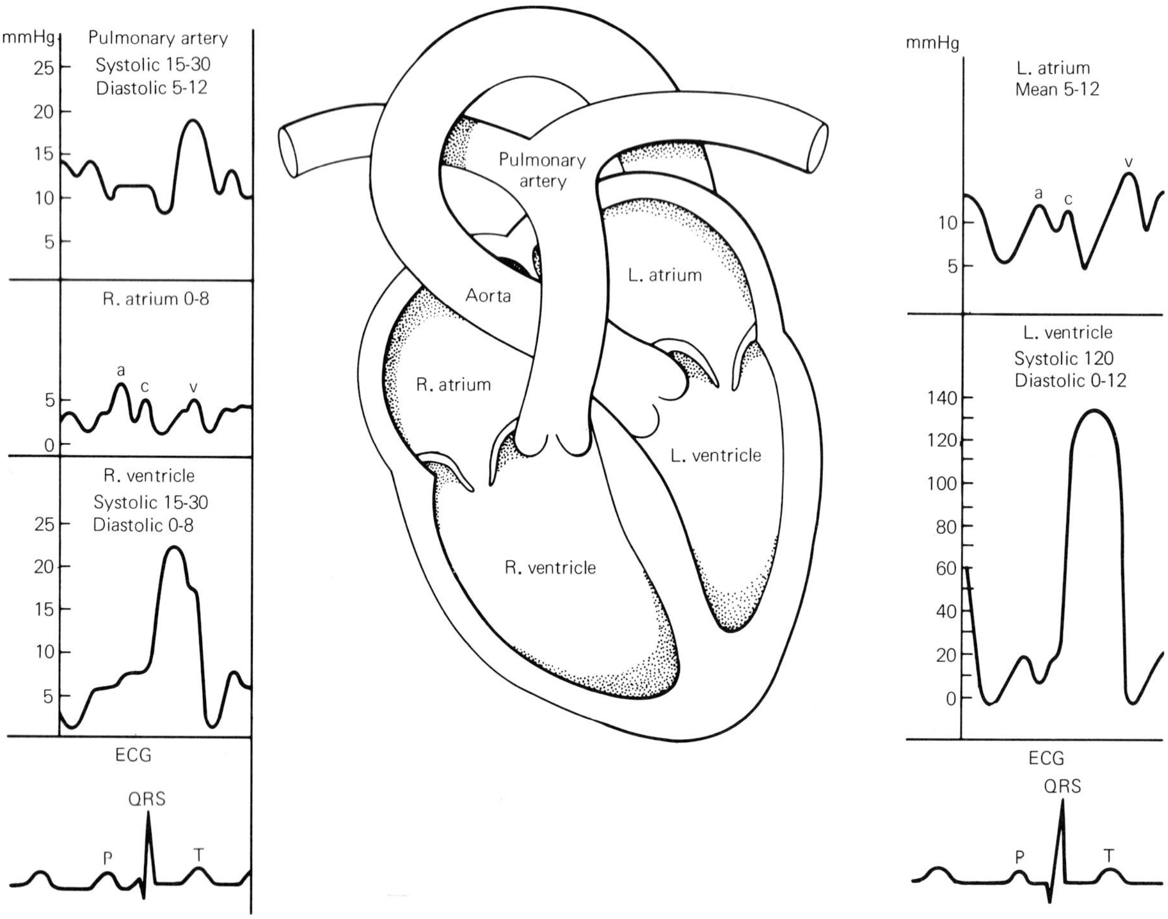

Figure 22-2 Adult circulation and normal pressure waves. (*After Netter, 1978.*)

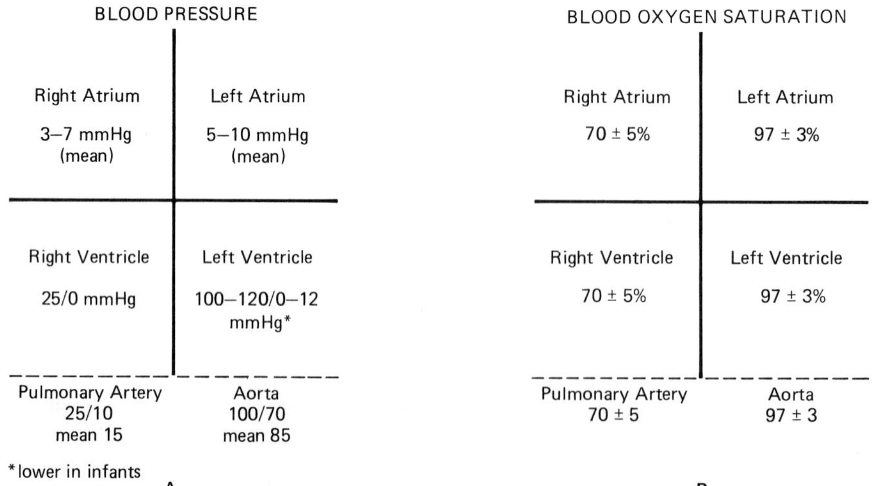

A. BLOOD PRESSURE

Right Atrium	Left Atrium
3–7 mmHg (mean)	5–10 mmHg (mean)
Right Ventricle	**Left Ventricle**
25/0 mmHg	100–120/0–12 mmHg*
Pulmonary Artery	**Aorta**
25/10 mean 15	100/70 mean 85

*lower in infants

B. BLOOD OXYGEN SATURATION

Right Atrium	Left Atrium
70 ± 5%	97 ± 3%
Right Ventricle	**Left Ventricle**
70 ± 5%	97 ± 3%
Pulmonary Artery	**Aorta**
70 ± 5	97 ± 3

Figure 22-3 Normal pressure and oxygen saturation of blood in the heart chambers.

diastole (relaxation). The left ventricular musculature is much thicker than the right and provides the required contraction pressure to force the blood through the aorta and out into the higher-pressure systemic circulation to perfuse the body. The blood circulates through the systemic capillary system that connects the arteries with the veins. In the capillaries the oxygen and nutrients move out of the blood to the cells in exchange for carbon dioxide and other metabolic waste products.

ASSESSMENT OF CARDIOVASCULAR FUNCTION

Accurate cardiovascular assessment is vital to the child with a congenital heart malformation. The assessment includes a nursing history, a physical examination, and diagnostic studies performed by specialized cardiologists and technicians.

The nursing history

A thorough admission history is obtained to provide a data base of the child's health and social history and to help caregivers meet the child's individual needs (see Chap. 14). The presenting problem (or chief complaint), the parents' history of heart disease and other pertinent illnesses, and patterns of daily living all provide information about a child with suspected or confirmed heart disease (Table 22-1).

Even though a tentative medical diagnosis is made prior to admission, it is important to determine the parents' and child's own understanding of why hospitalization is necessary. Asking what brings them to the hospital (chief complaint) and exploring what they think is the problem with the child's heart facilitate assessment of understanding and potential teaching needs.

Ask about past hospitalizations and illnesses, especially respiratory infections. Respiratory infections are frequently present in infants and,

Table 22-1 Outline of a History for a Child with Heart Disease

1. Chief Complaint or Presenting Problem

2. Past Medical History
Hospitalizations
Medications
Frequency of respiratory infections

3. Family History
Hypertension
Atherosclerosis
Myocardial infarction
Rheumatic fever
Others: diabetes mellitus, genetic diseases, birth defects

4. Maternal History
Previous childbirth history
Illness or complications during pregnancy
Exposure to x-ray therapy or rubella during pregnancy

5. Newborn
Weight
Gestational age
Length of labor
Apgar score
Need for resuscitation
Cyanosis at birth (transient or persistent)
Breathlessness
Grunting or wheezing respirations
Feeding difficulties

6. Infant or Toddler
Weight gain since birth
Diet and appetite
Feeding or sucking difficulties
Fatigue
Cyanosis
Developmental milestones:
- Holding head up (1 to 3 months)
- Sitting up without support (6 to 7 months)
- Crawling (8 to 10 months)
- Standing without support (12 to 14 months)
- Walking (by 18 months)
- Language development: sounds, words, sentences

7. Preschooler or School-Age Child
Daily activities:
- Hours of sleep
- Rest breaks
- Meals

Play tolerance:
- Running
- Climbing
- Riding a bicycle

Chest pain
Syncope
Fatigue
Breathlessness
History of rheumatic fever
Recent sore throat or upper respiratory infection:
- Joint pain
- Fever
- Loss of appetite

Days of school missed in last 6 months
Language development: sentences

less commonly, in older children with cardiac anomalies. Find out what medications the child has taken in the past and is presently taking, since the physician may want the child to receive these drugs while in the hospital. Record information regarding the dosage, frequency, side effects, and special precautions needed. Though the parents usually know the name of a drug that the child is taking, it is helpful to have them bring the prescription container to the hospital.

Inquire about family history related to heart disease, including cardiac defects, rheumatic fever, hypertension, atherosclerosis, sudden death, and myocardial infarctions. The presence of other disorders related to heart disease, such as genetic disorders, birth defects, and diabetes mellitus, should also be recorded in the family history.

If relevant, as in the case of a child less than 2 years old, investigate the maternal childbirth history, including illnesses, complications during pregnancy, use of medications, and exposure to x-ray therapy or rubella. Determine the type of labor and delivery, any complications, and the initial newborn assessment. Low birth weight, prematurity, need for respiratory assistance or resuscitation, cyanosis, or heart murmur may indicate the presence of a congenital heart defect.

Assessment of the general health of the child, patterns of daily living, and appropriate developmental milestones gives the nurse clues as to the severity of heart disease and the ability of the heart to function effectively. Ask objective questions. Ask the parents to clarify vague information by giving specific examples of the child's behavior.

Incorporate age-appropriate questions about activity tolerance into the parent's descriptions of usual patterns. Feeding difficulties, poor or weak sucking, and poor weight gain are common in infants with severe heart defects because eating requires increased energy and effort. They fatigue easily, become dyspneic, and may get cyanotic. Toddlers, preschoolers, and school-age children tire easily while playing and may become breathless. Identify the frequency of rest breaks by asking specific questions about usual age-related activities. For instance, ask how long the child plays outside and whether the child can run for a moderate distance, climb to "reasonable" heights, or ride a bike. Any difficulties should be noted, since activity tolerance is the most reliable indicator of cardiac status. Recently, graded exercise testing has helped assess cardiac status in individual children.

Chest pain, though usually pathological in adults, may occur during periods of stress and anxiety in children. Underlying cardiac pathology is rare except in pericarditis, an inflammation of the pericardial sac, where the major complaint is precordial chest pain. Generally, benign chest wall pain is common in school-age children and adolescents; however, a belief in the need for a thorough examination is increasing in the medical community.

Explore the impact of heart disease on the child and family to assess how the family as a unit and the individual members are coping with the child's illness. The parents can describe the child's relationship to them, to siblings, and to friends. An older child or adolescent may find it helpful to share feelings about having heart disease. If appropriate, once a therapeutic trusting relationship is established, explore how the parents felt when they learned about their child's heart problem. Some parents live in constant fear of sudden death, especially if the child shows overt effects of illness. Others may express feelings of guilt, grief, denial, and anxiety about the future. Collect data about other stress, financial or occupational, that the family is experiencing.

The physical examination

Inspection A major part of the physical assessment of a child with congenital heart disease is the inspection. A large portion of the inspection can be done without touching the child.

First, assess the child's general features. Evaluate general temperament for signs of irritability, restlessness, or lethargy that may indicate *hypoxia*, an inadequate supply of oxygen to body tissues. Assess growth by obtaining height and weight and plotting the values on a growth curve. Children with a congenital heart defect may be underweight for their age. Note the child's posture while standing or sitting. If possible, observe the child at play to note breathlessness, increasing cyanosis, or squatting to rest.

The nutritional status of the child should be evaluated, since feeding difficulties and poor weight gain are common in children with severe heart defects. Observe the child's level of alertness, brightness of eyes, and brilliance of hair. Redness of the gums may indicate a vitamin deficiency. Note the number of teeth the child has and whether they are deciduous or permanent teeth. Observe the child's gait for unsteadiness.

Observe the skin color when the child is at rest, agitated, or crying. The color may be difficult to assess if the child is anemic or jaundiced. In children with dark skin, subtle color changes are more difficult to assess. It is important to establish a baseline to aid in identifying cyanosis. The presence of *cyanosis,* a bluish discoloration of the skin, is indicative of oxygen-depleted blood circulating in the peripheral body tissues. Cyanosis occurs when the oxygen saturation (Sa_{O2}) is less than 85 percent or with 5 gm of reduced hemoglobin. The color of the nail beds, lips, and oral mucous membranes is the most reliable indicator of oxygen saturation in tissues. *Central cyanosis* involves the trunk, extremities, and mucous membranes. Cyanosis around the mouth (*circumoral cyanosis*) and around the eyes (*periorbital cyanosis*) may be observed in infants and young children and may or may not be related to heart disease. *Acrocyanosis* (blue-tinged hands and feet) is frequently observed in normal newborns and is not a reliable indicator of a heart problem. Besides cyanosis, note any pallor or diaphoresis (sweating). Flat, reddened, purplish pinpoint lesions called *petechiae* are also significant in children with suspected cardiovascular disease and may indicate blood-clotting disorders, circulatory stasis, or obstruction.

Inspect the nails of the fingers and toes for clubbing. *Clubbing,* a rounding of the tips of the fingers and toes with a convex curved angle, indicates chronic tissue hypoxia that accompanies severe heart or pulmonary disease (Fig. 22-4). Although the exact etiology is unknown, the cells expand in number to compensate for decreased oxygen saturation in peripheral tissues.

Assess respiratory status after removing the child's clothing. It is vital to observe respirations during periods of rest and activity, since problems in the cardiac system can affect respirations. Note the pattern of breathing. Normal infants typically use their abdominal muscles in breathing. Count the rate and note the depth and regularity of the respirations. Compare the values with the appropriate range for the child's age. (See Table 16-19.) Observe for signs of respiratory distress: (1) *tachypnea,* increased respiratory rate for a given age; (2) *dyspnea,* difficulty breathing; (3) *retractions,* use of the accessory muscles in the neck, clavicle area, sternum, and intercostal spaces; (4) *nasal flaring;* and (5) *audible breath sounds* such as inspiratory stridor and expiratory grunting.

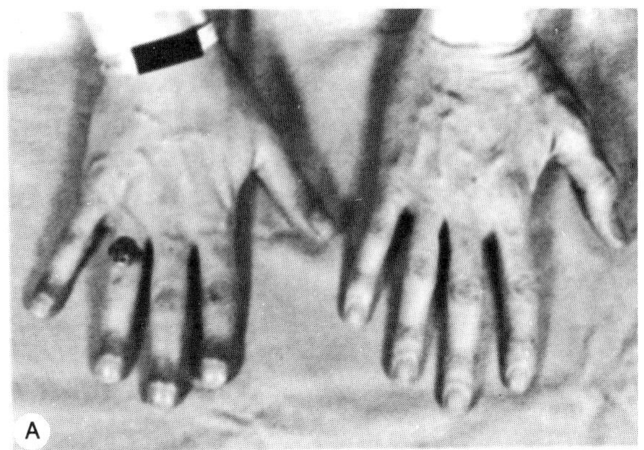

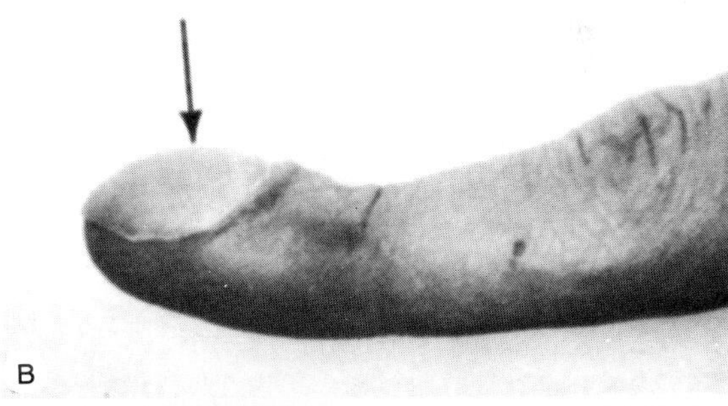

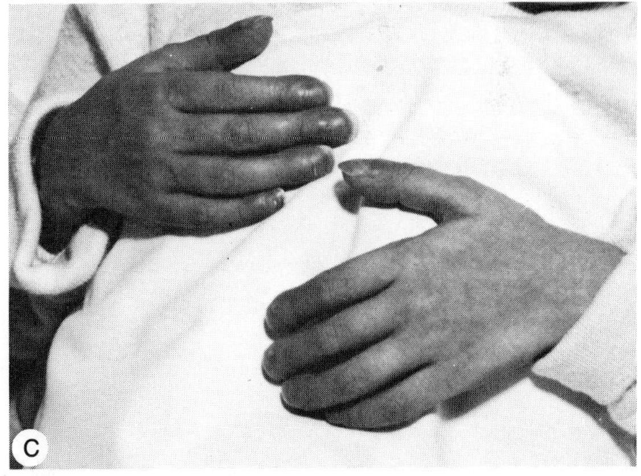

Figure 22-4 Clubbing. (*A*) Typical cyanosis and clubbing of the fingers in a young adult (left), compared with the fingers of a normal adult (right). (*B*) A close-up profile of clubbing (arrow). (*C*) Clubbing in a young child. (*[A] and [B] from Joseph Perloff, The Clinical Recognition of Congenital Heart Disease, 2d ed., Saunders, Philadelphia, 1978. Used with permission. [C] Courtesy of Robert W. Feldt.*)

Check for visibly bounding pulses in the neck

and in the chest over the point of maximum impulse. The point of maximum impulse is located at the fourth to fifth intercostal space to the left of the sternal border near the midclavicular line (Fig. 22-5). Visible pulsations (heaves) may indicate circulatory overload and ventricular hypertrophy. Thrills (low-frequency vibrations associated with murmurs) are best felt with the palm of the hand. The suprasternal notch can be palpated with a fingertip.

Palpation The use of palpation is essential in assessing cardiovascular status. The skin should be evaluated for temperature (warm or cool), moisture (dry or clammy), and turgor. The presence of "tenting" (the skin remains suspended when the skin over the abdomen is pinched and pulled taut) may indicate dehydration or electrolyte imbalance.

Body pulses should be evaluated for rate, rhythm, and volume. Palpate pulses in an orderly manner, beginning at the head and ending at the feet. Use a light touch, and palpate pulses on both sides of the body simultaneously. The temporal and carotid artery pulses may be weaker than in adults. Check brachial and radial pulses in the upper extremities and the femoral, popliteal, and dorsalis pedis pulses in the lower extremities. The following may be used as a guideline:

4+ Bounding
3+ Strong
2+ Palpable but weak
1+ Barely palpable
0 Absent

Note and record any alterations in the rhythm or quality.

Observe *capillary refill* time by pinching the tip of a finger or toe. Count the time in seconds that it takes for the blanched or whitened area to re-

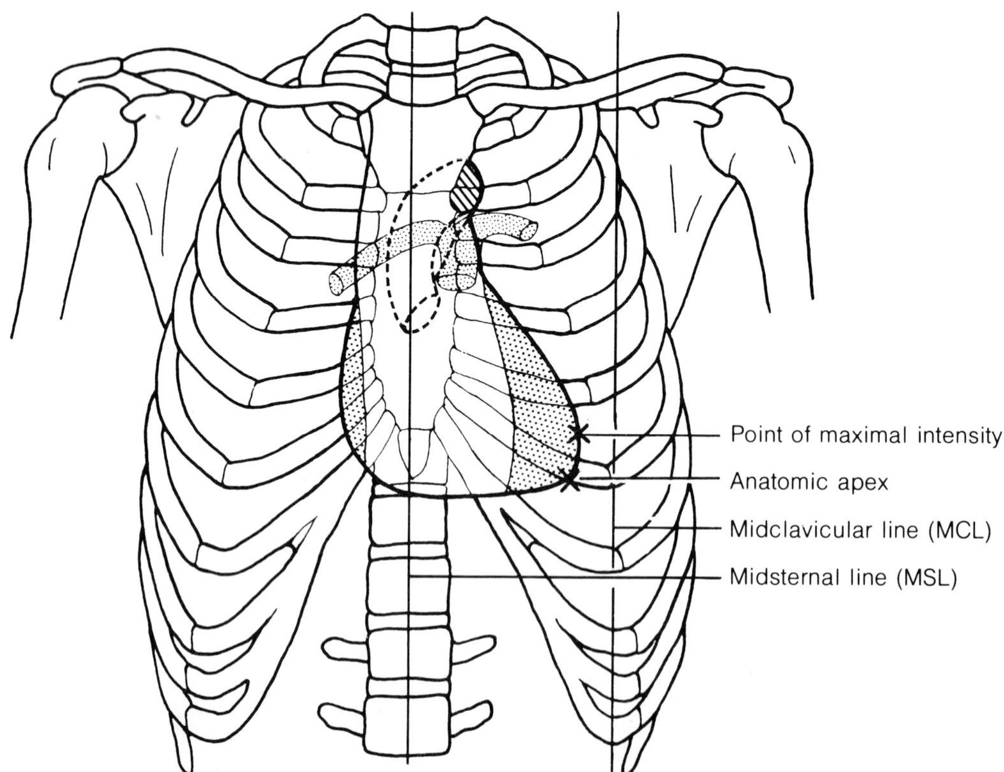

Figure 22-5 The point of maximum impulse. *(From E. Hochstein and A. L. Rubin, Physical Diagnosis, McGraw-Hill, New York, 1964. Used with permission.)*

sume its usual color. The color should return immediately if the heart is circulating blood effectively.

The child should be examined for evidence of edema. Fluid accumulation may occur in the interstitial tissues in heart failure, but evidence of overt peripheral edema is rarely seen in infants. In older children, dependent edema may be observed in areas affected by gravity and position. Check the ankles and sacral area for edema. Note whether the edema is pitting or nonpitting. Press the edematous area. If the press mark remains, note the time in seconds that it takes to lose the imprint. Pitting edema is frequently described on a scale from 1+ to 4+, with 4+ being the longest time that the edematous area takes to lose the press mark.

Advanced physical assessment skills include palpation of the liver and percussion of the borders of the heart. A discussion of these techniques is not within the scope of this text.

Auscultation The auscultation of blood pressure, breath sounds, and heart sounds is very important in cardiovascular assessment but is often threatening to young children, who sometimes fear that someone who listens to their heart can hear their private thoughts and wishes. The stethoscope and blood pressure apparatus are frightening, and the child interprets these instruments as intrusive and harmful to the body. Allowing the child to handle the blood pressure cuff and stethoscope before and after using them may help alleviate some fears of bodily harm (Fig. 14-3).

Blood pressure should be taken when the child is quiet, if possible, since anxiety may increase the blood pressure. Using an appropriate cuff size (see Table 16-21), take the blood pressure in all four extremities. In young infants, the blood pressure of the arms and legs should be equal. In children over 1 year of age, the blood pressure in the legs is normally 10 to 40 mmHg higher than that in the arms. Blood pressure in the legs lower than that in the arms may indicate coarctation of the aorta. Pressure should be released at a rate of 1 to 3 mmHg per second and allowed to fall to zero. Repeat each reading at least once.

With infants and young children, palpation of systolic blood pressure is much easier than auscultation. When possible, auscultate blood pressure to determine both the systolic and the diastolic components. Assessment of blood pressure using an electronic digital monitor is an accurate method. After obtaining the pressure values, compare them with normal ranges for the age of the child (Table 16-20). The *pulse pressure,* or the difference between the systolic and diastolic pressures, should be calculated. Although the normal pulse pressure spread is 20 to 50 mmHg, a greater pulse pressure may occur in hypertension, aortic regurgitation, arteriovenous malformation, or patent ductus arteriosus. A smaller pulse pressure may occur in tachycardia, severe aortic stenosis, pericardial effusion, or congestive heart failure. Abnormal blood pressure and pulse pressure findings should be noted and reported to the physician.

Auscultating breath sounds is important in the assessment of the cardiac and respiratory systems. Normally, breath sounds should be clear and equal bilaterally in all lobes of the lungs. Characteristically, breath sounds in the lower lobes are not as loud as those in the upper lobes, but they should still be heard. Any adventitious or abnormal sounds, such as rales, rhonchi, or wheezing, should be reported.

Normal heart sounds are condensed over the child's small chest area and are due to the combination of the closing of the valves, contraction of the heart, and vibrations of blood moving through the chambers. The first heart sound (S_1), *lub,* represents the closure of the mitral and tricuspid valves and is associated with the systolic portion of the cardiac cycle. It is heard over the entire precordium (the area of anterior chest wall overlying the heart) with the child in any position.

The second heart sound (S_2), *dub,* signifies the closing of the aortic and pulmonary valves and is associated with the end of systole and start of diastole, or the filling phase of the cardiac cycle. It can be heard over the entire precordium and is affected by respiration. A normal physiological splitting of S_2 into two components may be heard on inspiration. In newborns and infants, it may be difficult to ascertain the difference between S_1 and S_2, since their heart rate is so rapid. Light palpation over the carotid, apical, or femoral pulse area will help identify the first heart sound, since the pulses are synchronous with S_1.

A third heart sound (S_3) is present in half of normal children. It reflects transmitted vibrations during ventricular filling. The presence of S_3 can be heard best in the fifth intercostal space with the child in a supine position. The presence of S_3 may also indicate right heart failure or a systemic illness.

A fourth heart sound (S_4) is heard immediately before S_1 and, when audible, is heard best over the lower left sternal border. Though heard primarily in adults, S_4 represents an audible resistance to filling, as in aortic or pulmonary stenosis.

A nurse listening to the heart should first count the apical heart rate for a full minute when the child is resting or quiet. After this, identification of the audible heart sounds should be undertaken in a systematic manner—first, S_1; second, S_2; and third, S_3. Abnormal heart sounds are often difficult to auscultate, even by trained persons.

After counting the heart rate and comparing it with the normal range for the specific child, identify the rhythm, and record whether it is regular or irregular. An increased heart rate, *tachycardia,* or a decreased heart rate, *bradycardia,* should be reported.

Any noise heard between the heart sounds that is not characteristic of a specific heart sound is termed a *murmur.* The majority of murmurs heard in children are benign and do not represent underlying heart disease. They are called *functional murmurs* or *innocent murmurs* and reflect the normal blood turbulence transmitted through the child's thin chest wall. Murmurs are also caused by changes within the structure of the heart. Murmurs are heard when some resistance in the circulatory system is present that creates turbulence in blood flow. In congenital heart anomalies, a narrowed or incompetent valve, an altered structure, or a backflow of blood may produce a murmur.

Murmurs are characterized by six factors:

1. The *intensity,* or loudness, of a murmur is often rated on a scale ranging from grade I to grade VI. A grade I murmur is faint, and each grade successively increases in intensity. A grade VI murmur can be heard without a stethoscope.
2. The *frequency,* or pitch, of a murmur is related to the velocity of blood flow through or around the area of resistance. The greater the velocity of blood flow, the higher the pitch. Low-pitched murmurs are heard best using the diaphragm of the stethoscope, while higher-pitched murmurs are heard best using the bell portion.
3. The *configuration* of a murmur can be demonstrated, if diagramed, by a particular shape.
4. The *quality* of a murmur may be described as harsh, rasping, musical, whistling, rumbling, or blowing.
5. *Timing* in the cardiac cycle is one of the key diagnostic tools used to define a murmur. Murmurs are systolic, occurring between S_1 and S_2; diastolic, occurring between S_2 and S_1; or continuous, occurring throughout the entire cardiac cycle.
6. *Location,* or where a murmur is heard best.

Murmurs may radiate to other parts of the thorax. It is important to note whether a murmur can be auscultated through the posterior chest wall or palpated over the apical area, sternum, or posterior thorax. Also note whether the murmur changes with position or upon inspiration or expiration. Though detection of murmurs is difficult, the presence of even a loud murmur may not indicate a heart defect.

A *bruit* is a high-pitched murmur heard during systole over a specific part of the body other than the heart. Most bruits in children are not significant. Children with aortic or pulmonary stenosis, however, may have a systolic bruit heard over the carotid artery.

Diagnostic studies

Selected diagnostic studies may be done in conjunction with other components of cardiovascular assessment. The number and type of studies vary, depending on the clinical signs and symptoms present, the tentative diagnosis, and the plan of management of the particular problem.

Hematologic tests Hematologic studies measure specific blood components that may reflect cardiovascular function. The studies done and the normal ranges vary slightly from one institution to another (Table 22-2).

Serum electrolyte studies may be done as needed. Sodium, potassium, and calcium, which are important for intracellular and extracellular impulse conduction, have a significant effect on myocardial electrical conduction. Values within normal ranges are vital for efficient contractions of the muscular myocardium.

A complete blood count, including hemoglobin, hematocrit, and a white blood cell count, helps identify the quality as well as the quantity of the blood and plasma. An increased white blood cell value may indicate the presence of infection in the body. Children with cyanotic heart disease may have *polycythemia,* an increased number of red blood cells, as a result of elevated red blood

Table 22-2 Hematologic Values That May Reflect Cardiovascular Function*

Factor	Normal Range
Sodium	135 to 145 mEq per liter
Potassium	3.5 to 5.0 mEq per liter
Calcium	9 to 11 mg per 100 ml
Chloride	98 to 106 mEq per liter
White blood count	5000 to 10,000 per cubic millimeter
Red blood count	5,400,000 per cubic millimeter—males 4,600,000 per cubic millimeter—females
Hemoglobin	19 ± 5—newborns 14 ± 3—infants 12 ± 2—children 14 ± 2—adolescents
Hematocrit	40 to 52%—newborns 35 ± 5%—infants 35 to 37%—children 38 to 40%—adolescents
Blood urea nitrogen	10 to 20 mg per 100 ml
Creatinine	0.7 to 1.5 mg per 100 ml
Platelets	150,000 to 350,000 per cubic millimeter
Prothrombin time	11 to 16 s
Partial thromboplastin time	25 to 40 s
Cholesterol, total	120 to 230 mg per 100 ml—children and adolescents aged 1 to 19 years
Triglycerides	25 to 150 mg per 100 ml

*Values may vary slightly in different laboratories.

cell production. This increase reflects the body's attempt to compensate for the oxygen-depleted blood flow to peripheral tissues.

Coagulation studies may be done if there is a history of abnormal bleeding or bruising or a family history of bleeding or bruising tendency or as part of a screening procedure prior to invasive diagnostic studies or heart surgery. A platelet count, prothrombin time, and partial thromboplastin time are used to evaluate the essential components of the blood-clotting mechanism. Blood urea nitrogen and creatinine levels denote kidney function and may reflect the ability of the heart to perfuse the kidneys.

Blood gases may be measured depending on the diagnosis and specific cardiovascular disorder (Table 22-3). Venous, capillary, or arterial blood may be used, but an arterial blood gas sample is preferred since it is the most accurate.

Type and crossmatch studies done prior to a surgical procedure on the heart include an analysis of various blood factors necessary to prepare whole blood, packed red blood cells, and plasma. Special permission is required to infuse blood and should be obtained prior to heart surgery.

Children with congenital heart disease are subjected to multiple venipunctures, arterial punctures, and capillary finger sticks. Because of their level of cognitive development, children may lack the ability to understand the reasons for the repeated intrusive procedures. Helpful and necessary medical procedures and treatments are painful and are viewed as harmful to the body. Until children are 8 or 9, they think that the body is a hollow tube.[4] They fear that any hole made in the skin surface will result in blood loss. Adhesive strips used after various hematologic tests protect the "injured site" and help maintain the child's image of an intact body surface. Children need support during these procedures and comfort and reassurance afterward. The parents may choose not to be present during these procedures. The nurse must then provide the support the child requires.

Noninvasive studies Other diagnostic tests may involve noninvasive laboratory studies. One test or a combination of tests may be done, depending on the type of defect involved and the mode of treatment.

Anterior-posterior and lateral chest x-ray films are not taken routinely on admission. For children with suspected cardiac disorders, chest x-rays are important in evaluating pulmonary status and the presence of *cardiomegaly,* an enlarged heart.

An *echocardiogram* is a relatively new, non-

Table 22-3 Normal Arterial Blood Gas Values*

Factor	Normal Range
pH	7.35 to 7.45
P_{CO_2}	35 to 45 mmHg
P_{O_2}	80 to 100 mmHg
Carbonic acid	25 to 35 mmHg
Base excess	±2 mEq
Oxygen saturation	95 to 100%

*At normal body temperature.

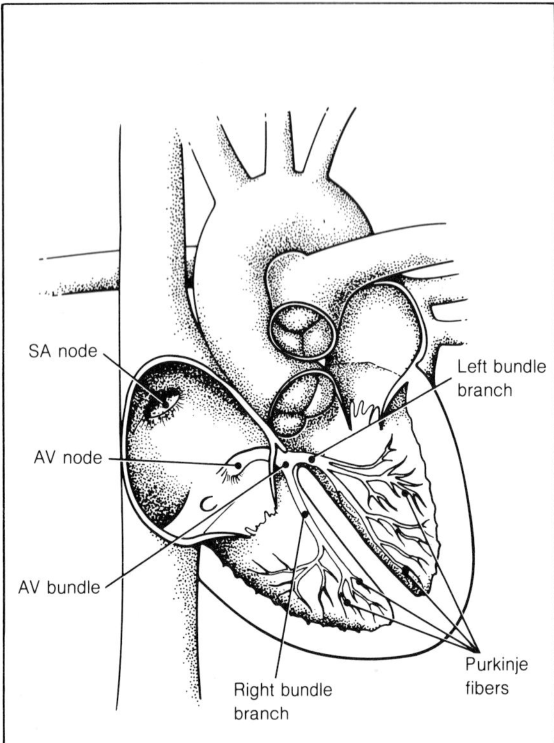

Figure 22-6 Electrical impulse conduction pathway in the heart. (*From D. A. Jones and J. S. Martin, in D. A. Jones et al. (eds.), Medical-Surgical Nursing, McGraw-Hill, New York, 1978. Used with permission.*)

traumatic diagnostic tool that employs an ultrasound technique. The picture that results is a reproduction of the image of sound echoes of the various structures of the heart and great vessels. An echocardiogram can be useful in detecting a cardiac defect. Doppler echocardiography provides information about the flow of blood within the heart chambers, across the valves, and in the great vessels.[5]

Phonocardiography produces a graphic representation of the sounds of blood flow in the heart and the great vessels. With the use of sound channels, an electrocardiography machine, and a pressure-recording device, a phonocardiogram can display normal and abnormal heart sounds. Audible and occasionally inaudible vibrations are recorded and provide more information regarding cardiac function.

An *electrocardiogram* (ECG) is a study of the electrical impulses created during cardiac contraction. The electrical activity of the heart is best measured by placing leads over the heart (chest leads) and the periphery (limb leads). The electrodes measure electric activity that is generated during a cardiac cycle.

Normally, the electric impulse originates in the *sinoatrial node,* located at the junction of the right atrium and the superior vena cava (Fig. 22-6). From there, the impulse travels to the *atrioventricular node,* located at the base of the atrial septum. The impulse is delayed slightly at the atrioventricular node. It then travels along the ventricular septum via a collection of special myocardial fibers called the *bundle of His.* The traveling impulse eventually passes through the *Purkinje fibers,* located in the right and left ventricles. Cardiac electric impulses are transmitted through the remainder of the body via the intracellular fluid. The electrocardiogram (ECG) is a reflection of the transmission of these impulses.

The waveforms usually recorded in an ECG represent the contraction and relaxation of the atria and ventricles (Fig. 22-7). The P wave represents *depolarization* (electric discharge) of the atria and is usually associated with atrial contraction. The QRS complex depicts the depolarization of the ventricle, or ventricular contraction. The P-R interval indicates the duration of conduction of the electric impulse from the sinoatrial node to the ventricles. The T wave represents the *repolarization,* or recovery period (electric charging), of the ventricles. A more detailed discussion of the ECG is beyond the scope of this text.

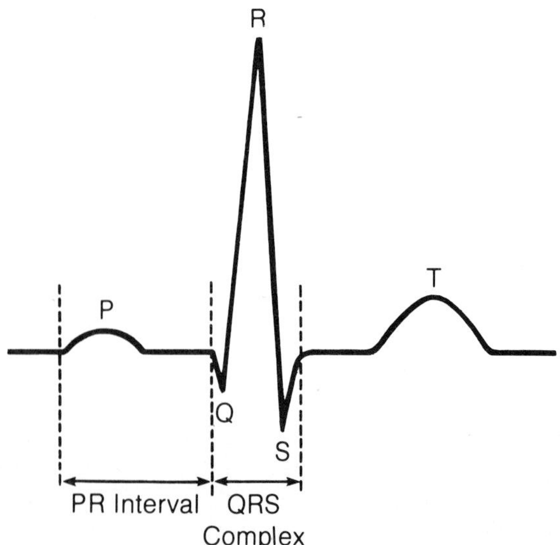

Figure 22-7 A normal electrocardiogram. Lead II pattern.

A *vectorcardiogram* can be helpful in the diagnosis of certain heart defects, such as aortic stenosis. Vectorcardiography accurately depicts the relationship between electric impulses and the degree of myocardium response. A vectorcardiogram is an alternative method to the ECG for displaying the electric activity and is usually obtained at the same time that the ECG is done.

Along with the standard ECG, a 24-h *Holter monitor* provides additional information about cardiac rhythm. The Holter monitor, a transistorized tape recorder attached to chest leads, tracks cardiac rhythm during the course of a typical day and night. The parents are given a 24-h diary in which they record times of normal activities and periods of stress. This device is helpful for a child who is suspected of having arrhythmias that are not readily detected by an ECG.

Sympathetic and parasympathetic nerve fibers influence the conducting tissues of the heart. Stimulation of the *sympathetic nerve fibers* accelerates the firing rate of the pacemaker (the sinoatrial node) and of abnormal pacemakers (ectopic foci) and speeds the rate of conduction, thereby increasing the heart rate. Stimulation of the *parasympathetic nerve fibers* produces an inhibitory effect (a vagal influence), depressing the firing of the pacemaker and slowing conduction.

Normal sinus rhythm represents a regular progression of the electric impulse through the heart at a rate appropriate for a given child's age. A child's ECG normally changes with age, especially during the first year. *Arrhythmia* and *dysrhythmia* are synonymous terms used to refer to cardiac rhythm irregularities. Arrhythmias can originate in any site within the heart, since each cell in the myocardium has the potential to discharge an electric impulse. Arrhythmias occurring along the conduction pathway are detected in the related area of the electrocardiographic tracing. A deviation in the P wave or P-R interval, for example, may suggest an abnormal contraction of the atria.

Although a wide variety of arrhythmias have been observed in children, they do not occur as frequently as in adults. The nurse should be alert for an irregular apical pulse signaling an arrhythmia. *Sinus arrhythmias,* commonly observed in healthy children, reflect a normal conduction pathway with an irregular rate that increases with inspiration and slows with expiration. *Sinus tachycardia* more specifically describes an increase in rate greater than a value appropriate for a child's age. The heart rate may be increased if the child is crying, anxious, or excited. The treatment for sinus tachycardia is symptomatic. Removing the cause will usually calm the child, and the heart will resume its usual rate.

An important disturbance in heart rate observed in children is *paroxysmal atrial tachycardia* (PAT). Its onset is heralded by a sudden increase in heart rate (more than 250 beats per minute) with signs of tachypnea and dyspnea. The heart rate may revert to normal spontaneously, or the child may require treatment. Prolonged episodes of PATs diminish cardiac output and predispose the child to congestive heart failure.

Sinus bradycardia is a heart rate lower than normal. It should be reported to a physician immediately, since treatment may be needed. It is important to remember that an adult's normal heart rate of 60 to 80 beats per minute would be considered bradycardic if auscultated in a newborn, whose pulse ranges from 120 to 160 beats per minute.

Many atrial and ventricular arrhythmias can be treated with medications that decrease the irritability of the foci by prolonging the *refractory period,* the time during which cells recover from an impulse discharge. Ventricular arrhythmias are more life-threatening than atrial arrhythmias, since they affect cardiac output more directly. Ventricular fibrillation is life-threatening and denotes a cardiac arrest situation. The ventricles are quivering, and cardiac output is nonexistent. Cardiopulmonary resuscitation must be initiated immediately. Defibrillation with electric shock stimulation, used in conjunction with emergency medications, may help restore normal sinus rhythm.

Invasive studies Invasive cardiac diagnostic procedures include cardiac catheterization and angiography. Both procedures carry additional risks to the child. Therefore, careful evaluation is required to ascertain that these tests are necessary.

Cardiac catheterization involves the passage of a thin, hollow radiopaque catheter into the cardiac chambers and great vessels. The route of entry depends on which side of the heart is to be visualized. To visualize the right side of the heart, the catheter is introduced via a cutdown into the antecubital fossa or percutaneously into a femoral vein. Left-sided cardiac catheterization carries more risks than right-sided catheterization because entry is made into the arterial system either through a brachial artery cutdown or percutaneously through the femoral artery. Major abnormalities can be visualized, and functions of the heart valves can be evaluated. Oxygen saturation of the blood can be measured as the catheter is advanced through the cardiac chambers. The location, magnitude, and direction of blood flow can be determined in part by the measurement of oxygen saturation in the various cardiac chambers. In addition, pressures in each chamber can be measured.

Preparation of the child and the family for cardiac catheterization is an important nursing responsibility. The procedure should be explained to the family and child (if appropriate for the child's age and level of understanding). Such visual aids as diagrams, photographs of the laboratory, a doll, and a miniature model of the laboratory equipment are effective teaching tools. A description of the sounds heard and the sensations felt is often helpful.

On admission to the hospital for the catheterization, vital signs, height, and weight are obtained. It is wise to make a comparison of the circulatory status of the right and left extremities before cardiac catheterization to establish a baseline for postcatheterization evaluation. The child is usually not given anything to eat or drink after midnight or 2 A.M. prior to the catheterization. Sedation may be used to help the child relax. Occasionally, general anesthesia is employed during the procedure. The room is darkened, and the large x-ray machine may be frightening. A familiar nurse should accompany the child to the catheterization lab to minimize anxiety and provide comfort.

After the catheterization, astute nursing management is of critical importance. Vital signs are taken every 15 to 30 min until stable and then frequently during the next 24 to 48 h. The pulse should be regular within limits appropriate for a given child. Report tachycardia or bradycardia to the physician. Observe the rate and depth of respirations, and note signs of dyspnea or tachypnea. Do not measure blood pressure on the affected limb. Check the systolic and diastolic readings against the precatheterization values, and note any significant change, such as *hypotension*.

Temperatures should be recorded with vital signs. Although contamination during the sterile catheterization procedure is rare, the nurse should keep the puncture site clean and dry and observe it for signs of infection. Special consideration should be taken to prevent contamination from excreta, especially at a femoral catheterization site in an infant or a young child.

In addition to vital sign checks, circulation is assessed frequently. A pressure dressing is placed over the puncture site to minimize the chance of bleeding and the formation of a hematoma. Record the type and amount of drainage on the dressing. If there is excessive oozing or bleeding, apply firm pressure directly on the dressing and notify the physician. Evaluate the circulation of the extremity used for the catheter entry. Adequate circulation is evidenced by a pale-pink color of the nail beds and skin of the affected extremity or by the precatheterization color in children with darker skin, a warm skin temperature, equal and regular pulses, and rapid capillary refill. Signs of compromised blood flow, such as cyanosis, coolness or mottling of the skin, numbness or tingling, and excessive bleeding from the puncture site, should be reported to the physician immediately.

Intake and output should be monitored to evaluate circulatory status and renal function. Decreased output or hematuria may result from the physiological response of the kidneys to the dye used for the catheterization x-ray studies.[6]

If no complications, such as hemorrhage, infection, arrhythmias, or allergic reactions, develop, the child will usually resume his or her normal diet as tolerated after the procedure. Activity may be limited after the catheterization but will return to normal after the puncture site has healed. If no other treatment is planned, the child is usually discharged from the hospital in 1 day. Dismissal teaching should include information regarding care of the puncture site. The child may need an opportunity to talk about the procedure, especially if it was very traumatic.

In *angiocardiography,* a radiopaque medium is introduced by catheter into a selected part or parts of the cardiovascular system. A series of x-rays or moving pictures are taken as the contrast medium is introduced into the body and flows through the heart. An angiogram shows anatomic detail of the heart structures and is usually done in conjunction with cardiac catheterization.

CONGESTIVE HEART FAILURE

Signs and symptoms of *congestive heart failure* at or soon after birth indicate that the heart of the newborn is unable to adapt to extrauterine life. *Cardiac failure*, or pump failure, is the inability of the myocardium to circulate sufficient oxygen and nutrients to meet the metabolic requirements of the body. *Congestive* refers to the symptoms related to fluid accumulation in various parts of the body. Congestive heart failure is the most frequent emergency problem occurring in children with cardiac disease.

Pathophysiology

Cardiac failure occurs when the heart is unable to keep up with its workload because of ineffective contractions, inability to fill properly, or hindrance in blood flow through the chambers of the heart. Congenital heart anomalies may cause cardiac failure either by hindering blood flow through a narrowed valve or by increasing the heart's workload. An increased workload occurs when blood is shunted from one chamber to another, leading to increased work for the affected chamber.

In order to supply enough blood to the body, the heart must maintain an adequate cardiac output. *Cardiac output* is the amount of blood ejected by the heart per minute. It is dependent on the heart rate and *stroke volume*, which is the amount of blood ejected from the heart with each contraction. A congenital heart anomaly that blocks effective blood flow forces the heart to respond with *compensatory mechanisms* that maintain or improve circulation to the tissues and organs of the body.

Increased sympathetic nervous system activity is an early compensatory mechanism. As the heart fails, reserves of norepinephrine, a neurotransmitter substance, become depleted, and circulating norepinephrine from the adrenal gland acts to constrict the blood vessels. This action returns more blood to the heart and augments the stroke volume. Another compensatory mechanism diverts blood from the stomach, intestines, and kidneys to the central nervous system and myocardium. The decreased blood volume through the kidneys leads to a decreased glomerular filtration rate. This stimulates the release of renin and aldosterone, causing sodium and water retention. Fluid and sodium retention aids cardiac output by increasing the volume of fluid returning to the heart. A third compensatory mechanism, hypertrophy and dilatation, increases heart size to maximize pumping effectiveness. Tachycardia also helps the heart compensate by increasing the rate to maintain an adequate cardiac output.

Manifestations

These mechanisms are unable to maintain the workload of the heart for long. *Cardiac decompensation* occurs, and the child exhibits signs of congestive heart failure. Since the body tissues and organs are deprived of sufficient oxygen and nutrients for metabolic needs, malaise or lethargy may be present. Tachycardia and a gallop rhythm are usually observed. Decreased urinary output (oliguria) may occur if renal perfusion is impaired. Weak peripheral pulses are present, and the extremities may be cool, mottled, and cyanotic because of peripheral vasoconstriction and diversion of blood to vital organs. An x-ray usually shows that the heart is enlarged, signifying the compensatory mechanism of hypertrophy and dilatation in response to the increased stress and workload.

In adults, cardiac failure may be predominantly right-sided or left-sided before the whole heart becomes involved. In children, it is usually impossible to make a clear distinction between right- and left-sided cardiac failure.[7] It is helpful, however, to consider the specific signs manifested in left-sided and right-sided cardiac failure in order to understand the total process and the effects on the body.

Failure which involves the left side of the heart is manifested by symptoms of altered respiratory function and respiratory distress. Tachypnea and dyspnea are the primary manifestations of left-sided cardiac failure. Wheezing, pulmonary rales, a hacking cough, and orthopnea (assuming an upright position to facilitate breathing) may also be present. A gallop rhythm is best heard with the bell of the stethoscope over the apex of the heart when the child is in a supine position. This signifies the decreased ability of the left ventricle to accommodate the increased blood volume. The presence of pink, frothy sputum and cyanosis would further indicate severely impaired gas exchange due to fluid accumulation in the alveoli. It is important to note that infants and young children do not verbally communicate their breathing difficulty. The astute nurse must look for other signs of respiratory distress, such as tachypnea, nasal flaring, retractions, wheezing, grunting, restlessness, and apprehension.

Right-sided cardiac failure is due to an increased volume of blood on the right side of the heart. The principal sign of right-sided cardiac failure is *hepatomegaly* (an enlarged liver) due to systemic congestion. Neck vein distention may be present in older children but is difficult to evaluate in newborns and infants because of their short necks. Peripheral edema is usually not present in young children, although scalp and facial edema or ascites may be observed. Fluid retention in an infant may be subtly reflected in a weight gain of a few ounces. Anorexia and abdominal pain may be present.

Nursing management

Nursing management of a child with congestive heart failure is directed toward increasing the efficiency of the heart and lessening the workload of the stressed myocardium. These goals are accomplished through the use of specific medications, rest, positioning, close observation, and fluid and nutrition balance.

The chief method of improving the strength of cardiac contraction is the administration of a digitalis preparation (Table 22-4). Although the types of preparations vary in terms of their onset and dosage, they all increase the force of contraction (inotropic action) and slow the heart rate (chronotropic action). These two effects enable the heart to empty more completely. In order to achieve a therapeutic blood level quickly, initial doses of the selected preparation are higher than usual (based on the child's weight).The administration of loading doses to achieve a therapeutic blood level is termed *digitalization*. After a therapeutic blood level is reached, lower maintenance doses are given twice a day. The administration of the correct dosage is crucial. Two nurses should always double-check the order and dosage, and compare the dosage with suggested dosage ranges for the child's weight. The elixir or liquid form of digitalis is useful for infants and young children. The nurse should take an apical pulse for a full minute before giving the medication. Although procedures vary slightly from one institution to another, the usual policy is to check with a physician before giving the drug if the pulse is lower than 100 in infants or below 60 in older children.

Oxygen therapy is employed to increase the amount of circulating oxygen in the blood and reduce the stress on the myocardium. For young infants, a hood may be used, while a face mask is used for older children. If oxygen is delivered with mist, as is frequently done, the nurse should make sure that the amount of mist is not so great as to increase the amount of fluid in lungs already filled with fluid. Aminophylline or a similar theophylline derivative (Table 22-4) may be used to dilate and relax the bronchioles and increase gas exchange.

Positioning is extremely important in the nursing management of a child with congestive heart failure. A semi-Fowler's position (45° elevation) helps decrease venous return of blood to the right atrium, prevents abdominal organs from placing pressure on the diaphragm, and allows fluid in the lungs to flow to the lower lobes. The surface area by which gas exchange takes place is increased. Car seats and infant seats are helpful in placing infants in an upright position. The position should be changed every 2 h to prevent complications of immobility, such as pressure sores and pneumonia. Promote skin integrity by applying lotion and avoiding such drying agents as harsh soaps.

Provide periods of rest. Observe activity tolerance to prevent overexertion. Alternate periods of such activity as bathing with rest breaks. Feeding difficulties are common, since infants with congestive heart failure are prone to dyspnea and fatigue. This can lead to frustration for the parents as well as the child. Use larger-holed nipples to minimize the energy needed for sucking. Formulas with increased calories per ounce may be helpful in providing optimal nutrition. Feed the infant in an upright position, and allow the baby to pull away from the nipple to rest. Such quiet, age-appropriate activities as playing with musical toys and rocking for an infant and reading and listening to music for older children are helpful. Small amounts of morphine sulfate (Table 22-4) may be given to relieve anxiety and excessive restlessness.

Vital signs are taken frequently, and respirations are assessed for rate, regularity, and depth. The presence or absence of cyanosis and the degree of edema should be accurately recorded. Although respirations and heart rate may be mechanically monitored (Table 22-5), the direct observation of the child must continue. The mechanical monitor is only an assessment aid.

Measure intake and output carefully. All in-

Table 22-4 Drugs Used to Improve Myocardial Efficiency in the Treatment of Congestive Heart Failure*

Medication	Usual Dosage	Pharmacological Action	Side Effects	Nursing Implications
Digoxin (digitalization)	Premature infants: 0.035 mg/kg PO Newborns: 0.05 mg/kg PO Children under 2 years: 0.05 to 0.06 mg/kg PO Children over 2 years: 0.03 to 0.04 mg/kg PO IM or IV: 75 to 80% of PO dose; one-fourth to one-third given in two divided doses in 24 h Maintenance dose: 25% of digitalizing dose	Strengthens myocardial contraction by stimulation of the vagus nerve to decrease the heart rate; improves cardiac output; has some use in the treatment of arrhythmias	Gastrointestinal irritation; "digitalis toxicity," especially bradycardia or tachycardia	Check apical pulse for full minute. Do *not* administer if pulse is less than 60 in adolescents and adults or 100 in infants. Check with the physician. Report low potassium level before digoxin administration. Report signs of digoxin toxicity.
Aminophylline	20 mg/kg per 24 h	Dilates pulmonary blood vessels to improve oxygen–carbon dioxide gas exchange; dilates the coronary arteries; increases cardiac output	Gastrointestinal irritation; central nervous system stimulation, especially in children: signs include headache, restlessness, and irritability; hypotension with IV administration	Report signs of nausea and vomiting related to the drug. Check signs of central nervous system stimulation. Check blood pressure every 5 min during IV infusion and for 1 h following infusion.
Lasix	1 to 3 mg/kg per 24 h PO IM or IV: 1 to 2 mg/kg per 24 h	Inhibits sodium reabsorption in the loop of Henle, promoting water excretion and thereby decreasing the circulating blood volume and reducing venous return as well as cardiac output	Hypokalemia	Monitor electrolyte levels, especially potassium. Encourage intake of foods high in potassium: orange juice and bananas.
Morphine sulfate	IM or IV: 0.1 to 0.2 mg/kg q4h to q6h, usually prn	Narcotic analgesic; relaxes smooth muscles and dilates pulmonary blood vessels Central nervous system depressant; relieves anxiety and restlessness	Depresses respirations and causes hypotension; causes constipation	Evaluate respiratory status and blood pressure frequently. Use additional safety precautions. Dangerous when used in children with underlying pulmonary disease.

**Digitalis preparations are being used with increasing caution in premature infants because of these infants' inability to metabolize the drug. This is related to liver and kidney immaturity.*

Table 22-5 Guidelines for the Care of a Child on a Monitor

1. Use grounded electric equipment *only*.
2. Set high-low pulse parameters appropriate for the child's age.
3. Apply electrode pads to clean, dry skin for a selected lead pattern. Lead II (RA, RL, LL) is a commonly used pattern.
4. Ensure a clear picture on the oscilloscope by:
   a. Checking electrode pads, wires, and cable for adequate electric function
   b. Reapplying electrode pads every 1 to 2 days and when necessary
5. Explain basic monitor function and alarm sounds to the child and the family.
6. Allow the child and the family to express their feelings about the monitor.

take (oral fluids, intravenous fluids) must be fairly equal to all output (urine, emesis, and stools). A principal tool in assessing fluid balance is accurately weighing the child twice a day. Weigh the child at the same time each day, usually before breakfast, with the same amount of clothing on. An infant should be undressed and protected from drafts. Disposable diapers are weighed before and after use, and the dry weight is subtracted from the wet weight to determine the quantity of urine output (1 ml equals 1 g). It is wise to have another nurse double-check a child's weight when there is a significant change from the previous weight. A 24-h fluid balance is calculated at midnight or 6 A.M. Any significant discrepancies between the amount of fluid taken in and the amount of fluid excreted should be reported. Diuretics such as furosemide (Lasix) are administered to promote sodium and water excretion (Table 22-4). Since potassium is excreted with sodium, it is important to encourage intake of foods high in potassium.

Long-term follow-up care and parental education are important, since many children with recurrent congestive heart failure will continue the therapeutic regimen after discharge. Parents should be given written instructions regarding the medications the child will be taking at home. Teach the parents to follow guidelines in administering the digitalis preparation. Double-check the dose, take the apical pulse before giving the medication, and check it against designated high and low pulse parameters. Occasionally, a child may miss a dose of digoxin. If more than one dose is skipped because of emesis, refusal to take it, or another reason, the physician should be consulted. Parents should encourage children who are taking diuretics to eat foods high in potassium. Include in discharge teaching the importance of positioning, feeding suggestions, prevention of infections, and anticipatory guidance for future episodes of congestive heart failure. Table 22-6 lists guidelines for teaching parents who must give digoxin to their child.

The prognosis for children with congestive heart failure depends on the cause and severity of the heart disease. Early diagnosis is a necessity. Accurate nursing assessment and appropriate intervention facilitate early recognition and prompt medical treatment.

The Nursing Care Plan at the end of this chapter is for an infant with congestive heart failure secondary to a congenital malformation, ventricular septal defect.

CONGENITAL HEART DEFECTS

There are many recognized types of *congenital heart malformations*. Nine common lesions represent 90 percent of all anomalies. Heart defects may be classified according to the presence or absence of cyanosis and the degree of pulmonary vascularity (blood flow to the lungs). The abnormality may be so minor that the individual is hardly affected. In other instances, it may be so major that other body systems must compensate

Table 22-6 Guidelines for Teaching Parents Whose Child Needs Digoxin

1. Explain to the parents the action and side effects of digoxin as well as the method of administration.
2. Tell the parents to give digoxin exactly as prescribed—usually every 12 h.
3. Instruct the parents to give digoxin 1 h before or 2 h after feedings.
4. Tell the parents that if the child vomits within 15 min after taking digoxin and they feel that most, if not all, has been lost, they can repeat the dose *one time*. Tell them that if more than 15 min has passed, they must not repeat the dose, and that if the child vomits two consecutive doses, they should call the doctor.
5. Instruct the parents to notify the doctor if the child becomes ill with anything that leads to loss of appetite, vomiting, diarrhea, or increasing difficulty in breathing.
6. Tell the parents to store digoxin in a safe place, preferably in a locked cabinet, out of children's reach.
7. Tell the parents to take anyone else who swallows digoxin to the nearest emergency room.

Source: Patricia Jackson, "Digoxin Therapy at Home: Keeping the Child Safe," *American Journal of Maternal-Child Nursing* **5**(2):106–107 (March–April 1979).

in some way for the defective structure. The severity of the defect directly influences the symptoms exhibited and the overall prognosis. The signs and symptoms that each child presents are merely a reflection of the hemodynamic alterations of the specific defect. Classification of congenital heart defects is difficult because of their variety and complexity. Traditionally, they are grouped into acyanotic and cyanotic categories, but it must be remembered that the types of lesions that usually cause cyanosis do not always do so; lesions that usually do not produce cyanosis will do so under special circumstances (Table 22-7).

Acyanotic heart defects

Acyanotic heart defects are those that usually do not cause cyanosis. Acyanotic heart disease is more common than cyanotic heart disease. In acyanotic heart disease, either there is no shunting, or diversion of blood, or else there is *left-to-right shunting,* in which blood is diverted from the left side of the heart (oxygen-enriched) to the right side (oxygen-depleted); therefore, only bright-red, oxygen-enriched blood enters the systemic circulation. Left-to-right shunting causes an increased amount of blood flow into the lungs and a tendency toward respiratory infections.

In patent ductus arteriosus, atrial septal defect, and ventricular septal defect, pulmonary vascularity is increased owing to the larger volume of blood in the lungs. Normal pulmonary vascularity exists in coarctation of the aorta and aortic stenosis; these types of acyanotic lesions are not associated with shunting.

Patent ductus arteriosus During fetal life, the ductus arteriosus maintains communication between the pulmonary artery and the aorta. Usually the ductus is essentially closed 10 to 15 h after birth. Failure of the ductus to close after birth allows that communication to persist (Fig. 22-8). *Patent ductus arteriosus* (PDA) is one of the most common congenital heart defects. Specific populations known to be at increased risk include:

1. Female and premature infants
2. Infants with respiratory distress syndrome or neonatal hypoxia
3. Infants born at high altitudes
4. Infants whose mothers had rubella during the first trimester of pregnancy

Blood flows from areas of higher to lower pressure. The direction of shunting through the ductus depends on the pressure difference between the aorta and the pulmonary artery. With the onset of respiration at birth, pulmonary vascular resistance begins to decrease. Separation of the placenta from the arterial system increases systemic vascular resistance, and aortic pressure rises. When aortic pressure exceeds pulmonary artery pressure, well-oxygenated blood is shunted

Table 22-7 Classification of Major Cardiac Defects

Acyanotic	Cyanotic	Pulmonary Vascularity
Left-to-right shunts:	**Admixture lesions:**	
Patent ductus arteriosus	Complete transposition of the great vessels	Increased
Atrial septal defect	Truncus arteriosus	Increased
Ventricular septal defect	Total anomalous pulmonary venous connection	Increased
Endocardial cushion defect		
Obstructive lesions:		
Coarctation of the aorta	None	Normal
Pulmonary stenosis	None	Normal
Aortic stenosis	None	Normal
	Obstruction to pulmonary blood flow with a defect:	
	Tetralogy of Fallot	Decreased
	Tricuspid atresia	Decreased

Source: James Moller, *Essentials of Pediatric Cardiology,* Davis, Philadelphia, 1978, p. 46.

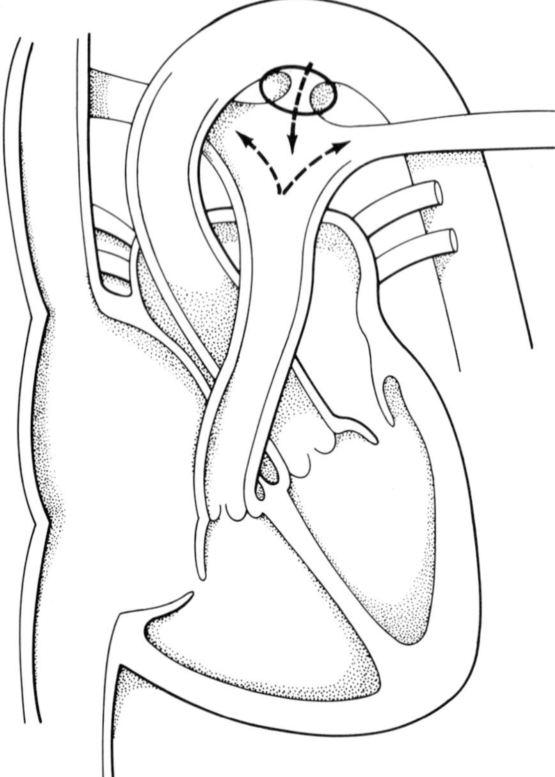

Figure 22-8 A patent ductus arteriosus. Oxygenated blood from the aorta flows through the patent ductus arteriosus and mixes with the unoxygenated blood flowing to the lungs in the pulmonary arteries. The incidence is 1:2000 live births.

from the aorta through the ductus to the pulmonary artery. The result of this increased flow is an increased volume load on the lungs, the left atrium, and the left ventricle. If the ductus is large, the right ventricle may have to generate higher pressures to eject its volume of blood into the pulmonary artery, since aortic pressures will be transmitted through the ductus to the pulmonary artery.

Presenting symptoms depend on the size of the ductus, the pressure difference between the aorta and the pulmonary artery, and the volume of blood flow through the ductus. In severe cases, congestive heart failure occurs. With small shunts, the presenting symptoms may be minimal. The rapid runoff from the aorta through the patent ductus decreases peripheral vascular resistance. This lowers the diastolic pressure and increases the pulse pressure. Features found on physical examination include a hyperactive precordium, bounding peripheral pulses, and a systolic or continuous murmur extending into diastole, heard best at the upper left sternal border and under the left clavicle. There may be a history of fatigue, weak cry, breathlessness, feeding difficulties, and increased susceptibility to upper respiratory infections. With large shunts, there is an increased risk of congestive heart failure, pulmonary hypertension, and bacterial endocarditis.

The correction of a PDA in the full-term infant has traditionally been done by surgical ligation. The small incision, or so-called "Band-Aid" surgery, does not require cardiopulmonary bypass, and the mortality rate is very low. Closure of the ductus restores normal circulation. Children whose PDA has been closed can look forward to a normal life.

Indomethacin, a prostaglandin synthetase inhibitor, is useful in producing closure of the PDA in premature infants.[8] Indomethacin stimulates the smooth muscle in the wall of the ductus to constrict, thus closing the opening. It is contraindicated in premature infants who have elevated bilirubin levels, bleeding, or decreased renal function.

Prostaglandin E_1 (PGE_1) is used to keep the ductus arteriosus open in newborns with certain congenital heart defects until surgery can be performed.[9] PGE_1 relaxes the smooth muscle of the ductus; it also causes peripheral vasodilatation and inhibits platelet aggregation. It is used in cyanotic defects with restricted pulmonary blood flow (pulmonary atresia, tricuspid atresia, and severe pulmonary stenosis) and in those with obstruction of blood flow to the systemic circulation (coarctation of the distal aortic arch and hypoplastic left heart syndrome).

PGE_1 is given intravenously through a large vein continuously until the defect is corrected surgically. The main side effects are apnea (10 to 12 percent in the first hour), fever (14 percent), seizures (4 percent), flushing (10 percent), bradycardia (7 percent), and hypotension (4 percent).[10] The infant who is receiving PGE_1 should be monitored closely, and special attention given to vital signs, blood gases, and cardiovascular and neurological status.

Atrial septal defect An *atrial septal defect* (ASD) is an abnormal opening in the atrial septum (Fig. 22-9). The two most common types are ostium secundum and ostium primum. An *ostium secundum* defect occurs in the midpor-

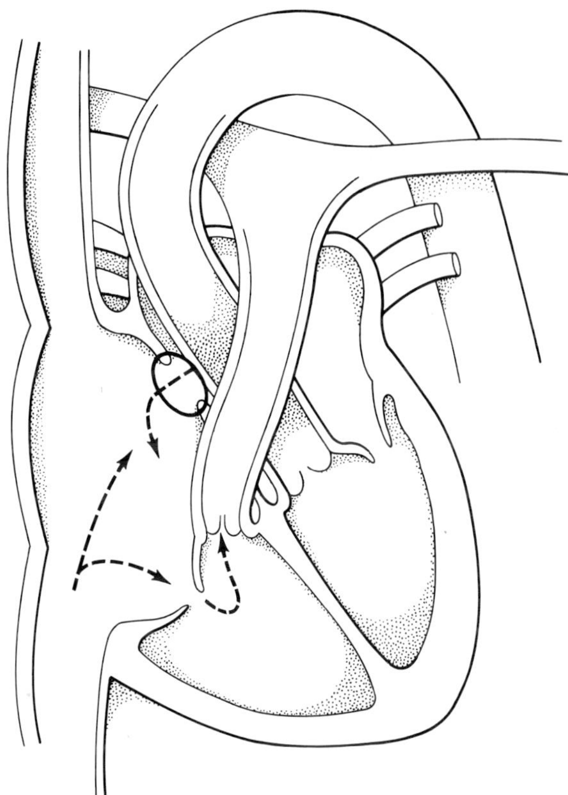

Figure 22-9 An atrial septal defect. Oxygenated blood is usually shunted from the left atrium to the right atrium. Mixed blood then flows to the right ventricle and into the pulmonary arteries.

tion of the septum and accounts for 10 percent of all congenital heart defects. An ostium secundum defect is more than just an anatomically open foramen ovale. The foramen ovale is normally held closed by left atrial pressure on a flap of septal tissue. An *ostium primum* defect is an abnormal opening low in the septum near the entrance of the superior vena cava into the right atrium. It is nearly always associated with a cleft or abnormality in the mitral valve that may render the valve incompetent. These defects involve the endocardial cushion. (See the section "Endocardial Cushion Defects.")

An ASD usually results in the shunting of blood from the left atrium to the right atrium because pressure is higher in the left atrium. The flow through the ASD may range from small to very large amounts. With anything other than an extremely small defect, right and left atrial pressures tend to equalize. Once this occurs, the degree of shunting is dependent on the relative distensibility of the ventricles. The right ventricle, being thinner-walled and less muscular than the left, accepts an extra volume load more readily. In diastole, during ventricular filling, the presence of an ASD allows all four chambers of the heart to communicate. At this point, the blood in the left atrium will take the path of least resistance and flow through the right atrium into the right ventricle.[11]

Shunting of blood from left to right through an ASD causes an increase in the workload of the right ventricle and increased blood flow through the pulmonary circulation. This eventually leads to right ventricular hypertrophy and may result in congestive heart failure. Heart failure is unusual in the infant or child with an ASD; it develops more commonly in untreated adults.

Most infants and children with an ASD are relatively asymptomatic, especially if the defect is of the ostium secundum variety. Typically, the splitting of the second heart sound is wide and "fixed" and is heard on expiration as well as inspiration. This is due to the increased stroke volume of the right ventricle, which delays closure of the pulmonary valve. The characteristic pulmonary ejection murmur is heard during systole at the left upper sternal border. Often the murmur is not present in the infant owing to the existence of normal right ventricular hypertrophy. Growth may be somewhat retarded but generally tends to fall within normal limits. There may be less than the normal tolerance for exercise, and the child may have frequent upper respiratory infections. If mitral regurgitation is associated with an ostium primum defect, there will be increased pressure in the left atrium and in the pulmonary vascular bed. Children with this condition are at greater risk for developing congestive heart failure.

In the presence of increased right atrial pressure due to alterations in heart structure or increased resistance to pulmonary blood flow, shunting will be from right to left. The same mechanism may cause right-to-left shunting through an anatomically patent foramen ovale. The child with right-to-left shunting is likely to manifest some degree of cyanosis. It should be noted that the newborn with an ASD may exhibit transient cyanosis. The right-to-left shunting in this situation is due to the high pulmonary resistance and the normal right ventricular hypertrophy found in the neonate.

Surgical correction of both types of ASD is

relatively simple. By utilizing cardiopulmonary bypass, repair of the septum is accomplished either by oversewing the small defect or by closing larger openings with a pericardial or Dacron patch. In the ostium primum defect, the cleft in the mitral valve is also repaired. Complications after surgery are minimal but include, on occasion, air emboli and transient heart block if suturing was done near the bundle of His.

The ideal age for surgical closure is approximately 5 years. Children whose defects are repaired before they reach the age of 20 are often able to lead normal, active lives. Survival rates are high. Surgical risk is lowest during the first 10 years of life and increases only slightly during the next decade. After this, the risk increases with age, as do the number of postoperative complications.[12]

Endocardial cushion defects The endocardial cushions form the lower portion of the atrial septum, the upper portion of the ventricular septum, and the septal leaflets of the endocardium.[13] Several developmental *endocardial cushion defects* are possible. A mild defect is the ostium primum defect (or incomplete atrioventricular canal) described above. A much more serious defect is a *complete atrioventricular* (AV) *canal*. Here the ostium primum defect is continuous with a larger defect in the ventricular septum and affects the septal leaflets of both the mitral and the tricuspid valves as well.

A child with an ostium primum defect may be asymptomatic or may develop congestive heart failure early in infancy, when a complete atrioventricular canal is present. Characteristic findings are left-to-right shunting, pulmonary hypertension, and mitral insufficiency. An apical pansystolic murmur, a pulmonary ejection murmur, and splitting of the second heart sound are also typical findings. Symptoms, when present, relate to congestive heart failure, poor growth, and frequent respiratory infections. For children with few or no symptoms, surgical correction is delayed until they are 5 to 10 years old. The defect is closed, and the mitral valve is repaired. In children with a complete atrioventricular canal, the mitral valve is frequently replaced, and the repair is done early in infancy, making the procedure a much greater risk than when the defect is mild.[14] There is a 20 to 30 percent risk of death in infants under the age of 3 months.[15]

Ventricular septal defect Incomplete development of the ventricular septum during fetal life will establish communication between the right and left ventricles and result in an abnormal blood flow pattern (Fig. 22-10). A *ventricular septal defect* (VSD) is the most common defect, accounting for almost 25 percent of all congenital malformations. If the defect is small or moderate in size, the amount of blood directed through it will be limited by its size. When the VSD is large, the relative resistance offered to flow out of the two chambers will determine the amount and direction of flow through it. The direction of flow is always determined by the difference in resistance to outflow from each ventricle. In the absence of other heart defects, the shunt is from the left ventricle to the right ventricle because pulmonary vascular resistance is lower than systemic vascular resistance.

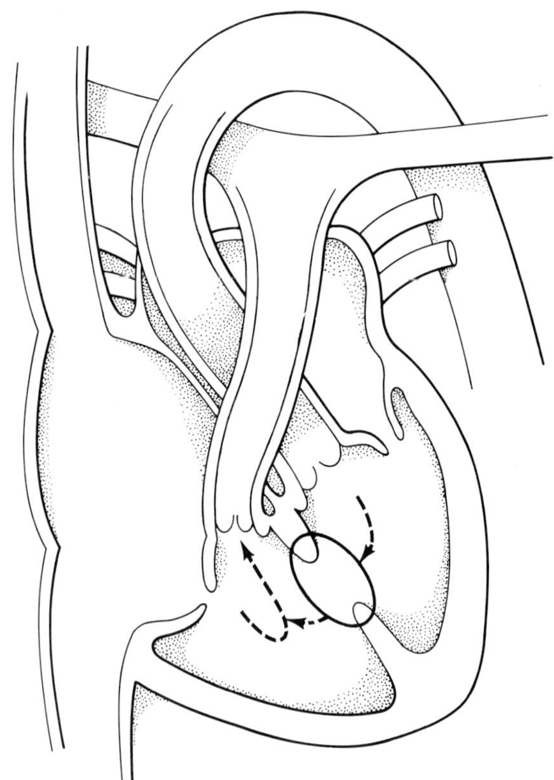

Figure 22-10 A ventricular septal defect. Oxygenated blood is usually shunted from the left ventricle to the right ventricle. Mixed blood then flows through the pulmonary arteries. The incidence is from 1.5:1000 to 2.5:1000 live births.

A small to moderate-sized VSD results in an increased volume in the right ventricle, pulmonary vasculature, left atrium, and left ventricle, whereas a large VSD results in both an increased volume and an increased pressure load. With large defects, the higher left ventricular pressures are transmitted to the right ventricle and pulmonary system. In response to this, pulmonary vascular resistance may rise, as nature's method of reducing the extra blood flow through the lungs.

The symptoms of a VSD vary with its size. Children with small to moderate-sized defects may be asymptomatic. Children with large defects present the classic signs of heart failure after the first month of life. These include increased respiratory rate, difficulty feeding, irritability, excessive perspiration, tachycardia, mild cyanosis, repeated pulmonary infections, and slow growth.

Management of children with a VSD is influenced by the knowledge that many of the defects of small to moderate size will close spontaneously in the early months of life. Prophylactic antibiotic therapy prior to and following dental care or operative procedures is used to prevent bacterial endocarditis. Asymptomatic children whose defects do not close spontaneously and those with large shunts should have them surgically corrected with a Dacron patch prior to starting school. If pulmonary hypertension is present, surgical repair before 2 years of age provides protection against irreversible damage to the small arteries of the lungs.

Symptomatic infants are treated with digoxin and diuretics. If this controls the symptoms, the operation is deferred until the infant is older and weighs 25 lb (11.3 kg). For infants who do not respond to medical management, either surgical closure of the VSD or a pulmonary artery banding to decrease flow through the pulmonary circulation may be indicated. Complete correction of the VSD is currently favored over banding, since many children who have had banding require reconstruction of the pulmonary artery at some future time.[16] Postoperative complications include primarily congestive heart failure and arrhythmias due to injury of the interventricular septum. Most children with a repaired VSD should reach adulthood with a good prognosis and lead normal lives.[17]

Coarctation of the aorta *Coarctation of the aorta* is a narrowing in the lumen of the aorta (Fig. 22-11). The constriction commonly occurs near the ductus arteriosus and is often described as *preductal* (before the ductus) or *postductal* (after the ductus). The resulting obstruction of blood flow through the aorta presents two major hemodynamic problems. First, the left ventricle must generate higher-than-normal pressures to eject an adequate stroke volume. Second, there is a reduced systolic pressure distal to the coarctation. In many cases, the body compensates for the obstruction to blood flow by developing collateral vessels to carry blood around the obstruction.

Presenting symptoms vary according to the severity of the defect, its anatomic location, and the presence or absence of associated cardiac

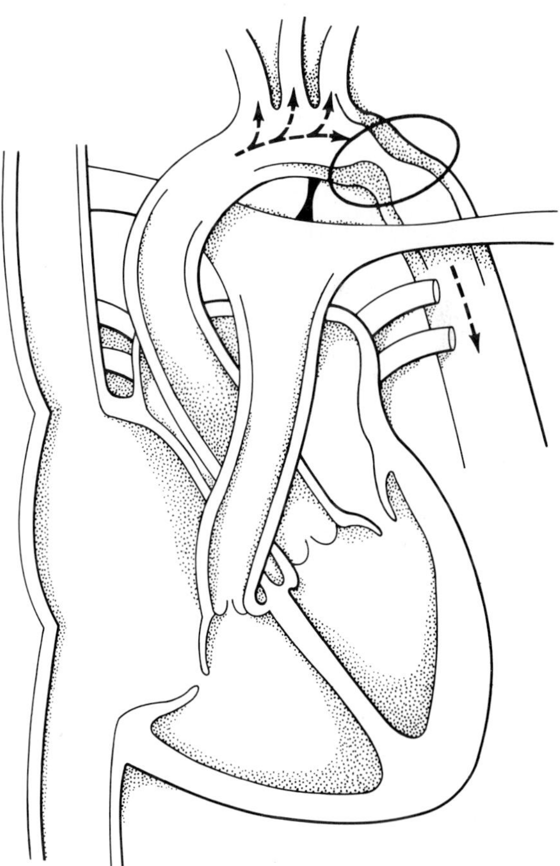

Figure 22-11 Coarctation of the aorta. Narrowing of the lumen results in increased systolic blood pressure proximal to the coarctation and decreased systolic blood pressure distally. The incidence is 1:13,000 live births.

anomalies. The typical patient with coarctation of the aorta is a male whose anomaly was discovered during a routine physical examination. When questioned, he may report episodes of sudden and unexplained epistaxis, frequent headaches, and leg fatigue. An examination frequently reveals full, bounding pulses in the upper extremities. This is due to the elevated pressure proximal to the narrowed portion of the lumen. Weak or absent pulses are found in the lower extremities, because of the reduced blood flow and pressure distal to the narrowed lumen. The systolic pressure may be equal in the four extremities or slightly higher in the arms than in the legs. Better development of the head and shoulders than of the hips and legs is possible. A comparison of the femoral and radial pulses will also show a delay in the femoral pulse. Pulsation is often seen, and a thrill palpated, in the suprasternal notch.

The murmur of coarctation of the aorta is systolic. It is heard posteriorly along the spine at the level of the obstruction. Both systolic and diastolic murmurs may be heard in other areas of the back and over the precordium. These are most often related to collateral circulation or to the coexistence of other cardiac anomalies.[18]

Congestive heart failure, poor weight gain, and feeding difficulties can occur early in the infant whose coarctation is severe. Other accompanying defects contribute to early congestive heart failure. The adult with an uncorrected coarctation is at risk for developing congestive heart failure, a dissecting aortic aneurysm (a blood-filled sac within the layers of the arterial wall), or an aortic rupture. Bacterial endocarditis may also occur. Systemic hypertension may lead to cerebral hemorrhage. Infants who manifest early congestive heart failure are often managed medically, and surgery is delayed until they are older. For those who do not respond to such treatment, surgical intervention provides the best chance for survival. Repair of the coarctation involves removal of the narrowed segment of the aorta with either end-to-end anastomosis or insertion of an aortic graft. More recently, patch graft enlargement of the narrowed segment has been done, using a cloth patch, the ligated and divided left subclavian artery, or Gore-tex, which is a soft, pliable synthetic material. Ideally, the operation is delayed as long as possible to allow the aorta to grow. Repair is done sometime between the ages of 3 and 10 years, before systemic hypertension becomes irreversible.

Postoperatively, hypertension is common and is easily treated with reserpine or sodium nitroprusside (Nipride). The prognosis is good for an asymptomatic child with a simple coarctation. Surgical repair in an infant, a child with severe symptoms, or an adult carries an increased risk. High mortality rates are associated with early repair in infants. Infants who survive may need additional surgery later in childhood, since stenosis can develop at the site of the anastomosis. Without correction of the defect, few people will live past the age of 50.[19]

Pulmonary stenosis The term *pulmonary stenosis* refers to any lesion that obstructs flow from the right ventricle to the lungs. The obstruction to flow may occur above or below the pulmonary valve, but in the majority of patients with isolated pulmonary stenosis, the obstruction is stenosis of the pulmonary valve itself.[20] Pulmonary stenosis accounts for 7 to 9 percent of all cardiac defects.

Blood flow through the pulmonary vasculature may be normal or diminished as a result of pulmonary valve stenosis. To maintain pulmonary blood flow, the right ventricle must produce a high systolic pressure. The right ventricle hypertrophies, and the thickened ventricle offers more resistance to filling. The right ventricle diastolic pressure then rises, with a corresponding rise in the right atrial pressure. If the pulmonary stenosis is severe enough to start this chain of events, the high right atrial pressure may reopen the foramen ovale. A right-to-left shunt through the foramen ovale will then occur.

On examination, a thrill and murmur, which radiate upward and to the left, are heard loudest in the second or third left interspace near the sternal border. The second heart sound is notably split.[21] Children with mild stenosis are usually asymptomatic. Infants with severe pulmonary stenosis will have profound congestive heart failure. The symptoms most frequently seen in moderate to severe stenosis are dyspnea and fatigue. Major symptoms frequently do not occur until just prior to death.

The treatment depends on the severity of the stenosis. Pulmonary stenosis is not a static process. Children diagnosed as having this type of defect need to be followed closely. Medical treatment may involve the use of *balloon angioplasty*. In a procedure similar to cardiac catheterization, a balloon is inflated across the stenotic valve, with minimal complications. Surgery is necessary in the case of a severe stenosis. Cardiopulmonary bypass is utilized, and a valvulotomy is performed.

Infants who present with congestive heart failure with pulmonary stenosis have a less favorable prognosis than those without failure. Children with mild stenosis have a normal life expectancy without surgical repair. The long-term results of a valvulotomy have been excellent. Without surgery, children with severe stenosis rarely live to their twenties.

Aortic stenosis *Aortic stenosis* has been identified in various forms. The largest percentage of children have valvular stenosis. The aortic valve may be bicuspid, unicuspid, or tricuspid.[22] In aortic stenosis, the left ventricle ejects its volume of blood through an orifice that is reduced in size. To accomplish this, the left ventricular systolic pressure rises, sometimes to as high as 250 mmHg. To generate these pressures, the left ventricle hypertrophies. The thickened ventricle offers more resistance to filling, and so diastolic pressure also rises. This rise in diastolic pressure in the left ventricle is transmitted to the left atrium, pulmonary vein, lungs, pulmonary artery, and right ventricle. The hypertrophy of the left ventricle leads to increased oxygen demand. Coronary artery blood flow may not be adequate to meet that demand, leading to chest pain, syncope, and ECG changes.

Males have a higher incidence of aortic stenosis than females. Most children with aortic stenosis develop normally and are asymptomatic. The presence of a murmur at the aortic area raises the suspicion of this congenital defect.

On examination, a thrill is present, and the cardiac impulse is heaving. The first heart sound is normal. The second heart sound is altered due to prolonged left ventricular ejection. The second heart sound may become single; the split may become narrow, or aortic closure may follow pulmonary closure. The murmur is systolic and is usually heard throughout the precordium.[23] A careful history may reveal symptoms of mild fatigue and dyspnea. Symptoms of angina or syncope, though they seldom occur, are important, as are signs of congestive heart failure in infants, since they may indicate the presence of significant stenosis.

There is an increased incidence of sudden death in the presence of severe aortic stenosis.[24] Children with moderate stenosis may not be allowed to participate in competitive sports. Children with mild stenosis are not limited in their activities. Follow-up management is required because the degree of stenosis may progress. Most children lead normal lives throughout childhood and adolescence. The signs and symptoms of the stenosis often do not become obvious until the fourth or fifth decade of life.

Surgery is indicated for children with significant stenosis with symptoms or severe stenosis in the absence of symptoms. The repair requires cardiopulmonary bypass. A valvulotomy, considered a palliative procedure, may be performed. Although it relieves the stenosis in the best way possible, usually some degree of stenosis or incompetence remains. An additional operation for valve replacement may be required at a later date.

Mitral valve prolapse *Mitral valve prolapse* occurs mainly in females and is usually recognized during adolescence. In this usually benign condition, one or both of the mitral valve leaflets prolapse back into the left atrium during ventricular systole. Diagnosis is made by auscultation when a blowing systolic murmur is heard. This person may be at risk for developing arrhythmias. No treatment is necessary except administration of prophylactic antibiotics before an invasive procedure (e.g., dental surgery, a tonsillectomy and adenoidectomy, or a bronchoscopy).

Cyanotic heart defects

As discussed earlier, cyanosis reflects the presence of reduced oxygen in the blood circulating through the tissues. A right-to-left shunt usually exists, allowing some of the systemic venous blood to bypass the lungs and reenter the systemic arterial circulation. Pulmonary vascularity may be increased (as in most children with transposition of the great arteries or in truncus arteriosus) or decreased (as in tetralogy of Fallot and tricuspid atresia), depending on the presence or absence of an obstructed blood flow between the heart and the lungs.

Cyanosis is typically associated with (1) clubbing of the fingers and toes (Fig. 22-4), due to lack of oxygen-enriched blood circulating in the periphery; (2) poor growth; (3) a tendency to develop cerebral abscesses; and (4) polycythemia. In polycythemia, the tissue hypoxia related to cyanosis stimulates bone marrow to increase red blood cell production for additional oxygen-carrying ability. Elevated hemoglobin and hematocrit values result. Infants, however, are prone to developing iron-deficiency anemia, which may disguise the elevated values. A low or normal hemoglobin value in children with cyanotic heart disease may reflect an iron deficiency requiring iron supplementation.

Complete transposition of the great arteries

Complete transposition of the great arteries involves reversal of the anatomic positions of the aorta and the pulmonary artery (Fig. 22-12). The aorta originates from the *right* ventricle, and the pulmonary artery originates from the *left* ventricle. Therefore, venous blood entering the right atrium will go to the right ventricle and return

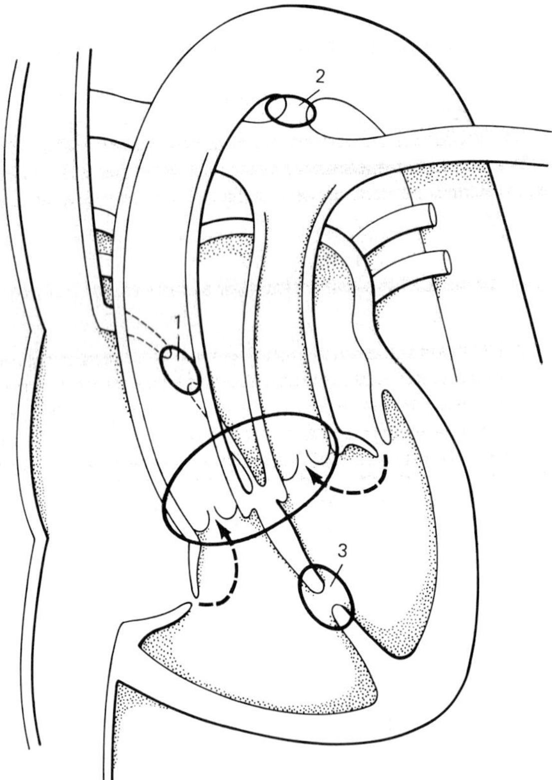

Figure 22-12 Complete transposition of the great arteries. Blood returning to the right side of the heart goes back to the body through the aorta, which arises from the right ventricle. Blood leaving the left ventricle goes out to the lungs through the pulmonary artery. Mixing of the oxygenated with the unoxygenated blood will not occur unless there is (1) an interatrial defect, (2) a patent ductus arteriosus, or (3) a ventricular septal defect.

to the systemic circulation via the aorta without having passed through the lungs to be oxygenated. Oxygenated blood entering the left atrium from the pulmonary circulation will travel to the left ventricle and return to the lungs without having supplied any oxygen to the body. Thus, two entirely separate circulatory systems are established.

The separation of the systemic and pulmonary circulations will result in death shortly after birth unless there is a communication between them. This communication is usually present in the form of a ventricular septal defect, an interatrial opening (a patent foramen ovale), or a patent ductus arteriosus. These, either alone or in combination, allow for the mixing of oxygenated with unoxygenated blood. In this way, the body receives enough oxygen to allow survival. Shunting of blood must be balanced, with equal amounts going in either direction, or overload of one or the other system will occur. With a patent ductus arteriosus, the upper extremities may be cyanotic, and the lower ones pink, until the ductus begins to close and cyanosis becomes widespread. Babies without a ventricular septal defect will also develop cyanosis during the newborn period.

The typical infant with a complete transposition is a male of normal or high birth weight who is visibly cyanotic. Tachypnea is often present due to pulmonary venous congestion. Closure of the ductus arteriosus can lead to a sudden deterioration in the condition of an infant who is dependent on that structure for a large portion of systemic oxygenation. Prostaglandin E_1 is given to delay closure of the ductus if the diagnosis is made early enough.

Auscultation may yield little information. It is possible that a variety of abnormal sounds may be heard, depending on the nature of the communication between the right and left heart. Conversely, there may be no murmurs. The arterial pulses may be full and bounding.

If the child survives early infancy, growth and development are generally retarded. Clubbing of the fingers and toes is seen. Polycythemia results and, if severe or prolonged, puts the child at risk for developing thrombosis, metabolic acidosis, and congestive heart failure. Respiratory infections are common.

If the infant is in severe distress, a palliative procedure is often done in the first few days or weeks of life. The objective is to allow better mixing of the oxygenated blood circulating through the lungs with the oxygen-depleted blood circulating through the body. The method preferred, because of its relatively low mortality rate and simplicity, is *balloon atrial septostomy* (the Rashkind procedure). During cardiac catheterization, a catheter with a balloon tip is passed from the right to the left atrium via the foramen ovale. The tip is then inflated and pulled forcefully through the atrial septum, tearing it. This procedure is repeated until the maximum effect is achieved. In many cases, arterial oxygen saturation is greatly improved. When atrial septostomy is not effective, an atrial septal defect may be created surgically.

An infant with a complete transposition accompanied by a large ventricular septal defect is subject to high pulmonary blood flow. In order to control congestive heart failure and prevent the development of increased pulmonary vascular resistance, a pulmonary artery banding may be done to decrease the amount of blood flow to the lungs.

The surgical corrections for transposition of the great vessels include artery switches and the Mustard procedure. An *artery switch* reverts the aorta and the pulmonary vessels to their normal position, while leaving the valves intact. This repair carries a high risk but is being done more frequently. Another corrective operation, the *Mustard procedure,* is accomplished by redirecting the blood flow inside the atria so that the blood from the inferior and superior venae cavae flows to the left ventricle and then to the lungs. The blood from the pulmonary veins then flows to the right ventricle and to the body. Thus, venous blood will be oxygenated in the lungs and carried to the body in the correct functional sequence, even though the right ventricle still pumps to the aorta and the left ventricle pumps to the pulmonary artery.

When the transposition is associated with a ventricular septal defect and pulmonary stenosis, the *Rastelli operation* provides both functional and anatomic correction. It involves tunneling blood inside the heart to connect the left ventricle to the aorta and using a conduit (tube) outside the heart to connect the right ventricle to the pulmonary artery.

Surgical repair of the transposition has significantly improved the prognosis of an infant with this defect. Problems encountered following surgery include arrhythmias and pulmonary vascular and venous obstruction due to baffle occlusion.[25] The ability of the right ventricle to continue to perform left ventricular work over a long period of time is difficult to determine.

Truncus arteriosus *Truncus arteriosus* is an uncommon lesion consisting of a large ventricular septal defect and a single artery that supplies the systemic and pulmonary circulations (Fig. 22-13). The truncus valve structure is frequently abnormal. Both ventricles eject their contents into the common artery, where oxygenated and oxygen-depleted blood mix. The oxygen saturation of this mixture is largely dependent on the relative volume of pulmonary blood flow. If pulmonary vascular resistance is high or the pulmonary arteries are small, arterial oxygen levels will be low. When the pulmonary arteries are of normal size and pulmonary re-

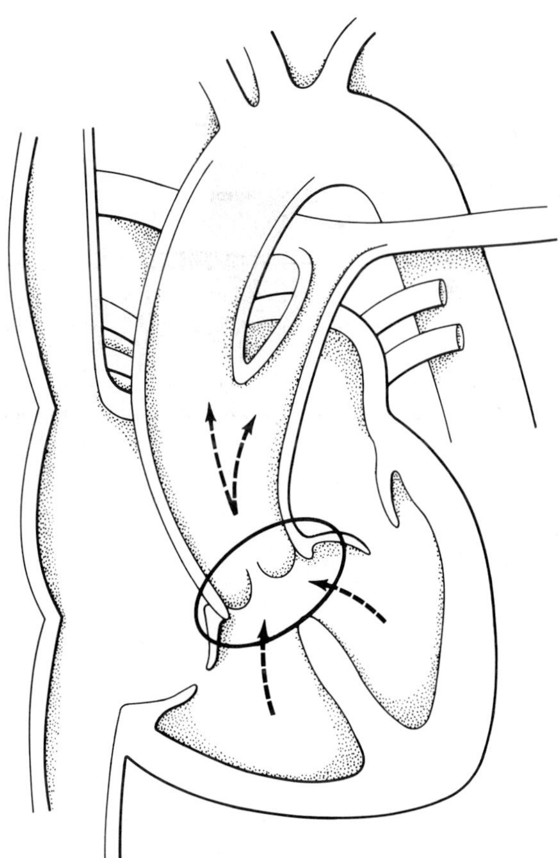

Figure 22-13 Truncus arteriosus with a ventricular septal defect. Oxygenated blood from the left ventricle and unoxygenated blood from the right ventricle flow through the single artery into the pulmonary and systemic circulations.

sistance is low, saturation of the truncus blood is greatly improved, and cyanosis is absent.

Infants with truncus arteriosus are characteristically ashen and cyanotic; the degree of cyanosis depends on which variety of the defect they have. Other symptoms frequently seen are dyspnea and fatigue associated with congestive heart failure. Generally, growth and development are retarded. A systolic murmur is usually present, and the second heart sound is single.

Most infants who present with this defect are very sick. Initial medical treatment is aimed at control of congestive heart failure, but for many, surgical intervention provides the only possibility for long-term survival. When a large pulmonary flow is present, the pulmonary arteries may be banded to prevent the development of high pulmonary vascular resistance. Complete correction closes the ventricular septal defect, leaving the truncus to serve as the aorta, and reestablishes communication between the right ventricle and the pulmonary arteries by means of a conduit. Mortality rates are high among children under the age of 2 years and when high pulmonary vascular resistance exists.[26] Nevertheless, the defect should be repaired before the child is 2 years old in order to prevent pulmonary vascular disease.

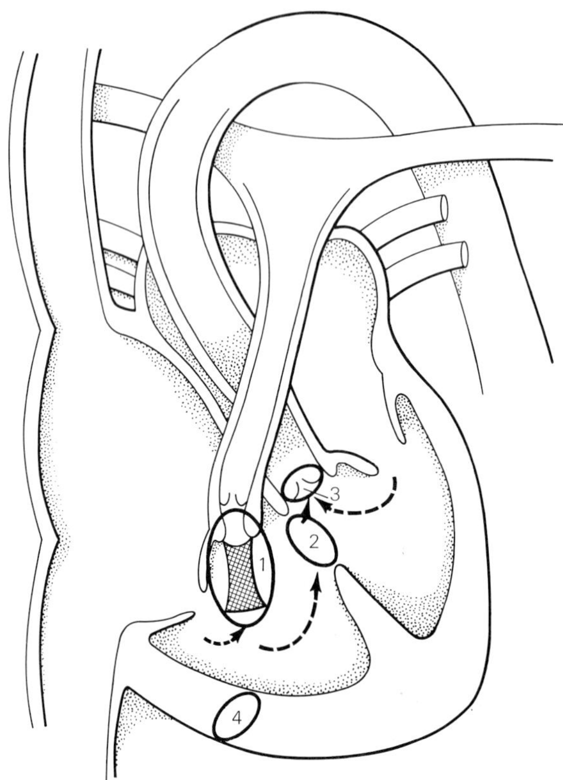

Figure 22-14 Tetralogy of Fallot. (1) Right ventricular outflow obstruction. (2) Ventricular septal defect. (3) The aorta overriding the ventricular septal defect. (4) Right ventricular hypertrophy. The incidence is 1:2000 live births.

Tetralogy of Fallot Four abnormalities are classically present in *tetralogy of Fallot*: (1) a right ventricular outflow obstruction, (2) a large ventricular septal defect (VSD), (3) overriding of the VSD by the aorta (dextroposition), and (4) right ventricular hypertrophy (Fig. 22-14). The obstruction to right ventricular outflow is due to tissue overgrowth in the infundibulum of the right ventricle (the smooth area directly below the pulmonary valve), stenosis in the pulmonary valve, or stenosis in the pulmonary artery or its branches. Pressures in the left and right ventricles are equal because of the large VSD. Since right ventricular pressures cannot exceed the left, blood flow through the pulmonary system is limited by the amount of resistance offered by the obstruction to pulmonary flow. The blood that is not ejected into the pulmonary circulation crosses the VSD and is ejected into the aorta. If there is mild pulmonary stenosis and mild right ventricular outflow obstruction, there may be a left-to-right shunt and no cyanosis. With growth, the stenosis grows, and eventually there is right-to-left shunting, causing cyanosis.

The right-to-left shunt and limited pulmonary blood flow are responsible for the outstanding clinical features of the disease. Cyanosis, which is usually not present at birth, appears sometime during the first year of life and generally becomes progressively severe. Clubbing of the fingers may be seen in older infants and children. The knee-chest position is frequently preferred by these children; squatting is characteristic following exercise or walking. They are frequently small for their age, and their activities are limited. A harsh systolic murmur, along the middle to upper left sternal border, and a single second heart sound will be heard on physical examination.[27]

Many of these children have hypoxic spells characterized by an increased rate and depth of respirations, accompanied by increasing cyanosis. This may progress to unconsciousness, seizures, and even death. These episodes may occur frequently, rarely, or never. Treatment of children who have hypoxic spells includes helping them squat by placing them in a knee-chest position; this increases the return of systemic venous blood to the heart and lungs and maximizes blood supply to the vital organs. The squatting position also minimizes possible respiratory acidosis by mechanically pushing the diaphragm up and forcing carbon dioxide out. Morphine sulfate, propranolol (Inderal), sodium bicarbonate, and even general anesthesia have been utilized to interrupt an attack.[28] Polycythemia develops early in children with tetralogy of Fallot to increase the oxygen-carrying ability of the blood. Over time, collateral circulation to the lungs may increase. Both the knee-chest position and polycythemia are mechanisms for relieving hypoxia.

Palliative shunt procedures are utilized to increase blood supply to the lungs until the child is older and is physically more able to undergo total correction, if there is pulmonary atresia, or if the child has severe hypoplasia of the pulmonary arteries (Table 22-8).

Complete correction includes relieving the obstruction of right ventricular outflow and closing the VSD. In some centers, complete correction is being done at earlier ages, thus avoiding the palliative shunt procedures. The immediate postoperative course following complete correction of tetralogy of Fallot may be difficult. Problems frequently encountered include hemorrhage, low cardiac output, heart failure, and arrhythmias (especially heart block).

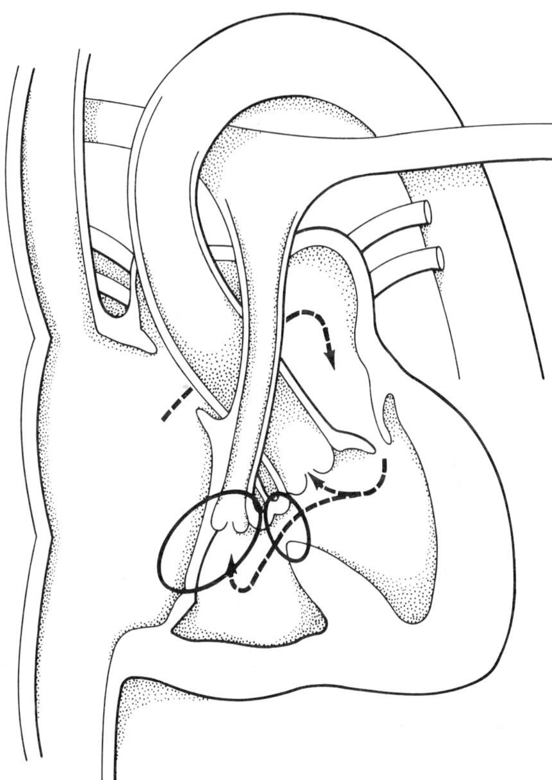

Figure 22-15 Tricuspid atresia. Unoxygenated blood flows from the right atrium to the left atrium. Blood flow to the pulmonary arteries arrives via the left ventricle, a ventricular septal defect, and the right ventricle.

Tricuspid atresia *Tricuspid atresia,* occurring in 2 percent of cardiac defects, is accompanied by a number of anatomic variations. The hallmark sign is absence of the tricuspid valve (Fig. 22-15). No direct communication between the right atrium and the right ventricle and pulmonary vasculature is present. Blood flows from the right atrium through the interatrial septum to the left atrium and into the left ventricle. Blood flow through the pulmonary vasculature usually occurs via a ventricular septal defect. In the absence of a ventricular septal defect, pulmonary blood flow is dependent on the ductus arteriosus or the bronchial artery collaterals. The right ventricle is small. The right atrium is usually enlarged, and congestive heart failure is common. Pulmonary edema is rare since pulmonary blood flow is usually diminished. As a result of the abnormal flow pattern, venous and arterial blood meet and mix in the left atrium. The left ventricle is enlarged and hypertrophied. Blood delivered to the general circulation is low in oxygen because of the mixing of venous and arterial blood in the left atrium.

Children with tricuspid atresia are sick from birth. They appear undernourished and are poorly

Table 22-8 Palliative Shunt Procedures for Children with Tetralogy of Fallot

Methods of Choice*

1. Blalock-Taussig procedure. An anastomosis between the subclavian artery and the pulmonary artery is established.
2. Modified Blalock-Taussig procedure. Gore-tex or Impra (polytetrafluoroethylene) is sewn between the subclavian artery or the aorta and the right or left pulmonary artery.
3. Waterston procedure. A communication between the ascending aorta and the right pulmonary artery is established.

*An infrequently used method is Potts' procedure. A communication between the descending thoracic aorta and the left pulmonary artery is established.

developed. Cyanosis is obvious except in the presence of adequate pulmonary flow. Dyspnea, fatigue, anoxic spells, clubbing, and signs of venous congestion are present. The first and second heart sounds are usually single. The murmur is variable or, in some cases, absent.[29] The prognosis for these children is poor, and death frequently occurs in the first year of life.[30]

Previously, a palliative shunt operation was all that was available. Now, a more corrective type of operation, the *Fontan operation,* is performed on children who do not have pulmonary hypertension. This operation involves connection of the right atrium to the small right ventricle or to the pulmonary artery, either directly or with a conduit. The blood then flows from the right atrium to the pulmonary artery without being pumped by a developed ventricle. Initial reports are encouraging, but long-term evaluation is not yet possible.[31] Although many children improve significantly after the operation, some continue to have problems with fatigue and fluid retention. Chances of success with surgery are decreased with mitral valve regurgitation, abnormal pulmonary vascular bed, and inadequate left ventricular function.

Single ventricle* When no partition exists between the two ventricles or when both the mitral and tricuspid valves empty into one ventricle and the other ventricle remains underdeveloped, a *univentricular defect* is present. The terms *double-inlet right ventricle* and *double-inlet left ventricle* are synonymous with *single ventricle*.[32]

The signs and symptoms are similar to those of a large ventricular septal defect (poor growth, frequent upper respiratory infections, and congestive heart failure). Some right-to-left shunting may occur because of the mixing of blood in the ventricle.[33]

Efforts to surgically create an artificial septum with a patch have not been encouraging. However, for persons with associated pulmonary stenosis, a modification of the operation described for tricuspid atresia has been successful. A patch is sewn, closing the orifice from the right atrium to the right ventricle. Then a drainage pathway is established directly from the right atrium to the pulmonary artery. Thus, right atrium blood flows directly into the lungs without passing through a ventricle, and the one ventricle now pumps blood only to the aorta. After surgery, problems such as a high right atrium pressure and other pulmonary difficulties (e.g., pleural effusions) complicate recovery.

Double-outlet right ventricle* This defect is similar to tetralogy of Fallot in that the aorta orifice overrides the ventricular septal defect. In double-outlet right ventricle, the aorta is so far displaced to the right that all or nearly all the aorta originates from the right ventricle. If the pulmonary artery continues to originate from the right ventricle as it normally does, then both great arteries have right ventricular origin. Pulmonary stenosis may or may not be associated with double-outlet right ventricle.

The signs and symptoms include frequent upper respiratory infections, S_3 heard at the apex of the heart, and a systolic thrill at the third and fourth intercostal spaces along the left sternal border.[34]

Repair is accomplished by closing the ventricular septal defect in such a way that the patch forms a tunnel which leads blood being ejected from the left ventricle through the ventricular septal defect and out the aorta.

Cardiac transplantation The many recent advances in medical therapy and surgical techniques are making heart and heart-lung transplantation in children a reality. These procedures are used in children with a destroyed myocardium, primary cardiac myopathy (dysfunction of the heart musculature), or rare congenital heart defects that cannot be repaired (e.g., hypoplastic left heart syndrome).[35]

Recent developments that have renewed interest in transplantation include safe endomyocardial biopsy methods to detect early cardiac rejection, better organ preservation through modern cardioplegia agents (cold chemicals circulated through a heart to conserve energy and preserve the myocardium), and the advent of a new immunosuppressive agent, cyclosporin A.

Organ procurement is a difficult problem because an adult heart is often too large for a child.[36] Although cyclosporin A is an improvement over conventional immunosuppressive therapy, it does not eliminate the hazards of rejection. Infection continues to be a major threat in any patient who has had immunosuppressive therapy. The 1-year survival rate in *adults* has improved from 42 to 63 percent, and now, with the use of cyclosporin A, it has increased to 81 percent.[37] Since few

*The authors wish to thank Dr. Dwight McGoon, of the Mayo Clinic, Rochester, Minn., for the information he provided in these sections.

transplantations have been done in children, no survival rates are available. See Chap. 26 for a brief discussion of the management of the child undergoing an organ transplant.

NURSING MANAGEMENT OF THE CHILD UNDERGOING HEART SURGERY

When such medications as digoxin and diuretics are no longer effective in treating a child with congenital heart disease, surgical intervention will be necessary. Surgery may be emergency or elective. Usually elective surgery is done before the child enters school, around 3 to 5 years of age. When a corrective procedure is done, it may be *palliative*—a temporary, partial correction done at birth, or soon after, to shunt blood and thus improve oxygenation until the infant gets older. A balloon septostomy, done in the catheterization laboratory to create a small opening between the atria, is an example of a palliative procedure. A total correction of a defect is attempted when the risks and possible complications of the surgical procedure are less than those of not having the surgery. Generally, the younger the child, the more risks are entailed in the surgery. This is especially true for newborns and infants.

Preoperative management

Assessment of a child who will have heart surgery is multifaceted. A cardiac catheterization may be performed prior to surgery. Studies done before surgery include a chest x-ray and a 12-lead ECG. A routine urinalysis is obtained.

Various blood studies are performed. Electrolyte and clotting studies are done, as well as a complete blood count. Blood gases may be drawn if the child has a cyanotic heart defect. All the studies done provide a data base for comparison during and after surgery.

On admission, it is important to obtain accurate baseline vital signs, including apical pulse rate and blood pressure in all extremities, and to assess respiratory status. Record the presence, severity, and location of cyanosis. Accurate measurements of height and weight are necessary, since amounts of future medications and intravenous fluids will be based on these measurements. Weigh the child without clothes. It is helpful to have another nurse double-check the weight if the infant or young child is agitated and moving around. Determine any allergies to food or medications, and record these in the chart, in the Kardex, and on the medication sheet. The child may be given a special allergy band (like an ID band) listing the drugs to which he or she is allergic. Loose teeth should be reported to prevent aspiration during intubation for surgery. Review the child's immunization status and possible recent exposure to any communicable diseases.

Preoperative teaching Include the child and the family in preoperative teaching. Assess their level of understanding about the heart defect and the impending surgical treatment. In the case of infants and toddlers, teaching is directed to the parents. Simple, direct explanations using diagrams, drawings, miniature models, and dolls help older preschoolers and school-age children learn. Teaching may be done in short, frequent sessions or condensed into one or two longer periods—depending on the child's age and condition.

Prior to teaching, discuss what type of procedure will be done with the surgeon. Identify anticipated complications to further enhance the teaching plan. Areas to cover in teaching include the anatomy of the heart and particular defect and preoperative, intraoperative, and postoperative procedures. Table 22-9 presents a useful checklist for teaching school-age children and adolescents.

Preoperative activities are often frightening and overwhelming to the child. Visits by the cardiac surgeon, the anesthesiologist, and, if possible, the primary intensive care unit nurse who will care for the child after surgery help clarify information that may be confusing or misunderstood. Explain that the child will not eat or drink after midnight before the surgery, emphasizing the importance of an empty stomach during the operation. Tell the older child about the morning preoperative medication and how it will make the child feel. The parents will be unable to go with the child to the operating room; therefore, stress that they will be waiting for the child's return. Knowing that loved ones are nearby and taking a favorite toy along help a child through this difficult experience (see Chap. 15).

When explaining the operative procedure, show the child as many items as possible that he or she will be exposed to in the coming days. Allowing the child to handle such equipment as surgical garments, anesthesia masks, and intravenous tubing facilitates the introduction of these

Table 22-9 Teaching Preparation for a School-Age Child or Adolescent Who Will Undergo Cardiac Surgery: A Checklist

Equipment for Teaching Kit
Doll
Soap
Foley catheter
Intravenous equipment
Monitor leads
Cardboard model of a monitor with a picture of the ECG on the screen
Oxygen mask or face tent
Balloons
Chest tube
Stethoscope
Syringes
Dressings or adhesive strips
Plain drawing paper and crayons or felt-tip pens
Heart models
Body outlines
Photographs
Books

Checklist for Teaching Sessions (Adapted to the Individual Child's Needs)
☐ Review of anatomy of heart and defect
☐ Understanding of surgical procedure
☐ Explanation of preoperative procedures:
1. Bath or shower with skin preparation
2. Visits by:
   a. Cardiac surgeon, Dr. ______
   b. Anesthesiologist, Dr. ______
   c. ICU nurse, ______
3. No food or drink in the morning
4. Transportation to the OR
5. Parents (where they will be)

☐ Operation
1. Showing equipment:
   a. Mask, hat, and gown
   b. Rubber face mask
2. Visiting the OR if possible
3. Explaining that anesthesia is a special sleep in which all body parts go to sleep
4. Giving assurance that no pain will be felt during the operation
5. Describing the incision (type, location, and size), using a doll

☐ Postoperative appearance and feelings
1. Feeling sleepy
2. Having a tube in the mouth connected to a breathing machine
3. Tubes (demonstrate on a doll):
   a. Nasogastric tube
   b. Chest tube
   c. Foley catheter
   d. Pacemaker wires
   e. IV in leg or arm
   f. Arterial pressure line
   g. RA or LA line
4. ECG monitoring that will show a TV picture of heartbeats
5. Suctioning, deep breathing, and coughing (blow balloons)
6. Pain medication
7. Oxygen mask (demonstrate on a doll)

☐ ICU routines
1. Visiting hours
2. Usual length of stay
3. Special nurse who will be with the child

☐ Surgical unit transfer
☐ Response to teaching
Child ______
______
Parents ______
______

Source: Adapted from "Pre-Op Teaching Checklist for Use with Children Undergoing Cardiac Surgery," prepared by Nancy Horvath, B.S.N., Instructor, Nursing Service—Pediatrics and Pediatrics Intensive Care Units, St. Mary's Hospital, Rochester, Minn. Used with permission.

new, intrusive devices in a nonthreatening manner. Some hospitals allow visits to the operating room and the intensive care unit to further decrease anxiety in older children. A videotape of the sights and sounds that the child will encounter on the way to the operating room may be helpful.

It is comforting to the parents and child to stress the care, attention, and close observation the child will receive during and after the operation. Emphasize the presence of the anesthetist or anesthesiologist during the operation. Tell the child that he or she will be in a "special" kind of sleep and will feel no pain during the operation. It is helpful to stress that the anesthesiologist will help the child wake up as well as go to sleep.

The size of the "cut" or incision is nearly always exaggerated in children's minds. Asking them to show how big they think the incision will be or draw a picture of it gives the nurse an idea of their fantasy level. Illustrating the location and size of the incision, sutures, or steri-strips on a doll or diagram may aid in the explanation.

Further teaching regarding the postoperative experience greatly depends on the child's age. It is important to stress that a nurse will always be nearby, that the child will feel sleepy or drowsy, and that medicine will be available for pain. Showing a doll with the various pieces of equipment used after surgery to monitor body functions (e.g., intravenous lines, an endotracheal tube, and a Foley catheter) helps prepare the child and the parents. Encourage the child to handle the equipment during and after the teaching sessions. Practice deep-breathing and coughing exercises with the child (Fig. 22-16). Balloons are useful to simulate lung inflation (inspiration) and deflation (expiration). A small pillow is helpful in demonstrating splinting, as is applying pressure to support the thoracic cavity while the child is coughing.

It is important to remember that children need to feel safe and secure. Fears of insecurity, impending danger, and bodily harm and mutilation, due to their lack of cognitive understanding, increase children's anxiety level and diminish their ability to cope with the surgical experience. Remember that it is far worse to give a child *too much* information during preoperative teaching than *too little*. Careful preparation and thoughtful preoperative teaching, appropriate for the particular child and family, promotes cooperation and makes the surgical experience less frightening.

Preoperative activities Some physicians may order a daily PhisoHex or Betadine shower or bath for 1 to 3 days prior to surgery. The skin is shaved in the operating room after the child is asleep. The night before surgery, the child may have a light supper. The child is not allowed to eat or drink after midnight, and so it is good to allow the child to have a cool drink before bedtime. Remove all fluids and food from the bedside table, and place a label at the foot of the bed saying that the child is not allowed to eat or drink. Vital signs are taken the evening before surgery and the morning of surgery. Any increase in temperature or sign of an upper respiratory infection should be reported to the physician. If there is any infection, surgery will usually be delayed until the child is better.

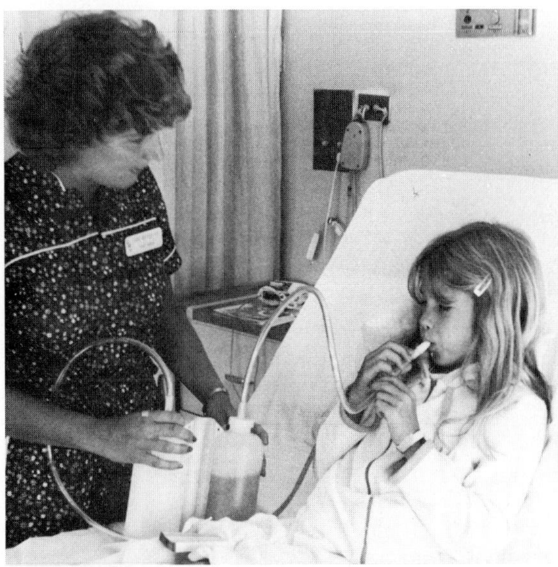

Figure 22-16 Preoperative teaching. These sessions prepare the child for procedures done before and after surgery. Blow bottles and devices such as balloons and Tri-Flow equipment make deep-breathing exercises fun.

Preoperative sedation helps relax the child and facilitate the induction of anesthesia. Medications used include various narcotic analgesics such as meperidine HCl, pentazocine HCl, or morphine sulfate. Occasionally, a narcotic sedative such as secobarbital or pentobarbital may be administered. Atropine sulfate or scopolamine is frequently given in conjunction with a narcotic analgesic or sedative. The nurse must double-check the ordered dosage of the preoperative medication against the child's weight before administering it and notify the anesthesiologist if there are any questions.

Sometimes parents are allowed to wait with their child before the surgery in a holding area outside the operating room. Encourage parents and other family members to wait in the designated area so they can learn immediately of the child's condition and speak with the surgeon after the operation.

The intraoperative period

Depending on the type of defect being repaired, the procedure is accomplished through either open or closed heart surgery. *Closed heart surgery* is done for relatively simple corrections of defects outside the heart, such as a patent ductus arteriosus ligation. *Open heart surgery* involves cutting into the myocardium and using a cardiopulmonary bypass machine, and it carries more risks than closed heart surgery.

During the surgery, vital signs are monitored closely. As soon as the child is asleep, various intravenous lines are inserted. Frequently, an intraarterial line is started percutaneously or through a cutdown in the radial artery or femoral artery. Then a *thoracotomy* or *sternotomy* incision is made, depending on the type of defect and the route of entry into the body needed to correct it.

Open heart surgery is accomplished in a bloodless field with the use of *extracorporeal* (outside the body) circulation. The right atrium is cannulated (a small tubular catheter is inserted). Blood then flows from the cannula through a cardiopulmonary bypass machine, where it is oxygenated with a membrane or bubble-type oxygenator. The machine acts as an artificial set of lungs. The warmed, filtered, and oxygen-enriched blood is returned through a cannula in the aorta and circulated throughout the body.

Deep hypothermia may be used in young children. During deep hypothermia, the child's body surface may be partially cooled with dry ice packs while appendages and genitals are protected. Then the blood vessels are cannulated, and the cardiopulmonary bypass machine centrally cools the blood and thus the body temperature to 12 to 20°C (53 to 76°F). At around 20°C, cardiac arrest occurs, and the surgeons correct the defect in a quiet, nonbeating heart. Cardiac arrest is limited to 60 to 90 min, and no brain damage occurs because the metabolic processes are considerably slowed. After the correction, the body is warmed gradually by warming the blood in the cardiopulmonary bypass machine. The heart usually begins beating on its own, but defibrillation may be needed if the rhythm is irregular.

Chest tubes are inserted during the suturing process, as are additional intravenous lines. A central venous pressure line, right and left atrial lines, or a pulmonary artery line helps to monitor cardiac function during the initial postoperative period.

Heart surgery is delicate and complicated and may take several hours. During the period of the child's surgery, the family should be informed of the child's progress at regular intervals.

Nursing management during the postoperative period

After surgery, the child is transferred directly to an intensive care unit or a similar critical care setting for 1 to 3 days or more until vital signs and related systems of the body are stable and functioning well. The goal of nursing management is the restoration and maintenance of optimal cardiovascular, respiratory, renal, and neurological function. It is vital that the nurse be able to identify subtle changes in the body systems which may herald impending complications. Intelligent assessment of children after cardiac surgery is especially important because their physiological reserves for compensating for physical insults like surgery are limited. To detect subtle symptoms of compromised reserves, each system is continuously monitored through careful nursing observations and mechanical recording devices.

There is great trauma to the body and heart during cardiac surgery as a result of manipulation and replacement of parts such as valves and patches and as a result of cutting through delicate impulse conduction and muscle fibers. The anesthesia used during surgery also depresses the contractility of the myocardium and affects ventilation capacity.

General assessment Vital signs are taken every 15 min for 1 h, every 30 min for 2 h, and then every hour for 24 to 48 h (Fig. 22-17). The apical pulse is auscultated for a full minute. The nurse must report an irregular heart rate, muffled or distant heart sounds, and murmurs or gallops. A cuff blood pressure may be taken in an arm or leg, and, if necessary, the sound may be amplified using an ultrasound device.

Temperature is monitored closely because young children, especially infants and newborns, have minimal stores of subcutaneous fat and immature thermal-regulating mechanisms. Initially, on admission to the intensive care setting, the child is *hypothermic* (has a low temperature) because of the cold operating room and, in some cases, as a result of the deep hypothermia used during repair of the defect. Warmed blankets or a heat lamp may be used to gradually increase the child's temperature to the normal range. *Hyperthermia* (an increased temperature) is common in the first 24 to 48 h after surgery because of the trauma of the surgery and cardiopulmonary bypass. Although antibiotics are given prophylactically, if a child's temperature remains elevated for longer than 48 h after surgery, cultures and sensitivities of the urine, blood, wound, and sputum are obtained to determine whether infection is present.

Cardiovascular function The child's vital signs are recorded by a cardiac monitor with modules depicting the ECG (usually lead II pattern), respiratory rate, and circulatory pressures. A pressure-sensing device is used to record arterial and venous pressure waves with corresponding nu-

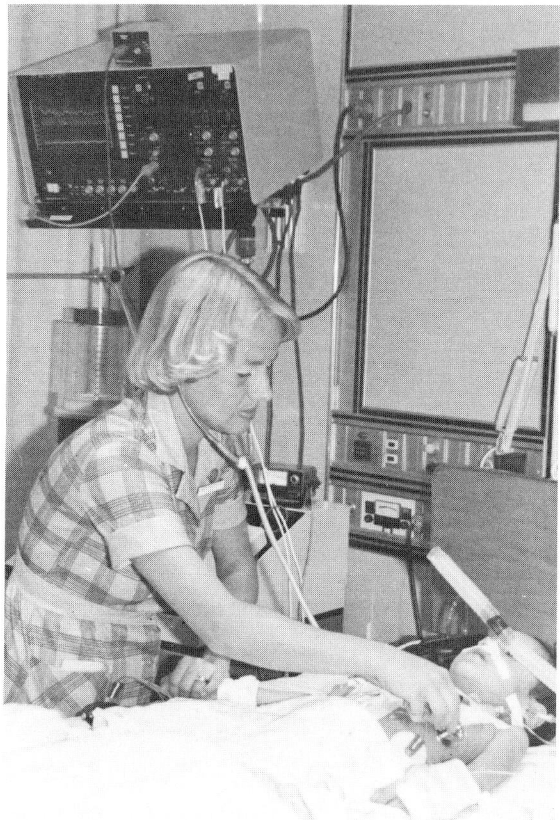

Figure 22-17 The immediate postoperative period. The child requires constant observation and support. Monitoring equipment facilitates assessment of cardiovascular status after surgery. (*Courtesy of Barbara Macpherson.*)

merical values visualized on an oscilloscope. These lines must not become kinked, since they are important in monitoring circulatory status within the chambers and great vessels of the heart. The mean arterial pressure, in addition to the systolic and diastolic values of the arterial pressure, is a valuable tool in assessing circulatory blood volume.

Assess the skin, primarily of the extremities, for color, temperature, moisture, and capillary refill. Palpate peripheral pulses on the right and left sides simultaneously. If all tissues are receiving an adequate blood volume and cardiac output is good, there will be (1) warm hands and feet; (2) equal, palpable peripheral pulses in all extremities; (3) pink or pale lips, oral mucous membranes, and nail beds; and (4) rapid capillary refill. Cyanotic or mottled skin and membranes, cool extremities, delayed capillary refill, and weak, thready pulses indicate decreased ability of the heart to pump oxygenated blood through the body tissues. Notify a physician immediately if signs of compromised circulation are noted.

Measurement of circulatory blood volume and cardiovascular function is accomplished with a central venous pressure (CVP) line. A CVP line is usually inserted into the right cephalic or basilic vein and is threaded into the right atrium, where the pressure is normally 0 to 5 mmHg. The placement of the CVP line is verified with a chest x-ray. The pressure reading is obtained with the child in a supine position. A low CVP value may indicate the need for fluid or blood replacement, while a high reading may indicate fluid overload, deteriorating cardiac function, or cardiac tamponade (bleeding into the pericardial sac).

Measuring chest tube drainage is essential to monitoring circulatory volume. Placement of chest tubes at the conclusion of surgery ensures proper drainage of blood from around the heart and pleural cavity, decreases the pressure around the heart and pulmonary structures, enhances the return of pulmonary function, and prevents infection in the pleural and mediastinal spaces. Underwater-seal chest drainage bottles were used in the past (Fig. 22-18). The one-bottle gravity system is an elementary water-sealed system. It is appropriate when the pleural cavity is used to drain air and only a small amount of fluid. When there is a need to drain large amounts of fluid, the two-bottle system is employed, the second bottle serving to hold any overflow from the first. Today such underwater-seal systems are employed only when pneumothorax is present or, in the older child, when drainage is expected to be minimal. Disposable chest tube drainage sets (Fig. 22-19) are capable of measuring drainage more accurately and are more popular than bottle systems.

The nurse must maintain patency of the chest tubes for proper drainage. There should be no kinks in the tubing, and connections between the chest tube and the drainage container must be intact and secured with adhesive tape (Fig. 22-20). The tubing should lie without tension to give the child room to move freely. Chest tubes are stripped or "milked" from the child to the drainage container every 15 min on admission and thereafter every 30 min and when necessary. The type of drainage and quantity (in mil-

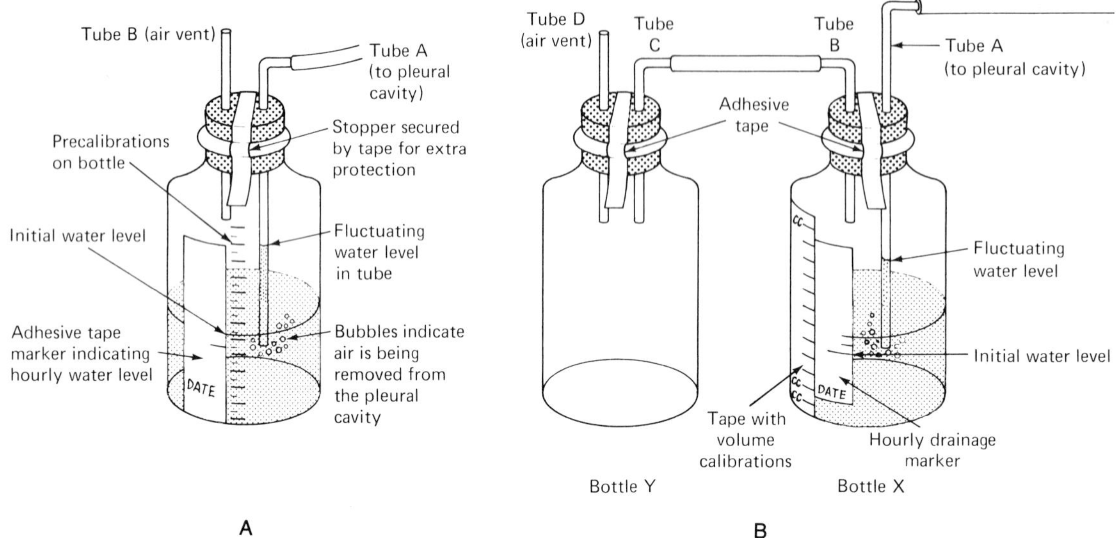

Figure 22-18 Water-seal drainage systems.
(*A*) The one-bottle gravity system. Note that tube A, from the patient's pleural cavity, is submerged in water. Some surgeons may elect to attach tube B to suction apparatus. (*B*) The two-bottle gravity system. If bottle X fills, the excess flows to bottle Y via tubes B and C. Fluid thus does not reenter the pleural cavity. Bottle Y is called the "trap" bottle. Some surgeons may elect to attach tube D to suction apparatus. (*From G. Scipien, M. U. Barnard, M. A. Chard, J. Howe, and P. J. Phillips* [*eds.*], *Comprehensive Pediatric Nursing, 3d ed., McGraw-Hill, New York, 1986, p. 974. Used with permission.*)

limeters) are recorded hourly. Initially, drainage will be sanguineous (bloody), then serous-sanguineous, and finally serous. Although drainage usually does not exceed 500 ml per 24 h, older children and those who have undergone surgery for transposition of the great arteries, tetralogy of Fallot, or truncus arteriosus experience increased sanguineous drainage. Any significant increase in the amount or type of drainage should be reported.

Chest tube drainage is computed as output along with all other body drainage. Two Kelly clamps or hemostats for each chest tube and petroleum gauze are kept at the bedside in case a chest tube becomes disconnected or falls out. A hissing sound alerts the nurse to a lack of patency in the tubing. *Never* clamp a chest tube that becomes disconnected when the child is on a respirator, however, because the child will develop a spontaneous tension pneumothorax.

Respiratory function Respiratory function has a twofold relationship to cardiac function. If arterial blood oxygenation is not maintained within required amounts, myocardial and tissue metabolism may be adversely affected, leading to decreased cardiac output, poor perfusion, metabolic acidosis, and further cardiac depression. The muscular work of respiration also depends on the oxygen supplied by an effectively pumping heart. Respiratory function is also affected by anesthesia, sedation, and incisional pain.

After heart surgery, mechanical ventilation assistance may be required. The child will have an oral or nasal endotracheal tube in place. The position of the tube is verified with a portable chest x-ray done routinely after the child is admitted to the unit. When children awake from the surgery, they should be told that they will not be able to talk. It is comforting to them to be instructed to shake their heads "yes" or "no" in order to communicate and to understand that a nurse is always nearby if they need anything. To keep the endotracheal tube patent, the child is suctioned (Table 21-5) every 1 to 2 h or when needed. Always ventilate the child with 100% oxygen before, during, and after suctioning. Initially, secretions may be blood-tinged as a result of the intubation process. If the child does not have an endotracheal tube, a face mask or oxygen hood will be used to deliver oxygen with mist.

General respiratory care includes noting the respiratory rate and depth and the presence of

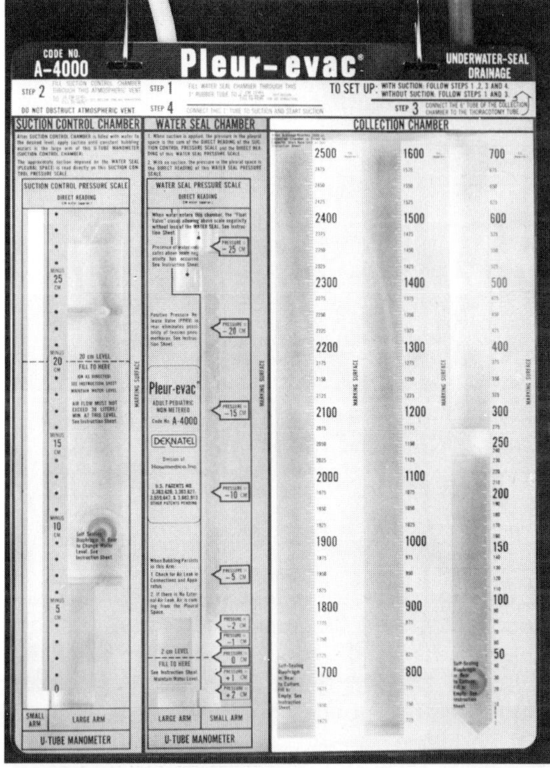

Figure 22-19 A disposable chest tube drainage system. Before use, the water-sealed chamber is filled to the 2-cm level to eliminate the possibility of airflow back into the pleural cavity. When suction pressure is desired, the suction control chamber is filled to provide the amount of negative pressure needed to facilitate drainage of the pleural cavity. When the collection chamber tubing is attached to the chest tube from the child, the drainage flows into the columns via the inlet tubing. The calibrated markings allow accurate measurement of drainage. If the drainage system fills to capacity, a new one may be attached to the chest tube or tubes. (*Photo courtesy of Deknatel, Inc., New York.*)

retractions. Observe the skin, lips, mucous membranes, and nail beds to assess oxygen saturation. Breath sounds are auscultated bilaterally, and absent or diminished sounds should be reported. Blood gases are drawn on admission to the intensive care unit and thereafter when necessary or after any change in oxygen concentration, tidal volume, or ventilatory rate. Position is changed, usually from side to side, every 2 h to prevent stasis of secretions and respiratory infection. The head of the bed may be flat for the first 24 h after surgery and then elevated to promote maximum lung expansion. Good skin care is vital, since children are not usually able to relieve pressures themselves until they wake sufficiently from the anesthesia.

Once the child is more awake, chest physiotherapy (see Fig. 16-34), coughing, and deep-breathing exercise are initiated every 2 h. A splint pillow is helpful to decrease the tension on the incision site as the child coughs. Nasotracheal suctioning may be done, if necessary, to stimulate the child's cough reflex.

Renal function Renal status is monitored carefully after heart surgery. Intake and output are accurately reported. Urinary drainage systems are used to facilitate close monitoring of urine output. Indwelling catheters may be used. In neonates and infants, blood taken for laboratory studies is counted as output.

The level of hydration is frequently assessed (Table 16-13). Skin turgor and the fontanels, lips, and mucous membranes are checked. Children are not overly hydrated after surgery in order to prevent fluid overload and myocardial stress. Intravenous fluids are infused at a rate appropriate for the child's body surface and usually contain a 10% concentration of dextrose for infants and children up to age 12.

Blood is monitored for blood urea nitrogen and creatinine levels. Urine specimens are tested for pH, glucose, ketones, protein, blood, and specific

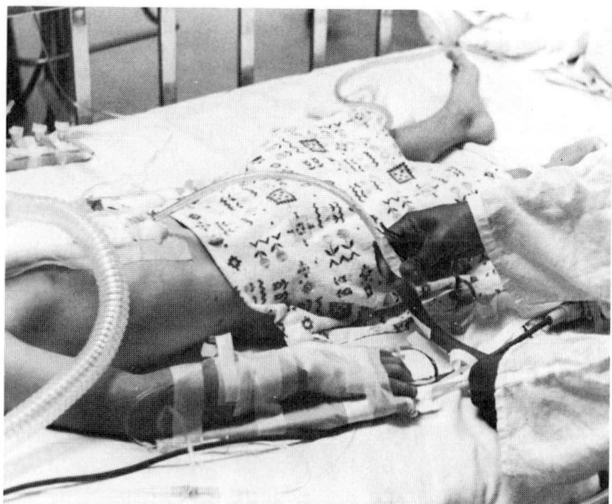

Figure 22-20 Chest tube care. Careful measures and precautions are vital in the nursing management of a child with chest tubes. The tube should be checked frequently for patency.

gravity. It is important to remember that circulatory status directly affects renal perfusion. The quantity of urine reflects circulating vascular status, whereas the quality of urine reflects renal function.

Neurological function The central nervous system is monitored closely after surgery. Cerebral blood flow may be hindered by a blood clot, or *embolus*, from the surgical procedure. A sleeping child should be easy to arouse, alert, and oriented. Although children are frequently confused and frightened in the intensive care unit, normal confusion must be distinguished from disorientation. Ask simple questions, and have the child say "yes" or "no" or nod his or her head. Wipe away the lubricating ointment placed in the eyes during surgery. Then check the pupils for size, equality, position, reaction to light, and accommodation. Muscle strength is evaluated by observing facial symmetry, hand grasp, and extremity movements. The response to pain can be assessed easily, since many procedures are being done simultaneously. Withdrawal from the direction of painful stimuli is an expected and appropriate response. It is important to have an accurate preoperative assessment recorded to compare with postoperative findings.

Hematologic studies Blood studies are simultaneously monitored to enhance assessment of the body systems. Blood-clotting studies are especially important, since heparin is administered to the child before extracorporeal circulation to minimize the chance of emboli. Serum electrolytes, hemoglobin, and hematocrit are evaluated closely, since a significant increase or decrease would directly affect cardiac function. Serum glucose levels may be increased because the cardiopulmonary bypass machine is primed with a parenteral glucose solution. Finger sticks can be done in infants to estimate serum glucose levels by placing a drop of blood on a test tape. A 50% dextrose intravenous solution is used for severe hypoglycemia.

Potassium levels are monitored closely, and potassium supplements are given to prevent arrhythmias from developing. Sodium and calcium levels must also be measured. Usually a continuous infusion of calcium is given during the immediate postoperative period.

The white blood cell count is evaluated for an increase due to infection. On the basis of the results of lab studies, vital signs, and chest tube drainage, blood is replaced using packed red blood cells, washed blood cells from the bypass machine, or plasma. As much as possible, a balance is maintained between blood lost and blood replaced.

Additional nursing care A nasogastric tube may be used to prevent aspiration and maintain decompression of the gastrointestinal tract while the child is not eating or drinking. After checking its placement, irrigate it with 10 to 15 ml of normal saline every 1 to 2 h to maintain patency. Record the amount, color, and consistency of the drainage hourly.

The child may be restrained during the immediate postoperative period. Use proper restraint techniques (Table 16-5) and provide good skin care.

The parents should be allowed to visit the child as soon as possible (Fig. 22-21). Although visiting policies vary, the parents' limited time with the child should be uninterrupted, if possible. Describe the child's appearance to the family beforehand. Explain that the child will look pale. Simple explanations such as "This tube helps your child breathe" are adequate. A chair by the bedside is helpful so that one member can sit,

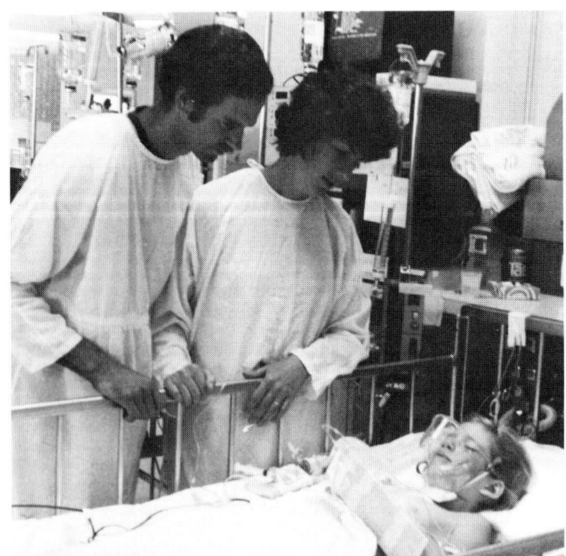

Figure 22-21 A postoperative parental visit. The nurse should describe the child's appearance to the parents in advance and provide support during visiting periods in the intensive care setting. The parents' presence is vital to the child during this difficult experience.

hold the child's hand, and talk to the child. The nurse should be aware that normally the parents are overwhelmed by the amount of tubes and monitoring equipment. It is helpful to plan well-spaced visits at times convenient for the family members in order to prevent severe emotional stress.

As the child wakes from the anesthesia, he or she may be restless and uncomfortable. If there are no signs of hemorrhage (increased chest tube drainage, decreased blood pressure, or increased pulse) and if neurological and respiratory difficulties have been ruled out, then the child is probably in pain. Narcotic analgesics are used cautiously after surgery. Controversy exists about the degree of pain that children perceive. Occasionally, morphine sulfate is administered intravenously in small doses to ease the child's discomfort yet avoid masking signs of complications. Morphine's relaxation effect on smooth muscles may cause the blood pressure to decrease slightly.

Drug treatment after cardiac surgery may include prophylactic antibiotic therapy for 4 to 10 days, electrolyte replacements such as calcium and potassium to promote optimal myocardial efficiency, and digoxin when indicated. In cases of hemodynamic instability, vasopressors such as dopamine HCl and nitroprusside are used cautiously.

As soon as the child can maintain satisfactory ventilation, the endotracheal tube is removed. After the tube is removed, tell the child that he or she will be hoarse and will have a sore throat for a few days. Continue to monitor respiratory status for any signs of respiratory distress. Coughing, deep-breathing, and ventilation exercises are continued. The nasogastric tube is removed when bowel sounds are heard, and the child can then begin taking sips of clear fluids according to the prescribed fluid regimen. Chest tubes are discontinued when there is minimal serous drainage. A chest x-ray is taken after the removal of the chest tubes to check for pneumothorax.

Complications may arise during surgery or in the immediate postoperative period (Table 22-10). The frequency and severity of the complications necessitate close observation and immediate attention. Respiratory problems are the most common complications following cardiac surgery.[38]

Cardiac arrest may occur following heart surgery and is usually a result of one or more complications. It may happen suddenly or may be preceded by subtle warning signs. Astute assessment of changes in skin color, vital signs, and blood gases, with subsequent appropriate intervention, may prevent cardiac arrest. An absence of pulse, respirations (if the child is not receiving ventilatory assistance), and blood pressure denotes an arrest. Prompt action is necessary to increase the child's chance of survival (Table 16-17). A patent airway must be obtained and maintained throughout the resuscitation procedures. Cardiac compressions at a rate appropriate for the age of the child are initiated by external or internal massage to maintain circulation. Once the arrest team is present (or if an arrest protocol is in existence), emergency cardiac drugs are administered to correct acidosis and stimulate the myocardium. Specific amounts of medications given are based on the child's weight. Guidelines should appear on the emergency equipment. The outcome of the arrest depends on the reason for the arrest, the status of the myocardium, and the timing of resuscitation.

Table 22-10 Postoperative Complications of Cardiac Surgery

Respiratory
Mucus accumulation
Pneumonia
Atelectasis
Pneumothorax
Pulmonary embolus
Cardiovascular
Arrhythmias
Cardiac tamponade
Hypovolemic shock
Heart failure
Embolus
Renal
Renal failure
Neurological
Embolus
Decreased cerebral blood flow
Infection
Mediastinitis
Wound infection

Convalescence

Once the child is transferred out of the intensive care area, the goals of nursing management focus on helping the child become stronger and preparing the child and family for discharge.

Coughing and deep-breathing exercises are continued, as well as auscultation of breath sounds. Fluids may continue to be restricted, and the child may be placed on a low-sodium diet. An ambulation schedule is followed, and the child is encouraged to alternate activities with rest breaks to avoid overexertion. External sutures, if present, and temporary pacemakers are removed before the child is discharged. When there are minimal postoperative complications, children are discharged 7 to 10 days after surgery.

Dismissal teaching should be initiated once the child is transferred from the intensive care setting. Families will need teaching about medications, activity, wound healing, and follow-up care. Important information should be written down and given to the family prior to discharge.

Directions given to parents should include the action, frequency of administration, and side effects of the medications the child will be taking at home. If the child is taking digoxin, instruct the parents to check the child's pulse, and give guidelines for withholding the drug or reporting an abnormal pulse. Similar information is necessary if the child will be taking a diuretic. Stress the importance of eating foods high in potassium, and provide the parents with a list of appropriate foods.

Activity limitations depend primarily on the type of repair done, the postoperative course, and the age of the child. Children under 2 years of age usually gauge their own activity level and sleep when they are tired. School-age children tend to overexert. They may return to school in 4 to 5 weeks, but they should not participate in physical education or vigorous sports for 1 to 3 months afterward. Some children who have had extensive surgical repairs may require as long as 6 months before they are able to tolerate demanding sports.

Instruct the parents to keep the incision site clean and dry and to observe for signs of infection around the suture line. Steri-strips may be kept on, but will fall off in a week or two. The child may complain of itching as the incision heals.

Make follow-up appointments before discharge. Usually, the child will visit the cardiac surgeon and the pediatric cardiologist. The parents must advise other health care professionals (such as the child's dentist, school nurse, and pediatrician) of the history of the child's heart disease. Prophylactic antibiotics such as penicillin, or erythromycin if the child is allergic to penicillin, should be given before and after dental procedures, genitourinary procedures, or any surgery or invasive procedure. This helps prevent *subacute bacterial endocarditis* (SBE), an infectious process usually caused by *Streptococcus viridans* and involving altered or malformed tissues of the heart. It can occur in children with congenital heart disease or as a complication of cardiac surgery.

After discharge, the child may have nightmares or temporary behavior changes. The nightmares usually disappear when the child becomes reaccustomed to the safe, nonthreatening environment of the home. Behavior changes range from hostile or aggressive actions to passive, dependent behavior; these disappear when the child has had an opportunity to release unresolved feelings regarding the surgical experience. Therapeutic play sessions before discharge may help a child overcome threatening, insecure feelings (Fig. 22-22). Younger children tend to regress and often need parental assistance with tasks they had previously mastered. Encourage the parents to allow the child to pass through these stages and to provide as much support as possible. They should allow the child to verbalize feelings about the experience. A follow-up visit to the surgical and intensive care units after discharge also helps the child deal with the experience.

Siblings may be envious of the increased attention the child receives before, during, and after hospitalization. In some instances, younger sib-

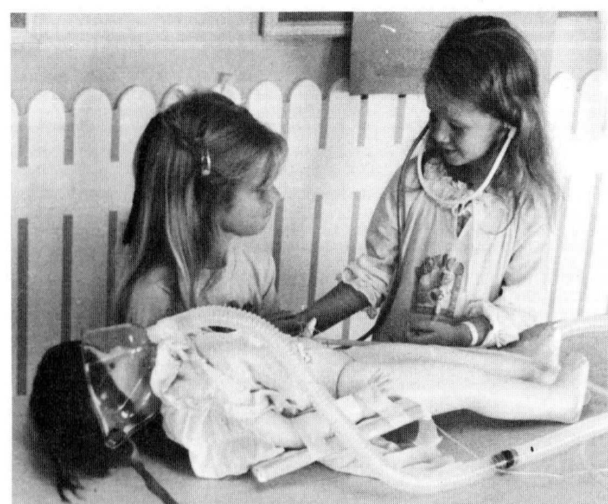

Figure 22-22 Therapeutic play. Planned play activities help children cope with threatening procedures and hospitalization.

lings may feel that they caused the child's bad experience through "bad" wishes or thoughts. Encourage the parents to deal with the siblings honestly and to maintain firm, realistic discipline policies within a loving, caring relationship.

Postperfusion syndrome is a long-term complication of heart surgery and extracorporeal circulation. The symptoms are vague and occur between the third and twelfth weeks after surgery, when the child is usually home. The symptoms include fever, malaise, arthritis, skin rash, and splenomegaly (an enlarged spleen). Treatment includes bed rest and administration of salicylates.[39]

Increasing numbers of children with congenital heart disease are now reaching adulthood. Both males and females will need to consider their cardiac status when planning to become parents.[40]

The risk during pregnancy is related to cyanosis. When cyanosis is not present and when the defect has been surgically corrected, this risk is not significant. When cyanosis or pulmonary hypertension is present, however, the risk increases and is related to fetal hypoxia.[41]

The method of contraception used by women with congenital heart disease must be chosen carefully. In the case of cyanosis or an obstructive lesion, oral contraceptives are contraindicated. Often a diaphragm is the safest choice.

The majority of congenital malformations fit the multifactorial inheritance pattern (see Chap. 6). Therefore, the incidence of congenital heart disease in children of those with most defects is probably double that of the normal population.[42]

ACQUIRED HEART DISEASE IN CHILDREN

Acute rheumatic fever

Acute rheumatic fever is the leading cause of postnatally acquired heart disease in children in the United States and western Europe.[43] Although the incidence varies with geographic area, age, and economic status, there is evidence of a decrease in new cases, due in part to improved living conditions. There may be a familial predisposition to the development of rheumatic fever and rheumatic heart disease. Crowded conditions, poor housing, dampness, and poor nutrition—often found among families in low socioeconomic classes and migrant groups—are believed to predispose children to rheumatic fever.

Rheumatic fever is a systemic, inflammatory collagen disease. It usually develops 1 to 3 weeks after a group A, beta-hemolytic streptococcal upper respiratory infection. There is a high prevalence following scarlet fever. Rheumatic fever affects primarily children between the ages of 5 and 15. There is a seasonal increase of rheumatic fever that correlates with the incidence of upper respiratory infections. Rheumatic fever peaks during spring on the east coast and during winter on the west coast.

Rheumatic fever seems to progress through four stages.[44] First there is the initial streptococcal infection, which goes undiagnosed or untreated. The second stage is characterized by a latent period of 1 to 3 weeks when the fever and infection seem to disappear but the individual may not quite return to normal. This is followed by phase three or the acute rheumatic episode, which may last 2 to 3 months. In the final phase, which exists for the rest of the child's life, all signs of rheumatic fever are gone, but varying degrees of residual heart disease may persist.

Manifestations The initial streptococcal infection is characterized by a sudden onset of a sore throat, a temperature of 38.4 to 40°C (101 to 104°F), and cervical and mandibular adenitis. Headache, abdominal pain, and vomiting may also be present. Diagnosis is by culture and history of recent exposure. As many as 20 percent of streptococcal infections may be asymptomatic. Treatment consists of intramuscular penicillin (1,200,000 units), oral penicillin (250,000 units four times daily for 10 days), or erythromycin (20 mg/lb per day for 10 days) when penicillin sensitivity exists.

The signs and symptoms of rheumatic fever involve target areas such as the joints, lungs, and heart. *Arthritis*, inflammation of the joints, is the most common complaint of children with rheumatic fever. Inflammation produces heat, redness, tenderness, swelling, pain, and limitation of joint movement. Such large joints as elbows, wrists, ankles, and knees may be involved, and the discomfort mistaken for "growing pains." Characteristic nonpainful subcutaneous nodules may be found over the joints, vertebrae, and skull. In the acute stage of rheumatic fever, the lungs may be the site of a pneumonia-type infection. *Carditis,* associated with congestive heart failure, is indicative of cardiac involvement. Cardiomegaly, demonstrated on x-ray, and pericarditis may be present with carditis. A friction rub, heard on auscultation, signifies pericarditis. As fluid accumulation increases in the pericardial sac due to the inflammation, the rub diminishes.

Permanent or transient ECG changes in the P-R interval, T wave, and QRS complex may occur if carditis is present. Sydenham's chorea demonstrates involvement of the nervous system and is manifested by emotional instability, involuntary muscle movements that disappear during sleep, ataxia, and muscle weakness. Chorea does not usually appear at the same time that carditis is present, but rather 2 to 6 months after the initial infection.[45] Nonspecific skin manifestations include urticaria, petechiae, and an erythematous rash. Epistaxis and abdominal pain in the right lower quadrant may also be present.

Diagnosis of rheumatic fever is made by using the modified Jones criteria. The diagnosis is positive if any *two major manifestations* or *one major and two minor manifestations* are present. Major manifestations include carditis, polyarthritis, chorea, subcutaneous nodules, and erythema marginatum. Minor manifestations include fever, an elevated erythrocyte sedimentation rate, a positive C-reactive protein, polyarthralgia, ECG changes, and a previous history of rheumatic fever.

The prognosis depends on the severity and treatment of the rheumatic fever. Carditis occurs in approximately 50 percent of the cases and increases the severity of the illness. Rheumatic carditis causes temporary insult and may lead to permanent damage to any of the three layers of the heart. Endocardial involvement is usually restricted to the mitral, tricuspid, and aortic valves. Edema and inflammation of the valves occur in the acute phase, and scarring may lead to valvular stenosis (constriction or narrowing of a valve lumen or orifice) or insufficiency (inability to perform a normal function, usually causing leakage). If acute inflammation progresses or recurs, scar formation and valvular damage may be permanent. Mitral insufficiency is the most common valvular lesion seen in the acute phase of rheumatic fever.

Treatment and nursing management The immediate goals of nursing management are directed toward maintaining optimal cardiac functioning and promoting the child's comfort. During the acute phase, the child is hospitalized if carditis is present, and intravenous antibiotics are given. Vital signs are taken frequently. The nurse should watch for the signs and symptoms of congestive heart failure. A systolic murmur, characteristic of mitral insufficiency, or a diastolic murmur due to aortic insufficiency may precede signs of heart failure. Since carditis may be fatal, it is imperative that the nurse report the presence of distended neck veins, pulmonary congestion, decreased urinary output, tachypnea, dyspnea, and tachycardia. Bed rest, which helps promote myocardial efficiency but has not been proved to affect residual heart disease, may be especially difficult for a young child. Periods of rest, alternated with passive activities appropriate for the child's age, are helpful. Ambulation is gradually increased on the basis of the child's well-being and the severity of carditis.

Maintenance of fluid balance and assessment of hydration are important components of nursing management. Record daily intake and output and weight to evaluate myocardial function. Determine hydration by checking the lips and mucous membranes, skin turgor, the fontanels, and the presence or absence of tears.

If chorea is present, additional safety precautions are instituted. Protect the child from the random, involuntary movements of the extremities. Siderails must be padded and remain up at all times. Restraints may be needed and should be applied when appropriate. Remain with the child when he or she is in a cart or wheelchair.

Medications are used to eradicate the infection and promote comfort. Salicylates are used for their antipyretic action, relief of joint pain, and treatment of mild carditis. Penicillin is the drug of choice. It is given orally, except when carditis is active. Then parenteral administration is used. Steroids help decrease the effect of the inflammatory process in moderate to severe carditis. Diuretics and digitalis products are used for congestive heart failure.

Long-term care and follow-up are essential to prevent recurrence. The parents need information regarding the disease, the treatment, and medication. Maintenance of prolonged bed rest is often unrealistic, and short periods of limited activity help decrease the frustrations of the child. Home visits by a public health nurse, social worker, and school tutor can help to continue meeting the needs of the child and family following hospitalization.

Streptococcal prophylaxis should be continued until age 18, until at least 5 years after the last rheumatic fever attack with no residual heart disease, and indefinitely in those with rheumatic heart disease. Recurrences take place in more than 50 percent of those not following streptococcal prophylaxis.[46] The surest method of prevention is the administration of penicillin G intramuscularly every 28 days; 400,000 units of potassium penicillin G can be given orally every day to the healthy, compliant child or adult.

Hypertension

Hypertension is an elevation of the systolic or diastolic blood pressure, or both, exceeding the normal range for a child of a given age and sex. Prolonged hypertension is associated with permanent changes in the blood vessels of the eye, heart, kidneys, and cerebrum. These changes predispose an individual to optic nerve damage, atherosclerosis, renal disease, and stroke.

Etiology There are two types of hypertension. *Primary,* or *essential, hypertension* has no known cause. *Secondary hypertension* is due to a pathophysiological process such as renal disease (acute or chronic pyelonephritis), endocrine disorders (adrenal disease), and cardiovascular disease (coarctation of the aorta). Hypertension in young children is most often secondary to a known cause, such as renal disease.

Although the actual incidence is not known, estimates of primary hypertension in children range from 1 to 11 percent. Persons at risk for hypertension are those in the 15- to 30-year-old age group. Hypertension in adolescents is most likely to occur in families with other hypertensive members. Blacks have a particularly high incidence of hypertension.[47]

Because of increasing recognition of the detrimental effects of sustained hypertension, more activities are now directed toward early recognition of hypertension and medical intervention. Evidence suggests that adults who are at risk for developing primary hypertension can be identified in childhood. Thus, more emphasis is being placed on early detection of persons with a greater tendency to develop hypertension and on children with higher-than-normal blood pressure values. Although the exact cause of primary hypertension has not been firmly established, heredity, obesity, and excess salt intake may be important contributing factors.

Blood pressure norms exist for definitions of systolic and diastolic hypertension in adults, but there is still some question about specific ranges in children. Systolic blood pressure in newborns rapidly increases from birth ($64 \pm 10/41 \pm 8$) to 1 month ($83 \pm 13/41 \pm 8$) to 3 months ($101 \pm 9/53 \pm 9$) and stabilizes there until about 4 to 5 years of age. Diastolic blood pressure seems to increase gradually up to 2 years of age and then levels off until age 5.[48]

Blood pressure in children is affected by their gene pool, age, lean body mass, fat, and maturation. Blood pressure tends to be higher in (1) older children than in younger children, (2) larger (heavier and taller) children than in smaller children, (3) obese children than in lean children, and (4) more sexually mature children than in less sexually mature children.[49] Ranges may vary (Table 16-20), but children who have persistent elevations in supine systolic and diastolic readings greater than the 90th percentile for their age and sex are considered to be borderline hypertensives.[50]

One of the reasons for lack of substantial data on hypertension in children is the difficulty in measurement. Current recommendations suggest that blood pressure be checked in any child over 3 years of age. Proper cuff size (Table 16-21) and a quiet, cooperative child are helpful in obtaining a proper pressure reading. Even then, it may be difficult to obtain a diastolic reading in infants and young children except through intraarterial pressure monitoring.

Manifestations The symptoms of hypertension vary. Usually a child with increased blood pressure does not demonstrate any overt symptoms. With severe disease, children may experience blurred vision, severe frontal headaches, generalized or focal seizures, epistaxis, and, on occasion, severe back or abdominal pain. Signs of hypertension seen on physical examination include retinal hemorrhages or exudates, constriction of the retinal arteries, and papilledema (edema of the optic disk).

To aid in the diagnosis of hypertension, it is vital that the nurse obtain an accurate history in order to evaluate the family history for frequency of hypertension, myocardial infarctions, renal disorders, diabetes or other endocrine disease, and strokes (cerebral vascular accidents). Such special diagnostic tests as abdominal aortography may be done if a tumor or other mass in the kidneys or adrenal gland is suspected of causing the hypertension. An intravenous pyelogram is frequently done to assess renal dysfunction. Through the injection of a contrast medium, aortography and an intravenous pyelogram allow the examination of the vascular system and the organs of the lower abdominal cavity. Various tests measuring urinary excretion of certain products are used to assess renal status. Hematologic studies include a complete blood count and tests of serum electrolytes, blood urea nitrogen, creatinine, and uric acid levels.

Treatment Medical management of the child or adolescent with definitive hypertension is varied. If secondary hypertension is diagnosed, the underlying cause is treated. If mild primary hypertension exists, follow-up care and monitoring are sufficient. Education of the child and family includes teaching about dietary modifications, such as decreased sodium, fat, and caloric intake; increased physical activity; medications; follow-up care; and promotion of compliance.

Dietary management is crucial. There is a positive correlation between increased salt consumption and the development of hypertension.[51] Avoidance of foods with a high sodium content has been established as an aid in decreasing blood pressure. Overweight children are counseled regarding diet, nutrition, and exercise. Family patterns and cultural practices regarding food are important considerations in dietary teaching.

Adequate exercise without excessive fatigue is important to promote optimal circulatory function. When encouraging proper activities, include information about the postural effects on blood pressure of several of the drugs used in treating hypertension. In addition, female adolescents with hypertension who are sexually active should be counseled about appropriate methods of contraception and planning pregnancies. Oral contraceptives should be avoided, since increased blood pressure due to use of these medications has been noted. For males, such antihypertensive drugs as methyldopa (Aldomet) and guanethidine (Ismelin) may cause impotence and inhibition of ejaculation.

At the present time, there is no single successful medication for the treatment of hypertension. Diuretics and vasodilating and neural regulating agents are used in combination. Diuretics are used to diminish plasma and extracellular fluid volume by acting on the renal tubules at different sites to inhibit reabsorption of sodium. Thiazide diuretics such as chlorothiazide (Diuril) and hydrochlorothiazide (Hydro-Diuril) are frequently used. Chlorthalidone (Hygroton), another oral diuretic, is a useful agent because it has a longer duration of action than chlorothiazide. Given in a single daily dose, it is good for use with children who have a difficult time remembering multiple-dose schedules.[52] More potent diuretics that act on the loop of Henle are furosemide (Lasix) and ethacrynic acid (Edecrin). These diuretics are restricted for use when significant fluid retention is present and hypertension does not respond to thiazide therapy. Nursing management includes monitoring serum electrolytes and promoting intake of foods high in potassium, such as orange juice and bananas.

Vasodilating agents directly affect smooth muscles by decreasing vascular tone and lowering peripheral resistance. Smooth muscle vasodilators include such drugs as hydralazine HCl (Apresoline), minoxidil (Loniten, which is currently used only for adults), and prazosin (Minipress).

Neural blocking agents act in various ways at the postganglionic nerve terminal to reduce the vasoconstricting responses elicited by stimulation of the sympathetic nervous system. Thus, the systemic blood pressure is lowered. Since the drugs decrease vasomotor tone, postural hypotension is a major side effect. Neural blocking agents include methyldopa (Aldomet), guanethidine (Ismelin), reserpine (Serpasil), propranolol (Inderal), and clonidine (Catapres).

Nursing management The nurse has an important role in identifying children at risk for developing hypertension and in promoting maintenance of therapeutic regimens designed to lower blood pressure. A community health nurse may be the first to note elevated blood pressure or to detect the symptoms of hypertension in a child or adolescent. Because a person with hypertension is often asymptomatic, compliance with a therapeutic regimen is difficult for anyone, especially adolescents. Since some medications cause postural hypotension, adolescents may feel worse while taking the drugs. Every effort should be made to maintain communication with the child and the parents. Discussions with the family should cover the therapeutic regimen, diet, and medications, their actions, and their side effects. Realistic goals should be set by the child and the family. Small group meetings for older children and adolescents who have hypertension may improve compliance and provide an opportunity to share experiences and feelings with peers.

Follow-up care should continue with the same nurse in order to maintain communication between the nurse and the family and to help develop a trusting relationship over a long period of time.

Atherosclerosis and lipid disorders

It is commonly accepted that coronary heart disease is the leading cause of death of adults in the United States. There is now evidence that one facet of coronary artery disease, *atherosclerosis,* begins in childhood and progressively worsens until symptoms appear in middle and late adulthood. *Atherosclerosis* is the accumulation of fatty deposits in the intimal layer of arteries, such as the aorta and the femoral, carotid, and cerebral vessels. The lesions narrow the lumen of the blood vessels, thereby decreasing the blood flow and predisposing the artery to thrombosis. A weakening in the wall of the affected artery may result in an *aneurysm* (a localized dilatation). The exact etiology of atherosclerosis is unknown. There is strong evidence that the progression and development of the disease are affected by heredity, sex, hypertension, diet, hyperlipidemia, obesity, physical inactivity, and smoking.

An elevated plasma lipid concentration is considered to be a major risk factor in the development of atherosclerosis in children as well as adults. It has been suggested that fatty streaks develop in the aorta as early as during the fetal period.[53] These streaks progress into hardened plaques during childhood, adolescence, and young adulthood and constitute potential atherosclerotic lesions.

Hyperlipidemia is a borderline high or increased plasma concentration of cholesterol, triglycerides, or both (Table 22-2). Since the majority of children with hyperlipidemia are asymptomatic and are rarely obese, a positive family history of coronary artery disease (before 50 years of age), elevated cholesterol or triglyceride levels in a parent or grandparent, or the presence of xanthomas (fatty fibrous nodules on the knees, elbows, face, and eyelids) provides clues that hyperlipidemia may be present.

There are five basic types of hyperlipidemia. Each type is defined by increased cholesterol or triglyceride levels (or both) and the elevation of a specific type of lipoprotein. Blood studies identify the specific type of hyperlipidemia.

Primary familial hypercholesterolemia (type II-A hyperlipoproteinemia) is the most commonly recognized type of familial hyperlipidemia in children. Laboratory tests show an elevated low-density lipoprotein (LDL) value with increased cholesterol levels. Although the exact etiology is unknown, the possibility exists that hyperlipoproteinemia is inherited as an autosomal dominant trait.

Serum lipid and lipoprotein normative levels are not yet firmly established, although guidelines for hyperlipidemia have been suggested.[54] Norms exist for values at the extremes. A fasting serum cholesterol level greater than 230 mg per 100 ml is indicative of the 95th percentile for American children.[55] Because of the need for early intervention, the higher the level of total cholesterol, the greater the effort that should be directed toward treatment if the family medical history is positive for atherosclerotic heart disease.[56] It is recommended that serum lipid levels be routinely monitored in hematologic studies on all school-age children.[57]

Treatment A modified dietary regimen is the main approach used to treat children with hyperlipidemia. Since it is not yet known whether one specific dietary factor is at fault in high lipid values, overall total caloric intake is reduced, and modifications based on the lipid value are made in the intake of saturated fats, cholesterol, and sugar.

If dietary treatment alone does not decrease serum lipid levels sufficiently and there is a definite family history of atherosclerotic heart disease, more stringent measures are instituted, and lipid-lowering drugs are used. The effect of a specific drug on a lipid disorder is related to its mode of action. Certain drugs, such as cholestyramine (Questran and Cuemid), reduce the plasma cholesterol levels by preventing the reabsorption of bile acids, while others, such as nicotinic acid (Clofibrate), alter lipoprotein production in the liver.[58]

Follow-up care is vital in promoting compliance. Clinic visits followed by home visits and telephone calls give the nurse an opportunity to evaluate the effectiveness and impact of a certain medical regimen. The family's compliance is promoted by recording accurate weights, undertaking hematologic studies to recheck cholesterol and triglyceride levels, and giving positive reinforcement. When necessary, the regimen can be altered to help the child and the family reach the desired goal. Mutual goal setting by the nurse and the family promotes compliance.

Kawasaki syndrome

Kawasaki syndrome (mucocutaneous lymph node syndrome) is an unusual and potentially fatal multisystem vasculitis that affects infants and children. The cardiovascular complications can be serious, although they occur in only a small percentage of cases. The fatality rate due to cardiovascular complications is 1 to 2 percent; the long-term prognosis for children with heart involvement is unknown, however.[59]

Kawasaki syndrome is increasing in incidence and occurs almost exclusively in infants and children under 5 years of age; the incidence is higher among boys than among girls. Asian children are affected more frequently than black or Caucasian children.[60] The etiology is unknown. There has been speculation that an environmental toxin, an immunologic process, or an infection is the cause. No viral or bacterial agents have been identified, although rickettsial-like bodies have been found in skin and lymph node biopsies.[61,62] Localized outbreaks point to an exogenous agent or toxin.[63] The disease does not appear to be communicable. There is a seasonal incidence, with the peak occurring in late winter and spring. A significant number of affected children have had a respiratory illness within 30 days prior to the onset of the disease.[64]

Manifestations The symptoms of Kawasaki syndrome, which are similar to those of scarlet fever, bullous erythema multiforme major, and infantile polyarteritis nodosa, make it a difficult disease to diagnose.[65] To make a diagnosis, the following symptoms should be present:

1. A fever lasting 5 days or more (38.5 to 40°C or 101.3 to 104°F)
2. Bilateral reddening of the conjunctivae without discharge
3. A change in the mucous membranes of the upper respiratory tract (e.g., a reddened pharynx; red, dry, fissured lips; or a strawberry-colored tongue)
4. Changes in the extremities (e.g., peripheral edema and erythema or desquamation of the hands and the soles of the feet)
5. A rash, primarily truncal, which can take many forms[66]
6. Cervical lymph node swelling (nonpurulent)

The clinical course of Kawasaki syndrome progresses in three stages. The onset of the acute febrile phase, lasting from 1 to 10 days, is heralded by an abrupt onset of fever and is followed in 1 to 3 days by many of the symptoms listed above. The subacute phase, which lasts from 10 to 25 days, begins when the fever subsides. There is desquamation of the fingers and toes, persistent anorexia, irritability, arthralgia and arthritis, thrombocytosis, and the beginning of myocardial dysfunction due to coronary thrombosis and aneurysm. The convalescent phase, lasting from 25 to 60 days or until the symptoms disappear, is manifested by the appearance of transverse grooves across the nail beds as well as by possible coronary thromboses and aneurysms. Neutropenia can last for 6 months or more. The third phase ends when the sedimentation rate returns to normal and all signs of illness have disappeared. Children at greatest risk for developing cardiac sequelae, especially aneurysms, are males under 1 year of age whose fevers lasted more than 15 days and whose rash and fever reappear.[67] Twenty percent of children with Kawasaki syndrome have some coronary artery involvement. The majority of the aneurysms regress in size and do not present problems. Some of the vessels, however, have a persistent abnormality or become stenotic. If the coronary arteries narrow in size, decreased blood flow to the myocardium and ischemia will result. Ischemic damage to the papillary muscle may cause mitral valve insufficiency. A simultaneous valvulitis can cause insufficiency of both the aortic and the mitral valves.

Because cardiac abnormalities occur or worsen 2 or more years after the onset of the disease, all children with Kawasaki syndrome must be followed closely. Symptoms of myocardial dysfunction and infarction include increased irritability, poor feeding, tachypnea, sweating, an ashen skin color, poor peripheral perfusion along with decreased blood pressure, and ECG abnormalities, such as S-T segment changes, premature ventricular contractions, and heart block. Serial echocardiograms are taken on children who exhibit signs of coronary artery abnormalities in order to monitor myocardial function.

Treatment and nursing management Since the etiology, epidemiology, and treatment of Kawasaki syndrome have not been fully established, the nursing and medical interventions are based on the symptoms. Meticulous physical and laboratory assessments are needed to determine the extent of the disease, myocardial function, and possible complications.

Children with coronary artery aneurysms are treated with salicylates and antiplatelet drug therapy to minimize coronary artery sclerosis. Surgery may be indicated with severe coronary artery stenosis or aneurysm. Although aneurysms of the aorta and branches often regress, they can rupture and cause sudden death. If echocardiograms show that an aneurysm is increasing in size or that arterial insufficiency is present, surgery may be necessary.

Nursing interventions are designed to provide comfort, rest, and relief of symptoms and to prevent complications. Fever and dry, reddened mucous membranes are managed with tepid sponges for a temperature over 38.4°C (101.2°F), clear liquids, intravenous therapy, and close observation of vital signs and of intake and output. Soap should not be used because of the inflammatory skin changes. Cool, moist compresses may help the skin rash. Oropharyngeal mucous membrane hyperemia makes eating difficult and causes anorexia. The child's nutritional requirements should be calculated, and high-calorie liquids or soft foods should be given. If the thrombocytopenia continues into the chronic phase, the child's physical activity may be limited.

Providing emotional support for the child and the family throughout the acute and chronic phases is essential. The child is miserable and very irritable. Explaining all the tests and procedures, providing play therapy, and encouraging the family members to stay with the child all help decrease anxiety and increase trust. The parents need to learn about the disease, know the signs and symptoms of myocardial dysfunction, and understand the importance of follow-up during the chronic phase of the illness.

Nursing Care Plan: Congestive Heart Failure

Patient: Manuel Oliverez **Age:** 6 months **Date of Admission:** 4/10

ASSESSMENT

The child was admitted to the pediatric unit with a diagnosis of congestive heart failure. Manuel had had one previous admission for pneumonia and circumoral cyanosis during feeding at 6 weeks of age. At that time, a cardiac catheterization was done, and he was diagnosed as having a ventricular septal defect. He was stabilized on digoxin and sent home 1 week later to await corrective surgery at 2 years of age.

One week prior to admission, Manuel had his routine 6-month checkup. At that time he weighed 6.1 kg, was eating well, and showed no signs of respiratory distress. Three days prior to admission, Mrs. Oliverez ran out of digoxin and did not think she had to renew it until today, when she brought her other two children into the clinic for immunizations. She mentioned to the nurse at the clinic that Manuel was not eating well today and seemed to be having trouble breathing. The nurse instructed Mrs. Oliverez to take Manuel to the emergency room immediately, and Manuel was admitted for treatment.

SOCIAL HISTORY

Mr. Oliverez works at two jobs in order to support his family of five and relies on public transportation to get to and from work. The family has no car. Because of the lack of transportation and the two preschool-age children at home, Mrs. Oliverez will not be able to visit Manuel every day. She tearfully stated that she hated to leave him and wished she could stay with him the entire time.

GENERAL APPEARANCE

The infant is irritable and restless. The mucous membranes are moderately cyanotic; the skin is pale and mottled. The anterior fontanel open: 1.5 cm; soft and full.

The authors gratefully acknowledge the assistance of Cindy S. Boehr, B.S.N., C.C.R.N., Children's Hospital of Los Angeles, Los Angeles, in revising this Nursing Care Plan.

PHYSICAL EXAMINATION

Weight: 6.4 kg. Temperature: 37.4°C (99.4°F), rectal. Pulse: 142, regular rhythm. Respiratory rate: 58, regular rhythm. Blood pressure: 98, palpation.

Cardiovascular function

Heart sounds are regular and loud. A loud holosystolic murmur is present. Heaves noted over the precordium. 2+ edema present on the dorsum of both feet and hands. Nail beds pale and cyanotic. Capillary filling time 5 s. Radial and pedal pulses present but are of fair quality.

Respiratory function

The respirations are shallow. Dyspnea is present, with audible expiratory grunting. Moderate subcostal and substernal retractions with moderate nasal flaring are present. There are equal bilateral breath sounds with scattered, coarse rhonchi.

Gastrointestinal function

The abdomen is round and full and tympanic to percussion. There are active bowel sounds in all quadrants.

DEVELOPMENTAL ASSESSMENT

Smiled at 7 weeks. Held head up at 6 weeks. Sat with support at $5\frac{1}{2}$ months. Does not yet sit without support. Reached for objects actively at 3 months. Makes isolated vowel sounds.

ADMISSION HISTORY

The primary nurse positioned Manuel in an infant seat and began O_2 at 2 liters of oxygen by nasal cannula. An IV was started in the saphenous vein of left foot, and medications were started. Blood for tests was drawn from an arterial stick after he had been on oxygen for 20 min. Within 2 h, Manuel had voided 120 ml of urine, color was more pink, and respiratory rate had decreased to 36 breaths per minute.

Mrs. Oliverez stayed in the room during the admission procedures. She phoned her sister and asked her to take care of the two older children. Mrs. Oliverez left to go home at 10:30 P.M. She told the primary nurse that it was reassuring to see Manuel resting more comfortably. The primary nurse gave her the unit telephone number and encouraged her to call whenever she wished.

PHYSICIAN'S ORDERS

1. Vital signs (temperature, pulse, respiratory rate, and blood pressure) q2h.
2. Elevate the head of the bed 45°.
3. O_2 2 liters by nasal cannula.
4. SMA 20 3 oz q4h if respiratory rate below 40.
5. Weigh bid.
6. Accurate intake and output.
7. IV of D5 0.2 NS with 3 mEq KCl per 100 cc at 10 cc/h.
8. Laboratory tests: serum electrolytes, complete blood count, blood urea nitrogen, and creatinine.
9. Furosemide (Lasix) 6 mg IM now; then give 6 mg orally bid starting in A.M.
10. Digoxin 0.04 mg IM now; then give 0.04 mg orally bid starting in A.M.
11. Heart monitor.

Nursing Diagnosis	Outcome Criteria	Nursing Interventions	Evaluation and Modifications
1. Alteration in comfort related to hypoxia and fatigue	☐ Manuel will not be irritable, but will be alert and responsive. ☐ Manuel will rest quietly in an upright position for at least three 2-h periods a day.	☐ Organize nursing care to provide periods of uninterrupted rest. Manuel usually naps at 10 A.M. and 2 P.M. ☐ Notify respiratory therapists and physicians of rest periods. ☐ Respond to Manuel's needs quickly to prevent him from becoming agitated. ☐ Encourage the mother to hold and rock Manuel. ☐ Elevate the head of the crib 45°. Prop the infant with blankets to keep him from falling sideways. ☐ Alternate his position with an infant seat and infant swing.	☐ Manuel demonstrates increased comfort by smiling in response to play and resting without signs of anxiousness.
2. Ineffective breathing patterns and airway clearance related to increased pulmonary congestion	☐ Manuel will expend less effort in breathing, as demonstrated by diminished retractions, grunting, and nasal flaring. ☐ Manuel will have less congestion, as demonstrated by a lack of productive coughing.	☐ Monitor respiratory rate, characteristics of respiration, and breath sounds q1h until stable; then monitor q2h. ☐ Ensure that Manuel is receiving oxygen therapy by taping the nasal cannula in place and checking the flow meter q2h. ☐ Observe and record respiratory changes during crying, feeding, and stooling.	☐ Manuel breathes at the rate of 30 to 40 breaths per minute. ☐ The chest was clear on auscultation. ☐ Respirations are easy.

Nursing Diagnosis	Outcome Criteria	Nursing Interventions	Evaluation and Modifications
		☐ Have no. 8 Fr. suction catheters available at the bedside, and suction at 80 mmHg. ☐ Do chest percussion and postural drainage q3h. Auscultate and record breath sounds before and after. Concentrate on the areas most in need of drainage.	
3. Potential for medication side effects related to Lasix administration	☐ Manuel's weight will return to its preillness level of 6.1 kg. ☐ Manuel will not have any evidence of fluid overload. His chest will be clear, and he will not have any edema. ☐ Manuel will not show any symptoms of dehydration—a depressed fontanel, dry mucous membranes, tachycardia, hypotension, or fever. ☐ Manuel will not display signs of electrolyte imbalance.	☐ Weigh the infant. Use the same scale each time. ☐ Calculate fluid balance q4h. Notify the physician if the imbalance is 100 ml. ☐ Keep Manuel bagged for accurate urine output measurement. Change the bag q8h. ☐ Measure urine specific gravity at every other voiding. ☐ Monitor hydration status q2h to q3h. Check: **a.** Mucous membranes **b.** Tearing **c.** Skin turgor **d.** Increased sucking on pacifier **e.** Heart rate, blood pressure, and temperature ☐ Monitor for signs of electrolyte imbalance. Indications of hypokalemia are premature ventricular contractions, increased effect of digoxin, and weakness and lethargy. Indications of hypocalcemia are decreased blood pressure (below 90), tetany, and irritability. ☐ Encourage high-potassium foods: bananas, strawberries, and orange juice (when the infant is eating).	☐ Manuel's urine output is approximately equal to his intake. ☐ Manuel does not display any signs of excess fluid retention, as evidenced by lack of periorbital and peripheral edema. ☐ Manuel is maintaining his electrolytes within normal limits.
4. Decreased activity tolerance related to decreased cardiac output and increased respiratory effort	☐ Manuel will be able to play for 10 min qid without showing signs of tiring—restlessness and distress. ☐ Manuel will show increasing interest in play, as evidenced by reaching for toys and smiling when playing verbal games.	☐ Plan a schedule for Manuel that allows time for play when he is most rested. ☐ Initially, provide toys for quiet, passive play—mobiles, small toys, music boxes, and stuffed animals.	☐ Manuel is getting adequate rest to supply energy for playing, eating, and breathing without fatigue or distress.

Nursing Diagnosis	Outcome Criteria	Nursing Interventions	Evaluation and Modifications
	☐ The parents will demonstrate an understanding of Manuel's activity tolerance by describing ways to modify his play when he is ill.	☐ Increase activity level as tolerated—using a walker or stroller, sitting in a high chair, and playing on the floor. ☐ Assess and record Manuel's response to activities, and stop activities at the first sign that he is tiring. ☐ Assess the parents' understanding of Manuel's need to play and rest in order to achieve normal development. ☐ Teach the parents ways to stimulate Manuel's development in each area—gross motor, fine motor, verbal, cognitive, and social—within the limits of his activity tolerance.	☐ The parents verbalized age-appropriate activities and the need for rest breaks.
5. Inadequate nutritional intake related to fatigue during feeding and respiratory distress	☐ Manuel will ingest 3 oz of SMA (low in sodium) q4h without emesis or increased respiratory distress. ☐ Manuel will require fewer rest periods during feeding. ☐ The parents will demonstrate their ability to feed Manuel by proper positioning and allowing adequate rest periods.	☐ Do not feed if the respiratory rate is above 40. ☐ Hold the infant in an upright position when feeding. ☐ Use a premature nipple with an enlarged hole. ☐ Burp the infant after every ounce to avoid abdominal distention. Allow him to pause and rest as needed. ☐ Feed or offer a pacifier to the infant at the first sign of hunger. ☐ Plan feeding times to correspond with the infant's schedule at home. ☐ Encourage the mother to be with the infant at feeding times.	☐ Manuel is maintaining his baseline weight during his hospitalization. ☐ Manuel tolerates his feeding times without a significant increase in respiratory rate (above 50) or heart rate (above 160).
6. Parental knowledge deficit related to the care of an infant with a ventricular septal defect	☐ The parents will be able to visit twice a week for a conference with Manuel's primary nurse. ☐ The parents will demonstrate an understanding of the therapeutic regimen regarding the following: ventricular septal defect, medication, activity, and feeding schedule.	☐ Assess the parents' understanding of the medical regimen. Reinforce their understanding, and deal with their concerns. Identify their teaching needs, and use appropriate audiovisual aids as necessary. ☐ Plan a schedule for teaching Manuel's parents the techniques for his home care.	☐ The parents are able to state the schedule, amount, and purpose of the medications. ☐ The parents verbalized their willingness to comply with the medical regimen. ☐ The parents can describe the signs and symptoms of recurring heart failure.

Nursing Diagnosis	Outcome Criteria	Nursing Interventions	Evaluation and Modifications
	☐ The parents will verbalize their understanding of the need for follow-up care.	☐ Teach the parents cardiopulmonary resuscitation techniques. ☐ Complete the community health nursing referral form. ☐ Make a follow-up telephone call to the family after discharge.	☐ The public health nurse will visit Mrs. Oliverez prior to discharge and will follow Manuel at home.

References

1. Moller, J. H., and W. A. Neal, *Heart Disease in Infancy,* Appleton Century Crofts, New York, 1981, pp. 1–11.
2. Moller, J. H., *Essentials of Pediatric Cardiology,* Davis, Philadelphia, 1978, p. 7.
3. Ibid.
4. Fraiberg, S., *The Magic Years,* Scribner, New York, 1959, p. 129.
5. Nishimura, R. A., F. A. Miller, M. J. Callahan, R. C. Benassi, J. B. Seward, and A. J. Tajik, "Doppler Echocardiography: Theory, Instrumentation, Technique, and Application," *Mayo Clinic Proceedings* **60**(5):321 (May 1985).
6. A. Rudolf, A., "Complications Occurring in Infants and Children," in E. Braunwald and H. Swan (eds.), *Cooperative Study on Cardiac Catheterization,* American Heart Association, New York, 1968, pp. 64–65.
7. Keith, J., "Congestive Heart Failure," in J. Keith, R. Rowe, and P. Vald (eds.), *Heart Disease in Infancy and Childhood,* 3d ed., Macmillan, New York, 1978, p. 167.
8. R. Rowe, "Patent Ductus Arteriosus," in Keith, Rowe, and Vald, op. cit., p. 443.
9. Stachura, L., "Care of the Infant with Ductus-Dependent Congenital Heart Disease Receiving Prostaglandin E," *Issues in Comprehensive Pediatric Nursing* **7**(4–5):203 (1984).
10. Ibid., pp. 210–211.
11. Perloff, J., *The Clinical Recognition of Congenital Heart Disease,* 2d ed., Saunders, Philadelphia, 1978, p. 280.
12. Keith, J., "Atrial Septal Defect: Ostium Secundum, Ostium Primum, and Atrioventricularis Communis (Common A-V Canal)," in Keith, Rowe, and Vald, op. cit., p. 398.
13. Moller, op. cit., p. 80.
14. Ibid., pp. 80–84.
15. Feldt, R. H. (ed.), *Atrioventricular Canal Defects,* Saunders, Philadelphia, 1976.
16. Graham, T., H. Bender, and M. Spach, "Defects of the Ventricular Septum," in A. J. Moss, F. H. Adams, and G. C. Emmanouilides (eds.), *Heart Disease in Infants, Children, and Adolescents,* 2d ed., Williams & Wilkins, Baltimore, 1977, p. 147.
17. Keith, Rowe, and Vald, op. cit., p. 398.
18. Perloff, op. cit., pp. 140–143.
19. Nadas, A. S., and D. C. Fyler, *Pediatric Cardiology,* 3d ed., Saunders, Philadelphia, 1972, p. 460.
20. Emmanouilides, G., "Obstructive Lesions of the Right Ventricle and the Pulmonary Arterial Tree," in Moss, Adams, and Emmanouilides, op. cit., p. 233.
21. Ibid., pp. 235–236.
22. Olley, P., K. Bloom, and R. Rowe, "Aortic Stenosis: Valvular, Subaortic, and Supravalvular," in Keith, Rowe, and Vald, op. cit., p. 698.
23. Ibid., pp. 700–701.
24. Ibid., p. 707.
25. Paul, M., "D-Transposition of the Great Arteries," in Moss, Adams, and Emmanouilides, op. cit., p. 333.
26. Mair, D., and D. Ritter, "Truncus Arteriosus," in Moss, Adams, and Emmanouilides, op. cit., p. 428.
27. Gunderoth, W., and I. Kwabori, "Tetrad of Fallot," in Moss, Adams, and Emmanouilides, op. cit., p. 281.
28. Ibid., p. 287.
29. Perloff, op. cit., p. 628.
30. Ibid., p. 625.
31. Rosenthal, A., "Tricuspid Atresia," in Moss, Adams, and Emmanouilides, op. cit., p. 298.
32. Elliott, L., P. Bream, and I. Gessner, "Single and Common Ventricle," in Moss, Adams, and Emmanouilides, op. cit., p. 380.
33. Ibid., p. 284.
34. Neufield, H., and P. Randall, "Double Outlet Right Ventricle," in Moss, Adams, and Emmanouilides, op. cit., p. 359.
35. Heimbecker, R., et al., "Heart and Heart-Lung Transplantation," *Heart and Lung* **13**(1):1 (January 1984).
36. Guttman, F., "Organ Transplantation in Children," *Pediatric Annals* **11**(11):910 (November 1982).

37. Oyer, P. E., E. B. Stinson, et al., "One Year Experience with Cyclosporin A in Clinical Heart Transplantation," *Heart Transplant* **1**:285 (1982).
38. Begglin, D. I., "Complications after Open Heart Surgery," *Nursing Clinics of North America* **4**(1):123–129 (March 1969).
39. Nelson, W., V. C. Vaughan, and R. J. McKay, *Textbook of Pediatrics,* 11th ed., Saunders, Philadelphia, 1979, p. 1327.
40. Davis, B. N., "Adolescents with Congenital Heart Disease Reaching Childbearing Years," *Issues in Health Care of Women* **4**(4–5):214 (July–October 1983).
41. Ibid., pp. 217–218.
42. Ibid., p. 219.
43. Wannamaker, L. W., and E. L. Kaplan, "Acute Rheumatic Fever," in Moss, Adams, and Emmanouilides, op. cit., pp. 515–532.
44. Diehl, A., "Clinical Aspects of Rheumatic Fever: An Update," *Comprehensive Pediatric Nursing,* **4**(2):67–76 (April 1980).
45. Wannamaker and Kaplan, op. cit.
46. Diehl, op. cit., p. 74.
47. Wood, J., "The Detection of Hypertension," in J. W. Hurst, R. B. Logue, R. C. Schlant, and N. R. Wenger (eds.), *The Heart: Arteries and Veins,* 4th ed., vols. 1 and 2, McGraw-Hill, New York, 1978, p. 1391.
48. Weidman, W., "Standards for Blood Pressure," in *Children's Blood Pressure,* Report of the Eighty-eighth Ross Conference on Pediatric Research, Ross Laboratories, Columbus, Ohio, 1985, p. 14.
49. Ibid., p. 16.
50. National Heart, Lung and Blood Institute's Task Force on Blood Pressure Control in Children, "Report of the Task Force on Blood Pressure Control in Children," *Pediatrics* **59**(suppl.):799 (May 1977).
51. Brock, D., "Decreasing Toddlers' Sodium Intake," *Pediatric Nursing* **11**(1):47 (January–February 1985).
52. Mirkin, B. L., and A. Sinaiko, "Clinical Pharmacology and Therapeutic Utilization of Antihypertensive Agents in Children," in M. I. New and L. Levine (eds.), *Juvenile Hypertension,* Raven Books, New York, 1977, p. 205.
53. Sinzinger, H., W. Feigl, C. Dadas, and J. H. Holzner, "Intimal Alterations of the Aorta and the Great Arteries of Newborns and Children," *Pathologica Microbiologica* **43**:129–133 (1975).
54. Srinivasan, S. R., R. R. Frerichs, and G. S. Berenson, "Serum Lipids and Lipoproteins in Children," in W. B. Strong (ed.), *Atherosclerosis: Its Pediatric Aspects,* Grune & Stratton, New York, 1978, pp. 102–103.
55. Blumenthal, S., M. J. Jesse, C. C. Hennekens, et al., "Risk Factors for Coronary Artery Disease in Children of Affected Families," *Journal of Pediatrics* **87**:1187–1192 (1975).
56. Srinivasan, Frerichs, and Berenson, op. cit., p. 103.
57. Ibid., p. 105.
58. Carter, G., and R. Lauer, "Atherosclerosis," in Moss, Adams, and Emmanouilides, op. cit., p. 715.
59. Kawasaki, J., F. Kasaki, et al., "A New Infantile Acute Febrile Mucocutaneous Lymph Node Syndrome Prevailing in Japan," *Pediatrics* **54**(9):271–276 (September 1974).
60. Bell, D. M., D. M. Morens, R. C. Holman, E. S. Harwitz, and M. K. Hunter, "Kawasaki Syndrome in the United States," *American Journal of Diseases of Children* **137**(3):211–214 (March 1983).
61. Lynch, M., and J. Gray, "Kawasaki Disease," *Pediatric Nursing* **8**(2):96 (March–April 1982).
62. Melish, M., et al., "Mucocutaneous Lymph Node Syndrome in the U.S.," *American Journal of Diseases of Children* **130**(6):599–607 (June 1976).
63. Bell, Morens, Holman, Harwitz, and Hunter, op. cit.
64. Ibid.
65. L'Orange, C., and M. Werner-McCullough, "Kawasaki Disease," *American Journal of Nursing,* **83**(4):558 (April 1983).
66. Yanagihara, R., and J. Todd, "Acute Febrile Mucocutaneous Lymph Node Syndrome," *American Journal of Diseases of Children,* **134**(6):603–614 (June 1980).
67. Melish, M., "Kawasaki Disease (Mucocutaneous Lymph Node Syndrome)," *Pediatrics in Review* **2**(4):107–114 (October 1980).

23

Joanette Pete James
Kathleen W. Hinoki

Hematologic function

Upon completion of this chapter, the student will be able to:

1 List the components of blood and their functions.

2 Distinguish between normal and abnormal levels of red blood cells, white blood cells, hemoglobin, and hematocrit for children from infancy through adolescence.

3 Identify the basic underlying pathology of the major anemias resulting from decreased production of cellular elements or increased destruction of cellular elements.

4 Describe three factors that may lead to iron-deficiency anemia.

5 Compare sickle cell trait, sickle cell anemia, and sickle cell disease.

6 Describe the most severe form of thalassemia.

7 Describe the coagulation process.

8 Compare and contrast the two major types of hemophilia.

9 Outline the instructions for a home infusion program for a child with hemophilia.

10 Write a nursing care plan for a child with hemophilia or sickle cell anemia.

11 Describe the major signs and symptoms of thrombocytopenic purpura.

EMBRYOLOGY OF BLOOD

The formation of blood cells, or *hemopoiesis*, begins as early as the fifteenth to the sixteenth day of embryonic life; the cells develop from undifferentiated stem cells called *hemocytoblasts*. The early cells, made by the yolk sac, bring nutrients and oxygen from the placenta to the embryo to promote growth and development of the fetus. By the second month of embryonic life, the liver, spleen, and lymph nodes begin to produce blood cells. Around the fourth month, the bone marrow becomes active in the production of blood cells. The ribs, sternum, and vertebrae produce a small amount of blood cells during intrauterine development, but shortly after birth all areas, except the red bone marrow, cease production of blood cells.

BLOOD COMPOSITION AND CHARACTERISTICS

Blood has two components: liquid (plasma) and formed cells (platelets and red and white blood cells). The cells normally constitute 38 to 52 percent of the total blood volume; the remainder is the straw-colored plasma, which is a complex mixture of 91 percent water and 9 percent solutes—proteins, electrolytes, hormones, and enzymes. The body contains approximately 90 ml of blood per kilogram of weight at birth. This decreases to approximately 75 ml of blood per kilogram of adult body weight, or about 5 to 6 liters of blood.

Blood has a slightly salty taste, a pH of 7.35 to 7.40, and a specific gravity of 1.055 to 1.065. Changes occur in blood volume and normal blood values as children get older. Table 23-1 lists the average blood values for the newborn, infant, child, and adolescent/adult.

MORPHOLOGY AND FUNCTION OF BLOOD

Erythrocytes

Erythrocytes, or *red blood cells* (RBCs), are biconcave, disk-shaped cells produced in the bone marrow and derived from the hemocytoblast. Figure 23-1 shows the maturation process of blood cells. At each stage of RBC development, greater quantities of hemoglobin and more and more cells are formed. Finally, after the cytoplasm of the normoblast has become filled with hemoglobin to a concentration of approximately 34%, the nucleus is autolyzed and absorbed. About 1 percent of circulating RBCs are *reticulocytes,* or immature erythrocytes; the rest are mature erythrocytes. The erythrocyte is very flexible, making it possible for the cell to bend and twist when squeezing through the narrowest of capillaries and then to regain its original shape when it enters larger vessels.

Erythrocyte production, or *erythropoiesis,* is stimulated by anything that decreases the amount of oxygen available to the bone marrow or body tissue. Hemorrhage, nutritional deficiencies, high altitude, physical activities, and endocrine disturbances may stimulate the kidneys to secrete *erythropoietin,* the hormone that regulates erythropoiesis.

The normal life span of erythrocytes is about 120 days. Old, worn-out RBCs are destroyed by phagocytes in the spleen, liver, and red bone marrow (the reticuloendothelial system). Normally, the rate of destruction of RBCs equals the rate of production, and so the number of circulating cells remains remarkably constant.

Hemoglobin The *hemoglobin* (Hgb) molecule is formed during the manufacture of the RBCs in the bone marrow. It consists of an iron-containing pigment—*heme*—and a simple protein—*globin.* Heme is an organic ring compound—protoporphyrin—to which iron is bound. It is the heme portion that combines with oxygen and carbon dioxide for transport. Hemoglobin carries 98 percent of the oxygen transported by the blood; less than 2 percent is carried in simple solution in the plasma.

Globin is formed by two pairs of polypeptide chains. When the chemical makeup of the globin chain changes, different kinds of hemoglobin are formed. Fetal hemoglobin, Hgb F, is composed of two alpha and two gamma polypeptide chains. Most hemoglobin is replaced by adult hemoglobin, Hgb A, during the first 6 months after birth. Hgb A is made up of two alpha and two beta chains. Abnormalities of these hemoglobin chains produce disorders of hemoglobin, or *hemoglobinopathies.* Because hemoglobin is a protein, hemoglobin type is a genetically controlled characteristic.

At birth, between 40 and 70 percent of the infant's hemoglobin is fetal hemoglobin. Fetal hemoglobin serves the fetus well because it has the ability to absorb oxygen at the low oxygen tensions found in fetal circulation. Hemoglobin disorders often do not appear until fetal hemoglobin is considerably reduced.

Bilirubin When RBCs are destroyed, either by natural cell aging and cell death or by disease, hemoglobin is set free and is broken down into globin and heme. Heme is further broken down into iron, which is reused by the marrow for manufacture of new RBCs, and protoporphyrin. Protoporphyrin is degraded, initially into unconjugated (fat-soluble) bilirubin and eventually into conjugated (water-soluble) bilirubin, which is then excreted in bile. The normal amount of circulating bilirubin in infants is 0.2 to 1.4 mg per 100 ml of blood. When the level rises above 5 mg per 100 ml (hyperbilirubinemia), as happens when RBCs are being destroyed at a rapid rate because of some abnormality, bilirubin escapes from the circulatory system and causes yellow discoloration (jaundice) of the body tissues.

Leukocytes

Leukocytes, or *white blood cells* (WBCs), are classified on the basis of size, shape of the nu-

Table 23-1 Average Range of Normal Blood Values

Measure	Newborn (Birth to 1 Month)	Infant (1 Month to 2 Years)	Child (2 to 12 Years)	Adolescent and Adult		Comment
				Male	Female	
Hemoglobin (g per 100 ml blood)	14 to 24	10 to 15	11 to 16	14 to 16	13 to 15.5	Chief means of transport for oxygen and carbon dioxide in blood
Hematocrit (ml packed cells per 100 ml blood)	43 to 63	30 to 42	34 to 37	42 to 52	37 to 47	Percent of blood made up of RBCs; the relative volume of cells and plasma
Red blood cells (millions per cubic millimeter)	4.8 to 7.1	4.5 to 5.1	3.8 to 5.5	4.8 to 5.5	4.4 to 5	
Reticulocytes (% of total RBCs)	4 to 6, decreasing to 0.5 to 1.6 by 2 weeks	0.5 to 1.6	0.5 to 1.6	0.5 to 1.6	0.5 to 1.6	Immature RBCs released from bone marrow within past 1 to 2 days
Erythrocyte Indices						
MCH (mean corpuscular Hgb), $\mu\mu g$	32 to 34	27 to 31	27 to 31	29 to 32	29 to 32	Amount of HGB in a cell $\text{MCH} = \frac{\text{Hgb} \times 10}{\text{RBC}}$
MCV (mean corpuscular volume), μm^3 per RBC	96 to 108	82 to 96	82 to 96	82 to 96	82 to 96	Volume of each RBC (size of cell) $\text{MCV} = \frac{\text{Hct} \times 10}{\text{RBC}}$
MCHC (mean corpuscular Hgb concentration, %)	32 to 33	32 to 36	32 to 36	32 to 36	32 to 36	Average Hgb content per deciliter packed cells $\text{MCHC} = \frac{\text{Hgb}}{\text{Hct}} \times 100$
White blood cells (number per cubic millimeter)	9000 to 30,000	5000 to 17,000	5000 to 10,000	5000 to 11,000		
Differential Count						
Neutrophils, %	40 to 80	30 to 50	55 to 60	38 to 70	38 to 70	Important in phagocytosis
Basophils, %	0 to 0.5	0 to 0.5	0 to 3	0 to 3	0 to 3	Release of heparin and histamine
Eosinophils, %	5	2 to 3	2	1 to 5	1 to 5	Phagocytosis plus plays a role in allergies
Lymphocytes, %	30 to 35	40 to 50	40 to 45	15 to 45	15 to 45	Key cells in immune responses
Monocytes, %	5 to 10	5 to 10	1 to 8	1 to 8	1 to 8	Capable of becoming macrophages
Platelets (thrombocytes, number per cubic millimeter)	140,000 to 300,000	200,000 to 473,000	150,000 to 450,000	200,000 to 400,000		Active in coagulation

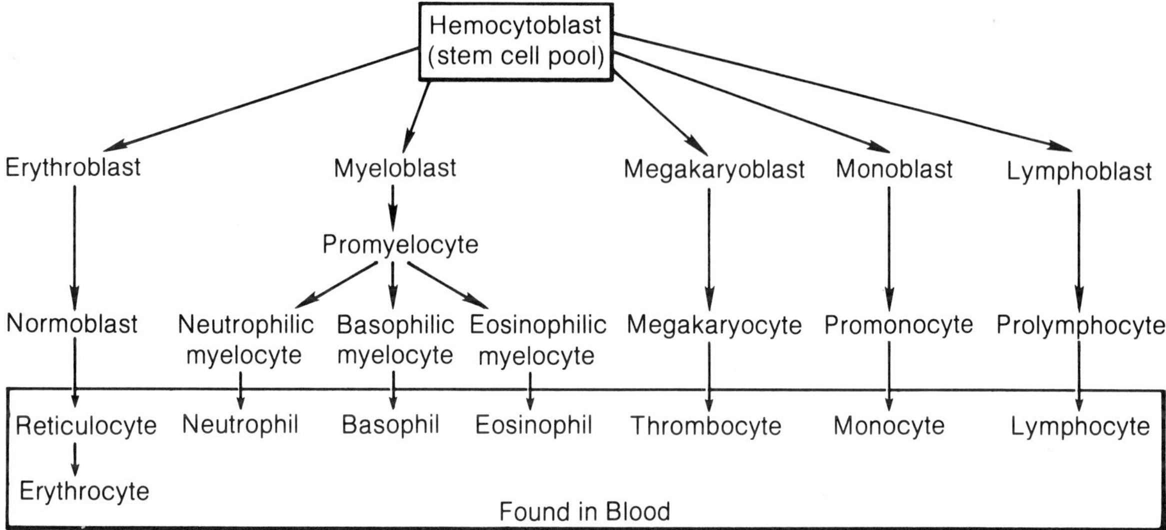

Figure 23-1 A diagrammatic summary of the orderly development of blood cells from a stem cell, or hemocytoblast.

cleus, and staining qualities of the cytoplasm. Granulocytes are the most numerous and include basophils, eosinophils, and neutrophils. The other major white blood cell (WBC) types are nongranulated lymphocytes and monocytes (Fig. 23-1).

Leukocytes are selectively attracted to areas where tissue has been invaded by microorganisms. Leukocytes are capable of engulfing (phagocytosis), neutralizing, and destroying bacteria and yeasts. They also digest inert foreign particles and inflammatory debris.

The total number and percentage of WBCs change with age (Table 23-1). Like the red blood count, the white blood count is highest at birth (approximately 12,000 per cubic millimeter) and decreases to an average of 7500 per cubic millimeter in adulthood.

Thrombocytes

Thrombocytes, or *platelets*, are the smallest and most fragile cells in circulating blood and originate from megakaryocytes, the largest cells in the bone marrow (Fig. 23-1). They are irregular in shape and are capable of ameboid movement. They are minute oval, nonnucleated, granular bodies whose primary function is clot formation.

When a blood vessel is damaged, platelets adhere immediately to the site of damage. They assume bizarre, irregular forms and have numerous points protruding from their surfaces. An accumulation of platelets and fibrin at the site of an injured vessel is called a *clot*.

Platelets also provide defense against infections. They are the first cells to interact with bacteria, viruses, and other foreign particles in circulating blood. In addition, platelets assist in *fibrinolysis*, or destruction of a clot. The normal concentration of platelets is lowest in the newborn (140,000 to 300,000 per cubic millimeter) and increases to 150,000 to 450,000 per cubic millimeter in the adult (Table 23-1).

Plasma

Blood *plasma* is a straw-colored solution of water (91 percent) and chemical compounds (9 percent), mainly proteins. Plasma is the medium by which the formed elements are transported in the blood vessels.

There are four major plasma proteins: albumin, globulin, fibrinogen, and prothrombin. *Albumin*, the most abundant, is important in maintaining the osmotic equilibrium of the blood. Since albumin cannot pass through the capillary wall, it remains in the bloodstream and exerts an osmotic pressure, attracting water from the tissue spaces back into the bloodstream. If dehydration or hemorrhage occurs, the plasma volume is reduced and shock may develop. In severe injuries, such as burns, albumin is able to escape from the capillaries, water cannot be retained, and blood volume drops. Infants are vulnerable to deficits in fluid volume because of their proportionately greater body fluid content and great extracellular fluid exchange.

Globulin is formed primarily in the liver. It combines with other proteins and transports them from one part of the body to another. The globulins also serve as antibodies (*immunoglobulins*) and provide immunity against some infections.

Fibrinogen and *prothrombin* are unstable proteins in the plasma that can split easily into smaller compounds, fibrin and thrombin. They are essential in clot formation.

The plasma proteins, which have low concentrations in early infancy, reach adult concentrations by 18 months. In a healthy person, the normal fluid volume of the plasma is maintained within relatively narrow limits.

The child who is suspected of having abnormalities of the blood or hemostasis will undergo many blood tests. Repeated punctures are upsetting. The nurse must be ready to explain the tests, support the child, and help the child and the parents cope with the procedures.

ALTERATIONS IN ERYTHROCYTES

Anemia

Anemia, a sign of an underlying pathological process, is a reduced RBC volume or a hemoglobin (Hgb) concentration below the normal range for the person's age. Children with anemia require a diagnostic search for the underlying cause.

A complete blood count (CBC) is the most valuable and most widely used laboratory test for the diagnosis and follow-up of anemia. A CBC includes all the cellular components of the blood (erythrocytes, leukocytes, and platelets). The RBC assessment includes both the number of erythrocytes and their shape (morphology). Morphology may also be determined by direct microscopic examination of a carefully prepared smear. Anemias may be classified according to the morphology of the erythrocyte size (microcytic, normocytic, or macrocytic) and the amount of hemoglobin pigment in the cells (normochromic or hypochromic). (See Table 23-2.)

The shape of the RBCs is important in making a diagnosis. In an anemic child, RBCs that are normocytic and normochromic point to the possibility of chronic infection, malignancy, endocrine hypofunction, marrow suppression, or blood loss. Macrocytic cells are caused by deficiencies of either folic acid or vitamin B_{12}. Erythrocytes that are microcytic and hypochromic are seen commonly in children with iron deficiencies but are also seen in children with thalassemia and lead toxicity. Other morphological distinctions, such as spherocytosis, fragmentation, and sickled cells, signal a hemolytic process. The amount of reticulocytes indicates how much the bone marrow is responding to an anemic state by increasing or decreasing the production of newly formed erythrocytes.

It is useful to classify the anemias further as resulting from either decreased production or increased destruction or loss of RBCs. To conceptualize them in this manner gives a better understanding of the underlying processes toward which the treatment is aimed.

Table 23-2 Erythrocyte Morphology and Related Conditions

Terminology	Description of Red Blood Cell	Condition in Which Found
Normocyte	Normal size and shape (biconcave disk)	Secondary anemia
Microcyte	Smaller than normal size	Secondary anemia, thalassemia
Macrocyte	Larger than normal size	Primary anemia due to folic acid and vitamin B_{12} deficiencies
Spherocyte	Slightly smaller than normal diameter; no central indentation or pallor	Hemoglobin C, thalassemia major
Normochromic	Normal pigmentation at edges of cell with normal central pallor	Acute blood loss; anemia due to extracorpuscular defects
Hypochromic	Pale-appearing cell with decreased color and accentuated central pallor	Any anemia
Anisocytosis	Variation in size of RBC	Any anemia
Poikilocytosis	Variation in shape of RBC	Any anemia

Other laboratory tests used in the diagnosis and follow-up of anemias are bone marrow aspiration and tests of bilirubin level, liver function, and hemoglobin electrophoresis. These and other tests are discussed later in relation to their use in specific disorders.

Signs and symptoms When the hemoglobin level drops to 7 or 8 g, signs or symptoms of physiological alterations begin to appear. Pallor of the skin and mucous membranes may become visible to the nurse. Anemias of about 8 to 11 g of hemoglobin are often detected on routine CBCs before surgery or during well-child examinations.

The body compensates for an anemic state by making adjustments to facilitate the transfer of oxygen. As the hemoglobin drops, cardiac output increases, heart rate increases, and the flow of blood is directed more to the vital tissues of the body. In addition, the affinity of hemoglobin for oxygen is reduced, allowing oxygen to be more freely taken up by the tissues. When the anemia is moderate to severe, the child may become weak or have shortness of breath upon exertion. After exertion, tachycardia may be marked. A baby may cry weakly and tire quickly after eating. Anorexia, irritability, and fatigability are noted by the parents of the anemic child.

Most anemias have an insidious onset and therefore give the body time to compensate for the loss of RBC mass. However, when there is a rapid loss of blood due to a major bleeding episode or a very rapid hemolysis (RBC destruction), the failure of the compensating mechanisms will eventually lead to congestive heart failure. Even anemia with a slow onset has the potential to cause cardiac failure when the hemoglobin level falls below 4 to 5 g. Dyspnea, increasing weakness, edema, and weight gain may warn of impending cardiac failure. Children with chronic diseases or other intercurrent problems such as respiratory disorders may develop congestive heart failure when the hemoglobin level reaches 4 to 6 g.

The history obtained from the parents and the nurse's physical assessment of an anemic child can be diagnostically helpful. Certain physical signs or clues in the history point to different etiologies for the anemia. For instance, increased bruising or nosebleed alerts the nurse to look for a bleeding disorder resulting in blood-loss anemia. A history of drug intake points to the possibility of toxic bone marrow suppression. Dark stools can mean blood loss into the intestinal tract, whereas a history of dark urine may mean that hemolysis is present and that bilirubin is being lost in the urine. Although various signs or symptoms are typical of certain disorders, many overlap and can complicate the diagnostic process. Laboratory confirmation is necessary to make a firm diagnosis.

Physiological anemia

Following birth, the normal infant's hemoglobin level drops from a high of around 19 g to a low of 10 to 11 g in 6 to 8 weeks. Premature and low-birth-weight babies may reach a low point of 7 to 9 g in 3 to 7 weeks because they have a smaller RBC mass at birth. The hemoglobin level declines because:

1. Rapid growth leads to an increase in blood volume and hemodilution.
2. RBCs survive for only about 90 days during this period.
3. Erythropoietin drops, causing a decreased production of new RBCs in the bone marrow.

Treatment No therapy is indicated unless this "normal" anemia is aggravated by nutritional deficiencies, infection, or other intercurrent problems. The administration of iron will not prevent the normal decline of the hemoglobin level. When the level reaches its low point, erythropoietin is spontaneously secreted to stimulate bone marrow production. The normal hemoglobin level will rise to about 12 g in the 1-year-old and will reach a mean of close to 13 g in the young teenager. Transfusions are used only in extreme cases, and then only with small amounts of packed cells. If larger transfusions are used, they can delay the spontaneous return of normal bone marrow production.

Nursing management The infant's diet should contain sufficient essential nutrients to prevent deficiencies of iron, folic acid, and vitamin E. Iron stores are adequate in the full-term infant until 6 months of age, but premature and low-birth-weight babies deplete their storage iron earlier. Cow's milk and breast milk are low in iron, and so supplemental iron is recommended after 4 months of age for full-term babies and earlier for premature infants. Ferrous iron preparations or iron-fortified formulas are given until cereals and meats, which are high in iron, can be introduced into the diet (usually at 6 months of age).

Iron-deficiency anemia

Iron-deficiency anemia occurs when total body iron is diminished. When a deficiency of iron begins, the hemoglobin level initially remains constant while the body uses up stored iron to make RBCs. As the iron stores become depleted, the level of circulating serum iron falls. The RBCs then develop the characteristic hypochromic, microcytic morphology (also seen in lead toxicity and thalassemia), and the hemoglobin level begins to fall. The plasma ferritin level can be tested in order to measure the stores of iron in the body. Low ferritin concentrations can signal an early iron deficiency before the iron stores are depleted and before the hemoglobin level begins to drop.

Etiology Iron-deficiency anemia is caused by four interrelated factors:

1. Deficient diet
2. Increased demand for growth
3. Blood loss
4. Poor absorption of dietary iron

In the newborn, iron-deficiency anemia can be caused by a premature birth, a twin pregnancy, fetal blood loss at the time of delivery, and being born to a severely iron-deficient mother. Most commonly in infancy, it is due to a diet that consists mainly of whole milk, without any other sources of iron. Periods of rapid growth and the onset of puberty make the adolescent female especially vulnerable to iron-deficiency anemia. Another cause is blood loss due to intestinal intolerance or hypersensitivity to whole milk, the ingestion of a particular drug (such as aspirin), or the presence of intestinal parasites. Malabsorption syndromes and prolonged bouts of diarrhea can also prevent iron from being absorbed by the body, despite an adequate dietary intake. Iron deficiency itself is associated with changes in the gut that promote blood loss. The mucosal lining is affected by the deficiency of iron, causing occult blood loss in the stool.

Incidence Iron-deficiency anemia is one of the most common disorders. It affects 10 to 30 percent of the world's population, most notably in underdeveloped countries. In developed countries it is the most common nutritional deficiency, usually affecting women, children, and the poor.

Manifestations The infant or child presents with few or many symptoms, depending on the severity of the anemia. Weakness, fatigue, irritability, dizziness, loss of appetite, stomatitis, dark stools, and skin pallor may be noted. In darker-skinned children, the nail beds, conjunctivae, and oral mucous membranes should be assessed rather than the skin itself. Iron-deficiency anemia may be associated with *pica,* or the ingestion of nonfood substances.

Diagnostic tests A hemoglobin level below 10.6 g in females and 12 g in males is suggestive of anemia. A hematocrit of less than 30 percent in either sex is significant. When a peripheral blood smear is done, a decrease in the plasma iron level and the total iron-binding capacity indicate a mild anemia. A decrease in mean corpuscular volume, mean corpuscular hemoglobin, and mean corpuscular hemoglobin concentration will not occur until the anemia is severe.

Treatment Medical management entails discovering the cause, treating it, and observing the response to treatment. The treatment of choice for the iron-deficient child is oral iron supplementation and diet counseling.

Normally, the body absorbs about 10 percent of the dietary intake of iron. When a child is iron-deficient, the absorption rises to around 20 percent. For this absorption to be of any consequence, a diet sufficient in iron must be provided. Various forms of ferrous iron are effective in correcting the anemia. Although a prompt response can be noted on the CBC within the first week, treatment should be continued for about 3 months after the hemoglobin level returns to normal in order to replenish the storage pool. The child's parents should be warned that oral iron supplements cause the stools to become black or dark green. Oral iron supplements are best absorbed in an empty stomach. Iron medication, like other medications, should be placed out of the reach of young children to prevent overdose poisoning. Normally, a reduced intake of cow's milk and the introduction of an adequate diet, along with oral iron therapy, are sufficient to correct the anemia.

Severe anemia with a hemoglobin level below 4 g may require a packed RBC transfusion and follow-up treatment with oral supplements. Intramuscular iron supplements may be needed when the parents fail to give the oral preparation or for a child who has intestinal malabsorption.

Nursing management When obtaining a history of the current illness, the nurse should note the presence of irritability, fatigue, weakness, and change in behavior. The usual diet should be described. Factors which may point to the cause of the illness should be noted—history of drug intake, exposure to environmental hazards, pica, or episodes of bleeding. Racial origin, a family history of anemia, jaundice, blood loss, and infection should be described.

Observations should include vital signs, color of the stools and urine, bruising or petechiae, and response to normal activities. To determine pallor, both the conjunctivae and the skin should be checked.

Anemic children need extended periods of rest and careful scheduling of nursing care to prevent undue fatigue. As the anemia is corrected, anorexia, irritability, and fatigue will lessen.

The severely anemic hospitalized child should be watched carefully for signs of congestive heart failure. Dyspnea, increasing weakness, edema, and weight gain are findings that warn of impending cardiac failure. A *slow* transfusion of packed RBCs can correct the cardiac dysfunction. Blood loss in the stool should be monitored by guaiac testing, since even a minor loss can worsen the anemia.

The nurse's role includes teaching. The parents should understand that the diet must contain sufficient amounts of iron-containing foods and that whole milk should be limited to 24 oz per day. Foods that are high in iron include liver, dried fruits, beef, veal, carrots, beans, spinach, peas, sweet potatoes, peaches, soybean products, green leafy vegetables, and fortified cereals. Pica is associated with iron deficiency, and the parents should be warned that the child may be eating dirt or paint chips, which can lead to worm ingestion or lead poisoning. Pica should decrease when the anemia is treated. Furthermore, parents who have been unable to meet the dietary needs of their infant often need counseling for other well-child care, such as immunizations and proper hygiene.

Prevention, of course, is the ideal way to handle the public health problem of iron-deficiency anemia. The nurse should counsel parents of newborns to provide an adequate diet and give supplemental iron as indicated for the age of the infant.

Aplastic anemias

Bone marrow aplasia is moderate to severe depression in bone marrow production of RBCs, WBCs, or platelets. The term *hypoplasia* is used when there is at least some production by the marrow. Any or all of the cellular elements may be decreased to any degree. In *pancytopenia*, all three cellular components are decreased in the peripheral blood. Aplastic anemia may be congenital or acquired.

Fanconi syndrome The commonest congenital aplastic anemia is *Fanconi syndrome*, a genetically transmitted anemia accompanied by microcephaly, limb deformities, heart and kidney anomalies, deafness, and short stature. The marrow aplasia is not evident until the age of 3 to 4 years, when bruising and nosebleeds appear. A bone marrow aspirate and biopsy reveal marked hypocellularity of the marrow, confirming the diagnosis. Treatment includes administering combined corticosteroids and anabolic steroids (methyltestosterone).

Blackfan-Diamond anemia Another congenital aplasia is *Blackfan-Diamond anemia*. This disorder is a pure RBC aplasia with normal numbers of circulating leukocytes and platelets. The bone marrow examination reveals markedly diminished to absent erythrocyte precursors. There is no known cause of this disorder, and there are no commonly associated anomalies. The presenting signs and laboratory data are those of severe anemia in infancy, with normocytic, normochromic RBCs and a marked decrease in reticulocytes (new, young RBCs). Approximately 10 percent of children with this disorder will at some time during childhood or puberty begin spontaneously to produce their own RBCs and will continue to do so. Corticosteroid treatment produces erythropoiesis in about 60 percent of children.

Acquired aplastic anemia *Acquired aplastic anemia* can be caused by damage to the bone marrow from the effects of drugs, toxins, infections, or radiation. Cancer chemotherapeutic drugs known to cause marrow damage include antimetabolites and alkylating agents. Radiation also severely depresses bone marrow production.

Other drugs associated with aplastic anemia include sulfonamides, quinicrine, phenylbutazone, mephenytoin, gold compounds, and, more important, chloramphenicol (Chloromycetin). Acquired aplasia can follow infection with measles, hepatitis, and possibly other viruses. Insecticides, as well as benzene and related hydrocarbons found in glues and petroleum distillate solvents, also cause marrow damage. Aplasia may be the presenting sign of acute leukemia or systemic lupus erythematosus. No cause is found in 50 percent of the cases.

Treatment However vigorous the therapy, the prognosis for children with aplastic anemia is poor without bone marrow transplantation. With acquired aplastic anemia, death may be the result of a rapid progression of the disease when supportive therapy is unable to keep up. In the more chronic forms, such as Fanconi syndrome or Blackfan-Diamond anemia, the prognosis is somewhat better with the proper use of supportive transfusions and antibiotics. Life is often extended into the second and third decades. For the acquired forms of the anemia, removal of the offending agent is most important. Both forms require supportive therapy to replace the necessary components of the blood.

Spontaneous bleeding may occur when the platelet count falls below about 30,000 per cubic millimeter; many children, however, have only occasional bleeding with counts even below 5000 per cubic millimeter. Platelet transfusions are necessary during surgery or to stop severe bleeding. Transfusions with packed RBCs may be needed after a bleeding episode or to maintain an acceptable hemoglobin level—8 to 10 g.

Children with Blackfan-Diamond anemia, who depend on monthly RBC transfusions, gradually accumulate iron in their bodies as a result of the large amounts of iron in packed RBCs. This iron overload becomes an increasing problem, since none of the extra iron received in the transfusion is lost through hemorrhage. The iron overload is deposited in the heart, liver, and pancreas and causes failure of these organs after years of transfusions. Deferoxamine (Desferal) therapy attempts to chelate the excess iron from the body. Deferoxamine, however, cannot usually keep up with the large amounts of iron deposited in the system.

A very low white blood count predisposes the aplastic child to infection—the major cause of death. Because WBC transfusions are difficult and costly, they are not done routinely. When infection is suspected, antibiotics should be started promptly, and the child must be hospitalized or watched closely as an outpatient.

Corticosteroids and androgenic steroids are used individually or in combination to stimulate bone marrow production. If this therapy is effective, it is sometimes 2 to 4 months before any improvement is seen. Among the side effects of corticosteroids are increased appetite with ensuing Cushingoid features, sodium retention, hypertension, and impairment of linear growth. The androgens cause masculinization of the child and a greater frequency of malignant hepatomas after prolonged therapy.

Bone marrow transplants have been of value in some children. Siblings who are histocompatible, as determined by tissue typing, are candidates to provide the marrow for the transplant. The 2-year survival rate with histocompatible sibling donors is about 85 percent. Tissue typing should be done immediately after the diagnosis is made because it becomes more difficult after transfusion therapy has begun.

Bone marrow transplantation Bone marrow transplantation is becoming more and more acceptable as a treatment for aplastic anemia as well as for leukemia. There are two types of bone marrow transplantation. In an *allogenic transplantation,* the marrow of a matched donor, often a sibling, is used, while in an *autologous transplantation,* the patient's own marrow is used. Several marrow specimens must be collected before the transplantation.

The child receives a chemotherapeutic agent or total body irradiation to suppress bone marrow function and reduce the chance of rejection. The marrow is transplanted, and the child is closely monitored and kept in a protective isolation unit with laminar airflow for 10 to 20 days.

Complications include infection, bleeding, and graft-vs.-host disease. Any blood products used must be irradiated. Peripheral blood counts begin to rise in about 3 weeks. The immune system and WBC level do not return to normal for nearly a year.

The whole bone marrow transplantation process is extremely stressful for the child and the family. Waiting for the graft to take (1 to 3 weeks), fear of rejection, and being very sick all take their toll. Nursing interventions include closely monitoring vital signs, intake and output, and body systems for signs of rejection. The child requires meticulous care and protection against infection, as well as support in coping with discomfort, intrusive procedures, and the fear of death. A further discussion of transplantation appears in Chap. 26.

Nursing management The assessment of the child with aplastic anemia is related to the deficiencies in platelets, WBCs, and RBCs. The parents and the child should be taught what signs to watch for and under what conditions they should come to the hospital for care or guidance.

The child should be monitored closely for increasing signs of anemia or blood loss. Nasal packing is necessary for nosebleeds. Contact sports should be avoided. Acetaminophen should be used instead of aspirin, which affects the function of platelets. Suppression of menstruation (by hormone therapy) may be necessary if blood loss is excessive.

Depending on how well the child's body compensates for the depression in RBC production, transfusions will occasionally be necessary to bring the hemoglobin back up to an acceptable level.

The nurse must be extremely vigilant during a transfusion. The child should be kept comfortable, and vital signs must be monitored closely. Signs of a transfusion reaction often occur within 10 min. Table 23-3 describes transfusion reactions and nursing responsibilities. When a transfusion reaction occurs, the blood should be stopped, the line should be kept open with intravenous fluid, and the physician should be notified.

The chance of overwhelming infection is a constant threat when the white blood count is very low. Parents should be instructed to seek medical care at the first sign of infection. With a serious infection, hospitalization and parenteral antibiotics are the safest way to manage the child. Avoidance of contact with ill children or adults and large crowds should be attempted.

Children and their families need help in dealing with the physical changes that are the common side effects of steroids. High-dose prednisone leads to increased appetite and weight gain, due to both caloric intake and water retention. To prevent massive weight gain, the parents can adjust the child's diet by providing low-calorie,

Table 23-3 Transfusion Reactions

Type of Reaction	Signs and Symptoms	Nursing Responsibilities
Febrile	Fever, chills, headache, nausea, vomiting	Check temperature q 30 min. Observe closely. Physician may elect to discontinue transfusion or give acetaminophen before transfusion.
Hemolytic	Fever, nausea, vomiting, abdominal and back pain, hematuria, oliguria, restlessness, flushing, tachypnea	Usually transfusion is discontinued, and blood samples are obtained. Monitor vital signs and intake and output. Encourage intake of fluids. Diuretics may be ordered. Check urine for hemoglobin.
Hypervolemic	Dyspnea, cough, cyanosis, pulmonary edema, pain, distended neck veins	Blood should always be administered evenly at the designated rate. Place child in upright position with legs dependent. Oxygen may help.
Hypersensitivity	Pruritus, urticaria, fever, asthma, hypotension, nausea, vomiting	Have epinephrine, antihistamines, and resuscitative equipment available. Monitor vital signs. Physician may order diphenhydramine before transfusion to alleviate allergic response. If reaction occurs, stop transfusion.
Bacterial contamination	Fever, chills, shock, coma, convulsions	Monitor vital signs, temperature, and neurological status. Emergency drugs need to be available—plasma expanders, corticosteroids, and vasopressors. Send sample of transfusion for culture and sensitivity.
Citrate intoxication	Tingling in fingers, cramps, tetany, convulsions, respiratory arrest	Infuse blood slowly. Stop transfusion, maintaining patency of line, and call physician.

highly nutritious foods. The masculinization caused by the androgens is also a troublesome problem. School-age girls are especially affected by increased hair growth, increased muscle mass, and masculinization of the features. Giving support and explanations to peers and school personnel may be helpful.

Although the anemia is of great concern to the caretakers of the child and is usually the most life-threatening condition, referral is necessary for the child with Fanconi syndrome in order to provide special education and follow-up for the accompanying problems.

Megaloblastic anemias

Deficiencies of folic acid or vitamin B_{12} cause the two megaloblastic anemias most common in children. In *megaloblastic anemias,* there are macrocytic RBCs as well as enlarged forms of leukocytes, platelets, and their precursors in the bone marrow. The large cells are produced in response to impaired DNA synthesis brought about by a lack of sufficient folic acid or vitamin B_{12}. Leukopenia and thrombocytopenia often accompany these deficiencies.

Vitamin B_{12} deficiency *Vitamin B_{12} deficiency* is rare in children and can be due to dietary insufficiency or to juvenile pernicious anemia. In pernicious anemia a glycoprotein, the *intrinsic factor,* which is normally secreted by the gastric mucosa to aid in the absorption of B_{12}, is missing. The Shilling test, using radioactive B_{12}, tests for B_{12} absorption by the stomach.

The typical symptoms of anemia plus a painful, smooth tongue are characteristic of vitamin B_{12} deficiency. Involvement of the nervous system causes tingling and numbness of the fingers and toes (paresthesias), ataxia, and impaired position sense. Treatment requires monthly injections of vitamin B_{12} throughout the child's life.

Folic acid deficiency Megaloblastic anemia is more often due to *folic acid deficiency* than to vitamin B_{12} deficiency. Impaired absorption, a diet deficient in folate, or an increased demand for folate is responsible for the developing anemia. Normal body stores of folate can sustain cell production for about 5 to 6 months after intake of folates stops. Therefore, the peak incidence of folic acid deficiency in infancy occurs at 4 to 7 months, when the prenatal supplies become depleted.

Folic acid is inefficiently absorbed in the child who has chronic diarrhea or celiac disease or who has undergone surgical resection of portions of the small intestine. Folic acid antagonists, such as methotrexate, cause megaloblastic changes. Rarely, this complication accompanies anticonvulsant therapy with diphenylhydantoin or phenobarbital. Poor dietary intake also causes a deficiency. Folic acid must be supplemented in the child who is drinking goat's milk.

Poor weight gain, irritability, diarrhea, and the symptoms associated with a low hemoglobin level are manifestations of folic acid deficiency anemia. The neurological effects of vitamin B_{12} deficiency are not seen in the folate-depleted child unless there is also a concomitant B_{12} depletion. Both forms of megaloblastic anemia, however, result in a smooth tongue that is sometimes painful and in gastrointestinal changes resulting in diarrhea.

Treatment and nursing management Children with folic acid deficiency respond well to oral doses of folic acid (100 to 200 mg daily). Therapy should be continued for at least 3 to 4 weeks to restore the storage pool. Folic acid administration can also partially correct anemia caused by vitamin B_{12} deficiency but will not correct the associated neurological symptoms.

The child with pernicious anemia and vitamin B_{12} deficiency will have to begin a lifelong therapy program. In most cases, the neurological symptoms disappear after the correction of the anemic state, but during the initial treatment the child will need to take safety precautions in order to compensate for neurological impairment. Impaired balance makes such activities as bicycling dangerous.

In the child with folic acid deficiency whose diet was deficient, after the folic acid stores of the body are replenished and the anemia is corrected to a normal hemoglobin level, no maintenance therapy is needed. However, unless a proper diet is followed, the anemia can recur. Good sources of folic acid are breast milk and cow's milk, fresh green vegetables, liver, kidney, beans, and nuts.

Blood-loss anemia

Rapid blood loss may result from a variety of disorders or trauma and can quickly lead to shock. Disorders of coagulation, such as hemophilia and a reduction in platelets, can cause serious acute bleeding. Excessive bruising or a petechial rash suggests coagulation abnormalities. During the fetal and neonatal periods, blood loss may be acute or chronic. Rapid blood loss can occur through the cord or the placenta or as a result of obstetric trauma. Chronic bleeding can be due to fetal-maternal or fetal-fetal transfusion in utero. Chronic blood loss in childhood usually occurs through the stools.

The erythrocytes in blood-loss anemia are normocytic and normochromic. Three to five days after an acute bleed, the bone marrow will produce a higher percentage of new reticulocytes. In the child with chronic bleeding, the reticulocyte count may be normal or increased, depending on how hard the bone marrow must work to replace the blood cells being lost. Blood-loss anemia does not affect the WBCs or platelets; however, decreased platelets may be the cause of the blood loss.

Treatment and nursing management Active bleeding must be stopped as quickly as possible by first-aid measures. If there is a known coagulation factor deficiency or severely decreased platelets, transfusions of the missing factor may be lifesaving.

Transfusions with packed RBCs are used to restore the oxygen-carrying capacity of the blood if the hemoglobin level falls dangerously low (e.g., 3 to 5 g). When the hemoglobin level is very low, transfusion with packed RBCs should be done slowly to avoid volume overload, which can cause congestive heart failure or pulmonary edema. The lower the hemoglobin level, the lower the number of milliliters per kilogram of body weight per hour in the transfusion.

Hemolytic anemias

Hemolytic anemias are characterized by premature destruction of erythrocytes (RBCs that survive less than 120 days); they are due either to a defect within the RBCs (corpuscular) or to damage outside the cell (extracorpuscular). Corpuscular hemolytic anemias are usually inherited, while extracorpuscular hemolytic anemias can be caused by mechanical factors, infections, toxins, drugs, and isoimmune disorders.

Manifestations With increased hemolysis, the bilirubin level becomes elevated. Many people with ongoing hemolytic disease have a yellowish tint in their sclerae which becomes more prominent as more rapid hemolysis occurs and which decreases as hemolysis decreases.

The child with hemolytic disease is subject to episodes of rapid hemolysis that can lead to very severe anemia and shock. Signs of increased hemolysis include increasing jaundice, fatigue, weakness, and pallor. Hemoglobinuria may appear as a red pigment in the urine and is indicative of a rapid hemolytic process.

The diagnosis of hemolytic disease is based on demonstration of shortened RBC survival time (less than 120 days), increased erythrocyte catabolism (increased bilirubin), and an elevated reticulocyte count.

The causes of extracorpuscular hemolysis can be grouped in five categories:

1. Mechanical factors: conditions involving deposits of fibrin in vessels due to thrombocytopenia or prosthetic heart valves
2. Infections, such as infectious mononucleosis, hepatitis, malaria, and *Clostridium welchii* infections
3. Toxins from snake bites
4. Drugs such as quinine and phenylhydrazine and substances such as lead
5. Isoimmune disorders, such as hemolytic disease of the newborn, and incompatible blood transfusions

Two major categories of corpuscular hemolytic anemias are those caused by enzyme deficiencies (e.g., pyruvate kinase deficiency and glucose-6-phosphate dehydrogenase deficiency) and those caused by membrane deficiencies (e.g., hereditary spherocytosis and hereditary elliptocytosis). The characteristics and treatment of diseases in these groups are reviewed in Table 23-4. Because these anemias have a genetic basis, their incidence is higher in some populations; for example, glucose-6-phosphate dehydrogenase deficiency is prevalent among Sephardic Jews, who frequently intermarry. A final group of hemolytic anemias can be traced to defects in hemoglobin structure (e.g., sickle cell disorders) or production (e.g., thalassemias). The sickle cell disorders are found most often among blacks, and the thalassemias (of the beta type) among people in or from Mediterranean countries. These hemoglobinopathies are summarized in Table 23-5.

Sickle cell hemoglobinopathies

Sickle cell hemoglobinopathies are a group of inherited RBC disorders characterized by the presence of sickle hemoglobin (Hgb S). Eight percent of the black population has sickle cell disease.

Table 23-4 Characteristics and Treatment of Hemolytic Anemias Due to Corpuscular Defects

Condition	Characteristics	Treatment
Enzyme Deficiency		
Pyruvate kinase deficiency	Symptoms range in severity from severe jaundice at birth requiring transfusions to a well-compensated hemolysis. Growth and development may be delayed.	Splenectomy. There will be some improvement after splenectomy, with less need for transfusions and better RBC production.
Glucose-6-phosphate dehydrogenase deficiency (G6PD)	Increased incidence among blacks (10 to 15%), Sephardic Jews, Orientals, and those of Mediterranean descent. May have mild congenital anemia, but usually hemolysis is precipitated by the ingestion of certain drugs that oxidize Hgb (antipyretics, analgesics, antimalarials, sulfonamides, and nitrofurans), infections, or ingestion of fava beans. Other signs: weakness, pallor, dark urine, scleral icterus.	Supportive treatment with transfusions. Control infection. Avoid drugs and fava beans.
Membrane Deficiency		
Hereditary spherocytosis	Autosomal dominant; incidence is 1:5000. Common in white population. Infant presents with anemia, splenomegaly, hyperbilirubinemia. Infection causes hemolytic crisis.	Supportive transfusions. Splenectomy. Splenectomy increases the child's risk of developing a pneumococcal infection; therefore, vaccine is needed. Prophylactic folic acid.
Hereditary elliptocytosis	Autosomal dominant; incidence is 1:2500. 90% have no symptoms. Otherwise, symptoms the same as in spherocytosis.	Same as spherocytosis.

Hgb S results from a change in the composition of the beta globin chains. This abnormal hemoglobin replaces all or part of the normal adult hemoglobin (Hgb A). This defect causes the RBC to sickle, i.e., to change from a round, biconcave disk to a crescent shape when oxygen is released to the tissues in the course of normal functioning. Hgb S is the most common of the more than 250 hemoglobin mutations in humans.

Hgb S is present in the homozygous state, as *sickle cell anemia,* in 1 percent of American blacks. It is present in the heterozygous state, as *sickle cell trait,* in 8 percent. Hgb S is also found in Spanish-Americans, Indians, and those of Mediterranean descent.

The child who receives one gene for normal Hgb A and one gene for Hgb S from his or her parents inherits the *sickle trait (Hgb AS).* If the child receives a gene for Hgb S from each parent, he or she inherits *sickle cell anemia (Hgb SS).* A gene for Hgb S in combination with another gene for abnormal hemoglobin also produces sickle cell disease, sickle celi C disease (Hgb SC), or sickle cell thalassemia (Hgb S-Thal). *Sickle cell disease* is the umbrella term used for all hemoglobin types in which Hgb S is present. See Table 23-5 for a comparison of hemoglobinopathies.

Figure 23-2 gives examples of mating between individuals with various types of hemoglobin. It is important to remember that the risk of having an affected child is the *same* for each pregnancy—no matter what happened in previous pregnancies.

Sickle cell trait *Sickle cell trait* (Hgb AS) is the carrier state for sickle cell anemia (Hgb SS). The *trait* has been confused with the *anemia* and also with other hemoglobin types that sickle. Persons with Hgb AS are not anemic, and their RBC survival time is normal. Only about 24 to 45 percent of their hemoglobin is Hgb S. Even though some of their cells do sickle, these individuals do not have the recurrent sickling crises or frequent infections that are associated with sickle cell diseases. Rarely, they experience pain-

Table 23-5 Characteristics of Hemoglobinopathies

Characteristic	Sickle Cell Trait	Sickle Cell Anemia	Hemoglobin SC Disease	Sickle Cell Beta and Thalassemia	Sickle Cell Beta O Thalassemia
Hgb type	AS	SS	SC	S-beta + thal. (SA + thal.)	S-beta O thal. (S + thal.)
Usual Hgb range	Normal	6 to 9 g	10 to 15 g	10 to 12 g	7 to 10 g
Course of illness	No illness	Severe anemia plus complications	Mild anemia and complications less frequent	Mild anemia, infrequent complications	Anemia plus complications
Spleen	Normal size	Usually not palpable, as in adult	Enlarged	Enlarged	Enlarged
Usual onset of crises	No crises	Early in life	Often adolescence and later	Often adolescence and later or none	Similar to SS
Amount of Hgb A present	More than 50%	No Hgb A	No Hgb A	Less than 40%	No Hgb A

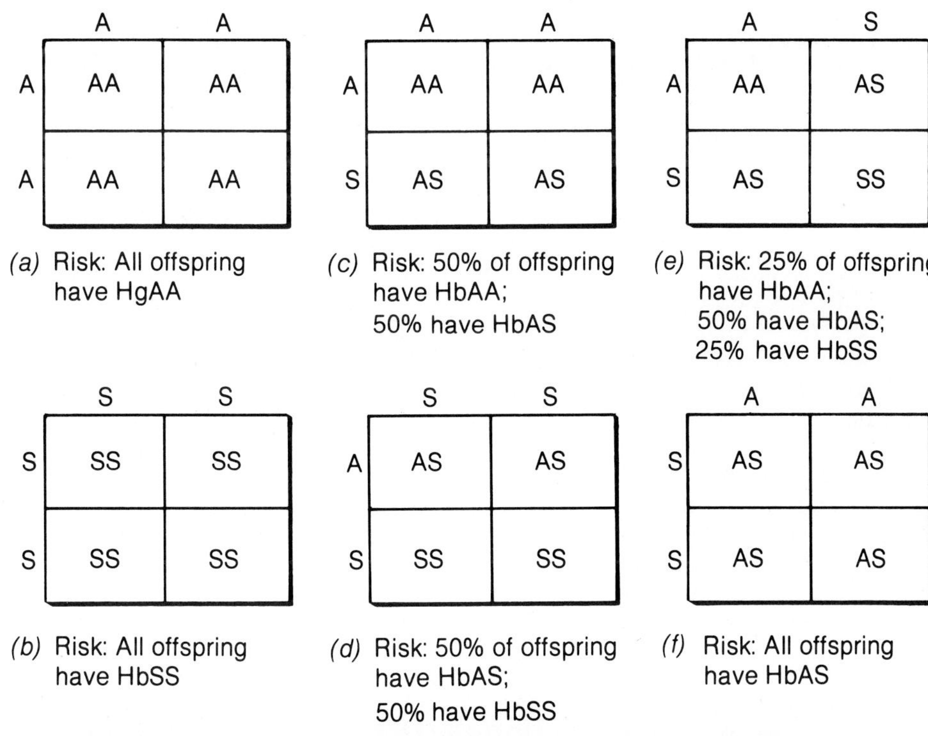

Figure 23-2 Inheritance from parents of normal and sickling hemoglobin. The hemoglobin types of one parent are shown in the left margin of each block, and those of the other parent are shown along the top. Each parent carries two alleles for hemoglobin. Because combinations at conception are random, the risk of each possible outcome in the zygote can be calculated according to statistical laws. Key: A, normal adult hemoglobin; S, sickling hemoglobin; AA, normal; AS, sickle cell trait; SS, sickle cell disease.

less hematuria or splenic infarcts. It is important for nurses to understand the difference between Hgb AS and Hgb SS in order to be able to explain the implications of each to parents and children and to the general public.

The common sickle cell hemoglobinopathies known to have abnormal hematologic findings and clinical manifestations requiring frequent medical attention are (1) sickle cell anemia (Hgb SS), (2) sickle cell C disease (Hgb SC), and (3) sickle cell thalassemia (Hgb S-Thal).

Sickle cell anemia Hgb SS is the most common form of sickle cell disease and has the most severe clinical manifestations. Its problems are related to rapid destruction of RBCs, vasoocclusion, and infection.

RBCs that contain Hgb S cannot be distinguished in appearance from normal RBCs until they sickle (Fig. 23-3). The sickle cell is rigid; its membrane is not as flexible as a normal RBC membrane. It becomes very fragile, with a life span of only 8 to 20 days. This results in chronic anemia. Under conditions of lowered oxygen tension, increased acidity, or increased viscosity, RBCs containing Hgb S will sickle, making it difficult for them to pass through the microcirculation (capillaries and sinusoids). Some remain in the irregular sickle shape; they are called *irreversible sickled cells* (Fig. 23-4). The sickling process tends to increase the blood viscosity, which then leads to stasis and more sickling. With each sickle cycle, the membrane of the RBC is damaged. Sickle-shaped cells wedge in the small blood vessels and block the flow of blood to body parts, producing ischemia and subsequent microinfarcts that cause tissue death.

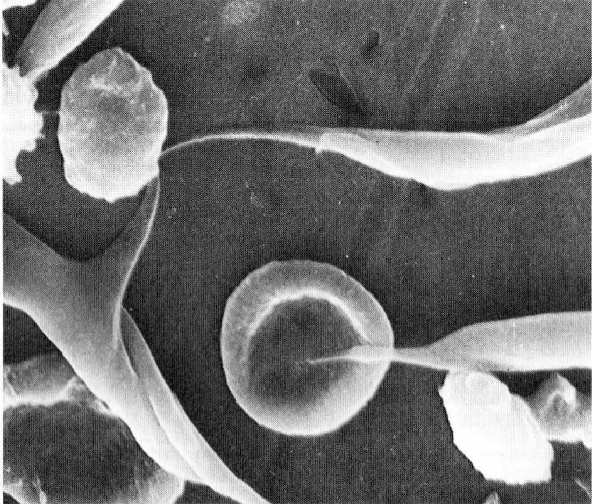

Figure 23-3 A scanning electron micrograph of human sickled RBCs in the deoxygenated state accompanied by one normal biconcave cell (× 10,000). (*Courtesy of R. F. Baker, Department of Microbiology, University of Southern California Medical School.*)

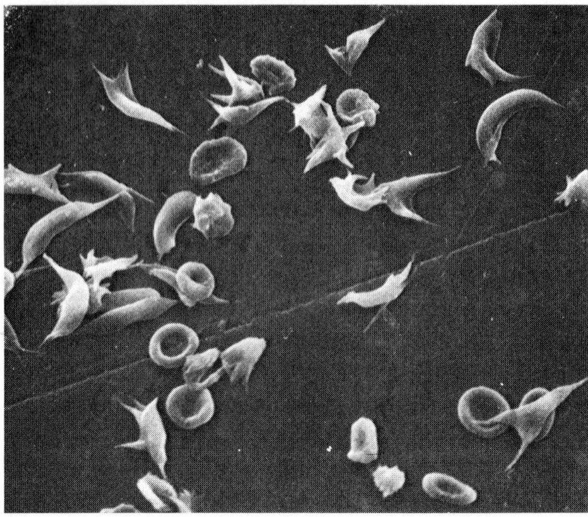

Figure 23-4 A scanning electron micrograph of a mixture of sickled human RBCs and normal human RBCs. (*Courtesy of R. F. Baker, Department of Microbiology, University of Southern California Medical School.*)

Manifestations Figure 23-5 diagrams the effects of Hgb S on various body systems. Over a period of time, major organs are affected, leading to severe malfunctioning and organ failure in various sites.

The *spleen* is one of the first organs to be affected. The gradual fibrosis and scarring generally produce autosplenectomy by age 7 to 8 years. Because of the abnormally functioning spleen, these children have an increased susceptibility to infections.

The *liver* becomes enlarged, firm, and tender. Liver damage affects the adult more than the child. The rapid breakdown of RBCs produces an excessive amount of bilirubin, causing jaundice, especially of the sclerae. Cholelithiasis may also contribute to jaundice.

A single episode of sickling in the *brain* can cause a cerebrovascular accident, seizures, or both. Cerebrovascular accidents occur most commonly under 10 years of age. Usually there

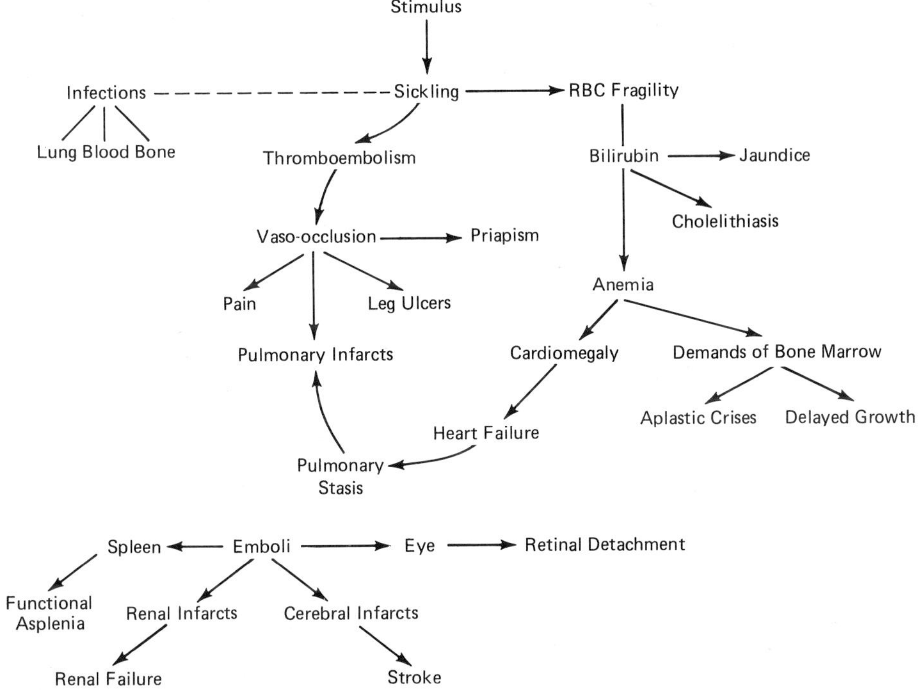

Figure 23-5 Potentially, every organ in the body can be affected by repeated episodes of sickling. (*Adapted from Ida Walters et al., "Complications of Sickle Cell Disease," Nursing Clinics of North America 8(1):140* [*March 1983*]. *Used with permission.*)

is no precipitating cause, although some are associated with hyperventilation.

The *heart* may become enlarged, with a murmur related to the anemia that exists.

Any infection in the *lungs* causes edema and stasis, which precipitate sickling. Pneumonia is common, and treatment is complicated by the impaired circulation. Pulmonary ventilation should be accomplished *without* hyperventilation. Therefore, the incentive spirometer, IPPB (Intermittent Positive Pressure Breathing apparatus) and blow bottles are all contraindicated.

In the *kidneys*, sickling and microinfarcts can cause permanent damage, manifested by hematuria and an inability to concentrate urine. Acute urinary tract infections can lead to pyelonephritis, particularly in older children and adults. Long-term sickling can destroy the glomeruli, leading to renal failure. Anuresis and nocturia are common.

Bone infarcts involving the small bones of the hands and feet are common in infants and young children. The resulting swelling and pain are the "hand-foot syndrome," or sickle cell dactylitis. These bones usually heal without deformity. Older people experience aseptic necrosis of the femoral and humeral heads and deterioration of thoracic and lumbar vertebrae.

Because of the chronic hypoxia, bones become very susceptible to infection. *Salmonella* osteomyelitis is common and often requires years of continuous antibiotic treatment.

The *eye* manifestations in sickle cell disease develop gradually and are common in Hgb SC and Hgb S-Thal. Proliferative sickle retinopathy can lead to blindness. Photocoagulation has proved helpful.

The chronic, recurring problem of *leg ulcers* usually begins during the middle to late teens. These painful ulcers are subject to local and systemic infection. Una boots provide protection and mobility.

Priapism, a persistent, painful erection of the penis, may occur at any age but is associated with the onset of puberty. The longer the erection lasts, the more difficult to relieve. Hypotonic fluids and a warm bath may help. The erection should be relieved within 2 h. Aspiration of the corpora cavernosa may be necessary.

The RBC containing Hgb S may not function for more than 8 to 20 days, considerably less than the normal 120-day life span. This hemolysis and resulting chronic anemia stimulate erythropoiesis, causing hyperplasia of the bone marrow.

In addition to the effects of sickling on the various body organs, the child will have a variety of complaints, such as fever, weakness, malaise, pain, anorexia, and vomiting. The disorder is not easily recognizable from the child's physical appearance, although the extremities may be disproportionately long.

Frequently, physical activities are restricted because of the lack of stamina. Children need to be allowed to set their own limits and not be pushed beyond them.

Sickle cell crises The child experiences painful sickling episodes, called *crises,* which are often brought on by dehydration and infections. In early adolescence, the child usually has fewer crises, but the frequency increases again during later adolescence and early adult life. Despite reports suggesting little survival into adulthood, life expectancy is unpredictable at this time. Some people live into their fifth and sixth decades.

Four events are described as sickle crisis: (1) vasoocclusive crisis, or pain crisis; (2) aplastic crisis, or reduction in RBC production; (3) splenic sequestration crisis; and (4) hyperhemolytic crisis, or hyperhemolysis.

Vasoocclusive crisis is the hallmark of the disease. The RBCs sickle and occlude the smaller blood vessels, producing pain due to lack of oxygen to the tissues. This may occur at any time after fetal Hgb diminishes sufficiently, usually at 3 to 6 months of age.

Painful episodes may be precipitated by dehydration, infection, stress, and exposure to extreme cold or heat. Pain may occur in the extremities, joints, back, or abdomen; older children and adults sometimes complain of pain everywhere. These episodes may last anywhere from 1 day to several days or weeks. They may follow a viral or bacterial infection and sometimes may be accompanied by local swelling and tenderness. Any fever should be evaluated as to the source and properly treated.

In *aplastic crisis* the rate of RBC production is severely or completely reduced. There are signs of increasing anemia, malaise, headache, and pallor. Aplastic crisis is thought to be precipitated by infections. When RBC production is severely reduced, the existing anemia becomes worse and requires transfusion support. Reticulocyte counts are used to determine the rate of RBC production, to make a diagnosis, and to manage aplastic crisis. RBC production usually resumes in a few days. Folic acid supplements are needed to aid in RBC production.

In *splenic sequestration crisis,* sickled RBCs get trapped, or sequestered, in the spleen, blocking blood flow. The spleen enlarges as more blood cells are trapped. Acute sequestration is often associated with septicemia. It is the leading cause of mortality in children with sickle cell disease. The infection and sudden worsening of the anemia are life-threatening. Transfusion is necessary as well as treatment for the infection. A splenectomy may be done after the child's first acute episode. The parents should be taught to check for signs of an enlarging spleen and increasing anemia, weakness, lethargy, and shock and should be instructed to seek immediate medical help if these symptoms occur.

In *hyperhemolytic crisis* RBCs are destroyed more rapidly than usual. It may occur in children while the spleen is still present, but in adults it probably either does not exist or is secondary to other complicating factors. An increase in reticulocytes suggests hemolysis, but there is not necessarily a decrease in the hemoglobin level. Hyperhemolytic crisis is painless, generally requires no treatment, and probably goes unnoticed unless it occurs in conjunction with another complication.

Diagnostic tests The hematocrit ranges from 18 to 30 percent. Hemoglobin electrophoresis reveals 80 to 95 percent Hgb S, 0 to 20 percent Hgb F, and a normal amount of Hgb A_2. Other sickling tests may be used as a follow-up.

Treatment Neither a cure nor an effective, safe treatment regimen is available for sickle cell disease. Treatment is directed toward relieving the symptoms and complications. Correction of dehydration, acidosis, and hypoxia is essential. Vasoocclusive episodes must be recognized as forerunners of more severe complications. Analgesics and transfusions for severe anemia are needed. Infection must be treated promptly with antibiotics. Pneumococcal vaccine is recommended for children over 2 years of age.

Probably the single most important treatment

for painful episodes is *water*—given intravenously and orally and applied locally. Hydration by means of increased fluid intake increases plasma volume and blood flow, dislodging sickled cells from the microcirculation. Water is applied locally in the form of warm, moist packs; tub baths or showers; or whirlpool baths or tanks.

The fluid requirements of a child in crisis are $1\frac{1}{2}$ to 2 times the maintenance amount. An oral fluid intake of 6 to 8 qt a day is recommended. A half-strength normal saline solution, with or without 5% dextrose, should be given intravenously to avoid sodium excess. Antibiotic therapy is used to treat or prevent infection. A folic acid supplement is often helpful when incorporated into the medical regimen. Effective pain management is best achieved by administering analgesics and giving supportive counseling, since it has been found that anxiety, depression, and fear may contribute to pain perception. Intravenous narcotics bring the quickest pain relief; it is best to start with a low-potency analgesic and progress to a higher-potency drug as needed. There is little indication that oxygen therapy is of any benefit, unless the arterial blood gas oxygen is 75 mmHg or less. Blood transfusions are indicated for priapism and severe pneumonia with hypoxia. They may be used prophylactically for the prevention of cerebrovascular accidents and for surgical patients, who often become hypoxic. Otherwise, transfusions are not recommended, since they carry the risks of iron overload, hepatitis, isoimmunization, acquired immune deficiency syndrome, and hyperviscosity.

Health maintenance through comprehensive care is very important to the child with sickle cell disease. The child should be seen every 6 to 12 weeks during childhood.

Nursing management The pathophysiology of Hgb SS has been described in detail to provide a firm basis for nursing care. The nurse must determine the problems experienced by the child and provide nursing intervention accordingly.

During a sickle cell crisis, the child will need meticulous nursing care based on a comprehensive approach and a caring attitude. Since dehydration, infection, overfatigue, prolonged exposure to heat and cold, and emotional stress may all contribute to sickle cell crisis, their prevention is a major goal for the nurse and the family.

Pain is a leading problem associated with the disease. Careful assessment, appropriate analgesia, and hydration are essential. Any swelling or painful area must be carefully described. Heat should not be applied to the abdomen unless appendicitis has been ruled out.

Oxygenation of tissues initially is achieved through bed rest with passive range-of-motion exercises and, later, progressive ambulation (Fig. 23-6). In addition, continuous moist heat, adequate hydration, pulmonary ventilation (by means of deep breathing and clearing of secretions), and prevention of infection contribute to oxygenation. Nursing care should be planned to allow adequate rest periods.

If blood transfusions are necessary, the nurse's responsibilities include observing for reactions and carefully regulating the transfusion rate to prevent hypervolemia.

Vital signs must be monitored closely to assess for impending shock, beginning infection, or problems with oxygenation. Gentle palpation of the spleen to check for enlargement may be helpful when splenic crisis is anticipated.

Children under 10 years of age who develop an increased temperature of 39°C (102°F) or above

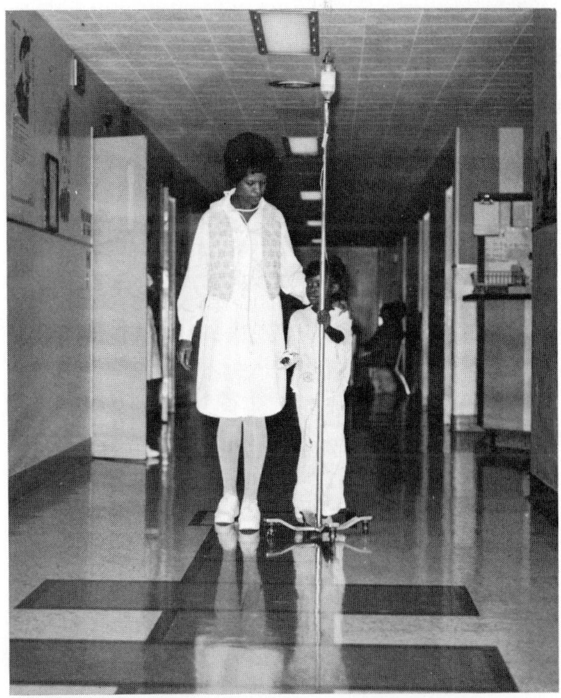

Figure 23-6 A child ambulating with the assistance of a nurse, receiving intravenous infusion, and pushing an intravenous pole for additional support.

should be hospitalized, cultured, and treated vigorously with antibiotics to protect them against pneumococcal pneumonia—a disease that can cause death within a few hours if untreated. The temperature should always be checked before any antipyretic analgesic is given.

To promote hydration, the nurse should offer oral fluids frequently—every 30 to 60 min. If the daily goal is 2400 ml, then a plan must be implemented to ensure that approximately 200 ml will be taken every waking hour during the day. Intravenous fluids require careful regulation. (Review the nursing measures described in Chap. 16 regarding oral and intravenous fluids.)

Another nursing goal is the prevention of acidosis. Hydration and well-balanced meals are useful in preventing this problem. The child's electrolyte balance should also be monitored, and changes reported to the physician. Daily weighing is helpful in checking for diuresis.

Because the kidneys do not concentrate urine well, fluids are easily lost. The child will need special protection in hot weather.

The child needs play activities that are appropriate for his or her age and condition. Occupational therapy visits are useful. If the child is missing school, the school program must be implemented in the hospital or the home.

Although puberty is often delayed in children with sickle cell disease, once it occurs they are usually fertile. The risk of producing offspring with the disease must be carefully explained. The nurse has an important role in giving these explanations and in providing birth control counseling. Neither oral contraceptives nor intrauterine devices are safe for the female with sickle cell disease. Barrier and chemical birth control methods, used carefully and competently, carry no risks of bleeding, infection, or emboli.

During pregnancy, there are increased risks for the mother with sickle cell disease and her baby. The pregnant patient needs careful follow-up; prompt, vigorous treatment of infection; and folic acid supplements. Some patients may be started on transfusion programs after a certain point in their pregnancy. Above all, the pregnant patient needs excellent care and the support of the health care team in the decision to have a child.

The parents especially need to understand that even with the best care, there will be periods of crises and setbacks. The risk of death is greatest in children under 5 years of age. The incidence of crises decreases thereafter. Nevertheless, the parents live constantly with the fear of losing their child.

Many parents feel guilty because of their genetic role in their child's disease. Methods of coping with those feelings vary. Helping them explore their feelings and learn to live with the situation positively are appropriate nursing responsibilities. Parents need to be encouraged to set reasonable limits for their children but to guard against overprotectiveness. Table 23-6 provides guidelines for teaching the parents of a child with Hgb SS.

Education, testing, and counseling, in that order, are important in identifying individuals who have the sickle gene. The federally funded sickle cell programs throughout the United States stress education first.

Education is especially important to those of childbearing age. General educational programs should also be directed toward other groups, such as employers, insurance companies, and school personnel in order to remove the stigma attached to having Hgb S.

Testing for Hgb S is a relatively easy procedure. The most accurate and definitive test is a test of hemoglobin electrophoresis. It should be used *initially* and should be followed by a sickling test, usually a solubility test, to distinguish Hgb S from other Hgbs that migrate in the same

Table 23-6 Guidelines for Teaching Parents of Children with Sickle Cell Disease

1. Encourage intake of 2000 to 4000 ml per day. Give the child something to drink every 30 to 60 min. Restrict cola drinks, coffee, and tea because of their diuretic qualities. Restrict cranberry juice because of acidosis.
2. Keep urine a light amber color through adequate fluid intake.
3. Any complicated illness with vomiting, diarrhea, pain, or elevated temperature of 39°C (102°F) or more should be treated in the hospital.
4. Encourage the child to eat a well-balanced diet high in folic acid.
5. See that the child gets plenty of rest and sleep.
6. Avoid situations that may contribute to crisis—dehydration, infection, prolonged stress (emotional or physical), fatigue, and prolonged exposure to heat or cold.
7. Have the child wear a medical alert tag, and keep people nearby informed of the illness.
8. Do not neglect regular health-maintenance care—immunizations, eye examinations, and dental care.
9. Avoid overprotectiveness and encourage the child to participate in age-appropriate activities as tolerated.

pattern. Hemoglobin electrophoresis distinguishes between sickle cell trait and sickle cell disease. Contrary to earlier thinking, Hgb S can be identified in the newborn by *microcolumn chromatography*. Hgb S can also be identified in the fetus by amniocentesis.

Counseling the person with sickle cell disease requires a special kind of expertise. Counselors should be aware that for some years there has been concern about the purposes and ethics of genetic counseling with regard to the disease. Some members of the black community have charged that counseling programs promote genocide and believe that their real purpose is to prevent blacks from reproducing.

The purpose and objectives of genetic counseling must be clearly defined to the clients. Genetic counseling should consist of giving information, correcting misconceptions, and providing support. It should also be nondirective and nonjudgmental. The goal should be to give information and support to individuals and couples that will enable them to make decisions about marriage and/or reproduction that they can live with. This approach, based on adequate information, shows respect for the clients' dignity and trust in their ability to make decisions that are best for them. See Chap. 6 for a further discussion of genetic counseling.

Sickle cell C disease *Sickle cell C disease* (Hgb SC) is the second most common sickle cell disease; it affects 2 to 3 percent of black Americans. It should not be confused with Hgb AS, even though a person with the disease has only one gene for sickle hemoglobin. A person with Hgb SC, which is a chronic disease, has *no* genes for normal adult hemoglobin. The clinical manifestations are often the same as those of Hgb SS, though less severe. Anemia and splenomegaly are present. Persons with Hgb SC are more prone to aseptic necrosis of femoral heads, *Salmonella* osteomyelitis, and sudden death due to fat embolisms than those with Hgb SS. Symptoms frequently do not begin until adolescence. The management of the disease and the precautions taken to prevent or treat problems are the same as those for sickle cell disease.

Sickle cell thalassemia The combined inheritance of Hgb S and thalassemia results in yet another sickle cell hemoglobinopathy. Thalassemias involve reduced production of a globin chain. In sickle cell thalassemia, the beta chain may be affected in one of two ways, producing either a mild or a severe form of thalassemia.

In the mild form, beta chain production is only mildly suppressed, resulting in some normal Hgb A formation. This is known as *beta + thalassemia*. The condition resembles Hgb SC but is frequently confused with Hgb AS. Because more Hgb S than Hgb A is present, a sickle cell hemoglobinopathy results.

When Hgb S and severe thalassemia genes are present in the same person, the onset, course, and prognosis of the illness are similar to those in Hgb SS. This condition is called *sickle cell beta 0* (no beta chain production) *thalassemia*. The hemoglobin level is approximately 9 to 11 g; the spleen, if present, may be enlarged.

Thalassemia

Etiology *Thalassemia* is an inherited disorder of hemoglobin synthesis in which there is either absent or diminished synthesis of one of the globin chains of Hgb A. This defect results in ineffective erythropoiesis and hemolysis of the RBCs. The four major hemoglobin chains involved are alpha, beta, gamma, and delta. The two major categories of thalassemia, alpha thalassemia and beta thalassemia, are discussed below. A person who has inherited one thalassemia gene and one normal gene is usually mildly affected and is said to have *thalassemia trait* or *thalassemia minor*. If a person has inherited two similar or identical thalassemia genes, the impairment of hemoglobin synthesis is severe, and the person is said to have *thalassemia major*. There appears to be a genetic basis for the varying degrees of severity. Beta thalassemia is seen more commonly in Mediterranean populations, while alpha thalassemia is more common in Oriental populations. Some alpha and beta thalassemias do occur in Africans and black Americans, however.

Manifestations *Alpha thalassemia* In *alpha thalassemias*, there is a partial or total decrease in alpha chain production. The alpha globin chain is necessary for the formation of *all* hemoglobin; therefore, any decrease in its production affects the formation of normal hemoglobin. Normally, four genes function to produce alpha chains; each gene is responsible for about 25 percent of alpha chain production. The activity of these four genes determines the severity of alpha thalassemia. The child with alpha thalassemia who is heterozygous can be asymptomatic, have a mild form of anemia, or have moderately severe anemia with splenomegaly and slight bilirubinemia.

Beta thalassemia In *beta thalassemia,* the excess beta globin chains, which are unable to participate in the formation of the hemoglobin molecule, precipitate inside the cell and damage the RBC membrane, shortening its survival time. Beta thalassemia is usually not detectable until around 6 months of age, when the fetal hemoglobin stores diminish. In the heterozygous form, *beta thalassemia minor,* there are no incapacitating signs or symptoms. The tip of the spleen may be felt on palpation.

The homozygous form, known as *beta thalassemia major* or *Cooley anemia,* is a more serious, life-threatening disease. It results when both parents have thalassemia minor. Growth retardation and severe anemia occur during the first year of life. Other manifestations are hepatosplenomegaly, mild jaundice, patchy skin pigmentation, anoxic leg ulcers, anorexia, and retarded mental development. The characteristic mongoloid facies result from a combination of signs related to anemia—thickened cranial and prominent cheek bones, a depressed nasal bridge, overgrowth of the maxilla, and periorbital puffiness. Cirrhosis of the liver eventually occurs, and gallstones are common.

Diagnostic tests Examination of blood reveals hypochromic, microcytic RBCs as well as target cells, elliptical cells, basophilic tippling, and an unbalanced production of globin chains. In the severe form, the hemoglobin level can be dangerously low.

Treatment The mild forms require no treatment. Beta thalassemia major, however, requires frequent transfusions to maintain a functional hemoglobin level (10 to 12 g). Unfortunately, the repeated transfusions make the patient susceptible to iron overload (hemosiderosis) and cardiac complications—cardiomegaly, arrhythmias, and congestive heart failure. Iron-chelating agents, such as deferoxamine, are given parenterally to prevent acute iron poisoning. The drug is given subcutaneously over a period of 10 to 12 h, five to six nights per week, using a pump. The excess iron is also deposited in the spleen; the spleen is usually removed by the time the child is 5 to 6 years old, which reduces the number of transfusions needed.

Children with thalassemia major die by the age of 2 or 3 years if they are not treated. The prognosis depends on the severity of the disease. Bone marrow transplantation is being studied as a possible treatment.

Nursing management Generally, the nursing care of children with thalassemia syndromes is supportive. There is no specific treatment, however, because transfusions are the mainstay of therapy. Most of the nursing measures, especially in terms of physiological needs, are dictated by the complications encountered. The nurse's ability to give proper support during the care and treatment of a child with a fatal illness is very important to the physical and emotional comfort of the child and his or her family.

The need for transfusions and their long-term effects should be explained well to the parents. As many treatments as possible should be done on an outpatient basis. Home treatment, using chelating agents, should be a part of the child's care as soon as the child and the parents are comfortable with the procedure and are willing to perform it. When a splenectomy has been done, the parents should be aware of the child's increased susceptibility to infections as well as the importance of compliance with the treatment regimen when prophylactic antibiotic therapy is instituted.

Improved methods of management are increasing the chances of survival. Therefore, the importance of health maintenance should not be overlooked. Health maintenance should focus on (1) education—including genetic information; (2) adaptation—daily activity with optimal exercise; (3) the child's self-concept—encouraging a positive self-image and being alert to manifestations of a poor self-image; and (4) referrals—the use of other agencies that will provide support services for the child and the parents.

Polycythemia

Polycythemia is characterized by an increase in the number of erythrocytes and an increase in blood volume; the cause is unknown. The bone marrow is dark red and intensely cellular. It is uncommon in children. The red blood count and the hemoglobin level may rise because decreased oxygen is reaching the tissues of the body. Cyanotic heart disorders create a need for more oxygen-carrying capacity as a result of poor circulatory dynamics. The newborn may become polycythemic secondary to either a maternal-fetal transfusion or an excessive amount of blood drained into the fetus from the placenta at birth. People who live for an extended time at high altitudes develop polycythemia to help compensate for the decreased oxygen.

An increase in the number of erythrocytes creates a higher viscosity in the blood. The high viscosity may cause headaches, lethargy, and pain in the extremities.

A child with polycythemia may require repeated phlebotomies to decrease the red blood count and the viscosity of the blood. In infants who have received maternal-fetal transfusion, the polycythemia will gradually resolve with growth and expanded vascular volume.

When the hemoglobin level rises above approximately 23 g, high blood viscosity can lead to respiratory distress, thrombosis, convulsions, or congestive heart failure as a result of volume overload. Knowing the normal hemoglobin concentrations for a child's age will enable the nurse to be alert to dangerously high levels.

MECHANISM AND ALTERATIONS OF COAGULATION

Coagulation, or clotting, of blood is a protective mechanism that guards against excessive loss of the body's life-sustaining fluid. At least 12 chemical substances, known as *blood factors,* are required for a clot to form (Table 23-7). These factors are present in the platelets and plasma or are produced during clotting reactions.

During the clotting process, blood loses its liquid quality and forms a jellylike mass at the injury site. Strands of fibrin appear, and together the mass and fibrin plug the hole in the vessel.

One type of clotting reaction starts when body cells as well as the vessel are damaged. The body cells release thromboplastin (factor III), which initiates a series of reactions. This process continues (Fig. 23-7) until thrombin has been converted from prothrombin and in turn causes activation of fibrinogen to fibrin. The reactions down to the creation of thrombin are known as the *extrinsic system* of clotting because the initiator, thromboplastin, is found outside (is extrinsic to) the blood.

A clot created without the stimulus of thromboplastin is also possible. The process employs only blood factors and other normal blood substances and hence is called the *intrinsic system.* In this situation, a roughened surface, typically due to a broken blood vessel, causes platelets to adhere. Platelets release factors of their own, and once again a series of blood factors undergo rapid activation (Fig. 23-7). The intrinsic and extrin-

Table 23-7 Coagulation Factors

International Name	Familiar Name	Characteristics
Factor I	Fibrinogen	Produced in liver; average 3000 mμ/ml
Factor II	Prothrombin	Vitamin K necessary for production in liver
Factor III	Thromboplastin	Present in tissues and platelets
Factor IV	Calcium	Present in plasma and serum
Factor V	Proaccelerin, labile factor, Ac globulin	Used up in clotting
Factor VII	Stable factor, convertin, SPCA	Produced in liver; not used up in clotting
Factor VIII	Antihemophilic factor (AHF) Antihemophilic globulin (AHG)	Synthesized by vascular epithelium Used up in clotting
Factor IX	Plasma thromboplastin component (PTC) Christmas factor Antihemophilic factor B	Produced in liver; not used up in clotting
Factor X	Stuart-Prower factor	Produced in liver with vitamin K
Factor XI	Plasma thromboplastin antecedent (PTA)	Present in serum and plasma
Factor XII	Hageman factor Antihemophilic factor D	Unknown site of production
Factor XIII	Fibrin-stabilizing factor Laki-Lorand factor	High levels in plasma

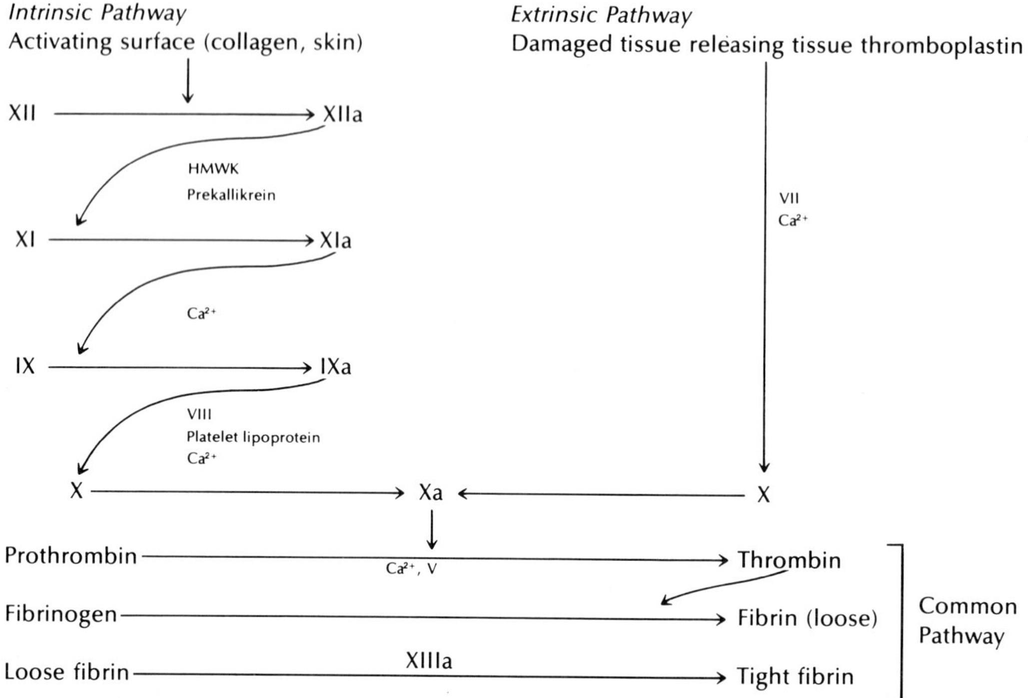

Figure 23-7 Extrinsic and intrinsic systems of coagulation. (*From Sylvia A. Price and Lorraine M. Wilson, Pathophysiology: Clinical Concepts of Disease Processes, 2d ed., McGraw-Hill, New York, 1982. Used with permission.*)

sic pathways end in a common pathway, in which thrombin and finally fibrin are created.

The complex mechanism of coagulation is well understood today. A malfunction or absence of a clotting factor causes some degree of bleeding tendency. The factors most frequently involved are VIII and IX. A few such disorders are discussed in the next section.

Various coagulation tests are used to determine impairment in blood-clotting factors. Because individual values vary among laboratories, the norms for each setting need to be determined by the nurse. Five common tests of coagulation are described in Table 23-8.

Hemophilia A

Hemophilia is the most common congenital bleeding disorder. The incidence of *hemophilia A* (a factor VIII deficiency) is estimated to be 80 per 1,000,000 people. It is an X-linked recessive disorder characterized by a deficiency of plasma factor VIII. The underlying defect is a congenital absence of the antihemophilic factor (AHF), which is vital in the formation of thromboplastin. Hemophilia A has a mutation rate of 25 percent per year.

The disorder is transmitted by clinically unaffected female carriers to male offspring. Approximately 85 percent of all persons with hemophilia have the classic variety. Hemophilia is generally classified according to the deficiency of AHF: mild, moderate, or severe. Table 23-9 describes the severity of bleeding tendency according to the factor VIII (AHF) plasma level. Normal levels range from 60 to 200 percent. A female carrier with a factor VIII of less than 30 percent may have excessive bleeding similar to that seen in hemophiliac males with the same level of factor VIII.

Manifestations The classic signs of the disorder are a prolonged coagulation time (up to 2 h or more) and a tendency to bleed into joints, muscles, and body cavities. Bleeding is characteristically a prolonged oozing or trickling, occurring spontaneously or after surgery or minor trauma. The diagnosis is usually made when

Table 23-8 Some Coagulation Test Values

Test	Newborn (Birth to 1 month)	Infant (1 month to 2 years)	Child (2 to 12 Years)	Adolescent and Adult	Characteristics
Bleeding time (min)	1 to 5	1 to 6	1 to 6	3 to 6	Usually normal if platelet count is above 100,000 per cubic milliliter. Time required for a 2.5-mm-deep puncture wound to stop bleeding.
Coagulation time (min)	2	5 to 8	9 to 12	9 to 12	Time it takes venous blood to clot in vitro. Involves every factor in coagulation mechanism
Prothrombin time (s)	12 to 20	12 to 14	12 to 15	10 to 13	Measures activity of prothrombin, fibrinogen, and factors V, VII, and X
Partial thromboplastin time (s)	90	90	90	90	Determines deficiencies of factors V, VII, VIII, IX, X, XI, and XII
Thrombin time (s)	3 to 5	3 to 5	3 to 5	3 to 5	Time for plasma to clot in presence of added plasma. Measures level of fibrinogen

prolonged bleeding occurs after circumcision or when there is severe bruising during the toddler period.

When the child reaches school age, he or she must cope with the most debilitating complications of the disorder, *hemarthrosis*, or bleeding into joints. Although any joint may be involved, the order of decreasing frequency of involvement is as follows: knee, elbow, ankle, hip, and shoulder. The child is usually limited in play activities because of tenderness, pain, and restricted motion. If bleeding progresses, the joint becomes swollen, hot, and immobile. The repeated presence of blood in joints causes degeneration of the synovial membrane with ankylosis, contractures, muscle weakness, and atrophy. If improperly treated, these changes can become permanent.

Because moisture is continually present in mucous membranes, bleeding there is often persistent, with considerable blood loss. Following a dental extraction, slow oozing may persist for

Table 23-9 Plasma Level of Factor VIII Related to Severity of Bleeding Tendency

Plasma Level of Factor VIII (AHF)	Degree of Bleeding	Symptoms
Less than 1%	Severe	Severe, spontaneous hemorrhage into large joints and deep tissues
1 to 5%	Moderately severe	Gross bleeding after minor injuries; some hemarthrosis and spontaneous bleeding
5 to 20%	Moderate	Bleeding after minor trauma or surgery
20 to 60%	Mild	Bleeding after major trauma or surgery
60 to 200%	Normal	No abnormal bleeding

up to 8 days. Bleeding can occur in any muscle but is seen most frequently in the calves, thighs, buttocks, and forearms. Retroperitoneal bleeding is fairly common; bleeding in the right iliopsoas region may mimic acute appendicitis.

Although it occurs infrequently, hemorrhage in the central nervous system is the major cause of death in hemophiliacs. Any trauma to the head or vertebral column should be treated immediately, and the child should be carefully observed for 24 h in a hospital.

Diagnostic tests Contrary to common belief, people with hemophilia do not bleed faster than others; they simply bleed longer. In patients with severe hemophilia, the coagulation time may range from 30 min to several hours. The partial thromboplastin time is significantly prolonged. Factor VIII is virtually absent from the plasma. When capillary fragility, bleeding time, prothrombin time, fibrinogen content, and platelet values are all within normal limits and the partial thromboplastin time is prolonged, a factor VIII assay should be performed, followed by a factor IX assay if factor VIII is normal. Accurate, timely diagnosis and reliable laboratory monitoring of treatment are fundamental to management of the child with hemophilia.

Treatment Modern hemophilia treatment consists of a comprehensive care approach based on the prevention or early treatment of bleeding. It addresses the medical, dental, orthopedic, educational, social, and behavioral problems encountered by hemophiliacs. In 1975, Congress established the Hemophilia Diagnostic and Treatment Center program. Twenty-five centers serve about half of the nation's 15,000 hemophiliacs. Each center utilizes the team approach.

Special efforts should be made to ensure a safe environment for an infant or a child. Cribs and playpens should be padded. As the child nears the toddler stage, large, hard toys and sharp pieces of furniture, such as end tables, should be removed to provide a safe area for exploration. As the child grows older, participation in noncontact sports, such as swimming, should be encouraged. Aspirin or aspirin-containing compounds should not be given, since aspirin inhibits platelet function. Acetaminophen, pentazocaine, propoxythene, or plain codeine can be used to alleviate pain.

Superficial abrasions and cuts usually stop bleeding if firm pressure is applied for several minutes. The treatment of choice for larger lacerations or internal bleeding is administration of lyophilized concentrates of factor VIII. The purpose is to raise the child's level of factor VIII to a certain percentage and to maintain it at that level until hemostasis is obtained. The half-life of AHF in the body is about 12 h.

Concentrates, listed in Table 23-10, are prepared by pharmaceutical companies from pools of human venous plasma from as many as 1000 donors. Concentrates cause few allergic reactions and are easy to reconstitute. Each unit of plasma utilized is nonreactive for hepatitis B surface antigen; unfortunately, this does not preclude the presence of the hepatitis virus.

Current research indicates that the hepatitis virus—as well as the human T-lymphotropic virus, type III (HTLV-III), and the lymphadenopathy-associated virus (LAV)—may be present in concentrates. Therefore, the child who receives a concentrate should be observed carefully for the signs and symptoms of hepatitis and aquired immunodeficiency syndrome (AIDS). (See Chap. 26.) Most commercial companies are heat-treating concentrates in the hope of reducing hemophiliacs' risk of contracting AIDS. Blood donors are also being screened for antibodies for AIDS. Approximately 1 percent of persons with AIDS are hemophiliacs or have other coagulation disorders.

Plasma from freshly drawn blood that is immediately frozen and then slowly thawed forms a precipitate that is a source of AHF. This product, *cryoprecipitate,* is the treatment of choice for the child who is rarely treated. Because cryoprecipitate requires few donors, the probability of transmitting infections with any one infusion is low. Carefully made cryoprecipitate contains about 100 units of factor VIII per bag. Blood

Table 23-10 Commercial Concentrates

Company	Name
Factor VIII	
Hyland	Hemofil
Courtland	AHG
Armour	Factorate
Alpha	Profilate
Cutter	Koate
Merieux	Actif-VIII
Factor IX	
Cutter	Konyne
Hyland	Proplex

type–specific cryoprecipitate should be given when large amounts of factor VIII are required, as in surgery. Both fresh frozen plasma and cryoprecipitate can cause severe allergic reactions.

Whether concentrate or cryoprecipitate is used, the child is given sufficient amounts to raise his or her AHF level by 30 to 100 percent, depending on the severity of the problem. To determine the number of factor VIII units needed to achieve a desired plasma factor VIII level, estimate the child's plasma volume (40 ml of plasma per kilogram of body weight) and multiply the plasma volume in milliliters by the desired increase in percent plasma factor VIII. For example, a child who has less than a 1 percent factor VIII level and weighs 38 kg has a plasma volume of 40 ml/kg × 38 kg, or 1500 ml. To raise the factor VIII level to 50 percent, the child will need 0.50 units per milliliter × 1500 ml, or 750 units of factor VIII.

It is usually difficult to control a hemorrhage in the mouth, tongue, or gums because the formed clot readily breaks down in the presence of saliva. In addition to factor replacement, which forms the clot, epsilon aminocaproic acid (Amicar), a fibrinolytic enzyme, helps preserve the clot until wound healing can occur. Parents should be instructed to give the aminocaproic acid every 6 h, not four times a day. This prevents the drug level from dropping during the night and the hemorrhage from recurring. Because of the possibility of disseminated intravascular clotting, aminocaproic acid is contraindicated in children who are suspected of having renal bleeding and in those who are receiving factor IX concentrate.

Inhibitors About 8 to 10 percent of children with severe classic hemophilia develop inhibitors to factor VIII. The antibody destroys the infused factor, rendering it ineffective in a clot formation. There is no way to predict who will develop inhibitors. Most inhibitors appear during childhood, but they may develop at any age in those who have frequently received plasma products. In most children the inhibitor level increases if additional factor VIII concentrate is administered; in a few, it remains low, despite further exposure to factor VIII. Porcine factor VIII concentrate, prothrombin complex concentrate, or anti-inhibitor coagulant complexes may be used; the latter are rarely given.

The treatment of children with inhibitors is difficult. Most institutions prefer to avoid plasma products for mild or moderate hemorrhages and rely on conservative methods, including ice packs, bed rest, and splinting.

Nursing management *Joints and muscles* The initial symptoms of a joint or muscle hemorrhage are pain, stiffness, and discomfort. If the child is treated with a 30 percent dose of concentrate at this time, the hemorrhage will usually stop, and there will be no need for joint aspiration or immobilization. Children with extensive hemorrhages in joints or muscles have swelling, increased warmth, and severe pain with motion; at this time a 50 percent dose will be required to stop the hemorrhage.

If the child has a painful effusion, aspiration may provide great relief of pain and lead to rapid recovery of function. Padded posterior molded splints may be applied for 3 to 4 days or until the swelling subsides. The child should be encouraged to exercise the involved joints as soon as the pain and swelling subside.

After any severe or prolonged hemorrhage, the nurse should evaluate the child for muscle atrophy or residual limitation of motion. Physical therapy should be instituted promptly, and a prophylactic dose (30 to 50 percent) of concentrate should be given each day before the exercise. If corrections are not made promptly, the stress of the abnormal distribution of weight during walking and the awkwardness of an abnormal alignment are likely to lead to further hemorrhage.

If a muscle or soft tissue hemorrhage presses on a nerve and decreases sensory or motor function, the child should receive repeated doses of plasma products until the swelling subsides. The nurse carefully assesses, records, and reports any progressive signs of sensory or motor loss. A hemorrhage in the iliopsoas muscle causes pain in the groin that sometimes radiates into the scrotum or lower quadrant of the abdomen. The hip is held in a flexed position, and extension is painful. Bleeding into the hip joint causes pain on hip rotation, while an iliopsoas bleed does not. The nurse should explain to the child that bed rest for 1 to 2 weeks and daily or twice-daily doses of plasma products are usually needed to achieve resolution of iliopsoas hemorrhages. When the pain has stopped and hip flexion is less than 25°, gentle exercises may be instituted in a pool. The nurse should encourage the child to progress slowly because iliopsoas hemorrhages recur easily. The use of crutches should also be encouraged until muscle strength returns.

Children with strong musculature have fewer hemorrhages than those with flabby muscles, because strong muscles support joints. From early childhood, a planned exercise program should be a part of the child's daily routine.

Hematuria The primary goal in treating *hematuria* is to *prevent* the formation of clots in the urine. Clots can block the urinary passages and cause further problems. The nurse who is caring for a child with hematuria should encourage the child to drink 6 to 8 oz of fluids every 2 to 3 h. The child should be taught to observe the color of the urine and to report any changes in color to the parents.

Emotional problems The diagnosis of hemophilia places stress on the family, particularly the parents and the affected child, but also on siblings and members of the extended family. From an early age, the child with hemophilia is expected to cope with untimely occurrences of painful hemorrhages resulting in immobilization, disruption of activities, hospitalizations, and joint deformities. At the same time, the child is expected to avoid dangerous endeavors, report hemorrhages promptly to his or her parents, reconcile these impulsive tendencies with wishes for independence, and ignore the many disruptions in educational plans. The current threat of being infected with the AIDS virus places an additional burden of fear on the child and the family. If the child is not helped to cope successfully with these problems, a broad range of crippling emotional problems may develop, including (1) low self-esteem and limited self-confidence, leading to excessive dependency and a failure to meet educational goals; (2) failure to accept the realities of hemophilia, leading to physical neglect; and (3) general prolonged immaturity and risk-taking behavior. Just as joint deformity can be minimized by prompt factor replacement therapy and exercise, crippling emotional problems can be prevented if they are recognized and treated in early childhood.

The most frequently observed problems among parents are (1) a tendency to overprotect the child or place undue restrictions on his or her activity, (2) a feeling of being burdened by the constant need to assess the child's health status and activity level, and (3) the father's lack of involvement in the child's care.

Common problems encountered by other family members are (1) siblings' feelings of being unloved, resentful, or envious of the attention that the parents give to the child with hemophilia; (2) carrier daughters' or sisters' fear of having children; and (3) grandparents' experiencing some of the stresses felt by the parents.

Emotional problems in children with hemophilia can be reduced if professional personnel and parents adopt attitudes and measures to help these children develop positive attitudes toward themselves and their disorder. Early in their lives, the following factors must be considered:

1. Emotional development is the same in all children. First, hemophiliac children are individuals; second, they have a disorder.
2. Interdependence requires the active participation of both parents.
3. Regardless of rigid supervision, they will hemorrhage as a result of some daily activities.
4. They should be allowed to discover appropriate activities during the preschool years.
5. They should be allowed to participate in their own care.
6. They should be included in decisions about their activities.
7. They should be given the maximum amount of information about their disorder.

Nurses can be most helpful in solving emotional problems if they readily refer children and their parents to appropriate counseling services as soon as a problem is detected. (See the Nursing Care Plan for a child with hemophilia A at the end of this chapter.)

Hemophilia B

Hemophilia B (Christmas disease, factor IX deficiency, or *PTC deficiency)* is an X-linked disorder resulting from a deficiency of factor IX coagulant activity. There are approximately seven cases of hemophilia A for every case of hemophilia B. The symptoms and management of hemophilia B are similar to those of classic hemophilia. It is important to distinguish between them in the laboratory because their treatment requires different replacement factors.

Home infusion programs

In the past, children with hemophilia experienced many hospitalizations with periods of extended bed rest for blood transfusions or other treatments. The availability of commercial concentrates, however, has made home infusion programs possible. Participants in a home infusion program are taught to recognize early symptoms of bleeding. With prompt treatment, most bleeding episodes are controlled quickly (Table 23-11). The following criteria must be met by participants in a home infusion program:

1. The family must indicate readiness to participate in the program.
2. The family must want to participate in the program.
3. The child must be 5 or 6 years old. Younger children may participate if they will sit still for venipunctures.
4. The veins must be large enough for successful venipuncture.
5. The child must require infusion at least once per week.
6. The parents must demonstrate maturity and be able to read instructions.
7. The parents and the child must have the emotional stability to accept the responsibilities of the program.
8. The parents must not have a frost-free freezer if the child will be receiving cryoprecipitate.
9. The family must participate in follow-up.
10. The child must have a complete physical examination.

When a family has been selected for a home infusion program in an outpatient setting, the nurse should individualize the instructions to meet the family's needs. Several sessions should be devoted to giving information about hemophilia as well as the technical aspects of performing the venipuncture. Emphasis should be placed on sterile technique and the signs and symptoms of bleeding and hepatitis, as well as on when not to treat the child at home. Adequate recording and follow-up should be stressed. Before beginning the program, the parents or the child must demonstrate several successful attempts at venipuncture (Fig. 23-8). The nurse must emphasize the fact that the home infusion program is not a substitute for continuous supervised medical care.

Thrombocytopenic purpura

Thrombocytopenic purpura is a deficiency of platelets (fewer than 100,000 per cubic millimeter) that occurs most often in 3- to 7-year-olds. The etiology is unclear, but thrombocytopenic purpura may result from such causes as destruction of platelets, infection, drug sensitivity, or exposure to ionizing radiation.

Drugs which destroy the platelets in both the mother and the fetus or which cause antibody formation against the fetal platelets are the thiazides, the sulfonamides, and quinine. These drugs should be taken with extreme caution during pregnancy.

The characteristic symptoms of thrombocytopenic purpura are spontaneous small hemorrhages (petechial lesions) into the skin or mucous membranes and bleeding from the nose, the gastrointestinal tract, or the urinary tract. The platelet count is always below 100,000 per cubic millimeter and may be as low as 10,000 per cubic millimeter.

Mothers who have thrombocytopenic purpura may give birth to infants with the disorder. Maternal antibodies cross the placenta and destroy the infant's platelets through a mechanism similar to that in Rh isoimmune disease. Thrombocytopenic purpura in newborns may also be caused by septicemia, congenital syphilis, or a congenital lack of megakaryocytes. In newborns the disorder is usually mild, and the platelet count rises within a short time after birth.

Acute thrombocytopenic purpura, which is characterized by a sudden onset, most often affects children and young adults, especially females. It may follow a mild respiratory infection or rubella. Fever and prostration are present. Spontaneous disappearance of the symptoms occurs in approximately 80 percent of children after a few weeks to a few months. Chronic thrombocytopenic purpura, which has a gradual onset, affects approximately 10 to 15 percent of the people with the disorder. It may start at any age but is seen infrequently in children. Clinical remissions and exacerbations occur, but the platelet count is always low. The size of the spleen is within normal limits. Children with the disorder have a tendency to bleed from many capillaries rather than from large vessels.

The diagnosis is confirmed with a series of coagulation tests related to platelet function. Platelets cannot be seen in a peripheral blood smear. WBCs are not affected; anemia, if present, is secondary, but partial thromboplastin time and prothrombin time are normal. Clot retraction is poor, since capillary fragility is greatly increased. Bone marrow is studied to rule out leukemia.

Treatment Corticosteroids are used to treat patients with moderately severe thrombocytopenic purpura of short duration, especially if the bleeding is from the gastrointestinal or genitourinary tract. The steroids produce a temporary increase

Table 23-11 Guidelines for the Home Infusion Instruction Program for the Child with Hemophilia

I. Venipuncture
   A. Anatomy—circulatory system
      1. Use anatomic diagrams to help the parents visualize appropriate veins. Allow for seven to ten instruction sessions.
   B. Actual practice of venipuncture
      1. Allay anxiety by allowing the parents to attempt venipuncture during each session.
      2. The child may be given a small amount of concentrate during each instruction session.

II. Concentrate preparation
   A. Concentrate
      1. Prescribed by the physician and dispensed by a pharmacy or blood bank.
      2. Price varies greatly, depending on geographic location and type of center.
      3. Average is 15 to 20 cents per unit for factor VIII. Slightly higher for factor IX.
   B. Dosage calculation
      1. Based on weight.
      2. Multiply the child's weight in kilograms by plasma volume (see example in text).
      3. Note: It is difficult to determine exact factor VIII units. Concentrate dosages are approximate and are rounded to the nearest hundred.
   C. Equipment needed
      1. Concentrate (see Table 23-10), diluent, 23-g scalp-vein needle, 30- to 50-ml syringe, antiseptic swab, tape, and bandage.
   D. Sterile techniques
      1. Stress throughout instruction sessions.
      2. Evaluate technique periodically.
   E. Storage of equipment
      1. Store equipment out of reach of children.
      2. Place concentrate in closed plastic container in refrigerator.
      3. Cryoprecipitate must not be stored in frost-free freezer. The temperature does not remain constant.
   F. Disposal of equipment
      1. Place entire syringe and used equipment in plastic or metal container.
      2. Return to center for disposal.

III. Hemophilia—related information
   A. Definition
      1. Give the parents a definition they can understand.
      2. Always include the child in the teaching.
      3. Include genetic information.
   B. Safety
      1. Proper storage and use of equipment.
      2. Hand-washing techniques.
   C. Dietary habits
      1. Prevent obesity.
      2. Encourage proper nutrition.
      3. Encourage intake of foods with high iron content.
   D. Exercise program
      1. Swimming.
      2. Bicycling.
      3. Gradual, gentle exercise program to strengthen all muscles.
      4. Refer to physical exercise program.
   E. Disciplinary actions
      1. Use appropriate measures that do not cause bleeding episodes.
   F. School habits
      1. Encourage school attendance.
      2. When the child is able to self-administer concentrate, get permission to keep one dose at school.
   G. Signs and symptoms of hemorrhages
      1. Discoloration, swelling, warmth, increasing immobility, and pain.
   H. Hepatitis
      1. Flulike symptoms, nausea, anorexia, malaise, fatigue, and moderate fever.
   I. Medications
      1. Instruct the parents to read medication labels to make sure they do not contain aspirin.
      2. Use acetaminophen for pain relief.

Table 23-11 Guidelines for the Home Infusion Instruction Program for the Child with Hemophilia (*Continued*)

- J. Allergic responses
  1. Instruct the parents to observe the child during each infusion for allergic responses.
     - a. Increased pulse and respirations.
     - b. Tingling sensation in the tongue and lips.
     - c. Flushes.
     - d. Itching, hives, or a rash.
  2. Increased pulse and respirations, tingling sensation in the tongue and lips, and flushes usually indicate that the rate of infusion is too rapid.
  3. If hives or a rash appears, stop infusion, record lot number, and report to the physician.
- K. When to contact the center or the physician
  1. After any head injury.
  2. When there is gastrointestinal bleeding.
  3. When there is neck or throat bleeding.
  4. When there is hemoptysis.
  5. When hemorrhage is not improved after three dosages of concentrate.
  6. When there is chest pain.
  7. When there is severe abdominal or back pain.
  8. When there is advanced joint or muscle bleeding (numbness or tingling or weakness of the extremities).

IV. Follow-up evaluation
- A. Review of venipuncture and preparation of concentrate
  1. Have a parent demonstrate the process at least once a year.
  2. Inform the parents of any new information.
- B. Evaluation of records
  1. Evaluate records for correlation with instructions.
  2. Note frequency and areas of bleeds.
  3. Make appropriate referral for persistent problems.

V. Termination from the program
- A. Poorly kept records
  1. Records must be accurate and complete.
  2. Concentrate and supplies must be accounted for.
- B. No annual physical examination
  1. Must have complete annual physical examination.
  2. Treatment regimen is altered if the child develops an inhibitor.
- C. Misuse of the program
  1. Records of hemorrhage indicate a delay in treatment.
  2. The parents fail to report certain hemorrhages to the center or the physician.
  3. There is drug abuse or use of supplies for other purposes.

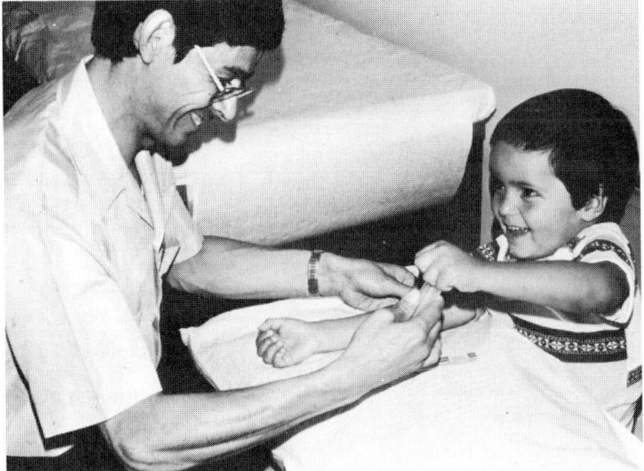

Figure 23-8 A father administering concentrate of factor VIII to his son at home.

in the platelet count and in some children will terminate the disorder within a few days. Transfusions of whole blood or platelets may be used when there has been substantial blood loss.

A splenectomy is usually the treatment of choice for patients with chronic cases of moderately severe thrombocytopenic purpura of more than 1 year's duration. It is also indicated in patients who do not respond to steroids or who have had two to three relapses with steroid therapy. The platelet count rises promptly following the splenectomy and often doubles within the first 24 h. Maximum values are reached 1 to 2 weeks postoperatively. A splenectomy is considered successful when the platelet count remains normal for at least 2 months. A splenectomy is curative in 70 to 90 percent of all patients.

Children with thrombocytopenic purpura should avoid trauma, contact sports, elective surgery, and tooth extraction. All unnecessary medications and exposure to potential toxins should be avoided. Children with mild thrombocytopenic purpura following viral infections do not require any treatment. They should be observed until petechiae disappear and the platelet count returns to normal.

Nursing management A primary concern in the nursing care of children with thrombocytopenic purpura is the concurrent bleeding tendency. The nursing assessment should begin with the prenatal history. A careful history of the mother's drug intake during pregnancy should be recorded. The nurse should observe the newborn's color and vital signs to detect the development of jaundice, ecchymoses, and petechial lesions. When the infant or child has an active period of bleeding, he or she should be observed closely for signs and symptoms of shock and possible internal and intracranial hemorrhage. If epistaxis (nosebleed) occurs, compression, packing, or hemostatic material may be utilized to control the bleeding.

The nurse must teach the child and the parents to assess the child's limitations and help the child adjust to them. Contact sports should be discouraged. The nurse should assist the child and parents in making the school and community aware of the child's limitations. When blood transfusions are indicated, the nurse should be supportive of both the parents and the child because they will be anxious at that time.

In planning for the child's discharge from the hospital, the nurse should teach the parents to recognize the signs of thrombocytopenic purpura, such as bleeding gums, petechiae, and ecchymoses. The parents should also be encouraged to continue medical supervision and to report any signs of bleeding to their physician immediately.

Nursing Care Plan: Hemophilia A

Patient: Roderick Wood **Age:** 5 years **Date of Admission:** 2/18 at 9 A.M.

ASSESSMENT

Roderick was admitted to the pediatric unit with a diagnosis of spontaneous massive right knee hemarthrosis secondary to hemophilia A.

GENERAL APPEARANCE

The right knee is tense, swollen, and hot. The overlying skin is shiny and red. The joint is slightly flexed, and range of motion is severely restricted. The pulse is irregular and weak. The skin is cool, clammy, and moist. He is anxious and frightened and is crying because the pain in his right knee is so severe.

PHYSICAL EXAMINATION

Weight: 27 kg. Pulse: 110. Respiratory rate: 24. Hemoglobin: 10 g. WBC: 10,800. AHF: below 1 percent.

HISTORY

Roderick's mother explained that he was diagnosed at birth as having severe hemophilia A. He has had only minor soft tissue bleeds. The family was on a camping trip when Roderick developed the spontaneous right knee hemorrhage. After the onset of mild pain, it took the family several hours to drive to the hospital. The nurse reported that the mother was visibly upset, stating that they should never have gone on a trip so far away from the hospital. She said that from now on they would stay home, even though the rest of the family loved to go camping.

PHYSICIAN'S ORDERS

1. 750 units of AHF concentrate IV q12h.
2. Elevate the right knee.
3. Apply an ice pack to the right knee.
4. Maintain absolute bed rest.
5. Meperidine 15 mg IM q4h prn for severe pain.
6. Acetaminophen 300 mg PO q4h prn for moderate pain.
7. Measure right knee circumference qd.
8. Vital signs q2h until stable.

Nursing Diagnosis	Outcome Criteria	Nursing Interventions	Evaluation and Modifications
1. Severe pain related to severe right knee hemorrhage	☐ Roderick will be more comfortable, as evidenced by: **a.** A decrease in frequency of administration of IM meperidine **b.** Cessation of crying **c.** Control of pain with Tylenol **d.** No complaints of pain with movement	☐ Administer IM meperidine regularly q4h while pain is severe (use small-gauge needle). ☐ Observe and record the effect of medication by asking Roderick whether his knee still hurts. ☐ Support bed covers over the knee. ☐ Change the ice pack prn. ☐ Support and elevate the right knee with a pillow. ☐ Prevent excessive movement.	☐ 2/18, 9 A.M.: Roderick stopped crying 20 min. after being given IM meperidine and said that his knee did not hurt 1 h after taking meperidine.

Nursing Diagnosis	Outcome Criteria	Nursing Interventions	Evaluation and Modifications
2. Severe spontaneous right knee hemorrhage related to hemophilia A	☐ Bleeding in the right knee will be controlled, as evidenced by: **a.** A reduction in the right knee circumference **b.** A reduction in the severity of pain **c.** An increase in range of motion **d.** A decrease in the temperature of the right knee **e.** A less shiny appearance of the right knee	☐ Immobilize the right knee. ☐ Administer concentrate as directed by the physician. ☐ Apply ice packs. ☐ Elevate the right knee. ☐ Administer pain medication as ordered. ☐ Maintain bed rest. ☐ Measure knee circumference q2h after injection of concentrate.	☐ Crying stopped. ☐ 4 h after concentrate injection, knee circumference was reduced by 2 cm. ☐ Roderick said that his knee does not hurt as much.
3. Potential for hemorrhage during nursing procedures related to hemophilia A	☐ Hemorrhages related to nursing procedures will be prevented, as evidenced by no hemorrhage.	☐ Take axillary temperature. ☐ Administer medications PO when possible. ☐ Rotate IM sites. ☐ Use small-gauge needles. ☐ Inject medication slowly. ☐ Apply pressure to the injection site. ☐ Maintain a safe environment.	☐ No evidence of hemorrhage.
4. Potential for continued bleeding related to inhibitor development to AHF	☐ Further bleeding will be prevented, as evidenced by: **a.** A decrease in the circumference of the right knee **b.** A decrease in the amount of pain experienced	☐ Measure the right knee circumference. ☐ Elevate the right knee. ☐ Keep an ice pack on the knee. ☐ Administer concentrate q12h. ☐ Check AHF level.	☐ Assay should reflect calculated rise in AHF level.
5. Potential fluid volume deficit related to blood loss into knee joint	☐ Adequate fluid balance will be maintained, as evidenced by: **a.** Oral fluid intake of at least 10 ml/h **b.** Urine output of at least 50 ml/h **c.** Urine specific gravity of 1.006 to 1.015 **d.** Moist oral mucous membranes **e.** Good skin turgor	☐ Encourage intake of fluids PO every 30 to 60 min. ☐ Record intake and output. ☐ Measure urine specific gravity at each voiding.	☐ 2/18, 12 noon: Oral intake was 300 ml; output was 225 ml; urine specific gravity 1.015.
6. Alteration in thermal regulation related to bleeding in right knee	☐ Temperature will be maintained within a normal range of 36 to 37.5°C (97.5 to 99.5°F).	☐ Monitor temperature q2h. ☐ Encourage intake of fluids PO every 30 to 60 min. ☐ Keep the bed dry, and the room cool. ☐ Administer acetaminophen q4h for temperature above 38.8°C (101°F).	☐ 2/18, 12 noon: Roderick is afebrile.

Nursing Diagnosis	Outcome Criteria	Nursing Interventions	Evaluation and Modifications
7. Fatigue related to pain and blood loss	☐ Fatigue will be decreased, as evidenced by: **a.** A relaxed state while resting **b.** A relaxed state when pain-free **c.** Sleeping 12 to 14 h per 24 h	☐ Schedule rest periods each day. ☐ Observe the quality and quantity of sleep. ☐ Administer analgesics prn. ☐ Schedule nursing care to include uninterrupted periods of rest. ☐ Limit visitors during rest periods. ☐ Monitor TV and radio use.	☐ 2/18, 2 P.M.: Roderick has had a 1-h nap and is resting quietly. His facial expression is relaxed.
8. Potential right knee contracture related to painful bleeding in right knee	☐ Permanent right knee contracture will be prevented, as evidenced by: **a.** Full range of motion in the right knee when pain and swelling subside **b.** Ambulation without pain	☐ Administer analgesics prn. ☐ Allow for gentle range of motion of knee during peak action of analgesics. ☐ Keep the right knee elevated and properly supported with pillows. ☐ Elicit the child's cooperation in straightening his knee as much as possible. ☐ Maintain the body in good alignment, and change position q2h.	☐ 2/18, 4 P.M.: There is improved extension of, and reduced swelling in, the right knee. Moves knee with greater ease. ☐ Plan for 2/20: Begin gentle passive exercise. Refer Roderick to physical therapy. Encourage water exercise, such as in a pool or a whirlpool bath.
9. Parental anxiety and guilt related to delay in getting medical assistance	☐ The parents will experience decreased anxiety and guilt, as evidenced by: **a.** Decreased self-blame **b.** Increased satisfaction with their role performance	☐ Assess the parents' anxiety level. ☐ Assess the parents' willingness to participate in a home infusion program. ☐ Assess and identify: **a.** The parents' feelings about hemophilia **b.** The parents' knowledge of their child's condition **c.** Familial relationships and support systems **d.** The coping mechanisms used by the parents ☐ Encourage the parents to: **a.** Permit the child to participate in activities **b.** Allow the child to participate in his care	☐ 2/18, 5 P.M.: The parents were asked whether they would like to be instructed in how to administer AHF to Roderick. They were assured that this would allow the family to continue to go on camping trips. ☐ The parents were told that this is a common occurrence and that if they had been able to treat Roderick at the first sign of a hemorrhage, they could have helped prevent the painful swollen knee that followed. ☐ The parents appeared eager to participate in the home infusion program. Instructions are to be scheduled by the nurse.

Bibliography

Baglini, Robert, "Laboratory Evaluation of Factor VIII and Factor IX," *American Journal of Medical Technology* **49**(12):857–862 (1983).

Beck, William S., *Hematology*, M.I.T., Cambridge, Mass., 1981.

Ciavarella, David, and Richard Counts, "Clinical Aspects of Hemophilia and von Willebrand's Disease," *American Journal of Medical Technology* **49**(12):850–854 (1983).

Embury, Stephen H., Andree M. Dozy, Judy Miller, J. R. Davis, Jr., Klara M. Kleman, Haiganoush Preisler, Elliott Vichinsky, William N. Lande, Bertram H. Lubin, Y. W. Kan, and William C. Mentzer, "Concurrent Sickle-Cell Anemia and α-Thalassemia," *The New England Journal of Medicine* **306**:270–274 (February 1982).

Fauci, Anthony, and Clifford Lane, "Overview of Clinical Syndromes and Immunology of AIDS," *Topics in Clinical Nursing* **6**(2):12–18 (July 1984).

Fischbach, Frances T., *A Manual of Laboratory Diagnostic Tests*, Lippincott, Philadelphia, 1984.

Gerald, Michael C., and Freda V. O'Bannon, *Nursing Pharmacology and Therapeutics*, Prentice-Hall, Englewood Cliffs, N.J., 1981.

Howes, Anne C., "Nursing Diagnoses and Care Plans for Ambulatory Care Patients with AIDS," *Topics in Clinical Nursing* **6**(2):61–66 (July 1984).

Koch, Barbara, Frank Galioto, Jack Kelleher, and David Goldstein, "Physical Fitness in Children with Hemophilia," *Archives of Physical Medicine and Rehabilitation* **65**:324–326 (1984).

Mears, J. Gregory, Herbert M. Lachman, Dominique Labie, and Ronald L. Nagel, "Alpha-Thalassemia Is Related to Prolonged Survival in Sickle Cell Anemia," *Blood* **62**:286–290 (August 1983).

Mooney, Nancy, "Hemophilic Arthropathy: A Literature Review," *Orthopedic Nursing* **2**(6):37–38 (1983).

Nagel, Ronald L., Mary E. Fabry, and D. K. Kaul, "New Insights on Sickle Cell Anemia," *Diagnostic Medicine* **7**:26–33 (May 1984).

Rapaport, Samuel I., *Introduction to Hematology*, Harper & Row, New York, 1971.

Rubinow, David, "The Psychological Impact of the Acquired Immune Deficiency Syndrome," *Topics in Clinical Nursing* **6**(2):26–30 (July 1984).

Ryan, Laura, "AIDS: A Threat to Physical and Psychological Integrity," *Topics in Clinical Nursing* **6**(2):19–25 (July 1984).

Schmalzer, Emily, Shu Chien, and Audrey K. Brown, "Transfusion Therapy in Sickle Cell Disease," *The American Journal of Pediatric Hematology/Oncology* **4**:395–406 (Winter 1982).

Sergis-Deavenport, Elaine, and James W. Varri, "Behavioral Techniques in Teaching Hemophilia Factor Replacement Procedures to Families," *Pediatric Nursing* **8**(6):416–419 (November–December 1982).

Smith, Peter, and Peter Levine, "The Benefits of Comprehensive Care of Hemophilia: A Five-Year Study of Outcome," *American Journal of Public Health* **74**(6):616–617 (June 1984).

Steinberg, Martin H., Wendy Rosenstock, Mary B. Coleman, Junious G. Adams, Ovidiu Platica, Marisol Cedeno, Ronald F. Reider, John T. Wilson, Paul Milner, and Stewart West, "Effects of Thalassemia and Microcytosis on the Hematologic and Vasoocclusive Severity of Sickle Cell Anemia," *Blood* **63**:1353–1360 (June 1984).

Trotter, Carol, and Duane K. Hasegawa, "Hemophilia B: Case Study and Intervention Plan," *Journal of Gynecological and Neonatal Nursing* **12**(2):82–85 (March–April 1983).

Vichinsky, Elliot P., Robert Johnson, and Bertram Lubin, "Multidisciplinary Approach to Pain Management in Sickle Cell Disease," *The American Journal of Pediatric Hematology/Oncology* **4**:328–332 (Fall 1982).

Walters, Ida, Monica S. Rozzell, Marva Hijazi, Becky Pack, Jane Luff, and Gloria Moore, "Complications of Sickle Cell Disease," *Nursing Clinics of North America* **18**(1):139–199 (March 1983).

24

Patricia J. Salisbury

Hormone regulation

Upon completion of this chapter, the student will be able to:

1 Describe negative feedback as it applies to the endocrine system.
2 List the glands in the endocrine system.
3 Describe the pathophysiology of hypopituitarism.
4 List four actions to be taken to assure proper administration of Pitressin.
5 Discuss the nursing care involved with a water-deprivation test.
6 Discuss the nursing care involved with a growth hormone stimulation test.
7 Discuss at least four areas of teaching to be covered with the family of a child with precocious puberty.
8 Identify at least five signs of hypothyroidism in infants.
9 Discuss the nursing care of a hypothyroid child when initially treated.
10 Discuss the nursing care of a hyperthyroid child when initially treated.
11 Discuss the nursing care of a child who has undergone a thyroidectomy.
12 Describe the functions of the hormones secreted by the cortex and medulla of the adrenal gland.
13 List at least five symptoms of hypoadrenocorticism.
14 Describe the pathophysiology of congenital adrenal hyperplasia.
15 List at least five physical symptoms of Cushing syndrome.
16 Discuss the nursing care of an adrenalectomy patient.
17 Describe the pathophysiology of diabetes mellitus.
18 Describe the pathophysiology of ketoacidosis.
19 Compare and contrast short-, intermediate-, and long-acting insulins.
20 Discuss the nursing care of a patient in ketoacidosis.
21 Compare first-void and second-void urines.
22 List at least four principles of insulin administration.
23 Compare and contrast hypoglycemia and hyperglycemia.

The endocrine system is composed of a number of glands located throughout the body that are responsible for growth, maturation, reproduction, metabolic processes, and the reaction of the body to stress. The endocrine system controls these processes through the secretion of *hormones,* which are chemical substances released directly into the bloodstream.

Some endocrine glands—the thyroid, parathyroids, thymus, pancreas, adrenals, and gonads (ovaries and testes)—work under the coordination of the pituitary gland, which for this reason is known as the *master gland.* This system is kept in equilibrium through negative feedback control. The pituitary gland secretes several *tropic* hormones, each of which stimulates a specific endocrine gland (called the *target gland* for that hormone). For example, the tropic substance thyroid-stimulating hormone (TSH) acts on the thyroid gland. Each target gland, in response to the pituitary hormone, releases its own hormones. In turn, elevated levels of the target gland hormone signal the pituitary to inhibit secretion of the tropic hormone. Likewise, the pituitary

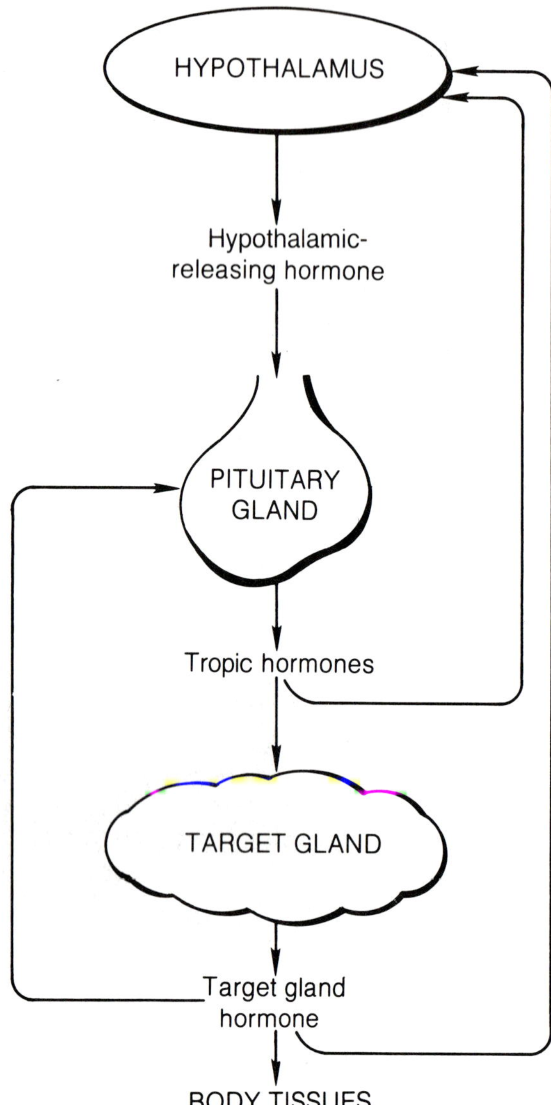

Figure 24-1 Negative feedback in the endocrine system.

detects low levels of the target gland hormone and then increases its tropic hormone secretion to cause increased secretion of the target gland hormone.

The *hypothalamus,* a portion of the brain located at the base of the skull, is also involved in hormonal secretion. A hypothalamic-releasing hormone (or factor) is secreted to regulate the secretion of each pituitary hormone. Similarly, high levels of pituitary hormone inhibit the release of hypothalamic hormones, and low levels of target gland hormone increase secretion. For example, in the case of the thyroid gland, the pituitary secretes TSH, which causes the thyroid to release thyroxine (T_4) and triiodothyronine (T_3). Elevated levels of T_4 and T_3 inhibit the release of TSH. When circulating levels of T_4 and T_3 fall, the hypothalamus secretes thyrotropin-releasing factor (TRF), which stimulates the pituitary, and the cycle is begun again (see Fig. 24-1).

Thus, when a problem develops in the endocrine system, it can be based at the level of the hypothalamus, the pituitary gland, or the target endocrine organ. Disorders of the endocrine glands are due mainly to hyperfunction and hypofunction; *hyperfunction* is excessive secretion of the hormone, and *hypofunction* is deficient secretion of the hormone.[1]

PITUITARY GLAND

Anatomy and physiology

The *pituitary gland,* or *hypophysis,* is an organ about the size of a fingertip located at the base of the brain and surrounded by the bony cup in the skull known as the *sella turcica.* Its connection to the hypothalamus is the hypophyseal stalk. The pituitary is divided into three sections: the anterior pituitary, or *adenohypophysis;* the intermediate lobe, or *pars intermedia;* and the posterior pituitary, or *neurohypophysis.*

The anterior pituitary secretes six identifiable hormones: (1) adrenocorticotropic hormone (ACTH); (2) thyroid-stimulating hormone (TSH), or thyrotropin; (3) growth hormone (GH), or somatotropin; (4) follicle-stimulating hormone (FSH); (5) luteinizing hormone (LH); and (6) prolactin (PRL), or luteotropic hormone. Their principal functions are listed in Table 24-1.

Hypopituitarism

Hypopituitarism occurs when the secretion of one or more pituitary hormones is deficient. As mentioned previously, this can result from a problem in the pituitary or the hypothalamus, although it is often difficult to identify where the problem originates. When all pituitary hormones are deficient, the condition is called *panhypopituitarism.* Although this condition is uncommon in children, it may occur as the result of a congenital defect or the development of a cra-

Table 24-1 Hormones of the Pituitary Gland

Hormone	Principal Functions
Anterior Pituitary Hormones	
ACTH (adrenocorticotropic hormone)	Stimulation of cortisol production by the adrenal cortex
TSH (thyroid-stimulating hormone)	Stimulation of thyroxine (T_4) and triiodothyronine (T_3) production by the thyroid
GH (growth hormone)	Developmental enlargement of body tissues via cell hypertrophy and hyperplasia
FSH (follicle-stimulating hormone)	Stimulation of ovarian follicle growth in the female and spermatogenesis in the male
LH (luteinizing hormone)	Stimulation of ovulation in the female and testosterone secretion in the male
PRL (prolactin)	Milk production in the lactating female
Intermediate Lobe Hormones	
MSH (melanocyte-stimulating hormone)	Involved in control of skin pigmentation
Posterior Pituitary Hormones	
ADH (antidiuretic hormone)	Functions in fluid and electrolyte balance by controlling reabsorption of water in the kidneys
Oxytocin	Milk ejection in the lactating female; uterine contractions

niopharyngioma. This nonmalignant cystic tumor of embryonic origin causes damage to the pituitary and hypothalamus through the accumulation of fluid in the tumor and the resulting pressure, rather than through metastasis. Children with hypopituitarism usually present with headaches, vomiting, and visual disturbance, because of the proximity of the pituitary and hypothalamus to the optic nerves. The past growth records of many of these children show a falling off on the growth grids as they became increasingly deficient in GH. If the child has reached adolescence, he or she may be most concerned about the failure to progress to normal puberty.

Single deficiencies in anterior pituitary hormones are not uncommon. The most frequently seen problem is isolated GH deficiency. This appears to be an inherited condition, often occurring in more than one child in a family.[2] GH causes growth of the cartilaginous parts of the bone and increases protein synthesis and the mobilization of stored fat in muscle and adipose tissue. Children with GH deficiency are of normal size at birth but develop growth retardation within the first 2 years of life. They are often below the 5th percentile or fail to grow more than 5 cm per year. Their growth curve, when plotted on normal growth grids (see Appendix B), appears to take a right turn somewhere before the age of 2. These children often have an infantile appearance (chubby bodies and round faces) and frequently show poor muscular development. If not diagnosed before their adolescent years, they will fail to attain normal puberty, even though they have normal pituitary sex hormones.

Diagnostic tests The diagnostic tests used to evaluate hypopituitarism are extensive, since each hormone must be evaluated. GH deficiency is evaluated by means of a stimulation test using exercise and a variety of substances such as arginine, insulin, estrogens, and L-dopa. Blood samples are obtained every 15 to 30 min over the course of several hours. All these substances appear to stimulate the release of GH, and a rise in GH level is expected in the normal patient. Thyroid and adrenal function are both evaluated through simple blood tests not involving stimulation, although these may be combined with a GH stimulation test. TSH levels are measurable in the blood. It is difficult to measure levels of ACTH, and therefore adrenal function is evaluated by measuring cortisol levels. LH and FSH can be measured directly in the blood. Recent technological advances have resulted in the isolation of gonadotropin-releasing hormone (GRH) and thyrotropin-releasing hormone (TRH). These substances are administered to individuals in an attempt to stimulate release of LH, FSH, and TSH, thereby differentiating pituitary and hypothalamic lesions. Frequently, bone age will be measured in order to evaluate a child's skeletal growth. X-ray pictures of the hands and wrists are taken, and the ossification of the child's bones is compared with standards for the child's sex and age.

Treatment and nursing management The role of the nurse in caring for children with pituitary problems can be extensive and may develop into a long-term relationship, since these children need continuing health care supervision. Often the nurse first becomes involved with a child and his or her family during the evaluation of the child's medical problem. This is usually an extremely stressful time for the family and the child because of the physical discomfort from the many blood tests that are ordered and the time required to reach a diagnosis. Anxiety is increased when the parents identify the problem as being "in the head" and envision craniotomy as the cure.

If craniotomy is the treatment of choice for a pituitary tumor, the nurse is involved with the child both before and after surgery. The child and the family need specific explanations of what will be done during surgery and what they can expect after surgery, since many fantasies are associated with surgery of the head. Because of the proximity of the optic nerves to the hypothalamic-pituitary region, blindness is always a danger in this type of surgery, and the family must be aware of this potential complication.[3] The nurse should be available and encourage the family and the child to discuss their fears of blindness. If there is decreasing vision after surgery, the nurse can help the child make some initial adjustments to the situation.

Two approaches are used for pituitary surgery: a frontal approach and a transsphenoidal approach. Postoperatively, the child is observed for signs of cerebral edema or increased intracranial pressure. Vital signs and neurological status are assessed frequently, and the dressings are observed. Leakage of cerebrospinal fluid may occur around the incision site in the frontal approach and from the nose in the transsphenoidal approach. A muscle graft is used to close the opening made for the exposure of the pituitary in the transsphenoidal approach, and the child is cautioned not to blow his or her nose in order to avoid moving the graft. The child is checked for signs of infection, since meningitis is a serious complication of surgery. Diabetes insipidus is a frequent transient problem after surgery. The nurse needs to observe the hourly urine output. The physician should be notified when the hourly output is over 100 ml or when the specific gravity is less than 1.010. Excessive fluid loss through the urine may result in dehydration. Postoperatively, the child may be required to undergo further testing to see whether pituitary function has been altered by surgery.[4]

Children with hypopituitarism and their families need a great deal of education following the diagnosis. A variety of medications will be used to replace the hormones that are now deficient. These may include thyroid, vasopressin, cortisone, mineralocorticoids, and estrogens or androgens. The parents need to know which specific drugs the child is receiving, why their child is receiving those drugs, and the importance of daily administration of the medications. This is especially important for children who are receiving cortisone replacement, since these children are adrenally insufficient. Stresses such as minor illnesses, fever, and accidents raise the child's cortisone requirements, which must be met by giving larger doses of medication. The nurse (in collaboration with dietitians and occupational and physical therapists) is responsible for teaching the parents how to meet the diversified needs of the child with hypopituitarism.

Children who are being evaluated for GH deficiency have special problems. Many of these problems are psychological. Older children are very short in comparison with their peers and as a result have usually taken a great deal of teasing. If their friends have entered puberty, then the teasing may center on sexual immaturity. Often these children are mistakenly believed to be much younger than they are, which can be most distressing to them. Younger children with severely impaired height have problems as well. They may be mistaken for infants, even though they are 3 or 4 years old, and may be babied or overprotected by those around them, leading to delays in development. The parents may be torn between finding an answer to the problem of the child's short stature and wanting to keep a delightful child dependent even longer. The child may also be ridiculed by peers because of the obesity that results from a lack of GH. Initial evaluation will include a GH stimulation test. During this test, the nurse needs to supervise the child closely. A heparin lock intravenous needle is inserted to reduce the number of venipunctures needed for drawing blood during the test. The nurse must ensure that the needle is well anchored so that it does not become dislodged. This is particularly important if exercise is used as part of the protocol for the GH stimulation test. Not only are repeated venipunctures painful, but they are also often difficult to accomplish in children who are exceptionally small for their age. The most frequently used substance in GH stimulation tests is insulin. When insulin is injected intravenously, profound hypoglycemia is expected to occur. The nurse needs to be in attendance at all times when this test is being performed in order to detect early signs of hypoglycemia so that the test may be terminated when they occur.

GH deficiency is treated with GH derived from pituitary extracts of human autopsy material, given as an intramuscular injection three times per week. The supply of GH has always been limited. The majority was available on a research basis, and candidates were screened extensively for admission to programs. Some GH was available for purchase; however, the price was prohibitive for most families. In 1985 all GH derived from human sources was removed from use after three patients died of a rare disease thought to be a contaminant of the GH. This only adds to the stress that the family and the child are undergoing, and the nurse needs to be fully aware of this situation. A limited amount of GH produced through gene-splicing techniques is now available. Because bioengineering techniques allow much greater production of GH, treatment of many more children will eventually be possible. If the child begins to receive GH, the family or the child is taught the injection technique. Rotation of injection sites needs to be stressed, since treatment often takes several years. Although the child and the family may be much relieved when GH injections have begun, they must be warned that the final height achieved may not be optimal, since some children develop antibodies to exogenous GH.

Diabetes insipidus

Diabetes insipidus (DI) is the most frequently occurring disorder associated with problems of the posterior pituitary. It results from an insufficiency in the production of antidiuretic hormone (ADH). ADH is produced in the hypothalamus and transported to the posterior pituitary, where it is released in response to an increased plasma osmolality and a decrease in extracellular fluid. ADH causes the renal tubules to reabsorb more fluid, resulting in retention of water in the body. True DI is a result of a deficiency of ADH, but a similar problem is caused by failure of the kidneys to respond to the action of ADH (nephrogenic DI) or compulsive water drinking (psychogenic DI).

DI may develop at any age. A central nervous system tumor, often a craniopharyngioma, is a frequent cause in children, although a significant number of children have idiopathic DI with no identifiable cause. DI may also be the result of congenital malformations of the central nervous system, histiocytosis X, or head trauma. Children with DI complain of polyuria and polydipsia. Infants often show a preference for water instead of milk. If the child has idiopathic DI, there will be no other symptoms. Headache, vomiting, and visual disturbance may indicate the presence of a central nervous system tumor, and there may be evidence of other pituitary deficiencies as well.

Diagnostic tests Since it is impossible to measure vasopressin levels, DI is evaluated by the individual's response to a water-deprivation test. The test is begun by giving the child nothing by mouth for 8 h. The urine specific gravity, urine volume, and body weight are then measured hourly. Serial determinations are obtained for sodium and urine and serum osmolality. Hematocrit and blood urea nitrogen may also be obtained. In a child with ADH deficiency who is losing large amounts of free body water, it is expected that the urine specific gravity will remain below 1.005, that the urine osmolality will remain below 150 mOsmol per kilogram, and that there will be no significant reduction in urine volume. Serum osmolality and sodium are expected to rise. Blood urea nitrogen and the hematocrit are used to evaluate whether the child received any water during the test.[5]

Treatment DI is treated with the administration of synthetic vasopressin. However, all forms of the drug now available involve difficulties in administration. Vasopressin tannate (Pitressin) in oil is a commonly used preparation. In this preparation, tiny flecks of the vasopressin are suspended in peanut oil, which makes even distribution of the drug in the oil very difficult. The duration of the effects of this preparation varies from individual to individual, and the administration schedule must be altered to meet the child's response. Most children require injections every 36 to 48 h. Lypressin (Diapid), a synthetic antidiuretic nasal spray, is easy to administer and is preferred by some older children. The duration of action varies from child to child, but most experience effects that last from 3 to 6 h. Frequent administration of the medication is a problem for some children, particularly at night. Absorption of the medication is also hindered by inflammation of the mucosa, and therefore it is less effective when the child has any upper respiratory infection. Desamino d-arginine vasopressin (DDAVP), a long-acting form of vasopressin nasal spray, is now the most popular preparation used. This form requires administration approximately twice a day. However, for many families, this medication may be prohibitively expensive.

Nursing management The child who is being evaluated for DI has some problems similar to those experienced by the child who is being evaluated for GH deficiency. The water-deprivation test is a long and difficult test for the child to endure. It is the nurse's major responsibility to assure that the child does not receive any type of fluid during the test period. Some children become obsessed with obtaining fluids and find devious ways to get them. Children have been known to drink from toilets, vases of flowers, and urinals. It is often a good idea to have a plumber turn off the water supply to the sink in the child's room while the test is being conducted. Some children require 24-h supervision during testing.

Accurate measurements of urinary output and urine specific gravity are essential during the test, as is accurate weighing. If the test continues during a change of staff, it is essential that the nurse coming on duty weigh the child in exactly the same manner as during the previous shift. If Pitressin is administered while the child is in the hospital, the nurse must observe for signs that the drug is diminishing in effectiveness, usually 36 to 48 h after administration. At this point, the child will begin to have increased urination, with a resulting increase in thirst. Before the child is discharged, the child and the family must be educated in the administration of vasopressin. If the child is placed on Pitressin, the family and/or the child must be taught the injection technique. The nurse and the family must be aware of the difficulties in administering Pitressin. Holding the vial under warm water will aid in drawing up the thick oil. Getting the flecks of vasopressin uniformly suspended is essential. This is best accomplished by vigorous shaking and flicking of the vial for 5 min. If the entire contents of the vial is not used at each injection, the remaining medication must be discarded, since there is no way to resuspend the preparation. Many children are allowed to decide when the next injection is due on the basis of increasing symptoms, rather than administering the drug according to a set schedule. Likewise, children who are placed on lypressin and desamino d-arginine vasopressin are taught to carry their medication with them so that they may use it when they have increasing urination.

Precocious puberty

Precocious puberty, or the development of secondary sex characteristics before the age of 8 or 9 years, is much more common in girls than in boys. Although central nervous system disorders, tumors, and adrenal disorders are causes of precocious puberty, the most common finding in girls is idiopathic precocious puberty. In these children there appears to be an early release of GRH from the hypothalamus, resulting in release of LH and FSH from the pituitary. These high levels of LH and FSH cause varying degrees of sexual precocity. The child may have precocious development of breast tissue (premature thelarche), which occurs most often in girls between the ages of 6 months and 2 years, or precocious appearance of sexual hair (premature adrenarche), which usually occurs in older girls, aged 5 to 8 years, or the child may progress to full puberty with menstruation.[6] With the onset of puberty, these children will have a corresponding growth spurt, which makes them taller than their peers during childhood but ultimately leads to early closure of the epiphyses with resulting short stature in adulthood.

Although organic causes of precocious puberty in the female are rare, the possibility of organic disease or tumor must be investigated. Initial diagnostic tests include skull x-rays, bone age films, 24-h urinary 17-ketosteroids to evaluate adrenal function, T_4 to evaluate thyroid function, and serum LH and FSH. The most traumatic part of the evaluation is often the bimanual abdominal-rectal examination. For the young child, sedation or even anesthesia may be necessary to accomplish this examination.

Treatment and nursing management A variety of drugs have been used to treat idiopathic precocious puberty with variable success. Provera (medroxyprogesterone acetate) is the most widely used drug. It appears to decrease gonadotropin secretion, which results in halting the progression of puberty and stopping menstruation; however, it does not alter the rapid growth rate of bone maturation.[7] Provera is used primarily with a menstruating young child when the problems of hygiene are not insignificant or when the child's and the family's anxiety level is very high. Provera is administered in the form of tablets taken daily or intramuscular injections given monthly; the injections have been found to be more effective. See also Chap. 25.

Caring for the girl with precocious puberty and her family can be a real challenge to the nurse. Many fears center on sexual problems. Parents are often afraid that the child's psychosexual development will be advanced because of precocious puberty, although this is not the case. It is not uncommon to see little girls who are sexually mature playing with dolls during the course of their evaluation. Fathers frequently fear that the child will be sexually molested. All these problems need to be explored and dealt with openly with the parents. If the girl has not begun to menstruate at the time of the evaluation, the family needs assistance in planning a discussion with her about impending menstruation in terms that she can understand. Unexplained bleeding can be frightening to a very young child. Hygiene also needs to be discussed with the family, since most parents are not used to caring for a young child who has a vaginal discharge, adult sweat patterns, and normal oily adult skin. The problem of height also needs to be discussed with the family. While the girl is growing, she may be much taller than her peers, which only increases her visibility as a child who is different. However, as she grows older, her peers will catch up and pass her, and she will face the problems of the adolescent with short stature. If the child is placed on medication in order to stop menstruation, the family needs to understand the importance of maintaining the schedule for injections. Since children who are given this medication are often very young, play therapy may be indicated in order to help them work through their frustrations and anger at having to have frequent injections for a condition they cannot understand.

THE THYROID GLAND

Anatomy and physiology

The *thyroid gland* is an H-shaped organ located in the neck, anterior to the trachea. The gland is not normally visible in children, although the isthmus or crossbar may be palpable. An enlargement of the thyroid gland is termed a *goiter.*

The thyroid gland is involved in control of metabolism. When foods containing iodine are ingested, the iodine passes into the circulation, where it is absorbed by the thyroid gland. This iodine then reacts with a protein called *thyroglobulin*, which is produced by the thyroid, to form the two thyroid hormones thyroxine (T_4) and triiodothyronine (T_3). These thyroid hormones act on all body tissues to increase metabolic activity by causing the body to burn available carbohydrates very rapidly, increasing the utilization of fats and depleting fat stores. These actions have very visible effects on some body systems. With the increased metabolic rate, all body tissues require increased quantities of nutrients. The cardiovascular system reacts by vasodilatation and increased cardiac output. T_4 also has a direct effect on the heart, increasing its metabolism as well as its rate and forcefulness of contraction. T_4 also greatly increases the reactivity of the nervous system, causing wakefulness with hypersecretion of the hormone and sleepiness with hyposecretion. Hypersecretion also causes a very fine but rapid tremor of the muscles. T_4 also increases the motility of the gastrointestinal tract and promotes a copious flow of digestive juices; therefore, hypersecretion may cause diarrhea. On the other hand, lack of T_4 has the opposite effects: sluggish motility and greatly diminished gastrointestinal secretion resulting in constipation. Excessive production of T_4 also causes a voracious appetite because of the rapid rate of metabolism. Inability to take in the needed nutrients can cause weight loss and vitamin deficiencies, particularly deficiencies of the B-complex vitamins.[8]

The thyroid gland, like other glands in the endocrine system, is kept in equilibrium through a negative feedback system. The hypothalamus secretes TRH, which acts on the anterior pituitary, causing it to secrete thyroid-stimulating hormone (TSH). High levels of TSH inhibit the hypothalamus from producing more TRH. The TSH produced acts on the thyroid gland to produce T_4 and T_3. High levels of circulating T_4 and T_3 will then inhibit secretion of TSH by the anterior pituitary.

Hypothyroidism

Hypothyroidism in children can take two forms: (1) congenital hypothyroidism, or cretinism, and (2) acquired hypothyroidism. Thyroid deficiency in cretinism is present at birth, although the disease may not become obvious for several months and occasionally is overlooked for years. *Ac-*

quired hypothyroidism is a thyroid deficiency that begins later in life, usually after the age of 2 years.

Congenital hypothyroidism results from malformation of the thyroid during embryonic development. The result may be a child with a total lack of thyroid tissue (*athyrotic cretinism*) or a child with a thyroid remnant, which may be located anywhere along the embryonic migratory tract of the thyroid—for example, in the mediastinum or under the base of the tongue. Presently, the causes of this malformation are not known. Other causes of congenital hypothyroidism include defective hormone synthesis, secretion, or utilization. The incidence of congenital hypothyroidism is approximately 1 in 4000 to 10,000 live births.[9, 10]

Manifestations Lack of sufficient thyroid tissue to produce adequate amounts of T_4 and T_3 results in a variety of symptoms. The athyrotic child who has had a lack of thyroid hormone prenatally will often show symptoms at birth. Because of the effects of thyroxine on neuromuscular control, athyrotic children are lethargic and seldom cry and may actually be thought of as extremely good babies. Their reactions are slow, and they often have feeding problems. They may have a low-pitched, gruntlike cry. Constipation is a common problem. Other problems frequently seen include cool, mottled skin; thick facial features; a thick tongue; umbilical hernia; dry skin; falling hair; and frequent respiratory infections. The child with a thyroid remnant may exhibit few, if any, symptoms during the newborn period. As the child grows and the amount of thyroid hormone being produced by the thyroid remnant becomes increasingly inadequate, symptoms slowly develop. In the older child, growth retardation may become apparent, and strabismus is frequently seen.[11] Children with either congenital or acquired hypothyroidism may be intellectually and developmentally delayed.

Diagnostic tests The diagnosis of hypothyroidism is made on the basis of several blood tests. T_4, T_3, and TSH are measured by radioimmunoassay (RIA). In the child with congenital hypothyroidism, T_3 and T_4 levels are low or nonexistent, and TSH levels are elevated. In the past, serum protein-bound iodine (PBI) was used to evaluate thyroid function. This test measures the amount of T_4 precursors in the blood; however, because of the technological advances of RIA, this test is no longer done. Bone age x-ray films are frequently ordered to assess the level of growth retardation. Thyroid scans using radioactive iodine are frequently performed on children with congenital hypothyroidism in order to detect thyroid remnants. However, these scans are usually delayed until the child is several years old. The child must be taken off the thyroid medication for a short period of time prior to the scanning, and therefore the scanning is delayed until major brain development has occurred. Cholesterol levels in older children may be markedly elevated because of the decreased utilization of fats.[12]

Treatment Treatment of congenital hypothyroidism consists of replacement of the deficient hormones with desiccated thyroid or a synthetic thyroid preparation, such as sodium levothyroxine (Synthroid). Progress is evaluated on the basis of serial T_4, T_3, and TSH levels and x-rays for bone age. Periodic psychological and developmental assessments are beneficial. The infant is evaluated frequently because medication needs to be increased as the child grows. Recently, screening of all newborn infants for congenital hypothyroidism has begun in many states. It is hoped that with this type of screening, the asymptomatic hypothyroid child will be identified before serious complications result.

The prognosis for children with congenital hypothyroidism is always guarded. Once these children are placed on medication, their physical symptoms are reversed (Fig. 24-2); however, the damage done to the developing central nervous system is often permanent. The result may be a child who is severely retarded or one with apparently normal intelligence but with developmental delays in one specific area. Speech problems are a common finding. Some children who receive thyroid replacement therapy develop normally, with no mental impairment; however, no guarantee can be made for any particular child.

Nursing management When the child is started on thyroid replacement medication, several weeks often elapse before the symptoms disappear. The nurse who is dealing with a hypothyroid child must understand that metabolism and general physical activity have been slowed down and that it will take longer for the child to accomplish most tasks. The nurse must also be aware that the child may be mentally retarded as a result of hypothyroidism, and communication with the child must be geared to the child's functional

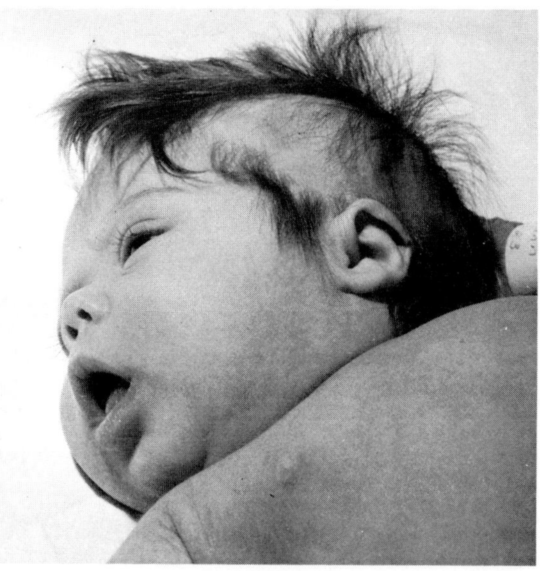

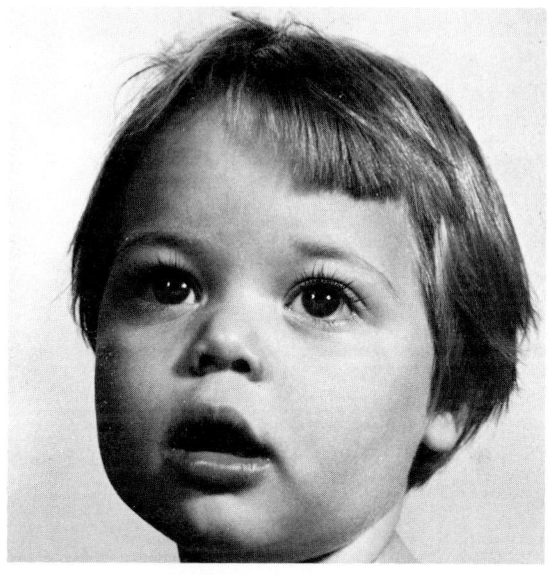

A B

Figure 24-2 Hypothyroidism. (*A*) A 10-week-old baby with the typical thickened facial features and fragile hair, which is falling out. (*B*) The same child after 16 months of treatment. (*From R. M. DeCoursey and J. L. Renfro, The Human Organism, 5th ed., McGraw-Hill, New York, 1980. Used with permission.*)

ability rather than his or her chronological age. Skin care is important. Avoiding soap and using skin lotions often help relieve some of the dryness that occurs. Feeding problems continue to cause difficulties. The nurse must remember that the child cannot be rushed and that a longer time must be allotted for feeding. The hypothyroid infant may need to be suctioned during feeding in order to remove mucous secretions, which may interfere with nursing. Constipation may continue. Offering the child increased amounts of fluid during the day will help keep the stools soft. For the older child, eating a variety of fresh fruits and vegetables may help stimulate the gastrointestinal tract. In severe cases, enemas may be needed.

The family of a hypothyroid child will need a great deal of support from the nurse. The nurse must help the family have realistic expectations concerning their child's development. They can neither label the child mentally retarded nor expect that there will be no problems in the future. Many mothers feel guilty, believing that something they did during the pregnancy caused the hypothyroidism; this needs to be discussed openly. The family needs a good understanding of the disease process, including the fact that the child will need to take medication for the rest of his or her life. Thyroid preparations come in tablet form only, and so the family must be told how to crush the tablets before giving them to a small child. The medication must not be given in the baby's bottle. The symptoms of hyperthyroidism must be explained to the family so that they can recognize any overtreatment in the child. It is not uncommon for symptoms such as a large tongue and strabismus to persist for many months after treatment has begun, and the family needs to be informed of this.

Hyperthyroidism

Hyperthyroidism, or *thyrotoxicosis*, in children is almost always secondary to Graves disease (also called *exophthalmic goiter*). Graves disease is a multisystem disorder composed of hyperthyroidism with thyroid enlargement and exophthalmos (protrusion of the eyeballs). In Graves disease, the thyroid produces large quantities of T_3 and T_4 without apparent stimulation from the pituitary. These large amounts of T_3 and T_4 suppress TSH production and block the pituitary's ability to respond to TRH. The etiology of Graves disease is unknown, although it occurs 5 to 6 times more frequently in girls than in boys. It is not uncommon to find many other family members who have a history of other thyroid problems. The incidence of Graves disease is approximately 4 per 1000 people in the general population.[13]

The course of Graves disease is usually slow, although there may be an abrupt onset. When questioned at the time of diagnosis, families often recall that there have been symptoms such as decreased school performance for the past year. The hyperthyroid period of Graves disease lasts for several years, although the time varies from child to child. A significant number of children will develop hypothyroidism later in life; therefore, it is important that these children have continuous follow-up.

Most children with Graves disease present with complaints of nervousness, decreasing school performance, heat intolerance, excessive sweating, and increased appetite with or without weight loss. They show tachycardia, systolic hypertension with markedly widened pulse pressure, mild exophthalmos, lid retraction and stare, tremors of the outstretched hand, and smooth, moist, warm skin. Almost all have an obvious goiter.[14]

The diagnosis of Graves disease is based on the history, physical examination, and laboratory findings. The levels of T_3, T_4, and TSH are measured. Ordinarily, T_3 and T_4 are elevated, and TSH is low; however, some children with hyperthyroidism have an elevated T_3 and a normal T_4. This entity, T_3 thyrotoxicosis, is another form of hyperthyroidism. When the diagnosis of Graves disease is questionable, a radioactive iodine uptake may be ordered. Iodine 123 or I^{131} is given by mouth. The radioactivity is then measured over the thyroid gland, usually at 4-, 6-, and 24-h intervals. The results are read as a percentage of the tracer dose taken up by the thyroid.

Treatment There are three modes of treatment for Graves disease, none of which is entirely satisfactory. The most commonly used form of treatment in children is the administration of oral medications. Propylthiouracil (PTU) and methimazole (Tapazole) block the production of thyroid hormones which produce the metabolic aspects of Graves disease, and they allow the disease to subside spontaneously. Drug therapy can have significant complications, the most serious of which is granulocytopenia. Rashes, fever, urticaria, arthritis, and a severe lupuslike syndrome have also been noted. Therapy is continued for 18 to 24 months. If signs of hyperthyroidism return, therapy may be reinstituted, or surgery may be recommended. A subtotal thyroidectomy is the second mode of treatment in Graves disease. Surgical treatment often involves significant complications. Vocal cord paralysis due to cutting the recurrent laryngeal nerves; hypoparathyroidism due to inadvertent removal of, or damage to, the parathyroid glands; hemorrhage necessitating a tracheostomy; and cosmetic disfigurement resulting from keloid formation are all complications. Since the surgeon can only estimate how much thyroid to leave intact in an attempt to keep the child euthyroid, the results are unpredictable. Most often the child will become hypothyroid after surgery, requiring the daily administration of thyroid replacement medication. However, if too little thyroid is removed, the child may still be hyperthyroid after surgery, requiring a second operation. Oral iodine (Lugol's solution or a saturated solution of potassium iodide) is given for 10 to 14 days preoperatively to control the hyperthyroidism and to reduce the vascularity of the thyroid gland. The third form of treatment of Graves disease is obliteration of the thyroid using radioactive iodine. This is a very popular form of treatment for adult patients; however, pediatricians generally limit its use to instances in which all other modes of therapy have failed or are contraindicated. Concerns center on exposure of the gonads of the young child to radioactivity, with subsequent genetic damage, and the development of thyroid cancer and leukemia. It is common for children to become hypothyroid after treatment with radioactive iodine. This condition may develop in the first year after treatment or may not become evident for many years.[15]

Hashimoto disease *Hashimoto disease*, or *chronic lymphocytic thyroiditis*, is the most frequently observed thyroid disorder in the United States. The disease is believed to have an autoimmune etiology. It appears that at some point the body begins to form antibodies against its own thyroid tissue. This causes an inflammatory response, leading to a moderately enlarged, firm, knobby goiter. This inflammatory response may have varied effects on the functioning of the thyroid. The individual may be euthyroid, hypothyroid, or hyperthyroid (the last condition is sometimes called *Hashitoxicosis*).

The diagnosis is based on the history, since the disorder appears to be a familial disease;

physical findings of the typical goiter; and laboratory data. Circulating thyroid antibodies—antithyroglobulin and antimicrosomal—are measured, as well as T_3, T_4, and TSH, to evaluate thyroid function. Treatment depends on thyroid function. Hypothyroidism, once present, is generally permanent and requires treatment with thyroid hormone. Hyperthyroidism is usually treated with oral medications, as in Graves disease, although the length of treatment may be shorter. For the euthyroid child, observation is all that is necessary; however, this is important, since many children will eventually become hypothyroid.[16]

Nursing management After starting oral medication, it may be 10 to 14 days before children with hyperthyroidism notice a change in their symptoms and 4 to 6 weeks before they become euthyroid.[17] Often these children are extremely agitated, and any stress, either physical or emotional, will exaggerate the hyperactive symptoms. Environmental stimulation should be kept to a minimum. This is especially true at night, since there may be an increased need for sleep and rest owing to constant fatigue caused by insomnia. Barbiturates may be ordered for sedation.

The effects of high levels of T_4 on the gastrointestinal tract may result in a need for a high caloric intake and produce a ravenous appetite. Small, frequent feedings with high-quality foods may be needed to meet the caloric needs and the increased need for the B-complex vitamins. Diarrhea may also be a problem at this time. Limiting the intake of fluid at meals may be of some benefit. The nurse must observe the frequency, color, consistency, and character of the stools. The goiter produced by hyperthyroidism may create a feeling of fullness in the throat. Because of this, the child may find that some foods are easier to swallow than others. These food preferences should be incorporated into the diet.

The child with hyperthyroidism loses tolerance to heat. The room should be well ventilated, and the temperature reduced if possible. Lightweight nightclothes should be provided. The child may be more comfortable without any covers on the bed. During the day, quiet activities should be encouraged rather than vigorous exercise in order to decrease the amount of body heat produced. Frequent bathing and sponging may also bring relief to the child who perspires heavily.

The child and the family need to be taught a great deal about their medications before the patient is discharged. Propylthiouracil (PTU) is rapidly removed from the circulation and therefore is given every 8 h. A common schedule is administration at 8 A.M., 4 P.M., and 12 midnight. This will necessitate waking the child to give a dose of medication. However, the parents need to understand that it is important to give the medication every 8 h rather than three times a day. PTU therapy has the possible side effect of agranulocytosis, and therefore many children will have routine white blood cell and differential counts while they are on therapy. The parents must report any signs of illness, particularly sore throat, skin eruptions, fever, headache, or general malaise. PTU is very bitter; however, the ability or inability to taste the medication is an inherited trait. Placing the pill on the back of the tongue and offering copious amounts of fluids may be of some help to children who are tasters. It is not uncommon to see children who are nontasters chewing PTU tablets. Often the parents will be asked to check sleeping pulses on their child once therapy has begun in order to assess how well the child is doing, and therefore they need to be taught this technique. Medication therapy may be so effective that the child becomes hypothyroid, and so the family is warned to report any signs of possible hypothyroidism.

The child who is to undergo a thyroidectomy needs to be given much information before surgery in order to alleviate fears and elicit cooperation. The child will be placed on an iodine preparation prior to surgery. Iodine preparations have a rather metallic taste and can be made more palatable by being diluted in large quantities of water or fruit juice. Having the child drink the preparation through a straw is also helpful. Postoperatively, the child is checked frequently for signs of hemorrhage, bleeding at the incision site, and changes in vital signs. Since severe hemorrhage may compress the trachea and obstruct breathing, a tracheotomy tray is kept by the bedside. Signs of hypoparathyroidism, such as tetany and numbness of the extremities, must be reported immediately. Treatment may include increasing the amount of calcium in the diet or administering calcium lactate or calcium gluconate.

Thyroid storm is a condition that results from the rapid release of thyroid hormone into the circulation. It can be precipitated by physical and emotional stress, infections, surgery, and radioactive iodine therapy. It is occasionally seen when hyperthyroid children are taken off antithyroid medications. Thyroid storm can be a life-threatening situation. The child progresses rapidly from fever and restlessness to delirium and shock. A nasogastric tube may be inserted to administer oral PTU. Intravenous fluids are started to combat shock. Medications include antipyretics, glucocorticoids, catecholamine-blocking agents, and vitamins.

THE ADRENAL GLANDS

Anatomy and physiology

The two *adrenal glands* are triangular-shaped organs located directly above each kidney. Each adrenal gland is divided into two sections—the medulla, or inner section, and the cortex, or outer section. Their functions are very different.

The medulla secretes two catecholamines, epinephrine and norepinephrine. When stress is placed on the body, either physical or psychological, the medulla responds with release of epinephrine and norepinephrine, which have a profound effect on all parts of the body. This *fight-or-flight response* prepares the body to deal with the stress. The combined activities of epinephrine and norepinephrine result in stimulation of the central nervous system, with increased alertness, increased cardiac output with increased force and rate of contraction, dilated coronary blood vessels, dilated blood vessels in skeletal muscle, elevated blood glucose, and an increase in free fatty acids (see Table 24-2). The adrenal cortex, or outer section, secretes three groups of hormones, all derived from cholesterol. These include mineralocorticoids, glucocorticoids, and adrenal androgens. Because of their chemical structure, adrenal androgens are also known as *17-ketosteroids*.

Although a number of mineralocorticoids are produced in the adrenal cortex, three are most common: aldosterone, corticosterone, and deoxycorticosterone. Aldosterone constitutes about 95 percent of the available mineralocorticoids. Their major function is to regulate electrolytes, particularly sodium, in the extracellular fluid. This is accomplished through the action of aldosterone on the renal tubules, causing reabsorption of sodium into the blood. Increased absorption of sodium causes a corresponding reabsorption of

Table 24-2 Adrenal Hormones

Type	Major Hormones	Action on Body
Hormones of the Cortex		
Mineralocorticoids	Aldosterone	Reabsorption of sodium by renal tubules
	Corticosterone	Reabsorption of chloride, leading to increased sodium chloride in extracellular fluid
	Deoxycorticosterone	Increases water absorption
		Increases interstitial fluid and blood volume
		Increases cardiac output
		Increases arterial pressure
Glucocorticoids	Cortisol	Elevates blood glucose through gluconeogenesis
		Increases circulating amino acids
		Decreases rate of glucose utilization by the cell
		Mobilizes fatty acids from adipose tissues
Androgens	DHEA	Unknown in males
		Pubic and axillary hair growth in females
		Maintenance of normal libido in females
Hormones of the Medulla		
Catecholamines	Epinephrine	Increases alertness through central nervous system stimulation
	Norepinephrine	Increases cardiac output:
		Increases force of contraction
		Increases heart rate
		Dilates coronary blood vessels
		Dilates blood vessels in muscles
		Elevates blood glucose
		Increases free fatty acids

chloride with a resulting increase of sodium chloride in the extracellular fluid. This elevation of salt in the extracellular fluid causes increased water absorption through osmosis and stimulation of osmoreceptors. The effects of aldosterone on electrolytes are an elevated interstitial fluid volume and blood volume and increased cardiac output. Excess blood flow causes local vasoconstriction and increased peripheral resistance, creating elevated arterial pressure.

The major glucocorticoid secreted is *cortisol*, also known as *hydrocortisone*. The major function of the glucocorticoids is to help the body resist physical stress. This is accomplished through effects on glucose, protein, and fat metabolism. As the name indicates, the glucocorticoids increase the glucose concentration in the blood through gluconeogenesis, the conversion of protein and fat into glucose. Protein metabolism is altered, allowing an increased quantity of amino acids to circulate. These amino acids are then available to provide energy or to repair tissue damage. This also causes a decrease in the rate of glucose utilization by the cells. Cortisol also affects mobilization of fatty acids from adipose tissue. This allows the body to utilize fat for fuel during periods of starvation or other stresses.

The role of adrenal androgens in normal physiology is unknown. The major adrenal androgen is the 17-ketosteroid dehydroepiandrosterone (DHEA). Although two-thirds of the ketosteroids in the urine of males come from adrenal sources, these adrenal androgens have no significant masculinizing effect in normal amounts. In females they are believed to cause growth of pubic and axillary hair and to be important in maintaining normal libido.

The mineralocorticoids, glucocorticoids, and adrenal androgens are all kept under control through negative feedback. Corticotropin-releasing hormone (CRH) is secreted by the hypothalamus. This is carried through the circulation to the pituitary, causing it to release ACTH. ACTH is transported by the peripheral circulation to the adrenal glands, where it causes steroid synthesis. Large doses of cortisol from the adrenal glands inhibit the release of CRH and ACTH, although this negative feedback can be overcome by stress. Large amounts of ACTH also feed back to inhibit CRH release. Aldosterone secretion is also regulated by angiotensin II, produced in the renin-angiotensin system, and is stimulated by increases in potassium concentrations.

Hypoadrenocorticism

Lack of adrenal hormones can result from primary adrenal failure associated with the adrenal glands themselves or from secondary adrenal failure related to insufficient ACTH secretion. Primary adrenal failure can be caused by a variety of conditions. Chronic adrenal insufficiency, termed *Addison disease*, is an uncommon condition in children. In the past, tuberculosis of the adrenal glands was a frequent cause of Addison disease; now, however, the majority of cases are attributed to idiopathic atrophy of the adrenal glands. In some cases, the disease may be the result of an autoimmune reaction, with the production of adrenal antibodies. This is frequently the case in children with multihormonal disorders. Congenital hypoplasia of the adrenal glands has also been reported as an inherited autosomal recessive trait.[18]

Infants with congenital hypoplasia of the adrenal glands and older children who present in adrenal crisis secondary to chronic adrenal insufficiency have nausea, vomiting, diarrhea, and dehydration. Hypoglycemia, hyponatremia, and hyperkalemia may be present as a result of the lack of mineralocorticoids and glucocorticoids. The child who is not in adrenal crisis may have weakness, anorexia, and weight loss. There may be hyperpigmentation of the skin owing to excessive secretion of ACTH and melanocyte-stimulating hormone (MSH). Alopecia and monilial infections of the skin and mucous membranes are common.

Evaluation of children for chronic adrenal insufficiency is based on several diagnostic tests. These include cortisol determinations during the ACTH stimulation test. The child is given synthetic ACTH (Cortrosyn) intramuscularly or intravenously, and the blood cortisol level is then measured every 30 min for $1\frac{1}{2}$ to 4 h. In the normal child, a rise in the cortisol level is expected to result from the stimulation of the ACTH. This test will tell whether there is adrenal function or not, but it does not differentiate between primary and secondary adrenal insufficiency. Two tests can be used to evaluate whether there is normal pituitary function or secondary adrenal insufficiency. These are the metyrapone test and the insulin tolerance test. In the *metyrapone test*, the child is given metyrapone either orally or intravenously, and blood samples are obtained for 11-deoxycorticoids. Metyrapone inhibits an enzyme needed for the formation of cortisol in the adrenal glands. The resulting low cortisol level stimulates the pituitary to secrete higher levels of ACTH. However, since the chemical process leading to the formation of cortisol cannot be completed, elevated levels of 11-deoxycortisol, the precursor of cortisol, result. In the child with secondary adrenal insufficiency, there is no rise in the level of 11-deoxycortisol, since the pituitary cannot be stimulated. The *insulin tolerance test* is conducted in the same manner as the GH stimulation test. Since hypoglycemia is a potent stimulus to ACTH release, an elevated cortisol level following hypoglycemia is considered a normal finding in this test (see the section "Hypopituitarism").[19]

Congenital adrenal hyperplasia

Another common cause of adrenal insufficiency in children is *congenital adrenal hyperplasia*, or *adrenogenital syndrome*. This inborn error of metabolism appears to be inherited as an autosomal recessive trait, and it is common to find that more than one child in a family has the condition, since each child has a 25 percent chance of being affected. The gene is found frequently in the normal population; the incidence may be as high as 1 in 35 individuals.[20]

In the formation of adrenal steroids from cholesterol, three pathways are used, leading to the formation of aldosterone, cortisol, and adrenal androgens. A variety of enzymes interact with precursor compounds to form these three substances. In congenital adrenal hyperplasia, one of the enzymes needed for aldosterone or cortisol production is missing, leading to overproduction of a precursor substance. This precursor then becomes part of the adrenal androgen pathway, leading to overproduction of androgens. Because insufficient amounts of aldosterone or cortisol are produced, the pituitary is stimulated through the negative feedback system to produce more ACTH. This ACTH stimulates the adrenal glands, causing adrenal hyperplasia and ultimately the production of more precursor substance.

The most common type of congenital adrenal hyperplasia is 21-hydroxylase deficiency. The absence of this enzyme affects both the mineralocorticoid pathway and the glucocorticoid pathway, leading to the overproduction of progesterone (a precursor of aldosterone) and 17-alpha hydroxyprogesterone (a precursor of cortisol). These two substances are then rerouted into the third pathway, causing an overproduction of adrenal androgens and virilization. The enzyme defect is usually not complete, allowing the formation of small amounts of aldosterone. In approximately half of affected children, the amount of aldosterone secreted is not sufficient to maintain the electrolyte balance, and salt-losing crises occur, usually early in infancy.

The second most frequently seen type of congenital adrenal hyperplasia is 11-hydroxylase deficiency. In this condition, the enzyme interferes with both mineralocorticoid production and glucocorticoid production, leading to the formation of 11-deoxycorticosterone (a precursor of aldosterone) and 11-deoxycortisol (a precursor of cortisol). Because 11-deoxycorticosterone is a potent retainer of salt, affected children do not have salt-losing crises but rather may have hypertension. These two substances feed back into the third pathway, and again there is overproduction of adrenal androgens. Several other types of congenital adrenal hyperplasia have been identified, although they are much less common.

Manifestations The effect of the increased adrenal androgens is virilization. The time at which this change occurs varies from child to child. Virilization may occur in utero, resulting in a female with ambiguous genitalia. There is often clitoral enlargement and labial fusion, and in extreme cases the urethra may open at the tip of what appears to be a phallus. The internal genitalia develop normally. Male fetuses may be virilized, although the effects are not usually visible. After birth, the male will continue to be virilized and will progress to what appears to be puberty—that is, increased height, with epiphyseal maturation; development of pubic, axillary, and facial hair; acne; lowering of the voice; and increased growth of the penis. In spite of this, the testes do not grow, and there is no spermatogenesis (Fig. 24-3). Female children also show signs of virilization, such as increased height and epiphyseal maturation, development of axillary and facial hair, and development of pubic hair with a male escutcheon, an enlarged clitoris, and hirsutism. If untreated, these children will be exceptionally tall during their early childhood years, but their epiphyses will close early, and ultimately they will be very short.

Congenital adrenal hyperplasia may become evident at any point in childhood. An infant may be evaluated at the time of birth because of ambiguous genitalia and be found to have congen-

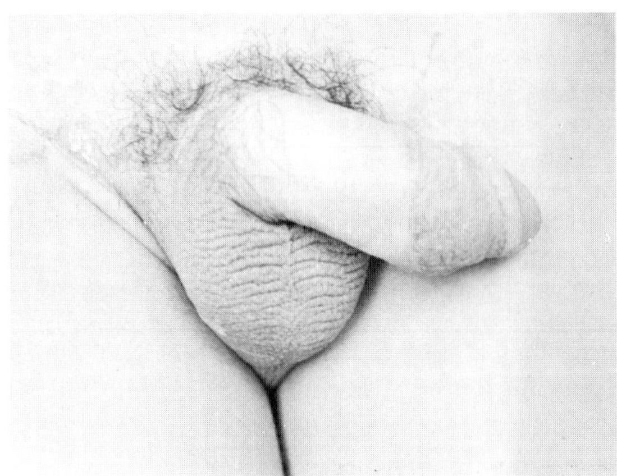

Figure 24-3 A 3-year-old boy with congenital adrenal hyperplasia, showing marked virilization at the time of diagnosis. His height was 108.5 cm, and his bone age was 10 years.

ital adrenal hyperplasia. Karyotyping may be done to identify the chromosomal sex of the child. The specific signs that alert the nurse to possible congenital adrenal hyperplasia are (1) a structure that looks like either an enlarged clitoris or a small penis with hypospadias, (2) a partial fusion of the labioscrotal skin that resembles an incompletely formed scrotum, and (3) the absence of gonads or a single gonad in an incompletely formed scrotum.[21] For further information on abnormalities of sexual development, see Chap. 25.

The child may first be seen later in infancy or childhood when the marginally adequate adrenal function becomes inadequate as a result of a stressful situation. Children with congenital adrenal hyperplasia who are salt losers may have few if any signs of virilization at the time of their diagnosis. On the other hand, occasionally children are seen late in childhood, when both males and females may be fully virilized. It is interesting to note that frequently parents do not question the appearance of secondary sex characteristics in very young children.

Diagnostic tests Several laboratory tests are used in the diagnosis and evaluation of congenital adrenal hyperplasia. Urine collections may be obtained for 17-ketosteroids and pregnanetriol; 17-ketosteroids are a general measure of increased adrenal androgen production, and pregnanetriol is the urinary metabolite of the excessive precursors in 21-hydroxylase deficiency. A 24-h urine collection for 17-hydroxysteroids may also be done in order to measure total cortisol production. In some areas a blood test is now available to measure serum 17-alpha hydroxyprogesterone. This is the easiest and most definitive test for 21-hydroxylase deficiency. In the older child, a bone age test may be ordered to assess the degree of skeletal maturation.

Treatment and nursing management If the child is admitted in an adrenal crisis, a medical emergency exists, and treatment will be vigorous, including intravenous replacement of fluids and electrolytes with the addition of glucocorticoids and mineralocorticoids. Once the child has stabilized, the treatment consists of the administration of glucocorticoids or glucocorticoids and mineralocorticoids. Cortisone is used as the glucocorticoid replacement. This can be given as intramuscular injections every third day or orally in tablet or liquid form (Cortef) every 8 h. Several preparations are available for mineralocorticoid replacement. Desoxycorticosterone acetate (DOCA) may be given as intramuscular injections or placed under the skin in pellet form for slow absorption. DOCA pellets are slowly absorbed and need to be replaced several times a year. They are used primarily in infants who have difficulty retaining medications orally. Nine-alpha-fluorocortisol acetate (Florinef) is also used as a mineralocorticoid supplement. It is given orally once daily in tablet form. Salt is needed for effective treatment with mineralocorticoids, and therefore some children may be given prescriptions for sodium chloride tablets.[22]

Some children with congenital adrenal hyperplasia may undergo surgery to repair their physical defects. Enlargement of the clitoris is a concern to parents. If the child is young, surgery may be deferred in the hope that as the child grows older, the labia will grow and surround the protruding clitoris. However, if the clitoris appears extremely hypertrophied, surgery may be indicated. Recent surgical advances have allowed resection of the shaft of the clitoris, resulting in a functional organ. However, not all attempts have been successful, and clitoral amputation may be the end result. In the past, clitorectomy was the only treatment available.

Virilization in male infants may be so extremely and irrevocably incomplete that the anatomy will prevent normal male functioning (intercourse, urination when standing, and development of secondary sex characteristics).[23]

Some physicians then recommend female sex assignment.[24]

Children with congenital adrenal hyperplasia may require surgery for correction of genital abnormalities. The age of the child will determine the type of preoperative teaching that can be done, although it must be remembered that all children have a fear of genital surgery.[25] Adjustments in glucocorticoid and mineralocorticoid dosages are made preoperatively to help the child deal with the stress of surgery. Postoperatively, the child will most likely have an indwelling catheter in place. Vital signs are monitored frequently to assess steroid replacement. Infants need to be restrained in order to prevent damage to the surgical area or removal of the indwelling catheter. The operative site needs to be checked for trauma, infection, necrosis, and other signs that skin grafts might not be taking. Good perineal hygiene is essential to prevent contamination of the area with feces.

Hyperadrenocorticism

Cushing syndrome, a form of *hyperadrenocorticism,* although fairly common in adulthood, is a rare syndrome in infancy and childhood. Because of the negative feedback system, overproduction of the adrenal hormones can be the result of problems at the level of the pituitary or the adrenal glands themselves. Increased ACTH production secondary to pituitary tumors results in bilateral adrenal hyperplasia. Adrenal tumors, either benign adenomas or highly malignant carcinomas, are also causes of Cushing syndrome. In children younger than 8 years of age, most cases of Cushing syndrome are due to malignant adrenal tumors.[26]

Manifestations The signs and symptoms of Cushing syndrome are caused by overproduction of glucocorticoids (cortisol). The utilization of body proteins for the formation of glucose (gluconeogenesis) causes retardation of body growth and a decrease in muscle mass, with muscle weakness. Alterations in carbohydrate and fat metabolism may lead to obesity and abnormal glucose tolerance test results. These changes result in a child who appears obese but has thin arms and legs. The fat may be deposited in the facial area, producing "moon facies," or across the shoulders and cervical area, leading to "buffalo hump." The skin is often thin with prominent capillaries, bruising, and purple striae. There may be electrolyte imbalance with subsequent weakness. Some children also have increased androgen secretion with resulting hirsutism and acne. Blood pressure may be elevated.

Diagnostic tests Diagnostic tests are used to differentiate between Cushing syndrome and exogenous obesity. In Cushing syndrome, 17-hydroxysteroids (a measure of total cortisol production) and 17-ketosteroids (a measure of total androgen production) are both elevated. Blood cortisol levels are also elevated, and their diurnal variation is absent. A dexamethasone suppression test may be conducted. Dexamethasone, which is a potent glucocorticoid, is administered orally in order to turn off ACTH production, and the production of cortisol is then suppressed. Blood cortisol levels and urinary17-hydroxysteroids are evaluated. The test may be conducted for 24 h or over the course of several days. Various x-ray procedures may be performed in an attempt to visualize an adrenal or pituitary tumor.[27]

Treatment For the child with an adrenal tumor, surgery is the treatment of choice. Since tumors suppress the normal pituitary-adrenal axis, preoperative and postoperative care includes hormonal replacement. Most children with adrenal adenoma regain their own adrenal function within 6 months after surgery and are entirely normal thereafter. The prognosis for the child with adrenal carcinoma, however, is poor. Radiation therapy and chemotherapy may be used in an attempt to elicit remission. The child with a pituitary tumor may receive pituitary irradiation, although a bilateral adrenalectomy is the most common form of treatment. In either case, the child will remain adrenally insufficient.

Nursing management The nurse has many opportunities to interact with the child with adrenal problems and his or her family. Often the first contact occurs when the child is hospitalized in adrenal crisis. This is a life-threatening situation, and administration of intravenous fluids at a uniform rate is critical. Careful monitoring of vital signs is essential, since children in adrenal crisis are often dehydrated. Signs of increasing dehydration or overhydration as a result of too vigorous medical management need to be evaluated. Accurate collection of 24-h urine specimens is essential, particularly if a diagnosis has not yet been made.

During the evaluation phase of adrenal disorders, the nurse needs to work closely with the child and the family in order to accomplish the testing with the least trauma to the child. The 24-h urine tests need to be collected accurately, beginning and ending at the time specifically ordered. The nurse must ensure that no urine is inadvertently lost. If the child is an infant and is not toilet-trained, proper placement and good adherence of the collection bag are a must. Young children must also be restrained in order to be prevented from dislodging the collection apparatus. Signs should be posted at the bedside and in the bathroom to prevent inadvertent discarding of urine that needs to be saved. When medications are used in suppression tests, it is essential that they be given at precisely the times ordered to obtain the desired results.

Once a diagnosis has been made, surgery may be performed. In Cushing syndrome, two approaches are used for surgery on the adrenal glands: an abdominal approach and a flank approach. Preoperatively, the child needs to be informed about what to expect after surgery, including the possible insertion of a nasogastric tube to relieve abdominal distention and an indwelling catheter to measure urine output. Preparation in coughing, deep breathing, and the use of blow bottles is helpful. Postoperatively, breathing is often painful because of the close proximity of the incision to the diaphragm.[28]

Following an adrenalectomy, the child's vital signs are monitored carefully. Hypertension is a complication due to mineralocorticoid release secondary to manipulation of the adrenals. Urine output is observed closely to detect impending shock. Parenteral cortisol is given to compensate for the deficiency in mineralocorticoid production.

It is difficult for any parent to understand adrenal disease. The nurse may need to discuss the pathophysiology of adrenal disease on many occasions. The physical changes that occur in adrenal diseases result in an altered body image. The child needs help in dealing with those changes which will be permanent and needs assurance that certain changes will disappear with therapy. For example, most children with Cushing syndrome will have lost all external appearances of the disease within 1 year after surgery.[29] Parents of children with congenital adrenal hyperplasia have many of the same concerns as parents of children with precocious puberty. Fears of sexual abuse need to be discussed openly. These parents may also harbor guilt feelings when the child's ultimate height is compromised as a result of late detection of the disease. This guilt may be exaggerated by the child's poor body image related to height.

Daily medications remain the major form of treatment for adrenal insufficiency, and the nurse has an opportunity to do a great deal of teaching in this area. The parents need to know what type of medication the child is taking and the importance of following the prescribed schedule. Glucocorticoids need to be given every 8 h in order to suppress the release of ACTH. Administration three times a day will not accomplish this. Children with adrenal insufficiency frequently have increased salt needs secondary to poor aldosterone production. The parents need to understand the physiology of this process and allow the child to use the salt shaker freely, particularly in the summer, when salt needs are increased as a result of sweating. Otherwise, the parents may limit the child's salt intake because they fear hypertension. Before discharge, the parents will be given instructions for medication dosage schedules when the child is sick. For minor illnesses or fever, the dose is usually doubled; for major illnesses or accidents, the dose may be tripled. When the child is not able to take oral medication, intramuscular cortisol is given. The parents and/or the child may be instructed in the injection technique. When any type of illness occurs, prompt medical attention is important. Wearing an identification (Medic Alert) necklace or bracelet is essential, since adrenal crisis is always a possibility.

THE PANCREAS: THE ISLETS OF LANGERHANS

Anatomy and physiology

The *pancreas* is both an endocrine and an exocrine gland. The endocrine portion consists of the *islets of Langerhans,* which are clusters of secreting tissues scattered throughout the pancreas. The alpha cells secrete *glucagon,* a substance that raises the blood sugar, and the beta cells secrete *insulin,* a substance that lowers the blood sugar. In the normal individual, insulin is secreted in response to an elevation in the blood glucose level. This rise in the insulin level causes a lowering of the blood sugar by facilitating the transport of glucose into the cells. This results in a nearly steady blood sugar level throughout the day. Without insulin, the body's cells are unable to utilize the glucose that is available to them. There are several exceptions, the most notable of which is the brain, which is able to utilize glucose directly from the circulation.

Insulin's major effect is on carbohydrate metabolism; however, it also affects fat and protein metabolism. Insulin also causes the transportation of fat into the fat cells, thus promoting fat storage. When insulin is not available, this transportation does not take place, and fatty acids are released into the blood. Protein metabolism is affected when glucose cannot be utilized for energy. Large quantities of protein and fat are utilized for energy in place of carbohydrates, with the result that fewer amino acids are available for the building of new cellular tissue.

Diabetes mellitus

Diabetes mellitus is a deficiency in insulin production. This disease is a multisystem disorder with cardiovascular, renal, ophthalmic, and neurological complications. There appear to be two types of diabetes: insulin-dependent diabetes mellitus (IDDM), which is usually diagnosed in children, and non-insulin-dependent diabetes mellitus (NIDDM), which is usually diagnosed in middle-aged or elderly adults.[30] Although these conditions have similar names, they are probably very different diseases.

Diabetes mellitus appears to be a multifactorial inherited disorder. That is, the individual inherits a predisposition for this disease; then, in the presence of certain environmental factors, unidentified at this time, some predisposed individuals will go on to develop the disease. Several theories exist concerning these environmental factors. It is speculated that some affected individuals have developed viral infections that attacked their susceptible pancreas. The Coxsackie virus, which causes one type of upper respiratory infection, is known to be involved in the development of diabetes. Another theory is that diabetes results from an autoimmune process. It has been noted that individuals with diabetes mellitus have an increased frequency of other autoimmune endocrine disorders, such as Hashimoto disease and adrenal diseases. Mature onset diabetes of the young (MODY) appears to be the only form of diabetes in which inheritance is clearly established; it is transmitted as an autosomal dominant disease. Characteristics include early onset of mild hyperglycemia and resistance to ketosis.[31]

In NIDDM, the pancreas produces an insufficient amount of insulin for normal metabolism. Many affected individuals who are overweight will have adequate insulin production if their weight is reduced, and this may be their only form of treatment. Others can be maintained on oral agents (pills) to stimulate the pancreas to produce more insulin. A small number of individuals will need to take insulin to supplement what their body is producing. In IDDM, however, the pancreas stops producing insulin totally. In fact, autopsies done on individuals with IDDM have shown that the beta cells have atrophied and disappeared. Thus, the only form of treatment that will be effective for individuals with IDDM is the administration of insulin. Other dissimilarities, such as the ability to develop ketosis, the types of complications, and the age at which complications develop, differentiate IDDM and NIDDM.

Although diabetes has been documented for thousands of years, relatively little is known about the disease. The incidence of IDDM in school-age children is about 1 in 600. It affects males and females equally. IDDM, unlike NIDDM, is uncommon in blacks. Diabetes may occur at any age, affecting children as young as 6 months, although it is most common in school-age children. It is most frequently diagnosed at 6 and 12 years of age.[32] If one child in a family has IDDM, a sibling's chances of developing it range from 2 to 6 percent.

Manifestations The onset of diabetes in children is rapid; most have the symptoms for 2 weeks or less before diagnosis. Lack of insulin in the body causes decreased utilization of glucose by the cells, with the resulting elevation in blood sugar. When the kidneys are no longer able to reabsorb the glucose, sugar begins to spill over into the urine (the so-called renal threshold is surpassed). This large amount of glucose pulls water with it through osmotic pressure, causing dehydration and thirst. This alteration in glucose metabolism leads to a conversion to fat and protein metabolism. This utilization of body mass for energy results in weight loss and a corresponding increased appetite. The metabolic changes result in the classic findings of uncontrolled diabetes: polyuria, polydipsia, and polyphagia.

If the child is not diagnosed at this time, the

signs and symptoms of ketoacidosis may develop. The body's dependence on fats and proteins for fuel leads to the formation of ketone bodies, a by-product of fat metabolism. The accumulation of ketone bodies—acetoacetic acid, β-hydroxybutyric acid, and acetone—causes a metabolic acidosis. As the level of ketones increases in the bloodstream, ketones begin to spill over into the urine. In an attempt to rid the body of the increasing quantities of carbon dioxide resulting from acidosis, the individual develops hyperpnea. Ketoacidosis also results in decreased peristalsis and stasis of fluid in the stomach, leading to nausea, vomiting, and abdominal distention. This loss of fluid combined with the osmotic diuresis leads to profound dehydration. At times the abdominal symptoms may be so severe that the child is thought to have appendicitis. If untreated, the child will become increasingly disoriented until coma develops. Renal shutdown may result, and ultimately death occurs.

The findings of hyperglycemia, glucosuria, and ketosis are considered sufficient evidence to make the diagnosis of diabetes mellitus in a child. Glucosuria and hyperglycemia occur occasionally with stressful situations such as head injuries and hypothalamic lesions, and glucosuria alone is associated with alterations in the renal tubular handling of glucose; however, these situations are rare.

Treatment The child who is admitted to the hospital with ketoacidosis may be moderately to critically ill. Blood is drawn for serum glucose, serum acetone, sodium, potassium, pH, and carbon dioxide measurements. Serum lipids may also be checked. Glucose levels will be elevated, sometimes as high as 1000 mg/dl, although the glucose level does not indicate the severity of the child's condition. Serum acetone levels are a measure of the level of ketones in the blood. They are reported as positive at 1:2, 1:4, and so on, indicating that there is a positive reaction on an Acetest tablet when a dilution of 1 part serum to 2 parts water or 1 part serum to 4 parts water is used. Therefore, the higher the number, the sicker the child; 1:16 is more serious than 1:4, for example. Potassium, an intracellular ion, is driven out of the cells in the initial phases of ketoacidosis, which may result in a falsely high serum potassium level. However, this potassium is soon removed from the system, leading to total body depletion of potassium. Blood lipids may be elevated because of the mobilization of fats for fuel, leading to falsely low electrolyte values. The pH and carbon dioxide measurements give the best indication of the child's state of acidosis. Children who are critically ill have been known to have a pH as low as 6.8 and a carbon dioxide level as low as 1.[33]

Once laboratory work has been done, parenteral fluids are begun to combat dehydration. Large amounts of fluids are administered rapidly, sometimes necessitating the use of two simultaneous intravenous lines. If there is any question of renal shutdown, an indwelling catheter may be inserted to monitor urinary output. Children are given nothing by mouth because of the decreased peristalsis, and some children may have a nasogastric tube inserted to decrease abdominal distention.

Low-dose continuous insulin infusion is the treatment of choice for ketoacidosis. An initial bolus of insulin is given intravenously, and then the continuous infusion is begun. Sodium bicarbonate may be administered to a severely acidotic child. A variety of intravenous solutions can be used to replace the lost electrolytes. Solutions containing glucose will be added to the intravenous insulin as the blood sugar begins to fall. Most children respond rapidly to this regimen and are chemically normal, eating well, and off intravenous maintenance within 24 to 48 h.

The nurse has a critical role in the management of the child in ketoacidosis. Vital signs and urinary output are checked frequently. The urine is also checked for the presence of sugar and acetone at each voiding. The child whose level of consciousness is decreased needs to be watched carefully for vomiting and possible aspiration. Neurological status should be checked, since cerebral edema may complicate the treatment of acidosis. Accurate measurements of intake and output are essential. If continuous insulin infusion is being used, the nurse must keep in mind that insulin disintegrates rapidly once it is mixed in solution, and therefore the insulin solution must be changed every 6 h. The rate at which the insulin is being administered must be kept steady, and a positive-pressure pump should be utilized. Infusing insulin too rapidly may cause hypoglycemia, and infusing it too slowly may delay the child's response. A cardiac monitor may be used to evaluate the child's potassium level. A flattening or absence of the T wave of the electrocardiogram may be the first indication of hypokalemia. A prolonged Q-T interval or the presence of depressed S-T segments also suggests hypokalemia. Once the child has stabilized and the intravenous insulin is to be discontinued, it is important to remember to give the first dose of subcutaneous insulin before discontinuing the intravenous insulin. Intravenous insulin is utilized very rapidly and will be virtually gone when the intravenous infusion is discontinued. If there is any delay between discontinuation of intravenous insulin and administration of the first dose of subcutaneous insulin, the child may slip back into hyperglycemia.

A variety of insulins are available for the treatment of diabetes. They are categorized as short-acting, intermediate-acting, or long-acting, according to their time of peak action and duration of action (see Table 24-3). Regular insulin is the only type that can be given intravenously; however, all insulin must be given by injection. Insulin is a protein and if taken orally would be digested by the individual's own digestive enzymes. Once a child has been taken off intravenous insulin, subcutaneous regular insulin is given three to four times a day. Once a dose has been established, the child is usually switched to short- and intermediate-acting insulins or an intermediate-acting insulin alone.

The majority of juvenile diabetics will experience a phenomenon known as the *honeymoon period* shortly after diagnosis. It appears that after an initial failing, the pancreas produces one last surge of insulin before it totally depletes itself. After the child is stabilized on the initial dose of insulin, during the honeymoon period the insulin needs will fall, and some children will need to be taken off insulin altogether. However, they will all need to go back on insulin eventually. The honeymoon period usually begins several weeks after diagnosis and may last 1 to 6 months, although there have been cases in which it lasted as long as 2 years. The parents need to be aware of this phenomenon, since the child who remains on a large dose of insulin may experience hypoglycemic reactions. This can also be a stressful time for children and parents who are having difficulty accepting the diagnosis. Often they feel that the physician has made an error and that the disease is actually going away. Some physicians will keep the young child on a token dose of 1 unit of insulin a day, rather than removing the child from insulin completely, because the psychological adjustment is so difficult.

The medical management of the child with IDDM varies greatly from physician to physician. More and more evidence is accumulating to show that tight control—i.e., the maintenance of normal or nearly normal blood sugar—will prevent the vascular complications of diabetes in the future. In general, the aim of management is normal growth and development, psychological well-being, and minimal hyperglycemia. Hyperglycemia is evaluated by a blood test that measures glycosolated hemoglobin or hemoglobin A_{1C}. This test is read as the percentage of hemoglobin attached to glucose and reflects the average blood sugar for the past 3 months. A desirable level is less than 8.5 percent.[34] The higher the hemoglobin A_{1C}, the more poorly controlled the child is.[35]

The course of the illness varies from child to child. Children who are ketosis-prone may have frequent hospitalizations or frequent absences from school as a result of ketoacidosis. However, many children are not ketosis-prone and will have no hospitalizations other than at the time they were diagnosed. The vascular complications of IDDM develop after long-standing diabetes, usually 20 years or more; this is not the case in NIDDM. These microvascular complications include retinopathy and possible blindness, nephropathy with possible kidney failure, and neuropathy. Some children develop complications during adolescence, although this is uncommon. Some never develop complications that are sig-

Table 24-3 Classification and Action Time of Insulins

Type	Example	Onset	Peak	Duration of Action
Rapid-acting	Regular	$\frac{1}{4}$ to 1 h	2 to 4 h	5 to 7 h
Intermediate-acting	NPH, lente	1 to 3 h	6 to 12 h	12 to 24 h
Long-acting	Ultralente, protamine zinc	4 to 6 h	14 to 24 h	36 h or more

Source: M. Wiener and G. Pepper, *Clinical Pharmacology and Therapeutics in Nursing*, McGraw-Hill, New York, 1985, p. 680.

nificant. It is impossible to predict the outcome for any particular child.

Nursing management The long-term management of the child with diabetes mellitus requires participation by all members of the health care team. The nurse has a vital role. After the initial diagnosis of diabetes is made, a great deal of information must be given to the child and the parents. It must be remembered that because of the shock, grief, and denial that families experience at the time of diagnosis, relatively little information may be retained at the beginning.

The family must learn several psychomotor skills during the hospitalization. The first of these skills is urine testing. Most children are able to accomplish this task by the age of 6 to 7 years. Two types of urine testing are done. One tests a first-void specimen; i.e., the child voids and tests this specimen of urine. The results will be an average of the sugar and acetone values since the child voided last, usually 2 h or more previously. The other type tests a second-void specimen; i.e., the child voids, waits approximately 15 min, and then voids again. The second specimen is then tested for sugar and acetone. This type of test reflects what is happening in the kidneys and therefore the circulation at the time of testing. Second-void specimens should be routinely tested when the child is hospitalized or anytime an insulin dose is being based solely on the results of urine testing. Most children test first-void specimens at home. Urine specimens are usually obtained before meals and at bedtime, although it is unrealistic to expect a child to test urine routinely while at school.

A variety of testing reagents are available for testing sugar and acetone. It is important to remember to utilize the proper color chart with each test, since they vary greatly. The American Diabetes Association has recommended that individuals with IDDM test with reagents that have an upper limit of 5 percent on the glucose scale. A variety of products are available, including both strip preparations and tablets. Strip preparations are preferred by most children because no equipment is needed. Strip preparations have the disadvantage of spoiling easily, particularly when the bottle caps are not replaced tightly. A few families prefer the 2-drop Clinitest tablets because they are inexpensive. If a child uses Clinitest tablets, the family must be warned of the pass-through phenomenon, which occurs when the urine contains more sugar than the test tablet can accurately indicate; the color in the test tube then passes through the bright orange at the top of the color scale and changes to a darker color, which may be misinterpreted as the lower end of the glucose scale. By watching the test tube constantly until the boiling reaction stops, the person doing the testing can see the full range of color that occurs and is not deceived by the pass-through phenomenon if it does occur. In the past, many preparations were graded according to pluses (+ to + + + +) rather than percentages. There is no consistency in the plus markings for different products. Therefore, it is now recommended that all tests be graded according to percentages rather than pluses.

Currently, more and more diabetic children (and their parents) are being taught to monitor blood glucose levels at home using a method such as a Chemstrip. An automatic lancet device punctures a fingertip, and a hanging drop of blood is transferred to the reagent area of the strip. After 60 s, the blood is wiped off with a cotton ball. After another 60 s (a total of 120 s), the color on the strip is compared with colors on the vial label (Fig. 24-4*A* and *B*). This reading gives the approximate blood glucose level. If a more precise reading is needed or if the parents or the child has difficulty interpreting the color chart, the strips may be used with a home glucose monitor, which is a machine that accurately reads the strips. It is interesting to note that many children find home glucose monitoring less objectionable than urine testing and are more compliant with this method. The child and the parents are taught how to adjust insulin, diet, and activity to maintain the blood glucose level between 80 and 120 mg/dl. Because the Chemstrip retains the color, strips can be saved and shown to the physician later for follow-up. A log of the test results and the insulin doses should be kept.

The insulin injection technique is taught to both the child and the parents. In the past, insulin was available in concentrations of 40, 80, and 100 units per milliliter. Now, only concentrations of 100 units per milliliter are normally encountered. If any of the older insulin is used, it is critically important that the type of syringe used (U 40, U 80, or U 100) be matched to the insulin concentration. Although the concentrations are different, 1 unit of U 40 equals 1 unit of U 80 or U 100. Insulin is stable at normal temperatures, but it must be protected from extreme heat and cold. The bottle or bottles in use

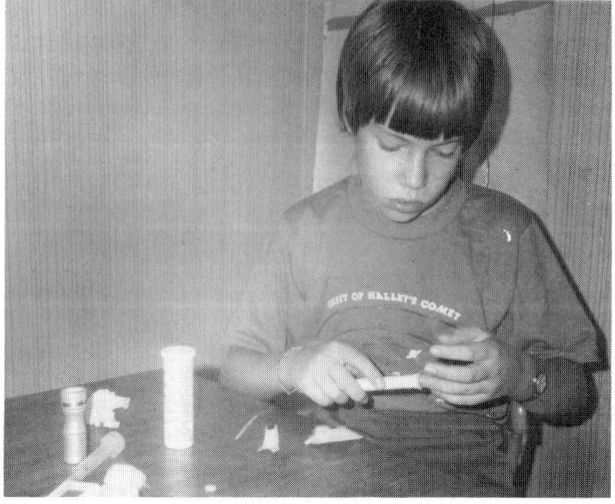

A

B

Figure 24-4 Home blood glucose monitoring. (*A*) This 9-year-old child is using an automatic lancet to puncture his fingertip to obtain blood. (*B*) The child times the procedure carefully before comparing the color on the Chemstrip with the color chart on the vial. (*Photos courtesy of Sharon Rising and Josh Rising.*)

should be kept at room temperature; this will make the insulin less irritating. Extra vials of insulin should be kept in the refrigerator. The injection technique is learned through demonstration and practice. A variety of different sites on the body are used in order to prevent atrophy or hypertrophy of the subcutaneous tissue, which interferes with insulin absorption. The same site should be used no more frequently than every 6 to 8 weeks. Sites commonly used are the posterior aspects of the arms, the deltoid regions, the upper outer quadrant of the buttocks, the abdomen, the thighs, and the calves. Often the best way to demonstrate the sites is to draw them on the child's body. This is far more effective than demonstrating on a teddy bear, for example, which has no anatomic landmarks. Children are able to master parts of the injection technique at a very early age, although there is some controversy as to how soon a child should be required to give his or her own injections (Fig. 24-5). Many people feel that the child should not be responsible for giving injections until adolescence. Others say that by the age of 10, the child has sufficient cognitive development and psychomotor skills to give injections. However, before then, the child and the parents should share in the experience. Some children are able to draw the insulin up into the syringe but are fearful of injecting themselves, while others are able to inject themselves easily but have difficulty drawing the insulin up into the syringe. In either case, the child should be allowed to learn and share the experience with the family. Many children will learn to give their own injections during the initial hospitalization. Both parents need to give the child at least one injection before discharge so that they will be capable of doing it in the event of an emergency.

Diet is an integral part of the therapy for the diabetic child. Diet plans vary from a regular diet, with the exception of concentrated sweets, to complicated diets based on divisions of calories into eighteenths of the total caloric intake. A common diet plan is based on American Diabetes Association exchange lists. All diet plans include snacks to cover peaks of insulin action and a bedtime snack to prevent nighttime hypoglycemia. Complete carbohydrates and foods high in fiber (whole-grain breads and cereals, fresh fruit and vegetables, and popcorn) are acceptable sources of fiber to children and can lead to better glycemic control than processed, refined foods.[36] Diets are also planned to promote normal growth and development and allow for the frequently changing activities of the child. It is important that the family understand the need for yearly diet revisions to accommodate the changing caloric needs of the growing child.

Many factors affect the control of diabetes in the child. Stress most commonly raises the blood sugar, although in some children it may cause hypoglycemic reactions. Exercise allows the passage of glucose directly into the cell without the addition of insulin, thereby lowering the blood sugar. On days when an unusually high level of physical activity is anticipated, insulin should be

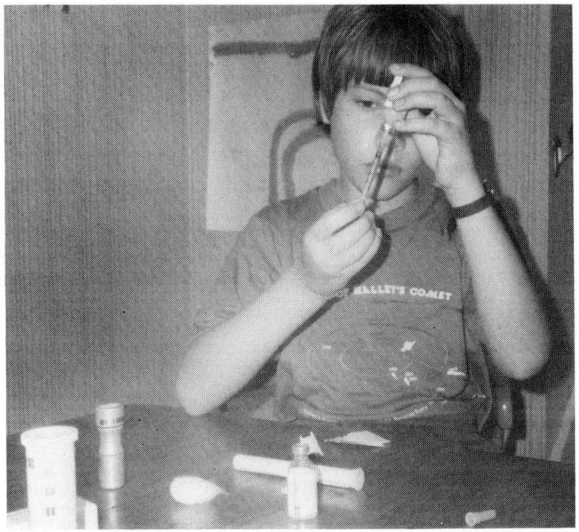

A

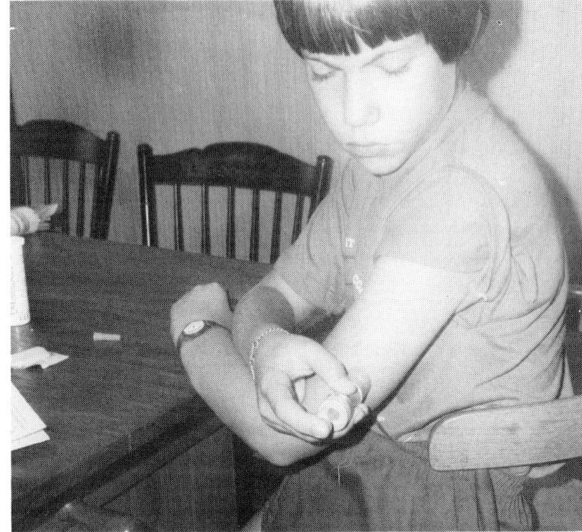

B

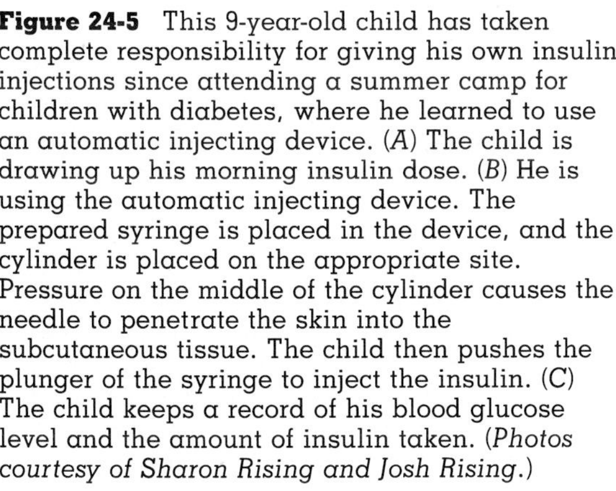

Figure 24-5 This 9-year-old child has taken complete responsibility for giving his own insulin injections since attending a summer camp for children with diabetes, where he learned to use an automatic injecting device. (*A*) The child is drawing up his morning insulin dose. (*B*) He is using the automatic injecting device. The prepared syringe is placed in the device, and the cylinder is placed on the appropriate site. Pressure on the middle of the cylinder causes the needle to penetrate the skin into the subcutaneous tissue. The child then pushes the plunger of the syringe to inject the insulin. (*C*) The child keeps a record of his blood glucose level and the amount of insulin taken. (*Photos courtesy of Sharon Rising and Josh Rising.*)

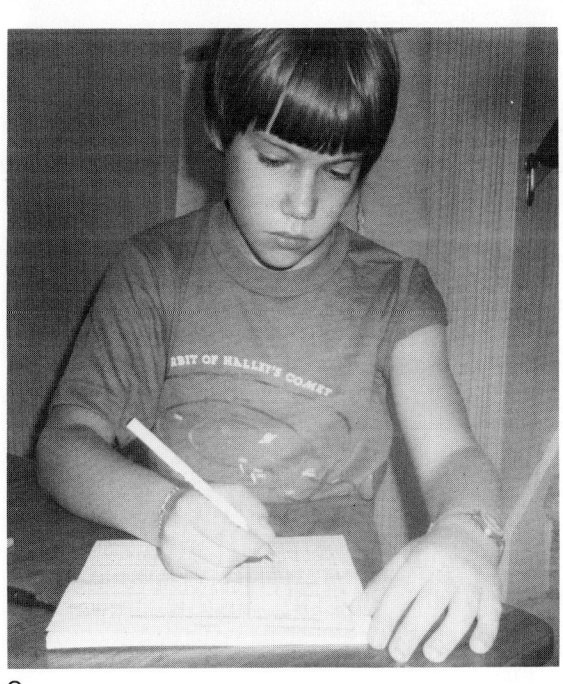

C

injected into the abdomen or buttock; uneven absorption can result from the increased blood supply to vigorously contracting limb muscles even though the insulin has been injected subcutaneously rather than intramuscularly. The production of GH and sex hormones in the growing child raises the insulin requirement. Day-to-day management fluctuates with each child, and the parents need to be able to differentiate between hyperglycemia and hypoglycemia (Table 24-4). Hypoglycemia is dangerous as well as embarrassing; repeated episodes may lead to brain damage. If the parents are in doubt as to whether the child is hypoglycemic or hyperglycemic, they are taught to treat the episode as hypoglycemia because feeding the child a small amount of sugar will not make hyperglycemia appreciably worse and because hypoglycemia is far more dangerous than hyperglycemia. Prescriptions for glucagon are given; these are kept at home in case

Table 24-4 Comparison of Hypoglycemia and Hyperglycemia

	Hyperglycemia (Acidosis)	Hypoglycemia (Insulin Reaction)
Clinical Features		
Onset	Slow (days)	Sudden (minutes to hours)
Symptoms	Thirst	Nervousness, irritability
	Headache	Headache
	Nausea	Fatigue
	Vomiting	Personality change
	Abdominal pain	Weakness
	Dim vision (myopia)	Blurred vision (diplopia)
	Dyspnea	Paresthesias
Signs	Flushing	Lethargy, stupor, convulsions
	Hyperventilation (Kussmaul respiration); rapid, deep breathing; eventual respiratory failure	Tremor
		Pallor
		Shallow respirations
	Dehydration (dry skin)	Sweating
	Rapid pulse	Variable pulse (early parasympathetic response, later sympathetic response)
	Soft eyeballs	
	Normal or absent reflexes	Positive Babinski reflex
	Acetone breath	Normal eyes
Chemical Features		
Urine	Glucose, acetone	No glucose in second voided specimen
Blood glucose	Above 240 mg/dl	Below 60 mg/dl

of hypoglycemia leading to unconsciousness. Glucagon works by mobilizing stored sugar from the liver, rapidly raising the blood sugar. However, if the sugar stores are depleted, the glucagon will have no effect, and the parents must seek help immediately. Before discharge, the parents need to know what to do if hyperglycemia or nausea and vomiting occur. During an illness, frequent blood testing may be needed if the child's appetite and intake are altered. Over-the-counter products with a high sugar content (e.g., cough syrups) should be avoided. With vomiting and diarrhea, medical care may be needed. Over time, most diabetic children and their families are able to learn to make minor adjustments in daily insulin doses to deal with elevated sugar and acetone levels.

Since the complications of long-standing diabetes do not occur in childhood, foot care and specialized skin care, which are taught to adult diabetics, are postponed for the child. Children with diabetes have no more foot problems, infections, or difficulty healing than other children. Therefore, the child needs to be taught normal good hygiene and normal first aid.

Some of the most difficult problems to deal with in a child with diabetes are the psychological effects of a chronic illness. Many parents are overprotective and fear that something will happen to their child. Others make the child's life so rigid that a normal childhood is impossible. Equally dysfunctional parenting occurs when the parents are either overindulgent or indifferent and rejecting. The parents continue to mourn the loss of their "normal" child. They, too, must make modifications in their life-style, such as *always* serving meals on time and bearing the large financial burden of monitoring and controlling their child's diabetes. Siblings may resent all the attention that the diabetic child receives. Adolescence can be a crisis period for the diabetic child and the family. Adolescents may use their diabetes as a way of acting out, resulting in poor control with frequent ketoacidosis and hospitalizations. In families where there are underlying family problems, diabetes tends to exacerbate them. The nurse needs to discuss these areas openly with the child and the family. It is far easier to prevent these problems than to deal with them in the future.

Nursing Care Plan: Diabetes Mellitus

Patient: Laurie Stewart **Age**: 14 years **Date of Admission**: 1/6 at 7:30 P.M.

ASSESSMENT

Laurie Stewart, a 14-year-old female, was admitted to the pediatric unit at 7:30 P.M. with a diagnosis of pharyngitis and diabetic ketoacidosis. The emergency room nurse who transported Laurie upstairs to the pediatric unit reported that Laurie was brought in by her mother at the advice of their doctor. Mrs. Stewart explained that the whole family had been sick with colds for the last week and that she herself had been confined to bed because of fever and cough for the last 3 days. Mrs. Stewart was unaware of Laurie's symptoms until late this afternoon, when Laurie "begged me to call the doctor."

Laurie explained that she felt well until 2 days ago, when she awoke with a sore throat. She felt progressively sicker during the day and had difficulty swallowing solid foods. This morning she took her normal dose of insulin, 17 units of regular and 35 units of lente. She was unable to eat any solid foods and had only small sips of Coca-Cola to drink, although she was very thirsty. By late this afternoon she was complaining of severe headache, abdominal pain, and difficulty breathing. Because Laurie had not tested her blood or urine since becoming ill, her physician advised her to come to the hospital for further evaluation.

ADMISSION ASSESSMENT

Upon arrival on the pediatric unit, the evening nurse made the following observations:

General appearance
Acutely ill-appearing and lethargic; answers questions but is somewhat disoriented.

Vital signs
Weight 43 kg (down approximately 2 kg from normal weight); temperature 38°C (100.4°F); pulse 88 per min; respirations 24 per min.

Skin
Pale and dry; minimal tenting and poor turgor.

Mouth
Mucous membranes dry, lips cracked and fissured, pharynx erythematous with white exudate on both tonsils.

Respirations
Deep Kussmaul respirations and strong odor of acetone on breath (smells like mixed-fruit-flavor gum).

Abdomen
Distended; no bowel sounds auscultated.

Urine
Five percent sugar, large acetone.

Blood sugar
By fingerstick > 800 mg/dl.

PHYSICIAN'S ORDERS

1. Test blood sugar, serum acetone, pH, carbon dioxide, and electrolytes stat.
2. Monitor blood sugar and serum acetone q2h × 4.
3. Do strep screen and Monospot.
4. Administer 2.5% IV dextrose and half-strength lactated Ringer's solution with 20 mEq of potassium chloride to run at 200 ml per hour.
5. Give 4 units of regular IV push insulin (done by physician).
6. Give 250 ml of IV normal saline with 100 units of regular insulin to run at 4 units per hour; connect to IVAC pump.
7. Maintain complete bed rest.
8. NPO except ice chips.
9. Monitor intake and output.
10. Weigh daily.
11. Take vital signs q2h.
12. Measure urine sugar and acetone with Chemstrip UGK at each voiding.
13. Place child on a cardiac monitor.

The physician started the IV, drew the blood for the work, and then gave the IV push insulin. While the evening nurse connected the cardiac monitor, she noted that Laurie moaned occasionally and complained of stomachache. Mrs. Stewart stayed in the room during these procedures and then announced that she had to go home because she had left her 11-year-old son in charge of the other children. The nurse gave her the unit telephone number and encouraged Mrs. Stewart to call to find out how Laurie was doing.

Shortly after Mrs. Stewart left, the nurse from the diabetes clinic arrived and related the following history. Laurie had been diagnosed as having diabetes 4 years ago. She is the oldest of seven children, and at the time of her diagnosis her mother stated that Laurie would have to take full responsibility for caring for her diabetes because she had too many other problems with the other children. Since her diagnosis, Laurie has not done particularly well and has had no family support. She has had a very difficult time following the clinic's recommendations. It is not uncommon for her to forget her insulin injections, and recently she stopped testing her blood and urine.

Nursing Diagnosis	Outcome Criteria	Nursing Interventions	Evaluation and Modifications
1. Alteration in glucose utilization secondary to infection	☐ Hyperglycemia will decrease, as evidenced by: **a.** Urinary glucose of 2 percent or less **b.** Negative urinary acetone **c.** Blood sugar 200 mg/dl or less **d.** Negative serum acetone	☐ Maintain IV insulin at 4 units per hour. ☐ Check urinary sugar and acetone at each voiding. ☐ Check blood sugar and serum acetone q2h. ☐ When blood glucose falls to 200 mg/dl, observe for insulin reaction.	☐ 1/6, 10:30 P.M.: IV is infusing well; urine is 5 percent sugar; negative acetone. ☐ 1/7, 12:30 A.M.: Urine is 2 percent sugar; negative acetone. ☐ Continue plan.
2. Fluid volume deficit and electrolyte imbalance related to osmotic diuresis	☐ Fluid and electrolyte balance will be restored, as evidenced by: **a.** Firm skin turgor **b.** Moist mucous membranes **c.** Urinary volume of approximately 1300 ml per 24 h **d.** Normal T wave formation **e.** Return to normal weight	☐ Maintain IV at 200 ml per hour with 20 mEq of potassium chloride. ☐ Apply Vaseline to lips q2h or prn; give ice chips prn. ☐ Record intake and output q2h. ☐ Monitor T wave q1h. ☐ Weigh daily.	☐ 1/6, 8:30 P.M.: IV is infusing well; normal T wave formation. Increased comfort from ice chips and Vaseline. ☐ 1/7, 12 noon: Weight is up to 43.5 kg. ☐ Continue plan.
3. Abdominal pain and distention with decreased peristalsis secondary to ketoacidosis	☐ Abdominal pain and distention will decrease, and normal peristalsis will be established.	☐ Provide measures to resolve ketoacidosis as outlined in nursing diagnoses 1 and 2. ☐ Give ice chips prn. ☐ Auscultate for bowel sounds q2h. ☐ Position child on side. ☐ Have child wear hospital gown without pants to bind at waist.	☐ 1/6, 9:30 P.M.: IV is infusing well; child is taking ice chips without increased distention; no nausea or vomiting. ☐ 1/7, 3:30 A.M.: Bowel sounds were auscultated. ☐ 1/7, 8 A.M.: Child is alert and hungry. ☐ Continue plan.
4. Alteration in breathing pattern: dyspnea related to metabolic acidosis	☐ Normal breathing patterns will be established, as evidenced by: **a.** Respiratory rate of 14 to 18 breaths per minute **b.** No acetone detectable on breath	☐ Provide measures to resolve ketoacidosis (nursing diagnoses 1 and 2). ☐ Elevate head of bed 45°.	☐ 1/6, 10:30 P.M.: Breathing has eased; child appears more comfortable. ☐ 1/7, 12:30 A.M.: No acetone was detectable on breath. ☐ Continue plan.

Nursing Diagnosis	Outcome Criteria	Nursing Interventions	Evaluation and Modifications
5. Fatigue and disorientation secondary to diminished cell utilization of glucose	☐ There will be reorientation of time and place and uninterrupted sleep between voidings.	☐ Provide measures to resolve ketoacidosis (nursing diagnoses 1 and 2). ☐ While child is awake, give short reminders of time and place. ☐ Evaluate physical signs without waking child. ☐ Offer ice chips when child is awakened for voiding.	☐ 1/7, 12:30 A.M.: Child is sleeping soundly. ☐ 1/7, 8:30 A.M.: Child is awake and oriented. ☐ Continue plan.
6. Lack of compliance with treatment regimen, leading to insufficient insulin intake and hospitalization	☐ Blood and urine tests will be done four times per day when child is confined to home because of illness.	☐ Begin education program to cover: **a.** Relationship of insulin needs to blood sugar and acetone **b.** Relationship of illness to insulin needs **c.** Psychomotor skills involved in blood and urine testing ☐ Give blood and urine testing equipment to child to take home. ☐ Review educational program with mother. ☐ Encourage mother to become involved with diabetes care, especially when child is ill. ☐ Introduce child to other adolescents with diabetes on pediatric unit. ☐ Suggest contacting Juvenile Diabetes Foundation children's group for support at home.	☐ 1/7, 12:30 P.M.: Child is testing blood and urine on her own. ☐ 1/7, 8 P.M.: Child is able to discuss relationship of illness, insulin, and blood sugar. ☐ Continue plan.

References

1. Williams, Robert H. (ed.), *Textbook of Endocrinology,* Saunders, Philadelphia, 1981, p. 4.
2. Bacon, George E., et al., *A Practice Approach to Pediatric Endocrinology,* Year Book, Chicago, 1982, p. 76.
3. Whaley, Lucille F., and Donna L. Wong, *Nursing Care of Infants and Children,* Mosby, St. Louis, 1983, p. 1024.
4. Ibid.
5. Bacon, op. cit., p. 254.
6. Ibid., p. 199.
7. Ibid., p. 200.
8. Williams, op. cit., p. 173.
9. Coody, Deborah, "Congenital Hypothyroidism," *Pediatric Nursing* **10**(6):342 (September–October 1984).
10. Bacon, op. cit., p. 139.
11. Ibid., p. 142.
12. Williams, op. cit., p. 172.
13. Ibid., p. 182.
14. Bacon, op. cit., p. 124.
15. Ibid., pp. 127–130.
16. Ibid., p. 134.
17. Ibid., p. 129.
18. Ibid., p. 164.
19. Ibid., pp. 169–170.
20. Ibid., p. 153.
21. Mazur, Tom, "Ambiguous Genitalia: Detection and Counseling," *Pediatric Nursing* **9**(6):417 (November–December 1983).
22. Williams, op. cit., p. 286.

23. Stanbury, J., J. Wyngaaren, D. Fredrickson, J. Goldstein, and M. Brown, *The Metabolic Basis of Inherited Disease,* McGraw-Hill, New York, 1983, p. 985.
24. Ibid.
25. Petrillo, Madeline, and Sirgay Sanger, *Emotional Care of Hospitalized Children,* Lippincott, Philadelphia, 1980, p. 17.
26. Bacon, op. cit., p. 167.
27. Ibid., pp. 168–169.
28. Whaley and Wong, op. cit., p. 1474.
29. Williams, op. cit., p. 269.
30. West, Kelly M., "Standardization of Definition, Classification, and Reporting in Diabetes-Related Epidemiologic Studies," *Diabetes Care* **2**:65–76 (1979).
31. Stanbury, Wyngaaren, Fredrickson, Goldstein, and Brown, op. cit., p. 102.
32. Green, Morris, and Robert J. Haggerty, *Ambulatory Pediatrics,* Saunders, Philadelphia, 1984, p. 394.
33. Bacon, op. cit., pp. 5–8.
34. Fow, Susan, "Home Blood Glucose Monitoring in Children with Insulin-Dependent Diabetes Mellitus," *Pediatric Nursing* **9**(6):439 (November–December 1983).
35. Ibid., p. 442.
36. Faro, Beverly, "Maintaining Good Control in Children with Diabetes," *Pediatric Nursing* **9**(5):371 (September–October 1983).

25

Rosalyn Podratz
Maureen DeMaio-Esteves
Julie A. Goodman

Reproductive function and adolescent sexuality

Upon completion of this chapter, the student will be able to:

1 Describe the anatomy and physiology of the male and female reproductive tracts.
2 Describe alterations related to dysfunctional uterine bleeding.
3 Describe the causal relationships between the embryological development of the reproductive tract and alterations such as ambiguous genitalia, Klinefelter syndrome, and monosomy X.
4 Identify several malformations of the male genital organs that affect normal urinary or reproductive function.
5 List the reasons why adolescents fail to use birth control methods.
6 Compare the effectiveness of temporary methods of birth control for teenagers.
7 Describe the teaching needed to prepare the teenage girl for her first pelvic examination.
8 Describe the social, psychological, and health-related problems associated with adolescent pregnancy.
9 Identify the predictors of success in young mothers.

Fertilization of an ovum by a sperm and continued embryological development occur in an ordered and systematic way. Genetic sex is determined at the time of conception by the presence of the X or Y chromosome in the sperm that fertilizes the ovum. When a sperm containing a chromosome complement of 23,X unites with an ovum containing a chromosome complement of 23,X a normal female, 46,XX, will result. When a sperm with a chromosome complement of 23,Y unites with an ovum with a chromosome complement of 23,X, a normal male, 46,XY, will result.

EMBRYOLOGICAL ORIGIN OF THE REPRODUCTIVE TRACT

Although an infant's sex is determined at conception, the reproductive system does not begin to develop until about the fourth week after fertilization.[1] Appropriate sexual development occurs if the subsequent steps in physical development proceed normally: first, differentiation of the bipotential gonad; second, differentiation and development of the internal reproductive system; and third, differentiation and development of the external genitalia (Fig. 25-1).[2]

During the first 6 weeks of gestation, the embryonic sex glands, or *gonads,* are undifferentiated in the male and the female. At this time the gonad is known as a *bipotential gonad* (able to form either testes or ovaries). It consists of a central medulla, which develops if the fetus is a male, and a cortex, which develops if the fetus is a female.

At about the seventh to the eighth week of gestation, differentiation into ovaries or testes takes place. The presence of the Y chromosome, with the H-Y gene on its short arm, is required for the development of testes.

The fetal internal reproductive structures de-

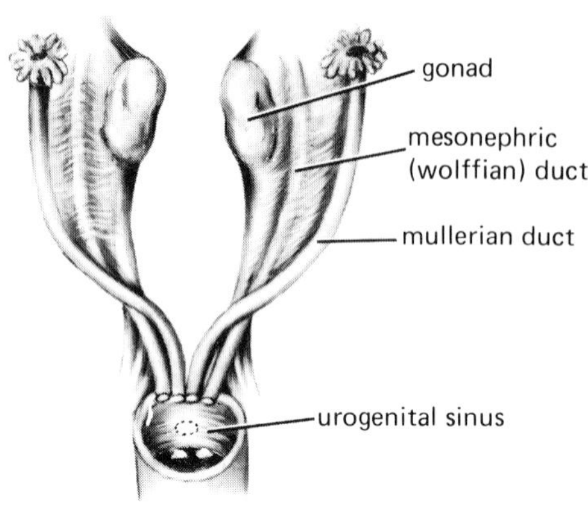

Figure 25-1 Differentiation of the bipotential gonad into testes or ovaries. (*A*) The primordial germ cells have colonized the peripheral region of the indifferent gonad. (*B* and *C*) Male germ cells migrate into the central mass of gonadal tissue. The periphery becomes free of cells, forming a connective tissue layer. (*D* and *E*) Female germ cells are surrounded by migrating gonadal cells to form primary follicles. (*From S. Ohno, Sex Chromosomes and Sex-Linked Genes, Springer-Verlag, New York, 1967, p. 163. Used with permission.*)

velop as female unless a masculinizing substance, androgens from the testes, is present. Under the influence of androgen and a nonsteroid substance produced by the fetal testes, the Wolffian ducts (male reproductive structures) develop into the epididymides, the vasa deferentia, and the seminal vesicles. At the same time, the growth of the Müllerian duct (a female reproductive structure) is inhibited, and the duct later degenerates.

The final stage of reproductive development is the differentiation of the external genitalia (Fig. 25-2). The fetus is clearly recognizable as a male or female by the third month. The external genitalia of both sexes develop from one set of structures. The beginnings of the external genitalia are found in the genital tubercle, the urethral folds, and the two genital swellings, or labioscrotal folds.

The external genitalia begin to develop sexual characteristics after 8 weeks of gestation. The *genital tubercle* elongates to form a central phallus. This extends to become either the penis or the clitoris. The *urethral folds* develop, and the *urethral groove* becomes the opening of the urogenital sinus, forming the lower vagina and urethral opening or the perineal and penile urethra. The two urethral folds fuse to become the skin that encloses the penile urethra and forms the foreskin. In the female, the unfused lips of the urethral folds become the labia minora and the hood of the clitoris. The genital swellings, or *labioscrotal folds*, fuse and become the scrotum in the male or remain unfused and become the labia majora in the female. If normal development fails to occur, the infant may be born with the genitourinary tract anomalies discussed in this chapter.

ANATOMY AND PHYSIOLOGY OF THE REPRODUCTIVE TRACT

The primary organs of reproduction are the *gonads:* the testes in the male and the ovaries in the female. The *germ cells*, or sex cells (the *gametes*), are the sperm in the male and the ova in the female. Reproduction is possible only when all the factors necessary for fertilization are present: the internal and external organs of reproduction, the appropriate hormones, and normal germ cell development.

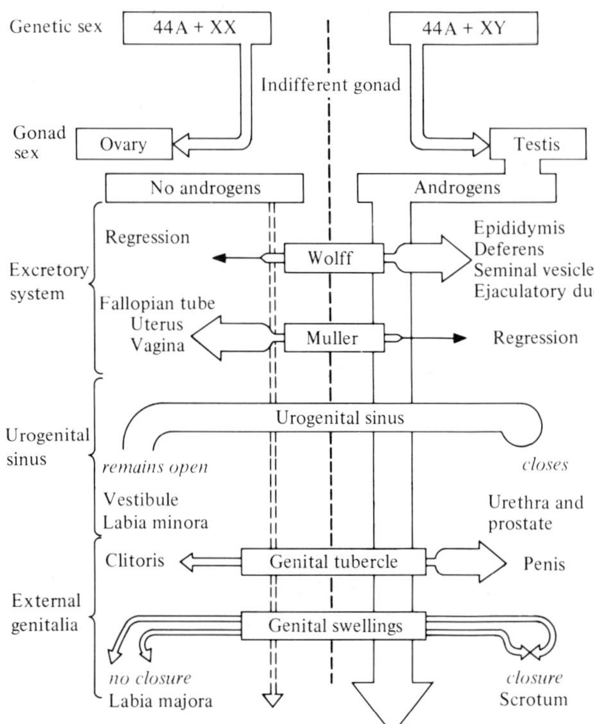

Figure 25-2 The developmental fate of the reproductive organs of the indifferent gonad and its hormonal regulation. (*From H. Tuchmann-Duplessis and P. Hagel, Illustrated Human Embryology, vol. 2, Organogenesis, Springer-Verlag, New York, 1974, p. 100. Used with permission.*)

Female reproductive anatomy

External female reproductive organs Figure 25-3 illustrates the external genitalia of the female. An understanding of the normal structures will facilitate an understanding of the visible external genital defects discussed later in this chapter. The *labia majora* are two folds of skin from the mons pubis that pass downward and disappear in the posterior portion of the vulva in front of the anus. They are analogous to the scrotum in the male. *Bartholin's glands* are located at the base on either side. These glands are responsible for the secretion of mucin, which keeps the surface of the labia moist. The *labia minora* are folds of skin and mucous membrane found between the labia majora. At the upper margin, the labia minora unite above the clitoris to form the *frenulum*. The *clitoris*, analogous to the penis in the male, has erectile tissue and sensory nerve endings and is covered by the prepuce. The *hymen*, a fold of mucous membrane, partially covers the external opening of the vagina. *Skene's ducts* are located on each side of the urinary meatus. Both the Skene's ducts and Bartholin's glands can harbor infection.

Internal female reproductive organs The *ovaries* are the active source of the female hormones, estrogen and progesterone. They consist of two layers: the *cortex*, or outer layer, contains the egg cells, or ova, and the *medulla*, or inner vascular layer, is the site of ova ripening. The *fallopian tubes*, each about 10 cm long, connect the ovaries to the uterus. These are narrower at the uterine end and have a funnel-shaped, fimbriated end over each ovary. Fingerlike folds of the inner muscle layer move by peristalsis, creating a current to transport the ovum through the tube toward the uterus.

The *uterus*, a muscular, pear-shaped organ located between the bladder and the rectum, has the ability to stretch to 500 times its normal capacity in full-term pregnancy and to return to near normal size. The *vagina*, or birth canal, is lined with mucous membrane that contains surface folds, or *rugae*, which facilitate stretching during childbirth. Figure 25-4 illustrates normal internal female reproductive anatomy.

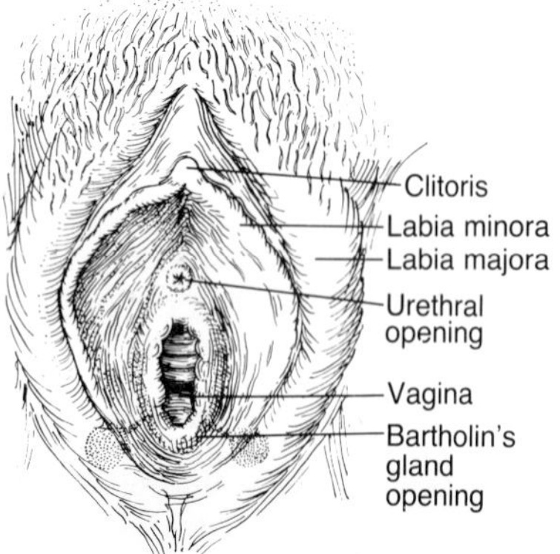

Figure 25-3 The external genitalia of the female. (*From Robert S. Hillman et al., Clinical Skills, McGraw-Hill, New York, 1981, p. 355. Used with permission.*)

Male reproductive anatomy

External male reproductive organs The external male reproductive organs are the *scrotum* and the *penis*. The scrotum contains the *testes* and is a continuation of the abdominal cavity. During fetal development, the testes develop in the peritoneal cavity. At about 36 weeks, the testes descend into the scrotal sac, and the canal connecting the sac to the abdominal cavity closes. The penis consists of *cavernous bodies* (erectile tissue) and the *urethra*. It is through the urethra that the seminal fluid is excreted. The cavernous bodies contain blood spaces that are empty when the penis is flaccid. When these spaces fill with blood, the penis becomes erect. The external urinary meatus is found in the *glans penis*. The glans penis is almost completely enclosed by a fold of skin called the *foreskin* or *prepuce*. This foreskin is removed when a circumcision is done.

Internal male reproductive organs The internal male reproductive organs are the testes, canal systems, and accessory structures (Fig. 25-5). The two testes in the scrotal sac contain the terminal portion of the *seminiferous tubules* (which eventually forms the tube of the *epididymis*) and interstitial tissue (which contains Leydig cells). The epithelial lining of the tubules consists of supporting cells and *spermatogenic* (sperm-producing) cells. The Leydig cells function in the production of androgens, especially testosterone. Production of sperm begins at puberty, and the seminiferous tubules undergo a gradual involution with advancing age.

PHYSIOLOGY OF REPRODUCTION

Puberty

The physical changes that occur during adolescence are characterized by maturation of the re-

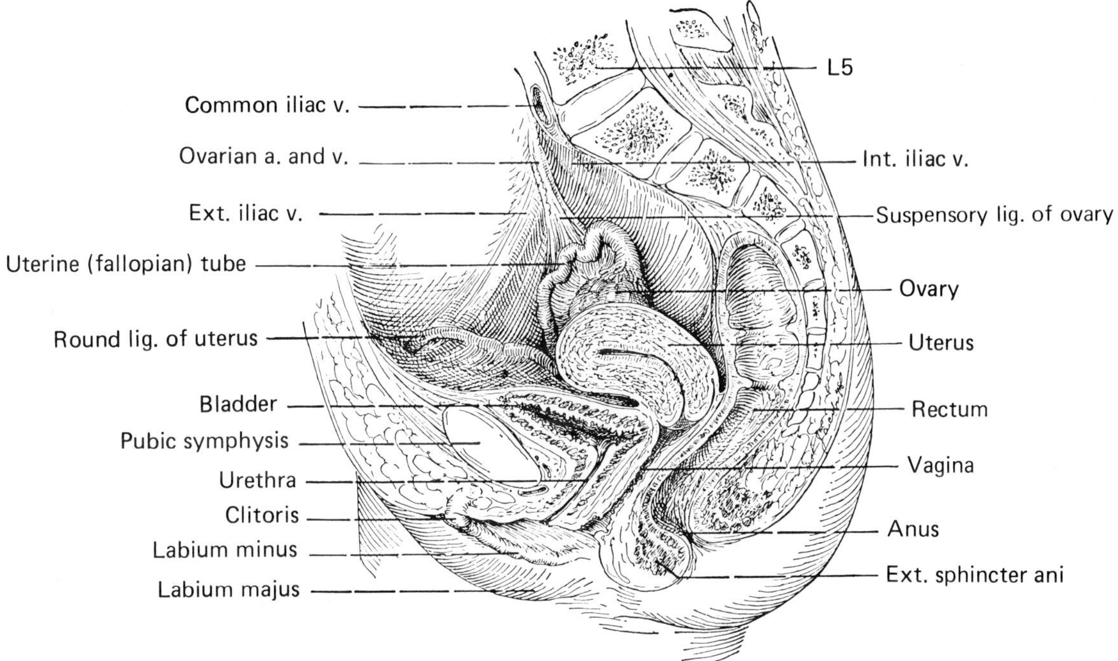

Figure 25-4 A midsagittal section through the female pelvis. (*From Charles E. Tobin and John J. Jacobs* [eds.], *Shearer's Manual of Human Dissection, 6th ed., McGraw-Hill, New York, 1981, p. 188. Used with permission.*)

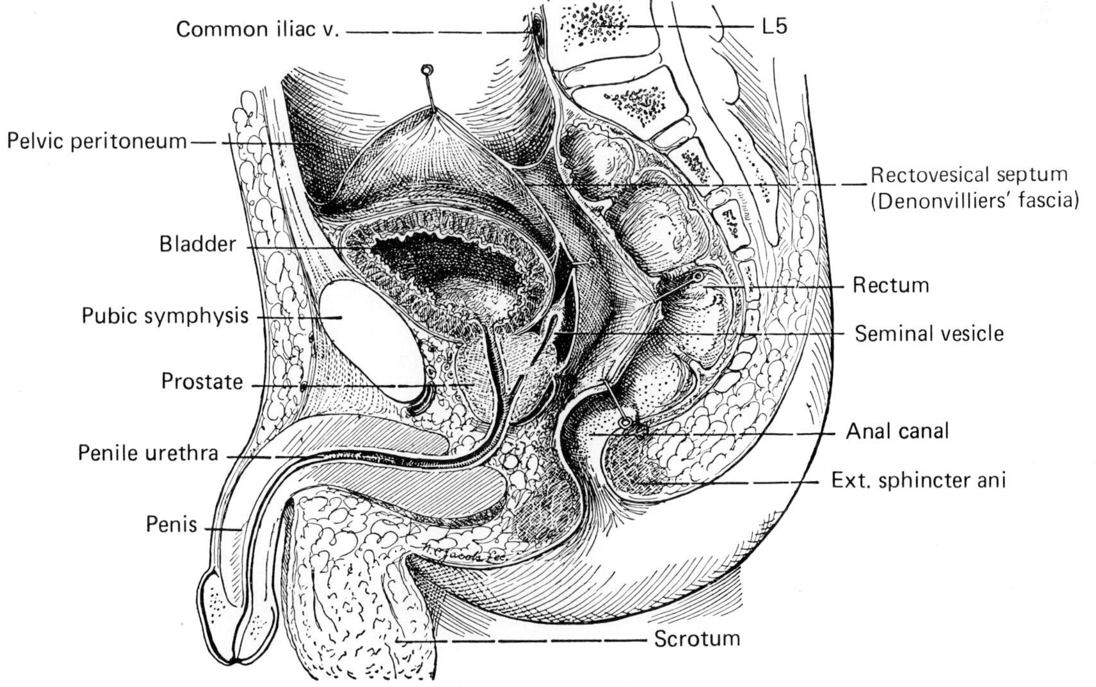

Figure 25-5 A midsagittal section through the male pelvis. (*From Charles E. Tobin and John J. Jacobs* [eds.], *Shearer's Manual of Human Dissection, 6th ed., McGraw-Hill, New York, 1981, p. 180. Used with permission.*)

productive organs, development of secondary sex characteristics, and a growth spurt that affects almost all the organs and tissues of the body. In boys, these changes occur from ages 12 to 20, and in girls they take place from ages 10 to 18.

During childhood, a low level of follicle-stimulating hormone from the adrenal cortex is present in both sexes. The hypothalamus is responsible for releasing factors to the pituitary that stimulate the release of gonadotropic hormones, which are responsible for pubertal sexual maturation. At puberty, there is a growth spurt in the male's testes and the female's uterus and an activation of pituitary and gonadal hormones (estrogens and androgens). Chapter 13 describes the changes and endocrinology of puberty.

The male hormonal cycle

The pituitary gland secretes two major gonadotropic hormones, which are responsible for male sexual function: follicle-stimulating hormone (FSH) and luteinizing hormone (LH). Androgens, principally testosterone, are secreted by the testes. FSH stimulates and regulates spermatogenesis in conjunction with testosterone. LH stimulates the interstitial Leydig cells to produce testosterone.

Female hormonal cycle

The ovaries contain all the primordial follicles (immature ova) at birth. They continue to grow slowly throughout childhood under the influence of low levels of follicle-stimulating hormone. At puberty, under the influence of higher levels of ovarian hormones, the follicles develop into mature ova. There is a cyclic production of estrogen for about 2 years prior to menstruation.

The menstrual cycle The *menstrual cycle* is determined by the cyclic interaction of releasing factors from the hypothalamus and hormones from the pituitary and the ovaries. The changes in the levels of estrogen and progesterone cause the uterine endometrial cells to proliferate, become secretory, and finally slough, resulting in menstruation. The average length of the menstrual cycle is 28 days, although cycles of 21-35 days are considered normal. The menstrual flow lasts about 3 to 7 days, and there is a blood loss of about 60 ml. Figure 25-6 shows the hormonal, ovarian, and uterine changes that take place during the menstrual cycle.

ABNORMALITIES OF SEXUAL DEVELOPMENT

An abnormality that occurs during any stage of embryological sexual development can lead to a defect that is present in the infant at birth. The following four mechanisms underlie most defects:

1. Abnormal sex determination due to faulty sex chromosomes
2. Failure of the bipotential gonad to differentiate
3. Incomplete development of the ductal system
4. Abnormal amounts of androgens or insensitivity of the male fetus to androgens[3]

Ambiguous genitalia

The first question normally asked by parents of a newborn is, "Is it a boy or a girl?" When the baby's genitalia are not clearly male or female, this question becomes difficult to answer. The presence of ambiguous genitalia should alert the physician or nurse to the possibility of associated defects in the internal reproductive tract. The abnormalities present in infants that cause the genitalia to appear ambiguous include (1) an enlarged clitoris or a small penis with hypospadias; (2) a partial fusion of the labioscrotal skin, which can look like an incompletely formed scrotum or a bifid scrotum; (3) the absence of gonads or a single testis in an incompletely formed scrotum; and (4) chordee tendineae (a downward bending of the penis, frequently associated with hypospadias).[4]

Hermaphroditism The condition of *hermaphroditism* is present when a female fetus is masculinized or a male fetus is incompletely masculinized. *True hermaphroditism,* in which both ovarian tissue and testicular tissue are present, is very rare. The chromosome complement is usually 46,XX but may be 46,XY. The choice of sex of rearing is determined largely by the external genitalia, with consideration given to which gonads are present.

Masculinized females *Masculinized females,* or *female pseudohermaphrodites,* have a chromosome complement of 46,XX, and the ovaries are present. The external genitalia resemble those of a male, even though the internal reproductive organs and the genetic components are female.

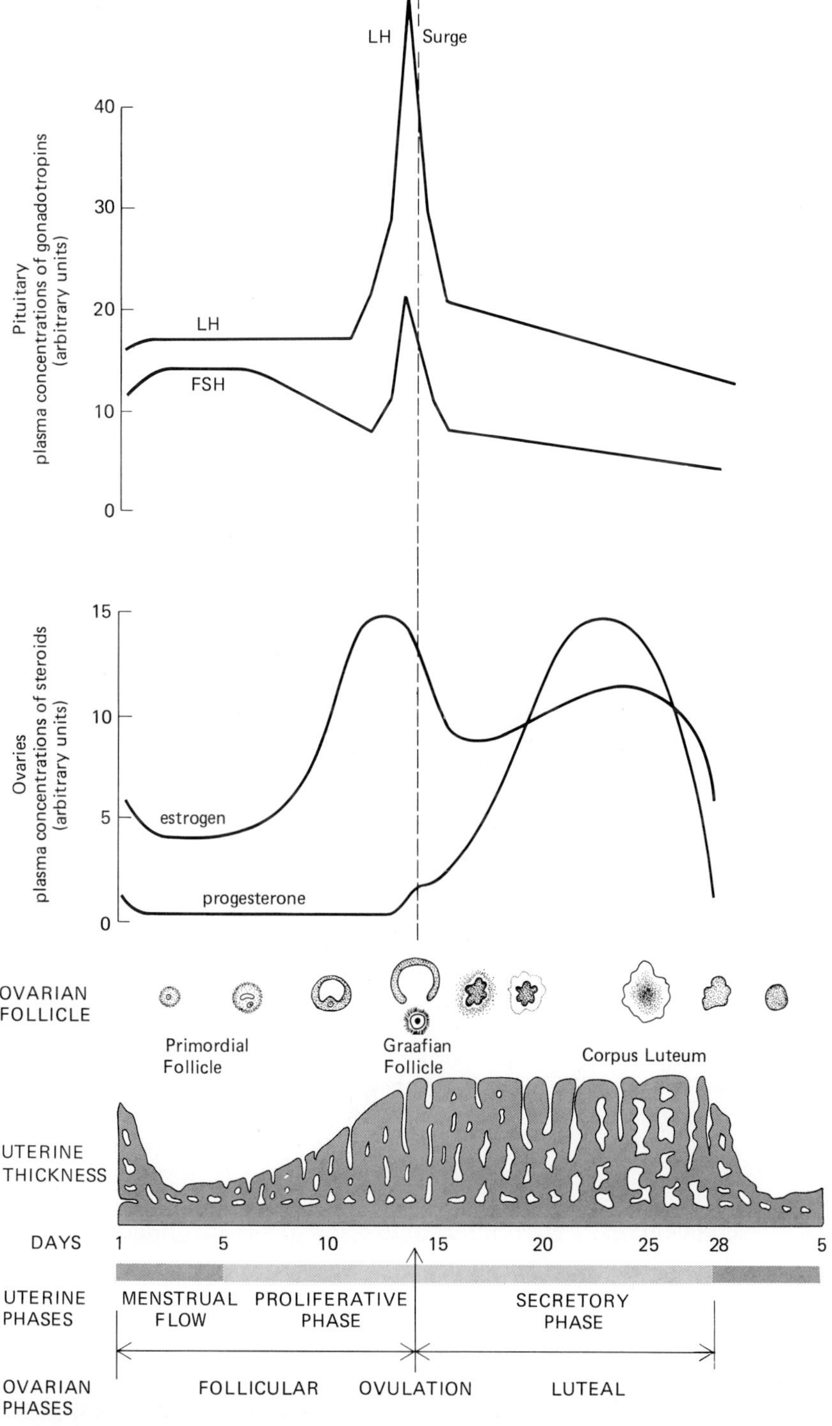

The cycle begins with day one of the menses and progresses in well-defined steps. The primordial follicle matures in the ovaries stimulated by pituitary and ovarian hormones and develops into the graafian follicle in the first 2 weeks of the cycle. At about 14 days, with the LH surge, ovulation occurs and the corpus luteum develops and produces large amounts of progesterone and estrogen.
The changes seen in the endometrial cycle are in direct response to the levels of estrogen and progesterone. The follicular phase, a period of rapid endometrial growth under the influence of estrogen, ends at ovulation. The luteal phase under the control of progesterone converts the endometrium into an actively secreting tissue. If no pregnancy occurs, the corpus luteum degenerates, with a drop in estrogen and progesterone that initiates the sloughing of the endometrium and the menstrual bleed.

Figure 25-6 A summary of plasma hormone concentrations, ovarian events, and uterine changes during the menstrual cycle. (*From Arthur J. Vander, James H. Sherman, and Dorothy S. Luciano, Human Physiology: Mechanisms of Body Function, 3d ed., McGraw-Hill, New York, 1980, p. 497. Used with permission.*)

The external genitalia have varying degrees of labial fusion and clitoral enlargement and resemble a penis and scrotum; however, no testes are palpable in what appears to be the scrotum. It is always important to differentiate female masculinization from undescended testes, a common occurrence in male infants.

Increased adrenal secretions are the most common cause of female fetal masculinization. This is called the *adrenogenital syndrome* and is discussed in Chap. 24. Recent medical literature has reported the development of ambiguous genitalia in infants whose mothers took Danazol for endometriosis during the first trimester of pregnancy. Steroids and progestational agents used during pregnancy cross the placental barrier and have an androgenic effect on the fetus's genitalia and urogenital sinus. They do not act on the Müllerian ducts. Therefore, the ovaries, tubes, and uterus are normal, while the external genitalia are masculinized. Surgical reconstruction of the labia, clitoris, and vagina is usually done during the first year. Estrogen cream may also be used for mild labial fusion, coupled with daily gentle, progressive manual separation. Cortisone therapy may enable a woman with this condition to bear children.

Incompletely masculinized males *Incompletely masculinized males*, or *male pseudohermaphrodites*, have a normal male chromosome complement of 46,XY. The testes may be undescended or atropic, and the external genitalia are affected. The penis may be small, hypospadiac, or fully formed, or a blind vaginal pouch may be present. Treatment with testosterone may be used to stimulate growth of the penis in some males.

Androgen insensitivity syndrome *Androgen insensitivity syndrome* is the result of a genetically male fetus that is unable to respond to androgen. The external genitalia are female, but undescended testes and a chromosome complement of 46,XY are present. The menstrual cycle does not begin during adolescence because the internal female sexual reproductive organs are absent. The child should be reared as a female, since the cells are unable to use androgen and therefore male sexual characteristics cannot be stimulated to develop.

Treatment When an infant has ambiguous genitalia, a complete diagnostic evaluation by a medical team made up of endocrinologists, urologists, and gynecologists is essential. A careful study of the chromosome complement, hormones, external genitalia, and internal reproductive organs is necessary before it can be decided whether a male or a female sex assignment will be best for the child. This decision is not always made on the basis of genetic sex. The functional genitalia and the predicted outcomes of medical and surgical procedures are also considered in the decision.

The first step in the evaluation is a complete maternal history, focusing particularly on hormones and medications taken during pregnancy, and a newborn physical examination. Any signs of hypospadias, undescended testes, an enlarged clitoris, labial fusion, or a small penis are noted. A buccal smear for nuclear chromatin (Barr body) is done. An X-chromatin-positive child is usually female, and an X-chromatin-negative child is a genetic male in 90 percent of the cases. Urinary steroid excretion is measured if adrenal cortex imbalance is implicated (see Chap. 24). Determination of the sex of gonads present is made by ultrasound and, if absolutely necessary, by exploratory surgery. Genitourinography (in which dye is injected to enable visualization of the genitourinary structures) will also help determine which internal reproductive structures are present, especially in the male.

Genital surgery is usually done at an early age. If the surgery is delayed or needs to be done in stages, the child is given age-appropriate information about the surgery. The most frequent surgical procedures are hypospadias repair, a clitoridectomy, and vaginal and penile reconstruction. Each child is approached on an individual basis, using the physical and genetic findings.

Counseling the parents of children with ambiguous genitalia should be done very carefully to avoid unduly frightening them, while making sure always to give accurate information. Mazure suggests that the parents should be told that the examination revealed "underdeveloped" or "unfinished" sex organs and that a more complete examination is needed to determine whether the internal sex organs are also underdeveloped and what the best course of treatment for the child is.[5] Explaining to parents that a fetus has the potential to be either a male or a female and giving them information regarding the differentiation of internal and external genitalia is helpful. They begin to understand that the process is complex and that sexual ambiguity can occur in any fetus if differentiation is interrupted.

After the gender has been ascertained, the condition should be fully explained to the parents. Pictures or sketches are used to illustrate exactly what happened during embryonic growth and what is present in their child. Correct anatomic terminology is used and defined. Emphasis should be placed on the fact that the child will not grow up with abnormal sexual desires and that sexual identity as a boy or a girl is greatly dependent on the sex of rearing. Sex orientation and gender role are established in the $1\frac{1}{2}$- to $2\frac{1}{2}$-year-old child, and sex assignment should be made before that time.

As the child grows older, the need for psychological guidance may become greater. Children with ambiguous genitalia will need explanations similar to those given to the parents so that they can understand their physical status as they become aware of their differences from other children. An honest approach to educating these children about their condition is important. They are all too aware that their genitals are the focus of attention; when children are known to be sterile, this should be shared with them, rather than letting them discover it later by themselves.

Delayed puberty

Adolescents who do not experience pubertal changes, especially when they compare themselves with others of the same age, may become very impatient and upset. Although most adolescents will develop normally, given time, during the waiting period they need to be treated with understanding. An underlying disease process, such as diabetes mellitus, malabsorption syndrome, anorexia nervosa, hypothyroidism, hyperthyroidism, and sometimes asthma, can delay puberty and should be considered. An error involving sex chromosomes can also result in failure to develop secondary sex characteristics. A general physical examination and the same diagnostic studies discussed earlier in this chapter may be necessary.

The onset of menstruation is given more attention in our society than any other sexual characteristic. Menstruation and secondary female sex characteristics serve as an indication of sexual development. The menarche (the onset of menstruation) requires normal functioning of the hypothalamus, pituitary, and ovaries; a normal uterus; and a patent lower genital tract. The average age at the onset of menstruation is from 9.1 to 17.7 years.[6] A delay much beyond the age of 14, if the girl has a short or immature stature and no secondary sex characteristics are present, indicates the need for evaluation of sexual development.

Klinefelter syndrome The chromosome complement of males with *Klinefelter syndrome* is usually 47,XXY. Klinefelter syndrome is not apparent until puberty, when normal male secondary characteristics fail to develop as a result of androgen deficiency. Instead, the boy begins to develop female characteristics, such as breast enlargement and fat deposits on the hips, and he retains a high-pitched voice. These males have a penis that is small to normal in size, small testes, and an absence of sperm in their seminal fluid, resulting in fertility problems. Mental impairment of varying degrees may also be present.

Treatment Treatment consists of oral administration of testosterone, subcutaneous implantation of testosterone (every 6 to 9 months), or stimulation of the testosterone-producing cells (Leydig cells) of the testes. Gonadotropin is used to improve male appearance.

Monosomy X *Monosomy X*, or *Turner syndrome*, results in the failure of normal female sexual development due to the absence of an X chromosome. There are several different karyotypes found in this disease, such as 45,X or 46 with an abnormal X. The ovaries are usually poorly developed or absent (female gonadal dysgenesis). The symptoms in puberty relate to estrogen deficiency: primary amenorrhea, scanty menstruation, lack of sexual development, and failure to grow (most affected girls are less than 150 cm tall). Some girls have a characteristic webbing of the neck due to the development of extra skinfolds, lymphedema of the legs, thin hair, ptosis (drooping of the eyelids), shield chest (tapering of the anterior chest wall with widely spaced nipples and poor breast development), and mental retardation. Congenital anomalies, especially cardiac defects, are frequently found with this syndrome.

Treatment Treatment of girls with monosomy X consists of estrogen replacement and psychological counseling. Initially, these children receive continuous estrogen therapy until the secondary sex characteristics have developed. Then cyclic estrogen therapy is begun (consisting of 3 weeks on the therapy and 1 week off), during which simulated menstruation occurs. Synthetic androgens may also be given to stimulate growth.

ALTERATIONS OF FEMALE REPRODUCTIVE FUNCTION

Dysfunctional uterine bleeding

Dysfunctional uterine bleeding may be characterized as excessive or prolonged (menorrhagia) or inadequate (oligomenorrhea). In girls between the ages of 10 and 20, most abnormal menstruation results from immaturity of the hypothalamic-pituitary-ovarian function; however, other sources must be excluded before this diagnosis can be confirmed.

In order for a cyclic menstrual flow to be maintained, four basic conditions must be present: (1) the hypothalamus must produce gonadotropin-releasing hormones, which regulate pituitary function; (2) the pituitary gland must release the gonadotropins, LH and FSH; (3) the ovaries must synthesize steroids, estrogen, and progesterone, in response to the gonadotropins; and (4) the cervix, vagina, and hymen must be patent and the uterus must have a cavity capable of endometrial development and shedding in response to the levels of ovarian steroids in the blood.[7]

Dysfunctional uterine bleeding is diagnosed by ruling out other causes of the bleeding. A complete evaluation includes a sexual and menstrual history, a pregnancy test, a culture for chlamydia and gonorrhea, a pelvic examination with a Pap smear, and a physical examination. Further testing done as indicated includes tests of adrenal, pituitary, and ovarian hormone levels; a complete blood count, including a platelet count; and coagulation studies to detect possible hematologic disease.

Typically, dysfunctional uterine bleeding is heavy, painless menstrual bleeding that occurs at abnormally long or abnormally short intervals. Estrogen causes the uterine endometrium to proliferate in the first half of the menstrual cycle, but it cannot convert uterine endometrium to secretory endometrium without progesterone and it cannot maintain the endometrium throughout the cycle. Insufficient ovarian production of progesterone thus results in patchy, endometrial sloughing with heavy, irregular bleeding as a result of estrogen breakthrough.[8]

Treatment Sources of heavy bleeding related to pregnancy, the presence of an intrauterine device, and sexually transmitted diseases such as chlamydia and gonorrhea infections, must be ruled out. Hematologic disease, with a history of bruising or prolonged bleeding and anemia, can result in irregular, anovulatory menses. Pituitary tumors may present with high prolactin levels, galactorrhea (secreting breasts in the nonpregnant, nonnursing woman), and adrenal tumors associated with androgenization (increased hair production on the face and back and acne). Elevated serum testosterone levels are indicative of increased ovarian output and an ovarian tumor. A pelvic examination is done to check for evidence of trauma or the presence of a foreign body, such as a forgotten tampon. The cervix is examined for changes, and the size and shape of the uterus are assessed; if the results of a manual examination are questionable, a pelvic ultrasound is done. Fibroids and polyps are a rare cause of dysfunctional uterine bleeding in young girls.

After other causes of menorrhagia have been ruled out, treatment is begun. If bleeding is minimal, the girl can be observed for 6 to 12 months to be certain that regular menstrual cycles are established. Anemia (a hemoglobin level below 10) indicates high blood loss and the need for hormonal treatment. High-hormone-level birth control pills are prescribed to stop the bleeding, followed by a lower dose for maintenance. Girls who do not want to take birth control pills can be given Premarin (conjugated estrogens) for about 21 days to stop heavy bleeding; then medroxyprogesterone (Provera, Amen, or Curretab) can be added for the last 10 days to induce a withdrawal flow. The therapy should continue for at least 3 months to prevent the dysfunctional uterine bleeding from recurring.

When dysfunctional uterine bleeding resists hormonal control or when it resumes after treatment has been discontinued, a dilatation and curettage (D and C) or further diagnostic studies may be needed to reveal the underlying cause of the bleeding. The uterine endometrium is scraped, and tissue specimens are sent for laboratory examination. The age of the child will determine her response to the D and C. The expected course and complications should be

Table 25-1 Dismissal Teaching Following a Dilatation and Curettage

Vaginal Bleeding	Hygiene	Pain	Infection	Contact Doctor for
Light, pinkish vaginal bleeding may continue for 1 week after surgery. Avoid heavy lifting and strenuous exercise for 1 to 2 weeks (may cause bleeding).	Cleanse perineum from front to back after elimination. Change perineal pad three to four times daily. Do not use tampons.	May experience mild abdominal cramps for 2 to 3 days following surgery.	Signs of infection: 1. Foul odor from vaginal discharge 2. Elevated temperature 3. Lower abdominal (uterine) pain	Signs of infection Severe pain or abdominal cramps Heavy, bright-red flow or clots Elevated temperature

explained in detail to both the child and the parents. Table 25-1 lists the plan for dismissal teaching.

Amenorrhea

Amenorrhea is the absence of menstrual periods. It is usually categorized as either primary amenorrhea or secondary amenorrhea. The initial history and physical examination must address each level of possible involvement, from the internal and external reproductive tract to the hypothalamus and pituitary. Drug intake, rapid weight loss, stress, strenuous exercise patterns, and severe nutritional deficiencies all may result in amenorrhea. Thc physical examination should assess patterns of development and growth, secondary sex characteristics, and the presence of normal internal and external genitalia, as well as an evaluation of the endocrine function of the ovaries, pituitary, adrenals, and hypothalamus.

Primary amenorrhea *Primary amenorrhea* is the condition in which no previous menstruation has occurred. Chromosomal abnormalities and genital tract malformations are more common when there is a history of primary amenorrhea. Forty percent of girls with primary amenorrhea and nearly all those without appropriate secondary sex characteristics have a genetic defect. Müllerian duct agenesis, with absence of the vagina, and testicular feminization are two of the most common causes of primary amenorrhea.

Imperforate hymen *Imperforate hymen* is an easily correctable cause of primary amenorrhea. The hymen covers the external opening of the vagina, thus preventing the menstrual blood from draining. This collection of blood is called *cryptomenorrhea*. The symptoms may include difficult urination, lower abdominal pain, and pain at the time of menstruation due to the increasing pressure in the vagina. The distended vagina appears as a lower abdominal and pelvic mass, with a bluish, bulging hymen. The treatment is partial incision with removal of the hymen. The retained blood is allowed to drain over a period of several days. Infection may be present because the retained blood is an excellent medium for bacterial growth.

Treatment After the less complex reasons for amenorrhea have been ruled out, endocrine and chromosomal disorders need to be evaluated. The presence of breast tissue indicates normal pituitary and ovarian function with the production of estrogen. The absence of breast tissue, but the presence of an intact uterus, indicates either a low level of follicle-stimulating hormone, with a pituitary or hypothalamic defect, or an elevated level of follicle-stimulating hormone, suggestive of ovarian failure (a Y chromosome and ovarian dysgenesis must be documented or ruled out). The presence of breast tissue and the absence of a uterus indicate the need to check for testicular feminization syndrome and perform a karyotype. The absence of both breasts and a uterus indicates the need for a karyotype; if the karyotype is XY, the gonads must be removed to prevent a possible malignancy as well as masculinization at puberty. Surgical and hormonal treatment was discussed earlier in the section "Ambiguous Genitalia."

Secondary amenorrhea *Secondary amenorrhea* is the cessation of menstruation after previous spontaneous menstrual bleeding has occurred. This disorder can have multiple causes. Endocrine disorders are the most common; however, systemic disease, excessive dieting, anorexia nervosa, Chron disease, ileitis, and frequent strenuous exercise all cause secondary amenorrhea.

Treatment Management begins with the physical examination and history, discussed earlier in this chapter. When other possible causes have been ruled out, endocrine function is evaluated. To determine whether a pituitary tumor is present, serum prolactin is tested; if this is normal, a progesterone challenge test is used to determine which organ—the ovaries, uterus, hypothalamus, or pituitary—is involved. Chapter 24 discusses endocrine disorders of the hypothalamus, pituitary, and adrenals.

Nutritional counseling, resulting in improved nutritional status, weight gain, and reduction of exercise for the strenuous exerciser will usually cause resumption of the menses. Replacement of estrogen and progesterone in cyclic fashion is the treatment for hypothalamic-pituitary or ovarian deficiencies. Polycystic ovary syndrome can be treated with oral contraceptives to repress the androgens, and fertility can be stimulated with clomiphene. A pituitary tumor is surgically removed or treated by suppressing prolactin secretion.

Dysmenorrhea The term *dysmenorrhea* should be reserved for fairly incapacitating, painful menstruation that is severe enough to cause the girl or the woman to try self-medication or to seek help from a physician. The amount of discomfort experienced during the secretory phase of the menstrual cycle is related significantly to the endometrial production of prostaglandins. These are increased both at the end of the menstrual cycle and at the onset of menstruation. It has been shown that primary dysmenorrhea is likely to be due to myometrial contractions induced by prostaglandins originating in the endometrium.

There are two major classifications of dysmenorrhea. *Primary dysmenorrhea* is unrelated to a pelvic abnormality. *Secondary dysmenorrhea* is usually related to specific organic pelvic pathology or an intrauterine device.

The common discomforts associated with dysmenorrhea include a sense of fullness in the pelvis, premenstrual tension, edema, enlargement and tenderness of the breasts, mild abdominal cramps, and backache.

The first step in dealing with dysmenorrhea is to consult with a physician to rule out the existence of pelvic pathology. This should include a complete gynecologic and pelvic examination. If no pathology is found, a second step might include a subjective assessment of the pain experienced; a patient questionnaire or rating scale can be given to the woman to fill out before, during, and after the menstrual cycle and can be used to evaluate the pain experienced.

Symptomatic relief may be provided by: routine genital hygiene, exercise, heat applied to the lower abdomen, vitamins, and teaching (including reassurance about the absence of serious pelvic disease and the likelihood that the pain will decrease after childbirth).

Further treatment may include the use of various drug regimens. Oral contraceptives which contain both estrogen and progesterone have been effective in treating dysmenorrhea because they inhibit ovulation. There is almost always complete relief of menstrual pain with this form of treatment. A drug regimen being used is the prostaglandin inhibitors. These drugs decrease prostaglandin production by inhibiting the enzyme system which synthesizes the prostaglandin compounds. By doing this, they inhibit the release of prostaglandin from the secretory endometrium, thus decreasing the pain of dysmenorrhea.

The specific drugs used for pain are nonsteroid, anti-inflammatory drugs such as salicylates (aspirin and phenacetin). Prostaglandin inhibitors, indomethacin, fenamoles (tolfenamic acid and mefenamic acid, e.g., Ponstel) naproxen sodium, and ibuprofen (Motrin) are also used for severe dysmenorrhea. The disadvantage of using the prostaglandin inhibitors is the severity of the side effects of the treatment. The side effects of prostaglandin inhibitors described in the literature include headache, blurred vision, drug rash, severe gastrointestinal disturbances, and aplastic anemia. Motrin has been cited as the safest inhibitor and has minimal side effects, but it is still under investigation for this purpose. The studies agree that when drug therapy is necessary, it should be started several (2 to 3) days prior to the onset of the menstrual flow and the symptoms of dysmenorrhea and continued until the flow and the symptoms disappear.

Table 25-2 Symptoms of Premenstrual Tension Syndrome

Gastrointestinal symptoms	Abdominal bloating, nausea, vomiting, constipation, food cravings, compulsive eating
Breast symptoms	Tenderness, engorgement, enlargement, heaviness
Genitourinary symptoms	Cystitis, enuresis, oliguria
Dermatologic symptoms	Acne, boils, hives, easy bruising, reoccurrence of herpes
Neurological and behavioral symptoms	Headaches, fainting, syncope, tension, depression, irritability, fatigue, lethargy, panic, suicide, assaults, child abuse

Premenstrual tension syndrome

Recently, *premenstrual tension syndrome* (PMT syndrome) has become recognized as a widely occurring phenomenon. The word *tension* is part of the name of this symptom complex because nervous tension is a symptom reported by all women with this syndrome. The symptoms are based on the relationship between the estrogen-progesterone and the renin-angiotensin-aldosterone systems. A disturbance in the hormone levels within these systems can result in PMT syndrome (Table 25-2).

Much has been written about the severity and variability of the symptoms experienced by women on an individual and on a month-to-month basis. Because of this variability, symptoms should be recorded for at least two to three menstrual cycles prior to the diagnosis and the start of any treatment protocol. This will establish a baseline of symptoms as a specific monthly pattern for the individual, which is one of the keys to diagnosis.

Abraham has divided PMT syndrome into several classifications and has suggested treatments for each classification.[9] These are listed in Table 25-3.[10,11,12]

INFECTION OF THE FEMALE REPRODUCTIVE TRACT

Vulvovaginitis

Irritation and inflammation of the vulva and vagina are frequently seen in young girls. The vaginal tissue is thin and unestrogenized and has a neutral pH, making it very susceptible to infections. The child may be reluctant to tell her parents what is wrong and may resist medical examination, making diagnosis difficult. The signs of vulvovaginitis are a red and edematous perineal area, itching, a foul-smelling or purulent vaginal discharge, and dysuria. Urinary tract infections often accompany vulvovaginitis, making it essential to obtain a clean catch urine specimen in addition to culturing the vaginal discharge.

The common causes of vulvovaginitis are chemical irritations, trauma, and infections. Bubble baths, masturbation, placing foreign objects into the vagina, and injury from falls may also cause vulvovaginitis. Infections are often re-

Table 25-3 Classifications of, and Suggested Treatments for, Premenstrual Tension Syndrome*

Classification	Symptoms	Suggested Treatments*
PMT-A (most common subgroup)	Anxiety, irritability, nervous tension, increased estrogen, decreased progesterone, excessive consumption of dairy products	Progesterone therapy, increased exercise, prostaglandin inhibitors, limited use of alcohol and tobacco.
PMT-H	Water and salt retention, nervous tension, abdominal bloating, breast tenderness, increased aldosterone levels	Dietary therapy: Sugar intake should be of complex carbohydrate variety (to help sustain the release of insulin) and should be 60 to 70% of the caloric intake.
PMT-C	Craving for sweets, increased appetite, food binges, fatigue, fainting spells, headache, altered glucose tolerance, nervous tension	Limit the use of caffeine-containing beverages (coffee, tea, and cola drinks); limit the use of chocolate; restrict sodium intake, consumption of dairy products, and simple sugar intake.
PMT-D (most serious symptom complex)	Depression, withdrawal, insomnia, confusion, forgetfulness, altered serum estrogen and progesterone levels, nervous tension	Restrict intake of animal fats; increase use of vegetable oils.

* The word *suggested* is used here because many different treatments are described in the literature.

lated to poor hygiene, especially wiping from the rectum toward the vagina and urethra. Pinworms, *Escherichia coli,* and other bacteria are common infectious agents. Chapter 28 discusses the common causes of vulvovaginitis, treatment, and nursing care. Sexual abuse is discussed in Chap. 38.

ALTERATIONS OF MALE REPRODUCTIVE FUNCTION

Hydrocele

A *hydrocele* is an accumulation of fluid anywhere within the course of the *processus vaginalis* (the pathway through which the testes, preceded by a fold of tissue, descend from the peritoneal cavity to the scrotum). Small scrotal hydroceles are commonly present at birth and are often associated with inguinal hernias.

Noncommunicating hydroceles are those in which the processus vaginalis has closed but in which fluid is trapped in the scrotum. These are usually stable, asymptomatic, and not reducible and can be transilluminated (to show presence of fluid and the testes). The peritoneal fluid trapped in the scrotum disappears slowly over a period of weeks or months. Most hydroceles resolve spontaneously during the first year of life, making surgical correction unnecessary.

Communicating hydroceles are those in which the processus vaginalis remains open and peritoneal fluid may be forced into the scrotum. The mother will usually notice a change in the size of the scrotum. It will be smaller in the morning, after the child has been asleep all night, and larger in the afternoon, after the child has been up most of the day. These hydroceles may be large enough to cause discomfort and herniation of the intestines. Surgical repair is required if they persist beyond the second year of life. Surgical repair of a hydrocele is similar to inguinal hernia repair and both defects are usually corrected at the same time.

Nursing Management Nursing management for a child who has had surgical repair of a hydrocele is similar to that for a child who has had inguinal hernia repair. Postoperative care involves placing an ice bag on the scrotum to prevent swelling, instituting voiding measures to avoid retention, keeping the area clean, and maintaining planned rest periods.

Cryptorchidism*

Etiology *Cryptorchidism* is a defect in which one testis or both testes fail to descend into the scrotal sac. In 95 percent of the cases of cryptorchidism there is true testicular nondescent; in 3 percent, one testis is present (monorchia); in 1 percent the testes are present, but are not in the scrotum (ectopic); and in 0.6 percent, there is an absence of both testes (anorchia).[13] At times it may be difficult to determine whether the testes are present, since retractile testes—testes that retract because of hyperactivity of the cremasteric reflex—may be difficult to palpate. While differentiation of the indifferent gonad into the testes occurs during the sixth or seventh week of fetal life, descent takes place in stages, and complete descent occurs during the last few weeks before birth.[14] Failure of the testes to descend is linked to deficient quantities of fetal testosterone, obstruction of the passageway to the scrotum, decreased intraabdominal pressure (e.g., lax abdominal musculature in prune-belly syndrome), and prematurity. (See Chap. 20 for a discussion of prune-belly syndrome.)

Incidence Cryptorchidism is directly related to the gestational age of the child. It occurs in approximately 30 percent of premature male infants, 3.4 percent of full-term male infants, and 0.8 percent of boys 1 year of age.[15] The incidence among adult men is about the same as that among 1-year-old boys, indicating that spontaneous descent rarely takes place after the age of 1 year.

Complications Risk factors associated with cryptorchidism include a potential for decreased fertility and an increased chance of developing testicular cancer. Temperatures are 1 to 2°C higher in the inguinal canal and abdominal cavity than in the scrotum. The higher temperatures are responsible for impaired spermatogenesis and may damage the undescended testis. Testicular biopsies have demonstrated irreversible changes in children as young as 2 years of age.[16] The potential for decreased fertility was demonstrated in a study in which 80 percent of the men with unilateral cyrptorchidism and 35 percent of those with bilateral cryptorchidism had fathered children.[17] Delaying treatment uniformly results in diminished fertility.[18]

*This section was written by Sheila Kramer, R.N., M.S.N.

In one study, it was shown that males with cryptorchidism are 20 to 50 times more likely to develop testicular cancer than unaffected males.[19] Interestingly, the testis on the other side in males with unilateral cryptorchidism is also at increased risk for the development of cancer. In a study of 93 patients with cryptorchidism, Batata found that no patient who had been treated prior to 2 years of age developed a testicular malignancy.[20] This underscores the need for early localization and treatment of undescended testes.

Localization technique Approximately 15 to 20 percent of children with cryptorchidism have nonpalpable testes. The testes themselves may be small, may be concealed by prepubic fat, and may be in the abdomen or absent. The testes can be best palpated when the child is examined while lying on his back in a frogleg position. Undescended testes are accurately diagnosed most of the time with the help of improved techniques, such as high-resolution ultrasound, gonadal venography and arteriography, herniography, and laparoscopy. Ultrasound has no known harmful effects and does not expose the child to radiation; it remains the procedure of choice for the diagnosis of nonpalpable testes.

Treatment There are three goals of therapy for cryptorchidism: (1) to bring the testes into an accessible position in order to enable early detection of malignancy, (2) to promote spermatogenesis and maximize fertility, and (3) to enhance psychological well-being and physical appearance, which are important to both the boy and his parents. These goals are accomplished through hormonal therapy and/or surgery.

Human chorionic gonadotropin stimulates secretion of testosterone from the testes and produces testicular descent in 20 to 30 percent of patients.[21] Nine doses of the hormone are given by intramuscular injection (one dose every other day). In studies done in Europe, gonadotropin-releasing hormone has been used to stimulate the pituitary gland to release luteinizing hormone and follicle-stimulating hormone, with a reported success rate of 80 percent.[22] At this time, however, the drug has not been approved by the FDA for use in the United States.

Surgical options include an orchiectomy or an orchiopexy. An *orchiectomy,* or surgical removal of one testis or both testes, is indicated in the postpubertal boy with unilateral cryptorchidism when the contralateral testis is normally descended. A variety of testicular prostheses are available that make physical appearance satisfactory.

Prepubertal boys who have not responded to hormonal therapy are candidates for an orchiopexy. It is recommended that an *orchiopexy,* or placement and fixation of the testes in the scrotum, be done between 1 and 2 years of age. When an orchiopexy is performed on a postpubertal boy with bilateral cryptorchidism, a testicular biopsy for cancer is done, and the boy is followed closely. Although the risk of developing testicular cancer is increased, the position of the testes allows the boy to retain endocrine function, and the testes are in a good position to be examined for cancer.

Surgical technique Cryptorchidism repair takes approximately 30 to 45 min and is performed on an outpatient basis. Eighty percent of children with cryptorchidism have associated inguinal hernias, which are also repaired at this time. An incision is made in the lower abdominal region. The spermatic cord and the testis are mobilized and dissected to achieve sufficient cord length for placement of the testis into the scrotum. A second incision in the scrotum creates a dartos pouch, into which the testis is placed and sutured. Dressings are not routinely applied. In the past, a rubber band was attached from the testis to the upper thigh to maintain the testis in the scrotum; this technique is seldom used today, since it has been replaced by formation of a dartos pouch and the use of sutures to maintain the testis in place. A return visit is scheduled for 10 to 14 days postoperatively; the physician examines the incision and ensures that the testis is remaining in the proper position.

Testicular autotransplantation may be necessary if the testes are intraabdominal. This technique involves division of the spermatic artery and vein with a reanastomosis to the inferior epigastric vessels, using an operating room microscope.[23]

Nursing management Parents whose child is found to be infertile may become anxious and feel guilty for not having sought medical attention earlier. If the child is old enough, he may also be aware that he is different from his peers and that his scrotum is not normal. Both parents and the child should be encouraged to express their concerns and feelings; they should be given clear explanations regarding the procedure and the prognosis and support in coping with this potentially emotional situation.

Testicular torsion

Testicular torsion occurs primarily in newborns and adolescents. In the newborn, torsion frequently occurs prior to birth, and the testes may already be infarcted before the first examination takes place. The fetal testes twist at the inguinal ring soon after entering the scrotum, when they are not attached to the scrotum and are rotating freely. This can also be caused by contraction of the cremaster muscle.

A second kind of torsion occurs as a result of anomalous suspension of the testes within the scrotum. Because the posterior attachments of the testes within the tunica vaginalis are missing, the testes hang by a small pedicle and can easily twist. Often there are no symptoms until the child reaches puberty, when the testes are heavy enough to cause twisting. Torsion most commonly occurs in boys aged 13 to 15, but it can happen at any age. The onset may have no obvious cause; torsion can follow normal activity or simple position changes during sleep. Initially, the venous blood flow is affected, but edema, congestion, and inflammation increase, with eventual impairment of the arterial blood flow and resulting testicular damage. Symptoms may include scrotal pain; nausea; vomiting; swollen and tender testes, which are palpated higher than usual in the scrotal sac because of shortening due to the twisting; and an inflammatory hydrocele.

Treatment Surgery done promptly after diagnosis is the treatment for testicular torsion. Allen states that a testis which is properly treated within 6 h of the onset of testicular torsion usually survives without significant injury. A testis that has been twisted for 24 h can rarely be salvaged.[24] Tests used to diagnose testicular torsion are a technetium TC 99m blood-flow scan to visualize the amount of blood flowing to the affected testis and a small-parts ultrasonography to visualize the structures within the scrotum. Surgery is relatively simple and carries a low risk. The scrotum is surgically explored, the twisting of the spermatic cord is corrected, and the testis is secured. After derotation, the testis appears blue and engorged, but the color should return to normal quickly. If there is doubt regarding the viability of the testis, it is covered with a warm, moist pack, and the surgical exploration of the other testis is completed. There is a high incidence of bilateral suspension anomalies, and so both testes should be examined, and any defect should be corrected. A testicular biopsy will be done if the testicular viability is still in question at this point. Nagler suggests that a clearly damaged testis should be removed, since it may adversely affect the normal testis through an autoimmune phenomenon.[25] Some surgeons prefer to insert a prosthetic testis into the scrotum at this time. The child may return home the same day with scrotal support and ice packs to prevent swelling.

ISSUES OF ADOLESCENT SEXUALITY

Adolescent sexuality

Understanding and dealing with sexuality in adolescence has become a major concern of many health professionals, educators, parents, and of adolescents themselves. However, a problem with this concern is the tendency to view adolescent sexuality in isolation. It must be viewed within the broader context of adolescence as a developmental phase as well as an individual experience. Within this framework, sexuality is considered in terms of the formation of personal identity, the maturation of interpersonal relationships, and self-esteem. Adolescent sexuality is for the most part experimental and is part of the process of defining the adolescent's identity. During the adolescent period, with its upsurge in hormonal and physical changes, adolescents' awareness of their bodies and concerns about their sexuality are heightened. The adolescent often voices these concerns with some familiar questions: "Who am I?" "Am I normal?" "Will I ever fall in love?" "Will anyone ever love me?"

Sexual identity Sexuality, which is one aspect of an individual's identity, begins with the formation of gender identity and sex role orientation during infancy. The patterns that emerge throughout childhood are refined during adolescence before culminating in adult sexual identity.[26] (See Chaps. 11 and 12.) The adolescent's sexuality and behavior in interpersonal relationships have a simultaneous, mutual influence on each other. Adolescents are continually defining their sexual identity in terms of how they relate to others. As this identity emerges, old beliefs and attitudes are often questioned, and the adolescent begins to separate from the family and come to terms with his or her own sexuality. Adolescents' sexual behavior is greatly influenced by their peers, and therefore it will to some extent reflect the attitudes and beliefs of the peer group. However, not all adolescents conform to peer pressure. Every adolescent makes an individual choice concerning the expression of his or her sexuality. The process of defining their own sexuality plays an integral role in the development of adolescents' self-esteem. How adolescents feel in terms of attractiveness or desirability is reflected in their self-esteem.

It is also important to understand the integral part that cognitive development plays in the way adolescents understand and express their sexuality. Adolescence is marked by the transition from concrete to formal operational thought, as defined by Piaget. Although the process of formal thought begins at approximately 11 to 12 years of age, it is not fully achieved until later adolescence. The adolescent's thoughts begin to extend from the actual toward the potential. Thus adolescents who have reached the stage of formal operationalized thought are able to delineate all possible consequences of a situation, and they try to discover which of these consequences really do occur. The adolescent who has yet to reach this cognitive stage or who reverts back to concrete thought when stressed becomes bound to phenomenal, here-and-now results. Another characteristic of concrete thinking is egocentricism. Adolescents are preoccupied with themselves and believe that everyone else is preoccupied with them.[27] Because of this inordinate amount of attention to the self and the perception that everyone else is interested in them, adolescents develop a feeling of uniqueness. This egocentric thought allows them to believe that they are very special and exceptional. For example, many adolescent girls may feel that even if they are sexually active, they will magically not become pregnant.[28] This egocentric thought also allows adolescents to become more experimental in their choices.

Ultimately, the adolescent will be forced to make many choices about defining and expressing sexuality. This must be done in an increasingly technological society characterized by rapid social change. The adolescent struggles with values, attitudes, and beliefs and does this without past experience to reflect on. Therefore, the nursing challenge is to understand the phenomenon of adolescent sexuality and help the adolescent through this transitional period.

Each adolescent has unique concerns regarding sexuality such as reactions to the physical changes in his or her body. Some adolescents welcome the outward signs of their development, while others do not want to accept their maturation. Adolescents may express anticipatory concerns about sexual intercourse, contraception, and venereal disease. However, they often will not express their concerns or thoughts about masturbation and homosexuality. Often adolescents need to be given permission to talk about these concerns.[29] All adolescents need to be assisted and educated in these areas, particularly as they relate to sexual exploration. For example, an adolescent's suspicion or fear that he or she is a homosexual must be differentiated from the actual presence of homosexuality. The adolescent needs to be reassured that erotic fantasies about, and emotional attachments to, someone of the same sex are not unusual and do not imply a homosexual orientation.[30] However, if an adolescent has been engaging in homosexual behavior for several years and does not wish to change this behavior, he or she may need support and guidance in making this choice.

Sexual activity Many adolescents choose to abstain from sexual intercourse or delay it until young adulthood. Others choose to express their sexuality through sexual intercourse. For some adolescents this is an active, well-thought-out decision, but for many it is a passive decision, which can lead to pregnancy and parenthood at an early age.

Trends in adolescent sexuality The most recent statistics show that 50 percent of young women aged 15 to 19 and 70 percent of young men aged 17 to 21 in the United States have had sexual intercourse. The average age of young women at the first sexual intercourse is 16.2 years, and that of young men is 15.7 years.[31]

Adolescents have many reasons for choosing to become sexually active: (1) to promote self-esteem,[32] (2) to experiment, (3) to conform to peer pressure, (4) to be loved, (5) to experience a rite of passage into adulthood, and (6) to rebel against authority. Major losses and family illness tend to be associated with decisions to become pregnant or to continue a pregnancy.[33] For most young men and women, the first experience with sexual intercourse seems to have been a spur-of-the-moment decision. In one study, only 17 percent of young women and 25 percent of young men said that they had planned their first act of intercourse.[34] Young women generally have sexual intercourse first with someone to whom they are committed in a relationship, whereas young men tend to have more casual relationships.

Use of contraceptives seems to be age-related, with young men showing the same pattern as young women. Those who are older at the first intercourse are more likely to use contraceptives than those who are younger. Adolescents who plan their first sexual intercourse, regardless of race or sex, are more likely to use contraceptives than those who do not plan it. There are no definite predictors for use of contraceptives; however some variables that are positively associated with contraceptive use are:

1. Self-confidence[35,36,37,38]
2. A sense of control in a heterosexual dyad[39]
3. An accurate knowledge of the risks of pregnancy and the reliability of various types of contraceptives[40]
4. A good education and high career goals[41]
5. Older age at the first coitus
6. Well-educated and/or working parents[42]
7. A steady sexual partner[43]

Variables that are inversely related to contraceptive use include episodic sexual relations and the belief, for one reason or another, that the girl cannot become pregnant or that contraceptives are neither safe nor desirable.[44] Embarrassment about using or buying contraceptives contributes to nonuse.[45] (Fig. 25-7.)

After an adolescent chooses a contraceptive method, there are often problems connected with the continuation of its use. Forty-three percent of adolescents who start to use a contraceptive do not continue to use it consistently. Most of the discontinuation of use appears to occur during the first 3 months.[46] The rate of discontinuation of use is related to the degree of satisfaction with, and the convenience of, the birth control method.

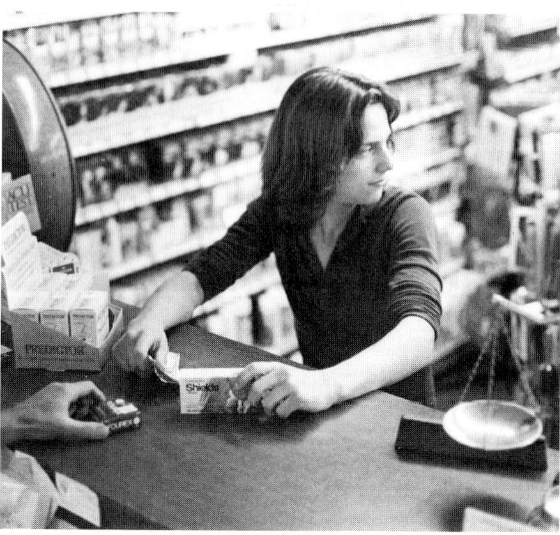

Figure 25-7 The teenager, who considers many ordinary things embarrassing, finds it very difficult to purchase condoms. (*Photo by Karel Bauer.*)

Choosing a birth control method

An adolescent's choice of a method of contraception should be safe and effective and should be one that the adolescent will feel comfortable using. The choice should be based on the adolescent's preference in conjunction with the health care provider's guidance. A detailed health history of the adolescent who is seeking contraceptives is obtained. Sexual partners and/or the parents should be included whenever possible. The history should include some of the following data:

1. Age at the first sexual intercourse
2. Frequency of sexual intercourse
3. Success with contraceptive methods used in the past
4. Sources of information regarding contraception and sexual activity (friends, parents, and classes)
5. Current level of understanding of contraceptive methods and their risks
6. Attitudes and beliefs regarding sexuality and contraceptives
7. Attitudes toward touching the body (e.g., whether a girl feels comfortable using tampons)
8. A complete family history
9. A history of the menstrual cycle: onset and problems (e.g., cramping, heavy flow, and vaginal discharge between menstrual periods) (Fig. 25-8)

Any young woman who is seeking a birth control method should have a complete physical ex-

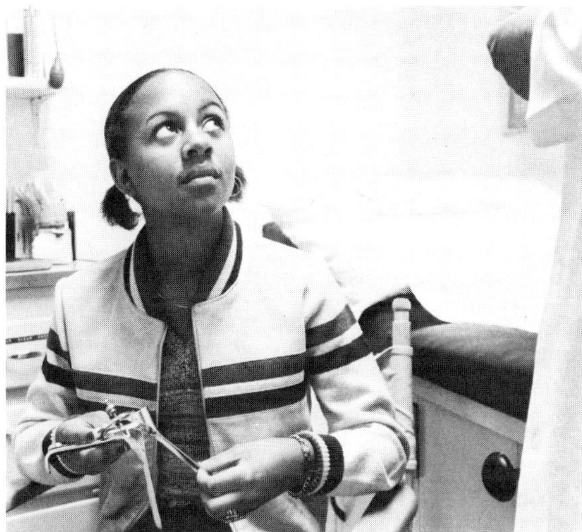

Figure 25-8 When a teenage girl has had the opportunity to become familiar with the equipment, the first pelvic examination is less frightening. (*Photo by Karel Bauer.*)

amination done to provide a baseline for future care and to detect present and potential health problems. The examination includes a blood pressure reading, a breast examination, and a pelvic examination with a Pap smear and testing for vaginitis as indicated by the physical findings. Laboratory tests that are routinely done are a hematocrit or hemoglobin test, a urinalysis, a culture for gonorrhea, and a serologic test for syphilis. Contraindications to the use of a birth control method, such as elevated blood pressure in the case of oral contraceptives or pelvic inflammatory disease in the case of an intrauterine device, should be evaluated. Return examinations, during which satisfaction with the method, correct use, and side effects are evaluated, are important. All young women should return in 3–6 months and again at least annually, and no prescription for an oral contraceptive should be for longer than 12 months. The complete assessment and examination, combined with information about the risks and benefits of each method of contraception, provide baseline data to help the adolescent choose the most appropriate method. (See Table 25-4.) Every effort should be made to include sexual partners in the counseling. It is important to stress to all adolescents that both males and females should take equal responsibility in matters pertaining to contraception.

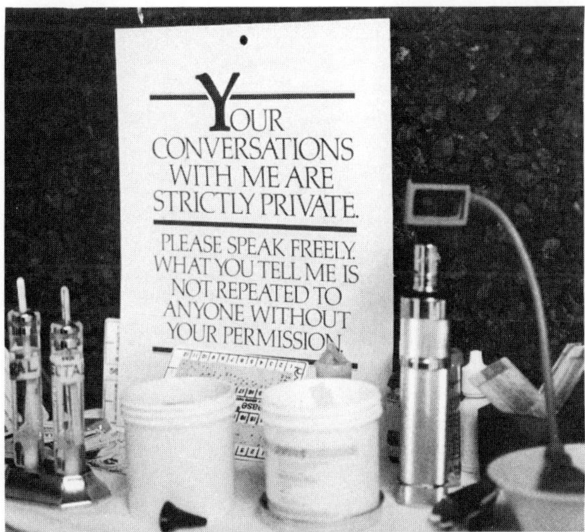

Figure 25-9 A teenager has the right to confidentiality and will talk more openly about health problems when he or she is assured that they will remain private. (*Photo by Karel Bauer.*)

Discussions about contraception can be held with individuals, couples, or peer groups. Adolescents benefit more from interactive communication with health care professionals, peers, and parents than from non-interactive communication. The highest level of birth control knowledge is associated with multiple sources of information. Although some parents object to sex education programs and birth control counseling outside the home, it has been found that girls who get all their information about sex and contraception at home have the lowest level of birth control knowledge. Adolescents need multiple sources of information and various educational strategies. Both the health care professional and the parents should be involved with these. It is well known that the parents influence a child's development of a sense of gender identity, gender-appropriate behavior, moral values, and ways of expressing affection. When both parents share equally in the responsibility of raising a child there may be a more favorable environment for learning about sex. Therefore, it is imperative for both the parents and the nurse to create an open-minded atmosphere in which the adolescent feels free to share concerns, anxieties, and needs.

No one birth control method should be advocated. By listening to the adolescent's needs and desires, the nurse can minimize error in use and prevent discontinuation of use.

Table 25-4 Temporary Methods of Contraception

Method	Description of Action	Instructions for Use	Effectiveness* Theoretical	Effectiveness* Actual in Adolescents
Oral contraceptives (the "pill")	Tablets containing varying doses of estrogens and progestogens. Main action is suppression of ovulation. They also alter cervical mucus (making it hostile to sperm), and lead to an unfavorable endometrial environment.	Take one pill daily for 21 days, at approximately the same time daily. Stop for 7 days. Menses will begin 1 to 4 days after pill has been stopped. Restart new pack of pills after 28-day cycle has been completed. Some pill packs contain 7 placebo or iron tablets, which can be taken instead of stopping for a week. Start on fifth day of menses; stop at end of pack. For early nausea, take at bedtime or with evening meal. For weight gain, reduce salt and caloric intake.	0.34	4 to 10
"Mini pill"	A tablet form of contraception which contains only low doses of progestogens. Ovulation is probably not inhibited, but hostile cervical mucus and an unfavorable endometrial environment provide contraceptive effect.	Take one pill daily, without stopping. Start on first day of menses; stop at end of pack. Use a second method for first few months.	1	3
Intrauterine device (IUD)	A plastic or polyethylene device in various shapes and sizes. It is inserted into uterus and usually remains there until user wishes it removed. Action of IUD is unknown, but it is thought to cause a local inflammatory reaction inside uterus, which prevents implantation of fertilized ovum. Copper and progesterone have been added to some IUDs for an extra antifertility effect.	Approximately $\frac{1}{2}$ in of IUD string will be in vagina. Insert finger to check for presence of string. (Can be checked by partner, also.) Notify health care provider if no string is felt, string feels much longer than after insertion, or plastic tip of IUD is felt protruding. Use another method of birth control until reexamined. Insert during menses; remove at any time during the cycle.	1 to 3	5
Diaphragm	A dome-shaped rubber cup on a circular metal spring. Used with spermicidal jelly or cream, it fits over cervix and blocks entry of sperm into uterus. Must be fitted by a trained health care provider. Diaphragms come in sizes from 55 to 105 mm in gradations of 5 mm and are	Prior to insertion put spermicidal jelly in cup and on rim of diaphragm. In lying, standing, or squatting position, ease diaphragm into vagina. Hook rim under symphysis pubis. Check to see that cervix is covered. If intercourse is repeated, add an applicator of foam or jelly without	3	17

*Number of pregnancies per woman-year of use.

Early Changes and Minor Side Effects	Other Possible Side Effects	Contraindications	Advantages and Disadvantages
Mild nausea; weight gain; breast tenderness†; spotting; breakthrough bleeding; shorter, lighter menses; missed or "silent" periods; mood changes; chloasma; acne	Depression; decreased libido; blood clots; heart attacks; hepatocellular tumors; prolonged amenorrhea after discontinuation; increase in yeast vaginitis; headaches; hypertension	History or present evidence of thromboembolic phenomena; heart disease; hypertension; sickle cell anemia; severe depression; pregnancy; liver dysfunction or disease; impaired cerebrovascular function; known or suspected carcinoma of the breast or genital tract; migraine headaches; epilepsy; lactation; ovarian dysfunction; diabetes; gall bladder disease	Advantages: Nearest to 100% effective; regular menstrual cycle, period predictable; decreased menstrual flow; decreased dysnemorrhea and premenstrual tension; decreased iron-deficiency anemia; not related to intercourse. Disadvantages: Increased susceptibility to VD; must take daily even if not having intercourse; must be started at specific time to be effective.
Irregularity in amount and duration of menses; spotting between periods; missed periods	None currently known	None currently known	Advantages: No estrogen-related side effects; not related to intercourse. Disadvantages: Irregular periods
Heavier and longer periods; cramps, spotting between periods	Spontaneous expulsion; perforation of uterus; embedding of IUD; pelvic inflammatory disease	Pelvic infections (acute, subacute, recurrent); severe dysmenorrhea; acute cervicitis; uterine abnormalities; allergy to copper; Wilson disease; cervical stenosis; small uterine cavity; abnormal cervical cytology; anemia; congenital or rheumatic heart disease; pregnancy	Advantages: Little maintenance or attention needed after insertion; not related to intercourse. Disadvantages: Higher rate of ectopic pregnancy; must be inserted and removed by health care provider (no self-involvement); repeated pelvic infections can lead to decreased fertility.
None	Allergy to rubber or spermicidal preparation	Damaged pelvic floor or relaxation, which prohibits a proper fit; prolapsed uterus; severe cystocele or rectocele; severe retroversion or anteversion of the uterus	Advantages: Few side effects; effective for infrequent intercourse; holds back menstrual flow during intercourse; good for learning about female anatomy. Disadvantages: Closely precedes sex act.

†Usually disappear within 2 to 3 months.

Table 25-4 Temporary methods of contraception (*Continued*)

Method	Description of Action	Instructions for Use	Effectiveness* Theoretical	Effectiveness* Actual in Adolescents
	inserted and removed by wearer.	removing diaphragm. Do not remove diaphragm or douche for 6 to 8 h after last intercourse. Wash with warm water, dry, and powder with cornstarch. Check for holes or tears periodically.		
Sponge	A soft, polyurethane foam sponge 2 in in diameter and 1.25 in thick, saturated with 1 g of nonoxynol-9. Releases spermicide over 24 h. Blocks cervix, absorbs sperm.	Moisten sponge with water to activate spermicide. Must be left in 6 hours after intercourse; not reusable.		15.8
Foams, jellies, and creams	Spermicidal preparations inserted into vagina. They slow down and kill entering sperm. Can be used alone or in conjunction with other methods.	Insert an applicator full of foam, cream, or jelly into vagina within 30 min of intercourse. Insert an additional application each time before intercourse is repeated. Do not douche; foam or cream is absorbed into skin. If douching is desired, wait 6 to 8 h after last intercourse. Use with condom for increased effectiveness.	3	20
Contraceptive suppository	Same as foams, jellies, and creams.	Unwrap and insert into the vagina 10 to 15 min before each intercourse. Do not douche for at least 6 to 8 h after intercourse.	3	20
Condom and spermicide	A thin rubber or skin sheath put over an erect penis. Creates a mechanical barrier which prevents sperm from getting into vagina.	Put condom on erect penis *prior* to penetration. If no tip on condom, allow ½-in slack in front to catch semen. Withdraw soon after ejaculation. Semen is more likely to leak out when penis is flaccid. Hold on to condom when withdrawing to prevent slipping off. If condom breaks during intercourse, insert an applicator of foam or jelly immediately. Use with foam for increased effectiveness.	1	Fewer than 5
Condom (rubber prophylactic)			3	10

*Number of pregnancies per woman-year of use.

Early Changes and Minor Side Effects	Other Possible Side Effects	Contraindications	Advantages and Disadvantages
			May become dislodged during intercourse; can be messy.
None	Possible risk of toxic shock syndrome; possible allergic reaction, including itching, irritation, and rash	None	Advantages: May be worn for full 24 h and used for multiple acts of intercourse; less likely to interfere with sexual spontaneity; is less messy and easier to insert than a diaphragm. Disadvantages: May become dislodged during intercourse; can be messy.
None	Allergy to spermicidal preparation	Allergy to spermicidal preparation	Advantages: Easily available, no prescription needed; helps prevent STD. Disadvantages: Can be messy; effective for only a short time.
None	Mild burning of vagina and penis related to allergy to spermicidal preparation	Allergy to spermicidal preparation	Same as for foams, jellies, and creams.
None	Allergy to rubber	Allergy to rubber	Advantages: Male method, allows for shared contraception; easily available; no prescription needed; provides increased protection against sexually transmitted diseases. Disadvantages: Requires interruption of coitus to put on; may reduce sensitivity of glans penis.

Table 25-4 Temporary methods of contraception (*Continued*)

Method	Description of Action	Instructions for Use	Effectiveness*	
			Theoretical	Actual in Adolescents
Rhythm	A pattern of abstinence from intercourse around the time of ovulation, or greatest time of fertility. Records must be kept of menstrual cycles, and calculations made for "safe days." New variations on this method include natural family planning and the Billings method, which add basal body temperature and evaluation of cervical mucus to the traditional rhythm system.	Keep record of menstrual cycles for 3 to 6 months. Subtract *18* from number of days in shortest cycle; subtract *11* from number of days in longest cycle. For example, cycles ranged from 28 to 30 days: 28 − 18 = 10; 30 − 11 = 19. Fertile or "unsafe" days are days 10 to 19 of cycle.	14	35 to 40
Hormonal implants, norplant system (being used on a trial basis)	Hormonal implants that provide continuous protection by releasing small amounts of levonorgestel (progestin) into the bloodstream.	Consists of Silastic capsule implants about 1.3 in long and 0.1 in in diameter. Six rods or 2 slightly longer rods; 30 mg of hormone is released. Inserted subcutaneously in inner aspect of upper arm or forearm.		Fewer than 1

*Number of pregnancies per woman-year of use.

Oral contraceptives *Oral contraceptives* (the "pill") are the most widely used birth control method among adolescents. Most adolescents who dislike barrier methods or rituals related to sexual activity tend to choose the pill.[47] Although the pill is theoretically the most effective method, it is less effective with adolescents than with adults. This is primarily the result of lack of motivation or of a misunderstanding of how to take the pill correctly. The pill is usually the contraceptive of choice for the adolescent who is involved in a steady relationship. Adolescents who have infrequent sex tend not to choose the pill. Some adolescent girls are afraid to take the pill because of the dangers associated with it, which have been publicized in the media. However, adolescent girls actually have a lower risk of developing complications related to the pill than adult females.[48] It is important to explore the adolescent girl's attitudes and concerns if she is considering using an oral contraceptive. (See Table 25-4.)

Barrier methods

Intrauterine devices An *intrauterine device,* which is a plastic device placed within the uterine cavity, is generally not recommended for adolescents. An adolescent who has never been pregnant will usually expel the device. All adolescents are at an increased risk for sterility, pelvic inflammatory disease, and severe cramping and bleeding. It is generally one of the least acceptable birth control methods for adolescents, but it may be chosen by some girls who have been pregnant before or who lack the motivation to use any other method of contraception.

Diaphragms A *diaphragm* might be an excellent choice for a highly motivated adolescent. It requires feeling comfortable about touching one's own body. Determining whether an adolescent girl has used tampons will give a clue as to her readiness to use a diaphragm. The girl must take the time to learn how to insert the diaphragm properly and must learn when she

Early Changes and Minor Side Effects	Other Possible Side Effects	Contraindications	Advantages and Disadvantages
None	None	Irregular cycles	Advantages: Acceptable for those who have moral or other objections to artificial birth control methods; promotes learning about bodily systems. Disadvantages: Irregular cycles make it difficult to follow successfully; abstinence may cause sexual frustration; problem if partner is not cooperative.
Tends to disrupt menstrual patterns; increases flow and length of menses (this effect subsides after a year); causes cervical mucus to thicken; limits the ability of the endometrium to support implantation.		Infection	Advantages: Provides up to 5 years of protection; 10 to 15 min for insertion; no serious error of insertion possible; return to fertility without compromise.

needs to be fitted for a new diaphragm. A new diaphragm is required after a pregnancy, after weight gain or loss of 10 lb or more, and after pelvic surgery.

Spermicidal sponges A *spermicidal sponge* involves some of the same considerations as a diaphragm, but it has some distinct advantages for the adolescent. The sponge can be used for multiple acts of sexual intercourse. It is easier to insert than a diaphragm and is less likely to interfere with sexual spontaneity. Since it is an over-the-counter product, it is easily available to the adolescent.

Condoms A *condom* combined with a *spermicidal agent* (a foam, jelly, or suppository) is almost as effective as the oral contraceptive pill. Condoms also have the added benefit of offering protection against some sexually transmitted diseases, such as gonorrhea, AIDS, syphilis, and herpes. Condoms and spermicidal agents are relatively inexpensive and are readily available without prescription. For these reasons, the majority of both men and women have reported that the condom was the method used at the first intercourse.[49] Disadvantages reported by male adolescents are the necessity of making a public purchase, a decrease in spontaneity during foreplay, decreased sensations, and the need for advance planning.[50] However, the adolescent can be taught how to overcome most of these problems.

Withdrawal *Withdrawal,* or *coitus interruptus,* is used by many adolescents who have no other means of protection. Its efficacy is limited, since sperm may be released prior to ejaculation. It also requires a high degree of motivation on the part of the male.

Rhythm method The *rhythm method,* or natural contraception, and the *calendar method,* which is based on cervical secretions, tend to be very ineffective in the adolescent because of the high degree of motivation needed, the irregularity of the adolescent girl's menstrual cycle and ovulation, and the keen awareness of body changes that is required. (See Table 25-4.)

Counseling The nurse educates the adolescent in the proper use of the chosen method and dispels any myths related to it. By assessing the adolescent's sources and level of information and by taking a nonjudgmental attitude, the nurse will be able to communicate and listen more effectively, and the adolescent will feel more comfortable discussing sexuality. Myths—such as that douching with vinegar will prevent pregnancy—can be discussed without fear or guilt.

For all men and women, the first act of intercourse is a milestone on the continuum of psychosexual development. It is an event that is always remembered. Some adolescents remember it with no regrets, but many remember it with guilt or worry. Most adolescents justify their decision to become sexually active by saying that they were in love. Each adolescent's decision should be viewed as unique. If an adolescent opts to abstain from being sexually active, that decision should be supported. Although the nurse sees a wide range of sexual expression—from total suppression to indiscriminate sexual behavior—it is important to keep in mind the significance of sexuality in the adolescent's life. Its importance can be underestimated or greatly exaggerated. Despite what is reported in the media, most adolescents are concerned primarily with school, sports, and other activities. However, adolescent sexuality should not be ignored by health professionals or parents. Promoting effective decision making in adolescents as well as providing comprehensive counseling and health care will aid in the prevention of unwanted pregnancies, sexually transmitted diseases, and misinformation.

Adolescent pregnancy

Nurses who work with pregnant adolescents must recognize the many personal and maturational differences among girls in the same age group. The large number of adolescent pregnancies reflects the complex problem being faced by health professionals, parents, and adolescents. Current statistics indicate that the pregnancy rate among adolescents has increased, while the actual birthrates are decreasing; 600,000 adolescent girls give birth each year, and 1.2 million become pregnant.[51]

Options These statistics reveal the choices that adolescents are making. When an adolescent girl becomes pregnant, both she and the young man must make difficult decisions that will affect the rest of their lives. Should the pregnancy be continued or terminated? If the pregnancy will be continued, should the baby be put up for adoption, should they raise it themselves, or should the grandparents raise it?

Options should be presented in an unbiased manner to ensure the adolescent's freedom of choice. In the process of making a decision, the adolescent will need time to talk and will require counseling, guidance, and support in dealing with the concerns related to the pregnancy. The decision that a young man or woman makes in regard to an unplanned pregnancy may result in a sense of loss and pain.

Abortion Some adolescents choose to terminate the pregnancy. Currently, approximately 30 percent of all abortions are obtained by adolescents. Approximately 41 percent choose to terminate their pregnancies with the highest abortion rate occurring among those aged 18 to 19 (61.1 abortions per 1000 young women).[52] For most young women, the sexual partner plays a prominent role in the decision to continue or terminate the pregnancy. Adolescents tend to be conservative in their attitudes toward abortion, favoring termination of the pregnancy only in particular situations.[53] The risk of complications with abortions is relatively small and generally relates to the gestational age of the fetus. The adolescent who delays making a choice or who cannot make up her mind makes a passive decision to have the baby. Once the decision is made, either passively or actively, to continue the pregnancy, the adolescent is faced with the decision regarding whether to keep the baby or place it for adoption.

Adoption Few adolescents choose to place the baby for adoption; only 4 percent make that decision.[54] Adolescents with limited financial and/or family support are more likely to place the baby for adoption. The feeling of loss that the adolescent girl experiences is very strong. It is now generally believed that separation will be facilitated if she mourns the actual loss rather than the fantasy loss. For this reason, some agencies encourage interaction between the adopting parents and the mother in order to balance the grief of the loss with the knowledge that the infant will receive continued care and nurturing. The adolescent mother is not the only one who mourns the loss of a child. Many adolescent fathers feel the impact of the loss, as do many of the families of the young mothers and fathers. Some families mourn the loss of a grandchild, the loss of their child's innocence, and the loss of trust.

Keeping the Baby Many young pregnant women decide to continue the pregnancy and keep the child, despite the difficulties they will face. In today's society, the stigma of being a pregnant adolescent or an adolescent mother has decreased, as the incidence of pregnancy among adolescents has increased. Whereas at one time pregnant adolescents were banished from their families, schools, and communities, now they usually find some support and acceptance. In some communities the pregnant adolescent is still stigmatized, but changes are occurring. In the past, teenagers were not allowed to stay in school; now they can remain and continue their education. Some schools have set up prenatal and parenting classes to meet the needs of pregnant adolescents and their partners. Having and keeping the baby does not mean living "happily ever after," as so many teenagers expect. Often they are unwilling to listen to what adults tell them about the realities of parenthood and will continue to deny the impact that the baby will have on their lives. Hearing teenage parents talk about the demands and rewards of parenthood is sometimes more palatable to them. Adolescents should make long-term plans regarding who will provide financial support and housing and who will raise and care for the child. Marriages entered into to "make the baby legal" are very fragile, have a high divorce rate, and should be approached cautiously.

If an adolescent is part of a group in which pregnancy is frequent and accepted, not being pregnant may make her different. If she is part of a group in which pregnancy is not usually accepted, she may find that being pregnant is very stressful, since it will interfere with career goals, and she may decide to terminate the pregnancy.

Counseling the pregnant adolescent

Whether the decision is made to terminate or continue the pregnancy, the adolescent, her sexual partner, and their families will need counseling and health education from a nonjudgmental, interested professional. Most pregnant adolescents, their partners, and their families need to express feelings about the pregnancy and develop confidence concerning their decisions relating to it. For some adolescents, group sessions may be easier than individual sessions. Others prefer individual counseling. Cultural differences will influence counseling needs during pregnancy. Counseling for the pregnant teenager should include plans for future birth control, preparation for childbirth, prenatal needs and concerns, and parenting skills. The nurse should be keenly aware of his or her own sexual attitudes and beliefs and separate them from those of the adolescent. Only then can the nurse be therapeutic.

Issues of adolescent parenthood Over 1.2 million adolescent girls are currently bearing children each year, and 1.33 million children are now being raised by adolescent mothers.[55] Because they are adolescents, these mothers have limited resources for promoting their own and their infants' development.[56,57,58]

Most early research indicated that pregnancy in adolescence constituted a risk factor for the newborn, both physically and developmentally. Recent research has shown that it is not the mother's age but rather the socioeconomic status and other related factors that affect the infant's development.[59] In terms of physical development, low birth weight has typically been associated with younger maternal age. The exact reasons for the higher incidence of low-birth-weight infants among adolescent mothers have not been clearly established. In the past, physical immaturity and poor nutrition were suggested as the causes of low-birth-weight infants, but recent research has found that this is not true.[60,61] Although it is not entirely clear whether biological or socioeconomic inadequacies are the cause, it is becoming more evident in the research that adolescent mothers, as a group, present with a greater preponderance of risk factors, such as low weight gain, drug use, and low socioeconomic status, requiring more careful management. These risk factors are amenable to interventions by the nurse and other health professionals. Therefore, the focus of nursing interventions should include not only providing quality prenatal health care but also assisting adolescent mothers in preventing repeat pregnancy, increasing knowledge about child development, and responding appropriately to their infant. The knowledge and skills acquired by the adolescent should be continually reassessed and reinforced during the first two critical years of their child's development.

For many adolescents, parenthood thrusts new conflicts and roles into an already complex world and often disrupts the developmental tasks of adolescence. The adolescent father needs to become aware of his critical role in the development of the child, be encouraged to be involved in the birth process, and become aware of his rights and responsibilities. The nurse should support the young father in realistically meeting the needs of the child and the child's mother and his own needs. At the same time, the adolescent father will need guidance and support as well as time to explore his emotional feelings about the pregnancy. All too often the young man and his feelings are not acknowledged by the pregnant adolescent, the family, or the health professionals.

Both the adolescent mother and father will be faced with some very stressful issues:

1. Need for acceptance by their peers
2. Possible interruption of educational or career goals
3. Stressed relationships with boyfriend/girlfriend
4. Strained relationships with their families
5. Unrealistic expectations about their infant
6. Accepting her changing body
7. Accepting their new roles as parents
8. Continued dependence on their families for support

Parental behavior of adolescents The stressful events that accompany pregnancy and parenthood in adolescence have caused many to question the ability of adolescents to provide quality parenting. Recent research has indicated that there may be qualitative differences between the parental behavior of adolescent mothers and adult mothers. Most adolescent mothers prefer physical rather than verbal interactions with their infants. It has been suggested that interactions which are only physical in nature are less nurturing than those combining physical and verbal interactions. To develop a secure attachment with her infant, the adolescent mother must practice sensitive parental behaviors, such as the ability to perceive the child's cues, interpret them, and respond appropriately.

The issue of parental behaviors also involves potential child abuse. Currently there is much controversy concerning abuse and suboptimal development of children of adolescent parents. It has been found that 3 to 9 percent of adolescent parents abuse their children during their own adolescence. When child abuse is related to maternal age at the birth of the first child the statistics are more alarming, showing that approximately 28 to 38 percent of abusing parents were in their teens when the first child was conceived. It is believed that as the young parents raise their children and are faced with a myriad of financial and sociological problems, they become prone to abusing their children. For this reason, it is very important to provide appropriate interventions during adolescence. Although some studies have indicated that young maternal age has an adverse effect on a child's cognitive development, new research has suggested that psychosocial factors associated with pregnancy during adolescence have the major influence. Thus the nurse must realize that not all adolescents are at risk for parenting failure. Close emotional support given by family members during the pregnancy to the new parents and their child can smooth the transition to quality parenthood and provide the basis for optimal child development.

Management Some of the goals of nursing care for the pregnant adolescent, the father of the child, and their families include:

1. Helping promote a physically safe and emotionally satisfying pregnancy
2. Encouraging early and continued prenatal care
3. Providing a supportive environment
4. Providing counseling and health education concerning contraception and parenting skills and dispelling myths
5. Using innovative educational strategies, e.g., role playing and parenting and sexuality games developed by professionals, such as Humanopoly
6. Providing follow-up for the care of the adolescent and the child

Adolescents want health care professionals who are genuinely interested in them and willing to listen to them. The nurse should build a trusting relationship with the adolescent, bearing in mind that adolescents will often "test" the nurse to see whether he or she is really concerned. Communication between the adolescents and their families can be enhanced by helping adolescents develop communication skills and make responsible decisions about sexuality. The nurse who works with adolescents should develop competence and confidence in answering sensitive or potentially embarrassing questions and should be able to defuse embarrassment.

Clarifying values, exploring adolescents' attitudes and beliefs, assessing their coping strategies, and helping them develop realistic goals are necessary components of nursing intervention. It is also important for the nurse to assess the adolescent's cognitive and developmental level, interpersonal relationships with peers and family members, and self-esteem. Educational strategies and counseling need to be innovative, age-appropriate, and effective for adolescents. Nurses who work with adolescents will find the experience a very challenging one that demands expertise in adolescent physical and cognitive development, an ability to communicate, and a desire to enhance emotional and interpersonal growth.

References

1. Langman, J., *Medical Embryology,* 3d ed., Williams & Wilkins, Baltimore, 1975, p. 175.
2. Whaley, Lucille, and Donna Wong, *Nursing Care of Infants and Children,* Mosby, St. Louis, 1979, p. 419.
3. Summit, R. L., "Differential Diagnosis of Genital Ambiguity in the Newborn," *Clinical Obstetrical Gynecology* **15**:112–139 (1972).
4. Mazur, Tom, "Ambiguous Genitalia: Detection and Counseling," *Pediatric Nursing* **9**(6):417 (November–December 1983).
5. Ibid., p. 420.
6. Gibbons, William E., "Diagnosis: Amenorrhea," *Hospital Medicine,* p. 57 (December 1983).
7. Ibid., p. 57.
8. Demarest, Colleen B., "When the Teen Has Irregular Periods," *Patient Care,* p. 152 (October 1984).
9. Abraham, Guy E., "Nutritional Factors in the Etiology of the Premenstrual Tension Syndromes," *Journal of Reproductive Medicine* **28**:446–464 (July 1983).
10. Wilson, Mary Ann, "Menstrual Disorders: Premenstrual Syndrome, Dysmenorrhea, Amenorrhea," *Journal of Gynecologic Nursing* (Suppl.):11s–19s (March–April 1984).
11. Zaven, H., and M. D. Chakmakjian, "A Critical Assessment of Therapy for Premenstrual Tension Syndrome," *The Journal of Reproductive Medicine,* **28**(8):532–538 (August 1983).
12. Wilhelm-Hass, Elaine, "Premenstrual Syndrome: Its Nature, Evaluation, and Management," *Journal of Gynecologic Nursing* 223–229 (July–August 1984).
13. Kramer, S. A., "Cryptorchidism: Current State of the Art in Diagnosis and Treatment," *Continuing Education for the Family Physician* **8**:737–741 (1983).
14. Rajfer, J., et al., "Testicular Descent: Normal and Abnormal," *Urologic Clinics of North America* **5**:223–235 (1978).
15. Scorer, C. G., et al., "Congenital Anomalies of the Testes," in J. H. Harrison et al. (eds.), *Campbell's Urology,* 4th ed., Saunders, Philadelphia, 1979.
16. Hadziselimovic, F., et al., "Surgical Correction of Cryptorchidism at 2 Years: Electron Microscope and Morphometric Investigation," *Journal of Pediatric Surgery* **10**:19 (1975).
17. Hezmall, H. P., et al., "Cryptorchidism and Infertility," *Urologic Clinics of North America* **9**:361 (1982).
18. Gilhooly, P. E., et al., "Fertility Prospects for Children with Cryptorchidism," *American Journal of Diseases of Children* **138**:940–943 (1984).
19. Martin, D. C., "Malignancy in the Cryptorchid Testis," *Urologic Clinics of North America* **9**:371 (1982).
20. Batata, M. A., et al., "Testicular Cancer in Cryptorchidism," *Cancer* **49**:1023–1030 (1982).
21. Gob, J. C., et al., "Hormonal Therapy of Cryptorchidism with HCG," *Urologic Clinics of North America* **9**:405–411 (1982).
22. Hadziselimovic, F., "Treatment of Cryptorchidism with GnRH," *Urologic Clinics of North America* **9**:413–420 (1982).
23. Wacksman, J., et al., "Technique of Testicular Autotransplantation Using a Microvascular Anastomosis," *Surgery, Gynecology, and Obstetrics* **150**:399–400 (March 1980).
24. Allen, Terry D., "Testicular Torsion: To Avert a Tragedy, Don't Wait for a Diagnosis," *Consultant* 302 (March 1984).
25. Nagler, H. M., et al., "The Effect of Testicular Torsion on the Contralateral Testes," *Journal of Urology* **128**:1343 (1942).
26. Money, J., and A. A. Ehrhardt, *Man and Woman, Boy and Girl,* Johns Hopkins, Baltimore, 1972.
27. Cobliner, G. W., "Pregnancy in the Single Adolescent Girl: The Role of Cognitive Functions," *Journal of Youth and Adolescence* **3**(1):17–29 (1974).
28. Elkind, D., and I. Weiner, *Development of the Child,* Wiley, New York, 1978.
29. Mims, F., and M. Swensen, *Sexuality: A Nursing Perspective,* McGraw-Hill, New York, 1980.
30. Katchadovrian, H., "Adolescent Sexuality," *Symposium on Adolescent Medicine* **27**(1):17–28 (1980).
31. Zelnik, M., and F. Shah, "First Intercourse among Young Americans," *Family Planning Perspectives* **15**(2) (1983).
32. Sorenson, R., *Adolescent Sexuality in Contemporary*

America, World Publishing, Cleveland, 1973.
33. Carlson, M., et al., "An Exploratory Study of Life Change Events, Social Support and Pregnancy Decisions in Adolescents," *Adolescence* **19**(76):765–779 (Winter 1984).
34. Zelnik and Shah, op. cit.
35. Herold, W., M. Godwin, and D. Lero, "Self-Esteem, Locus of Control and Adolescent Contraception," *Journal of Psychology,* **101**:83 (1979).
36. Hornick, J., et al., "Premarital Contraception Usage among Male and Female Adolescents," *Family Coordinator* **28**:181 (1979).
37. Reiss, I., et al., "Premarital Contraceptive Usage: A Study and Some Theoretical Exploration," *Journal of Marriage and the Family* **37**:619 (1975).
38. Babikan, H. M., et al., "A Study of Teenage Pregnancy," *American Journal of Psychiatry* **128**:755–760 (1971).
39. MacDonald, A., "Internal-External Locus of Control and the Practice of Birth Control," *Psychology Report* **27**:206–209 (1970).
40. Luker, K., "Taking Chances: Abortion and the Decision Not To," *Contraception,* University of California Press, Berkeley, 1975.
41. Jorgenson, S., S. King, and B. Torrey, "Dyadic and Social Network Influences on Adolescent Exposure to Pregnancy Risk," *Journal of Marriage and the Family* **42**:141 (1980).
42. Furstenberg, F., Jr., et al., "Contraceptive Continuation among Adolescents Attending Family Planning Clinics," *Family Planning Perspectives* **15**(5):211–217 (1983).
43. Strahle, W., "Premarital Coitus among Female Adolescents," *Archives of Sexual Behavior* **12**(1) (1983).
44. Chilman, C., *Adolescent Sexuality in Changing American Society,* U.S. Department of Health, Education, and Welfare, Washington, D.C., 1978.
45. Zelnik, M., and J. Kanter, "Sexual and Contraceptive Experience of Young Unmarried Women in the U.S.: 1976 and 1971," *Family Planning Perspectives* **9**:55–71 (1977).
46. Furstenberg et al., op. cit.
47. Turetsky, R., and V. Strasburger, "Adolescent Contraception," *Clinical Pediatrics* **22**(5):337–341 (1983).
48. Ibid.
49. Zelnik and Shah, op. cit.
50. Greydanus, D. E., "Contraception in Adolescence: An Overview for the Pediatrician," *Pediatric Annals* **9**:52–63 (1980).
51. *Teenage Pregnancy: The Problem Hasn't Gone Away,* A. Guttmacher Institute, New York, 1981.
52. Henshaw, S., and K. O'Reilly, "Characteristics of Abortion Patients in the United States," *Family Planning Perspectives* **15**(1):5–7 (1983).
53. Zelnik, M., and J. Kanter, "Sexual and Contraceptive Experiences of Young Unmarried Women in the U.S.: 1976 and 1971," in Furstenberg et al. (eds.), *Teenage Sexuality, Pregnancy and Childbearing,* University of Pennsylvania Press, Philadelphia, 1981.
54. Mercer, R., "Assessing and Counseling Teenage Mothers during the Prenatal Period," *Nursing Clinics of North America* **18**(2):293–301 (1983).
55. *Teenage Pregnancy.*
56. Baldwin, W., and V. S. Cain, "The Children of Teenage Parents," *Family Planning Perspectives* **12**(1):34–43 (1980).
57. Horowitz, J. A., C. B. Hughes, and B. J. Perdee, "Parenting Reassessed: A Nursing Perspective," Prentice-Hall, Englewood Cliffs, N.J., 1982.
58. Philliber, S. G., and E. H. Graham, "The Impact of Age of Mother on Mother-Child Interaction Patterns," *Journal of Marriage and Family* **44**(2):355–366.
59. Roosa, M. E., et al., "A Comparison of Teenage and Older Mothers: A Systems Analysis," *Journal of Marriage and the Family* **44**(2):367–377.
60. Horon, I. L., Strobin, and McDonald, "Birth Weights of Infants Born to Adolescents," *American Journal of Obstetrics and Gynecology,* **146**(4):444–449 (1983).
61. Zuckerman, B., et al., "Neonatal Outcome: Is Adolescent Pregnancy a Risk Factor?" *Pediatrics* **71**(4):489–493 (1983).

26

Margaret A. Brady

The immune system

Upon completion of this chapter, the student will be able to:

1 Describe the specific function of each type of cell and tissue of the immune system.
2 Discuss the meaning of the term *antigen*.
3 Describe the body's response to an antigen.
4 Differentiate between the two main types of immunity.
5 Write a plan for the early recognition and treatment of anaphylaxis.
6 Identify the pathophysiological changes commonly seen in allergic rhinitis and atopic dermatitis.
7 Distinguish between hypersensitivity and hyposensitization.
8 Describe the steps in the environmental and physical assessment of an allergic child.
9 Identify the major pathophysiological changes seen in autoimmune diseases.
10 Describe the function of the human leukocyte antigen system.

ANATOMY AND PHYSIOLOGY OF THE IMMUNE SYSTEM

Immunity and specific immunity

The body has both passive and active systems to protect it against harmful substances. Passive types of defenses include the skin and mucous membranes, which act as physical barriers, and gastric secretions, which act as biochemical protectors. Active defenses are the inflammatory reaction and the immune system response. Briefly, the immune system is composed of specific cells, tissues, and organs that maintain body defenses against substances considered foreign or harmful. It also removes worn-out "self" components, such as red blood cells, and destroys abnormal cells, which constantly arise as a result of mutation.

Drugs, radiation, malnutrition, and illness are capable of disturbing the normal function of the immune system. An alteration can predispose the body to infection or malignant growths; it may also bring about immune system diseases.

CELLS, TISSUES, AND ORGANS OF THE IMMUNE SYSTEM

The *cellular elements* serving the immune process are located throughout the body and are both fixed (attached) in tissues and floating in blood and lymph. The three most important cell types are:

1. *Macrophages* Cells that are highly specialized to ingest and destroy particulate matter by phagocytosis.
2. *Lymphocytes* White blood cells that differentiate into T cells and B cells, which are the types active in immune responses. B cells produce antibody. T cells carry out a direct attack on antigen. Natural killer cells are lymphocytes that lack typical T- or B-cell characteristics. They kill tumor cells.
3. *Mediator cells* Mast cells, basophils, neutrophils, and platelets (cell fragments). These release chemicals such as kinin protease, histamine, serotonin, slow-reacting substance of anaphylaxis (SRS-A), and vasoactive amines during inflammatory reactions and immune reactions (see Table 26-1).

The *tissues* of the immune system are:

1. *Lymph* The fluid that flows through lymphatic vessels, nodules, and nodes and carries foreign substances and T and B cells.
2. *Lymph nodes* Masses of lymphoid tissue surrounded by a capsule and placed in the path of lymphatic vessels so that lymph must circulate through them, where it is filtered and antigen is trapped for contact with lymphocytes.
3. *Peripheral lymphoid tissue* Tiny masses of lymphoid tissue without capsules. Nodules are scattered throughout the body, but dense collections are found near body surfaces in the submucosal tissues of the respiratory, genitourinary, and intestinal tracts. They function to trap invading particles.

Table 26-1 Chemical Mediators and Their Pharmacological Action

Mediator	Action
Histamine	Increased permeability of capillaries Contraction of bronchiolar and other smooth muscle Increased gastric, nasal, bronchial mucus, and lacrimal secretions
SRS-A (slow-reacting substance of anaphylaxis)	Sustained smooth-muscle contraction
Serotonin	Increased vascular permeability Smooth-muscle contraction
Kinin protease	Increased vascular permeability, contraction of smooth muscles, increased secretion of mucous glands

Organs that serve the immune system include the following:

1. *Bone marrow* Produces cells destined to become T or B cells. Bone marrow is also believed to be where lymphocytes differentiate into B cells.
2. *Thymus* The organ where lymphocytes become T cells.
3. *Spleen* The filtering organ of the blood, where foreign particles may be trapped for encounter with lymphocytes.

THE IMMUNE RESPONSE

One of the system's powerful active defenses is the *immune response*. This is a chain of reactions tailored to the unique characteristics of the harmful substance. It is therefore called a *specific defense*.

Antigens

The term for a substance to which the immune system responds is *antigen*. An antigen is usually a protein or polysaccharide but is more broadly defined as any substance capable of stimulating an immune response. Antigens include substances foreign to the body as well as constituents of the body that for some reason the immune system recognizes as foreign.

Sequence of immunologic events The steps in an immune response are (1) recognition of an antigen, (2) production of an antibody and cells prepared to attack that antigen, and (3) destruction of the antigen. Immunity against the antigen, sometimes lasting throughout life, is usually the outcome of such an immune response. Immunity is a quicker, stronger, more effective response to the same antigen if it is detected by the immune system again.

By virtue of its molecular weight and composition, each antigen is unique. One hypothesis concerning the mechanism underlying the immune response suggests that each antigen serves as a template (pattern) for the production of the antibody or cells capable of attacking it. This "lock and key" idea explains why each antibody fits only one antigen.

An invader that penetrates the barriers of the skin, mucous membranes, and lymph nodules, or an internally arising "foreign" element, either will be eliminated by macrophages or will find itself in the lymph. Lymph flows through lymphatic vessels to lymph nodes, where foreign matter (the antigen) is filtered from the lymph, trapped, held for contact with T or B lymphocytes, and phagocytized. T or B lymphocytes multiply in the lymph node after contact with the antigen. This causes the lymph node to enlarge from 2 to 5 times in size and become palpable when there is infection in the area of the node.

If the antigen escapes the lymph node, it is carried by the lymph through the thoracic duct and into the bloodstream. Blood can also be invaded directly through capillaries and venules. The spleen, by filtering blood, provides another arena for antigen-lymphocyte contact. Phagocytic elements in the spleen attempt to destroy the invader. The spleen is essential in the avoidance of overwhelming infection.

TWO TYPES OF SPECIFIC IMMUNITY

Immediate immunity

Immunity produced by the B lymphocytes is called *immediate immunity* because of the speed of the reaction. It is also known as *humoral immunity* (the term *humoral* is derived from the Latin word meaning "to be moist") because the antibody floats freely in body fluids.

B lymphocytes, when stimulated by exposure to an antigen, differentiate into *plasma cells*, which produce antibodies specific to the antigen. Other B lymphocytes that have encountered this antigen divide to produce a population of identical B cells, *memory cells*, which are primed to recognize this antigen in the future. These cells are responsible for immunologic memory. They "remember" the antigen when they encounter it again and produce a rapid, strong antibody response called the *secondary antibody response*.

The antibodies produced by the transformation of the B lymphocyte float freely in body fluids. For this reason, an antibody can quickly reach an antigen located almost anywhere in the body. *Immunoglobulins* (Ig) include all known antibodies; there are five classes of immunoglobulins, each with a specific biological function. Table 26-2 summarizes the five classes of immunoglobulins. Chapter 9 discusses immunoglobulin levels in the newborn.

Cell-mediated immunity

When an antigen triggers an immune response by a T lymphocyte, the T lymphocyte multiplies. It produces a population of effector T cytotoxic and T memory cells identical to the T lymphocyte that first encountered the antigen, but with the same antigen receptor specificity as their parent T cells. Effector T cytotoxic cells attack only those cells bearing their specific antigens

Table 26-2 Classes of Immunoglobulins

IgG
The most abundant immunoglobulin in serum. Predominant antibody response in second exposure to an antigen; crosses the placenta to provide the fetus and newborn with short-term immunity; used for passive immunization when a preformed antibody is injected into a susceptible host exposed to a disease such as hepatitis

IgM
The first class of antibody to respond to infection, especially in extravascular spaces

IgA
Defends exposed body cavities; found in seromucous secretions of the lacrimal, salivary, and mammary glands and the gastrointestinal genitourinary, and respiratory tracts

IgE
Responsible for immediate hypersensitivity, including anaphylaxis; responsible for allergic symptoms; fixes to surface of mast cells; induces release of vasoactive amines; is produced in greater quantities in allergic than nonallergic children

IgD
Functions unknown; may operate to activate or suppress lymphocytes

Table 26-3 Summary of the Two Types of Immune Response

Type	Characteristics	Gives Immunity to:	Is Responsible for:
Humoral	Circulating antibody B cells Immediate reactions Persists months to years	Staphylococci Streptococci *Hemophilus influenzae* Pneumococci Rubeola, varicella, hepatitis (initial protection only)	Anaphylaxis Hay fever Asthma Hemolytic disease Autoimmune disease
Cellular	Sensitized lymphocytes T cells Delayed reactions Persists for a lifetime	Acid-fast bacteria (TB) Rubeola Varicella Herpes Cytomegalovirus Fungi	Organ and tissue transplant reactions Contact dermatitis
Both humoral and cellular	Formed in lymphoid tissue Antigen specific Stimulated by antigen Memory cells formed		

by direct cell contact. This is called *cell-mediated immunity.*

Whether the T-lymphocyte or B-lymphocyte system is stimulated by an antigen depends on the characteristic of the specific antigen. Table 26-3 summarizes the two types of immunity and includes examples of types of antigens that stimulate them.

HOW ANTIBODIES WORK

Antibodies have a wide range of functions, including stimulating growth and promoting cytotoxicity (cell destruction). They can combine with antigens, promoting an immunologic effect, or bind with other cells in a nonimmunologic manner. Antibodies neutralize antigens through a process called a *primary immunologic reaction.* Antibodies can also work in conjunction with amplification systems to increase their destructive powers. The complement system (a system of serum proteins) is the best known amplification system. Because other substances (complements) are required for the antigen-antibody response to occur, it is called a *secondary immunologic reaction.* Antibodies may also be absorbed onto the surface of T cells and act as T-cell receptors for antigens.

ANTIGEN-ANTIBODY REACTIONS

When an antigen is encountered by the immune system for the *first* time, it takes up to 2 weeks for the immunologic events of recognition, antibody production, and antigen destruction to function optimally. This is called the *primary response.* It is the *secondary, anamnestic,* or *memory* response—when a specific antigen is encountered for the second time, for the third time, or at a subsequent time—that can produce tissue-damaging reactions. Specific antibodies quickly appear in the serum. Usually the secondary response is beneficial to the child and represents normal immune function. Vaccination works because of this secondary response. However, in some children dangerous malfunctions occur—tissue-damaging reactions, which can be divided into four major types.

Type I reactions

Type I reactions, or *anaphylactic reactions,* are the most immediate and acute reactions. Certain children have a genetic predisposition to produce large amounts of IgE that attaches itself to the surface of mast cells (in tissue) and basophils (in blood). When an antigen combines with the antibody on the mast cell surface, the cell bursts and releases histamine, kinin protease, serotonin, and SRS-A. These pharmacological agents are responsible for three major events: the contraction of smooth muscle, especially the bronchiolar muscles; capillary dilation; and stimulation of mucus-secreting cells.

In its most severe form a type I reaction causes *systemic anaphylaxis,* which can rapidly result in death if treatment is not initiated immediately.

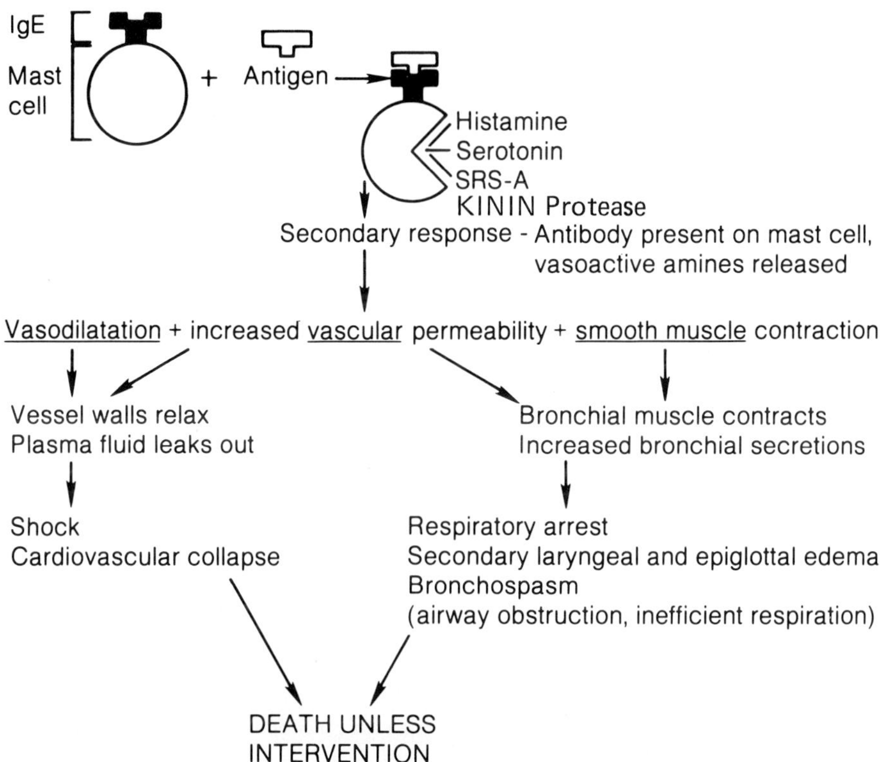

Figure 26-1 A diagrammatic representation of anaphylaxis.

Local anaphylaxis occurs in allergic asthma (in the lungs), rhinitis (in the nose), hay fever (in the nose), and rash (on the skin). Allergens causing anaphylaxis can be ingested, inhaled, or injected. Drugs, insect bites, foods, and inhalants can be responsible for anaphylaxis. See Fig. 26-1 for a diagrammatic representation of anaphylaxis. The signs, symptoms, and treatment of anaphylaxis are presented in Table 26-4. *Systemic anaphylaxis is a medical emergency, and the nurse must be able to recognize it and initiate treatment immediately.* All the responses occurring in anaphylaxis are reversible by drug therapy if initiated immediately. This type of immune reaction represents hyperreactivity of the immune system and does not occur in all children. It is also called *reaginic hypersensitivity.*

Type II reactions

IgG and IgM are responsible for *type II reactions,* also known as *cytotoxic reactions*. The antigen is on the surface of a body cell, and the antibody is free-floating. When the antibody attaches to a cell-bound antigen, the cell breaks open and is destroyed. Autoimmune hemolytic anemia (a condition in which a child's own red blood cells are destroyed by antibodies), transfusion reactions (each person possesses naturally occurring antibodies to blood group antigens different from his or her own), and organ transplant rejection reactions (the antigens on the surfaces of the transplanted tissue are immediately recognized as foreign and are attacked) are examples of type II antigen-antibody reactions. The type II reactions to blood transfusions and tissue transplants would be expected to occur in any immunologically competent child. Autoimmune hemolytic anemia is an immune disorder.

Type III reactions

Type III reactions, or *immune complex reactions,* occur in body and tissue fluids. The antigen-antibody complexes deposit on small vessel walls, causing vasculitis, or in the dermis, epidermis, joints, choroid plexus of the skull, or

Table 26-4 Nursing Care in Anaphylaxis

Whenever You Give a Drug:

1. Always check for history of allergy of any type.
2. Always check for previous exposure to the agent being used.

Watch 20 to 30 Min for:

1. Generalized feeling of warmth
2. Itching palms, soles, and throat
3. Tingling sensations on the face or mouth
4. Hoarseness
5. Dysphagia
6. Tightness in the chest and throat
7. Wheezing, dyspnea, and cough
8. Urticaria
9. Signs and symptoms of shock

If Symptoms Occur:

1. Report to physician.
2. Administer:
   a. *Antihistamine*—Benadryl intravenously (blocks effects of histamine)
   b. *Epinephrine*—Adrenalin intravenously or intramuscularly (action is the opposite of that of histamine) to stimulate the myocardium, increase cardiac output, increase blood pressure, and relax smooth muscle of the respiratory tract
   c. *Aminophylline* (bronchodilator)
3. Gather:
   a. Oral airway
   b. Endotracheal tube
   c. Tracheotomy set
   d. Tourniquets
   e. Ambu bag
   f. Oxygen setup
   g. Parenteral fluids and tubing
4. Monitor blood pressure, pulse, and respiration every 3 to 5 min.
5. If antigenic insult is on extremity, apply a loose tourniquet near and above site of antigen. Occlusion should be sufficient to obstruct venous flow and *must be relaxed* for 1 min every 3 min. (Use timer if necessary.)

glomeruli. Tissue damage is caused by proteolytic (protein-destroying) enzymes liberated during attempted phagocytosis of the complexes. Thus it involves complex-mediated injury. Rheumatoid arthritis and glomerulonephritis are examples of diseases that can be caused by type III reactions.

Type IV reactions

Type IV reactions, or *delayed hypersensitivity reactions,* are mediated by sensitized lymphocytes. Receptors on the surface of the sensitized lymphocyte recognize and combine with the antigen. This causes the sensitized lymphocyte to release products known as *lymphokines,* which trigger an inflammatory reaction that helps in the destruction and elimination of antigen and can cause tissue damage. This reaction is responsible for contact dermatitis, transplanted tissue rejection (a delayed reaction), the prolonged reaction of insect bites, tuberculous lesions in the lung, Hashimoto disease, and lesions seen in cell-mediated coccidioidomycosis and histoplasmosis. This cell-mediated reaction causes a positive skin test for tuberculosis. If a person tested has been previously infected with tuberculosis, an area of induration and edema will develop at the injection site after several hours and will persist for 48 h (see Table 26-3).

ALTERATIONS INVOLVING A DEFICIENCY OR EXCESS OF IMMUNE SYSTEM CELLS OR TISSUES

Deficiency in immune response

Immune deficiency diseases in children can be the result of a deficiency of the B cell, the T cell, or both. Rarely occurring primary immunodeficiency diseases in infants and children are sometimes difficult to recognize. The symptoms or complications of the diseases may not appear for several months or even years after birth. Frequently symptoms will begin at about 3 months of age, when maternal immunity, transmitted prior to birth, is on the decline.

Manifestations While the clinical diagnosis and treatment are specific to each disease, the nurse who takes the child's history should be aware of common clinical features suggestive of immunodeficiency disease. Failure to grow may be a result of the repeated insults of these diseases. The history of past illnesses will frequently reveal infections or unusually severe responses to agents that do not normally produce such responses in children. The child is extremely susceptible to upper respiratory infections and has a predisposition to chronic pulmonary disease and sinusitis. Recurrent skin infections or abscesses, intractable eczema, conjunctivitis (secondary to a *Hemophilus influenzae* infection), chronic gastrointestinal distress, and diarrhea, as well as cytomegalovirus, rubeola, and *Candida* infections (monilial and yeast infections), are increased in incidence. Lymphoid cancers are also more frequent. Known allergies should be recorded, and the child's immunization status and reaction should be determined. Immunization using live viruses is contraindicated in a child with T-cell deficiency because the child may develop an overwhelming infection from the agent.

Diagnostic tests The diagnosis of immunodeficiency disease is made by measuring the level of serum immunoglobulins. High levels of maternally derived IgG can make diagnosis during the first 3 months of life difficult. Normal levels of IgA and IgM will virtually rule out the presence of significant immunodeficiency disease. The presence of palpable inguinal lymph nodes and visible tonsillar tissue will also help rule out immunodeficiency disease. Bone marrow aspiration is sometimes used as a diagnostic measure to determine whether plasma cells are present.

Treatment Treatment of immunodeficiency disease includes intramuscular or intravenous administration of immune serum globulin. Pain at the site of an intramuscular injection can be controlled by mixing a small amount of local anesthetic with the immune serum globulin in the syringe. Large doses of immune serum globulin for adults and older children may require an intravenous route. Another treatment, usually for T-cell deficiency, is bone marrow transplantation; ideally, marrow aspirated from a matched sibling is used. A complication of T-cell deficiency may be a graft-vs.-host reaction as a result of blood transfusions and bone marrow transplantations. Blood products should be irradiated prior to administration to destroy the transfused T cells.

Nursing management includes support for the families of these children, since they have a poor prognosis and significant health problems. Chapters 34 and 35 discuss the care of children with long-term disease processes and aspects of family support. The parents are told to reduce exposure to infectious disease by avoiding crowds and persons known to be ill. Many of the diseases are X-linked or result from autosomal recessive traits. See Chap. 6 for information on genetic disease transmission, evaluation, and counseling. Table 26-5 describes primary immunodeficiency disorders and lists the causes and treatment.

Panhypogammaglobulinemia

There are four forms of *panhypogammaglobulinemia,* also called *congenital agammaglobulinemia*: an X-linked form (Bruton disease), an autosomal recessive form, a sporadic form, and a "late onset" form. Infantile sex-linked agammaglobulinemia renders an infant incapable of mounting a humoral response (a B-cell deficiency). The child cannot produce free-floating antibodies and therefore is subjected to repeated bacterial infections, particularly from *Staphylococcus, Pneumococcus,* and *Hemophilus influenzae.* Cell-mediated responses (T-cell responses) are normal. Since it is female carriers who pass the defect on to their sons, the disease is usually seen in young boys. The age at diagnosis varies from 3 months to 4 years, depending on when the symptoms are manifested. Treatment is frequent injection of human gamma globulin. This is used up in antigen-antibody reactions and cannot be replenished by the child, and so it must be repeatedly injected.

Thymic hypoplasia

Children with *thymic hypoplasia,* also called *Di George syndrome,* have a T-cell deficiency and cannot mount an effective immune response to a fungal or viral illness. They can be overwhelmed by routine viral immunizations. These children can also have a weakened humoral system response. The cause of this condition is failure of the fetal thymus to develop and "process" the T cells. A spontaneous cure may occur. If the cellular immune defect persists, a fetal thymus transplant is recommended. Associated failure of the parathyroid to develop will often result in hypocalcemia and symptoms of tetany in the infant. Calcium gluconate is administered concurrently with vitamin D until normal serum calcium levels are attained.

Combined immunodeficiency disease

In *combined immunodeficiency disease,* both the T-cell and the B-cell systems are deficient. It is apparent within the first weeks of life, and the child usually dies by the age of 2 years as the result of overwhelming infections. Bone marrow transplantation has been successful when marrow from histocompatible siblings has been used.

Table 26-5 Primary Immunodeficiency Disorders

Deficiency Disorder	Cause, Description, and Treatment
Bruton disease	X-linked panhypogammaglobulinemia; defective B-cell function; recurrent invasive infections; recurrent sinopulmonary infections; malabsorption; eczema; can be treated with IgG injections.
Di George syndrome	Deficiency in T-cell mechanism; absent or deficient thymus; tetany secondary to hyocalcemia; normal to deficient B-cell function; increased susceptibility to fungal and viral infections; can be treated with fetal thymus transplant.
Combined immunodeficiency disease	Both T cells and B cells are deficient; X-linked autosomal recessive, sporadic forms; apparent in first few weeks of life; causes death by age 2 from overwhelming viral or bacterial infections, infant gastroenteritis, malabsorption, pulmonary infection, or failure to grow.
Ataxia-telangiectasia	Deficiency of IgA and IgE; autosomal recessive; chromosomal breakage syndrome; ataxia; oculocutaneous telangiectasia; recurrent sinopulmonary infections.
Wiskott-Aldrich syndrome	X-linked recessive inheritance; bleeding secondary to thrombocytopenia; eczema; marked susceptibility to infection; IgM deficiency—child is prone to gram-negative infections; child is prone to lymphoreticular malignancies; median survival—6.5 years.
Chédiak-Higashi syndrome	Autosomal recessive; decreased pigmentation in skin, hair, and eyes; skin and bowel infections; malignancies develop in children who survive.
Transient hypogammaglobulinemia of infancy	Delay in initiation of infant's production of IgG for 15 to 30 weeks; infant is highly susceptible to infections; treated with IgG injections.

Partial immunodeficiency diseases

Partial immunodeficiency diseases related to prematurity are more common than the three severe immunodeficiency diseases discussed above. Premature infants may have a problem with transient hypogammaglobulinemia. Normally, there is a delay in the production of gamma-G globulin (IgG) by the infant for 15 to 30 weeks while the mother's IgG, which is transferred transplacentally, is used up. In the premature infant, the full amount of maternal antibodies is not transferred, and the baby's own immune response is delayed. The child is highly susceptible to infection but can be treated with human IgG injections.

Acquired immunodeficiency syndrome

Acquired immunodeficiency syndrome (AIDS) is a newly described disease occurring in adults and children. It is a condition in which a previously healthy person develops a defect in part of the immune system. This life-threatening illness is blood-borne and viral in origin and involves defective cell-mediated immunity caused by alterations in the T lymphocytes. The HTLV-III (AIDS) virus has been found in blood, semen, breast milk, and saliva.[1]

Incidence Children at increased risk for acquiring AIDS are (1) children who have household contacts with high-risk adults or whose parents are high-risk adults (AIDS victims, male homosexuals, intravenous drug users, and hemophiliacs); (2) children who are given transfusions, especially sick newborns and premature infants; and (3) hemophiliacs (factor VIII and factor IX deficiencies). Epidemiological data have confirmed that the AIDS virus is transmitted during heterosexual or homosexual sexual relations, by sharing contaminated needles, through blood transfusions or clotting factors (that have not been heat-treated), and by transplacental passage to the fetus. (Blood products for hemophiliacs have been heat-treated to kill the AIDS virus since about 1980. A national recommendation for heat treatment of blood products was published in 1984.) No cases have documented that the disease is spread by sharing meals, sneezing, or coughing or through other casual contacts.[2]

Manifestations The diagnosis of AIDS is difficult in the early stages because no specific signs are present and the incubation period ranges from a few months up to 5 years. No test is available for diagnosis, but an antibody screening test, the enzyme-linked immunosorbent assay (ELISA), can be used to screen blood donors. Children with AIDS are vulnerable to serious infections from opportunist organisms such as *Pneumocystis carinii pneumonia, Candida,* the herpes simplex virus, and cytomegaloviruses. Certain malignancies, such as Kaposi sarcoma and Burkitt lymphoma, and other nonspecific conditions, such as failure to thrive, generalized lymph node swelling, and chronic diarrhea, are also found in children with AIDS.

Treatment Although the ELISA test is available, no laboratory test can provide a completely reliable diagnosis of AIDS at the present time. Diagnosis is based primarily on a medical history of chronic unexplained lymphadenopathy, the absence of any current illness or drug use known to cause lymphadenopathy, and the presence of reactive hyperplasia in a lymph node when a biopsy is performed. There is no cure for this eventually fatal disease, and treatment is directed toward preventing and controlling infection from opportunist organisms and giving supportive care. AIDS patients are usually on blood, needle, enteric, urine, and secretion precautions, and gloves should be worn when handling any of these sources of infection.

Nursing management Since AIDS attacks multiple body systems, the nurse must realize the importance of a holistic approach to a patient's care. The primary role of the nurse who is working with a child with AIDS is to provide an atmosphere of understanding and acceptance for the child and his or her family and guidance in providing comfort care (see Chap. 35), and to prevent the spread of the disease. Since AIDS disease is ultimately fatal, the psychological impact is overwhelming, and counseling should be provided at the time of diagnosis. Families are taught precautions to prevent the spread of the disease (see Table 26-6).[3] Since AIDS in children is often transmitted from their parents or from blood products, there is a great deal of guilt connected with the transmission of the disease. Nurses must also assess and evaluate methods of improving nursing care and family support, while safeguarding their own health by keeping abreast of the latest research findings on AIDS transmission. Support groups for caregivers are essential to help them overcome the fear of caring for patients with this disease.

Table 26-6 Recommendations for the Individual Judged to Have an HTLV-III (AIDS) Infection to Prevent Spread of the Disease

1. Refrain from donating blood, plasma, body organs, tissue, or sperm.
2. Be aware of the risk of infecting others through sexual intercourse, sharing needles, and possible oral-genital contact. Condoms may reduce the possibility of transmission.
3. Do not share toothbrushes, razors, or other articles that can become contaminated with blood.
4. Be aware that women who have a seropositive test or whose partner has a seropositive test are at increased risk of acquiring AIDS and can transmit AIDS to their offspring if they become pregnant.
5. If accidental bleeding occurs, clean contaminated surfaces with a freshly mixed solution of 1 part household bleach and 10 parts water.
6. Have devices that have punctured the skin steam-sterilized by autoclave, or whenever possible use disposable needles and equipment.
7. Inform medical and dental caregivers of the disease so that precautions for appropriate prevention of transmission to others can be taken.
8. If drugs are used, do not let others use needles you have used, and do not use someone else's needles; do not leave needles where others may pick them up or accidentally be pricked by them.

Neoplasms

Neoplastic changes can occur in a child's immune system. *Neoplasms*, termed *lymphomas*, are cancers involving the immune system tissues, while in *leukemia*, neoplastic lymphoid cells appear in large quantities in the blood. Immunodeficiency states are associated with an increased risk of developing lymphomas during childhood.

ALTERATIONS PRODUCING TISSUE-DAMAGING REACTIONS

The immunologic disorders causing tissue-damaging reactions are much more commonly encountered in children. This category of immunologic alterations includes allergy, antigen-antibody complex diseases, histocompatibility problems, and the development of autoantibodies.

Allergy

The alteration in the immune system that is most commonly found in children is the tissue-damaging antigen-antibody reaction. This is caused by immunologic "memory," coupled with an excessive production of the immunoglobulin IgE. The antibody attaches itself to mast or basophil cells that release histamine, serotonin, SRS-A, kinin protease, or all of them when they break open. When the antigen encounters its specific IgE antibody on a mediator cell, the chemical mediators are released, and tissue damage occurs.

The terms *hypersensitivity, atopy,* and *allergy* are used interchangeably to indicate a situation in which a child is sensitized (has had a previous experience with an antigen) and subsequent contact with the antigen causes tissue damage. When the antibody formed to an antigen is from the humoral (B-cell) system, the hypersensitivity reaction is *immediate*. In allergy, adverse physiological responses occur as a result of antigen-antibody reactions induced by certain antigens (allergens).

Chemical mediators are released in the target organ, causing clinical manifestations of the disease. Allergic or atopic children differ from normal children in that they *overproduce* IgE antibodies. Everybody produces IgE to some antigens, but atopic children form IgE antibodies in large amounts when exposed to such common environmental substances as house dust and pollen.

Atopic children have the following characteristics:

1. Hereditary or familial patterns of allergy
2. Production of IgE antibodies on exposure to common environmental substances
3. Hyperactivity of the airways
4. Hyperactivity of the skin
5. High levels of eosinophils in the blood and tissue secretions.

Common forms of childhood atopy include allergic rhinitis, hay fever, asthma, atopic dermatitis, and food allergy.

Any child who is suspected of having an allergic problem should have a complete physical examination and diagnostic workup. A thorough

Table 26-7 History for Suspected Allergy

Environment	Attempt to Relate Child's Symptoms and Their Absence (Periods When Child Is Symptom-Free) to:
Activity	Physical exercise, sleep, play (i.e., are symptoms increased or decreased during activity and sleep?)
Place	School, country, friends' homes, child's home: new or old, woolen rugs, furniture, blankets, feather pillows, stuffed toys, aquariums, smokers, plants, family's hobbies (e.g., painting, furniture refinishing), household cleaning products, sprays, type of heating and cooling system, presence of pets, child's bedroom
Time of day	At night, in the morning, after meals, after snacks
Season of year	Cold, humidity, wind, spring, summer, fall, winter, type of clothing, sweating
Animal contact	Schoolroom, at friends' houses, at home
Diet	Breast- or bottle-fed, length of time, introduction of foods, maternal food allergies and intolerances, other family food allergies, frequency of nausea, vomiting, diarrhea, rash, colic, stomachache
	Complete diet history: everything in the mouth, including toothpaste, especially ingestion of cow's milk, milk products, eggs, wheat, cereals, chocolate, fish, nuts (these foods are frequent allergic agents)
Medications	Use of any type of medication, length of time, reactions, time since last used

medical history of the family and the child is essential. The child, the family, and the environment must be considered. Table 26-7 outlines the areas to be included in the history to help identify suspected allergies. Table 26-8 presents common physical findings seen in the child who is suspected of having an allergy. Table 26-9 summarizes diagnostic laboratory tests.

There are three principles in the treatment of allergic children: remove the allergen, relieve the symptoms, and prevent future attacks. Table 26-10 discusses some methods of environmental and food management that are helpful to the parents of allergic children. Sometimes removal of the allergen will also prevent future attacks.

Table 26-8 Physical Assessment: Indicators of Possible Allergic Problem

Eyes*	"Allergic shiner"—discoloration, dark circles, and swelling under lower lid—from edema and venous stasis. Spasm of upper lid muscle—from edema and venous stasis. Conjunctivitis; upper lid is red, itchy, swollen; blepharitis; tearing.
Ears	Hearing loss, pain, discharge, dizziness, bulging tympanic membrane, frequent otitis.
Nose*	Transverse nasal crease from rubbing tip of nose upward to relieve itching. Facial grimaces from wrinkling of nose to relieve itching, sinusitis. Nasal congestion, discharge.
Mouth*	Mouth ulcers, mouth breathing, high arched palate from mouth breathing, sore throat.
Chest	Deformities—pectus excavatum, barrel chest, use of accessory muscles to breathe, wheezing, shortness of breath, frequent colds and pneumonia, cough.
Skin	Presence of rash, evidence of scratching. Note color of rash. Observe for presence of lesions and urticaria. Observe back of knees, behind ears, antecubital fossae (front of elbows), crawling surfaces on babies, scalp, cheeks. Observe for patches of hair loss.
Central nervous system	Headache, irritability, fatigue, depression.
Gastrointestinal	Frequent diarrhea, vomiting, stomachaches, flatulence, cramps.

*See also Fig. 26-2.

Table 26-9 Laboratory Investigation of Allergic Disorders

Blood count	Eosinophilia—total eosinophil count is elevated in allergy.
Radioallergosorbent test (RAST)	Used to estimate quantity of IgE antibody produced to cow's milk, egg, fish, nuts, pollens, house dust, mites, animal dander, molds, insect stings, penicillin. The test identifies the specific antibody the child is producing.
Serum immunoglobulins (antibody titers)	Specific antibody level can be measured.
Skin testing	Skin exposure to minute quantities of suspected allergens, followed by observation of skin for type of reaction. See text.
Challenge testing	Under carefully controlled conditions, the child is exposed to the suspect allergen, and results of the exposure are observed. Used to identify allergens.

Once symptoms have occurred, they must be treated. In some cases, allergic symptoms are short-lived and reverse themselves when the allergen is removed. When this is not the case, medication must be used.

The most frequently used drugs in allergy are *antihistamines*. These drugs work by competing with histamine for combination with cell receptors in tissues. The antihistamine has a high affinity for these receptor sites (it gets there rapidly and holds on tight), preventing the cell from responding to histamine. The physiological effects of histamine (increased capillary permeability and smooth muscle contraction) cannot occur. The antihistamine drugs, because of the way they work, must be present before or early in an allergic reaction. These drugs cannot reverse allergic reactions once they have occurred. Antihistamine treatment is temporary and relieves only symptoms. It does not treat the cause of the allergy, and every attempt should be made to identify the allergen and remove it.

If removal of the allergen is not possible, such as in ragweed or pollen allergies, *hyposensitization* or *desensitization* may be tried. The allergen must be identified and verified by *skin testing* (introducing minute quantities of the

Table 26-10 Management of the Environment of an Allergic Child

Removal of the Allergen

1. Avoid contact with pets that have fur or feathers.
2. Keep house as dust- and mold-free as possible.
3. Remove dust-collecting items—venetian blinds, knick-knacks, and books.
4. Dust three times a week with damp mop or cloth.
5. Clean frequently; do not use fans; close doors and windows.
6. Cover mattress and pillow with plastic casings (not plastic bags, which can suffocate the child).
7. Use synthetic pillows and blankets—no wool, feathers, or horsehair.
8. Use foam rubber furniture.
9. Remove wool rugs and cotton-stuffed toys from bedroom.
10. Avoid forced-air heating and cooling.
11. Close vents, cover with cheesecloth, and clean frequently.
12. Use portable air filter and space heater (can be rented), taking precautions against fires and burns.
13. Avoid mold—damp basements, house plants, vaporizers, and bathroom mold.
14. Avoid wood piles, leaf piles, and unkempt buildings.
15. Avoid cut grass, smoke, and perfumes if they trigger symptoms.

Restricted Diet

1. Eliminate all suspect foods. Read all labels for products containing the allergen*.
2. Frequently implicated foods are nuts, fish, shellfish, legumes, milk, eggs, corn, citrus fruits, melons, berries, chocolate, seeds, and nondairy substitutes containing caseinate.

*Consider everything the child ingests, including drugs, toothpaste, mouthwash, candy, soft drinks, and chewing gum.

suspected allergen into the skin of the forearm or back in children and reading the reaction by recording its size, shape, and character) or by means of the radioallergosorbent test (see Table 26-9). Subcutaneous injections of dilute extracts of the identified allergen are given weekly or monthly, and the dose is gradually increased.

Hyposensitization works by causing IgG antibodies to be formed in response to injection of the allergen. IgG has a higher affinity for the allergen than IgE and therefore combines with it first. The allergen is destroyed by the IgG before it comes in contact with IgE. Thus the problems of a Type I hypersensitivity reaction are avoided. Hyposensitization can work only if the specific allergen can be positively identified. Because children who are undergoing skin testing and hyposensitization are atopic, emergency precautions should always be taken. Epinephrine should be available during testing and hyposensitization injections in the event of an anaphylactic reaction. Occasionally, children will have delayed symptoms later that day. Treatment is usually continued for approximately 3 years in children who show clinical improvement. Stressing the importance of compliance with the treatment regimen is therefore an important aspect of patient education.

The family and the child with an allergy should be well informed about the allergic problem. They should understand the cause and the treatment, especially if it may lead to a local or systemic anaphylactic reaction. When allergy problems are severe or potentially fatal, the child should wear a necklace or bracelet that gives the names of the known allergens. An alternative is to pin a card giving the important information to the child's clothing. The Medic Alert Foundation, P.O. Box 1009, Turlock, Calif. 95380, is a charitable, nonprofit organization which for a small fee will supply a Medic Alert bracelet or necklace. The emblem, which is recognized around the world, has the medical problem and the wearer's file number engraved on the back. Medic Alert maintains a central file, accessible 24 h a day by telephone, with specific information about the wearer's problem. Children with severe allergies can benefit from this service.

Atopic dermatitis

Atopic dermatitis, or *eczema,* is not a single disease, but rather a state of hyperactivity of the skin. It can be a tiny localized lesion or can cover the entire surface of the body. *Atopic dermatitis* occurs predominantly in infants, and frequently develops between the second and sixth months of life. Fewer than 50 percent of these children are free of the disease by the age of 18 months. In most cases, the disease becomes quiescent by age 5. For some children, mild to moderate atopic dermatitis persists into adolescence and adulthood. The cause of the disease is not known, but its development is influenced by immune, genetic, pharmacological, and environmental factors. Many affected children have high levels of serum IgE.

Both abnormal humoral and cellular immunity are believed to be responsible for atopic dermatitis, although the exact pathological mechanism is not fully understood. There is a known decreased pruritic threshold and abnormal skin reactivity. The release of histamine causes vasodilatation, and the epidermis is invaded by inflammatory cells, causing edema. *Lichenification,* or the loss of the stratum corneum, with thickening, scaling, and erythema of the skin, results from the chronic irritation caused by prolonged scratching.

Manifestations The first lesions of infantile atopic dermatitis are usually on the cheeks; then they spread over the face, behind the ears, and to the scalp. The trauma and irritation caused by crawling result in involvement of the crawling surfaces of the forearms and legs. The flexure areas of the elbow (the antecubital fossae) and behind the knee (the popliteal fossae) are also affected. Children with eczema have excessively dry skin, and the active lesions are initially pruritic and erythematous. The severe itching leads to continual rubbing or scratching, which causes the skin to weep, crust, and scale. The lesions are not contagious but are susceptible to secondary bacterial infection from staphylococci, B-hemolytic streptococci, and the herpes simplex virus. Infection can lead to the complication of cellulitis. Vaccination for smallpox and contact with anyone who has recently been vaccinated are *absolutely contraindicated.* Vaccinial infection is no longer a great problem in the United States, since routine smallpox vaccination has been discontinued.

Treatment Management of eczema depends on an accurate diagnosis and a careful identification of the characteristics of the particular child's eczema. Effective treatment includes avoiding contact with anything that makes the eczema worse and implementing a plan to break the itch-scratch-itch cycle. While there is controversy concerning the role of food allergies in initiating or maintaining atopic dermatitis, cow's milk, egg white, wheat, citrus fruits, and chocolate are systematically tested for an allergic reaction. Extremes of temperature must be avoided. The child should wear lightweight cotton rather than clothing made of wool and other rough, harsh fabrics that hold heat. The goal is to prevent sweating, since it seems to aggravate the disease. Providing skin care that relieves dryness and minimizes itching is another major goal. Table 26-11 lists guidelines for the care of eczema in childhood.

Table 26-11 Management of Eczema in Childhood

Hygiene

Prevent infections by frequent, careful hand-washing. Keep fingernails short and clean. The child may need mittens at night to prevent scratching. Frequently cleanse the diaper area with plain tepid water.

Diet

Systematically eliminate suspect food from the diet. Encourage mothers to breast-feed future babies. Use special soybean- and meat-based formulas for infants with milk allergies.

Clothing

Avoid clothing that causes sweating. Use cotton fabrics or soft synthetics. Avoid wool and heat-holding synthetics. Do not overdress.

Play

Encourage normal activities. Apply lubricating cream before swimming. Cool, sunny days when the humidity is low are especially good for outside play.

Skin care

Avoid hot bathwater; use warm water instead. Minimal bathing is recommended. Do not give bubble baths or use fragrant oils. Use mild, superfatted soaps or no soaps. Rehydrate skin with lubricants such as Eucerin after baths. Give colloid baths (2 cups of cornstarch added to bathwater) to relieve itching. Pat the skin dry. Apply cool, wet compresses during the acute stage. Use Cetaphil (a nondrying cleansing lotion) if baths exacerbate the eczema.

Management during the acute phase can include applying cool, wet compresses; giving oral antibiotics to control secondary infection; and applying a topical high-potency steroid cream. Corticosteroids are anti-inflammatory, immunosuppressive, and vasoconstricting and should not be used in the presence of infection. They should be used sparingly because systemic absorption occurs. Antihistamines are administered to stop the itch-scratch-itch cycle and promote sleep during an exacerbation of a child's eczema.

Parents should be taught how to apply wet compresses. A solution, often Burow's solution (aluminum acetate solution), is ordered by the physician. Soft, clean, nonirritating materials such as layers of gauze or old cotton sheets are used for the compress. They are soaked in the solution, wrung out so that they are wet but not dripping, and applied to the involved area. Evaporation of the solution plays an important role in drying the weeping eruption. If the compress is covered with plastic, evaporation cannot take place. Therefore, bath towels or triple layers of sheets should be used instead to prevent chilling. A typical application schedule is $\frac{1}{2}$ to 1 h on and 2 to 4 h off for about 2 to 3 days. After the compress is removed, an emollient cream is applied. A gradual drying of the weeping process will begin within 24 h. Seborrheic dermatitis, which is a common problem during infancy and may be confused with atopic dermatitis, is discussed in Chap. 27.

Allergic contact dermatitis

Allergic contact dermatitis involves a type IV mechanism of delayed hypersensitivity mediated by sensitized T lymphocytes. The etiologic agent is a simple chemical or other compound. Plants (e.g., poison ivy, poison oak, and poison sumac), cosmetics, industrial products, detergents, topical medications (e.g., neomycin and Mycolog creams), clothing, food, and metals (e.g., nickel) have all been implicated. These agents produce their effect by combining with tissue protein to form an antigen complex. Intracellular edema of the epidermis is the underlying cellular change that occurs.

The lesions that are produced in allergic contact dermatitis are localized and restricted to the area of contact. They are characterized by redness; they may be papules, vesicles, or bullae in the acute stage; and they itch intensely. Thickening, scaling, and lichenification result if there is chronic exposure to the offending substance. Treatment is directed at removing the offending substance and reducing the inflammatory response.

Poison ivy dermatitis

Poison ivy dermatitis is a common allergic contact dermatitis seen in children. Poison ivy grows in most parts of the United States, along with its cousins, poison oak (found in the west) and the relatively rare poison sumac (found in the east). Poison ivy is an attractive plant; it has clusters of three shiny leaves grouped in a triangular pattern and in the summer produces red berries, which turn white during the winter; the foliage is bright red in the fall. Reactions to poison ivy, poison oak, and poison sumac are similar. They contain a heavy oil—urushiol—in the canals inside the leaves, stems, and roots; an undamaged plant has no urushiol on its surface. However, the leaves are easily bruised, allowing the urushiol to escape. A drop of urushiol the size of a pinhead can cause severe allergic reactions and can be carried on animals, coats, clothing, shoes, and tools for many years after the contact. Poison ivy is difficult to destroy and should not be burned. Breathing smoke from burning poison ivy can produce head-to-toe dermatitis, lung infections, and severe laryngeal edema; this plant has become the scourge of forest fire fighters.[4]

Manifestations The skin eruption caused by contact with urushiol is an allergic reaction. Most children become sensitized between 5 and 10 years of age; after this, their immune system will be reactivated each time they come in contact with poison ivy. The urushiol penetrates the outer skin layer and binds itself to the skin cells. This sets up an antigen-antibody response, and the area fills up with white blood cells that release so much toxin that they cause the skin to separate, creating blisters. Poison ivy dermatitis varies from a mild to a severe reaction. Intense itching causes the child to scratch; the fingers then become contaminated and transfer urushiol to other parts of the body. It is important to wash the child's hands and clothing, any item that has come into contact with poison ivy, and the affected areas thoroughly with soap and water.

Within 24 h the skin becomes swollen, and large blisters appear, break, and drain. Crusting, swelling, and pruritus last several weeks in severe cases. Characteristic locations for the rash are exposed areas, such as the hands, face, and legs, but it can affect any part of the body, often appearing in linear streaks caused by the child's scratching.

Treatment Mild cases of poison ivy dermatitis can be treated with a topical corticosteroid preparation applied judiciously to localized areas. Oral antihistamine such as diphenhydramine (Benadryl) may also relieve the itching. With a severe eruption, systemic cortisone therapy is necessary for relief. Prednisone (1 to 2 mg per kilogram of body weight given orally) can be used for several weeks until the eruptions disappear. Scratching can cause secondary bacterial infections, necessitating additional treatment.

There is controversy concerning the various ways of reducing a child's allergy to poison ivy. Desensitizing agents are available for oral and subcutaneous administration, but studies do not show that the protection is predictable, and the agents often produce undesirable side effects. If used at all, they should be given only to children who are extremely sensitive to urushiol.

Allergic rhinitis

Allergic rhinitis can be seasonal (e.g., hay fever) or nonseasonal. The child often has a positive family history of allergy and has been sensitized after exposure by inhalation or ingestion early in life with subsequent IgE development. Allergic rhinitis is more common in young boys than young girls and is characterized by partial or complete nasal obstruction, sudden and recurrent episodes of sneezing and itching in the nose and upper throat, a watery nasal discharge, and watering, itchy, red, swollen eyes.

The pathophysiology is due to the effects of histamine on the nasal mucosa, causing vasodilatation and increased capillary permeability with leakage of fluid into the nasal passages, excessive mucus secretion, and swollen mucous membranes that close nasal passages. Eosinophils predominate in both nasal secretions and tissue. Figure 26-2 illustrates the facial characteristics of allergic rhinitis.

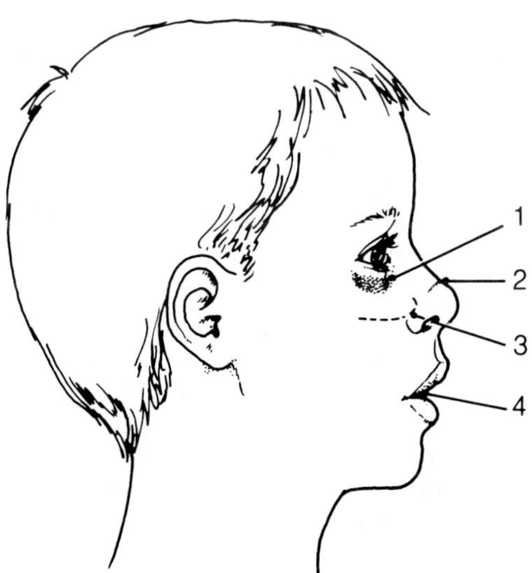

Figure 26-2 The facial characteristics of a child with allergic rhinitis. (1) An allergic shiner, a dark discoloration of the orbitopalpebral groove. (2) A transverse nasal crease due to constant rubbing of the nose upward (allergic salute). (3) Enlargement of the inferior turbinates. (4) Mouth breathing due to nasal obstruction. (*After J. A. Kuzemo, Allergy in Children, Priory House, Standford, England, 1978. Used with permission.*)

The management of the allergic child's environment has been discussed earlier (Table 26-10). Medication includes nose drops or nasal sprays that decrease nasal stuffiness by causing nasal vasoconstriction. These drugs should be used only for short-term treatment, not for prevention. Overuse causes vasodilatation (a rebound phenomenon), requiring increasing doses to produce a therapeutic vasoconstriction. Antihistamines can prevent a full-blown attack and are effective in relieving itching, rhinorrhea, and sneezing when begun early and used on a regular basis. Intranasal cromolyn sodium used prophylactically is effective when applied regularly. It stabilizes mast cell membranes and granules. Hyposensitization may be useful when the allergen can be accurately identified.

Stinging-insect allergy

The stings of yellow jackets, wasps, hornets, and honeybees, listed in the order of the insects' aggressiveness, pose a threat, ranging from a mild nuisance to a severe, life-threatening problem. In the south, the sting of the fire ant can also be dangerous. At least 50 people die annually in the United States as a result of insect stings. Children and young adults are especially likely to be stung.

Manifestations The venom injected by stinging insects has many components. If the child is allergic to stings, one or more of these components may trigger a reaction, which is for the most part IgE-mediated.

Localized reactions A normal reaction to a sting is swelling, redness, and pain at the site, which disappear in a day or two. The mildest form of allergic reaction is a very large swelling around the site of the sting persisting as long as a week.

Systemic allergic reactions In a systemic allergic reaction, symptoms occur at areas remote from the sting, usually within 15 min. At times only the skin is involved, and there is urticaria or a more severe reaction, angioedema. Chest tightness, difficulty breathing and swallowing, fainting, and loss of consciousness may occur. In the most dangerous life-threatening reactions, the sting causes shock or airway obstruction. The shock reaction, anaphylaxis, results as blood vessels throughout the body dilate and body fluid leaks from the vessels into the tissues, causing edema and circulatory collapse. The heart is unable to maintain the blood pressure because of the decreased venous blood returning to it. Vital organs such as the brain become anoxic, and the child begins to lose consciousness. If the condition is not reversed, vital organs of the body are severely damaged, and the child can die. Airway obstruction is caused by laryngeal edema (swelling of the air passages). This happens more quickly in small children because their airways are smaller and can be blocked more quickly by swelling. (See Table 26-4 and Fig. 26-1.)

Treatment Localized reactions can be treated by applying ice to the sting to limit the swelling and reduce pain. An oral antihistamine can be used to help relieve the itching and swelling. Honeybees have a barbed stinger, and it—along with a venom sac about the size of a pinhead—stays in the skin. The stinger should be removed by scraping the skin surface with a fingernail or a flat surface, such as the blade of a knife. Squeezing will release more venom into the area and should be avoided.[5]

The best treatment is prevention of bee stings. Children should be taught to avoid situations in which they are likely to be stung. They should wear shoes outside at all times to protect their feet from stinging insects and should stay away from flower beds and areas where food is present, including picnic areas, places where garbage is kept, and orchards where there is fallen fruit. Perfumes and scented preparations attract insects, and dark-colored clothes attract them more than light-colored clothes. Children should be instructed to leave an area if a stinging insect appears threatening. Undue excitement or slapping at the insect may cause it to sting.

Allergic children can be stung, despite great efforts to avoid this. The drug of choice for more severe reactions is epinephrine 1:1000 (Adrenalin). The subcutaneous dose differs according to the child's age and size (0.1 or 0.5 ml) and is repeated in 20 min if necessary. Early treatment will usually reverse the systemic reaction. For children who are in shock and who do not respond to epinephrine, rapid intravenous administration of a saline solution or other solution will usually replace the depleted blood volume and allow the heart to resume normal circulation. A tracheostomy may be necessary if laryngeal edema has blocked the airway.

If a child has experienced an allergic reaction to a sting, there is a risk that the next sting will have a more severe effect. Emergency anaphylaxis kits containing premeasured doses of epinephrine prepared for injection, an antihistamine tablet, and a tourniquet to use if the sting is on an extremity are readily available for self-treatment of severe reactions. Children and their parents must be carefully instructed in the use of these kits. They must be familiar with the contents, know the indications for the use of the drugs, and be skilled in the technique of subcutaneous administration of epinephrine. A reaction can occur a few minutes after a sting. Injected epinephrine begins to work within minutes of administration. Antihistamine tablets can be used for local reactions, but they take much longer to be dissolved and absorbed and must not be thought of as the first line of defense. An identification bracelet (Medic Alert) should be worn at all times and the emergency kit kept nearby.

Immunotherapy For the allergic child who is in danger of having a severe reaction, purified venom preparations are available for use in hyposensitization. Purified venom is injected by the physician weekly until a maintenance level is reached. Monthly injections may need to be continued indefinitely because it is not known how long the immunity provided by the injections lasts. This is a complicated, long-term, expensive, and somewhat dangerous form of therapy, but it does provide protection against a severe reaction that is not provided by any other form of treatment.

Food allergy

The symptoms of food allergy mimic the symptoms of many other disorders. Gastrointestinal symptoms such as diarrhea, vomiting, occult gastrointestinal bleeding, and failure to thrive are the most common reactions to ingested food proteins. The underlying mechanism may be hypersensitivity response or a nonimmunologic adverse reaction, for example, lactose intolerance. Immediate hypersensitivity reactions can also be due to foods. These IgE-mediated responses characteristically have a rapid onset; upon exposure of the child to food allergens, they may present as angioedema of the lips, mouth, uvula, and glottis or as asthma. *Angioedema* is swelling similar to urticaria but involves deeper subcutaneous or submucous tissues.

Table 26-12 Symptoms Sometimes Attributable to Food Allergy

Headache	Tension
Abdominal pain	Learning problems
Otitis media (serous)	Hyperactivity
Epigastric distress	Drowsiness
Emotional lability	Prostration
Rhinitis	Sweating
Enuresis	Irritability
Muscle aches	Pallor
Fatigue	Nasal congestion
Poor dexterity	Circles under the eyes

Food allergy can occur in someone who has a positive family history of allergy or who has had an allergy to something else. Children can be allergic to corn sugar coatings on, or dyes in, medications. Diabetics can react adversely to insulin prepared from pig pancreas (protamine insulin). Table 26-12 lists other symptoms that are sometimes attributed to food allergy.

Identifying a food allergy is extremely difficult because of delayed symptoms, multiple ingredients in foods, irregular exposure to the allergen, and difficulty in documenting the immunologic nature of the signs and symptoms attributed to food ingestion. During infancy, diet—especially cow's milk—is often blamed for common symptoms such as colic, constipation, diarrhea, frequent vomiting, and various skin rashes. It is important to differentiate secondary responses to environmental factors (e.g., lactase or sucrose-isomaltase deficiencies) from adverse reactions associated with an immunologic response. When these enzyme deficiencies occur, gastrointestinal symptoms are due to an intolerance to a particular substance, not to an allergic response.

While difficult, prevention of attacks is somewhat easier in food allergy than in inhalation allergies because an elimination diet can be used. Foods are eliminated one at a time for several days, and the reaction is noted. Chief dietary offenders in infants and young children are cow's milk, egg albumin, wheat, chocolate, and citrus fruits. A double-blind food challenge test may be needed to prove unequivocally that a food is responsible for the adverse reaction. In a double-blind food challenge test, the child and usually the parents do not know whether the feeding contains the substances thought to cause the allergy. A registered dietitian should be consulted to help in the diagnostic process and in planning a long-term elimination diet that will provide the child with proper nutrition. The dietitian provides assistance in keeping an accurate diet history and can give the parents recipes that will keep the child interested in food. Some infants and small children who have been shown to be highly intolerant to certain foods "outgrow" these intolerances as they get older. Why or how this happens is unclear. Later, the foods may be reintroduced, depending on the severity of the original symptoms, and the child is observed for signs of recurring allergies.

When cow's milk is the offending agent in an infant, alternative formulas are used. Initially, a soybean-based formula (Isomil, ProSobee, or Neo-Mull-Soy) is given. If the child is also allergic to soybeans, a meat-based formula, such as Nutramigen, Pregestimil, or Vivonex, may be used. The infant is kept on the milk-free diet for about a year.

HISTOCOMPATIBILITY (TISSUE COMPATIBILITY)

The immune system recognizes components of the body as "self" by recognizing histocompatible antigens (antigens that are compatible with tissue) on the cell surface of most human cells. There are certain configurations on a child's cells that enable the body to recognize "self" components and distinguish them from "nonself," or "foreign," components. The immune response is launched against the foreign components.

This self-recognition system, known as the *human leukocyte antigen system* (HLA system), is located on an area on chromosome no. 6, called the *major histocompatibility complex*. The major histocompatibility complex is unique to each individual. It controls for the synthesis (formation) of transplantation antigens, influences immune responses to infectious attack, and provides information about disease association, such as childhood arthritis, and about disease linkage, such as congenital adrenal hyperplasia.

ALTERATIONS IN HISTOCOMPATIBILITY

Organ and tissue transplantation

Organ transplantation began many years ago with skin grafting. Today, transplantation is the accepted treatment of choice for certain disease states, and in some instances it offers the only

Table 26-13 Basic Elements of Transplantation

Indications for transplantation	The treatment of choice when a vital organ is irreparably damaged or defective. Factors to consider are age of the child, especially small size of an infant, psychoemotional status, presence of generalized infection, and multisystem disease.
Graft types	*Allografts*—donor and recipient are of the same species but are genetically not identical. *Isografts*—donor and recipient are identical twins.
Allografting procedures*	Blood transfusions Renal transplantations—may be done for end-stage renal disease; 77% of patients are functioning after 1 year. Average cost is $25,000.* Bone marrow transplantations—done for aplastic anemia, leukemia, and certain immune diseases. Average cost is $130,000. Bone transplantations—most common grafts today to replace bone destroyed by tumors, trauma, and infection and to avoid amputations. Cost is from $4500 to $5000. Pancreas transplantations—done for diabetes. Average cost is $35,000. Corneal transplantations—average cost is $3000. Liver transplantations—done for biliary atresia or liver disease. Average cost is $120,000. Heart transplantations—done when there is cardiac muscle damage and the heart no longer functions. Average cost is over $100,000. Skin transplantations—done for severe burns. Thymus transplantations—done for Di George syndrome.
Tissue typing	Necessary to determine tissue or organ HLA compatibility and avoid disparity in HLA antigens. The greater the HLA match between donor and recipient, the lower the dose of immunosuppressives required, and the fewer the complications (fatal opportunistic infections, diabetes mellitus, or malignancy).
HLA system	The major histocompatibility HLAs that humans produce are HLA-A, B, C, D, and DR; these distinct antigens are carried on cell membranes of nucleated cells.
Rejection phenomenon	The main danger in transplantation is rejection of donor tissue. Allograft rejection is an immune reaction mediated by sensitized T lymphocytes and their products. Response is stimulated by differences in HLA antigens between donor and recipient.
Renal rejection	*Hyperacute rejection* occurs immediately, in minutes to hours, as a result of preformed antibodies against donor's HLA or ABO (blood) antigens. Marked by irreversible vascular injury and thrombosis, caused by previous transfusions or transplants. *Acute rejection* occurs within 30 to 90 days. Marked by intense mononuclear infiltration of the kidneys; reversible with immunosuppresive therapy. *Chronic rejection* occurs after months or years. Marked by chronic mononuclear infiltrate buildup and gradual occlusion of renal blood vessels, difficult to manage; poor prognosis.
Immunosuppressive therapy	The goal is to inhibit moderate to weak rejection reactions with immunosuppressive therapy: corticosteroids, azathioprine, cyclosporine, and others, such as antithymocyte globulin (bone marrow) and pregraft blood transfusions (renal grafts from cadaver donors).
Potential consequences of immunosuppressive therapy	Increased susceptibility to infection, development of neoplasms, and graft-vs.-host disease (the donor's lymphoid cells transplanted along with the graft become sensitized and launch an unchallenged immune attack against the host).

*Cost estimates are from an unpublished Mayo Clinic fact sheet (April, 1985).

hope of survival for children who would otherwise be doomed to die. Prior to 1968, infants with severe combined immunodeficiency disease invariably died within the first year of life. Today, with bone marrow transplantation, 8-year survivals have been reported in 30 percent of young infants with the disease who have undergone this procedure. Similarly, children and adolescents with aplastic anemia who are treated with bone marrow transplantation have a greater than 50 percent chance of surviving more than 1 year.[6] Liver transplantation for the treatment of congenital biliary atresia has provided from months to years of added functional life for many children, especially since the advent of cyclosporine; heart transplantations for the treatment of selected congenital defects have recently been attempted in children.

Children who undergo transplantation and their families require the long-term support of all members of the health care team as they struggle to cope with issues such as: (1) the child's ability to reach normal psychosocial, cognitive, and emotional developmental milestones; (2) the child's need to cope with his or her altered physical appearance; (3) stress within the family due to either the financial burden of the illness or the emotional strain caused by a chronic, life-threatening situation; and (4) the moral and ethical dilemmas associated with the underlying disease process or the transplantation.

Basic principles of transplantation When tissue is transplanted, the HLA system antigen on the cell surface of the donor tissue is recognized as "foreign" by the recipient, and the immune system responds by destroying the tissue. When tissue transplantations are planned, every effort is made to find a donor whose HLA configurations are compatible with the recipient's. There is the highest probability of success with transplanted tissue when the tissue of family members, especially siblings, is used, because genetic similarity exists. The long-term survival of people who undergo transplantation is associated with similar HLA-A, B, C, and DR antigen matchings.

The use of immunosuppressive therapy helps prevent graft rejection. The agents used are nonspecific and interfere with either the induction or the expression of the immune response. Immunosuppression or immunologic depression is accomplished with corticosteroids, azathioprine, and cyclosporine. Immunosuppression and immunologic depression are also unwanted effects of irradiation, exposure to cytotoxic chemicals, poor general health and nutrition, and some diseases. Table 26-13 lists the basic elements of transplantation.

AUTOIMMUNE DISEASES

The body's system of recognizing components as "self" can break down. If this happens, the body forms antibodies against its own "self" components (autoantibodies), and the resulting condition is an autoimmune disease. The lesions of autoimmune diseases are the result of inflammatory destruction of the target tissue, usually connective tissue of the skin, glomeruli in the kidneys, joints, serous membranes, and blood vessels.

The pathophysiology of these diseases is tissue damage due to an antigen-antibody reaction that results in inflammation; deposition of immune complexes (Ag-Ab complexes) in small vessels of the involved area, causing stasis, edema, and inflammation; or both inflammation and deposition. In rheumatoid arthritis, enzyme products liberated at the site of inflammation cause chronic synovitis. This leads to destruction of joint cartilage and results in structural alterations of joints. Other autoimmune diseases that occur in childhood include systemic lupus erythematosus, dermatomyositis, autoimmune hemolytic anemia, autoimmune thrombocytopenic purpura, and Hashimoto disease, which is the most common cause of thyroid disease in children and adolescents. The lesions of juvenile insulin-dependent diabetes, which occur in the islets of Langerhans in the pancreas, have the pathological appearance of the lesions of an autoimmune disease. Glomerulonephritis is now recognized as a disease that results when autoantibodies attack the basement membrane of the glomeruli or when Ag-Ab complexes cause vasculitis when deposited in the glomerular capillaries.

SYSTEMIC LUPUS ERYTHEMATOSUS

Systemic lupus erythematosus (SLE) affects many parts of the body, chiefly the kidneys, hemopoietic tissue, the skin, and the cardiovascular system. The cause is unknown but altered immune reactivity is involved. Serum immunoglobulin levels are elevated. Antibodies are also present that react with various nuclear constituents (antinuclear antibodies). The presence of circulating immune complexes is associated with tissue inflammation and injury. Vasculitis is a major pathological finding.

The onset or exacerbation of SLE appears to be related to intercurrent infections thought to be caused by an increased susceptibility to infection. SLE is sometimes familial, and 20 percent of the cases begin in children over the age of 8. SLE in children is generally a more severe disease than it is in adults. It is a progressive disease, but may remit spontaneously or be quiescent for many years. Common symptoms in children include fever, malaise, arthritis or arthralgia, and rash. The "butterfly rash"—which consists of reddish-blue or red scaly patches on the cheeks and extending over the bridge of the nose, in the shape of a butterfly—is one cutaneous manifestation of this disease. Most children with SLE develop renal involvement. Nephritis, central nervous system complications, infections, and pulmonary lupus are major causes of death in children with SLE. Nursing management includes long-term support for these children and their families. (See Chap. 34.)

References

1. Centers for Disease Control, "Provisional Public Health Service Inter-Agency Recommendations for Screening Donated Blood and Plasma for Antibody to the Virus Causing Acquired Immunodeficiency Syndrome," *Morbidity and Mortality Weekly Report* **34** (1):5 (January 1985).
2. Ibid.
3. Centers for Disease Control, "Information about the Test for Antibodies to the HTLV-III Virus," *Morbidity and Mortality Weekly Report* **34** (1):11 (January 1985).
4. Vietmeyer, Noel, "Science Has Got Its Hands on Poison Ivy, Oak and Sumac," *Smithsonian* 89 (August 1985).
5. ——— "Insect Stings." *Mayo Clinic Health Letter* 6 (August 1985).
6. Bellanti, Joseph A., *Immunology,* vol. III, Saunders, Philadelphia, 1985, p. 61.

27

Madeleine Lynch Martin

Integument

Upon completion of this chapter, the student will be able to:

1 List the four functions of the skin.
2 Describe the essential areas to be covered during an interview for assessment of a child with a skin disorder.
3 Assess a child for skin integrity and disorders.
4 Describe the causes of, and treatment for, seborrheic and diaper dermatitis.
5 Describe the process of the development of acne.
6 Identify the methods of treatment used for acne.
7 Describe the physical, emotional, and social significance of a burn injury in the life of a child and the child's family.
8 Describe the initial physiological alterations which accompany a burn injury.
9 Identify alterations in the body systems which develop as a response to a thermal injury.
10 Describe the normal process of wound healing.
11 List the steps in intitial first aid for a thermally injured child.
12 Discuss appropriate nursing intervention during the acute care management of a burned child.
13 Describe a thermal injury based on depth of tissue damage, amount of body surface area involved, and type of injury.
14 List the steps and goals of burn care.
15 List four commercially available topical antimicrobial agents, including their advantages and disadvantages.
16 List the goals of physical and emotional rehabilitation of a burned child.

The *integumentary system* can be defined as the outside covering or shell of the body. This external surface of the body is formed by the skin and its associated structures. These are often called *skin appendages* and include hair, nails, glands, and sensory skin receptors. The skin is the single largest organ of the body. It provides a supple, protective covering; serves as a barrier to loss of internal body fluids and electrolytes; and is a regulator of heat. The skin grows, changes, and renews and repairs itself efficiently. The appearance of the skin reflects the child's general state of health.

EMBRYONIC ORIGIN

The epidermis is formed from the embryonic *ectoderm* (the outer layer). By 7 weeks of gestation, the epidermis is a single layer of cuboidal cells covering the embryo with primitive skin. It thickens to two layers by 11 weeks of gestation and continues to thicken to five layers, and it closely resembles mature skin at birth. It is thin at birth, about 1 mm, and increases to about twice that thickness at maturity.

The dermis is derived from the *mesoderm* and forms the connective tissue layer underlying the epidermis.

The skin appendages have a separate developmental timetable. The sebaceous glands are functional during fetal life and are responsible for the secretions that combine with dead epithelium to form vernix caseosa. From birth through infancy they gradually decrease in size and remain relatively inactive until puberty. The *eccrine* sweat glands appear during the fifth month of fetal life but are not functional. The *apocrine* sweat glands, which are associated with the hair follicles, are present at birth but do not mature until puberty. Nails appear at about 16 weeks of gestation, and hair at about 20 weeks.[1]

STRUCTURE OF THE SKIN

The epidermis

The *epidermis,* the outer layer of the skin, is composed of five epidermal layers resting on a basment membrane (basal cells). These basal cells produce new epidermal cells, which constantly replace the older exterior cells by being pushed outward toward the skin surface. The *stratum corneum,* the most superficial skin layer, contains a layer of dead, flat, scalelike cells filled with keratin. These are shed continuously and are rubbed off by contact with clothing, by washing, and by exposure to the environment. The lower layer of the epidermis contains melanocytes, whose function is to form the melanin, or pigment, of the skin. It is the degree of activity of these cells, not the number of melanocytes, that gives the skin its characteristic light or dark color[2] (see Fig. 27-1).

The dermis

The *dermis* is directly under the epidermis. It is thicker; is composed of tough, elastic, connective tissue; and provides the structural and nutritional layer for the epidermis. It contains a network of blood vessels, nerves, and lymphatics that nourish the skin cells. The hair follicles and glands originate deep in the dermis. These glands invaginate into the dermal layers, incorporating epidermis as gland linings.

The subcutaneous layer

The *subcutaneous layer,* found under the dermis, is composed mainly of fat and loose connective tissue, with larger blood vessels, nerves, and lymph channels than the dermis. This layer provides fat and body fluid storage, acts as the body insulator against the elements, and provides for safety by cushioning the body.

THE SKIN FUNCTIONS

The skin has four essential functions; protection of underlying parts, heat regulation, prevention of water and electrolyte loss, and reception of sensory stimuli.

Protection

The epidermis contains keratinized (horny) cells that resist penetration by bacteria, chemicals, and parasites and protect the body from cold, heat, and injury. The sebum, oily secretions of the sebaceous glands, lubricates the skin, keeping it supple and decreasing fluid loss. These secretions provide a surface film of water, lipids, acids, and polypeptides that have a bacteriostatic effect.

The thickness of the epidermis varies in different parts of the body. The hands and feet are subjected to heavy use and have thick skin, about 5 to 6 mm. The thinnest skin is found in sensitive areas of the body: on the eyelids, the eardrums, and the penis, where it is about 1 to 2 mm thick. The epidermis and dermis are thin and loosely connected at birth. Thus in young children minimal friction can cause separation of the dermal and epidermal layers, resulting in blisters. The thin outer layer of skin in infants can easily be rubbed off, making them very susceptible to skin breakdown. The epidermal layer gradually thickens and becomes tougher with age.

At adolescence, sex hormone secretion increases, causing skin changes. Estrogen in the female thickens the skin, making it soft and smooth and increasing dermal fat and vascularity. Androgens in males cause the characteristic thickening and darkening of their skin.

Heat regulation

The skin helps maintain the important function of temperature control of the body. This is accomplished by regulation of heat loss through

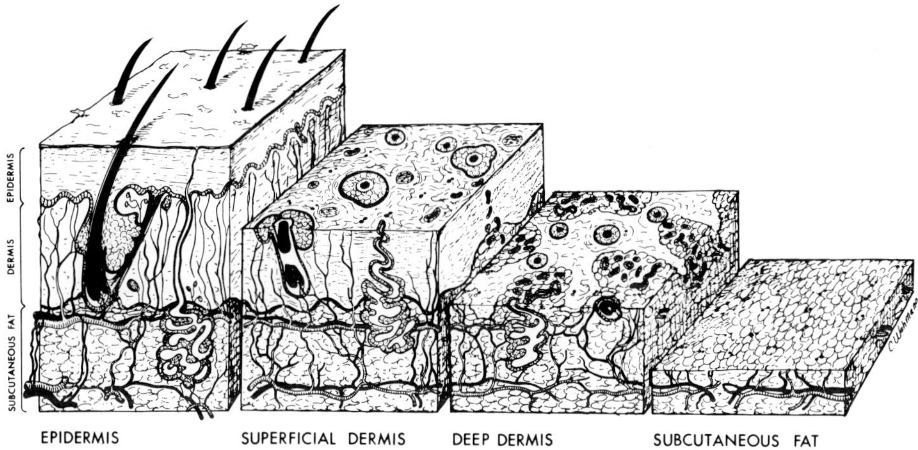

Figure 27-1 Anatomy of the skin and subcutaneous fat.

sweating and cutaneous vascular changes. Sweating and vasodilatation decrease the body temperature; vasoconstriction, shivering, and muscle activity raise the body temperature. The eccrine glands are responsible for sweating in response to thermal stimuli. Children sweat much less than adults, and thus it is more difficult for them to regulate body temperature by sweating. Surface heat loss is also greater in children than in adults because children have a larger proportion of body surface area and less body fat with blood vessels closer to a thin skin surface.

Prevention of water and electrolyte loss

The intact skin is a relatively impermeable membrane that retards the exchange of liquids between the internal body and the outside environment. The intact skin effectively prevents excessive loss of essential body constituents. It does permit some water loss when water is evaporated on the skin surface to cool the body. The skin's effectiveness as a fluid barrier is clearly apparent when the profuse fluid and electrolyte loss following disruption of the skin by a burn is observed.

The skin as a sense organ

The skin is the major contributor to the touch sensation and can be described as a tactile organ. Touch, pressure, pain, cold, and heat are all sensations experienced through the skin. The skin conducts impulses to the brain, and these impulses are used to adjust the body to relieve uncomfortable sensations. Often these sensations are protective devices and permit the body to alter its position before damage to tissue occurs. Positive impulses are just as important as negative protective impulses. Pleasurable touch stimulates and motivates behavior from fetal life through adulthood.

THE INTERVIEW AND HISTORY FOR SKIN ASSESSMENT

A child presenting with a skin rash or skin lesions needs careful evaluation. Skin disorders may be the result of dry skin, which is often caused by excessive bathing and exposure to the sun, water, and wind; they may be due to inadequate skin care related to poor hygiene; or they may have multiple complex etiologies. The caregiver's first step in assessing the child with a skin problem who comes to a clinic or hospital is to obtain a careful history. The following areas should be covered in the interview.

The skin and lesions

When the skin problem first appeared
The signs that were present and the way the skin felt
If a rash is present, whether it spread and how it is distributed
Other symptoms of illness, such as fever, headache, vomiting, and pain, that were associated with the onset of the skin disorder
How the child was treated

(See Chap. 28 for a discussion of the skin lesions commonly seen in communicable diseases, the inflammatory response, and the many diseases that cause secondary skin reactions.)

Contacts, exposure, and history of the skin problem

Communicable diseases that the child has had in the past
Whether the child has had any recent illnesses or been exposed to persons with communicable diseases
Whether anyone else in the family is sick
Whether the child has been exposed to an unsanitary environment, contaminated drinking water or food, or disease-carrying insects (especially ticks and mosquitoes), as could happen during a trip to a foreign country or on a camping trip

Drug history

Whether the child has taken any prescription or nonprescription drugs

Allergies: the family history and the child's history

Whether the child or the family has a history of allergies
Whether the allergies are seasonal, contact-related, job-related, or associated with stress
Whether the child was exposed to plant, animal, or food substances that could have caused the skin problem
Whether powders, oils, lotions, makeup, or cleansing agents are used on the child's skin
What shampoos, rinses, or coloring agents are used and whether there has been a recent change to different products

(Chapter 26 discusses the hypersensitive response involved in eczema, food allergies, insect stings, and exposure to plant allergens. Guidelines for testing, environmental considerations, treatment, and skin care are presented in Tables 26-10 to 26-12.)

Multiple bruises, cuts, and injuries

Unexplained bruises, fractures, and cuts may be an indication of an abusive living situation or of a disease. Assessment for child abuse is discussed in Chap. 38. Multiple bruises, falls, and fractures may accompany diseases such as leukemia, hemophilia, and bone cancer and diseases that affect balance and mobility.

PHYSICAL ASSESSMENT OF A CHILD WITH A SKIN DISORDER

During an examination for a skin-related complaint, it is important to undress the child and examine the entire body. While this is easily accomplished with a newborn, the nurse must be aware of an older child's concerns about modesty and should cover the body parts that are not being examined. The examination should be conducted in a systematic manner, beginning with the head, neck, arms, and legs and then proceeding down the trunk. A good source of light during the examination is essential. Taking the simple precaution of washing the hands before and after the examination is basic to preventing the spread of a disease from one child to the next and from one caregiver to another.

Skin characteristics as they relate to the child's age must be considered. A newborn, for example, has many deviations of the skin that would be considered abnormal in an older child. It is important to note the presence of birthmarks—such as nevi, hemangiomas, mongolian spots, and port-wine stains—and their specific characteristics. While most birthmarks are benign, the presence of pigmented nevi may indicate a neurological disorder; the parents must be told what will happen to a birthmark and should be informed of any ramifications of treatment. Hemangiomas, for example, can be quite disfiguring, and parents are anxious to have them removed; however, surgical removal of a hemangioma can leave a large scar, and often the best course of action is to wait for natural involution. Chapter 8 discusses birthmarks and skin characteristics; a knowledge of these is essential when an infant is being examined. The nurse must also keep in mind the other characteristic changes that occur in older children. For example, the skin becomes more oily, and acne is common in adolescents.

The skin is generally assessed for surface characteristics (color, moisture, turgor, temperature, and hygiene) and for the presence of alterations in skin integrity (bruises, lesions, cuts, and rashes). Healthy skin can vary in *color*—it can be black, red, yellow, white, or any combination of these. Marked pallor, redness, jaundice (especially in the eyes), and cyanosis are signs of disease processes. The *texture* of the skin is usually smooth and soft, and the skin is normally warm to the touch. Dryness, cracking, and excessive coolness or heat should be evaluated for the cause, and preventive skin care initiated. Since the fatty subcutaneous layer has a high fluid content, the state of *hydration* can be determined on the basis of the skin turgor and tone. In young children, the upper abdomen is a good place to check skin turgor. In older children, the area under the clavicle is often used. Healthy skin will "snap" back into place when it is pinched up between the thumb and forefinger and then released. The word *tenting* is used in relation to skin which remains elevated when pinched up or which returns to normal very slowly. Tenting is a sign of poor skin turgor and dehydration. Dehydration is discussed in Chap. 18; Fig. 18-7 shows how to test skin turgor.

Care of the skin and *good hygiene* are especially important for children who wear diapers; however, poor hygiene can lead to abrasions, lesions, and infections in children of all ages. The skin should be clean and free of odor. When body hair is examined, it is inspected for quantity, texture, and the presence of parasites. Body and hair lice are especially prevalent in children who live in unsanitary environments and who practice poor personal hygiene, but they can also be communicated through contacts at school and in public places. Table 28-11 lists parasitic infections and their treatment.

Skin lesions are categorized as either *primary lesions*, which are a response to a particular disease, or *secondary lesions*, which are caused by scratching, itching, and a resultant secondary infection. The primary lesions of chickenpox—papules, vesicles, and then pustules, which are very itchy—are a common example. When these are scratched, a secondary lesion consisting of an infection with organisms transmitted by the child's hands develops.

ASSESSING SKIN LESIONS

Lesions are described according to type, size, color, consistency, texture, distribution, location, configuration, cause, and communicability.[1] Tables 28-5 and 28-6 describe the primary and secondary lesions of the skin seen most often in infectious diseases. Table 27-1 lists additional types of lesions not covered in those tables.

Table 27-1 Additional Terminology Commonly Used in Skin Assessment

Types of Lesions

1. *Petechiae* Small, flat, round purple spots caused by bleeding; later turn a yellow or greenish color
2. *Purpura* A condition in which hemorrhages cause petechiae, ecchymoses (larger than petechiae), and hematomas (the largest)
3. *Patches* Flat, circumscribed lesions of the skin or mucous membranes, larger than 1 cm
4. *Plaques* Solid, elevated, circumscribed superficial lesions, more than 1 cm in diameter
5. *Fissures* Cracks in the skin
6. *Ulcers* Excavated areas in the skin

Patterns or Configurations of Lesions

1. *Discrete lesions* Individual lesions, separated from one another by patches of skin
2. *Confluent lesions* Lesions that are blended or joined and look like one large mass
3. *Anular lesions* Lesions with a ringlike pattern (ringworm)

The rashes of most diseases have a typical pattern (distribution). Often the extension is from the trunk to the extremities over a predictable period of time. For example, a rash that develops in response to a drug will occur suddenly and is often generalized (it appears over the body). In contrast, the rash in rubeola (measles) begins as individual papules on the first day of the rash and then progresses to confluent maculopapules that make the skin appear flushed and red by the third day. The rash is concentrated mainly on the head and trunk and is less extensive on the extremities.

MANAGEMENT OF SKIN PROBLEMS

Inspecting the skin and describing the lesions are essential steps in managing skin problems. A specimen from a wet lesion can be obtained with a cotton swab and then cultured. Skin biopsies are done, or skin scrapings are gathered, cultured, and examined microscopically. The procedure for allergy skin testing is described in Chap. 26.

Dryness of the skin can be responsible for itching that causes rashes and skin breakdown. It can be prevented or treated by using a humidifier, bath oils, and lubricants after bathing. Nonalkaline skin cleansers, such as Aveeno Bar, Basis superfatted soap, and Lowila Cake, are less drying and cause fewer skin reactions than regular or perfumed soaps.

Other treatments for skin diseases include bathing and the use of topical products and oral medications. For example, 8 oz of colloidal oatmeal or 4 to 16 oz of cornstarch added to tepid bathwater can relieve itching and inflammation. Coal tar products are sometimes used for psoriasis, but should not be used when the skin is acutely inflamed or excoriated. Oral antihistamines may be used when there is severe itching or when itching interferes with sleep. The child is begun on a low dose of diphenhydramine (Benadryl), and the dose is increased gradually as needed. Antihistamines such as Benadryl will make the child sleepy.

Topical drugs are more evenly absorbed through well-hydrated skin; absorption through skin that has been altered by disease is sporadic and uncontrollable. Topical therapeutic agents are used to alleviate itching, restore hydration, cleanse or debride the area, stop infection, reduce inflammation, and protect the skin. An inflamed dermatitis with no signs of infection may be treated using a 1% hydrocortisone ointment or cream. A more potent drug should not be used on the face or anogenital area because it may induce atrophy. Bacterial infections should be treated with the medication indicated by the clinical findings or laboratory culture. Medications used for the care of burns are discussed in detail later in this chapter.

DISORDERS OF THE SKIN

Diaper dermatitis

Diaper dermatitis, or *diaper rash*, is usually caused by chemical irritants, heat, moisture retention, inadequate cleansing of the perineal area, or a bacterial infection of the perineal area. A contact dermatitis may be due to irritation from urine, feces, soaps, or friction. Applying a diaper too tightly and using tight plastic pants or having the plastic on a disposable diaper next to the skin can cause rubbing and excessive heat due to moisture and ammonia retention. A rash on the waist and upper thighs is often caused by irritation from plastic or rubber waistbands and bands around the legs. Applying an occlusive ointment can prevent air from reaching a rash and may seal urine and organisms next to the skin, actually promoting diaper rash if the skin is not completely clean and dried prior to application.

A diaper rash caused by contact agents is usually seen in the areas touched by the diaper, and the groin creases are unaffected. A diaper rash that is not treated immediately will spread to the fold areas (intertrigo) and often becomes secondarily infected. Although yeast infections are the most common, staphylococcal and (somewhat less commonly) streptococcal infections can also occur in the diaper area.

If miliaria, or prickly heat, is the cause of a diaper rash, clusters of red vesicles and papules will be seen over the chest, axillae, neck, and forehead as well as in the diaper area. Miliaria is usually the result of dressing a baby too warmly or of hot, humid weather.

Treatment Diaper rash is usually managed by changing the diaper as soon as it becomes wet or soiled. It is also helpful to wash the diaper area with a wet cloth or to give a partial bath when the stool is difficult to remove, patting the area dry and being sure to include the creases. Creating too much friction when drying should be avoided, since this can actually cause blisters or rub off the baby's skin, creating an open lesion. The perineal area can also be exposed to air and light three to four times a day to hasten healing. Changing the diapers before the parents retire will reduce the length of time that the baby is wet, and placing an absorbent pad on the bed and using double or triple cloth diapers will eliminate the need for plastic pants. While most parents use disposable diapers, in the case of a severe diaper rash, cloth diapers are better, unless they are used with plastic pants. However, cloth diapers must be either commercially laundered or laundered at home; if they are laundered at home, they should be thoroughly prerinsed in a solution that will counteract the ammonia; washed with a mild soap, such as Dreft or Ivory; and then thoroughly rinsed several times to remove all the soap.

When the diaper area appears infected with pustules or whitish-looking lesions, the area should be cultured for yeast and bacteria. Specific treatments for yeast, streptococcal, and staphylococcal infections are discussed in Chap. 28.

Seborrheic dermatitis

Seborrheic dermatitis, also known as *cradle cap,* is a chronic inflammatory disease. It can begin within the first month of life and most often involves the scalp, the face, and the skin creases. Salmon-colored, scaly plaques are present on the scalp and extend to the eyelids, the external ear, the axillae, and the inguinal and perineal areas.

Seborrheic dermatitis sometimes occurs in the diaper area with a secondary *Candida* (yeast) infection. The condition is reactivated in some people later in life as a result of stressful situations, poor hygiene, or excessive perspiration. Secondary infections with *Candida* are especially common.

Treatment Cradle cap can be controlled by rubbing warm mineral oil into the scalp at night, washing it out with a mild shampoo, and then gently combing out the scales with a fine-tooth comb. Rubbing the head gently with a textured washcloth during routine shampooing will help prevent the buildup of scales. Perfumed oils should not be used, and oil should not be applied to the baby's head every day and left on. Shampoos containing selenium sulfide—or, for severe cases, tar—can be used, being careful to keep it from getting into the baby's eyes. Topical low-potency hydrocortisone is sometimes applied to reduce severe itching and inflammation. Other skinfold areas are dried using preparations containing mild coal tar or salicylic acid.

Acne vulgaris*

Acne vulgaris, or "pimples," is the most common skin disorder of people in their early teens and twenties. It causes inflammation of conspicuous areas of the body: the face, the shoulders, the chest, and the back. When acne is active, the *comedones* (blackheads and whiteheads), papules, pustules, nodules, and cysts are unsightly. After the acute process has subsided, the skin is often left scarred.

In most persons, acne begins in puberty and subsides at about 22 to 23 years of age. However, it can begin as early as 5 years of age and continue to be active into the forties.

Both males and females are affected by acne, and the pattern of appearance in a family indicates that acne is a dominant trait. Many factors point to androgenic hormone stimulation of the skin as a prime factor in its development. Acne seems to be aggravated by emotional stress, winter weather, some stimulant drugs, and body changes during the premenstrual period. Regardless of the cause, acne is a complex, chronic problem that brings discomfort and mental distress to 80 to 90 percent of adolescents.

Etiology Pilosebaceous glands are found in large numbers on the face and in smaller, but significant, numbers on the back, chest, and shoulders. These glands are composed of a hair follicle and a large sebaceous (oil-producing) gland. At puberty, under the influence of the increased androgenic hormone secretions from the adrenal glands and gonads, the glands mature. Their size and secretions increase, and the cells lining the ducts grow more rapidly and are shed in greater numbers. The oily gland secretions are called *sebum,* which is composed of keratin, lipids, and fatty acids and contains bacteria. In the person without acne, the increased secretion of sebum, mixed with large numbers of gland-lining cells, is extruded from the pilosebaceous glands onto the skin.

In acne, the cells shed from the lining of a pilosebaceous gland block the opening to the skin surface. This plug prevents the gland from emptying its contents onto the skin. The melanin content of the plug gives it a dark color. If the pore is open to the air, the sebum also darkens through the oxidation process. Therefore, with the passage of time, the part of the plug at the skin surface develops a black pigmentation. This is called an *open comedo,* or blackhead. If the comedo maintains its opening to the skin surface, the contents of the gland can be slowly and continuously discharged without causing much damage. However, the pore containing the comedo often dilates, and the blackhead becomes larger.

If the skin covers the pore, it is called a whitehead, or *closed comedo.* Beneath the plug, the gland continues to produce hair and sebum, causing progressive gland enlargement. This enlargement turns the gland into a distended sac, which can be ruptured. The contents of the ruptured sac are irritating and cause inflammation around the gland.

Sebaceous glands that rupture and cause inflammation near the surface of the skin produce

*This section was written by William F. Walsh, M.D.

a pustule (a pus-filled pimple). Ruptures deeper under the skin produce papules. These papules can become pus-filled and are prone to the development of nodules, cysts, and scar formation.

Living in the pilosebaceous glands are bacteria called *Corynebacterium acnes*. The enzymes of the bacteria split the sebum into free fatty acids. These fatty acids are the most irritating part of the sebum and significantly increase the inflammatory response around the ruptured gland.

Thus the acne process involves plugging of a pilosebaceous gland and glandular enlargement if the plugging is complete, followed by rupture and the release of irritating glandular contents. These irritating substances, especially the free fatty acids released by the *C. acnes* bacteria, cause an inflammation as the body utilizes its defenses to remove the ruptured gland material. A secondary infection with staphylococci, due to picking or squeezing the lesions, can complicate the problem.

Manifestations The comedo is the most characteristic lesion of acne. If the gland maintains its opening to the skin surface, blackheads, or open comedones, appear on the face. If the skin grows over the surface opening of the gland, a whitehead, or closed comedo, appears. With enlargement of the gland, a papule is formed. Enlargement and rupture cause swelling, and the area becomes red and tender. Pustules and cysts are formed as a result of this process. In more severe cases, scarring occurs with healing. The degree of scarring varies, depending on the person and the severity of the acne. The scars may be depressed pits in the skin or may become nodules if the person is susceptible to *keloid* (scar) formation.

Treatment *Diet* Recent control studies show no evidence that diet has any influence on the course of acne. Some individuals believe that sweets and greasy foods make the process worse and should be avoided.

Topical treatment Various drying and *exfoliating* (peeling) agents are used in the treatment of acne. These include abrasive soaps, astringents, ultraviolet light, sulfur, resorcinol, and salicylic acid. Sulfur (1 to 5%) and resorcinol (1 to 10%) dry and peel existing comedones, papules, and pustules and allow them to empty, but fail to prevent closed comedones, or whiteheads. The most potent topical agents currently in use are benzoyl peroxide and tretinoin.

Topical medications *Benzoyl peroxide* has been in use since 1934. Only recently have effective lotions and gel forms been developed. Benzoyl peroxide produces a fine *desquamation* (peeling) that helps to allow expression of the comedo. It also inhibits *C. acnes* and the formation of free fatty acids, which this bacterium promotes.

Benzoyl peroxide can be irritating and drying, and its use must be introduced gradually, especially in people with sensitive skin. Depending on the individual, a thin film of benzoyl peroxide is rubbed into the skin gently, either daily or every second or third day. As the skin develops a tolerance for this treatment, the strength of the preparation and the frequency of application can be increased. This usually takes 2 to 3 weeks. If the skin becomes irritated or dry, the preparation can be discontinued for several days, and lubricants can be used until the irritation subsides. Skin irritation from benzoyl peroxide is reduced or avoided if the preparation is introduced and used cautiously.

Tretinoin (vitamin A acid) began to be used for topical treatment in 1969. Its use increases cell turnover within the pilosebaceous gland and decreases the "stickiness" of the cells that are shed into the sebum. It causes a thinning of the epidermis, which promotes extrusion of the comedo and decreases comedo formation. It also aids in the penetration of benzoyl peroxide and topical antibiotics into the pilosebaceous gland.

Tretinoin and benzoyl peroxide are both irritating. Treatment with tretinoin is begun cautiously, according to a schedule similar to that used for benzoyl peroxide. A mild soap should be used to wash the area, no more than two or three times a day, and the person should wait at least 30 min after washing before applying tretinoin. Sunscreens should be used if prolonged exposure to the sun is anticipated. The therapeutic effect of these medications is enhanced by using them in combination (one in the morning and one at night).

Salicyclic acid (5 to 10%) is less effective than either tretinoin or benzoyl peroxide. It is sometimes used for teenagers with mild acne who have problems with tretinoin or as an alternative to tretinoin in combination with benzoyl peroxide.

Topical antibiotics Topical tetracycline,

erythromycin, and clindamycin can suppress the growth of *C. acnes*.

Systemic treatment Systemic antibiotics are helpful in treating inflammation, pustules, and cysts. They suppress the growth of *C. acnes*, causing a reduction in the irritating free fatty acids produced by the bacterial reaction. They are used less often now than in the past because of the effective topical treatment currently available.

Tetracycline is the most commonly used oral antibiotic because it is effective and inexpensive and has few side effects. Therapy often begins with a dosage of 500 to 1000 mg per day; this is gradually decreased to the lowest dose that produces a good response. This may be 250 mg every day or every other day. Usually a minimum of 3 to 4 weeks of treatment is necessary, and low-dose therapy is continued for months. Complications include vaginal moniliasis, gastrointestinal irritation (nausea and vomiting), and allergy. Tetracycline must be taken on an empty stomach and not with milk, since it combines with calcium. It is not used in children younger than 12 years of age or during the first trimester of pregnancy because of the possibility of tooth discoloration in the child.

Erythromycin is often used for long-term acne treatment. When a person does not respond sufficiently to tetracycline or erythromycin, clindamycin or minocycline can be used. *Clindamycin* can cause pseudomembranous ulcerative colitis, and systemic use should not be continued over a long period. *Minocycline* causes a high incidence of headache and dizziness.

Management The person with acne vulgaris feels that each "zit" or acne lesion is an unsightly blemish and is self-conscious about it. This is especially true of the impressionable teenager, whose adult personality is being formed. This conspicuous and disfiguring process is traumatic to the personality and to self-esteem. The nurse must approach the teenager with kindness and understanding. A sympathetic approach will often elicit the trust and cooperation necessary to carry out a treatment program. The nurse begins with gentle questioning about the skin problem. A treatment plan should then be formulated. The plan begins with education concerning the cause and treatment of acne. Topical medication must be explained carefully, and the teenager should be followed while using it. When inflammation is prominent, systemic antibiotics are added to the program.

Sometimes removal of the comedones is advocated, and instructions are given. The adolescent should wash his or her face two to three times a day, wash the hair frequently, and keep the hair off the face to help reduce oiliness. Keeping the hands away from the face is also important: "picking" and resting the face in the hands are to be avoided because they predispose to infection and scarring.

Instruction and encouragement are vital. The treatment can take weeks, and often there are some unpleasant side effects, including erythema, superficial peeling, and at times a temporary worsening of the acne process. A nurse who has established a good rapport with an adolescent will be able to give emotional support that will encourage compliance with the long-term treatment regimen necessary for control.

BURNS

Management of the pediatric burn patient presents the nurse with a demanding and challenging opportunity to implement all aspects of nursing care. The stress involved in a burn injury cannot be overstated. Every major physiological organ system is potentially involved. Psychologically and socially, the burn represents a major life event with dramatic effects. Furthermore, in a pediatric burn patient these physiological and psychosocial changes are interrelated with the accomplishment of necessary developmental tasks. As a primary caregiver on the burn care team, the nurse must have an understanding of the responses of the child to the injury. Such knowledge, combined with skill in accepted burn care techniques, serves as the basis for planning, implementing, and evaluating the care of the pediatric burn victim.

Scope of the problem

Approximately 2 million individuals are burned annually in the United States. It is estimated that 30 percent of these are children. While some 6000 children still die annually as a result of burns, improved care techniques have greatly increased children's chances of survival. Just 15 years ago, a child with a 40 percent third-degree burn had only guarded chances of survival. Now, a child with this same burn injury has an 80 percent chance of recovery.

Certain types of thermal injury appear to be associated with selected age groups. Flames and house fires are common causes of burns in infants. As children begin to crawl and explore the environment, they may chew on exposed electric cords, causing injury to the mouth, lips, tongue, and teeth. Preadolescent and adolescent boys have a relatively high incidence of burns due to gasoline, as a result of working with engines or throwing combustible liquids on an open fire. Boys in this age group also sustain frequent electrical injuries from high-voltage power sources. Girls in this age group are more often burned while cooking or while tending such home heating sources as wood stoves and fireplaces. The majority of all burns in children occur when they are unattended or are in the care of babysitters.

Burns can be prevented. The importance of supervising children and of leaving children in the care of a responsible person must be stressed to parents. Flameproof clothing greatly reduces the extent of injury from flame burns. Proper safety measures should be observed around combustible liquids and electric appliances. Screens should be used with sources of open flames in the home. Fire exit drills should be practiced with children. Programs of fire and burn prevention that include these facts and other safety measures should be developed for public education. The nurse must take every opportunity to educate families in the basics of burn prevention.[3]

Assessment of the injury

Care of the injury begins with an assessment and description of the burn. Burns are best described according to (1) type of injury, (2) amount of body surface involved, and (3) depth of tissue damage.

Type of injury The type of injury depends on the source of the tissue damage. The nurse should determine whether the child has sustained an electrical burn, a chemical burn, frostbite, a scald, or a direct-flame injury.

Electrical injuries result in extensive tissue destruction. Skin damage is seen at the point of entry of the electric current and the point of exit. Such surface burns are usually circumscribed, deep, charred, depressed wounds involving cutaneous and subcutaneous tissue (Fig. 27-2). When the body acts as a conductor from the source of electricity to the ground, electricity passes through the body. As the electric current passes through the body, it encounters resistance, and electric energy is converted to heat energy, causing internal thermal tissue destruction. The current usually follows the path of least resistance, making blood vessels and nerve passages most susceptible to injury. However, damage to muscle and bones is frequently seen. Damage to major vessels may result in spontaneous hemorrhage during the post-injury period. The child must be observed carefully for evidence of internal damage and ischemia, which may not be immediately apparent. Amputation may be necessary if there is extensive muscle and bone involvement. In addition to thermal damage to the skin and internal structures, the initial electrical contact may cause corresponding physiological disruption. The cardiopulmonary system is especially vulnerable, and cardiac and respiratory arrest may result, demanding immediate resuscitation.

Although *chemical burns* are more frequent among adults and are usually associated with industrial accidents, chemical burn patients are also encountered by the pediatric nurse. Fireworks, flares, and improperly stored household chemicals may result in injury to a child. The chemical reaction of the agent on the skin results in tissue damage similar to that seen in other types of burns. Treatment focuses on removing the source of damage. Flushing with copious amounts of water or saline is indicated

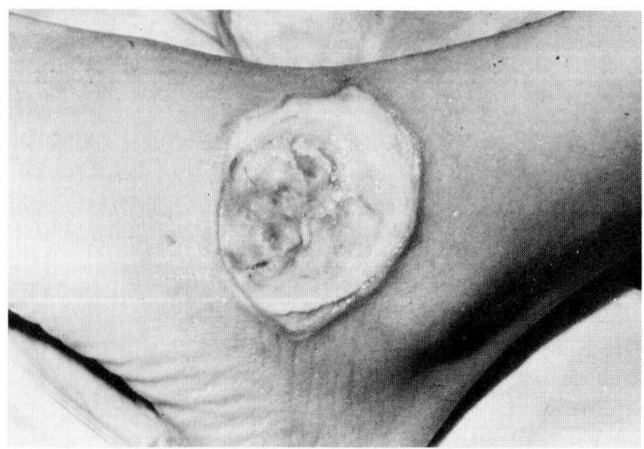

Figure 27-2 An ulcerated area caused by an electrical injury.

for most chemical burns. Water is contraindicated in phosphorous injuries because it activates phosphorus. A 1% copper sulfate solution as a washing agent is recommended in such cases.[4]

Scalds, flame injury, and *sunburn* cause tissue damage as a result of excessive heat. The physiological response is similar in all these injuries and will be discussed in detail later in this chapter. The most important factor in limiting tissue destruction is removing or extinguishing the source of heat as quickly as possible.

In some regions, *cold injury,* or *frostbite,* may also be encountered by the pediatric nurse. Such injuries are due to excessive cold rather than excessive heat. The tissue destruction is similar to that in burns, however, and warrants inclusion in a discussion of the care of a thermally injured child.

The most important factors causing tissue damage are wind, temperature, and humidity. Tissue damage results from direct freezing of tissue and extreme vasoconstriction, causing local ischemia. First aid for frostbite is directed toward quick recognition and warming of the affected part. Warm, moist heat applied by means of immersion or wet packs is effective. The nurse must recognize that a person with a cold injury frequently experiences insensitivity to touch, pain, temperature, and other stimulation and cannot respond to the temperature of the warming agent. A moderately warm solution, 39°C (103°F), is recommended so as not to cause further tissue damage.

Amount of body surface involved The second factor used in describing a thermal injury is an estimate of the percentage of total body surface area. Generally, the greater the amount of body surface area damaged, the more serious the injury. The Lund and Browder technique, which is a convenient and useful tool for assessing a child's burn, allows for modifications based on the child's physical development and body proportions, but the nurse must be aware of normal growth and development as they relate to body surface area. For example, an infant, who has a large proportion of body surface area in the head and trunk, will present a very different burn profile from that of a 10-year-old child, who has relatively more body surface area in the extremities (Fig. 27-3).

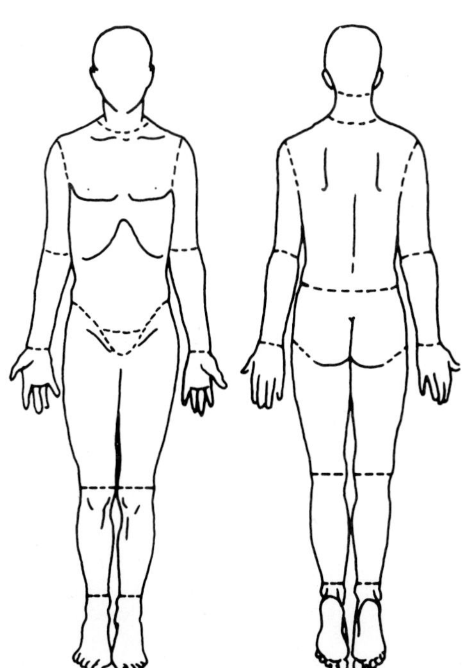

AREA	1 Yr.	1-4 Yrs.	5-9 Yrs.	10-14 Yrs.	15 Yrs.	Adult	2°	3°
Head	19	17	13	11	9	7		
Neck	2	2	2	2	2	2		
Ant. Trunk	13	13	13	13	13	13		
Post. Trunk	13	13	13	13	13	13		
R. Buttock	2½	2½	2½	2½	2½	2½		
L. Buttock	2½	2½	2½	2½	2½	2½		
Genitalia	1	1	1	1	1	1		
R.U. Arm	4	4	4	4	4	4		
L.U. Arm	4	4	4	4	4	4		
R.L. Arm	3	3	3	3	3	3		
L.L. Arm	3	3	3	3	3	3		
R. Hand	2½	2½	2½	2½	2½	2½		
L. Hand	2½	2½	2½	2½	2½	2½		
R. Thigh	5½	6½	8	8½	9	9½		
L. Thigh	5½	6½	8	8½	9	9½		
R. Leg	5	5	5½	6	6½	7		
L. Leg	5	5	5½	6	6½	7		
R. Foot	3½	3½	3½	3½	3½	3½		
L. Foot	3½	3½	3½	3½	3½	3½		
TOTAL								

Figure 27-3 The Lund and Browder method of calculating burn size. (*From C. P. Artz and J. A. Moncrief, The Treatment of Burns, 2d ed., Saunders, Philadelphia, 1969. Used with permission.*)

Table 27-2 Classification of Burn Depth

Traditional Terminology	Anatomic Terminology	Depth of Involvement	Depth of Anatomic Involvement
First-degree burn	Epidermal	Partial thickness	Stratum corneum of the epidermis
Second-degree burn	Intradermal: Superficial Deep dermal	Partial thickness	Dermis to a variable extent
Third-degree burn	Subdermal	Full thickness	Subcutaneous adipose tissue, fascia, muscles, and bones

Source: G. Scipien, M. U. Barnard, M. A. Chard, J. Howe, and P. J. Phillips (eds.), *Comprehensive Pediatric Nursing*, 3d ed., McGraw-Hill, New York, 1986, p. 1333. Used with permission.

Depth of tissue damage In addition to estimating the amount of body surface area involved and identifying the type of injury, the nurse also describes the depth of tissue destruction. Burns can be classified as first-, second-, or third-degree injuries (Table 27-2). A *first-degree burn* involves the covering layer of epidermis. The skin becomes red but does not blister, and the person has normal or increased pain sensation. First-degree burns are due to overexposure to such heat sources as the sun. Healing occurs spontaneously and rapidly.

A *second-degree burn* results in damage to all or most of the epidermis and some of the dermis. None of the underlying tissue structure is involved, however, and epithelization and spontaneous healing can occur. Such a burn has a moist, pink to cherry-red appearance, is painful, and frequently blisters. A second-degree injury can become a third-degree injury if infection occurs that causes further tissue destruction (Table 27-3).

In contrast to first- and second-degree burns, a *third-degree burn* destroys the entire epidermis and dermis down to the underlying fat. In a severe injury, fat, muscle, and bone may be damaged, but there is no pain sensation because the nerve endings are damaged. The burn is cherry red to black or gray and may be either wet or dry and leathery. Healing is not spontaneous, and grafting is required for wound coverage. (See Fig. 27-1.)

Pathophysiology

Immediate body response The initial physiological alterations which accompany a burn injury are commonly referred to as *burn shock* and occur during approximately the first 48 h after the burn. This phenomenon occurs in people in

Table 27-3 Characteristics of Depth of Injury

Depth of Injury	Appearance	Pain Sensitivity	Edema Formation	Healing Time	Scarring	Cause
First degree	Pink to red	Painful	Very slight	3 to 5 days	None	Sunburn, flash, explosives
Second degree	Red to pale ivory and moist; may have vesicles and bullae	Extremely painful	Very edematous	21 to 28 days (variable)	None	Flash, scalds, flame, brief contact with hot objects
Third degree	White, cherry red, or black; may contain bullae and thrombosed veins; dry and leathery	Painless to touch	Marked edema may require escharotomies	Requires grafting	Yes	Flame, high-intensity flash, electrical, chemical, hot object, scalds in infants and the elderly

Source: G. Scipien, M. U. Barnard, M. A. Chard, J. Howe, and P. J. Phillips (eds.), *Comprehensive Pediatric Nursing*, 3d ed., McGraw-Hill, New York, 1986, p. 1334. Used with permission.

all age groups; however, the child is at a special risk during this period. Immature kidneys, an unstable peripheral circulation, high metabolism, and a larger body surface area in proportion to body weight are factors which increase the risk in the younger child; children under 2 years of age are especially vulnerable. Generally, the older the child, the better the body systems can respond to the injury. In children, there is usually a systemic response to burns which cover more than 20 percent of their total body surface area. Infants and very young children may suffer a systemic response to burns which cover 10 to 15 percent of their total body surface area.[5]

A major component of the burn shock response is the alteration of fluid balance. Approximately 50 to 70 percent of the body weight is water, which is distributed in the intracellular and extracellular spaces. The *intracellular fluid* constitutes the majority of body fluid weight. The *extracellular fluid* consists of the interstitial fluid, which bathes the cells, and the *intravascular fluid*, or plasma. Thus the normal system is represented as having three compartments: the intracellular, interstitial, and intravascular compartments. Through the process of diffusion and filtration, fluids within these compartments are constantly interchanging. Nutrients carried in the blood pass through the interstitial spaces to the blood, where they are filtered through the kidneys.

Following a thermal injury, there are disruptions in this distribution of body fluid. As a result of a marked increase in capillary permeability, plasma leaks into the tissue, causing generalized edema or blistering. Red blood cells, which are larger, remain in the vessels. This loss of fluid in the vascular spaces results in decreased circulatory blood volume, which in turn causes a fall in blood pressure. The hematocrit rises because of hemoconcentration. Further, as plasma protein leaks into the tissue, there is a loss of the colloidal osmotic pressure difference between the capillaries and the tissue fluid, resulting in alterations in electrolyte balance. Potassium, which is contained primarily within cells, is lost into the interstitial spaces. Sodium passes into these spaces, contributing to edema and further fluid loss from the vascular system.

Resuscitation by fluid replacement must be monitored carefully to avoid either dehydration or overhydration.[6] As circulating blood decreases, renal vasoconstriction occurs, decreasing the glomerular filtration rate. This will elevate the blood urea nitrogen and creatinine levels. Permanent renal damage can be avoided by providing adequate fluid replacement, although very young children are especially prone to permanent kidney damage. In addition, the child cannot excrete large volumes of nonelectrolytic fluid and may suffer from fluid overload.

The most acute response is seen in the first 18 h. The response gradually decreases, and after 48 to 72 h the capillaries generally heal. As permeability decreases, fluid shift occurs as fluid from the tissues returns to the circulatory system. Throughout this period, urinary output should be monitored carefully, and an hourly urine output of 10 to 30 ml should be maintained. Individual output is based on the child's age. Parenteral therapy may be decreased as the circulatory status improves and as urinary output increases (Table 27-4).

Alterations of other body systems *Pulmonary damage* Damage to the respiratory system associated with thermal injury has only recently been recognized as a major factor in morbidity among burn patients. A burned child may exhibit respiratory involvement at the time of the injury, in connection with the acute burn shock response, or as a later complication during the postinjury course.

Direct respiratory damage at the time of the injury is rare because the moist air in the respiratory tract dissipates the heat and has a cooling effect. However, indirect respiratory damage due to lack of oxygen in the burning environment may result in severe respiratory damage or death, even in cases where minimal or no cutaneous injury is present. Also, when a victim is trapped in an enclosed space, such as an automobile, toxic fumes from burning materials can cause damage to the respiratory tract. The nurse should observe for singed nares or facial hair, a sooty tongue, blistering of the oral mucosa, and signs of products of combustion in the sputum, since these are strong indicators of respiratory involvement. Because initial postburn x-rays are frequently negative, repeated x-rays are indicated when a patient is suspected of having sustained respiratory damage.

During the initial postburn period, decreased circulating blood, resulting in hypovolemic shock and shunting of unoxygenated blood, can cause alterations in the child's respiratory status. Signs of early respiratory compromise include shallow,

Table 27-4 Signs and Symptoms of Fluid Deficit and Overload

	Extracellular Fluid Volume			
	Deficit		Excess	
	Moderate	Severe	Moderate	Severe
Cardiovascular	Orthostatic hypotension Tachycardia Collapsed veins Collapsing pulse	Cutaneous lividity (gray color) Hypotension Distant heart sounds Cold extremities Absent peripheral pulses	Elevated venous pressure Distention of peripheral veins Increased cardiac output Loud heart sounds Functional murmurs Bounding pulse High pulse pressure Increased pulmonary second sound Gallop	Pulmonary edema
Tissue signs	Soft, small tongue with longitudinal wrinkling Decreased skin turgor	Atonic muscles Sunken eyes	Subcutaneous pitting edema Basilar rales	Anasarca Moist rales Vomiting Diarrhea
Metabolism	Mild decrease in temperature (97 to 99°F) (36.1 to 37.2°C)	Marked decrease in temperature (95 to 98°F) (35 to 36.7°C)	None	None

rigid breathing; disorientation; restlessness; and copious mucus secretions. Treatment should be aimed at increasing alveolar oxygen, increasing the ability of the lungs to utilize available oxygen, and minimizing tissue oxygen requirements. Thus, humidified oxygen and gentle frequent suctioning are indicated. Careful precautions should be taken to avoid aspiration of oral intake or vomitus. If not monitored carefully, fluid therapy at this time can result in pulmonary edema. The importance of maintaining adequate fluid replacement while monitoring the acid-base balance and avoiding fluid overload must be stressed. If facial and neck edema are present or expected, early intubation should be considered. Such early intubation may avoid the necessity of performing an emergency tracheotomy, with the accompanying risk of infection. Pain and thick, binding eschar (dead, burned tissue) may also inhibit adequate ventilation.

The child should be made as comfortable as possible and should be reassured about his or her condition. There remains much controversy concerning the use of pain medications in children. Some institutions administer intravenous analgesics. Others believe that such analgesics alter cardiac and respiratory functioning and are contraindicated. The nurse should be familiar with the philosophy of his or her institution. It is imperative that during the emergent period of capillary permeability, all such analgesics be administered intravenously rather than intramuscularly. During periods of increased capillary permeability and edema, medications administered intramuscularly pool in the tissue. If a fluid shift occurs, such medications enter the circulatory system and can result in severe overdose or death.

If the eschar, which is frequently leathery and binding, is a circumferential band around the chest wall, an escharotomy should be considered (Fig. 27-4). An escharotomy involves a surgical incision through the eschar only to release pressure. Because the incision goes only through the destroyed tissue, the patient experiences no pain, and bleeding should be minimal.

Forced immobility and sepsis are two frequent causes of respiratory distress during the later postburn course. Turning, coughing, and deep breathing, as well as active and passive exercises and early ambulation, improve ventilation and counter the effects of immobility. Infection control mandates the use of both topical and systemic antibiotics and aseptic technique, including wearing gloves, a gown, and a mask and using sterile linens.

Renal damage A variety of renal changes are associated with a burn injury. Such changes can be permanent or temporary. An initial decrease in glomerular filtration rate, which results from hypovolemia and renal vasoconstriction, was discussed earlier. Permanent renal damage can result in a patient with a history of renal disease or in a very young child if fluid replacement is not adequate. The most frequent causes of such renal damage are hypovolemia and the circulating by-products of muscle necrosis and red blood cell destruction. While adequate fluid resuscitation is vital, osmolarity should be monitored. For example, an increased urine output accompanied by an increased urine specific gravity may indicate renal damage rather than inadequate fluid resuscitation. In such cases, further fluid resuscitation will result only in fluid overload to the circulatory system, with little assistance to the kidneys. Mannitol may be administered as an osmotic diuretic. Occasionally, renal dialysis is necessary.[7]

Glycosuria may be seen during the first week after the burn. This condition is usually part of the overall physiological stress response to the trauma. Such glycosuria is usually accompanied by a release of catecholamines and an altered insulin response, which allows the carbohydrate metabolism to shift from energy storage to utilization. Assessment of glucose metabolism by means of blood and urine testing is essential for proper burn management. Although glycosuria usually clears spontaneously, administration of insulin, fluid replacement, and dietary management must be considered in care planning.

A urinary tract infection is a potential complication following a serious burn. The child's defenses are weakened, and frequently a urinary catheter is in place. Scrupulous care of the perineal area and removal of the catheter as soon as the circulatory status has stabilized are indicated.

Gastrointestinal damage Gastric dilatation and paralytic ileus usually occur early in the postburn period, but the nurse should observe for signs of gastric distress throughout the recovery period. Stress ulcers, frequently referred to as *Curling's ulcers,* are also associated with burn trauma and are similar to acute stress ulcers seen in the general hospital population. The nurse must be alert for (1) an unexplained falling hematocrit, (2) a distended abdomen, (3) occult blood in the stool (black stools), and (4) brown or red returns from the nasogastric tube.

In the case of large burns in children, it is often wise to insert a nasogastric tube attached to suction. Such a tube will prevent vomiting and aspiration, increase the child's comfort, and allow for easier, more accurate examination of the abdomen. It will also help prevent the com-

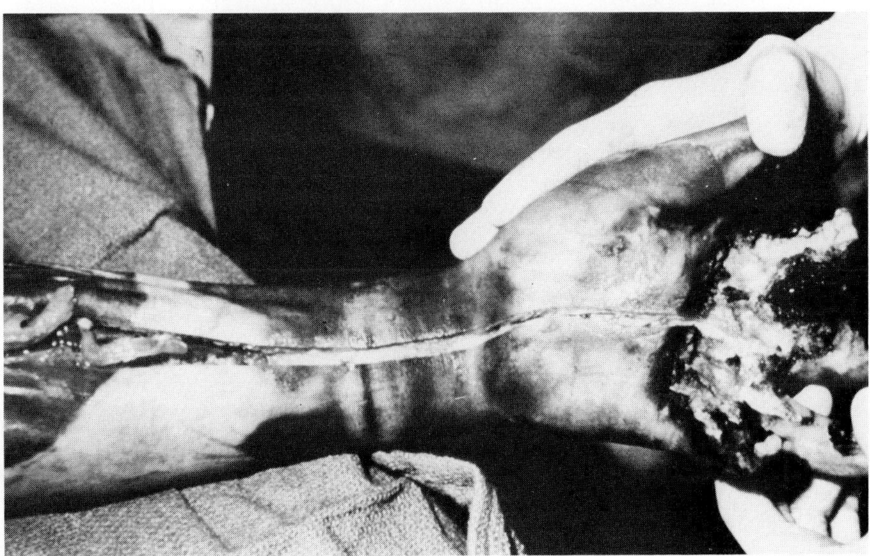

Figure 27-4 An escharotomy, which is a surgical incision through the eschar only to relieve pressure on underlying structures.

mon complications of gastric dilatation and paralytic ileus. An antacid regimen is usually initiated by mouth or nasogastric tube. Antacids are frequently prescribed every 2 h and alternated with milk or tube feedings so that something is given every hour. Knowing that prophylaxis is the best treatment for Curling's ulcer will help the nurse realize the importance of adhering to the time schedules for administering such medication. After there has been adequate fluid resuscitation and when bowel sounds have returned, the nasogastric tube is removed.

Integumentary healing Following thc initial shock response, capillaries begin to heal, edema is reabsorbed, and damaged tissue can be distinguished from living tissue. Epithelization begins, and fibroblasts appear. At this point, four main processes of wound healing begin: (1) separation of dead tissue (eschar), (2) regeneration of connective tissue and vasculature, (3) epithelization, and (4) contraction.

Eschar separation occurs primarily as a result of natural separation, surgical removal, or infection. Natural separation is slow and increases the risk of wound infection. Bacteria speed separation of eschar, but they also damage underlying tissue. Thus, early surgical excision has become the treatment of choice. After the eschar has separated, blood vessels redevelop in the wound. Fibroblasts, microphages, and collagens begin to form. New collagen tissue formation begins at the edge of the wound, slowly advancing for total coverage. In a third-degree injury, this process is slow. New tissue formed in the center of the wound is of poor quality, and the wound requires surgical grafting.

Scar formation presents additional problems in severe burns. As collagen advances, it thickens and then shrinks, causing contractures. Good nursing care is essential in contracture prevention. Splints applied properly to maintain the joints in positions of function are also essential. Elastic pressure garments also help eliminate some of the thickening of the scar tissue. If contractures do develop, surgical release is frequently necessary. The nurse should remember that a scar may not "mature" until 8 to 12 months after the injury. The patient is discharged with splints and pressure garments, which must be reassessed and refitted during regular clinic visits.

Excessive scar formation (*hypertrophic scarring*) may also occur after a burn and presents special cosmetic problems for the burned child. Prevention of inflammation and full-thickness skin grafts may eliminate much hypertrophic scarring. However, in some cases surgery is again required. Hypertrophic scarring should not be confused with keloid formation. *Keloids* are large, elevated masses of connective tissue which develop in certain individuals in spite of optimum medical and nursing care. While hypertrophic scars soften and decrease in time, keloids continue to grow unless treated with hormones and/or surgery.

Treatment

First Aid The initial step in first aid for burns is to stop the burning process. This involves separating the person from the heat source by smothering the flames or stopping the electric current. Then all smoldering clothing and such articles as metal belt buckles or rings, which retain heat, should be removed. If clothing adheres to the skin, it should be dampened to extinguish any heat and left in place for removal at the hospital. With small surface burns, the affected part is immersed in cool water. Specific first aid for chemical and electrical burns was discussed earlier. As a final step, the victim should be wrapped in clean sheets for transport to a physician or hospital.

After these steps are taken, minor burns can be treated by washing the wound with a solution of mild soap and peroxide, sterile saline, or both. The area may then be allowed to heal exposed, or a sterile sheet of fine-mesh gauze may be applied and held in place with a light bandage dressing. In selected cases, topical antibacterial ointment, such as ampicillin, is applied to the wound, but this is not routinely indicated. The parents of the burned child may wash and dress the wound at home on a daily basis, depending on the area of the body involved and the amount of drainage. However, the dressing should be changed every 3 days by a professional so that he or she can observe healing and check for signs of infection.

A brief medical history, including allergies, immunizations, and relevant medical conditions, is important for treatment. If the last tetanus immunization was given more than 3 years previously, prophylactic tetanus toxoid must be administered on admission. Medical conditions such as diabetes, hypertension, and allergies will affect treatment plans and decisions concerning the necessity of hospitalization.

Table 27-5 Steps in Acute Care of a Child with a Large Burn

1. Maintain an adequate airway.
2. Institute IV therapy—fluid resuscitation.
3. Insert a nasogastric tube.
4. Monitor ouput; insert a catheter.
5. Control pain.
6. Give tetanus toxoid if needed.
7. Take infection control measures.
8. Weigh the child.
9. Provide emotional support for the child and the family.

In the case of more serious burns, more extensive measures should be taken. In the young child, second-degree burns over 15 percent of the body, deep second- and third-degree burns, third-degree burns over 2 percent of the body, and burns of the face, neck, hands, perineum, and feet usually require hospitalization. In addition, children with fractures and respiratory involvement, children with electrical burns, and children with such preexisting conditions as renal disease or diabetes should be initially admitted.[8] Table 27-5 lists the steps in the acute care of a child with a large burn.

Acute care On admission of the child to the hospital, edema must be anticipated, and preventive measures should be taken to ensure *adequate ventilation* if the child has suffered a major burn or burns of the face and neck. Endotracheal tubes, if inserted early, may prevent the need for a subsequent tracheostomy. Suctioning equipment and humidified oxygen should be available.

Fluid resuscitation is a major consideration in the acute care phase of treatment. *Intravenous therapy* is directed toward maintaining the cardiocirculatory system. If possible, a large vessel in an unburned area should be selected for the cutdown in order to avoid contamination and possible sepsis. Formulas for fluid resuscitation vary from institution to institution, and the nurse should be familiar with the protocol in his or her hospital. Most formulas involve some calculation of percent of burn and body weight in kilograms. Colloids such as blood, plasma, and albumin are usually avoided during the first 24 h, when vascular damage is greatest, since colloids leak from the vascular spaces. A nearly isotonic solution, such as lactated Ringer's solution, is often the solution of choice. A formula of 3 ml of fluid per combined percentage of second- and third-degree burn multiplied by the child's weight in kilograms is a useful formula for calculating the total fluid needs for the first 24 h. (All burns that cover more than 40 percent of the body are calculated at 40 percent, and no higher.) One-half of this calculated amount is administered during the first 8 h after the burn. One-fourth of the total calculated fluid needs is then administered during the second and third 8-h periods. It is important that fluid replacement calculations be based on the time of injury, not on the time of admission to the hospital. Table 27-6 presents the fluid replacement formula.

During the second 24 h, fluid replacement includes addition of colloid solution or plasma. The total amount of solution needed during the second 24-h period is usually about one-half the amount of solution calculated for the first 24-h period. This calculated amount is administered throughout the second 24-h period unless an alteration in urinary output indicates a need to increase or decrease fluid therapy. Sodium, potassium, and chlorides are also added. Subsequent fluid replacement depends on the physiological response of the child and on any complications that develop. Anemia may occur as a response to red blood cell breakdown. Blood specimens should be obtained to measure hematocrit, hemoglobin, and blood urea nitrogen, and for type and cross-matching for transfusions.

Also at the time of admission, a Foley catheter should be inserted. Vital signs and urinary output should be monitored hourly to evaluate the adequacy of fluid replacement. The hourly output should be 5 to 10 ml in children under 1 year of age, 10 to 20 ml in children between 1 and 10 years of age, and 15 to 30 ml in children over the age of 10 and in adults.[9] Urine specimens are obtained in order to measure pH, sugar,

Table 27-6 Fluid Replacement Formula*

Figuring Fluid Amount

3 ml × kg body weight × percent of combined second- and third-degree injury up to 40% = total 24-h fluid needs

Example:

3 ml × 30 kg × 40% = 3600 ml

Figuring Rate of Administration

$\frac{1}{2}$	$\frac{1}{4}$	$\frac{1}{4}$
First 8 h	Second 8 h	Third 8 h
1800 ml	900 ml	900 ml

*Used with permission of Shriners Burns Institute, Cincinnati.

and acetone levels. A nasogastric tube attached to suction is useful in avoiding gastric distress. Table 27-7 summarizes nursing interventions.

During the admission procedure, the wound is washed with a solution of saline, peroxide, and mild detergent. For larger burns, when the equipment is available, wound cleansing may be more effectively done in a whirlpool tank. A gentle washing technique should be used to remove loose skin and foreign materials. Following a complete cleansing and rinsing, a more accurate assessment of the extent of the burn is possible, and,

Table 27-7 Summary of Nursing Interventions

Child's Needs	Nursing Action
First Aid	Stop the burning process. Do cardiopulmonary resuscitation as needed. Evaluate for other injuries and stabilize as necessary. Remove loose clothing from burned area. Cover with clean, dry wraps. Give nothing by mouth. Insert IV lines. Transport or admit as indicated.
Immediate Care	
General nursing considerations	Assess severity of burn. Initiate fluid therapy to control burn shock. Insert nasogastric tube. Insert Foley catheter for fluid titration. Do baseline ECG, take x-ray, and do blood work.
Respiratory support	Assess for signs of respiratory involvement. Support ventilation with oxygen, frequent suctioning, positioning, and intubation as needed. Monitor blood gases. Reassure the child.
Hair removal	Shave hair from wound areas. Shave beards (if adolescent male). Keep hair clean and away from wound or cut.
Escharotomy	Perform escharotomy if necessary to relieve respiratory distress and prevent circulatory occlusion. Explain procedure to the child and the family. No pain medication should be necessary.
Positioning	Place the child in a semi-Fowler's or high Fowler's position to prevent aspiration and reduce workload of the heart. Elevate the arms on pillows.
Support measures	Give all pain medications intravenously. Support the family and the child. Let the family talk with the child before separation or before insertion of the endotracheal tube, since there may not be a chance for verbal interaction for some time.
Acute Care	
General nursing measures	Insert nasogastric tube. Control pain. Control infection. Weigh the child. Give fluid resuscitation to maintain adequate output. Provide emotional support for the child and the family. Allow for rest. Give wound care.
Promoting wound healing	Clean and debride the wound. Utilize appropriate techniques of open or closed dressing procedures. Prevent trauma to healing tissue. Give nutritional support to maintain anabolic phase of metabolism.

Table 27-7 Summary of Nursing Interventions (*Continued*)

Child's Needs	Nursing Action
Management and prevention of complications	Attach nasogastric tube to suction; give antacids q2h. Titrate fluids. Observe for signs of respiratory compromise. Have the child turn, cough, and deep-breathe.
Infection control	Use good aseptic technique. Administer topical and systemic antimicrobials as ordered. Do routine wound cultures. Support the immune system. Give adequate nutritional support.
Positioning and comfort measures	Maintain proper body alignment. Turn the child frequently. Provide for exercise (active and passive). Give relaxing massages. Prevent deformity, such as foot-drop.
Hygiene	Give mouth care. Bathe unburned areas and shampoo to control infection and maintain healthy unburned tissue.
Nutrition	Observe for signs of poor nutritional management, including weakness; fatigue; poor healing; derangements of fat, carbohydrate, and protein metabolism; anemia; and weight loss. Offer frequent feedings. Give high-protein, high-calorie supplements. Offer foods appropriate to the child's developmental stage and personal preferences. Conserve energy and body heat.
Emotional Support	Minimize regression. Encourage interaction with others and the environment. Develop a one-on-one relationship with the primary nurse. Support the family. Modify nursing approach as the child and the family move through the psychological response phases of impact, retreat, acknowledgment, and reconstruction. Explain procedures. Be honest and consistent.
Pain Assessment and Management	
Assessment	Be aware that pain is an individual, subjective feeling for each child. Assess indicators of pain, including physiological manifestations, verbal statements, vocalizations, facial expressions, body movements, and responses to the surrounding environment.
Treatment	Administer drugs. Provide diversional activities. Give trance and hypnotic therapy. Involve the child in treatment procedures. Hold and stroke the child.
Rehabilitation	Begin rehabilitation at the time of injury. Provide early mobilization. Provide active and passive exercises. Provide games and play exercises. Supply individually fitted splints and braces, applied properly and evaluated and modified regularly.
Discharge Planning	Include the family early in the treatment program. Provide resource identification and coordination. Hold predischarge interagency planning conferences. Provide information and age-specific teaching plans for home care procedures. Arrange for appropriate follow-up processes prior to discharge. Ensure the availability of supplies and equipment. Encourage the parents' and the child's verbalizations of concerns and questions.

if necessary, alterations are made in fluid therapy. All solutions used for wound care should be warmed to body temperature. The importance of strict aseptic technique throughout the admission procedure must be stressed.

Infection In a thermal injury, the skin, which is the body's first line of defense against infection, has been destroyed. During the overwhelming stress response, the immunologic response of the body is taxed to the extreme, and infection is a major threat to the burned child. Maintaining the overall physiological status of the child through optimum nursing and medical care helps the body resist infection. It is practically impossible to maintain a sterile burn wound. Common organisms which may colonize the burn wound are *Candida, Staphylococcus aureus, Streptococcus, Providencia stuartii,* and *Pseudomonas.* Although there have been great advances in controlling burn wound infection with antibiotic therapy during the past decade, resistant strains of organisms have developed. Therefore, prophylaxis through meticulous nursing care is still essential. Penicillin is sometimes given on admission as a prophylactic against *Streptococcus* and *Staphylococcus* organisms, which are normal skin flora. Routine wound cultures done twice weekly for organism identification and antibiotic sensitivity are useful in determining the antimicrobial of choice. Many commercial antimicrobials are available, and the nurse must be aware of the indications for these agents and of the dosages and routes of administration.[10]

The patient and the patient's environment are also sources of infection, since normal skin bacteria may be present in hair follicles and on unburned skin. Other patients, personnel, and equipment are also possible sources of contamination. Good aseptic technique, prevention of cross-contamination, support of the patient's immune system, and constant monitoring for bacterial growth in wounds are essential for infection control. Table 27-8 lists factors associated with the development of wound infections.

Table 27-8 General Factors Associated with Development of Wound Infections

Depressed cellular and humoral host resistance factors
Recurrent or remote infection
Malnutrition
Prolonged preoperative hospitalization
Obesity
Shock
Antibiotic therapy preceding an operation
Certain chemotherapy such as cytotoxic drugs and steroids
Extremes of age
Certain diseases such as diabetes mellitus, advanced malignant disease, and lupus erythematosus

Wound care There are several generally accepted goals of wound care, including (1) minimizing infection, (2) removing dead tissue, (3) preventing conversion of a partial-thickness injury to full-thickness damage, (4) allowing for drainage from the wound, (5) preparing the wound for homografting and autografting, and (6) decreasing the severity of scars and contractures.

There are two major types of dressing procedures: open (or exposed) and closed.

Open method In the *open method,* after careful cleansing, the wound is left exposed to the air, and a dry, cool, clean environment is provided. A crust forms over the wound that serves as a protective layer for underlying tissue and prevents bacterial growth. This method may be modified by the topical application of antimicrobial ointments or creams, applied either directly on the wound or impregnated in fine-mesh gauze.

Closed method When the *closed method* is used, the wound must also be carefully cleaned and rinsed prior to each dressing application. At least twice daily the wound is thoroughly cleaned of all exudate, creams, and ointments and is examined visually. After washing and rinsing and before applying the dressing, cultures should be obtained twice a week to determine a sensitivity profile for selection of topical antibiotics. Cleansing is done at the bedside with sterile basins of washing solution (described earlier) or in a whirlpool tank. Manual debridement should be done at this time, and all loose eschar should be removed. A single layer of gauze, impregnated with the topical agent of choice, is applied to the wound. A useful hint for the application of topical agents is to use fine-mesh gauze for impregnating with ointments and coarse-mesh gauze for impregnating with creams. The wound is then wrapped with several layers of coarse-mesh gauze bandage to absorb drainage and protect the wound. When the impregnated gauze layer is applied, it should not be wrapped circumferentially around the extremity or trunk. If it is wrapped circumferentially, as edema forms or as drainage saturates the gauze and dries, constriction may result, leading to circulatory impairment. Rather, vertical strips should be placed next to one another, and overlapping of strips and contact with unburned tissue should be avoided. When necessary, the gauze should be cut to match the approximate size of the wound, since topical agents can cause irritation to healthy skin. Mesh may be used as a final layer to secure the dressing in place.

Topical agents There are several commercially available *topical agents*. The agent chosen should not produce electrolyte imbalance, should cause minimal discomfort to the child, should promote eschar separation, and should have antimicrobial effects.

Silvadene (silver sulfadiazine), a silver substance in a water-soluble cream base, is an effective inhibitor of gram-negative, gram-positive, and *Candida albicans* organisms. It acts on the cell wall and membrane. Its advantages include little delay in eschar separation, no pain or burning on application, and no known electrolyte imbalance. It is applied directly to the wound by "buttering" or may be impregnated in coarse-mesh gauze (Fig. 27-5).

Sulfamylon (mafenide acetate) is also used as a topical antimicrobial. It is effective against gram-positive and gram-negative organisms, diffusing through the eschar for infection control. It is usually applied twice daily and is thoroughly removed before reapplication. Because Sulfamylon is a carbonic anhydrase inhibitor, the renal buffering system may be inhibited. When used on children with respiratory impairment, care should be taken to observe for acid-base imbalance. Children may complain of stinging when the cream is initially applied. In addition, some children may develop a rash, which should be noted and reported. The method of application is as discussed for Silvadene. Care should be taken with all topicals to avoid contact with healthy skin.

Betadine (providone-iodine) has broad-spectrum germicidal action against common organisms. It is nonirritating, does not block air from the site of application, and is easily washed off skin and natural fibers. It has the advantage of being available in an assortment of forms—ointments, solutions, sprays, foams, and swabs. The foam form is especially convenient for the nurse, since it is water-soluble, adheres and conforms to the shape of the wound, and has little runoff while providing protection. Betadine is applied topically in a manner consistent with the form selected, and a dressing may be applied. As must be done when using other topical agents, the wound should be washed once or twice daily, and fresh Betadine must be applied.

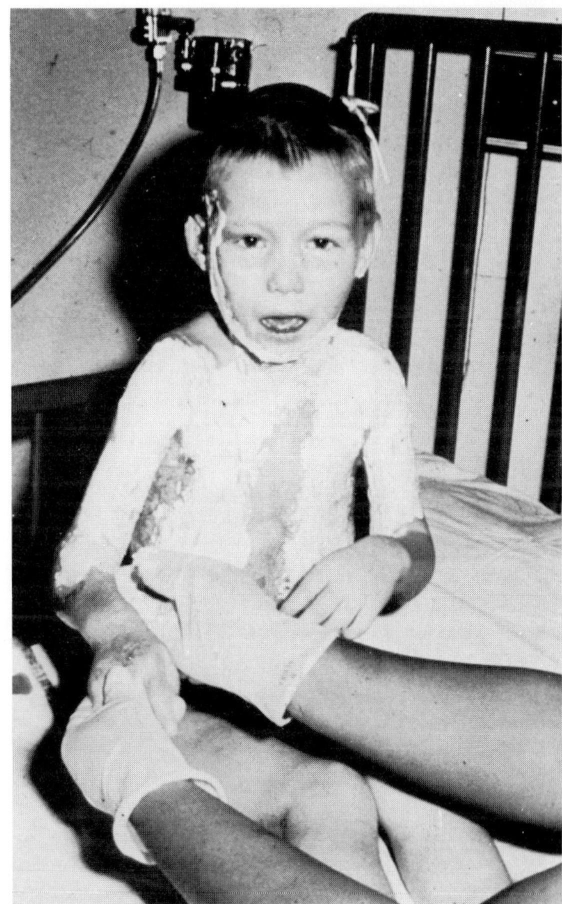

Figure 27-5 Application of silver sulfadiazine to the burn wound of a child with a 50 percent burn. (*From G. Scipien, M. U. Barnard, M. A. Chard, J. Howe, and P. J. Phillips* [*eds.*], *Comprehensive Pediatric Nursing, 3d ed., McGraw-Hill, New York, 1986, p. 1336. Used with permission.*)

Silver nitrate is a liquid which is applied to a burn wound as a continuous wet dressing, similar to saline soaks. The silver ion is considered bactericidal, but the solution can penetrate only 1 to 2 cm of burn eschar and is not effective on already deeply colonized wounds. Since the dressing must remain saturated, several layers of gauze dressing are saturated and held in place by stretch gauze wrap. While the child is usually very comfortable with this solution, evaporative heat loss from the wet dressing is a problem. The child should be covered with a blanket to minimize heat loss, and bed linens should be changed as they become wet. Children should be monitored carefully for loss of sodium and potassium ions, and supplements should be given by mouth or intravenously, as tolerated. This type of dressing is especially tedious for the nurse. The child's bed must be kept dry, while the dressings must be kept saturated to avoid drying and concentration of the silver ion on the skin. In addition, the solution stains everything with which it comes in contact black. Walls, uniforms, and linens should be protected, since special stain removers are required.

Gentamicin is a broad-spectrum antibiotic and is highly effective in the treatment of primary and secondary bacterial infections of the skin. Bacteria susceptible to the agent include sensitive strains of streptococci (including group A beta hemolytic), *Pseudomonas*, and *Klebsiella*. It is a bactericidal agent and has the same advantages as silver sulfadiazine. It may be "buttered" directly onto the wound, or fine-mesh gauze can be impregnated with gentamicin and then applied.

Surgical procedures (excision and grafting)

Excision Removal of eschar is essential for ultimate wound closure, and the decision may be made to surgically remove (excise) the eschar rather than wait for natural sloughing. Such surgical excision may lower the risk of mortality, facilitate early rehabilitation, and shorten the time of hospitalization. Some removal of eschar may be done by the nurse at the bedside or in a whirlpool tank, but only that tissue which can be removed with limited bleeding should be removed. Blunt, sterile scissors are used to clip away devitalized tissue. A gentle scrubbing motion is also effective in removing eschar. Aggressive scrubbing or probing with scissors and forceps is unnecessary and may damage the underlying wound bed, which is important for grafting.

Extensive removal of eschar is done in the operating room under anesthesia. Excision includes all deep dermal and full-thickness burned tissue down to the normal tissue layer. Because blood loss may be extensive during surgery, transfusions are often indicated on the day of surgery. The nurse should thus be aware of the risks, complications, and needs of the child in regard to the use of blood products.

Grafting If possible, the wound is closed with autografts at the same time that excision is performed. *Autografts* are skin grafts taken from an uninjured or healthy area on the child. Such grafts may be of partial thickness (0.010 to 0.035 in) or full thickness (greater than 0.035 in). Partial-thickness grafts are usually used for greater area coverage, because when full-thickness grafts are taken, the donor site itself must be grafted for closure. Full-thickness grafts are indicated for selected reconstructive cases, such as on the hands, where tissue strength is needed, and on the face, for cosmetic purposes. Partial-thickness grafts are expanded by passing the tissue through a mesh dermatome. Expansion in this manner allows for added coverage when limited good tissue is available for wound closure. It also decreases the size of the donor site needed. For expansion, the mesh dermatome makes small slits in the tissue. When expanded, these small slits become small diamond-shaped openings within the sheet of tissue, making it possible to expand the skin to from 2 to 3 times its original width. These small openings can then epithelize from the margins of surrounding skin. These small openings also allow for adequate drainage of serum from the wound (Figs. 27-6 and 27-7).

Care should be taken when changing dressings on grafted areas. An accepted procedure is for no dressing change to be undertaken until 3 days after grafting. The initial dressing change on the third day is then done by the physician,

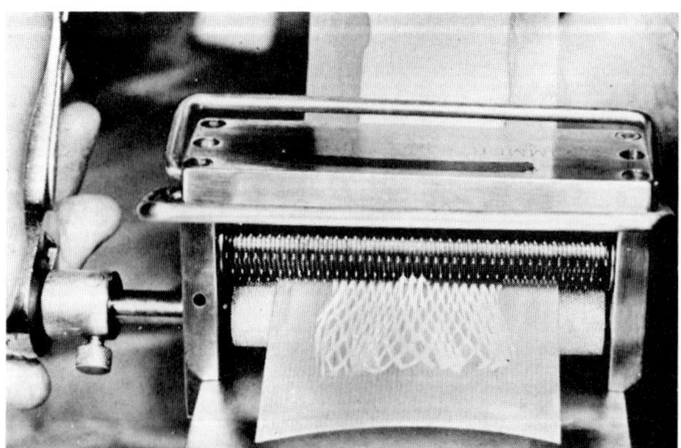

Figure 27-6 Mesh dermatome reduces the size of the tissue needed for grafting by making slits to allow for expansion of the graft. (*Shriners Burn Institute, Cincinnati. Used with permission.*)

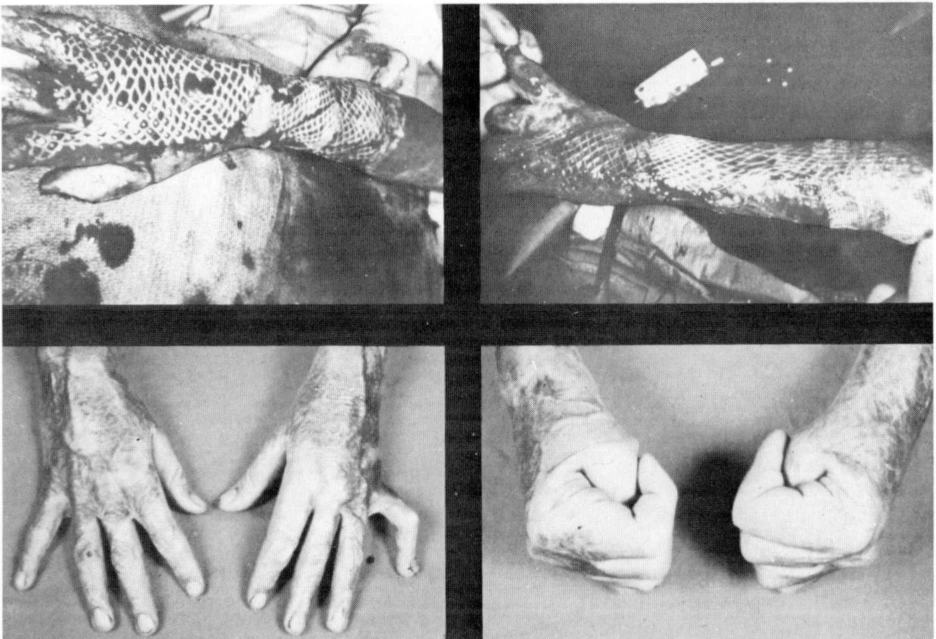

Figure 27-7 Hands showing the use of mesh autografts and progressive stages of healing. (*Shriners Burn Institute, Cincinnati. Used with permission.*)

who examines the area for graft take. As the nurse resumes dressing change procedures, he or she must be careful not to damage epithelizing tissue. Strict aseptic technique is continued in order to prevent infection, which can destroy the graft and result in the need for another grafting procedure.

Frequently, the severely burned child has limited areas available for donor sites. In such cases, homografts or heterografts are used. *Homografts* are skin taken from a person other than the patient, usually cadaver skin available through tissue banks. *Heterografts* are taken from an animal, such as a pig or a dog. Pigskin dressings are frequently encountered by the nurse. They are applied in much the same way as dressings using topical antimicrobial agents. Heterografts and homografts decrease water and electrolyte loss from the burn wound and protect the area either until it is ready for autografting or until donor sites are available. They are changed every 2 to 3 days. When the underlying tissue is pink and vascularization has occurred, the wound bed is ready for autografting.

The donor site itself represents a second-degree injury and requires optimal nursing care. At the time of surgery, the donor site is covered with a single sheet of fine-mesh gauze. This remains in place, and the wound is exposed to air and allowed to dry. As the wound heals, edges of the gauze will loosen and should be clipped away with scissors by the nurse. Preventing infection and minimizing moisture and pressure on the donor site are important.

Nutritional support Burn hypermetabolism continues to be a major concern in nursing care. Evaporative water loss, elevated temperature, and increased catecholamines may all contribute to the increased metabolic rate. The exact cause is still debated. Carbohydrates, as the main source of energy for muscle work and body heat production, are rapidly metabolized. Carbohydrate metabolism is shifted from energy storage to energy utilization. Body stores of fat and protein are depleted through catabolism. The dietary requirements of a child who has suffered a burn may be 2 to 4 times as great as those of a normal child and are essential for tissue repair and survival. A diet high in protein, calories, vitamins B and C, and iron is needed.

The nurse, the dietitian, the family, and the

child must all be involved in meeting these requirements. The child's food likes and dislikes should be determined. Foods which taste good can be served attractively. Between-meal snacks, such as milk shakes and ice cream, and electrolyte solutions, such as Gatorade, are all readily available. Nutritional supplements given by feeding tube or by mouth are helpful, as are supplements of vitamins and minerals. Commercially produced high-protein and high-calorie mixtures are available and may be served between meals. Such mixtures tend to be hypertonic, pulling water into the gastrointestinal tract, and so the nurse should observe for diarrhea. Supplemental vitamins, potassium, and calcium are frequently calculated into the nutritional regimen. Total caloric intake is recorded, and the child is weighed frequently. During the acute phase when edema is present, the child should be weighed daily. During the healing period, the child is weighed twice weekly to evaluate weight loss and adequacy of caloric intake. Treatments should be planned so that they do not interfere with mealtimes. The nurse should make every effort to assist in conservation of the child's energy and body heat by avoiding unnecessary exposure of the burn wound, by properly applying the dressings, and by maintaining a comfortably warm environment.

Emotional needs

No matter how small the burn surface is, the injury represents a change in body appearance and requires a process of adjustment. The nurse should not minimize the significance of the altered body image and should recognize the child's attempt, over time, to deal with the alteration.

Trauma response pattern A pattern of response, which can be anticipated after a burn injury, has been described.[11] An understanding of this response helps the nurse better meet the emotional needs of the child and his or her family.

Impact The initial response, or *impact*, is one of shock and disbelief. The child may be confused and frightened. Lack of oxygen, electrolyte imbalance, and strange surroundings all contribute to restlessness and disorientation.

Depersonalization *Depersonalization* also occurs at this time. Often children perceive what is happening, but do not experience the event as happening to them. The family is also confused and frightened. They have no understanding of the severity of the injury or of the expected treatment. They are overwhelmed by the many decisions which must be made. The nurse's intervention should be structured to decrease the family's anxiety. Procedures are explained to the family and the child in a supportive, honest manner. Short, simple explanations are given in a calm tone. Honesty is essential, since this is the beginning of the trust relationship, which must develop between the staff, the child, and the family.

Retreat As the shock begins to lessen, a second response, a period of *retreat*, or withdrawal, may be observed. During this period a mechanism occurs whereby the child and the family attempt to negate the seriousness of the situation and avoid it through repression and suppression. This denial brings a sense of relief, and it will persist until the child and the family are faced with reality. The nurse accepts this but does not reinforce it. Rather, the nurse presents reality in small amounts and in a supportive manner, maintaining a relationship with the child and the family.

Acknowledgment As the family begins to recognize the significance of the illness, there is a period of *acknowledgment* and mourning. The child and the family have experienced many losses, and both anger and depression are common at this time. The child has lost independence, body image, and previous roles, such as that of a sibling or a sixth-grader. The child must begin to assimilate the new role of patient. The nurse's acceptance of the child will support the child's self-acceptance. Even if the burn is not fatal, the family has lost the child as they knew him or her before the injury, and they may have to give up some of the expectations they once had for the child's future. They may experience feelings of guilt, anger, and depression, which may cause them to avoid the child at a time when loving and caring are needed. Additional conflict may result as the staff members perform many of the functions that were previously performed by the family. The delegation of authority from the family to the staff is often nonverbal and anxiety-provoking. The nurse should encourage the family to recognize and express their feelings. The nurse's support at this time can allow the family to maintain emotional contact with the child as they move toward planning for the future. The nurse should include the child in the treatment plans and should be available to talk with the child.

The reconstructive phase The family and the child move toward the *reconstructive* phase. This is a time for new approaches to life. Doubts and fears of failure emerge, as the child tries new ways to manage the environment when confronted with his or her limitations. The nurse reinforces realistic goals through encouragement, acceptance, and collaborative planning.

The nurse should be aware that the burned child experiences a significant amount of both acute and chronic pain. The child's pain often has psychological implications. Chronic pain is associated with the loss of skin and exposed nerve endings. The most frequently encountered acute pain is during dressing changes and debridement. Fear, anxiety, and the absence of the parents often contribute to the pain response. Because pain is a subjective experience, the nurse should attempt to assess pain levels more objectively by eliciting the child's own report of pain, observing the child's behavior, and assessing preinjury behavior patterns. For care of the child in pain, see Chap. 34.

While little can be done to make such painful procedures as dressing changes, debridements, whirlpool baths, and physical therapy pleasant, the nurse can take steps to help the child. Explaining the procedure and its purpose may decrease anxiety. Giving skilled nursing care and removing dressings as quickly and painlessly as possible are also important. Supporting children's expressions of feelings and allowing them to participate in debridement and dressing removal give them a feeling of some control over what is happening to them and a sense of importance.

Play therapy is especially helpful in a pediatric burn unit. Play can be classified as therapeutic or diversional, and both are useful. *Diversional play* allows relaxation as children endure long weeks of hospitalization. *Therapeutic play* is more structured and serves several purposes: (1) it permits expression of feelings such as aggression and fear; (2) it clarifies distorted perceptions; (3) it allows assessment of the child's emotional developmental level and degree of regression; (4) it provides stimulation; and (5) it prepares the child for discharge.

The burn team To meet the emotional needs of the child and the family, the nurse must be in touch with his or her own feelings. Caring for children with burns is emotionally difficult. Nurses frequently see their role as that of helping others, relieving distress, and returning the child to society. Providing nursing care to burned children, however, includes performing nursing care procedures which result in pain, and the child may be discharged with scars and the prospect of further reconstructive surgery. In severe burns, death is an ever-present threat. The patient care team forms a mutual support group in which feelings can be shared and accepted. Through such support and acceptance of their own feelings, those on the burn team can help the family and the child to reach optimal physical and emotional rehabilitation.

Good emotional care includes observing, assessing, interacting, and intervening. In some units a mental health team consisting of a nurse, a psychiatrist, a physical therapist, and a social worker may be formed. In other units, a mental health specialist is available for consultation. In all settings the nurse must remember that good emotional support is not the responsibility of one individual. It is the responsibility of all who come in contact with the child and his or her family.

Rehabilitation

Rehabilitation begins early in the nursing process; the goal is to promote optimal physical, social, and emotional adjustment in the child. For example, if allowed to heal without proper positioning, exercises, and splinting, a third-degree burn can cause complete immobilization of a joint in a nonfunctional position, and surgical release will be required.

Early mobilization is one of the best methods of preventing many complications. Active and passive exercises are used to strengthen the child and maintain joint function. An excellent time to perform such exercises is during tubbing procedures. The soothing action and the buoyancy of the water help the child exercise with less pain. Passive exercises are performed by the nurse, the physical therapist, and the parents early in the hospitalization. As the wound is grafted and heals, the child can engage in more active exercise. Children can be encouraged to exercise while they watch television. Such gross motor activities as ball throwing or gymnastic-type games also provide exercise and social stimulation. Formal exercise must be done at least twice a day.

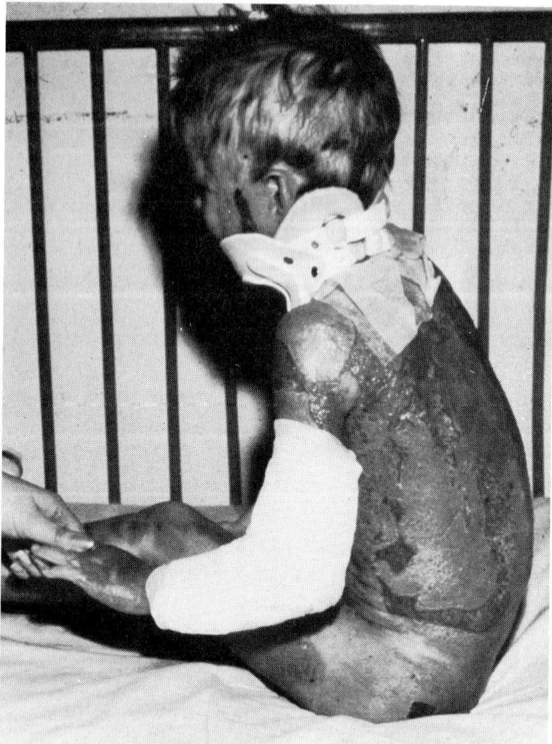

Figure 27-8 The use of neck and elbow splints to prevent further contractures in a child with a 50 percent burn. (*From G. Scipien, M. U. Barnard, M. A. Chard, J. Howe, and P. J. Phillips* [eds.], *Comprehensive Pediatric Nursing, 3d ed., McGraw Hill, New York, 1986, p. 1343. Used with permission.*)

Individually fitted splints and braces help maintain joint function. Some are worn 24 h a day and are removed only for washing, dressing changes, and exercise. Others are used only when the child is in bed or is out of bed, depending on the purpose of the device. The nurse must see that these appliances are worn in the correct manner and at the times specified. A well-made splint accomplishes nothing if it is allowed to be stuffed in a bag of toys or in a bedside table rather than being worn by the child (Fig. 27-8).

Some of the frequently encountered problems that the family faces at discharge are itching, the appearance of the scar, unhealed wound tissue, and splints and braces. The scar may be rough and red; as the scar matures over time, this usually decreases. Itching and flaking of the scar should be discussed with the parents. Scratching can damage the tissue and cause infection. Mild cream can be applied at home and massaged into the tissue. It will help eliminate itching and will soften the scar.[12]

There may be small unhealed areas when the child is discharged, and a small dressing may be needed. Optimal cleansing and bathing should be stressed. A few days prior to discharge, the person who will be responsible for the child's home care should come to the unit and begin performing these activities, with the staff present for support and guidance. The parents are also instructed in the proper fit and application of splints and braces. They are encouraged to report any problems to the unit or a physician.

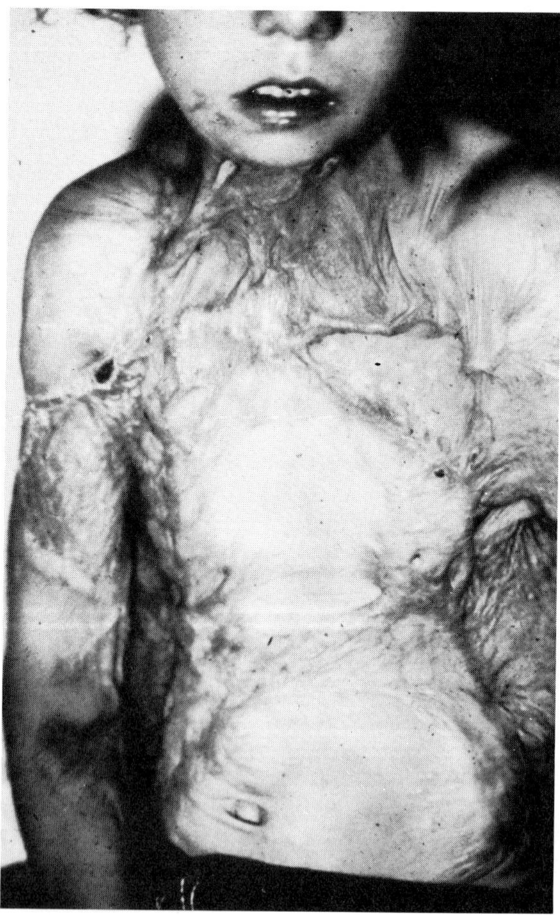

Figure 27-9 Contractures resulting from inadequate follow-up care after a 50 percent burn. This photograph was taken 2 years after the injury. (*From G. Scipien, M. U. Barnard, M. A. Chard, J. Howe, and P. J. Phillips* [eds.], *Comprehensive Pediatric Nursing, 3d ed., McGraw-Hill, New York, 1986, p. 1345. Used with permission.*)

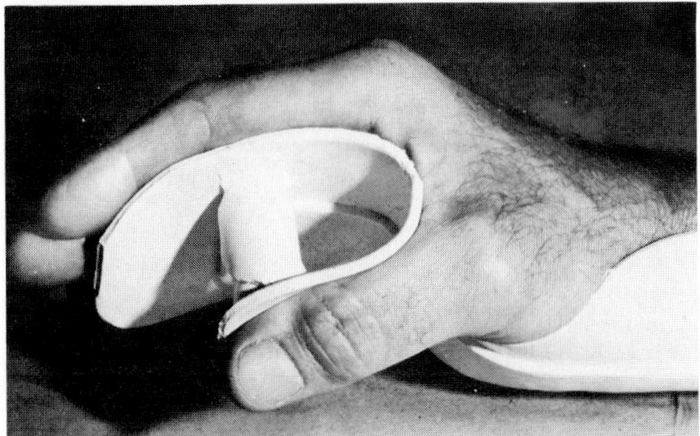

Figure 27-10 A molded hand splint demonstrated on a therapist. (*Shriners Burn Institute, Cincinnati. Used with permission.*)

Even with optimal care, some dysfunction or cosmetic problems cannot be prevented, and surgery will be necessary. This is especially true of children in whom scar tissue growth does not coincide with muscular and skeletal development (Fig. 27-9). The scar is often allowed to mature for 1 year before surgery is performed. The child should understand at the time of discharge the need for future surgical admissions. Most surgical contracture releases involve excision of the scar and inlay of a graft. Splints, molded appliances to maintain position, and special braces may be necessary for a short period following surgery to maintain the functional position obtained (Fig. 27-10).

As the child matures, physical deformities will present unique problems at each phase of growth and development. Adjustment to school requires collaboration between the child, the family, the teacher, and the school system. Adolescence brings a preoccupation with physical attributes, and social service agencies should be called on to prevent psychological maladjustment. In addition, physical growth spurts and sexual development may necessitate surgery. If a child's chest wall has been extensively burned, with resulting inelastic scar tissues, for example, surgical release may be necessary for breast development.

The goal of rehabilitating the child so that he or she can be an optimally functioning member of society is the responsibility of all members of the burn team. Collaboration between the child, the family, community agencies, and the family physician should be ongoing.[13]

Nursing Care Plan: Burn

Patient: Joey Martino *Age:* 2 years *Date of Admission:* 1/15 10:30 A.M.

ASSESSMENT

Joey Martino, 2 years old, was burned when his older sibling threw gasoline on burning trash. The flames quickly ignited the front of Joey's sweater. The child's parents immersed him in cool water immediately and summoned an ambulance.

Upon arrival at the emergency room, Joey was crying with pain, and he was obviously frightened. Both parents were distraught. Loud wheezing was audible (without the aid of a stethoscope) between Joey's sobs. Since Joey had burns around his head and neck, an endotracheal tube was immediately inserted to ensure a patent airway. An intravenous cutdown was performed in an unaffected lower extremity, and a Ringer's lactate infusion was initiated. Joey's weight was 28 lb (12.7 kg) on admission to the emergency room. Vital signs were stable and within normal limits.

The physicians determined that Joey's burns covered 35 percent of his body. He had second-degree burns on his face, ears, neck, upper anterior trunk, parts of both upper and lower arms, and both hands. He also suffered third-degree burns on both upper and lower arms and on a small portion of the anterior trunk (see Burn Evaluation Chart). Fluid resuscitation and wound treatment were started in the emergency room. Before Joey was transferred to the pediatric unit, a central venous pressure line, a nasogastric tube, and a Foley catheter were inserted.

Joey responded well to therapy, and diuresis began 51 h postburn. His weight is now $29\frac{1}{2}$ lb (13.4 kg). Much of the facial and neck edema that resulted from his burns has subsided, but some periocular edema remains. He has full range of motion of his neck. Joey's endotracheal tube and Foley catheter were removed 24 h ago. His respirations are regular at 28 to 30 per min. Scattered bilateral wheezing is audible on auscultation. His other vital signs are stable and within normal limits. Joey's bowel sounds returned 44 h postburn, and the nasogastric tube was removed 12 h later. Full range of motion of burned extremities can be elicited during dressing changes. Joey is generally cooperative, but he protests vigorously during dressing changes. Partial-thickness skin grafts will be applied to areas that suffered third-degree burns. This surgery will be performed in approximately 4 days.

Joey lives with his parents, his $3\frac{1}{2}$-year-old brother, and his 5-year-old sister. Prior to his injury, Joey was in good health and demonstrated growth and development appropriate for his age. His immunizations are up to date, and he has no known drug sensitivities or allergies. He has not had any communicable diseases. There is no family history of heart disease or diabetes mellitus. At least one of Joey's parents has remained at his bedside since admission.

Burn Evaluation Chart

Area	Percent of Total Body Surface Area*	Percent Burned	
		2°	3°
Head	17	5	0
Neck	2	1.5	0
Anterior trunk	13	6.5	4
Right upper arm	4	2	2
Left upper arm	4	2	2
Right lower arm	3	1.5	1.5
Left lower arm	3	1	2
Right hand	2.5	2	0
Left hand	2.5	2	0

*The percent of total body surface area in a child between the ages of 1 and 4 years.

The author acknowledges the assistance of Arlene Church Miller in preparing this Nursing Care Plan.

Nursing diagnosis	Outcome Criteria	Nursing Interventions	Evaluation and Modifications
1. Potential for ineffective breathing pattern related to neck and facial edema and to restricted chest expansion	☐ Respiratory rate will be between 28 and 32 per min. ☐ Breath sounds will be clear. ☐ There will be symmetrical chest movements during respirations. ☐ The skin and mucous membranes in unaffected areas will remain pink.	☐ Monitor respiratory rate and rhythm q1h and record. ☐ Auscultate lungs q1h; note abnormal sounds (rales, rhonchi, wheezing). ☐ Do nasal and oropharyngeal suctioning prn; notify physician if Joey requires tracheal suctioning to remove secretions. ☐ Observe for labored breathing, hoarseness, stridor, restlessness, paradoxical chest movement, cyanosis, and sudden high fever. ☐ Notify physician of abnormal breathing patterns.	☐ Respiratory rate stable; averages 28 to 30 per min. ☐ Wheezing substantially diminished in last 24 h; faint bilateral scattered wheezing audible upon auscultation only; Joey is able to cough effectively.
		☐ Keep oropharyngeal airway, endotracheal tube, and oxygen at bedside.	☐ Continue plan.
2. Impairment of skin integrity related to second- and third-degree thermal burns	☐ The burn wounds will heal (revascularization and reepithelization).	☐ Provide wound care: **a.** Apply continuous wet silver nitrate dressings to arms and anterior trunk; redress q8h (9 A.M., 5 P.M., and 1 A.M.) and rewet q8h (1 P.M., 9 P.M., and 5 A.M.). **b.** Apply silver sulfadiazine and gauze dressing to face, neck, and hands q8h (9 A.M., 5 P.M., and 1 A.M.). ☐ Provide meticulous care of the face, eyes, ears, and hands. ☐ Handle wounds gently. ☐ Avoid pressure by frequent turning and positioning. ☐ Observe and record the appearance of wounds at each dressing change. ☐ Administer a sedative or analgesic, as ordered, prior to dressing changes. ☐ Carry out actions for potential infection.	☐ Even blood supply observed during dressing changes.
	☐ Joey's ears will return to a normal appearance.	☐ Apply warm, wet compresses to ears, as specified by physician. ☐ Use sufficient layers of gauze to separate skin layers and facilitate drainage.	☐ Ears are returning to normal appearance; some edema and redness remain.

Nursing diagnosis	Outcome Criteria	Nursing Interventions	Evaluation and Modifications
		☐ Examine ears q8h; observe pinna for edema, tenderness, pain, and redness. ☐ Position Joey to prevent pressure on ears.	☐ Continue plan.
3. Pain related to second-degree burns	☐ Joey will obtain sufficient relief from pain, enabling him to: **a.** Sleep at least 4 continuous h. **b.** Perform active range-of-motion exercises. **c.** Withstand dressing changes.	☐ Observe frequently for signs of pain (irritability, crying, "guarding" of affected areas, withdrawal, and rocking or rhythmic movements). ☐ Communicate to other staff members Joey's pattern of pain expression. ☐ Coordinate care activities to allow for periods of uninterrupted sleep. ☐ Administer analgesic, prn, as ordered. ☐ Coordinate administration of analgesic with dressing changes whenever possible; administer medication approximately 1 h prior to treatment.	☐ Acetaminophen elixir, 120 mg, appears effective; requires medication q5 to 6 h. ☐ Falls asleep within 45 min after receiving medication. ☐ Continue plan.
4. Potential for infection related to thermal burns	☐ Burn wounds will remain free of infection.	☐ Use strict aseptic technique; sterile gown, gloves, and mask. ☐ Employ reverse isolation. ☐ Explain reasons for precautions to parents. ☐ Teach parents how to don and discard gown, gloves, and mask. ☐ Provide wound care as specified. ☐ Culture wounds twice a week. ☐ Prevent Joey from touching and picking at wounds and dressings. ☐ Change soiled dressings immediately. ☐ Administer antibiotic as prescribed by physician.	☐ No exudate observed in wounds. ☐ Negative wound cultures. ☐ Continue plan.
5. Potential fluid volume deficit related to burn sequelae	☐ Vital signs will be within normal limits, as evidenced by: **a.** Rectal temperature between 36.7 and 38.2°C (98° and 100.8°F) **b.** Pulse between 100 and 140 per minute	☐ Monitor and record vital signs and central venous pressure q2h.	☐ Vital signs were stable during previous 24 h. Temperature: 37.2 to 38.2°C (99° to 100.8°F). Pulse: 110 to 122 per minute. Respirations: 28 to 30 breaths per minute. Blood pressure: 90/56 to 96/60. Central venous pressure: 4 to 6 cm.

Nursing diagnosis	Outcome Criteria	Nursing Interventions	Evaluation and Modifications
	c. Respirations between 28 and 32 breaths per minute **d.** Blood pressure between 88/54 and 98/60 **e.** Central venous pressure between 3 and 10 cm		
	☐ 24-h fluid intake (IV and PO) will be equivalent to amount specified by physician.	☐ Maintain IV infusion at rate specified by physician and record amount infused q1h. Give sips of clear liquids after removal of nasogastric tube; increase oral intake gradually, as tolerated.	☐ Intake during previous 24 h was 2450 ml (IV, 1900 ml; PO, 550 ml).
	☐ Urinary function will be within normal limits, as evidenced by: **a.** Urinary output of at least 15 ml/h **b.** Urine specific gravity between 1.002 and 1.028	☐ Notify physician if hourly oral fluid intake exceeds 40 ml for 3 h; regulate IV rate accordingly. ☐ Measure and record intake and output q2h. ☐ Use pediatric urine collection device to obtain *accurate* output. ☐ Monitor and record urine specific gravity q4h.	☐ Urinary output during previous 24 h was 1934 ml. ☐ Urine specific gravity during previous 8 h 1.007 to 1.012.
	☐ Joey will return to his preburn weight of 12.7 kg within 4 to 10 days postburn and will maintain his preburn weight thereafter.	☐ Weigh q8h (*after* dressings have been removed). ☐ Observe for signs of fluid volume overload (increased central venous pressure, marked increase in urinary output, dyspnea, rales, irritability, seizures). ☐ Observe for signs of fluid volume deficit (decreased urinary output, thirst, dry mucous membranes, urine specific gravity above 1.030, tachycardia, poor skin turgor). ☐ Notify physician of abnormal signs or symptoms, prn.	☐ Weight is 13.4 kg (29½ lb); no change in last 24 h. ☐ Continue plan.
6. Potential alteration in thermoregulation related to burn sequelae	☐ Rectal temperature will be stable between 36.7 and 38.2°C (98° and 100.8°F).	☐ Monitor rectal temperature q2h and record. ☐ Observe for shivering and excessive diuresis. ☐ Apply warm silver nitrate and saline prior to dressing changes and treatments.	☐ Temperature was stable during previous 24 h, ranging between 36.7 and 38.7°C (98° and 101.6°F).

Nursing diagnosis	Outcome Criteria	Nursing Interventions	Evaluation and Modifications
		☐ Avoid extremes in environmental temperatures, drafts, and damp clothing or linens. ☐ Maintain adequate calorie intake. ☐ Notify physician of temperature liability.	☐ Continue plan.
7. Impaired mobility related to burn injury	☐ Joey will have full range of joint motion in his upper extremities and fingers.	☐ Encourage active motion of fingers and arms during waking hours. ☐ Encourage Joey to feed himself. ☐ Play games requiring use of arms and hands at least qid (Joey likes Inky-Dinky Spider and Simon Says). ☐ Do passive range-of-motion exercises tid, during dressing changes (9 A.M., 5 P.M., and 1 A.M.). ☐ Splint hands in position of function when Joey is asleep. Bandage fingers carefully, preventing contact between skin surfaces. Tell Joey that the bandages are like "big mittens."	☐ Joey demonstrates full range of motion in fingers while eating and at play; full range of wrist, elbow, and shoulder was elicited during dressing changes. ☐ Continue plan.
8. Potential nutritional deficit related to burn sequelae	☐ Oral intake will be at least 1980 kcal per 24 h. ☐ Protein intake will be at least 73 g per 24 h.	☐ Do daily calorie count. ☐ Do daily weight and record. ☐ Arrange meeting between Joey's mother and nutritionist to plan meals and snacks consisting of Joey's favorite foods. ☐ Gradually increase diet once Joey has been able to tolerate clear liquids for 8 h. ☐ Provide milk shakes, ice cream, and other high-caloric, high-protein supplements between meals and at bedtime. ☐ Provide finger foods, such as hot dogs and small pieces of fruit. ☐ Encourage but do not force Joey to eat. ☐ Give small, frequent feedings. ☐ Reward with praise when he does eat.	☐ Joey's caloric intake for the last 24 h was 1650 kcal. ☐ Weight is 13.4 kg (29½ lb). ☐ Joey has been taking liquids and soft foods for the last 16 h; will begin regular foods today. ☐ Joey needs much encouragement; takes only small amounts at one time.

Nursing diagnosis	Outcome Criteria	Nursing Interventions	Evaluation and Modifications
		☐ Plan care and activities to allow a rest period before and after meals. ☐ Administer supplemental vitamins and iron as ordered by physician.	
	☐ Joey will maintain normal bowel sounds and gastrointestinal function.	☐ Measure and record abdominal girth q4h. ☐ Test all stools for guaiac. ☐ Observe for "coffee-ground" vomitus, abdominal distention, and decreasing hematocrit and report to physician promptly. ☐ Administer antacid as ordered by physician.	☐ Bowel sounds returned 44 h postburn and remain audible upon auscultation. ☐ Abdominal girth is 55 cm; unchanged for last 48 h ☐ No bowel movements since nasogastric tube was removed. ☐ Continue plan.
9. Alteration in vision related to periocular edema	☐ Joey will regain his preburn visual ability.	☐ Identify self upon entering room until Joey's visual ability returns. ☐ Give short, simple explanations of procedures just prior to carrying them out. ☐ Irrigate eyes and instill ophthalmic ointment q4h, as prescribed. ☐ Observe and record condition of periocular skin and extent of edema; note any exudate. ☐ Tell Joey he will be able to see better when his eyes "open up."	☐ Eyelid edema is subsiding; clear exudate is easily removed by irrigation; no redness or purulent exudate. ☐ Joey can open his eyes about halfway. ☐ Continue plan.
10. Potential separation anxiety related to injury and hospitalization	☐ Joey will demonstrate behaviors expected of a toddler separated from his parents (crying and protesting when parents leave and negativism).	☐ Encourage rooming-in or frequent visiting by parents. ☐ Encourage parents to participate in Joey's care when they feel ready to do so. ☐ Minimize the number of staff caring for Joey (consistency). ☐ Keep all explanations simple and honest. ☐ Provide physical contact, such as holding and rocking, as much as possible. ☐ Allow Joey to demonstrate independence whenever appropriate (putting on slippers, selecting juice, selecting a toy for a play period, etc.).	☐ Joey continues to protest when parents leave and during treatments. ☐ Joey maintains interest in his surroundings and interacts with the environment.

Nursing diagnosis	Outcome Criteria	Nursing Interventions	Evaluation and Modifications
		☐ Expect some regressive behaviors (preference for a bottle, toilet "accidents," etc.). ☐ Suggest that parents leave a small personal item with Joey until they return. ☐ Suggest that siblings send drawings and little handmade projects to Joey. ☐ Suggest a short visit by siblings.	☐ Continue plan.
11. Alterations in family processes related to child's injury	☐ Parents will be able to: **a.** Verbalize their feelings about Joey's injury and hospitalization **b.** Identify ways they can assist siblings to express their feelings about Joey's injury	☐ Provide parents with time and privacy so that they can verbalize their concerns. ☐ Explain all treatments to parents. ☐ Answer parents' questions honestly and patiently; refer them to physician when appropriate. ☐ Suggest visits by grandparents or other adults who know Joey so that parents can spend time with siblings. ☐ Encourage parents to get enough sleep, to eat meals regularly, etc. ☐ Assure parents that nurses will be with Joey when they cannot be present.	☐ Parents were able to discuss the accident and their feelings with nurse on one occasion; further verbalization should be encouraged. ☐ Parents are willing to allow grandparents to relieve them for short periods.
		☐ Discuss methods of assisting siblings to express their feelings about Joey's injury. **a.** Tell parents that it is normal for the siblings to feel guilty, not only because of the accident, but also because it is normal for children to "wish" that their siblings would "go away." **b.** Suggest storytelling; a parent starts a story about a child, *not* named Joey, who was accidentally hurt while playing with his brother and sister; the parent then encourages the siblings to continue the story and fill in the rest of "what	☐ Parents are receptive to storytelling and other methods suggested by nurse; parents verbalized intention to try suggestions.

Nursing diagnosis	Outcome Criteria	Nursing Interventions	Evaluation and Modifications
		happened." Explain that the parents can use a story to explain what is happening to Joey now, to assure the siblings that he will come home, how accidents can happen, etc. **c.** Keep siblings informed about Joey's progress and his treatment (in simple terms). **d.** Have Joey send some little items home to his siblings. ☐ Before Joey is discharged, and when parents seem ready, introduce subject of accident prevention (do *not* blame parents); provide anticipatory teaching.	☐ Continue plan.

References

1. Fleming, Juanita W., "Common Dermatologic Conditions in Children," *Maternal-Child Nursing* **6**:347 (September–October 1981).
2. Hansen, Ronald, et al., "Perennial Problems, Disposing of Diaper Rash," *Patient Care* 59 (October 1984).
3. MacMillan, Bruce, and Daniel Friedberg, "Special Problems of the Pediatric Burn Patient," in R. Hummel (ed.), *Clinical Burn Therapy,* John Wright, Boston, 1982, p. 431.
4. Jacoby, Florence Greenhouse, *Nursing Care of the Patient with Burns,* Mosby, St. Louis, 1976, p. 99.
5. Ibid., p. 95.
6. Jacoby, Florence Greenhouse, *The Burn Patient: Management and Operating Room Support,* Ethicon, p. 6.
7. Rudowski, Weitald, et al., *Burn Therapy and Research,* Johns Hopkins, Baltimore, 1976.
8. Jacoby, *The Burn Patient,* p. 6.
9. Howard, Rosanne, and Nancie Herbold, *Nutrition in Clinical Care,* McGraw-Hill, New York, 1978, p. 534.
10. Polk, Hiram, and Harlan Stone, *Hospital-Acquired Infections in Surgery,* University Park Press, Baltimore, 1977, pp. 39–50.
11. Ragiel, Cornelia, "The Impact of Critical Injury on Patient, Family and Clinical Systems," *Critical Care Quarterly* **7**(3):73–78 (December 1984).
12. Stoddard, Jean, "Rehabilitation of the Burn-Injured Patient," *Critical Care Quarterly* **1**:30–33 (December 1978).
13. Johnson, C. L., E. J. O'Shoughnessy, and C. Ostergren, *Burn Management,* Raven Books, New York, 1981.

28

Sally J. Valentine

Infectious processes

Upon completion of this chapter, the student will be able to:

1. Describe the nurse's role in controlling infection and caring for children with communicable diseases.
2. List specific and nonspecific defenses against infection.
3. Describe types of immunity and how each is acquired.
4. Describe the cycle of infection transmission.
5. State measures that can be used to decrease the likelihood of transmission of a foodborne illness.
6. List the nursing management for manifestations of communicable infections.
7. Describe the lesions of rashes.
8. Identify the properties of the following types of communicable diseases: bacterial, viral, rickettsial, parasitic, and fungal.
9. Describe the common childhood diseases and their specific characteristics.
10. Describe the treatment, symptoms, and transmission of sexually transmitted diseases.
11. Explain the consequences of untreated sexually transmitted diseases in the male and the female.

The child's body must constantly defend itself against invasion by microorganisms to remain in a state of health. The nurse who works with children can expect recognition, control, and prevention of infection to be a part of the care of every child.

Familiarity with the language used to describe the process of infection is basic to the nurse's understanding of the transmission of disease. The language describes the conditions of, and relationships between, the *host* (the child), the *agent* (the organism), and the *environment* that result in infection. Preventing the transmission of infection is a major function of the nurse. Understanding the process of infection helps the nurse identify points at which intervention would interfere with the spread of disease.

Not every contact between an infectious agent and a host results in infection. For infection to occur, there must be:

1. An adequate *dose* (quantity of the infectious agent)

2. Adequate *virulence* or *pathogenicity* (strength of the infectious agent)
3. Adequate exposure time
4. A susceptible host
5. Entry by the infectious agent into the host via the appropriate portal

Most organisms prefer a particular location in the body for growth, but the majority *enter* through the digestive and respiratory tracts.

When an infectious agent successfully invades a host and multiplies, infection results. If the infection provokes an *immune response* (the production of antibodies) but no signs or symptoms of disease are evident, the infection is *inapparent* or *subclinical*. This is also known as the *carrier state:* the host is not sick, but is harboring the organism and can transmit it to others. The carrier state occurs in many infectious diseases during the *incubation period* (the time between the host's exposure to the organism and the appearance of symptoms). Disease exists when there are overt clinical manifestations of infection, such as pain, swelling, redness, rash, and fever.

THE NURSE'S ROLE IN CHILDHOOD INFECTION

It is the responsibility of the nurse to prevent, recognize, and control infection. Educating the child and the family about promoting and maintaining health is the primary prevention role of the nurse. Good hygiene and immunization are the most effective infection-prevention measures. The ability to recognize infection or the potential for infection enables the nurse to limit the spread, initiate early treatment, and avoid complications of the infection. Special factors in the recognition of infection in children are discussed below in the section "Childhood Predisposition to Infection." The basic mechanisms for controlling infection are:

1. Early recognition of infectious disease and appropriate isolation of the host
2. Identification and follow-up of contacts
3. Hand-washing between contacts with patients
4. Screening for susceptible children who have been exposed to infectious disease before hospital admission. The nurse should:
   a. Not admit a child who is to undergo an elective procedure.
   b. Isolate the child.
   c. Determine the susceptibility status of other patients.
   d. Provide protective isolation for other children who are highly susceptible. (See Chap. 16 for information about isolation.)

The nurse's role in caring for a child with an infection includes:

1. Observing for signs of infection, the spread of infection, and impending complications
2. Assessing the child's and the family's health practices to determine why the child acquired the infection
3. Assessing the health status of contacts
4. Providing optimal hydration and nutrition
5. Providing rest for the child, the infected body area, or both
6. Providing comfort measures for manifestations of the infection (itching, pain, dry skin, dry mouth, sensitive eyes, anxiety, etc.)
7. Providing control measures for fever, cough, nausea, vomiting, and diarrhea
8. Protecting the child against a secondary infection
9. Educating the child and the family about the infection and its treatment and prevention and about prevention of further infections

CHILDHOOD PREDISPOSITION TO INFECTION

Children have a high incidence of infection because of their high risk of exposure and their physiological and immunologic immaturity. The young child is ill equipped to resist infection. Air passageways are shorter and narrower, permitting rapid entry of organisms. The short, straight eustachian tube of the young child allows a throat infection to spread via the tube to the middle ear. Contamination of the urethra, which is also shorter in the young child, facilitates entry of microorganisms into the bladder. The use of diapers causes fecal contamination of the urethra and predisposes the skin to breakdown (diaper rash) and infection. The diaper area promotes the growth of organisms because it is rich in nutrients and is moist and dark. Scratching in the diaper area introduces microorganisms from the hands. When the fingers become contaminated with fecal organisms, the organisms are spread to the nose, mouth, eyes, ears, and skin.

Sebaceous skin secretions are limited in children, causing the skin to be dry and easily injured. Skin injury permits entry of organisms. Excessive salivation during teething and when the child is thumb-sucking breaks down the skin around the mouth, facilitating the entry of microorganisms. Contaminated fingers and foreign objects introduce microorganisms into the mouth and onto the skin around the mouth. Some young children insert foreign objects into the nose and ears, predisposing them to infection in these areas. Poor nutritional status can also make a child more susceptible to infection. The young child's dependence on milk products, which are a good medium for bacterial growth, increases the likelihood of infection.

The young child's immune system is not completely developed, compromising the ability to react to infection. Immunity to many infectious agents develops only after exposure to them through illness or vaccination. The newborn and the infant are largely unexposed to infectious agents. Increased social contact as the child grows older provides exposure to many different pathogenic organisms.

The anatomic and physiological immaturity of the child becomes apparent when illness does occur. The cardiac sphincter of the stomach is more relaxed, predisposing the young child to vomiting. Marked elevation of temperature and convulsions indicate central nervous system immaturity. Fluid and electrolyte balance is easily upset by fever, diarrhea, or vomiting. The child becomes sick very rapidly, demonstrating how quickly children's defenses can be overcome. Young children are generally less able than older children to clearly communicate the presence of pain, enabling an infection to progress unnoticed.

Children spend much of their day in close contact with other children, which facilitates the transmission of microorganisms. They often exchange clothing or toys and share food that may be contaminated, especially with saliva and nasal secretions. Siblings frequently share toilet articles (toothbrushes, combs, and washcloths) and even bathe together.

These are only some of the reasons why infection occurs so frequently in children and why the pediatric nurse can expect to be concerned about infection with every pediatric patient.

DEFENSES AGAINST INFECTION

Nonspecific defenses

Barriers to infection The child has defenses that protect against invasion by microorganisms. Nonspecific defenses protect against invasion of any sort. The first line of defense is the epithelium that covers the exterior of the body and lines the internal surfaces. The intact epithelium provides a mechanical barrier to invasion. Other mechanical barriers result from the cleansing action of the flow of tears, urine, and saliva. The hairs in the nose filter and trap inhaled organisms, and the mucus and cilia in the respiratory tract trap and propel organisms upward to be expelled by coughing, sneezing, or swallowing. The normal flora of the skin, mouth, and lower gastrointestinal tract provide a biological defense by competing with pathogens for nutrients, thus inhibiting their growth. The acidity of gastric secretions and of the skin also chemically inhibits the growth of pathogens. Lysozyme, which is present in tears, nasal secretions, and saliva, breaks down the bacterial cell wall, causing chemical destruction. All these nonspecific defenses protect the child against the invasion of the body by microorganisms.

Phagocytosis The child also possesses nonspecific defenses that protect against infection once invasion has occurred. These defenses are the white blood cells that ingest and destroy invading agents. This protection is known as *phagocytosis*. The most highly phagocytic cells are *macrophages*. *Fixed macrophages* line the sinuses of the liver, spleen, bone marrow, and lymph nodes and are attached to the walls of the alveoli and the lymph and blood channels. As microorganisms travel through these areas in the blood or lymph, they are removed by being engulfed by macrophages. Macrophages in the liver remove invaders that have entered the portal circulation by traveling through the gastric mucosa. There are also *floating macrophages*, which circulate in the blood and travel to the site of infection. When microorganisms have penetrated into the tissue of the body, floating macrophages move to the site, proliferate, and "wall off" the infection from surrounding tissue, limiting its ability to spread.

Specific defenses

Immunity, the body's powerful adaptive response to invasion by microorganisms, must be developed specifically for each microorganism. Each microorganism or toxin has a unique chemical and physical composition that allows the cells of the immune system to identify it on first encounter and recognize it on subsequent encounters. Agents that stimulate a response by the immune system are termed *antigens.*

The immune response is the production of *antibodies,* which work to destroy invading agents by creating conditions that enhance phagocytosis. Phagocytosis is facilitated when an antibody either covers the surface of an antigen or attacks the cell wall of an agent, causing the agent to rupture. This antigen-antibody complex then either clumps (agglutinates) or precipitates.

Complement system The antigen-antibody complex activates still another system of defense, the *complement system.* This is an amplification system; it increases the efficiency and effectiveness of antibodies. The complement system consists of nine enzymes located in plasma and other body fluids that, when activated, attack invading organisms by one of the following means:

1. *Lysis* Digesting the cell membranes, causing the cell to burst
2. *Opsonization* Coating the surface of the agent to make it more easily phagocytized
3. *Chemotaxis* Attracting phagocytic cells to the area
4. *Agglutination* Causing antigens to stick together
5. *Neutralization* Attacking the molecular structure of a virus

In addition, complement enzymes initiate a local inflammatory response that prevents movement of the agent through the tissue. The inflammatory response is discussed later in this chapter.

Specific response to invaders, *immunity,* is an effective means of destroying invading agents and removing them from the body, and it is clearly essential to the survival of the child.

The immune response

The body does not respond immediately with the production of antibodies on the first exposure to an antigen. The antigen, or invading agent, is transported to the lymphoid tissue, where most of it is destroyed by white blood cells. If the antigen reaches the circulating blood, up to 90 percent may be removed on the first passage through the liver and spleen. This type of nonspecific immune destruction occurs during the first 4 to 7 days after the organism enters the host. After the first exposure to an antigen, the antigen-specific immune response takes almost 2 weeks to become functional. This is why children usually become ill if they are exposed to an infectious disease not previously encountered. Invasion has occurred by an agent unknown to the body, and although the nonspecific defenses work to their capacity to destroy the invader, they are less effective than the specific immune system.

When an agent is able to invade the body a second time, it is recognized by the immune system. This *secondary response,* which takes place much faster than the response to the first encounter with the agent (the *primary response*), is known as the *anamnestic response* or *memory response.* Larger quantities of antibodies are produced much sooner than at the first exposure. The invading agent is destroyed before it can multiply enough to cause illness. See Fig. 28-1.

Development of antibodies

Lymphocytes are responsible for immune responses. When they encounter an antigen, they produce clones, i.e., identical cells all derived from a single cell. In a *humoral immune response,* the offspring cells produce antibodies, which circulate in body fluids and eliminate the antigen. A different kind of antigen stimulates a *cellular immune response.* In this case, the clones are specially prepared cells that carry antibodies on their surface. When these cells come into contact with the antigen, they release lethal substances against it. The two types of immunity—cellular and humoral—are discussed in Chap. 26, and their distinct characteristics are summarized in Table 26-3. The types of antibodies are described in Table 26-2.

Understanding immunoglobulins and their development gives the nurse a basis for understanding infection and immunization schedules in childhood. Children are especially prone to infection because their immune systems are not entirely developed and they have not been exposed to many antigens. Therefore, little specific

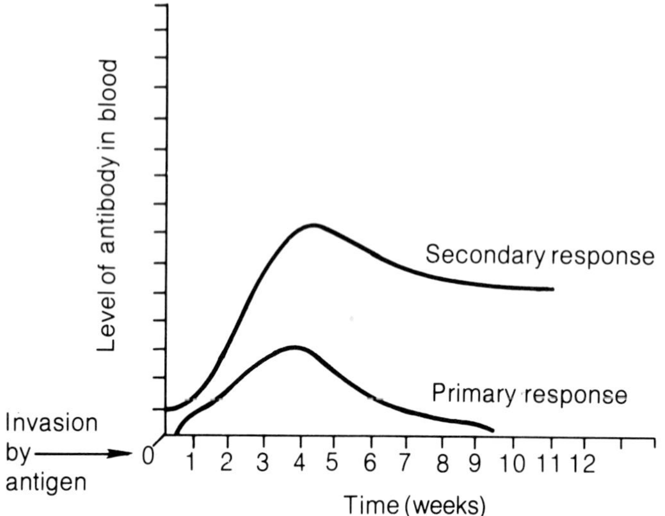

Figure 28-1 Primary and secondary immune responses. The primary response has the following characteristics: (1) antibody production is delayed for several days, (2) it takes 2 to 3 weeks to increase antibody levels, and (3) after many weeks, antibodies are largely used up, and only low levels remain. The secondary response has the following characteristics: (1) the period between exposure and full antibody production is shorter, (2) higher levels are attained, (3) antibody levels remain higher, and (4) the second and subsequent exposures to an antigen require smaller doses of the antigen to provoke a full response.

immunity has built up. Infants are born with some antibody protection—gamma-G globulin that has crossed the placenta—but these antibodies are quickly used up or are broken down by the body.

Immunization

The two principles underlying childhood immunization schedules are (1) to wait until the child's antibody-forming mechanisms are mature enough to respond and (2) to avoid immunization when maternal antibodies remain in the child, which would neutralize the antigenic stimulus. The immunity received from the mother through the placenta is called *passive immunity* because the baby's immune system was not involved in the production of the antibodies; they came preformed from the mother's system. Immunization is begun early so that the child's system can *actively* produce its own antibodies. The child is immunized with antigenic material (bacteria and viruses or their by-products) from major childhood infections (diphtheria, pertussis, tetanus, polio, measles, mumps, and rubella). The antigen used in immunizations has had its pathogenicity (ability to produce disease) weakened or destroyed, but the immune system recognizes it as an antigen. With the first immunization, low levels of antibodies are produced. *Booster doses,* second and third immunizations, cause a secondary response in which high levels of antibodies are produced that will persist for years to protect the child. The three main reasons for giving booster doses are:

1. To elicit a secondary, or memory, response in the immune system (Fig. 28-1)
2. To make sure that maternal antibodies have not prevented the child's immune system from responding (Fig. 28-2)
3. To challenge the child's continuously developing immune system

The immune response in immunization is similar to the response that occurs during a *naturally acquired* infection, but the child does not get the disease. The development of immunity is an *active process* on the part of the child's immune system and results in *acquired immunity* against a disease. Immunization is not a totally natural process because the natural phenomenon of acquiring the disease has been altered by reducing the ability of the organism to cause the disease and by *purposely* introducing the organism into the host. Therefore, immunization produces *artificially acquired immunity.* The American Academy of Pediatrics, in its *Report of the Committee on Infectious Diseases, 1982,* stated that active immunization is the most effective tool in preventing infectious disease. See Table 14-5 for immunization schedules and Table 28-1 for a summary of the mechanisms of defense against infection.

Factors that depress defenses

There are factors that interfere with the child's defenses against infection. Mechanical obstruction causing stasis of some drainage system of the body (e.g., the bladder, sinuses, skin pores,

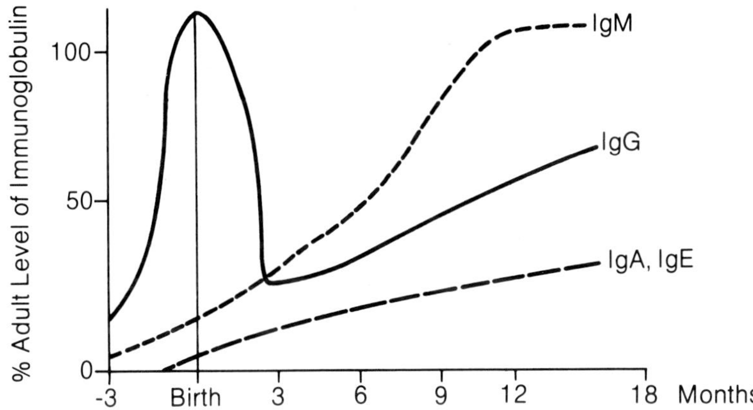

Figure 28-2 Immunoglobulin development in the young child. At birth the infant has more than 100 percent of the adult level of IgG, having received IgG from the mother across the placenta and also having produced his or her own IgG for several months before birth. Maternal IgG is used up or broken down by the child's body by about 4 months. *(From Ivan Roitt, Essential Immunology, Blackwell, London, 1971, p. 56.)*

or tear ducts) creates conditions favorable for infection. These, plus circulatory disturbances (ischemia or congestion and edema of an area or shock), interfere with the movement and function of white blood cells. Nutritional deficiencies, debilitating diseases, concurrent infections, and endocrine imbalance can adversely affect defenses. Steroid and radiation therapy depress the immune system and predispose the child to infection.

THE PROCESS OF INFECTION

Once an infectious agent has successfully invaded the tissues of a host, there are three main patterns of the spread of infection: to the lymphatic vessels, through the body spaces, and via the blood.

Organisms that produce a local infection spread by means of the lymphatic vessels to the local lymph nodes. This spread can cause *lymphangitis*, or inflammation around the lymphatic vessels, which, if superficial, appears as red streaks under the skin. Organisms that reach the lymph nodes cause *lymphadenitis*, or swelling and tenderness of the node. If the organism is not stopped in the lymph node, it travels through the lymphatic vessels, through the thoracic duct, and to the blood.

The presence of bacteria in the blood is known as *bacteremia;* the presence of viruses in the blood is called *viremia*. Bacteria in the blood are attacked by white blood cells. When the bacterial agent is engulfed but not destroyed, it can proliferate within the white blood cells. Eventually, the white blood cells rupture, releasing massive numbers of organisms into the blood, overwhelming the defenses of the host, and causing *septicemia*. Bacteremia is a laboratory finding confirming the presence of bacteria in the blood, while septicemia is a clinical diagnosis indicating bacteremia with a serious clinical status.

Bacteria in the blood can be responsible for metastatic foci of infection. The direction and means of spread of an invading agent determine what the disease will become. A streptococcal sore throat can become acute otitis media or a brain abscess, depending on the direction and means of invasion of a particular strain of streptococcus.

Infection can also spread directly through tissue spaces, such as the peritoneal cavity and the pleural, subarachnoid, pericardial, and joint spaces, and through the tubes of the respiratory,

Table 28-1 Summary of the Mechanisms of Defense against Infection

Type	Example
Nonspecific Defenses	
Mechanical barriers	Mucus and cilia, skin, flow of tears and urine
Biological barriers	Competing organisms
Chemical barriers	Lysozyme and acidity
Nonspecific Immunity	Interferon (see section "Viral Infections")
Specific Immunity	
Active:	
Naturally acquired	Infection
Artificially acquired	Immunization
Passive:	
Naturally acquired	Maternal IgG in baby
Artificially acquired	Preformed antibody injected, RhoGAM, gamma globulin

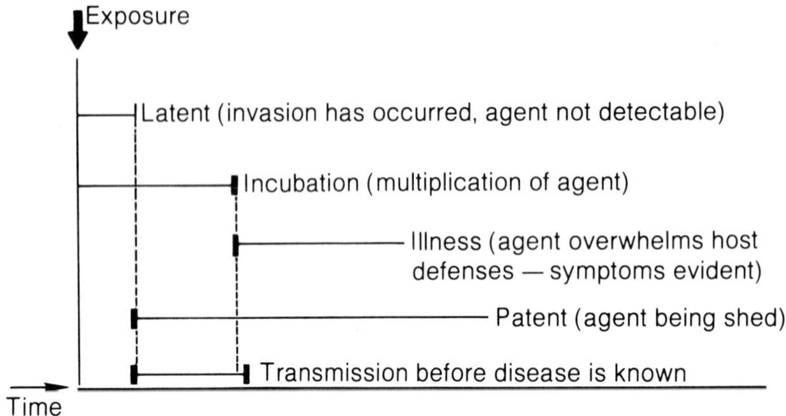

Figure 28-3 General scheme of the stages of infection.

genitourinary, and gastrointestinal tracts. Movement of the body or the infected part facilitates the spread of infection.

When an agent has entered the body but is not yet detectable, the infection is *latent*. The agent is not being shed by the host, and the host is not clinically ill. When the agent begins to multiply and reach numbers sufficient to produce signs and symptoms of disease, the *incubation period* ends and illness occurs. Between the time of exposure and the onset of illness, the agent can be transmitted. The period of communicability has begun. The infection is said to be *patent* when the agent is being shed by the host and can be transmitted. Figure 28-3 shows the relationships of these stages of the disease process to one another and to time.

The period of communicability continues until the end of the patent period, which varies greatly from disease to disease. The greatest spread of communicable disease occurs between the end of the latent period and the onset of the illness. The host is asymptomatic and hence is unaware of the multiplication of the organism in his or her body, and the organism is present in sufficient numbers to begin to be shed by the host. The host unknowingly spreads the disease.

TRANSMISSION OF INFECTION

Transmission is the movement of microorganisms from their *source* to a new host. The *source* is the person, place, or thing from which the infectious agent passes to the host by *direct contact* or *indirectly* through a vehicle or a vector. Table 28-2 lists the methods by which communicable diseases spread from one person to others.

Infection may also be transmitted through food that is contaminated by bacteria, parasites, or viruses. Causative agents may originally be carried by animals and be transmitted to the child through the oral-fecal route. Proper food handling and preparation—including hand-washing by food handlers, refrigerating foods, and thoroughly cooking foods—can prevent foodborne diseases. Foods that are susceptible to contamination are listed in Table 28-3.

In many infections of childhood, the route of exit of the agent from the host is the source of

Table 28-2 Means of Transmission

Contact Spread
Direct:
Touching, physical contact between source and host.
Indirect:
Host contacts a contaminated intermediate object.
Droplet:
Agent is expelled from source during talking, sneezing, coughing; most must be close by for disease transmission.

Common Vehicle
A *fomite* (contaminated inanimate object) which can deliver an agent to one or many hosts (e.g., through contaminated food, combs, towels).

Airborne Agent
Agent becomes suspended in air, droplets, or dust particles; travels in air movement, ventilation systems.

Vector-Borne Agent
Agent is transported by an animal, such as infected household pets, mites, mosquitoes, or wild mammal *(vector)*.

Table 28-3 Foods Susceptible to Contamination and the Most Common Contaminants

Food Types	Contaminant Organisms
Pork, products containing pork	*Trichinella spiralis* or *Salmonella*
Eggs and egg products, milk	*Salmonella*
Home or commercially canned foods low in acid (e.g., meats, creamed soups, mushrooms); fish, fruits, vegetables, honey	*Clostridium botulinum*
Custards, sauces, gravy, soups, salads (especially those made with mayonnaise)	*Staphylococcus aureus*
Meats	*Clostridium perfringes*
Raw shellfish, food handled by person carrying the virus	Hepatitis virus A

transmission of the infection. It is important to know the portals of exit of the major infectious agents so that disease transmission can be interrupted.

The portals of exit of the agents that cause the major childhood illnesses are the respiratory and gastrointestinal tracts, the skin, wounds, and blood. Table 28-4 lists the sources of several childhood illnesses. See Table 16-10 for isolation precautions required for children with various infectious diseases.

MANIFESTATIONS OF INFECTION

Inflammation

The inflammatory response is a sequence of events aimed at limiting the invasion of microorganisms. The tissue trauma that results when microorganisms metabolize and multiply stimulates damaged host cells to liberate histamine. Histamine increases local blood flow and the permeability of capillaries at the site. The increased blood flow brings white blood cells to the area, and the increased permeability permits fluid and fibrinogen to leak into extravascular spaces. The area becomes "walled off" because both tissue spaces and lymph vessels are blocked, which reduces movement and fluid flow and therefore limits the spread of the agent. A cavity may form at the site of the infection and become filled with dead white blood cells and other necrotic material, or pus. Eventually, either the cavity breaks open at a body surface and releases the pus, or the pus is *autolyzed* (absorbed by surrounding tissue until it is gone).

The physiological purpose of inflammation is to destroy an agent, remove it and its products, limit its extension, and set into motion the mechanism for repair and replacement of damaged tissue. The clinical signs of inflammation are redness, swelling, and heat. Symptoms include pain and impaired movement.

Since infection can be spread by movement of the tissue fluids in the infected area, *rest of the area is essential*. Heat administered by compresses, soaks, or lamps promotes healing by increasing circulation to the area. Cold is used to limit swelling. The application of either heat or cold may decrease pain associated with inflammation. Pharmacological treatment of infection includes the use of analgesics, antipyretics, and organism-specific antibiotic therapy.

Fever

Fever is generally considered to be a sign of infection when it is above 38°C (100.4°F) orally or 38.3°C (101°F) rectally. An elevated temperature is an objective sign that something is wrong. Fever may indicate the presence of infection and provide a measure of the severity of disease, the response to therapy, and the return to a normal level of health. Dehydration can also elevate the temperature.

The child's body regulates temperature by balancing heat production and loss. When fever occurs, there is both increased heat production and decreased heat loss. In infectious disease, fever can be caused by substances called *pyrogens*, which are secreted by toxic bacteria or degenerating tissue. Pyrogens work by causing the

Table 28-4 Portals of Exit for Several Childhood Illnesses

Feces	Mouth, Nose, and Respiratory Secretions
Salmonella infections	Pertussis
Polio	Pneumonia
Infectious hepatitis	Scarlet fever
	Meningitis
	Measles
	Mumps
	Polio
	Influenza
	Encephalitis

hypothalamic thermostat to be set at a higher level than normal. The body then works to raise the body temperature to this higher level by means of heat conservation and increased heat production.

When fever is due to dehydration or when pyrogenic substances cause the temperature setting to increase, it takes several hours for the body temperature to reach the new setting. Because the blood temperature is lower than the reset hypothalamus setting, the child feels cold or has chills. When the body temperature reaches the level of the new setting, the child feels neither cold nor warm. A child who "feels cold" may be in the process of temperature elevation and should be checked at frequent intervals. The nursing care of a child with a fever is discussed in Chap. 16.

Rashes

Rashes are frequently seen in childhood infections. A skin eruption or rash is called an *exanthema*. A rash on the mucous membrane is called an *enanthema*. How rashes occur is not completely understood, but two pathological events take place. First, capillaries near the skin surface are damaged by toxins, infectious agents, or antigen-antibody reactions. Skin cells are also damaged, and the eruptions that are seen are local inflammatory reactions.

The terminology used to characterize rashes is important in communicating findings (Tables 28-5 and 28-6) and describing primary lesions of the skin. When observing a child with a rash, it is important to note the following:

1. The specific characteristics of the lesions, such as size, shape, color, and extent and whether they are raised or flat
2. The precise location on the body
3. How the rash progresses on the body, including where it is spreading and whether the lesions are changing in character

Precision is essential in describing a child's rash. Note whether the rash is red, salmon-colored, pink, purple, or brown; whether it has some characteristic that is predominant, like raised borders or an unusual distribution; whether it itches; and whether the child feels ill. Ask the child or the parents whether they know what may have caused the rash and whether they know anyone else with a similar rash. Ask about recent exposures to others with communicable diseases. Establish the medication history of the child. Rashes caused by antibiotics or other medications can occur during or after drug administration. The child may not feel ill with a drug rash but will probably feel ill with measles or another rash due to infection. It is also important to note any other clinical signs or symptoms that have preceded or are occurring with the rash.

Nursing management of rashes is aimed at prevention of scarring and a secondary infection due to scratching. Table 26-11 describes the management of eczema in children in terms of hygiene, diet, clothing, play, and skin care. Some lotions are helpful, and systemic medications such as Benadryl can sometimes control itching. Clothing should be kept clean and changed frequently. When lesions are open, sterile linens may be used for the hospitalized child to prevent a secondary infection.

Once the reason for a child's rash has been established, the expected progression of the rash should be explained to the child and the parents. They should be taught the importance of not scratching, rubbing, or breaking open any lesion because of the danger of a secondary bacterial infection and scarring. The family of a child with a rash should be carefully interviewed to determine whether the family members have been immunized against the childhood diseases that are currently preventable by immunization.

AGENTS OF CHILDHOOD INFECTION

There are five major categories of microorganisms that cause infection in children: bacteria, viruses, parasites, rickettsiae, and fungi.

Bacterial infections

Characteristics Bacteria have several characteristics that enable them to cause disease. They are encapsulated, which inhibits phagocytosis. Some have flagella (tails), which aid in motility, or pili (hairlike structures), which facilitate attachment to body tissues and other surfaces. They form spores when nutritional conditions are poor, permitting survival and making them highly resistant to physical and chemical attempts to destroy them.

Bacteria cause damage to the host by interfering with the body's attempt to "wall off" the invasion, interfering with phagocytosis, directly

Table 28-5 Primary Lesions of the Skin

Type	Definition	Example	Diagram
Macule	A flat circumscribed area of color change in the skin without surface elevation. Size: 1 mm to 2 cm	Freckles, vitiligo, purpura, petechiae, flat moles, ecchymosis	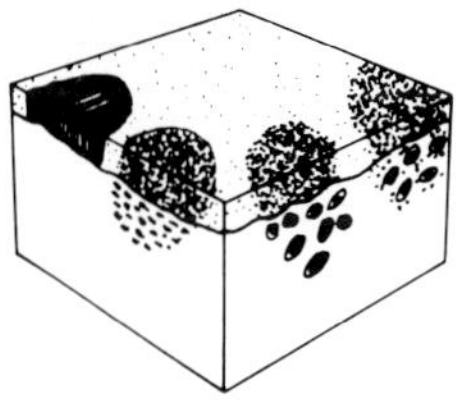
Papule	A circumscribed solid and elevated lesion. Size: 1 mm to 1 cm	Ringworms, acne, psoriasis, warts	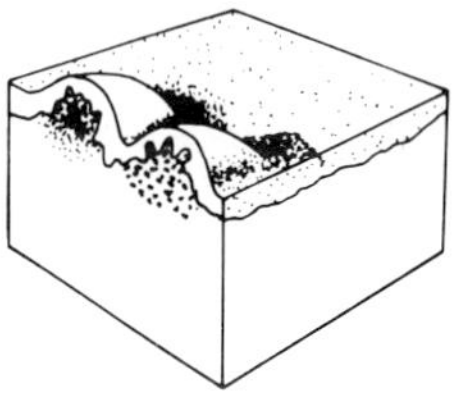
Nodule	A solid, elevated lesion extending deeper in the dermis. Size: 1 to 2 cm	Erythema nodosum	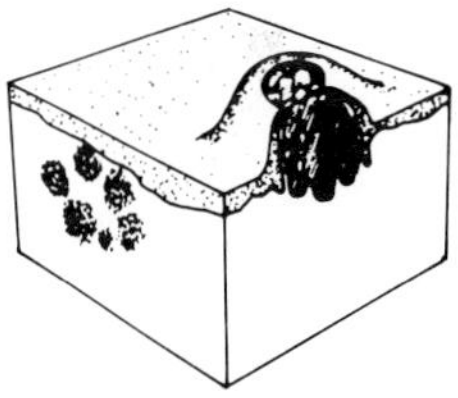
Tumor	A solid mass larger than a nodule. Size: over 2 cm	Basal cell epithelioma	
Cyst	A papule or nodule containing fluid or viscous material. Size: 1 mm or over	Sebaceous and epidermal cysts	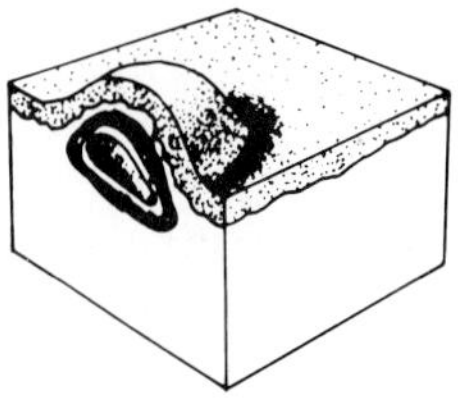
Wheal	A clustering of papular-type lesions creating an edematous plaque. Fluid in upper layer. Size: 1 mm to several cm	Mosquito bites, urticaria	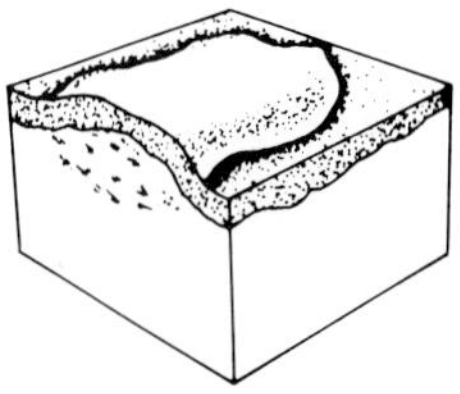
Vesicle	A bulging, small, sharply defined lesion filled with serous fluid or blood. Size: less than 1 cm	Herpes simplex, herpes zoster	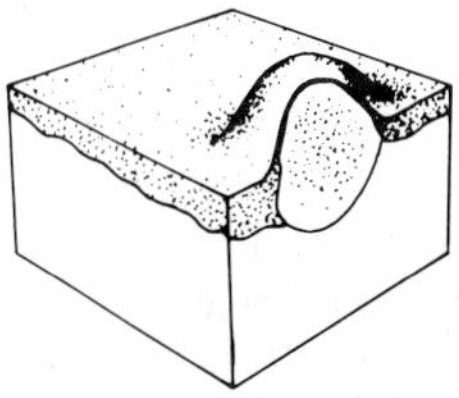
Bulla	Larger than a vesicle. Size: over 1 cm	Pemphigus, second-degree burns	
Pustule	A vesicle or bulla filled with pus. Size: 1 mm to 1 cm	Impetigo, acne vulgaris	

Source: M. Kinney et al. (eds.), *AACN's Clinical Reference for Critical-Care Nursing*, McGraw-Hill, New York, 1981, pp. 265, 266. Used with permission.

Table 28-6 Secondary Lesions of the Skin

Type	Definition	Example	Diagram
Crust	Dried serum, blood, pus, or sebum which forms on the surface of any vesicle or pustule lesion when it ruptures	Infectious dermatitis, eczema, impetigo	
Scale	Dried fragments of sloughed, dead epidermis	Exfoliative dermatitis, seborrheic dermatitis	

Source: M. Kinney et al. (eds.), *AACN's Clinical Reference for Critical-Care Nursing*, McGraw-Hill, New York, 1981, p. 266. Used with permission.

destroying body tissues, and causing reactions that result in fever. Some bacteria produce toxins. *Exotoxins,* toxins released by the bacterial cell into the surrounding tissue and spaces, are antigenic; a specific antibody, known as an *antitoxin,* is formed.

Exotoxins that are inactivated by formaldehyde still retain their antigenicity. *Toxoids,* or inactivated toxins, are used to stimulate an immune response. Diphtheria and tetanus toxoids are routinely used for this purpose. A preformed antitoxin is used when exposure has occurred or is suspected to have occurred. Tetanus antitoxin is given after a puncture wound.

Diagnosis The preferred methods of diagnosis in bacterial infections are a *culture* and a *smear* of infected tissue or fluid. The purpose is to identify the organism and its particular biological and biochemical activities. Because drying destroys many bacteria, care must be taken to provide a sterile nutrient broth for the specimen. Prompt delivery to the laboratory is essential. When obtaining a specimen of blood, urine, spinal fluid, or other body fluid, extreme care must be taken to avoid contamination of the specimen. A contaminated specimen can result in an incorrect diagnosis; as a result, the child may be put through a unnecessary course of anti-infective therapy, or the wrong medication may be prescribed.

Treatment Bacteria are remarkably able to adapt to environmental conditions. The clinical significance of this is the increased tolerance of bacteria for antibacterial drugs. Strains of bacteria have become resistant to antibiotic drugs because of inadequate treatment of an infection with an antibiotic. When treatment is inadequate, in terms of either dosage level or length of time that the drug is administered, the weaker organisms are destroyed, while the stronger ones survive, multiply, and create a more resistant strain.

Antibiotics, when used to treat an identified infection, should be administered for a full 10 to 14 days. When a culture is taken and an antibiotic is started before the culture results are available, it is appropriate to discontinue the drug if the organism is not one for which the antibiotic is specific and to change to an effective antibiotic. Table 28-7 presents the common bacterial diseases of childhood. Discussion of the body system affected and the nursing management appears in the appropriate chapter.

Viral infections

Viruses can complete their life cycle only within a living cell. Once a virus has invaded a cell, normal cell function ceases, and the cell's machinery is used by the virus to reproduce itself. The host cell is fatally damaged when it either

Table 28-7 Common Bacterial Diseases of Childhood

Agent	Source	Disease	Comments
Streptococcus pyogenes	Everywhere. Skin, nasopharynx	Streptococcal pharyngitis	One of the most common infections of children 5 to 15 years old. Spread from person to person by nasal droplets or saliva; also by contaminated foods. Crowding enhances spread. Food- or water-borne outbreaks are explosive. Not all infected children will have symptoms; some have mild illness for a few days. Elevated temperature (38.3°C [101°F]), sore throat, nausea and vomiting, abdominal pain, redness, edema, coryza, petechiae of mucosa. Diagnosis by positive throat culture. Antibiotics for 10 to 14 days. Penicillin G is most effective. Child returns to school after 24 h of antibiotic therapy. In hospital, secretion precautions taken until 24 h effective therapy has been administered.
		Scarlet fever, scarlatina (milder rash in children given penicillin)	Clinical symptoms are the same as those of streptococcal pharyngitis, but on second day red rash, "blush," blanches on pressure, circumoral pallor, "strawberry" tongue. High fever: 39.5°C (103°F). Treatment is the same as treatment of pharyngitis. Desquamation occurs usually after a week; extent and duration are related to intensity of the rash.
		Complications of streptococcal infection: acute rheumatic fever, acute glomerulonephritis	Suspected cases of strep must be cultured, and positives treated for 10 to 14 days to prevent complications. Siblings and contacts of infected person must be cultured.
Streptococcus pneumoniae	Upper respiratory tract		Resistant to phagocytosis. Produce toxins.
		Pneumococcal pneumonia	Rapid growth to lungs; bronchopneumonia after aspiration; associated with anesthesia, seizures, coma.
		Otitis media	More than one-third of otitis is strep. Most children have first attack by age 6. Recurrent attacks lead to hearing loss and learning problems. Penicillin or erythromycin is the drug of choice.
		Mastoiditis, sinusitis, meningitis, endocarditis	One of the three most common agents in bacterial meningitis. See related chapters for nursing management.
Staphylococcus aureus	Skin, nose, gut, part of normal flora; nasal carriers common. Improperly refrigerated cream- or egg-based food	Boils, wound infections, septicemia, endocarditis, osteomyelitis, impetigo, furuncles, styes, pneumonia, meningitis, food poisoning	Antibiotic-resistant strains exist in hospitals, where many children become infected. Prevention: 1. Wash hands after exposure and before working with susceptible persons. 2. Isolate patients with staph. a. Strict isolation for persons with lung abscesses or pneumonia as well as for those with large draining wounds that cannot be contained.

Table 28-7 Common Bacterial Diseases of Childhood *(Continued)*

Agent	Source	Disease	Comments
			b. Drainage and secretion precautions for persons with wounds with drainage that can be adequately controlled with dressings. c. Enteric precautions for persons with staphylococcal food poisoning. 3. Permit self-care when possible, especially new mother and baby. 4. Nurses are frequent carriers of resistant strains of staph in nose and skin. 5. Be alert to any skin infection, especially in people with IV, indwelling catheter, or shunts; skin infection can lead to septicemia and should be treated. 6. Antibiotic treatment must be continued for 2 to 4 weeks. a. Methicillin, nafcillin, or oxacillin. b. Local care may suffice for superficial lesions. c. Symptomatic management for food poisoning.
		Impetigo (can be caused by *Streptococcus* as well as *Staphylococcus*)	Lesions begin as vesicles and progress to pustules containing cloudy yellow fluid; rupture easily, leaving red oozing lesion that crusts and spreads by extension. Usually on face or other exposed areas. Most common in spring and summer in conditions of poor hygiene and nutrition. Contagious—*itchy*. Treatment: systemic and, less effectively, local antibiotics. Avoid scratching and secondary infection. Scabs may be removed to facilitate cleaning, treatment, and healing; saline soaks or compresses two to three times daily. Keep personal articles, washcloth, and towel separate. Check family and close contacts for disease. Isolate from other children. Wash hands meticulously.
		Staphylococcal infections, scalded skin syndrome	Caused by the staphylococcal exfoliative toxin. Incubation period is 1 to 10 days. Is more commonly seen in younger children. Antibiotic therapy is helpful. Rash develops, making skin appear scalded.
		Toxic shock syndrome	Is seen predominantly in adolescent and young adult females and is often associated with the presence of the menstrual period and the use of tampons. Symptoms include high fever, rash similar to a sunburn, diarrhea, vomiting, and shock. Wash hands before handling tampons. Do not use superabsorbent tampons. Change tampon every 4 to 6 h. Alternate use of pads and tampons, especially at night. Teach signs of toxic shock syndrome; if signs occur, remove tampon and see a doctor.

Table 28-7 Common Bacterial Diseases of Childhood *(Continued)*

Agent	Source	Disease	Comments
Corynebacterium diphtheriae	Infected persons—intimate contact required for spread. Droplets from nasopharynx; also fomites, animals, milk; carriers exist	Diphtheria	Incubation period is 2 to 4 days. Fever, if present, is a low-grade one. May be symptomless or rapidly fatal; location of infection varies: anterior nasal, tonsillar, pharyngeal, laryngeal, bronchial. Pseudomembrane forms, obstructing breathing. Systemic effects on heart secondary to toxin. High fatality rate. Strict isolation, antibiotics (penicillin and erythromycin are effective), and bed rest are very important because of complication of myocarditis. Suction equipment at bedside is important in maintaining a patent airway. Other supportive measures include mist tents for persons with laryngeal involvement, maintenance of hydration, and medication for pain. Treatment includes DAT (diphtheria antitoxin skin test first for sensitivity to horse serum). Is *preventable* by active immunization in childhood. Booster is required every 10 years. Care to prevent infection secondary to pneumonia is required. All carriers should be treated with antimicrobial therapy.
Neisseria meningitidis	Nasopharynx; carriers exist; respiratory transmission	Meningococcemia	Abrupt onset of fever, malaise, and rash. Disseminated intravascular coagulation, shock, coma, and death may occur, despite appropriate therapy. Rash is petechial; hemorrhagic lesions.
		Meningococcal meningitis	Circle area on skin and count lesions every hour to monitor progression. Major worldwide health problem. High fatality rate. Respiratory isolation until 24 h after effective therapy has begun. Rifampin prophylaxis for contacts and affected child if appropriate (see Table 28-8).
Pseudomonas aeruginosa	Soil, water, vegetation	Infections of urinary tract, surgical wounds, burns; pneumonia	Opportunist pathogen (does not cause disease in healthy persons). Most frequent cause of death in patients with leukemia, cystic fibrosis, or extensive burns. Resistance to drugs is common.
Salmonella	Infected feces; urine from humans; contaminated poultry, eggs, beef, pork, raw and powdered milk, pet turtles. Asymptomatic carriers	Intestinal: Gastroenteritis Extraintestinal: Bacteremia, osteomyelitis, meningitis	Sudden onset of abdominal pain, diarrhea, nausea and vomiting, dehydration, and fever lasting several days. Proper hand-washing and food handling can prevent it. Refrigeration prevents multiplication of organisms. In uncomplicated gastroenteritis, antimicrobial therapy does not shorten the course and may lengthen the carrier status time. Enteric isolation precautions are required for duration of illness (5 to 7 days). Dispose of diapers carefully.

Table 28-7 Common Bacterial Diseases of Childhood *(Continued)*

Agent	Source	Disease	Comments
	Contaminated water supply, inadequate sewage disposal, feces or urine of infected human	Typhoid fever	Headache, malaise, diarrhea (occasionally constipation instead), fever, abdominal pain and distention, and rose spots on abdomen and chest. Danger that intestinal lesions (Peyer's patches) will perforate or hemorrhage. All cases must be reported. Treatment by antimicrobials is useful (ampicillin and chloramphenicol). Enteric isolation until three consecutive negative cultures are obtained after antibiotic therapy is completed.
Shigella	Person-to-person contact; feces of infected human; contaminated food, water, or inanimate objects. May be carried by flies	Bacillary dysentery (incubation period: 3 days)	Problem in young school-age children—they contaminate hands touching toilet seat and then toys, bedclothes, etc. Excessive fluid loss from diarrhea and vomiting; high fever (up to 40.6°C [105°F]). Acute onset of abdominal pain, cramping, diarrhea with mucus; feces may be blood-tinged. Diagnosis should be confirmed, and treatment instituted to eliminate reservoir of infection. Enteric isolation until three negative cultures are obtained after antibiotic therapy. Symptoms resolve in 5 to 10 days. Bacteria are shed in 1 to 4 weeks. Bacteria enter distal small intestines and colon and multiply, releasing endotoxin.
Hemophilus influenzae	Nasopharynx of healthy or ill carriers	Otitis media, pneumonia	Second leading cause of otitis media in children. Symptoms may be vague.
		Meningitis, bacteremia, cellulitis, epiglottitis, pericarditis	Meningitis should be treated with both ampicillin and chloramphenicol until susceptibility of the organism is established. Contacts are prophylactically treated with rifampin (see Table 28-8). Respiratory isolation until 24 h of effective therapy has been administered. Secretion precautions for persons with draining lesions. Exposed children who become febrile should be medically evaluated. *H. influenzae* vaccine has not been shown to be effective in children under the age of 18 months.
Bordetella pertussis	Respiratory discharges of infected human	Whooping cough	Stage 1, catarrhal: Slow onset of common cold symptoms; cough becomes more severe, nocturnal; lasts 10 to 14 days. Stage 2, paroxysmal (4 to 6 weeks): Violent, sharp cough followed by inspiratory whoop—face and neck veins distended, and face cyanotic during cough; vomiting of mucus. Can lead to exhaustion and malnutrition. Stage 3, convalescent: Gradual decrease in cough over 2 months. Fatality rate high in children under 1 year old. Most common in late winter and early spring. Observe for airway obstruction; provide bed rest and maintain hydration. Antibiotic therapy

Table 28-7 Common Bacterial Diseases of Childhood *(Continued)*

Agent	Source	Disease	Comments
			may decrease the communicability of the disease, and if given in the catarrhal stage may decrease the intensity of the disease. Respiratory isolation until erythromycin has been administered for 7 days; with no erythromycin, isolate for 3 weeks. Immunization available; must begin at 6 to 8 weeks, and series must be completed. Immunity is not lifelong or complete. Booster doses are given to household contacts and other close contacts under 7 years of age who have previously been immunized. Side effects of the pertussis vaccine are *common* and include slight fever, tenderness at the site, and malaise. Reactions that contraindicate continuation of the immunization schedule for pertussis include seizures, encephalitis, excessive screaming (persisting for 3 h or longer), and an elevation in temperature greater than 40.5°C (105°F). In general, the benefits of pertussis immunization outweigh the side effects.
Clostridium tetani	Soil contaminated by feces of domestic animals and humans	Tetanus	Organism is normal inhabitant of the gut, but becomes dangerous when introduced into a wound where anaerobic conditions exist (puncture wounds and under the crusts of burns). Tetanus neonatorum—unhealed umbilicus contaminated with feces. Organism produces a powerful neurotoxin. Hyperirritability of muscles, especially in the face, neck, and trunk; spasms of strong muscle groups produce lockjaw and opisthotonos (arched back), headache, fever, convulsions; difficulty with breathing, swallowing, and urinating due to muscle spasm. Treatment includes human tetanus immunoglobulin. If this is not available, tetanus antitoxin may be given (testing for sensitivity to horse serum is necessary prior to administration). Antibiotics; tranquilizers, sedatives, and muscle relaxants; indwelling catheters for urine; IV fluids with electrolytes; a tracheostomy; suctioning; and oxygen are used in the care of a patient with tetanus. Nursing care includes reducing all stimuli, especially sound, light, and touch, which may precipitate spasm; flatus-minimizing diet. Immunization available. A booster dose is given every 5 to 10 years. Human tetanus immunoglobulin in conjunction with tetanus toxoid is given when wounds are very dirty or injuries are severe or crushing.

Table 28-7 Common Bacterial Diseases of Childhood *(Continued)*

Agent	Source	Disease	Comments
Campylobacter fetus	Contaminated milk, foods, infected humans or animals. Fecal-oral transmission	*Campylobacter* enteritis	Rapid onset of diarrhea. Stools may be bloody; child is febrile; pain is located in the abdomen. Antibiotic therapy may be used. In mild cases only supportive management may be used. Maintain enteric precautions until stool cultures are negative.
Clostridium botulinum	Food contaminated with spores of *C. botulinum*. Due to improperly prepared home-canned foods. Not usually caused by commercially canned foods	Botulism	Symmetrical paralysis, especially of the respiratory muscles; double vision; normal temperature. In infants, there may be floppy, weak suck and a weak cry. Onset of symptoms usually occurs between 6 h and 8 days. Antitoxin is available. Observation and supportive respiratory management are important features in the treatment of botulism.
Clostridium perfringens	Undercooked meat; symptoms produced by toxins	Perfringens (food poisoning)	Cramping; watery diarrhea; no elevation in temperature. Onset of symptoms is from 8 to 24 h after ingestion of undercooked meat. No treatment or isolation is necessary.

bursts open or slowly leaks new virus. The newly synthesized viruses move on to infect other host cells.

Viruses reach the human host by means of droplets, direct contact, and animal or arthropod vectors. The virus causes diseases predominantly through cell destruction. Viruses are responsible for the common cold, measles, mumps, chickenpox, polio, and many other diseases.

Viruses are generally prevented from invading the host by intact skin and mucous membranes. Once the host has been invaded, the inflammatory process resulting from cell injury can prevent the spread of the infection. Raising the local temperature and increasing the acidity of the chemicals released by damaged cells cause unfavorable conditions for viral growth. Viruses induce the host cells to produce *interferon,* a protein that inhibits viral multiplication, and *virus-specific antibodies.*

Viral diseases can be controlled through public health measures, including proper sanitation and hygiene, and some of them are preventable by immunization. Sanitary disposal of human feces, hand-washing by food handlers, and insect and rodent eradication programs have contributed to the control of many viral diseases. Immunization has worked well in reducing the number of cases of smallpox, polio, measles, mumps, and rubella. The common cold and some influenza viruses change their antigenic characteristics so frequently that vaccines are not useful.

Prevention of viral illnesses is very important because treatment measures are limited. Only symptomatic treatment can be given. Antibiotics are not useful. Antiviral therapy is difficult because the drug must destroy the virus without destroying the host's cell that it is inhabiting. Drugs that will block the movement of a virus into the cell and drugs that will stimulate the host's cells to produce interferon are currently being developed.

Viruses are difficult to grow in the laboratory, and therefore the diagnosis of viral illness is based on the clinical presentation of the disease and on *antibody titers,* or measurements of the host's blood levels of a virus-specifc antibody. An antibody titer is routinely done on women during the first trimester of pregnancy to determine whether they have levels of antibodies against rubella sufficient to protect the fetus if they should be

Table 28-8 Rifampin Prophylaxis when Children Develop *Hemophilus Influenzae* or *Neisseria Meningitidis Infections*

1. Prophylactic administration of rifampin is recommended for all household contacts (both adults and children) when at least one of these contacts is under 4 years of age.
2. Household contacts are defined as individuals who reside in the same home with a child who has developed either a *Hemophilus influenzae* or *Neisseria meningitidis* infection. These persons should have about 4 h of contact with the affected child on five of the last seven days prior to hospitalization. When the parents or other family members are not sure whether they have had 4 h of exposure to the child, ask whether the suspected contacts eat meals with the child. If they eat meals together, they most likely have had about 4 h of exposure time.
3. When more than two children in a day-care setting develop an infection with the same organism in a 2-month period, rifampin prophylaxis is advised for all children and adult contacts.
4. The hospitalized child receives rifampin prophylaxis beginning just prior to discharge. Appropriate antibiotic therapy for the infection does not eliminate the carrier state of the child.
5. Pregnant women are not treated with rifampin because safe use of this drug during pregnancy has not been determined.
6. A dose of rifampin, 20 mg per kg of body weight, is given orally *once daily* for *4 days* for *H. influenzae* contacts. A dose of 10 mg per kg of body weight is given *twice daily* for 2 *days* for *N. meningitidis* contacts. Maximum dose is 600 mg.
7. A liquid form of rifampin is not available. For infants and young children, tablets are crushed, weighed, and packaged for single-dose administration by the pharmacist.
8. For best drug levels, administer rifampin on an empty stomach (1 h before or 2 h after meals).
9. Rifampin stains urine, stool, sweat, saliva, and tears a red-orange color. Parents are informed of these expected results. Contact lens wearers are told that rifampin stains soft contact lenses permanently and that they should not be worn during treatment.
10. Women taking oral contraceptives need to consider alternative birth control methods, since rifampin increases metabolization of these drugs.
11. Parents are recommended to seek prompt medical evaluation for febrile episodes in exposed children.

Sources: American Academy of Pediatrics, Committee on Infectious Diseases, "Revision of Recommendation for Use of Rifampin Prophylaxis of Contacts of Patients with Haemophilus Influenzae Infection," *Pediatrics* **74**:301–302 (August 1984); L. E. Govoni and J. E. Hayes, *Drugs and Nursing Implications,* 4th ed., Appleton Century Crofts, New York, 1982, pp. 945–947; and D. Wink, "Bacterial Meningitis in Children," *American Journal of Nursing* **84**:456–460 (April 1984).

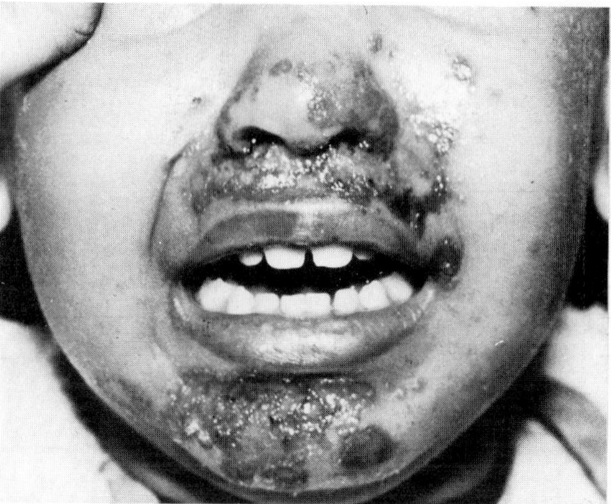

Figure 28-4 Classic impetigo with superficial oozing and crusted ulcers. Note the involvement of the nares; the nose is the likely site of the infective organism. (*From R. A. Hoekelman et al. [eds.], Principles of Pediatrics: Health Care of the Young, McGraw-Hill, New York, 1978, p. 1371.*)

exposed to rubella during the pregnancy. Table 28-9 presents the common viral infections of childhood.

Rickettsial diseases

Rickettsiae are microorganisms that need a host cell to multiply. Their reservoir is some species of mammal. They are transferred to humans by lice, fleas, ticks, and mites; therefore, the diseases they cause are known as *arthropod-borne diseases*. The arthropod either injects the agent when it bites the host or deposits the agent on the host's skin as it defecates during biting. The host scratches and inoculates the agent into broken or irritated skin.

Rickettsiae establish themselves in the lining of small blood vessels in the host. The small vessels of the skin are most frequently involved, causing the characteristic rash associated with rickettsial diseases. The vascular lesions result from edema and obstruction and can also occur in the lungs, heart, liver, kidneys, and central nervous system. Infection by *rickettsiae* stimulates the development of rickettsia-specific antibodies, and immunity is generally lifelong.

Diagnosis is made on the basis of clinical signs and symptoms, serologic tests, and isolation of

Table 28-9 Common Viral Infections of Childhood

Disease	Source and Means of Transmission	Manifestations	Treatment	Nursing Management	Control	Complications
Chickenpox (varicella): Agent: Varicella zoster. Incubation period: 12 to 21 days. Is communicable. Isolation period: 1 to 2 days before onset of the rash and until all lesions are crusted. Strict isolation for 7 days after onset of the rash or until all lesions have dried.	Contact with discharges from the skin of an infected person. Airborne transmission has also been documented. Most commonly seen in late winter and early spring.	Prodromal phase: mild fever, malaise. Then a rash develops. The rash starts on the trunk as crops of reddened macules that progress to fluid-filled vesicles that crust. The rash is pruritic.	Only supportive therapy is available at present. Acyclovir and Vidarabine are being tested. Topical and systemic antipruritics may be given. Aspirin should not be given for fever management because of its relationship to the development of Reye syndrome later.	Assess the skin for development of new crops of lesions. Give a daily bath, clip the nails short, and administer antipruritics to decrease itching. Instruct the child not to scratch the lesions. Provide age-appropriate diversional activities and a restful environment.	Immunization is being developed but currently is not available. Varicella zoster immune globulin (VZIG) should be given to children at high risk for developing progressive disease.	Secondary bacterial infections and scarring related to scratching. Meningitis, encephalitis, arthritis. Pneumonia—rare in the normal child. Progressive varicella (where lesions continue to develop into the second week) is seen in the immunocompromised child. Congenital varicella may occur when maternal varicella occurs during the first or second trimester of pregnancy. Limb and other deformities may result; no isolation is necessary.

Rubeola (red measles): Agent: rubeola virus. Incubation period: 9 to 12 days. Is communicable. Isolation period: 4 days before onset of the rash and 4 days after the rash begins. Respiratory isolation.	Contact with the respiratory tract secretions, blood, or urine of an infected person. Also, less commonly, airborne transmission.	Slow onset of symptoms of a cold, including nasal discharge, tearing, and sneezing. Fever occurs, reaching as high as 40 to 40.6°C (104 to 105°F) on the third or fourth day of the rash. Koplik's spots (pink macules with a bluish spot in the center) are found in the mouth about 2 days after onset of the first symptoms. Two days later, a dusty-red rash appears; initially it is maculopapular and then coalesces, starting on the upper neck and forehead and spreading to involve the face, trunk, and extremities. The child is sickest on day 3 or 4 of the rash. The rash resolves in 6 to 8 days.	Supportive management.	Isolate the child from susceptible family members. Provide a restful environment. If photophobia occurs, prevent exposure to bright lights and sunlight. Darkening the room is usually unnecessary. Temperature should be monitored by the parents every 4 to 6 h. Fevers are managed with tepid baths and acetaminophen. Encourage intake of fluids to prevent dehydration when the child is febrile.	Live measles vaccine is available; children should be immunized at age 15 months. The course may be prevented or modified by administration of gamma globulin, which may give passive temporary immunity.	Rare; usually secondary bacterial infections, otitis media, or pneumonia. Very rarely encephalitis develops.

Table 28-9 Common Viral Infections of Childhood (*Continued*)

Disease	Source and Means of Transmission	Manifestations	Treatment	Nursing Management	Control	Complications
Rubella (German measles or 3-day measles): Agent: rubella virus. Incubation period: 14 to 21 days. Is communicable. Isolation period: 7 days before to 5 days after onset of the rash. Infants with congenital infection may shed the virus for a year or more. Strict isolation for infants with congenital infection. Respiratory isolation for others.	Droplets or contact with the nasopharyngeal secretions, blood, or feces of an infected person. Peak incidence is late winter to early spring.	Variable; may be headache, coryza, sore throat, malaise, mild conjunctivitis, fever and lymph node enlargement and tenderness; usually a pale pink rash appears at the hairline and spreads downward; symptoms and the rash may appear together, or the rash may be delayed; the rash is gone in 1 to 5 days.	No specific therapy.	Nursing personnel caring for hospitalized rubella patients should be immune to the disease. The child may return to school after the rash has been present for 5 days.	Live virus vaccine is given at age 15 months or if the child is not immune (girls). Pregnant women and nursing personnel are tested to determine immunity.	Rare; may include encephalitis and a mild arthritis which may last for 3 to 28 days (more common in older persons). Maternal rubella during the first 3 months of pregnancy has a teratogenic effect on the fetus. Signs of classic rubella syndrome include low birth weight, deafness (not always detected in the neonatal period), blindness due to congenital cataracts or glaucoma, jaundice, hepatosplenomegaly, cardiac involvement, and cerebral defects (mental retardation and microcephaly).
Mumps (parotitis): Agent: paramyxovirus. Incubation period: 12 to 25 days. Is communicable. Isolation period: 7 days before	Contact with the saliva of an infected person or with droplets of saliva. Most commonly seen in late winter and spring.	Sudden onset of headache, myalgia, earache, fever, anorexia, or parotid swelling; may be unilateral or bilateral. Swallowing may	No specific therapy. Analgesics and antipyretics may be helpful.	Provide bed rest to decrease swelling. Warm or cool compresses may decrease discomfort associated with swollen parotid	Live virus vaccine is available. Children should be immunized at age 15 months, with mumps vaccine alone or in combination	Rare in prepubertal children. Meningoencephalitis and postpubertal orchitis and oophoritis have been noted. The latter two com-

and up to 9 days after onset. Inapparent infection is common. Respiratory isolation is required for hospitalized children until swelling has subsided (usually by 9 days).		be difficult.		glands. Avoid foods which require lots of chewing and which are either sour or acidic, since these may increase pain. Observe for central nervous system changes such as a change in level of consciousness or nuchal rigidity.	with measles and rubella vaccine.	plications rarely lead to sterility.
Smallpox (variola): Agent: variola virus. Incubation period: 12 to 14 days. Is communicable. Isolation period: 2 days before onset until all crusts have dropped off (about 3 to 4 weeks).	Contact with an infected person or fomites. Lesions and crusts are infectious.	Abrupt onset of severe headache, chills, malaise, and high fever. A macular rash begins on the third or fourth day on the face and then spreads to the body and mucous membranes. The rash becomes papular, and the fever drops. Lesions appear in a single crop and progress at the same rate. Papules become vesicular in 24 h and pustular in about 5 to 6 days. At about the ninth day, lesions begin to dry, and crusts drop off at the end of 3 to 4 weeks, leaving scars in many cases.	No effective treatment. Vaccination is no longer required in the United States. (No cases of the disease have been reported since 1977.)	Maintain strict isolation. Give supportive therapy. Prevent dehydration and secondary infection. Provide good nutrition. Give skin care.	Has been controlled in most of the world by vaccinations. Vaccination is required for travel to countries where the disease may still exist.	Secondary bacterial infection of lesions. In persons with eczema, the disease can spread to eczematous skin and become systemic. Allergic encephalitis after vaccination.

Table 28-9 Common Viral Infections of Childhood (*Continued*)

Disease	Source and Means of Transmission	Manifestations	Treatment	Nursing Management	Control	Complications
Influenza: Agent: type A, B, or C orthomyxovirus. Incubation period: 1 to 3 days. Is communicable. Isolation period: 24 h before and after onset of symptoms. Virus shedding may continue up to 7 days. Respiratory isolation with secretion precautions necessary for hospitalized children for 5 days after onset of symptoms.	Direct contact with the nasal or throat discharge of an infected person. Small-droplet and airborne transmission are unlikely.	Acute onset of fever, chills, myalgia, cough, sore throat, and headache.	Generally supportive. Amantadine has been recommended for children with underlying illness who might be adversely affected by development of this disease.	Provide for adequate fluid intake by offering soothing fluids that the child prefers. Take cooling measures and administer antipyretics if needed for fever control.	Immunizations are available; their usefulness is limited, since the virus frequently changes its antigenic characteristics. May be useful for high-risk groups in time of epidemic influenza (especially for immune-impaired persons, e.g., those undergoing cancer therapy).	Pneumonia, bronchitis, and bronchiolitis.

Roseola infantum: Agent: an unidentified virus. Incubation period: 5 to 15 days. Communicability is unknown. Isolation of child is not required.	Source and means of transmission are unidentified.	A high fever (40 to 40.6°C [104 to 105°F]) for 3 to 4 days. When the fever goes down, a maculopapular rash appears first on the trunk and then spreads to the rest of the body. The rash fades in 1 to 3 days and is often confused with rubella and allergies.	No specific therapy. Fevers are managed with acetaminophen. Phenobarbital may be given to infants with a history of convulsive seizures.	Monitor temperature every 4 to 6 h. Take cooling measures and administer antipyretics as needed for fever management.	None known.	Febrile seizures.
Fifth disease (erythema infectiosum): Agent: an unidentified virus. Incubation period: 6 to 14 days. Communicability is uncertain. No isolation is required.	Contact with an infected person.	Erythema on the face, primarily on the cheeks, gives the "slapped face" appearance; lasts 1 to 4 days. Red maculopapular spots appear on the face and upper and lower extremities, lasting about a week. The rash may reappear as a result of heat, cold, or trauma.	None needed.	Take comfort measures for the rash. Explain the benign nature of the illness to the parents.	Limit direct contact.	Uncommon.

Table 28-9 Common Viral Infections of Childhood (*Continued*)

Disease	Source and Means of Transmission	Manifestations	Treatment	Nursing Management	Control	Complications
Poliomyelitis (infantile paralysis): Agent: polio virus types 1, 2, and 3. Incubation period: 7 to 14 days. Is communicable shortly before onset and during the first week of illness. Enteric precautions are required for duration of the hospital stay. The virus may be shed in the stools for 6 to 8 weeks.	Contact with droplets and with pharyngeal or intestinal excretions of an infected person that are spread to the mouth of the host.	Abortive poliomyelitis: abrupt onset of headache, low fever, anorexia, nausea, and vomiting, lasting 24 to 48 h. Nonparalytic poliomyelitis: same as in abortive form but intensified, with central nervous system involvement, stiff neck, and pain on movement. Paralytic poliomyelitis: same as in nonparalytic form, but the child is acutely ill; paralysis may be the first sign; paralysis determines clinical signs; may affect the respiratory system, extremities, bladder, circulatory system, or pharynx.	Supportive measures related to the extent of the disease.	Complete bed rest and an environment conducive to this are critical. Passive range-of-motion exercises are done to avoid development of contractures. Position the child in a way that will prevent footdrop. Hot baths or compresses may be comforting for aching or tight muscles. If respiratory function is affected, adequate oxygenation needs to be assured by maintaining a clear airway (provide percussion, postural drainage, and suctioning as needed). Emotional support of the child and the family is also important.	Oral live virus vaccine is available and should be given in infancy. This vaccine should not be given to immunodeficient children or their family members because the live virus is shed by the person who receives the live virus immunization. In these cases, inactivated poliovirus vaccine is given.	Respiratory or circulatory failure, bacterial infections, and emotional disturbances. Permanent paralysis.
Rabies: Agent: rabies virus. Incubation period: 9 days to several months.	Contact with the saliva of a diseased animal through bites or scratches.	Occurs in three stages and affects the central nervous system; damages the	All wounds must be cleansed with soap and water. Prophylaxis after exposure to ra-	Give supportive care. Avoid self-contamination with the child's saliva. Cleanse	Immunization of dogs and cats. Persons in high-risk groups (e.g., veterinarians	Death will occur unless antirabies vaccines are begun shortly after exposure.

Is communicable. The virus is shed 3 to 5 days before onset of the disease and throughout its course. Strict isolation for the duration of the illness is essential.	Skunks, bats, and bat excreta are common sources. Dogs, cats, coyotes, foxes, and raccoons are also infected. The animal that inflicted the bite is confined for 14 days for observation.	pons, medulla, brainstem, and thalamus. Prodromal stage: headache, malaise, fever, and numbness and tingling at bite; lasts 2 to 4 days. Excitation stage: increasing nervous irritability and apprehension; severe spasm of muscles of swallowing and respiration. Paralytic stage: muscle spasms stop; stupor, coma, and death may follow.	bies includes rabies immune human globulin and an inactivated virus vaccine.	all wounds with 20% tincture of green soap.	and animal handlers) may have preexposure immunization.	
Infectious mononucleosis: Agent: Epstein-Barr virus diagnosed by Mono-Spot blood test. Incubation period: 10 to 50 days. Is communicable during shedding of the virus, which continues for several months. Secretion precautions should be maintained for saliva of the child during hospitalization.	Intimate contact with an infected person and blood transfusions.	Malaise, anorexia, and fatigue. Sore throat, fever, cervical lymphadenopathy, hepatosplenomegaly, and enlarged tonsils with exudate.	No specific therapy is available. Antibiotics are used to treat underlying bacterial diseases. Clinical trials using acyclovir and interferon are in progress.	Bed rest is important. Encourage adequate fluid intake. Manage fevers. Advance activity as tolerated; the child should avoid strenuous physical activities for the first few months and avoid contact sports for a few more months.	Persons with a recent history of Epstein-Barr infections should not donate blood.	Splenic rupture. Aseptic meningitis, Guillain-Barré syndrome, and encephalitis are central nervous system complications. Rashes may occur and have been associated with the administration of ampicillin.

Table 28-9 Common Viral Infections of Childhood (*Continued*)

Disease	Source and Means of Transmission	Manifestations	Treatment	Nursing Management	Control	Complications
Infectious hepatitis: Agent: hepatitis virus A. Incubation period: 15 to 40 days. Is communicable 2 weeks prior to onset of jaundice. Enteric precautions are necessary for a week after onset of jaundice for children who are not yet toilet-trained or who have poor hygiene or diarrhea. There are no chronic carriers.	Fecal-oral transmission from contaminated water or food (e.g., shellfish). Crowded conditions, poor personal hygiene. Control and screening of food handlers are necessary.	Acute illness characterized by fever, anorexia, nausea, and fatigue. Jaundice with dark-colored urine and clay-colored stools may also occur, although jaundice is not as common in children with infectious hepatitis.	No specific treatment.	Good hand-washing technique and personal hygiene are essential to prevent transmission. Most cases are managed at home. Allow activity as tolerated. The child may tolerate frequent small meals better than a few large meals.	No specific measures are known. Prophylaxis of close contacts with gamma globulin is recommended.	Chronic sequelae have not been identified.
Serum hepatitis: Agent: hepatitis virus B. Incubation period: 60 to 180 days. Chronic carriers may be asymptomatic and are considered capable of communicating the disease. Health professionals who are carriers do not increase the risk of serum hepatitis in patients they care	Transfusion of blood and blood products of infected persons. Transplacental transmission does occur (see Chap. 17). Intimate contact (saliva, semen, and vaginal secretions).	Same as in infectious hepatitis. A rash and joint pain also occur occasionally early in the course of the disease.	No specific treatment.	Same as for infectious hepatitis.	A vaccine is available and is recommended for members of high-risk groups (including nurses who handle IV equipment and all others who come into contact with blood frequently). Hyperimmune globulin is given when there is known exposure to blood positive	Chronic liver disease.

to slightly over a week. The virus may be shed for up to 3 weeks in some cases. Exact communicability is not known. Respiratory and oral secretion precautions should be maintained if the child is hospitalized.		may be poor feeders, and older children may have anorexia.		nursing management.	nel with respiratory illnesses should avoid caring for infants during times of respiratory syncytial virus epidemics to decrease nosocomial spread of this disease.	
Gastroenteritis: Agents: rotavirus, Norwalk agent, and echo virus. Incubation period: 1 to 3 days. Communicability is unknown. Probably shedding of the virus begins at onset of symptoms and continues for a week. Enteric precautions are recommended.	Fecal-oral contamination.	Nausea, vomiting, and diarrhea are the most common symptoms. Fever and abdominal discomfort may also occur.	Supportive management, which includes rehydration orally or parenterally if dehydration occurs.	Assess fluid and electrolyte balance. See Chap. 18 for additional nursing management.	Hand-washing and good personal hygiene.	Dehydration and subsequent electrolyte imbalance.

Table 28-9 Common Viral Infections of Childhood (*Continued*)

Disease	Source and Means of Transmission	Manifestations	Treatment	Nursing Management	Control	Complications
Herpes simplex: Agent: Herpes Type I usually causes oral lesions; Type II usually causes genital lesions and neonatal disease. Incubation period: 2 to 20 days. Is communicable. The length of communicability is not known; the virus may be shed weeks after recovery. Secretion precautions should be maintained for the duration of the illness when the child is hospitalized. If infection is limited to the central nervous system, no isolation precautions are needed. (Genital herpes is discussed later in this chapter.)	Person-to-person contact. The exact mechanism is unknown. Intimate contact with the secretion of an infected person. Genital lesions: sexual contact. In newborns, contact with genital lesions during birth. Direct inoculation causes lesions of herpetic whitlow.	Depend on the portal of entry of the virus and factors such as the child's immune status and age. *Oral lesions* are often accompanied by fever, anorexia, irritability, and a sore mouth. The lesions are located on mucous membranes and are vesicular initially, with crusting in about 5 to 7 days. *Genital lesions* are rare in children before puberty, and if they occur, sexual abuse should be considered. The lesions are similar to oral lesions. The perineal area is usually reddened, edematous, and white, and vesic-	Depends on the severity of the illness. In general, topical steroids are contraindicated. Vidarabine used for herpes encephalitis and neonatal lesions of the skin and mucous membranes is effective. Other antiviral agents are currently being tested.	Provide supportive management. With oral lesions, offering cool, nonacidic fluids frequently around the clock may prevent dehydration. Maintain good oral hygiene. Genital lesions and their management are discussed later in this chapter.	No immunization is available. Delivery of an infant by cesarean section when the mother has cultures positive for herpes simplex virus or has clinical lesions before rupture of membranes eliminates spread of lesions of the lower genital tract. Cesarean section should be considered if membranes have been ruptured less than 6 h (exposure of the unborn child has probably taken place if membranes have been ruptured for longer than 6 h). Nursing personnel with herpetic whitlow lesions should not	Systemic infection involving the lungs, central nervous system, or liver. Local neurological illnesses may occur. Half of newborns affected with herpes during the neonatal period are born prior to the thirty-eighth week of gestation. Dehydration and excessive bleeding of the lesions may also be complications. Bacterial infections may occur in eczema herpeticum but rarely occur in acute oral lesions.

ular lesions are seen. These lesions crust in 10 to 14 days. *Herpetic whitlow* lesions are vesicular and are usually located on the hands or fingers. *Eczema herpeticum* vesicular lesions that become crusted are imposed on atopic eczema. The child may develop fever and irritability before crops of lesions appear. The herpes simplex virus remains latent in nerve endings and is activated by fever, sunlight, stress, or trauma. Recurrent infections that develop are usually localized lesions ("cold sores") without generalized symptoms. Many herpes infections are subclinical.

perform activities related to patient care. Staff members with active oral lesions should not kiss infants or children with eczema. How much of a risk they pose to the children they are caring for is unknown at present.

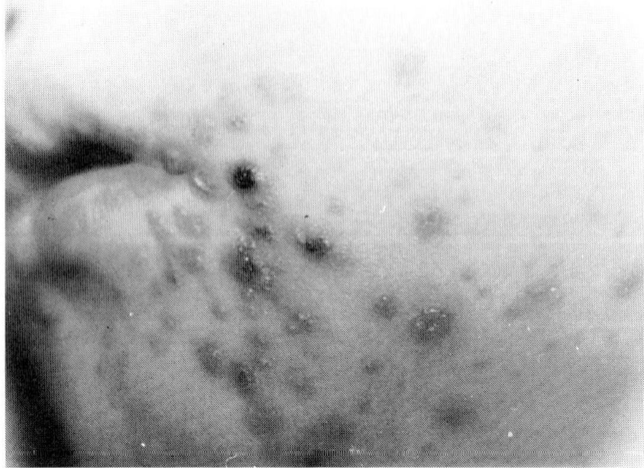

Figure 28-5 A child with the typical lesions of chickenpox (varicella). The chickenpox rash presents in "crops," with papules, vesicles, and crusts appearing in that order and with new lesions occurring after the original eruption.

the organism. Treatment is symptomatic. Rickettsial infections respond to administration of adequate amounts of either chloramphenicol or tetracyclines. Tetracyclines should not be given to children under the age of 9. Tetracyclines and chloramphenicol suppress the organism so that the child's immune processes can destroy the infection. Table 28-10 presents the major rickettsial infections of childhood.

Parasitic diseases

Parasites depend on humans to complete some stage of their life cycle. They cause damage to humans by using nutrients that the body needs for their growth. Some parasites cause anemia by feeding on blood, and others cause local tissue inflammation and destruction by taking up space or by producing a toxin. Some parasites cause the host to have an allergic reaction. Many parasites have elaborate life cycles involving several hosts. Generally, parasites are either *endoparasites,* which live inside the body, or *ectoparasites,* which live outside the body. The most common endoparasites in children are the helminths, or worms. The most common ectoparasites are lice.

Trichinae (*Trichinella spiralis*) and *tapeworms* (*Taenia saginata*) are two parasitic food contaminants. Trichinosis is generally associated with pork. It is spread when a hog eats garbage containing the trichina larvae, which then become embedded in the animal's muscles. Cooking the garbage before it is fed to hogs will prevent the spread of the parasites to the animals. When pork is prepared for human consumption, it should be thoroughly cooked (whitish gray in color, with no evidence of pink remaining). This will kill the parasites and prevent their spread to a human host.

Like trichinae, tapeworms are spread through garbage and can also be spread when cattle graze in polluted pastures. When humans eat raw or undercooked meat (beef or pork) which contains tapeworms, the organisms mature and continue their life cycle in the intestinal tract. Thorough cooking of meat will prevent the spread of this organism to humans. Table 28-11 presents the major parasitic infections of childhood.

Fungal diseases

The study of fungal diseases that affect humans is known as *medical mycology.* The two major groups of fungi are yeasts and molds. Mycotic infections can be either superficial infections, known as *dermatophytoses,* which involve the skin and nails, or deep mycoses, producing systemic infection.

The superficial mycoses are acquired by direct personal contact. The dermatophytes cause disfigurement by digesting the keratin of the skin, hair, or nails. *Ringworm,* so called because of the sharply demarked red, ringlike border of the lesions, is a superficial mycotic infection. The specific fungus can be identified by microscopic examination of skin scrapings. Local antifungal treatment is usually effective. See Fig. 28-6.

The deep fungal infections are transmitted by inhalation of airborne or dust-borne spores. These fungi are weak antigens, and they do not produce toxins. They cause damage by provoking a hypersensitivity reaction by the host against their proteins. The most commonly occurring systemic mycosis in children is *histoplasmosis.* The diseases caused by these agents are serious and can be fatal. They sometimes occur when the host's resistance is lowered or when the normal flora are altered as a result of prolonged antibiotic therapy. Deep fungal infections are difficult to treat, and there are few specific antifungal agents. Amphotericin B is sometimes used. Table 28-12 presents the common fungal infections of childhood.

Table 28-10 Major Rickettsial Infections of Childhood

Disease and Agent	Source and Means of Transmission	Incubation Period	Manifestations	Treatment	Nursing Management	Control	Complications
Epidemic typhus (*Rickettsia prowazekii*)	Body lice. Feces of the lice are scratched into the skin.	7 to 14 days	High fever, headache, and generalized aches and pains. A maculopapular rash appears by days 4 to 6, first on the trunk near the axillae; the face, palms, and soles of the feet are spared. The rash progresses from maculopapular to hemorrhagic, and finally brown pigmented areas develop.	Tetracycline or chloramphenicol until the child is afebrile for at least 3 days.	Close supervision is necessary if the child is stuporous. Maintain hydration. Take nursing measures and give medication for fever control. Instruct the parents to wash the child's clothing in hot water to kill lice and eggs.	Delouse the child with insecticides and isolate until this has been accomplished. Exposed persons need to be deloused if indicated. Vaccine is no longer available in the United States.	Coma, delirium, or mental changes may occur. In cases of severe disease, there may also be cardiac manifestations.
Endemic typhus (*Rickettsia mooseri* or *typhi*)	Rat fleas. Feces of the fleas are scratched into the skin.	7 to 12 days	A milder version of epidemic typhus; the rash is rarely hemorrhagic.	Tetracycline or chloramphenicol until the child is afebrile for at least 3 days.	Maintain close supervision if the child is stuporous. Maintain hydration. Take nursing measures and give medication for fever control. Instruct the parents to wash the child's clothing in hot water to kill lice and eggs.	Eradicate rodents and rat fleas. No isolation is necessary. Vaccine is no longer available.	Complications rarely occur.

Table 28-10 Major Rickettsial Infections of Childhood (*Continued*)

Disease and Agent	Source and Means of Transmission	Incubation Period	Manifestations	Treatment	Nursing Management	Control	Complications
Rocky Mountain spotted fever (*Rickettsia rickettsii*)	Tick bites (from ticks on dogs and wild rodents).	1 to 10 days	Early symptoms are muscular aches, headache, malaise, and anorexia; then a high fever develops, and early symptoms are accentuated. A rash, consisting of bright-red macules, begins at the ankles and spreads to the palms, soles, back, arms, thighs, and chest.	Tetracycline or chloramphenicol until the child is afebrile for at least 2 or 3 days.	Educate the parents about the disease, including what to do if ticks are seen. Provide nutritious foods and beverages to maintain hydration status. Manage fevers.	Remove ticks, protecting the hands and not crushing the ticks; no isolation is necessary; an enduring immunity develops after the disease.	Complications are infrequent if the disease is treated; they are severe or fatal in untreated cases: disseminated intravascular coagulation, gangrene, deafness, and encephalitis.
Q fever (*Rickettsia burnetii*)	Harbored in domestic farm animals and transmitted by inhalation of infected dust or consumption of contaminated raw milk.	2 to 4 weeks	Sudden onset of fever, chills, and weakness. Within a week, chest pains and a cough develop. There is no rash.	Tetracycline or chloramphenicol until the child is afebrile for 2 or 3 days.	Provide for adequate nutrition. Give supportive care.	No isolation is necessary. Adequate pasteurization of milk is required to kill the organism.	Pneumonia is a common complication. Endocarditis, hepatitis, meningitis, and nephritis are reported complications, generally lasting from 1 to 4 weeks.

Lyme disease (*Borrelia burdorferi*)	Tick bites. Small mammals are hosts to immature ticks; the white-tailed deer is the preferred host for the adult tick. Geographically in United States has occurred in upper Midwest, Pacific Northwest, and northeastern coast. Seasonal; occurs between May and October.	Variable; several days to weeks	Systemic symptoms: malaise, fatigue, fever, headache, and stiff neck and muscles. The typical cutaneous rash, *erythema chronicum migrans* (ECM), is a large, round, erythematous skin rash. The lesion begins with a macule or papule at the site of the tick bite and expands several days or weeks later, developing a bright-red border. Secondary lesions may develop several days after the first ECM lesion.	Early institution of antibiotics reduces complications and shortens ECM; it also decreases the arthritic complications. Penicillin is recommended in children younger than 5. Tetracycline appears to be most effective in preventing major sequelae in adults.	Educate families about the disease. Provide comfort measures for arthritis. Assist with medication.	Avoid tick-infested areas; avoid overpopulation of white-tailed deer. Inspect household pets who may be tick carriers.	Arthritis, neurological abnormalities such as meningitis and cranial neuropathies (Bell's palsy), and cardiac abnormalities (atrioventricular block) may occur.

Table 28-11 Major Parasitic Infections of Childhood (*Continued*)

Disease and Agent	Source and Means of Transmission	Incubation Period	Manifestations	Treatment	Nursing Management	Control	Complications
Endoparasites; helminths							
Roundworm (*Ascaris*)*	Soil, with infected eggs from human feces. Ingestion of eggs from soil-contaminated food, toys, hands, water, and dust.	8 to 10 weeks	Larval stage: lung symptoms, asthma, wheezing, itching, malaise, and fever. Worm stage: abdominal pain, nausea, vomiting, malnutrition, dehydration, electrolyte imbalance, and anorexia.	Treat with anthelmintics (pyrantel-pamoate stains stools red).	Instruct the child and the family about the disease and the treatment; good hand-washing is important.	Appropriate handling of enteric secretions is important; decontaminate toys; wash the hands thoroughly. Isolation of the child is not necessary.	Adult worms may migrate and block the pancreatic and bile duct; intestinal obstruction.
Pinworm (*Enterobius vermicularis*)	Infected humans; contaminated hands, food, and air (from shaking infected bedding or clothing).	2 to 6 weeks	Eggs stick to perianal skin; intense itching, may lead to loss of sleep, irritability, nausea, and vomiting. Worms lay eggs at the anus. Pressing cellophane tape on the anus will pick up eggs or worms for inspection under a microscope.	Treat family members as well as the child with anthelmintics.	Reassure the family that the infection is not the result of poor sanitation; the disease is easily treated and is not a serious problem. Recommend keeping the fingernails short, frequent hand-washing, and having children sleep alone. Linens, pajamas, and underwear should be laundered and should not be shaken.	Infection in families common, especially in temperate and colder climate where children live and play closer together. Reinfection is common unless all family members are treated at the same time. Isolation precautions are not necessary.	Complications are rare.

*Adult roundworms lay eggs in the intestines. The eggs pass to soil, incubating there in 2 to 3 weeks. When eggs in soil are swallowed, larvae penetrate the intestines and move to the lungs and back to the gastrointestinal tract.

					A thorough housecleaning is necessary, including damp-mopping floors and cleaning the vacuum cleaner.		
Hookworm (*Necator americanus; Ancylostoma duodenale*)	Soil contaminated with human feces. Larvae penetrate unbroken skin (usually on the feet), enter the blood, migrate to the lungs, and then are swallowed.	6 weeks	Symptoms depend on the number of worms; worms feed on the host's blood, causing anemia, pain, diarrhea, and itching. Physical and sexual development may be delayed with chronic infestation.	Treat the child and the family with anthelmintics.	Educate the family and the child regarding appropriate disposal of human feces, wearing of shoes, and adequate dietary intake.	Improve sanitation.	With severe infestation, there may be palpitations, tachycardia, edema, and congestive heart failure.
Trichinosis (*Trichinella spiralis*)	Pigs fed garbage that is not cooked are the most common source. Humans are infected through ingestion of insufficiently cooked pork.	5 to 7 days	Symptoms depend on the amount ingested and the stage. Intestinal stage: nausea, vomiting, diarrhea, fever, and urticaria. When in general circulation: edema of the face and eyelids, fever, cardiac or respiratory symptoms, muscle aches, and chest pain.	Treat with thiabendazole during the intestinal phase; its effectiveness in later stages is questionable.	Teach the family to cook pork thoroughly, until it is whitish gray in color. Maintain bed rest. Give analgesics for fever and discomfort.	Boil garbage before giving it to pigs.	Cardiac failure and death are rare; with central nervous system invasion, headache and stiff neck occur.

Table 28-11 Major Parasitic Infections of Childhood (*Continued*)

Disease and Agent	Source and Means of Transmission	Incubation Period	Manifestations	Treatment	Nursing Management	Control	Complications
Ectoparasites							
Pediculosis (*Pediculus humanus capitis*: head lice; *P.h. corporis*: body lice; *Phthirius pubis*: pubic lice, "crabs")	Close contact with infested persons or articles.	Days to weeks	Head lice are most common in children. Eggs attach to hair shafts (louse is on the scalp), causing intense itching and excoriation.	Improve personal hygiene; shampoo and bathe with gamma benzene hexachloride (e.g., Kwell) or pyrethrin-based products. If on eyelashes, apply petroleum jelly to the area; remove lice manually.	Educate the child and the family about the transmission of the disease and the treatment. Fomites play a role in transmission; therefore, encourage the child to use his or her own combs, brushes, hats, etc.	Prevent close contact with infected persons; treat all family members at the same time if appropriate. Launder linens in hot water. Re-treat if the first treatment was not effective, but no more often than twice in 1 week. The child may return to school the morning after the first treatment.	Secondary bacterial infections are common.
Scabies (*Sarcoptes scabiei*: "itch mites")	Close contact with infested persons.	2 to 6 weeks	Intense itching in areas between fingers and toes and on the wrists, abdomen, axillae, and genitalia. Mite burrows under the skin, leaving eggs and feces in blackish-red bumps.	Treat the skin with gamma benzene hexachloride (e.g., Kwell). Wash clothing, bedding, and personal articles in hot, soapy water.	Educate the child and the family about the disease, including the role of families in transmission and necessary precautions. Nurses wear gowns and gloves when caring for the child before and during treatment.	All family members should be treated simultaneously, even if asymptomatic. Isolation is not required after treatment.	Secondary bacterial infections are common.

					Careful hand-washing is also important. Instruct the parents to launder bedding and clothing.		
Giardiasis (*Giardia lamblia*), a protozoan	The cyst form of giardiasis is ingested. The organism inhabits the mucosa of the duodenum and upper jejunum. Spread by person-to-person contact, or waterborne or foodborne; spread in day-care centers from non-toilet-trained children.	2 to 3 weeks	Most infected persons are asymptomatic. Diarrhea may alternate with constipation, abdominal cramps, anorexia, nausea, vomiting, headache, low-grade fever, weight loss, malaise, and flatulence.	Untreated infections usually resolve spontaneously in 4 to 6 weeks. Chronic infections have been documented. Treat with quinacrine hydrochloride (Atabrine) 2 mg/kg three times daily for 5 days for children (maximum, 300 mg/day); for adults, 100 mg three times a day for 5 days. Adults may be treated with metronidazole (Flagyl) 250 mg three times a day for 5 days. Use in children if other drugs fail or are	Good hand-washing, especially after diaper changes.	Diagnose from stool specimen for cysts. Follow good hygienic practices in day-care centers, especially proper diaper disposal. Thorough hand-washing is important. Avoid drinking untreated or improperly treated surface water.	None known.

Table 28-11 Major Parasitic Infections of Childhood (*Continued*)

Disease and Agent	Source and Means of Transmission	Incubation Period	Manifestations	Treatment	Nursing Management	Control	Complications
				not tolerated; dosage is 5 mg per kg of body weight three times daily for 5 days. Furazolidone (Furoxone) is available in suspension; for children, the dose is 1.25 mg per kg of body weight four times a day for 7 days; for adults, the dose is 100 mg four times a day for 7 days. None of these drugs are recommended in pregnancy. Paromomycin, 30 mg per kg of body weight, may be given 3 to 4 times daily for 7 days.			

Table 28-12 Common Fungal Infections of Childhood

Disease and Agent	Source and Means of Transmission	Manifestations	Treatment	Nursing Management	Control	Complications
Tinea capitis (scalp ringworm)	Close contact with infected humans and animals.	Small reddened scaling areas on the scalp, often associated with alopecia.	Topical antifungal agents alone are of little value in treating an active infection. Systemic griseofulvin for 4 to 8 weeks is usually effective.	Griseofulvin should be given after meals to increase absorption and to decrease gastrointestinal disturbances. Educate the child and the family regarding transmission of the disease. Tell the child not to share hats or combs with others.	Destroy or decontaminate hats, combs, etc. Provide a protective covering for the area until therapy is initiated.	Complications are rare. May include fever and lymphadenopathy.
Tinea corporis (body ringworm)	Close contact with infected humans and animals.	Circular lesions that are slightly raised and red at the periphery are found on smooth, nonhairy skin. Itchiness and scaling are common.	Topical miconazole or clotrimazole is effective. Extensive disease can be treated with griseofulvin systemically.	Give griseofulvin after meals. Educate the child and the family about the disease. Advise against sharing hats and combs.	Decontaminate or destroy clothing.	Complications rarely occur.
Tinea cruris ("jock itch")	Direct contact with the skin, clothing, or towels of infected humans.	The lesions are similar to those of tinea corporis except that they are limited to the groin area.	Topical antifungal, lotions are effective.	Keep the area clean and dry. The child should wear loose clothing and cotton underwear and should not share towels. Educate the child and the family regarding disease transmission.	Decontaminate or destroy clothing.	Complications rarely occur.
Tinea pedis (athlete's foot)	Contact with the skin or desquamated skin of infected persons	Vesicular lesions occur between the toes and on the soles; the	Topical antifungal lotions, ointments, and powders are ef-	Have the child wear clean, dry socks and avoid sweating feet;	Infected persons should not use public showers or other public	Complications rarely occur. Griseofulvin treatment may

	or with colonies of fungi present in damp areas (especially public pools, showers, and locker rooms).	skin becomes macerated and peels, and fissures form. The lesions are frequently pruritic.	fective. Systemic griseofulvin may also be used.	change socks as needed. Dry well between toes after bathing. Encourage the child to wear sandals to decrease perspiration on the feet.	facilities. Public areas need to be adequately cleaned. Clogs should be worn in public showers.	fail if foot hygiene is poor.
Candidiasis (moniliasis, yeast, and thrush)	Contact with infected persons. Newborns may be infected during birth. Hands, bottles, and nipples become contaminated with yeast.	Transient infection in the mouth—white, curdy oral patches (thrush)—may be caused by systemic antibiotic therapy. Infants may develop infections in wet, macerated areas such as the diaper area and neck creases. The rash has a red base with a white exudate that turns grayish if dried.	Oral and topical antifungal agents are effective. Amphotericin B is the drug of choice for systemic infections. Nystatin liquid is given po four times daily. Apply antifungal ointment to clean, dry diaper area after each diaper change.	With the oral disease form, encourage the parents not to share bottles or spoons with siblings or other children. Wash bottles and nipples with hot, soapy water and brush. When the disease is in the neck folds, rinse with hot water. Cleanse the area, especially after meals, and keep it as dry as possible. When the disease is in the diaper area, change the diapers when wet and air-dry if possible. Wash hands carefully.	Hand-washing between contacts with patients is important, especially when caring for an infected child. Infants with the oral disease form do not need water isolation. Older children with mucous membrane lesions should be maintained on drainage and secretion precautions.	The disease may disseminate, generally in immunocompromised children.
Histoplasmosis	Inhalation of airborne spores from soil with a highly organic content (around chicken coops, bat caves, etc.).	Symptoms appear 10 to 14 days after exposure; they may be benign. The child may be asymptomatic or may	Amphotericin B is the drug of choice. The minimum length of treatment is 6 months.	Manage fevers with nursing measures and medication as ordered. Encourage intake of foods high in	Spray to reduce dust, and investigate outbreaks for common sources.	The disease may disseminate, which is potentially fatal. Symptoms of disseminated disease may in-

Table 28-12 Common Fungal Infections of Childhood (*Continued*)

Disease and Agent	Source and Means of Transmission	Manifestations	Treatment	Nursing Management	Control	Complications
		have symptoms due to a lung lesion—fever, malaise, cough, chest pain, and weakness—lasting 4 to 6 weeks. A very serious disease with a high fatality rate. The acute, disseminated form of the disease is most frequent in children under 2 years of age. The chronic form is uncommon in children.		potassium, since treatment with amphotericin B may lead to hypokalemia.		clude hepatosplenomegaly, fever, diarrhea, skin lesions, and pneumonitis.
Coccidioidomycosis (San Joaquin Valley fever)	Inhalation of dust containing arthrospores of *C. immitis*. Occurs in the western United States, northern Mexico, and parts of Central and South America.	The symptoms of primary disease are mild and flulike. Some children have more severe symptoms, including fever, cough, anorexia, aches, and a sore throat. An erythematous rash on the trunk, which may spread over the body, is not uncommon.	Primary disease is mild and self-limited and requires no therapy. Amphotericin B is the drug of choice; the minimum length of treatment is 6 months.	Give supportive care. Determine whether the child has traveled if the disease is not commonly seen in the area. Depending on the degree of dissemination, some isolation precautions may be indicated.	No effective immunization has been developed.	Dissemination may occur, although rarely, within 6 months of development of primary disease. Dissemination is unlikely after 1 year. Affected areas may include the bones, joints, lymph nodes, skin, and meninges. Meningitis is a more common complication in children than in adults; without treatment, it results in death.

gonococcal infections, child abuse must be considered.

Gonorrhea ("clap," "dose," or "drip") is caused by *Neisseria gonorrhoeae,* an anaerobic gram-negative diplococcus bacterium whose growth is enhanced in the presence of carbon dioxide. *N. gonorrhoeae* is sensitive to light, air, and temperature and can penetrate only mucous membranes such as those found in the cervix, urethra, mouth, throat, and anus; it lives in the submucosa. It is transmitted only by sexual contact or during the birth process, not by contact with toilet seats or dirty towels.

Infection A gonococcal infection in boys usually causes urethritis (pain on urination) and a thick, creamy discharge (penile drip) within 2 to 14 days of infection. These symptoms cause most boys to seek treatment. The symptoms may spontaneously decrease after 2 to 8 weeks. However, the disease is still present and can spread to a sexual partner or invade the posterior urethra, epididymis, and prostate gland. As many as 50 percent of infected males may remain totally asymptomatic; 50 percent of females may have no symptoms or such mild discharge, dysuria, or pelvic tenderness that they do not seek medical care. Symptoms in girls seeking care usually include a yellow, irritating vaginal discharge; perineal irritation; and painful urination.

Diagnosis A definitive diagnosis in both males and females may be made by using a culture of Thayer-Martin medium (TMM, chocolate agar) or modified Thayer-Martin (MTM, chocolate agar plus antibiotics that inhibit the majority of the normal flora). A cotton swab is used to culture the cervix in females or the urethra, rectum, and mouth in males and females. The plate is then incubated in a carbon dioxide environment. The first ounce of freshly voided urine from the male will contain pus cells. This can be collected and centrifuged, and the sediment used for a culture. Immediate diagnosis in males can be made using urethral discharge to do a Gram stain. Positive findings show polymorphonuclear cells with gram-negative intracellular diplococci. A Gram stain is not reliable in females because the cervix has gram-negative bacteria as normal flora.

In 1976, a new type of gonococcus—*penicillinase-producing Neisseria gonorrhoeae* (PPNG), which is resistant to penicillin therapy and usually ampicillin—was recognized in the United States. Although there are few cases of PPNG in the United States, posttreatment culturing of every patient with gonorrhea is very important. This is best done 3 to 7 days after the course of antibiotics is complete. If the repeat culture is positive, a test to detect the penicillinase enzyme can be done by the local health department. See Table 28-13 for treatment schedules.

Complications

Pelvic Inflammatory Disease More than 1 million females develop pelvic inflammatory disease (PID) each year in the United States, and 16 to 20 percent of them are adolescents. Risk factors include use of an intrauterine device, a current *N. gonorrhoeae* or *C. trachomatis* infection, and a past history of gonococcal PID. In gonococcal PID, the organism spreads from the cervix to the fallopian tubes by way of the lymphatics. The onset of symptoms is often abrupt, and the symptoms may include abdominal pain and fever. Some infections are subclinical, and no signs or symptoms are present.

Pertinent physical findings are exquisite bilateral lower abdominal pain, pain on gentle motion of the cervix (Chandelier sign) during a vaginal examination, a positive gonorrhea culture, an increased white blood count, and an increased erythrocyte sedimentation rate. Hospitalization is required only for severe infections. Gonococcal PID must be differentiated from ectopic pregnancy, appendicitis, endometritis, pyelonephritis, and torsion of *adnexa* (tubes and ovaries), which cause similar signs. *Fitz-Hugh–Curtis syndrome* (acute perihepatitis) causes right upper quadrant abdominal pain, hepatic tenderness, and abnormal liver function. Tubal-ovarian abscesses and tubal strictures due to gonococcal PID are the leading cause of infertility in women and also predispose them to ectopic pregnancy.

Disseminated Gonococcal Infection Gonococci can cause systemic disease by spreading via the bloodstream and lymphatics. Arthritis is the most common complication of the spread of a gonococcal infection. The arthritis-dermatitis syndrome involves the wrists, knees, ankles, and small joints of the hands and feet. A typical rash with papular, petechial, and pustular skin lesions occurs primarily on the distal extremities. Sometimes the gonococcal organisms have been cultured from the skin lesions. Endocarditis and meningitis seen in response to a systemic infection occur, but are rare.

Table 28-13 Recommended Treatment for Gonococcal Infections

Diagnosis	Therapy	Alternatives
Uncomplicated gonorrhea: Child weighing more than 45 kg	Procaine penicillin, 4.8 million units IM at two sites with 1 g of probenecid PO	*Tetracycline, 0.5 g PO qid for 5 to 7 days (total dose: 10 g); ampicillin, 3.5 g with 1 g of probenecid PO; amoxicillin, 3 g with 1 g of probenecid PO
Child weighing less than 45 kg	Amoxicillin, 50 mg/kg PO, plus probenecid, 25 mg/kg PO, or aqueous penicillin G, 100,000 units per kilogram IM, plus probenecid, 25 mg/kg PO	If child is allergic to penicillin, spectinomycin, 40 mg/kg IM
Gonorrhea in pregnancy	Amoxicillin, 50 mg/kg PO, plus probenecid, 25 mg/kg PO, or aqueous penicillin G, 100,000 units per kilogram IM, plus probenecid, 25 mg/kg PO	If allergic to penicillin, erthromycin, 1 g PO, followed by 0.5 g qid for 4 days; cefazolin, 2 g IM plus 1 g of probenecid; or spectinomycin, 2 g IM
Treatment failures or penicillinase-producing strains	Spectinomycin, 2 g IM in single injection	If infection is resistant to spectinomycin, cefoxitin, 2 g IM, plus probenecid, 1 g PO
Pelvic inflammatory disease (outpatient)	Tetracycline, 0.5 g qid for 10 days	Procaine penicillin, 4.8 million units IM, or ampicillin, 3.5 g PO, or amoxicillin, 3 g PO, plus probenecid, 1 g PO, followed by ampicillin or amoxicillin, 0.5 g PO qid for 10 days
Pelvic inflammatory disease (hospitalized patient)	†Penicillin, 20 million units IV per day until improvement; then ampicillin, 0.5 g PO qid for 10 days	Tetracycline, 0.25 g IV qid until improvement; then 0.5 g PO qid for 10 days
Disseminated gonococcal infection	Penicillin, 10 million units IV per day until improvement; then 0.5 g ampicillin qid for a total of 7 days	Ampicillin, 3.5 g PO, or amoxicillin, 3 g PO, plus probenecid, 1 g PO, followed by ampicillin or amoxicillin, 0.5 g PO qid for 7 days. Tetracycline, 0.5 g PO qid for 7 days. Spectinomycin, 4 g per day in two doses IM for 3 days, is the drug of choice for penicillinase-producing *N. gonorrhoeae*.
Disseminated gonococcal disease (infants)	Penicillin G, 75,000 to 100,000 units per kilogram per day in two to three doses for 7 days	
Gonococcal ophthalmia, peritonitis, or arthritis (child weighing less than 45 kg)	Penicillin G, 100,000 units per kilogram per day IV for 7 days	
Meningitis (child weighing less than 45 kg)	Aqueous penicillin G, 250,000 units per kilogram per day in six doses IV for 10 days	
Infant	Penicillin G, 100,000 units per kilogram per day IV in three to four doses for 10 days	
Gonococcal ophthalmia (neonatal disease)	Penicillin, 50,000 units per kilogram per day in two doses IV for 7 days	

*Tetracyclines should not be used during pregnancy or in children under 9 years of age.

†Long-acting penicillins (such as benzathine penicillin G) and penicillin V are *not* recommended in the treatment of gonorrhea.

Sources: Adapted from CDC guidelines and American Academy of Pediatrics, Committee on Infectious Diseases, *1982 Red Book*, Evanston, Ill.

Ophthalmia Neonatorum (Conjunctivitis) This infection of the newborn's eyes is acquired during passage through the birth canal of an infected mother. Often bacteria are harbored in Bartholin's glands. The incubation period is 2 to 4 days. If symptoms of purulent conjunctival discharge and edema are not treated, blindness can result.

Silver nitrate drops or tetracycline or erythromycin ointment is routinely administered to infants at birth to prevent this infection. In most cases, infants born to mothers with an active infection do not develop conjunctivitis with this treatment. However, a single intramuscular dose of penicillin is recommended for these infants because occasional cases of gonococcal conjunctivitis and of infection of organs such as the liver, heart, and brain have been reported.

Preadolescent Gonococcal Infection In young girls, symptoms of gonococcal infection are labial redness and swelling and purulent vaginal discharge. Boys have the same symptoms as adult males. In the first year of life, gonococcal vulvovaginitis is most frequently acquired nonsexually, especially when the infant shares a bed with an infected parent or when hygiene is poor. After the age of 1 year, most infections in children result from sexual abuse (rape, sexual assault, or incest). Young children who are suspected of having STDs should have cultures of the pharynx and rectum as well as the vagina and urethra.

Syphilis

Syphilis ("lues," "siff," "pox," or "bad blood") is caused by *Treponema pallidum,* an aerobic spirochete which enters the body during sexual contact through mucous membranes or a cut in the skin. Syphilis may also be transmitted transplacentally from an affected mother to the unborn fetus. This fragile organism dies quickly outside the body and is easily killed by drying and common bacterial agents. There is a very low incidence of the disease in persons under the age of 19.

During the incubation period of 10 to 90 days (the average is 21 days), the person has no symptoms. The *primary stage,* during which a *chancre* (a hard, painless ulcer) appears at the site of infection (usually the penis, cervix, vulva, mouth, or rectum), begins about 21 days after contact. The chancre may not be noticed because there is no pain. If it is not treated, it will last for 3 to 5 weeks or more and then disappear.

The secondary stage begins 6 weeks to several months after the infection and lasts for a few days to a year, but it may recur up to 2 years later. Symptoms of secondary syphilis are:

1. Skin eruptions: a generalized rash that is bilaterally symmetrical; *mucous patches,* lesions in the mouth; and *condylomata lata,* warts on the genital area. All these skin lesions are infectious.
2. Systemic symptoms: low-grade fever, headache, malaise, and baldness (alopecia).
3. Adenopathy or swollen glands.
4. A positive serology test for syphilis.

These symptoms mimic those of other diseases and resolve slowly and spontaneously even without treatment.

The latent period, during which there are no overt symptoms, begins with the resolution of the secondary symptoms and may last for a few years or for the remainder of the person's life.

After 10 to 20 years, *tertiary syphilis* develops; it may be benign or result in blindness, heart disease, paralysis, organic brain disease, or even death, depending on which body system the spirochetes affect. The lesions in tertiary syphilis are called *gummas;* they affect any body system, but particularly cardiovascular tissue. *Neurosyphilis* is a syphilitic infection of the nervous system. *General paresis* is a form of central nervous system syphilis in which the nerve roots are affected. In *tabes dorsalis,* the dorsal roots of the spinal cord are affected.

Congenital syphilis In congenital syphilis, the disease is transmitted from an infected pregnant woman to her unborn infant. It was previously thought that the spirochete crosses the placenta only after the eighteenth week of pregnancy. It is now known that the fetus can be infected at any gestational age, although exactly when fetal damage occurs is questionable. A general rule is: The longer the duration of the untreated maternal infection before pregnancy, the less likely it is that the fetus will be stillborn or damaged. Latent or tertiary syphilis is less likely to cause stillbirth and severe infection than primary or secondary syphilis. Treatment of the mother should be initiated as soon as she is diagnosed. Penicillin crosses the placenta and also cures the

Table 28-14 Signs of Congenital Syphilis

Early Signs (Newborns)
Skin lesions—small, dark-red, copper-colored spots, often bullous
Snuffles—profuse nasal discharge with resulting rhagades (facial scars or fissures)
Hepatosplenomegaly—enlarged liver and spleen
Abnormal cerebrospinal fluid findings
Osteochondritis—femur and humerus affected
Late Signs (Children over 2 Years of Age)
Interstitial keratitis (blindness)
Hutchinson teeth (widely spaced, notched central incisors)
Saddle nose (destruction of cartilage of nasal septum)

infected fetus. Treatment will not reverse prior damage. As a result of early screening of pregnant women, congenital syphilis is very rarely seen. See Table 28-14 for the signs of congenital syphilis.

Diagnosis When a lesion or rash is present in primary, secondary, or congenital syphilis, the diagnosis may be made by visualizing the organism (*T. pallidum*) from the lesion under a dark-field microscope. The serological tests—VDRL, FTA, and RPR—will be negative during the incubation period of syphilis, but positive during the primary, secondary, latent, and tertiary stages.

Treatment Primary, secondary, and latent syphilis infections of less than 1 year's duration are treated with 2.4 million units of long-acting benzathine penicillin given intramuscularly in a single injection. If an adolescent is allergic to penicillin, the treatment is a total dosage of 30 g of tetracycline or erythromycin. Syphilis of more than 1 year's duration is treated with 2.4 million units of benzathine penicillin given intramuscularly weekly for 3 successive weeks. Cerebrospinal fluid examination is advisable for all patients with syphilis of more than 1 year's duration to rule out neurosyphilis. All sexual partners are treated in the same way as the person with the active infection.

Adolescents who are being treated for syphilis should be warned of the possibility of experiencing a Jarisch-Herxheimer reaction, which occurs in 50 to 90 percent of people within a few hours of treatment and lasts for 24 to 48 h. The reaction consists of headache, chills, fatigue, and transient fever. Its cause is unknown, but it may be due to an allergic reaction or to a release of endotoxins from the killed treponemata. The treatment is rest and aspirin.

Follow-up care includes repeat VDRLs at 3-month intervals during the first year and treatment of suspected contacts.

Vaginitis

Vaginitis is a common ailment that is not necessarily dangerous but can be very uncomfortable, painful, and anxiety-producing. Vaginitis is a special problem for adolescents, who may keep silent and feel guilty because they associate it with venereal disease. Antibiotic therapy, long-term steroid therapy, irritation caused by foreign bodies or masturbation, chemical irritation (douching), diabetes, pregnancy, use of birth control pills, and sexual contact predispose individuals to vaginitis.

Normal vaginal discharge is transparent or slightly milky in color; a vaginal infection is characterized by an increased amount of discharge that is foul-smelling, irritating, and purulent. The infection may spread from the vagina to include the vulva and cervix. Another agent that causes vaginitis is *Chlamydia trachomatis,* which was discussed earlier in this chapter. The symptoms of most vaginal infections are similar: vulvovaginal itching, redness, and soreness; burning on urination; and pain during intercourse. Variations in types of vaginal discharge help differentiate the infections.

Monilial infections Monilial infections are caused by an overgrowth of a fungus, *Candida albicans,* which may be found in the normal vaginal flora. There is a thick, white discharge, sometimes resembling cottage cheese. The vagina is intensely itchy, and the perineum appears inflamed and sore. Approximately one-third to one-half of all vaginal infections are caused by *C. albicans*. Some predisposing factors for overgrowth of the fungus in adolescents include poorly controlled diabetes, antibiotic therapy, steroid treatment, poor health, poor hygiene, use of oral contraceptives, and pregnancy. Monilial infections can also be sexually transmitted.

Because *C. albicans* needs a dark, warm, moist area for growth, males who are circumcised or who practice good hygiene usually do not develop symptoms. A local, red, itchy rash may develop on the penis after contact with the infected discharge. Treatment of males consists of using

Table 28-15 Symptoms, Diagnosis, and Treatment of Vaginal Infections

Infection	Symptoms	Diagnosis	Treatment
Moniliasis (*Candida albicans*)	Itching; thick, cheesy, white discharge; erythematous vulva and vagina; not malodorous; dyspareunia (pain on intercourse); dysuria	Use vaginal discharge material in potassium hydroxide on glass slide examined under microscope or Nickerson culture.	Nystatin (Mycostatin), 1 to 2 suppositories daily for 2 to 3 weeks inserted high in vagina (continue during menstruation to complete therapy). Monistat cream, one applicator daily for 7 to 10 days.
Trichomoniasis (*Trichomonas vaginalis*)	Malodorous, frothy, yellow-green discharge; itchy, erythematous vulvovagina and cervix; strawberry cervix; dyspareunia; dysuria	Use normal saline with vaginal discharge on glass slide examined under microscope (moving protozoa are seen).	Flagyl, 2 g orally in single dose. Reinfection: Flagyl, 250 mg PO tid for 10 days. Not used during pregnancy. Avoid alcohol until 2 days after treatment.
Nonspecific (*Gardnerella vaginalis*); "clue cells"	Thinnish, grayish-white discharge, malodorous; itchiness rare; dysuria; dyspareunia	Vaginal material and normal saline on glass slide examined under microscope, then cultured.	Flagyl, 2 g PO in single dose. Reinfection: Flagyl, 500 mg PO bid for 7 days.
Herpes genitalis (herpes simplex virus, types 1 and 2)	Early symptoms may include itching, burning, or tingling, followed by appearance of fluid-filled vesicles which rupture 1 to 2 days later, and then painful, small, round, shallow ulcers with red base that may last up to 1 to 3 weeks; dyspareunia and dysuria. With recurrent infection, symptoms milder—last 4 to 10 days	Viral cultures. Tzank test. Positive viral titers for herpes simplex.	No cure. Analgesics for pain; warm sitz bath. Acyclovir, when available in oral form, may become the drug of choice to prevent and/or minimize episodes.

a nystatin ointment on the rash and abstaining from sexual contact (or wearing condoms). Treatment of females includes using a fungicidal or antibiotic vaginal cream or suppositories. Taking sitz baths and wearing loose clothing and cotton underwear may help. Decreasing the amount of free carbohydrates in the diet is also suggested. Table 28-15 presents the symptoms, diagnosis, and treatment of vaginal infections.

Trichomoniasis Trichomoniasis is caused by the protozoan *Trichomonas vaginalis*. Human beings and other mammals, insects, fish, and fowl are known to serve as hosts to these flagellated parasites. They normally are carried in the intestinal tract. *Trichomonas* accounts for up to 28 percent of genital infections in adolescent girls and may be responsible for as much as 15 percent of urethritis in boys. Trichomoniasis may be transmitted through sexual contact or by self-infection through contamination from the rectum. The discharge is usually very irritating, thin, foamy, and yellowish green in color.

Males are usually asymptomatic (carriers) but can spread the infection to sexual partners through the ejaculate. Therefore, both sexual partners should be treated with Flagyl. Alcoholic beverages should be avoided for 2 days after treatment with Flagyl, since it has a minor Antabuse effect (alcohol causes nausea). Flagyl should not be used during pregnancy (Table 28-15).

Nonspecific vaginitis *Nonspecific vaginitis* is a term used for vulvovaginitis when gonococci, yeast, trichomonas, *Chlamydia*, or an allergic reaction is not the cause. *Gardnerella vaginalis*, a bacterium, is responsible for more than 90 percent of nonspecific vaginitis. Although adolescent boys are usually asymptomatic, gardnerella may be transmitted during sexual contact. Therefore, with recurrent infections, both partners should be treated to prevent reinfection. *G. vaginalis* responds well to treatment with Flagyl (Table 28-15).

Herpes Twenty-five to fifty percent of all persons with herpetic infections are teenagers. Herpetic lesions, papules, blisters, and craterlike open sores on the perineal area, the vagina, or the penis may be either type 1 (oral herpes) or type 2 (genital herpes). Type 1 is transmitted by oral-genital contact, and type 2 by genital contact. There is no significant difference in the clinical manifestations of the two types. There is no cure for herpes; however, medications are available to relieve the pain that occurs. In addition, topical antiviral agents and oral acyclovir may be used, although their exact actions are not known. Sexual intercourse during periods of active infection will aggravate the lesions and spread the herpes.

After the sores have healed, the virus remains in the nerve cells, preventing the body's immune system from eliminating it. Since the herpes virus stays alive in the body, it can remain dormant or become active at any time. The recurrence rate is variable, but herpes is more likely to recur during periods of stress. Some persons will have only one outbreak; others will have lesions periodically throughout their lives. Recurrent herpes infections increase the risk of cervical cancer, and so regular Pap smears are advised (Table 28-15).

Venereal warts Venereal warts (condylomata acuminata), like skin warts, are caused by **human papillomavirus**. They are found in the moist, warm areas around the vagina, labia, and rectum and on the penis and can be spread by sexual contact. They should not be confused with condylomata lata, which are extremely infectious wartlike manifestations of syphilis. They are usually discovered by the individual, who then goes for treatment.

Podophyllin, which is poisonous if ingested, is used to paint the warts. The normal skin around the wart is protected with petroleum jelly. Podophyllin should be washed off after 1 or 2 h or when burning is felt. Multiple treatments, two to three times weekly, are required before the warts dry up and fall off. Large warts may be more easily removed with surgery or cryosurgery.

Acquired immunodeficiency syndrome Acquired immunodeficiency syndrome (AIDS) was first described in 1981 and was seen predominantly in Los Angeles, New York City, and San Francisco, where the victims were male homosexuals and intravenous drug users.

As of June 16, 1986, 21,420 cases of AIDS had been reported to the Centers for Disease Control (CDC). The CDC predicts that the number of cases in the United States will double annually. Three hundred and six cases of AIDS have been reported in children under the age of 13. Seventy percent of the reported cases in children under 13 years of age have been fatal.

Much research is being done on AIDS, and new developments are constantly occurring. The original CDC definition of AIDS is based on clinical signs and symptoms. A child who has been infected by an opportunist organism or who has a malignancy that indicates an underlying cellular immunodeficiency, when other causes of immunodeficiency have been ruled out, is considered to have AIDS. The most common opportunist pathogens responsible for infection are cytomegalovirus, *Pneumocystis carinii,* and *Candida*. Kaposi sarcoma in a person under 60 years of age is a malignancy that indicates an underlying immunodeficiency and the presence of AIDS.

The human T-cell lymphotropic virus type III (HTLV-III) was identified in 1984, after the initial CDC definition of AIDS. It is *thought* to be the causative agent of AIDS; exactly how it causes the immunodeficiency is still not understood.

Transmission AIDS is transmitted by sexual contact or by parenteral inoculation (such as when blood or blood products are infused and when needles for intravenous drug use are shared). Casual transmission is thought to be rare, since none of the non-sexually-involved household contacts of AIDS victims have contracted the disease to this date.

Six groups of people are considered to be in the high-risk category for developing AIDS: homosexual or bisexual males, intravenous drug abusers, Haitians, hemophiliacs, persons who receive blood or blood products, and the sexual partners of infected persons. The majority of children who develop AIDS either have a parent who has AIDS or who is at risk for developing AIDS or have received a transfusion of blood or blood products.

Incubation The incubation period for AIDS is thought to be of long duration, ranging from several months to several years. The symptoms seem to appear sooner in a child who was born to a mother with the disease than in a child who acquired the disease as a result of a blood transfusion.

Manifestations An AIDS-related complex (ARC), or prodrome, has been identified. The child presents with weight loss or failure to thrive, recurrent infections (such as meningitis or otitis media), and general lymphadenopathy. There may also be chronic diarrhea, persistent oral candidiasis, or interstitial pneumonitis. The child is in the high-risk group for developing AIDS but has no malignancy or signs of opportunist infection. Development of an opportunist infection or a malignancy with a cellular immunodeficiency leads to the diagnosis of AIDS.

Diagnostic tests Laboratory findings in the diagnosis of AIDS reveal an absolute lymphopenia. There is a decreased number of helper T cells and an increased number of suppressor T cells, and consequently the helper-cell/suppressor-cell ratio is reversed. Serum immunoglobulins are greatly increased. The child with AIDS has absent delayed hypersensitivity to skin tests placed with recall antigens. There is also a decreased response to mitogens.

Antibodies to HTLV-III are found in the serological tests of those with the disease and also in some asymptomatic members of high-risk groups. A chronic carrier state may exist.

Treatment Treatment of the child with AIDS centers on early diagnosis and control of the opportunist infection or malignancy. No treatment is currently available that will correct or prevent the immunodeficiency. There is no cure.

In some centers, intravenous immunoglobulins are administered in an attempt to decrease the incidence of sepsis and meningitis.

Nursing management Nursing management of the child with AIDS and his or her family must be comprehensive. Nurses focus their energies on preventing infection in the susceptible child, providing for adequate nutritional intake, giving psychosocial support to the child and the family, and providing an environment and activities that foster normal development of the child.

Preventing Infections The first nursing goal is to prevent infections in the child with AIDS. The prompt administration of antibiotic regimens ordered is necessary, and explaining these to the family facilitates compliance if the child continues therapy at home. Adequate hydration loosens secretions of the respiratory tract, making them easier to eliminate by coughing. Respiratory tract infections are not uncommon in the child with AIDS.

Children with AIDS tend to be prone to oral candidial infections; these are treated with topical medication. Rashes in the diaper area are also not uncommon; when they occur, leaving the area open to air permits drying to take place.

Staff who care for a child with AIDS should not have skin lesions that could be transmitted to the child. Using aseptic technique and washing the hands thoroughly between patients help prevent the spread of infection to the child. The parents and other family members need to know the importance of hand-washing.

Providing Adequate Nutrition Often children presenting with AIDS have lost weight or are considered to be failing to thrive. A diet high in protein and calories is necessary so that weight may be regained.

The diet history is obtained. It is essential to have information about the child's food preferences and usual mealtime routines. Serving more frequent, smaller meals or giving nutritional supplements may be helpful. Planning the diet with the person who will be cooking for the child at home increases the likelihood of compliance.

At times, nasogastric feedings or total parenteral nutrition is appropriate for the child with AIDS.

Providing Psychosocial Support for the Child and the Family Consistent care is essential in providing support to the family of a child who has AIDS. Primary and associate nurses provide continuity and give appropriate information to the family members. Support is essential for a family that is coping with a disease that has such an uncertain, and usually poor, outcome.

The family must deal with the social stigma of belonging to a high-risk group. Others may not want to associate with the child and the family because they are afraid of contracting the disease. The decision regarding school attendance is especially difficult, and this problem is far from being resolved.

Educating the family and the child in a manner that they can understand is another task of the health care team. Giving age-appropriate explanations to children helps increase their understanding.

Providing an Environment and Activities That Foster Normal Development Age-appropriate toys that can be easily washed are best for the hospitalized child; all children need sensory stimulation on a regular basis. Whether children with AIDS should be allowed to go to day-care centers or attend school is a controversial issue, and the CDC has not yet issued specific guidelines on this matter.

Control At the present time there are no immunizations for AIDS or any other means of preventing the disease. Since AIDS is transmitted through sexual contact and through contact with infected blood or body fluids, precautions concerning blood and body fluids must be taken while the child with AIDS is in the hospital. This means that if contact with blood is likely, gloves should be worn. If clothing is likely to be contaminated, a gown should also be worn.

Nurses should not recap or crush needles used with AIDS patients because of the possibility of self-inoculation. Care must be used when handling sharp objects, such as scalpels, that have been contaminated by secretions from an AIDS patient. Any blood or secretions that are spilled (at home or in the hospital) should be cleaned up using a solution consisting of 1 part bleach to 10 parts water, and gloves should be worn.

Thorough hand-washing is important for both the staff and the family as a means of reducing the risk of spreading the infection.

Nursing management of STDs

The nurse is in an important position to educate adolescents about STDs. Many adolescents, especially girls, who suspect that they have an STD will go to a nurse rather than their parents. An assessment should be made concerning the adolescent's understanding of normal body functions and general hygiene. Adolescents need to understand the infection they are being treated for and the relationship of STDs to gynecological problems. Their ability to carry out the prescribed treatment should also be assessed. Contacts will need to be identified, traced, and treated.

Laws concerning the treatment of minors in all 50 states have enabled public and private health care agencies to check and treat adolescents for STDs in complete confidence. Many adolescents will come for treatment sooner if they know that their parents will not be notified.

To help the adolescent feel at ease, the nurse should be open, honest, able to listen, and nonjudgmental. Having a same-sex examiner and involving a minimum of persons in the examination help put the adolescent at ease. Explaining the pelvic examination may lessen the adolescent girl's fear of this procedure. Making reading material and visual aids available may be useful for adolescents who find it difficult to verbalize their concerns. Ideally, all adolescents

Table 28-16 Suggestions for Adolescents concerning Maintenance of Reproductive Tract Health

1. Get enough sleep and exercise.
2. Eat a well-balanced diet.
3. Reduce sugar in the diet (sugar is a factor in some forms of vaginitis).
4. Avoid douches (the vagina continuously cleanses itself).
5. Avoid harsh soaps, bubble baths, feminine hygiene sprays, and deodorized tampons (can produce irritations)
6. Wipe from front to back after a bowel movement.
7. Wear cotton underwear (allows more air circulation and less bacterial growth).
8. Begin yearly pelvic exams and Pap smears if sexually active.
9. Learn the symptoms of STDs and seek medical help early.

Table 28-17 Guidelines for the Adolescent Being Treated for an STD

1. The most important preventive factor is care in selecting a sexual partner. (Multiple partners raise the risk of contracting an STD.)
2. Using condoms reduces the risk of contracting an STD. Foams and diaphragms may have some, but less, preventive effect. Pills and IUDs provide no protection.
3. Douching and washing with soap are of questionable value for preventing STDs.
4. Sexual partners should be checked and treated, if necessary.
5. Use sitz baths for vaginal and perineal irritation.
6. Eliminate stimulants—caffeine, tea, cola drinks (may be irritating to the inflamed area).
7. Take all medication as prescribed, even if symptoms disappear before the medication is completed.
8. If symptoms do not go away after all medication is completed, return for further examination and treatment.
9. The risks and complications of STDs are so great that the teenager should understand them and provide protection through the use of condoms. (Both boys and girls should carry their own supply.)

should be required to take courses in family life and sex education that include factual information on STDs.

The nurse may be asked to interview the child or the family when an infection in a preadolescent is being treated. Since a gonococcal or syphilitic infection may be connected with sexual abuse, the nurse must be an alert and objective listener. Assessing how an infection may have been contracted and whether the child or the family needs counseling is important. Role playing with a doll sometimes elicits more information during an interview with a child.

Table 28-16 lists some suggestions that the nurse can give to adolescents concerning the maintenance of reproductive tract health. Additional instructions for an adolescent who is being treated for an STD are listed in Table 28-17.

When seeking medical care, adolescents have the right to *privacy, dignity,* and *confidentiality* and the right to *understand* the treatment prescribed and to *consent* to it or *refuse* it. They also have responsibilities: to *be honest, follow the treatment plan, report changes,* and *keep appointments*. These rights and responsibilities are essential for optimum care.

Bibliography

Acquired Immunodeficiency Syndrome (AIDS) Weekly Surveillance Report—United States AIDS Activity, Centers for Disease Control, Center for Infectious Diseases, Atlanta, Aug. 19, 1985.

Academy of Pediatrics, Committee on Infectious Diseases, *1982 Red Book,* American Academy of Pediatrics, Evanston, Ill., 1982.

———, "Revision of Recommendation for Use of Rifampin Prophylaxis of Contacts of Patients with Haemophilus Influenzae Infection," *Pediatrics* **74**:301–302 (August 1984).

Bell, T. A., "Common Sexually Transmitted Diseases of Children and Adolescents," in J. D. Nelson and G. H. McCracken (eds.), *Clinical Reviews in Pediatric Infectious Disease,* Mosby, St. Louis, 1985, pp. 261–274.

Bettoli, Elena J., "Herpes: Facts and Fallacies," *American Journal of Nursing,* **82**:924–929 (June 1982).

Boland, Mary, and Teresa D. B. Gaskill, "Managing AIDS in Children," *American Journal of Maternal-Child Nursing* **9**:384–389 (November–December 1984).

Borkowsky, William, "Viral Infections in Immunocompromised Children," *Pediatric Annals* **13**:682–692 (September 1984).

Brunell, P. A., "Enteroviral Infections," *Pediatric Infectious Disease* **4**:S46–S47 (May–June 1985).

Bryson, Yvonne J., "The Use of Acyclovir in Children," *Pediatric Infectious Disease* **3**:345–348 (July 1984).

Cates, W., and J. L. Rauh, "Adolescents and Sexually Transmitted Diseases: An Expanding Problem," *Journal of Adolescent Health Care* **6**:257–261 (July 1985).

Coleman, Deborah Ann, "TB: The Disease That's Not Dead Yet," *RN* :49–60 (September 1984).

Coward, Doris Dickerson, "The Other Herpesviruses: Epstein-Barr and Cytomegalovirus," *Nurse Practitioner* **8**:13–18 (April 1983).

Daum, R. S., and D. M. Granoff, "A Vaccine against Haemophilus Influenzae Type B," *Pediatric Infectious Disease* **4**:355–357 (July–August 1985).

DeLiberti, John H., and Stefan Tedrow, "Bone and Joint Complications of Haemophilus Influenzae Meningitis," *Clinical Pediatrics* **22**:7–10 (January 1983).

Devore, Nancy E., V. M. Jackson, and S. L. Piening, "TORCH Infections," *American Journal of Nursing* **83**:1660–1665 (December 1983).

Drutz, David J., and Antonino Catanzaro, "Coccidioidomycosis," *American Review of Respiratory Disease* **117**:559–585 (1978).

Friedman, Harvey M., M. R. Lewis, D. M. Nemerofsky, and S. A. Plotkin, "Acquisition of Cytomegalovirus Infection among Female Employees at a Pediatric Hospital," *Pediatric Infectious Disease* **3**:233–235 (May 1984).

Greaves, Wayne L., A. B. Kaiser, R. H. Alford, and W. Schaffner, "The Problem of Herpetic Whitlow among Hospital Personnel," *Infection Control* **1**:381–385 (1980).

Grose, C., "The Many Faces of Infectious Mononucleosis: The Spectrum of Epstein-Barr Virus Infection in Children," *Pediatrics in Review* **7**:35–44 (August 1985).

Hammerschlag, Margaret R., "Infections Due to Chlamydia Trachomatis," *Pediatric Annals* **13**:673–681 (September 1984).

Jackson, Marguerite M., "Viral Hepatitis," *Nursing Clinics of North America* **15**:729–746 (December 1980).

Jemison-Smith, Pearl, "Understanding the Acquired Immune Deficiency Syndrome," *NITA* **7**:114–116 (March–April 1984).

———, "Preventing Hepatitis B," *NITA* **8**:283–288 (July–August 1985).

Kahn, A., and D. Blum, "Factors for Poor Prognosis in Fulmination Meningococcemia," *Clinical Pediatrics* **17**:680–687 (September 1978).

Long, Sarah S., "Botulism in Infancy," *Pediatric Infectious Disease* **3**:266–271 (May 1984).

McCarthy, Paul L., G. W. Grundy, S. Z. Spiesel, and T. F. Dolan, "Bacteremia in Children: An Outpatient Clinical Review," *Pediatrics* **57**:861–000 (June 1976).

Massey, K., "Rocky Mountain Spotted Fever: A National Disease," *American Journal of Maternal-Child Nursing* **7**:104–109 (March–April 1982).

Minster, Julia, "Nursing Management of Patients with Scabies and Lice," *Nursing Clinics of North America* **15**:747–756 (December 1980).

Nahmias, Andre J., and Richard J. Whitley, "Herpes Simplex Virus Encephalitis in Pediatrics," *Pediatrics in Review* **2**:259–266 (March 1981).

Nichols, Arlene O., "Taking the Fear out of Rabies Treatment," *Nursing 83* **13**:42–43 (June 1983).

San Joaquin, V. H., and M. I. Marks, "New Agents in Diarrhea," in Nelson and McCracken, op. cit., pp. 201–218.

Scheld, W. Michael, "Theoretical and Practical Considerations of Antibiotic Therapy for Bacterial Meningitis," *Pediatric Infectious Disease* **4**:74–83 (January 1985).

Schluttenhofer, Nancy, "The Special Challenge of Empyemas," *Nursing 84* **14**:57–60 (December 1984).

Tobin, B. K., "Nursing Life's Guide to Hidden Hazards on the Job, Part I: Infectious Diseases," *Nursing Life* **5**:18–23 (July–August 1985).

Todd, James K., "Office Laboratory Diagnosis of Skin and Soft Tissue Infections," *Pediatric Infectious Disease* **4**:84–87 (January 1985).

Whettam, J., "Update on Toxic Shock: How to Spot It and Treat It," *RN* **84**:55–60 (February 1984).

29

Stephanie Wright
Phyllis J. D'Ambra

Mobility

Upon completion of this chapter, the student will be able to:

1 Briefly describe the embryological development of the musculoskeletal system.
2 Identify on a human skeleton the skull, vertebral column, clavicle, humerus, radius, ulna, femur, tibia, fibula, and hip acetabulum.
3 Define and/or describe bone, cartilage, tendon, ligament, diaphysis, epiphysis, metaphysis, periosteum, joint, synovial membrane, and callus.
4 Demonstrate flexion, extension, abduction, adduction, internal rotation, external rotation, pronation, and supination.
5 List five areas to be assessed by the nurse before planning care for a child with an alteration in mobility.
6 Name the seven items to be assessed when checking the neurovascular status of an extremity.
7 Identify the five effects that immobilization has on a child and his or her family.
8 Describe the preparation of a child for cast application.
9 Describe the skin care of a child in a cast.
10 Describe how to keep a cast clean and dry.
11 Describe the preparation of a child for cast removal.
12 List four basic rules for caring for a child in traction.
13 Name two of the major causes of trauma to the musculoskeletal system in children.
14 Describe two ways of preventing injury to the musculoskeletal system.
15 Identify and describe five conditions that cause alterations in mobility in children.

ORIGIN, STRUCTURE, AND FUNCTION OF THE MUSCULOSKELETAL SYSTEM

Bones and cartilage make up the supportive and protective framework of the body. Bones also provide the surfaces to which the muscles, tendons, and ligaments are attached. Bones and muscles work intimately together to provide for support and motion in the human body.

Origins of muscles and bones

The musculoskeletal system begins to form during the third week of embryonic life. It arises from the mesodermal layer (or middle germ layer), which appears in the developing embryo at about this time. The embryo, at this stage in development, has a primitive trunk support called the *notochord*. From the mesoderm, blocks of tissue appear called *somites*. The somites develop specialized cells which migrate toward the notochord and surround it. These cells develop into the backbone and ribs by about the sixth week of embryonic life. From the somites, specialized tissue also develops that is the precursor of muscles. These cells differentiate and develop into separate muscle groups, beginning at about the fifth week of embryonic life, and eventually form the trunk muscles.

Meanwhile, arm buds and then leg buds have appeared in the embryo at about the fourth week. Growth occurs very rapidly; the fingers develop by the sixth week. The growth of the lower extremities lags about a week behind, with the toes appearing at about the seventh week. Refinement of the limbs continues until, by the end of the third month, the shape and form of the hands and feet are completed. The bones and joints of the limbs develop from the mesodermal layer at that location, and the muscles develop around the bones. By the end of 8 weeks of development, a complete miniature skeleton has been formed, comprised of cartilage and fibrous membrane. Muscle development continues, and by the beginning of the third month of intrauterine life, the baby begins to move spontaneously.

The skeleton of cartilage and fibrous membrane provides a support system which can grow rapidly with the developing embryo. The cartilage begins to be replaced by bone during the eighth week. The bony skeleton is needed for more substantial support as the baby grows. This process, called *ossification,* will continue throughout intrauterine life and childhood. By 16 weeks of gestation, enough of the baby's developing skeleton has been replaced by bone so that the skeletal structure can be seen on an x-ray of the mother's abdomen. At birth, the central portions of most of the larger bones have ossified, although the ends are still mainly cartilage. Figure 29-1 illustrates how ossification proceeds in a long bone.

The bones of the face and skull do not develop from cartilage. Bone is laid down directly over a fibrous membrane, and therefore these bones are

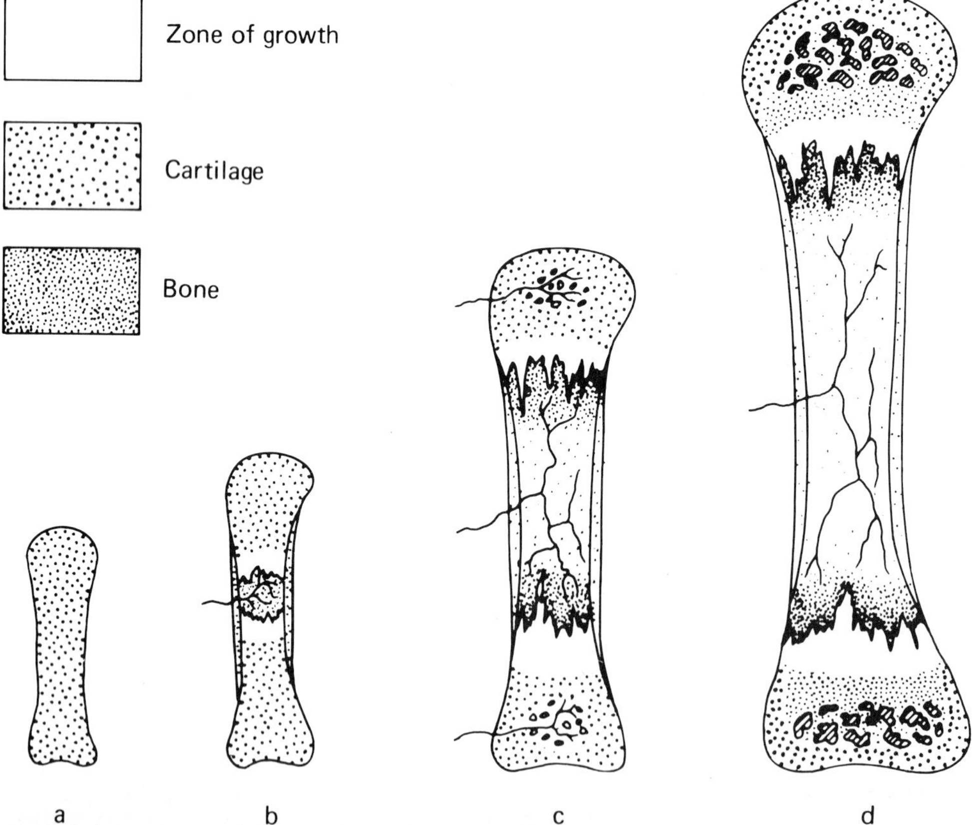

Figure 29-1 Ossification of a long bone. Ossification begins in the central shaft, or diaphysis. Separate ossification centers develop in the epiphysis. (*From R. M. DeCoursey, The Human Organism, 3d ed., McGraw-Hill, New York, 1968. Used with permission.*)

referred to as *membranous bones,* rather than cartilaginous bones. Ossification of the skull also is only partially completed at birth. The skull is still composed of separate bones, separated by the sutures. The fontanels, or soft spots, are apparent at the corners of the adjoining membranous bones. Ossification is not completed until later in childhood, when the skull becomes one solid bony structure.

Anatomy and physiology of bone

There are generally considered to be four classes of bones: (1) long bones, (2) short bones, (3) flat bones, and (4) irregular bones. *Long bones* are found in the limbs and the fingers and toes. They are easily identified by their long central shaft. *Short bones* are found in the wrists and ankles (carpals and tarsals). Short bones are generally cuboidal in shape. *Flat bones* are thin and may be somewhat curved (the bones in the skull and ribs). *Irregular bones* are all those not included in the first three groups. The vertebrae are examples of irregular bones.

Figure 29-2 shows the major divisions of a typical long bone. The *diaphysis* is the central shaft. Ossification of long bones begins in this area and spreads outward. This area is often referred to as the *primary ossification center.* The ends of the long bones are the *epiphyses.* A separate secondary center of ossification begins here. Most of the secondary centers of ossification appear after birth. Between the diaphysis and epiphysis is a line of cartilage, the epiphyseal line or plate. It is from this area that all growth in length takes place. The epiphyseal line tends to become smaller as growth and ossification proceed. For this reason, x-rays of bones, particularly those of the hands, can be used to establish a "bone age" for a child. This is a helpful tool in diagnosing certain endocrine disorders that affect bone growth. The epiphyseal line does not disappear or close until all growth is completed. The area on the central shaft directly adjacent to the epiphyseal plate is the *metaphysis.*

Bone is a living tissue. It consists of approximately two-thirds inorganic material, mainly calcium phosphate, which provides for hardness. The remainder is organic material. The *osteocytes,* or bone cells, maintain the structure of the bone and are found scattered throughout the bone, separated by intercellular substance, which is composed of inorganic salts and collagen. The osteocytes produce and maintain intercellular substance, continually exchanging the inorganic materials within the bone. There are two types of bone tissue: compact bone, which is extremely dense, and spongy bone, which has a more open texture.

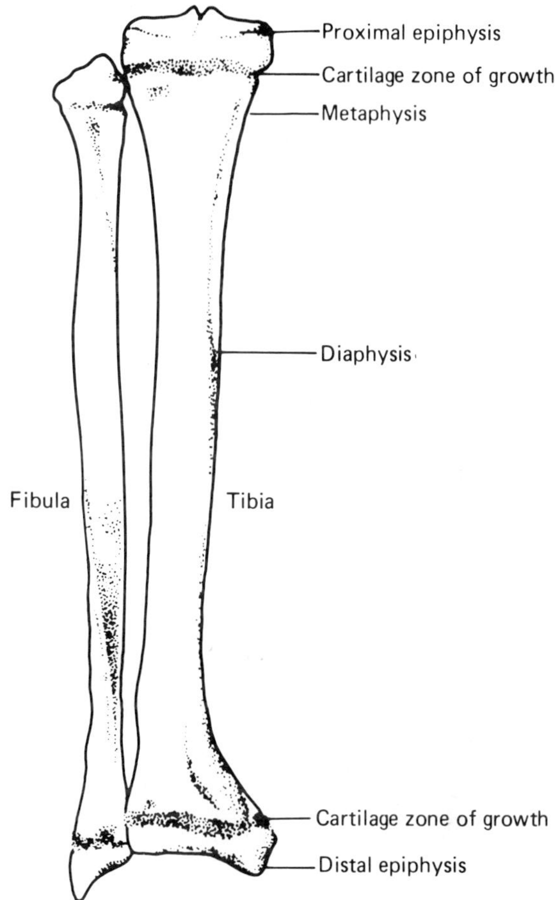

Figure 29-2 A typical long bone. (*From R. M. DeCoursey, The Human Organism, 3d ed., McGraw-Hill, New York, 1968. Used with permission.*)

Bones are covered by a membrane, the *periosteum.* The blood supply for the osteocytes originates in the periosteum and reaches the cells through small pathways in the bone called *haversian canals.* The periosteum is divided into a fibrous outer layer and an osteogenic inner layer. The osteocytes originate in this inner layer and form intercellular substance around themselves. As they do this, growth in bone diameter occurs.

Joints and body motion

The junction of two bones is a *joint,* or articulation. Joints may be nonmovable or movable. At a movable joint, the bone end is covered with a thin layer of cushioning articular cartilage. The joint is surrounded by a capsule of fibrous tissue, which helps hold the bones together. Bones may also be directly joined by ligaments. The joint capsule is lined with the synovial membrane, which provides lubrication for the joint. Further stability is provided by overlying muscles and tendons. Joints may be further classified according to the shape of their surfaces and the type of movement of which they are capable.

Muscles give motion to joints. Muscles are structures of specialized cells that are capable of shortening. Muscle attached to the skeletal system is under voluntary control. Most muscles have two or more attachments to the skeleton. Some are attached directly to the periosteum, while others are attached to the bone by tendons. The more fixed attachment is the muscle origin; the more movable is the insertion. When the muscle contracts or shortens, the two attachments come closer to each other, producing movement at a joint.

ASSESSMENT OF CHILDREN WITH ALTERATIONS IN MOBILITY

Nursing assessment related to the musculoskeletal system is done in a variety of settings. The nurse who cares for newborns and uses a newborn assessment guide may be able to discern early alterations in mobility. Public health nurses and school nurses often utilize their assessment skills in these areas. Alterations in mobility are seen in any pediatric screening program or pediatrician's office as well as by nurses who deal primarily with children who have musculoskeletal disorders. In the hospital orthopedic setting, nurses will encounter primarily children who fall into two broad categories: those with long-term disabilities and those who are victims of trauma. Assessment should be tailored to the special needs of children in these two quite different groups.

Nursing history

The nurse begins the assessment by getting the child's view of the problem or, if the child is too young, by obtaining information from the parents. The child's view is extremely important, not only in isolating and identifying the individual aspects of the physical care needed, but also in assessing the impact of the problem on the child's life. Adolescents are frequently encountered in an orthopedic setting and should be given the opportunity to supply the history. Respecting their independence creates a favorable climate for establishing a working relationship. Children with long-term physical disabilities are often extremely knowledgeable about their condition. Allowing them to supply as much information as possible fosters some autonomy in a situation in which opportunities for developing competence may be limited.

History of the musculoskeletal problem *Gross motor and fine motor development* Determine whether the child reached gross motor and fine motor developmental milestones at the appropriate times.

Presence of congenital deformity, birth injury, or disease requiring hospitalization or surgery These conditions include congenital hip dysplasia, clubfoot, fractures related to a traumatic birth, deformities related to intrauterine position, and a breech delivery. Determine the following:

What physical limitations are imposed by the condition or conditions?
What are the social, developmental, and emotional effects of the physical changes?
What effect have these problems had on the child's life-style?
What is the child's pattern of daily living?
What changes in daily living patterns must be included in the plan for hospital routines and used to set goals for rehabilitation?
Does the child use special orthopedic devices or equipment (orthopedic shoes, braces, splints, crutches, or prostheses)? How much assistance does the child require to use this equipment? These devices should be included in the nursing care plan for the child while he or she is hospitalized.
Has the child had orthopedic surgery?
What is the history of any disease process that is present?

Traumatic injury or accident Obtain a clear account of the nature of the traumatic injury or accident and the first-aid measures that were taken, and determine the means of transportation that were used after the injury or accident. Also determine whether the child is conscious and alert by talking to the child and observing his or her behavior. In most cases of serious injury, children are admitted to the emergency department. (See Chap. 33 for additional information on treating children who have suffered traumatic injuries.)

Family relationships Determine the nature of the parent-child relationship by noting the following:

Are the parent-child interactions appropriate for the child's age and developmental level?
Does the parent allow the child to express his or her feelings and points of view during the interview?
Does the parent express feelings of guilt, especially in the case of a traumatic injury, or does the parent blame the child for the accident?

School and peers Assess the effect of the injury or accident on the child's school attendance and peer relationships by determining the following:

Will the hospitalization require a prolonged absence from school?
Has the child been attending a regular classroom, and at what grade level?
Is the grade level appropriate for the child's age, and how are the child's grades?
Have plans been made to continue the child's education away from school?
Can peers visit the child in the hospital?
Do peers understand the problem?

Diet history During prolonged periods of hospitalization, increased fluids and roughage are needed. Determine the child's food preferences.

Review of systems Determine the child's bowel and urinary habits, cardiovascular and musculoskeletal status, and the condition of the skin. The effects of immobilization are discussed later in this chapter.

Emotional impact The emotional impact of a traumatic injury or accident is discussed later in this chapter.

Pain Determine the following:

Is the child currently in pain?
Where is the pain, and are signs of swelling, trauma, or fractures present?
What increases the pain, and under what circumstances does the pain occur?
What pain medications or treatments were administered prior to the assessment?
The findings of the physician's physical examination and the physical therapist's evaluation must also be reviewed and included in the data base.

Physical examination

Measurements and observations The physical examination includes measurements of height and weight and observation of stance, posture, ability to walk, gait, and symmetry of the body and limbs. Muscle strength is compared on both sides of the body, and the normal appearance and movement of the joints and limbs and the normal limb and body alignment are noted. Measuring the extremities may be necessary if one limb appears smaller or shorter than the other. Check for any limitation in range of motion.

Skin Check for the presence of bleeding, contusions, breaks in the skin, or swelling. The skin should be intact before cast application, since skin lesions can be a source of infection.

Neurovascular status Check the extremities for the presence of a fracture or residual effects of a previous injury. (The neurological assessment provides a baseline for checking neurological function and circulatory status after surgery.) It is also important to test for sensation; note the color, temperature, and pulses of the extremities distal to the injury; and determine whether edema is present. Check circulatory status by pressing the skin or a nail bed. The area will blanch, but the color should return quickly when pressure is released and the capillaries refill with blood. Observe for evidence of impaired motor or sensory function, lack of spontaneous movement, and inability to wiggle the fingers or toes.

Accident or traumatic injury In the case of an accident or traumatic injury, splint an extremity if there is evidence of a fracture or dislocation before moving the child. Do not encourage movement of the extremities until after spinal x-rays have been taken and it has been determined that no spinal injury exists. Check the level of consciousness and pupil response. If a spinal cord injury is suspected, immobilize the body as a unit. Turn the child by logrolling, moving the body as a rigid unit. It is also important to observe for signs of impaired neurovascular status, as described above; to observe for shock; and to check vital signs.

Diagnostic studies

X-rays X-rays are the most common diagnostic tool used with children who have a musculoskeletal disease. They may be repeated at frequent intervals in order to reassess the status of bone healing.

CT scans CT scans are used in addition to x-rays when further diagnostic information is necessary. A bone scan may be used with children to detect tumors or bone infection. A bone scan involves injecting a radioactive material and follow-up scanning several hours later.

Arthrograms Arthrograms involve injecting a radiopaque dye into a joint; they are used in combination with x-rays to diagnose joint disease.

Biopsies and arthroscopies These surgical procedures are employed for diagnostic purposes. A bone or muscle biopsy is performed to remove a piece of tissue for pathological examination. An arthroscopy enables the orthopedic surgeon to visualize a joint directly through an arthroscope, which is a special optical device.[1]

IMMOBILIZATION

Disorders of the musculoskeletal system often require immobilization of a body part during the treatment regimen. Healthy children are by nature active beings and immobilization of a child may not be easy to accomplish. It invariably has some ramifications. The degree of immobilization will influence the effects: The greater the extent of immobilization and the longer the time period that it is required, the more pronounced the side effects will be.

Physical effects

Body systems commonly affected by immobilization are: the urinary, digestive, cardiovascular, skin, and musculoskeletal systems. In the *musculoskeletal system*, immobilization is used to place a body part at rest and to place a body part in normal alignment for a sufficient period of time for healing to occur. While this is occurring, certain undesirable changes are taking place. Any muscle group that is not being used is subject to atrophy. This is usually quite apparent when a cast is removed. The casted extremity is smaller than the uncasted extremity because of disuse atrophy. Any joints encased in plaster will have lost some of their mobility. This means that strength and range of motion must gradually be restored to that extremity through exercise. Since the flexors of a joint are generally stronger than the extensors, any joint not held in position by plaster or traction will be subject to a flexion contracture. Areas particularly vulnerable to this are the hip, knee, and foot.

Loss of some of the mineral portion of the bone begins to occur with disuse of a body part. Although this change is more pronounced in older persons, it also occurs in children who experience great degrees of immobilization for prolonged periods of time.

Every attempt should be made to minimize these effects on body parts by movement and exercise of any body part whose immobilization is not necessary for treatment. Preferably this movement should be actively performed by the child. A physical therapist can work with the child to establish a daily exercise program. The nurse who is working with the child can usually establish a simple daily exercise program. Observe the movement of the child. Young, healthy children often exercise all their mobile extremities without prompting (Fig 29-3). Take note of the areas

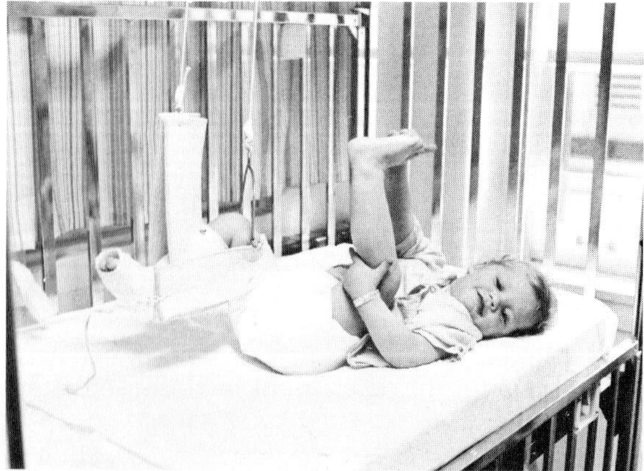

Figure 29-3 This 22-month-old in skeletal traction illustrates why young, healthy children may not need an exercise program.

for which an exercise program is needed. The following are important:

1. Have the child perform active range-of-motion exercises whenever possible.
2. When a child cannot actively move a part or when the child is too young to follow instructions, put the joints through passive range-of-motion exercises.
3. Have the child exercise the quadriceps muscle over the anterior portion of the thigh. Quadriceps setting is done by pressing the back of the knee down onto the bed. When done on a regular basis, this helps prepare the muscles of the leg for ambulation.
4. Encourage the child to strengthen the upper extremities by the use of a trapeze attached to the bed.

The duration and frequency of exercise sessions will need to be based on the child's general condition and strength. Often it is good to begin with two sessions a day. To encourage the continuation of an exercise program, it is helpful to establish a regular routine and make the program enjoyable. Establish certain goals for the child. Make the exercises playlike whenever possible; for example, include a throwing game, or have the child kick an object attached to the bed frame.

If possible, avoid having the hip or knee continuously flexed. This is often a comfortable position for the child, but the hip and knee need regular extension to prevent the development of flexion contractures. For children with traction applied to a lower extremity, a support for the foot should be provided to prevent equinus deformity of the foot.

All the vital functions tend to slow with immobilization. Circulation may be sluggish. This, along with pressure on the skin, makes skin breakdown more likely. Changing position or massaging areas subject to pressure helps reduce the likelihood of skin breakdown. Healthy, well-nourished children with a normal layer of subcutaneous fat will have fewer problems with skin breakdown.

Decreased motility of the gastrointestinal tract due to lack of activity may produce constipation. A record should be kept of the child's bowel function. A dietary regimen that includes fresh fruits and vegetables, other sources of fiber, and adequate amounts of liquid will often eliminate the necessity for stool softeners, enemas, and suppositories. Appetite may be diminished, but this problem is often related to the unfamiliarity of the food in the hospital and may be remedied temporarily by providing some familiar foods from home until the child has an opportunity to adapt. Smaller, more frequent feedings may be more attractive to a child when there is little physical activity to stimulate appetite. Allowing the child as much choice as possible in diet is always beneficial. Demineralization of bone during prolonged bed rest produces an increased concentration of calcium in the urine, which makes the immobilized child more prone to the development of renal calculi.[2] Increasing fluid intake and maintaining an acid pH of the urine will help prevent this occurrence. Although the child needs normal calcium intake for bone healing, excessive amounts of milk should be avoided, since too much milk further raises the serum calcium level.

Emotional effects

The emotional reaction of the child to immobilization will be influenced by the child's age, the amount of preparation provided for the experience, and the circumstances surrounding the event. Older children can obviously be better prepared when immobilization is anticipated. Discussion of what it will be like to be in a cast or traction should be instituted by the parents. The family can prepare favorite activities, books, and games to pass the hours. When immobilization is not foreseen, as in the case of an accident, the child must do all his or her adapting after the fact.

Some children, particularly young ones, show an immediate reaction to being immobilized. It is common for older children to accept their imposed restraints quietly during the first few days and then to experience some reaction. Depression, withdrawal, and disobedient and aggressive behavior are seen in children as reactions to immobilization and hospitalization. Some sort of reaction should be considered usual and the normal result of immobilizing a healthy child. Physical capabilities are a part of each person's identity. Immobilization of a child limits these capabilities, alters the child's self-image, and may threaten the child's self-esteem. Also, many children use physical activity as a means of discharging feelings of anger and hostility. This normal and healthy way of handling emotional energy is denied them once they are immobilized. Although an uncooperative child is more difficult for the parents and staff to handle, the child needs freedom to express his or her feelings within certain bounds. These bounds need to be clearly defined for the child. Most children will show signs of making a good adaptation to their limitation of activity and their surroundings within a week.

If a child physically resists immobilization to the point where it interferes with treatment, then some sort of restraint may be required. Restraints are to be avoided, if at all possible, since they may be traumatic to the child. However, sometimes restraints relieve the child of the burden of maintaining a position by acting as a gentle reminder that certain movements are not allowed. Restraints should never be used in a punitive fashion. The child needs to understand that they are a necessary part of treatment to ensure that healing takes place.

Achievement of normal developmental goals for the child's age must be stimulated. Appropriate toys are an important part of this planning. See Chaps. 15 and 16 for some of the basic needs of the hospitalized child.

Environmental stimulation might include decorating the room, bed, or traction apparatus with toys, posters, or cards. A child's bed should be positioned to provide as much of a view of the surrounding activity as possible; a view out the window or down the hall will help lessen the feeling of isolation. Whenever possible, the child should be moved out of his or her room. Children in casts can be moved on a stretcher, wagon, or cart or in someone's arms. Moving a child may be time-consuming and hard work, but it is definitely worth the time and trouble. A trip to the playroom or another area for a meal may stimulate the appetite. Just having the opportunity to observe activity in the hall provides diversion and stimulation. This also allows for more contact between children. Making friends may prove to be the most therapeutic measure of all in assisting the child to adjust to illness and limitation of activity, and it may even make the illness a personal growth experience. Many of these friendships continue long after hospitalization and the completion of treatment.

Care of a child in a cast

The types of casts used in the treatment of children are illustrated in Fig 29-4. A cast may be used for gradual correction of a deformity, as an initial treatment to provide immobilization for a fracture, as a follow-up to traction, or as a means of immobilization following surgery on bones, joints, or muscles. Many casting materials are available, and new ones are continually being developed; however, the two most commonly used materials are plaster of paris and fiberglass.

A plaster cast is made from a gauze bandage impregnated with plaster of paris. During application, the plaster bandage is wet and then applied over an underlying layer of padding or a piece of cotton stockinette. Figure 29-5 shows a plaster cast being applied to a leg. During application of a plaster cast, the chemical reaction that takes place generates heat, and the cast feels warm. Complete drying of a plaster cast takes 24 h or longer.

Fiberglass casts are applied in a similar manner. The bandaging material is a fiberglass knit, which is coarser in texture than the plaster bandaging material. It is wet at the time of application in order to activate the polyurethane resin impregnated in the fabric. It is usually applied over a piece of stockinette made of polypropylene, which dries more rapidly than cotton. Fiberglass sets quickly, usually within 15 min, and generates little heat.

The choice of casting material is determined by the type and amount of displacement of the fracture, cost considerations, and the personal preference of the applicator. Fiberglass is preferred because it is lighter in weight and stronger and is not damaged by water. Plaster is the least expensive casting material; it costs one-fifth as much as fiberglass. Plaster can be shaped and molded to the extremity with greater ease, and for that reason it is often preferred for the initial casting of a displaced fracture.[3]

Preparation for casting Care of the child begins with preparation for casting, when the child should be awake. In an emergency situation, there may be little time for preparation, but every child needs to have certain things explained:

1. The steps in cast application
2. The extent of pain or discomfort and what will be done to help
3. The warmth of the cast during application
4. What the cast will look like and what area it will cover

It is helpful to have the child look at a drawing of the cast or to see a similar cast on another

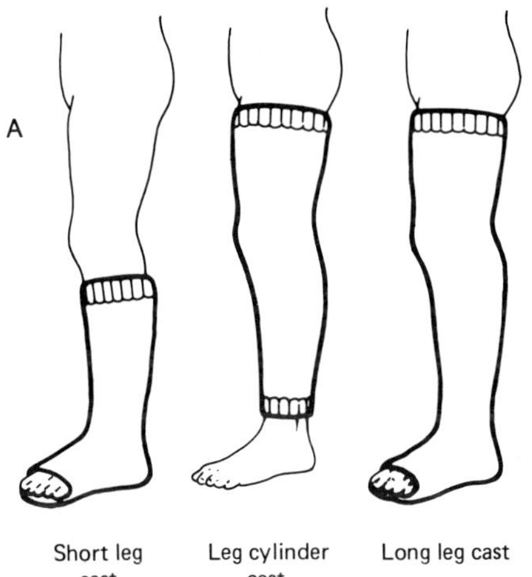

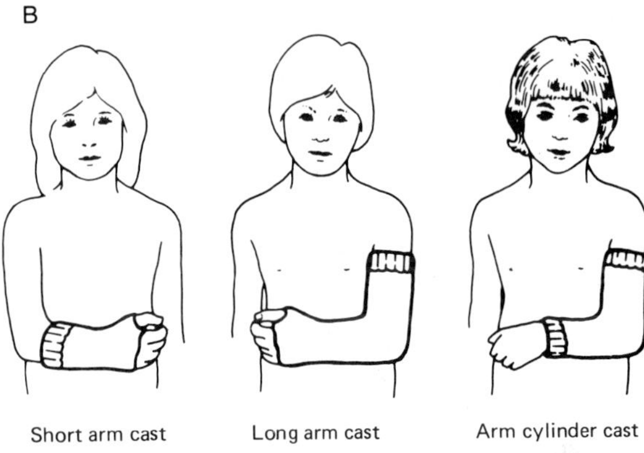

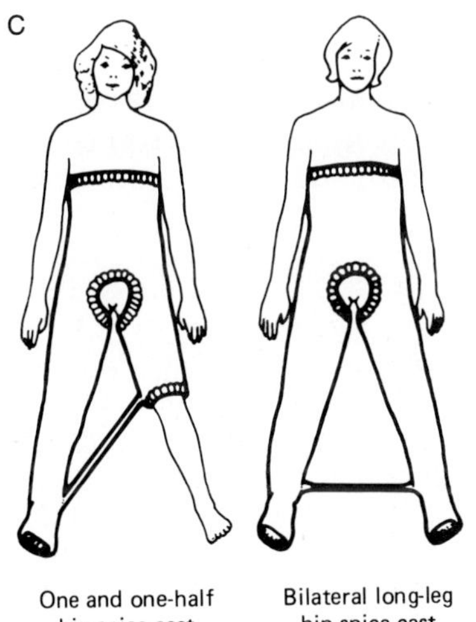

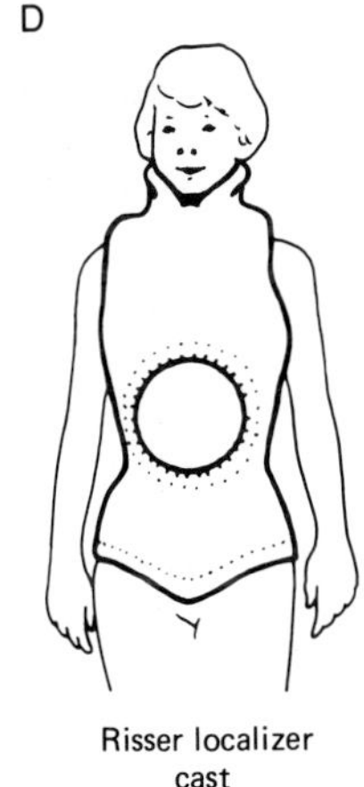

Figure 29-4 Casts commonly used in the treatment of children. (*From Nancy E. Hilt and William Schmitt, Jr., Pediatric Orthopedic Nursing, Mosby, St. Louis, 1975. Used with permission.*)

child. The child may apply a cast or see one applied to a doll. The apprehension of some older children may be allayed by talking with another child who has had a cast application. Books are excellent ways to help prepare children for casting or to help them express their feelings about it afterward.

Physical preparation should include an assessment of skin areas to be covered by plaster. If a piece of stockinette is to be used under the cast, this will need to be applied.

Once the cast is applied, care must be taken not to dent or damage it until drying is completed. Plaster casts require more careful handling during the initial 24 h after application than fiberglass casts. When lifting the cast, avoid indenting the plaster with the fingers by lifting the cast with the palms of the hands. Plaster casts should not be covered during the initial 20 to 24 h after application, since covering them will slow the drying process. The child needs to be turned regularly to allow all surfaces of the plaster cast to dry.

Neurovascular status A cast must be snug enough to provide the necessary immobilization without interfering with circulation. Every cast application carries with it the risk of circulatory

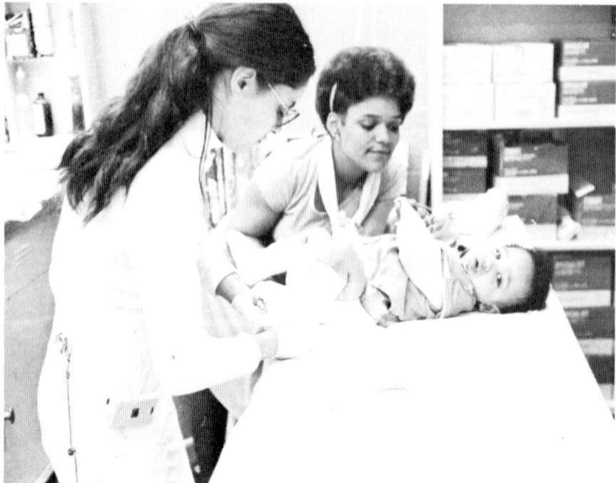

Figure 29-5 Application of short leg casts made of plaster.

impairment. Since impairment of circulation can result in irreparable damage and even permanent loss of function, the checking of neurovascular status is of extreme importance. If an injury or a surgical procedure preceded cast application, swelling may further compromise circulation.

Using the initial assessment of neurovascular status prior to cast application as a baseline, the nurse begins assessing the area immediately following application and hourly for about 12 to 24 h. The length of time that hourly checks are continued depends on the amount of swelling and the rapidity with which neurovascular status returns to normal. Following the initial hourly checks, neurovascular status should be assessed every 4 h. Each check should include an assessment of temperature, color, capillary refill, amount of edema, sensation, motion, and pain in the area distal to the cast application (Fig. 29-6). If the appropriate areas of the extremity are accessible, pulse should also be included in the assessment. If there is impairment of circulation, there will be edema, coldness, pallor or cyanosis, and poor capillary refill. If circulatory compromise continues, there will be pain, numbness, and loss of sensation and motion. When an arm or leg is casted, each finger and toe should be checked individually, since impairment to some fingers and toes can occur without impairment to others.

When edema is present, elevating the casted extremity above the level of the heart is often indicated to help reduce swelling. Coldness of the extremity may be due partially to the contact with the wet cast. It is not uncommon for one or two signs of slowing of circulation to appear. The nurse must then carefully check for any other signs.

The physician should be aware of the child's neurovascular status and should be apprised of any changes. For example, if a child's extremity following casting is slightly edematous and cool, with a rapid color return after blanching and normal sensation and motion, the nurse should observe carefully for any deterioration in return of color or in sensation and motion. Pain may be more difficult to assess, since some pain normally accompanies a fracture or surgery. Extreme pain or pain that is poorly relieved by medication should be reported. Pain is usually confined to the operative or fracture area. Pain in other areas should be investigated. In small children, only the amount of pain can be assessed, and other signs of neurovascular status must be relied on. If circulation is compromised, cutting or removing the cast may be necessary to restore circulation. Some orthopedic units employ a separate chart for recording checks of neurovascular status (Fig. 29-7). Each check of neurovascular status should be carefully noted

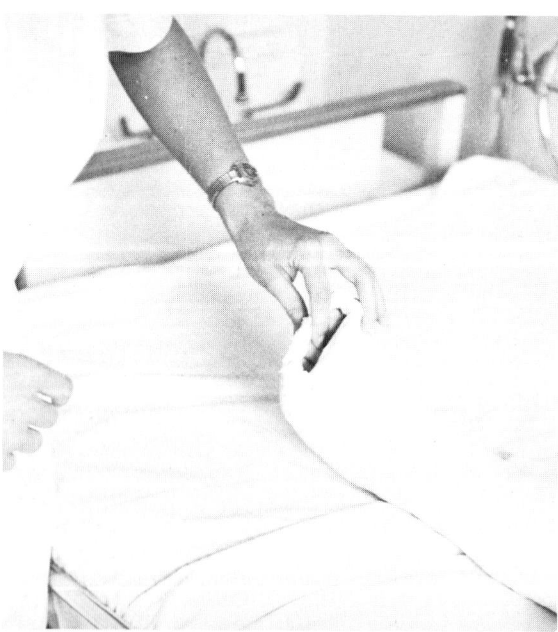

Figure 29-6 The nurse is checking the neurovascular status of a casted extremity. When the cast covers most of the extremity, good lighting is essential. A flashlight may be necessary.

Procedure:											
Date:											
Time:											
SKIN TEMPERATURE											
Warm											
Cool											
Cold											
SKIN COLOR											
Normal											
Pale											
Dusky (bluish)											
Red											
CAPILLARY REFILL											
Normal											
Sluggish											
Faster											
EDEMA											
Not present											
Mild											
Moderate											
Severe											
SENSATION											
Touch											
Sharp (to pin)											
Dull (to pin)											
Tingling											
Numbness											
None											

Date:											
Time:											
MOTION											
Present											
Absent											
Foot											
Dorsiflex											
Plantarflex											
Fingers											
Flexion											
Extension											
Abduction											
PAIN											
None											
Mild											
Moderate											
Severe											
PULSES											
Pedal											
Tibialis											
Radial											

Figure 29-7 Neurovascular status checklist.

on the child's chart. This facilitates the detection of any changes in the child's condition.

Skin care Care of the skin includes daily inspection of all visible skin at the edges of the cast and as far under the cast as possible (using a flashlight) for signs of redness or skin breakdown, which can occur as a result of pressure or abrasion from the cast edge. Following cast application, all plaster particles need to be removed from under the cast edges. The cast edges should be finished and smoothed to minimize skin abrasion. If the cast is lined with stockinette, this can be stretched over the cast edge and secured with tape or plaster. The cast edges can also be finished with adhesive tape or moleskin. This is commonly referred to as a *petaling* because the tape or moleskin is cut into petal shapes and applied to the cast edges as illustrated in Fig. 29-8. Finishing of the cast edges in this manner should be delayed until the cast is dry.

Skin edges adjacent to the cast should be kept clean and dry. If the cast indents adjacent skin areas, some trimming of the cast following application may be necessary for comfort. The nurse must first check with the physician to be certain that trimming will not affect the therapeutic value of the cast. A piece of padding may be placed under an edge that is uncomfortable for the child. Applying alcohol to the skin around the cast edges may help toughen the skin and may also provide some relief from itching.[4]

The cast may exert pressure on skin areas under the cast that are not visible. The pressure may be sufficient to produce skin breakdown. This is most likely to occur over bony prominences. The main indicator of pressure and skin breakdown is pain. It is continuous and intense at the location of the pressure. An older child

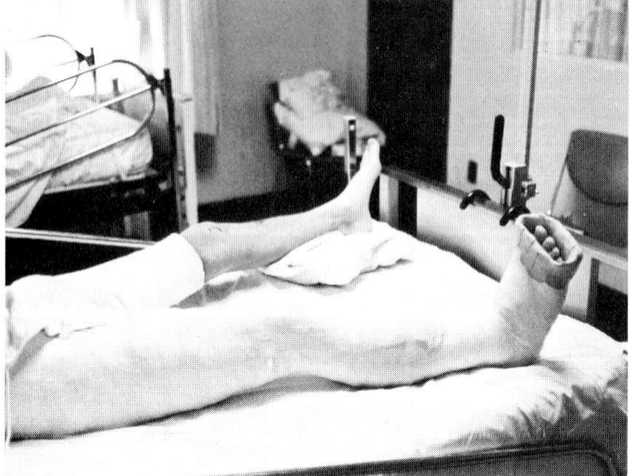

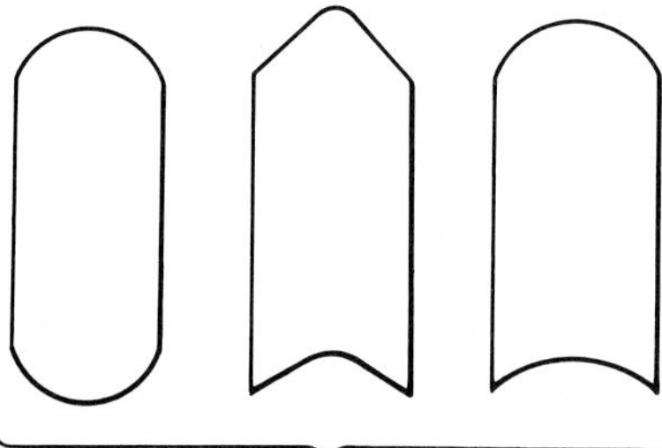

Figure 29-8 Petaled cast edges. The cast edges on the right foot are finished with moleskin, while the edges above the left knee are petaled with tape. The picture also shows three common petal shapes. Cast edges are petaled to protect the skin from rough edges and crumbling cast edges.

will be able to pinpoint the painful area. A younger child will be fussy and irritable beyond the time usually required for cast adjustment. Pain over a period of days followed by sudden relief may indicate that breakdown has progressed through the full skin thickness and sensation has been lost.[5] If skin breakdown occurs, there may be an unpleasant odor. Smelling the cast may provide a clue.

When a pressure area exists or is suspected of existing, removing the cast or "windowing" (removing a piece of the cast over the pressure area) may be required. This may be done to inspect the area and then determine what action needs to be taken. The removed piece may be reapplied with plaster.

Skin care includes frequent turning of all children who are not ambulatory. In the case of older children with large, heavy casts, this may require several persons. Parts of the cast should not be used for lifting or turning, since this may damage the cast.

Keeping the cast clean The cast must be kept clean and dry. If moisture penetrates a plaster cast, it will soften and may need to be replaced. While fiberglass casting materials are not harmed by water, the lining of the cast must be thoroughly dried to avoid maceration of the skin. This can be accomplished using a hair dryer on a warm setting; usually 30 to 60 min of drying time is required. A clean, relatively odorless cast will be more pleasant for the child and those who care for the child. The two main causes of soiling of a cast are eating and elimination. When the child is eating, the cast can be protected with bibs or a towel. Protecting the cast from the products of elimination is more difficult when the cast approaches the perineal area.

In children who have bowel and bladder control, the cast is protected at the time of toileting. This is best accomplished by putting a piece of plastic over the cast edges. With a long leg cast, plastic placed over the top of the cast and tucked inside will suffice. When a child is wearing a plaster jacket and must remain flat, care must be taken to prevent soiling of the posterior cast edge and to prevent urine from running up inside the cast. Boys can use a urinal and have fewer problems with toileting than girls. Some children find a fracture pan more comfortable because of its lower height. A standard bedpan may be used satisfactorily if the upper torso is elevated slightly with pillows to prevent urine from running into the cast.

The following technique usually provides good results. Roll the child onto one side. Tuck a sturdy piece of plastic about 12 in wide into the back of the cast. Place a pillow or two behind the shoulders and the upper portion of the cast for elevation, if necessary. Place the bedpan under the child's buttocks and roll the child back onto the pillows and the bedpan. Tuck the lower edge of the plastic into the bedpan and tuck a similar piece of plastic under the front edge of the cast and into the bedpan between the child's legs. The plastic will help funnel the products of elimination into the bedpan. Always check to see that the upper torso is not lower than the perineal area. After elimination is completed, remove both pieces of plastic and place them in the bedpan. Turn the child onto one side and remove the bedpan and pillows.

The technique for toileting a child in a spica

cast is similar, but since the cast also covers the inner thigh area, the entire cast edge around the perineal area must be protected. This may take several pieces of plastic, all of which are funneled into the bedpan. Encourage children to request the bedpan before elimination becomes urgent, since some time is required for proper preparation.

When a child does not have bowel and bladder control, maintaining cast cleanliness is more difficult. For children with long leg casts, the usual diapering techniques can be utilized, with frequent changes. Children in plaster jackets or spica casts will usually require a split Bradford frame for protection of the cast (Fig. 29-9). Use of the frame is indicated in any child who has poor bowel or bladder control. The frame is elevated on blocks on the bed and is secured, with the head slightly higher than the perineal area to prevent urine from entering the cast. The child is placed either prone or supine on the frame with the perineal area over the opening. The child is secured to the frame. A piece of linen placed around the frame and the child's casted torso and secured with several safety pins usually works well. A piece of plastic is tucked into the cast edges and funneled into a bedpan under the frame. All products of elimination drain into the bedpan, and the cast remains clean and dry. The bedpan and the plastic need to be changed frequently to control odor. The child's perineal area can easily be washed at this time. It is usually convenient to do this when turning the child on the frame and as often as needed between turning.

A piece of disposable diaper can be tucked into the perineal opening of the cast for short periods of time. This is convenient when transporting the child from one area to another. The piece of diaper must be changed very frequently to avoid wetting or soiling the cast. A small piece of sanitary napkin tucked inside the diaper will provide more absorbency and allow for longer periods between changes without wetting the cast.

Activity for casted children Casted children should be permitted as much activity and mobility as possible. Children who cannot ambulate should be provided with another means of transportation (Fig. 29-10).

When planning diversionary activities for a child in a cast, care must be taken that small children do not drop or place small objects down

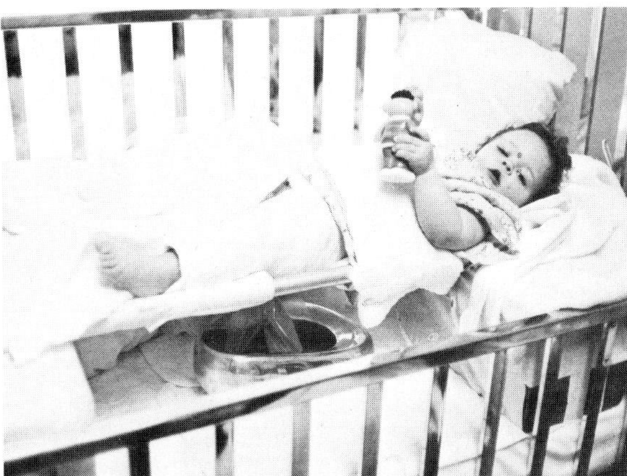

Figure 29-9 A child in a hip spica cast on a split Bradford frame. Note that the upper body and legs are supported by two canvas strips and that the buttocks are in the open space over the bedpan.

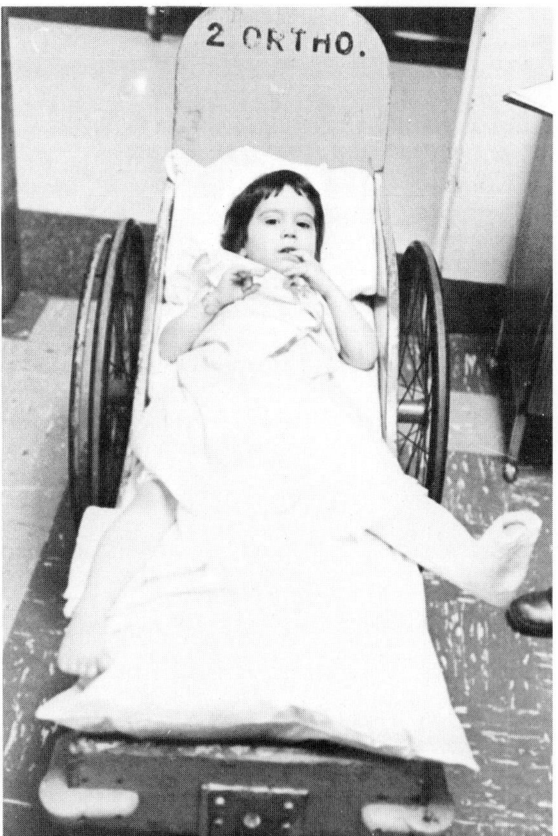

Figure 29-10 A child with a hip spica cast can be placed in a cart to permit movement outside the bedroom.

inside the cast. Children should be instructed not to place anything except the fingers inside the cast.

Removal of a cast The cast may be removed after healing is completed or for purposes of assessing the healing process, after which a new cast is applied. Casts are usually removed with a vibrating cast cutter or cast saw, as shown in Fig. 29-11. Children should be shown the cast cutter and told that it will cut the cast, not them. Cast cutting is noisy, and many children are frightened by it, even with adequate preparation. Distracting the child with toys may be helpful. The child may be fearful that the casted part will be painful without the support of the cast.

The child and the parents need preparation for the appearance of the casted part. The skin area under the cast will be covered with dead skin cells that would normally have been sloughed but remain in place under the cast, where they form a yellow scale. Muscle areas will appear flabby. The casted extremity will usually look smaller than the uncasted one.

The child may experience some discomfort as movement is resumed after the cast is removed. The previously casted area needs gentle handling, with movement instituted slowly. An exercise program will be prescribed by either the physician or the physical therapist to restore normal function to the part. In many hospitals a trip to the physical therapy department is a routine part of cast removal.

Cleansing of the skin should be done gently. The best method of removing accumulated dead skin is soaking the area with mineral oil and then gently rubbing. Vigorous scrubbing will damage the skin beneath the scaly outer layer.

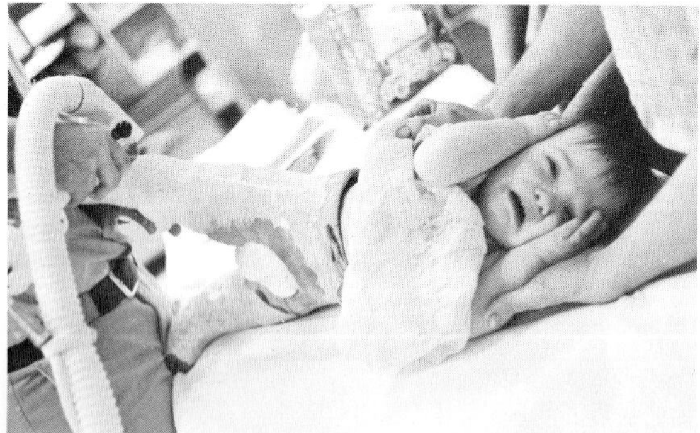

Figure 29-11 Removal of a hip spica cast. The noise of the cast cutter is very frightening. Children need explanations prior to cast removal and much reassurance during the process.

Home care of a child in a cast Instruction for the parents begins when the cast is applied and as they observe the care of the child. The parents of hospitalized children should be encouraged to assume as much responsibility for care as they are willing to. This instruction should include positioning, skin care, toileting, and checking circulation, since all these will be continued after discharge. When a child has been cared for on a Bradford frame, this may be continued at home. The parents need to know how to set the frame up as well as how to place the child on the frame and care for the child.

The parents must receive thorough instructions concerning the child's exercise program and what activities are permitted. The child needs to be a part of family activities at home and should not be confined to a bedroom, if at all possible. Small children can easily be carried from one room to another or up and down stairs. Older children may need to have their sleeping quarters relocated. A wagon or other wheeled vehicle may be adapted for use at home. Parents are often ingenious at finding ways to allow a child to be more mobile. A large skateboard-type vehicle may be constructed. This permits a child in a spica cast to move about on the abdomen, using the hands for self-propulsion.[6] Many types of commonly used baby equipment can be successfully adapted for an infant in a spica cast.[7]

Oral instructions followed by complete written instructions are given. At the very least, the parents should receive written guidelines about conditions that should be reported to the physician, including any signs of circulatory impairment, skin breakdown, or weakening of the cast (see Table 29-1).

Care of a child in traction

Traction is the application of a pulling force, manually or mechanically, to a part of the body. The essential components are *traction* (the pulling force in the direction in which the bone is to be aligned), *countertraction* (the resistance of the muscle and the body weight to moving in the direction of the traction), and *friction* (the force exerted between the patient and the bed). Traction is used in the treatment of fractures to align the bone fragments, immobilize the parts

Table 29-1 General Guidelines for Cast Care

1. Avoid getting the cast wet, unless instructed otherwise by the physician.
2. If the cast edges are rough and cause irritation, pad them with a soft material, such as cotton, or cover them with adhesive tape or moleskin.
3. If the cast becomes soft, cracked, or loose, notify the physician.
4. If swelling occurs, place the hand or foot in a highly elevated position. If there is no improvement within several hours, notify the physician.
5. The onset of numbness or tingling (a pins-and-needles sensation) should be reported to the physician.
6. If you have had surgery, check your temperature twice a day (in the morning and in the evening), and notify the physician if it is above 100°F.
7. If you have steadily increasing pain which is unrelieved by pain medication or elevation of the extremity, notify the physician.
8. Exercise the affected extremity frequently. Notify the physician if you notice a progressive inability to move the fingers or toes.
9. If you notice a progressive feeling of coldness or a change in the color of the affected limb, call the physician.
10. Do not put **anything** under or inside the cast.
11. Use pain medication cautiously, since it may alter your ability to react safely.

until they are healed or stabilized in another way (with a cast or splint), and overcome the muscle spasms that cause pain and the displacement of the bone ends. Traction is also used to decrease spinal curvature (scoliosis), immobilize joint dislocations, and overcome muscle contractures.

Manual traction *Manual traction* is the application of a pulling force with the hands on the part that is to be realigned. This is commonly done during surgery or in the emergency department prior to the application of traction or casting.

Mechanical traction *Mechanical traction* involves a system of weights, ropes, and pulleys mounted on a frame that is secured to the bed; it is used to apply a force that pulls the part in the direction established by the physician. It is applied to the skin or to the skeleton. The *line of pull* is adjusted up or down, or the part is suspended in a direction that will realign the part. The amount of weight applied and the number of pulleys determine the forward pull. Two pulleys will exert double the amount of pull. Thus multiple pulleys reduce the amount of weight needed to produce the same amount of force. Countertraction must be applied if traction is to be effective.

The initial application of traction is usually done by the physician. Traction may also be applied by the nurse, depending on the type of traction, the reason for its application, and the experience of the nursing personnel.

Skin traction *Skin traction* applies the mechanical pulling force directly to the skin through the use of adhesives and wraps. It is generally used in situations that require light or intermittent traction and a moderate amount of force for a relatively short time. This type of traction is often appropriate for use with children who have fractures with little bone displacement and mild muscle spasms. Skin traction is also used with children because their fractures heal quickly and do not require heavy traction. Before skin traction is applied, the condition of the skin is assessed. The skin should be intact, without signs of vascular insufficiency, neurovascular compromise, or rashes and no history of sensitivity to the adhesives that are used to secure the traction to the limb. Skin traction should not be used on fractures that require more than 5 to 7 lb of weight or when the length of treatment is expected to exceed 3 to 4 weeks. If rotation of a limb needs to be controlled to align the fracture, skin traction is not used.

Buck's extension Buck's extension is applied by using a sponge-rubber boot or adhesive straps. The pulling force is applied through a single pulley, with the leg in a straight line. The weights are usually under 8 lb. The foot of the bed may be elevated 6 in to provide countertraction. The child can be carefully turned from side to side, making sure that the affected leg is kept in alignment. Buck's extension is often used to treat children who have fractures or contractures of the hip or who have Legg-Calve-Perthes disease.

Russell's traction Russell's traction is applied with a sponge-rubber boot or adhesive straps. A two-pulley system is used at the foot, and another force is applied to a sling under the knee attached to an overhead pulley. The weight rarely exceeds 4 lb; however, the two-pulley system at the foot doubles the amount of traction force. Countertraction is provided by elevating the foot of the bed about 6 in. Figure 29-12 shows a child in a split Russell's traction.

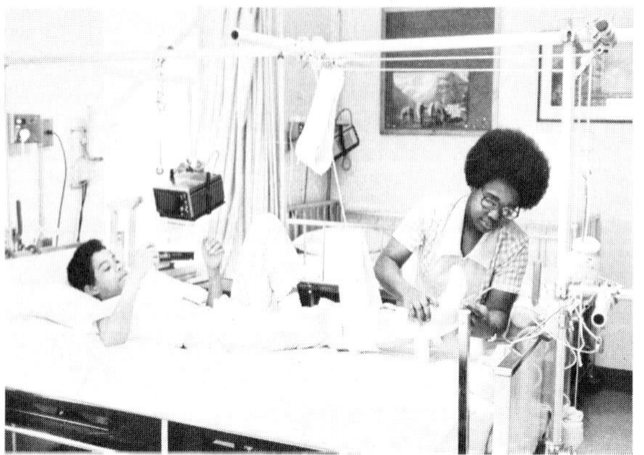

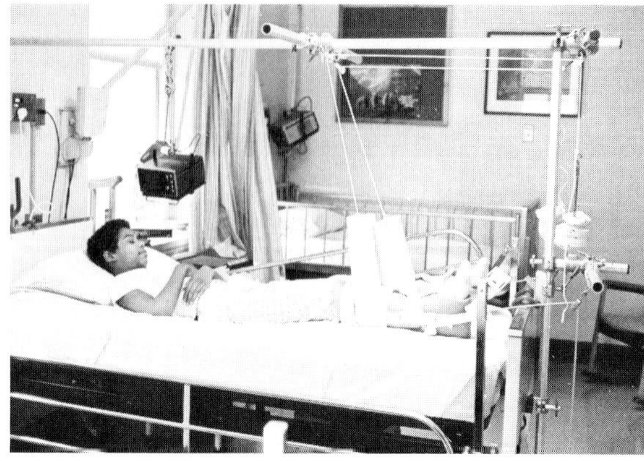

Figure 29-12 A child in split Russell's traction. This skin traction is nonadherent and is periodically removed and reapplied by the nursing staff.

Bryant's traction In Bryant's traction, adhesive traction strips are applied to both legs. The legs are wrapped to the hips. The knees are left slightly flexed to avoid stretching the popliteal muscle and causing compression of blood vessels to the foot. The ankle bones are well padded, care is taken to prevent undue pressure on the achilles tendon, and a small notch is cut in the tapes at the ankle to allow the child to move the feet more easily. The foot plate is padded and is placed so that the toes will just touch the plate if extended. Both legs are suspended vertically, with the hips flexed at a 90° angle from pulleys on an overhead bar attached to weights. The weights are usually less than half the weight of the child. The buttocks should clear the bed so that the nurse's flat hand will fit under them. Countertraction is provided by the weight of the child, and a jacket restraint or a T-strap around the waist may be needed to keep the child in place. Bryant's traction is used only with children under 2 years of age and weighing less than 30 lb, whose weight is not sufficient to provide countertraction for other types of traction. It is not suitable for use with older children because postural hypotension and tight hamstrings cause circulatory problems. The child must be carefully assessed in both the affected and the unaffected extremity for pain and neurovascular status every 2 h. If circulatory impairment develops, the dressings are loosened, traction is reduced, and the legs are taken out of traction. Complaints of pain may indicate vascular insufficiency and should never be disregarded. *Tight bandages have the potential to cause compartment syndrome and ischemic necrosis of the lower extremities*. Bandages are rewrapped daily so that the vascular condition of the legs can be checked. Bryant's traction is used in the treatment of congenital hip dislocation. It is infrequently used to treat fractures of the femur because circulatory complications have been documented in the nonaffected leg. Figure 29-15 shows a child in Bryant's traction.

Skeletal traction *Skeletal traction* applies the force through the insertion of pins or wires directly into the bone. Tongs applied directly to the skull are used for cervical traction. Insertion of these devices is a surgical procedure, and the child is anesthetized. Skeletal traction can be used with 20 to 30 lb of force and for as long as 3 to 4 months. It will also control the rotation of a part. Skeletal traction is the treatment of choice when a fracture is fragmented, muscle spasms are severe, or cervical spine injury is present. Figure 29-17 shows overhead skeletal arm traction.

Overhead 90-90 traction Overhead 90-90 traction is usually used to treat fractures of the humerus or femur. The elbow or knee is suspended and flexed at a 90° angle. The forearm or foot and calf are supported in a sling connected to an overhead pulley. While this type of traction can be applied using skin traction, it is most often applied using skeletal traction. The weights rarely exceed 12 lb in skeletal traction and 6 lb in skin traction. The weight of the body provides countertraction. Figure 29-16 shows 90-90 traction for treatment of a fractured femur.

Dunlop's traction Dunlop's traction is used to reduce supracondylar fractures of the humerus. While skin traction can be used, it is more usual to insert a pin into the humerus so that greater pulling force and better alignment of the elbow can be attained. The arm is extended straight out from the shoulder (90° angle of abduction), and the elbow is usually bent to 45°. The angle is adjusted by the physician as needed to reduce the fracture. The pull is in two directions. With skeletal traction the force is applied laterally to the elbow and the upper arm, stretching the bicep muscle, and from the hand to the elbow, aligning the forearm. With skin traction a sling with a weight pulling downward is placed on the upper arm just above the elbow. Countertraction is provided by elevating the side of the bed on the same side as the traction.

Crutchfield tongs and halo traction devices Crutchfield tongs and halo traction devices are inserted directly into the skull when traction on the spine is needed. The insertion of the tongs or the pins is a surgical procedure. The area of insertion is shaved and anesthetized. With halo traction the pins are inserted and then attached to the halo ring. This traction is used primarily to straighten the spine and is discussed in the section "Scoliosis" later in this chapter. Tongs are used to stabilize the vertebrae, to prevent additional damage in the case of serious spinal injuries, and to permit healing of the injury. The traction pull is in line with the spine, but the direction of the pull is altered by the degree of extension or flexion of the neck. The weight applied is adjusted to reduce the dislocation and overcome the muscle spasms and is carefully monitored, using x-rays and the condition of the patient as a guide. Countertraction can be provided by elevating the head of the bed on shock blocks. The patient is logrolled for linen change and back care. Traction is often attached to a turning frame, such as a Stryker frame, to facilitate care. Potential complications are pin tract infections, skin breakdown on the back of the head, and loosening of the pins and the traction device.

Preparation for traction application

Traction itself is not usually painful. Traction helps alleviate some of the pain caused by the fracture by overcoming the muscle spasm that accompanies it. The child can usually be reassured that pain from a fracture will be decreased once traction is applied. When traction is used for stretching or straightening, as in children with scoliosis, discomfort may occur when it is applied and when weight is added. Children need reassurance that medication is available for relief of pain. The cause of severe pain should be evaluated carefully, since it can be a warning of nerve compression and compartment syndrome.

Nursing care of a child in traction *Maintaining the traction* Traction should be continuous. It should never be interrupted unless specifically ordered by the physician. The nursing personnel who are caring for the child should routinely check to make sure that the weights are hanging free; that the ropes are correctly positioned in the pulleys, footplates, and spreader blocks; that knots are not present in the pulleys; that the tapes and bandages have not slipped; that the pin screws are tight; and that the bed linens are not interfering with traction. Nonadherent skin traction is periodically removed and reapplied. Adherent skin traction and skeletal traction should never be interrupted.

Safety of the system The weights should hang free and should not be touching the floor. Frayed ropes should be replaced. Never add or remove weights without a specific order from the physician. Keep the weights out of the child's reach and make sure that they can be easily inspected. If possible, position the weights so that they are less apt to be bumped.

Friction Anything that increases friction will reduce the efficiency of the traction and decrease the pull. Friction can be increased by pressure of the bedclothes, if the footplate touches the end of the bed, or if the heels dig into the bed.

Positioning The effectiveness of traction often depends on countertraction, or pull in opposition to the pull of the traction created by the child's body weight. The child must be periodically moved to the top of the bed, since sliding to the bottom of the bed interferes with countertraction in some types of traction. Countertraction is maintained by the child's body weight and by raising the head or foot of the bed on shock blocks (usually 6 in high) and keeping the child in a flat position. To avoid reducing countertraction, the child is usually not allowed to sit up, and if the head of the bed is raised at all, it is raised no more that 20° for short periods of time. A firm mattress or bed boards are essential for correct positioning. The body should be kept straight in bed, since bending to one side will change the line of pull.

Activity The amount of movement allowed will be determined by the physician. The child needs clear instructions concerning position and activity. The child in traction should be moved carefully, using smooth, steady movements to minimize muscle spasm and pain. Bumping the bed or using jerky movements can cause severe pain. More than one person may be needed to give back care and to change the bed linen. When moving the child, lift from the unaffected side. If turning is allowed, it should be done very carefully. A child in Buck's traction can be turned from side to side. A child in cervical traction will need to be logrolled or turned on a specially designed bed such as a Stryker frame.

Restraints should be used only when explanations and reminders have not been effective. A Bradford frame may be used as a means of positioning to provide countertraction as well as for toileting purposes. Providing restraint by securing the child to a Bradford frame also prevents excessive movement, which may interfere with traction.

Exercise A trapeze is often attached to the bed frame when a child is in traction. This permits the child to assist in lifting when toileting and is helpful when giving skin care and changing the bed linen. A trapeze allows an older child to do beneficial exercises and strengthen the arm and shoulder muscles. The trapeze bar should hang slightly below the child's shoulders and should be long enough so that the elbows are flexed about 20° when the bar is grasped. Trapezes are not used with children in cervical traction. They should be used with caution, since they can be a safety hazard for young children.

All joints that are not directly involved in traction should be positioned to maintain function and should be put through the full range of motion. The lower extremities can also be exercised by means of dorsiflexion (pulling the toes toward the knees), plantarflexion (extending the ankles and pointing the toes), quadriceps setting (tightening the thigh muscles and pushing the knees into the bed), ankle circling, and straight leg raising. The upper extremities are usually exercised by using the hands and arms for eating, bathing, and brushing the hair. The arms, hands, and fingers must be put through the full range of motion.

Skin care Maintaining skin integrity in the areas subjected to long-term pressure requires vigilance. Inspect the skin for pressure areas and massage the areas three to four times a day. The skin over bony prominences is most likely to break down (the skin on the back, heels, ankles, sacrum and coccyx, and elbows). A piece of sheepskin will reduce the irritation caused by the bed linen, and foam cushions may alleviate pressure on the heels and elbows. The child who has little subcutaneous fat or who will be in traction for a long time may need an alternating-pressure mattress. The bed should be free of wrinkles, and the child should be kept clean and dry.

Pin site care Care of the insertion site for skeletal pins or wires differs from one institution to another and from one physician to another. Some physicians want no care to be given to pin sites, while others want daily cleansing, Betadine scrubs, antibiotic ointments, and sterile dressings around the pin site. Whatever the routine, regular observation of the site is important. Inflammation of, or discharge from, the area should be reported to the physician. The position of the pin should be noted on a daily basis, and any sign of slippage should be reported to the physician.

Neurovascular status Fractures and the application of casts and traction can affect neurovascular status. Neurovascular checks were discussed in the section "Care of a Child in a Cast" and are discussed further in the section "Fractures"; the checks described in those sections should be done for a child in traction. Bandages are checked for excessive tightness.

General care Children in traction have large areas of skin exposed and can become very cold. The room temperature may have to be raised so that the child, not the family or the nursing personnel, is comfortable. It may be difficult to cover the child without interfering with the traction, but often a pair of warm socks or a towel placed on the extremities increases the child's comfort.

Changing the bed linen and toileting may require some ingenuity and improvisation. Sometimes it is more convenient to change the bed linen from the top to the bottom rather than from side to side. A fracture bedpan requires less lifting and movement and may be more comfortable than a regular bedpan.

Psychological needs Traction looks uncomfortable, and the child and the parents need time to adjust to the appearance of all the equipment. They need to understand the purpose of various parts of the traction device. The parents need to know exactly how much movement is allowed. As the parents and the child become accustomed to the traction, the parents usually become actively involved in the child's care if they receive some encouragement and instruction from the staff. Particular attention should be paid to the child's immediate environment. A child in traction often cannot be moved, but stimulation can be provided through cheerful decorations, which may also serve to camouflage some of the traction equipment.

TRAUMA

Trauma to the musculoskeletal system is a common occurrence. Children who are very active and athletic are especially likely to find themselves in situations in which trauma may occur. Motor vehicle accidents are a common cause of trauma to muscles and bones. Children are injured both as pedestrians and as passengers. Other causes of musculoskeletal trauma in children are falls, sports injuries, and lawn mowers.

While parents are becoming more conscious of automobile safety and the importance of proper restraint systems for children, more public education is needed concerning safety in sports. Those in charge of school-run athletic programs are usually fairly conscientious about safety, but children are frequently unsupervised during other sports activities. Skateboarding is a good example of an activity that has resulted in many arm, leg, and head injuries.[8] Many children are also not aware of the dangers posed by power lawn mowers. Young children are most frequently injured by falling into the path of a lawn mower or falling from a riding mower.[9] These children have extremely mutilating injuries, frequently with loss of a limb or a portion of it.

Nurses must take every opportunity in every setting to talk about safety to help parents prevent fractures and other injuries.

Sprains and dislocations

A *sprain* is trauma to one of the ligaments that stabilizes a joint. In children, sprains are most likely to occur as a result of sports activities. Pain and swelling commonly occur. Treatment usually consists of some degree of immobilization until the swelling begins to subside and then gradual return to use of the joint. Elastic bandages are commonly used to provide support to the joint during the healing period. Ice may be used initially to reduce the swelling and pain following injury. Warmth may be used once the initial swelling has subsided to provide comfort, to increase circulation, and to promote healing.

Dislocations and *subluxations* as a result of trauma are not particularly common in children, with the exception of the elbow. A dislocation of a joint occurs when the two bone surfaces that come together to form the joint are completely separated from each other. A subluxation occurs when the bones are displaced but not completely separated.

"Pulled elbow" is a subluxation of the elbow that occurs in small children as a result of a sudden pull on the extended arm. This might occur when a child suddenly pulls away from an adult who is holding his or her hand or when an adult lifts a child by the arm. Sometimes a click can be heard as the joint is displaced. The child experiences immediate pain and will refuse to use the arm, often holding it next to the body with the other arm. Once the subluxation is reduced, immediate relief of pain is experienced. Usually no other treatment is necessary. The parents should be cautioned to avoid pulling on the arm to prevent recurrence of the injury.

FRACTURES

Because a child's skeletal structure is different from that of an adult, the patterns of fractures, problems associated with them, and methods of treatment are different in adults and children. Generally, a child's skeletal structure can withstand a greater degree of bending without fracture than an adult's. This is not because of significantly less bone calcification in a child but because of a decreased density of young bone, due in part to the fact that haversian canals (longitudinal canals that contain the blood vessels, lymph systems, and nerves of the bone) constitute a greater part of a child's bone. A break in a child's bone is more often incomplete because it does not spread by extension as easily as a break in the more dense bone of an adult. The haversian canals in the bone stop the break from extending, much as a hole in a piece of glass will prevent a crack from spreading beyond it. Compression fractures are also more common in children because of the porous nature of their bones. The periosteum in a child is much thicker and less readily torn than that in an adult and has greater osteogenic properties, producing callus faster than in an adult. Thus displacement of fractures is less frequent, healing occurs more rapidly, and nonunion is rare.

Types of injuries and fractures

Fractures in children tend to occur in the long bones and in the areas where bone growth is occurring—the epiphyseal plates.*

Epiphyseal plate injuries The growth cartilage, or epiphyseal plate, found at the ends of the long bones of growing children has the consistency of hard rubber. The epiphyseal plate provides some cushioning for the joint surface and some protection against traumatic injury to the joint. It is also the site from which bones grow and remodel themselves. The epiphyseal plate is the weakest area of the long bones and is susceptible to displacement or fracture, but it usually heals quickly. As the child grows older, the bones gradually calcify. The point where the calcified and uncalcified portions of the epiphyseal plate meet is the most susceptible to injury. It is called the *plane of separation*. This area is bloodless, and so an epiphyseal separation at this junction produces little swelling or deformity and thus is often difficult to diagnose. The growing part of the epiphyseal plate is called the *germinal layer;* if much of this layer is disturbed, the result can be longitudinal bone growth arrest, asymmetrical limb length, or deformity.

Injuries to the epiphyseal plate include tearing of the ligaments, displacement of a bone fragment in the joint, and a comminuted compression fracture. The most common cause of epiphyseal separation or fracture is a twisting or sideways force on a joint; frequently the elbow, knee, or ankle is injured in this way, often while the child is engaged in a sport or strenuous play. Osgood-Schlatter disease and tennis elbow are examples of stress-induced fractures of the epiphyseal plate. These conditions require resting the affected part for about 12 weeks in order for healing to occur. Slipped femoral epiphysis and Osgood-Schlatter disease are discussed later in this chapter.

*The following discussion of types of fractures is based on Mercer Rang, *Children's Fractures,* Lippincott, Philadelphia, 1983.

Normal healing of uncomplicated epiphyseal plate separation takes place in about 1 to 2 weeks. The space between the calcified and uncalcified layers fills with fibrin, widening the gap in the cartilage for about 2 weeks, when revascularization begins. Good alignment of the displaced epiphyseal plate fragments will result in a small scar but no growth disturbance. Pins or screws passed through the center of the plate to hold fragments in alignment will not disturb growth unless they are too close to the margin of the epiphyseal plate. Passive, continuous motion can be used to stimulate healing and prevent adhesions.

Interrupting the blood supply to the germinal layer will cause avascular necrosis of the epiphyseal plate and the epiphysis. Growth disturbances also result when the plate is crushed or infected, improper conjunction of the parts with nonunion exists, a hyperemic response to the injury produces local overgrowth, or a callus bridge forms between the epiphysis and the metaphysis. A callus bridge is bone formation between the two fragments that blocks the normal bone growth in the area where it forms. Angular deformity results when only one side of the epiphysis continues to grow. The bone bridge must be surgically removed and is replaced with autogenous fat or rubber, after which future growth is normal.

Buckle fractures A buckle fracture is a compression fracture that pushes up the bone, producing an elevated ring or ridge at the fracture site. A buckle is seen in the porous bone where bone growth is occurring near the epiphyseal plate. This area of the bone does not have the strength of the more solid structures around it and tends to be subject to injury.

Traumatic bowing of a bone Children's bones will bend as much as 45° before fracturing. A bend will straighten itself in a few minutes; however, the bone will not be completely straight. Bowing occurs most commonly in the ulna and fibula in association with breaks in the radius and tibia. Bowing is not a true fracture and is referred to as *plastic deformation of the bone*. Since no hemorrhage is present and no new bone forms, the deformity is not remodeled.

Greenstick fractures A greenstick fracture typically occurs in the wrist of a young child who falls on an outstretched hand. In a greenstick fracture the bone is bent beyond its limits. A severe angulation deformity is present, as one side breaks and the other side is compressed (bends). A strong hinge of periosteum holds the bone on the compression side. Complete closure of a greenstick fracture may be prevented by the rough edges of the bone itself or by the muscle pull. When the angulation of the bone is too great, the fracture will be completed by the physician, and the bone straightened. If this is not done, a permanent deformity of the bone may remain.

Complete fractures There are many different kinds of fractures (see Fig. 29-13). Comminuted fractures are very rare in children because their bones are flexible. The bone edges in a complete fracture are often held in place by the periosteum, since it remains intact more often in children than in adults. Thus displaced fractures are less common in children. When a fracture is displaced, a hinge of periosteum may remain and can assist by holding the bone fragments in place, or it can have the opposite effect and make reduction more difficult by interfering with bone replacement.

Bone healing

When a bone is broken, there is always some trauma to the soft tissues surrounding the fracture, causing swelling. This can be the result of the force that caused the fracture or the movement and displacement of the fractured bone ends that caused trauma to the soft tissues. Of particular concern is trauma to the major blood vessels or nerves which may occur as a result of fracture, particularly in the area of the elbow.

When a fracture occurs, the periosteum is torn and pulled away from the bone, and bleeding occurs. This results in the formation of a hematoma around the fracture site. Osteoblasts are released from the broken ends of the bone into the area surrounding the fracture. The bone ends that have lost their blood supply become necrotic and degenerate. The hematoma around the bone ends changes to a fibrous connective tissue bridge

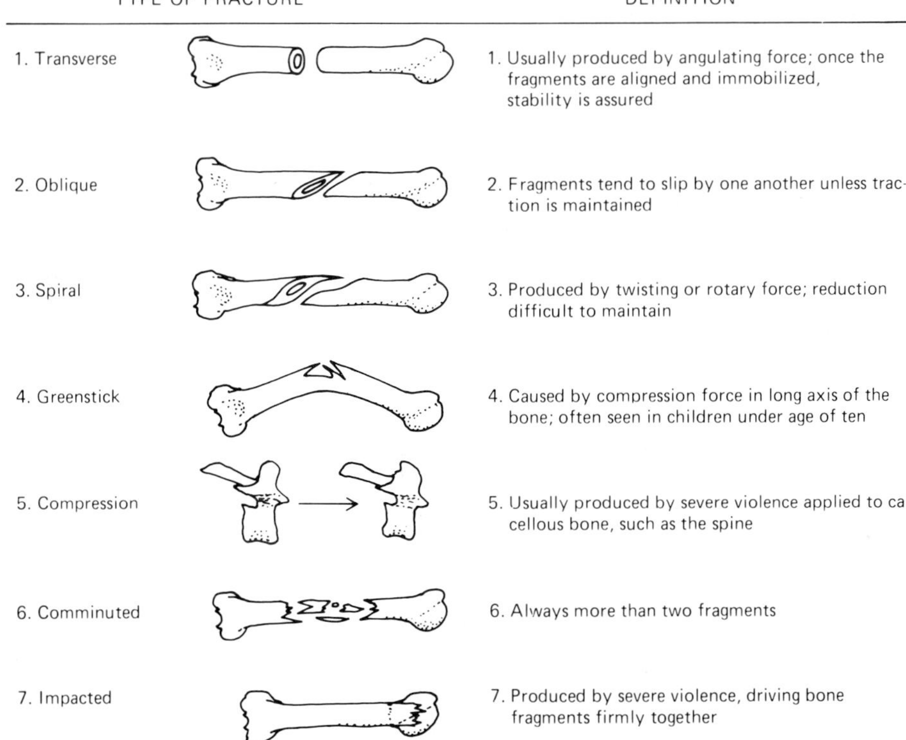

Figure 29-13 General classifications of fractures. (*From J. Barry, Emergency Medicine, McGraw-Hill, New York, 1978, p. 319.*)

and then into cartilage and bone through the action of the osteoblasts. This initial union of the bone ends is called *callus formation*. As callus is gradually changed into solid bone, remodeling and reshaping of the fracture will occur.

Children's bones heal quickly, and therefore bones should be realigned early to prevent them from healing in a faulty position. During the period of healing, the bone must be immobilized to maintain the correct position of the bone ends and to allow for solid healing of the bone before it is subjected to normal stress. The younger the child, the more rapidly bone healing takes place. A femoral fracture in a newborn may heal in 2 to 3 weeks, while in an adolescent this same degree of healing may take 8 to 10 weeks. This means that the period of immobilization required is generally shorter in children, especially young children.

Growth remodeling

A fracture in a long bone that is not in perfect alignment may be remodeled as the child grows. This means that a bony deformity caused by imperfect repair will often correct itself as growth occurs. In remodeling, the deformity of malunion is corrected by periosteal reabsorption on the protruding side, and the opposite concave side is filled out with new periosteal bone. The younger the child and the closer the break is to the epiphyseal plate, the more correction takes place.

Overgrowth

In children, a limb that has had a fracture of the long bone may grow about 1 cm longer than the unaffected limb over the course of 1 to 2 years after the break. Stimulation of longitudinal bone growth is due to increased blood supply to the growth cartilage in the injured limb. Overgrowth usually compensates for the length lost (about 1 cm) through the overlapping of bone ends at the fracture site.

Complications of fractures

Nursing care of a child in a cast and a child in traction and the vascular and neurological assessment were discussed earlier in this chapter. While the nurse must be immediately concerned about a tight cast that impairs circulation, it is also important to remember that a cast that is too loose or that fits improperly will allow the fracture to displace or angulate. The cast should be molded and applied in the position desired to keep the fracture reduced in good anatomic position. Squeezing the cast or changing the position of a part after the cast has been applied only results in occluding circulation and creating an improperly fitted cast. If a cast is so loose that a hand can be placed inside it and the cast moved up and down, the cast may need to be replaced.

Emboli Immobility and incorrectly applied casts or traction can cause local pressure on a vein. A child with a fracture, especially of the lower extremities, who is on prolonged bed rest is predisposed to venous stasis and formation of a blood clot. The clot can become detached and be carried to a lung, the brain, or the heart and may be life-threatening. Nursing interventions to prevent emboli include exercising the extremities, avoiding pressure on the popliteal space, using antiembolic stockings, taking care not to massage the calves, and preventing casts or traction appliances from constricting circulation.

Fat emboli are often associated with traumatic fractures of the long bones and multiple fractures and appear 12 h to 3 days after the trauma. The effects range from mild and transient to life-threatening and prolonged. There are two theories regarding the origin of fat emboli: (1) that they result when fat droplets are released from the bone marrow into the bloodstream and (2) that they result from a change in the metabolism of fat in response to trauma. The major clinical sign is acute respiratory failure due to the capillary occlusion and escape of fluid into the lungs, resulting in hemorrhagic pneumonitis. Fat droplets may also occlude the cerebral circulation, decreasing oxygen to the brain. Changes in mental state such as memory loss, restlessness, confusion, an elevated temperature, and a headache should prompt investigation. Petechiae around the neck, upper chest, and shoulders; in the conjunctivae; or in the mouth are late signs of a fat embolism. Carefully immobilizing the child and avoiding movement at the fracture site during the acute phase may help prevent the release of fat into the bloodstream. Oxygen, steroids, anticoagulants, and low-molecular-weight dextran are included in the care plan.

Compartment syndrome Compartment syndrome is a progressive interference with the blood flow to a portion of an extremity. The increased pressure in the compartments can be caused by trauma, hemorrhage, exertion, traction, a tight cast or dressing, and/or burns. If left untreated, it will result in the permanent death of muscle groups and peripheral nerves and a contracted, paralyzed, and nonfunctioning extremity.

A compartment consists of a fascial sheath that surrounds a muscle or a muscle group and the vessels and nerves that pass through it. It is large enough to allow the passage only of main arteries, nerves, and tendons. Edema inside the closed spaces of the tissue compartments can obstruct venous circulation and cause arterial occlusion, resulting in compromised circulation and ischemia of the part. The common feature of cases of compartment syndrome is the mechanism by which they develop. This is the ischemia-edema cycle: muscle swelling leads to venous arterial compression, which leads to arterial occlusion, which in turn causes muscle ischemia.[10]

Compartment syndrome of the forearm is known as *Volkmann ischemic contracture* and is associated with fractures of the humerus and the elbow. It can produce a paralyzed, deformed arm with a clawlike hand. In the lower extremities it is often referred to as *anterior compartment syndrome,* although three compartments—anterior, lateral, and posterior—are present in the leg. The outcome is a clubfoot deformity with loss of motion at the ankle.

The signs and symptoms of compartment syndrome are progressive. Early detection is essential to save the function of the limb. Clinical evaluation consists of nerve and circulation checks, documentation of progressive pain, and an increase in pain on passive range of motion or a sudden absence of pain. The patient will experience severe pain, which will progress to numbness, tingling, loss of sensation, and inability to flex or extend the fingers or move the toes. The extremity may become very edematous, and the child may feel pressure. The last stages of compartment syndrome consist of paresis and absence of a pulse. If the pain is greater than the pain caused by the primary problem, such as a fracture, burn, or contusion, and is not relieved by standard medication, a possible compartment syndrome should be considered.

Pressure within the muscle is measured by inserting a catheter to measure intracompartmental pressure. The normal range of pressure is 16 to 20 mmHg. Pressures exceeding 30 mmHg prevent perfusion with blood. If left untreated, high pressure can result in impaired circulation and necrosis of the skin, fascia, and muscles, which can lead to ulceration and gangrene of the muscle. There are two phases of treatment. The first phase is medical and consists of releasing the pressure (cutting casts, removing dressings, and reducing the weight on traction), straightening a flexed elbow, elevating the extremity, and using ice and diuretics. The second phase is surgical intervention, which is required if the pressure cannot be reduced to a safe level. A fasciotomy opens the fascia along the entire length of the muscle (in the arm from the elbow to the palm). A fasciotomy within 8 h of the onset of compartment syndrome almost always returns function to normal immediately.

Nerve damage Peroneal nerve palsy or footdrop can be due to the trauma of the injury itself or to damage caused by excessive traction, pressure, or impaired circulation related to treatment. The child is unable to dorsiflex the foot. The ability to walk is impaired, and the child must wear a brace indefinitely or until the function returns. Nerve damage is prevented by making sure that traction does not cause pressure over the lateral surface of the knee. The nurse should avoid having the child lie with the leg externally rotated, since this will put pressure on the head of the fibula. If a sensory deficit to touch, pinprick, and movement is noted, the physician should be informed immediately.

Treatment of fractures

A child is usually brought to the physician by a parent who suspects that there is a fracture because an accident has occurred or the child is complaining. Sometimes the diagnosis is obvious and is based on the presence of swelling, hematoma, deformity, diminished function of the part, pain, or (less frequently) protrusion of the bone or crepitus, which is a grating sound made by movement of the bone fragments. Sometimes the signs in a child are more subtle because the fracture is held in place by the periosteum or is in the growth cartilage. Any child who is suspected of having a fracture will first have the part x-rayed. The child may be in considerable pain and needs to be handled gently during the procedure. The fracture site should be splinted prior to the x-ray to reduce pain and prevent displacement of the bones. Unnecessary movement and palpation of the part should be avoided. To prevent missing fractures in the same limb, the joints above and below the fracture should be included in the x-ray. Since nerves and blood vessels can also be damaged, neurovascular status must be assessed. (See the earlier sections "Care of a Child in a Cast" and "Complications of Fractures.")

Once the fracture is diagnosed, the goals of care are to regain good alignment and length of the bone through reduction of the fracture and to immobilize the fracture in that alignment through the use of casts, traction, and fixation devices. The ultimate goal is to restore the full function of the injured part.

Closed reduction or manipulation is the most frequent method of fracture reduction in children. It is accomplished through a combination of manual traction and force applied with the hands to push the bone ends into position. In a closed reduction of a displaced fracture, the physician may use a process of retracing the path of the fracture (moving the limb through the path it took during the break) to put the fracture in alignment and make certain that the periosteum and soft tissues are not caught in the break.[11]

Bone fragments are more often overlapping in closed reductions. A 1-cm overlap of the bone is acceptable because overgrowth of the bone will usually compensate for this loss in length. If the child has less than 2 years of growth remaining, the overgrowth may be less and a smaller degree of overlap is acceptable. Closed reduction of fractures with acceptable results becomes more difficult as the child becomes older.

Local or general anesthesia may be used, but the child must receive some kind of analgesic and sedative medication to reduce the amount of pain during the reduction and in the period immediately afterward. A cast is molded to the part during application to keep the fracture reduced.

Open reduction involves exposure of the bones through a surgical incision. It is always done under general anesthesia, and some type of internal-fixation device (a rod, screw, plate, or nail) is inserted to stabilize the fracture. Open reduction is used if alignment cannot be obtained by the closed method. It is the first choice in displaced intraarticular fractures of the humerus, femur, olecranon, and patella. Displaced fractures in the middle of the shaft of a bone that are grossly shortened, angulated, or rotated; fractures that cross the epiphyseal plate at right angles; and multiple fractures usually require open reduction and internal fixation.

Once a fracture has been reduced, its position can be maintained by the use of a cast, traction, internal-fixation devices, or an external-fixation (Hoffmann) device (see Fig. 29-14). External-fixation devices are most likely to be used with open fractures or when there is extensive skin loss associated with the fracture.[12] For complete immobilization, a cast usually incorporates the joint above and the joint below the fracture site. Traction is more likely to be needed in fractures of bones where large muscles pull on the bone fragments. In such cases, a cast may not hold the bones in the correct alignment. When traction is needed, it is used until callus formation provides sufficient stability to the fracture so that a cast can be applied.

Fractures that can be treated with a closed reduction and casting may not require that the child be admitted to the hospital. Sometimes

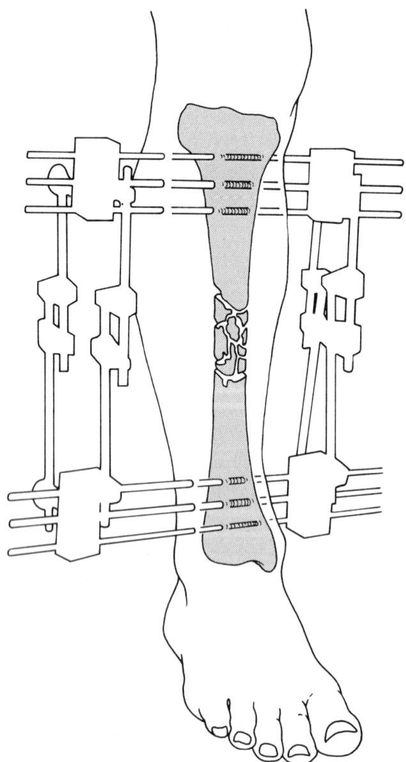

Figure 29-14 An external-fixation device in place for treatment of a comminuted fracture of the tibia. *(From A. Brooker et al., Principles of External Fixation, Williams & Wilkins, Baltimore, 1983.)*

children are admitted for the purpose of observing neurovascular status for a period of time, particularly if there is extensive swelling. Children whose fractures require traction, surgery, or an external-fixation device will require hospitalization, sometimes for extended periods of time.

Nursing care of a child with a fracture If the fracture is untreated, the basic rule of first aid is to splint the fracture as it lies. The principle is to avoid movement at the fracture site, since this may cause further injury to the limb. The child may arrive for treatment with the fracture splinted. Whether the fracture has been treated or not, assessments of neurovascular status should begin immediately and continue hourly for at least 24 h.

The child is usually in pain and will require regular pain medication for the first days following the injury.[13] Children are often fearful of being cared for by the nurse because any jarring or moving of the affected extremity causes considerable pain. When the child is in traction, caution should be taken to avoid bumping the bed or any part of the traction apparatus. All moving of the child for physical care needs to be done with extreme gentleness to prevent increasing discomfort in the period immediately following the fracture. As callus formation begins and the swelling subsides, pain will decrease, and the child will be better able to tolerate being moved for physical care.

In emergency situations children and parents need accurate explanations of procedures to be performed. These explanations may be brief because of the need for prompt medical attention. The child's pain may interfere with his or her understanding of any information that is given. The parents are often visibly upset when trauma has occurred. Their ability to process any information given to them under these circumstances may also be limited. This means that detailed explanations of the nature of the injury and the treatment may be more meaningful after the initial crisis has passed. It is best not to assume that the parents have received or understood much information given in emergency situations.

Parents often feel responsible or guilty after a traumatic injury has occurred. Some parents express these feelings, while others find these feelings so painful that they avoid discussing them and choose to concentrate on the physical problems. Some parents attempt to blame or rebuke the child, especially if disobedience had anything to do with the injury. Staff members usually have difficulty accepting this type of reaction from parents. Indeed, they may feel angry with the parents for having allowed the accident to occur. Parents need to express these feelings without being judged. In the period following an injury, the parents may be extremely solicitous or overprotective of the child in an attempt to relieve these guilt feelings.

The child's response to the injury can include any of the usual responses to illness. A sudden, unexpected injury carries with it a threat to physical well-being that may manifest itself in fearfulness or phobic reactions in the child following the injury. This is a very understandable reaction. Usually these fears can be resolved by allowing the child to express his or her feelings without being ridiculed. Many children need to talk at length about the circumstances surrounding an accident. This helps dissipate some of the anxiety associated with the event.

Fracture of the clavicle The clavicle is one of the most frequently broken bones in children. A fracture can occur at birth because of pressure on the shoulders during delivery. A fracture of the clavicle commonly occurs when a child falls from a bed or high chair and lands on an outstretched arm, an elbow, or a shoulder. While older children may complain of pain, in infants the only symptom may be lack of spontaneous movement on the affected side.

When a fracture of the clavicle occurs at birth, healing and remodeling of the bone take place easily and rapidly. No treatment at all may be utilized, or the affected arm may be immobilized by using tape or by pinning the sleeve of the shirt to the shirt body. For older children, a figure-eight bandage may be used to brace the shoulders back and prevent the bone ends from overlapping. This is usually worn for several weeks.[14]

Leg fractures Fractures of the tibia and fibula can often be treated with reduction and casting. Fractures of the femur often require traction to maintain reduction. In children under 2 years of age, Bryant's traction is commonly used (Fig. 29-15). For older children, several types of traction are used, depending on the nature of the fracture. One commonly used type is called *90-90 traction,* which is illustrated in Fig. 29-16.

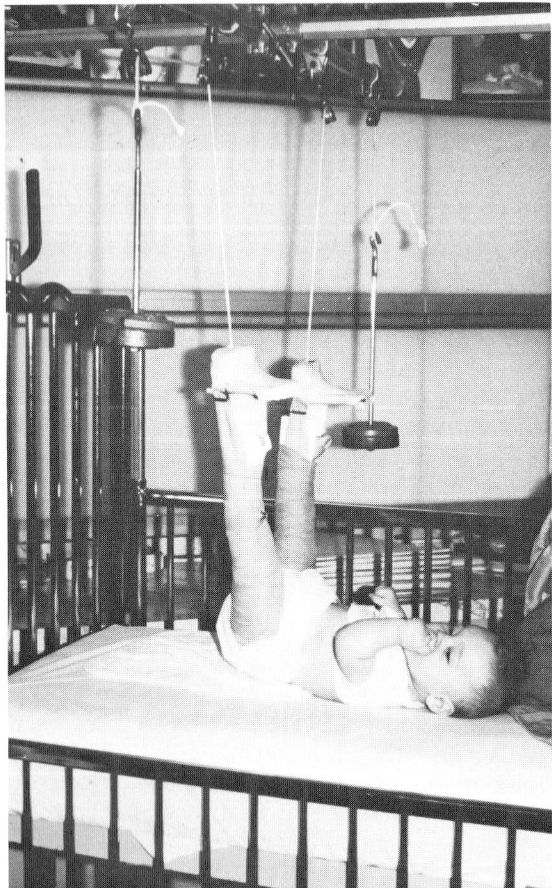

Figure 29-15 Bryant's traction for treatment of a fractured femur in a 6-month-old infant.

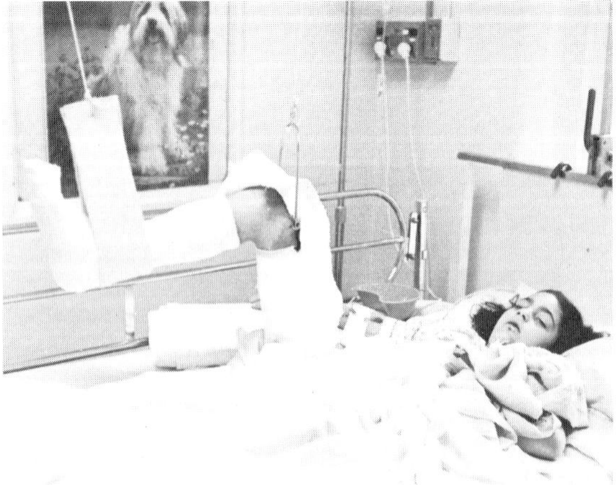

Figure 29-16 90-90 skeletal traction for treatment of a fractured femur in a 7-year-old child.

The traction is applied to a pin placed in the distal fragment of the femur. Three or four weeks of traction are often required before casting can be done. Fractures of the femur require a hip spica cast for immobilization following traction.

Arm fractures Falls are the most common cause of arm fractures. Many can be treated with reduction and casting. Of particular concern are fractures near the elbow because there is considerable danger of damage to, or compression of, the brachial artery and the radial, ulnar, or median nerves.[15] The *supracondylar fracture* of the humerus, a common fracture in children, is a fracture in which the distal humerus just above the elbow fractures. Supracondylar fractures may be treated using closed reduction and casting or open reduction with internal fixation. Some require skin or skeletal traction (Fig. 29-17).[16] The method of treatment depends on the amount of displacement of the fracture fragments, the amount of swelling, and the neurovascular status of the arm. In every case, assessment of neurovascular status is of primary importance because of the high incidence of neurovascular complications in fractures in the elbow area.

If undetected, trauma to the brachial artery can result in *Volkmann's contracture*, which is a disabling and permanent loss of function in the hand. It is produced by ischemia to the muscles of the forearm as a result of injury to, or spasm of, the brachial artery. Within 24 h, swelling and compression can produce permanent damage to the muscles and nerves. The child can be left with paralysis of the muscles of the wrist and fingers. Symptoms of disruption of circulation and neurological function include pain in the forearm, pallor of the hand, absence of the radial pulse, and inability to extend the fingers or wrist. If neurovascular compromise occurs, cast removal or immediate surgery may be necessary to prevent permanent damage.

In cases of supracondylar fracture, the physician may establish a specific protocol for assessing neurovascular status. If not, the nurse should assess neurovascular status hourly. This assessment should include checking for radial pulse and checking the child's ability to extend the wrist and all fingers. Any change warrants immediate attention from the physician.

Skull fractures Trauma to the head may result in a skull fracture. Usually the skull fracture itself is not the main concern, but rather injury to the brain beneath, which can be caused by a blow that is forceful enough to produce a fracture. The fracture will heal without treatment unless a fragment of the skull is depressed or displaced. Surgery may be required to elevate the bone fragment. (The treatment of head injuries is discussed in Chap. 30.)

Spinal cord injuries Accidents are the major cause of spinal cord injuries in children. Automobile accidents, diving accidents, falls, gunshot wounds, and accidents while playing sports are some of the causes of spinal cord injuries. Cervical fractures can occur following occipital blows (flexion) or facial blows (extension). Vertebral compression fractures are the most common cause of spinal cord damage. Vertebral dislocation and severing of the cord are less common than compression. Increased compression of the spinal cord due to edema and hemorrhage can cause ischemia of the spinal cord with necrotic damage for a few days to a week after the injury.

Immediate care of a suspected spinal cord injury includes avoiding twisting or pulling, which can further damage the spinal cord. The head, neck, and back must be stabilized in straight alignment prior to transfer. The child should not be allowed to walk or sit, and a pillow is not used under the head if a spinal cord injury is suspected. A flat, stable surface such as a door is used for transport. In a diving accident, spinal cord damage often occurs when the child is dragged out of the water. Stabilizing the spine before removing the child from the water can prevent further spinal cord damage.

Respirations should be evaluated, since respiratory distress can occur with a cervical injury. The child should be asked not to move the extremities before being x-rayed because this can cause further spinal cord damage. The nurse observes for complaints of numbness, tingling, or loss of sensation and evaluates the strength of hand grasps.

Skeletal traction is used to immobilize the spine, prevent damage from bone fragments, relieve pressure from compression, and prevent further damage while edema and hemorrhage resolve. (See the previous section "Traction.") After 2 to 4 weeks the cervical traction is removed and the spine is stabilized with a brace, such as a halo brace or the Peterson brace.

A surgical fusion may be done if the back remains unstable or causes pain. Fusion is the process of stabilizing the vertebrae by taking bone from another part of the body, often the iliac spine, and grafting it to the spine. A posterior fusion is

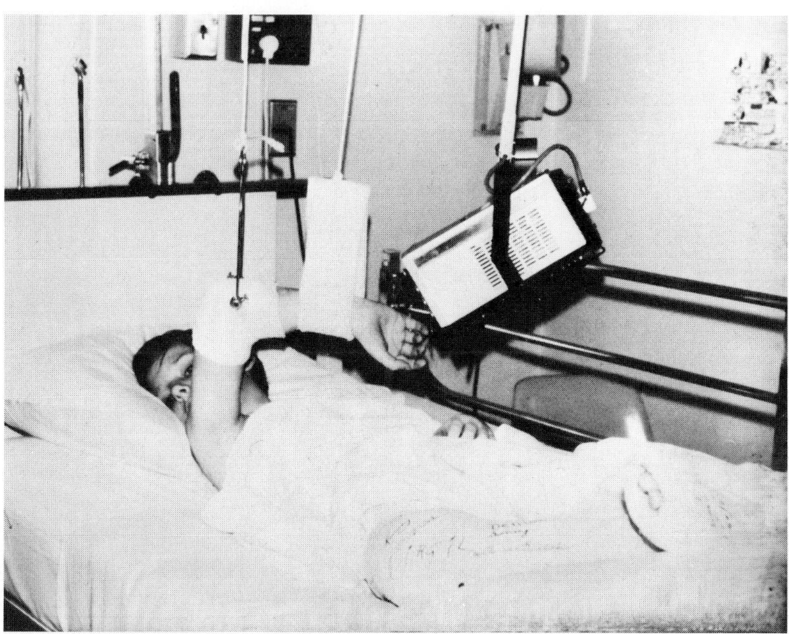

Figure 29-17 Overhead skeletal arm traction for treatment of a fractured humerus.

done from the back, while an anterior fusion is placed on the front side of the spine. After a spinal fusion, a body brace or cast is worn for 6 more weeks. Spinal fusion is discussed in the section "Scoliosis."

Traumatic amputations

Loss of a body part in children is most likely to occur as a result of a motor vehicle accident or a lawn mower injury. Treatment is aimed at making the limb as functional as possible with the use of a prosthetic device.

This type of injury has a devastating effect on the parents, and they may be incapacitated with guilt. The grief reaction of children to the loss of a body part varies with age. Younger children often make an amazing adaptation, both physically and emotionally, to the profound change in body function and body image. Older children experience longer periods of mourning and adjustment. The parents and the child require the maximal support possible in order for the child to make a healthy adjustment.

CARE OF THE CHILD WHO UNDERGOES ORTHOPEDIC SURGERY

Common orthopedic surgical procedures used with children include:

1. Various corrective procedures on bones themselves, such as surgical procedures for congenital dislocation of the hip
2. Muscle or tendon transplants to improve function of a part that has been damaged as a result of trauma or other cause
3. Removal of bone tumors
4. Spinal fusion for scoliosis

Healing following surgical trauma usually requires some degree of immobilization. Most children who have undergone orthopedic surgical procedures have casts applied immediately following the surgical procedure while they are still anesthetized.

Preoperative care

Preoperative diagnostic work consists mainly of x-rays and routine blood work. Preoperative nursing care concentrates heavily on preparing the child and the family for the surgery and the postoperative routine. See Chap. 15 and the section "Care of a Child in a Cast." The nurse should tell the child the details of the preoperative routines, explain the surgery in appropriate language, indicate the site of the incision, and describe the appearance and "feel" of the cast.

The child and the parents need a thorough discussion of the degree of immobilization that will follow surgery. The parents may express concerns about their ability to care for the child if the child is to be discharged in a cast. They need answers to specific questions and reassurance that they will receive thorough instructions once the surgery has been performed.

Physical preparation includes shaving the incisional area. Care must be taken not to damage the skin in any way. Any skin lesion or break should be pointed out to the surgeon, since this increases the chance that infection will be transmitted to the bone. Usually, preoperative injections are not given near the operative area.

Whether the child requires preoperative teaching of coughing and deep breathing or using the incentive spirometer depends on the extent of the surgery and the degree of immobilization. Children who will undergo spinal fusion for scoliosis require careful teaching in this area.

Both the parents and the child need to be prepared for postoperative pain. Orthopedic surgery is physically traumatic because the manipulation of bone requires much physical force, including sawing and chiseling. Orthopedic surgical procedures are accompanied by a considerable amount of pain. Besides pain in the immediate surgical area, children may complain of muscular aches and pains in other areas. Trauma to muscle may also produce muscle spasm following surgery. Morphine or Demerol is the usual postoperative pain medication used with orthopedic procedures. Most children require it regularly for 12 to 24 h after surgery and then are given a milder pain medication. A muscle relaxant may be required for the relief of muscle spasm as well.

Postoperative care

Assessment of vital signs should always include assessment of neurovascular status. The same procedure is used as when a cast is applied. Some swelling accompanies surgery and is to be expected. Postoperative elevation of an extremity is indicated to help prevent and reduce swelling (Fig. 29-18). When elevating an extremity, care should be taken to keep the cast well supported, since it may be wet when the child returns from surgery. Elevation on several pillows is often effective. Suspension of an extremity with slings and weights may also be used.

In most cases the incisional area and wound dressing are covered with plaster. Once blood saturates the dressing, it will be absorbed by the cast. Some staining of the cast with blood immediately over the incision is usual. If the staining is increasing, it is common to outline the stain with a ballpoint pen and mark the time on the cast. When the nurse or physician returns to recheck the child, he or she can see how much more staining has occurred in that period of time. The nurse should also describe the intensity of the staining, just as would be done with any surgical drainage. This staining can be covered with more plaster before discharge to improve the appearance of the cast.

During the postoperative period, the parents need to learn to care for the child in preparation for discharge. The instructions given are the same ones that any parents would receive when their child is being discharged with a cast. The parents of children who have undergone surgery also need to be aware of the signs of infection: temperature elevation, staining of the cast by wound drainage, and a foul odor emanating from the cast.

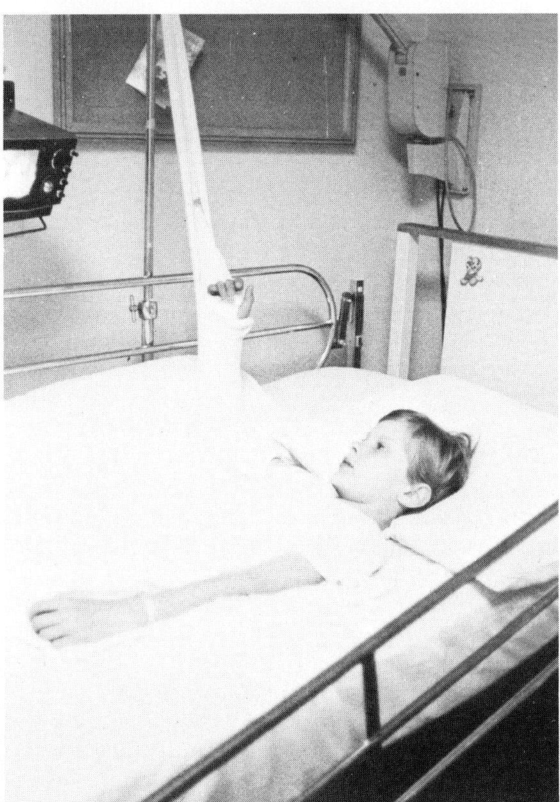

Figure 29-18 Elevation of an extremity following surgery to reduce swelling.

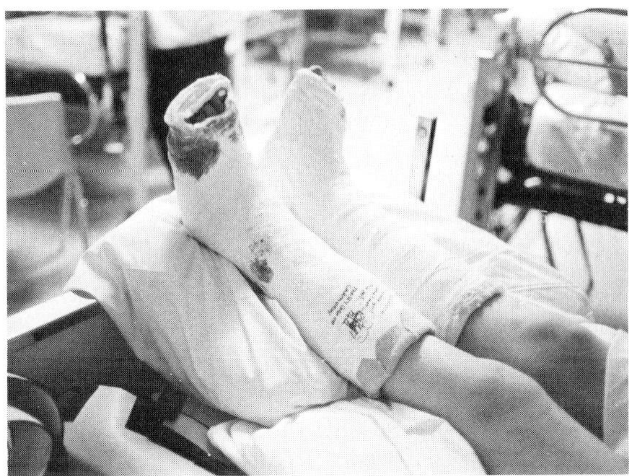

Figure 29-19 Staining of casts with blood following surgery.

Children may return to the surgeon's office for cast removal. Children who have undergone more extensive procedures may be readmitted to the hospital for cast removal and physical therapy.

CONGENITAL DISORDERS

Clubfoot

In *clubfoot* (talipes equinovarus), the foot is adducted, and there is inversion and equinus (plantar flexion) of the foot. A clubfoot is illustrated in Fig. 29-20*A*. A true clubfoot has an anatomic deformity of the muscles and bones that prevents it from being manipulated into a normal position. In contrast, some infants are born with a positional deformity of the foot simulating clubfoot, but with manipulation this foot can be placed in a corrected position. The most common method of treating clubfoot is serial casting. Starting shortly after birth, plaster casts are applied to gently and gradually correct the deformity. These are changed at weekly intervals until correction is achieved, usually within a few months. Once the condition has been corrected, the parents are instructed in exercises for the

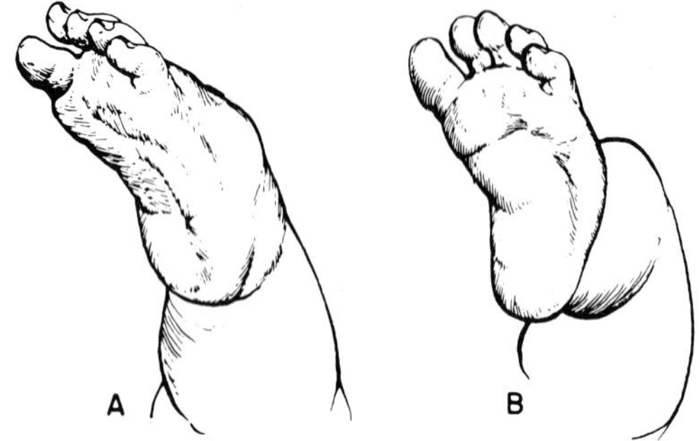

Figure 29-20 Congenital foot deformities. (*A*) Clubfoot. (*B*) Metatarsus adductus. (*Courtesy of Craig Gosling, Indiana University School of Medicine, Department of Medical Illustration.*)

feet. Bivalved casts may be used to hold the foot in the corrected position during sleep. These are casts that have been applied, dried, and split into anterior and posterior halves. They may be reapplied periodically and held in place by wrapping them with elastic bandages. Corrective shoes may also be used for maintaining correction. They may be used in conjunction with a Dennis-Browne bar. This is a metal bar, fastened to the soles of the shoes, that helps maintain the feet in the desired position.

Most infants have good correction with treatment. A small percentage may require more extensive surgical treatment, such as a tendon transplant, to prevent recurrence of the problem.

Metatarsus adductus

In this condition, also called *metatarsus varus*, the forefoot is adducted in relation to the posterior portion of the foot (Fig. 29-20*B*). In some infants the condition can be passively corrected by holding the hindfoot and pressing the forefoot into a normal position. In these cases, corrections can be obtained through an exercise program as the parents regularly place the forefoot in the normal position. Straight-last or reverse-last shoes may be used to achieve or maintain correction. Normal shoes have a last that curves inward at the forefoot. A straight-last shoe has no curve, while a reverse-last shoe curves outward at the forefoot. The shoes may be placed on a Dennis-Browne bar at night so that the child sleeps with the feet turned outward.

If the feet cannot be placed in the correct position passively, a true bony deformity exists. This usually requires serial casting. Following casting, straight-last shoes may be worn to maintain correction.

Congenital dislocation of the hip

Dislocation of the hip at birth is just one extreme of a problem usually referred to as *congenital hip dysplasia*. This condition consists of an instability of the hip joint in which (1) the head of the femur may be easily dislocated, (2) the head of the femur may be subluxed or rides higher in the hip socket than usual, or (3) the head of the femur may be dislocated or actually out of the hip socket (or acetabulum). All gradations of the problem require immediate treatment in order that the hip may develop normally.

The exact cause of congenital hip dysplasia is not known. There is some familial tendency, and the condition is more prevalent in females. There may be some relationship between relaxation of the hip capsule (the ligaments that surround and stabilize the hip) and congenital hip dysplasia. The position of the baby in the mother's uterus and a breech birth may contribute to the condition as well.

The hip joint at birth is still largely cartilage. It is necessary that the head of the femur be in the correct position in the hip socket so that the socket develops a normal shape and configuration as growth and ossification proceed. If the condition is left untreated, as the child begins to walk, the hip joint will flatten. Once this has occurred, treatment is much more difficult. For this reason, early diagnosis and treatment are extremely important.

Every newborn assessment includes an assessment of the hips. Commonly described signs of congenital hip dysplasia are unequal skin folds on the thigh or buttocks, unequal height of the knees when the infant is lying on a firm surface with the hips and knees flexed, and limitation of abduction of the affected hip. Figure 29-21 illustrates checking for these three classic signs. These signs may not be present in newborns because their development depends on muscular changes which occur over time. A more accurate assessment involves grasping the femur with the hip and knee flexed and abducting and lifting the femur. If the hip is dislocated, the femoral head will reenter the acetabulum, and a click will be felt or heard (Ortolani's sign).[17]

Barlow's test is the reverse of the test using Ortolani's sign. If the femoral head is in the acetabulum at the time of the examination, Barlow's

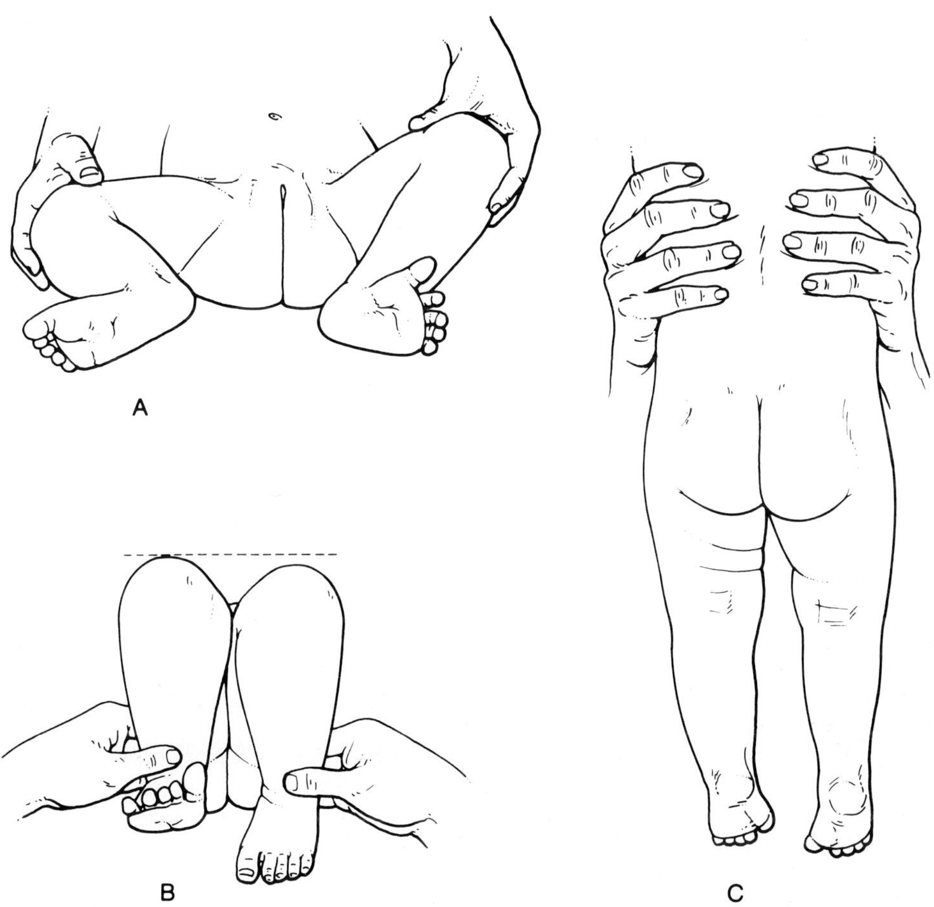

Figure 29-21 Checking for signs of hip dysplasia. (*A*) The nurse checks abduction of the thighs (there is full abduction on the right and limited abduction on the left). (*B*) The nurse checks the relative height of the knees (the right knee is higher than the left). (C) The nurse checks the symmetry of the skinfolds in the gluteus and thighs (the skinfolds are asymmetrical). *(From G. Scipien, M. U. Barnard, M. A. Chard, J. Howe, and P. J. Phillips [eds.], Comprehensive Pediatric Nursing, 3d ed., McGraw-Hill, New York, 1986, p. 1273. Used with permission.)*

test is used to test the stability of the hip. The presence of any of these signs should be reported to the physician and usually indicates the need for x-rays of the hips.

If some degree of hip dysplasia is present, treatment in early infancy is relatively simple. The goal of treatment is to keep the head of the femur in the acetabulum. In very mild cases of hip dysplasia, triple diapering is still used to hold the legs in abduction. Other modalities that are used in the early stages of treatment are the Palvik harness, the Ilfeld splint, and the Frejka splint. The Palvik harness is secured over the shoulder and is used to keep the hip flexed and in the abduction position. The Ilfeld splint is used for the same purpose. The design is somewhat less complicated, and there is less range of motion at the hip joint. It is worn over both legs and is secured by a strap to maintain hip abduction (see Fig. 29-22*A* and *B*). Regardless of the choice of device, the primary goal of treatment of a dislocated hip in early infancy is positioning the hip in abduction and providing for flexion and some external rotation.

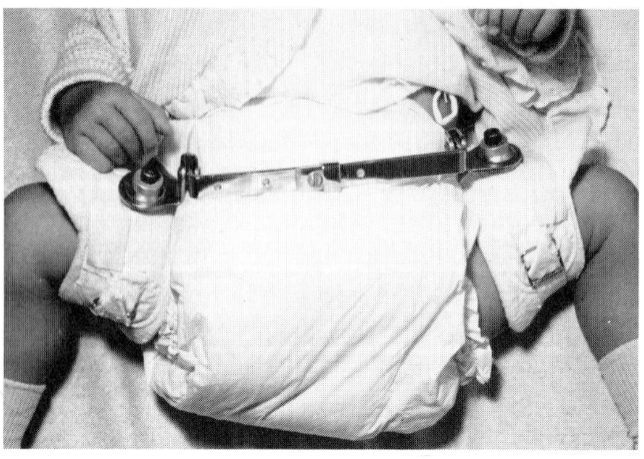

A

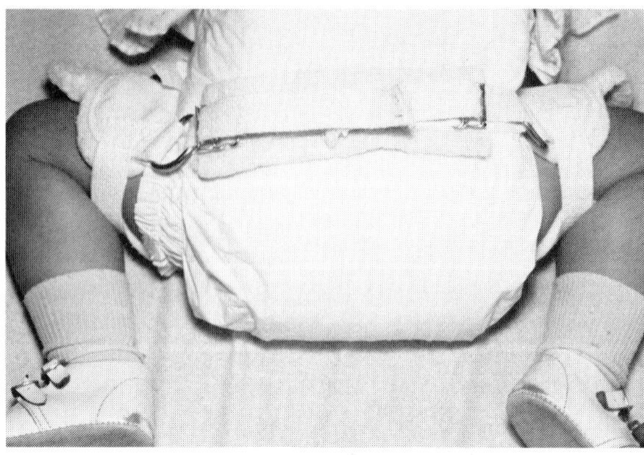

B

Figure 29-22 The Ilfeld splint is one of the newer apparatuses used to keep the hips abducted in a frog position for the child with congenital dislocation of the hips. (*A*) Front view. (*B*) Back view.

When the condition is more severe, the position of the hip may be maintained by a hip spica cast. The length of treatment is determined by the progress of the hip on x-ray. Usually within several months the hip is developing normally.

Children with undiagnosed and untreated congenital dislocation of the hip develop an abnormal gait when they begin to walk, which may cause the parents to seek medical attention. When the child puts weight on the affected hip, the pelvis drops on the opposite side. When dislocation is bilateral, this results in a waddling gait. The longer congenital hip dysplasia goes undetected, the more difficult the treatment is. Walking tends to increase the upward displacement of the head of the femur. Older infants and children may require traction to bring the head of the femur down to the level of the acetabulum. Older children may require traction and surgical reduction to place the head of the femur in the acetabulum. These treatments are followed by immobilization in a spica cast. The success of treatment decreases as the child's age increases. If treatment is not completed in childhood, total hip replacement may be done in young adulthood.

Torticollis

Contraction and fibrosis of the sternocleidomastoid muscle produce a condition known as *torticollis*, or *wryneck*. The shortening of the muscle causes the head to be tilted toward the affected side and the chin to be rotated to the opposite side. There may also be a fibrous mass within the affected muscle. The cause of this congenital condition is not known. Torticollis may be evident at birth or may not appear until several weeks after birth.

Treatment consists of gradual stretching of the contracted muscle with exercise. The parents are also encouraged to position the child so that when they get the child's attention, he or she will turn the head toward the affected side; this helps stretch the muscle. If these exercises are started early and continued faithfully, most children will obtain good correction within a few months. A small number of children may require surgical treatment.

Congenital amputation and phocomelia

Infants are born with all degrees and varieties of absence and deformity of the extremities. Various terms are used to describe these conditions. *Syndactylism* is the joining of two digits. *Polydactylism* is the presence of extra digits. *Amelia* is the absence of an extremity (sometimes called *congenital amputation*), and *phocomelia* is the attachment of a limb directly to the trunk with an intervening portion missing. The severity of limb deformities varies from the presence of a small extra digit to the complete absence of all four extremities.

All these conditions arise during embryonic life when the limb buds are developing. Drugs administered in the first 3 months of pregnancy may induce these defects, as occurred in Europe with the use of the drug thalidomide.

Treatment is aimed at allowing the child to

develop as much normal function of the involved extremity as possible. This may include surgical procedures. Extra digits may be surgically removed. Attachments, or webbing, between digits may be removed or reduced. A finger may be moved to serve as a thumb. In some cases, amputation of a deformed limb is necessary to permit the use of a prosthetic device that will allow the child to function more normally.

Nursing management Initial nursing care is aimed at helping the parents deal with the grief response that accompanies the diagnosis of a congenital problem. Although musculoskeletal problems are not usually life-threatening, they may have long-term effects on the child's physical mobility and life-style. They are also quite visible to others. Parents often have questions about the long-term effects: Will the child be able to run and play normally or participate in sports? How will the problem affect the child's appearance? These may seem like minor concerns to some, but they are of major importance to the parents.

The parents need careful explanations of treatments, especially those to be continued at home. The nurse must take into consideration that the parents are just learning to care for a newborn. Caring for a newborn in a cast may seem overwhelming at first. If an exercise regimen is part of the treatment plan, the parents should have the opportunity to demonstrate correct execution of the exercises several times; the success of the treatment may depend upon this.

DEVELOPMENTAL PROBLEMS

Shoes for normal feet

Parents often have questions about shoes for their children. Shoes basically protect the feet from physical trauma and temperature extremes. Children with normal feet do not need shoes for support. Usually a baby needs shoes when beginning to stand or walk outdoors, where foot protection and warmth are needed. Infants' shoes are made somewhat higher around the ankle so that the child will keep them on the foot. In infants the heel tends to be rounded, and a shoe with a lower cut will easily slip off the foot. No ankle support is needed. When the heel is sufficiently developed so that a regular oxford or sneaker will stay on the foot, these may be worn. Shoes do not need to be expensive, but they must fit properly, allowing some room for growth.

Flatfoot

Flatfoot is a condition in which the medial arch of the foot is absent when the child is standing. This causes the foot to pronate, or roll toward the medial, or inward, side. Infants almost always assume this position when they first stand or walk with the feet wide apart. There is very little medial arch apparent on an infant's foot. As the child gradually brings the feet closer together, the body weight is shifted toward the center of the foot. With growth and redistribution of body fat, the medial arch becomes more developed.

In older children, flatfoot requires treatment if the condition causes the child discomfort or limits his or her physical activity. Often the foot has a normal-looking medial arch when no weight is put on it, but the arch disappears when the child stands on the foot. This may be caused by weakness or laxity of the foot ligaments. Children with flatfoot may toe-in because this changes the weight distribution on the foot and alleviates foot strain.

The treatment consists of supporting the medial arch. A shoe with a heel will sometimes improve the weight distribution on the foot. Some sort of medial arch support is often prescribed. A Thomas heel, which has a forward extension on the medial side, is commonly used.

Toeing-in and toeing-out

There are many reasons why children walk with the toes pointing in or out. It can result from problems with the foot itself or problems elsewhere in the leg, including the hip. The position of the knee indicates whether the problem is above or below the knee. If the knee is in the midline position while the foot turns, the problem is below the knee. If the knee deviates as well, the problem is above the knee. Most causes of toeing-in and toeing-out correct themselves with growth and maturation.

Internal torsion, or twisting, of the tibia is a fairly common occurrence in infants. It causes a toeing-in gait but is self-correcting within the first few years of life. It usually requires no treatment. Torsion of the tibia or femur and the associated toeing-in or toeing-out gait may be associated with persistent postures assumed by the child: sleeping with the legs turned inward or sitting on the floor with the knees bent and the feet turned outward. Discouraging assumption of these positions may help correct the problem.

Bow-legs and knock-knees

Both bow-legs and knock-knees occur normally during the process of growth and development of the lower extremities. Infants often appear bow-legged, but by the age of 3 they may appear knock-kneed. The degree to which these conditions occur is influenced by hereditary factors. By age 7 or 8, most children's legs are straight.

Pains in the musculoskeletal system

Pain in the muscles and joints is a common occurrence in children. It may be due to excessive activity. Growth itself places some stress on bone and muscle. Many children experience what are commonly called "growing pains." These typically occur during the night. The child awakens complaining of pain. There is no redness or swelling, and the pain does not seem to increase with joint motion. It is usually relieved by rubbing or by applying heat or cold. The pain is gone in the morning. Any pain that is regular and persistent or does not follow this pattern needs to be investigated by a physician.

HEREDITARY DISORDERS

Muscular dystrophy

Etiology Muscular dystrophy is a genetically determined disease, and the primary changes that it causes are muscular and are not secondary to any disorder in the peripheral nervous system or the central nervous system. The types described differ in respect to age at the onset, the muscles involved, and the rate of progression. The disease is insidious, with periods of progression and remission, eventual incapacitation, and finally death. The classifications usually accepted are (1) Duchenne muscular dystrophy, or pseudohypertrophic (autosomal recessive); (2) limb-girdle muscular dystrophy (autosomal recessive); and (3) facioscapulohumeral muscular dystrophy (autosomal dominant).

Duchenne muscular dystrophy Duchenne muscular dystrophy is the most common form of the disease and is transmitted in a sex-linked autosomal recessive pattern. This means that the vast majority of victims are boys. The child appears normal at birth, and the onset of the disease is usually prior to 5 years of age. There is a characteristic enlargement, or *pseudohypertrophy,* of certain muscles, especially of the calves and shoulders. While the muscles appear large, they are actually weakened because of infiltration with fat. As the disease progresses, children frequently fall, have difficulty keeping up with their peers, and are unable to climb stairs or rise from the floor without using the arms, owing to increased weakness of the extensor muscles of the lower extremities and pelvic girdle. Children with Duchenne muscular dystrophy get up from the floor by rolling to a prone position, pushing themselves to a kneeling position with the arms, and then standing up by placing the hands against the shins, knees, and thighs. This method of standing by "walking the hands up the legs" is known as *Gower's sign*. Characteristically, children with Duchenne muscular dystrophy stand with lumbar lordosis (curvature of the lumbar spine) and extended knees; they have enlarged calves and may have difficulty standing because of equinus deformity (clubfoot). The hypertrophic calf muscles are stronger than the anterior leg muscles, and eventually this results in a pattern of toe-walking caused by the contraction of the heel cords. Later there is wasting of the shoulder muscles and development of kyphosis and scoliosis. Respiratory muscle failure and cardiomegaly are frequently related to complications causing death. Ambulation often becomes impossible by about 12 years of age, and death by age 20 is frequent.

Limb-girdle muscular dystrophy This is a less common autosomal recessive type, and the onset is from about age 10 to age 50. Weakness occurs gradually in the scapulohumeral girdle (shoulders) and/or the pelvic girdle, and severe disability develops within a 20-year span, leading to death.

Facioscapulohumeral muscular dystrophy This disease is autosomal dominant and affects males and females equally; the onset is in the second decade of life. The facial muscles are affected first, causing speech problems and an expressionless face. Next the muscles of the shoulder girdle are affected, and the child is unable to raise the arms over the head. Most children with this disease have significant disability, but remain ambulatory and can look forward to a normal life span.

Management During the diagnostic phase, the nurse's main concerns are preparing the child for diagnostic testing and assisting the family members as they confront the diagnosis of muscular dystrophy and its long-term ramifications.

The diagnosis of muscular dystrophy is confirmed by serum enzyme measurements, an electromyelogram (EMG), and a muscle biopsy. The creatine phosphokinase serum enzyme level is very elevated. The EMG shows decreased strength of muscle contraction (a decrease in amplitude) and decreased speed of muscle response. A positive muscle biopsy reveals degeneration of muscle fibers and replacement with fat and connective tissue.

An EMG involves insertion of needles into the muscle mass to measure electrical activity; it is a painful test for a child. A muscle biopsy is also painful and requires anesthesia and preparation for surgery. Preparing the child and the parents will not decrease the pain but will help them understand and accept the procedures.

There is no effective treatment for this disorder. Since children with muscular dystrophy tend to develop complications as a result of muscular weakness and spinal deformities, the goal of care is to keep them as active as possible in order to prevent physical deterioration. A vigorous program of exercise is prescribed to help prevent or delay contractures, disuse atrophy of the muscles, obesity, and respiratory problems. Braces may be used for support, and the surgical release of contractures may prolong the ability to ambulate.

Home care of children with chronic diseases is discussed in Chap. 34. The parents of children with muscular dystrophy may also receive support, both emotional and physical, from the Muscular Dystrophy Association, which provides a support network, help in diagnosis, and necessary equipment. The parents need to understand the pattern of transmission of muscular dystrophy and the possibility of bearing other children with the disorder. Genetic counseling should include testing of male siblings for the presence of the disease and of female siblings for the carrier state.

Osteogenesis imperfecta

This condition is characterized by fragile bones which fracture easily. Also, the child with osteogenesis imperfecta characteristically has blue sclerae. Some children with this condition also develop deafness later in life. Osteogenesis imperfecta is thought to be a dominant hereditary trait.

Two forms are recognized. In children with the congenital form, fractures occur in utero or at birth, and the disease is usually severe and produces a great deal of deformity or death. In children with the late form of the disease, fractures may not appear until several years after birth. The disease is usually milder with fewer fractures, and the tendency to fracture disappears after puberty. Children with osteogenesis imperfecta have some degree of growth retardation, depending on the severity of the disease.

Treatment of the disease is aimed at preventing deformity due to the frequent fractures. In children with severe osteogenesis imperfecta, the use of rods, surgically placed within the long bones, may prevent further fracture and deformity.

Management Caring for children with osteogenesis imperfecta requires delicate and gentle handling to avoid breaking a bone. Usually the parents or the children can give excellent instructions in this regard because they know just how much stress the bones can tolerate.

During the period of diagnosis, the parents need genetic counseling concerning the risks to future offspring and the risk factors for their children when they reach childbearing age. In some areas there are parent support groups for parents of children with this condition.

ACQUIRED ALTERATIONS IN MOBILITY

Juvenile rheumatoid arthritis

Juvenile rheumatoid arthritis (JRA) is the most common rheumatic disease of childhood. The highest incidence occurs in children between the ages of 1 and 3 years.[18] Although the etiology of JRA is not yet established, it is known to be an autoimmune disease.

Manifestations The term *arthritis* implies inflammation of the joints. This is evidenced by joint swelling, tenderness, pain on motion, decreased range of motion, and increased warmth and redness of the involved joint or joints. Stiffness, particularly in the morning, is also common and is often related to the activity of the arthritis. During exacerbations increased fluid is present in the joint, and the synovial lining which contains the fluid in the joint space also becomes thickened. To help decrease pain and discomfort, children often hold involved joints in a flexed position, which encourages such problems as flexion contractures. Fortunately, the disease has a cyclic nature, with varying periods of exacerbations and remissions.

Although no two cases are alike, three subtypes of JRA are generally recognized: the systemic onset type; the pauciarticular onset type; and the polyarticular onset type. These are distinguished on the basis of clinical and laboratory findings present during the first 6 months of the disease. The *systemic onset type* (also known as *Still disease*) occurs with equal frequency in boys and girls. Children with systemic onset JRA often have high-spiking fevers, which tend to occur in the late afternoon or evening and disappear in the night and early morning. They also have a maculopapular rash which comes and goes, often with the fevers. Enlargement of the lymph nodes, liver, and spleen are common, as are high white blood cell and platelet counts, significant anemia, and high sedimentation rates. Pericarditis occurs in about 20 percent of these children. Joint involvement may or may not be present in the beginning stages of the disease. Children with this type of JRA can be acutely ill.

In *pauciarticular onset type* of JRA, four or fewer joints are involved during the first 6 months. Sometimes only one joint is involved, such as a knee, ankle, or elbow. Children with this type of JRA may have a positive antinuclear antibody test; those who do are at high risk for developing an insidious inflammation of the front part of the eye, called *iridocyclitis*. Because this inflammation occurs without early symptoms, slit-lamp eye examinations every 3 months are necessary to help detect this problem. Early treatment can significantly reduce the permanent visual loss.

The *polyarticular onset type* of JRA is similar to the adult form of rheumatoid arthritis. Five or more joints are involved during the first 6 months, frequently including the small joints in the hands and feet. Both the pauciarticular and the polyarticular onset types of JRA are more common in girls than in boys.

The general prognosis for children with JRA is good. Some children recover completely within a few years, and many are in permanent remission by adolescence. The long-term effects depend on the severity and length of activity of the disease and on the treatment.

Treatment Treatment of JRA is aimed at controlling inflammation, promoting normal function, and preventing deformity of the joints. Aspirin or other anti-inflammatory medications such as tolmetin are prescribed. Children who continue to have significant problems may require treatment with gold or, less frequently, with corticosteroids. Surgery is rarely necessary. A home exercise program to promote extension and strengthening and other physical therapy measures, such as splinting, may be instituted. Problematic morning stiffness can be reduced with a warm bath or shower or hot compresses. Contact sports should be discouraged, but bicycling, swimming, walking, frequent changes of position, and participation in age-appropriate activities of daily living are recommended except during acute exacerbations. Daily attendance at a regular school is also advised, with modifications as necessary.

The lack of any known cure and the unpredictable course of JRA make this a frustrating and frightening disease for the parents and the child. All family members need continual support and encouragement, particularly during the crisis periods of diagnosis and exacerbations. Occasionally, hospitalization is necessary for acute problems or rehabilitation.

The parents of children on long-term aspirin therapy must be educated about the signs of aspirin toxicity, the need for occasional tests of salicylate levels and liver function, and the potential for gastrointestinal upsets. This latter problem can be reduced by administering the aspirin with meals or antacids. In addition, the parents must understand that in order for aspirin to have its anti-inflammatory effect, it must be taken several times a day, not just on an as-needed basis.

During acute episodes, an exercise program is often prescribed to be carried out by the nurse or physical therapist. Whenever possible, active motion of the joint by the child is best. Hot compresses applied to joints and warm baths may be used to help alleviate stiffness. Night splints may be used to hold joints in extension and help prevent flexion contractures. Since movement produces pain, the child is afraid of movement. Gentleness in handling and moving is indicated.

Many parents turn to unproven remedies in an effort to decrease their child's discomfort. The nurse who maintains a good rapport with the family members can often encourage them to continue with the recommended treatment program. Finally, teachers and other caregivers must be adequately informed about the needs of the child with JRA.

Osteomyelitis

Infection in the bone, or *osteomyelitis*, arises from one of three sources: contamination of a fracture, introduction of infection during a surgical procedure, or blood-borne infection secondary to infection elsewhere in the body. The causative organism is usually streptococcus or staphylococcus.

When the condition is blood-borne, it tends to localize in the bone metaphyses, but may then spread to other parts of the bone. The initial symptoms are fever, pain, and decreased movement of the affected part. There may be swelling, redness, or heat, depending on the extent of the infection. The child may be seriously ill with septicemia.

The treatment is intravenous antibiotics for a period of several weeks, combined with immobilization of the extremity by limitation of activity or the use of splints, bivalved casts, or skin traction. Many infections respond well to this treatment. Surgical drainage of the infected area may be necessary. Treatment is aimed at preventing the spread of the infection to other areas of the bone. Inadequate treatment can lead to a chronic osteomyelitis, which may resist treatment.

Chronic osteomyelitis causes extensive bone tissue damage, requiring numerous surgical procedures that drain and debride the wound. If the bone remains unstable, a bone graft from either the child or a bone bank can be used to restore bone stability.

Treatment The child is immobilized for several weeks and receives intravenous antibiotic therapy. Protection and care of the intravenous injection site will ensure that the child receives antibiotics at regularly scheduled intervals.

If the infected area is open or has been surgically drained, careful precautions must be taken to avoid the spread of organisms to other patients or visitors.

Children with osteomyelitis are discharged on oral antibiotics, often to be continued for a period of months. The family must understand the importance of regular, long-term administration of antibiotics, even when symptoms are absent.

Synovitis of the hip

Synovitis is an acute inflammation of the hip that is self-limiting and of short duration. It may occur secondary to trauma. When there has been no trauma, there has often been an acute respiratory illness for 1 or 2 weeks before the appearance of the hip symptoms. The disorder usually occurs in males between 3 and 10 years of age.[19]

The child complains of pain, sometimes in the knee, and may limp. A fever is often present. The range of motion of the joint is limited, and there is usually a flexion contracture of the hip. The joint may be tender when palpated.

The hip is immobilized with traction, often split Russell's traction. This usually provides relief of pain and corrects the hip flexion contracture. Within a few days, full motion of the hip without pain has returned. Sometimes weight-bearing is limited for a short period after initial treatment with traction.

Legg-Perthes disease

Etiology The symptoms of first-stage Legg-Perthes disease, or aseptic necrosis of the head of the femur, are much like those of synovitis of the hip, and it must be differentiated from that disease. Legg-Perthes disease may be preceded by synovitis of the hip, or there may have been no previous hip problems. The onset is less acute than in synovitis of the hip. Usually, the child complains of knee pain and limps for a period of weeks. There is also limitation of motion and muscle atrophy with hip flexion contracture. Legg-Perthes disease occurs most commonly in children aged 3 to 12,[20] and most cases are diagnosed in children between 4 and 8 years of age. Males are affected 4 times as frequently as females.

Manifestations The development of this disease is related to a decreased or absent blood supply to the head of the femur. In the process of normal bone development, a good blood supply is needed to nourish the epiphyseal plate so that it can grow. Synovial fluid, which is similar to plasma, nourishes the outside of the head of the femur, and blood vessels develop to nourish the inside. During development, the vessels to the head of the femur are somehow cut off, and the cartilage dies. After a few weeks, the blood supply is restored through the spaces left by the cartilage, and the dead tissue is absorbed and is gradually replaced with bone. The process of restoring the tissue is Legg-Perthes disease.

The disease generally progresses in three stages: (1) the period of onset, lasting several weeks, during which there is pain, a limp, swelling and edema of the joint, and atrophy of the muscle; (2) the period of necrosis of the head of the femur, lasting from months to a year or longer, during which the head of the femur becomes soft and x-rays show the secondary ossification center in the head of the femur as an opaque spot; and (3) the period of regeneration of the head of the femur, which can take several years.

Legg-Perthes disease is usually discovered in the second stage, when the dead tissue of the hip is very spongy and provides little or no support to the head of the femur. The head of the femur can collapse unless weight is taken off the hip while the bone regenerates.

Treatment The main focus of the treatment plan is keeping the hip abducted and internally rotated and putting the head of the femur in the acetabulum, thus helping it maintain its shape as it hardens. Initial treatment is bed rest and immobilization with traction. This relieves pain and restores motion to the hip. The traction is removed when the child has achieved a good range of motion, and the child may then be permitted to ambulate without bearing weight on the affected hip. If this is not accomplished in 7 to 10 days, an adducted tenotomy is performed to gain full range of motion. The child is then placed in a bilateral Petrie cast (a hip spica cast with a brace), which makes it possible for the child to ambulate and still provides rest for the head of the femur. Depending on the severity of the disease, the child might use a Scottish Rite brace instead to prevent weight-bearing on the head of the femur. A number of orthopedic appliances have been devised that allow non-weight-bearing ambulation. Whatever method is used, it is continued until the regenerative phase of the disease is well under way, usually for about 2 years. Bearing weight prior to that time results in flattening of the head of the femur and permanent distortion of the hip joint.

Surgical intervention may be needed if the conservative measures do not adequately maintain the head of the femur in the acetabulum or if treatment is expected to be especially prolonged. An osteotomy is performed to surgically maintain coverage of the femoral head.

It is extremely important that the parents understand the course of the disease. Successful treatment of Legg-Perthes disease is based on long periods without weight-bearing. It is the parents who must be diligent in enforcing strict compliance with the prescribed regimen. They need to plan how to adapt the child's daily living pattern to make the adjustment to this change in mobility easier. Ways of helping a child deal with immobilization were presented at the beginning of this chapter.

Osgood-Schlatter disease

This condition, which is common among older school-age children and young adolescents, causes knee pain and is due to separation and fragmentation of the tibial tubercle. It is thought to be similar to Legg-Perthes disease because there is an avascular necrosis of the tubercle, similar to the changes that take place in the femoral head in Legg-Perthes disease. Pain is aggravated by any activity that causes the patellar tendon to pull on the tibial tubercle: running, climbing stairs, and bicycling. The disease is usually self-limited, but may cause enough pain to require some limitations on activity or immobilization of the knee. It can occur bilaterally. Children with Osgood-Schlatter disease do not usually require hospitalization.

Slipped femoral epiphysis

In a growing child the epiphyseal plate represents a weak area in the bone. Stress to this area can result in slippage across the epiphyseal line, displacing the epiphysis from its usual position. The most common place for this to occur is at the upper femoral epiphysis. Figure 29-23*A* shows a normal hip, and Fig. 29-23*B* shows one in which a medial slip of the femoral head has occurred.

This condition occurs most commonly in boys between 10 and 17 years of age. Girls are less frequently affected.[21] It occurs more frequently in overweight children and in children who are thin and have recently had a period of rapid adolescent growth.

The onset of symptoms is insidious. The child complains of pain in the hip, knee, or thigh over a period of time and may have a limp. The leg tends to externally rotate, and range of motion may be limited. The diagnosis is made by x-ray visualization of the slip.

Once the condition is diagnosed, weight-bearing is immediately stopped and the child is placed in traction. The most common treatment is surgical; a compression screw is inserted through the epiphyseal line to secure the epiphysis and prevent further slippage. Care must be taken during treatment and surgery that no further trauma to the epiphyseal plate occurs and that the blood supply to the femoral head is not disturbed. Interference with the blood supply can result in necrosis of the head of the femur.

Postoperatively, the child is placed in traction and is progressed to partial weight-bearing with crutches for discharge. The child is then gradually progressed to full weight-bearing. The pin is removed after the epiphysis has closed, which may be as long as several years after surgery.

Nursing management This condition greatly changes the life-style of a very active, athletic adolescent. The nurse needs to explore how the

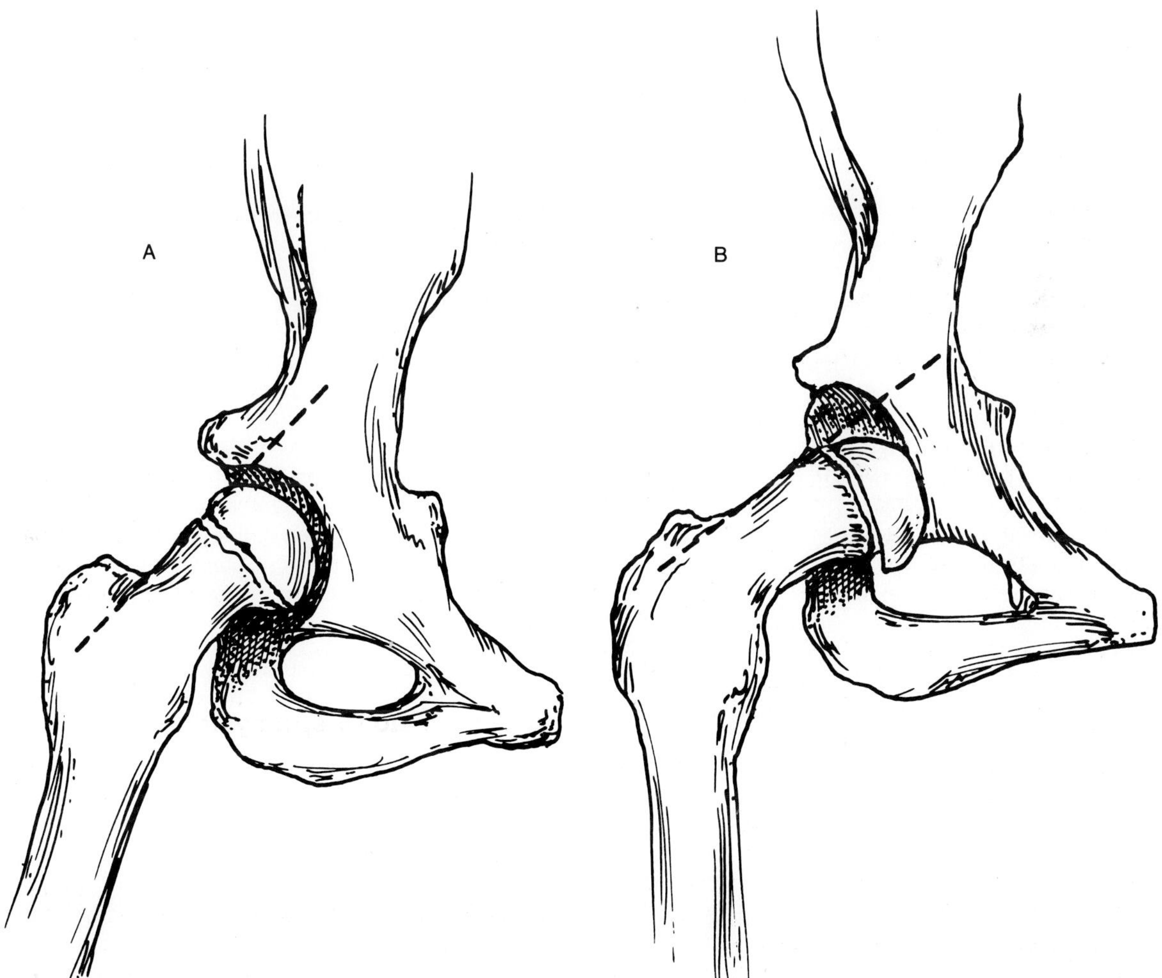

Figure 29-23 (*A*) A normal hip. (*B*) A medial slip of the head of the femur. (*From R. A. Hoekelman et al. [eds.], Principles of Pediatrics: Health Care of the Young, McGraw-Hill, New York, 1978. Used with permission.*)

child and the family are responding to this anticipated change. Some families and some adolescents place great emphasis on athletic achievements and may find this a difficult adjustment. The child and the family must understand the rationale for, and the importance of, limitations on activity.

If the adolescent is overweight, a consultation with a dietitian and a discussion of weight control are needed. Extra body weight places more stress on the epiphyseal plate.

During follow-up care, the other hip is observed for signs of slippage, since some children develop the condition bilaterally. The family and the child need to be aware of this possibility.

Kyphosis

Kyphosis, or humpback, is a condition in which there is an increased posterior protrusion, or rounding, of the spine. It may be congenital, secondary to a fusion between the anterior portion of the vertebral bodies.

Etiology Excessive kyphosis can be the result of poor posture. The most common form occurs in developing adolescents and is known as *Scheurmann disease, adolescent roundback,* or *juvenile epiphysitis.* Kyphosis occurs less commonly than scoliosis, and it affects males and females almost equally. Although the etiology is unknown, the deformity develops as the result of bony fragmentation and irregularity of vertebral end plates, which produces disk space narrowing and anterior wedging of the vertebral body. The most common location for this process is in the thoracic spine, but it may occur in the lumbar region.

Manifestation Occasionally, the child complains of mild backache, but often there are no symptoms. The child with Scheurmann disease has increased thoracokyphosis which is fixed and structural. A child with poor posture may have the same appearance as one with Scheurmann disease, but the deformity is supple and easily reversible.

Treatment Untreated Scheurmann disease can result in a significant kyphotic cosmetic deformity. The most common treatment is use of a brace, either a Milwaukee brace or a TSLO brace with external extension. The principle is to distract the spine through the use of pads, making the child extend the spine and stand tall. The brace is usually worn full time for 1 year and then at night for 1 year. An exercise program is incorporated as part of the treatment. Exercise does not prevent the progression of the disease, but it keeps the muscles firm and in tone. Surgical intervention may be required in some cases.

Scoliosis

Etiology and pathology Scoliosis is a lateral curvature of the spine and always involves some rotation of the vertebrae. There are two basic types: functional scoliosis and structural scoliosis.

Functional scoliosis Functional scoliosis is a curve that develops secondary to another abnormality, usually in the hip or lower extremity. A common form seen in children is a functional curve secondary to unequal leg length. Attention to the underlying problem will correct the spinal curvature.

Structural scoliosis Structural scoliosis is a curve that cannot be voluntarily corrected by the child. The curve is typically S-shaped and results from a defect in the boney-supporting structures of the spine. Some of the curvature of the spine is an attempt by the body to compensate for the change in posture that is resulting from the scoliosis. Figure 29-24 shows an x-ray depicting scoliosis. The curvature of the spine compresses the lungs and puts pressure on the heart, thus impairing respiratory and cardiac function. There are three classifications of structural scoliosis based on etiology and structural deformity: congenital scoliosis, neuromuscular scoliosis, and idiopathic scoliosis.

Congenital scoliosis Congenital scoliosis results from congenital malformations of the bony vertebral column. The vertebral bodies develop an anomaly, usually during the third to the fifth weeks of gestation. There is a 20 percent incidence of other congenital anomalies as well, including cardiac anomalies and urinary problems, that require workup. Children with congenital scoliosis may require bracing or surgery early in life to stabilize the spine and prevent progression of the curvature.

Neuromuscular scoliosis Neuromuscular scoliosis is caused by neuropathic and myopathic diseases such as cerebral palsy, muscu-

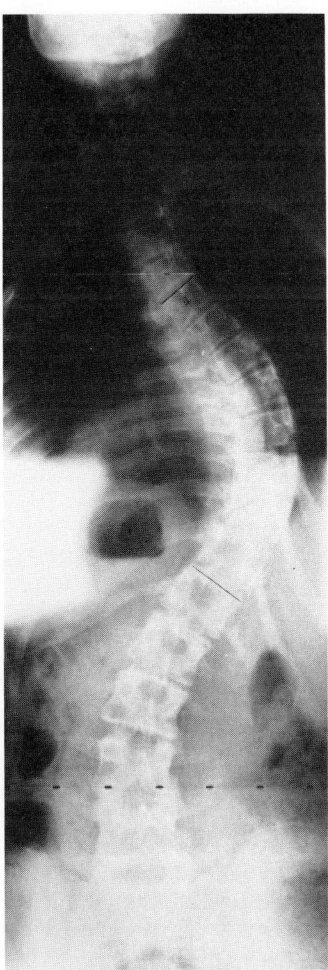

Figure 29-24 An x-ray showing the severe lateral curve of scoliosis.

lar dystrophy, poliomyelitis, and myelomeningocele. Although the etiology is unknown, it is assumed that the deformity results from paralysis of the paraspinal and trunk muscles or alteration of balance mechanisms. Muscle weakness collapses the spine and impairs respiratory and cardiac function. Bracing can be used to stabilize the curve and help the child gain trunk balance. Luque instrumentation of the spine (spinal fusion) has been used to stabilize progressive curves.

Idiopathic scoliosis Idiopathic scoliosis is the most common form of structural scoliosis and usually occurs between the ages of 10 and 13, at the time of the adolescent growth spurt. The etiology of idiopathic scoliosis, which can produce a severe deformity in a healthy child, is unknown. The sudden awareness of this deformity in an adolescent can be devastating to the entire family. About 85 percent of affected adolescents are girls. A family history is important, since there is a strong familial tendency in scoliosis. Siblings and other relatives are at high risk for developing scoliosis.

Idiopathic scoliosis tends to occur in otherwise healthy, active children, and the symptoms usually go undetected. Adolescents are shy and modest and are rarely seen unclothed by their parents. Improperly fitting clothes or a crooked hemline may sometimes prompt the parents to examine the child's body more closely. The curve may be detected during a routine physical examination at school or by the family physician. Early diagnosis of the curve, before it becomes severe, increases the chance that a nonoperative means of correction will be successful. All children aged 10 to 13 (grades 5 to 8) should be screened yearly for scoliosis. Both boys and girls should be examined, since recent research has shown that scoliosis occurs in both sexes, al-

Table 29-2 Examination of the Back as Done during Routine Scoliosis Screening

Position of the Student	Observations by the Examiner*
1. Stands erect, feet together and arms hanging straight down. (The examiner is seated, observing the student's back.)	1. Shoulder level unequal? 2. Hip level unequal? 3. Waistline uneven? 4. Spine curved? 5. One shoulder blade more prominent than the other? 6. Distances between the arms and body unequal?
2. Bends forward at the waist, back parallel with floor, feet together, knees unbent, arms hanging freely, and palms together. (The examiner is seated, observing the front and rear of the student.)	1. Difference in level between the two sides of the back? 2. Hump on one side of the upper back? 3. Compensating hump on other side of the lower back?
3. Stands erect and then bends forward (swayback). Assumes positions described above, with persisting side to the examiner. (The examiner is seated, observing the side view of the student.)	1. Thoracic gibbus (hump)? 2. Lumbar lordosis? 3. Thoracic gibbus on forward bending?

*If findings are positive, there is a possibility of scoliosis.

Source: Adapted from "Scoliosis Screening for Early Detection," Multi Video International, Minneapolis, Minn., 1975.

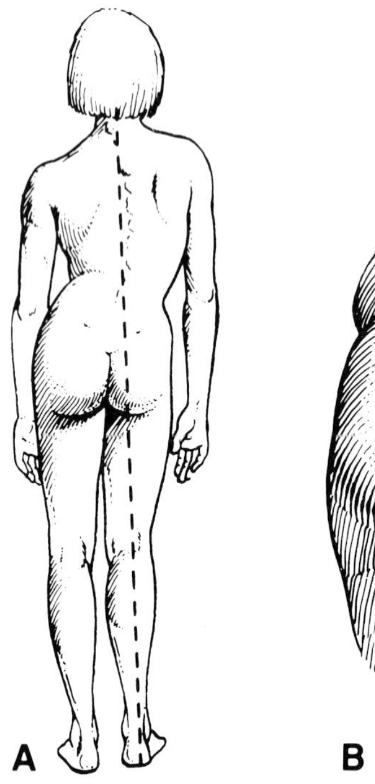

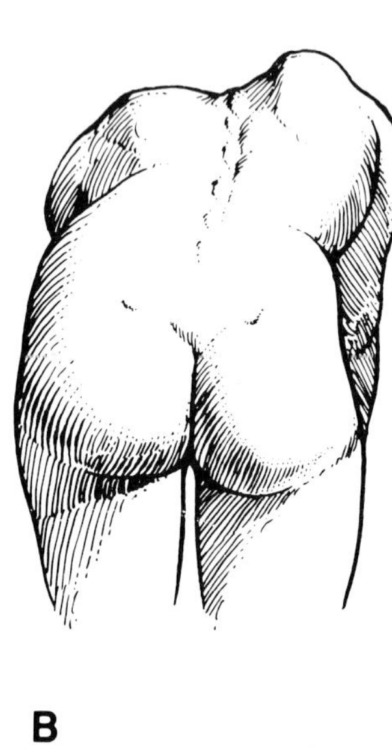

Figure 29-25 Spinal deformities. (*A*) Scoliosis—standing. Note the uneven shoulder heights, the protrusion of the left hip, and the unequal arm lengths. (*B*) Scoliosis—bending. Note the protrusion of the right shoulder blade. (*Modified from G. Scipien, M. U. Barnard, M. A. Chard, J. Howe, and P. J. Phillips* [eds.], *Comprehensive Pediatric Nursing, 3d ed., McGraw-Hill, New York, 1986, p. 1300. Used with permission.*)

though hormonal changes seem to accelerate scoliosis in girls at adolescence. It is appropriate to use a gym class to conduct this examination. Boys are asked to strip to the waist, and girls are examined in a bra and shorts or a bathing suit. Nurses or trained examiners do the screening. Eighteen states have adopted school screening programs for the detection of scoliosis. Table 29-2 lists guidelines for examination of the back in scoliosis screening. Figure 29-25 shows spinal deformities in scoliosis. In Delaware, the school screening program has been so successful that surgery has not been required for school-age children.

Treatment Children with positive findings are referred to a physician for diagnostic studies. Usually there is lateral curvature of the spine, which produces changes in the vertebrae and ribs as it becomes greater. The shoulders are not level, and a hump on the affected side of the back is present. With increased involvement, the lungs and heart become compressed; if severe kyphosis is also present, it may be difficult for the child to eat.

Usually an x-ray is done to determine the degree of curvature. Treatment is based on the measurement of the lateral curve on x-ray. A mild curve of 10 to 20 percent is followed with regular x-rays to observe for progression of the curve. A curve of 20 to 40 percent is treated either with a brace or with electrical stimulation (Fig. 29-26*A* and *B*). A curve above 40 percent requires surgical intervention. Many cases never progress to the point where treatment is required. The pattern of progression of a curve is unpredictable, but often an increase in curvature accompanies a growth spurt. Once growth is completed, minor curves usually do not progress. The child with a mild to moderate curve should always be alerted to the possibility of further curvature. Spinal curvature may increase during pregnancy and should be closely observed.

Nonoperative treatment Nonoperative treatment is based on the use of a Milwaukee brace, a Boston brace, or electrical stimulation in conjunction with an exercise program. The most common brace used is the Boston brace (Fig. 29-27). A much older brace, the Milwaukee brace (Fig. 29-28), is still used in some areas. The brace is usually worn 23 h a day and must be worn until growth is completed. The exercise program is tailored to the child and depends on the location of the curve. The program consists of pelvic tilts, shifting in the opposite direction

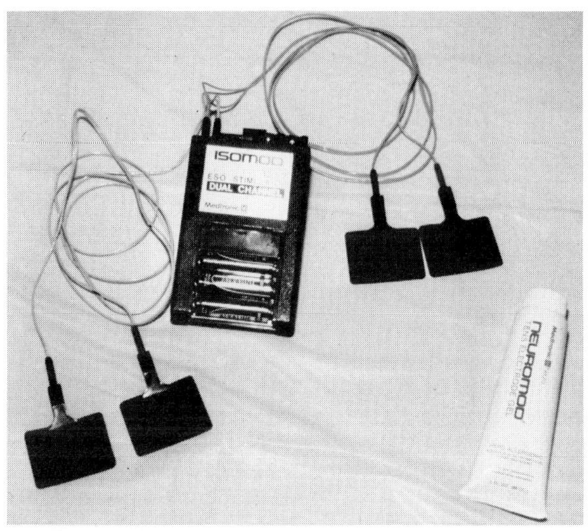

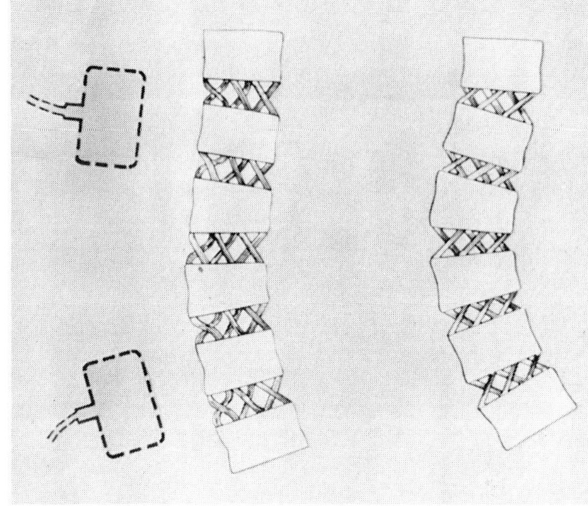

Figure 29-26 (*A*) The equipment used for electrical stimulation in the treatment of scoliosis. (*B*) The stimulation plates are in place next to the spine. Note how the vertebrae move in response to stimulation.

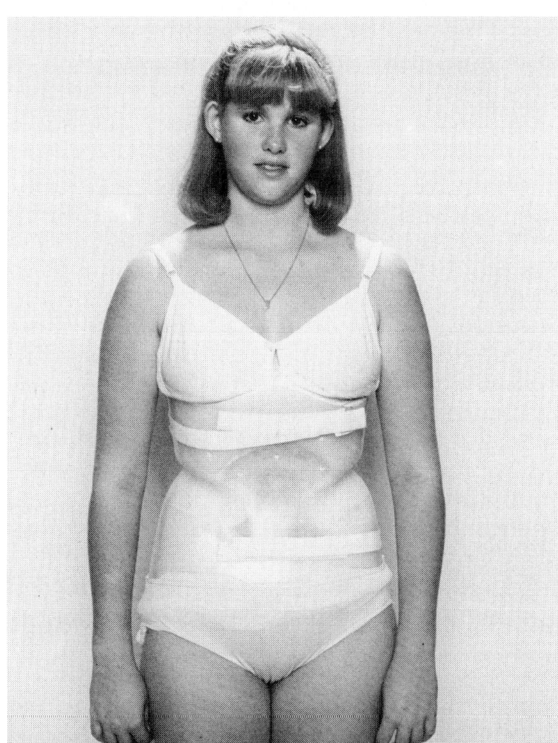

Figure 29-27 An adolescent with scoliosis wearing a Boston brace. Notice the Velcro closures, which make application and adjustment easier. The Boston brace is now widely used as a substitute for the more cumbersome Milwaukee brace.

of the curve, and abdominal strengthening exercises. If the curve progresses despite brace treatment, surgical intervention is required.

Management of the child in a brace includes giving skin care, maintaining the brace itself, and helping the child adjust to his or her appearance while wearing the brace, which im-

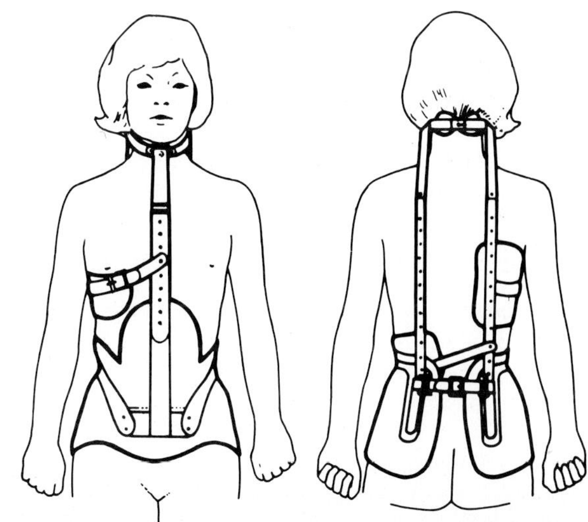

Figure 29-28 The Milwaukee brace has been used for scoliosis for many years and is still used in some areas. (*From Nancy E. Hilt and William E. Schmitt, Jr., Pediatric Orthopedic Nursing, Mosby, St. Louis, 1975. Used with permission.*)

proves compliance with the treatment regimen. The skin needs to be kept clean and checked each day for pressure sores. A cotton undergarment or a cotton body stocking may be used to prevent rubbing and absorb perspiration. It is important to maintain the prescribed exercise program in order to prevent muscle weakness and atrophy. The brace must be kept clean, and the screws and straps must be tightened as needed. A positive self-image is necessary for compliance. The parents should be encouraged to shop for clothing that is attractive and fits over the brace. The opportunity to talk to other adolescents who have undergone this treatment in a support group or on an individual basis is invaluable.

Electrical stimulation (ESO) is surface stimulation, performed under Food and Drug Administration controls. It is used in the management of early, progressive scoliosis under the same conditions in which a brace would be prescribed. The system consists of a stimulator, a pair of electric cables, and a pair of electrodes. The stimulator produces electrostimulation through the skin to the back muscle. The stimulation of the appropriate muscles can arrest or correct the curvature. The system is used for the same length of time as bracing, but only while the child is asleep.

Surgical treatment Surgical treatment involves straightening the spine. The most commonly performed procedure is the Harrington rod spinal fusion. In this procedure, a stainless steel rod is placed along the posterior spinal column and is anchored on the concave side of the curve. A less frequently used procedure is Luque wires (thin, cliplike, flexible wires), which are wrapped around the fusion site and a rod. Surgery is accompanied by spinal fusion involving correction of the twisting of the vertebrae by derotation of the posterior elements and the use of a bone graft. Small pieces of bone taken from the child's iliac crest are placed over the area of fusion. Postoperatively, as the bone heals, it fuses into a solid mass of bone.

An *anterior fusion* may be done several weeks prior to the posterior fusion in children with very severe scoliosis. A thoracotomy incision is made, and the anterior portions of the vertebrae are removed. Grafts from a rib or sometimes a portion of the fibula are used to stabilize the spinal column. If the child is young, usually under 10 years of age, the periosteum is stripped away from the fibula as the piece of bone is removed; the bone usually repairs itself if the periosteum is left intact. After the anterior incision has had time to heal, a posterior fusion is done.

Halo femoral traction may be used in the treatment of very severe curves for more gradual correction. Skeletal pins are inserted into the skull and are attached to a metal halo encircling the head and into the distal femurs. These pins are attached to traction, and the spine is gradually pulled into a straight position. After surgery, the halo apparatus may be incorporated into a cast. Often one of the other surgical procedures for posterior fusion, such as the Harrington rod spinal fusion, is used after the halo traction has been used for initial straightening.

Nursing management Adolescents with scoliosis face a frightening ordeal. Wearing a brace for a year or more is not easily accepted by an adolescent. Use of a brace does not guarantee that surgery will not be necessary. Caring for adolescents with scoliosis who have undergone spinal fusion procedures requires incorporation of all the principles of nursing care related to immobilization, traction, and orthopedic surgery. They are challenging patients.

Scoliosis occurs at a time when adolescents are trying to gain independence from adults, adopt peer codes and life-styles, and develop their own identity. A brace affects adolescents' developmental process by making them dependent on their parents and physicians for medical care. A brace does not conform to peer standards and causes a distortion of body image. The parents' guilt may prevent them from giving the needed emotional support. Nursing intervention is essential at this time to help the adolescent and the parents deal with their feelings, to promote an understanding of scoliosis and brace use, and to encourage the adolescent to accept responsibility for his or her body.

Skeletal traction apparatuses look painful and frightening. However, children seem to experience little pain from the skeletal pins. They may experience pain or muscle spasm as weights are applied to the traction or weights are increased.

Postoperative care Postoperative teaching should include specifics regarding the care that is recommended in the nurse's particular institution. This usually includes logrolling after surgery until the cast or brace is applied, or the child may be placed in a Stryker frame. Teaching must also include respiratory care, the use of a catheter or bedpan, insertion of a nasogastric tube, and administration of pain medication, as well as orientation to the intensive care unit if the child will be moved there.

Correction of scoliosis involves extensive surgery with significant blood loss, often requiring transfusion. Careful and frequent assessments of vital signs and neurological function are necessary. Spinal fusion always carries with it some risk of disruption of the blood supply to the spinal cord or spinal nerves, which can interfere with neurological function below that point. Postoperatively, the neurovascular status of both lower extremities should be regularly checked. Noting the child's ability to void is also of special importance in ensuring that neurological function of the bladder has not been impaired.

Prevention of atelectasis needs special attention for several reasons. If the child had a severe curve, this may have interfered with pulmonary function through lung compression. The child has had a long period of general anesthesia and will be on bed rest for 3 to 4 days. Intermittent positive-pressure treatments may be indicated for lung expansion, in addition to using an incentive spirometer or coughing and deep breathing.

Most children will have a nasogastric tube in place for a day or so following surgery, and there will be pain as a result of the large incision at the fusion site.

In the past, the only alternative after a fusion was a full body cast after the surgical incision had been allowed to heal for at least 10 days. A postoperative fusion brace (Fig. 29-29*A* and *B*) is now available for use after surgery and has revolutionized postoperative care. A plaster mold is made soon after surgery, and the brace is made while the child is still lying on the Stryker frame. Usually it takes 3 to 4 days for the brace to be completed. Before the child wears the brace, a body stocking is put on by the nurse to prevent unnecessary exposure; the brace is then secured in place, and ambulation begins immediately. The child usually goes home ambulatory and returns to school and resumes normal activity within 2 weeks. The fusion brace is worn for 5 to 6 months. Home care is greatly simplified because the child is able to shower. Once healing is completed, the brace is removed; the only activities that are per-

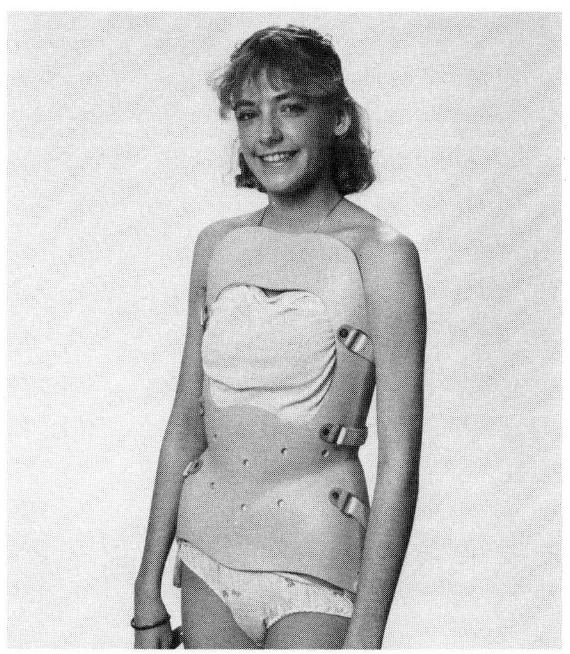

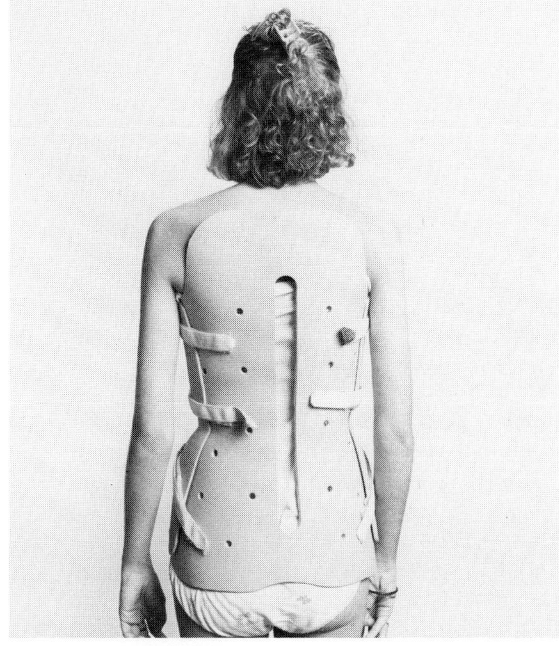

Figure 29-29 (*A*) Front view of a postfusion brace, which replaces the cast after fusion for scoliosis. (*B*) Back view of a postfusion brace.

manently restricted are high diving and doing gymnastics.

Ambulatory children need assistance with physical care as they recover from surgery and become adjusted to daily life in a brace. The Nursing Care Plan at the end of this chapter presents the details of postoperative care following the insertion of a Harrington rod.

Adolescents are always concerned about the effect of the treatment on their appearance. The correction of the curve will improve their general appearance, and this has a very positive effect on their acceptance of the treatment. They may have specific questions about scarring from surgery or at pin sites. They are always concerned about being accepted by their peers. Long-term contact with adolescents with scoliosis enables the nurse to get to know them well and makes nursing care an enjoyable and rewarding experience.

Nursing Care Plan: Surgery for Scoliosis Repair

Patient: Janet Myers *Age:* 16 years, 2 months *Date of Admission:* 4/27, 9:30 A.M.

ASSESSMENT

Janet Myers, a 16-year-old girl, was accompanied by her mother and father on admission for spinal fusion to straighten her back. She appears to be a healthy and well-nourished adolescent. Her weight is appropriate for her height. She appeared neatly dressed in jeans and a sweater.

HISTORY

Janet has had no prior hospitalization. She has no allergies. Her health has been good; the only previous illnesses that required treatment were respiratory illnesses. She has a history of recurrent middle ear infections, but the last episode was several years ago. Her regular physician has given her the usual childhood immunizations. He noted the beginning of scoliosis 2 years ago and referred her to an orthopedist, who has followed the case since then. She has been wearing a Milwaukee brace for almost 2 years, but during the past 6 months her scoliosis has worsened, despite the brace and exercises. She was admitted for fusion with insertion of Harrington rods. She was not wearing the brace upon admission.

PHYSICAL EXAMINATION

Height: 5 feet 4 in. Weight: 110 lb. Temperature: 36.7°C (98.0°F). Pulse: 80. Respirations: 24 breaths per minute. Blood pressure: 102/74.

Diet and elimination

Eats three meals a day plus a snack after school. Eats most foods. Describes her appetite as good. Likes pork chops and lasagna. Dislikes cauliflower. Liquid intake at home consists of milk, tea, fruit juice, and occasional soft drinks. Has had no problems with elimination.

Dental history

Is wearing braces. Sees dentist and orthodontist on a regular basis.

Reproductive history

Menarche occurred 6 months ago. Menstrual periods have been somewhat irregular. Last menstrual period was about 3 weeks ago. Experiences some cramps on first day of menstrual period. Some breast development is apparent, and she wears a bra.

Skin

Appears intact and healthy. Face breaks out occasionally. Skin over back is clear.

Musculoskeletal system

Limbs appear equal in size. Gait appears normal. Scoliosis is apparent. Left hip is higher than right. Shoulders appear of even height. Is able to move all body parts normally. Plays volleyball at school. Scoliosis has not interfered with normal activity. Has had no pain. Has normal response to touch and prick in extremities. Lower extremities appear pink and warm and evidence good capillary filling.

Daily patterns

Arises at 7 A.M., dresses, eats breakfast, and catches school bus at 7:40 A.M. Attends school from 8 A.M. until 2:30 P.M. Often visits with friends after school. Sometimes helps with dinner preparation. After dinner, does homework or watches TV. Usual bedtime is 10 P.M.

Hobbies and activities

Enjoys reading, painting, and listening to music. Art is her favorite subject at school.

Reaction to illness

Feels scoliosis is becoming noticeable. Is concerned about brace appearance and what clothing she will be able to wear over the brace. Expressed no explicit concerns about the surgery itself. Wonders how she will feed herself and care for herself in a brace. Parents had numerous specific questions about how surgery is performed and about preoperative and postoperative routines.

Nursing Diagnosis	Outcome Criteria	Nursing Intervention	Evaluation and Modification
1. Knowledge deficit related to surgical procedure and postoperative care.	☐ Patient will understand: **a.** Sequence of treatment and procedure **b.** Amount of discomfort with surgery	☐ Assess patient's and parents' level of understanding. ☐ Complete patient information sheet in 24 h; assign a primary nurse. ☐ Assess and identify: **a.** Patient's and parents' feelings and reactions to the surgical procedure **b.** Parents' knowledge of patient's condition **c.** Parent and child relationship **d.** Patient's and parents' coping mechanisms ☐ Include all family members and support structure.	☐ 4/27: Primary nurse was assigned. ☐ Parents express their fears about anesthesia, possible paralysis, and the pain their child will experience. ☐ Patient is concerned about the pain, her incision, and fear of anesthesia. ☐ Physician spoke with parents about their concerns and reviewed the surgery. ☐ Primary nurse reviewed preoperative routine, postoperative care, use of ICU, and Stryker frame and included all members of family, including support people.
2. Potential for ineffective breathing patterns related to postanesthesia state and postoperative immobility	☐ Patient will understand: **a.** Coughing and deep-breathing techniques **b.** Sequence of treatments ☐ Patient's lungs will remain clear to auscultation.	☐ Assess and document: **a.** Coughing and deep breathing preoperatively **b.** Coughing and deep breathing q2h postoperatively for 24 to 48 h and then q4h. **c.** Respiration rate, depth, and character	☐ 4/28: Coughing and deep breathing need encouragement; family is helping motivate patient to deep-breathe. ☐ 4/29: Lungs are clear; patient is less apprehensive.
3. Potential for hemorrhage related to surgical intervention	☐ Patient's blood pressure, temperature, and pulse will remain within normal limits. There will be no unusual amount of bloody drainage from the wound.	☐ Check vital signs and drainage q1h for 12 h. ☐ Check vital signs and drainage q2½ h. ☐ Check vital signs and drainage q4h thereafter.	☐ 4/28: Vital signs are stable. ☐ Small amount of bright-red bloody drainage was noted on dressing. ☐ 4/28–4/29: Vital signs are stable. No increase in drainage was noted.
4. Potential for impaired physical mobility related to surgical intervention and treatment restrictions	☐ Neurovascular status of the lower extremities and bladder function will remain normal following surgery.	☐ Check neurovascular status with each check of vital signs following surgery. ☐ Encourage patient to void following surgery. Measure urine output at each voiding. Check bladder for distention.	☐ 4/28: Neurovascular check q1h. Motion and sensation are intact. ☐ 4/28: Patient was unable to void; bladder was distended. In and out catheterization was done—600 ml. ☐ Six hours following catheterization, patient voided 500 ml with no further retention.
5. Potential for skin integrity impairment related to tissue trauma and application of brace	☐ Patient's skin will be intact, comfortable, and normal in color.	☐ Examine pressure points (heels, elbows, buttocks, etc.) for pressure. ☐ Turn patient as ordered. ☐ When brace is applied, check all edges for pressure on skin.	☐ 4/28: Heels were elevated off bed; area was reddened. Resolved within ½ h. ☐ 4/28: Patient was turned q2h; skin was monitored carefully. Ted stockings were removed for evaluation of skin.

Nursing Diagnosis	Outcome Criteria	Nursing Intervention	Evaluation and Modification
			☐ 5/1: Brace was applied. ☐ Skin was checked; reddened area was noted over buttocks. Orthotist was called, and adjustments were made. ☐ 5/5: Is ambulating well; no skin irritations.
6. Alteration in comfort: pain related to surgical intervention	☐ Patient will be comfortable.	☐ Administer pain medication promptly when required. ☐ Explain to parents the need for medication and support.	4/28: Administered pain medication. Requires pain medication q4h to q6h for first 24 h. ☐ Mother stayed with patient and helped to relieve anxiety. ☐ 4/30: Pain medication requirement is reduced. ☐ Parents and patient are less anxious and anticipating brace application.
7. Total self-care deficit related to activity restrictions	☐ Patient will accept temporary dependency but will gradually regain independence.	☐ Elicit patient's feelings about being confined to bed and being dependent. ☐ As she progresses, encourage self-care, such as washing hands and face, combing hair, and eating. ☐ Ambulate patient after bracing. ☐ Assist patient with walking when braced.	☐ 4/28: Accepts care of parents and nurses but attempts to help when possible. ☐ 4/30: Is brushing her teeth and attempts to feed herself liquids. Asked for her makeup. ☐ 5/1: Assisted with ambulation. ☐ 5/2: Was ambulatory with no assistance. ☐ 5/3: Is ambulating well and doing self-care. ☐ 5/3: Raised toilet seat was used to give total independence.
8. Diversional activity deficit related to immobility	☐ Patient will engage in stimulating activities once physically able.	☐ Explore activities and interests. ☐ Invite friends to visit. ☐ Encourage other adolescents on unit to visit with patient.	☐ 4/27: Was introduced to activities coordinator on adolescent unit. ☐ 5/1: Is using prism glasses to watch TV. ☐ 5/2: Is able to ambulate to activity area. ☐ 5/3: Painting was organized by activity director.
9. Anticipating anxiety about school related to prolonged absence from school	☐ Patient will keep up with schoolwork. ☐ Patient will maintain contact with peers.	☐ Classes started in hospital for credits. ☐ Encourage visits from peers. ☐ Encourage contact with other adolescent patients.	☐ 4/20: Parents have made arrangements for a teacher at home for 2 weeks. ☐ 4/27: Was introduced to hospital teacher. ☐ 4/30: Friends from school visited and brought posters and letters from friends.

Nursing Diagnosis	Outcome Criteria	Nursing Intervention	Evaluation and Modification
10. Potential disturbance of self-concept related to brace	☐ Patient will be comfortable with her appearance.	☐ Try to elicit patient's specific concerns about her appearance. ☐ Emphasize the positive effect upon appearance that the correction of scoliosis will have. ☐ Discuss clothing that patient can wear with the brace. ☐ Encourage patient to take an interest in her appearance.	☐ 4/27: Is concerned about appearance of the brace. Was introduced to patient wearing a postfusion brace. ☐ 5/3: Was visited by classmates. Their reactions helped her self-confidence. ☐ 5/3: Mother brought clothes. When patient saw herself in the mirror, she stated, "It's not as bad as I thought." ☐ 5/3: Applied makeup; is anxious to start showering.
11. Potential alteration in parenting related to unfamiliar treatments	☐ Parents will be comfortable with treatment regimen and with their child's progress. ☐ Parents will feel confident in their ability to care for their child.	☐ Involve parents in care as soon as possible. Discuss adaptations to be made at home for care. ☐ Give parents home care instructions prior to discharge so that they will be prepared for home care. ☐ Arrange for parents to call following discharge, if needed.	☐ 4/28: Parents were given home care instructions to review and were asked to bring questions at time of discharge. ☐ 4/28: Parents are assisting with care. ☐ 5/1: Mother has made arrangements for a raised toilet seat for home use, evaluated a bed for home use, and arranged with a neighbor to borrow station wagon for trip home. ☐ 5/5: Mother has taken 2 weeks off to help with transition. ☐ 5/5: Brace care was reviewed, including showering techniques. ☐ 5/6: On discharge, parents felt comfortable and confident and said they will call if any problems arise.

References

1. Hamilton, Helen (ed.), *Diagnostics,* Springhouse, Hicksville, N.Y., 1981, pp. 698–707.
2. Browse, Norman L., *The Physiology and Pathology of Bedrest,* Charles C Thomas, Springfield, Ill., 1965, p.64.
3. Lane, Patricia L., "New Synthetic Casts: What Nurses Need to Know," *Orthopedic Nursing* **1**:13–20 (November–December 1982).
4. Hilt, Nancy, and Shirley Cogburn, *Manual of Orthopedics,* Mosby, St. Louis, 1980, p. 486.
5. Turek, Samuel L., *Orthopedics: Principles and Their Application,* Lippincott, Philadelphia, 1984, p. 1219.
6. Hilt, Nancy, and E. William Schmitt, *Pediatric Orthopedic Nursing,* Mosby, St. Louis, 1975, p. 117.
7. Holland, Suzanne, "Up-to-Date Home Care of a Baby in a Hip Spica Cast," *Pediatric Nursing* **9**:114–115 (March–April 1983).
8. Jacobs, Robert, "Skateboard Accidents," *Pediatrics* **59**:939–942 (June 1977).
9. Ross, Paul, Edward Schwentker, and Hugh Bryan, "Mutilating Lawn Mower Injuries in Children," *Journal of the American Medical Association* **236**:480–481 (August 1976).
10. Eatron and Green, "Compartment Syndrome," *Orthopedic Clinics of North America* **3**(1):175 (March 1972).
11. Ibrahim, Kamal, "An Overview of Children's Fractures," *Pediatric Nursing* **10**:57–65 (January–February 1984).

12. Tolo, Vernon T., "External Skeletal Fixation in Children's Fractures," *Journal of Pediatric Orthopedics* **3**:435–442 (September 1983).
13. Farrell, Jane, "Orthopedic Pain," *American Journal of Nursing* **84**:466–487 (April 1984).
14. Tachdjian, Mihran O., *Pediatric Orthopedics*, Saunders, Philadelphia, 1972, p. 1545.
15. Gosling, Harry R., and Stephen L. Pillsbury, *Complications of Fracture Management,* Lippincott, Philadelphia, 1984, p. 338.
16. Katz, Jacob, and Yasoma Challenor, "Childhood Orthopedic Syndromes," in *Disorders of the Musculoskeletal System and Injuries,* Saunders, Philadelphia, 1974.
17. Ferguson, Albert, *Orthopedic Surgery in Infancy and Childhood*, Williams & Wilkins, Baltimore, 1981, p. 171.
18. Cassidy, James T., *Textbook of Pediatric Rheumatology,* Wiley, New York, 1982, p. 174.
19. Ferguson, op. cit., p. 347.
20. Ibid., p. 242.
21. Ibid., p. 226.

30

Susan Steiner Nash

Neurological function

Upon completion of this chapter, the student will be able to:

1 Describe the protective mechanisms of the brain.
2 Identify five neurological functions and the methods used to evaluate them in a nursing assessment.
3 Describe the nurse's responsibility before, during, and after neurological diagnostic tests.
4 List six signs and symptoms of increasing intracranial pressure.
5 Contrast two types of partial seizures and two types of generalized seizures.
6 Describe the nursing management of a child with a myelomeningocele.
7 Contrast communicating and noncommunicating hydrocephalus.
8 Describe three types of cerebral palsy.
9 Explain the nursing implications of dyslexia.
10 Describe the nursing management of a child with bacterial meningitis.
11 Describe the nursing management of an unconscious child.
12 Describe the differences between concussion and contusions.
13 Describe the signs of spinal shock.
14 Discuss the nursing management of a child with spinal cord injury.
15 Identity the signs and symptoms of lead poisoning.

EMBRYOLOGY OF THE NERVOUS SYSTEM

The foundation of the nervous system is established with the appearance of the *primitive streak* late in the second week of gestation. The primitive streak, formed from the ectoderm, establishes the longitudinal axis of the embryo. Cranial thickening of the primitive streak leads to development of a column of cells known as the *notochord*. The ectoderm overlying the notochord in the midbody region thickens and is known as the *neural plate*.

The neural plate thickens, widens, and develops a groove. Its sides pull inward and gradually fuse, forming the *neural tube*. The cephalic part of the neural tube begins to enlarge as the tube closes, and it expands to form the embryonic brain. The remaining and longest part of the neural tube becomes the spinal cord. The *lumen* (cavity) of the neural tube forms the central canal of the spinal cord and the *ventricles* (hollow chambers) of the brain. Genetic miscoding or exposure of the embryo to teratogenic agents (drugs, infection, or radiation) during the third to the fourth weeks may result in failure of the neural tube to close, leading to serious defects such as spina bifida and anencephaly.

During the fifth week of gestation, the brain begins to separate into three major sections: (1) the forebrain (cerebrum), (2) the midbrain, and (3) the hindbrain (cerebellum and brainstem). The hindbrain further develops to form the *pons* and *cerebellum* and later the *medulla oblongata*. Cavities develop within the three sections and later become the ventricular system. The vertebral arches develop from the mesoderm at the same time.

During the eighth to the twelfth weeks, the cerebellar hemispheres become evident. The growth of the head slows down as the body begins to catch up. The ventricles (which contain the choroid plexuses), the medulla, and the midbrain continue their development.

ANATOMY AND PHYSIOLOGY OF THE NERVOUS SYSTEM

The central nervous system

The *central nervous system* (CNS) has two major components: the brain and the spinal cord (Fig. 30-1). The brain is made up of the cerebrum, the cerebellum, and the brainstem.

The *cerebrum,* or cerebral cortex, is divided by a longitudinal fissure into the right and left hemispheres. Each hemisphere is further di-

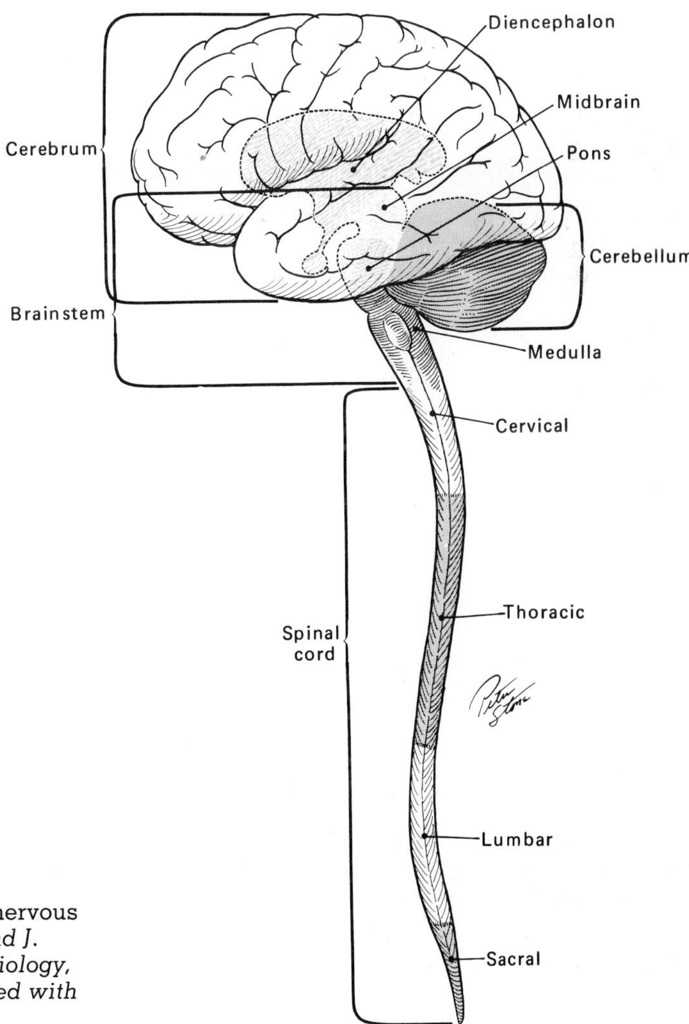

Figure 30-1 Lateral view of the central nervous system. *(From L. L. Langley, I. Telford, and J. Christensen, Dynamic Anatomy and Physiology, 5th ed., McGraw-Hill, New York, 1980. Used with permission.)*

vided (Fig. 30-2) into the frontal, parietal, temporal, and occipital lobes and the insula, which lies deep within the brain.

The *cerebellum* lies between the cerebrum and brainstem. Acting on information coming into it through the spinal cord and brainstem, it controls smooth and coordinated movements by refining signals from the cortex.

The *brainstem* lies between the cervical vertebrae and the cerebellum. It is made up of the medulla, pons, midbrain (mesencephalon), and diencephalon. The brainstem manages the basic life-support systems of the body. Within the brainstem is the *reticular formation*. It has con nections to the rest of the brain and controls the overall degree of CNS activity. Its main function, performed by the *reticular activating system* (RAS), is control of wakefulness, sleep, and attention.[1]

The cylindrical spinal cord is an elongated mass of nerve tissue descending from the foramen magnum two-thirds of the distance down the spinal column. CNS input and output move to and from the cord along nerve fibers that travel bundled together as *spinal nerves*. Thirty-one pairs of spinal nerves emerge from the spinal cord. Each spinal nerve consists of a dorsal (sensory, afferent) and a ventral (motor, efferent) root. Each root is composed of many nerve fibers. The spinal nerve is formed just outside the spinal cord by the dorsal and ventral roots. Spinal nerves are named according to the vertebral level at which they leave the spinal canal. Thus there are 8 pairs of cervical nerves, 12 pairs of thoracic nerves, 5 pairs of lumbar nerves, 5 pairs of sacral nerves, and 1 pair of coccygeal nerves.

The peripheral nervous system

The nerves connecting the CNS with the "periphery" are, for convenience, described as belonging to a *peripheral nervous system* (PNS). The periphery consists of everything outside the CNS, including sensory receptors, muscles, and glands. There are both afferent and efferent fibers within most of these nerves. Some of these fibers connect the CNS to glands, the heart, and smooth muscle. Fibers with these functions are considered part of the *autonomic nervous system* (ANS). The ANS is even further divided (Fig. 30-3). The nerve fibers that leave the spinal cord at the cervical, thoracic, and lumbar levels are

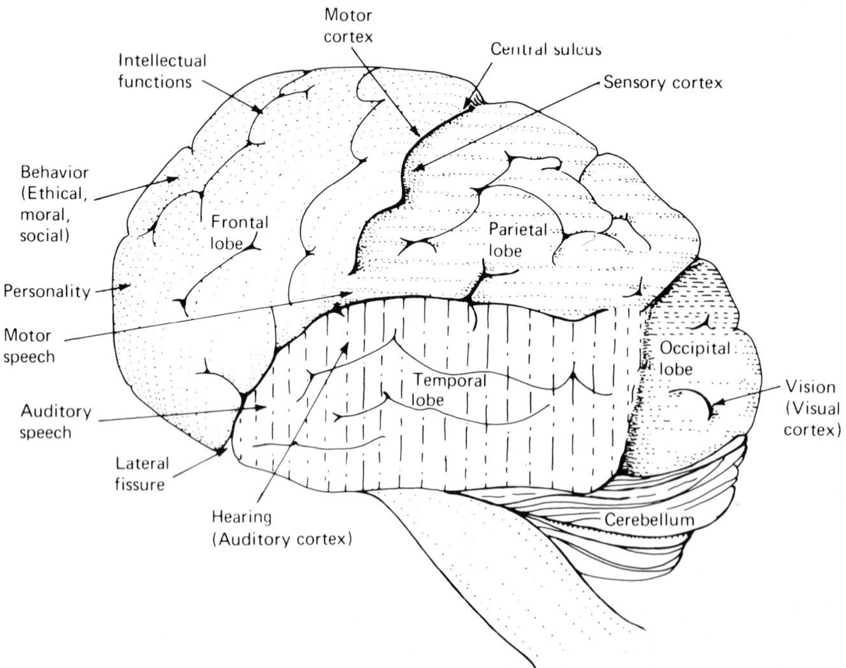

Figure 30-2 Lateral view of the cerebrum. (*From G. Scipien, M. U. Barnard, M. A. Chard, J. Howe, and P. J. Phillips* [eds.], *Comprehensive Pediatric Nursing, 3d ed., McGraw-Hill, New York, 1986, p. 759. Used with permission.*)

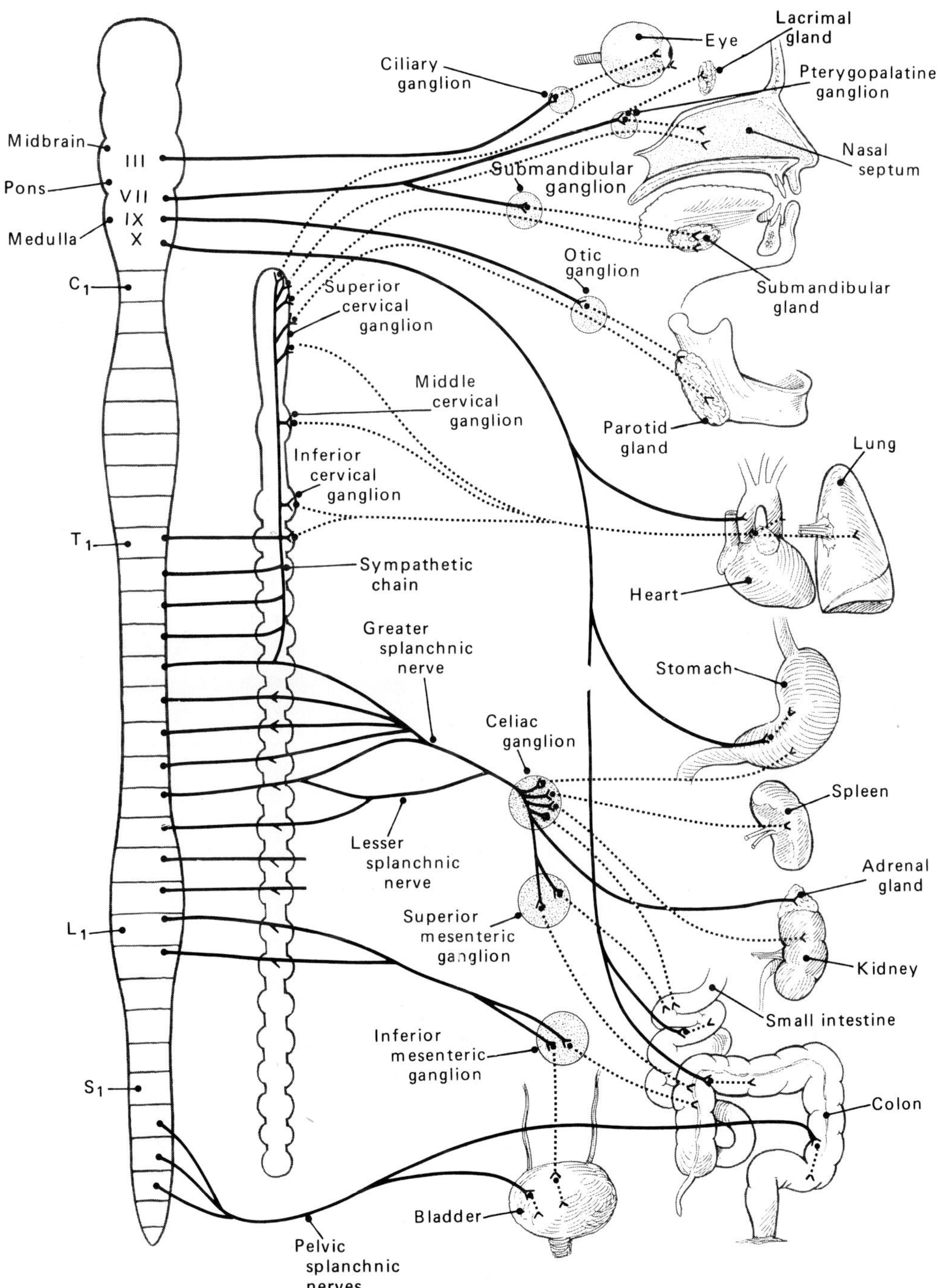

Figure 30-3 The autonomic nervous system, schematic view. The nerves emerging from the brainstem and from sacral levels are parasympathetic. The nerves emerging from T1 to L2 are sympathetic. (*From L. L. Langley, I. Telford, and J. Christensen, Dynamic Anatomy and Physiology, 5th ed., McGraw-Hill, New York, 1980. Used with permission.*)

sympathetic fibers. Those which leave the brainstem and the sacral level of the spinal cord are *parasympathetic* fibers. Although the ANS network is anatomically different from the rest of the PNS and although the ANS nerve fibers give rise to different effects, the various systems (the ANS, PNS, and CNS) work together, not in isolation. Table 30-1 summarizes the divisions and functions of the nervous system.

The neuron

The basic cell of the nervous system is the *neuron*. It is composed of a cell body and fibers. The fibers conducting impulses to the cell body are called *dendrites;* those carrying impulses away from the cell body are known as *axons*. Neurons are incapable of reproducing themselves and die if deprived of oxygen for as little as 4 or 5 min. Loss of the neuron is permanent if the cell body dies. Regeneration is possible for neurons outside the CNS if the damage is to an axon or dendrite. For example, in the case of a severed finger that is carefully sutured back together, regeneration of the axons is possible. This happens slowly—at the rate of 1 cm per month. Nerve fibers within the CNS do not regenerate. A severed portion of the spinal cord, for example, remains nonfunctional.

Neurons form circuits that integrate all functions of the nervous system. About 75 percent of neuron cell bodies are found in the cerebral cortex, the outermost layer of the cerebrum. There are other important clusters of cell bodies as well. Clusters of cell bodies are called *nuclei* when located in the CNS and *ganglia* when located in the PNS.

Table 30-1 Divisions of the Nervous System

- **I.** Central nervous system
  - **A.** Brain
    1. Cerebrum
       - a. Cerebral cortex—controls voluntary motor and sensory function. Center for behavior, emotions, and speech
       - b. Cerebral nuclei or basal ganglia—help control muscle tone and tremor; inhibit movement
    2. Cerebellum—coordination of all muscular activity, muscle tone, position sense (proprioception), and reflexes
    3. Brainstem
       - a. Diencephalon
         - (1) Thalamus—organizes sensory messages, emotions, and expression
         - (2) Hypothalamus—maintains homeostasis
       - b. Midbrain—relay station for motor and sensory fibers
       - c. Pons—relay station for motor and sensory fibers
       - d. Medulla—contains vital centers (cardiac, respiratory, and vasomotor)
  - **B.** Spinal cord
- **II.** Peripheral nervous system (includes cranial and spinal nerves)
  - **A.** Afferent system—carries information from sensory receptors (*to* the CNS)
  - **B.** Efferent system—carries impulses to muscles (*away from* the CNS)
    1. Somatic nervous system—supplies motor and sensory fibers to skin and skeletal muscles
    2. Autonomic nervous system—supplies smooth muscle, cardiac muscle, and glands in viscera. The fibers of these systems have opposing effects and work to maintain homeostasis.
       - a. Sympathetic—emergency mobilization of energy
       - b. Parasympathetic—stimulates visceral functions during relaxation

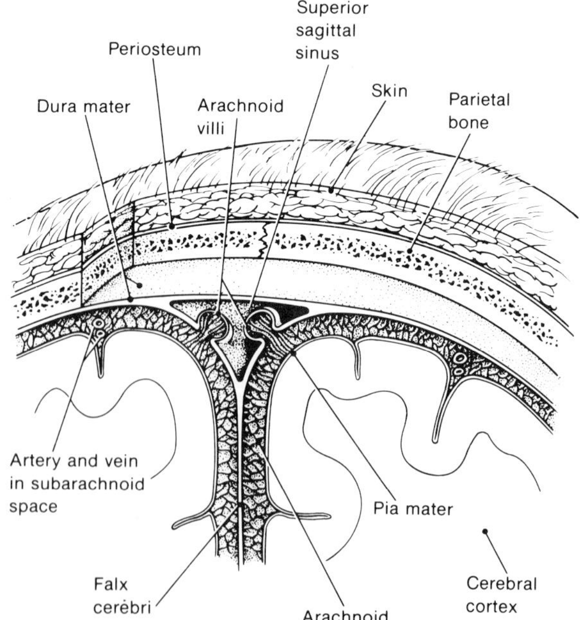

Figure 30-4 A section of the brain and skull showing the meninges and associated structures. (*From G. Scipien, M. U. Barnard, M. A. Chard, J. Howe, and P. J. Phillips [eds.], Comprehensive Pediatric Nursing, 3d ed., McGraw-Hill, New York, 1986, p. 802. Used with permission.*)

The meninges

The brain and spinal cord are encased in three connective tissue membranes—the *meninges* (Fig. 30-4). The inner layer next to the brain, the *pia mater,* is a delicate membrane filled with a network of tiny blood vessels that nourish neural tissue. The *arachnoid* is a thin, transparent layer that forms a cobweblike structure between the pia mater and the *dura mater,* the outermost layer. The dura mater has two extensions. The *falx cerebri* divides the right and left cerebral hemispheres, and the *tentorium cerebri* separates the cerebral hemispheres from the cerebellum.[2]

Cerebrospinal fluid

Cerebrospinal fluid (CSF) is a cushion of colorless fluid that fills the ventricles and surrounds the brain and spinal cord. It protects the brain from jarring movements of the head. CSF contains minute traces of white blood cells, protein, and glucose.

CSF is formed in clusters of blood vessels, the choroid plexus, of the ventricles. It flows from the lateral ventricles through the interventricular foramen (foramen of Monro) to the third ventricle through the cerebral aqueduct and into the fourth ventricle (Fig. 30-5). It passes from there

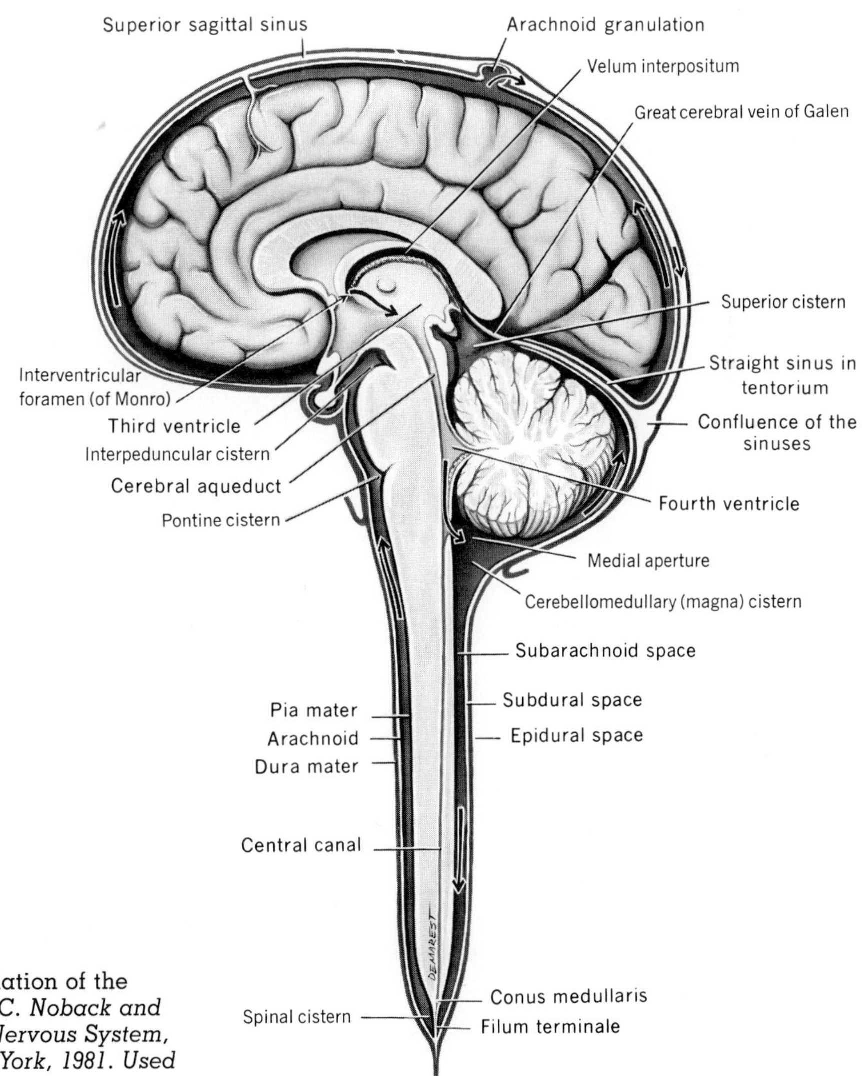

Figure 30-5 Normal circulation of the cerebrospinal fluid. (*From C. Noback and R. Demarest, The Human Nervous System, 3d ed., McGraw-Hill, New York, 1981. Used with permission.*)

Table 30-2 Neurological Diagnostic Tests

Test	Purpose	Procedure	Nursing Care (before Test)	Nursing Care (after Test)
Electroencephalogram	To examine brain waves and electrical activity to: Identify damaged or nonfunctioning areas Identify seizure disorders Follow progress of child after encephalitis, encephalopathy, or head injury	Multiple electrodes are placed on various areas of head with adhesive. Readings are taken sleeping, awake, and hyperventilating. May be done on outpatient basis.	Explain purpose to parents and child. Explain placements of electrodes and say that EEG is not painful. May shampoo hair to remove oils that would interfere with electrode readings. Do not give coffee, tea, caffeinated soda, or alcohol on the day of the examination (contain stimulants or depressants). Do not give medications unless specifically ordered. Sleep-deprive 8 to 10 h prior to study if ordered.	Wash electrode paste from hair. Allow child to rest. Provide means of resolving feelings, e.g., therapeutic play.
Skull series	To study bone configuration of skull to identify: Skull fractures Developmental disorders of bony growth, e.g., premature or postmature closing of fontanels Tumors or hemorrhage Presence of old fractures to rule out child battering	X-ray is taken of head. May be done on outpatient basis.	Explain to parents and child x-ray equipment, which may be frightening; explain that there is no pain and describe procedure. Remove glasses, hearing aids, dentures, barrettes, hairpins, etc., from mouth or head.	Allow child to express feelings created by procedure.
Pneumoencephalogram	To demonstrate shape, size, symmetry, and position of ventricular system and subarachnoid spaces to identify: Space-filling abnormality of brain and meninges (except hydrocephalus) Tumors or masses	Air is injected into subarachnoid space from lumbar or cisternal site. X-rays are taken of head. General anesthetic is given. Hospitalization is required.	Explain to parents and child the procedure, NPO for 6 to 8 h prior to study, preoperative and postoperative occurrences.	Keep child flat, at rest, and check neurological signs q$\frac{1}{2}$h four times and then q1h to q2h as appropriate. Observe and care for headache, vomiting, irritability, fever, meningeal irritation, intracranial pressure.

				Encourage fluids if not contraindicated to assist in repletion of CSF. Provide for means of resolving feelings when condition is satisfactory.
Brain scan	To identify brain tumors, some vascular lesions, and masses	Iodinated human serum (^{131}I HSA) or ^{203}Hg Neohydrin is given IV 2 h prior to scan. X-rays are taken of head. May be done on outpatient basis.	Explain to parents and child procedure and its purpose; explain that IV medication is given; describe x-ray equipment.	Rarely done. Allow child to express feelings, e.g., through therapeutic play.
Ventriculogram	To visualize ventricles of brain to identify: Hydrocephalus Masses, lesions	Air is injected into ventricles. X-rays are taken during and after. General anesthetic is given. Hospitalization is required.	Explain to parents and child reasons for NPO for 6 to 8 h prior to study, medication, preoperative and postoperative occurrences.	Keep child flat, at rest, and check neurological signs q½ h four times and then as appropriate. Severe headache likely for 12 to 48 h—provide comfort. Encourage fluids to replenish CSF. Observe for alteration in intracranial pressure. Provide for therapeutic play when condition is improved.
Myelogram	To visualize subarachnoid space of spinal cord to identify: Tumors, masses Interference in flow of CSF Fractures, dislocation, foreign bodies	Air or iodinized contrast medium is injected into subarachnoid space via lumbar or cisternal puncture. X-rays are taken. Iodinized medium is removed. Hospitalization is preferred.	Explain to parents and child procedure, purpose, reasons for NPO for 6 to 8 h prior to study, sedative prn.	Keep child flat, at rest. Observe for headache, alterations in intracranial pressure, temperature for 24 to 48 h. Provide comfort. Encourage taking fluids. Provide for therapeutic play to resolve feelings.

Table 30-2 Neurological Diagnostic Tests (*Continued*)

Test	Purpose	Procedure	Nursing Care (before Test)	Nursing Care (after Test)
Angiogram	To identify: Vascular anomalies, lesions Hemorrhage Tumors, masses	Radiopaque substance is injected into carotid, brachial, vertebral, or femoral artery or vein or a dural sinus. General anesthetic is given. Surgical exposure of vessel to be injected may be necessary. Hospitalization is required. X-rays are taken.	Explain to parents and child reasons for NPO for 6 to 8 h prior to procedure, sedative, preoperative and postoperative procedures.	Observe for complications of transient hemiplegia, seizures, petechiae, transient loss of vision, thrombus at injected site, hemorrhage or hematoma at injected site (emergency tracheostomy may be needed if jugular was used), alterations in intracranial pressure, and level of consciousness. Manage complications if they occur. Provide comfort. Help resolve feelings with therapeutic play.
Lumbar puncture	To identify: Intracranial pressure Culture, sensitivity, cell count, sugar, protein of CSF Hemorrhage in CNS To reduce intracranial pressure	Needle is inserted into lumbar area of subarachnoid space. Manometer is attached to determine pressure. Queckenstedt test is performed. CSF is collected in tubes which have to be numbered and labeled accurately. May be done on outpatient or inpatient basis.	Explain to parents and child procedure, purpose, need for sedation, and that some pain is encountered. During procedure: Position child on side with knees flexed on abdomen and head flexed on chest to open lumbar space. Hold child firmly. Provide constant verbal support. Observe child for tolerance of procedure. Label and number tubes of CSF in order of their collection.	Keep child flat, at rest. Observe and care for headache. Encourage taking fluids. Provide therapeutic play.

Subdural tap	To identify: Subdural effusions Subdural or ventricular hemorrhage Bacteria in subdural or ventricular spaces To obtain fluid for laboratory analysis To relieve intracranial pressure To instill medication	Needle is inserted into subdural space or ventricle through open anterior fontanel or during craniotomy. Hospitalization is usually required.	Explain to parents and child procedure and need to consent concerning shaving area on head. Shave the hair over open anterior fontanel. During procedure: Position child on back with head facing forward. Hold head securely. Observe child for tolerance of procedure. Label tubes in order they were collected. Tape tubes of fluid to the child's bedside unit and label tubes according to day and time of collection.	Keep child flat, at rest. Observe for alterations of intracranial pressure and leakage of fluid from tap site.
Ventricular tap (procedure is the same as for a subdural tap)				
Computerized transaxial tomography (CAT scan)	To identify by a combination of computer and x-ray techniques slight differences in density of tissue of intracranial structures: vascular anomalies, lesions, hemorrhage, tumors, masses, ventricular size	Patient is placed in supine position on special couch that moves into scanning unit. To facilitate study, area to be scanned is placed in soft latex material, eliminating air between head and diaphragm of machine and permitting x-ray beams to penetrate more effectively. Patient must remain motionless during procedure, which takes up to about an hour.	Explain to parents and child the procedure, its purpose, and that IV medication may be given. Describe the equipment. Keep the child NPO, if so ordered prior to the study. Explain the need for sedation, if the patient is an infant or young child.	Allow child to express feelings created by procedure. If contrast material was injected, observe for thrombi at injection site.

Table 30-2 Neurological Diagnostic Tests (*Continued*)

Test	Purpose	Procedure	Nursing Care (before Test)	Nursing Care (after Test)
		In some instances, the physician may choose to inject a contrast medium into a vein and repeat the scanning procedure to obtain additional information. May be done on outpatient basis.		
Intracranial pressure monitoring	To monitor increased intracranial pressure in cases of extremely high intracranial pressure	A burr hole is made behind hairline of forehead. After nicking the dura, a Richmond screw is placed 1 mm below the dura into the subarachnoid spaces. Screw is connected to tubing that is connected to a graph.	Explain to parents the need and procedure. Shave hair at hairline. During procedure: Position child on back with head facing forward. Hold head securely. Carefully monitor graph readout. Assess for leakage around site and connecting tubes.	Keep child flat, at rest. Observe for alterations of intracranial pressure and leakage of fluid from burr hole site.

Source: Adapted from G. M. Scipien, M. U. Barnard, M. A. Chard, J Howe, and P. J. Phillips (eds.), *Comprehensive Pediatric Nursing*, 3d ed., McGraw-Hill, New York, 1983, p. 770–773. Used with permission.

through the medial aperture (foramen of Magendie) out to the subarachnoid space of the brain and spinal cord. Aided by circulatory, respiratory, and postural changes, it flows to the top of the outer surface of the brain. There it is absorbed into the vascular system through one-way valves in the arachnoid villi.

The blood-brain barrier

The *blood-brain barrier* is a protective mechanism that controls both the *kinds* of substances entering the extracellular spaces of the brain and the *rate* of entrance. It regulates the electrolyte and nutrient composition of the neurons and protects the neurons from undesirable substances (some drugs) in the bloodstream. Oxygen, carbon dioxide, water, and lipid-soluble drugs enter the brain freely.

Under normal conditions 15 percent of total cardiac output flows to the brain. The brain consumes more oxygen than any other single organ of the body. Much of that oxygen is used for oxidation of glucose, the brain's chief source of energy. The brain first ceases to function when there is inadequate glucose, oxygen, and enzymes and then catabolizes itself, causing destruction of its substance.[3]

DIAGNOSTIC TESTS

Table 30-2 describes frequently used diagnostic tests and appropriate nursing interventions for alterations of the nervous system.

If the child is prepared for the sensations that will be experienced during diagnostic testing, his or her anxiety will be reduced. A tape recording of the sounds in the x-ray room may be helpful. If a lumbar puncture is needed, the nurse can describe the quiet of the room, the coolness of the antiseptic solution on the lower back, the little stick of the needle through which local anesthetic is injected, and the pressure the child will sense during needle insertion. All these will help prepare the child for the actual experience. However, preparation must be timed to avoid creating needless anxiety in the child.

After a procedure a child needs verbal praise and reassurance about the handling of pain. Further approval can be shown by awarding a sticker, which serves as a "badge of courage," gives recognition to the fear or pain that the child faced, and helps the child assimilate the experience.

NURSING ASSESSMENT OF NEUROLOGICAL FUNCTION

An important part of newborn assessment is estimation of gestational age. (See Chap. 8.) As an infant matures, developmental progress should be monitored closely. By 4 months the Denver Developmental Screening Test (described in Chap. 14) can be used to assess developmental progress. As the child becomes older, the neurological examination more closely resembles that given to an adult because myelinization of the nerves and fiber tracts is complete.

The physician uses the medical neurological exam to aid in differential diagnosis and locate the origin of the disease.[4] Nurses assist in the data collection process. In addition, nurses assist people with the basic needs and activities of daily living. Data related to the neurological dysfunction are assessed to determine the effect that any alteration may have on those activities and needs. The nurse monitors neurological status to aid in the detection of life-threatening illness. A modified neurological assessment is used to determine problems in self-care experienced by the child.

The nurse's assessment of neurological function can be structured around the integrated functions of eating, communication, thinking, moving, and elimination. Lyons has described five functions to be evaluated by the nurse: (1) consciousness, (2) mentation (including language), (3) motor function, (4) sensory function, and (5) bowel and bladder function.[5] Table 30-3 provides an outline for evaluating these functions and the parts of the nervous system that control them.

Assessment of the child's neurological status begins with data collection and a thorough history. This can be done on admission or during daily care. An interview provides the basis for evaluating thinking, memory, language, and the child's perception of his or her own abilities and condition.

In order to make reliable and relevant nursing assessments and to interpret the data gathered, the nurse must have a background knowledge in neuroanatomy and physiology. That knowledge must be combined with an understanding

Table 30-3 Neurological Dysfunctions and Nursing Assessment Methods

Functional Category	Origin in Nervous System	Methods of Evaluation
1. Consciousness		
	Reticular activating system	State of alertness (see later description of altered level of consciousness) Reaction to pain, noise, stimuli Vital signs
2. Mentation		
Thinking Feeling Memory Perceptual disorders	Cerebral hemispheres	Oriented to time, persons, place Recognition of family members Recognition of simple objects, color Recent and past memory (e.g., what was eaten for supper last night)
3. Language and Speech		
Dysarthria (defects in articulation, enunciation, and speech rhythm)	Brainstem, cerebellum Cranial nerves VII, IX, X, XII*	What is the child's cry like? Child must be old enough to talk. Have child repeat a phrase.
Dysphonia (abnormal sounds)		Look for a hoarse voice.
Aphasia (inability to use and understand written word)	Temporal and parietal lobes	Child must have learned to speak (2 to 3 years). Child must have learned to read (6 to 8 years). A child who has been in school 2 years should be able to send and receive written messages.
Agnosia (inability to recognize objects by means of touch, sight)	Parietal, temporal, occipital lobes	Have child close eyes. Place a familiar object in child's hand and ask child to identify it when eyes are shut.
4. Motor Function		
Expression	N. III	Look at symmetry of smile, frown, raising of eyebrows; blow out candle.
Eating, swallowing	N. V, IX, X, XII	Check ability to chew and swallow and presence of gag reflex.
Eye movements	N. III, IV, VI	Check extraocular movement (ability to follow examiner's finger). Check pupil size, reaction to light, accommodation. Is double vision present? Do eyes move rhythmically side to side or up and down (nystagmus)?
Movement (posture, balance, gait)	Cerebellum, spinal cord	Posture of newborn is flexion. Have child walk across room by putting one foot directly in front of the other. Balance—have child stand with eyes closed and feet together.
Muscle strength		Test hand grip, each side.
Muscle tone		Check flexion and extension of forearms, upper arms, legs, hips.
5. Sensory function		
Vision	N. II Occipital lobe	Check with Snellen eye chart.
Smell	N. I	Can child detect familiar odors (e.g., coffee and peppermint)?
Hearing	N. VIII	Whisper or use ticking of watch.
Taste	N. VII, IX	Check taste of sugar or salt on tongue.
Sensation: pain, temperature, touch, proprioception	Peripheral nerves plus brain N. V	Note paresthesias or abnormal sensations such as numbness, tingling, or burning. Check sensation on face, corneal reflex.
6. Elimination		
Bowel	Spinal nerves S3 to S5	Check for incontinence, fecal impaction.
Bladder	Autonomic nerves	Check for urinary incontinence.
	Spinal nerves T9 to L2, S2 to S4	Check for urinary incontinence due to flaccid or spastic bladder.

Source: Adapted from Marilyn Lyons, "Recognition of Neurological Dysfunction," *Nurse Practitioner* **4**(5)35–37 (September–October 1979).

*Names of cranial nerves:

I—Olfactory	IV—Trochlear	VII—Facial	X—Vagus
II—Optic	V—Trigeminal	VIII—Acoustic	XI—Spinal accessory
III—Oculomotor	VI—Abducens	IX—Glossopharyngeal	XII—Hypoglossal

of normal growth and development. For example, incontinence in a 6-year-old may indicate pathology. In a 6-month-old, incontinence is normal and indicative only of immaturity of the nervous system.

Assessment of consciousness

Disturbances of consciousness are caused by anything that interferes with the functioning of the cerebral cortex or reticular activating system. There are many classification systems for describing progressive changes in consciousness. One example is given below:

Level 1—consciousness The child is alert and responsive to stimuli.
Level 2—lethargy and drowsiness There is clouding of consciousness. The child's senses are dulled, and he or she may fall asleep even when the conditions are not conducive to sleeping. After arousal, the child will make appropriate verbal and motor responses to painful stimuli.
Level 3—delirium In this state the child experiences disorientation, fear, irritability, and sensory distortions. Agitation, loud talking or crying, and suspiciousness may be present. The child may be incontinent.
Level 4—stupor The child may be restless, but purposeful physical and mental activities are minimal. The child barely responds to verbal stimuli and reacts to strong stimuli by reflex withdrawal, grimacing, or unintelligible sounds. Spontaneous movements are common. The child may be incontinent.
Level 5—coma or semicoma In light coma, the child may respond semipurposefully to painful stimuli. Reflex reactions may be present, but the plantar reflexes maintain an upward flare. The child is usually incontinent.
Deep coma This is a profound state of insensibility. The child does not respond to painful stimuli. The child's muscles are flaccid, and he or she is incontinent.

A more precise scale, known as the *Glasgow coma scale,* has been developed to measure level of consciousness when impairment is suspected. This scale has been proved to be an accurate and reliable tool that allows standardization of observations (Table 30-4 and Fig. 30-6).[6] Because one-third of the scale is based on verbal responses, however, its use is limited to children who can talk.

Whenever disturbances of consciousness are present in children, other, related disturbances are also present and must be monitored by the nurse.

Breathing patterns Children who are comatose may experience one of the abnormal respiratory patterns described below.[7]

1. *Cheyne-Stokes respirations* Rapid, deep breathing alternating with slow, shallow breathing or apnea
2. *Central neurogenic hyperventilation* Sustained, regular, rapid, deep breathing
3. *Apneustic breathing* Breathing in which prolonged inspiratory phases alternate with expiratory pauses, causing irregular rhythm

Other breathing patterns are characterized by apnea, irregular rhythm and depth of breathing, hiccups, and yawning.

The eyes The pathways of the sympathetic system that control pupil size lie alongside those areas controlling consciousness. Pupil size and reactivity are closely related to level of consciousness. The nurse must observe the equality, size, and reactivity to light of each pupil.

To assess the corneal light reflex, ask the child to look straight ahead. Bring a penlight in from the side of the face. Note the response of the pupil into which the light is shone (the direct response) and the response of the opposite pupil (the indirect response). Dilatation of the pupil is a result of sympathetic nerve activity; constriction is a parasympathetic response.

Assessment of mentation

An initial assessment of the child's mentation includes level of awareness, general behavior and appearance, and facial expression. Are they appropriate for the child's age and condition? To assess language and memory and thinking process, the nurse must know what is normal behavior within each child's age range.

Assessment of motor response

Purposeful motor function is assessed by observing the child during eating, feeding, ambulating, and playing. Is the child's spontaneous behavior restless, agitated, or calm? Are strength, muscle

Table 30-4 Glasgow Coma Scale

Category of Response	Appropriate Stimulus	Response	Score
Eyes open	Approach to the bedside	*Spontaneously*	4
	Verbal command	*To speech*. Eyes open to name or to command.	3
	Pain (pressure on the proximal nail bed)*	*To pain*. Does not open eyes to previous stimuli, but does to pain.	2
		None. Does not open eyes to any stimulus.	1
Best verbal response	Score best response child makes with maximum arousal. Painful stimulus may be needed.	*Oriented*. Converses; knows who he or she is; where he or she is; year and month.	5
		Confused. Converses but is disoriented in one or more spheres.	4
		Inappropriate words. Without sustained conversation; words disorganized or inappropriate (e.g., cursing).	3
		Incomprehensible. Makes sounds (e.g., moaning), but no recognizable words.	2
		None. No sound even with painful stimuli.	1
Best motor response	Verbal command (e.g., "Raise your arm; hold up two fingers.")	*Obeys command*.	6
	Pain (pressure on proximal nail bed)	*Localizes pain*. Does not obey, but "finds" offending stimulus and attempts to remove it.	5
		Flexion withdrawal.† Flexes arm in response to pain, without abnormal flexion posture.	4
		Abnormal flexion. Flexes arm at elbow and pronates, making a fist.	3
		Abnormal extension. Extends arm at elbow; usually adducts and internally rotates arm at shoulder.	2
		None	1

*Produces the least interrater variability.

†Added to the original scale by many centers.

mass, and coordination similar in each side of the body?

Specific changes in motor function help pinpoint the origin of any disease process. Localized lesions usually do not affect consciousness but may cause motor or sensory changes. A serious injury or insult to the cerebrum results in the child's being without a cerebrum. This is known as a *decerebrate* state and is evidenced by extension posturing. An injury which interferes with the signals sent from the cortex results in a *decorticate* state. This is characterized by flexion of the elbows and wrists and extension of the legs and feet.[8,9] A child in a coma will usually exhibit abnormal motor responses. Early reflexes that normally are gradually replaced by voluntary muscle activity are described in Chap. 8. Persistence of the Babinski sign, or its reappearance after age 2, indicates an abnormal response.

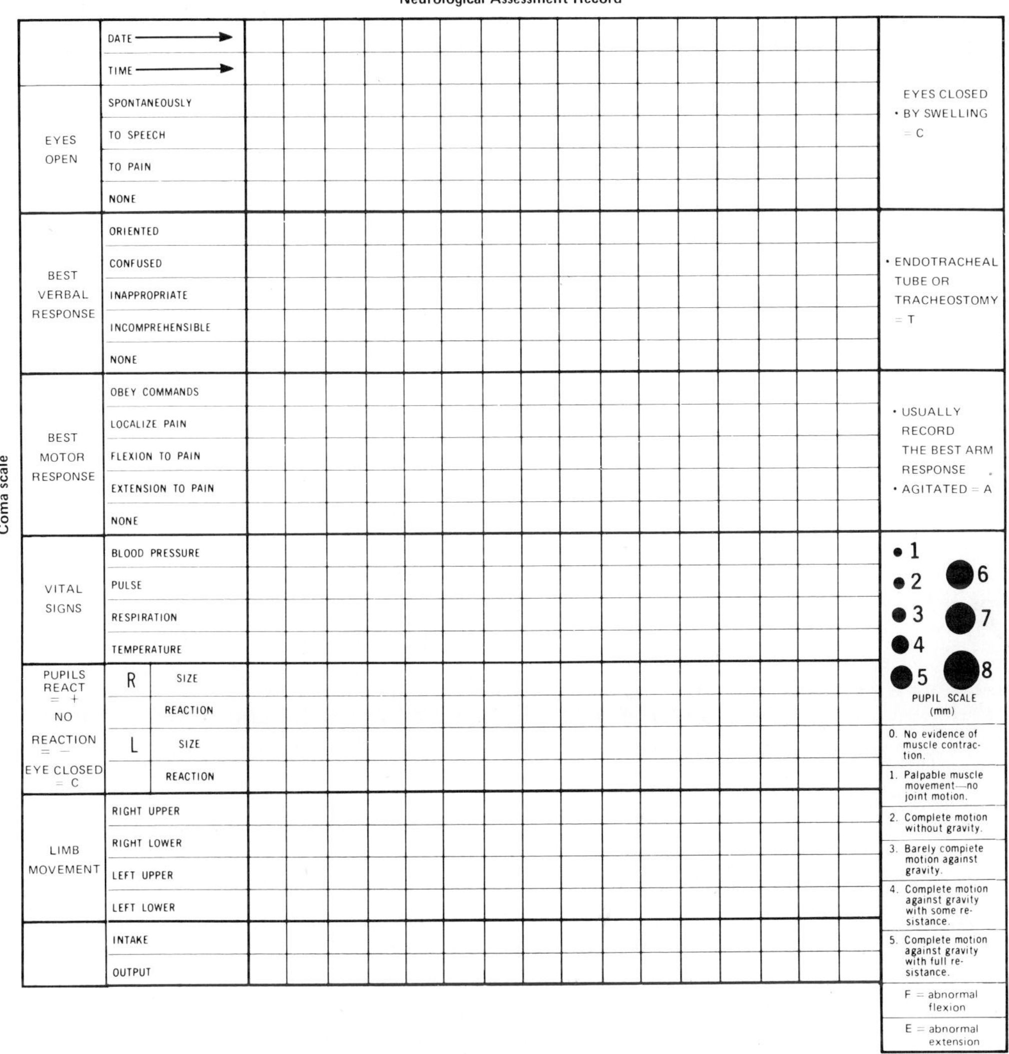

Neurological Assessment Record

	DATE →		
	TIME →		
Coma scale — EYES OPEN	SPONTANEOUSLY		EYES CLOSED • BY SWELLING = C
	TO SPEECH		
	TO PAIN		
	NONE		
Coma scale — BEST VERBAL RESPONSE	ORIENTED		• ENDOTRACHEAL TUBE OR TRACHEOSTOMY = T
	CONFUSED		
	INAPPROPRIATE		
	INCOMPREHENSIBLE		
	NONE		
Coma scale — BEST MOTOR RESPONSE	OBEY COMMANDS		• USUALLY RECORD THE BEST ARM RESPONSE • AGITATED = A
	LOCALIZE PAIN		
	FLEXION TO PAIN		
	EXTENSION TO PAIN		
	NONE		
VITAL SIGNS	BLOOD PRESSURE		PUPIL SCALE (mm): 1, 2, 3, 4, 5, 6, 7, 8
	PULSE		
	RESPIRATION		
	TEMPERATURE		
PUPILS REACT = + NO REACTION = − EYE CLOSED = C	R	SIZE	
		REACTION	
	L	SIZE	0. No evidence of muscle contraction.
		REACTION	1. Palpable muscle movement—no joint motion.
LIMB MOVEMENT	RIGHT UPPER		2. Complete motion without gravity.
	RIGHT LOWER		3. Barely complete motion against gravity.
	LEFT UPPER		4. Complete motion against gravity with some resistance.
	LEFT LOWER		5. Complete motion against gravity with full resistance.
	INTAKE		F = abnormal flexion
	OUTPUT		E = abnormal extension

Figure 30-6 A neurological assessment record employing the Glasgow coma scale (reduced from its original size). An operational definition of coma is a score of 7 or less (no eye opening, no comprehensible verbal response, and no motor response to command). *(From M. Kinney et al. [eds.], AACN's Clinical Reference for Critical Care Nursing, McGraw-Hill, New York, 1980.)*

Assessment of sensory function

The nursing history must carefully describe the sensory loss or abnormality in terms of location, duration, frequency, and aggravating or alleviating factors. With his or her eyes shut, the child can be asked questions like the following. "Tell me when you feel something by saying 'now.' " "Do you feel something hot or cold?" "Do you feel something sharp or dull?" "Is your finger moving up or down?" Other methods of checking cranial nerve sensation are described in Table 30-3. Disturbances of sensation may be evident in terms of pain, numbness, tingling, or loss of the sense of touch, pressure, or pain.

Assessment of elimination

Because a child's maturational level is so important in assessing neurological function, the significance of incontinence depends on the child's age. Any change in bowel or bladder control should be carefully described. Nursing management must focus on preventing incontinence and keeping the child clean and dry. Distention should be avoided, and impactions or infections prevented.

Nursing the neurological patient

Because children experience the world around them through the nervous system, any neurological dysfunction places them at risk. Nursing care must be planned and administered to protect children when they are helpless and vulnerable. Nursing care must also provide the human interaction and environmental support that will enable children to make the best possible adaptation to their illness.

Many children with an alteration in neurological function will need long-term care. They then become particularly dependent on the willingness and ability of others because they are helpless.

The safety of children is of paramount importance to the nurse. When children lose sensation in a body part, they may forget to protect that part. No warning system exists to remind them to move that part away from a dangerous object. Children who are in bed may not feel a small toy under the body. The nurse must check the bed, keep it smooth and clean, and schedule a routine inspection of all vulnerable areas.

Nursing care cannot be given haphazardly, without attention to planned outcomes and desired results. Scientific principles must be translated into intelligent nursing interventions that are consistently carried out to enhance the child's recovery and adjustment. The following sections of this chapter outline the nursing management of each alteration.

INCREASED INTRACRANIAL PRESSURE

Assessment

Diligent assessment of the signs of increasing intracranial pressure (ICP) is essential when caring for the pediatric neurological patient (Table 30-5). Bleeding, growing tumors, and a buildup of cerebrospinal fluid all can raise ICP. Compression of cerebral blood vessels may result in brain anoxia. The functioning of vital centers that control heart rate, respiration, and consciousness may be disrupted by brainstem compression.

Open suture lines accommodate increasing pressure by spreading apart in children less than 18 to 24 months of age. The head circumference increases, and the fontanels become tense and bulge. Head circumference and chest circumference normally enlarge at approximately the same rate during the first 2 years of life and are almost the same (a difference of 1 to 2 cm). Therefore, if increased ICP is suspected, both the head and the chest are initially measured. Head circumference is measured daily and is compared with baseline chest circumference to validate markedly accelerated growth rate of the head.[10] See Fig. 30-7.

Table 30-5 Signs and Symptoms of Increased Intracranial Pressure

Early Symptoms	Intermediate Symptoms	Late Symptoms
Irritability	Projectile vomiting	Decreased level of consciousness
Restlessness	Tense, bulging fontanel in child under 18 months of age	Decreased reflexes
Anorexia	Severe headache	Decreased rate of respirations or change in pattern
Headache	Sluggish, unequal response of pupils to light	Elevated temperature
Nausea	Papilledema (edema of optic disk)	Herniation of optic disk (creates blindness)
	Blurred vision	Dilated pupils
	Diplopia (double vision)	Sunset eyes
	Decrease in pulse and increase in systolic blood pressure	Decerebrate rigidity
	Seizures	Death

Source: Adapted from G. M. Scipien, M. U. Barnard, M. A. Chard, J. Howe, and P. J. Phillips (eds.), *Comprehensive Pediatric Nursing,* 3d ed., McGraw-Hill, New York, 1986, p. 777. Used with permission.

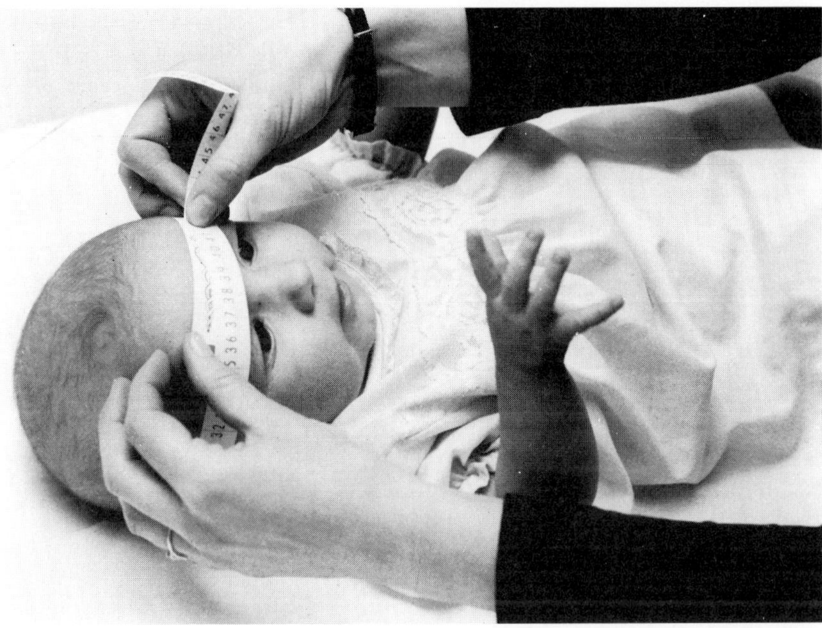

Figure 30-7 Measuring head circumference. (*From M. Alexander and M. Brown, Pediatric History-Taking and Physical Diagnosis for Nurses, McGraw-Hill, New York, 1979. Used with permission.*)

Increased ICP makes the infant irritable and lethargic. The infant's cry becomes high-pitched and weak. Early reflexes used to evaluate the neurological status of the neonate and infant are described in Chap. 8.

One place where increased pressure in or against the cerebrum will seek release is at the tentorial incisure after the cranium becomes rigid with the closing of the fontanels by 18 to 24 months of age.

The tentorium cerebri, an extension of the dura, acts as a floor for the occipital area of the cerebrum and as a roof for the cerebellum. Its inner free border fits around the midbrain, and the area within this ring is the *tentorial incisure*. A rise in intracranial pressure may cause tentorial herniation, with brain tissue forced over the edge of the incisure and down against the midbrain (Fig. 30-8). Lesions below the tentorium cause pressure on the cerebellar tonsils and compress the medulla.

Signs of tentorial herniation include dilatation of the pupil on the same (ipsilateral) side as the lesion due to pressure on the oculomotor nerve. Dilatation of the pupil and sluggish reaction to light may precede, accompany, or follow a decrease in consciousness. The child becomes restless, cannot remember names of people, and is hard to arouse. As the brain is increasingly shifted and as more pressure is applied to the brainstem, Cheyne-Stokes respirations develop and a positive Babinski reflex is present. The respiratory pattern changes to hyperventilation, inspiration length increases, and finally an irregular pattern leads to cessation of respirations. The pupils become dilated. The nurse *must* become familiar with the signs of tentorial herniation because it can rapidly bring about permanent brain damage and even death.

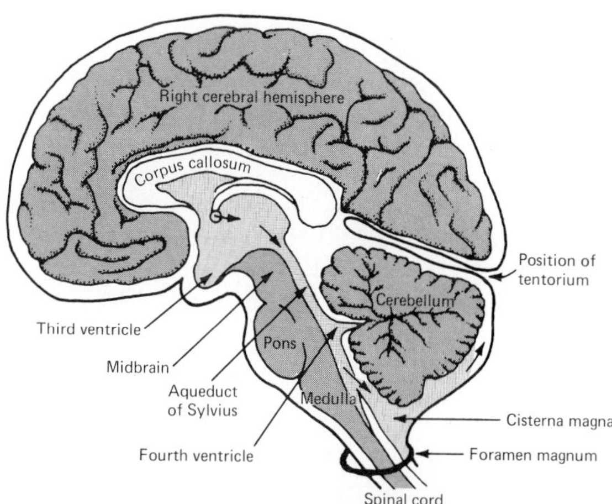

Figure 30-8 The brain and brainstem, sagittal section. (*From M. Kinney et al. [eds.], AACN's Clinical Reference for Critical Care Nursing, McGraw-Hill, New York, 1980. Used with permission.*)

The sole outlet of the cranium after closure of the fontanels is the foramen magnum, where the brainstem and spinal cord merge. Increased ICP creates a special hazard with a procedure such as lumbar puncture. A sudden release of pressure may cause the brainstem to be sucked down (herniate) through the foramen magnum, which would be lethal.

Rapidly increasing ICP is a medical emergency. Medical management includes fluid regulation, hypertonic drug therapy (Table 30-6), ICP monitoring, and surgical intervention.

Nursing management

Children who experience increasing ICP may also experience nausea and weakened suck responses and therefore may have difficulty eating. Extra encouragement to eat may be necessary. Intake and output must be carefully measured and recorded. A quiet environment is needed. Loud television should be prohibited. Bumping of the bed should be avoided. Every effort should be made to prevent undue stimulation that might cause seizures. A padded tongue blade should be available at the bedside, and padded siderails should be used in case of seizures.

Regular neurological assessment includes evaluation of (1) level of consciousness, (2) pupillary response and eye movement, (3) motor and sensory function, and (4) vital signs and patterns of respiration. All are assessed at 15-min to 2-h intervals.

A patent airway must be maintained. Suctioning is used for this as needed. Chest physiotherapy (see Chap. 16) is done regularly, at least every 2 h. Blood gases must be routinely monitored when artificial ventilation is necessary. Hyperventilation may be used to reduce cerebral blood flow and give the brain room to expand.

The head of the bed is elevated 20 to 30° to reduce cerebral edema and discomfort. The neck is kept straight to improve venous return. Straining when stooling elevates cerebral pressure and must be avoided.

Increased ICP can lead to loss of consciousness. If this happens, the principles of care are those which would be followed for any unconscious child, regardless of cause. The child requires meticulous nursing care with careful attention to observing, recording, and evaluating neurological signs and to maintaining a patent airway.

Unconscious children need careful skin care and bathing. Massaging and turning, every 1 to 2 h, prevent skin breakdown. Often a urinary catheter is left in place to protect the skin when there is incontinence and to allow accurate measurement of output. Range-of-motion exercises help maintain muscle tone and circulation.

Intravenous fluids (usually normal saline), tube feedings, or hyperalimentation are used to provide hydration and nutrition. Fluids are often restricted to prevent fluid overload in the brain.

Nurses must remember that the child's sense of hearing is often the last to be lost and the first to return. The nurse should speak to the child in a caring voice and encourage the parents to do the same. The child can be held gently and rocked.

The parents are extremely frightened and concerned when their child is unconscious. They feel guilt, fear, extreme anxiety, and even anger. They must be helped to express their feelings and given support. They are worried about their child's normalcy and future development. Remember that children often have amazing recoveries from trauma that causes unconsciousness. The nurse must help the parents not to give up hope too soon.

HEADACHES

Forty percent of children will have experienced a headache by the age of 7.[11] Causative factors include systemic illness or infection, neurological disease, tension, or migraine. Headache may also accompany increased ICP.

A detailed history of the headache pattern is necessary. The child and a parent should be asked to describe its onset, character, location, severity, frequency, and duration and any aggravating or alleviating factors. Accompanying symptoms of dizziness, nausea, vomiting, or pallor should be described.

Diagnostic tests will be used to look for the cause. Headaches due to increased ICP may be aggravated by lying down, coughing, or sneezing. The underlying cause must be treated quickly in these children.

Migraine headaches occur in 4 percent of all children.[12] Although children can be affected from age 3 to 17 years, they usually experience migraine headaches around age 12. There is often a family history of migraine. The child may experience a visual disturbance, or *aura,* before

Table 30-6 Commonly Used Hypertonic Drugs

Drug	Indications and Actions	Dosage	Nursing Actions	Side Effects
Mannitol	Used in emergency situations (not satisfactory for long-term use). Give as rapidly as possible—usually in 10 to 20 min.	Parenteral administration, 50 to 200 g qid (20% solution), flow rate adjusted to urine output.	Assess cardiovascular baseline. Maintain patent urinary catheter—careful assessment of urinary output, check mannitol for crystallization; 20% mannitol needs filter. Do not give directly with blood transfusion.	Congestive heart failure, rapid breathing, cough, hyponatremia, apprehension, twitching, convulsions
Urea (Urevert)	Used in emergency situations (not satisfactory for long-term use).	Parenteral administration, no more than 120 g per day, infuse slowly, 4 ml/h or 30% solution.	Maintain IV site and patent urinary catheter. Hazardous in patients with renal, hepatic, or cardiac failure.	Skin necrosis at IV site, hypokalemia, weakness, irritability, elevated blood ammonia levels
Glycerol	Slow-acting; useful in long-term treatment.	Oral administration or through nasogastric tube, 0.5 g per kilogram of body weight q3h to q4h.	Mix with iced lemon juice or other juice to make it taste better.	Hypernatremia, agitation, dry membranes, dehydration
Corticosteroids (Decadron and prednisone)	Useful in local and generalized cranial edema.	Oral or IV administration, 10 to 16 mg dexamethasone qd, 100 to 200 mg prednisone qd	Observe for signs of infection.	Decreased immune response

the headache. Some headaches will cause changes in electroencephalogram (EEG) patterns and even improve with anticonvulsant medications. Children who have occasional migraine headaches usually respond to Tylenol and bed rest.[13]

Occasionally tension headaches will cause real disruption in the child's life. Support, reassurance, and the use of methods designed to reduce stress have proved helpful. The child will need help in learning to cope with anxiety in a more healthful manner.

SEIZURE DISORDERS

Epilepsy, also called *convulsive disorder,* is a chronic condition in which there are recurring seizures. The seizures are characterized by sudden sensory, motor, and/or behavioral changes caused by abnormal electrical discharges in the brain. A seizure is a symptom that indicates an underlying disorder, just as a fever indicates an infection.[14] The area of electrical or chemical abnormality in the brain determines the nature of the seizure.

All humans are susceptible to seizures if the circumstances are right. Factors that can precipitate a seizure include:

1. A lowering of blood sugar quickly below 40 mg/ml
2. An abrupt decrease in blood pressure below a critical level
3. Insufficient oxygen to meet the body's needs
4. A rise in body temperature above 40.5°C (105°F).[15]

Individuals with chronic recurrent seizure disorder have a lowered seizure threshold and are more sensitive to minor changes in the brain's electrical activity. The risk of having a seizure at some time in one's life is 10 percent. The risk of developing epilepsy is approximately 1 percent or less. Approximately one-third of all convulsive disorders appear during the first 5 years of life, one-third during the elementary school years, and one-third during adolescence and young adulthood.[16]

A single seizure may be due to high fever, metabolic alterations, toxins, hemorrhage, drug withdrawal, tumors, or anoxia. Recurrent seizures, or epilepsy, may be genetic, idiopathic (the cause is unknown), or secondary (organic) to trauma or conditions that cause a single seizure. In approximately half the cases of epilepsy, the cause is unknown.[17] Confirmation of the diagnosis of epilepsy is made on the basis of a careful history of the onset of seizures, characteristic behaviors during seizures, and coincidental brain wave alterations indicated in the EEG. A computerized tomographic (CT) brain scan is also used in selected cases. See Table 30-2 for a review of diagnostic tests.

Seizures in newborns

Newborns are quite susceptible to seizure activity because of nervous system immaturity. Metabolic alterations such as hypocalcemia, hypoglycemia, anoxia, uremia, and infection can irritate the newborn's sensitive nervous system. Infants of diabetic mothers and drug-dependent mothers and other high-risk infants are particularly prone to seizures.

Nursing interventions include measurement of blood glucose and assessment of neurological status. It is essential to distinguish between seizure twitching and normal random movements or reflexes.

Febrile seizures

Because of a lowered seizure threshold, children between the ages of 6 months and 6 years (but especially those under 3 years of age) are susceptible to seizures when their temperature rises above 38.8°C (101.8°F). Temperature thresholds vary with each child, but dehydration, allergies, and a history of birth trauma seem to be contributing factors to febrile seizures.

Epilepsy occurs in 2 to 3 percent of children with febrile convulsions. Children who are at high risk for developing recurrent nonfebrile seizures include those who:

1. Experience their first seizure before 15 to 18 months of age
2. Demonstrate associated neurological abnormalities
3. Experience complex seizure patterns
4. Have family members with a positive history of seizures
5. Are normal but have had two febrile seizures[18,19,20]

Children with two or more risk factors have a 13 percent chance of developing epilepsy before the age of 7 years.

Management of epilepsy centers on the treatment of acute convulsions followed by treatment of the potential chronic state. Diazepam (0.2 mg per kilogram of body weight) may be given intravenously for immediate control of a seizure. The dose may be repeated every 15 min, if needed, up to four times. Sodium phenobarbital (10 mg per kilogram of body weight), given intravenously or intramuscularly, is another option.

Phenobarbital is used for prophylactic treatment of febrile seizures in children who have two or more of the risk factors listed above. Phenobarbital dosage is 3 to 5 mg per kilogram of body weight for at least $2\frac{1}{2}$ asymptomatic years. At the end of this time, the medication should be gradually discontinued over a period of 1 to 2 months.[21,22]

Initially, the nurse obtains a careful history. If the seizure occurred outside the hospital (as it usually does), the parents are asked to describe the events leading up to the seizure and the child's behavior during and after the seizure.

The key nursing responsibility is prevention of febrile seizures by carefully monitoring the child's temperature, administering acetaminophen or aspirin in appropriate dosages, and, if necessary, sponging with tepid water.

The parents should be taught to watch their child for signs of infection and dehydration, such as listlessness, fussiness, poor urine output, nausea, and vomiting. The child should be given antipyretic medications every 4 h for a minimum of 24 h after the onset of a fever (37.8°C [100°F]). The parents should be reminded not to put the child in a tub of cold water, since this can stimulate shivering and thus precipitate a seizure.

Epilepsy

Seizures have been classified according to their etiology, site of origin in the brain, and characteristics. The International Classification of Epileptic Seizures (idiopathic or organic chronic seizures) uses four major categories based on the location of excessive neuronal discharge in the brain as shown by the EEG:

1. Partial seizures—seizures beginning locally
   a. Simple symptoms (generally without impairment of consciousness)
      (1) Motor symptoms
      (2) Sensory symptoms
      (3) Autonomic symptoms
      (4) Compound forms
   b. Complex symptoms (generally with impairment of consciousness)
      (1) Impairment of consciousness only
      (2) Cognitive symptoms
      (3) Affective symptoms
      (4) Psychosensory symptoms
      (5) Psychomotor symptoms
   c. Partial seizures that become generalized
2. Generalized seizures—bilaterally symmetrical without local onset
   a. Absences (petit mal)—brief loss of consciousness with no change in muscle tone
   b. Bilateral myoclonic—sudden brief contractures of a muscle or group of muscles
   c. Infantile spasms—brief, symmetrical muscle contractions, usually associated with cerebral abnormalities
   d. Clonic—jerking spasms alternating with relaxation
   e. Tonic—sustained contraction of all body muscles
   f. Atonic—lack of muscle tone
   g. Akinetic—sudden momentary loss of muscle tone and posture control
3. Unilateral seizures—usually in children
4. Unclassified epileptic seizures—due to incomplete data[23]

Partial seizures *Partial seizures* begin locally and may or may not become generalized. There are two primary forms: Jacksonian seizures and psychomotor seizures. *Jacksonian seizures* are focal motor seizures that generally do not involve loss of consciousness. The characteristic "Jacksonian march" begins with localized motions of the thumb, hand, or foot and progresses in clonic, marchlike movements to involve the same side of the body. It may end in a generalized tonic-clonic seizure. This seizure is associated with organic brain lesions and is uncommon in children. *Psychomotor seizures,* or *temporal lobe seizures,* are present in about one-third of chronic seizure disorders and may occur at any age. *Temporal lobe* seizures involve the most complex patterns of behavior and high levels of cerebral motor and sensory function. Altered behavior includes chewing, changes in color perception, and arrest of activity with staring, picking at clothing, and wandering. Since some aspects of memory originate in the temporal lobe, the child may not remember the seizure. It may last several minutes or several hours. The child should not be restrained. A soft, calm voice should be used to reorient the child to the environment.

Generalized seizures *Generalized seizures* have diffuse effects on cerebral functions. Characteristically, the child does not experience an *aura*, a peculiar sensation or *warning* such as a strange taste or smell, or "butterflies" in the stomach.

Absences *Absences*, formally known as *petit mal seizures*, may go unrecognized because the only clue may be a teacher's complaint that the child does not pay attention in school. Petit mal epilepsy rarely occurs before the age of 2 or after the age of 14. This state of absence, or unawareness, can occur 50 to 200 times per day if the child is untreated and is most often seen in children between the ages of 6 and 14. The child may demonstrate staring spells, rapid eye blinking, small twitching movements, or daydreaming lasting 3 to 30 s. Following the seizure the child resumes the interrupted activity as if nothing had happened.

Myoclonic infantile spasms *Myoclonic infantile spasms* usually appear in the 4- to 8-month-old as brief spasms of the head or brief periods of opisthotonos. Initially these spasms last only a few seconds. Gradually the head-bobbings increase in frequency and power and may progress to a generalized seizure. Spasms occur 20 to 300 times a day, usually during periods of awakening or falling asleep. Ninety percent of children with myoclonic infantile spasms have some form of preexisting neurological abnormality.

Adrenocorticotropic hormone (ACTH) and corticosteroids have been shown to be approximately 87 percent effective in seizure control. Clonazepam, valproic acid, and a ketogenic diet have also been used with minimal success. The developmental outcome is not affected by treatment with ACTH. Children with this diagnosis have a poor developmental prognosis.[24]

Generalized tonic-clonic seizures *Generalized tonic-clonic seizures*, formally known as *grand mal seizures*, are the most dramatic form of epilepsy. The child experiences a sudden loss of consciousness and alternating tonic and clonic movements. The facial muscles begin jerking, and the jaws clamp shut. There may be frothing of saliva, dyspnea, and bowel and bladder incontinence. Respirations are irregular, pharyngeal secretions are increased, and tachypnea and hypertension are also present. Following the seizure the child enters a drowsy, calm period called the *postictal state*. During this period the child is not easily aroused or else may awaken in about 5 min and be confused. Often the child sleeps for several hours after the seizure.

Status epilepticus *Status epilepticus* is characterized by recurrent seizures, usually grand mal, with no interval or relatively short intervals between them. This condition constitutes a medical emergency, since successive tonic and clonic seizures lead to exhaustion, respiratory failure, and death. Vital functions must be supported, the seizures stopped, the cause determined, and further seizures prevented. Diazepam or intravenous phenytoin is used to stop the seizures. High doses, used to reach therapeutic blood levels quickly, produce cardiac and respiratory side effects. Meticulous monitoring of vital signs is essential.[25,26]

Treatment Medical treatment is aimed at determining the type and cause of the seizures the child has experienced. A complete medical examination includes a detailed history and neurological exam, electroencephalography, computerized axial tomography, and skull x-rays.

Epilepsy is managed most effectively with anticonvulsant therapy. Anticonvulsants raise the seizure threshold or prevent the spread of abnormal electric discharges through the brain. The selection of an anticonvulsant is influenced by:

1. The type of seizure experienced
2. The dosage required to achieve therapeutic blood levels
3. The number of side effects produced
4. The availability of an alternative drug in case the first drug fails[27]

A comparison of the most commonly prescribed anticonvulsants, indications for use, usual dosages, therapeutic serum levels, and side effects appears in Table 30-7. With proper use of drugs, 50 percent of people with epilepsy can have their seizures completely controlled, and another 30 percent can have them nearly controlled.

An anticonvulsant is absorbed through the gastrointestinal tract and metabolized in the liver. A steady state is achieved within the body when the amount of drug absorbed equals the amount excreted. Children usually metabolize drugs faster than adults do.[28]

Drug therapy is begun using one medication at a time until a therapeutic blood level is established. Another drug is added if seizure control is not achieved with one drug. Children and parents need to understand that a therapeutic drug program can take months to establish.

Follow-up examinations include complete blood counts, liver studies, and measurements of blood serum levels. Drug therapy must be

Table 30-7 Common Anticonvulsants

Drug	Indications	Usual Dosage	Therapeutic Serum Level	Side Effects or Adverse Reactions
Carbamazepine (Tegretol)	Complex partial: psychomotor, temporal lobe Generalized: grand mal	7 to 20 mg/kg per day in children	4 to 12 μg/ml	Nystagmus, slurred speech, drowsiness, dizziness, blurred or double vision, lethargy, decreased white blood cells and platelets, liver toxicity
Clonazepam (Clonopin)	Generalized: absences, akinetic, myoclonic	0.1 to 0.2 mg/kg per day maintenance in children	0.13 to 0.72 μg/ml	Lethargy, drowsiness, dizziness, nausea and vomiting, ataxia, behavior changes, hypersalivation
ACTH	Myoclonic infantile spasms	40 to 80 units per day IM for 28 days Gradually tapering doses for 28 days		Increased appetite, Cushingoid obesity, facial acne, muscle weakness, peripheral edema, increased blood pressure, increased irritability, increased susceptibility to infection
Phenytoin (Dilantin)	Generalized: grand mal	5 to 10 mg/kg per day in children	10 to 20 μg/ml	Ataxia, nystagmus, drowsiness, gum hyperplasia, rash, gastric distress, deformed teeth in children in predental ages, acne, increased hair growth. Dilantin suspension form may be difficult to measure in the small amounts necessary for infants. Careful parental teaching required
Phenobarbital (Mebaral or Luminal)	Generalized: grand mal, petit mal Partial: all forms	1 to 5 mg/kg per day in children	10 to 40 μg/ml	Drowsiness, ataxia, nystagmus, rash, hyperactivity, megaloblastic anemia
Primidone (Mysoline)	Generalized: grand mal Partial: psychomotor (temporal)	10 to 20 mg/kg per day in children	6 to 12 μg/ml	Drowsiness, nausea, ataxia, nystagmus, rash, anemia
Valproic acid (Depakene)	Partial simple and complex Absences Multiple seizures	10 mg/kg per day initially 40 mg/kg per day maximum	50 to 100 μg/ml	Anorexia, nausea and vomiting, diarrhea, drowsiness, temporary hair loss, hepatic toxicity, decreased platelets
Ethosuximide (Zarontin)	Generalized: absences, minor motor	20 to 30 mg/kg per day in children	40 to 100 μg/ml	Nausea and vomiting, abdominal pain, headache, drowsiness, dizziness, hiccups, blood dyscrasia

References: 37, 38, 39.

reevaluated during periods of rapid growth, during times of physical or emotional stress, and when the child has been seizure-free for 2 to 3 years.

When to terminate anticonvulsant therapy is controversial. Because of the potential for serious long-term side effects, anticonvulsants should be terminated as soon as feasible. Medication can be gradually reduced after about 2 years of seizure control.[29] If the seizures had an early onset, a relapse is more likely.

A ketogenic diet, biofeedback, and surgery are used to treat selected cases of epilepsy when drug therapy has been unsuccessful. The most successful treatment for epilepsy, however, is anticonvulsant therapy.

Seizure assessment The type of seizure is determined by the site of the abnormal electric discharges in the brain. The onset and progression of the seizure may help the physician determine the brain area involved. It is the nurse's responsibility to carefully describe the child's behavior prior to, during, and following the seizure.

Questions to be answered regarding the onset include:

What happened immediately before the seizure?
Was the child restless or calm before the seizure?
What was the child doing before the seizure?
What was the first sign of the seizure?

The nurse should always document the child's behavior during the seizure:

When did the seizure start? Was there jerking or twitching? Did it spread to other parts of the body?
What was the position of the child's body during the seizure? Did it change?
What were the child's breathing pattern and color during the seizure?
Were there pupil changes? (If a seizure is of focal origin, the eyes may point away from the irritating focus.)
In an older child, was there bladder or bowel incontinence during the seizure?
How long did the seizure last?

The nurse should make note of the child's behavior following the seizure:

Was the child sleepy or groggy?
Was the child's speech clear? If not, what changes in speech occurred?
Could the child move all the extremities?
Were the reflexes normal after the seizure?
Did the child complain of an unusual feeling in any body part?
Was the child fearful, irritable, or confused?

Nursing management Providing a safe environment for the child who has a seizure disorder is one of the most important nursing goals. The nurse must consider the child's age and developmental needs as well as the type and frequency of the seizures. A protective helmet may be appropriate for a child who has frequent seizures so that he or she can ambulate and play freely. The crib and the siderails should be padded, and only soft, safe toys should be allowed in bed. The child, the parents, and nurses must work together to identify cues that indicate that a seizure is imminent. A padded tongue blade should be available at the bedside and kept near the child when he or she leaves the room. It can be inserted only at the beginning of a seizure—*before* the jaws are clenched.

A seizure is dramatic and may be frightening to those around the child. When a generalized seizure occurs, certain precautions are essential for the safety of the child:

1. Keep calm. The seizure cannot be stopped once it has begun. Do not try to wake the child. The child is not in pain. The nurse's goal is to maintain a safe environment and carefully observe the seizure pattern. Note the *time* of onset. *Do not leave the child.*
2. Prevent the child from falling. If the child is standing or is sitting in a chair, gently ease the child to the floor. Loosen any constricting clothing around the neck.
3. Use a padded tongue blade to prevent laceration of the tongue and cheeks. It is inserted between the teeth if the jaws are *not* clenched. The nurse *should not force open* clenched jaws or *put his or her fingers into the mouth.* Forcing objects into the child's mouth can precipitate vomiting, and the fingers can be badly bitten.
4. Keep the child's head and body from striking hard or sharp objects. The crib and the siderails should be padded. A towel or blanket can be tucked under the child's head. Maintain the child's airway by hyperextending the neck and head. Do not physically restrain the child; restrictions of movement contribute to muscle strain and may cause dislocation or fracture.
5. Once the child is quiet, turn the child to a side position with the face pointed downward so that saliva or vomitus can drain out. This decreases the chance of aspiration. Carefully evaluate the need for pharyngeal suctioning.
6. Allow the child to rest, preferably in bed.
7. Be honest: "You had a seizure. I will stay with you awhile." Help the child become reoriented to the environment.
8. Document the pattern and length of the seizure and the child's response.

When the child is being regulated on a drug, the nurse is responsible for assessing its effect. The nurse looks for idiosyncratic side effects that are related not to the amount of the drug taken but rather to the body's response outside the central nervous system. The skin, gums, liver, and bone marrow may be involved.

Dose-related toxicity is usually manifested in the central nervous system. Signs of toxicity include drowsiness, ataxia (incoordination of voluntary muscle activity), diplopia, and mental dullness. The following tests are helpful in assessing drug toxicity:[30,31]

1. Test the eyes for *nystagmus* (rhythmic oscillation of the eyeballs) by asking the child to follow your finger as it is moved from one lateral extreme of the visual field to another. Nystagmus with diplopia suggests toxicity. Describe your observations.
2. Check *coordination* by asking the child to touch a finger to the nose and to walk by placing one foot directly in front of the other. Difficulty with balance when walking or an inability to maintain an upright position with the eyes closed and the feet together (Romberg's sign) may be evidence of ataxia and drug toxicity.

Compliance with the prescribed treatment plan is essential for successful management of seizures. Some people have difficulty remembering when to take their medication. Others experience side effects, such as drowsiness, which interfere with their life-style. Still others fear "drug addiction." Antiepileptic medications are not effective if they are not taken as directed. The nurse must assess the child's and the parents' understanding of how the drugs work and why they must be taken as prescribed. The nurse must also determine whether the family has established a workable, consistent schedule for administration of the medications and whether the child and the parents know what to do if the child forgets to take the drug according to schedule. Stress the importance of *never* stopping the medication without consulting the physician.

Individuals differ in their ability to absorb, distribute, metabolize, and excrete drugs. Seizure control is achieved with varying doses and types of anticonvulsants. Other medications that the child is taking may also affect the action of the anticonvulsants. The serum level of phenytoin, for example, can be decreased by phenobarbital, dexamethasone, digitoxin, and ethanol.[32] Oral contraceptive drug levels are lowered by such drugs as phenytoin, phenobarbital, primidone, and carbamazepine.[33] The nurse must be familiar with the other medications that the child is taking so that appropriate counseling and education can be made available.

Infants who receive daily ACTH for infantile spasms become cranky and irritable and very hungry. They may benefit from early introduction of solids and dilution of formula based on recommended dietary requirements. If acne develops, washing with warm water and baby soap is helpful. Infant stimulation programs and physical therapy should be implemented when delayed motor development exists. Blood pressure must be checked weekly, since hypertension occurs in 50 percent of children who receive ACTH.[34]

The nurse's role with the parents Epilepsy requires major adjustments on the part of the child and the family. It is a chronic condition. Some aspects of the disorder cannot be altered, no matter how much one understands or accepts. Some children will have seizures all their lives.

Unlike other chronic conditions, epilepsy is episodic. The onset is sudden, and there is little or no warning. Even if the child senses an aura, the seizure cannot be prevented. For this reason, high hurdles must be overcome in adjusting to epilepsy. A child who is well controlled on medications may still be fearful of having a seizure. This fear can be lessened if the child feels that proper care will be given during a seizure and that continued acceptance will follow after the seizure.[35]

The diagnosis of epilepsy is complicated by the fact that in a majority of cases the cause is unknown and the child will need to take anticonvulsant medications over a prolonged period. The parents respond in many ways to the diagnosis of epilepsy. An overwhelming sense of grief is very common. Denial, fear, and guilt are also common.

Epilepsy has historically been viewed with suspicion, fear, and overprotection. It is not surprising that parents experience a sense of grief and fear. Many misconceptions still exist regarding the impact of epilepsy on the child's intelligence and potential. The child's self-esteem is dramatically affected by rejection from the family or peers. Lowered self-esteem decreases the child's chances of making a healthy adjustment to the disorder.

The parents need help in understanding the nature of their child's seizure disorder and the medical treatment indicated. They are told the facts and are helped to develop realistic expectations for their child. The nurse who expects that the parents can care for the child and can cope with the situation will usually elicit this behavior in the parents. The nurse should identify the family's strengths and build on them.

The parents can help their child by being honest and open when discussing epilepsy. The child should be helped to anticipate problems and should know what to do if a seizure occurs. If the epilepsy is not totally controlled, the people around the child must know his or her seizure history, the medications that the child uses, and what to do during a seizure.

The nurse must stress to the parents that a major goal is to make sure that their child takes the proper amount of medication at the correct time. A written record of seizure activity and medication use is desirable. Compliance with the drug regimen is essential for the control of epilepsy. Parents and children must be familiar with the action of drugs and their side effects. Children with epilepsy need to learn to be responsible for the management of their disorder. Taking medications and making decisions about physical and other restrictions must gradually become the responsibility of the child, not the parents or the school personnel.

The parents can help their child by providing a structured, supportive home environment in which the child is assured of adequate rest and nutrition. The child will also benefit from regular physical exercise. There is no "safe" situation, and if the child is to learn, some risks must be taken. The most positive effect of exercise for the child with epilepsy may be that it teaches the child that he or she is less likely to have a seizure while exercising. People with epilepsy should avoid dangerous sports, since even a minor seizure could result in disaster. Swimming is safe if the seizures are controlled by medications and a qualified adult is supervising. Exercise fosters a sense of well-being by affirming that the child is capable of performing and competing.[36]

It is important for the parents to divide their attention and concern equally among all the children in the family. Giving special attention to the child with epilepsy and assigning the child fewer responsibilities than siblings must be avoided. The child should be encouraged to develop as normally as possible and discouraged from using epilepsy as an excuse or a "crutch" to avoid responsibility.

The nurse should encourage the parents to get in touch with other parents of children with a similar seizure disorder. An older child will benefit from contact with another child who is coping well with a similar problem. Local and state epilepsy organizations sponsor support groups, provide information, and offer classes in the medical, psychosocial, and vocational aspects of living with epilepsy.

The nurses may be called on to educate children and teachers in school so that they will be better able to support and accept their classmate with epilepsy. The nurse may also act as a patient-advocate in the community and in employment settings. State and national epilepsy programs can provide information about affirmative action rights in the workplace, social security benefits, driver's licenses, and workers' compensation. See Chap. 34 for a further discussion of chronic illness and related issues.

BRAIN DEATH

Brain death is irreversible brain damage resulting in a coma and requiring artificial support of pulmonary and cardiac function. The child lacks spontaneous movement and does not respond to any visual, auditory, or cutaneous stimulation. The diagnosis is made on the basis of (1) absence of cerebral functions; (2) absence of brainstem functions, including spontaneous respirations; and (3) irreversibility of the state. Two consecutive 30-min EEG recordings done 6 h apart confirm the diagnosis. It should be understood, however, that the clinical and EEG criteria for brain death in infants and young children are not well established. A flat or silent EEG in the absence of profound hypothermia or drug intoxication is a valuable indicator of cerebral death. Nursing care focuses on data collection and providing emotional support for the family, while maintaining life-support systems.

CONGENITAL ALTERATIONS OF THE CENTRAL NERVOUS SYSTEM

Faulty closure of the neural tube or bony protection of the central nervous system leads to mild defects, such as spina bifida occulta, or to severe defects that are incompatible with life, such as anencephaly. Table 30-8 describes types of neural tube malformations. These defects make up a significant proportion of all congenital anomalies and affect 3 to 4 infants among every 1000 born.[40]

Table 30-8 Neural Tube Malformations

Cranium bifidum or encephalocele:	Defect in closure of bones of skull.
Occult cranium bifidum	Bony defect of skull only.
Simple cranial meningocele	Meninges and cerebrospinal fluid protrude through skull defect.
Encephalomeningocele	Brain tissues, meninges, and CSF protrude through skull defect.
Anencephaly	Absence of skull, brain, and other vital tissues.
Spina bifida:	Defect in closure of vertebral column.
Spina bifida occulta	Bony defect of vertebrae only; no external sac.
Meningocele	Meninges and CSF protrude through defect (normal spinal cord usually).
Myelomeningocele	Meninges, CSF, and abnormal spinal cord protrude through defect.
Rachischisis	Incomplete closure of vertebrae, meninges, and spinal cord. Not repairable. Death usually results from infection.

Source: Adapted from Sherrilyn Passo, "Malformations of the Neural Tube," in Diane McElroy and Gayle Davis (eds.), *Nursing Clinics of North America* **15**(1):6 (March 1980).

When a child is born with a neural tube defect, the risk of recurrence increases in relation to the family history. With a negative family history the risk of having another child with a neural tube defect is 1 in 20, or 5 percent. With a positive family history the risk increases to 1 in 10, or 10 percent. An affected adult or a sibling of an affected person is also at greater risk for producing a child with a neural tube defect than the general population.[41]

Open neural tube defects (anencephaly, meningocele, and myelomeningocele) can now be diagnosed during the second trimester of pregnancy by amniocentesis, and measurement of *alpha fetoprotein* (AFP) and acetylcholinesterase levels in the amniotic fluid. The presence of rapidly adhering cells is also a diagnostic help. Larger lesions may show on a serial sonogram. Closed defects (spina bifida occulta) do not communicate with the amniotic fluid, and the AFP level does not rise. Because most children with neural tube defects are born to families with no previous history of the problem, efforts are under way to develop a screening program for pregnant women to measure their serum AFP level at 16 to 18 weeks of gestation. Two tests that show an increased serum AFP level suggest a defect and the need for amniocentesis and examination of the amniotic fluid.[42]

Cranial malformations

Encephalocele A defect associated with a cleft in the cranium—or *encephalocele*—can occur anywhere in the skull but is most common in the occipital area. In *occult cranium bifidum,* only the bone is affected; there is no involvement of the CNS, and thus the infant has a good prognosis. When the nervous tissue, meninges, and CSF are involved, as in *encephalomeningocele,* brain damage is inevitable, and seizures, hydrocephalus, and mental retardation are frequent complications. The diagnosis is usually readily made on the basis of the protruding sac. Palpation and transillumination aid in the differential diagnosis.

In the case of a severe defect, the decision may be made not to repair it surgically. Whether surgery is done or not, the sac must be carefully protected. Pressure on an encephalocele can cause impaired consciousness, impaired respirations, and bulging fontanels.

Anencephaly *Anencephaly* is a severe neural tube defect that is immediately evident at birth. The protective cranial skull and cerebral hemispheres are absent. Most fetuses with anencephaly are aborted early in pregnancy or are stillborn. Some may live a short time if the brainstem functions. Reflex reactions of respirations, swallowing, and sucking may keep the child alive for a few days.

Nursing management Parents whose child has a severe cranial malformation must be supported in their grief and disappointment. Usually seeing the baby helps them come to terms with reality and prevents even worse imaginary visions. The parents will need accurate information and support in their decision making regarding surgical treatment. (See Chap. 4.)

When surgical repair is feasible, special care must be taken by the nurse to keep the sac clean and to prevent rupture.[43] Vital functions are monitored closely. Postoperatively, the wound must be kept free of any contamination. The parents are encouraged to help with care. They will need nursing support to learn the best methods of feeding and bathing their child. Long-term management requires a team approach to the many physical, social, emotional, and financial problems associated with an encephalocele. The parents will need to know the signs of infection and of hydrocephalus and the risk of bearing other children with the disorder.

Microcephaly Microcephaly is a condition characterized by a head that is significantly smaller than normal. The baby has a long, narrow, receding forehead; a small cranium; and a flat occiput. Brain weight may be less than 1000 g, or one-fourth the normal size. The fontanels are either small or closed.

Careful assessment of microcephaly is necessary to rule out *craniostenosis* (premature closure of sutures). Craniostenosis is due to faulty bone growth, not to faulty brain growth, as in microcephaly. Surgical treatment is done on the closed sutures for cosmetic reasons, to relieve pressure, and to allow normal brain growth.

The impaired brain growth in microcephaly may be due to an autosomal recessive disorder, a chromosomal abnormality, or a teratogenic insult during pregnancy. The degree of neurological abnormality and mental retardation varies from mild to severe.

Nursing management The major objective of care is to promote the highest level of development possible for the child. Nursing care is directed toward helping the parents adapt to the situation. A multidisciplinary approach is necessary, with continued family support available as choices are made regarding the child's care and education. Genetic counseling may be helpful to the family if more children are desired.

Spinal malformations

Spina bifida occulta *Spina bifida occulta*, or an incomplete fusion of the vertebrae, may be signaled by an overlying dimple or tuft of hair. Neuromuscular disturbances of bladder and bowel control and paraparesis (partial paralysis) can occur in rare instances (Fig. 30-9*A*).

Meningocele A *meningocele*, which can be as small as an acorn or as large as an orange, contains meninges and CSF. It generally occurs in the lumbar area and is covered by abnormal skin or meninges. Because no nervous tissue is present, a light can be shone through it (transillumination). Early surgical repair is done to prevent infection. Neurological complications are less severe than when nervous tissue protrudes into the sac, but hydrocephalus can develop (Fig. 30-9*B*).

Myelomeningocele A *myelomeningocele*, also called a *meningomyelocele*, is more severe than a meningocele because it contains meninges, spinal fluid, *and* neural tissue. The sac may be as large as a grapefruit and is prone to leakage through the thin membrane or skin that covers it (Figs. 30-9C and 30-10). The spinal cord and nerve roots may stop at the sac, ending motor and sensory function below that point. Paralysis, sensory loss, and bowel and bladder dysfunction are common and are determined by the level of the lesion.

A lesion at the thoracic level causes total lower extremity paralysis. If the lesion is at T12, pelvic flexion is possible. Thoracic lesions are rarer than lumbar and sacral defects. If the lesion is at L1 or L2, hip flexion is possible. Children with these defects will ordinarily be confined to a wheelchair. When L3 and L4 levels of paralysis are present, the child has potential knee movement and may become ambulatory with long or short leg braces and crutches. Lesions at L5 or below allow varying degrees of foot and ankle movement. Some of these children may be ambulatory without braces (see Table 30-17).

Treatment A comprehensive program requires a team of specialists to:

1. Complete a thorough neurological examination, paying particular attention to lower extremity motor function
2. Provide counseling and emotional support in the decision-making process regarding the issue of surgical intervention

X-rays of skull, spine, hips, and chest are done. Cultures determine the presence of infection. Developing hydrocephalus is monitored by daily measurement of head circumference, palpation of the fontanels, and computerized axial tomography.

There is controversy regarding when to close the sac. "Early" closure (within 48 h) is advocated by physicians in most cases and is viewed as essential when the back lesion is actually leaking CSF. Some researchers contend that "delayed" closure (between 3 and 7 days) or even "late" closure (between 1 week and 10 months) may not pose the risk that there will be further nerve damage related to subsequent exposure to

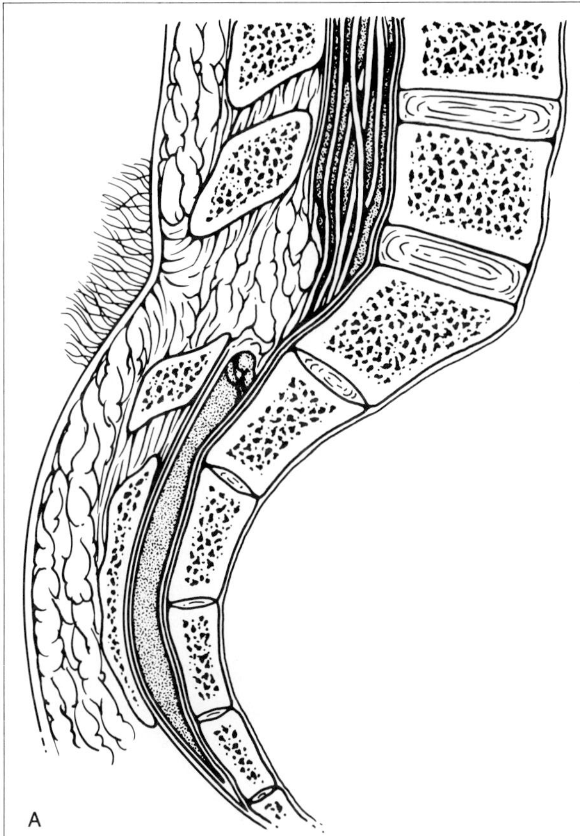

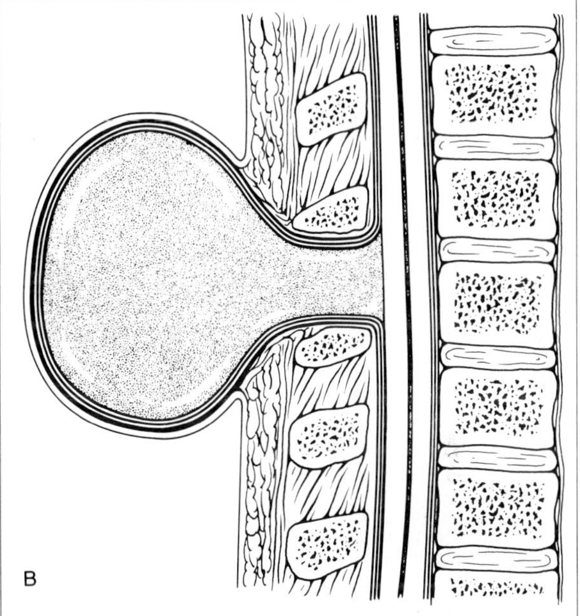

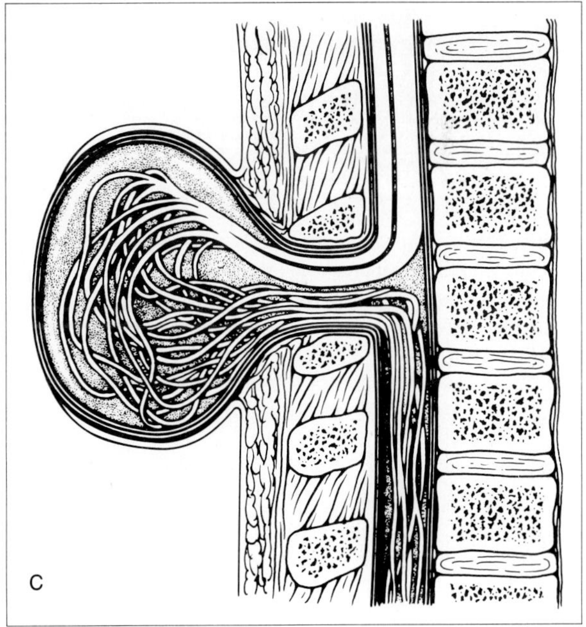

Figure 30-9 Congenital malformations of the spine. (*A*) Spina bifida occulta, an incomplete fusion of the vertebral arches without an external sac. A dimple or tuft of hair may signal its presence. (*B*) Meningocele. The external sac contains meninges and CSF. (*C*) Myelomeningocele. The external sac contains meninges, CSF, and immature spinal cord tissue. (*From Beverly A. Bowens, "The Nervous System," in M. Armstrong et al. [eds.], McGraw-Hill Handbook of Clinical Nursing, McGraw-Hill, New York, 1979. Used with permission.*)

extrauterine environmental stressors such as infection.[44,45,46]

There is also controversy among physicians regarding the most appropriate treatment for children born with a myelomeningocele. If the child has other severe defects as well as infection and hydrocephalus, some physicians recommend no intervention. Others advocate repair of every defect.[47,48] The parents must be involved in the decision-making process and supported in their choice. Giving them as much information as possible helps them make decisions. The courts may become involved when issues of sanctity vs. quality of life are raised. Chapter 4 discusses moral considerations in pediatric nursing.

Once surgical repair is done, the goals of the health care team include (1) maintenance of renal function, (2) control of bladder and bowel

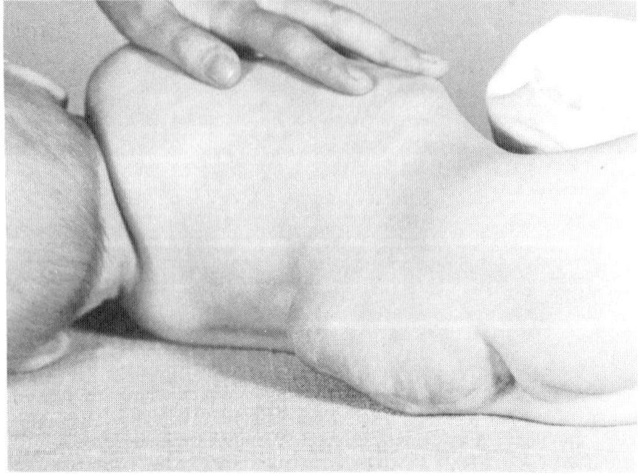

A

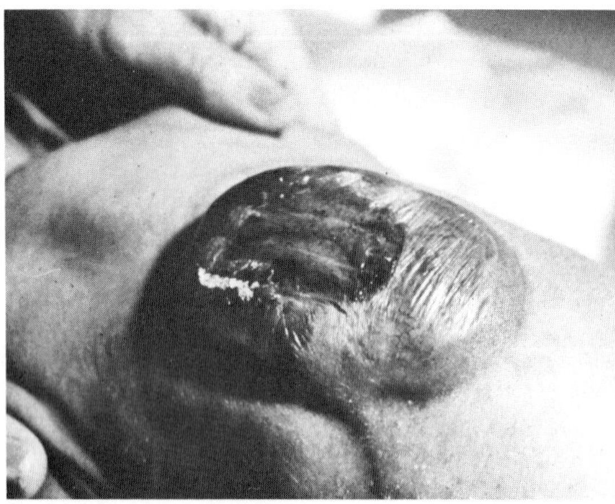

B

Figure 30-10 Myelomeningoceles. (*A*) With skin covering. (*Photo courtesy of D. Jack Mayfield, Department of Orthopaedic Surgery, University of Minnesota.*) (*B*) With thin, abnormal membrane covering. (*Photo courtesy of Dr. Edward R. Laws, Mayo Clinic, Rochester, Minn.*)

function, (3) promotion of independent locomotion, (4) independence in activities of daily living, and (5) achievement of social acceptance. With vigorous early treatment and careful follow-up, a large percentage of children with myelomeningoceles can meet these goals.[49,50,51]

Nursing management Nursing care of the child with a meningocele or myelomeningocele can be divided into the acute and chronic phases. The immediate problems relate to preoperative and postoperative care. Long-term care includes management of the associated complications (Table 30-9).

Acute care Nursing care is directed toward observing neurological status, recognizing complications, and providing for basic needs during the preoperative and postoperative periods.

Table 30-9 Complications of Myelomeningocele

Hydrocephalus—occurs in 75 to 90% of children with lumbar myelomeningoceles
Impaired bladder and bowel control
Motor impairment: partial or complete paralysis
Sensory impairment: skin disturbances, decubitus ulcers
In utero joint deformities:
Flexion or extension contractures
Talipes valgus or varus (clubfeet)
Congenital hip dislocation
Kyphosis or scoliosis
Osteoporosis: leads to spontaneous fractures
Obesity
Hydrosyringomyelia (dilatation of the spinal cord central canal by CSF pressure with formation of fistulas within spinal cord tissue): scoliosis, spasticity, weakness and paralysis, personality changes

The nurse should observe the baby for spontaneous movement, usual position, and response to body stimulation. Voiding and defecation patterns are monitored for amount and frequency. The presence or absence of the *anal reflex* (constriction of the sphincter upon stroking) is determined.

In rare instances, the physician may order manual compression of the bladder over the suprapubic area to promote complete emptying (Credé method); this may result in reflux. (See Chap. 20.)

Hydrocephalus is a secondary complication in at least 80 to 90 percent of children with a myelomeningocele. The nurse must measure the head and chest daily to assess for increasing ICP. The fontanels are palpated often for fullness and bulging. Increasing lethargy or irritability and other signs of increasing ICP should be noted.

The nurse must watch for signs of infection. Meningitis is a common complication, although early surgery and prophylactic antibiotic therapy have reduced its frequency. Restlessness, irritability, increased sensitivity to noise and light, excessive crying, and fever may indicate meningitis.

Care of the sac is extremely important. Correct positioning in a *prone* position is achieved through use of the Bradford frame or with small rolls and sandbags. Usually a low Trendelenberg position is favored to decrease pressure in the sac. The baby's head is turned to the side, and the legs are abducted to counteract hip subluxation. Pressure on the sac must be avoided because rupture could cause a sudden loss of CSF, leading to herniation of the brainstem and pressure on vital centers.

The sac is carefully observed for leakage or abrasions. Dressings, although seldom used, are applied with aseptic technique. A plastic wrap may be applied below the spinal defect to protect it from stool, which can spurt out erratically (Fig. 30-11).

Since early repair is the norm, feeding may not be begun until after surgery. However, if feeding is indicated, it will be difficult if the infant cannot be held or is irritable. The head should be elevated slightly and turned to the side if possible. A soft nipple and chin support will help if the baby has difficulty sucking. Feeding should be a time of fondling and stimulation by touch. The baby can be touched gently on the head, arms, and upper back. The normal cuddling situation should be imitated as closely as possible for the infant who must be fed lying on his or her abdomen. Intake is recorded accurately; daily weights may be ordered, depending on the baby's progress.

Following surgical closure of the sac, nursing care is similar to that described above. Special emphasis is given to observing for shock, development of increased ICP, hydrocephalus, wound leakage, infection, and adequacy of respiratory status and neurological function. Precautions are used to prevent contamination of the wound from feces or urine.

The infant may be placed on the abdomen or side. The head may be elevated if hydrocephalus is present. If leakage of CSF occurs, the head is lowered to reduce pressure on the wound.

The parents need a great deal of psychological support. Usually the baby has been rushed from the local hospital to a large medical center, leaving the new mother behind. Anxiety and fears are great. The mother may experience some guilt and ask herself, "What did I do to make this happen?" Once the parents are assured that the baby will survive surgery, they begin to realize how extensive their child's problems may be. Surgical intervention is the first step in a long series of future hospitalizations, surgeries, and crises.

The nurse is responsible for assessing the parents' level of understanding regarding the defect, what surgery involves, and how to cope with the child's impairments. Table 30-10 is a teaching guideline that can be used postoperatively to prepare the parents for discharge and long-term care of their child.

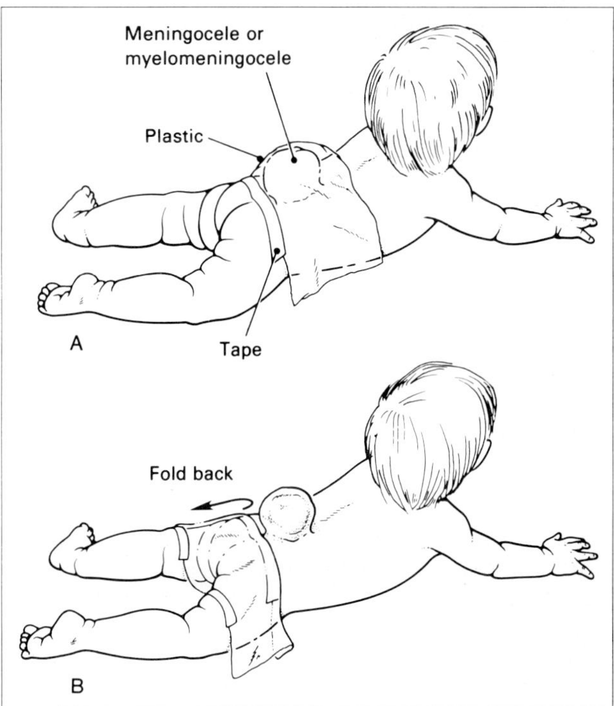

Figure 30-11 Use of ordinary kitchen-variety plastic wrap to protect a spinal defect from contamination. When the plastic wrap is folded back to expose the area, it can be taped to the thighs. (*From Beverly A. Bowens, "The Nervous System," in M. Armstrong et al. [eds.], McGraw-Hill Handbook of Clinical Nursing, McGraw-Hill, New York, 1979. Used with permission.*)

Table 30-10 Checklist for Teaching and Dismissal Planning Following Repair of Myelomeningocele

________	Feeding
________	Skin care
________	Positioning
________	Wound care
________	Elimination:
	Bladder drainage program
	Bowel
________	Range-of-motion exercises
________	Stimulation program
________	Orthopedic problems
________	Complications to watch for:
	Hydrocephalus
	Fontanels
	Head circumference
	Infection
	Temperature
	Other signs

Long-term care Long-term management includes providing a balanced diet and maintaining adequate fluid intake. With decreased mobility, the child is predisposed to constipation. Milk is recommended for the young child but may be restricted in the adolescent to decrease formation of renal calculi.

Children with a myelomeningocele are at high risk for becoming overweight. They may require a lower caloric intake because of the decreased mobility associated with long-term orthopedic management. If the nurse combines instruction about nutrition and exercise with behavioral interventions, weight control can be a realizable goal.[52]

Since urinary reflux and infection can cause permanent renal damage, bladder dysfunction is the most threatening of the child's long-term problems. Continued monitoring of urologic status is essential. Prophylactic antibiotics and bladder training may be used. Chapter 20 provides a more complete discussion of bladder management in myelomeningocele. The neuropathic (neurogenic) bladder is one of the most difficult problems associated with myelomeningocele. Bladder control becomes more important once the child enters school. Artificial sphincters are an option, but they occasionally cause erosion of tissue.[53] Ileal conduits have also been used, but they can produce significant long-term complications. In contrast, clean intermittent catheterization has been shown to be safe and effective.[54,55] The child is gradually taught the steps in the procedure until total independence is achieved. Indwelling catheters and external collecting devices are also used. When decisions are made concerning the management of urine collection, however, consideration must be given to the need for adaptation when the child becomes sexually mature.

Bowel training is established through chemical and mechanical stimulation. Prune juice at bedtime may be helpful to the older child. A suppository before a meal, warm fluid after the meal, and planned time on the potty-chair or toilet are helpful. Sometimes a stool softener is necessary. A balanced diet high in bulk and fiber and adequate fluids help maintain the consistent stool necessary for regulation.

Usually, children with myelodysplasia become independent in bowel and bladder function much later than nonhandicapped children.[56] Independence is adversely affected by mental retardation and by higher lesions. The emotional consequences of incontinence include a poor self-image, lack of motivation, lack of opportunities for heterosexual intimacy, and poor sexual identity.

Long-term orthopedic management includes exercise, casting, traction, braces, and surgical correction of deformities. By the age of 1 year the child should be equipped with appropriate braces and should be weight-bearing. Lightweight sport wheelchairs and other adaptive equipment allow the child to participate more fully in sports and to move easily about a court or a track (Fig. 30-12).

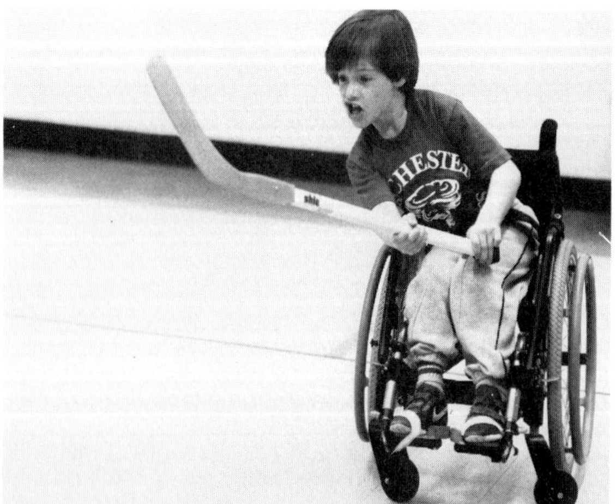

Figure 30-12 Lightweight sport wheelchairs allow children to participate in a wide variety of sports. (*Photo courtesy of Rochester Post-Bulletin.*)

The developmental changes of adolescence bring new or greater concerns to the child regarding body image, sexual identity, and peer acceptance. Scoliosis and kyphosis are common complications in adolescents, especially in those with higher defects. Typically, girls with myelodysplasia mature earlier than their peers.[57] The child will need information about sexuality and his or her sexual potential. The sexual potential of males varies according to the height of the lesion. Whether erection is possible or not, few males will be able to father a child.[58] Females ordinarily are able to experience intercourse, pregnancy, and delivery. Both males and females may experience problems with hygiene because of immobility and incontinence, but these can be worked out.

The parents need help in understanding how important it is to promote independence in their child. Children from 4 to 6 years of age can take some responsibility for bowel and bladder care as well as for other activities of daily living. The parents can benefit from the support of parent groups of the Spina Bifida Association of America. The child should be encouraged to participate in organized activities, such as the Special Olympics, and to develop social skills. Successful handicapped people provide useful role models for these children. Adolescents need to become responsible for recognizing their problems and doing something about them.[59]

Providing for the emotional needs of the family is important. Each developmental hurdle that is not mastered by the child reactivates their grief. The grief process is a cyclic process. The parents can be given anticipatory guidance and assurance that the feelings they experience are normal. By teaching the parents about the malformation and its implications and management, the nurse returns a sense of control to the child and the family. Plans are made jointly with the parents and the child.

Hydrocephalus

Pathophysiology *Hydrocephalus* is an abnormal accumulation of CSF in the brain caused by excessive production, inadequate reabsorption, or obstruction of circulation of CSF through the ventricles. The incidence of congenital hydrocephalus is 1:1000 infants.

Noncommunicating hydrocephalus (internal or obstructive) is due to blockage in the ventricular system that prevents CSF from flowing to the subarachnoid spaces of the brain where it is absorbed. Most cases of noncommunicating hydrocephalus are due to developmental malformations, neoplasms, infections, or trauma. *Arnold-Chiari* malformation, a *noncommunicating* obstruction of the fourth ventricle, results from the downward displacement of the lower brainstem and cerebellum into the cervical canal. It is associated with myelomeningocele and abnormal development of the cerebral hemispheres.

In *communicating* hydrocephalus, an excessive amount of CSF moves freely through the ventricles but is not absorbed by the arachnoid villi. Nonabsorption, caused by fibrosis of the arachnoid villi, is often the result of hemorrhage or infection. Communicating hydrocephalus is the most common type.

The infant with hydrocephalus displays bulging fontanels, an enlarging head, prominent scalp veins, a fixed downward gaze of the eyes with the sclerae visible above the irises *(sunset eyes)*, and eventual thinning of the scalp (Fig. 30-13). In the older child whose sutures have closed, leaving no room for head expansion, the signs and symptoms of increased ICP include headache, nausea, vomiting, papilledema, seizures, and decreasing levels of consciousness.

Diagnosis is possible in utero through the use of ultrasound. After birth, transillumination, neurological evaluation, measurement of head circumference, and computerized axial tomography are used.

Treatment The treatment of hydrocephalus is almost always surgical. The obstruction to circulating CSF is reduced if possible. More often, a shunt is introduced into the ventricular system to reroute CSF and facilitate its absorption. A burr hole is drilled into the skull, and the tip of a thin polyethylene catheter is inserted into the ventricle. The catheter is threaded behind the ear into the jugular vein and into the right atrium or peritoneal cavity (Fig. 30-14). A one-way valve in the catheter allows fluid to drain off when pressure increases. Some valves require "pumping" or pressing several times a day to keep the tube patent and draining. Several shunt revisions or replacements, usually every 20 to 24 months, may be necessary during childhood because:

1. The child develops bacteria.
2. The catheter becomes clogged.

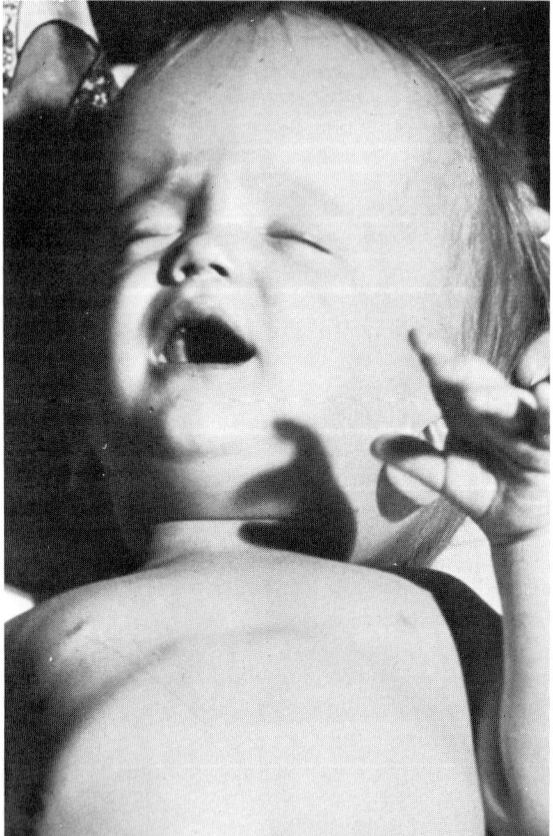

Figure 30-13 An 11-month-old infant with hydrocephalus. (*Photo courtesy of Dr. Robert W. Feldt, Mayo Clinic, Rochester, Minn.*)

3. The pumping mechanism fails.
4. The catheter tubing becomes too short as the child grows.
5. One end of the catheter becomes dislodged.[60,61]

Untreated hydrocephalus has a 50 to 60 percent mortality rate. With treatment, 80 percent of affected children survive and one-half to one-third are intellectually and neurologically normal. Persistent infections and shunt revisions are emotionally, physically, and financially draining to both the child and the family.

Despite its effectiveness, shunting is associated with considerable complications. Medical therapy with acetazolamide (10 mg per kilogram of body weight per day) and furosemide (1 mg per kilogram of body weight per day) has been proved effective as an alternative to shunting in selected cases. The progression of hydrocephalus is controlled until the sutures can become fibrosed and spontaneous arrest can occur.[62]

Nursing management The observations of the child before surgery are the same as those described for the child with increased ICP. Head circumference and the fontanels are monitored closely in the infant. Eating may be difficult because the child is lethargic and irritable. If the head is large, it must be carefully supported and protected from developing pressure areas. The parents will need support and education in regard to the purpose of surgery and expected care following surgery.

Postoperatively, the child is positioned on the unoperative side and kept flat to avoid sudden reduction of ICP. The dressing is observed closely, and neurological status is monitored at least every 15 min. Total intake and output are measured. Because salt and fluid are lost through drainage of CSF, electrolyte replacement is done carefully. Signs of irritability, bulging fontanels, decreasing levels of consciousness, and increasing temperature are reported promptly. Prophylactic antibiotic therapy is routine.

Before discharge, the parents must be taught how to recognize the signs of increasing ICP, infection, and other signs indicating shunt malfunction. Usually the child will need to avoid contact sports but can participate in most other activities. Sharing information helps allay parental anxiety and prevents overprotection of the child.

Infection, often due to *Staphylococcus epidermidis* or *Staphylococcus aureus*, usually requires removal of the shunt and replacement. Shunt revisions are more common in children than in adults. The earlier a shunt is placed, the more likely it is that it will need to be revised. Increased frequency of infection and revision mean a poor long-term prognosis for the child.

ALTERATIONS IN BRAIN FUNCTION

Cerebral palsy

Pathophysiology *Cerebral palsy* (CP) is a nonprogressive central motor deficit in which voluntary muscles are poorly controlled. It is a common crippling condition of childhood, affecting at least 1 to 2 out of 1000 children.

Interference with oxygen supply before, during, or after birth increases the risk of develop-

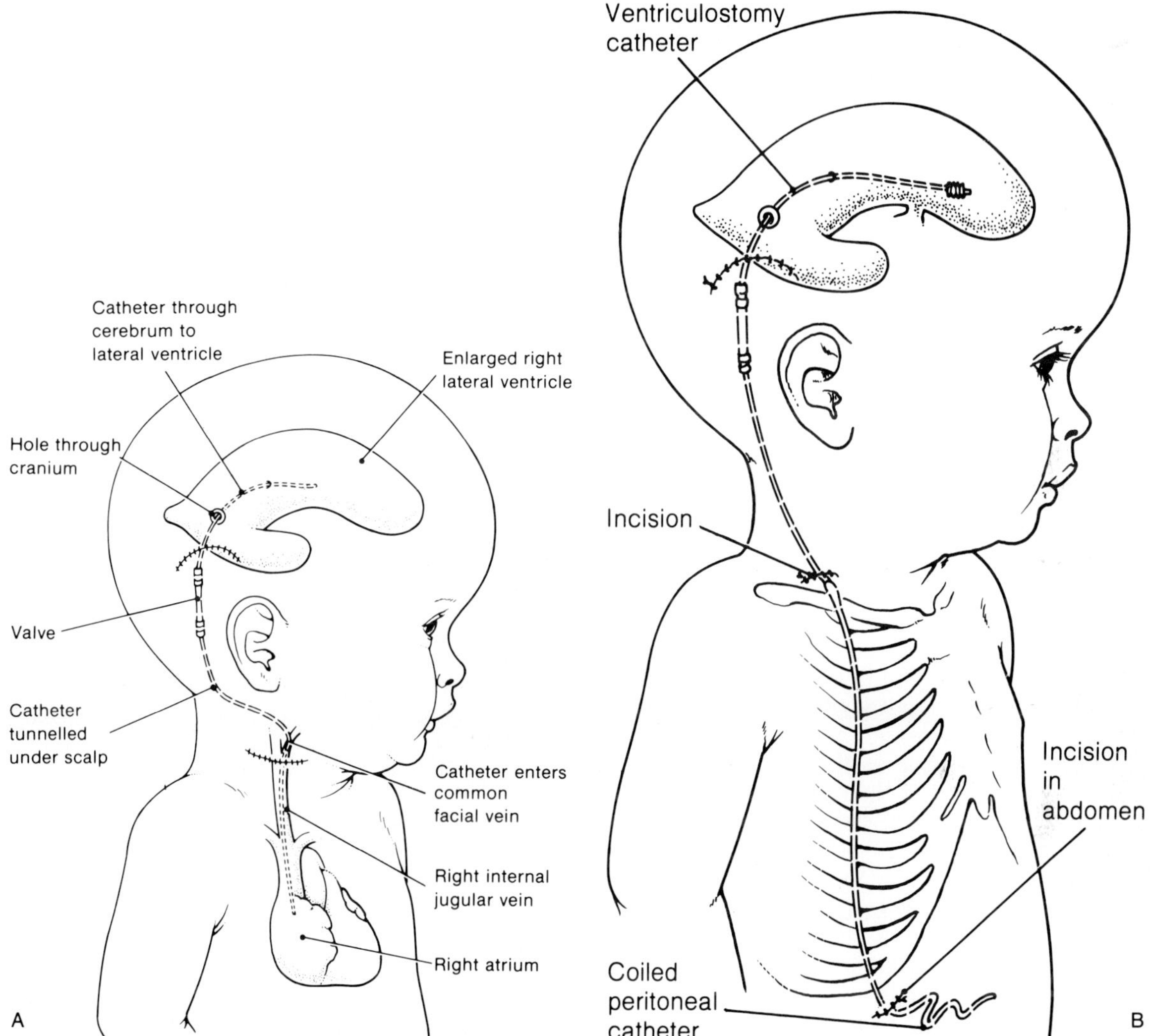

Figure 30-14 Shunts used in hydrocephalus. (*A*) A ventriculoatrial shunt. The catheter is inserted into the anterior horn of the lateral ventricle, passed through a tunnel under the scalp, and connected to a catheter previously inserted into the atrium. (*B*) A ventriculoperitoneal shunt. The ventricular catheter is threaded subcutaneously down the occipital-parietal area toward the anterior portion of the neck. There it is connected to the peritoneal catheter, which has been passed up the anterior abdomen and chest to the neck. (*From G. Scipien, M. U. Barnard, M. A. Chard, J. Howe, and P. J. Phillips* [*eds.*], *Comprehensive Pediatric Nursing, 3d ed., McGraw-Hill, New York, 1986, p. 784–5. Used with permission.*)

ing CP. The severity of neuromuscular involvement depends on the stage of fetal development and the duration of the anoxia. Maternal factors associated with an increased risk of CP in an offspring are age (under 18), diabetes, intrauterine infection, and toxemia. CP is 3 times as common in premature infants as in full-term infants. Premature infants, especially those who are small for gestational age, seem to be at the highest risk.[63]

Neonatal signs that are strongly predictive of an increased risk of CP are Apgar scores of 3 or less at 10 min and beyond, neonatal seizures, and abnormal neurological status in the newborn period.[64] In 20 to 30 percent of cases of CP there is no apparent cause.[65]

Detection Severe cases of CP may be detected at birth. A feeble cry, general weakness, and difficulty eating alert the nurse to a CNS problem. Prior to 1 year of age a definite diagnosis of CP is extremely hard to make. In contrast to the hypotonic infants, other children with CP are dramatically hyperextended, and the legs are crossed in a scissor position. These infants are difficult to hold and cuddle. Other infants with CP may roll from a prone to a supine position very early.

Usually CP is diagnosed because the child is delayed in reaching developmental milestones and because of abnormal continuation of newborn reflexes (the Moro, tonic neck, startle, and grasp reflexes). Twenty percent of infants with CP show persistence of the tonic neck reflex after 6 months. As the nervous system matures, deficits become more apparent. Delays in learning to roll over, sit, crawl, walk, and talk signal the parents and the nurse that something is wrong. Exaggerated reflexes and asymmetry of the limbs and muscles are warning signs. The parents may notice that their 4-month-old infant uses only one hand when reaching out. Normally, hand preference is not seen until 1 year of age or later. Involuntary movements, accompanied by spasticity, athetosis, or ataxia, make their appearance by $1\frac{1}{2}$ to 2 years of age.

One-third of children with CP have some degree of mental retardation, and one-half have seizures. Vision and hearing impairments frequently increase the child's difficulty with communication. Other disabilities associated with CP include learning disabilities, communication disorders, skeletal deformities, and carious teeth. Children with CP who can sit alone by 2 years of age will usually be able to walk. Those who are not sitting alone by age 4, however, seldom walk independently (Fig. 30-15).

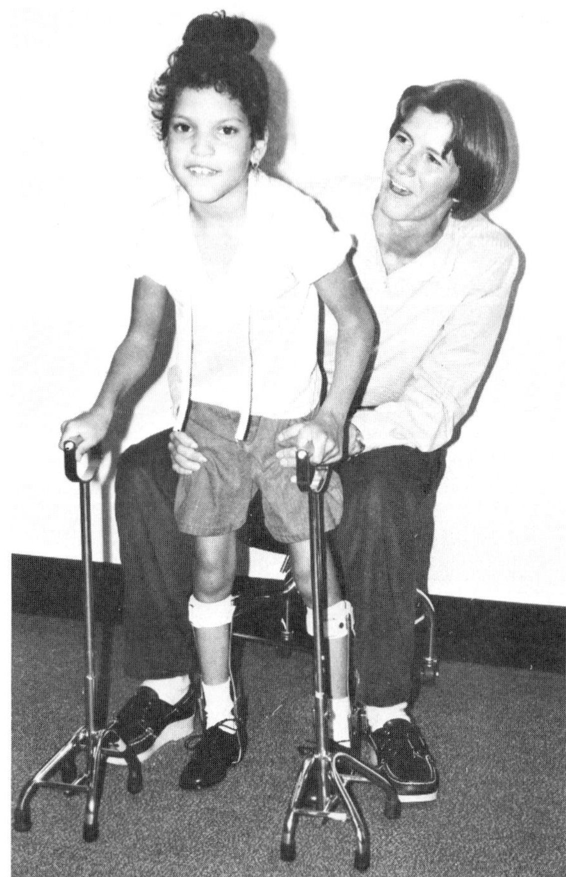

Figure 30-15 Use of a four-point walker helps the child learn balance and to walk. (*Photo courtesy of Dr. Daniel Halpern, Department of Physical Medicine and Rehabilitation, University of Minnesota.*)

Classification CP can be classified into three types: (1) spastic, (2) dyskinetic or athetoid, and (3) ataxic. Table 30-11 lists the incidence and main characteristics of the three types of CP.[66]

Spastic CP is characterized by exaggerated reflexive movements of one or more limbs. Initially there may be hypotonicity in the affected extremities, with hypertonicity gradually appearing. Muscle groups become tight, shortened, and contracted. Reflexes are exaggerated. Difficulty in swallowing and drooling indicate head and neck muscle involvement. Communication difficulties due to muscle impairment may be misinterpreted as retardation in these children.

Athetoid or *dyskinetic CP* is characterized by involuntary slow, writhing (athetoid), random movements of all extremities, the head, and the face. Muscle hypertrophy can result from the constant motion. Usually muscle tone is decreased. The writhing, athetoid movements do not usually appear until 18 months, suggesting that a certain maturity of the CNS is necessary.

Ataxic CP is manifested by disturbances of balance, uncoordinated arms, hypoactive reflexes, and often a horizontal nystagmus. The infant exhibits little leg movement and may drag the legs when beginning to crawl.

Treatment Medical treatment is determined primarily by the extent of neuromuscular involvement. A comprehensive, interdisciplinary team approach provides the services needed to

Table 30-11 Characteristics of Cerebral Palsy

Type	Frequency	Characteristics
Spastic:	50 to 75% of all children with CP	Hypertonic muscle spasm, varying from facial muscle to total body involvement. Poor control of posture, balance, and fine movement
Hemiparesis		One side of body affected, with greater involvement of upper extremity
Quadriplegia		All four extremities involved to some degree
Diplegia		All four extremities affected, but lower extremities involved to greater degree
Triplegia		Three extremities involved
Dyskinetic:	25% of all children with CP	Difficulty performing voluntary movements
Athetosis		Slow, random writhing movements that disappear during sleep and are aggravated by stress
Dystonia		Decreased muscle tone
Ataxia:	Less than 10% of all children with CP	Hypotonic state with intention tremor and muscle incoordination, especially of upper extremities. Loss of posture and balance
Congenital ataxia		Hypotonic reflexes with balance disturbances
Ataxic diplegia		Spasticity in lower extremities in addition to ataxia

help the child achieve the highest possible level of neuromuscular functioning and independence. Goals of the treatment of CP are summarized in Table 30-12.

Nursing management The nurse is an integral member of the interdisciplinary team caring for the child with CP. Care plans designed by the team will be implemented by the nurse in the hospital, community, clinic, or school.

Many children with CP have a communication problem. It may take several minutes for them to express themselves. It is essential that nurses be patient, attentive, and interested. The nurse cannot assume that a child with CP is retarded simply because difficulty in communication is present. Hearing aids, spelling symbol or picture boards, typewriters, and sign language can help improve expressive and receptive communication.

Table 30-12 Goals of Cerebral Palsy Treatment and Approaches to Treatment

Goal	Approach	Description
Maintain normal tone	Range-of-motion exercises (active and passive)	Movement of joints to their fullest capacity
	Stretching exercises	Physical exercises designed to extend muscles to their fullest capacity
	Careful positioning	Braces, corsets, head halter, splints, appliances, and right-angle placement of all extremities
Increase voluntary control and inhibit involuntary random movement	Medications (used infrequently)	Maintenance levels of Valium may be administered
	Motor-point block	Injections of phenol with electrical stimulation Drug therapy
Prevent contractures	Range-of-motion exercises	Movement of all joints to their fullest capacity
	Intermittent stretching	Daily short-term traction, bracing, or inhibitive casting of extremities to stretch muscles
Correct contractures	Surgical release	Prevent complete immobilization
Develop adequate communication skills	Visual exam and correction	
	Hearing exam and correction	To determine whether child is deaf, rather than mentally retarded
	Learning and practicing movements of speech	Purposeful movements involving swallowing, lip movement, and chewing to improve speech patterns

Children with CP may need assistance with eating, elimination, and other basic activities. Sometimes swallowing difficulties or tongue movements impair eating. Choking may be a problem.

The nurse compensates for these problems with adaptive equipment (Fig. 30-16), individualized feeding programs, and careful upright positioning. Mealtimes provide an opportunity for promoting and reinforcing more normal sensorimotor patterns.[67]

Handling children with CP can prove difficult. The family is taught techniques to promote normal movement, balance, and posture in the young child. Careful positioning while carrying the child helps develop and strengthen equilibrium and maintaining behaviors. Carrying techniques include:

1. Carry the child prone to strengthen head control.
2. Carry the child in a sitting position while controlling arm and leg movements to assist in flexion.
3. Carry the child with an arm between the child's legs to compensate for tight adductors.
4. Bend the child with spasticity forward at the hips and sit the child up before lifting.[68,69]

The older child and the child with athetosis should be lifted from behind by placing the arms under the child's upper arms and grasping the inner aspects of the thighs. The nurse's chest supports the child's back and promotes a forward head position.

When the child wears braces, meticulous skin care is essential. The skin needs to be checked every 4 h for redness, wrinkling, blistering, or cyanosis. Brace cuffs are sufficiently tight when two fingers can be placed inside them.

Emphasis is placed on helping the child develop independence in locomotion and activities of daily living. If a child is hospitalized, the home treatment program must be adapted so that progress will continue. Parents are essential in helping the nurse develop an appropriate care plan.

The parents will need continued support and help as they face the constant demands of caring for and raising a handicapped child. Discipline may be difficult. Siblings must be considered. The parents will need help in understanding their child's abilities and assets, how to parent a handicapped child, and how to keep the family system strong and supportive. They will need to understand the developmental and educational needs of their child as well as how to meet them. The parents and the child have the ultimate responsibility for the child's rehabilitation and for meeting the goals of optimum development, independence, and emotional adjustment. See Chap. 34 for more information on chronic illness.

Developmental dyslexia*

Developmental dyslexia is a specific language learning disability characterized by difficulty

*This section was written by Marcia K. Henry, M.A.

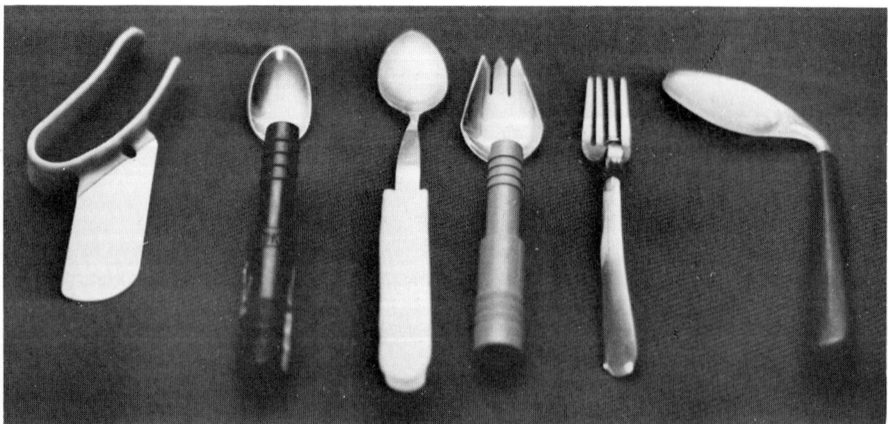

Figure 30-16 Special utensils for the handicapped. (*From Virginia F. Strange, "Dietary Assistance," in L. M. Shortridge and E. Lee [eds.], Introductory Skills for Nursing Practice, McGraw-Hill, New York, 1980.*)

learning to read, spell, and write. The term is used in reference to children and adults who have normal or above-normal intelligence, conventional educational opportunities, and no primary emotional problems but who have difficulty learning to read, despite good performance in other areas. Other names for the disability include *specific language disability, developmental reading disability,* and *word blindness;* it is incorrectly termed *attention deficit disorder* and *minimal brain dysfunction.*

No single cause has been found for developmental dyslexia, but possible causes are often grouped into three broad categories: educational, psychological, and biological. New research at Harvard's Beth Israel Hospital on the brains of dyslexics studied during postmortem examinations has revealed characteristic disorders of brain development. It seems likely that these disorders are an important cause of a significant number of cases of severe dyslexia.

It is estimated that 5 to 15 percent of school-age children are dyslexic.[70] According to Duane, the "frequency of specific reading retardation (developmental dyslexia) appears to equal or exceed the combined frequency of mental retardation, cerebral palsy, and epilepsy."[71] Obviously, developmental dyslexia is an important public health problem.

Symptoms Children with dyslexia show marked differences; their only uniform characteristic is a reading level significantly below what one would expect for their age and intelligence. Two of the most significant characteristics of dyslexia are that it affects many more boys than girls and that genetic factors play a role. Dyslexia seems to run in families; 50 percent or more of affected children have family histories of the disorder.[72]

Samuel Torrey Orton, one of the first major researchers in the area of dyslexia, identified the dyslexic errors most widely known today.[73] These include:

1. Difficulty learning and remembering printed words
2. In some cases, reversal of orientation of letters (*b* for *d* and *p* for *q*) or numbers (*6* for *9*)
3. Reversal of the sequence of letters in words (*tar* for *rat* and *quite* for *quiet*) or numbers (*12* for *21*)
4. Omission or addition of entire words while reading
5. Difficulty understanding the sound values of letters and their combinations (confusion of vowel sounds and substitution of one consonant for another)
6. Persistent spelling errors
7. Difficulty writing

Orton also pointed out that a large proportion of dyslexics are left-handed or ambidextrous or have trouble differentiating between right and left. Certain other common symptoms that may not relate only to dyslexia include (1) delayed or inadequate spoken language, (2) difficulty finding the "right" word when speaking, (3) confusion about directions in space or time (right and left, up and down, and yesterday and tomorrow), and (4) motor disorders such as clumsiness and cramped, illegible handwriting.

A child with dyslexia may have a deficit in visual processing, auditory processing, or both. *Visual processing* refers to the integration and expression of visual images in the brain after the eyes receive them. When a defect in visual memory occurs, the child has difficulty recognizing, reading, spelling, recalling, or memorizing written words.

Auditory processing refers not to actual hearing but to what happens to the impulses in the brain. Children with below-average auditory memory may have difficulty pronouncing words, remembering a series of directions, and memorizing dates, word definitions, and multiplication tables. Children with dyslexia may have difficulty following oral instructions or comprehending written material, even though they can read it.

Fortunately, very few children exhibit all these features, but dyslexics share enough problems in common to distinguish them as a group with unique educational needs.

Detection and treatment Early detection is essential to prevent the child from being labeled as a slow learner, retarded, lazy, immature, or a daydreamer. In addition to having a complete medical evaluation, children who are having problems learning to read and to spell in school should be tested by trained educational specialists or psychologists. The specialist will pay particular attention to motor skills, handedness, language development, error patterns in reading and spelling, auditory and visual processing, and school and social behavior. After careful examination of the error patterns demonstrated in a variety of tests, the diagnostician will make specific recommendations for special help, such as tutoring, summer school, speech therapy, or placement in special education classes.

The diagnostician may also recommend specific remedial approaches, since the treatment of dyslexia is educational. It is likely that no one method will work for all children, but a structured, sequential, multisensory approach is often beneficial. The child learns to "feel" letter shapes by tracing them and to be cued by the movement of the lips and tongue when sounding and writing words. The student sees, hears, feels, and says the letter symbol and sound. The child learns phonics, or the relationship of symbol to sound, as well as spelling rules and patterns and the structural properties of prefixes, suffixes, and word roots, for example. In essence, the logical structure of the English language must be learned.

A classic example of spelling errors made by a dyslexic child is shown in Fig. 30-17. To achieve full academic potential, a dyslexic child must devote hours to drill, repetition, and reinforcement of correct responses and must practice reading. Progress depends on early intervention and appropriate treatment, innate intelligence, and individual motivation. Medication is not appropriate for a dyslexic child. Psychological symptoms that interfere with remediation or development may indicate the need for counseling. Academic failure can reduce the child's self-esteem and increase vulnerability to other stresses. In addition, behavior may become disruptive or delinquent. In an unpublished study of adolescents seen in Minnesota juvenile courts, Dennis Hogenson, a psychologist, found that one-third were reading 2 or more years below grade level, despite average or above-average intelligence.

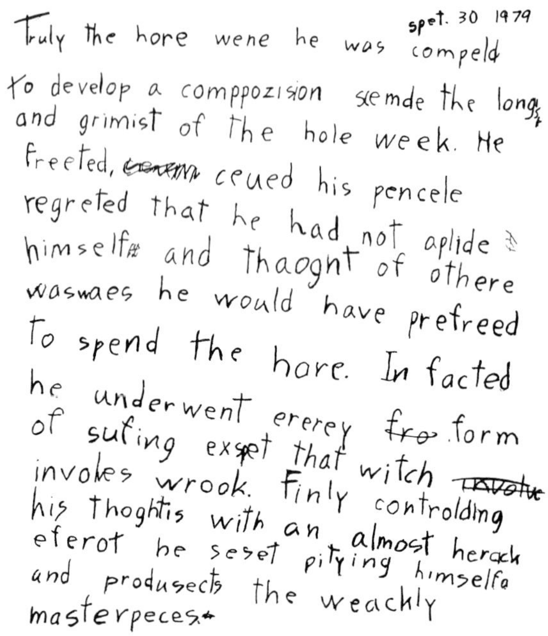

spet. 30 1979
Truly the hore wene he was compeld
to develop a comppozision semde the long
and grimist of the hole week. He
freeted, ceued his pencele
regreted that he had not aplide
himself and thaognt of othere
waswaes he would have prefreed
to spend the hore. In facted
he underwent ererey form
of sufing exspt that witch
involes wrook. Finly controlding
his thoghtis with an almost herack
eferot he seset pitying himselfa
and produsects the weackly
masterpeces.

Figure 30-17 A sample of the handwriting of a boy with developmental dyslexia. This sample was written by a boy aged 12 years and 4 months as his language therapist dictated from the quote below. This boy's IQ tested as 170 (Binet), and he was in the seventh grade (grade 7, 2 months). Quote: "Truly the hour when he was compelled to develop a composition seemed the longest and grimmest of the whole week. He fretted, chewed his pencil, regretted that he had not applied himself earlier, and thought of other ways he would have preferred to spend the hour. In fact, he underwent every form of suffering except that which involves work. Finally, controlling his thoughts with an almost heroic effort, he ceased pitying himself and produced the weekly masterpiece." (*Courtesy of Marcia K. Henry.*)

Nursing management The main responsibilities of the nurse in the area of developmental dyslexia are to recognize, teach, support, and refer. The decoding (word recognition and identification) and reading comprehension levels of the child should be assessed if reading materials are used in patient education. The nurse should ask the child to read aloud. If either decoding or comprehension is difficult, the text should be read to the child. The nurse must also clarify written instructions. Are they understood? Can the child repeat them in his or her own words? The child should be encouraged to use a "hands-on" approach, i.e. to act things out. Because a dyslexic child may have a short attention span and visual and auditory processing difficulties, several return demonstrations may be necessary when a procedure must be learned.

Pediatric and community health nurses play an increasingly important role in referring a child for evaluation if a receptive, retentive, or expressive written or spoken language problem is noted. Additional information on dyslexia, along with the location of diagnostic and remedial centers throughout the country, can be obtained from the Orton Dyslexia Society, 724 York Road, Baltimore, Md. 21204, or the Association for Children with Learning Disabilities, 5225 Grace Street, Pittsburgh, Pa. 15236.

ALTERATIONS DUE TO INFECTION

Meningitis

Meningitis, or inflammation of the meninges, is a very serious disease and requires immediate treatment to prevent a rapid, fulminating course ending in death. With early recognition and treatment, most children recover. There are three different clinical entities of meningitis: bacterial meningitis, viral meningitis, and neonatal meningitis.

Bacterial meningitis *Pathophysiology* *Bacterial meningitis* can follow any infection of the head or face (otitis media, mastoiditis, or a sinus infection), a gastrointestinal disturbance, or contamination of the meninges as a result of penetrating head wounds or neural tube defects. Most cases in children over 2 years of age are caused by *Hemophilus influenzae* Type B; *Neisseria meningitidis* types A, B, C, and Y (meningococcus); or *Diplococcus pneumoniae* (pneumococcus).

H. influenzae type B (HIB) accounts for more than 60 percent of cases of meningitis in children younger than 6 years of age.[74] Administration of HIB polysaccharide vaccine has been recommended for all children aged 2 to 5 years. Children who attend day-care facilities are at particular risk for acquiring systemic HIB disease. Initial vaccination at 18 months of age for these children should be considered.[75] Use of HIB vaccine in children younger than 18 months is not advised, since serum antibodies induced by vaccination are short-lived in children younger than 18 months of age.[76]

The symptoms of bacterial meningitis vary greatly according to age. Children over 2 years of age develop the classic signs of meningeal irritation: headache, neck stiffness (nuchal rigidity) and pain, and resistance of flexion of the neck and head. Neurological findings include:

1. *Brudzinski's sign* Brisk flexion of the knees occurs when the supine child's neck is flexed.
2. *Kernig's sign* Resistance to knee extension occurs when the supine child's thigh is flexed at right angles to the trunk.

Opisthotonos occurs as the disease gets worse. Other classic symptoms of meningitis include fever, malaise, lethargy, chills, photophobia, vomiting, and seizures.

Infection in the brain causes hyperemia, brain edema, and formation of a purulent exudate. The flow of CSF may be obstructed by thick pus, fibrin, or even adhesions. Brain abscesses may develop. When the infection spreads to the cranial nerves, hearing, vision, and facial movement may be impaired.

Infants over 28 days of age often present with fever, vomiting, and irritability. As the disease progresses, seizures, a high-pitched cry, and a full, tense fontanel indicate increasing ICP.

Treatment Immediate hospitalization, a lumbar puncture and analysis of CSF, vigorous antibiotic therapy, and supportive care are necessary to ensure the best possible outcome for the child.

CSF typically shows an increase in white blood cells and protein and a decrease in glucose. The fluid is examined microscopically, and a culture and sensitivity are done. Table 30-13 contrasts normal CSF analysis with that typical of meningitis and encephalitis.

The child is placed in respiratory isolation for at least 24 h. Intravenous antibiotic therapy is begun using large doses of broad-spectrum antibiotics until the exact pathogen is identified. Specific antibiotics and daily dosages are listed in Table 30-14. Fever is reduced. Ventilation, reduction of increased ICP, control of seizures, and management of bacterial shock are all important elements of medical care. Subdural effusions are treated by repeated removal of small amounts of fluid from the subdural space.

Fluid deficits are corrected, but *overhydration* must be avoided to prevent additional cerebral edema. When *inappropriate antidiuretic hormone syndrome* occurs, as it does in 50 percent of patients with meningitis, water is retained, leading to greater cerebral edema. When this happens, as little fluid as possible is used to administer antibiotics and electrolytes (800 to 1000 ml/m^2 per day).[77,78]

Viral meningitis *Viral meningitis,* or *aseptic meningitis,* is most often caused by enteroviruses or is the sequela of mumps, measles, or herpes. The onset may be abrupt or gradual with symptoms of headache, fever, malaise, nausea, vomiting, and other signs of meningeal irritation. The course is not as progressive as that in bacterial meningitis. Maculopapular rashes are associated with the echo viruses. Examination of CSF may reveal a slight elevation in pressure

Table 30-13 Cerebrospinal Fluid Analysis

	Normal	Bacterial Meningitis	Encephalitis
Pressure (mmH_2O)	40 to 200	Increased	Normal or moderately increased
Appearance	Clear	Cloudy	Clear
White cells (per cubic millimeter)	0 to 5	1000 to 4000	Above 500
Protein (milligrams per 100 ml)	20 to 40	60 to 100 or more	Slightly increased
Glucose (milligrams per 100 ml)	50 to 90	Decreased or absent	Normal
Culture	Negative	Positive in 80 to 90% of untreated children	

and the white blood count, but the CSF is otherwise normal. Medical treatment is symptomatic. Nursing care is essentially supportive. Usually the child has an uncomplicated illness and a good recovery.

Neonatal meningitis *Neonatal meningitis* is a serious problem in newborns, accounting for 70 percent of all deaths from bacterial meningitis.[79] The mortality rate is high, varying from 40 to 80 percent. Preterm infants are twice as susceptible as full-term infants. Gram-negative organisms such as *Escherichia coli, Klebsiella, Pseudomonas, Salmonella,* and group B streptococcus are the usual causative bacteria.

Diagnosis is difficult because infants do not show the classic signs of meningitis. They may have an elevated temperature or one that is below normal. They may be lethargic or hyperactive. Typically they are septic, feed poorly, have loose stools, and experience respiratory distress. Seizures, hepatomegaly, and jaundice may be present.

Neonates with meningitis are critically ill and need intensive nursing care and multiple support systems. Many will experience neurological damage after recovery.

Table 30-14 Antibiotic Management of Bacterial Meningitis in Children

Antibiotic	Daily Dosage per Kilogram of Body Weight
Penicillin G	150,000 to 300,000 units
Ampicillin	100 to 400 mg
Chloramphenical	100 mg
Cefotaxime	50 mg
Oxacillin	200 mg
Gentamicin	5 to 7.5 mg
Vanocomycin	40 mg
Methicillin	50 mg

References: 80, 81, 82.

Nursing management Because meningitis affects so many children, it is frequently encountered by nurses. Nurses in community settings must recognize the symptoms that suggest meningitis. The nurse who cares for the ill child must be highly skilled and knowledgeable in order to provide the needed nursing care.

Nursing care centers on assessing neurological status, supporting the child during diagnostic procedures, providing for basic needs, and protecting the child from injury. Observations of vital signs and blood pressure, sensory and motor function, and level of consciousness are made frequently.

The child with bacterial meningitis remains in respiratory isolation (Table 16-9) for at least 24 h. Children who are suspected of having meningitis are placed in respiratory isolation for 24 h while the physician awaits the culture results. Only cases caused by *N. meningitidis* require respiratory isolation. The parents must be taught the appropriate isolation procedures. They need opportunities to express their fears and to receive encouragement and support from those who are caring for their child. They may feel guilty because they did not seek medical help earlier. In some cases they may experience anger if a visit to a health professional for an upper respiratory infection did not result in the diagnosis of meningitis. They need help in understanding why the initial symptoms are often indistinguishable from those of other minor infections that children often acquire.

When a lumbar puncture is done, the nurse must prepare the child and the parents for the procedure with a simple explanation of what will occur. The child is positioned on a bed or a flat surface with the back next to the edge. The child lies on the side with the head flexed, the knees drawn up on the abdomen, and the back rounded (Figs 16-13 and 16-14). This position widens the space between the lumbar vertebral spines, making puncture of the subarachnoid space easier. By holding the child with one arm behind the neck and one behind the thighs and locking the hands in front of the child, the nurse can help the child maintain the flexed position. Talking softly to the child throughout the procedure can be calming.

A lumbar puncture is a sterile procedure. After skin preparation, the physician injects a local anesthetic and then inserts the needle. After the stylet is removed, a few drops of CSF are allowed to drip out before the manometer is attached. Pressure is recorded at the point where CSF stops rising. Appropriate samples of CSF are taken in sterile containers. Closing pressure is measured, and the needle is withdrawn. An adhesive bandage is applied at the site.

The nurse must always be alert for respiratory complications when the child's head is flexed. If CSF pressure is very high, herniation of the brainstem through the foramen magnum is possible with sudden release of pressure upon puncture. The *Queckenstedt test* (manual compression of the internal jugular veins, which normally causes a rise in CSF pressure) is contraindicated when CSF pressure is elevated.

The child's room should be kept cool and quiet, and all environmental stimuli should be reduced. Photophobia requires dimming a bright light. If the child has seizures, or is unconscious, the previously discussed nursing measures should be taken. Measures to reduce fever are used (see Chap. 16).

Accurate measurement of intake and output is essential. If oral food or fluids are allowed, feedings may be very slow. A patent intravenous line will be needed for several days, making it essential to protect and preserve the infusion site. The nurse must observe for side effects of antibiotics used in therapy. The urine specific gravity is monitored and there is a careful balancing of intake and output. Daily weights must be ordered.

Grouping nursing care activities together allows the child periods of uninterrupted rest. Play and other diversionary activities are provided as recovery begins.

Encephalitis

Encephalitis is a complex inflammation of the central nervous system. It is often associated with mumps, rubeola, chickenpox, herpes, and mosquito-borne viruses (California, eastern or western equine, and St. Louis encephalitis). Encephalitis due to mumps or rubeola can be prevented by immunization. The virus cannot be identified in more than half the cases of encephalitis.

The onset may be slow or rapid. Characteristically there is headache, fever, and drowsiness with a progressive decrease in consciousness. Nausea,. vomiting, malaise, and signs of increased ICP point to cerebral involvement. CSF studies may show a slight elevation in pressure and white blood count (Table 30-13). Seizures are likely in an infant.

Medical and nursing care is primarily supportive. The acute stage is often a medical emergency, and conscientious nursing care is essential. Careful monitoring of cerebral edema, fever, respiratory and neurological status, and fluid and electrolyte balance is important. Medications may be used to control increased ICP.

The prognosis is guarded. Death is not unusual. Recovery may be dramatic or may take several weeks. Mental retardation, seizures, or motor impairment may follow encephalitis. Family support, teaching, rehabilitation, and follow-up care depend on the outcome of the illness.

Reye syndrome

Pathophysiology In selected incidents a minor viral illness results in a severe encephalopathy called *Reye syndrome*. This massive physiological crisis strikes with frightening swiftness and frequently has fatal consequences. Children are affected from the age of 6 months through adolescence. Incidence is greatest between the months of November and March.[83]

Reye syndrome is the result of an internal buildup of ammonia in the blood (more than 50 μg/ml) and a rapid form of liver damage due to fatty tissue degeneration. Cerebral edema causes coma, hyperventilation, tachycardia, brain damage, or death. With vigorous medical intervention, 60 to 80 percent of children recover.[84]

The child develops severe, persistent vomiting after an apparent recovery from influenza (often type B) or chickenpox (varicella). Soon the child complains of fatigue, drowsiness, or general listlessness. A few hours to a few days after the vomiting develops, the first signs of encephalopathy appear. The child may become disoriented and combative and may hallucinate and lose consciousness.

The diagnosis is based on a history of viral illness, evidence of cerebral dysfunction (electroencephalographic changes), and a liver biopsy showing fatty degeneration. Laboratory tests reveal hypoglycemia, elevated ammonia, elevated levels of serum glutamic oxaloacetic transaminase and serum glutamic pyruvic transaminase, and a prolonged prothrombin time—all reflecting a decrease in liver function. There is usually a combined respiratory alkalosis and metabolic acidosis.[85]

There is an apparent relationship between the use of salicylates and Reye snydrome.[86] Research suggests that ingestion of salicylates in combination with viral illness may cause the structural damage seen in Reye syndrome.[87,88]

Treatment Medical treatment varies from conservative approaches based on supportive care to dramatic interventions involving total exchange transfusions or total body washouts. Management is based on staging of the disease according to level of consciousness and EEG findings. Various clinical stages have been described and are used to determine the severity of the illness and the aggressiveness of treatment (Table 30-15). The child who progresses rapidly through these stages or who goes beyond stage 3 has a poorer prognosis than others with less severe disease.

Table 30-15 Criteria for Staging in Reye Syndrome

Stage I	Drowsiness, lethargy, vomiting, temperature elevated; grade I EEG
Stage II	Disorientation, combativeness, hyperventilation, tachycardia, purposeful response to pain; grade 2 or 3 EEG
Stage III	Deepening coma, decorticate posturing in response to pain—dilated pupils. Response to light; grade 3 or 4 EEG
Stage IV	Deepening coma, spontaneous decerebrate posture, dilated pupils, temperature elevated; grade 3 or 4 EEG
Stage V	Cessation of spontaneous respirations, temperature elevated; grade 5 or silent EEG

Sources: Adapted from Peggy Dalgas, "Reye's Syndrome Update," *MCN* **8**:346–347 (September–October 1983); and Martha Rogers et al., "National Reye Syndrome Surveillance, *1982*," Pediatrics **75**(2):261 (February 1985).

Medical treatment includes constant monitoring of (1) fluid and electrolytes, (2) central venous pressure, (3) arterial blood gases, (4) liver function, (5) ventilation, and (6) ICP. Drug therapy may be used to sterilize the bowel in order to decrease ammonia formation and also to decrease cerebral edema. Exchange transfusions and total body washouts are some of the methods used to remove toxins and ammonia and provide needed clotting factors.

Nursing management The child who is severely ill with Reye syndrome requires intensive nursing care to support vital functions. Basic supportive care and accurate assessment of neurological status are essential. A nasogastric tube, an endotracheal tube, a urinary catheter, an intravenous line, and other equipment for monitoring pressures, gas exchange, and vital functions may be used.

Providing emotional and psychological support for the family is a nursing priority. A sudden illness of such serious consequence is a terrifying experience. Care must be taken when explaining the important function of each piece of equipment and when helping the parents support their child. They may be afraid to stay in the room with the child, much less touch the child.

Although the mortality rate is high, recovery can be very rapid and often occurs without any neurological damage. Usually the child experiences stress and anxiety when he or she awakens in a strange, frightening environment with no idea of what has happened. The child needs orientation to the surroundings and the illness. Above all, the child needs the parents present during this difficult period.

ALTERATIONS DUE TO TRAUMA: PHYSICAL OR CHEMICAL

Head injuries

An injury to the head can cause a skull fracture or damage to the soft tissue of the brain, leading to bruising, edema, or hemorrhage. Children are especially prone to head injuries as a result of birth injury, falls, motor vehicle accidents, sports injuries, or physical abuse. One-half of all children who die from accidents have some kind of head injury. Children's resilient skulls, however, are more able to absorb and withstand a blow than those of older individuals. Yet because children's tissues are fragile and more easily damaged, long-term effects are more likely.

Pathophysiology The skull varies in thickness from 2 to 6 mm; the thinnest part is in the temporoparietal area. Fractures running through the grooves under the skull can cause tearing of blood vessels and severe hemorrhage. Most skull fractures are *linear* (there is no displacement of bone) and can be asymptomatic. *Depressed skull fractures* (broken pieces of bone pushed inward) are unusual in children under 3 years of age and usually follow a high-velocity blow. A basal skull fracture with dural tears can allow seepage of CSF out of the nose (rhinorrhea) or ear (otorrhea).

Soft tissue injury to the brain is due to the forces of acceleration, deceleration, and deformation. These forces cause stress to brain tissue through movement of the brain within the cranium.[89]

The term *coup* is used to describe the bruising of the brain at the site of trauma. Because the skull moves faster than the brain when hit, it also stops moving sooner. The slower-moving brain rebounds off the skull and is injured on the opposite side; this injury is termed a *contrecoup*.

Shearing stresses, due to this unequal movement of brain tissue, negative pressure, stretching, and compression, act to cause shock, laceration with hemorrhage, increased CSF, and cerebral edema. Regardless of the cause, the physical damage to the brain produces several clinical entities.

A *concussion* is the most frequent type of closed head injury in children. It is characterized by a transient and reversible neuronal dysfunction leading to a brief loss of consciousness. Memory loss of events before (retrograde amnesia) or after (anterograde amnesia) the injury is common. Damage is diffuse, with shearing of many axons in the brainstem and subcortical areas.[90] The signs and symptoms include headache, pallor, vomiting, apathy, and irritability.

Cerebral *contusions* or lacerations are more severe types of injuries, causing hemorrhagic lesions and tears in the brain tissue. They are deemed major head injuries and are considered a medical emergency. Contusions can cause focal neurological disturbances or more widespread damage when cerebral edema is present. Unconsciousness may last for a longer time than with concussion, and abnormal neurological signs are present. The posttraumatic period is characterized by more severe symptoms—mild fever, vomiting, headache, somnolence, and confusion—lasting for a longer time than in a concussion.

When the brain injury is severe, a hematoma may result. Hematomas are classified according to their location as follows:

1. *Extradural* Between the dura and the skull
2. *Subdural* Between the dura and the arachnoid
3. *Subarachnoid* Bleeding into the subarachnoid space
4. *Intracerebral* Within the cerebral tissues themselves

An *extradural hematoma* frequently follows a skull fracture that causes tearing of the middle meningeal artery (Fig. 30-18*A*). Brain compression occurs rapidly because of arterial bleeding, and tentorial herniation is likely. (See the section "Increased Intracranial Pressure" earlier in this chapter.) Treatment is the removal of the clot. The mortality rate is 25 percent.

A *subdural hematoma* (Fig 30-18*B*) occurs 10 times more frequently in children than other hematomas.[91] It is usually bilateral and due to venous bleeding. A great deal of blood can accumulate in the young child's skull before signs of increased ICP occur (Table 30-5). Subacute and chronic subdural hematomas are frequently found in abused children (Fig 30-18*B*). Subdural hematomas occur most frequently in children under 2 years of age.

An *acute subdural hematoma* is associated with meningeal tears, severe head injury, and cerebral edema. The mortality rate is over 50 percent. Symptoms of a *subacute subdural hematoma* appear within 3 days to 3 weeks after the injury. Symptoms of a *chronic subdural hematoma* appear within 3 weeks to 6 months.[92] Subtle mood changes, irritability, drowsiness, seizures, and decreasing consciousness are signs of a subdural hematoma. The very young child will have bulging fontanels and mild head enlargement.

Repeated subdural taps over a 10-day period are used to treat chronic subdural hematomas in infants. Excess blood is removed and accurately measured. Surgery is necessary if bleeding does not stop or in older children if the sub-

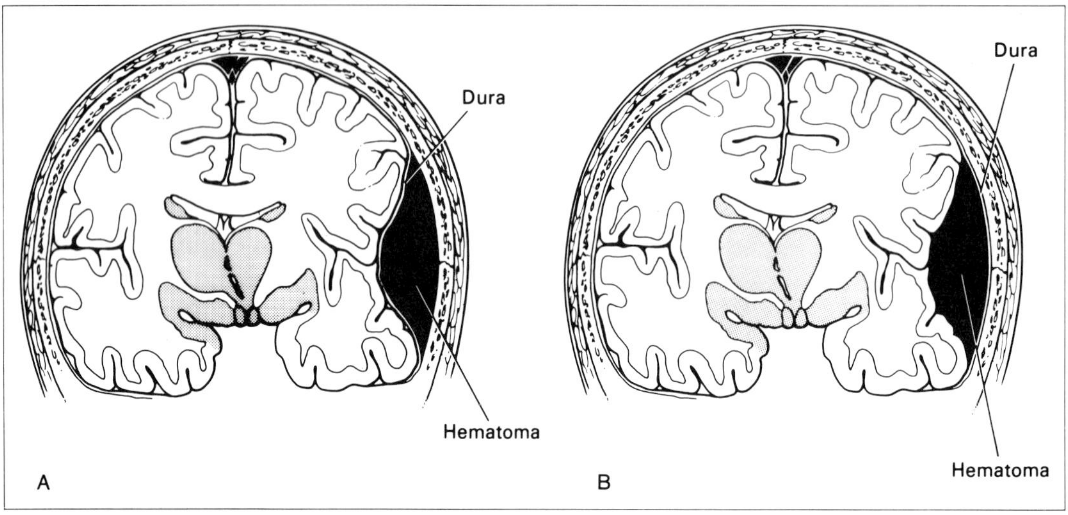

Figure 30-18 Hematomas. (*A*) Extradural. (*B*) Subdural. (*From Beverly A. Bowens, "The Nervous System," in M. Armstrong et al.* [eds.], *McGraw-Hill Handbook of Clinical Nursing, McGraw-Hill, New York, 1979. Used with permission.)*

dural space cannot be reached by subdural puncture. A shunt, similar to that used in hydrocephalus, is often put in place to treat communicating hydrocephalus, a frequent complication.

Diagnosis of head injuries is based on a complete neurological assessment, a skull x-ray, a CAT scan, an echoencephalogram, or angiographic studies. Lumbar punctures are not done if any signs of increased ICP are present.

Treatment Treatment of a head injury is based on the severity of the injury. With a mild concussion and loss of consciousness for less than 5 min, the child may be observed closely at home for 24 h. Indications for at-home observation include stable alertness, normal vital signs, normal neurological assessment, no more than three vomiting episodes, and parents who can be relied on to observe the child carefully.

The parents may wonder about letting their child sleep. They need careful instructions about how to observe their child and what signs indicate danger. The parents should be instructed to check their child every hour in the following ways:

1. Wake up the sleeping child. Is it easy to wake the child? Is the child alert and oriented to time, place, and other people?
2. Check the child's pupils for size, equality, and reaction to light.
3. Check the movement and strength of the extremities. Are the child's hand grasps of equal strength?

The parents are instructed to bring their child to the hospital if drowsiness is worse, if the child does not respond, if vomiting or headache increases, if one-sided weakness develops, or if the pupils appear unequal in size or reaction to light.

More serious head injuries are characterized by longer periods of unconsciousness or a period of alertness followed by decreasing consciousness, seizures, or repeated vomiting. Treatment is based on assessment of neurological status and other injuries (Table 30-16). The child must be hospitalized.

Fluids are restricted to 75 percent of normal because of cerebral edema. Cerebral edema is also managed with corticosteroids (dexamethasone), hypertonic solutions (short-term usage), and hyperventilation via controlled ventilation. Hyperventilation, with the Pa_{CO_2} kept at 25 to 30 mmHg, will reduce cerebral blood flow. Less blood flow, and therefore less volume and pressure, will give the swollen brain more room. Blood gases are monitored closely if a respirator is used. ICP monitoring may also be done.[93]

Laboratory tests are done to monitor kidney

Table 30-16 Checklist for Head Injury Assessment

Airway
Head:
  Lacerations
  Depressed skull fracture
  Drainage from ears, nose, mouth
Neurological status:
  Level of consciousness
  Vital signs
  Pupils, size, reaction, movement
  Motor and sensory function
  Breathing pattern
Bleeding
Broken bones
Bladder, bowel control

function and sepsis. A urinary catheter is used to monitor output. Occasionally a cooling blanket is necessary if fever is difficult to control.

Clear drainage from the nose or ear should be checked with Dextrostix for the presence of glucose, which identifies the drainage as CSF. Antibiotics are used with any penetrating injuries to prevent infection.

Surgical treatment is used for depressed fractures and removal of hematomas. A Jackson-Pratt drain is often placed in the epidural space to drain off excess blood after surgery. It must be recharged periodically as it fills with blood. Since its suction decreases as it is filled, the bulb should be emptied frequently using sterile technique. The blood is measured accurately and may be replaced (by transfusion) with whole blood on a volume basis.

Nursing management The neurological examination forms the baseline for all future observations of the child and may be considered in the decision concerning surgical intervention. Level of consciousness remains the most sensitive indicator of neurological condition. Pupillary responses and vital signs must also be checked frequently.

It is imperative that nurses document their assessments clearly, accurately, and completely. Objective evidence is essential to document a trend or change in the child's condition. Vital signs are often checked every 15 min for 4 h and then every hour. As the child improves, the frequency is decreased.

The child who is unconscious needs meticulous nursing care. Hypoventilation must be prevented, and an airway maintained. The child is turned and suctioned as necessary. The head and neck should be kept in straight alignment, and the head of the bed elevated 30° to increase venous return from the head. With any fluid loss or drainage from a laceration, it is important to estimate the amount on the dressing. Dressings should be reinforced or changed before they become wet on the outside to prevent entrance of a pathogen into the wound. Catheter care, accurate measurements of intake and output, and daily weights are important. Passive range-of-motion exercises and elastic stockings aid in venous return.

The child may be confused and combative. A screaming child is difficult to manage and may cause the nurse such unwelcome feelings as frustration and anger. The nurse must remember that bruising of the brain causes the irrational behavior. Restraining the child can lead to agitation, and thus increased ICP, and should be avoided if possible.

It is helpful to talk soothingly to the child. A calm, gentle touch and voice will be reassuring. The child's parents should be encouraged to keep contact with the child. The nurse should also remain with the child as much as possible.

The nurse should make another neurological assessment and look for changes if the child's condition changes. Any localizing signs should be noted. A child may need to be checked every 3 to 4 min so that a detailed report can be given to the attending physician. Nursing care focuses on early recognition of complications.

Children recover from head injuries amazingly well, although long-term rehabilitation may be necessary after severe injuries. Posttraumatic amnesia, or loss of day-to-day memory, is related to the degree of brain damage and length of unconsciousness. Memory may be one of the last functions to return. The child can be expected to experience 2 days of posttraumatic amnesia for each day of decreased level of consciousness.[94]

Some children develop the *posttraumatic syndrome:* severe headache, dizziness, tinnitus, double vision, difficulty focusing, slight ataxia, personality changes, poor coordination, depression, and learning difficulties. Ordinarily, children experience fewer problems than adults. By the end of a year, these symptoms usually disappear.

Posttraumatic seizures develop more frequently in children than in adults—usually within 1 to 3 months. Prophylactic anticonvulsant therapy is sometimes begun during hospitalization and is tapered off in a few years if no seizures occur.

Spinal cord injuries

Spinal cord trauma in childhood is most often the result of an accident or a sports injury. Damage to the bone or cord and nerve roots can be caused by fracture, dislocation, interruption of vascular supply, compression, contusion, or laceration. Hyperextension, flexion, and rotation forces can all cause various degrees of damage. The sites most often affected in children include C1 to C2, C5 to C6, and T11 to L2.

Pathophysiology A cervical spinal injury can produce paralysis of all four extremities (quadriplegia) with involvement of respiratory muscles. Injury at C1 to C2 is usually incompatible with life. With a thoracic-level spinal cord injury, the muscles of the lower extremities, bladder, and rectum are involved. Usually automatic urinary activity is possible. With a lumbar-level spinal cord injury, flaccid paralysis of the lower extremities, bladder, and rectum results, with no automatic bladder activity. Table 30-17 lists the expected activities of daily living that a child (or adult) can eventually manage, according to the level of injury.

When injury occurs, edema, inflammation, and ischemia develop in the spinal cord at the site of the injury. The immediate signs of compression are loss of movement and sensation below the level of the injury, urinary retention, absence of reflexes, and pain at the injury site. *Spinal shock* occurs with the sudden disruption of central and autonomic pathways and leads to a *flaccid* paralysis, lack of reflexes, vasodilatation, and hypotension.

When spinal shock is present and reflexes are absent, there will be (1) atrophy of both the paralyzed and noninvolved muscles, (2) an atonic bladder and urinary retention, (3) respiratory difficulty with a higher lesion, (4) calcium loss, (5) great risk of pressure sores, and (6) inability to regulate body temperature (with higher lesions). Spinal shock lasts from 1 day to 6 weeks, when autonomic reflex activity returns. Usually the shorter the period of spinal shock, the greater the degree of recovery. With the return of some reflex activity, there may be muscle twitching, increased muscle tone, and involuntary muscle movement. This increase in activity may give false hope to the child and the family concerning a complete recovery.

The return of spinal reflexes can lead to contractures and *autonomic dysreflexia*. Autonomic dysreflexia constitutes an emergency. The increase in sympathetic activity causes systolic blood pressure to rise to over 200 mmHg. The child experiences a severe headache, sweating, shivering, flushing of the face and upper extremities, piloerection, and cardiac arrhythmias. Seizures and retinal or cerebral hemorrhages may be precipitated. Treatment consists of removing the stimulus and reducing the blood pressure.

The usual causes of autonomic dysreflexia are an overdistended bladder, fecal impaction, and other types of sensory overload such as leg spasms, a decubitus ulcer, or overdistention of the stomach. Treatment is immediate removal of the cause. The bladder should be emptied gradually, since sudden decompression can cause a quick drop in blood pressure. Careful, gentle manual removal of an impaction followed by a suppository is a reasonably safe approach for fecal impaction.

Initially the child should be placed in a sitting position (if possible), and the physician notified. Ganglionic blocking agents may be necessary. The best treatment is prevention by immediate investigation of early signs of distress (gooseflesh, restlessness, and perspiration) and prevention of triggering events. Both the child and the nurse must be alert for the development of this complication.

In the final stages of cord injury, neurological signs stabilize. Young children with high thoracic and cervical lesions are prone to develop curvature of the spine because of unequal muscle tension and spasticity. Reflex activity in the child with a high injury reaches its maximum in about 2 years and then diminishes.

Treatment The initial care of a cord-injured child is very important. A coordinated team trained in stabilization and transfer techniques should move the child. Early management is supportive of vital functions. The last normal cord segment is used to classify the injury. A child with complete C7 function level has a functioning C7 root but no function below that level and should be able to bend and straighten the elbow (Table 30-17).

X-rays and a neurological exam are done. Oxygen, assisted respiration, maintenance of blood pressure, nasogastric suction, intravenous dexamethasone, prophylactic heparin in chil-

Table 30-17 ADL Functional Ability Associated with Level of Spinal Injury

Level	Motor Innervation	Spared	Quick Check of Function after Injury	Independence	Equipment and Abilities
C_3	C_1 to C_3: neck trapezius	Head rotation	—	No	Respirator or electrophrenic implant—quadriplegia
C_4	Diaphragm	Neck stability, diaphragm (respiratory insufficiency)	—	No	Electric wheelchair propulsion, puff control, externally powered devices
C_5	Deltoid, biceps	Elbow flexion, supination	Lifts elbow to shoulder	Variable	Electric wheelchair or rim projections, assisted sliding board transfer, pressure relief, powered wrist-hand orthosis—assisted with bladder and bowel management.
C_6	Extensor (carpi) radialis	Wrist extension, elbow pronation, fair shoulder stability	—	Independent in feeding, grooming, dressing, upper extremity; may be independent in wheelchair	Wrist-driven flexor hinge orthosis prehension; wheelchair hand rim projections to relieve skin pressure; wheelchair driven with cuff and hand controls; lift for transfer. May do self-catheterization
C_7	Triceps; extends elbow, wrist, hand	Finger and elbow extension, weak finger flexion	—	Independent in wheelchair	Bed and car transfer, electric typewriter. Drives with hand control. Travels on plane. Does self-catheterization
C_8 to T_1	Flexor digitorum	Hand intrinsics	Grip	Independent in wheelchair	Standard wheelchair rims. Writes, touch-types, drives with hand control
T_2 to T_{12}	Intercostals, thoracic and abdominal musculature	Trunk stability	—	Independent in wheelchair	Bath transfer, wheelchair to 6-in curbs and into car. Drives car with hand control
L_1 to L_3	Abdominal musculature	Hip flexion, weak knee extension	—	Home ambulation with knee-ankle-foot orthosis, crutches	Bladder management program necessary
L_4	Quadriceps	Knee extension	Lifts leg or flexes hip	Community ambulation	Bladder management program necessary
L_5 to S_2	Gastrocnemius, bowel and bladder, ankle, foot	Hip abduction and extension, foot dorsiflexion, strong plantar flexion	Extends knee, pushes toe downward; ankle jerk	Ambulation with ankle-foot orthosis or none, possibly cane	Bladder management program necessary. Travels on bus

Source: Adapted from Gabriella Molna, *Pediatric Rehabilitation,* Williams & Wilkins, Baltimore, 1985, p. 287.

dren 10 years and older, and traction may be indicated.[95] Surgery is done only if one of the following conditions is present:

1. There is an increasing neurological deficit.
2. Bone is impinging on the cord or nerve root.
3. There is an opening in the dura.
4. Abdominal wounds are communicating with the spinal cord.

Nursing management Children with spinal cord injuries require excellent long-term nursing care. Although the care is similar to that required by the infant with a myelomeningocele, it differs considerably because of the child's age (usually the child is an adolescent) and the suddenness of the injury.

When motor dysfunction is present, the nursing care goals are to maintain physiological functioning; to prevent complications of immobility; to help resolve issues of grief, dependency, and body image; and to promote adaptation.[96]

Initially, vital functions must be maintained. Flexion of the neck must be avoided to prevent airway obstruction. Decreased vital capacity, oxygen distribution, and respiratory reserves all contribute to respiratory difficulty or arrest. Assisted ventilation and suctioning may be necessary. Some children will be helped with incentive spirometers. Chest physiotherapy may be done every 2 h. Assisted coughing is helpful with higher lesions. In assisted coughing, the child breathes in and out at least three times. Then the nurse pushes in and up on the diaphragm to help the child cough. This procedure may be necessary every 2 to 3 h with a new lesion.

Children with spinal cord injuries are at increased risk for pressure sores because they lack vasomotor control and sensation and have decreased peripheral circulation. Normal pressure from body weight can cause tissue ischemia in 30 min. It is imperative that these children be turned at least every 1 to 2 h; their skin must be kept clean and dry. Vigorous rubbing and soap should be avoided. Children should be lifted, not dragged, across the sheets. Foam elbow, heel, and sacrum protectors and gentle massage are helpful. Alternating pressure mattresses are used frequently.[97] Donuts and rubber rings should never be used. When children are immobilized, their healing powers are diminished because cell breakdown is greater than cell production. If a decubitus ulcer develops, the child can lose up to 50 mg of protein a day. Maintaining intact skin requires much less nursing care time than caring for a decubitus ulcer.

The child should be properly positioned in bed as well as turned frequently. Once the acute phase is over, active and passive range-of-motion exercises are begun. If spasticity is present, the limb should be positioned in opposition to the position of contraction. Keeping the child in a prone position with the limbs straight for several short periods each day helps prevent contractures. A great deal of care must be taken when moving a child with a flaccid paralysis in order to protect the limbs from strain or injury.

Nutritional needs are increased, and the child requires a diet high in vitamins, calories, and protein. Weight should be measured and monitored as soon as possible. Fluids should be maintained at 1500 to 2000 ml a day as soon as peristalsis returns. Inactivity and calcium loss from bones predispose the child to renal calculi. Urine is checked for color, clarity, specific gravity, and amount.

Remobilization of the child begins after the acute phase to minimize osteoporosis. Gradually the child is raised from a lying position to a sitting position and then to an erect position. Mobilization involves the following:

1. Proper fit and application of external spinal mobilization appliances
2. Gradual elevation of the child's head and trunk
3. Careful monitoring of vital signs and assessing for hypotension and syncope
4. Pressure relief techniques
5. Stable transfer and bed mobility techniques[98]

Eventually wheelchairs, braces, and adaptive devices will be selected to allow the child to gain maximum mobility and independence.

Damage to the cord results in a neuropathic (neurogenic) bladder and bowel. Normally, cerebral control provides an inhibitory influence over the micturition reflex when the bladder fills to keep it from emptying spontaneously. When upper motor neuron damage occurs, this control is gone, and the bladder will empty automatically, but often incompletely, once reflex activity returns. If the conus medullaris or peripheral nerves to the bladder are damaged, the bladder has no innervation and will overdistend. Eventually this causes overflow incontinence. It is also possible to have mixed lesions that produce varying degrees of these conditions.

Because bladder function may not always be

predictable on the basis of the cord-level injury, each child must be evaluated urologically. Reflex tests, blood tests, and kidney and bladder studies are performed to establish functional ability and to determine a baseline for future evaluation. Since renal failure due to repeated infections is the most common cause of death in the post-acute phase of spinal cord injury, bladder management is extremely important.

Bladder training is achieved through methods such as intermittent catheterization, triggering mechanisms, pharmacological agents, and sometimes urinary diversion. (Bladder training is discussed in greater detail in Chap. 20.) Fluids are regulated, and intake and output are measured carefully. The urine may be kept acidic with ascorbic acid (1 to 4 g daily) and cranberry juice to minimize the formation of stones.

Bowel training is based on a high-roughage diet, fluids, use of suppositories and stool softeners, activity, and manual stimulation. The rectum should be stimulated with a gloved, lubricated finger prior to insertion of a suppository. The tip of the finger is inserted into the rectum, and the finger is gently rotated for 15 to 30 s. Usually, regular bowel movements and good control can be established by following a consistent routine. Table 30-18 summarizes the components of a bowel management program.[99,100]

Table 30-18 Components of Bowel Management Programs

Strategy	Action
Diet management	Nutritious diet high in fiber and bulk; alters stool consistency
Colace (dioctyl sodium sulfosuccinate)	Softens stool
Metamucil	Alters stool consistency; forms soft, bulky stools
Senna	Mild laxative action
Digital stimulation	Causes sphincter to relax so stool can be expelled
Suppositories:	
Bisacodyl	Irritates bowel and initiates reflex peristalsis
Vacuetts	Releases carbon dioxide, distends bowel, initiates peristalsis
Glycerine	Softens stool and stimulates reflex peristalsis
Positioning:	
Sitting position	Preferred; peristalsis is greater, gravity assists in stool elimination
Lying position	Left side-lying position
Abdominal massage	Stimulates peristalsis
Offer liquid 15 min prior to initiation of bowel routine	Increases peristalsis

Self-control in bowel and bladder functions is an important symbol of autonomy and self-control. "Accidents" can damage children's self-esteem and increase their sense of isolation. Including children in plans and goal setting increases their sense of participation and self-control.

The nurse must recognize that the child and the family are totally unprepared for the effects of spinal cord injury. At first the situation may be too much for them to comprehend in all its ramifications. Shock, disbelief, and denial are common. During the acute phase, the child may appear tense, jittery, and apathetic. Dependency needs are increased. Loss of control of body functions and abilities causes tremendous changes in body image and self-concept. Day by day, the child and the family are forced to face the impact that the injury will have on the child's future life.

After the initial acute phase subsides, anxiety, anger, and depression may become more evident. As the child is confronted with reality, issues of mobility and self-care arise. The child is faced with learning new skills when self-image and self-esteem may be at a low ebb. The family is confronted with financial problems and long-term rehabilitation needs.

As in any grieving process, the emotional and physical changes that occur will cause the child to fluctuate among many emotional states. The nurse will need to be knowledgeable about the tentative nursing prognosis so that preparation of the child and the family for the future can be accomplished. Appropriate communication shows concern and caring and emphasizes hopeful signs without giving false reassurance.

As recovery proceeds, the child and the family gradually become ready for more information. The nurse must guard against overwhelming them with all that must be learned.

Slowly, children and adolescents become curious about what their bodies can do. They decide that life is worth living after all and can then make amazing progress toward self-care.

Problems with self-concept can become particularly important in adolescents. Adolescents normally are sorting out their identity, establishing their independence, and exploring their sexuality. Suddenly all is changed. Depression is normal, as they grieve over this major loss.

Adolescents will have many concerns about sexuality. While a primary concern of young children is mobility, mature adolescents will give high priority to sexual function.[101] They will have many questions and concerns, which they may not be able to share. Information must be provided about what can be expected.

Sexual function in girls is usually unimpaired, except that genital sensation and reflex vaginal lubrication are decreased. Menstruation may cease for about 6 months and then return. A female with a spinal cord injury can usually become pregnant and deliver vaginally.

Sexual function in the male is unpredictable and much more likely to be altered. Reflex erection is possible with a high lesion and an intact sacral cord. Erection and ejaculation may be possible with incomplete lesions. Erection is not possible with cauda equina lesions. Ordinarily, males will be impotent. Intrapenile devices that provide a controlled erection are now available, making intercourse possible for more males. The male with a penile implant, however, is sterile.

Openness in communication with adolescents will help allay their fears and encourage sharing of anxieties. Sexual counseling should include helping adolescents learn how to express intimacy and how to be sexual human beings within the limitations placed on them. Nurses should examine their own attitudes toward sexuality and be familiar with all the ways in which individuals can find sexual gratification. When children's sexual role is altered, testing will occur with those around them. The nurse may have to set limits on behavior. The nurse keeps communication lines open and should understand the child's basic need to define his or her sexuality. The nursing care plan at the end of the chapter pertains to an adolescent male with a spinal cord injury.

Lead poisoning

Lead poisoning (plumbism) poses a serious health hazard to children under age 6, but especially to those between 1 and 3 years of age. Lead poisoning is usually due to the ingestion of nonfood substances (pica). It is an outgrowth of the toddler's curiosity and hand-to-mouth behavior.[102]

Until the 1940s, interior house paint contained lead. Young children often chewed on their painted cribs or window sills or ate paint chips. (A very small number of paint chips may contain up to 100 mg of lead.) Federal legislation was passed in 1973 prohibiting the use of lead-based paint in homes. Unfortunately, many older homes and apartment buildings have underlying layers of lead-based paint and plaster. Often these dwellings are in deteriorating slum areas, where children have limited environmental stimuli and poor diets and families are under social and economic stress.

Other sources of lead poisoning are improperly fired lead-glazed pottery, water from lead pipes, lead-based paints or toys, lead-sealed containers used for storage, and batteries. Recent studies indicate that soil and dust in areas surrounding heavily traveled inner-city highways have elevated lead contents as a result of the settling of atmospheric lead from automobile exhausts. Children who live near congested highways have higher lead concentrations in their blood than those who live in rural areas.[103] Children who "sniff" leaded gasoline can also be poisoned. Current data indicate that 4 percent of all American children under the age of 6 years have elevated blood lead levels.[104]

Pathophysiology The effect of lead on body systems is due to inhibition of certain enzymatic reactions that are essential to the transport of substances across cell membranes. Usually bone marrow is affected first. The production of heme is altered, leading to a hemolytic anemia, one of the initial signs of the disease. Although lead damages the cells of renal tubules and bone marrow, its effects on these tissues are reversible.

The effects of lead on the central nervous system are the most significant because they are probably irreversible. Symptoms range from mild neurological disability to acute encephalopathy manifested by hypertension, increased ICP, cerebral edema, stupor, seizures, coma, and even death. See Table 30-19 for classifications of lead poisoning.

Symptoms of chronic lead poisoning may not appear for several months and depend on the amount of lead ingested. Even when symptoms do occur, they may mimic those of viral infections or behavioral disturbances. Common symptoms are anorexia, abdominal pain, anemia, constipation, nausea, and vomiting. Behavioral changes include clumsiness, irritability, apathy, and lethargy. The young child may have difficulty with fine or gross motor skills that were mastered months before. Low-level lead poison-

Table 30-19 Classification of Lead Poisoning

	Mild	Moderate	Severe
Exposure	Soil or dust	Paint ingestion, predisposing iron deficiency, positive family history	Paint ingestion, secondary iron deficiency
Symptoms	None	Usually none; may be loss of appetite	Lethargy, fever, hepatosplenomegaly
Sequelae	Cognitive involvement	Behavioral and cognitive involvement	Ataxia, seizures, coma, increased ICP, neurological abnormalities
Lead levels	25 to 49 μg per 100 ml	49 to 70 μg per 100 ml	Above 70 μg per 100 ml
Complete blood count	Normal	Mild anemia	Basophilic stripping, anemia
EP levels	35 to 135 μg per 100 ml	125 to 250 μg per 100 ml	Above 250 μg per 100 ml

Source: Adapted from John W. Graef and Thomas E. Cone, Jr. (eds.), *Manual of Pediatric Therapeutics*, 3d ed., Little, Brown, Boston, 1985, p. 113.

ing may go undetected and manifest itself in underachievement in school. This is a national concern.

Detection Screening procedures for lead poisoning are based on measurement of the amount of lead or the erythrocyte protoporphyrin (EP) level in blood. In high-risk communities, the EP level is used for routine screening because it requires only a fingerstick.

Normal blood lead levels range from 15 to 40 μg/100 ml. When the blood level of lead is above 40 μg/100 ml, further diagnostic study is indicated, and chelating (ability to bind with a metal) treatment becomes mandatory at levels over 50 to 60 μg/100 ml. EP levels above normal (40 to 75 μg/100 ml) may indicate anemia but are almost always caused by lead poisoning when they exceed 190 μg/100 ml. Usually several diagnostic tests are combined, and clinical symptoms evaluated, before a course of treatment is begun.

Other signs of lead poisoning include:

1. Increased density in long bones at the metaphysis
2. Lead in the urine and hair
3. A blue lead line in gums
4. Increased protein and traces of lead in CSF

Treatment Treatment of lead poisoning is based on six principles:[105]

1. Removal of the child from the source of lead
2. Maintenance of adequate urine output while avoiding overhydration
3. Administration of chelating agents to remove the lead
4. Prevention of seizures and increased ICP
5. Detection of the source of lead and removing the lead from the source, if possible
6. Careful follow-up

Acute lead poisoning (encephalopathy) or chronic lead poisoning with high blood lead levels requires immediate treatment with chelating agents. These combine with lead in the blood and enhance excretion in the urine. Calcium disodium edetate (Ca EDTA) and dimercaprol (BAL) are two chelating agents used as antidotes for lead and other heavy-metal poisoning.[106] Penicillamine is an oral chelating agent used for children who do not tolerate Ca EDTA or BAL. (See Table 30-20.)

Symptomatic treatment involves control of seizures, oxygen and respiratory support, close observation of neurological status and kidney function, and monitoring of calcium and phosphorus levels. Chelating agents, especially Ca EDTA, also remove calcium and can be toxic to the kidneys.

Nursing management Ideally, nursing care focuses on the prevention of lead poisoning by identifying and helping screen children at risk. Prevention is especially important, since the prognosis following lead poisoning is not very good. The mortality rate can be as high as 25 percent following acute encephalopathy. Even with treatment, children with prolonged exposure to lead show residual effects such as mental

Table 30-20 Antidotes for Lead Poisoning

Antidote	Dose	Comments
Dimercaprol (BAL)	3 to 5 mg/kg q4h IM for 2 days, then 2.5 to 3 mg/kg q6h IM for 2 days; then q12h for 7 days	Observe for fever, myalgia, hypotension or hypertension, pulmonary edema. Also used for arsenic poisoning.
Calcium disodium ethylenediamine-tetraacetate (Ca EDTA)	50 to 75 mg/kg per day IM or IV in three to six divided doses up to 5 days with encephalopathy or blood lead levels 100 mg per 100 ml or more	Given till urine returns to nontoxic levels. Can cause renal tubular necrosis, and so fluid must be given in adequate quantities.
Penicillamine	100 mg/kg per day up to 1 g per day in divided doses up to 5 days	Do not give if allergic to penicillin. Monitor for proteinuria. Antidote for copper, lead, and mercury.

Source: Adapted from M. Wiener, G. Pepper, G. Kuhn-Weisman, and J. Rimano, *Clinical Pharmacology and Therapeutics in Nursing*, McGraw-Hill, New York, 1985, p. 995.

retardation, seizure disorders, and behavioral disturbances.

For those children who are acutely ill, the nurse must carry out the designated medical regimen and administer chelating agents. When Ca EDTA and BAL are administered concurrently through an intramuscular route, a child can receive up to 12 injections per day or 60 injections in 5 days. Any child who receives that many injections will need careful preparation, an opportunity to "check off" each one on a chart, and play therapy to help work out his or her feelings about this invasive therapy.

Injections must be rotated carefully. If each site is divided into four corners and a center and if six muscles are used (right and left vastus lateralis, ventrogluteal, and gluteus maximus), each specific location will be used only twice. A local anesthetic may be added to the medication and injected first so that pain is reduced.

Nursing care includes careful neurological assessment, measurement of intake and output, and support of basic needs. Seizure precautions are necessary because of cerebral edema. All aspects of nursing care described earlier for the unconscious child are appropriate for the child with acute encephalopathy.[107]

Before the child leaves the hospital, the home environment must be evaluated and made lead-free if possible. All possible sources of lead must be removed, and close supervision guaranteed to keep children away from sources that cannot be eliminated.

The health department and the medical social worker often must be involved, along with other members of the health care team. With increased awareness of symptoms, effective screening programs, and quick intervention, there should continue to be a decline in the incidence of lead poisoning in children.

Nursing Care Plan: Spinal Cord Damage*

Patient: Tim Jones | *Age:* 16 years | *Date of Admission:* July 6

ASSESSMENT

Date: September 4
Diagnosis: Fracture dislocation of C5-6
Sex: Male
Religion: Catholic
Weight: 62 kg
Parents' Marital Status: Married
Siblings: 3 sisters—14, 13, 12 years
Allergies: None known

PHYSICAL EXAMINATION

Temperature: 38.5°C (101.3°F). Respiration: 30 breaths per minute. Pulse: 92. Blood pressure: 100/60.

GENERAL APPEARANCE

Tim gives the appearance of a well-developed 16-year-old boy. He cannot move his lower extremities and lacks any sensation below the nipple line. He has gross movement of his upper extremities but lacks fine finger movement and has spotty areas of sensation in arms. His skin is in good condition with no pressure areas. His lungs are congested, and upon auscultation scattered rales and rhonchi are heard throughout both lung fields. He said, "I'm going to walk out of here; you just wait and see."

HISTORY OF PRESENT ILLNESS

Tim is a 16-year-old white male who suffered a fracture dislocation of C5 and C6 when he dived into shallow water at a gravel pit. Shortly after admission, Tim underwent a cervical fusion and is now stabilized with a Philadelphia collar. Tim's motor and sensory levels are intact at C7. After spending 4 weeks on a neurology unit, Tim was transferred to a rehabilitation unit 1 week ago.

As Tim's primary nurse, you assess that he is depressed, sometimes refuses his nursing care, and is unmotivated to learn about, or participate in, self-care.

Although Tim's family lives 150 mi away, Tim's mother is with him from early morning until late at night and is available for all his needs. Tim and his father were very close before the accident. His father now visits Tim on the weekends with the rest of the family.

PHYSICIAN'S ORDERS

1. Bladder retraining program:
   a. 1800-ml fluid program—400 ml at meals (8 A.M., 12 noon, and 6 P.M.) and 200 ml at 10 A.M., 2 P.M., and 4 P.M.
   b. Tap bladder q3h (automatic or upper motor neuron bladder)
   c. Intermittent catheterization q6h (immediately after every other bladder tapping)
   d. Urine culture and sensitivity every week
   e. Sulfamethoxazole, trimethoprim (Septra) 1 bid
2. Bowel retraining program:
   a. Dulcolax suppository qod
   b. High-fiber diet
   c. Colace 100 mg bid
3. Respiratory program:
   a. Chest physiotherapy and postural drainage q4h
   b. Deep breathing and supportive cough q1h to q2h while awake
4. Skin maintenance program:
   a. Turn q2h
   b. Sheepskin—full-length
   c. Up in wheelchair 1 to 2 h tid as tolerated—with a cushion
5. Nutrition
   a. High-protein, high-fiber diet
   b. Weigh weekly
6. Physical therapy
7. Occupational therapy
8. Recreational therapy

*Prepared by Kathy Orth, R.N., M.S. Formerly head nurse, Neuro-Rehabilitative Unit, St. Mary's Hospital, Rochester, Minn.

Nursing Diagnosis	Outcome Criteria*	Nursing Interventions	Evaluation and Modifications
1. Respiratory congestion related to neuromuscular impairment and decreased ability to move secretions	☐ Tim will not show any signs of congestion in 1 week, as evidenced by: **a.** Lungs clear upon auscultation **b.** Clear secretions or no secretions brought up with supportive cough, q1h while awake and q3h at night **c.** Respiratory rate within normal limits (fewer than 26 breaths per minute) ☐ Tim will describe the signs and symptoms of respiratory congestion.	☐ Auscultate lungs q4h before and after chest physiotherapy and postural drainage. ☐ Do chest physiotherapy and postural drainage q4h. ☐ Encourage deep breathing and assist with supportive cough q1h while Tim is awake. ☐ Voldyne q1h throughout the day. ☐ Observe for signs of respiratory distress: tachypnea, restlessness, and cyanosis. ☐ Teach Tim the importance of deep breathing and supportive cough. ☐ Teach Tim the signs and symptoms of respiratory congestion (increased temperature, productive cough, shortness of breath, and increased respiratory rate).	☐ Tim continues to show slight respiratory congestion. ☐ Tim's lungs were auscultated q4h. Scattered rhonchi in the bases of both lungs were noted. ☐ Deep breathing, supportive cough, and chest physiotherapy often result in no productive cough; when secretions are brought up, they are clear. ☐ Respiratory rate is consistently 20 to 24. Continue plan until the lungs are clear of congestion and then auscultate once a day. ☐ Continue EOCs (expected outcome criteria) and nursing interventions.
2. Alterations in bladder elimination: neurogenic bladder	☐ In 6 weeks Tim will demonstrate adherence to a bladder retraining program by emptying his bladder by suprapubic tapping of the bladder q3h.	☐ Instruct Tim in bladder retraining program: **a.** Reinforce the importance of completely emptying the bladder using an effective tapping technique to decrease residual urine volumes. Do intermittent catheterizations within 15 min after tapping is completed. **b.** Assist with tapping as needed—encourage Tim to tap his own bladder. **c.** Do intermittent catheterizations q6h until residuals are less than 75 ml for 3 consecutive days.	☐ Tim is cooperative and adheres to his bladder retraining program with reminders from the nursing staff. ☐ Tim is beginning to tap himself; he tires after 3 min and requires assistance. Urine volumes with tapping range from 75 to 150 ml. ☐ Residual urine volumes are running 150 to 250 ml.
	☐ Tim will maintain a fluid intake of 1800 ml—400 ml at meals (8 A.M., 12 noon, and 6 P.M.) and 200 ml at 10 A.M., 2 P.M., and 4 P.M.	☐ Make sure that Tim has access to fluids at the specified times. Encourage him to keep track of his own intake and output.	☐ Tim is adhering to the 1800-ml fluid program and is keeping track of input and output himself.

*For this patient, long-term goals (outcome criteria) are appropriate.

Nursing Diagnosis	Outcome Criteria*	Nursing Interventions	Evaluation and Modifications
	☐ Tim will help with perineal hygiene bid.	☐ Explain the importance of washing the perineal area bid to help prevent urinary tract infections. ☐ Assist Tim as needed with perineal hygiene.	☐ Perineal hygiene was performed by the nurse in the morning and before Tim went to sleep. The physical therapist will be contacted for assistive devices to aid Tim in this task.
	☐ Tim will describe the effects and side effects of Septra.	☐ Administer medication and describe how the medication helps keep the urine free from bacteria.	☐ Tim stated that he was taking Septra to help prevent urinary tract infections.
	☐ Tim will describe the signs and symptoms of urinary tract infections.	☐ Describe the signs and symptoms of urinary tract infections to Tim, including: **a.** Incontinence **b.** Difficulty obtaining results by tapping bladder **c.** Cloudy and/or foul-smelling urine **d.** A rise in the pH (↑ 7.0) of the urine (not always reliable) **e.** Temperature and chills **f.** Nausea	☐ Tim stated the signs and symptoms of an impending urinary tract infection: a rise in temperature, chills, incontinence, nausea, cloudy or foul-smelling urine, an increased pH in urine, and difficulty getting results when tapping the bladder. ☐ Continue plan.
3. Alterations in bowel elimination: neurogenic bowel	☐ In 4 weeks Tim will demonstrate how to empty his bowels at regularly scheduled intervals by adhering to a bowel retraining program.	☐ Instruct Tim and explain the bowel retraining program. Encourage an optimal level of independence.	☐ 9/18: Tim has been continent of bowel since beginning his bowel retraining program.
	☐ Tim will empty his bowels according to a regular schedule.	☐ Determine with Tim the preferred time of day to complete bowel evacuation—preferably after a meal. Stress the importance of establishing a regular schedule qod. Assess for problems with constipation or impaction.	☐ Tim is currently performing bowel care every other day after breakfast.
	☐ Tim will administer a Dulcolax suppository with the help of an assistive device.	☐ Explain the purpose and action of Dulcolax suppositories. Observe Tim's response to Dulcolax (when evacuation occurs after insertion of the suppository) and the nature of the results. Contact the occupational therapist to obtain an assistive device for inserting the suppository. ☐ Evaluate how effective the assistive device is.	☐ Tim still needs some help using his assistive device when inserting suppositories.

Nursing Diagnosis	Outcome Criteria*	Nursing Interventions	Evaluation and Modifications
	☐ Tim will eat at least eight fiber-containing foods daily.	☐ Explain the importance of bulk and fiber in the diet. Give Tim a list of foods that are high in fiber.	☐ When planning his daily menu, Tim chooses at least eight foods containing fiber and eats them consistently.
	☐ Tim will maintain a fluid intake of 1800 ml.	☐ Explain how fluid intake affects the bowels. Encourage Tim to keep his fluid intake up to 1800 ml per day.	☐ Intake is consistently 1800 ml.
	☐ Tim will describe the effects and side effects of Colace and Metamucil.	☐ Give Colace, 100 mg bid, for constipation first. ☐ Give Metamucil, 1 tsp bid. ☐ Explain the purpose and action of Colace (a stool softener) and Metamucil (a bulk-forming medication).	☐ Tim is able to describe the effects and side effects of Colace and Metamucil. ☐ Continue plan.
4. Self-care deficit related to neurological impairment	☐ Tim will reach an optimal level of independence in activities of daily living by the time of discharge. ☐ Tim will learn how to direct cares that he is not able to perform physically. ☐ With the help of assistive devices, Tim will be able to brush his hair, brush his teeth, wash his face and upper body, dress his upper body, and follow a similar pattern for bathing and dressing his lower extremities.	☐ Follow up and encourage Tim to use what he has learned in occupational therapy and physical therapy. ☐ Help Tim use assistive devices, orthotic (splinting) devices, or prosthetic devices, when performing activities of daily living. ☐ Emphasize independence by instructing Tim to direct his activities of daily living. ☐ Encourage mother and other family members to support Tim's independence. ☐ Teach the mother and other family members the skills needed to assist Tim in home care.	☐ 9/18: Tim is beginning to perform some activities of daily living with the help of assistive devices. ☐ Tim is not able to direct his own cares at this point. ☐ Tim is able to brush his hair using an assistive device. ☐ Tim is able to brush his teeth using an assistive device. ☐ Tim is able to wash his face, but he still needs assistance with the rest of his upper body. ☐ Tim is not able to dress his upper body yet or to wash or dress his lower extremities. ☐ Continue plan.
5. Potential for skin breakdown related to loss of sensation and decreased mobility	☐ Tim will describe the importance of following a skin care program and will not develop any areas of skin breakdown during and after hospitalization.	☐ Assess the skin for redness, rashes, and dryness at every turning. Turn Tim and rub the skin surfaces q2h when Tim is in bed. Use a cushion in the wheelchair and a water mattress in bed.	☐ 9/18: No skin breakdown noted.
	☐ Tim will describe the principles of preventing skin breakdown.	☐ Instruct Tim in the principles of good skin care.	☐ Tim is beginning to understand the principles of skin care. He does not know all the pressure points (bony prominences).
	☐ Tim will list the signs of impending skin breakdown.	☐ Describe the signs and symptoms of skin breakdown (e.g., a reddened area that does not blanch).	☐ Tim was able to verbalize the warning signs of skin breakdown.

Nursing Diagnosis	Outcome Criteria*	Nursing Interventions	Evaluation and Modifications
	☐ Tim will inspect his skin (especially areas prone to injury) bid.	☐ Provide a long-handled mirror so that Tim can begin to inspect his own skin. ☐ Identify bony prominences to Tim. ☐ Assist Tim as needed.	☐ Tim is not able to use his mirror effectively to inspect his skin; he needs practice.
	☐ Tim will eat a high-protein diet consistently.	☐ Help Tim choose a high-protein, high-fiber diet.	☐ Tim consistently eats a high-protein diet.
6. Potential joint contractures of upper and lower extremities related to muscle spasm and decreased mobility	☐ Tim will achieve and maintain optimum joint mobility as evidenced by: **a.** Absence of joint deformity **b.** Absence of contractures	☐ Maintain body alignment. ☐ Support and assist in the physical therapy program (PROM, AROM, etc.). ☐ Inspect the joints for impending contractures. ☐ Apply splints as ordered.	☐ Maximum joint mobility was noted. ☐ There were no complaints of joint stiffness. ☐ No contractures were noted.
7. Sexual dysfunction related to neuromuscular impairment	☐ Tim will display an optimum level of sexual health as evidenced by: **a.** Expressing feelings to the nursing staff about change in sexual function. **b.** Describing the separation of sexual function from sexuality.	☐ Assess Tim's concern about his sexuality. ☐ Display an attitude of acceptance and willingness to discuss sexual concerns. ☐ Explore Tim's feelings about loss of masculinity. ☐ Provide an opportunity for Tim to acquire information about expected sexual function and fertility.	☐ Tim has not expressed his feelings regarding his sexuality to the staff. His girlfriend visits regularly on weekends. ☐ Tim remains hesitant to discuss his feelings regarding sexuality. He must open up before this objective can be accomplished.
8. Grieving related to loss of neurological function	☐ Tim will come to accept his disability through: **a.** Verbalizing his feelings about his spinal cord injury and loss of function **b.** Exploring his future and changes in his life-style with the nurse, family, and friends	☐ Encourage Tim to look at his injury realistically and focus on his abilities rather than his disability. ☐ Display acceptance of Tim's behavior. ☐ Assist Tim in developing his independence and self-reliance. ☐ Provide an environment that is conducive to nurse-patient interaction. Spend time with Tim. ☐ Encourage Tim to share his feelings about his injury and his expectations in life. ☐ Encourage Tim and his family and friends to discuss their feelings with one another. ☐ Provide an opportunity for Tim to become involved in group discussions with other patients.	☐ Tim still feels that he will "walk out of here" and is not realistic about his disability. ☐ Tim is beginning to verbalize his feelings about his injury. ☐ Tim has not discussed any future expectations at this time. ☐ Continue plan.

References

1. Adams, Raymond D., and Maurice Victor, *Principles of Neurology,* 2d ed., McGraw-Hill, New York, 1981, p.235.
2. Taylor, Joyce, and Sally Ballenger, *Neurological Dysfunctions and Nursing Interventions,* McGraw-Hill, New York, 1980, p. 51.
3. Ibid., p. 307.
4. Berg, Bruce O. (ed.), *Child Neurology: A Clinical Manual,* Jones, Greenbrae, Calif., 1984, p. 179.
5. Lyons, Marilyn, "Recognition of Neurological Dysfunction," *Nurse Practitioner,* **4**(5):34 (September–October 1979).
6. Jones, Cathy, "Glasgow Coma Scale," *American Journal of Nursing* **79**(9):1551–1553 (September 1979).
7. Adams, op. cit., p. 240.
8. Ibid., p. 241.
9. DeJong, Russell, *The Neurological Examination,* Harper & Row, New York, 1979, p. 472.
10. Mayo Clinic and Mayo Foundation, *Clinical Examination in Neurology,* Saunders, Philadelphia, 1981, p. 40.
11. Berg, op. cit., p. 241.
12. Ibid., p. 246.
13. Ibid., p. 248.
14. *Epilepsy: Medical Aspects,* Comprehensive Epilepsy Program, University of Minnesota, Minneapolis, 1984, p. 1.
15. Feldman, Robert G., "Epilepsy in Adolescents and Adults," in Frederick C. Barett et al. (ed.), *1981 Current Therapy,* Saunders, Philadelphia, 1981, p. 772–773.
16. *Epilepsy: Medical Aspects,* p. 1.
17. Berg, op. cit., pp. 179–180.
18. Dodson, W. Edwin, "Epilepsy in Childhood," in Barett et al., op. cit., p. 784.
19. Rabe, Edward F., "Febrile Convulsions," in Sidney S. Gellis and Benjamin M. Kagan (eds.), *Current Pediatric Therapy,* vol. II, Saunders, Philadelphia, 1984, pp. 75–77.
20. Berkowitz, Carol D., and Chris R. Jones, "The PNP's Role in Evaluation and Management of Febrile Seizures," *Pediatric Nursing* **9**(6):434 (November–December 1983).
21. Berg, op. cit., p. 194.
22. Ibid., p. 182.
23. Gastault, H., "Clinical and Electroencephalographical Classification of Epileptic Seizures," *Epilepsia* **11**:102–113 (1970).
24. Singer, William, "Infantile Spasms," in Gellis and Kagan, op. cit., pp. 77–78.
25. Chee, Claire M., "Seizure Disorders," in Diane McElroy and Gayle Davis (eds.), *Nursing Clinics of North America* **15**(1):76 (March 1980).
26. Menkes, John H., "Seizure Disorders," in Gellis and Kagan, op. cit., p. 74.
27. Feldman, Robert G., "Epilepsy in Adolescents and Adults," in Barett et al., op. cit., p. 772.
28. Hahn, Anne, Robert L. Barkin, and Sandy Oestreich, *Pharmacology in Nursing,* 15th ed., Mosby, St. Louis, 1982, pp. 210–230.
29. Feldman, op. cit., p. 73.
30. Hawken, Margarethe, and Judith Ozunar, "Practical Aspects of Anticonvulsant Therapy," *American Journal of Nursing* **76**(6):1065 (June 1979).
31. Hahn, Barkin, and Oestreich, op. cit., p. 1067.
32. Hawken and Ozunar, op. cit., p. 1067.
33. Ibid., p. 1066.
34. Singer, op. cit., p. 78.
35. *Epilepsy and the School Age Child,* Comprehensive Epilepsy Program, University of Minnesota, Minneapolis, 1980, p. 1.
36. Spack, Norman P., "Medical Problems of the Exercising Child: Asthma, Diabetes, and Epilepsy," in Lyle J. Micheli (ed.), *Pediatric and Adolescent Sports Medicine,* Little, Brown, Boston, 1984, pp. 124–127.
37. Parrish, Mary Ann, "A Comparison of Behavioral Side Effects Related to Commonly Used Anticonvulsants," *Pediatric Nursing* **10**(2):149–150 (April 1984).
38. Beran, John A., and Jeremy H. Thompson, *Essentials of Pharmacology,* 3d ed., Harper & Row, New York, 1983, pp. 287–293.
39. Hahn, Barkin, and Oestreich, op. cit., p. 210.
40. Berg, op. cit., p. 30.
41. Passo, Sherrilyn, "Malformations of the Neural Tube," in McElroy and Davis, op. cit., p. 8.
42. Kousseff, Boris G., "Sacral Meningocele with Conotruncal Heart Defects: A Possible Autosomal Recessive Trait," *Pediatrics* **74**(3):395–398 (September 1984).
43. Passo, op. cit., p. 10.
44. Ibid., p. 20.
45. Badell-Ribera, Angeles, "Myelodysplasia," in Gabriella E. Molnar (ed.), *Pediatric Rehabilitation,* Williams & Wilkins, Baltimore, 1985, pp. 176–180.
46. Charney, Edward B., et. al., "Management of the NBZM: Time for a Decision Making Process," *Pediatrics* **75**(1):63–64 (January 1985).
47. Gross, Richard H., et al., "Early Management and Decision for the Treatment of Myelomeningocele," *Pediatrics* **72**(4):453–454 (October 1983).
48. Feiwell, Earl, "Selection of Appropriate Treatment for Patients with Myelomeningocele," *Orthopedic Clinics of North America* **12**(1):103 (January 1981).
49. Sousa, Jan Carr, et al., "Developmental Guidelines for Children with Myelodysplasia," *The Journal of the American Physical Therapy Association* **63**(1):26–29 (January 1983).
50. Myers, Gary J., "Myelomeningocele: The Medical Aspects," *Pediatric Clinics of North America* **31**(1):165–175 (February 1984).
51. Badell-Ribera, op. cit., pp. 187–202.
52. Killam, Patricia E., "Behavioral Pediatric Weight Rehabilitation for Children with MMC," *MCN* **8**(4):280 (July–August 1983).

53. Cass, A. S., et al., "Management of the Neurogenic Bladder in 413 Children," *The Journal of Urology* **132**(3):524 (September 1984).
54. Crooks, K. Kenny, and Benedicta G. Enrile, "Comparison of the Ileal Conduit and Clean Intermittent Catheterization for Myelomeningocele," *Pediatrics* **72**(2):203 (August 1983).
55. Perez-Marrero, R., et al., "Clean Intermittent Catheterization in Myelomeningocele Children Less than 3 Years Old," *The Journal of Urology* **128**:779 (October 1982).
56. Sousa, J. C., L. H. Gordon, and D. B. Shurtleff, "Assessing the Development of Daily Living Skills in Patients with Spina Bifida," *Developmental Medicine and Child Neurology* **18**(Suppl. 37):134–142 (1976).
57. Hayden, P. W., S. L. Davenport, and M. M. Campbell, "Adolescents with Myelodysplasia: Impact of Physical Disability in Emotional Maturation," *Pediatrics* **64**(1):53–59 (July 1979).
58. Passo, op. cit., p. 20.
59. Shurtleff, D. B., P. W. Hayden, W. H. Chapman, J. B. Broy, and M. L. Hill, "Myelodysplasia," *Western Journal of Medicine* **122**(3):199–205 (March 1975).
60. Jabbour, J. T., "Hydrocephalus," in Gellis and Benjamin, op. cit.
61. Berg, op. cit., pp. 42–43.
62. Shinnar, S., et al., "Management of Hydrocephalus in Infancy: Use of Acetazolamide and Furosemide to Avoid CS Shunts," *The Journal of Pediatrics* **107**(1):31 (January 1985).
63. Taft, L. T., "Cerebral Palsy," *Pediatrics in Review* **6**(2):35 (August 1984).
64. Davis, Gayle Tart, and Patty Maynard Hill, "Cerebral Palsy," in McElroy and Davis, op. cit., pp. 47–48.
65. Taft, op. cit., p. 65.
66. Stanley, Fiona, and Eva Alberman, *The Epidemiology of the Cerebral Palsies*, Lippincott, Philadelphia, 1984, p. 48.
67. Kosowski, Margaret Mary, and Deborah Lee Sopczyk, "Feeding Hospitalized Children with Developmental Disabilities," *Maternal-Child Nursing* **10**(3):190–194 (May–June 1985).
68. Steele, Shirley, "Young Children with Cerebral Palsy: Practical Guidelines for Care," *Pediatric Nursing* **11**(4):259 (July–August 1985).
69. Stern, Francine Martin, "Motor Development Difficulties during and after Hospitalization: Recognition and Intervention," *Developmental Interventions in Neonatal Care,* Contemporary Forums, Washington, D.C., 1985, pp. 174–175.
70. Critchley, M., and E. A. Critchley, *Dyslexia Defined,* Charles C Thomas, Springfield, Ill., 1978.
71. Duane, D. D., "A Neurological Overview of Specific Language Disability for the Non-Neurologist," *Bulletin of the Orton Society* **24**:5–36 (1974).
72. Hermann, K., *Reading Disability,* Munkgaard, Copenhagen, 1959.
73. Orton, S. T., *Reading, Writing, and Speech Problems in Children,* Norton, New York, 1937.
74. Fraser, D. W., "Haemophilus Influenza in the Community and the Home," in S. H. Sell and P. F. Wright (eds.), *Haemophilus Influenza: Epidemiology, Immunology, and Prevention of Disease,* Elsevier Biomedical, New York, 1982, pp. 11–21.
75. ———, "Polysaccharide Vaccine for Prevention of Haemophilus Influenza Type B Disease," *Morbidity and Mortality Weekly Report,* **134**(15):201–205 (April 1985).
76. American Academy of Pediatrics, Committee on Infectious Disease, "Revisions of Recommendation for Use of Rifampin Prophylaxis of Contacts of Patients with Haemophilus Influenzae Infection," *Pediatrics* **74**(2):301–302 (August 1984).
77. Barett, op. cit., pp. 46–47.
78. Gaddy, Debra S., "Meningitis in the Pediatric Population," in McElroy and Davis, op. cit., p. 90.
79. Ibid., p. 92.
80. Ibid., p. 90.
81. Jacobs, Richard F., et al., "A Prospective Randomized Comparison of Cefotaxime vs. Ampicillin and Chloramphanicol for Bacterial Meningitis in Children," *Journal of Pediatrics* **107**(1):129 (July 1985).
82. Schwartz, James F., "Infections of the Nervous System," in Berg, op. cit., p. 128.
83. Dalgas, Pegg, "Reye's Syndrome Update," *MCN* **8**:345 (September–October 1983).
84. Barett, op. cit., p. 33.
85. Rodgers, Martha, et al., "National Reye Syndrome Surveillance, 1982," *Pediatrics* **75**(2):260 (February 1985).
86. U.S. Department of Health, Human Services and Public Services, Food and Drug Administration, Publication no. FDA 85-3149, Rockville, Md., 1985.
87. Starko, K. M., and F. G. Mullick, "Hepatic and Cerebral Pathology Findings in Children with Fatal Salycilate Intoxication," *Lancet* **1**:326–329 (January 1983).
88. Quint, Peter A., and Frank D. Allman, "Differentiation of Chronic Salicylism from Reye Syndrome," *Pediatrics* **74**(6):1117 (December 1984).
89. Jennett, Bryan, and Graham Teasdale, *Management of Head Injuries,* Davis, Philadelphia, 1981, pp. 21–22.
90. Taylor and Ballenger, op. cit., pp. 401–402.
91. Walleck, Connie, "Head Trauma in Children," in McElroy and Davis, op. cit., p. 120.
92. Ibid., pp. 118–119.
93. Jennett and Teasdale, op. cit., pp. 241–243.
94. Taylor and Ballenger, op. cit., p. 404.
95. Perrin, Jane C. S., "Spinal Cord Injuries," in Molnar, op. cit., pp. 272–274.
96. Taylor and Ballenger, op. cit., p. 235.
97. Staas, William E., and Janet G. LaMantia, "Decubitus Ulcers," in Asa P. Ruskin (ed.), *Current Therapy in Physiatry,* Saunders, Philadelphia, 1984, pp. 410–412.
98. Perinchief, Judith M., et al., "Rehabilitation of the Spinal Cord Injury," in Molnar, op. cit., p. 426.
99. Staas, William, and Janet G. LaMantia, "Bowel Function and Control," in Ruskin, op. cit., pp. 407–409.
100. Perrin, op. cit., p. 280.
101. Ibid., p. 284.

102. Dietrich, Kim N., et al., "Contribution of Societal and Developmental Factors to Lead Exposure during the First Year of Life," *Pediatrics* **75**(6):1118 (June 1985).
103. LeFeverkee, Joyce, *Laboratory Diagnostic Tests with Nursing Implications,* Appleton Century Crofts, New York, 1982, pp. 165–166.
104. Graef, John W., and Thomas E. Cone, Jr. (eds), *Manual of Pediatric Therapeutics,* 3d ed., Little, Brown, Boston, 1985, p. 110.
105. Needleman, Herbert, "Increased Lead Absorption and Acute Poisoning," in Gellis and Kagan, op. cit., pp. 662–663.
106. Graef and Cone, op. cit., p. 113.
107. LeFeverkee, op. cit., p. 166.

31

Carol J. Hill

Special senses

Upon completion of this chapter, the student will be able to:

1. Describe the normal appearance of external eye structures.
2. Describe two methods for obtaining the cooperation of a toddler during an eye examination.
3. List five suggestions the nurse can make to parents concerning prevention of eye trauma.
4. Describe the procedure for instilling eye medications.
5. Contrast congenital glaucoma and congenital cataracts.
6. List three manifestations of strabismus.
7. Describe the preoperative preparation for a child who will undergo eye surgery.
8. Construct a plan of care to meet the needs of a child during the period following eye surgery.
9. Describe the passage of a sound wave from the external ear to the brain.
10. Identify two methods for testing the hearing of a child.
11. List the steps involved in instilling ear drops.
12. Describe nursing measures to increase the comfort of a child with otitis media.
13. List five nursing interventions to increase the security of a sensory-impaired child who is hospitalized.

Alterations in the special senses of vision and hearing can occur prenatally and at any time throughout childhood, although certain alterations are most apt to occur at specific times. Specific alterations will be considered in this chapter after a review of the development, anatomy, physiology, and assessment of the eye and ear.

EMBRYOLOGICAL DEVELOPMENT OF THE EYE

From its first appearance in the fourth week of fetal life, the eye develops rapidly, and by the sixteenth week it appears to be a fairly typical human eye. The first portion to develop is called the *optic vesicle*, from which the retina later develops. By the sixth week, the nervous and pigment layers of the eye and the lens are being formed. The structures of the sclera, cornea, iris, ciliary body, choroid, and eyelids form between the sixth and the twelfth weeks. Maternal disease, radiation, and drugs have the most disastrous effect on eye development from the fourth to the eighth weeks of gestation. From 16 weeks of gestation until birth, further refinement of eye structures occurs. Initially the eyes are located on each side of the head; as the head and facial areas broaden, the eyes converge, which enables them to function together, resulting in binocular vision and depth perception.

Development of the eye is not complete at birth. The eyes of the newborn are sensitive to light; blinking and pupillary reflexes are present. The newborn has peripheral vision and is able to follow objects to the midline. Visual acuity is approximately 20/400 at birth and 20/100 by 6 months. The macula matures over the first 4 to 6 months, making central vision possible. By the age of 2, vision is well developed, but it continues to mature until the child is approximately 6 years old. See Tables 9-5 and 10-1.

Table 31-1 Parts and Functions of the Eye

Part	Function
Surrounding Structures	
Extrinsic ocular muscles	Six muscles connecting eyeball to orbit to provide lateral, up-and-down movement
Eyelids, lashes	Protect eyeball from foreign objects, intense light, blunt force
Conjunctiva	Mucous membrane lining inner eyelid and outer eyeball
Lacrimal apparatus	Lacrimal gland and series of ducts; produces and drains away tears.
Eyeball	
Sclera	Outermost layer of eyeball; supports and protects eye
Cornea	Anterior one-sixth of eyeball; serves as principal refracting medium for light rays
Choroid	Vascular middle layer of eyeball; provides nourishment for retina
Ciliary body	Anterior extension of choroid consisting of ciliary processes, which secrete aqueous humor, and ciliary muscles, which regulate lens shape
Iris	Muscular, colored diaphragm which controls amount of light admitted to inner eyeball through pupil
Lens	Biconvex, transparent structure which refracts light rays on retina by changing shape
Aqueous humor	Alkaline, watery fluid filling anterior and posterior chambers; nourishes lens and cornea
Vitreous body (humor)	Jelly-like substance making up four-fifths of eyeball; maintains eyeball shape
Retina	Provides conversion of light rays to nerve impulses
Optic nerve	Transmits nerve impulses from retina to visual area of occipital lobe in brain

ANATOMY OF THE EYE

The eye is situated within the orbital cavity, which is made up of skull bones and provides some protection for the eyeball. The major structures of the eye and their functions are summarized in Table 31-1 and Fig. 31-1.

PHYSIOLOGY OF THE EYE

To be visualized, an object must go through several processes: refraction, accommodation, transformation of the visual images into nerve impulses, and transmission to the brain. When light rays are refracted, they are bent so that the light from a large area can be focused on a small area. Light rays are bent successively by the cornea, aqueous humor, lens, and vitreous body. Each refracting surface converges the light rays slightly more until the image of the object is formed on the retina.

In order for close objects to be projected on the retina, accommodation must take place. The lens provides this function by changing to a more convex shape. Pupillary constriction and the convergence of both eyes are also part of the accommodative process. When viewing distant objects, the lens resumes its usual biconvex shape.

The image formed on the retina is transformed into nervous impulses by the photosensitive cells of the retina, the rods and cones. Cones are sensitive to day vision and colors. They are most numerous at the center of the retina in the area known as the *macula*. Rods are sensitive to dim light. They are found outside the macula. The impulses generated by rod and cone cells pass along the optic nerve, out of the orbital cavity, and to the visual area within the occipital lobe, where the image is interpreted.

ASSESSMENT OF THE EYE

Assessment of visual function includes a thorough history from the parent accompanying the child, inspection of the eyes for observable alter-

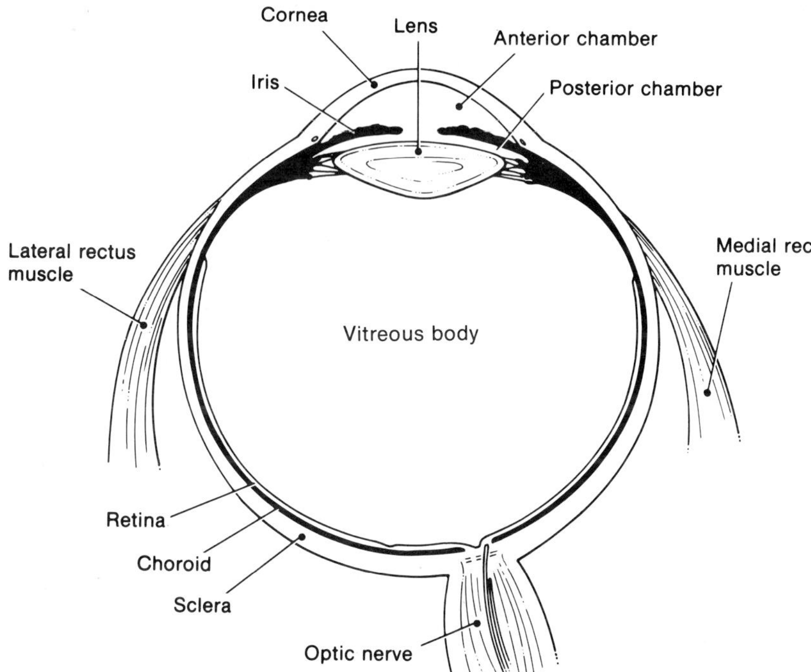

Figure 31-1 Anatomy of the eye. (*From G. Scipien, M. U. Barnard, M. A. Chard, J. Howe, and P. J. Phillips [eds.], Comprehensive Pediatric Nursing, 3d ed., McGraw-Hill, New York, 1986, p. 1367. Used with permission.*)

ations as outlined in Table 31-2, measurement of visual acuity, and assessment of extrinsic muscle balance. Evaluation of the internal structures of the eye is generally performed by a physician who has experience in this area. Any deviation from normal will also be referred to an ophthalmologist for further evaluation and possible treatment.

The history obtained from the parents or other caretakers should include both symptoms and functional alterations of the eyes. These areas are summarized in Table 31-3.

Nursing measures to facilitate assessment

The nurse can facilitate assessment of the eyes in several ways. Obtain the history first, before handling the child. While obtaining the history, assess as much as possible indirectly, e.g., symmetry of the eye position and how the child uses the eyes. Avoid sudden or hurried movement. Infants and young children feel most secure on the parent's lap. Use of a bottle or pacifier may keep an infant relatively quiet. To check the red reflex, have the parent hold the infant over the shoulder while the examiner approaches the child from behind. The *red reflex* is the reddish-orange circular glow which normally fills the pupil when a light is shone into the eye. If necessary, an infant or a young child can be restrained by placing the child on the back on the parent's lap, with the head facing the examiner. The parent can hold the hands of the child and restrain the body at the same time, with the child's legs placed around the parent's waist and restrained by the parent's elbows.[1]

To gain the cooperation of an older child, use positive suggestions, such as "Look at the picture of the dog," rather than "Will you look straight ahead?" Allow the child time to become familiar with the penlight or ophthalmoscope. Ask questions of the child rather than talking over the child to the parent. The older child can be examined while seated on a chair or the examining table.

Assessment of visual acuity

Procedures used to assess visual acuity depend on the age of the child. Table 31-4 lists assessment tools useful for children in various age groups. An infant can also be tested with Visually Evoked Potentials. Electrodes placed on the infant's occiput record electric signals following a visual stimulation. When checking the visual acuity of a preschooler with the E test, a better response may be elicited if the E is referred to

Table 31-2 Examination of the Eye by Inspection

Part	Normal Appearance	Abnormal Appearance
Surrounding Structures		
Orbit	Proportionate with other facial features; eyes aligned with each other	Edema, discoloration
Eyebrows		Thick, bushy, joined; scaliness, crusting
Eyelids, lashes	Lids open completely; lids open simultaneously	Drooping, discoloration, edema, excessive blinking or squinting, upward slant, sties, discharge, lice, masses, absent eyelashes, absent or excessive tearing
Ocular muscles	Eyes move up, down, laterally, obliquely; equal corneal light reflex	Crossing of eyes
Conjunctiva	Moist, smooth, nonreddened	Redness, pallor, jaundice
Eye Proper		
Cornea	Clear, equal size	Scarring, ulcerations, opacities
Sclera	White color	Jaundiced, reddened
Iris	Same color in both eyes; forms complete circle	Dull color
Pupils	Round, equal, react to light; constrict on accommodation	Nystagmus
Lens	Red reflex present	Sunken
Globe		Blank-looking, protruding

as a table and the child is asked which way the legs point. Asking the parents to practice with the child the day before the test is also helpful. The Titmus Optical Tester is a machine in which the child sees letters or E's projected onto a screen. This machine helps minimize distraction and memorization.

Table 31-3 Information about Visual Function Gathered by Interview

Symptomatic Alterations
Presence of reddened eyes
Discharge from lids or eyes
Pain, discomfort, itching in or around eyes
Excessive tearing
Crossed eyes
Blurring of vision
Presence of spots before eyes
Swelling of eyelids
Rubbing eyes, squinting, frowning
Oversensitivity to light
Recurring sties

Functional Alterations
Parent suspects child cannot see
Holding objects very close to eyes
Covering one eye while playing with toy or reading
Difficulty seeing chalkboard at school
Headaches after doing close work at school
Skipping over words when reading out loud
Stumbling over objects
Tilting head when looking at objects

Extrinsic muscle balance testing

Testing the function of the ocular muscles can be accomplished by use of the Hirschberg test and the cover test. Both these tests require fixation of the eyes on an object. This is more easily achieved in a child if the object is visually interesting, such as a small toy.[2] When performing the Hirschberg test, the examiner shines a pen-

Table 31-4 Methods Used to Assess Visual Acuity

Infants and Toddlers
History: parent believes child can see
Ability to fixate on an object
Pupillary response to light
Visually evoked potentials

Preschoolers
Snellen illiterate E chart, cards, or Titmus Optical Tester

School-Age Children and Adolescents
Snellen letter chart
Color vision plates

light into the child's eyes; the light should reflect on the same spot on both corneas.

The cover test is performed by covering one eye with a card or the examiner's hand while watching the uncovered eye for movement. Then the eye is uncovered and is watched for movement. After the child rests for a few minutes, the test is repeated on the other eye. Any movement of the eyes indicates muscle imbalance. Another test for muscle function involves telling the child to follow the examiner's finger through the directions of gaze; small finger puppets may hold the child's attention.

Peripheral and color vision

Peripheral vision can be difficult to assess in infants, but the following method can be used for gross assessment. Attract the child's attention to an object straight ahead, such as the examiner's face. After the child's vision is fixed, introduce another object, such as a large toy or a flashing light, from one side until the child refixes vision on the new object. Assess peripheral vision on the opposite side in the same way.

Assessment of color vision in young children is not routine unless optic nerve disease is suspected. Toddlers can be asked to match identically colored objects.[3] Older children can be tested using the Ishihara pseudoisochromatic plates, which are used to test adults. These plates contain a series of numbers made up of dots of various colors and sizes. The dots are superimposed on backgrounds made up of similar dots.[4] The child can be asked to trace the numbers with a dry paintbrush.[5]

NURSING MANAGEMENT: EDUCATION ABOUT EYE CARE

The teaching role of the nurse focuses on providing information to the parents and the child about maintaining healthy eyes, obtaining medical advice in case of injury or illness, and carrying out specific treatments, such as instillation of eye drops or ointments.

Maintaining healthy eyes

A child's eyes should be examined as a minimum at the following times: as a newborn, at age 3, before entering grade school, midway through elementary school, before entering high school, and at 2-year intervals thereafter.

Most eye injuries are preventable; most blindness is a result of trauma. Providing guidance to parents about prevention can be facilitated by using a developmental approach, i.e., by determining which risks are greater at certain developmental stages and providing suggestions on how those risks can be minimized or prevented. Table 31-5 presents guidelines for preventing eye injuries.

When to seek medical advice

The information given in Table 31-3 is useful for teaching parents when to seek medical advice. Parents should also be alert to the following symptoms: the presence of photophobia, enlargement of the eye, growths on the lid or surface of the eye, irregularities in pupil shape, and the presence of white reflections from behind the pupil.

Eye treatment by parents

Before the parents examine the child's eyes, their hands should be washed. Discourage use of over-the-counter drops for eye irritation because the drops may mask symptoms of disease and delay proper treatment; these drops are unnecessary for normal eye hygiene. Caution the parents to refrain from using an antibiotic prescribed for a child for a previous eye condition if symptoms recur. Drugs prescribed for another child with similar symptoms should not be used. Some of these medications lose their effectiveness after a period of time. Use of the wrong medication can be dangerous as well as delay essential medical treatment.

The nurse demonstrates to the parents the proper procedure for instilling eye drops or ointments. Cleanliness of the parent's hands and the medication is important. The dropper or tip of the ointment tube should not touch the eye or any other surface. Several methods can be used to insert the medication. Rather than forcing the lids apart, the drops can be placed at the inner canthus; when the child opens the eyes, the drops will roll in. The child may need to be mummied or placed on the bed with the head stabilized between the parent's legs. If the child is a sound sleeper, arranging the schedule so that one dose is given at night may be successful. With the child in a supine position, gently pull down the lower lid and insert the drops in the lower conjunctiva (Fig. 31-2).

To instill eye ointments, place a thin ribbon

Table 31-5 Guidelines for Prevention of Eye Injuries in Children

Developmental Stage	Risk	Preventive Measures
Infancy	Pokes self or others with sharp objects	Dispose of broken toys. Child should not play with Popsicle sticks, pencils, Tinkertoys, etc.
Toddlerhood	Falls while carrying objects	Child should not run with pencils, lollipop sticks, etc.
	Drinks antifreeze	Keep antifreeze (all poisons) locked up in cabinet.
	Throws sand or dirt	Supervise outdoor play.
Preschool age	Waves sharp objects	Provide blunt-tipped scissors. Have child sit quietly at table when using scissors. Teach child to walk holding point of scissors down.
	Experiments with aerosol cans, perfumes	Place out of reach.
School age	Fireworks	Supervise rigidly if allowed at all.
	Missiles such as BB guns, arrows	Allow supervised use only.
	Football, hockey, baseball injuries	Provide playground supervision, explain risks.
Adolescence	Same as for school age, plus contact lenses	Clean properly, remove at bedtime, do not overwear.
	Motorcycle accidents.	Use safety helmets.
	Eye makeup—infection	Remove eye makeup with petroleum jelly or mineral oil at bedtime; do not share makeup with friends.
All ages	Automobile accidents	Infants and toddlers—use dynamically tested car restraint. Preschoolers and older children—use seat belts when over 40 lb or 4 years, shoulder harness when over 55 in.
	Power lawn mowers—can throw objects such as rocks	Do not allow child to play nearby when lawn mower is in use.
	Direct sunlight	Teach child not to look at sun.

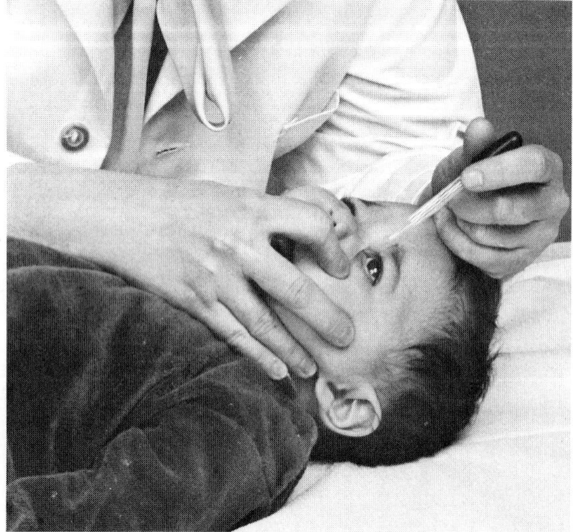

Figure 31-2 Instillation of eye drops.

along the inner margin of the lower lid without pressing the eyeballs or forcing the lids against the bony rims of the orbits. An ointment may be prescribed because a crying child tends to force drops out by squeezing the lids and dilutes the drops with tears.[6]

CONGENITAL ALTERATIONS OF THE EYE

Cataracts

Pathophysiology A *cataract* is a unilateral or bilateral opacity of part or all of the lens as a result of heredity or an environmental insult. The opacity of the lens makes it impervious to light. The most common environmental cause is maternal rubella during the first trimester of pregnancy. When an infant with cataracts is examined, the red reflex is absent or does not fill the pupil; a white glow may be seen behind the pupil when cataracts are far advanced.

Treatment If cataracts are not extracted early, further visual development may be impaired. Bilateral complete cataracts are often removed by the time the child is 1 to 3 months of age. Each eye is operated on within a week of the other. The lens is broken up, aspirated, and irrigated through an incision at the junction of the cornea and sclera. *Phacoemulsification,* a procedure in which the lens is broken up by high-frequency sound waves, is also used.

Postoperatively, the eye is patched until photophobia has diminished, and then an eye shield is worn for approximately 1 week. The child may be discharged on the day of surgery and seen in the outpatient clinic the following day. Steroid and atropine sulfate drops are instilled two or three times each day for 4 to 6 weeks to prevent glaucoma, which can result from the adhesion of the iris to residual lens matter.

Several weeks postoperatively, after inflammation has decreased, the child is fitted for glasses or contact lenses to replace the missing lens. Introduction of contact lenses in infancy has been successful; the lenses are modified as the eye changes with the child's growth. A 7- or 8-year-old can often be taught how to insert the lenses.[7] (See the section "Contact Lenses" later in this chapter.)

The prognosis varies, but vision may be improved only to 20/100 or 20/200.[8] Complications include glaucoma and retinal detachment, both of which may occur years after surgery has been performed. The coexistence of other eye anomalies, such as microphthalmia and poor retinal function, also affects the prognosis.

Glaucoma

Pathophysiology Congenital or infantile glaucoma is a result of inadequate drainage of the aqueous fluid from the anterior portion of the eye. Normally, aqueous fluid leaves the eye through a trabecular meshwork located at the junction of the sclera, cornea, and iris. Obstruction of the flow of aqueous fluid in children is usually due to faulty development of the trabecular meshwork. The obstruction results in increased pressure within the eyeball, eventually leading to atrophy of the optic nerve. Most infantile glaucoma is apparent within the first 12 months of life. Early symptoms include extreme sensitivity to light and excessive tearing due to the irritation of the corneal epithelium. The photophobia may be so severe that the infant keeps the eyes closed even when eating.[9] As the disease progresses, the cornea enlarges and becomes hazy; the eyeball itself enlarges if the child is under age 3. (See Fig. 31-3.)

Glaucoma may be hereditary or may result from congenital rubella, retinopathy of prematurity, retinoblastoma, or trauma. In many cases the cause is unknown. If the child is born with enlarged eyes, the vision may not be salvageable. If manifestations of glaucoma occur after birth but within the first year of life and if treatment is begun promptly, the prognosis is excellent for 90 percent of these children,[10] although increased intraocular pressure may recur years after surgery is performed.[11]

Treatment The treatment of congenital or infantile glaucoma is surgery. Preoperatively, the child may be given pilocarpine hydrochloride eye drops to keep the pupils constricted and acetazolamide to lower the intraocular pressure and reduce corneal edema. The usual surgical procedure is a *goniotomy,* in which a fine knife is introduced through the cornea into the anterior chamber to incise the trabecular meshwork. The length of hospitalization may be 1 or 2 days. Complications of a goniotomy are uncommon but include hemorrhage and infection. The child is

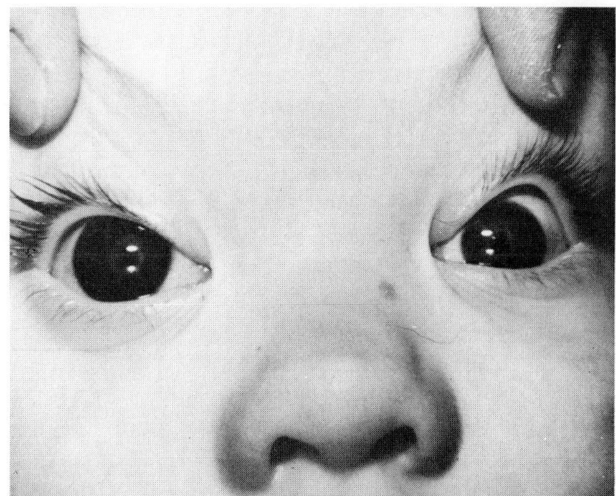

Figure 31-3 Congenital glaucoma. Note the enlargement of the cornea of the right eye. *(Courtesy of Dr. J. Olson, United Hospital, Grand Forks, N. Dak.)*

examined under anesthesia 4 to 6 weeks postoperatively to measure intraocular pressure and examine the retina. Follow-up examinations are scheduled for every 3 to 4 months during the first year, every 6 months during the second year, and then yearly.[12] Several goniotomies may need to be performed to halt the disease.

Nursing management When caring for a child with cataracts or glaucoma, the most important considerations for promoting the security of the child are consistency of routine and the presence of the parents. An infant or a very young child cannot be prepared for the experience. Obtain a thorough history from the parents at the time of admission, including sleeping and feeding routines and skills the child has mastered, and record this information on the Kardex. Assure the parents that their presence throughout the child's hospital stay is welcome and helpful for their child.

Postoperatively, the nurse focuses on assessing the child's recovery from anesthesia, preventing injury to the eye that was operated on, maintaining the child's fluid and electrolyte balance, and promoting the ability of the parents to comfort and care for their child. The child will have bandaged eyes. Elbow restraints can be applied to prevent pulling at the bandages or rubbing the eyes. A very young child usually needs to be distracted and comforted rather than told not to pull at the bandages. Preoperative preparation for an older toddler or a preschooler is similar to that used for a child having strabismus repair. (See the section "Strabismus" later in this chapter.) The child usually has a scratchy sensation in the eye that was operated on rather than actual pain. While recovering from the anesthesia, the child is often restless. Crying will increase intraocular pressure; holding and gently rocking the child, especially by the parents, may decrease the crying. If possible, position the child who has glaucoma on the side that was not operated on to enhance serous drainage. Start oral fluids cautiously as soon as the child is awake; vomiting also increases intraocular pressure. Return to the child's room frequently during the early postoperative period to assess the child's condition and the parents' need for assistance, especially with a restless, crying child. Increasing restlessness may indicate intraocular hemorrhage.

The role of the nurse as a teacher includes preparation for discharge. Show the parents how to instill the prescribed eye drops following cataract surgery and, if possible, assist them in actually carrying out this procedure while the child is still hospitalized. Stress the importance of using the drops until they are discontinued by the ophthalmologist.

Provide suggestions concerning prevention of injury to the eye that was operated on. The surgeon may suggest use of a lightweight patch over the eye at night to prevent rubbing. Applying elbow restraints at home may help prevent rubbing when the child is not being held. Depending on institutional policy, the parents might be able to take home the tongue-blade restraints used in the hospital, or they can make their own using rolled-up newspapers or magazines. Remind the parents to remove the elbow restraints periodically to prevent skin irritation and to exercise the arms. Suggest to the parents that they provide for quiet play rather than active play. Long periods of crying should be avoided in order to prevent increased ocular pressure. The child may show increased sensitivity to light and will be more comfortable if he or she is not exposed to direct light. If pain, increased swelling, or discharge in the eye occurs, the parents should seek medical advice. An appointment with the child's physician should also be made.

Treatment of cataracts and glaucoma requires ongoing long-term care. The nurse can help the family express their concerns about the child's visual deficit and the continuing care necessary to preserve remaining visual function. The nurse can also assist the parents in understanding the physician's explanations or suggest that the physician talk with the parents again if a lack of understanding is apparent.

The nurse also has a role in the early detection of children with glaucoma. Newborns who appear to have photophobia, tearing of the eyes, or large corneas should be promptly referred to a physician.[13]

ACQUIRED ALTERATIONS OF THE EYE

Retinopathy of prematurity

Pathophysiology *Retinopathy of prematurity,* also called *retrolental fibroplasia,*[14] occurs as a response of the immature retina of a premature infant to high levels of oxygen and other, unknown factors. It can also occur in full-term infants and premature infants who have not had oxygen; the cause in these cases is unknown.

In the presence of high oxygen levels, the retinal vessels constrict; the resulting decreased oxygen levels lead to dilatation of the vessels and new vascular growth extending into the vitreous body. Hemorrhages of these new, delicate vessels result in retinal detachment. In the most severe cases, the retrolental space (the space behind the lens) is filled with fibrous tissue, the eyes appear small and sunken, and the child is blind. If the process is not complete, the child has retinal scarring with reduced visual acuity. Retinal detachments can occur even into adolescence as a result of the retinal scarring. Strabismus and amblyopia may also occur in children who had mild retinopathy. Injections of vitamin E are being tried for prevention and treatment.

Nursing management In providing care to a premature infant, the nurse monitors arterial oxygen levels closely as long as an umbilical catheter is in place. Safe arterial oxygen levels and the length of oxygen therapy which produces retinopathy have not been established, but it is believed that the least amount of oxygen needed for optimal central nervous system oxygenation should be used.[15] The nurse's observations of the infant's behavior are important in establishing required oxygen levels. Oxygen should be given only when essential and should be discontinued, reduced, or given intermittently as soon as possible.[16]

After the arterial catheter is discontinued, the oxygen levels in the Isolette should be kept below 40 percent. All newborns who receive oxygen therapy should have their eyes examined when oxygen is discontinued, before discharge, at 7 to 9 weeks of age, and between 3 and 6 months following discharge. Infants who have any degree of retinopathy should have their eyes reexamined until the eyes are stable and then at 6- to 12-month intervals.[17] The nurse can help the parents understand the necessity of frequent eye examinations.

The parents of a premature infant are faced with acceptance of the premature birth and possible loss of the child. It may be difficult for them to accept that their child has defective vision or is blind as a result of treatment given to save the child's life. The nurse can and should provide opportunities for them to express their feelings.

Strabismus

Pathophysiology *Strabismus,* or crossing of the eyes, results from abnormal coordination of eye movements. (See Fig. 31-4.) It can be bilateral or unilateral. The eyes may turn in (*esotropia*), out (*exotropia*), or up or down (*vertical strabismus*). It may be congenital—i.e., present before 6 months—or acquired later in early childhood. The most common cause is an imbalance of the extraocular muscles, which control eye movement, but strabismus can also result from a difference in refractive ability of the two eyes. Aside from its effect on the child's appearance, which may result in teasing from peers as early as age 3, strabismus can result in suppression of vision in the deviating eye. This is known as *amblyopia*. When the eyes do not function together, the image seen by the child is not fused; this lack of fusion results in *diplopia*. To eliminate the confusing or double image, the brain suppresses the cells of the macula so that visual stimuli are not registered; in time this leads to atrophy of the macula. This visual deficit tends to be more common in esotropia. The older the child, the longer treatment is necessary to reverse amblyopia. After the age of 6, treatment is generally not successful in restoring vision.

Symptoms indicating the presence of strabismus include, in addition to apparent deviation,

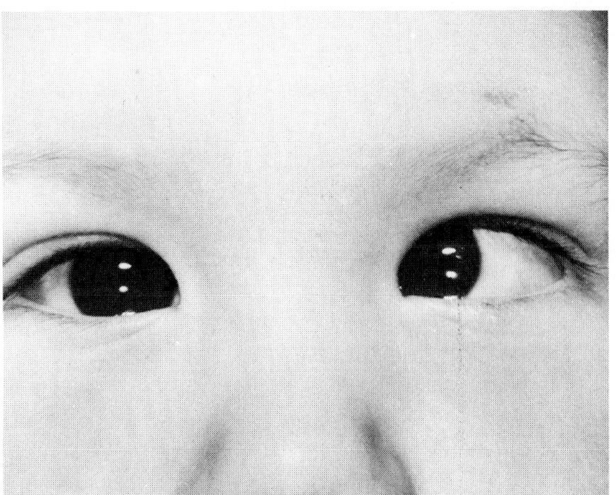

Figure 31-4 Bilateral strabismus—esotropia. (*Courtesy of Dr. M. Mariano, United Hospital, Grand Forks, N. Dak.*)

complaints of double vision, difficulty reading, and unusual head positions, such as turning or tilting the head. Occasionally an infant is suspected of having strabismus, but in reality the appearance is due to the presence of epicanthal folds and the wide bridge of the nose. This *pseudostrabismus* is rechecked at 6-month intervals to be certain that true strabismus is not present.

Treatment Treatment of strabismus usually involves correction of amblyopia if present, surgery for muscle imbalance, and glasses to correct differences in refraction.

Amblyopia is treated by patching the normal eye in order to force use of the deviating eye. In the 1-year-old child, correction may be obtained in less than 2 weeks, while in the 6-year-old child, correction may take 6 months. The child is examined frequently to be certain that the patched eye does not become amblyopic from disuse.

Surgery is performed after amblyopia has been corrected and involves resection or recession of one or more ocular muscles. Resection results in a shortened muscle, which strengthens it; recession weakens the muscle by lengthening it. Surgery may need to be performed more than once.

Surgical correction often takes place between 6 and 24 months of age. The child is generally admitted the day before surgery and is discharged the day following surgery. The eye is patched until the evening of the day of surgery. Strabismus surgery can also be performed on an outpatient basis.[18] The child is usually discharged with prescriptions for an antibiotic and a steroid ointment.

Nursing management In the outpatient clinic the nurse can teach the child and the parents to correctly utilize patching for amblyopia. The parents need to know which eye is to be patched. They must understand that the patch is to remain on at all times. Elastoplast patches, which are available in most drugstores, can be applied with tincture of benzoin, which helps decrease skin irritation and increase adherence. The child often resists the patch because it is hot and uncomfortable, decreases the ability to see, and sets the child apart from peers. The parents may need to apply mittens or elbow restraints to prevent an infant from pulling off the patch. Older children can be told that it is a "pirate's patch." An older child may have difficulty reading. Encourage the parents to keep their child's appointments with the physician; the progress of the amblyopic eye as well as the other eye needs to be monitored closely to prevent disuse amblyopia. When the vision in the amblyopic eye is close to normal, the child may be weaned from the patch. Because amblyopia can recur until about age 9, frequent examinations are still necessary after vision has been corrected, and part-time patching may be continued.

Preoperative teaching Preoperative care of a child who will undergo strabismus surgery is the same as that for any child who will undergo surgery. In addition, the child can be told that the eye is going to be fixed and that when he or she wakes up, the eyes will be covered. Assure the child that after the patches are removed, the child will be able to see. Blindfold the child the evening before surgery so that he or she can experience not being able to see. Attach a call light to the bed and have the child practice using it when blindfolded.

Postoperative care When the child returns from surgery, suggest that the parents hold the child and assist them in doing so. Even when prepared, the child may panic when sight is not possible. Before the nurse touches the child or talks with the parents, his or her identity should be made known to the child. It is helpful if the same nurse who prepared the child preoperatively cares for the child postoperatively so that the child hears a familiar voice.

Remain with the parents until they seem confident of their ability to comfort the child, and return frequently to provide assistance as well as to check on the child's general condition. Although the possibility of increasing intraocular pressure is not a concern with this surgery, start oral fluids cautiously to keep the child more comfortable by preventing vomiting. A small amount of serous drainage from the eye that was operated on is expected. Elbow restraints may be needed to prevent the child from pulling at the patch or rubbing the eyes. When the child is fully awake, usually distraction is enough to prevent eye rubbing. The child may enjoy putting a patch on a doll or stuffed animal; provide toys for quiet play. Before the eye patch is removed, prepare the parents for a swollen, reddened eye.

Before discharging the child, demonstrate to the parents how to insert the eye drops or eye ointment and explain the purpose of the medication. Alert them to symptoms of possible infection, such as increased drainage which becomes purulent or increased swelling. Explain the necessity for a return appointment with the surgeon and encourage them to call the surgeon at any time before that if they have questions. The eye may remain reddened and edematous for several days. A school-age child may have to endure some teasing about the reddened eye and the loss of eyelashes. Any activity which may damage the eye, such as contact sports, should be avoided.

Refractive errors

Pathophysiology There are three common types of refractive errors in children: *hyperopia* (farsightedness), *myopia* (nearsightedness), and *astigmatism*. (See Fig. 31-5.) Refractive errors are often familial and related to anatomic deviations in the eyeball. In hyperopia, the eyeball is shorter than normal; thus the light rays converge behind the retina when the child views close objects, resulting in blurred vision. Many preschool children are slightly hyperopic and do not need corrective lenses. As the eyeball lengthens during growth, the problem may be outgrown. If there is a significant difference between the visual acuity of the two eyes, glasses will be needed to prevent the development of amblyopia. A contact lens may be used in the hyperopic eye.

Myopia frequently develops after the age of 8. In this condition, the eyeball is too long, and light rays are focused in front of the retina. Myopia tends to increase in severity as the eyeball lengthens during childhood. Myopic children need corrective glasses and should be checked yearly. Unilateral myopia can result in amblyopia. A child who is nearsighted may complain of not being able to see the chalkboard or may be observed looking at distant objects with partially closed eyes.[19]

Astigmatism occurs because the cornea is curved irregularly; thus some light rays are focused in front of the retina, and others behind it. As a result, vision is blurred. Astigmatism is hard to detect before a child is 5 years old. Blurred vision results in complaints of headaches after

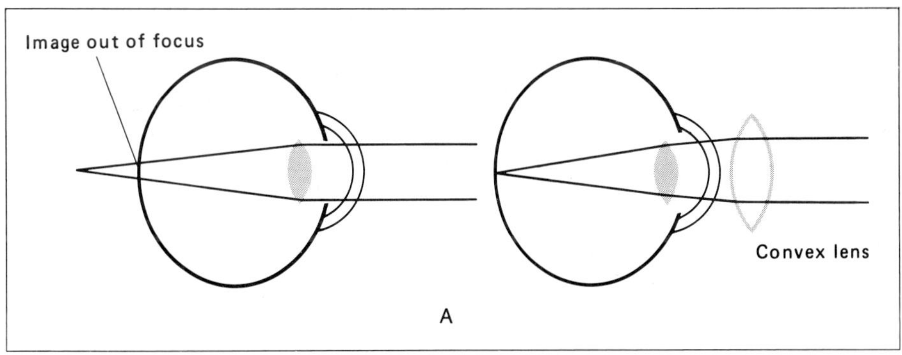

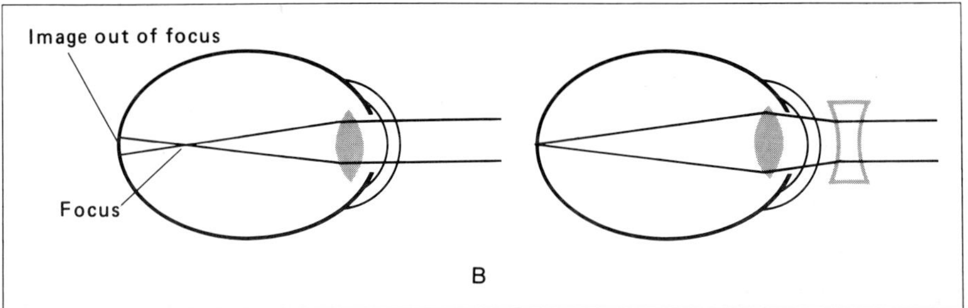

Figure 31-5 Hyperopia and myopia. (*A*) At the right, hyperopia is corrected with a biconvex lens. (*B*) Myopia. At the right, myopia is corrected with a biconcave lens. (*From L. L. Langley, I. Telford, and J. Christensen, Dynamic Anatomy and Physiology, 4th ed., McGraw-Hill, New York, 1974. Used with permission.*)

doing close work. Glasses are necessary for correction.

Contact lenses Contact lenses may be used in place of glasses to correct refractive errors. The primary advantage of contact lenses is cosmetic; contact lenses also provide more normal vision than glasses because the lenses are fitted right to the cornea and move with the eyes. There are no frames to block peripheral vision.

The child of 7 or 8 is able to insert and care for contact lenses but will need parental supervision in following wearing schedules and maintaining strict cleanliness.[20] Teenagers, because of their increased interest in improving their appearance, are more likely to tolerate the initial discomfort during the adjustment period. They are also more dependable about caring for the lenses.

Two types of contact lenses are readily available. The hard lens, which has been in use the longest, is made of a hard plastic material. This lens may provide better vision, since it can correct for the irregularities of the corneal surface. Hard lenses are less expensive and resist wear and tear better than soft lenses. The soft lens, which is made of a flexible plastic material, is easier to adjust to, and the wearer is less likely to develop eye infections. However, soft lenses are more expensive, are more difficult to clean, and have a shorter life span. Soft lenses also absorb eye medications and aerosols such as perfume and hair spray; these substances can damage the lens and can continue to irritate the cornea when it is in contact with the lens.[21]

Hard lenses are generally used for children under 2 because they are easier for the parents to handle. Children over 2 generally accept soft lenses better.[22] Extended-wear lenses are not used routinely for children.

When a child is fitted for contact lenses, the nurse ensures that the child and the parents understand how to wear and care for the lenses. The nurse needs to know what instructions have been given to the child and the parents. Written instructions are helpful. The child should carefully follow the schedule established by the doctor during the initial adjustment period. A special solution and procedure are necessary for cleaning the lenses. The child should be cautioned against using saliva to clean or reinsert a lens, since this may result in eye infection or in swallowing of the lens. Contact lenses should not be worn when the child is sleeping because this decreases the amount of oxygen that the cornea receives and may lead to corneal abrasions. Contact lenses should not be worn when the child is swimming; they are easily lost underwater, and soft lenses may absorb the chlorine in water. Contact lenses should also be kept away from high temperatures; for example, they should not be placed on a car dashboard or on a television set.[23] Contact lenses should be inserted before eye makeup is applied, and using excessive eye makeup should be avoided. The child's eyes should be examined every 6 months. It is advisable for the child to carry identification indicating that he or she is wearing contact lenses.

The most common complications of contact lens wear are corneal abrasions, which are very painful, and ocular infection, which can lead to loss of vision. If the child follows the prescribed instructions carefully, these complications will rarely occur. Symptoms indicating a need for evaluation include pain when wearing the lenses or after removing them, inability to keep the eyes open, markedly increased light sensitivity, hazy vision, and extremely reddened eyes.[24]

Glasses Glasses should be shatterproof. Plastic frames are more desirable than metal ones because metal bends out of shape too easily. Plastic lenses are lighter in weight, but they may be unsuitable for children because they are so easily scratched. Athletic straps or headbands are useful in keeping glasses in place. An older child can be taught to clean his or her glasses with warm water and a soft cloth. To prevent scratching, glasses should not be laid down on the lenses. To prevent breakage, they should be kept in a case when not being worn. Glasses should fit well to prevent irritation of the bridge of the nose and behind the ears; the child is more likely to wear the glasses if the skin is not irritated. Once the child realizes how much better vision is with glasses, he or she is likely to keep them on. Persistence on the part of the parents may be necessary to keep glasses on an infant or toddler. Glasses require an initial period of adjustment; the child may complain of headaches for a few days. If headaches persist, the lenses should be rechecked by the prescribing physician to be certain that the correction is accurate. Older children may need an opportunity to talk about feelings related to a change in appearance that makes them look different from their peers.

Nursing management of children with refractive errors The functions of the nurse include encouraging frequent eye examinations in children, especially if visual difficulties have already been determined; providing follow-up referral of children detected in vision screening clinics; and providing information to the parents and the child about the care and wearing of glasses or contact lenses.

Infectious processes

Ophthalmia neonatorum Any type of conjunctivitis in the newborn is referred to as *ophthalmia neonatorum.* The most common cause is a chemical reaction to the silver nitrate drops instilled after birth to prevent gonococcal conjunctivitis.

The newborn who develops a copious mucopurulent discharge from the eyes 2 to 5 days after birth usually has gonococcal conjunctivitis. If untreated, this infection can lead to corneal ulceration and ultimately blindness. The infant is isolated and treated with systemic penicillin and topical tetracycline or erythromycin. Before instilling the topical medication, irrigate the involved eye with normal saline. Restrain the infant so that rubbing the eyes is not possible. If only one eye is involved, avoid contaminating the uninvolved eye. Open the involved eye frequently to release the pus. The pressure of the accumulating discharge can lead to corneal ulceration. Wearing protective glasses will prevent contamination of the nurse's eyes. Allow the mother to verbalize her feelings; she may express guilt because the infant has picked up an infection from her. With prompt penicillin treatment, loss of vision usually does not occur.

Inclusion conjunctivitis is caused by an organism similar to the one that causes trachoma. It is also picked up during the birth process. Symptoms of mucopurulent discharge usually appear 5 to 10 days after birth. Inclusion conjunctivitis may result in conjunctival scarring and corneal ulcers, which usually heal without permanent effects if properly treated.[25] This type of conjunctivitis is usually treated with oral erythromycin and topical tetracycline for 10 days.

Conjunctivitis in the older child Conjunctivitis in the older child may be due to drug reactions, allergies, disease of the cornea, or viral and bacterial infections. Most conjunctivitis is a result of infections. Symptoms include tearing and a mucopurulent discharge, which may result in morning lid-sticking and a sandy feeling in the eyes. Conjunctivitis due to a bacterial infection, often staphylococcus or *Hemophilus influenzae,* produces more discharge. Instillation of antibiotic ointments or drops, preceded by cleansing the eyes with sterile water, is used to treat bacterial infections.

Viral conjunctivitis is usually accompanied by other symptoms of an upper respiratory infection and is usually self-limiting. Many eye specialists recommend undertreating conjunctivitis, especially if the origin is viral. Antibiotic ointments may be used to prevent secondary infection. The use of steroid ointments can mask herpes virus or fungal infections, which can result in corneal ulcerations and scarring. Viral conjunctivitis is readily spread from one child to another.

Nursing management The nurse can suggest that the parents avoid over-the-counter remedies and seek medical advice for persistent conjunctivitis. The parents may need to be taught the instillation of eye drops or ointments; careful hand-washing before and after should be emphasized. Towels and washcloths should not be shared; swimming and bathing with siblings should be discontinued until the infection subsides.

Trachoma *Trachoma* is a chronic disease affecting both the conjunctiva and the cornea; it is caused by *Chlamydia trachomatis,* a viruslike organism. Trachoma may be one of the leading causes of preventable blindness. Poor hygiene favors its spread. In the United States it is uncommon except in the southwest. The infection is fairly mild in school-age children but is increasingly severe in adolescents and adults. Early symptoms include a mild amount of mucopurulent discharge and reddened eyes. As the disease progresses, the conjunctiva becomes scarred, resulting in malformed lids, which may ulcerate the cornea. Inflammation of the cornea itself leads to vascularization and blindness. Treatment consists of oral tetracycline or erythromycin and a topical antibiotic. Tell the parents or the child to irrigate the eyes before the medication is instilled. Edema can be reduced by using cold compresses, and photophobia is diminished by decreasing the amount of light in the room. Emphasize the need for careful follow-up.

Hordeolums *Hordeolums*, or *sties*, are red, painful swellings due to infection of the sebaceous glands or hair follicles at the margin of the eyelids. Sties tend to occur in crops and can be spread from one hair follicle to the next by the fingers. The cause is usually staphylococcus. Sties are treated with topical antibiotics and warm, moist packs applied several times a day. Sties usually drain spontaneously; occasionally they need to be drained surgically. Sties that recur call for further investigation. Extension of the infection to other parts of the eye is also possible.

Chalazions *Chalazions* are painless cysts which form in the connective tissue supporting the eyelid. They may disappear spontaneously within a month or may be surgically removed. They can become secondarily infected.

Trauma

Trauma to the eye can be caused by foreign bodies, corneal abrasions, chemical burns, blowout fractures, lacerations, perforations, and hemorrhage of the globe. The causes of accidental injury have already been discussed. Children with eye injuries, except for the simplest type caused by a foreign body, should be examined and treated by an ophthalmologist. Visual acuity should be determined whenever possible after an injury.

Nursing management Foreign bodies in the lower or upper lid can usually be removed with a cotton swab. Visible nonmetallic foreign bodies on the sclera or cornea can be irrigated off with normal saline or water.

Chemical burns can cause serious eye damage. Alkalis are most destructive because they penetrate rapidly through the cornea and deep into the eyeball. For a chemical burn, immediately flush the injured eye with large amounts of water for at least 15 minutes. In the emergency room, an intravenous normal saline solution and tubing work well.

Whenever a child is admitted to the hospital for an eye injury, the child will probably be placed on bed rest with one or both eyes patched. If a younger child is very apprehensive, only the injured eye may be patched. Place the child in a quiet room away from the activity of the nurses' station. Decrease the room lighting if one eye is not patched. Sensory deprivation and fear of loss of vision may concern the child most. The parents' presence is reassuring. The nurse can provide appropriate diversion and sensory stimulation by such means as reading to the child, providing a radio, and visiting with the child.

The child may feel that the accident was a punishment for misbehavior. The accident may have occurred when the child was doing something he or she had been told not to do. Provide the child with the opportunity to express feelings either through play or through talking. Assure the child that the accident was not a punishment. The parents may express guilt because they feel that they should have supervised the child's activity more closely.

Some eye injuries may require months before visual acuity, full or partial, is restored. If the child is of school age, the nurse can contact the hospital social services department to arrange for a tutor. Such complications as glaucoma, cataracts, and retinal detachment can occur years after an injury. Encourage the parents to continue regular eye examinations after the eye has healed so that complications can be detected early.

VISUAL IMPAIRMENT AND BLINDNESS

Blindness may be partial or total. Legal blindness is the inability to see at 20 ft, even with corrective lenses, what a person with normal vision sees at 200 ft. Few persons are totally blind; most have some degree of light perception.

Congenital visual impairment

An infant may be diagnosed as being blind in the hospital soon after birth, or the parents may suspect that the child does not see. Whenever a child is diagnosed as being severely visually handicapped, the parents will go through a grief process similar to the grieving that follows any loss. The nurse can support the parents in whatever phase of grieving they exhibit. They may ask for information about the cause and severity of the visual impairment and the availability of treatment. They need assistance in accepting the idea that their child is first of all a child and secondarily a child with impaired vision. They need information about available resources within or outside the local community. Social service agencies should be able to provide referrals to state agencies and to community health agencies. In many states, teachers and counselors associated with a school for the blind can help the parents plan a home program to ensure full development of the child's potential. The community health nurse can work with the counselors and parents in implementing the program.

The infant who is blind from birth is at risk because most early learning takes place through visual cues. In addition, parent-infant bonding occurs primarily through eye contact. The blind infant obviously cannot establish eye contact, and the parents may feel rebuffed. The parents will need to learn different cues for interpreting the infant's feelings of pleasure or displeasure. The infant who is not stimulated will not develop mentally or emotionally but will withdraw. A blind child will need to be taught all the tasks that a sighted child learns by visual imitation. Visually impaired children may crawl and walk later than sighted children because there is no visual incentive for them to move. They will be unable to read braille unless they develop finger dexterity. When they reach school age, a decision will have to be made concerning whether they will benefit most from a residential school for the blind or a regular school system with special visual devices and teachers. The current trend is for visually impaired children to attend public schools whenever possible. With support from professionals and the family, the blind child can adapt well to a seeing world. Table 31-6 lists suggestions for promoting a blind child's development.

Rearing a congenitally blind child requires considerable emotional and physical investment on the part of the family. The needs of the other family members can become forgotten or secondary. An alert nurse can encourage the other family members to consider their own needs as well. (See Figs. 31-6 and 31-7.)

Acquired visual impairment

A child who has lost his or her sight as a result of an illness or injury may assume that the loss is a result of misbehavior and needs to be given the opportunity to express those fears. The child may show regressive or openly hostile behavior. While hostility resulting in failure to cooperate with treatment or in aggressive behavior cannot be tolerated, the child does need the opportunity to express resentment at having lost his or her sight. Not until then can the child accept any assistance toward rehabilitation. Counseling may be necessary. The nurse can refer the family to social services for information about local rehabilitation services such as mobility training. The child's independence should be maintained as

Table 31-6 Methods of Promoting the Development of Blind Children

Infants	1. Tell them when you are picking them up. 2. Hold and touch them frequently. 3. Carry them from room to room in an infant carrier on the parent's back. 4. String a cradle gym across the top of the crib. 5. Prop them in a sitting position to teach head control. 6. Teach hand usage by playing pat-a-cake and splashing in water. 7. Avoid leaving them in a crib for long periods. 8. Teach them to smile by lifting the corners of the mouth gently when a familiar person talks. 9. Place articles of different shapes, sizes, and textures in the hand. 10. Offer finger foods. 11. String large beads on a stiff cord. 12. Use noisemaking toys to encourage mobility and location of sounds.
Toddlers	1. Read stories, especially children's books with touch or smell inserts. 2. Place the same type of food in the same spot on the plate each time. 3. Use bowls with suction cups for feeding. 4. Describe sounds. 5. Provide large beads to string, zippers to zip, and sewing cards. 6. Describe what is happening while dressing. 7. Teach the body parts. 8. Avoid playpens. 9. Involve them in household tasks. 10. Teach them to turn toward a person they are talking to. 11. Interest them in walking by placing objects on a couch near them.
Preschoolers	1. Provide play opportunities with sighted children. 2. Sew tags on the back of clothing to facilitate dressing. 3. Explain where things come from, e.g., that water comes from a faucet. 4. Teach differences in textures—sandpaper, buttons, clay, etc. 5. Draw simple shapes on paper with school glue to form raised patterns.
School-age Children and Adolescents	1. Encourage skating and swimming. 2. Teach use of a typewriter and tape recorder; teach braille. 3. Encourage activities with sighted friends. 4. Assist in vocational testing and in making career choices.

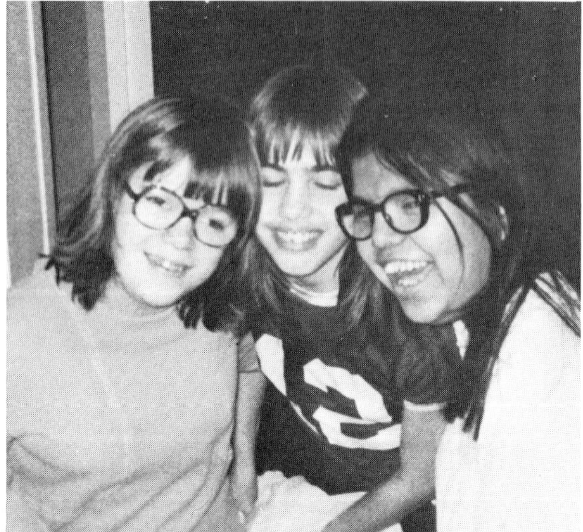

Figure 31-6 Visually impaired children from a residential school. (*Courtesy of North Dakota State School for the Blind, Grand Forks, N. Dak.*)

much as possible; this may be difficult for the parents, who may express their feelings of guilt and concern by trying to do everything possible for their child. If a sibling is responsible for the injury, that child may need assistance in working through feelings. Siblings may also feel that a similar accident could happen to them.

As soon as medically possible, the child should be ambulated. Help the child learn the placement of objects in the room and practice going from one object to the next. Make use of whatever residual vision, such as light perception, is present. Encourage the child to feed, bathe, and dress himself or herself.

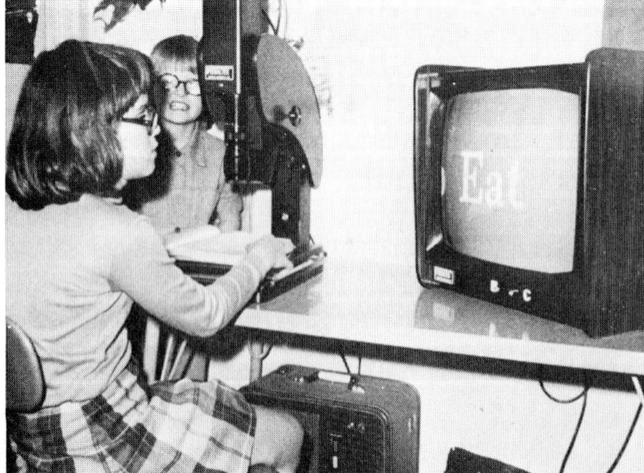

Figure 31-7 A visually impaired child using a closed-circuit television magnifier. (*Courtesy of North Dakota State School for the Blind, Grand Forks, N. Dak.*)

Admission of a blind child to the hospital

A blind child may be admitted to the hospital for an eye examination or for an unrelated illness. When admitting the child, obtain a thorough history from the parents, including the length of time the child has been blind; what self-help skills, such as feeding and dressing, the child performs at home; what limits are set at home; what kinds of activities are enjoyed; and whether the child has been hospitalized previously. Encourage the parents to remain with their child and participate in care; they can act as interpreters and security givers in a strange environment. Orient the child to the room and to the placement of objects, such as the bed and the bathroom door. Walk the child around the unit several times. Explain the sounds the child may be hearing, such as the noise when a call light is pushed and the beep of a monitor or an intravenous pump. If possible, put the child in a room with another child of the same age. A blind child can become easily disoriented in a new environment and withdraw.

Before carrying out any procedure, explain it thoroughly and allow the child to handle the items if possible. Explain that siderails will be up when the child is in bed; keep the bed at its lowest height. Return objects in the room to the same place and guide the child's hands to them. Unless essential for safety, avoid hand restraints; the child needs the hands to stay in touch with reality. Help the child remain as independent as possible; for example, set up the meal tray, but encourage self-feeding.

If the child leaves the unit for any reason, tape a note to the chart or pin a note on the gown. When a child will undergo surgery, a parent or another familiar person can stay with the child until he or she is asleep and be present in the recovery room when the child awakens. Use the information contained in the nursing history to help the child carry out as many self-care activities as possible. When entering or leaving the room, tell the child that you have arrived or are going. Provide play activities appropriate for the child's age. Spend time with the child other than when procedures are being done. Assess the interaction of the child and the parents and the child's developmental level. Provide referral to community health nursing services or social service as appropriate.

EMBRYOLOGY OF THE EAR

Development of the ear begins at around 3 weeks of gestation. Each portion of the ear—external, middle, and inner—develops separately and follows its own timetable. The internal ear is the first portion to begin developing. By the eighth to the tenth week the semicircular canals are present; the cochlea is complete by 12 weeks. By the end of the eighth week an auditory tube is developing: this will become the middle ear. The tympanic membrane is not formed until 28 weeks of gestation.

The external ear is obvious by 8 weeks of gestation. By 11 weeks the ear begins to resemble the typical adult ear. Initially the external ear lies level with the lower jaw, but by the sixteenth week it rises to its higher position on the side of the head. At 20 weeks of gestation portions of the ear begin to ossify.

The ears of the newborn are functional at birth, but the infant is deaf until amniotic fluid drains from the ears and the pressure within the ear is equalized. This is usually accomplished within a few hours after birth. The newborn responds to noise by blinking or exhibiting the Moro reflex. Although the hearing mechanism is developed completely at birth, it undergoes maturation throughout early childhood.[26] (See Table 9-6.)

ANATOMY OF THE EAR

The ear consists of three parts: the external ear, the middle ear, and the inner ear. The anatomy and functions of the various parts are summarized in Table 31-7 and Fig. 31-8.

Table 31-7 Anatomy of the Ear

Part	Function
External Ear	
Auricle	Thin cartilage structure which collects sound waves and channels them into external auditory canal
External auditory canal	S-shaped structure which brings sound waves to middle ear and helps protect and lubricate ear with cilia and cerumen
Middle Ear	
Tympanic membrane	Thin, transparent membrane which vibrates when struck by sound waves
Auditory ossicles	Three small bones which move sound waves from tympanic membrane to fluid-filled inner ear across oval window
Eustachian tube	Small tube connecting middle ear to nasopharynx; made partially of cartilage; maintains equal air pressure between middle ear and external ear and prevents contents of nasopharynx from entering middle ear
Inner Ear	
Oval window	Transmits sound waves from stapes into fluid of inner ear
Round window	Expands and contracts as fluid waves in inner ear change and serves as a relief valve
Vestibule	Central portion of inner ear
Semicircular canals	Maintain sensation of equilibrium and balance
Cochlea	Snail-shaped object in which sound waves are changed to nervous impulses by hair cells contained within it
Organ of Corti	Lies within the cochlea and contains the nerve cells which are sensitive to sound vibrations
Auditory nerve	Transmits nervous impulses to the auditory center within the upper part of the temporal area in the brain

PHYSIOLOGY: SOUND CONDUCTION

Sound waves are caught and carried to the tympanic membrane by the auricle and the external auditory meatus. Sound waves set the tympanic membrane in motion in harmony with their frequency. This vibration is passed on to the auditory ossicles within the middle ear. The third ossicle communicates with the oval window and sets it in motion. The vibration of the oval window creates waves within the fluid of the inner ear. These fluid waves are carried to the basilar membrane within the cochlea. The movement of the fibers of the basilar membrane stimulates the hair cells of the organ of Corti, which lies on

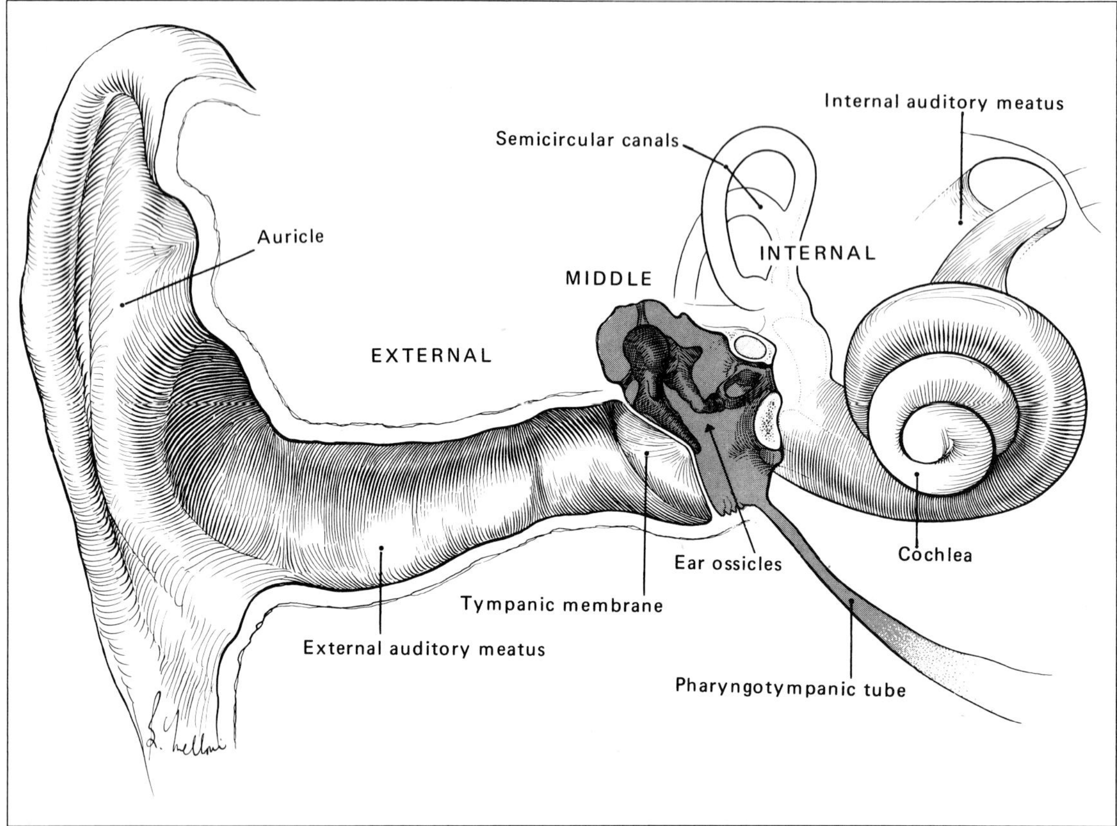

Figure 31-8 Anatomy of the ear. (*From L. L. Langley, I. Telford, and J. Christensen, Dynamic Anatomy and Physiology, 4th ed., McGraw-Hill, New York, 1974. Used with permission.*)

top of the basilar membrane. The result is the stimulation of the axon fibers that make up the auditory nerve. The impulses are then transmitted to the auditory area within the temporal lobe of the brain, where the sounds are interpreted.

When sound is transmitted by bone conduction through the skull, the waves are transmitted to the inner ear, bypassing the external ear and the middle ear.

ASSESSMENT OF THE EAR

Inspection

Assessment of the ear is done primarily by careful inspection and palpation. Table 31-8 summarizes the major points that should be checked. An infant or small child can easily be examined on the mother's lap. In order to examine the eardrum, the child will need to be restrained to prevent any movement which could injure the ear. The mother can hold the child against her body, tucking one arm behind her and holding the other arm while placing the child's legs between her knees. She can then hold the child's head against

Table 31-8 Assessment of the External Ear

Auricles
Well-shaped and complete, absence of skin tags or fistulas
Lie flat against the head
Proportionate to rest of head
Pinna crosses line drawn from outer canthus of eye to occipital prominence
Flesh-colored
Absence of tenderness behind ear
External Ear Canal
Appears patent
Absence of furuncles and foreign objects in canal
Absence of odor
Absence of dried or free running discharge

her body to stabilize the head. The child can also be examined on the examining table with the head turned to one side and the mother or nurse standing at the head of the table holding the child's arms up against the head to stabilize it. Evaluating the tympanic membrane requires experience. The examiner will be looking for the color, mobility, the presence of the light reflex, and evidence of perforation, retraction, or bulging of the tympanic membrane. Before using the otoscope, familiarize the child with it by showing the child the instrument, allowing the child to "blow out the light," shining the light on the child's hand, or describing it as a flashlight.

Hearing tests

A child's hearing ability can be partially assessed by careful interviewing of a parent. The questions should relate to the sequence of growth and development. (See Table 31-9.) A hearing inventory can also be used to elicit information from parents. (See Table 31-10.)

Formalized testing of newborns has been carried out in some hospitals with a device called a *Crib-O-Gram*. This device consists of a transducer which is sensitive to motion, a strip chart recorder, a timing system, and a loudspeaker. The newborn lies on the transducer, and a record is made of responses to sounds.[27] A newer method of testing hearing in the newborn is the *Auditory Response Cradle*, which is a cradle that supports the head and the body and monitors and records the infant's head, trunk, and limb movements after auditory stimulation is presented through ear probes.[28]

Table 31-9 Assessment of Hearing Ability During an Interview

Infants
Respond to noise
Stop activity when someone enters room

Toddlers and Preschoolers
Language development

School-Age Children and Adolescents
Described by teacher and parents as being inattentive
Complain of difficulty hearing in school
Excessive volume on radio or television
Complain of ear pain, dizziness, ear ringing

Children of All Ages
History of frequent ear infections
History of ear discharge

Children aged 2 months to 1 or 2 years can be tested by using various toys, such as a rubber squeeze toy with a whistle or a bell or rattle with a known intensity and frequency. The child is distracted with a toy, and the examiner then makes a noise and evaluates the child's response.[29]

For the toddler and the young preschooler, play conditioning techniques can be used. The child is taught to carry out a specific task when a sound is heard. The child will need to become familiar with the toys and the task first. Examples of tasks include placing a ring on a peg and putting toy animals back into a toy barn. Each correct response is rewarded socially as well. The whisper test can also be used with preschoolers. Tuning fork tests are difficult to explain to young children.

The 4- to 5-year-old and the school-age child can be tested with pure-tone audiometry. The audiometer provides a graphic chart of the child's hearing ability at various frequencies and intensities of sound. The record is made in terms of decibels (dB); 0 dB is the intensity of sound heard 50 percent of the time by a person with normal hearing. Each ear is tested separately; the child is taught to respond to each sound heard by raising one hand. (See Fig. 31-9.)

Several specialized tests are also available for use with children who are too young or who have behavioral problems which limit cooperation. In auditory brainstem evoked-response testing, electrodes are placed on the child's head, and an electroencephalogram is recorded which detects changes when a sound stimulus is presented.[30] Electrocochleography is performed under general anesthesia. A needle electrode is placed through the eardrum, and introduction of a sound results in stimulation of the cochlea.[31]

Nursing management

A child's hearing ability should be assessed at birth, at every well-child visit during the first 3 years, and then every 2 to 3 years.[32] Formal testing is not done; the assessment indicates whether there is a need for further testing.

Normally, ear hygiene consists only of washing the external ear and the edge of the ear canal with a soft washcloth. Cerumen (earwax) serves a protective function and does not need to be removed under most circumstances. Remind parents not to use bobby pins, paper clips, or cotton-tipped applicators to remove earwax. Us-

Table 31-10 Hearing Inventory

Parent ______________________ Child's Name ______________________

Address ______________________ Age ______ Birth Date ______________________

Phone ______________________

Doctor ______________________

Please answer the first questions and then complete the section in your child's age group.

Section 1

	(Circle)	
a. Are you concerned that your child might have a hearing loss?	Yes	No
b. Do you know of any of your child's blood relatives who have a hearing loss? If yes, who (relationship)? ______________	Yes	No
What caused the loss? ______________		
Did he or she wear an aid or attend a special school for the deaf?	Yes	No
c. During your pregnancy, did you have 3-day measles, rubella, or rash with a fever?	Yes	No
d. Did your child weigh 3 lb $5\frac{1}{2}$ oz or less at birth?	Yes	No
e. Was your child in the intensive care nursery?	Yes	No

Section 2

Find the section listing your baby's age and check behavior you have noticed in your child.

3 to 6 months: Date ______________ Your baby:	Yes	No	Don't Know
a. Is awakened from sleep by loud noises	____	____	____
b. Cries unusually loud and very frequently	____	____	____
c. Turns head toward familiar noises like the phone and kitchen sounds	____	____	____
d. Cannot be soothed by voice or music	____	____	____
e. Coos and babbles (makes baby noises)	____	____	____
6 to 9 months: Date ______________ Your baby:			
a. Responds when talked to	____	____	____
b. Sleeps soundly through loud noises	____	____	____
c. Turns head when name is called	____	____	____
d. Does not make baby sounds	____	____	____
e. Likes to shake rattles and bells	____	____	____
9 to 12 months: Date ______________ Your baby:			
a. Imitates his or her own sounds when you say them	____	____	____
b. Ignores quiet sounds and voices	____	____	____
c. Is starting to talk with baby sounds or first words	____	____	____
d. Needs to be yelled at to get his or her attention	____	____	____
e. Listens when talked to	____	____	____
12 to 15 months: Date ______________ Your baby:			
a. Is saying first words	____	____	____
b. Does not pay attention	____	____	____
c. Follows simple directions like "Come to Mama" and "No"	____	____	____
d. Misbehaves and does not understand directions	____	____	____
e. Responds to his or her name when called from another room	____	____	____
16 to 20 months: Date ______________ Your baby:			
a. Says 6 to 20 words	____	____	____
b. Is hard to handle and needs directions repeated often	____	____	____
c. Responds when spoken to with back turned	____	____	____
d. Points to express wants, seldom using words	____	____	____
e. Talks and plays with other children	____	____	____
f. Pulls at people for attention	____	____	____

Note: This form can be completed by the parent at 3-month intervals.

Source: G. Scipien, M. U. Barnard, M. A. Chard, J. Howe, and P. J. Phillips (eds.), *Comprehensive Pediatric Nursing,* 3d ed., McGraw-Hill, New York, 1985, p. 623.

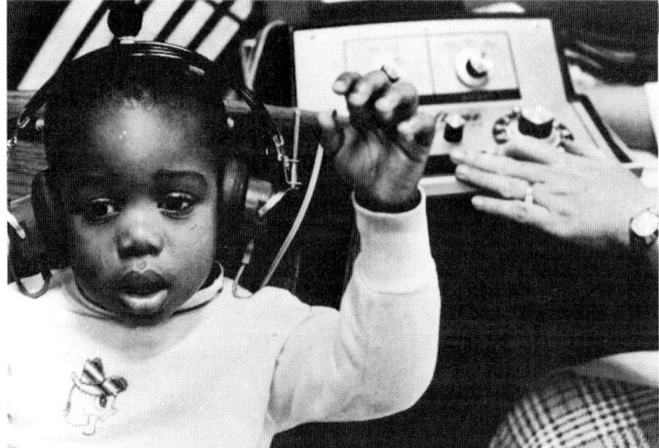

Figure 31-9 Testing the hearing of a 4-year-old child with an audiometer. [*From Pediatric Nursing*, **2**(5) (1976). *Reprinted with permission*.]

ing these instruments usually results in pushing the wax further into the ear canal against the tympanic membrane or in injuring the canal itself.

Symptoms of ear disease for which parents will need to seek medical advice include pain in the ear or behind it, especially if accompanied by fever; any discharge from the ear; any evidence or suspicion of decreased hearing ability; and complaints of dizziness or loss of balance.

If instillation of ear drops has been prescribed, demonstrate to the parents how this is done. For an infant, it is often easier if one parent holds the child while the other parent instills the drops. The medication should be at room temperature to prevent dizziness. Instruct the parents to have the child lie on the side, straighten the ear canal by pulling down for an infant or young child and pulling up for an older child, and put in the required number of drops. After instillation, the child should remain on the side for a few minutes. The child may complain that the drops tickle, but there should be no pain. (See Fig. 31-10.)

Ear irrigations tend to be messy and time-consuming procedures which children dislike, but occasionally they are necessary for removal of excessive earwax. Either an ear syringe or a Water Pik on the low setting can be used. The Water Pik helps break up the wax.[33] A mixture of warm water and hydrogen peroxide is often used. The solution is squirted forcefully into the ear canal and allowed to run out into a basin held below the ear. The fluid should be directed back and up against the wall of the ear canal to prevent pushing the earwax further against the tympanic membrane. The procedure should be stopped if the child feels pain.[34] The procedure is repeated until the ear canal is free of enough wax so that the tympanic membrane can be visualized.

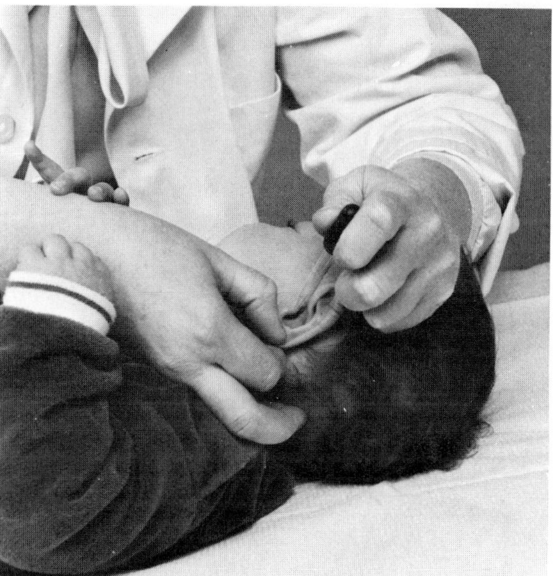

Figure 31-10 Instillation of ear drops.

DEAFNESS

Pathophysiology

Hearing impairment varies from mild to profound. Losses are classified by decibels; a hearing loss ranging from 25 to 45 dB is a mild loss, and one over 95 dB is a profound loss. (See Table 31-11.) A child who has a hearing loss before the age of 2 or 3 cannot develop normal language skills. Hearing impairment can have a conductive or sensorineural basis. *Conductive loss* is due to an abnormality of the external or middle ear that prohibits a transmission of sound waves to the inner ear. *Sensorineural loss* may involve the cochlea, auditory nerve, brainstem, or central nervous system. Hearing impairment can also be a combination of conductive and sensorineural or mixed loss.

Deafness may be due to hereditary factors, prenatal rubella infection, prematurity, hyperbilirubinemia, mumps, measles, meningitis, and trauma. Medications known to impair hearing include kanamycin, gentamicin, neomycin, and streptomycin. The acutely ill infant in an intensive care setting is bombarded with a variety of continuous and sudden noises such as those made

Table 31-11 Handicapping Effects of Hearing Loss

Average Hearing 500 to 2000 Hz (ANSI)	Description	Condition	Sounds Heard without Amplification	Degree of Handicap (If Not Treated in First Year of Life)	Probable Needs
0 to 15 dB	Normal range	Serous otitis, perforation, monomeric membrane, tympanosclerosis	All speech sounds	None	None
15 to 25 dB	Slight hearing loss	Serous otitis, perforation, monomeric membrane, sensorineural loss, tympanosclerosis	Vowel sounds heard clearly; may miss unvoiced consonant sounds	Mild auditory dysfunction in language learning	Consideration of need for hearing aid, lip reading, auditory training, speech therapy, preferential seating
25 to 40 dB	Mild hearing loss	Serous otitis, perforation, tympanosclerosis, monomeric membrane, sensorineural loss	Hears only some louder voiced speech sounds	Auditory learning dysfunction, mild language retardation, mild speech problems, inattention	Hearing aid, lip reading, auditory training, speech therapy
40 to 65 dB	Moderate hearing loss	Chronic otitis, middle ear anomaly, sensorineural loss	Misses most speech sounds at normal conversational level	Speech problems, language retardation, learning dysfunction, inattention	All the above plus consideration of special classroom situation
65 to 95 dB	Severe hearing loss	Sensorineural or mixed loss due to sensorineural loss plus middle ear disease	Hears no speech sounds of normal conversation	Severe speech problems, language retardation, learning dysfunction, inattention	All the above plus probable assignment to special classes
95 dB or more	Profound hearing loss	Sensorineural or mixed loss	Hears no speech or other sounds	Severe speech problems, language retardation, learning dysfunction, inattention	All the above plus probable assignment to special classes

Source: Jerry L. Northern (ed.), *Hearing Disorders*, Little, Brown, Boston, 1976. Used with permission.

by incubators, respirators, apnea monitor alarms, and intravenous pump alarms; these noises may contribute to hearing loss.[35]

Treatment

The child who has a congenital anomaly of the outer or middle ear is checked for inner ear function. If the inner ear is normal, the child is fitted with a bone conduction hearing aid. Reconstructive surgery is usually performed when the child is around 5.

Medical treatment is of no benefit to the child with a sensorineural loss. The child is fitted with a hearing aid as early as 6 months if hearing loss is over 50 dB. Introduction of hearing aids is most successful in infants and helps prevent the language deprivation to which deaf infants are prone. Hearing aids which transmit the sound to both ears (binaural hearing aids) are generally used. Infants go through periods of rapid growth and require regular refitting of hearing aids.[36] Hearing aids that are attached to the body are used for children 3 years old and under because the pinna is not strong enough to support a postauricular hearing aid and because the child's short neck makes that type of hearing aid uncomfortable.[37] An older child may be unwilling to wear a hearing aid that is attached to the body. Recently a cochlear implant has been tested in a few children over $3\frac{1}{2}$ years of age with positive results. While a cochlear implant does not enable the child to understand speech, it does provide auditory stimulation.[38]

Nursing management

When the diagnosis of hearing impairment is made, the parents will need information regarding the cause and treatment as well as support. Contact with parents who are successfully rearing hearing-impaired children may provide the most support. The parents may express guilt, resentment, and anxiety about how to care for their child.

If the child is fitted for a hearing aid, the parents will need to be taught how to insert the hearing aid and maintain proper function. They will be taught to check the hearing aid daily for function, perform simple repairs, and replace the batteries. The hearing aid must fit well to prevent ear irritation and squealing or whistling noises. It will be refitted as the child grows.

Referral by the nurse to an agency that can provide a program of education and stimulation for the child and the audiological services necessary for evaluation of hearing impairment is essential. Hearing loss may be progressive, especially when it is due to rubella syndrome and hereditary diseases.[39] Unless the family lives near a major city, the child and the parents may have to travel many miles to get the assistance they need.

It is essential for normal brain development that the child be able to use residual hearing as early as possible and be stimulated fully. Ideally, the infant is involved in a home program as soon as the diagnosis of hearing impairment is made. The parents are taught how to talk to the child and stimulate normal development. They also receive the support they need to express their feelings about the child and the stresses imposed on the family by the child's hearing impairment. After the age of 3 the child may be enrolled in a nursery school where he or she can learn further communication and socialization skills.[40] When the child reaches school age, the parents will have to decide whether to send the child to a public school that provides special tutoring or to a residential school for the deaf. There are several types of communication systems for the hearing-impaired; which type is best remains controversial (Fig. 31-11). Some educators believe that children should not be taught any type of sign language until they can read lips well,

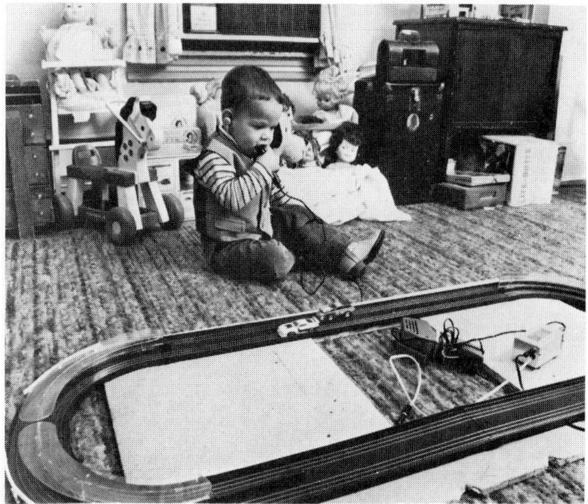

Figure 31-11 Teaching a deaf 2-year-old to speak. The racing car moves on the track when the child talks into the microphone. The set was made by the Telephone Pioneers Organization of Western Electric. (*Courtesy of Western Electric.*)

which may be after the elementary school years; others believe in total communication, which includes lip reading, using sign language, finger spelling, and using residual hearing.

Hospital care of a deaf child When a deaf child is admitted to the hospital, the nurse assesses thoroughly the child's capabilities and needs, just as is done for a blind child who is hospitalized. Hearing loss isolates the child from the external world. It is difficult for a hearing-impaired child to comprehend such abstract concepts as pain. During the admission interview, ask how long the child has been deaf, whether deafness occurred before language ability was attained, what type of communication system the family has been using, and whether the child uses hearing aids.

During the admission procedure, teach the child how to call a nurse by having a nurse outside the door come into the room each time the child presses the call button. This may need to be repeated several times.

To maintain consistency, plan a time schedule for daily events and record it in the Kardex. The child will be more comfortable with the communication patterns that have been developed with the parents; encourage the parents to stay with the child, and use the parents as much as possible when talking with the child or when explaining events or procedures. Assign one nurse to care for the child. To allow for scheduled days off, arrange for the primary nurse and the nurse who is caring for the child to work together for a day.

When entering the room, always touch the child before beginning to talk. Face the child from a distance of 3 to 4 ft. A female nurse can wear lipstick so that the child can read the lips more easily. When it is necessary to perform a procedure behind the child, such as an enema, arrange for another person to stand in front of the child and explain the procedure as it is being carried out.

Use pictures or models of the actual objects to explain procedures or carry out preoperative teaching. If the child can read, use written communication as much as necessary.

Use every opportunity to orient the child to the new environment. Call attention to objects in the area and events that are occurring there; allow the child to explore areas within the hospital with nursing personnel. Introduce the child to other children on the unit.

Words are easily misinterpreted by the hearing-impaired child; more cues are picked up by facial expressions and body language. A frown or a look of disgust or worry conveys more to the child than what the nurse says.

If the child uses a hearing aid, be sure that the batteries are working and that the hearing aid is clean and intact. If the child leaves the unit for any reason, the hearing aid should be in place.

For a child who will undergo surgery, the experience is less threatening if the parents can accompany the child to the holding room and if surgery personnel leave their masks off until the child is asleep. The hearing aid should remain in place until the child is anesthetized; as soon as the child is brought to the recovery room, the hearing aid should be put back into place. To ensure that the hearing aid is not misplaced or damaged, the circulating nurse can label it and send it to the recovery room as soon as it is removed from the sleeping child. When the child returns to the unit, it is helpful to have the parents present.

The care provided by the nurse to the hospitalized deaf child is presented in the Nursing Care Plan at the end of this chapter.

ACQUIRED ALTERATIONS OF THE EAR

Acute otitis media*

Pathophysiology *Acute otitis media* is an infection of the middle ear which occurs frequently following an upper respiratory infection in young children because of the anatomy of the eustachian tube. In infants the eustachian tube is wider, shorter, and placed more horizontally than in older children. The supine position of the infant also promotes the introduction of bacteria from the pharynx through the eustachian tube and into the middle ear. Older children often have enlarged lymphoid tissue which obstructs the eustachian tube; they also have more frequent upper respiratory infections, predisposing them to otitis media. The most common causative organisms are *Hemophilus influenzae,* streptococci, and pneumococci.

An infant may have vague symptoms such as irritability, prolonged crying, fever, vomiting, and diarrhea following a cold. The child may pull at the involved ear. In an older child, infection also

*This section, which appears on pages 676–677, is repeated here for the reader's convenience.

follows a cold, and the child complains of ear pain in addition to having a fever. Pain is due to the edema of the tympanic membrane.[41] On examination, the tympanic membrane may appear red and bulging, and the light reflex may be muddled. Mobility of the tympanic membrane may be decreased.

Treatment Treatment is usually carried out at home unless an infant becomes dehydrated. Oral ampicillin is usually prescribed for 10 days; decongestants or antihistamines may also be given, although their value has not been substantiated. The physician may reevaluate the child in several days. A *myringotomy,* which is a small incision in the tympanic membrane, may be performed to relieve the pressure and permit drainage from the middle ear. Two weeks after the infection, the ears should be examined again, and the child checked for hearing loss.

Complications of acute otitis media include the development of a chronic form of otitis, mastoiditis, or meningitis. The child with chronic otitis media has recurring episodes of middle ear infection, which can lead to mastoiditis or to hearing loss as a result of immobilization of the ossicles and damage to the cochlea.

Nursing management Teaching the parents how to care for a child with otitis media includes giving instructions about administration of ampicillin and comfort measures. Ampicillin is absorbed best when given 1 h before meals. The medication should be continued for the full 10 days. It is tempting to discontinue the medication after symptoms are relieved, especially if giving it involves a struggle. Occasionally, administration of ampicillin results in the appearance of a maculopapular rash or diarrhea. The physician should be notified; in most instances the medication will be continued.

For relief of pain, aspirin or acetaminophen can be given. Occasionally, the child will require codeine. Suggest to the parents that they place the child with the head turned to the affected side and put a heating pad on a low setting underneath the ear. When using heating pads with small children, constant supervision is necessary to prevent burns. If pain persists or increases, if the temperature rises, or if the child becomes lethargic and appears to have a stiff neck, the physician should be notified. Tell the parents the importance of returning to the physician for evaluation after the infection has subsided. Teach the parents that allowing an infant or a toddler to have a bottle in bed may predispose the child to otitis media because of the position of the eustachian tube.

Serous otitis media*

Pathophysiology Serous otitis media is the most common cause of hearing loss in school-age children and is usually the result of eustachian tube dysfunction or adenoidal hypertrophy. Allergy may also be involved. Chronic middle ear disease early in childhood may significantly delay the child developmentally, especially in word and sentence usage. It is unknown whether this delay persists or whether there is a catch-up period.[42]

The most common symptoms of serous otitis media are a fluctuating hearing loss reported by the teacher or parents, mild intermittent pain, and a feeling of fullness in the ear. Blockage of the eustachian tube results in a negative middle ear pressure, which leads to increased mucoid secretion and increased permeability of the middle ear capillaries. On ear examination, the tympanic membrane will appear retracted, making the landmarks more visible, and dull or blue; a fluid level or air bubbles may be seen behind the drum. A tympanogram is a graph which represents the mobility of the tympanic membrane by measuring the air pressure on either side of the tympanic membrane; in serous otitis media, the tympanic membrane is immobile.

Treatment Medical treatment usually consists of antibiotics, antihistamines, and decongestants. The child is taught exercises such as blowing balloons to reopen the eustachian tube. If treatment is not successful within 4 weeks, a small Teflon tube which resembles a small dumbbell may be inserted into the tympanic membrane. The tube acts as a substitute eustachian tube by providing aeration into the middle ear. The tube works itself out into the external ear canal within 6 months. It may need to be reinserted if the condition has not resolved by then. An adenoidectomy may be performed at the time the tube is inserted. A complication of tube insertion is a permanent perforation of the tympanic membrane.

Nursing management Insertion of ventilating tubes into the tympanic membrane may be performed in the emergency outpatient department. The child is discharged several hours after

---

*This section, which appears on pages 676–677, is repeated here for the reader's convenience.

the procedure when he or she is taking oral fluids and has voided. The child may be admitted to the pediatric unit if he or she lives some distance from the hospital or if an adenoidectomy is to be performed.

When the child is admitted, ask the parents whether the child has decreased hearing, and if so, note it on the Kardex. Postoperatively, the child returns to the unit awake and alert. Slight serous or mucoid drainage may be noted in the operative ear; the discharge can be wiped away, but cotton balls should not be inserted into the ear.

The nurse's role in preparing the child and the parents for discharge includes demonstrating the procedure for instilling ear drops and teaching the special precautions necessary as long as the tube is in place. Steroid ear drops may be prescribed to reduce inflammation. The medication should be discontinued if the child complains of pain. The parents will note hearing improvement when the drainage from the ear subsides.

Since the ventilating tube provides an open pathway into the middle ear, no water should be allowed in the ear. For bathing or shampooing, a cotton ball coated with petroleum jelly can be inserted into the ear. Showering should be avoided until the tube is out. The child's hair should not be shampooed in the bathtub in order to prevent contaminated bathwater from entering the ear. Swimming may be permitted if the child has a well-fitting earplug. It is best if the child avoids swimming underwater. Diving is contraindicated without an intact tympanic membrane; the change in pressure that takes place when diving may rupture the oval or round window, leading to permanent deafness.

The parents should contact the doctor if hearing again decreases or if drainage increases. The child will be rechecked about 2 weeks after tube insertion and every 3 or 4 months until the tube is out. Frequent ear examinations after that will be continued to monitor recurrences.

Mastoiditis

Pathophysiology and treatment *Mastoiditis* occurs when the bony partitions between the mastoid air cells are destroyed and the area fills with purulent material. This complication is rare with the use of antibiotics. Symptoms include a dull ache behind the affected ear, a low-grade fever, increased irritability, and the appearance of a red, edematous area behind the ear. A mastoidectomy may need to be performed. The incision is usually made behind the pinna and is covered with padding and a head bandage. Drains may be inserted to prevent hematoma formation. The child may be dizzy and nauseated if the balance apparatus has been disturbed during surgery. Following a simple mastoidectomy, the child may be discharged the day after surgery.

Postoperative nursing management Increasing pain, swelling, and large amounts of serosanguineous drainage from the incision should be noted. Drooling from the mouth or drooping of the corner of the mouth on the operative side may indicate injury to the facial nerve. Begin oral fluids cautiously to prevent vomiting. Position the child on the unaffected side. Change the position of the child and ambulate the child slowly to decrease dizziness. The child will probably receive antibiotics which will be continued at home. Drains and packing may be removed on the third or fourth postoperative day. When discharging the child, send home enough dressings so that the parents can keep the surgical area clean and dry and show the parents how to change the dressing as needed. Shampoos and showers should be avoided until the surgical site is completely healed.

Otitis externa

Otitis externa is an inflammation of the external ear canal, often referred to as *swimmer's ear* because it frequently results when contaminated water enters the ear. *Pseudomonas* is usually the causative organism. The child complains of pain due to the edema of the skin in the external ear canal. When the tragus of the ear is moved, the child will feel pain. The child should be seen by a physician to differentiate between otitis externa and otitis media. Treatment usually consists of local heat and aspirin for pain relief plus antibiotic ear drops containing a combination of polymyxin B, neomycin, and bacitracin. Water should be kept out of the ears until the infection has subsided; swimming is usually contraindicated. This condition can become chronic, although the chronic form is generally not seen in children.

Ear trauma

Trauma to the ear can result from foreign bodies, penetration of the ear canal or tympanic membrane with a sharp object, a blow to the head, and loud noise.

Foreign objects that can cause trauma to the ear include insects and small objects such as peas, beads, matchsticks, and pieces of chewing gum. Small children frequently poke objects into their own or their friends' ears. The child may complain of pain, and decreased hearing may be noted. The attempt to remove the object may result in more damage because the object may be pushed up against or through the tympanic membrane, dislocating the ossicles and pushing the stapes into the oval window. It is best to bring the child to the physician's office for removal of the object. Unless the object is a vegetable such as a pea or a bean, which will swell, or unless the tympanic membrane appears to be perforated, the object may be removed by irrigation. An insect will be killed first by instilling a few drops of alcohol. Suction or forceps may also be used to remove the object. A small child may need a general anesthetic to prevent movement during removal.

Lacerations to the external auditory canal or the tympanic membrane are frequently the result of too vigorous ear cleaning. These lacerations usually heal spontaneously.

A blow to the head caused by a fall, a slap, or a firm kiss on the ear can rupture the tympanic membrane, or the round or oval window, or dislodge the cochlea, resulting in pain, partial deafness, and middle ear infection. Sudden loud noises such as capgun explosions can also damage the ear, as can prolonged listening to amplified music.[43] Children who have had an ear injury should have their hearing checked several weeks after the incident. Slapping the child across the side of the head is not an acceptable form of discipline. The parents may need counseling to learn more effective discipline techniques and to express guilt feelings if slapping has resulted in hearing loss.

THE DEAF AND BLIND CHILD

Characteristics

Congenital rubella is the most common cause of both deafness and blindness in a child. The coexistence of other medical problems such as hydrocephaly, microcephaly, and cerebral palsy is common. It is difficult to determine whether these children are developmentally delayed because of injury to the brain or because the knowledge necessary for testing and stimulating development is lacking.

Everything that sighted, hearing children learn visually and through sound must be taught to deaf and blind children. Intersensory stimulation cannot be coordinated by these children; it is difficult for them to learn what is external to themselves. Characteristics of the deaf and blind child may include hyperactivity, inability to distinguish between night and day, and addiction to light stimulation expressed by gazing at a light or moving the fingers in front of the eyes. The child is apt to resist any type of physical contact and has to learn to enjoy being held and touched.[44]

Effect on the family

The parents may react to their deaf and blind child by trying to meet all the child's needs or by ignoring the child and refusing to develop any type of communication system. It is difficult for the family members to achieve a balanced integration of the child into their lives, and there are as yet few professionals available to help them.[45] Even with professional assistance, rearing the child to take advantage of opportunities rather than withdrawing may require an investment that few families can undertake without significant changes in their life-style and damage to their own physical and mental health.

Nursing management

The parents need professional intervention as soon as their child is identified as being deaf and blind. The nurse should initiate a referral through the social services department and community health agencies as soon as possible and should provide opportunities for the parents to express their concerns.

When a deaf and blind child is hospitalized, it is usually because of an associated medical problem. Obtain a careful history from the parents or other caretakers. Institutional caretakers will not be able to stay with the child, and although the parents may be requested to stay, they may legitimately need a break from the constant pressure of caring for the child. Determine what, if any, communication system the child is learning; use of finger spelling is common. For safety, a small child may need to be in a crib with a safety top. Take the child out of the crib frequently for holding, touching, or walking around the unit to prevent regression and withdrawal. Ask what play activities the child enjoys and continue them, and determine what skills the child has learned, such as feeding or dressing. If possible, the same nurse should be assigned to provide for consistency; the nurse will be frustrated as well as challenged, however, and will need some relief. Assess the parents' acceptance of their child and the assistance they are receiving, and, if appropriate, suggest other sources of help. Provide the parents the opportunity to verbalize their frustrations and discouragement.

As a member of the community, the nurse can encourage all parents to have children immunized for rubella and encourage all women who are considering becoming pregnant to be checked for rubella. In some states, rubella screening is part of the premarital blood work required to obtain a marriage license.

Nursing Care Plan: Hearing-Impaired Child

Patient: Sara *Age:* 8 years *Date of Admission:* 8/12

ASSESSMENT

Sara, age 8, was admitted to the hospital because of severe abdominal pain. After observation and laboratory study, the cause was diagnosed as acute appendicitis. Soon afterward the surgeon removed an inflamed appendix. Sara's mother was with her in the operating room until Sara was asleep. The girl's hearing aids were left in place until then and were replaced in the recovery room.

Sara wears binaural body-type hearing aids and has had moderate hearing loss since age 4, when she had meningitis. Hearing loss is in the range of 40 to 60 dB, where she misses most conversational speech. Since her impairment occurred after development of language, her grasp of abstract terms is greater than would be the case if the loss had preceded speech.

Sara is in the second grade and does well in school, but she is about 1 year behind in academic skills. She receives special help from a resource teacher every school day. Sara is being trained to read lips and is in speech therapy. Her speech is understandable.

Sara's mother stays with her during hospital visiting hours. Her father visits when he can, and her grandmother manages the household, which includes a sister of 10 and a brother of 4. Sara's hospital roommate is a girl of 10 who is in traction because of a fractured femur.

Sara's birth history and development were normal. She has been well except for meningitis at 4 and chickenpox at 6, and she contracts a few upper respiratory infections each year. This is her first hospital admission since the age of 4. Immunizations are up to date. Both her mother (age 34) and father (age 38) are well, as are her siblings. Her maternal grandmother has mature-onset diabetes, and her paternal grandfather died of lung cancer at 65.

Sara weighs 55 lb (25 kg) and is 50 in (127 cm) tall, both of which place her in the 50th percentile by age.

Her father manages a local men's clothing store. Her mother is not employed outside her home. Both parents hold college degrees. Sara shares a bedroom with her sister. Sara's family has accepted her hearing impairment. She has several playmates in the neighborhood and is a Brownie Scout. The family is active in church.

Nursing Diagnosis	Outcome Criteria	Nursing Interventions*	Evaluation and Modifications
1. Inability to hear normal conversation related to hearing loss	☐ Sara will be able to communicate with hospital personnel, as evidenced by: **a.** Responding to instructions **b.** Appropriately using call light to summon nurse	☐ Tape over intercom button at nurses' station. ☐ Note degree of hearing impairment on Kardex. ☐ Teach Sara that nurse will come when call button is pushed by having a nurse stand outside the room and come into the room immediately when the call light goes on; repeat until Sara understands. ☐ Avoid approaching Sara from behind.	☐ Mother is staying with Sara and caring for hearing aids with Sara's assistance. Sara is able to cooperate with procedures.

*The author acknowledges the assistance of Keith Ellen Ragsdale in formulating the nursing interventions.

Nursing Diagnosis	Outcome Criteria	Nursing Interventions	Evaluation and Modifications
		☐ Touch Sara before talking to gain her attention. ☐ Be certain light is on nurses' face; stand in front of Sara within 3 to 4 ft with face turned toward Sara; if female nurse, use dark or contrasting lipstick. ☐ Use mother as communication source, but avoid directing all conversation to mother. ☐ Print simple statements or words if necessary. ☐ Make certain hearing aids are functioning, batteries are working, and ear molds are clean and intact. Ask mother how hearing aids are cared for at home.	
2. Potential feeling of insecurity and isolation related to hearing impairment and newness of environment	☐ Sara will feel secure in hospital environment, as evidenced by: **a.** Calling for nurse when needed **b.** Initiating conversation with nursing personnel **c.** Asking questions about surroundings **d.** Maintaining interests she enjoyed at home **e.** Talking and playing with roommate	☐ Place Sara in room close to nurses' station. ☐ Encourage parents to stay with Sara; provide cot; also provide break time for parents. ☐ Ask parents, if necessary, to interpret Sara's needs. ☐ Assign same nurse to care for Sara each day; 2 days prior to assigned nurse's day off, introduce person who will be caring for Sara. ☐ Follow the same time schedule each day as much as possible so that Sara will know when routines occur and when a nurse will be with her. Give Sara a brief written plan for each day.	☐ Sara uses call button to request nursing assistance. Sara smiles when nurse is present, asks questions of nurse about hospital routines, and talks with nurse about home and school. She is observed carrying on animated conversations with parents and roommate.
3. Decreased ability to understand environmental activities related to hearing impairment	☐ Sara will understand what is happening to her, as evidenced by: **a.** Being able to repeat accurately what she has been told **b.** Assisting nursing personnel when caring for her	☐ When entering room, explain what nurse will be doing; remember that Sara is very aware of facial expression and body movement. ☐ Explain to Sara what is happening when caring for her roommate. ☐ Make requests such as "Sit on this chair" rather than "sit over there." ☐ Use pictures, actual equipment, and concrete words to explain routines and procedures. Avoid abstract terms such as *pain*.	☐ Sara is able to explain procedures back to nurse and cooperates with nurse when care is being provided.

Nursing Diagnosis	Outcome Criteria	Nursing Interventions	Evaluation and Modifications
		☐ When it is necessary to perform treatments or procedures behind Sara, have another person stand in front of Sara to explain what is happening.	
4. Potential to regress in developmental level related to stress of hospitalization	☐ Sara will maintain her developmental level, as evidenced by: **a.** Talking and playing with her roommate **b.** Playing with other hospitalized children in the playroom **c.** Participating in daily cares such as bathing **d.** Reading simple stories	☐ Place Sara in room with child Sara's age, introduce Sara to her roommate, and tell the roommate that Sara is unable to hear well. ☐ Add to Kardex that room assignment should not be changed. ☐ Call attention to surroundings and explain equipment in the room. ☐ When Sara is ambulatory, show her around unit and allow her to explore under supervision; if possible, allow her to leave unit accompanied by mother or nurse. ☐ Take Sara to playroom and introduce her to children playing there. Stay with her until she seems secure and return as necessary. Suggest that mother accompany her to playroom at first. ☐ Supply equipment for diversional activities, such as paper and crayons, clay, and books at second-grade level. ☐ Arrange to play cards or table games with her or set up game with roommate who is in traction. ☐ Practice academic skills, such as printing and adding numbers.	☐ Sara appeared shy at interacting with roommate at first, but now enjoys card games with her. Roommate asks Sara about her hearing impairment, explains new occurrences, and enjoys her company. Sara has been reluctant to go to the playroom. ☐ Sara assists with her bath, brushes her teeth, and chooses new nightgowns. ☐ Revise plan by arranging specific times to take Sara to the playroom and arranging for other children Sara's age to be in the playroom at that time.
5. Potential postoperative complications related to anesthesia and abdominal surgery	☐ Sara's physiological functions will return to preillness or prehospitalization state, as evidenced by: **a.** No symptoms of an upper respiratory tract infection **b.** No symptoms of infection: heat, edema, pain, or redness	☐ See Chap. 19 for specific actions related to caring for child who has had abdominal surgery. ☐ Demonstrate deep breathing and coughing in presence of mother. ☐ Determine if she is in pain by pointing to incisional area and watching facial expressions rather than by asking about pain.	☐ Sara is taking a soft diet well. There is no abdominal distention. Sara had a bowel movement on the third postoperative day. The incision is healing, lungs are clear, and Sara is ambulating well. She dislikes injections; oral medication controls incisional discomfort.

References

1. Bunic, J. Raymond, "Ocular Examination in Infants and Children," in John S. Crawford and J. Donald Morin (eds.), *The Eye in Childhood*, Grune & Stratton, New York, 1983, p. 29.
2. Ibid., p. 20.
3. Ibid., p. 24.
4. Newell, Frank W., *Ophthalmology: Principles and Concepts*, 5th ed., Mosby, St. Louis, 1982, p. 251.
5. Moody, Everett A., "Ophthalmic Examination of Infants and Children," in Robison D. Harley (ed.), *Pediatric Ophthalmology*, 2d ed., Saunders, Philadelphia, 1983, p. 122.
6. Ellis, Phillip P., "Eye," in C. Henry Kempe, Henry K. Silver, and Donough O'Brien (eds.), *Current Pediatric Diagnosis and Treatment*, 7th ed., Lange, Los Altos, Calif., 1982, p. 206.
7. Halberg, G. Peter, "Contact Lenses for Infants and Children," in Harley, op. cit., p. 1287.
8. Calhoun, Joseph, and David A. Hilnes, "Cataracts and Intraocular Lens Implantation," in Harley, op. cit., p. 564.
9. Nelson, Leonard B., *Pediatric Ophthalmology*, Saunders, Philadelphia, 1984, p. 114.
10. Walton, David S., "Glaucoma in Infants and Children," in Harley, op. cit., p. 596.
11. Kolker, Allan E., and John Hetherington, *Becker-Shaffer's Diagnosis and Therapy of the Glaucomas*, Mosby, St. Louis, 1983, p. 337.
12. Ibid., p. 500.
13. Wassenberg, Cathy, "Common Visual Disorders in Children," *Nursing Clinics of North America* **16**(3):479–485 (September 1981).
14. Committee for the Classification of Retinopathy of Prematurity, "An International Classification of Retinopathy of Prematurity," *Archives of Ophthalmology* **102**(8):1130–1134 (August 1984).
15. Chisholm, Lionel, and Morris Shusterman, "Retina and Vitreous," in Crawford and Morin, op. cit., pp. 297, 301.
16. Newell, op. cit., p. 286.
17. Chisholm and Shusterman, op. cit., p. 301.
18. Wright, Kenneth W., "An Update on Amblyopia and Strabismus," *Consultant* **22**(11):97–113 (November 1982).
19. Brent, Henry P., and Maria Arstikaitis, "Correction of Refractive Errors," in Crawford and Morin, op. cit., p. 37.
20. Halberg, loc. cit.
21. Lowther, Gerald, *Contact Lenses: Procedures and Techniques*, Butterworths, Boston, 1982, p. 313.
22. Brent, Henry P., "Contact Lenses," in Crawford and Morin, op. cit., p. 536.
23. Lowther, op. cit., p. 283.
24. Ibid., p. 301.
25. Kuzdan, Jerome, and Maria Arstikaitis, "External Ocular Diseases," in Crawford and Morin, op. cit., p. 218.
26. Nelms, Bobbie Crew, and Ruth G. Mullins, *Growth and Development: A Primary Health Care Approach*, Prentice-Hall, Englewood Cliffs, N.J., 1982, p. 186.
27. Northern, Jerry L., and Marion P. Downs, *Hearing in Children*, 3d ed., Williams & Wilkins, Baltimore, 1984, p. 247.
28. Ibid., p. 249.
29. Ibid., p. 250.
30. Ibid., p. 210.
31. Ibid., p. 216.
32. Leith, Leslie, "Well Child Care," in Jane A. Fox (ed.), *Primary Health Care of the Young*, McGraw-Hill, New York, 1981, p. 140.
33. Watkins, Sue, Teresa H. Moore, and Jean Phillips, "Clearing Impacted Ears," *American Journal of Nursing* **84**(9):1107 (September 1984).
34. Harkass, Carol Kennell, "Clearing the Occluded Auditory Canal," *Pediatric Nursing* **8**(1):23–25 (January–February 1982).
35. Northern and Downs, op. cit., p. 67.
36. Behrman, Richard E., and Victor C. Vaughan, *Nelson's Textbook of Pediatrics*, 12th ed., Saunders, Philadelphia, 1983, p. 1024.
37. Hasenstab, M. Suzanne, and John S. Horner, *Comprehensive Intervention with Hearing-Impaired Infants and Preschool Children*, Aspen, Rockville, Md., 1982, p. 49.
38. Eisenberg, Laurie, and William F. House, "Initial Experience with the Cochlear Implant in Children," *Annals of Otology, Rhinology, and Laryngology* **91**(Suppl. 2, Part 3):67–73 (March–April 1982).
39. Northern and Downs, op. cit., p. 243.
40. Hasenstab and Horner, op. cit., p. 355.
41. Sorenson, Henning, "Therapy in Acute Otitis Media," in Basharat Jasbi (ed.), *Pediatric Otorhinolaryngology: A Review of Ear, Nose, and Throat Problems in Children*, Appleton Century Crofts, New York, 1980, p. 55.
42. Teele, David W., Jerome O. Klein, and Bernard A. Rosner, "Otitis Media with Effusion during the First Three Years of Life and Development of Speech and Language," *Pediatrics* **74**(2):282–287 (August 1984).
43. Sataloff, Robert Thayer, "Pediatric Hearing Loss," *Pediatric Nursing* **65**(5):16–18 (September–October 1980).
44. McInnes, J. M., and J. A. Treffry, *Deaf-Blind Infants and Children: A Developmental Guide*, University of Toronto Press, Toronto, 1982, pp. 2–3.
45. Ibid., p. 267.

32

Gladys M. Scipien

Cellular proliferation

Upon completion of this chapter, the student will be able to:

1. Discuss the incidence of cancer in children, rates of survival, and mortality rates.
2. Discuss the differences between malignant and nonmalignant neoplasms.
3. Cite at least three factors implicated in the etiology of cancer in children.
4. Name and describe at least three types of malignant neoplasms that affect children.
5. Discuss the principles underlying the three treatment modalities for cancer in children.
6. Discuss the impact that cancer may have on the child, the parents, and siblings.
7. Describe specific nursing responsibilities entailed in caring for children with various forms of cancer.

CANCER IN CHILDREN AND ADOLESCENTS

Incidence

There is nothing more demanding, more challenging, or more emotionally draining than working with children who have cancer. These children and their families must cope with a disease process which, after accidents, is the leading cause of death in persons under 15 years of age. The incidence of childhood cancer is estimated to be 10 per 100,000 children, or approximately 6000 new cases each year. There has been a slight decline in its incidence since 1970. Although cancer affects children of all races, there are differences in frequency and survival rates among different races. See Table 32-1 for the incidence of common malignancies in children.

Survival

In the early 1950s fewer than 20 percent of children with common forms of childhood cancer

Table 32-1 Major Forms of Malignancies in Children under 15 Years of Age

Form	Incidence, %
Leukemia (all types)	39
Brain tumors	11
Neuroblastomas	8
Wilms tumors	7
Non-Hodgkin lymphomas	6
Hodgkin disease	5
Rhabdomyosarcomas	4
Ewing sarcomas	3
Osteogenic sarcomas	3
Retinoblastomas	3
Other types of tumors	11
	100

Source: Adapted from Mary J. Waskerwitz and Kathy Ruccione, "An Overview of Cancer in Children in the 1980's," *Nursing Clinics of North America* **20**(1):6 (March 1985).

could be expected to live for 2 years. Advancements in treatment modalities have resulted in dramatically improved survival rates. At the present time, about 50 percent of all children with some form of malignancy can expect to be cured of the disease.[1] Unfortunately, not all childhood cancers are responsive to treatment. The survival rates of children with brain tumors or neuroblastomas have not improved substantially over the years. Cancer should be viewed as a chronic illness which is controllable, if not curable.

Mortality

Cancer continues to be the leading cause of pediatric deaths due to illness, but the mortality rate has decreased over the last 30 years. In 1950, there were 8 deaths per 100,000 children; by 1976, there were 5 per 100,000. The American Cancer Society estimates that about 1600 pediatric deaths occur annually.[2] Until the cause of cancer is known, slow progress will be made in lowering this statistic further.

Diagnosis

Primary pediatric caregivers need to be alert to signs of cancer in the children whom they see for routine and apparently insignificant problems. Many asymptomatic cancerous tumors are detected during routine physical examinations. Early diagnosis of cancer is vital if the best possible results of available cancer treatment are to be realized. It is important for medical caregivers to know that the signs of cancer in children are not those seen in adults. Fernback lists the following common symptoms as the seven warning signs of cancer in children:

1. *Fever* Children who have a persistent fever without an identifiable cause are often seen at an oncologist's office with undiagnosed cancer.
2. *Pain* Fifteen to twenty percent of children with leukemia and bone tumors complain of bone pain. Headaches and vomiting, especially early in the morning, may be a sign of an intracranial tumor.
3. *Masses* Abdominal masses are often not noticed until they become very large; any growing mass in a child is regarded as abnormal. An enlarged lymph node should be biopsied in an asymptomatic child if it increases in size after 2 weeks, fails to decrease in size after 4 to 6 weeks, or fails to return to normal size after 8 to 12 weeks. Enlarged lymph nodes associated with fever, weight loss, or an abnormal chest x-ray are likely to be associated with a serious disease and should be regarded with suspicion. When nodes other than the anterior cervical chain are enlarged, they should be regarded with suspicion.
4. *Purpura* Increased bruising or a petechial eruption may be a sign of thrombocytopenia caused by bone marrow compromise due to leukemia or a metastatic tumor. Periorbital ecchymosis may be a sign of metastatic neuroblastoma.
5. *Pallor* A pale appearance due to anemia may be the result of bone marrow compromise caused by a metastatic tumor.
6. *Changes in balance, gait, or personality* Brain tumors are the second most common form of cancer in children. The symptoms are subtle and may be difficult to recognize. There may be seizures, or the parents may notice personality changes. The signs of increased intracranial pressure frequently develop very slowly.
7. *Changes in the eye* A whitish reflection through the pupil is the classic sign of retinoblastoma. The child may also squint, as if he or she were having trouble seeing.[3]

PATHOPHYSIOLOGY OF MALIGNANT NEOPLASMS

Types of neoplasms

Neoplasms, also known as *tumors,* are masses of cells that proliferate abnormally. This rapid cell growth may be benign or malignant. *Benign* neoplasms are generally not life-threatening, but they sometimes exert pressure on adjacent structures. A benign brain tumor, for example, may exert pressure on vital centers in the cranium. *Malignant* neoplasms consist of cancer cells that have the ability to spread to adjacent and distant structures. Thus, malignant neoplasms are potentially life-threatening.

There are several types of malignant neoplasms. A *carcinoma* is a malignancy that consists of epithelial cells found in the skin, the linings of lungs, and other body cavities. Carcinomas are seen predominantly in adults. An *adenocarcinoma* is a malignant, mixed mesodermal tumor, with glandular elements, which arises from the parenchyma of such glands as the breast, thyroid, or prostate. A neoplasm derived primarily from lymphocytic or histiocytic elements of lymphoid tissue is called a *lymphoma*. At the present time, lymphomas are further subdivided into (1) Hodgkin disease and (2) non-Hodgkin lymphoma. A highly malignant tumor that consists of embryonic connective tissue arising in the mesoderm is called a *sarcoma*. It can involve bone, cartilage, muscle, blood vessels, and lymphoid tissue and takes its name from the predominant tissue of origin. For example, osteosarcoma is a bone tumor, and a lymphosarcoma is a tumor of lymphoid tissue. A malignancy that occurs only in children is an *embryonic* tumor. It is a mixed mesodermal tumor arising from embryonic cells and manifested as a Wilms tumor or a teratoma. *Leukemia* affects the hematopoietic tissue, causing a proliferation of leukocytes, their precursors, or both. This proliferative process can involve myeloid tissue (red bone marrow) responsible for manufacturing granular leukocytes (eosinophils, neutrophils, and basophils). Leukemia can also affect red blood cells, platelets, and lymphatic tissue which produces nongranular leukocytes (lymphocytes and monocytes). The specific leukemic process is identified according to the tissue that is primarily involved. Lymphoid tissue, for example, is affected in lymphocytic or lymphatic leukemia.

Etiologic factors

While cancer in adults can occur in the bowel, bladder, lungs, and skin, with specific causes related to length of exposure to a variety of carcinogenic and environmental agents, the cause of cancer in children is unknown. Most adult tumors arise in surface organs or glands, while malignancies in children frequently occur in deep tissue, the bone marrow, the blood, skeletal bone, neural crest tissue, muscle, or the kidneys. The danger signs of cancer in adults usually are not evident in children.

The high incidence of malignancies in the first 4 years of life (41 percent of all types of childhood cancers) points to the embryonic nature of some tumors. They may have been present at birth or during the postnatal period, but the tumor cells never matured. The rapid proliferation of these cells is similar to the growth of embryonic tissue.

Although the origin of cancer in children is unknown, there are several variables that seem to be implicated in some way. Perhaps when the etiology is eventually identified, researchers will find that there are a number of interrelated causes.

Intrauterine exposure to carcinogens Between 1940 and 1970, diethylstilbestrol (DES) was often prescribed for pregnant women to prevent spontaneous abortions. It is now known that DES can result in vaginal or cervical adenocarcinomas and other abnormalities in female offspring 14 to 22 years later. Male offspring can demonstrate abnormalities that may predispose them to testicular malignancies. Since this drug demonstrates the ability to cross the placental barrier, it is assumed that other carcinogens can affect the embryo and fetus in utero. While many agents are suspected, the effect of physical and chemical substances is unclear at present.

Physical carcinogens Diagnostic radiation of pregnant women increases the incidence of leukemia and other malignancies in their children. Several years ago, therapeutic doses of radiation were used on the necks of infants and toddlers who had thyroid enlargements; this has resulted in a higher-than-average incidence of cancer of the thyroid.

Genetic influence There is no established genetic cause of cancer in children, but some congenital defects are associated with malignancies. Examples are aniridia in Wilms tumor and neurofibromatosis in connection with brain tumors. Leukemia has a higher incidence among children with certain chromosomal aberrations. Perhaps the best example of a heritable single-gene disorder is retinoblastoma, described later in this chapter. Some think that children with common malignancies may have inherited a predisposition through a single-gene disorder.

During the last few years, in applying recombinant DNA techniques to cancer biology, some investigators have obtained evidence which suggests that mutations in DNA cause neoplasms. According to Nienhuis, "By mutation, translocation, recombination or other genetic mechanisms, these normal genes—called proto-oncogenes or cellular oncogenes—may acquire the ability to contribute to, or cause the neoplastic phenotype."[4] Precisely how this occurs is unknown; however, researchers are detecting these abnormalities with increasing frequency.

In one study, abnormal chromosomes were identified in 75 percent of patients with acute nonlymphocytic leukemia.[5] Other investigators have found aberrations in the tumor cells of children with Wilms tumors[6] and acute lymphocytic leukemia.[7] A Roswell Park Memorial Institute study detected chromosomal anomalies in 59.5 percent of children with acute lymphocytic leukemia. Translocation was the most common structural aberration noted in the abnormal karyotypes.[8] In some research centers, these advancements have resulted in the incorporation of cytogenetic studies into the diagnostic workup of all children admitted with malignancies.

Immune defects Some authorities believe that the body has a surveillance system that identifies and destroys neoplastic cells by immunologically reacting to them before they are able to proliferate and develop into a detectable tumor. However, a malfunction of the surveillance mechanism could permit continued cellular division. Children with a number of immunodeficiencies are more prone to developing lymphoid malignancies. Individuals who are immunosuppressed for organ transplantations also have a higher-than-normal incidence of malignancies. Although not a direct cause of cancer in children, the immunosuppression is implicated in some way.

Viruses Investigative work is being done to determine whether an oncological virus is involved in the development of malignant neoplasms. A viruslike substance extracted from tumors of animals has produced leukemia, sarcomas, and other malignancies in mice. In addition, herpes simplex types I and II and cytomegalovirus have been shown to be responsible for malignancies in animals; however, that capability has not been demonstrated in humans.[9] There is no conclusive basis for a virus-cancer etiology at this point. The Epstein-Barr virus has been identified in Burkitt lymphoma, a non-Hodgkin type of lymphoma. Some researchers think that the interaction of viruses and certain chemicals may cause chromosomal damage, which in turn results in malignancies. Although there is a great deal of speculation about viruses, their role in childhood cancer is unknown.

Characteristics of malignant tumors

Malignant neoplasms are composed of poorly differentiated cells with observable abnormalities of the nucleus and cytoplasm. The majority of tumors in children are malignant, and some of them have characteristics that make them unique to the pediatric population.

Rapid growth Normally, such cellular operations as replication, orderly growth, differentiation, maintenance of a repair system, and cessation of activities on maturation are controlled by some internal regulatory process. For example, when a wound occurs, healing epithelial cells divide at its margins and migrate across the wound in order to complete the repair. Once the wound heals, cellular division and motility cease. In malignant cells, signals that halt such activity either are ignored or are ineffective in controlling proliferation. For example, in acute lymphocytic leukemia, the immature cells crowd out normal blood elements, inhibiting their production. It is the disregard for bodily need that typifies malignant cells as they proliferate erratically.

Tissue invasion As these cells multiply, they invade and destroy normal tissue surrounding the tumor. Malignant tumors are not encapsulated, have irregular shapes and nondefined borders, and infiltrate along lines of least resistance, e.g., into soft tissue. Cartilage, fascia, and ligaments are more resistant than softer tissues to this type of invasion. It is thought that malignant cells secrete toxins or enzymes that injure normal cells by breaking down the tissue matrix, thereby permitting an easy infiltration.

Two unique properties appear to enhance the ability of malignant cells to spread to adjacent or distant sites. Surface membranes of malignant cells reduce the ability of nearby normal cells to adhere to one another. This *decreased adhesiveness* allows the shedding of cells from the primary neoplasm and permits the development of foci in other sites. The second property is *loss of contact inhibition*. Contact inhibition is the normal cessation of cellular division and migration of cells when contact with other cells is established, as occurs in wound healing. When contact between malignant cells is made, chaotic proliferation continues. Normal and abnormal cells compete for essential nutrients, and eventually the normal cells are destroyed. This localized, pathologically altered tissue is termed the *primary tumor*.

Metastasis After a local infiltration has occurred, malignant cells establish satellite foci of the same cell type as the primary lesion. This process is known as *metastasis*. (This feature distinguishes malignant tumors from benign neoplasms.) Malignant cells often spread through the *lymphatic* system. Cell "emboli" break away from the primary lesion and move to a lymph node, where a secondary site develops. As these cells multiply and involve the entire node, other malignant cells move on to the next group of nodes.

Another common route for metastasis in children is a *hematogenous spread,* which affects the circulatory system and such vascular organs as the lungs, liver, or bone. Infiltrating small veins, or capillaries, free-floating neoplastic cells held together by fibrin penetrate the wall of a blood vessel, entering the surrounding tissue to establish a secondary site. A third type of metastasis seen in children occurs with abdominal neoplasms. The malignancy extends along tissue planes to adjacent organs. Cells may also be detached from the surface of a malignant neoplasm mechanically, by a surgeon doing a resection or biopsy, or during palpation of an abdominal mass. Just a single transplanted malignant cell has the potential for establishing another site.

TREATMENT OF MALIGNANT NEOPLASMS IN CHILDREN AND ADOLESCENTS

Malignancies in childhood can be treated by chemotherapy, radiotherapy, or surgery. In some instances, one modality may be effective, while in other situations, two or possibly all three approaches may be utilized. Many factors determine treatment, including the child's age, the tumor, the extent of disease at the time of diagnosis, and the unique tumor cell characteristics. It is not unusual for aggressive treatment to involve a combination of modalities. The sole purpose of therapy is to destroy or remove malignant cells which jeopardize a life.

Chemotherapy

General principles in therapy In the last 12 to 15 years, great strides have been made in treating malignancies systematically. As a result of the development of new agents and the use of combinations of several drugs, both remissions and survival rates have increased significantly. The advantages of using drugs in combination include (1) a decrease in resistance to one drug, (2) a lessening of the severe side effects of massive doses of a single agent, and (3) breakdown of the tumor cell cycle at multiple sites.

Malignant cells tend to proliferate at a steady rate, regardless of the body's need for those particular cells. However, it is important to remember that only a small percentage of all the tumor cells multiply at any given time. A tumor mass consists of four compartments with cells moving freely between them. The first compartment consists of temporarily differentiated cells, the bulk of the tumor. The second is a proliferating compartment, which is the target for chemotherapy and a source of metastasis. The third is a stationary differentiated compartment, which often becomes filled with differentiated cells of the host's tissue without further division. The fourth is the compartment of dying cells. Cytotoxic agents are most effective when cells are proliferating.

Chemotherapeutic drugs are categorized according to their effectiveness in specific phases of a cell's generation time, and therefore it is necessary to know a cell's life cycle. See Table 32-2. Agents capable of destroying malignant cells only when they are in a specific phase of division are called *cell-cycle-specific* drugs. Some examples are vincristine, which inhibits mitosis, and methotrexate, which affects the synthesis of DNA. Others destroy proliferating cells without regard to their generational phases, and they are considered to be *cell-cycle-nonspecific* agents. The antibiotic and alkylating agents are examples.

Most children and adolescents receive these cytotoxic drugs over varying periods of time. Initially, when treatment is most intense, large doses are administered in an effort to destroy as many proliferating cells as possible. Later, a mainte-

Table 32-2 Cellular Generation Time

Phase	Activity	Dynamics
G_0	Resting or out-of-cycle phase.	Cell remains in this stage until called to replenish cell population.
G_1	When signal is received, RNA and protein synthesis occurs.	Length of time in this phase varies and is dependent on, and proportional to, individual cells. Rapidly growing cells have a short G_1.
S	DNA synthesis occurs.	Chromosomes double and transcribe genetic material to RNA, including sequence for cellular function and renewal.
G_2	This is quiet phase in preparation for mitosis.	Here, protein synthesis provides material for mitotic spindle apparatus.
M (mitosis)	Cell passes through four phases (prophase, metaphase, anaphase, and telophase).	Results in two identical daughter cells, each with 46 chromosomes.

nance dose is given at specific intervals. It is extremely difficult to predict the length of treatment, the duration of a drug's effectiveness, or the individual patient's response to chemotherapy. That is one reason why treatment protocols are almost constantly changing.

Agents The drugs most often used in chemotherapy are divided into seven broad categories based on either their origins or their actions. These classifications are presented in Table 32-3.

Since almost all these drugs are specific for neoplastic chemotherapy, it is necessary for the nurse to know the action of these medications, their side effects, and the nursing implications of each one of them. The most commonly used agents are listed in Table 32-3. The table does not include experimental drugs that a child may receive.

Safety in administration and the treatment of extravasation A great deal of concern has centered on the consequences to handlers of drugs used in chemotherapy. While urine samples of patients are expected to demonstrate significant levels of mutagenic activity, similar findings have been detected in urine samples of nurses and pharmacists. A mutagen is "a substance that produces a permanent, inheritable change in the genetic material of a cell,"[10] and therefore its presence in the urine of health care providers is significant. Although there are no conclusive results, many institutions have taken steps to protect their employees. Nurses need to adhere to established guidelines until potential risks are confirmed.

Individuals involved in preparing or administering these antineoplastic drugs should receive proper instruction beforehand. All these substances need to be handled safely, cautiously, and respectfully. If a powder is being reconstituted or a solution is being diluted, a mask, disposable gloves, protective eye gear, and a surgical gown with ribbed, knitted cuffs should be worn. If the solution comes in contact with the skin, the entire area needs to be washed thoroughly with soap and water. After the gloves have been discarded, the hands should be washed. Since air contamination presents the possibility of risk by inhalation, these agents should be prepared *only* in a vertical laminar flow hood which carries particles away from the individual.

Precautions also need to be taken when any material is spilled accidentally and should include the contaminated external surfaces of syringes and intravenous bottles. Contaminated needles and syringes are left intact and disposed of in leakproof and punctureproof containers. This prevents any aerosol generation, which occurs when needles are cut. All the equipment used in preparing and administering these drugs, and the materials used to clean spillage, are placed in a specifically designated container that is sealed and incinerated.

These drugs are excreted by the child. Therefore, vomitus, urine, and feces must be considered highly contaminated waste. Gloves should be worn whenever these excreta are handled.

While some authorities believe that exposure over time results in chromosomal damage, no conclusive results have been obtained.[11] Until that determination is made, it is most important to take precautions to decrease the risk of this occupational hazard.

Table 32-3 Common Chemotherapeutic Drugs (*Continued*)

Drug	Route	Diseases in Which Drug is Effective	Common Side Effects	Nursing Implications Peculiar to This Drug
Alkylating Agents These cell-cycle-nonspecific drugs attach themselves to nucleic acid and interfere with mitosis.				
Busulfan (Myleran)	PO	Chronic myelogenous leukemia	BMD*; rare N/V†; renal toxicity; hyperpigmentation of skin; interstitial pulmonary fibrosis with prolonged use; wasting syndrome	Check child frequently for anorexia or weight loss, which may indicate wasting syndrome.
Carmustine (BCNU)	IV	Brain tumors; NHL; neuroblastomas; leukemia with CNS disease	Pain along vein and a flushed feeling during its administration; tissue necrosis if infiltrated; BMD 3 to 5 weeks after dose; N/V 6 h after dose; diarrhea; renal toxicity; mild hepatotoxicity	Drug darkens skin and hardens veins along sites used for injection. Warm soaks to hands and arms tid helps. Giving drug on IV drip can prevent burning during infusion.
Cytoxan (cyclophosphamide)	PO IM IV	Retinoblastomas; NHL; neuroblastomas; ALL; ANLL; rhabdomyosarcomas; ovarian tumors; Hodgkin disease; Ewing sarcoma; tumor; osteosarcoma	Hemorrhagic cystitis; stomatitis; liver dysfunction; BMD 1 to 14 days after dose; N/V 3 to 6 h after dose; facial flushing and hyperpigmentation of skin; sterility (amenorrhea and aspermia)	Good hydration is essential. Force fluids $1\frac{1}{2}$ to 2 times maintenance for 24 h prior to and 48 h after dose. Have child void qH for 24 h after receiving dose. The medication should be given in the morning to decrease time in the bladder.
Dacarbazine (DTIC)	IV	Hodgkin disease; neuroblastomas	BMD 2 to 4 weeks after dose; alopecia; pain along vein and a metallic taste during administration; N/V 1 to 2 h after administration; flulike syndrome with headache and malaise up to 10 days after dose; mild hepatotoxicity; renal toxicity	Give medication on IV drip to prevent burning on infusion. The drug should be protected from the light by a covering bag during infusion. If the IV infiltrates, tissue necrosis will occur at the site.
Lomustine (CCNU)	PO	Brain tumors; Hodgkin disease	N/V 2 to 6 h after dose; BMD 4 to 6 weeks after dose; hepatotoxicity	Child needs to be instructed to take medication on an empty stomach to decrease the likelihood of N/V.
Nitrogen mustard Mechlorethamine Mustargen	IV IT‡	NHL; Hodgkin disease; ovarian carcinomas; chronic leukemia; solid tumors	N/V 1 to 6 h after dose; alopecia; BMD 2 to 3 weeks after dose; hepatotoxicity; tinnitus and decreased hearing	Mix this drug cautiously; avoid contact with skin and eyes. If contact occurs, severe burns will result. If the IV infiltrates, tissue necrosis will occur at the site.

*Bone marrow depression.

†Nausea and vomiting.

‡Intrathecal.

Table 32-3 Common Chemotherapeutic Drugs (*Continued*)

Drug	Route	Diseases in Which Drug is Effective	Common Side Effects	Nursing Implications Peculiar to This Drug
Plant Alkaloids				
These natural products are obtained from the periwinkle plant and stop cell division in metaphase of mitosis, interfering with spindle formation and synthesis as well as processing for RNA.				
Vinblastine (Velban)	IV	Hodgkin disease; NHL	Some N/V; diarrhea; BMD to 4 to 11 days after dose; neurotoxicity; alopecia; mental depression	If the IV infiltrates, there will be tissue necrosis at the site. Vinca drugs are metabolized primarily by the liver; therefore, hepatotoxicity is possible.
Vincristine (Oncovin)	IV	Wilms tumors; retinoblastomas; Ewing sarcomas; ANLL; osteosarcomas; rhabdomyosarcomas; neuroblastomas; ALL; NHL; Hodgkin disease	Constipation; jaw pain, alopecia, stomatitis; neurotoxicity—ptosis; paralytic ileus; loss of deep tendon reflexes; tingling or numbness of hands and feet	Child needs to be checked frequently for signs of neurotoxicity. The drug may cause decreased spermatogenesis; the physician should tell an adolescent boy and his parents this before beginning treatment.
Antimetabolites				
These agents resemble cell metabolites so closely that they are absorbed by a cell and inhibit certain biochemical reactions required for RNA synthesis and cellular growth.				
Cytosine arabinoside (Ara-C) (pyrimidine analog)	IV IM IT SC	CNS leukemia; NHL; Hodgkin disease	N/V; BMD 7 to 14 days after dose; diarrhea; stomatitis; esophagitis; hepatotoxicity; upper gastrointestinal ulcerations	Often administered as an SC injection on several consecutive days at home. Instruction is critical, as is follow-up regarding administration of drug and care.
Hydroxyurea (Hydrea)	PO	NHL; chronic leukemia; ovarian carcinomas	N/V; diarrhea; BMD with rapid leukopenia; stomatitis, gastrointestinal ulcerations; rash, pruritus; renal toxicity	Should be given cautiously to a child with some renal dysfunction.
Methotrexate (MTX) (folic acid analog)	PO IV IM IT	ALL; ANLL; NHL; osteosarcomas; CNS leukemia; solid tumors	Stomatitis; gastrointestinal and mucosal ulceratons; N/V; diarrhea; BMD delayed; alopecia; renal toxicity; hepatic fibrosis	The child and the family need to be instructed to avoid vitamins or other drugs because this drug is a folic acid antagonist.
5-Azacytidine (5-Aza C)	IV	ANLL	N/V; diarrhea; BMD	This drug shold be infused slowly in order to decrease the severity of N/V.
6-Mercaptopurine (6-MP) (purine analog)	PO	ALL; ANLL	BMD 1 to 4 weeks after dose; renal toxicity; N/V; stomatitis and jaundice (rarely)	The effect of 6-MP is potentiated when given with Allopurinol. Therefore, 6-MP dose should be decreased when both drugs are given together.
6-Thioguanine (6-TG)	PO	ANLL; NHL; ALL; chronic granulocytic leukemia	N/V; diarrhea; BMD; hepatotoxicity; stomatitis; skin rash; photosensitivity; unsteady gait	Blood counts must be monitored because of the cumulative effect that 6-TG has on bone marrow. These patients may need assistance when ambulating because of unsteady gait.

Table 32-3 Common Chemotherapeutic Drugs (*Continued*)

Drug	Route	Diseases in Which Drug is Effective	Common Side Effects	Nursing Implications Peculiar to This Drug
Antineoplastic Antibiotics				
These cell-cycle-nonspecific drugs are natural products of some soil fungi. They form stable complexes with DNA and inhibit DNA and sometimes subsequent RNA synthesis.				
Adriamycin (doxorubicin)	IV	Osteosarcomas; ALL; ANLL; NHL; Hodgkin disease; neuroblastomas; Ewing sarcomas; Wilms tumors; rhabdomyosarcoma; ovarian carcinomas	BMD; fever; stomatitis; N/V; alopecia; cardiomyopathy after cumulative doses above 550 mg/m^2	If the IV infiltrates, there will be tissue necrosis at the site. This drug colors urine red for approximately 24 to 48 h after dose is administered, and child needs to be forewarned of this.
Bleomycin (Blenoxane)	IV IM SC	Hodgkin disease; NHL; testicular carcinomas	Anaphylaxis; allergic reaction may occur up to 3 to 5 h after dose; fever; hypotension; N/V; chills; stomatitis; darkened nail beds, palms, feet; macular rash of fingers and hands; anorexia; pulmonary fibrosis	First dose should be a *decreased* test dose. Observe child for such pulmonary symptoms as dyspnea, coughing, or fever, which can occur immediately or gradually. Pulmonary fibrosis or pneumonitis is more likely when radiation therapy is concurrent or has been completed.
Dactinomycin (actinomycin D)	IV	Rhabdomyosarcomas; embryonic tumors; Ewing sarcomas; Wilms tumors	N/V 4 to 5 h after dose; stomatitis; BMD 1 to 2 weeks after last dose; alopecia; acne; diarrhea; hepatotoxicity	If the IV infiltrates, there may be tissue necrosis at the site. If radiotherapy has been or is being given, this drug potentiates its effect.
Daunorubicin (rubidomycin; daunomycin)	IV	ALL; ANLL; NHL	BMD; fever; N/V; stomatitis; alopecia; cardiomyopathy after cumulative doses above 550 mg/m^2	If the IV infiltrates, there will be tissue necrosis at the site. This drug colors urine red for approximately 24 to 48 h after dose is administered, and child needs to be forewarned of this.
Enzymes				
Extracellular supplies of the amino acid asparagine, essential for survival of malignant cells, are destroyed, killing the neoplastic cells.				
L-Asparaginase (Elspar)	IV IM	ALL; ANLL and NHL	Anaphylaxis; chills; fever; hypotension; dyspnea; N/V; malaise; anorexia; hepatotoxicity; pancreatic toxicity with hyperglycemia; protein and coagulation abnormalities	When mixing the drug, swirl vial slowly; *do not shake*. The first dose should be a low test dose to determine sensitivity. Steroids, Adrenalin, and antihistamines should be drawn up and at bedside when this drug is administered.

Table 32-3 Common Chemotherapeutic Drugs (*Continued*)

Drug	Route	Diseases in Which Drug is Effective	Common Side Effects	Nursing Implications Peculiar to This Drug
Hormones				
Corticosteroids have a cytotoxic effect on protein receptors inside neoplastic cells.				
Corticosteroids (prednisone, dexamethasone)	PO	Hodgkin disease; ALL; ANLL; NHL	Increased appetite; weight gain; personality changes. Long-term side effects: moon face, obesity; fluid retention; muscle weakness, osteoporosis; facial flushing; euphoria; hypertension; gastric irritation; immunosuppression	Explain effect of drug on appetite, weight, and personality changes. Antacid may be needed. Encourage the intake of foods rich in potassium—bananas and orange juice. Monitor blood pressure, urine (glucose, albumin), and stools (occult blood). Observe child for potential infection.
Miscellaneous				
Synthetic substances whose cytotoxic properties are unknown and inorganic substances whose cytotoxic actions are unknown.				
Procarbazine (Matulane)	PO	Hodgkin disease; NHL	N/V; BMD 2 to 5 weeks after dose; mild CNS toxicity; stomatitis; diarrhea; drowsiness; chills; fever; weakness; fatigue	This drug is a monamine oxidase inhibitor; therefore, foods such as ripe bananas, cheese, and alcohol, as well as such drugs as antidepressants and sympathomimetics, must be avoided. Otherwise, an Antabuse type of reaction may occur.
cis-Platinum	IV	Neuroblastomas; rhabdomyosarcomas; testicular carcinomas; osteosarcomas; Ewing sarcomas	N/V; renal toxicity; ototoxicity; BMD 3 weeks after dose	Since renal damage is possible during excretion, the child should receive IV fluids prior to, during, and after the infusion of medication (at least $1\frac{1}{2}$ maintenance). Strict monitoring of intake and output and of vital signs q1h during infusion is essential. Tissue necrosis can occur if the IV infiltrates.

Source: Adapted from D. Fochtman, J. Fergusson, N. Ford, and A. Pryor, "The Treatment of Cancer in Children," in J. Fochtman and G. V. Foley (eds.), *Nursing Care of the Child With Cancer,* Little, Brown, Boston, 1982, pp. 191–205; and A. S. Pryor, "Cancer Chemotherapy in Children," *Issues in Comprehensive Pediatric Nursing* **3**(5):50–55 (November 1978).

While proper handling and correct administration are essential, it is critical for the nurse to know the unique properties of drugs that children receive, especially those classified as vesicants. Specifically, a *vesicant* is "an agent which, when accidentally infiltrated into the skin, causes local tissue breakdown and necrosis."[12] Therefore, an accidental extravasation is a major concern of a nurse who is administering such a medication. Some drugs which cause such a tissue response are carmustine, Adriamycin, vincristine, and vinblastine.

The site must be monitored carefully. If the child complains of a burning or a stinging pain or if there is the slightest indication of an infiltration, administration *must* stop. Initially, the child experiences pain, followed by a tissue response of swelling, redness, and vesicle formation. Subsequently, the ulceration and necrosis may necessitate a skin graft to close the significant craterlike damage to the site.

Treatment protocols for an extravasation vary among hospitals. All facilities recommend stopping the flow, disconnecting the tubing from the needle, and leaving the needle in place so that an aspiration can be done (to remove any interstitial medication). After this point, protocols differ. Some institutions utilize 0.9 percent sodium chloride to dilute the remaining infiltrate, and others infuse a cortisone preparation. Many oncology treatment centers have extravasation kits available. They contain antidotes in order to decrease the tissue damage. Ice packs or cold packs should be placed over the site. The physician also needs to be notified.

Complications of therapy Selectivity is not a characteristic of these extremely potent cytotoxic drugs. As a result, normal cells are affected, especially those which have a high rate of proliferation. That is why gastrointestinal mucosa, hair follicles, and bone marrow respond as they do to these agents.

Toxic side effects demonstrated by the gastrointestinal tract include stomatitis, ulcerations, diarrhea, nausea, and vomiting, while alopecia is characteristic of damage done to hair follicles. Patients are closely monitored for bone marrow depression (leukopenia, thrombocytopenia, agranulocytosis, and anemia), which can create a life-threatening situation. White cells and platelets evidence toxic effects much more quickly than red cells. Precipitous drops in either count may indicate the necessity for discontinuing a drug. This is why complete blood counts and bone marrow aspirations must be done frequently. Drugs can have a cumulative effect on the bone marrow, and subsequent depression can occur weeks or months after treatment. Therefore, follow-up clinic or office visits are imperative.

Another potential complication is drug-induced *immunosuppression,* which results in overwhelming infection. The extent of infection depends on many factors, such as the dose, route, schedule, duration, type, and number of agents being administered. It is almost impossible to predict the effect of these drugs on the immune response of human beings because they range from no obvious ill effects to substantial inhibition.

The infection frequency increases when combinations of chemotherapeutic agents are being administered. In addition, cyclophosphamide and adriamycin appear to be most immunosuppressive. Fortunately, this tremendously increased susceptibility to infection is a reversible phenomenon.

Radiotherapy, which is an important treatment in some types of malignancies, is also immunosuppressive, primarily because a bone marrow field is almost always included in the site to be irradiated. Total body irradiation (TBI) in preparation for a bone marrow transplantation may result in a fulminating bacterial, viral, fungal, or protozoan infection which culminates in death.

Radiotherapy

Principles of treatment Radiotherapy is sometimes used in treating neoplasms in children in combination with chemotherapy, surgery, or both. Its objective is to destroy malignant cells by an ionization process which damages the nucleus and eventually kills these cells, but it can also be used to arrest the growth of a tumor or for palliative purposes.

The dosage is determined in *rads* (radiation absorbed dose), which refer to the quantity delivered to the site. The dosage is divided into small doses and given over a period of weeks, with treatments on weekdays and rest from the treatments on weekends, until the predetermined amount has been administered. The actual duration of treatment is very short, and the parents can expect the child to be finished in less than 15 min. Scheduling the treatment for the same time every day allows the child to establish a routine, which is helpful in coping with side effects. If the white blood count is so dangerously suppressed that infection becomes a threat, treatments are stopped until the white blood count returns to a safe level. The time factor is important because malignant cells are unable to recover from the irradiation damage, while normal cells have an opportunity to do so.

Malignant cells demonstrate varying degrees of sensitivity to irradiation. Wilms tumors and Ewing sarcomas are most sensitive, rhabdomyosarcomas are moderately sensitive, and osteosarcomas are least sensitive.

Normal body cells are selectively altered in this treatment. It is especially important to remember that in children, growing tissue is involved. Radiotherapy can result in severe orthopedic deformities as the child grows. However, if radiation can destroy a neoplasm, then it may be necessary to take that risk.

Body marking and shielding Before radiation therapy is started, the child is seen in the radiology department, where the radiologic oncologist identifies the specific structures to be irradiated. The child's skin is marked with an indelible ink so that the target area is the same at each treatment. Body marking and simulation takes about 1 h. The parents and the child need to understand the purpose of this procedure. It is important to stress that the indelible markings are not to be removed or altered until treatment has been concluded. From time to time the radiology technician will touch up some of the markings, since normal showering and wearing of clothes tend to lighten them. Most agencies also use the first visit to go through a simulated treatment, when the child and the family have an opportunity to ask questions about the equipment and to meet the staff members who will be involved in the therapy. At this time the pattern for the molds in which the lead shields are formed will be made. Individualized lead shields are made for each child using x-rays and the markings on the child's body (Fig. 32-1).

After this initial visit, the child begins the radiation therapy. Once treatment begins, the lead shield is used to protect the areas that are not being treated. Every effort is made to protect the gonads, the lungs, the heart, the spinal cord, and other vulnerable organs from radiation if they

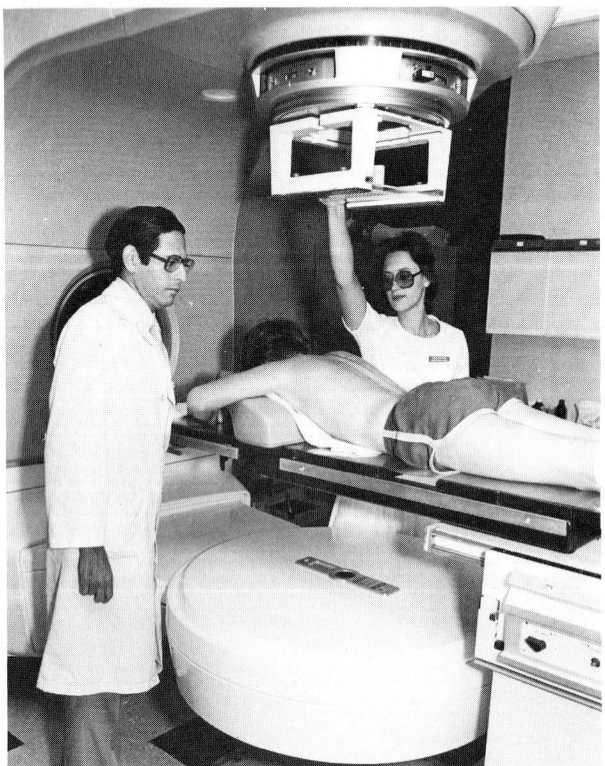

Figure 32-1 Preparing a child for spinal axis radiation therapy. (*Courtesy of the North Shore University Hospital—Cornell Medical Center. From G. Scipien, M. U. Barnard, M. A. Chard, J. Howe, and P. J. Phillips* [eds.], *Comprehensive Pediatric Nursing, 3d ed., McGraw-Hill, New York, 1986, p. 815. Used with permission.*)

are not the target area. A thin lead beading is placed over the spinal cord to protect it from radiation, if it cannot be otherwise shielded.

Complications of radiation There are many local and systemic responses to radiation. They vary according to the treatment and the age of the child. *Alopecia* frequently occurs over the part of the cranium that is being irradiated (Fig. 32-2). The hair begins to fall out after several weeks of treatment, is lost over a period of a few days, and grows back approximately 8 to 10 weeks after treatment is concluded. When large doses of radiation are given, as in the case of a child with a brain tumor, hair loss may be permanent.

Hair loss has a tremendous impact on body image and self-esteem. Children, and especially teenagers, feel a great sadness and depression during the time when the hair is falling out. It is important to have them shop for a wig or decide what kind of head covering they will use before the baldness actually occurs. For a child who receives only partial radiation of the head, such as a child whose lymph node region is being irradiated to treat Hodgkin disease, it is important to have a good hairstylist shape the hair. The top layer of hair can be left long so that it will hide the bald area at the base of the head. When the hair grows back, there may be some differences; previously curly hair may be straight, and the texture and color may be slightly different.

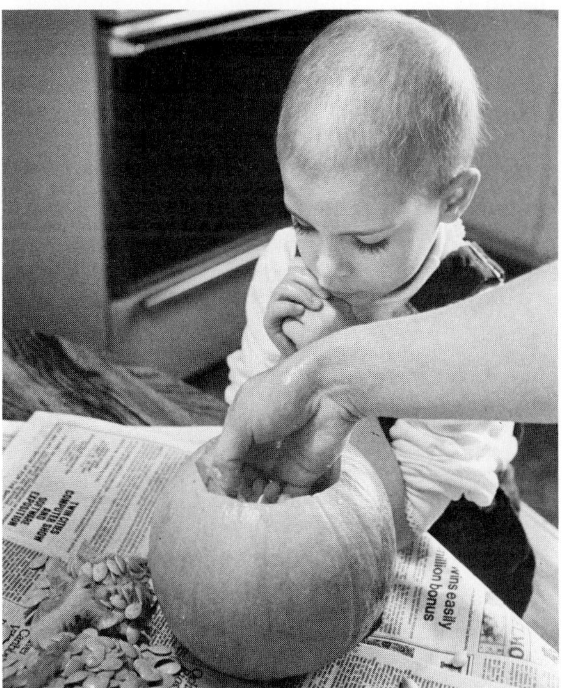

Figure 32-2 This 5-year-old girl has alopecia caused by radiation therapy given prior to a bone marrow transplantation. (*Used with permission of the Minneapolis Star and Tribune.*)

Skin irritations are common local responses, especially if the child is also receiving actinomycin D or doxorubicin, since these drugs potentiate skin reactions. The skin begins to show a pink blush, which over a period of weeks gradually looks like a sunburn. Near the end of treatment, after approximately 4 weeks, the skin looks and feels more brown and leathery. It may crack in the crease areas in the axillae and groin and may become painful and bleed. Once treatment is terminated, the skin will peel and gradually heal; the new skin will be pink and more normal in appearance, but it may still have a rough texture. The skin in the area that was treated will be sensitive to sun and to cold. A sunblock will need to be used to protect the skin against sunburn, and a covering should be used to prevent frostbite. Skin care during treatment includes using neither deodorants nor commercial baby powders because they contain metal and their use will cause a severe axillary burn. Since radiation damages the sweat glands, sweat is not produced, and the odor that adolescents worry about is largely nonexistent. If the armpits are included in the radiation field, they should not be shaved. After treatment is in progress this is no longer a problem, since the hair will be lost. Bathing should be done in warm water, not hot water, using a little mild soap or no soap; the body is patted dry, and cornstarch is applied in the groin and axillary areas to prevent chafing and a prescribed topical cortisone preparation should be used for cracking and redness.

With head and neck radiation, the eyes may become dry or tear excessively. Artificial tears may be used to relieve red, itchy eyes. Saliva is decreased in amount and becomes very thick, causing a dry, sticky mouth. A dry mouth makes it difficult to eat and talk and increases tartar formation on the teeth. Dental care should be discussed with the radiologist, since very careful brushing and flossing and more frequent scaling of the teeth may be needed to prevent decay.

Stomatitis may make it difficult to eat, and a sore throat may make it difficult to swallow. It is important to have the child weigh in at least several times a week if the upper gastrointestinal tract is in the radiation target area. Viscous zylocaine, mouthwashes, and pain medications may be needed to reduce the mouth and throat pain so that the child can eat. When the stomach and abdomen are the target of treatment, nausea, vomiting, and/or diarrhea may occur. Antiemetics should be taken several hours before treatment, and the child should experiment with different time intervals and different medications in an effort to prevent nausea. Once vomiting has begun, it is extremely difficult to stop.

If an extremity is being irradiated, there is an increased danger of pathological fractures, but there are few other systemic side effects. Bone marrow depression can precipitate some major problems such as anemia, infections, and bleeding. Exposure to infections should be avoided, since the immunosuppression is severe and infections can be fulminating.

Radiation over joints and muscles can cause a constriction of the muscle sheath and cartilage and lead to muscular pains and aches. These improve with moderate stretching and exercise, but continue to be a long-term complaint.

Although treatments last only a short time, the effects last throughout the day. Many children are exhausted by the treatment and sleep for several hours afterward. Intermittent vomiting is common; as one teenage girl graphically explained when asked what she was doing, "I'm just hanging around hugging the porcelain." Nausea usually becomes worse from Monday to Friday, resolves somewhat over the weekend (when no treatments are given), and intensifies as the weeks go by. Most radiation treatment is done on an outpatient basis. The length of treatment varies, but if more than one field is irradiated and if breaks are required to allow the white blood cell production to increase, treatment may take from 1 to 3 months. Going to the treatment center every day becomes very exhausting, tiresome, and costly for both the child and the family.

Long-term effects of treatment

The goal of aggressively treating a child with cancer is to realize a cure; a person who has been cured of cancer is defined as someone who is disease-free after 5 years, is mentally healthy, is functioning at an appropriate developmental level, and is a productive member of society. Successful treatment has increased the number of survivors, and health care providers are now more knowledgeable about the toxic effects of these approaches months and years after therapy has been completed, especially when both chemotherapy and radiation therapy have been used. Nurses must know the diverse long-term physical and psychosocial effects so that they will be more effective in their work with these children and their families and will be aware of the consequences of successful management.

Physical effects The skeletal system can be affected by radiation therapy; the deformities vary, depending on the site, the child's age at the time, and the dose given. For example, irradiating one side of the spinal column can result in asymmetrical growth, and scoliosis or kyphosis becomes evident during the adolescent growth spurt. While irradiating the head and neck can cause an altered growth pattern of facial bones, treating long bone neoplasms increases the tendency to fracture, heal poorly, or develop osteonecrosis.[13] Prolonged use of methotrexate has the same effect.

Long-term use of cyclophosphamide can result in vesicoureteral reflux and chronic bladder fibrosis.[14] Radiation in conjunction with actinomycin D can result in severe kidney damage.[15] Radiation nephritis may persist and lead to chronic renal failure.[16]

Radiation to the chest, even though most of the heart and lungs is shielded, can cause permanent scarring that is visible on chest x-rays. The child may find that his or her stamina is greatly reduced and that physical activities result in much shortness of breath. This problem gradually improves, although fibrotic areas may continue to be seen on chest x-rays. Some long-term pulmonary problems include pneumonitis, fibrosis, and, ultimately, pulmonary insufficiency. As many as 30 percent of children who receive chest radiotherapy develop early signs of acute pericarditis.[17] Late effects are ventricular dysfunction and congestive heart failure, which is sometimes reversible. Children who have received radiation therapy in conjunction with adriamycin are susceptible to cardiotoxicity.

Some drugs, such as adriamycin, methotrexate, and 6-mercaptopurine, have been implicated in gastrointestinal disorders, especially nonspecific hepatic fibrosis. Radiation has caused the development of obstructions and strictures and has affected enzyme levels, thus impairing absorption.[18]

The signs and symptoms of chronic encephalopathy are evident in children who have received prophylactic central nervous system radiation for leukemia. These manifestations include lethargy, dementia, seizures, and spastic quadriplegia. In children who also received methotrexate, disabilities extend to headaches, abnormal EEGs, and gait disturbances,[19] as well as learning disorders that encompass motor, perceptual, behavioral, and language problems.[20]

Thyroid problems after radiation include hypothyroidism or hyperthyroidism, nodules, and carcinomas. According to Schimpff, the incidence can be as high as 66 percent in children with Hodgkin disease who were treated with "mantle" radiation (radiation of the mediastinal, hilar, cervical, supraclavicular, and axillary areas).[21]

Problems in the reproductive system range from amenorrhea and diminished spermatogenesis to infertility and sterility. Menopausal symptoms—sweating and hot flashes—result from decreased estrogen production. Estrogen supplementation, often in the form of birth control pills, is prescribed. The teratogenic effects of some drugs, as demonstrated in laboratory studies of animals, have prompted concern regarding similar effects in the offspring of treated females. However, chemotherapy *before conception* or *after the first trimester of pregnancy* does not appear to result in major congenital anomalies in offspring.[22, 23, 24]

Children who survive after radiation therapy are 20 times more likely to develop a second malignancy than children in the general population.[25] Leukemia, bone sarcomas, and cancer of the thyroid are the most common malignancies in children who have had extensive radiation.[26] The combination of antineoplastic drugs and radiation is far more oncogenic than either treatment alone. Survivors of Hodgkin disease who receive both treatments have the highest incidence of subsequent malignancies.[27]

Psychosocial effects Children who have been treated for cancer are subjected to the stress and anxiety of living with a chronic, life-threatening disease. Its toll is evident psychologically, socially, behaviorally, and developmentally. The negative responses of peers, the social isolation, and the thought of living with a disease whose outcome is unknown, or of facing death, affect personality development, contribute to low self-esteem, and necessitate an almost constant adaptation. As a result, these children are at far greater risk for developing emotional problems than children with non-life-threatening chronic health problems.[28]

School-related problems are significant. Absenteeism is common, and while much of it can be attributed to outpatient follow-up visits or to complications, school phobias also may be responsible for some absences.[29] Children with acute lymphocytic leukemia may do poorly because their IQ scores are lower than those of their peers, which some investigators have attributed to cranial irradiation.[30] Feeling sick because of body aches and fatigue may cause short attention spans and learning disorders that affect performance. Teachers tend to have lower expectations for children who have completed their therapy, and as a result, these students do not function up to their potentials.[31] (See Chap. 34.)

When they look for employment, these young people contend with job discrimination, which may be as high as 40 percent.[32] Employers fear excessive absenteeism and anticipate increased insurance premiums. Young people have difficulty purchasing insurance because companies are hesitant to insure someone who has had cancer. When they are able to buy insurance, they pay higher premiums, and individual health insurance policies contain clauses that restrict coverage for those who have a history of cancer.[33] The American Cancer Society has been instrumental in passing legislation making it discriminatory not to hire a person because he or she has had cancer. However, it is very difficult to prove this discrimination.

These problems interfere with the quality of life of childhood survivors of cancer. Psychological support and open communication systems between the child, the family, and health care providers need to be maintained over time because these measures help the child cope more effectively and adjust more readily.

Surgery

Complete removal of a malignancy is the most effective treatment, but it is not always possible. In all too many children, diagnosis is made after the cancer has metastasized. At this point, the malignant cells cannot be completely removed. Chemotherapy, radiation, or both may precede an operation in order to decrease the size of the tumor and make surgical dissection possible.

In those instances in which surgery is performed, the micrometastases which remain can be destroyed by antitumor drugs, radiotherapy, or both. Surgical intervention is palliative when there is regional or advanced tissue involvement. Specific surgical procedures which may be performed on children are discussed later in this chapter.

Nutrition

As was previously mentioned, the chance that children with cancer will be cured or go into long-term remission is greatly improved. Malnutrition is an acute problem, however, and is present in about half of the children with cancer. Some children have lost their appetites and significant amounts of weight by the time they are diagnosed. Others begin to have nutritional problems when radiation therapy or chemotherapy treatments are started. Table 32-3 lists the side effects of commonly used chemotherapeutic agents; most of the gastrointestinal symptoms are described in the earlier section "Complications of Therapy." An underlying cause of malnutrition is the high metabolism of the rapidly reproducing tumor cells. Tumor cells consume the nutrients necessary for normal growth and development.

Frequently the diets of children with cancer are inadequate in protein and carbohydrates, and fluid intake is low. Foods do not taste good, and nausea, vomiting, diarrhea, and chemotherapy-induced intestinal lesions cause fluid imbalances and anemia. The control of diarrhea and the maintenance of fluid and electrolyte balance are discussed in Chap. 18. It is essential for these children to have adequate amounts of protein to counteract the bone marrow suppression and low red blood cell production that is common in many cancers. Essential amino acids are needed to produce red blood cells—23 g of protein for 2-year-olds and 34 g for 10-year-olds. Carbohydrate intake is increased to provide calories and prevent weight loss. Lack of carbohydrates can cause diaphoresis, nervousness, irritability, tremors, headaches, and listlessness. Good sources of carbohydrates that are favorites of many children are cereals, pastas, fruits, milk shakes, ice cream, and puddings. The child who is undergoing chemotherapy needs adequate fluids to flush the toxins through the kidneys. The younger the child, the higher the fluid requirement per kilogram of body weight. A formula for determining fluid requirements is given in Chap. 18.

Other ways to improve food intake include offering small servings of high-quality food at frequent intervals (six times a day), letting children help plan their diets, and paying special attention to providing foods that will help with specific problems, such as constipation or diarrhea, sodium retention or depletion, and potassium depletion.

The nurse and the family should keep a record of the child's intake, since it is easy to overestimate the amount of food eaten. It is also important to keep track of the number of stools and the number of times the child vomits, since these will indicate whether there is a danger of dehydration. The best objective measure of nutritional status is weight; the child should be weighed at least once or twice weekly and should be weighed daily if weight loss and dehydration are severe.

ASSESSMENT OF THE IMPACT OF CANCER

The child

Many factors influence a child's responses to cancer. A major one is his or her stage of development. Younger children (toddlers and preschoolers) react very differently from the way school-age children and adolescents react, in spite of the fact that all these children know they are not feeling well and want to know why.

Young children While toddlers and preschoolers do not comprehend a great deal, they realize that their lives are changing and correctly perceive their parents' emotions. They can pick up cues from health professionals too. Whispering in small groups, tearfulness, and showers of gifts are mystifying and convey that something is dreadfully wrong. The child's anxiety is related to mutilation, immobilization, and bodily changes. The principles described in Chap. 15 should be used to prepare the child for painful procedures and to promote coping.

Older children Older children are shocked and angry about their illness and the changes it imposes, and they demonstrate emotions similar to those of their parents. "Why me?" is a question they often ask. Some children believe they are being punished for wrongdoing. Adolescents may not wish to talk about what they are experiencing. Withdrawal and depression are common. Parents may not answer the questions that adolescents raise because they cannot bear the pain associated with sharing the information. Adolescents need love, security, and support in addition to thorough explanations because they are old enough to understand. A family's reluctance to respond to these queries compounds the problem for adolescents because they have no recourse. When they are denied an opportunity to discuss their fears about their illness or its treatment, they supply their own answers. Often, these are more bizarre than the truth. Adolescents lose control at the very time when they are striving for independence. Therefore, allowing them some control over decision making helps them immensely.

Older children have probably thought about career choices. They may need to alter their plans in view of the diagnosis. Extracurricular activities, especially contact sports like football, may not be possible, but alternatives, such as managing the team, may be acceptable. It is no wonder that adolescents demonstrate their anger so frequently. They seem to be losing so much.

Pain is one consequence of the disease that affects all children. It may be a direct result of the metastatic process or secondary to surgery or diagnostic tests, such as bone marrow aspiration. Children who are being treated for cancer live in constant fear of pain. Emotional outbursts and kicking and screaming can be expected if, for example, a decision is made to obtain a sample of marrow. The child must know that all efforts will be made to relieve his or her discomfort. Pain management is discussed in Chaps. 34 and 35.

It is essential to develop a trusting relationship with the child and the parents, but the honesty on which it must be based can be excruciating. Whether to tell a child the diagnosis or not is a difficult decision for the parents. The problem is not a major issue when a child is unable to comprehend what is being said. However, children are extremely perceptive, and it is difficult to deny the diagnosis in the case of an older child or an adolescent. Although the decision not to inform a child of the diagnosis may be an easy one initially, the reasons for follow-up blood examinations, bone marrow aspirations, or a relapse are hard to explain. Subsequent deceitful explanations often generate more hostility in the child.

The child's understanding of death is related to his or her cognitive development. Four-year-olds consider it a temporary state because they see an actor on television get shot and die and appear again next week in another movie. Teenagers understand that when death occurs, life ceases. Their frustration and anger need resolution so that they can accept the inevitable. Children's understanding of death and their responses to fatal illness are discussed in Chap. 35.

The family

The parents The parents are devastated by the news that their child has a malignancy. They are shocked and angry and cannot believe what is being said. During this initial period, the nurse must often reiterate the facts because the parents may repeatedly ask the same questions, hoping to get different answers.

When the diagnosis is confirmed, there should be a frank, honest discussion with the parents and other members of the family in order to provide them with as much information as they can absorb at that time. An overview of the course of the disease, the treatment, and the prognosis is essential, even though the family may not be ready to hear what is being said. Unwarranted optimism or pessimism is inappropriate at this time and can be detrimental to the overall management of the child. Although the physician is responsible for informing the parents about the child's diagnosis and treatment, the nurse also has an important role at this time. Often the nurse participates in the physician's discussion with the parents. After the physician has explained the child's illness and treatment, it is important that the nurse confer frequently with the parents. They may have unanswered questions and may need clarification of information that the physician has given them. It is most important to maintain open lines of communication, in spite of the time required for this. How a family copes with this stressful situation often depends on the nurse's communication and support.

It is not unusual for the parents to think that the diagnosis is wrong and to verbalize a desire to take the child to another doctor, another city, or another medical center for a second opinion.

Although having another consultation is the parents' right, it is important to point out the added cost and disruption of the home that may result. The parents should not be deterred from seeking another opinion unless the diagnosticians are *absolutely* positive of the diagnosis and seeking another opinion will only waste valuable time.

Consent to begin treatment is obtained after a complete discussion of protocols available for the primary cell type involved. Honest information about the side effects of radiation therapy or chemotherapeutic agents must be provided by the physician.

It is not unusual for the parents to raise the issue of alternative methods of treating the malignancy. Media coverage of certain children who have been given "alternative" treatment is widespread. Laetrile, krebiozan, and other drugs; dietary regimens; and electrical gadgets do not cure cancer, despite the fact that medical quacks are eager to persuade people otherwise. The parents are vulnerable to the appeal of alternative treatment. They need reassurance regarding the legitimate research efforts being conducted by the public sector (the National Cancer Institute, the Food and Drug Administration, and the U.S. Public Health Service) and the private sector (medical centers and drug companies).

The family must cope with innumerable emotional and economic stresses almost immediately. Accepting the reality of the diagnosis takes time. Treatment is begun immediately, however, usually in a specialized medical center. Therefore, a move to another city may be necessary. Unless there are friends or relatives in the area, food and lodging become a substantial expense, especially when the parents remain with their child. The parents are usually not compensated for their absence from work.

Other children in the family may have to stay with relatives while their sibling is hospitalized. This displacement is disruptive, especially for young children. While these problems are most substantial in the initial phase of the illness, they may continue after the child's discharge. Follow-up visits for a physical examination, x-ray, blood and urine analysis, or bone marrow aspiration are repeated for an indefinite period. A relapse catapults the entire family into another stressful cycle.

Financial burdens contribute to the family's woes. There may be no income as a result of absences from work. Health insurance plans seldom cover all medical costs. Cytotoxic drugs are expensive, and those used in maintenance may be needed for years. Bone marrow transplantation costs about $50,000. Transportation expenses for follow-up visits and special foods for a child who has stomatitis or gastrointestinal side effects must also be considered. An economic drain occurs rapidly in the presence of this catastrophic illness and can financially ruin a family for many years.

Support systems help families cope with what appear to be overwhelming circumstances. Parents who have a strong marriage and healthy perceptions of themselves in their roles as partners and parents are often drawn closer together by the illness. Families with strong religious beliefs can often sustain trying times. Extended families and grandparents can provide assistance, often in the form of financial support. Grandparents may assume responsibility for care of siblings, and they may also relieve parents during their hospital vigils.

A special bond unites the parents of children who have cancer. A national group, "Candlelighters," consists of parents who have or who have had a child with this disease. They can assist in many ways, whether by finding living accommodations in a distant city or helping the child's parents resolve a particular problem. They are invaluable advisers because they have experienced similar situations.

Health care providers can give support throughout the course of the illness. By establishing a relationship based on honesty and trust, health care providers help enhance a family's coping skills and decrease their stress. Keeping the parents informed of the child's progress and permitting them to exercise their parenting responsibilities by providing physical care for the child are important. Showing concern for and respecting the parents' privacy, while also being available to answer their questions, serves to decrease their apprehension and also demonstrates the extent to which the nurse cares about them and their child.

Several issues must be discussed before the child is discharged after the initial treatment. Follow-up visits and compliance with drug or treatment regimens which continue after discharge are absolute imperatives. Children often determine their own activity levels, doing as much as they desire. One topic frequently raised by parents is discipline and what to do in a situation which demands a form of punishment. A child is more secure when parental expectations are very clear. Infringements of family rules should not be allowed, and the child should be disciplined as he or she was before the illness was diagnosed. The child is often eager to return to school, primarily because of peer group interactions. Advising the parents to meet with the school nurse (to give information about medications the child is taking), the teacher, and classmates before the child returns can help avoid severe consequences. They need to be told about body changes such as weight gain, alopecia, and a prosthesis; activities in which the child can participate; and the child's limitations. This anticipatory action may make it easier for the child to resume classroom activities.

Siblings When a child's malignancy is first diagnosed, he or she becomes the center of family life. The siblings resent the new focus of attention. They become angry because established family routines are cast aside and because their parents spend most of their time at the hospital. In addition, very little, if any, information is shared with them. The ill child is showered with gifts, is no longer responsible for chores, and is no longer punished for wrongdoings. This turn of events can be most frustrating for siblings who are not old enough to understand what is happening. Not only do healthy siblings resent the parents' preoccupation but they also interpret it as a rejection of themselves. They may have a variety of problems at home and in the classroom setting, ranging from disruptive behavior to refusal to attend school. Their creative imaginations may lead them to think that they, too, have a fatal illness.

A healthy sibling's friends can create added pressures if they make fun of the bodily changes evident in the ill brother or sister; this may increase the well child's anger or guilt. Often, the climate in the home prevents the siblings from going to the parents with these problems.

In some instances, a one-on-one confrontation between the ill child and a healthy sibling can precipitate a verbal encounter which allows the latter to share his or her feelings, clears the air, and promotes greater understanding. It is important that the parents take the time to offer thorough, comprehensible explanations to siblings, who may then assume greater responsibilities with regard to the physical care of the ill child or supervision during play; their cooperation can bring strength and cohesiveness to the family.

The nurse

A nurse is committed to helping children return to optimum levels of health. This is reasonably easy to achieve when a child is admitted for a ruptured appendix, for example. However, in oncology, the "unknown" factor is the nature of the child's response to therapy. Providing nursing care to children with cancer is challenging, exciting, gratifying, and frustrating.

It is natural for a compassionate nurse occasionally to become discouraged, angry, and depressed because of the extent of the child's disease or disappointed in the effectiveness of treatment. Coping strategies for nurses are discussed in Chap. 35.

Developing a strong relationship with the child and the family enables the nurse to make suggestions about the child's care. For example, if grandparents are available, the parents can be encouraged to spend a day with the other children or by themselves. They need to get away, to talk, and to put things into perspective.

The nurse can help the family members learn about the disease, the child's care requirements, and the importance of returning for follow-up visits. The importance of preventing infection and the signs of infection must be stressed. In order to be an effective teacher, the nurse must assess the child's and the parents' needs and determine their readiness to learn before using basic teaching-learning principles. Discharge teaching begins soon after admission, not the day before the child leaves the hospital. The child's and the parents' learning can often be evaluated during future clinic or doctor's office visits. Changes in the treatment protocol can be reviewed with the parents or the child and instituted at home. Home care is discussed at length in Chap. 34.

MALIGNANT NEOPLASMS AFFECTING CHILDREN AND ADOLESCENTS

Leukemia

Leukemia is the most common type of cancer in children and accounts for about one-third of all types of cancers seen in the pediatric population.[34] It is a primary disorder of bone marrow in which normal blood cells in the marrow are replaced by immature cells (blast cells) as a result of an uncontrollable proliferation of leukocytes. In the process of multiplying, the blast cells, which do not mature, accumulate in the marrow. This inhibits the production of other cells, such as erythrocytes and platelets.

While the cause of leukemia is unknown, several factors appear to have some relationship to its development. Exposure to ionizing radiation received a great deal of attention after a high incidence of leukemia occurred among survivors of atom bomb blasts. The role of viruses in the etiology of leukemia has been demonstrated in mice. The similarities between animal and human leukemia are such that some investigators assume that viruses are implicated. A genetic basis is suspected too because (1) the incidence of leukemia in siblings is 4 times the normal rate, (2) there is a high incidence in children with chromosomal abnormalities like trisomy 21, (3) leukemia is present in children with genetically determined disorders such as congenital agammaglobulinemia, and (4) if a child has a homozygous twin with leukemia, there is a 20 percent chance that he or she will also develop leukemia within a year.

Types of leukemia Leukemia is classified according to the specific predominating cell found in the peripheral blood smear and bone marrow aspiration. Two forms are most common in children: (1) acute lymphocytic, or acute lymphoblastic, leukemia (ALL) and (2) acute nonlymphocytic leukemia (ANLL), which includes myelocytic leukemia, monocytic leukemia, and erythrocytic leukemia. About 80 percent of leukemic children have ALL, while the remainder have ANLL. ALL is usually diagnosed in children over 1 year of age, especially those between 2 and 5 years of age, and more males develop the disease than females. ANLL is usually seen in older children and affects males and females equally.

Manifestations The clinical manifestations are common to *all* forms of acute leukemia (ALL *and* ANLL), and a diagnosis is difficult to make because the symptoms may appear in isolation or in various combinations. Their presence depends on the amount of bone marrow compromise as well as on the extent and location of extramedullary infiltration (disease in organs other than bone marrow). Petechiae and bruising are commonly noticed by the parents. Bone pain and arthralgia, which are common, may be confused with the symptoms of other musculoskeletal disorders. Fever and pallor may be present. With an extensive marrow invasion, there is anemia, fatigue, dyspnea, and tachycardia. The central nervous system (CNS) can be infiltrated, and the child is irritable and lethargic, vomits, and has headaches.

Diagnostic tests Since this disease involves the hemopoietic system, extensive blood tests are imperative. A complete blood count and a platelet count are done, hemoglobin and hematocrit are tested, and differential and uric acid levels are measured. In addition, cultures of the urine, blood, nose, throat, and gingiva are ordered. A *bone marrow aspiration* is mandatory for a diagnosis and for differentiation between ALL and ANLL. This technique enables the physician to obtain samples of bone marrow for microscopic cell examination. The posterior iliac crest is most often used as the aspiration site because it contains active bone marrow, is easy to locate, and permits easy restraint of the child. The nurse administers sedation prior to the procedure (if ordered) and positions the child. When the posterior iliac crest is the site, the child is placed in a prone position with a pillow or towel roll under the hips. The nurse also restrains the child as necessary and provides soothing words of support during the procedure. A bone marrow aspiration is extremely painful for individuals of all ages.

Chest x-rays, long bone surveys, an intravenous pyelogram, and a variety of other kidney and liver function tests help in identifying extramedullary sites and in assessing the hepatic and renal systems, which will play a vital role in the detoxification and excretion of cytotoxic agents. The high frequency of central nervous system involvement makes a lumbar puncture necessary so that the cerebrospinal fluid can be examined.

Treatment At the present time, the goal of treating children with ALL is cure, and it is reached through the use of radiation therapy and chemotherapy in the minimum amounts that are capable of producing therapeutic results. After combinations of agents began to be used, there was a drastic reduction in deaths from leukemia, as well as an increase in the number of remissions and prolonged periods of remission.

A child with ALL is usually treated in three stages. The first stage centers on *remission induction;* the total number of leukemic cells in the body is reduced, which permits the return of normal bone marrow production. It takes about

4 weeks for a remission to occur; the drugs most frequently used are prednisone and vincristine, although some medical centers also incorporate L-asparaginase. About 95 percent of children respond to this treatment. The second stage focuses on *prophylaxis*, or a method of destroying leukemic cells located in the CNS. The CNS is often a sanctuary for malignant cells shielded from the chemotherapeutic agents because of the physiological blood-brain barrier. Specifically, the cranial vault is irradiated, and methotrexate is administered intrathecally. However, because of the long-term sequelae of CNS therapy, some medical centers now use different strategies. For example, cranial irradiation is not used for children who have good diagnoses, and reduced amounts are given to others. There are no data available yet regarding the effectiveness of these alternative methods.[35] The last stage is concerned with *remission maintenance*. When remission is successfully accomplished, the child takes methotrexate and 6-mercaptopurine to maintain this status. Sometimes vincristine and prednisone are used. Children can remain in remission for an indefinite period of time. Medications are usually discontinued after 3 years of remission. Approximately 80 percent of children who sustain remission for 2 to 3 years continue to remain in remission and appear to be cured.

A *relapse* occurs when the drugs being used are no longer effective and abnormal cells reappear. The first relapse is especially significant because it indicates a very poor prognosis. Every effort is made to prevent its occurrence. A relapse means that it is no longer possible to control disease. Therefore, cytosine arabinoside and Adriamycin, and possibly some investigative agents, are often incorporated into the drug regimen in an effort to extend the effectiveness of the drugs available. After a relapse, each remission becomes shorter and shorter until death occurs.

Treatment of a child with ANLL focuses solely on the use of drugs. There are a variety of inductive protocols, including cytosine arabinoside, 5-azacytidine, and either doxorubicin or daunorubicin. Other drugs may or may not be used. Unfortunately, ANLL has not been as responsive to treatment as ALL. CNS prophylactic radiation does not seem to help children with ANLL.

Two other treatment modalities need brief elaboration: *bone marrow transplantation* and *immunotherapy*. Unfortunately, donors for bone marrow transplantations are not easily found, the cost is high, massive doses of chemotherapy and total body irradiation are required, and transplantation is not yet done except in research settings. As a result of the radiation, children who receive bone marrow transplantations are susceptible to even the weakest strains of infections. They also may develop graft-vs.-host disease. Transplantation appears to be more successful when children with ALL are treated during the second remission rather than later. Some medical centers perform bone marrow transplantations on children with ANLL 1 month after they enter their first remission. While the results are encouraging, there are no reliable data as yet.[35]

Immunotherapy seemed to be a promising approach when it was found that BCG vaccine could stimulate immunity against leukemia-associated antigens. It has not, however, generated or maintained remissions in many patients who have been studied. Some investigators do not believe that immunotherapy should be a treatment for ALL.

Supportive measures A number of standard supportive measures play an important role in the care of the child with leukemia. Transfusions are essential in the presence of anemia and thrombocytopenia. To prevent volume overload, packed red blood cells are administered instead of whole blood. White blood cell and platelet transfusions are used frequently, especially in the presence of drug-induced depressed bone marrow. Without them, combating sepsis and hemorrhage is an overwhelming and, in some instances, impossible task.

Diminished humoral and cellular defense mechanisms, secondary to immunosuppression, make these children most susceptible to infections. In fact, about 75 percent of deaths from leukemia can be attributed to invading pathogens. Therefore, children are isolated or placed in laminar flow units to combat this serious complication of leukopenia. Hemorrhage is the second most common cause of death because of the depressed marrow and thrombocytopenia.

Prognosis Survival rates have improved substantially, especially among children with ALL, but extramedullary infiltration is more common. Sites such as the kidneys, ovaries, testes, and CNS may be invaded. Monitoring closely is imperative if disease control is to be achieved.

The overall prognosis of the child with ALL is favorable, but the eventual outcome depends on a number of variables, such as the child's age, the initial white blood count, and the presence or absence of extramedullary disease. Children between the ages of 2 and 10 years in whom extramedullary invasion is not present and whose white blood counts are below 100,000 have the best prognosis. On the one hand, about 90 to 95 percent of children with ALL go into an initial remission, and 50 to 60 percent survive for at least 5 years, a statistic which seems to be improving annually. Until recently, the prognosis for children with ANLL was poor. For many years, the rate of initial remission was only 40 to 50 percent, and remission seldom lasted longer than 6 months. Recent improvements in treatment protocols have, however, resulted in remission rates of about 70 percent, and remissions last approximately 2 years. Ongoing research in the treatment of ANLL may provide a more promising prognosis in the future.

Response to therapy varies among children. It depends on the type of malignant cell present, the extent of involvement (local or disseminated), the child's age, treatment modalities available, and general physical health status, especially kidney and liver function.

Nursing management When a child who is suspected of having leukemia is hospitalized, the symptoms are usually minimal. The battery of tests essential for diagnosis are invasive and painful. Explaining them honestly, and precisely, will help develop a relationship which elicits the child's cooperation. Both a lumbar puncture and bone marrow aspiration are painful (the latter is more so). They are important procedures which will be repeated in the future in order to assess response to chemotherapy or the extent of relapse. Being present when they are performed, reassuring the child, and using local anesthetics can decrease both anxiety and discomfort.

When chemotherapy begins, the side effects of cytotoxic agents cause many problems which can generate a number of complications. Corticosteroids, which are an exception, contribute to feelings of euphoria and a marked increase in appetite. Drugs may also result in alterations in body image. Normal eating patterns are disrupted because of mechanical problems due to oral lesions and gingival bleeding. See Fig. 32-3. The nurse is called upon to demonstrate creative ability in providing a high-protein, high-calorie diet to a child who is experiencing pain and an unpleasant taste. Supplemental high-calorie liquids can be used. The nutritionist should be consulted, and the parents may be asked to bring foods prepared at home. Children from various ethnic groups may have an improved dietary intake when food is brought in from home. The parents, who feel frustrated and helpless be-

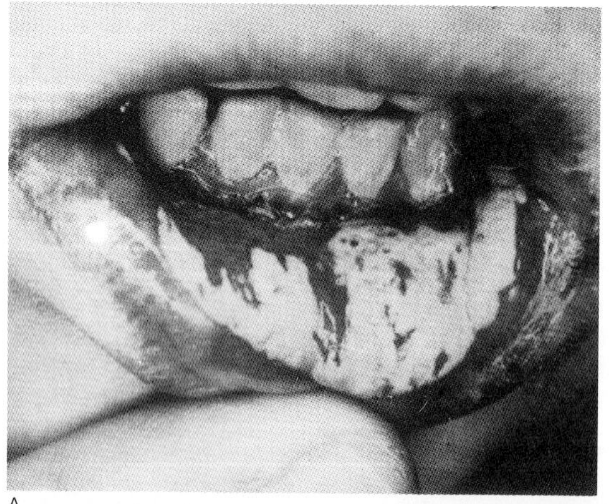
A

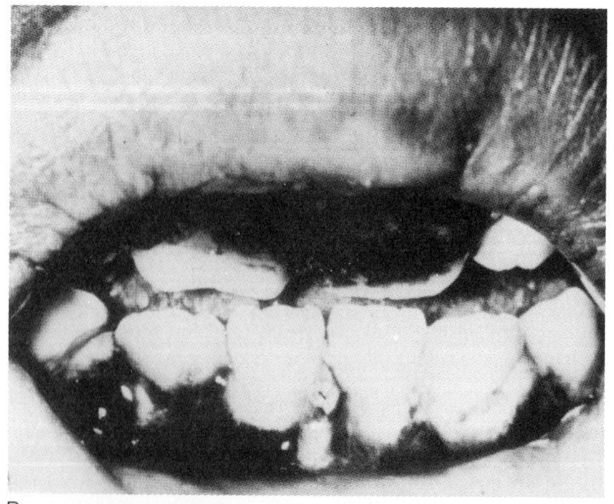
B

Figure 32-3 Oral lesions seen in children with leukemia. (*A*) Oral candidiasis, or thrush. (*B*) Bleeding of the gums and gingival infiltration, which are common in ALL. (*From G. Scipien, M. U. Barnard, M. A. Chard, J. Howe, and P. J. Phillips* [eds.], *Comprehensive Pediatric Nursing, 3d ed., McGraw-Hill, New York, 1986, p. 1023. Used with permission.*)

cause of the diagnosis, are pleased to help. Allowing children to select food they wish to eat may stimulate their interest.

Brushing the teeth may be difficult if lesions are present, and so the nurse needs to use good judgment in providing oral hygiene. A Water Pik cleans the teeth and provides gingival stimulation similar to chewing. Lemon and glycerine swabs or hydrogen peroxide mixed with saline or sterile water, used as a mouthwash, is effective. Water rinses may be the only alternative for severely affected children. The use of forks, spoons, and straws may be curtailed to prevent further injury.

Without exercise or foods high in bulk, these children have bowel problems, especially when they are receiving vincristine, which exhibits a neurotoxic sign in constipation. Increasing fluid intake and giving stool softeners can prevent a potential problem.

The gastrointestinal side effects of some drugs may result in the development of rectal ulcers, which begin as small, tender, red lesions. Assessing the anal area frequently and providing good skin care are effective in preventing necrosis. Leukemic children need to be turned and positioned frequently. A piece of sheepskin or an alternating pressure mattress should be used if available. Rectal temperatures are *not* taken, and ointments, which tend to trap organisms (enhancing an infection), are never used. The child should be bathed after voiding or having a bowel movement to decrease the likelihood of introducing contaminants.

Because infection is the leading cause of death, all efforts need to be directed toward lessening this possibility. Meticulous hand-washing by the nurse, the parents, and the child is essential. While venipunctures are necessary and can be a source of infection, injections are avoided, if possible, in an attempt to maintain skin integrity. A private room and protective isolation measures (see Chap. 16) or a laminar flow unit may be used to decrease the likelihood of infection. In the event that an infection does not respond to antibiotics, a white blood cell (granulocytes) transfusion can be done. Some children may develop chills and an elevated temperature, particularly after repeated transfusions. These are monitored, recorded, and reported; however, the transfusion is not discontinued.

When a child is in the remission induction phase of treatment, blood transfusions are given to correct anemia. Transfusions are *not* administered prior to bone marrow aspirations or the confirmation of diagnosis, even in the presence of severe anemia. The administration of blood elements masks the true hematologic picture. Nursing responsibilities during a blood transfusion are directed toward observation of the child and maintenance of a patent site. It may be necessary to immobilize the child (see Chap. 16). It is important to make the child as comfortable as possible for the next few hours. The rate of blood flow is monitored closely to prevent circulatory overload. Since the risk of complications increases with successive transfusions, it is imperative that the nurse observe for signs of *transfusion reaction*. Most reactions occur during the first 10 min. They include chills, fever, restlessness, irritability, hematuria, and oliguria. When reaction is suspected, the transfusion *must be stopped*, and a physician is called. If a double setup is used, saline can be infused in the interim, retaining patency. The remaining blood is sent back to the blood bank, where it is cultured and examined. A specimen of the child's blood is drawn and sent for culture.

Hemorrhage is also a very serious problem in leukemic children. Their bodies must be examined often to determine the presence of (and increase in) ecchymosis and petechiae as well as bleeding into soft tissue, which is a superb medium for infection. Platelet transfusions may be given during active bleeding episodes, such as uncontrollable epistaxis, or in the presence of low platelet counts (20,000/mm^3). A temperature elevation can occur during a platelet transfusion. Simple measures often control minor local bleeding effectively. Ice or cold compresses and gentle pressure may be used. A dry tea bag can be applied to control gingival bleeding. Salt pork, trimmed to size, acts as an astringent and provides pressure to control epistaxis. The removal of a salt pork pack (usually 12 to 24 h later) causes less disruption to the mucosa than removal of a sterile gauze pack.

The child must cope with many bodily changes which accompany the illness and treatment. They should be free to select diversional activities, but the nurse needs to help them cope with the emotions they are experiencing. Play provides that opportunity. Pounding toys, storytelling, and role playing are all effective avenues of expression (see Chap. 15).

Teaching is a high priority for the nurse. Both the child and the parents must anticipate radiation- or drug-induced alopecia, and the child should be prepared to wear a wig, baseball cap, or scarf. They also need to be reassured of regrowth in 2 to 4 months. Because the risk of infection is high, activities which bring the child in contact with crowds (e.g., in stores and at movie theaters) may need to be curtailed. This is especially true in the winter. Explaining the signs and symptoms of drug toxicity and the correct dose makes the parents more relaxed in relation to discharge. See the Nursing Care Plan for a child with acute lymphoblastic leukemia at the end of this chapter.

Brain tumors

The CNS is the most common site of solid tumors in children. About 60 to 70 percent are located in the posterior fossa, and the rest are located in the anterior portion of the brain.

In general, tumors occur in both males and females, but there are exceptions. (These will be discussed in relation to specific tumors.) Brain tumors are diagnosed most frequently in children 5 to 10 years of age. The incidence decreases toward adolescence. Although there are specific ages at which the incidence peaks, it is important to remember that they can occur in children of *all* ages.

Diagnosis of brain tumors It is extremely important to identify and treat brain tumors as early and as effectively as possible because a significant number are compatible with long-term survival. In addition, early recognition decreases the likelihood of residual neurological or visual disturbances which may be caused by the tumor.

Obtaining a careful history and attending to what a parent may consider inconsequential symptoms (e.g., clumsiness, persistent inability to get the ball over home plate, or the evolution of a behavior problem in a formerly delightful, cooperative child) are of great importance in data collection.

Symptoms indicative of a CNS mass vary according to its anatomic site and rate of growth and the child's age and stage of development. Perhaps the most important nonlocalizing sign is increased intracranial pressure (ICP). This occurs because the lesion obstructs ventricles or displaces tissue by its growth. The latter is especially significant in children whose cranial sutures are closed. This symptom is not present in an infant or toddler (birth through age 2) whose sutures are not closed and whose head expands to accommodate the growing lesion. This fact underscores the importance of doing routine head measurements on young children.

A frequent complaint is a generalized, intermittent headache, which is worse on rising from a recumbent position (after sleeping or napping). It is also intensified by coughing, sneezing, or straining. The diagnosis may be delayed in the case of a young school-age child who complains of a headache which is misinterpreted as a classroom problem or a ploy to avoid school. Headaches are often accompanied by nausea and forceful vomiting as well as lethargy and irritability.

Eye problems are also evident in children with brain tumors; they include diplopia, strabismus, nystagmus, squinting, and tilting the head in a peculiar manner to improve visual acuity. Children have an incredible ability to compensate for these changes. As a result, they unknowingly complicate and, in some instances, delay the diagnosis.

Once all the subjective data have been collected, the child undergoes a wide variety of neurological tests in order to locate, identify, and confirm the presence of a brain tumor. These tests include a lumbar puncture, cerebrospinal fluid analysis, anterior-posterior and lateral skull x rays, EEGs, CAT scans, brain scans, ventriculograms, myelograms, arteriograms, pneumoencephalograms, and echoencephalograms. Nuclear magnetic resonance is a new noninvasive imaging technique that makes it possible to identify a brain tumor as small as 2 mm. These tests are discussed in detail in Chap. 30.

Cerebellar astrocytoma A *cerebellar astrocytoma* is a benign tumor whose cells resemble astrocytes. The onset is insidious, and it affects boys and girls equally, primarily those between the ages of 5 and 8 years. It has a very slow course and hence is capable of doing a significant amount of neurological damage before it is discovered.

Diagnosis and treatment The symptoms include increased ICP, tremors which indicate a focal disturbance, hypotonia, and diminished reflexes. Papilledema can result in nystagmus, optic atrophy, and blindness. A gait disturbance is present.

Several radiological studies can be used in making a diagnosis, but a CAT scan has replaced many of them. Treatment involves surgical removal of the mass. A total excision can result in a 90 percent cure. When the mass is inaccessible or when minimal amounts are resected, radiation therapy is started. In these cases, the prognosis is poor. The abnormal gait and the tremors, which were present before surgery, persist. These symptoms improve over time and are not disabling.

Medulloblastoma A *medulloblastoma,* which is the malignant tumor found most frequently in children, is a highly malignant, rapidly growing lesion whose cells are similar to those in the primitive medullary tube. It tends to metastasize readily along the cerebrospinal fluid pathways, and it is this rapid invasion which makes excision so difficult. It occurs most commonly in 3- to 6-year-olds and is found twice as often in boys as in girls.

Diagnosis and treatment Initially, the clinical symptoms include early-morning headaches, anorexia, vomiting, and an unsteady gait. As the tumor grows, ataxia develops, along with nystagmus, papilledema, and drowsiness.

This neoplasm must be removed to facilitate the flow of cerebrospinal fluid; however, total excision is almost impossible. Since this tumor is highly susceptible to radiation, therapy is started very shortly after surgery. In addition, two chemotherapeutic agents are started: vincristine and cytoxan. The prognosis is poor. Most affected children survive for only 1 or 2 years.

Brainstem glioma A *brainstem glioma* is a malignant lesion, usually consisting of astrocytomas and, less frequently, glioblastomas; it is particularly infiltrative because of its cellular makeup. Its location makes it capable of affecting vital control centers, such as those responsible for respirations and heartbeat, and so it is not amenable to surgery.

Diagnosis and treatment The presence of a brainstem glioma is signified by a myriad of cranial nerve palsies (involving cranial nerves V through X), ataxia (indicating pyramidal tract involvement), and nystagmus. There is a positive Babinski reflex and hyperreflexia, as well as a slow increase in ICP.

This tumor is inoperable because of its attachment to strategic centers. Palliative radiotherapy decreases the size of the tumor. Few children survive beyond 18 months.

Ependymoma An *ependymoma* is a slow-growing mass originating from the lining of the spinal cord canal and cerebral ventricles; it most frequently involves the floor of the fourth ventricle. As it extends upward, it blocks the flow of cerebrospinal fluid, resulting in obstructive hydrocephaly. The peak incidence is between birth and 3 years of age.

Diagnosis and treatment The symptoms include increased ICP, headache, nystagmus, nausea, vomiting, and an unsteady gait. The presence of cranial nerve palsies and a positive Babinski reflex can indicate brainstem infiltration. Young children with open cranial sutures may have head enlargement. An early sign is vomiting, but it is the episodes of *repeated* vomiting that are especially significant. Vomiting results from pressure on the emetic center, the site of the mass.

The location of this lesion makes the prognosis poor, in spite of its slow growth. The surgical treatment is removal of the bulk of the tumor. It cannot be removed completely because it is inseparable from the floor of the ventricle. A shunting procedure allows the cerebrospinal fluid to circulate. Because the neoplasm is radiosensitive, radiation therapy is done. Children with this tumor can live for as little as 12 months or as long as 10 years.

Craniopharyngioma A *craniopharyngioma,* located near the pituitary gland, arises from squamous epithelial cells which are remnants of the embryonic Rathke's pouch. Its growth characteristics resemble those of a benign neoplasm. It is associated with endocrine dysfunction, but it is also capable of producing a deformity of the sella turcica. A craniopharyngioma can be diagnosed anytime in childhood or adolescence; boys and girls are equally affected.

Diagnosis and treatment The clinical manifestations include increased ICP (early), endocrine dysfunction, and alterations in personality and memory. If the tumor appears in adolescence, there is delayed sexual maturation. With compression of the optic chiasma and optic atrophy, there are a variety of eye problems, ranging from asymmetrical field deficits to the gradual loss of visual acuity. Unfortunately, the child is usually unaware of his or her decreasing vision.

Both a CAT scan and a cerebral angiography are helpful procedures in making a diagnosis. Complete removal is not possible because of the neoplasm's adherence to a structure such as the optic chiasma. Although a majority of the tumor may be removed, subsequent surgery is sometimes necessary because the remaining cells continue to proliferate. Although the tumor is radiation-resistant, the future growth of the mass can be controlled by radiation therapy.

Postoperatively, the symptoms of diabetes insipidus may be severe, and electrolytes need to be monitored very closely. It is a lifelong problem that necessitates hormonal replacement therapy, including antidiuretic hormones and corticosteroids. However, children with a craniopharyngioma can live relatively normal lives for many years.

The visual problems will remain. If repeated surgical excisions are necessary, visual acuity will deteriorate with each episode.

Management of brain tumors When a child who is suspected of having a brain tumor is admitted to the hospital, it is most important for the nurse to collect data which will serve as a basis for comparison during the hospitalization. This information should include the child's previous health status, the presence of any allergies, the achievement of developmental milestones, and a nutritional history, as well as the child's height and weight. Vital signs, taken every 4 h, should include the pulse pressure. The head circumference of an infant is measured and recorded, and this should be done on a daily basis thereafter.

Headaches need to be assessed for presence, severity, location, and duration. Small children who are unable to convey their discomfort should be observed for increased irritability, holding their heads, or rocking in bed.

Seizures also may occur as a result of the expanding mass or an increase in ICP. These children should be placed on seizure precautions, and oxygen and suctioning equipment should be at the bedside.

Neurological assessments are done every 4 h and include levels of consciousness, deep tendon reflexes, and cranial nerve function, as well as changes in speech or memory. When coordination, muscle strength, and gait are tested or observed, any deviations, abnormal patterns, or asymmetrical responses are particularly noteworthy.

Nausea and vomiting are major complaints. The nurse must identify when nausea and vomiting occur and must measure the amount expelled. Sometimes fluid restrictions are instituted, and therefore records of intake and output are essential. Urine specific gravity is monitored routinely, and the stools should be observed for constipation. Straining while stooling can increase ICP and also precipitate headaches.

When assessing eye changes, the nurse records the size and equality of the pupils, their reaction to light, and their ability to accommodate, as well as the presence of nystagmus. Subtle clinical changes are difficult to detect, and in some medical centers ICP monitoring may be done using a device such as an epidural sensor.

When being examined for the presence and location of a brain tumor, the child undergoes a myriad of strange procedures and is exposed to frightening equipment. Children need explanations and the presence of a familiar person to allay their fears. A most distressing test is the pneumoencephalogram, which leaves the child with a headache. Even though the child must lie flat, the headache is likely to persist for 24 h.

The parents are anxious about all aspects of the diagnosis because the brain is involved. Many express feelings of guilt because they ignored the child's complaints and delayed the visit to the physician. Listening can relieve their anxiety and promote a therapeutic relationship, which will be helpful in the months to come.

Most neoplasms of the brain are treated using surgery, radiation therapy, or both. When a craniotomy will be performed, the child and the parents need to be prepared for the head shave, which is very upsetting to the child. They must expect a bulky dressing after the operation. The parents are also told that their child will have facial edema and will be comatose upon return to the unit. The day of surgery is extremely difficult for families, and they are grateful for any news that the nurse can communicate from the operating room.

After recovering from anesthesia, the child is transported to the intensive care unit, where the nurse monitors vital signs closely until they are stable. Both pupillary responses are assessed frequently. Sluggish, unequal, or dilated pupils are promptly reported. The type of fluid infusing is checked, and the rate of flow is meticulously observed to prevent increased ICP. Placing the child on the unaffected side with the head of the bed elevated reduces edema and decreases ICP.

The head dressing is examined frequently for drainage. When drainage is present, the color, amount, and odor are recorded. The drainage area is circled with a pen or pencil, and the time is noted, so that the rate of increase can be monitored. A felt-tip pen is *never* used because of its rapid absorptive qualities. Serosanguineous drainage is common, but if the amount increases substantially, it is necessary to reinforce the bandage with sterile dressings and notify the neurosurgeon. Infection is a prime concern because the incision provides a direct pathway to the brain. Sometimes a child attempts to remove the dressing, and so it may be necessary to use mitts on the hands. If that intervention is ineffective, elbow restraints may be necessary (see Chap. 16). Under no circumstances should other types of restraints be used. If the child resists them, the ICP increases.

Facial and intracranial edema are normal consequences of surgery. The eyelids are edematous, but edema can extend to the neck. Since there is a potential for airway obstruction, both respirations and the extent of edema must be evaluated periodically. The child's blinking reflex is depressed, and so methylcellulose eye drops are used to prevent corneal damage.

The trauma of neurosurgery and the edema increase nervous tissue irritability and can affect the respiratory control center, necessitating mechanical ventilation. The temperature control center is easily irritated, too, resulting in fever. Since fever is a common postoperative response, hypothermia blankets are applied shortly after surgery. Because the elevated temperature is secondary to a CNS disturbance, it responds poorly to antipyretics. The nurse should remove the bed covers and lower the room temperature in addition to using hypothermia. When the child's condition is stable, the child is returned to his or her room.

Positioning and giving skin care every 2 h are essential because the child is unconscious. It is important to avoid jarring the bed. Turning is best done by two nurses, who can maintain the child's alignment. Although the child is unconscious, hearing is not impaired. It is therefore important to be mindful about conversations in the child's presence.

Once the child wakes, alertness increases steadily. Levels of consciousness, general behavior, responses to stimuli, and the gag, blink, and swallowing reflexes must be noted. Any deterioration to a lower level of consciousness warrants notifying a physician.

Once the swallowing reflex has been verified, clear oral fluids may be started. The diet is progressed gradually. Intravenous fluids are usually continued until the patient is eating and drinking well.

Some residual neurological damage may be evident when the child is allowed out of bed. It is probably due to edema or trauma. Gradually, there will be a steady improvement in strength and an increase in physical activity.

The head dressing remains in place until healing is complete. Later, hats, scarves, caps, or wigs are worn until the hair grows back. Padded football helmets are used for young children, who may fall.

The nurse needs to coordinate discharge planning. A referral to the local visiting nurses' association should be made, and the visiting nurse should be informed of the teaching done in the hospital and of the child's and the family's needs.

Malignant tumors of the eye

Rhabdomyosarcoma A *rhabdomyosarcoma* is a sarcoma that originates in the striated muscle and in lymphatic, vascular, or connective tissue. There are four types: (1) embryonic, (2) alveolar, (3) pleomorphic (very rare in children), and (4) a mixed type, which can be a combination of the other three.

Embryonic rhabdomyosarcomas are seen most frequently in children, and although the primary sites are the head, neck, abdomen, and genitourinary tract, the majority are confined to the head and neck. About 60 percent are orbital in origin.

Rhabdomyosarcomas occur in boys and girls equally; children between the ages of 2 and 6 years are most frequently affected. Some patients are less than 1 year old, which suggests that an intrauterine factor is a causative agent.

The child's symptoms vary according to the structures involved. Symptoms of middle ear involvement, which are often mistaken for symptoms of chronic otitis media, include pain and drainage. Hence, a delay in diagnosis is not unusual because the clinical manifestations can resemble those of a more common childhood problem. If there are neoplasms on the trunk or an extremity, they appear as painless, firm swellings attached to underlying tissues, which cannot be explained. An abdominal mass is most difficult to diagnose because it produces no symptoms until there is fairly extensive metastasis. This malignancy metastasizes easily to regional tissue lymph nodes, or there may be hematogenous dissemination to the lungs, bone, and marrow, often before it is recognized.

Diagnosis and treatment The clinical symptoms depend on the site and rate of proliferation. When the orbit of an eye is affected, there is no optic atrophy and vision is not impaired. The first sign indicating a mass within the orbit is *proptosis*, a forward protrusion of the eye caused by the proliferating neoplasm. This neoplasm metastasizes early. Hence, at the time of diagnosis about two-thirds of the children have an extension of the disease to regional tissues or lymph. Dissemination in the blood to the lungs, bone, or bone marrow is also possible.

The diagnostic tests include a complete blood count, a chest x-ray, a metastatic survey, bone marrow aspiration, tomograms, and an extensive ophthalmologic examination. The diagnosis is confirmed only by a histological analysis.

The combination of surgery, radiotherapy, and chemotherapy has resulted in a great improvement in survival rates. The prognosis is especially favorable when the tumor is confined to the orbit and can be completely excised. For children whose tumors are removed, a variety of agents can be used to suppress the growth of micrometastasis: vincristine, dactinomycin, doxorubicin, and cyclophosphamide. It is important to remember that the prognosis is directly related to the extent of the disease at the time of diagnosis. In the presence of disseminated disease when the child is initially seen the chances of survival are less than 20 percent.

Optic nerve glioma *Optic nerve gliomas* account for the largest percentage of tumors which affect the optic nerve, and about 95 percent are diagnosed in children. Their cellular composition consists of astrocytomas, which are benign and grow slowly. There is a strong association with neurofibromatosis, or von Recklinghausen disease, and multiple café au lait spots are present on the bodies of about 25 percent of children with these tumors. Males and females are affected equally. These tumors usually occur in the first 10 years of life.

Strabismus and nystagmus appear early, but it is possible for months to elapse before the correct diagnosis is made. When the glioma is confined to one orbit, exophthalmos and impaired vision can develop. If the lesion grows posteriorly, the optic chiasma and the other optic nerve are involved, resulting in bilateral eye problems. Should the foramen of Monro become obstructed, there is increased ICP. Optic nerve atrophy occurs because of constant compression exerted by the growing tumor.

Diagnosis and treatment Diagnostic tests are usually conducted by an ophthalmologist. If the optic chiasma is affected, a neurosurgeon is involved in the diagnosis and subsequent treatment. The tests include measuring both visual fields and visual activity, skull x-rays, an intracranial pneumogram, and a funduscopic examination.

If the glioma is confined to a single orbit, a total resection may be feasible. This technique preserves the globe as a natural prosthesis. Reflex actions are controlled by the unaffected eye. Vision is lost because the optic nerve has been removed. If the bilateral optic nerve is involved or if the chiasma is infiltrated, one of two approaches is used. A significant portion of the tumor can be removed to restore flow of cerebrospinal fluid, or a ventricular shunt which circumvents the mass can be utilized. Radiation may be used postoperatively to decrease the size of the tumor even further.

Retinoblastoma A *retinoblastoma* is the most common intraocular tumor in children; it is a congenital lesion consisting of embryonic retinal cells. Although it may be present at birth (1 per 15,000 to 20,000 births), it is usually detected during infancy or before the age of 3 years.

Retinoblastomas are usually unilateral and nontransmittable to offspring. Children who have bilateral involvement will transmit it as an autosomal dominant gene to 15 percent of their offspring. Retinoblastomas can also be accompanied by a chromosomal aberration.

A retinoblastoma produces very few clinical signs or symptoms. The normal red reflex of the retina is missing. The pupil has a whitish appearance known as cat's-eye reflex. Strabismus is common. The eye may be red and painful, with or without glaucoma. Vision may be impaired or even lost, but it is difficult to assess because of the child's age.

Diagnosis and treatment The diagnosis is determined by ophthalmic examination under anesthesia and with x-rays, a CAT scan, and ultrasonography. Visualization of the tumor's calcified surface and seeding of the vitreous are characteristic, confirming findings.

Staging done by an ophthalmologist refers to the survival of the eye in reference to vision and *not* to the prognosis as it affects preservation of life. A group I tumor is one small tumor, or there may be several very small tumors, and the outcome is most favorable. Group V tumors are large tumors with vitreous seeding, and the prognosis is very poor.

When the tumor is unilateral and small, all attempts are made to preserve the child's vision. Radiation, cobalt implants, light coagulation with a laser beam, or cryotherapy may be used. If there is optic nerve involvement, an enucleation is done to decrease the likelihood of micrometastasis, and chemotherapy (vincristine, cyclophosphamide, or Adriamycin) may be instituted.

If there is bilateral involvement, the eye affected most severely is removed. The remaining eye may be treated with radiation and light coagulation. Chemotherapy generally is used for the treatment of extensive local or metastatic disease. With the refinement of treatment protocols, the prognosis for children with a retinoblastoma has improved to the point where more than 90 percent survive.

Management Malignant neoplasms which affect the eye catapult a family into crisis because of (1) a delay in diagnosis, (2) parental guilt about transmitting the gene, and (3) the loss of vision. It is important for the nurse to help the parents cope with the guilt they are experiencing. Whenever possible, the nurse should emphasize positive aspects. For example, cases of retinoblastoma have a more favorable outcome than cases of some other malignancies in children. If involvement is unilateral, vision in the unaffected eye remains intact. However, bilateral involvement compounds the difficulty of the situation.

It is especially difficult for the parents if they have been asked to give consent for an enucleation. Granting permission for surgery is an agonizing process for the parents. It is crucial for the nurse to spend time with the parents, allowing them to verbalize their fears about coping with the enucleation, the child's future resentment regarding their decision, and possible disfigurement. If consent for an enucleation is given, the child must be prepared for the vision changes that will result from surgery. When an eye prosthesis is planned, this should also be discussed with the child. These topics are difficult to talk about, but the child's and the parent's fears and anxieties must be explored if resolution is to occur. The nursing care of children who undergo eye surgery is discussed in Chap. 31.

Neuroblastoma

A *neuroblastoma,* which is the most common solid malignant tumor in children, arises from primitive sympathetic neuroblasts of neural crest origin. The primary sites are the adrenal glands and areas anywhere along the sympathetic chain. Therefore, lesions may be found in the retroperitoneal area, the neck, the abdomen, or the chest. Unfortunately, metastasis occurs in about two-thirds of affected children before a diagnosis is made.

This lesion is found slightly more often in males than in females. While neuroblastomas are usually detected in the first 5 years of life, the majority are found in children under 3 years of age.

The symptoms are related to the anatomic site involved. If a cervical ganglion is implicated, there is a painless mass in the neck. If the chest is the primary site, dyspnea or a cough may be present. An abdominal mass can be detected by a parent or during a routine physical examination. A pelvic lesion usually causes a change in bowel habits, urinary frequency, or retention. Systemic signs are irritability, anorexia, fatigue, anemia, and a low-grade fever. Distant metastasis has occurred if the child has periorbital swelling, periorbital ecchymosis, and exophthalmos.

Diagnosis Diagnostic procedures include a physical examination, a complete blood count and platelet count, and CAT scans of the chest, abdomen, and pelvis. An intravenous pyelogram is done when an abdominal tumor is suspected. Urine collections to detect the presence of catecholamines and metabolic by-products, especially vanillylmandelic acid (VMA), are vital in confirming the diagnosis of a neuroblastoma. Bone marrow aspiration is important in determining infiltration and, hence, staging. The diagnosis is confirmed by a histological examination at the time of excision or when a distant tumor is biopsied.

Staging Neuroblastomas are classified according to *stages*. These enable investigators to determine the effectiveness of treatment modalities and estimate prognoses in relation to tissue involvement:

Stage I The tumor is confined to the organ or structure of origin.
Stage II The tumor extends beyond the organ or structure of origin, but it does not cross the midline; regional lymph nodes on the ipsilateral side may be involved.
Stage III The tumor extends beyond the midline with bilateral regional lymph node involvement.
Stage IV There is evidence of remote disease in soft tissue, parenchymatous organs, the skeleton, and distant lymph node groups.
Stage IV-S The child would be classified as in stage I or stage II except for remote disease confined to the liver, spleen, or bone marrow. There is no evidence of metastasis on skeletal survey.

Treatment A complete excision is performed when the child has a localized neuroblastoma. This procedure generally results in a cure without further treatment. If the lesion cannot be totally removed, the residual regional disease is irradiated. Since the tissue is radiosensitive, favorable results can be achieved. The high incidence of metastasis necessitates the use of chemotherapeutic agents because surgery and radiation are no longer effective. The most effective drugs seem to be cyclophosphamide, vincristine, and dacarbazine (DTIC).

Prognosis The prognosis depends on the child's age and the degree of dissemination at the time of diagnosis. The best overall prognosis is for children under 1 year of age. About 90 percent survive in stages I and II, while those in stage IV have survival rates of less than 10 percent. If the neuroblastoma can be excised or if there is microscopic residual regional disease amenable to radiation, a cure is possible. Children over 1 year of age with either regional or distant metastasis may have a clinical response to drug therapy; however, a cure is very rare. Whether they are treated with surgery alone or with surgery in combination with radiation therapy or chemotherapy, urine must be collected periodically to detect the presence of catecholamines and VMA in order to monitor their bodies' responses to treatment.

Management The unpredictable nature of this malignancy and its poor prognosis contribute to the anxiety and apprehension of the parents. They feel guilty because the child was not seen earlier and occasionally demonstrate this as hostility.

The large number of radiological studies and the 24-h urine collections need to be explained in detail. Since the parents will collect urine for examination for months after discharge, involving them preoperatively can help them learn the necessary skills. Many of these children are not toilet-trained, which complicates the collection process. Surgical sites may be abdominal, thoracic, or cervical. The parents may be taught to do dressing changes using sterile technique.

Wilms tumor (nephroblastoma)

A *Wilms tumor* is the most common abdominal tumor found in children. Derived from primitive renoblasts, it arises in the parenchyma of the kidney and grows by expanding into the renal cavity. Occurring equally in boys and girls, it is usually diagnosed before the age of 5 years; the majority of these tumors are seen in 2- and 3-year-olds.

Often, this nontender lesion is first discovered by the parents or is palpated by a physician doing a routine physical examination. Symptoms develop late and include anorexia and pain. Hematuria and hypertension are late findings. When metastasis to the lungs is present, children have such pulmonary problems as dyspnea or a cough.

Diagnosis and treatment Radiographic studies include a chest x-ray, a bone survey, an inferior vena cavagram, and an angiogram. An intravenous pyelogram demonstrates a distorted caliceal system indicative of a mass. Renal function is assessed through blood urea nitrogen, creatinine, creatinine clearance, and uric acid determinations. A complete blood count and a battery of liver function tests are performed to detect infiltration by this neoplasm. In addition, tests of total protein, serum glutamic oxaloacetic transaminase, serum glutamic pyruvic transaminase, lactic dehydrogenase, and alkaline phosphatase are done.

Once the diagnosis is made, a histological confirmation is essential. Therefore, surgery is scheduled 24 to 48 h later. Staging is done to precisely identify the extent of the tumor and facilitate the selection of an effective treatment protocol. Table 32-4 lists stages, modes of treatment, and prognoses. In the course of the transabdominal exploratory laparotomy, a nephrectomy is performed, the contralateral kidney and

Table 32-4 Stages, Treatment, and Prognosis of Wilms Tumor

Stage	Extent of Involvement	Treatment	Prognosis
I	Tumor confined to renal capsule; completely resected	*Surgical:* Nephrectomy *Chemotherapy:* Vincristine and dactinomycin	About 90% of patients can be cured.
II	Tumor extended through renal capsule; completely resected	*Surgical:* Nephrectomy *Chemotherapy:* Vincristine and dactinomycin *Radiotherapy:* To renal bed	About 60% of patients can be cured.
III	Tumor extended into or beyond renal bed	*Surgical:* Nephrectomy *Chemotherapy:* Vincristine, dactinomycin, and doxorubicin	About 60% of patients can be cured.
IV	Hematogenous metastasis to lungs, liver, bone, or brain	*Radiotherapy:* Radiation to residual areas of tumor	About 50% of patients survive.
V	Bilateral renal involvement, either initially or later	*Surgical:* Removal of most affected kidney *Chemotherapy:* Vincristine, dactinomycin, and doxorubicin *Radiation:* To remaining kidney	Long-term disease-free control can be achieved in about 50% of patients.

Source: James G. Hughes, *Synopsis of Pediatrics,* 5th ed., Mosby, St. Louis, 1980, p. 770.

liver are examined, and lymph nodes are inspected (and biopsied), while other structures are all carefully scrutinized.

Subsequent treatment depends on the stage assigned. Usually, radiation therapy treatments begin immediately after surgery. All children receive some form of chemotherapy. The drugs used most frequently are dactinomycin, vincristine, and doxorubicin. Approximately 90 percent of these children have favorable prognoses.

Nursing management These children should have signs at the head of their cribs or beds reading "Do Not Palpate Abdomen." There is a risk of rupturing the renal capsule during palpation. This can cause malignant cells to break away from the primary mass. The nurse should tell the parents of a child who will have a nephrectomy for Wilms tumor that there will be a large incision, which is necessary because internal organ examination is essential during the laparotomy.

Postoperatively, intake and output are monitored closely because parenteral fluid replacement is necessary. The patency of the nasogastric tube is maintained by normal saline irrigations every 2 h. Abdominal girth measurements are done every 2 h to check for distention. The location at which abdominal girth measurements are taken should be marked so that all nurses will measure the same circumference and the results will be valid. Dressings are checked for excessive drainage. Vital signs and rate of the intravenous flow are monitored and recorded.

These children recover rapidly from surgery and begin radiation therapy and chemotherapy shortly thereafter.

Bone tumors

Malignant tumors of the bone usually appear in the second decade of life. The child frequently appears well when he or she is seen initially for a traumatic injury such as a fracture, which is identified as pathological in nature. Osteogenic sarcoma and Ewing sarcoma are the two most common malignancies which involve bone. The same bones are usually implicated in both disorders. Any bony structure may be involved, but the long bones of the skeleton are often affected.

Osteosarcoma An *osteosarcoma,* or *osteogenic sarcoma,* arises from bone-forming osteoblasts, and as a result this neoplasm contains primitive cells that are forming the matrix of true bone. As the lesion grows within the medullary cavity, it eventually penetrates the periosteum and extends into soft tissue. There is destruction of preexisting bone. Any major long bone can be affected, especially the metaphysis of the lower end of the femur or upper end of the humerus.

Most children are between 10 and 15 years of age at the time of diagnosis. This lesion affects both sexes equally at a young age, but almost twice as many males are afflicted during adolescence. The increased incidence may be due to the rapid growth spurt which occurs at this stage of development.

Osteosarcomas have been diagnosed in children following exposure to irradiation. They are also seen in some who have survived a retinoblastoma.

While a pathological fracture may be the first indication of a problem, some children also complain initially of intermittent pain, which later becomes intense and continuous. Local swelling and tenderness follow. An x-ray of the affected limb usually reveals bone and periosteal destruction, new bone formation, and a soft mass with some calcification (see Fig. 32-4). Metastasis to the lungs is common and rapid.

Diagnosis and treatment Extensive radiological studies are necessary to evaluate the lesion, determine its extensiveness, and screen for metastasis. They include a bone scan, a bone survey, a chest x-ray and tomograms, a urinalysis, a complete blood count, and a platelet count. Liver function tests, including tests of alkaline phosphatase, transaminase, and protein electrophoresis, are also performed. Absolute confirmation of the diagnosis requires a histological examination.

An amputation of the affected limb, with a sufficient margin of normal bone to ensure complete removal of the tumor, was the treatment of choice until very recently. Now it is controversial. That drastic approach is utilized when no alternatives are available. Another surgical intervention may be a wedge resection of a lung in the presence of metastasis.

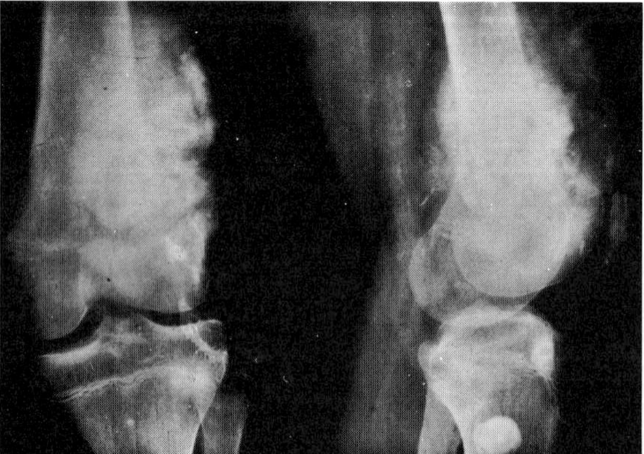

Figure 32-4 This x-ray demonstrates the bone destruction, soft tissue mass, and new bone in a patient with osteosarcoma of the femur. (*From S. Swartz et al., Principles of Surgery, 2d ed., McGraw-Hill, New York, 1974, p. 1778.*)

Some medical centers are trying to avoid the need for amputating a limb, which is a traumatic procedure for a child or an adolescent to experience. In those settings chemotherapy is started prior to surgery; then the neoplasm is resected, and a reinforcing prosthesis (made of metal or of a bone graft from the child or a cadaver) is inserted into the affected bone. This approach is a promising one.

Chemotherapy is given for up to 2 years. The drugs most commonly used are high-dose methotrexate, cisplatin, and doxorubicin. The prognosis has improved over the last decade. At the present time, about 50 percent of school-age children and adolescents with this disease are surviving.[36]

Ewing sarcoma *Ewing sarcoma* has an affinity for such long bones as the femur or tibia, but such flat bones as the ribs or scapula can also be primary sites. Arising from primitive bone marrow cells, myeloblasts, this neoplasm is capable of metastasis to the lungs and other bone. It appears primarily in the second decade of life, and for some unexplained reason it affects males twice as often as females.

The initial findings—localized pain in the affected bone, followed by tenderness, swelling, and heat—are very similar to those seen in children with osteosarcomas. An x-ray of the involved part demonstrates bone destruction and a soft tissue mass, with a characteristic "sunburst" sign of calcification.

Diagnosis and treatment Some of the initial studies are tests of hemoglobin and hematocrit, a white blood count, a platelet count, and tests of serum glutamic oxaloacetic transaminase (SGOT), alkaline phosphatase, and uric acid, in addition to a urinalysis. A 24-h urine collection for VMA and catecholamines is done to rule out neuroblastoma. Radiological studies include a chest x-ray, a bone survey and scan, tomograms, and an x-ray of the involved area. The diagnosis is confirmed by a biopsy.

Surgical intervention, either excision or amputation, has not improved the survival rate for children with this sarcoma, and therefore radiation therapy and chemotherapy are used in an effort to extend life. Combinations of vincristine, dactinomycin, doxorubicin, and cyclophosphamide have been especially effective. Some oncologists use doxorubicin in the protocols of children with advanced disease.

The prognosis can be very favorable for about 50 percent of children who did not demonstrate any signs of metastasis at the time of diagnosis.

Nursing management of children with bone tumors For children who have had these neoplasms excised, postoperative care is comparable to that provided for any patient with an orthopedic problem. Amputation of an extremity necessitates additional support and counseling. Amputating the limb of a child with an osteosarcoma is a drastic intervention for which the child must be prepared. School-age children and adolescents are able to convey their fears and anxieties about the operation. The alteration in body image initiates a grieving process, which is normal. The nurse should expect anger, depression, hostility, or withdrawal. All these are legitimate responses. The nurse must allow the child an opportunity to vent his or her feelings. Issues related to the prosthesis, peer group reactions to the amputation, or environmental handicaps can affect the success of rehabilitation.

Some orthopedic surgeons apply a temporary prosthesis after surgery, which can prevent serious complications such as contractures, stump edema, and phantom limb pain. However, the presence of this appliance prevents observation of the pressure dressing, which can be displaced, affecting both the incision and stump healing. An elastic bandage is used to decrease edema formation. For the first 24 h after surgery, the stump (with or without a prosthesis) is kept elevated to improve venous return and decrease the edema. If the child does not have a prosthesis, specific exercises are done to condition the stump for receiving one.

Early ambulation is essential. The physical therapist begins to work with the child early, teaching the child to use the prosthesis or to crutch-walk.

The nurse assumes responsibility for coordinating these rehabilitative activities. The nurse's observations are important in assessing the child's readiness for crutch-walking. A team conference is held to evaluate the child's overall (physical and emotional) progress and to identify activity levels. Discharge planning and consultation with appropriate nurses in the community begin soon after surgery. A community health nurse who is knowledgeable about services available to the family and a school nurse who can evaluate physical barriers which will confront the child when he or she returns to school are important resources.

Chemotherapy is used for children with either osteosarcomas or Ewing sarcomas. The instructins that are given to the family are similar to those previously described. Discharge teaching emphasizes compliance with the treatment regimen (office or clinic visits, medications, and restrictions on activities) and a gradual resumption of activities to allow the child to work toward functioning at his or her maximum potential.

Lymphomas

Hodgkin disease *Hodgkin disease* is characterized by a progressive, painless enlargement of lymph nodes, predictable extension to adjacent nodes, and subsequent extralymphatic metastasis. The cause of this lymphoma is unknown. There are four histological types: (1) lymphocytic predominance, (2) nodular sclerosis, (3) mixed cellularity, and (4) lymphocytic depletion. The first two classifications have the most favorable prognosis, while the last has the poorest.

Hodgkin disease is found predominantly in males and is rare before 5 years of age. It increases in frequency during the school-age period, and the incidence rises sharply between the ages of 15 and 34 and after the age of 50.

Initially, there is a firm, rubbery, movable nontender mass. About half of these neoplasms are found in cervical lymph nodes; the rest occur in the axillary, inguinal, and mediastinal nodes. As the disease spreads, it affects the retroperitoneal nodes and extends to the spleen, liver, and bone marrow. Tumor enlargement can cause serious complications, such as tracheobronchial compression and subsequent airway obstruction, when the tumor is present in the mediastinum. Compression of the esophagus can affect swallowing. Although most pediatric patients do not have evidence of systemic disease at the time of diagnosis, the manifestations include fatigue, anorexia, an intermittent fever, nausea, pruritus, and weight loss. These symptoms become significant during the staging process because the presence of night sweats, unexplained fever, or weight loss results in classification of the disease in subcategory B of a particular stage. Classification in subcategory A is done when systemic symptoms are absent. An enlarged spleen is present early, but there are no common hematologic abnormalities if the disease process is localized.

Diagnosis and treatment Clinical staging, confirmed by pathological examination, is imperative for defining the progress of the disease and planning treatment. After a detailed history is obtained, a complete physical examination is done. Blood is drawn for a complete blood count and for measurement of sedimentation rate and the serum copper and iron levels. Suspicious lymph nodes are biopsied. If the biopsy is positive, a pelvic bone marrow biopsy is performed. A battery of radiological studies are necessary to determine bone and other organ involvement. A chest x-ray, an inferior vena cavagram, a lymphangiogram, and a CAT scan are also done. In the presence of hilar adenopathy, whole lung tomograms furnish information about the extent of the lymphoma. If there is a risk of extensive involvement, an intravenous pyelogram and liver function tests are essential.

Since a definitive diagnosis can be made only on the basis of a histological examination of tissue from an involved node, a staging laparotomy is performed if the disease is thought to be in an early stage. A splenectomy is done at this time because the spleen is a common site for early Hodgkin disease. A metal clip is put on the spleen stump as a marker that can be visualized for radiation treatment. Multiple lymph nodes along the aortic node chain and the liver are biopsied. If the inguinal nodes are involved, the ovaries are moved during the laparotomy to a position behind the bladder so they can be shielded during radiation therapy.

After the procedure is completed and tissue is examined, the disease stage is determined (see Table 32-5). The presence of a unique type of

Table 32-5 Stage, Treatment, and Prognosis of Hodgkin Disease

Stage	Extent of Involvement	Treatment	Prognosis
I	Limited to one anatomic region or two contiguous anatomic regions on same side of diaphragm	Irradiation to an extended field.	With a favorable histology, long-term disease-free control (more than 10 years) can be achieved in 90% of patients.
II	Present in more than two regions or two noncontiguous regions on same side of diaphragm	Irradiation to an extended field. Some centers may institute chemotherapy.	With a favorable histology, long-term disease-free control can be achieved in about 80% of patients.
III	Present on both sides of diaphragm but not extending beyond involvement of lymph nodes, spleen, or Waldeyer's ring	Irradiation therapy to an extended field and/or total nodal (mastoid to groin); may be given chemotherapy: **a.** Mustargen, Oncovin, prednisone, and procarbazine (MOPP); Cyclophosphamide, Oncovin, prednisone, and procarbazine (COPP); or a combination of the above agents, also including vincristine, bleomycin, and vinblastine **b.** With evidence of recurrence, BCNU, Adriamycin, or DTIC may be used effectively.	With a favorable histology, about 60% of patients can expect long-term disease-free control.
IV	Involvement extends to bone marrow, lung parenchyma, pleura, liver, bone, skin, gastrointestinal tract, or any tissue or organ in addition to lymph nodes, spleen, or Waldeyer's ring		About 25 to 40% of patients survive for about 5 years.

Subdivisions

A: No symptoms at the time of diagnosis

B: Symptoms at the time of diagnosis, including unexplained fever, weight loss, and night sweats

Source: Phillip Lanzkowsky, "Diseases of the Blood and Childhood Malignancies," in Robert A. Hoekelman et al. (eds.), *Principles of Pediatrics*, McGraw-Hill, New York, 1978, p. 1049.

cell, called the *Reed-Sternberg cell,* is essential for the diagnosis of Hodgkin disease. The ultimate prognosis depends on the stage of disease at the time of diagnosis and the histological type of cell.

The overall cure rate has improved substantially. Irradiation and combinations of cytotoxic drugs which are effective in combating this lymphoma have resulted in long-term disease control, even in children with more disseminated disease.

Non-Hodgkin lymphoma *Non-Hodgkin lymphoma* (NHL) is 3 to 4 times more common in children than Hodgkin disease. The NHLs are a large group of heterogenous malignant disease entities, including lymphosarcoma, reticulum cell sarcoma, American Burkitt lymphoma, African Burkitt lymphoma, and stem cell lymphoma. These neoplasms all arise from the lymphoid components of the immune system, and while their etiology is unknown, there is speculation that some of them may be viral in origin. The Epstein-Barr virus has been implicated in African Burkitt lymphoma. Recently, these malignancies were categorized as NHLs because of difficulties and confusion in classifying and comparing them individually.

The Rapport classification, which is categorized according to the predominant cell involved, subdivides NHL as follows: lymphocytic, histiocytic, and mixed or undifferentiated. Each is also subdivided into a nodular or a diffuse type. The mixed as well as the nodular types have a good prognosis, but they are very rare in children.

NHL can occur at any age, but most cases are diagnosed in children and adolescents between 5 and 15 years of age. It is more common in boys than in girls.

The common sites are abdominal areas (the ovaries, liver, spleen, appendix, distal ileum, cecum, lymph nodes, and kidneys) and mediastinal areas. However, other structures may also be involved (e.g., the head, neck, and testes). The clinical manifestations depend on the site and the extent of involvement. Usually a painless enlargement, which has proliferated rapidly, is discovered. If the primary site is the retroperitoneal area, there may be signs of abdominal obstruction with pain, diarrhea, and vomiting. The child may demonstrate distention, weight loss, irritability, anorexia, and fever.

Diagnosis and treatment Blood and bone marrow infiltration is common, which may make it difficult to distinguish this neoplasm from ALL. In many instances, the diagnosis is made after dissemination to other sites has resulted in some obvious complaints.

Tests used to confirm the diagnosis of NHL are similar to those used to determine the presence of Hodgkin disease. A complete blood count, blood chemistries, a urinalysis, and Epstein-Barr virus titres are done. In addition, liver, bone, and gallium scans, as well as an intravenous pyelogram, are performed. Bone marrow aspiration and a lumbar puncture for analysis of spinal fluid are done to assess the possibility of extranodal dissemination. Liver, spleen, brain, bone, and whole-body scans, along with a lymphangiogram, also can reveal other sites.

Staging is not done in NHL. The malignancies which compose this group of diseases have very different courses, complications, and histological classifications. Therefore, treatment is not based on this process.

While confirmation of the diagnosis is based on a tissue examination, there is great controversy as to whether a laparotomy should be done. In any case, a biopsy *must* be performed. If complete excision is possible, then it should be done. Extensive surgical procedures are not indicated, however. They do not increase the chances of survival and can be responsible for "seeding," or spreading malignant cells through the circulatory system to distant sites. These malignancies are sensitive to radiation, and therefore radiation therapy and chemotherapy are the two most effective treatment modalities.

While chemotherapy varies according to a center's protocol, an extensive number of agents are utilized, including methotrexate, prednisone, cyclophosphamide, vincristine, daunorubicin, thioguanine, carmustine, and L-asparaginase. The combination used depends on the child's status at any time. Intrathecal methotrexate or cytosine arabinoside is also administered. These children are also started on allopurinol.

The treatment of NHL is aggressive, and the numbers of different treatment modalities are significant; however, survival rates have improved as a result. They can be as high as 75 percent.

Nursing management The diagnostic procedures are frightening unless they are thoroughly explained to the child. After a biopsy, routine postoperative measures are instituted. Since these children are treated with radiation therapy and chemotherapy, teaching should center on those treatments. Although treatment may be started in the hospital, it is done primarily on an outpatient basis.

Follow-up visits are vital for children with NHL. Leukemic conversion is possible. Teaching related to that complication should be delayed until it appears. Activities should be limited or expanded, depending on how the child feels. With the improved prognosis, planning for college should be encouraged.

Malignant tumors of the reproductive tract

Adenocarcinoma An *adenocarcinoma* can occur in the children of women who took DES during pregnancy. The primary site is the vagina; however, it can be found in the cervix or ovaries. A majority of patients are adolescents or young adults (14 to 22 years old). The most common symptom is prolonged, persistent, irregular bleeding. It is often confused with the irregular bleeding which occurs with the onset of the menarche. The tumor consists of tubules and glands lined with glycogen and "hobnail" cells. It is sometimes called *clear cell carcinoma*.

Diagnosis and treatment A vaginal mass is discovered upon examination. The necessary vaginal and rectal digital examinations are most anxiety-provoking for an adolescent. Diagnostic tests include a complete blood count, a urinalysis, abdominal x-rays, and tomograms. The diagnosis is confirmed by a histological examination.

If the site is within the ovaries, a radical hysterectomy is done. Uterine involvement is treated with a radioisotope implantation, followed by a radical hysterectomy. While these tumors are relatively uncommon, the prognosis depends on early diagnosis and aggressive treatment.

Teratomas A *teratoma* is a true neoplasm and is composed of bizarre, chaotically arranged tissue. It is histologically and embryologically foreign to the area in which it is found.

Ovarian teratomas *Ovarian teratomas* are the most common tumors found in young females. They are also called *dermoid cysts* or *benign cystic teratomas*. A variety of well-differentiated cells, such as squamous epithelium and sebaceous and sweat glands as well as hair, bone, and teeth, are found in these tumors. About 50 percent of these ovarian neoplasms are benign. They occur during infancy, childhood, and adolescence.

Abdominal pain is a common symptom. In children, the ovaries are considered abdominal (rather than pelvic) organs because the child's body is small (see Fig. 32-5). Hence, the neoplasm produces pain because of its pressure on other abdominal organs. Consequently, Wilms tumor and neuroblastoma need to be ruled out. Nausea and vomiting, suggestive of appendicitis, are also present. A pelvic mass can be palpated.

Diagnostic tests include a complete blood count, urinalysis, and pelvic and rectal examinations. X-rays of the abdomen and of the kidneys, ureter, and bladder complete the radiological assessment.

Treatment Treatment consists of removing the neoplasm surgically. To preserve ovarian tissue, an ovarian cystectomy is done. The prog-

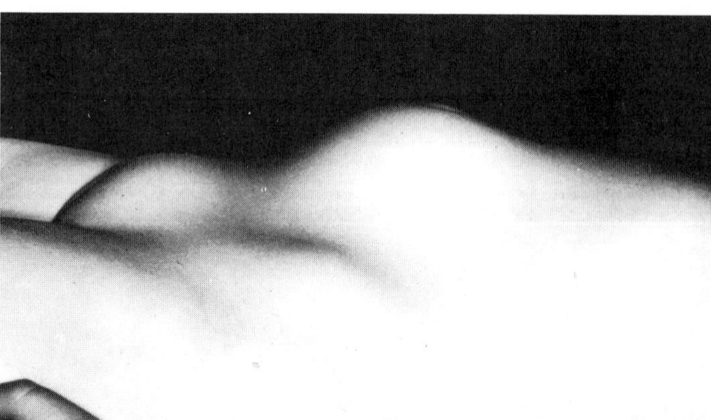

Figure 32-5 An ovarian mass in a four-year-old. The nurse must remember that the ovaries are abdominal organs in childhood. (*From R. A. Hoekelman et al.* [eds.], *Principles of Pediatrics: Health Care of the Young, McGraw-Hill, New York, 1978, p. 1331.*)

nosis is excellent. If a pathological examination reveals malignant changes, surgery is more radical, followed by chemotherapy. The drugs most commonly used are actinomycin D, vincristine, and cyclophosphamide. Cure is possible if there is no evidence of metastasis. With metastasis, the prognosis is doubtful.

Testicular teratomas *Testicular teratomas* may be found at birth or during infancy or early childhood. They are benign neoplasms, detected by enlargement of the testes. Testicular teratomas are often misdiagnosed as hydroceles.

Histologically, the tumor involves all three germ layers. It is not unusual to find cartilage, bone, and adipose and lymphoid tissue in a testicular teratoma. A diagnostic workup includes a complete blood count; a urinalysis; x-rays of the kidneys, ureter, and bladder; and a rectal examination. The teratoma is removed when an orchiectomy is performed. The prognosis is excellent.

Management Children who are suspected of having teratomas need support when procedures are done. Vaginal and rectal examinations are frightening to young children. A nurse's explanations and presence can be instrumental in obtaining the child's cooperation.

Since the majority of these neoplasms are benign, the anxiety and stress experienced by these families is substantially less. However, providing time for them to discuss the medical problem and seizing opportunities to teach are still important nursing functions.

Nursing Care Plan: Acute Lymphoblastic Leukemia

Patient: Joseph "Skip" Jasinski **Age:** 4 years, 1 month **Date of Admission:** 5/3 at 6 P.M.

ASSESSMENT

Joseph Jasinski, a 4-year-old whose nickname is Skip, was admitted to the pediatric unit on 5/3 after an earlier visit to his pediatrician. His parents accompanied him, along with his only sibling, a 6-year-old sister. This preschooler has had no previous serious illnesses or hospitalizations. The admitting diagnosis was to rule out acute lymphocytic leukemia.

GENERAL APPEARANCE

Skip is pale and listless and has ecchymotic areas on his body.

PHYSICAL EXAMINATION

Weight: 18.2 kg (40 lb). Temperature: 38.8°C (101.8°F). Pulse: 136. Respirations: 45.

HISTORY

Skip was well until about 3 weeks ago, when his mother noticed that his appetite was not as good as it had been. Several evenings later, while giving him his bath, she found black-and-blue marks on his body. When she asked Skip how he got them, he said that he did not know but that he had not hurt himself. When his activity levels decreased and he started to "mope around the house" and complain of "hurting all over," Mrs. Jasinski decided to take him to the pediatrician. After examining him, the pediatrician decided that hospitalization was necessary because he had always been a very active, healthy boy and his current complaints justified a complete blood workup, which could be done best in the hospital.

The physical examination revealed enlarged lymph nodes, a moderate hepatosplenomegaly, and ecchymotic areas scattered over the body. The blood work done in his pediatrician's office revealed a white blood count of 13,000 mm^3, a hemoglobin of 10 g/dl, a platelet count of 45,000 mm^3, and an elevated uric acid level. The next afternoon, after a bone marrow aspiration and spinal tap, the results indicated that the marrow aspirated was hypercellular with 85 percent blasts; however, the spinal fluid indicated that there was no central nervous system infiltration. The diagnosis of acute lymphoblastic leukemia was confirmed, and Skip was started on his chemotherapy, which consisted of prednisone, vincristine, and L-asparaginase. He remained on protective isolation because of the case mix on the unit at the time.

PHYSICIAN'S ORDERS

1. Admit to 7 North.
2. Protective isolation.
3. Hematology precautions (soft toothbrush, no rectal temperatures, no suppositories, no injections, etc.).
4. Vital signs q4h and more frequently if warranted.
5. Temperature q1h when febrile.
6. Spinal tap at 9 A.M. on 5/4.
7. Bone marrow aspiration following tap on 5/4.
8. CBC, differential blood count, hgb, hct, and uric acid levels.
9. Routine urinalysis.
10. Urine, nose, throat, gingiva, and blood cultures in A.M.
11. Regular diet as tolerated.
12. Restricted activity in room.
13. Intake and output.
14. Daily weights.

Nursing Diagnosis	Outcome Criteria	Nursing Interventions	Evaluation and Modifications
1. Blood volume deficit related to therapy-induced myelosuppression	☐ Skip will remain hemorrhage-free.	☐ Monitor vital signs q4h and assess for signs of hemorrhage. ☐ Avoid IM injections.	☐ Vital signs have been stable since admission; no signs of hemorrhage since admission.
2. Alteration in blood constituents related to therapy-induced myelosuppression		☐ Use firm, gentle pressure for at least 5 min to control bleeding at venipuncture and injection sites. ☐ Post "Bleeding Precautions" sign at bedside.	
		☐ Avoid play activities which could result in accidental injury.	☐ 5/21: Out of isolation; needs supervision when with others.
	☐ Skip will demonstrate: **a.** No increase in ecchymotic areas	☐ Inspect skin q8h for evidence of ecchymoses and petechiae. ☐ Handle Skip gently to prevent bleeding.	☐ No new ecchymoses or petechiae since admission.
	b. Intact gingival, oral, nasal, and rectal mucosa with no evidence of bleeding	☐ Check nasal, oropharyngeal, and rectal mucosa q8h. ☐ Control local bleeding prn: **a.** Dry tea-bag compress to oral mucosa	☐ 5/5: Gingival bleeding at 9:30 A.M.; tea bag effective.
		b. Ice or cold compress and gentle pressure for at least 10 min to area or nostril	☐ 5/6: Episode of epistaxis at 2 P.M.; salt pork effective.
		c. Salt pork topical application to nasal mucous membranes	☐ No bleeding since 5/6.
3. Alteration in body defense mechanisms related to therapy-induced myelosuppression	☐ Skip will remain free of infection.	☐ Put Skip in private room; take reverse isolation precautions, including gown and mask.	☐ 5/3: Reverse isolation was instituted; procedures were explained.
		☐ Require careful, thorough hand-washing by all who enter room. ☐ Limit visitors to parents and necessary personnel. ☐ Encourage parents' presence as much as possible. ☐ Exclude anyone with evidence of infection.	☐ One parent remains with Skip at all times, assisting with care and providing diversions.
	☐ Skip's temperature will remain below 38.3°C (100.8°F).	☐ Monitor temperature orally q4h, or q1h if temperature is 38.2°C (100.8°F). ☐ Report temperature elevation to physician promptly. ☐ Use alcohol and iodine prep prior to venipunctures and injections.	☐ Skip's temperature ranges from 37.7 to 38°C (99.8° to 100.4°F). ☐ No signs of infection have been noted since admission.

Nursing Diagnosis	Outcome Criteria	Nursing Interventions	Evaluation and Modifications
		☐ Assess for infection in target areas, such as venipuncture sites, skin, oral mucous membranes, and perianal area. ☐ (See related nursing actions listed with nursing diagnoses 4, 9, and 13.)	☐ 5/21: Reverse isolation was discontinued; private room and strict hand-washing maintained; continue other measures specified in plan.
4. Potential impairment of skin and mucous membrane integrity related to therapy-induced myelosuppression and mechanical pressure	☐ Skip will maintain an intact integument.	☐ Maintain meticulous skin and scalp cleanliness. ☐ Avoid use of drying soaps. ☐ Apply lotion and gentle massage to pressure areas q8h.	
	☐ Skip will experience minimal mucosal disruption due to oral lesions. ☐ Skip will experience minimal mucosal disruption due to perianal lesions.	☐ Oral hygiene before and after eating and at bedtime: **a.** If no lesions are present, use soft toothbrush and gentle strokes. **b.** If lesions are present, use cotton swab. **c.** Use 4 parts sterile water and 1 part hydrogen peroxide for mouthwash. **d.** Use Water Pik, if possible; let Skip select temperature of solution.	☐ 5/13: Three lesions, approximately 0.3 to 0.4 cm, on lips; four lesions on oral mucous membranes (three on right and one on left), measuring approximately 0.4 cm. ☐ 5/13: Skip is eager to use Water Pik with warm solution.
		☐ Avoid introducing sharp instruments into mouth. ☐ Use caution with drinking straws. ☐ Do not take rectal temperatures. ☐ Wash perianal area with hexachlorophene and water frequently and after every voiding and bowel movement. ☐ Change position frequently; avoid pressure on sacral area; use sheepskin or alternating-pressure mattress. ☐ Expose lesions to air and heat lamp for 20 min three to four times a day (nap times are best).	☐ 5/16: Skip says his mouth feels better; lesions appear smaller and less inflamed. ☐ 5/22: Lesions on mucosa are almost healed; one lesion, approximately 0.1 cm, remains on left lower lip. ☐ 5/14: Three small lesions, approximately 0.7 cm in diameter, in anal area. ☐ 5/16: Lesions still approximately 0.7 cm. ☐ 5/18: Lesions approximately 0.3 cm. ☐ 5/20: Perianal lesions resolved; discontinue heat lamp; continue preventive measures.
5. Fatigue related to anemia	☐ Skip will be able to tolerate activities of daily living and moderate activity without fatigue.	☐ Observe Skip's tolerance of activities of daily living and other activity. ☐ Discourage active play until hgb and hct improve.	☐ 5/4: Played with truck in room for about 1 h, with fatigue (hgb, 8.8; hct, 28). Activity was terminated, and storytelling and drawing were substituted.

Nursing Diagnosis	Outcome Criteria	Nursing Interventions	Evaluation and Modifications
		☐ Encourage foods high in protein and calories. (Skip likes ice cream, milk shakes, yogurt, tuna fish, and peanut butter.)	
	☐ Skip will have at least two 1-h naps or rest periods per day. ☐ Skip will get at least 8 to 10 h of sleep per 24 h.	☐ Schedule 1-h nap for 11 A.M. to 12 noon and for 3:30 to 4:30 P.M. ☐ Plan meals and treatments around rest periods. ☐ Maintain "quiet" even if Skip cannot or will not sleep. (He likes puzzles, books, cards, drawing, and TV.)	☐ 5/7: Skip usually sleeps during rest periods and all night.
	☐ Skip will experience few or no side effects from the administration of blood products.	☐ Administer blood products cautiously. **a.** Double-check blood type, blood slips, and ID band with another nurse before hanging blood. **b.** Use Y-type infusion set with NS as alternative infusion, in case of reaction. **c.** Take temperature before starting transfusion, q1h during transfusion, and 1 and 2 h after transfusion. **d.** Observe Skip closely for first 10 to 20 min of transfusion. **e.** *Stop* transfusion if chills, fever, urticaria, headache, low back pain, dyspnea, or wheezing occurs. **f.** Run transfusion no faster than 3 h.	☐ 5/5: Packed cells, 100 ml, were administered between 5 and 8 P.M. Temperature was 37.7°C (99.8°F) to 38°C (100.4°F). No reaction was observed.
6. Potential nutritional deficit related to anorexia, nausea, vomiting, and oral lesions	☐ Skip will be able to ingest at least 1800 cal a day.	☐ Fortify custards, puddings, and milk shakes with powdered milk supplement. ☐ Add polycose to all liquids. ☐ Place small snack of a favorite food in front of Skip q2h. ☐ Make foods visually appealing ("faces," shapes, and colors). ☐ Encourage parents to assist Skip with meals. ☐ Permit Skip to choose menu as much as possible.	☐ 5/6: Poor intake due to nausea and vomiting. ☐ 5/9: Snacks eaten erratically; Skip likes "white" (vanilla) the best. ☐ 5/12–5/14: Nausea and vomiting; poor intake despite medication. ☐ 5/17: Eating is much improved; drank 1790 ml.

Nursing Diagnosis	Outcome Criteria	Nursing Interventions	Evaluation and Modifications
		☐ Administer antiemetic 30 to 40 min before meals when nausea and vomiting are present. ☐ Obtain order for local anesthetic for oral lesions if they interfere with po intake. ☐ Try cool, bland foods when Skip's mouth is sore. ☐ Provide meals in peer group setting when isolation is discontinued.	☐ 5/13–5/16: Anesthetic not necessary; nausea and vomiting seem to interfere with eating. ☐ 5/21: Began eating meals with peers; appetite has improved.
7. Potential alteration in renal function related to chemotherapy-induced hyperuricosuria	☐ Skip will have: **a.** Urinary output of approximately 85 to 100 ml/h **b.** Fluid intake of 1900 to 2100 ml per day **c.** Urine specific gravity between 1.004 and 1.015 **d.** Urine pH between 7.5 and 8.5	☐ Measure intake and output. ☐ Report urinary output which is 200 ml or more below intake for a 24-h period. ☐ Offer fluids which promote alkalinization of urine, such as milk and orange juice. ☐ Administer IV fluids if oral intake is insufficient and during periods of nausea and vomiting. ☐ Measure urine specific gravity at each voiding; notify physician if it is higher than 1.020 or lower than 1.002. ☐ Check urine pH at each voiding; notify physician if it is below 7.4 or above 8.6. ☐ Visually examine all urine in good light for sediment or particles. ☐ Strain all urine. ☐ Administer prophylactic allopurinol as ordered.	☐ 5/4–5/10: Intake averages 1970 ml per day; output averages 1935 ml per day. ☐ 5/11–5/17: Intake averages 2057 ml per day; output averages 1983 ml per day. ☐ 5/18–5/24: Intake averages 2036 ml per day; output averages 1978 ml per day (see daily intake and output sheets). IV fluids necessary on day of vincristine therapy and for about 2 to 3 days following therapy. ☐ 5/4–5/24: Urine specific gravity is 1.007 to 1.011. ☐ 5/4–5/24: pH ranges between 7.6 and 8.1
8. Alteration in metabolism related to steroid therapy	☐ Skip will: **a.** Maintain balance between fluid intake and output **b.** Remain infection-free	☐ Assess for side effects of prednisone (moon face, red cheeks, protuberant abdomen, fluid retention, and supraclavicular fat pads). ☐ Weigh daily, before breakfast. ☐ Measure intake and output. Observe for fluid intake in excess of output. (See nursing intervention 2 for nursing diagnosis 7.) ☐ Observe for signs and symptoms of infection; steroids can mask fever.	☐ 5/4: Prednisone therapy was initiated. ☐ 5/9: Appetite has not improved; moon face and red cheeks are apparent. Skip does not appear concerned about these changes. ☐ 5/9–5/10: Fluid intake was 197 ml above output. ☐ 5/11–5/12: Intake and output were approximately equal. ☐ 5/14: Intake and output continue to balance.

Nursing Diagnosis	Outcome Criteria	Nursing Interventions	Evaluation and Modifications
		☐ Take advantage of increase in appetite, which can result from therapy.	☐ 5/16: Protuberant abdomen evident, no signs of infection, and no change in appetite.
9. Potential alteration in social behaviors related to steroid therapy and isolation	☐ Skip will: **a.** Maintain a social interaction pattern similar to his previous pattern. **b.** Be able to tolerate periods of 1 to $1\frac{1}{2}$ h alone in room if parent or nurse cannot be present.	☐ Observe for mood swings and euphoria. ☐ Provide company (parent or nurse) and diversional activities. ☐ Set limits on behavior if necessary; involve parents in limit setting. ☐ Visit with Skip in his room for 20 min q1h to q$1\frac{1}{2}$ h during waking hours when parent not present. ☐ Supervise type and amount of interaction with other children when reverse isolation discontinued (euphoria may cause him to overdo). ☐ Provide guidance to parents regarding activity with peers.	☐ 5/7: After a period of nausea and vomiting passed, Skip became "happy," constantly chattering and calling out to all passing in corridor ("Hi ya!") and laughing deliberately at only slightly humorous incidents. ☐ 5/12–5/16: Rapid change in behavior; weepy and quiet during period of nausea and vomiting. ☐ 5/20: Can tolerate about 55 min alone, if given something to "finish" before parent or nurse returns, such as a drawing. ☐ 5/21: Is out of isolation; mother is supervising activity.
10. Potential alteration in elimination related to vincristine therapy	☐ Skip will have normal, formed bowel movements at least qd.	☐ Record frequency and consistency of bowel movements. ☐ Administer stool softener. ☐ Maintain fluid intake.	☐ 5/4–5/10: Normal bowel movements qd. ☐ 5/11–5/17: Normal bowel movements qd. ☐ 5/18–5/23: Normal bowel movements qd.
11. Potential alteration in perception and coordination related to therapy-induced neuropathy, leukemic invasion of the central nervous system, or both	☐ Skip will: **a.** Report normal sensation in extremities **b.** Demonstrate equal strength in extremities which is adequate to perform activities of daily living **c.** Demonstrate normal gait **d.** Demonstrate normal joint mobility **e.** Maintain normal body alignment **f.** Demonstrate orientation to time, place, and person	☐ Check extremities for weakness bid. ☐ Ask Skip how his hands and feet "feel" to assess for tingling, numbness, or both. ☐ Institute foot board prn. ☐ Assess gait and mobility qd. ☐ Keep padded tongue blade, airway, and oxygen at bedside. ☐ Observe for irritability, lethargy, or headache. ☐ Report all symptoms suggesting neuropathy to physician. ☐ Maintain fluid intake between 1900 ml and 2100 ml during chemotherapy. ☐ Curtail activities prn.	☐ 5/12: Foot-drop was noted; foot board was instituted. ☐ 5/16: Numbness and weakness in right hand. ☐ 5/18: Weakness and numbness have subsided. ☐ 5/18–5/23: No ataxia or abnormal gait was observed; continue observations.

Nursing Diagnosis	Outcome Criteria	Nursing Interventions	Evaluation and Modifications
12. Potential alteration in comfort related to pain	☐ Skip will be able to report: **a.** That he is comfortable and free of pain **b.** A minimal number of painful episodes	☐ Change position at least q2h. ☐ Move body parts gently. ☐ Avoid pressure on bony prominences or painful sites. ☐ Assess for jaw pain caused by vincristine therapy. ☐ Administer nonsalicylate analgesics prn. ☐ Provide quiet, pleasing environment.	☐ 5/4–5/11: Is moving self about; is pain-free. ☐ 5/12–5/19: Remains pain-free. ☐ 5/20–5/24: Remains pain-free; continue observations and plan.
13. Parental lack of knowledge about ALL and its treatment	☐ Parents will be able to: **a.** Verbalize correct information regarding Skip's illness and his treatment	☐ Assess parents' understanding of information given by physician. ☐ Correct misinformation and misunderstandings verbalized. ☐ Provide explanations about Skip's illness and treatment. ☐ Keep sessions short (30 to 45 min). ☐ Do not overload parents with too much information at one time; observe their responses. ☐ Allow sufficient time for parents to ask questions; answer questions frankly; refer parents to physician for further information prn. ☐ Content of teaching: **a.** Alteration in blood constituents; role of platelets in blood; rationale for curtailing potentially vigorous play. **b.** Reason for protective isolation and importance of good handwashing and excluding persons with infections. Encourage parents to visit as much as possible; suggest appropriate diversions; assure parents that isolation will be discontinued when Skip's white blood count approaches normal.	☐ 5/3: Hand-washing and gown-and-mask technique return demonstration by parents was satisfactory. ☐ Parents were able to repeat information regarding alterations in blood, potential for bleeding, anemia, and Skip's reactions to isolation during A.M. discussion. ☐ 5/4: Parents were able to repeat information discussed during P.M. discussion: Skip's need for increased fluids and effects of prednisone. Parents are asking many questions about Skip's reaction to illness. Parents are still upset, but seem to comprehend information.
		c. Need for good skin care; skin lesions may occur as a side effect of therapy despite preventive	☐ 5/5: Preventive skin care and nutritional needs were discussed with Skip's mother; she was able to ac-

Nursing Diagnosis	Outcome Criteria	Nursing Interventions	Evaluation and Modifications
		measures. Measures to minimize discomfort and help resolve lesions will be used. **d.** Skip's fatigue and the need for adequate rest. **e.** Anorexia, nausea, and vomiting are frequent side effects of therapy; measures which may help Skip eat an adequate amount of nutrients; enlist parents' cooperation. **f.** Necessity for high fluid intake and, possibly, IV fluids. **g.** Side effects of prednisone therapy; euphoria may alter Skip's behavior and cause him to overdo; mood swings from "happy" days to "blue" days can occur. **h.** Other side effects of therapy: constipation, neurological changes, alopecia, pain. **i.** Potential stressful impact of illness, hospitalization, and treatment on Skip. **j.** Prior to discharge, discuss Skip's limitations and abilities, i.e., avoiding crowds, need for a head covering, fatigue, preschool attendance, and discipline. ☐ Repeat all explanations prn, as parents' comprehension may be affected by their own stress.	curately repeat information to Skip's father later in the day. Side effects of therapy were discussed with both parents in P.M.; both appeared distressed and expressed concerns. Parents concluded that side effects can be endured if the therapy can help Skip. ☐ 5/6: Explanation of need for high fluid intake during therapy was repeated prior to starting IV infusion; mother verbalized understanding. ☐ 5/7: Side effects of therapy and Skip's responses to illness and hospitalization were discussed; parents verbalized understanding correctly.
14. Potential alteration in body image related to therapy-induced alopecia	☐ Parents and Skip will be able to: **a.** Verbalize their understanding of the reason for the hair loss **b.** Verbally acknowledge that the hair will grow back **c.** Formulate an explanation for children and	☐ Prepare Skip and parents for hair loss. ☐ Acknowledge that hair loss is upsetting to most people. ☐ Give careful daily scalp care. ☐ Expose scalp to air as much as possible when in room or at home.	☐ 5/15: Moderate amount of hair was lost as Skip's mother was combing his hair; mother was initially dismayed, but nurse reminded her that hair loss will be temporary. Skip is aware of hair loss, but does not seem concerned.

Nursing Diagnosis	Outcome Criteria	Nursing Interventions	Evaluation and Modifications
	adults who ask questions about Skip's appearance	☐ Suggest use of "doctor's" cap, baseball cap, or other head covering when Skip is with others, at school or at play. ☐ Stress that hair will grow back in 3 to 6 months, but its color and texture may differ. ☐ If repeated therapy with the same drugs is necessary, hair loss may be less severe.	☐ 5/16: Skip's father brought him a baseball cap with the emblem of Skip's favorite team; Skip wants to sleep with it on.
		☐ Prepare Skip and parents for others' questions, which may be blunt and upsetting. Children, in particular, may say things that upset Skip or his sister.	☐ 5/19: Parents have decided that a short, truthful answer would be best, and then the subject should be changed. ☐ 5/23: Skip told inquiring children in the hospital that his medicine made his hair fall out, adding "It doesn't bother me, though, cause it's gonna grow back."
15. Emotional stress related to hospitalization and invasive procedures	☐ Skip will be able to: **a.** Tolerate necessary procedures **b.** Use acceptable means to discharge his anger, tension, and fear	☐ Explain each procedure to Skip just prior to and during the procedure (explaining procedures too far in advance will increase his anxiety). ☐ Use words to describe the sensations Skip will experience during the procedure, such as "sting" from an injection. Be honest; *do not* say it will not hurt if it will hurt. ☐ Use simple, clear words in all explanations. ☐ Ask Skip to tell "what comes next" in the procedure to distract him. ☐ Tell Skip he can cry if it hurts, but he must remain still. ☐ Tell Skip that the nurse or his parents will help him to hold still so the doctor can finish and the hurt will be over sooner. ☐ Allow parents to be present, if they wish, and encourage them to comfort Skip after painful proce-	☐ 5/10: Explanations are ongoing; both parents and Skip appear to have less fear and stress. ☐ 5/6: Skip cried during venipuncture for IV infusion, but remained still; he is able to do the same during blood tests.

Nursing Diagnosis	Outcome Criteria	Nursing Interventions	Evaluation and Modifications
		dures and praise his bravery. ☐ Do not allow parents, visitors, or health care providers to carry on conversations about Skip or any other matters within his hearing since he may misunderstand and fantasize unnecessarily. ☐ Tell Skip's parents that his need to express himself and release tension is normal and expected. ☐ Suggest suitable means of play and expression to help channel Skip's feelings; activities might include toy workbench and hammer, punching bag, water play, and play with character dolls (doctor, nurse, and family members), syringes, IV tubing, and bandages. ☐ Use storytelling to elicit Skip's fears and fantasies.	☐ 5/10: Through play, Skip "vigorously" performed a bone marrow aspiration on an astronaut doll. ☐ 5/18: Tolerated bone marrow aspiration better than previously. Skip often jumps right into a story and takes over, relating frightening episodes, such as bone marrow aspiration.
	☐ Parents will be able to allow Skip to express his feelings in an acceptable manner and impose limits when necessary.	☐ Caution parents that unacceptable behaviors should be limited, just as they would be ordinarily. Overindulgence should be avoided.	☐ 5/21: Initially, maternal grandmother was very overindulgent. Parents better understand consequences of this now, and grandmother has refrained from excessive indulgence when she visits.
16. Parental stress related to the suddenness and seriousness of Skip's illness	☐ Parents will be able to: **a.** Verbalize their fears to the nurse **b.** Ask the nurse questions they may have about Skip's condition and his care **c.** Express their anger and tension in an acceptable manner **d.** Provide Skip with supportive physical and emotional care	☐ Initiate discussions with Skip's parents regarding his illness and their feelings; do *not* wait for parents to ask questions. ☐ Provide a private place for discussions. ☐ Acknowledge that it is upsetting for parents to find out that their child has leukemia; this helps them verbalize their feelings and fears. ☐ Assure them that there is *nothing* they could have done to prevent Skip's illness. ☐ Remind parents that the physician has given them a hopeful prognosis for Skip.	☐ 5/3: Met with both parents after Skip's admission; both were upset but able to understand basics of Skip's diagnosis; further discussion deferred because of parents' obvious anxiety and fatigue. ☐ 5/4: Parents were tearful during meeting and kept asking why this happened to Skip. After initial release of feelings and tears, parents began asking questions about Skip's illness and treatment. ☐ 5/5: Skip had first dose of vincristine while mother was present. After the procedure, mother confided to

Nursing Diagnosis	Outcome Criteria	Nursing Interventions	Evaluation and Modifications
		☐ Encourage parents to ask any questions they may have; tell them that *no* question is a silly question. ☐ Provide parents with a private place to vent their feelings after they have assisted Skip during a traumatic procedure, such as a bone marrow aspiration. ☐ Assure parents that the nurse is available to speak with Skip's sister and grandparents. ☐ Expect that parents may not always be able to control their feelings; they may become hostile, angry, or critical of health care providers or the hospital. They may also become tearful or upset in front of Skip. Provide parents with a private place to express themselves if these episodes occur. ☐ Initiate private conferences with parents at least every other day. Focus on positive aspects of Skip's progress, but allow parents to discuss distressing side effects that Skip is experiencing. These conferences are essential, since the success of remission induction cannot be determined for several weeks. ☐ Encourage parents to spend a quiet evening together on occasion. Assure them that the nurses will take care of Skip.	the nurse: "It hurt me, too." Both parents were able to ask questions freely. ☐ 5/6–5/16: Discussions are held with parents every day or every other day; parents have good rapport with nurses. ☐ 5/13: Met with maternal grandparents and answered their questions. ☐ 5/18: Skip is much improved after 3 days of nausea and vomiting; parents went out to celebrate their ninth wedding anniversary (which was the day of Skip's admission) upon urging of nurse and Skip. Skip said, "I'll be okay with the nurse!" ☐ 5/20: Met with Skip's sister and parents; she is afraid Skip won't come home. Discussed Skip and explained that the doctors and nurses are helping Skip get well enough to go home. After being prepared for changes in Skip's appearance, sister visited with Skip for about 30 min. She told him that she is keeping his room neat for when he comes home and that all the neighborhood kids can't wait for him to come home. Visit with Skip seemed to benefit all family members.

References

1. Klopovich, P. M., and R. C. Trueworthy, "Adherence to Chemotherapy Regimens among Children with Cancer," *Topics in Clinical Nursing* 19–24 (April 1985).
2. *Cancer Facts and Figures,* American Cancer Society, New York, 1984.
3. Fernback, Donald J., "The Role of the Family Physician in the Care of the Child with Cancer," *Ca—A Cancer Journal for Clinicians,* **35**(5):258 September–October 1985).
4. Nienhuis, A. W., "Genetic Mechanisms in Neoplasia," *Blood* **64**(5):949–950 (1984).
5. Grier, H. E., and H. J. Weinstein, "Acute Non-Lymphocytic Leukemia," *Pediatric Clinics of North America* **32**(3):653–668 (June 1985).

6. Kondo, K., Chilcote, H. S. Maurer, and J. D. Rowley, "Chromosomal Abnormalities in Tumor Cells from Patients with Sporadic Wilms Tumor," *Cancer Research* **44**:5376–5381 (November 1984).
7. Kocova, M., J. R. Kowalczyk, and A. A. Sandberg, "Translocation 4:11 Acute Leukemia: Three Case Reports and Review of the Literature," *Cancer Genetics and Cytogenetics* **16**:21–32 (March 1985).
8. Kowalczyk, J. R., et al., "Cytogenetic Findings in Childhood Acute Lymphoblastic Leukemia," *Cancer Genetics and Cytogenetics* **15**:47–64, (1985).
9. Foley, G. V., and P. Yenske, "Common Issues in Pediatric Cancer," in D. Fochtman and G. V. Foley (eds.), *Nursing Care of the Child with Cancer,* Little, Brown, Boston, 1982, pp. 1–16.
10. Reich, S. D., "Antineoplastic Agents as Potential Carcinogins: Are Nurses and Pharmacists at Risk?" *Cancer Nursing* **4**:500–502 (December 1981).
11. Mattia, M. A., and S. L. Blake, "Hospital Hazards: Cancer Drugs,"*American Journal of Nursing* **83**(5):759–762 (May 1983).
12. Stagg, R. J., C. S. Viele, and R. J. Ignoffo, "Neoplastic Disorders," M. B. Weiner and G. A. Pepper (eds.), *Clinical Pharmacology and Therapeutics in Nursing,* McGraw-Hill, New York, 1985, p. 751.
13. Jaffe, N., "Late Sequelae of Cancer Therapy," in W. W. Sutow, D. J. Fernbach, and T. J. Vietti (eds.), *Clinical Pediatric Oncology,* Mosby, St. Louis, 1984, pp. 810–832.
14. Schein, P. S., and S. H. Winokur, "Immunosuppressive and Cytotoxic Chemotherapy: Long-Term Complications," *Annals of Internal Medicine* **82**:84–95 (1975).
15. Ruccione, K., and J. Ferguson, "Late Effects of Childhood Cancer and Its Treatment," *Oncology Nursing Forum* **11**(5):54–64 (1984).
16. McCalla, J., "A Multidisciplinary Approach to Identification and Remedial Intervention for Adverse Late Effects of Cancer Therapy," *Nursing Clinics of North America* **20**(1):117–131 (1985).
17. Byrd, R. L., "Late Effects of Treatment of Cancer in Children," *Pediatric Annals* **12**(6):450–459 (1983).
18. Ibid., p. 459.
19. Jaffe, op. cit., p. 830.
20. Byrd, op. cit., p. 454.
21. Schimpff, S. G., C. H. Diggs, and J. G. Wiswell, "Radiation Related Thyroid Dysfunction: Implications for the Treatment of Hodgkin's Disease," *Annals of Internal Medicine* **92**:91–98 (1980).
22. Blatt, J., et al., "Pregnancy Outcome Following Cancer Chemotherapy," *The American Journal of Medicine* **69**:829–831 (November 1980).
23. Kolnits, P. H., et al., "Pregnancy Outcomes in Patients Treated for Hodgkin's Disease," *Proceedings of American Association for Cancer Research and American Society of Clinical Oncology* **22**:381 (1981).
24. Horning, S. J., et al., "Female Reproductive Potential after Treatment for Hodgkin's Disease," *The New England Journal of Medicine* **304**:1382 (1981).
25. McCalla, op. cit., p. 117.
26. Meadows, A. T., et al., "Declines in I.Q. Scores and Cognitive Dysfunctions in Children with ALL Treated with Cranial Irradiation," *Lancet* 1015–1018 (November 1981).
27. Nelson, D. F., et al., "Second Malignant Neoplasms in Patients Treated for Hodgkin's Disease with Radiotherapy or Radiotherapy and Chemotherapy," *Cancer* **48**(11):2386–2393 (December 1981).
28. Koocher, G. P., et al., "The Special Problems of Survivors," in G. P. Koocher and J. E. O'Malley (eds.), *The Damocles Syndrome,* McGraw-Hill, New York, 1981, pp. 112–129.
29. McCalla, loc. cit.
30. Meadows et al., op cit., p. 1015.
31. Ferguson, J. H., "Cognitive Late Effects of Treatment for ALL in Childhood," *Topics in Clinical Nursing* **3**:21–29.
32. Koocher et al., op. cit., p. 112.
33. Ibid., p. 1120.
34. Waskerwitz, M. J., et al., "An Overview of Cancer in Children in the 1980's," in Fochtman and Foley, op. cit., pp. 1–16.
35. Grier and Weinstein, op. cit., p. 657.
36. Ettinger, L. J., "Osteosarcoma," *Pediatric Annals* **12**:374–382 (1983).

33

Bonnie Westra

Emergencies in children

Upon completion of this chapter, the student will be able to:

1 Identify the appropriate roles of the emergency department nurse in caring for children who have experienced emergencies.

2 Establish priorities in caring for children who have suffered multiple trauma.

3 Apply the nursing process to children who have experienced accidents and injuries.

4 Describe the care of the family whose child has died of sudden infant death syndrome.

5 Develop a nursing care plan for a sexual assault victim.

The term *emergency department* immediately conjures up a variety of images. To the lay person, the emergency department (ED) is often a frightening scene of traumatic injuries, upset families, and fast-moving, all-knowing nurses and doctors. To health professionals, the ED can mean a tense, stressful atmosphere; a challenge to skill and knowledge; and often, a fight for life over death. However, the ED is much more than this. Nurses who care for patients in this setting have a multifaceted role; they do more than just race down the hall with resuscitation equipment. In the emergency setting, the nurse uses assessment skills, performs complicated procedures, and communicates with numerous people. Giving emotional support and teaching are important parts of the ED nurse's role. Often, the nurse must carry out several of these activities within a short span of time.

Acutely ill children in the ED, whether their families are present or not, add unique dimensions to the functions and responsibilities of the nurse. Although the nursing principles are the same, children are not little adults, and emergency care of pediatric patients presents special challenges. There are physiological as well as emotional and developmental differences among children of different ages which require a special approach and response. This chapter will discuss some common pediatric emergencies not dealt with elsewhere in this book and the nurse's role in providing care for children and their families in specific emergency situations.

Contact with children and their families in the ED is often brief and hurried. It is generally not conducive to a full range of nursing interventions. At the same time, the situation demands that the nurse meet numerous patient needs by utilizing a variety of nursing interventions. The nurse in the ED is often the first health care professional and hospital representative whom the child and his or her family encounter during an acute illness. The manner in which the nurse greets and treats them in the ED may influence their opinions of the entire hospital experience.

ROLE OF THE NURSE

Triage

Assess and prioritize Many types of patients seek care in the pediatric ED. The following are typical examples: a school-age girl with asthma who is audibly wheezing and in slight respiratory distress; a 2-month-old infant with a fever; a toddler with an upper respiratory infection; an unconscious teenager with multiple trauma suffered in a motorcycle accident; and a 6-year-old boy who has fallen from a tree and is crying because of pain in his arm. If these children came to the ED at the same time, the nurse could not possibly attend to all of them at once. Therefore, as a manager of patient care, the nurse begins with triage. *Triage* is a system according to which priorities of medical treatment are assigned on the basis of urgency or chance for survival. In order to set priorities accurately, the nurse makes an initial assessment of each patient. The assessment needs to be quick and thorough and must serve as a tool for determining the immediate needs of the patient. The focus of the initial assessment is on airway, breathing, and circulation—the ABCs (see Table 33-1). With this type of assessment, the nurse will immediately recognize life-threatening situations and be able to deal with them by initiating appropriate action.

If a child is not in immediate danger, the nurse then assesses in more detail other body systems and assigns priorities for medical attention and treatment. A quick review of body systems, beginning with neurological function, is an organized, efficient approach. Other valuable information is obtained by talking with the child and the family. This interviewing can be done while completing the systems assessment. The knowledge obtained from the brief medical history can be used as a partial basis for triage decisions. Questions such as "Why did you bring your child to the hospital?" "How long has your child been like this?" and "How is your child acting differently from usual?" will elicit needed information about the duration and seriousness of the illness.

Nelson's index for rating the severity of acute nontraumatic illness (Table 33-2) in pediatric patients can be used as a screening device for triage in an ED.[1] Children with a score of 10 are judged "not sick," those with a score of 8 or 9 are judged "moderately sick," and those with a score of 7 or less are judged "very sick." Table 33-2 can be used by the ED nurse as an aid in deciding which pediatric patient should be attended to first.

Coordinate care In addition to setting priorities for medical treatment, the nurse doing triage in the ED maintains close contact with the other health care professionals. The nurse alerts them to the number of children who are waiting, informs them of the findings of the brief assessments, and discusses with them the possible treatments which may be needed. The families and the children who are waiting are not left unattended. The nurse explains to them briefly the system of priorities and tries to establish when they will be seen. The nurse returns to the child and his or her family periodically to reassure them that they have not been forgotten and that they will be taken care of as soon as possible.

Initiate diagnostic tests While children are waiting in the ED, the triage nurse may use standing orders to initiate diagnostic tests. For instance, children who present with a fever of unknown origin or who may be experiencing symptoms of a urinary tract infection could have a midstream urine collected when they are able to void. Possible fractures will require x-rays, which the triage nurse may obtain before the child sees the physician. By initiating diagnostic tests, the triage shortens the time that the child spends in the ED. Information is provided to the

Table 33-1 Triage for Victims of Multiple Trauma

Priority Order of Care	Assessment	Intervention
Airway	Air movement—Look, listen, and feel. Check to see whether tongue is back in throat over trachea.	Place head in nose-up or "sniffing" position. Do not hyperextend neck in case of neck fracture.
	Presence of mucus, blood, emesis, or foreign body in mouth.	Wipe away or suction out foreign matter.
	Inability to maintain adequate airway.	Assist with placement of airway device: nasopharyngeal or oropharyngeal device; cricoid puncture; endotracheal intubation.
Breathing	Inadequate or asymmetrical chest expansion; absent breath sounds.	Begin rescue breathing and oxygen therapy.
	Open chest wound.	Apply gauze soaked with petroleum jelly to seal hole. Assist with chest tube insertion.
	Inadequate arterial blood gases.	Begin oxygen therapy.
Circulation	Absent carotid pulse.	Start closed-chest cardiac massage.
	Areas of bleeding.	Control external bleeding with sterile compression dressing. Elevate extremity that is bleeding; apply MAST trousers.
	Inadequate vital signs. Infants: pulse above 160. Preschoolers: pulse above 140. Older children: pulse above 120. Blood pressure below 70 mmHg.	Insert two IV lines, assist with fluid and blood replacement, and administer vasopressor drugs as prescribed. Fluid bolus of 20 cc per kg of body weight. Blood replacement of 10 cc per kg of body weight.
	Skin temperature and color.	Provide measures as above; maintain body warmth as much as possible.
	Urine output.	Insert Foley catheter—metered output.
Consciousness	Level of consciousness—comatose, stuporous, drowsy, alert, or anxious.	Increase frequency of observation for changes in mental status; observe for patient safety.
	Increased intracranial pressure.	Elevate head of bed. Administer steroids and diuretics as prescribed.
	Pupillary response: size, equality, reaction to light.	Increase frequency of observation if changes occur.
	Movement and sensation of extremities, hand grasp, elbow lift, hip and knee flexion, toe wiggle.	Increase frequency of observation if changes occur.
Major organ system	Signs of abdominal trauma: contusions, abrasions, wounds, and increasing pain. Auscultation for bowel sounds. Palpation for tenderness. Nausea, vomiting, distention, rigidity, and guarding.	Assist with procedures: nasogastric tube placement, application of mast trousers, diagnostic tests (x-rays, etc), laboratory tests, paracentesis, examination of pelvis and rectum.
	Decreased urine output, hematuria.	Measure output. Check for specific gravity. Observe for injuries.
Skeletal system	Pain, pulses, paresthesias, paralysis or movement, and pallor of extremities. Pulses distal to injury. Movement and sensation. Swelling, deformity, and asymmetry.	Immobilize body part and elevate it. Place ice over injury. Assist with x-rays of affected part including one joint above and one joint below injury. Assist with splinting, taping, or casts.

physician in a timely manner, enabling a diagnosis to be made and treatment to be prescribed.

Promote public relations The ED nurse strives to create an atmosphere of calm and reassurance. The nurse is not only a manager but also a caregiver who realizes that the children and their families are under stress. Families who have brought a sick or injured child to the ED are in a strange environment and are fearful about their child's welfare. The nurse is usually the first health care professional they encounter. If the nurse greets the child and the family in a hurried, insensitive manner, their anxiety is increased and their attitude toward the entire experience can be colored. Once a negative reaction has developed, it is difficult to overcome. One of the most important roles of the nurse in the ED

Table 33-2 An Index of Severity for Acute Pediatric Illness

Variable	Point Value 0	1	2
Respiratory effort	Labored or absent	Some distress	No distress
Color	Cyanotic	Pale, flushed, mottled	Normal
Activity	Delirium, stupor, coma	Lethargy	Normal
Temperature	Below 36.4 or above 40°C (below 97.4 or above 104°F)	38.4 to 40°C (101.1 to 104°F)	36.4 to 38.4°C (97.4 to 101°F)
Play	Refusal to play	Decreased play activity	Normal play activity

Source: Kathleen G. Nelson, "An Index of Severity for Acute Pediatric Illness," *American Journal of Public Health* **70**(8):804–807 (August 1980). Used with permission.

is to provide the physical and emotional support required to assist a family through the anxieties and stress of such an experience.

Provide care One area in which the nurse attempts to provide physical support is the performance of therapeutic procedures. In the ED there are vital signs to be taken, medications to be given, intravenous infusions to be started, and dressings to be applied. The nurse carries out these procedures in a competent, calm manner. Despite the urgency of the situation, accuracy and safety are indispensable. It would be of no value to hurriedly draw up and administer an emergency medication, only to have it seriously jeopardize the child's life because the dose is incorrect. To prepare a medication for a child requires strict and careful mathematical calculation, even in the tense atmosphere of an ED.

Other nursing procedures, in addition to medication administration, require safety measures and caution. Preparing a struggling 2-year-old for a lumbar puncture is greatly different from instructing an alert 17-year-old how to bend for the same procedure. It is the nurse's responsibility to prepare the child adequately for procedures in order to ensure the safety of the child and the accuracy of the treatment.

Communicate and counsel In the role of caregiver, the nurse provides competent physical care and a safe and reassuring environment for the family, but it is in the role of communicator and counselor that emotional support becomes the nurse's primary focus. This role is often easily sidestepped in a busy ED. The rapid succession of injured and ill children and their families makes it difficult to establish a significant nurse-patient relationship. Because of the tension and excitement associated with a life-threatening situation, a lower priority seems to be given to the feelings and emotions of the people involved. It is not only possible but also essential for ED personnel to provide emotional support for children and their families.

Any situation or event becomes stressful when it is perceived as a threat. The stress produces feelings of anxiety. An ED situation is stressful to almost everyone involved. A health emergency may threaten a life as well as physical well-being. It can threaten security, stability, and love. It places people in an environment where they have little control over what happens to their own bodies or those of their loved ones.

Anxiety There are different levels of anxiety. At a low level, a person becomes more alert and more aware of the surroundings and is open to learning and understanding. As anxiety increases, perception decreases. Listening and comprehension become more difficult. At the panic level, the inner turmoil is so great that perception of external stimuli is almost impossible. A knowledge of the levels of anxiety and the effects of anxiety is essential for a nurse who communicates with children and their families in an ED. This knowledge will determine the type of explanation given and the method of instruction used, as shown in the following examples.

Example: An 8-year-old girl has been driven to the ED by her mother. She has twisted her ankle while roller-skating. The ankle is swollen and painful. Both she and her mother are nervous but think that it is not a serious injury. After the x-rays have been taken and the foot has been examined by the doctor, a diagnosis of sprain is made. The nurse begins to explain how the foot will be bandaged and how it should be cared for at home. Both the mother and the child listen attentively and ask pertinent questions about when the child can go to school and how long the ankle will hurt. They are functioning at a low level of anxiety: Their perceptions are sharpened and their responses are appropriate and show interest. They may experience such bodily reactions as increased pulse and respirations or nervousness, but they are in control of their reactions.

Example: Far greater anxiety is exhibited by the young parents of a 5-month-old boy who has died from sudden infant death syndrome. The mother is crying almost hysterically. The father sits with his head bowed and his face in his hands. The physician is explaining the causes. The parents are unable to respond. They are at a panic level of anxiety and have very little perception of what is going on around them. These parents require brief, simple explanations and direct, basic instructions. Explanations will need to be repeated more than once because their grief prevents them from grasping what is said to them.

Aware of the way anxiety affects the level of comprehension, the nurse will need to verify the child's and the family's understanding of what they have been told. This is not done by simply asking, "Do you understand what I have just said?" An automatic response would be "yes." To determine whether the child and the family really did comprehend, the nurse can ask them to repeat the information that has just been given. This alerts the nurse to their anxiety level and to the effectiveness of the communication that is taking place. When a person is in a state of panic, it is often necessary to give instructions to another person who is not so immediately involved, such as a friend or another relative; to provide written instructions to be taken home; to make a referral to another professional for future follow-up; or to do all these things. Chapter 15 discusses additional methods for helping parents reduce anxiety.

Developmental level In addition to tailoring communication to the anxiety level of the child, the nurse who works with children must realize that such communication also needs to be age-specific. The developmental level of a child determines to a great extent what the child wants to hear and how it needs to be said. A 3-year-old wants an explanation of what is happening. It should, however, be brief and pertain to what is going on in the child's immediate surroundings—what is going to be done—what it will feel like, and how the child will be positioned. A school-age child, who is inquisitive, might like to be told the reasons for treatments and to be given basic explanations of anatomy. A teenager wants to be treated like the adult that he or she is becoming and to be given choices. An adolescent is concerned about body image and the future implications of an injury or illness. A knowledge of the developmental stages of childhood is as essential for the ED nurse as it is for the nurse in a pediatric unit.

Family theory Along with an understanding of developmental stages and anxiety levels, the nurse in the ED also utilizes an awareness of family theory. Children are usually accompanied by their families and friends, who are concerned and closely involved. Everything that happens to the child affects the family also. Therefore, nurses need to realize that they are caring not for just one individual but for several, if not many. Nursing actions are more effective if the nurse is aware of the close bond that exists between the child and the primary caregiver (usually the mother or father) and if the nurse provides for close and prolonged contact between the child and the primary caregiver.

The parent should be allowed to be with the child during procedures and needs to have a clear explanation of what to expect and how to help the child cope. Emotionally, the parent and the child are linked very closely. A child is sensitive to a parent's feelings. These feelings are often transmitted to the child without a word. The child may sense fear in the person who has always been strong and protective. The child may then be afraid simply because the parent is. A child who is afraid and anxious often becomes restless, squirms, and even thrashes about. This may complicate the injuries or the illness. Calming the child can be accomplished at least to an extent by calming the parent. A parent who is given complete explanations and honest information becomes less anxious and is better able to focus on the child's fears and to help the nurse support the young patient. Direct involvement of the parents continues throughout the entire time that the child is being treated in the ED. Equipment is demonstrated, procedures are explained, and plans are discussed, in an effort to keep the family included in the care.

It is reassuring to parents to be with their child during a stressful experience. They are able to actually observe what is happening. Parents imagine many horrible things in a waiting room while their child is behind closed doors. Parents who are permitted to stay often remark, "Is that all there is to it? I thought it would be much worse." Somehow, reality is far less frightening than the imagination. Several institutions have discovered that allowing the families to remain, even in life-threatening situations, is beneficial to both them and the child. Allowing the parents to remain with the child also seems to relieve them of some of the guilt they experience because they were not able to prevent the illness or injury. The nurse should ask the parents to sit down during procedures because some may become faint.

Every parent is an individual, and the members of every family have unique ways of relating to one another. The nurse adapts care to the needs of each specific family and child. Not all parents want to stay with their children during treatment. Some prefer to wait outside the room. Their decision should be accepted and supported. The parents should inform the child where they will wait. The nurse then provides support for the child during the treatment.

Some parents are not emotionally able to remain in attendance during medical treatments. The nurse should be able to assess the coping abilities of the parents and to determine whether it would be detrimental to the welfare of the child if they remained. If, after receiving reassurance and explanations, the parents are still unable to focus on what is being said or are still extremely agitated, the nurse should ask them to leave. They should be told where to wait and reassured that their decision is appropriate and good for both them and their child. Communication with parents who remain in the waiting room continues throughout the time the child is being treated. The nurse gives the parents frequent information concerning the condition of their child and what is being done. The child also needs to know where the parents are, that they are concerned, and that they will be waiting when the treatment is finished.

Occasionally a child is admitted to an ED without any family member present. The child may have been brought from camp or from school or by ambulance from the scene of an accident. Except in life-threatening situations, emergency personnel may be legally unable to provide any type of treatment without the express permission of the parents or guardian. What can be done depends on state laws and hospital policy. It is frequently the nurse who must contact the parents and inform them of what has happened to their child. It is important to be aware of the impact that this communication will have on parents. Simple, accurate information will be most clearly understood. The parents may also need to be told how to locate the ED and to be reminded to drive carefully. If it is true, the nurse reassures them that their child is in no danger and will be waiting for them when they arrive.

Patient education

In addition to the roles of triage nurse, care-provider, and communicator-counselor, the ED nurse is an educator. Although the time families spend in an ED is short, it is a period during which they become a captive audience, and sometimes they are both receptive and responsive. Because the nurse knows the effect of anxiety on perception, he or she is aware that a person under stress often becomes more alert and perceptive; teaching is most effective when a person is experiencing a low level of stress. The majority of children who enter an ED have minor illnesses and injuries. They are usually eager to understand what has happened and what they can do to facilitate recovery. The parents often suffer guilt feelings, assuming that it was their neglect or their actions that caused the injury or illness. They want to learn how to prevent further problems and how to care for their child. However, because they do not wish to display what they assume is poor parenting or ignorance, many parents do not speak up; they do not ask questions. The nurse must recognize a parent's needs and intervene to meet them. Every encounter with a health care provider should be a learning experience for both the child and the parents.

Several categories of teaching are pertinent to the ED setting: (1) instructions regarding follow-up care for the present problem, (2) general health care teaching, and (3) anticipatory guidance. Table 15-5 presents a four-step approach to patient teaching which can be used by the ED nurse.

Follow-up care

Instructions for follow-up care are important because much of the treatment initiated in the ED can be undone if care is not continued at home. Instructions given hurriedly or offhandedly can easily be misunderstood by the most well-meaning parent. Once at home, the parent may wonder, "Did the nurse say to use ice the first day and then warm compresses or heat the first day followed by ice?" The following guidelines will facilitate effective teaching:

1. Assess the educational background and intellectual level of the parents and their prior experience with the health care system; then teach them at an appropriate level.
2. Instructions should be clear and simple and phrased according to the parents' and the child's level of understanding.
3. Essential instructions should be written down and sent home with the family.
4. The parents should be asked to repeat in their own words what they have been told.
5. After repeating the instructions, the parents should also be asked to state how they will use the information.
6. Familiar measurements, such as teaspoons or tablespoons, should be used.
7. The parents should be urged to call the ED to check on the instructions or to ask questions. Include a written telephone number.

Compliance with instructions is often very low. One reason usually cited is lack of understanding. Once the nurse has clearly taught a procedure that must be performed at home, it is usually beneficial to explain the purpose of it, including simple physiology and the effects of the procedure. Most children and their families will respond better when they understand what they are doing and why. Children and their families are partners in health care.

Further actions that the nurse can take to ensure compliance with prescribed treatment include matching verbal instructions with written ones. If there is a discrepancy between them, the child and the parents may become confused. Involving the child and the parents in care, such as holding a dressing or applying an ointment, shows them that the ED nurse thinks they are capable of performing the procedure. Compliance with prescribed treatments can be further reinforced by asking the child and the parents how or when they will carry out certain activities, such as taking or administering medications.

General health care

The nurse in the ED also has many opportunities to provide general health care teaching. For example, while taking a history from the mother of a 4-year-old, the nurse learns that the child has never been immunized. After attending to the problem which brought the mother in, the nurse talks with her about immunizations, explaining what they are, how they protect the child, and where to get them. The nurse discovers that the mother has no pediatrician and that evidently no one had ever really explained immunizations before. The immunizations were not the reason for the visit to the emergency room, but the child's need was recognized, and appropriate nursing intervention followed.

Anticipatory guidance

Along with general health care teaching, anticipatory guidance is often a function of the ED nurse. Anticipatory guidance is preparation for the future care of the child. It focuses on growth and development. In the ED, a primary goal of anticipatory guidance is prevention of accidents. For example, as the mother of a toddler with an upper respiratory infection is preparing to go home, the nurse may begin a discussion of accidental poisonings and ways to "child-proof" the home. Concrete, simple suggestions that the parent can put into practice at home should always be included in any type of preventive teaching.

Finally, the nurse in the ED must remember that no matter what brings the child to the hospital, careful and accurate documentation is required. Baseline data, procedures, and reaction, all follow-up care and instruction, and the child's and the family's understanding of follow-up care should be written in the child's record.

ACCIDENTS AND INJURIES

Accidents and traumatic injuries are the chief causes of children's visits to EDs. Accidents are the leading cause of death in children 1 to 14 years of age, and they also cause large numbers of nonfatal injuries that require treatment and hospitalization.

As children grow and develop new skills and abilities, the type of accident to which they are susceptible changes accordingly. A breakdown of specific accidents by age reveals the progression of developmental stages and physiological growth (Table 33-3).

An infant is most likely to be injured by falling or by being improperly restrained in an automobile. As the child becomes mobile, he or she may suffer injury or death in a motor vehicle accident as either a passenger or a pedestrian. Later the adolescent is involved as a driver.

No matter how accidents happen, they can lead to multiple injuries, fractures and sprains, lacerations, burns, poisonings, and drownings. They have a significant physical, emotional, social, and financial impact on the child and the entire family.

Multiple trauma

Motor vehicle accidents frequently result in multiple trauma injuries. Several major organs of the body may sustain serious damage. The nurse in the ED quickly assesses the child with multiple traumatic injuries. Evaluation of the life-support systems—airway, breathing, and circulation—is a primary focus. Then a more detailed assessment of damage to other organs is performed. Head injuries, abdominal trauma with internal hemorrhage, and fractured bones are the most common sequelae of motor vehicle accidents. Table 33-1 outlines a triage system of assessment and intervention for multiple trauma.

Respiratory distress

Etiology and clinical manifestations Children who experience multiple trauma are at risk for developing respiratory distress. Blockage of the airway can occur when the tongue falls back in an unconscious child, or foreign particles and excess mucus can block the airways. Breathing can be compromised as a result of neurological damage, chest trauma, or metabolic abnormalities. Circulatory problems further complicate an inadequate respiratory status. Table 33-1 presents the signs and symptoms that the ED nurse must assess.

Treatment and nursing management Cardiopulmonary resuscitation (CPR), as described in Table 16-7, should be implemented whenever the ED nurse cares for a child who is not breathing and has no pulse. Advanced cardiac life support (ACLS) may be required if CPR is not effective. ACLS includes establishing an intravenous line, preparing for endotracheal intubation, cardiac monitoring, preparing for administration of drugs, and possible defibrillation.

Establishing an intravenous line should receive high priority in ACLS. With circulatory collapse, placing an intravenous line becomes more difficult. Whenever possible, this should be done prior to a cardiopulmonary arrest.

During ACLS, airway management is facilitated by intubation. Table 33-4 provides guidelines for selection of endotracheal tubes and suction catheters. The ED nurse assists with intubation by selecting the correct endotracheal tube, suctioning excess secretions, and managing the airway once the endotracheal tube is in place. In some hospitals, however, code teams perform these functions.

Table 33-3 Types of Accidents by Specific Age

Birth to 1 Year	1 to 4 Years	5 to 14 Years
Falls	Motor vehicle accidents	Motor vehicle accidents
Poisoning	Poisoning	Drowning
Burns	Burns	Burns
Aspiration of foreign objects	Drowning	Firearms
		Bicycle accidents

Table 33-4 Guidelines for Selection of Endotracheal Tubes and Suction Catheters

Age	Endotracheal Tube Size (mm)	Suction Catheter
Newborn	3.0	6F
6 months	3.5	8F
18 months	4.0	8F
3 years	4.5	8F
5 years	5.0	10F
6 years	5.5	10F
8 years	6.0	10F
12 years	6.5	10F
16 years	7.0	10F
Adult woman	8.0 to 8.5	12F
Adult male	8.5 to 9.0	14F

Source: K. M. McIntyre and A. J. Lewis: *Textbook of Advanced Cardiac Life Support*, American Heart Association, Dallas, 1981. Used with permission.

Placing the child on a cardiac monitor provides the ED nurse with information about the effectiveness of CPR and whether the child's heart has begun functioning on its own. Both medications and defibrillation may be used to increase the heart's effectiveness. Table 33-5 lists the medications used for ACLS. If defibrillation is required, it should be done using paddles of the correct size. For infants, 4.5-cm paddles are used, and 8-cm paddles are used for older children. Electrode paste and saline-soaked gauze or defibrillation pads are placed over the skin to improve electrical conduction from the paddles to the heart. One paddle is placed to the right of the sternum at the second rib, and the other is placed at the left midclavicular line, at the level of the xiphoid process. Two watt-seconds per kilogram of body weight should be used initially and the dose doubled if further defibrillation is required.[2]

Hypovolemic shock

Incidence and etiology Children who have experienced multiple trauma are at risk for going into hypovolemic shock. A loss of more than 25 percent of circulating blood volume causes hypovolemic shock. Blood volume is estimated by calculating 80 ml per kilogram of body weight. Hypovolemic shock results from excessive external fluid loss, such as arterial bleeding, or from excessive internal fluid loss, causing inadequate blood flow to vital organs. Blunt trauma to the abdomen is most frequently the cause of internal bleeding, which affects major body organs, such as the liver, spleen, or kidneys. Shock causes inadequate tissue perfusion, leading to metabolic abnormalities. If it is not rapidly corrected, death will result.

Pathophysiology When the body rapidly loses blood volume—e.g., following a major trauma—it tries to compensate. Initially, venous and right heart pressures are decreased as a result of loss of blood volume. Vasoconstriction occurs to preserve the blood pressure. The heart rate increases to compensate for the lost blood volume. The arterial blood pressure decreases because of decreased blood volume. However, the diastolic pressure may increase, reflecting vasoconstriction. Decreased tissue perfusion occurs,

Table 33-5 Drugs Used in ACLS for Infants and Children

Drug	Dose	How Supplied	Remarks
Atropine sulfate	0.01 to 0.03 mg/kg	0.1 mg/ml	
Calcium chloride	0.3 ml/kg	100 mg/ml (10%)	Give slowly
Dexamethasone sodium phosphate	0.3 mg/kg per 24 h	4 mg/ml	
Dopamine hydrochloride	2 to 10 μg/kg per minute	40 mg/ml	α-receptor dominate at ≥ 10 μg/kg per minute
Epinephrine	0.1 ml/kg	1 : 10,000	1 : 1000 must be diluted
Epinephrine infusion	Start at 0.1 μg/kg per minute	1 : 1000 (1 mg)	Usual effect ≤ 1.5 μg/kg per minute
Furosemide	1 mg/kg per dose	10 mg/ml	
Isoproterenol hydrochloride	Start at 0.1 μg/kg per minute	1 mg per 5 ml	Usual effect 0.1 to 1.0 μg/kg per minute
Lidocaine	1 mg/kg per dose	10 mg/ml (1%) 20 mg/ml (20%)	
Lidocaine infusion	30 μg/kg per minute	10 mg/ml (1%) 20 mg/ml (2%) 40 mg/ml (4%)	
Norepinephrine	Start at 0.1 μg/kg per minute	1 mg/ml	Titrate to desired effect
Naloxone hydrochloride	0.01 mg/kg per dose	0.4 mg/ml 0.02 mg/ml	Short half-life
Sodium nitroprusside	Start at 0.5 μg/kg per minute	10 mg/ml	Usual effect at 1 to 10 μg/kg per minute
Sodium bicarbonate	1 to 2 mEq/kg per dose 0.3 × kg × base deficit	1 mEq/ml	Should be diluted in newborns

Source: K. M. McIntyre and A. J. Lewis, *Textbook of Advanced Cardiac Life Support*, American Heart Association, Dallas, 1981. Used with permission.

especially in the extremities, as the body attempts to maintain vital organs, such as the brain and kidneys. Anaerobic metabolism and acidosis result. Hypovolemic shock is life-threatening to a child who has experienced multiple trauma. Understanding the pathophysiology helps the ED nurse anticipate the child's needs.

Clinical manifestations Frequent observations of vital signs, mentation, skin, urinary output, and pain help the ED nurse anticipate impending shock. In an older child, blood pressure less than 70 mmHg with tachycardia indicates a 25 percent blood volume loss and the existence of shock. In children, vital signs vary with age. The following is a quick rule of thumb for estimating parameters:

The upper limits of *normal pulse* are 160 beats per minute for infants, 140 beats per minute for preschool children, and 120 beats per minute for older children.
The *systolic blood pressure* is estimated as 80 plus 2 times the child's age.
The *diastolic blood pressure* is about two-thirds of the systolic blood pressure.[3]

As blood volume decreases, the child becomes anxious and agitated. Eventually, depressed mentation occurs, leading to unconsciousness. The ED nurse, however, must not assume that mentation is related to hypovolemia, since head trauma frequently occurs in multiple trauma. Pale, ashen skin that is cold and sweaty should prompt the nurse to consider hypovolemic shock. Urinary output also decreases with hypovolemia. Changes in pain, especially in the abdomen, may signify increasing bleeding as a result of organ damage.

Treatment and nursing management The goal in hypovolemic shock is to maintain adequate circulation until the underlying problems can be corrected. Management of the respiratory system is the first priority. Next the nurse should ensure that the circulation is adequate. Placing the child in a Trendelenburg position is contraindicated in head injury, but should be considered otherwise. Intravenous fluid replacement with normal saline or Ringer's lactate is begun as soon as possible by establishing at least two intravenous sites. Application of antishock (MAST) trousers increases the blood volume by one-tenth to one-fifth within 2 minutes. One leg of an adult suit can be used if pediatric trousers are not available. Maintaining an adequate urinary output is facilitated by insertion of a Foley catheter. Urine should be monitored in children every 30 min. Pharmacological agents and blood replacement are usually ordered. Cardiac monitoring, as well as frequent measurements of vital signs, is essential for evaluating the child's unstable condition.

The parents will be very anxious, which is normal when any life-threatening emergency occurs. When possible, they should be allowed to be with their child. If this is not possible, one of the ED nurses or another support person, such as the chaplain, should be with them. A child who is in hypovolemic shock should be transferred to an intensive care unit for close observation. The parents must be informed prior to the transfer about what to expect and should be reassured that everything possible is being done for their child.

Head injury

Twenty-five to fifty percent of all accidents involve head injury. Many head injuries are minor, resulting in a brief loss of consciousness, and cause no serious damage. Others involve damage to brain tissue and can lead to sudden deterioration and death. The ED nurse must be able to evaluate the seriousness of a head injury and use appropriate interventions. The severity of a head injury depends on the involvement of the soft brain tissue. A skull fracture alone is of little consequence. The nurse performs a thorough neurological examination to determine the extent of the injury and to document the child's condition for future reference. Evaluation of level of consciousness and detection of any signs that indicate location of brain damage are of primary importance. A neurological checklist is very helpful and ensures consistent examinations by different personnel over a period of time (Tables 30-3, 30-4, and 30-18). Children with minor head injuries are usually discharged and are observed at home by their parents. The parents should be given clear instructions about the importance of evaluating the alertness of their child. They should be informed of changes that could indicate a problem and told what to do if the changes take place (Chap. 30).

Damage to major organ systems

Etiology A child with a head injury rarely goes into shock. Therefore, if the ED nurse detects symptoms of shock (hypotension; a rapid, thready pulse; and cold and clammy skin), causes other than the head injury must be suspected. A frequent cause of shock is internal bleeding due to abdominal injuries. The mortality rate from abdominal trauma is relatively high in comparison with that from other types of injuries. The organs most frequently injured as a result of abdominal trauma in a child are the spleen, the liver, the kidneys, and the intestines. The primary symptoms are abdominal pain, tenderness, distention, and rigidity and vomiting. Occasionally, shock may be the only important sign. Children frequently vomit after trauma, and so vomiting is significant only in conjunction with other symptoms. At times, bleeding from abdominal injuries is gradual, and the development of an acute abdomen is insidious. Children with multiple trauma require close observation for several days to rule out the possibility of significant but covert injuries. Because of the child's small blood volume, it is important for the nurse to correctly calculate actual blood loss. In a child, hemorrhage may seem insignificant until it is compared with total blood volume.

Nursing management The nursing care plan for a child with possible abdominal injuries consists of frequent evaluations of vital signs, consistent measurements of abdominal girth, and accurate monitoring of urinary output with a retention catheter. Children often develop paralytic ileus after trauma, and so a nasogastric tube is inserted and connected to intermittent suction while the child is still in the emergency room. Then careful nursing observation for signs of physiological deterioration continues as the child is transferred to an inpatient unit. During this time, the nurse must be aware that both the child and the parents are very frightened. The nurse should explain procedures and provide emotional support.

Fractures, sprains, and strains

Falls frequently result in a visit to an ED. Although falls can lead to a multiplicity of injuries, fractures (broken bones), sprains (partial tearing of a ligament), and strains (overstretching of a muscle) are the most frequent consequences. (See Chap. 29 for a discussion of sprains and types of fractures.)

Treatment and nursing management When a child comes to the ED with a history of an injury and with pain localized to a particular area of bone, a fracture should be suspected. The nurse's first responsibility is to assess the child for respiratory and circulatory status and then for the following local and systemic signs of fracture:

1. Deformity—shortening, angulation, or rotation.
2. Local pain and tenderness
3. Grating or crepitation
4. Swelling
5. Bruising and discoloration
6. Loss of function or abnormal mobility
7. Appearance of fragments
8. Shock

A careful history should describe the kind and amount of trauma involved, when it occurred, the direction of force, other possible injuries, and any emergency treatment at the scene. All other organs need to be examined to avoid missing other injuries.

Several basic principles of care should be followed. With a suspected fracture, unnecessary handling must be avoided, and the area immobilized. Splints are used to prevent further damage to skin, muscles, nerves, and blood vessels. Clean dressings should be applied to any wounds, and hemorrhage should be controlled with direct pressure. The nurse should be familiar with the five P's of vascular occlusion distal to the injury and check for them: *pain, pulselessness, paresthesia, pallor,* and *paralysis*. It is often helpful to compare the injured extremity with the uninjured one.

Once the injured part has been initially evaluated and protected by splinting, x-rays are taken to provide a definitive diagnosis. In children, the uninjured extremity may also be x-rayed if a comparison of epiphyseal growth plates is desired.

The child with an orthopedic injury experiences fear, anxiety, and pain. The nurse will need to establish rapport quickly to make an assessment possible. Gentle, firm handling is necessary while the child and the family are prepared for what will happen next. If the possibility of surgery exists, the child is given nothing orally. Intramuscular pain medications are best (Demerol, 1 mg per kg of body weight, works well). The time the child last ate, allergies, and any significant medical or surgical history should be determined.

Teaching Severe strains and sprains respond to immobilization of the joint with splinting, wrapping or taping, application of ice, and elevation (Fig. 33-1). Ice should be applied for the first 24 to 48 h after an injury to reduce swelling. After 48 h, heat is used to aid healing. Sometimes splints are applied, and the child is instructed to return in 2 to 5 days for application of a plaster cast. If crutches are necessary, the child will need instruction in their correct use.

When a plaster cast is applied, the child and the family should be given written instructions to take home regarding cast care and warning signs and symptoms. The following is an example of appropriate instructions:

1. Your cast will require 24 to 48 h to dry. Walking casts are not ready for walking until they are dry.
2. Report any of the following to the emergency department: excessive swelling above or below the cast; continuous color change after elevation of the extremity for 30 min; an excessively loose cast; marked pain if someone moves their fingers or toes; irritation or a rubbing sensation of the skin around or under the cast leading to redness or blisters; decreased ability to move the fingers or toes; and increasing pain that is not relieved by medication.
3. Do not cover your cast with paint, since it must be able to "breathe."

The nurse, too, must remain alert for changes in color, warmth, sensation, and motion following cast application. (A more extensive discussion of orthopedic injuries and their treatment, including cast care, appears in Chap. 29.)

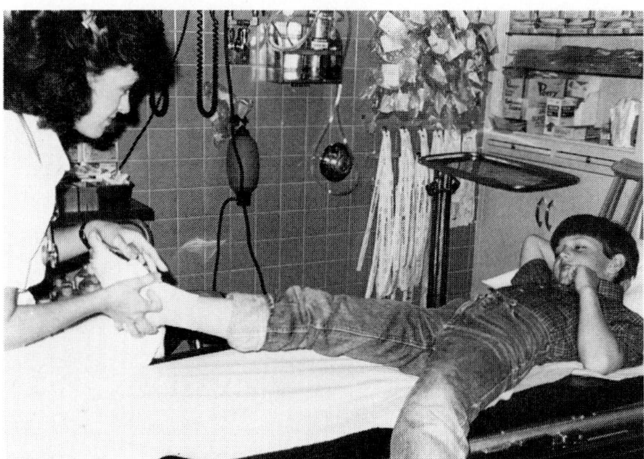

Figure 33-1 Immobilization of a sprained ankle. (*Photo courtesy of Linda Olivet.*)

Lacerations

Lacerations occur commonly in children. They usually affect only the skin and fatty tissue beneath it. Sometimes muscles, tendons, blood vessels, ligaments, or nerves are cut. Minor lacerations are often treated at home. Usually cuts on the trunk or face should be examined by the physician in the ED. The parents may also bring their child in after a laceration has begun to show signs of infection.

Treatment and nursing management The nurse will first determine when and how the laceration occurred. Other important historical data include the date of the last tetanus immunization, allergies, and significant medical conditions, such as bleeding or circulatory problems. The size and depth of the laceration should be described, and the amount of bleeding and accompanying injuries noted. Vital signs are documented.

If there is profuse bleeding, pressure applied with a sterile compress, elevation, and ice are indicated. Minimal bleeding may be controlled with a sterile compress (Fig. 33-2).

If the child has symptoms of infection, a culture should be done before the wound is cleansed. The nurse should also determine whether wood splinters are present in the wound. Wounds containing wood should never be soaked, since wood expands when wet.

Next the wound should be cleansed. (It may be wise to check for allergies again.) A sterile 4- by 4-in pad and a Zephiran solution are often used for facial lacerations. Hands and feet may be soaked in a basin of cool water to which Betadine soap solution has been added. Betadine soap solution and sterile 4- by 4-in pads are used to cleanse other areas.

After the wound is cleansed, it can be protected with a sterile towel until treatment is begun. X-rays may be taken to detect the presence of a foreign body, such as fragments of glass, wood, or metal (Fig. 33-3).

The wound is then dressed or stitched. The nurse is responsible for maintaining a sterile field, providing necessary equipment, and assisting in holding the child still during the procedure. Xylocaine (1 percent) is frequently used for anesthesia. Epinephrine may be added if control of

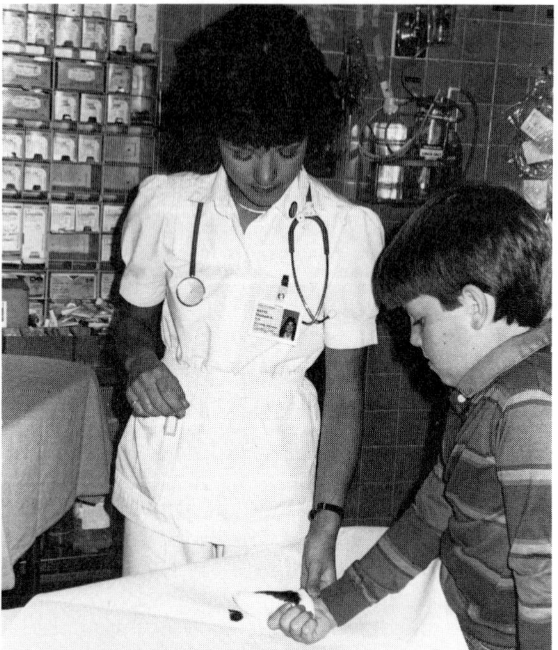

Figure 33-2 A sterile compress used to control bleeding. (*Photo courtesy of Linda Olivet.*)

bleeding is important. Epinephrine is never used on fingers, toes, ears, the nose, or the penis, since vasoconstriction could cause circulatory impairment.

Any significant laceration threatens the child's sense of body integrity. It is always helpful to ask the child what he or she expects to happen. There is often time after the wound is cleansed, and before stitches are placed, to read a story to the child, such as "Becky Gets Stitches."[4] If the parents read the story or hear it, they too are prepared for this experience. The child should be encouraged to express his or her feelings about the entire experience.

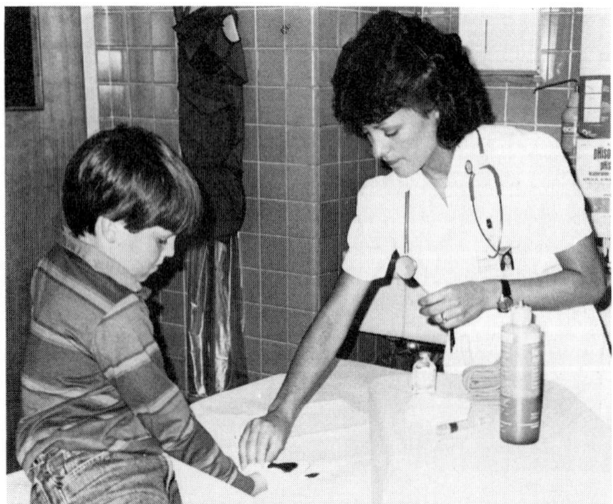

Figure 33-3 Preparation of a wound for stitches. (*Photo courtesy of Linda Olivet.*)

Tetanus prophylaxis is necessary in most lacerations, puncture wounds, and open fractures and in any case of multiple injury. If the wound is "dirty" or was made by a rusty object, a tetanus booster is given if the last immunization was given more than 2 to 3 years before the injury. If the wound is "clean," the last tetanus injection is usually considered adequate for 5 to 8 years. Antibiotic therapy may also be given if deemed appropriate. Table 33-6 gives an example of written instructions that can be given to the parents and the child regarding care of a laceration after discharge from the ED.

Burns

Incidence and etiology Burns, whether thermal, electrical, or chemical, are a major source of accidents among children. The consequences can be devastating, with treatment and hospitalization ranging from 6 weeks to 2 years. Electrical burns are particularly serious because passage of the electric current through the body can

Table 33-6 Instructions to Parents: Care of a Child with an Open Wound

After initial emergency care of a wound, it is as important to care properly for the injury until healing is complete:

1. Keep the wound clean and dry.
2. Notify the doctor if any of the following signs of infection appear:
   a. Redness, particularly if increasing and streaking from the area of the wound
   b. Pain, especially if increasing in severity
   c. Heat or warmth in the area of the wound
   d. Swelling
   e. Drainage, especially if there is a bad odor or there is pus
   f. Chills, elevated temperature, or both

Keep your outpatient visit appointment.

Doctor ______________________

Phone ______________________

Source: City of Boston, Department of Health and Hospitals.

cause cardiac arrhythmia, aneurysm, or late cataracts.

Burns are now one of the five leading causes of death in children. There are approximately 200,000 burn cases in the United States yearly. About one-half of these are children. Of the total, 80 percent are avoidable accidents, and of that number, 50 percent are the result of the child's actions and 15 percent are the result of carelessness or neglect on the part of the caretaker. Only 15 percent involve the child as an innocent bystander. In only about 10 percent of all burns are children intended victims. These burns are classified as child abuse.

Treatment and nursing management When a burned child arrives in the ED, the major goals of treatment are (1) to assess respiratory status, (2) to begin fluid replacement, (3) to evaluate the extent and depth of the wounds, and (4) to initiate cleansing measures.

Smoke inhalation accounts for 80 percent of the deaths associated with burns. The ED nurse immediately determines patency of the airway. Initially, respiratory status may be unaffected, but edema of the respiratory tract due to burns or smoke inhalation can lead to airway obstruction any time from 4 to 24 h after the actual burn. Signs of smoke inhalation, such as burned or singed areas of the face and throat, smoky-smelling breath, charcoal in the sputum, or any symptoms of respiratory distress, should alert the nurse to the possibility of future airway obstruction.

The extent and depth of burns form a basis for type of treatment and calculation of fluid replacement (Fig. 27-2). It is generally agreed that any child with second- to third-degree burns over 10 to 15 percent of the body requires hospitalization. Burns of the hands and feet are also usually treated on an inpatient basis to ensure correct splinting of the extremity and to prevent contractures.

First-degree burns cause red skin that is extremely painful. In the case of first-degree burns that result from the spilling of grease, a degreaser should first be applied to clean the skin. The skin should then be cleansed. Usually cold, wet towels are the most comfortable bandage. Greasy dressings, such as a piece of gauze to which ointment has been applied, are difficult to remove and may retain moisture and therefore encourage the growth of bacteria.

Second-degree burns require sterile technique. They are best treated by removing *broken* blisters, cleansing the area with saline, and applying Silvadene cream and a Xerofoam gauze dressing with a layer of absorbing gauze over it. It is important to check the child's allergies again before applying Silvadene, since it contains sulfa.

More severe burns are initially cleansed with warmed saline and then dressed with an ointment application such as providone-iodine (Betadine) or Silvadene. Care must be taken to prevent hypothermia, since heat loss occurs with severe burns. Vital signs, including temperature, are monitored frequently.

Fluid loss begins immediately after any burn. Therefore, fluid replacement is a priority of treatment. Initially, a solution of Ringer's lactate may be started while calculation of fluid replacement is determined. A cutdown in an unaffected part of the body is preferred because it provides stability for long-term intravenous therapy and a large lumen for colloid infusion, if needed. A urinary retention catheter is necessary for accurate measurement of urine output in order to determine adequate fluid therapy. The burned child is weighed, if at all possible, or a close estimation of weight is obtained from the family. Tetanus toxoid is also administered to the burn victim in the ED.

The immediate treatment for a chemical burn is to flush the area with large amounts of warm water for approximately 20 min. If the eyes are burned, they too are flushed with water. A shower works well for burns covering large areas of the body. Then the child is transported to the ED, where the burns are washed again. Burned eyes should be flushed with physiological saline. If only one eye is involved, it is important to rinse the fluid away from the other eye. No attempt is made to neutralize the chemical because neutralization produces heat, which can cause further damage. Chemical burns may continue to cause damage for some time, and so multiple washings may be ordered. Most household containers stress the need to flush a contact area with water, but parents may need to be reminded to read labels for warnings and treatment as they are making purchases. Some items may be so dangerous that they are not advisable for use in homes with children. The care and treatment of burns is discussed in Chap. 27.

Poisoning

Incidence Poisoning is the number one acute emergency in children. Sixty-five percent of the more than 5 million yearly ingestions of poison in the United States occur in children under 5 years of age and are accidental.[5] When poisonings occur after the age of 5, the nurse must be alert to this "cry for help," or suicide attempt, which indicates a need for careful investigation and intervention.

Toddlers and preschoolers are prone to accidental poisoning because of their rapid motor maturation and newfound mobility. Compared with the infant, the 18- to 36-month-old seems to be everywhere and into everything. The child touches and pokes, listens, sees, smells, and frequently tastes and swallows.

Etiology Children will taste and swallow almost anything that is within their reach. The availability and frequency of use of substances determine which ones are most commonly ingested. Soaps, detergents, and cleaners are the number one agents in poisonings. They are followed by plants, vitamins and minerals, and aspirin.[6] Child-proof bottle caps have removed aspirin from its former position as the number one child poisoner. Prescription medications belonging to anyone in the family are a potential risk. Children love to explore purses, where visitors may have their medications. Small children may also take an overdose of their own medications, e.g., lanoxin. Because the parent gives the child a medication every day, the drug may seem as harmless as food to the child. Other commonly ingested poisons include bleach, paint thinners, insecticides, and petroleum distillates. Baby powder ingestion accounts for 1 percent of all calls to poison control centers for children under 3 years of age.[7]

While in the past it was generally assumed that the child who ingested poisonous substances came from a home that was not adequately safe, recent studies seem to conclude that stress in the family plays an important part.[8] Accidental poisonings in young children may be seen as their effort to cope with the family disorganization that surrounds them. Such crises as divorce, pregnancy, academic difficulties, illness, and death may precipitate an accidental poisoning in a young child or a deliberate self-poisoning in an older child. Once a child has had an ingestion episode, there is a 50 percent chance that he or she will repeat the episode within 1 year. Many poisonings occur between 4 P.M. and 6 P.M. while dinner is being prepared. The nurse must understand that a variety of factors, including stress and availability, interact to precipitate the incidence of accidental and deliberate self-poisonings.

Treatment and nursing management Many parents and caretakers call the ED when they suspect that a child has ingested a substance that is potentially poisonous. The triage nurse must carefully assess the situation. If there is ever *any* doubt, the child should be brought to the ED. The parents should be advised to bring the empty container (or plant) to the hospital.

Some ingested substances are considered "nontoxic." They include such things as antacids, chalk, deodorant, glue, ink, lipstick, laxatives, latex paint, perfume, shampoo, toothpaste, and vitamins. To designate an ingestion as nontoxic, the substance must be absolutely identified, there must be no warning on the container ("Danger," "Call physician immediately," or "Caution"), the amount ingested must be known, and the victim must be free of symptoms. For the average drug, 5 times the average dose is toxic.

When the poison is unknown, the nurse or physician will have to investigate thoroughly to determine the culprit. The following are indications that a poisoning has occurred:

1. The onset of signs and symptoms is abrupt.
2. The child is in the "at risk" age group (1 to 4 years).
3. The child has a previous history of poison ingestion.
4. There is multiple organ system involvement.

The nurse can ask specific questions in an attempt to determine the type of substance that was ingested: "What was the child doing before the symptoms developed?" "Where was the child playing? In the garage? In the kitchen? In the bathroom?" "What types of substances are stored there?" "What types of containers are they in?" "When did the child become symptomatic?" "How much of the product was available and in what form?" In any case of poisoning the nurse considers the possibility that other children may also have ingested the substance. Children are known to share their discoveries.

The emergency management of poisoning is aimed at preventing absorption of the poison beyond that point which the body can safely detoxify or that can be effectively antagonized by antidotes. When a child is known, or thought, to have ingested a poisonous substance, the treatment begins immediately—at home, if possible. Before vomiting is induced, the local ED, a physician, or a poison control center should be called. Induction of vomiting is generally the most immediate, effective method of removing the poison if the child's vital signs are stable. Mechanical methods, such as placing a finger at the back of the throat, are often ineffective and a waste of time. Ipecac is the recommended emetic and may be purchased by parents without a prescription. It is a drug which should be kept in all homes with small children. The dose is 15 ml for a child aged 1 to 5 years and 30 ml for an older child, followed by at least 200 ml of any fluid. Ipecac is not recommended for children under the age of 1 year. If there is no vomiting within 15 min, the same dose may be repeated. No further doses of ipecac should be given, since the drug is cardiotoxic and may have dangerous side effects when administered in large doses. The "universal antidote" of burned toast, milk of magnesia, and charcoal is usually not effective, and valuable time is spent trying to persuade the child to swallow these things.

Vomiting should never be induced if a child (1) has ingested a corrosive alkali or acid, (2) has swallowed a petroleum product, (3) is unconscious or has lost the gag or cough reflex, or (4) is having seizures. An alkali or acid such as bleach or drain cleaner damages the mucous membrane of the esophagus as it is swallowed, and vomiting may cause further damage. Even one drop of a drain cleaner will severely burn the esophagus. If a child who has ingested a petroleum product such as paint thinner or furniture polish vomits, there is an increased danger of aspiration and of the development of lipoid pneumonia, which is very difficult to treat. Any person who is unconscious or having a seizure and vomits has an increased risk of aspiration and possible airway obstruction. ED personnel will find it useful to have a poison treatment chart available for quick reference, since many frightened parents call a hospital when their child has swallowed a dangerous substance. (See Appendix E.)

Once a child who has ingested poison is brought to the ED, treatment is basically supportive. Few of the harmful substances have specific antidotes, and unless information is readily available, medical care should be begun without it. The parents should be advised to bring the empty container to the hospital and should be asked to estimate how much was ingested. The volume of a swallow in a $1\frac{1}{2}$- to 3-year-old is 4.5 ml; in an adult it is 15 ml. Medical treatment is more precise if the type and amount of the ingested substance are known. Table 33-7 describes major treatment considerations in cases of poisoned or overdosed patients.

If the substance is unknown, the nurse must observe the child carefully for signs and symptoms that will aid the physician in the differential diagnosis. These signs and symptoms are listed in Table 33-8. Poisonous substances that are known to have specific antidotes are listed in Table 33-9, along with their specific antidotes.

The goal of treatment in the ED is removal of the poison. Syrup of ipecac is given if indicated. When vomiting has been initiated in the home, the results are evaluated in the ED. The parents should be instructed to bring all emesis with them.

Although gastric lavage is not as effective in removing gastric contents as emesis, it can be used as long as the child is not convulsing or if the child has an endotracheal tube in place. A no. 22 to 26F Ewald or Jacques orogastric tube is used for a child, and a no. 34 to 36F is used for an adult. When the tube is in place, the stomach contents are aspirated, and the initial material is saved for toxicological study. The lavage fluid is half-normal or normal saline used in quantities of 50 to 100 ml for children. When returns are clear, the lavage is stopped. Often, activated charcoal and later a cathartic are given by stomach tube and left in the stomach. The tube must be pinched off before it is withdrawn.

Activated charcoal is being used increasingly in the treatment of poisoning. It may be the most potent general antidote available. It is an *adsorbent* that inactivates many poisonous substances in the stomach. It decreases the amount of the poison available for absorption into the blood supply. The charcoal should not be given before syrup of ipecac because charcoal will absorb the ipecac and drastically reduce its effectiveness. It may be given after the child has vomited. Charcoal is given orally or by tube in doses of 2 g per kilogram of body weight mixed with 60 ml of water.

Throughout the treatment of a child who has experienced an accidental poisoning, the nurse maintains close observation of vital signs and neurological status. A child may arrive in the ED crying loudly but within 1/2 h begin to exhibit signs of serious respiratory depression. Sedation is rarely administered to a child after a poison

Table 33-7 Major Treatment Considerations in Poisoned or Overdosed Patients

Agent	Comments	Treatment Considerations
Sedative-hypnotics (Valium, Librium, Tranxene, Serax, Ativan, Xanax, Dalmane, phenobarbital, Nembutal, Seconal, Noctec, Doriden, Noludor, Placidyl, Quaalude, and various others)	Central nervous system depression, coma, hypotension, hypoxia, and respiratory and cardiac failure are seen. Withdrawal with hyper-irritability and serious, life-threatening seizures can occur 16 to 24 h following discontinuance. Simultaneous ingestion with other depressants (alcohol) is common. In severe acute sedative-hypnotic overdose, prolonged absence (24 h) of brain activity and function may be reversible with favorable outcome. Nonbarbiturate sedative-hypnotics (chloral hydrate, glutethimide, meprobamate, methylprylon, and ethchlorvynol) produce a clinical picture similar to that produced by barbiturates (secobarbital, pentobarbital, amobarbital, and phenobarbital). They may be much more toxic than barbiturates, and duration of coma much longer. Benzodiazepines (diazepam, chlordiazepoxide, flurazepam) are often involved in overdoses. While inherent lethality is low when they are taken alone, combination with alcohol and other sedative-hypnotics greatly increases risk.	Treatment is supportive. Forced diuresis and alkalinization of urine to remove drug may be beneficial in long-acting barbiturate overdose. In view of the number of overdoses involving barbiturates, there is a remarkably high recovery rate. Respiratory assistance, rehydration, management of hypotension, and maintenance of adequate urine output are important treatment considerations. Do *not* use respiratory stimulants in an attempt to arouse overdosed patients from coma. The effects of these drugs are unpredictable and can produce seizures. The effectiveness of forced diuresis and dialysis is insignificant for most nonbarbiturate hypnotics because of their protein binding and affinity for lipids. The use of resin hemoperfusion systems may prove effective for severe barbiturate overdoses with prolonged coma as more experience with this method is gained. If physical dependence on sedative-hypnotics is established, treatment for withdrawal should be closely supervised and carried out in a hospital setting.
Ethanol	Severe hypoglycemia may occur in children following ingestion of large quantities. Mouthwashes, over-the-counter prescription cough and cold preparations, perfumes, and colognes are common sources of ethanol ingestion in children. Varying degrees of intoxicated behavior are seen. Ethanol should always be suspected as a contributory cause in acute overdoses when the patient appears to have ingested agents with central nervous system depressant effects.	Treatment is supportive and symptomatic. Convulsions associated with hypoglycemia are seen and can be treated with glucose and diazepam.
Aspirin	In acute overdose, peak salicylate levels may not occur until 6 to 10 h after ingestion. Severity of overdose estimated on basis of blood salicylate level and interval between ingestion and measurement. Metabolic acidosis, which will enhance salicylate distribution to the brain, should	Removal of aspirin by emesis or lavage has been successful even 10 h after ingestion. Activated charcoal can be a useful adjunct to treatment. Alkalinization of urine promotes elimination of salicylates. Administration of potassium and fluids can facilitate attempts at alkalinization of urine.

Table 33-7 Major Treatment Considerations in Poisoned or Overdosed Patients (*Continued*)

Agent	Comments	Treatment Considerations
	be avoided. Hyperventilation, tinnitus, fever, acidosis, and hypoglycemia are symptoms often seen in mild to moderately severe overdose. Serum salicylate levels, electrolytes, blood gases and pH, and renal and cardiac function must be monitored.	
Acetaminophen (Tylenol, Datril, and various others)	Commonly available and widely promoted over the counter; seen increasingly and frequently in overdoses. Can be a serious liver toxin in acute overdose.	Treatment of choice is prevention of further absorption of drug. Supportive care and close monitoring are required for 3 to 5 days, with particular attention to liver function and symptoms of jaundice and to impending ecephalopathy. N-acetylcysteine is now being used investigationally in its treatment.
Narcotics (propoxyphene [Darvon], pentazocine [Talwin], diphenoxylate [Lomotil], codeine, and various others)	Opiate overdose patients classically present with pinpoint pupils (unless anoxia has caused dilation), areflexia, respiratory depression, and cyanotic, clammy pallor. Immediate cardiopulmonary resuscitation provided if needed, with protection of airway and vital functions. Opiate-dependent user may experience severe abstinence syndrome during recovery from acute overdose, or this may be precipitated by use of narcotic antagonist.	Comatose patients with small pupils, bradycardia, depressed respiratory function, and hypotension should be given narcotic antagonist. Naloxone is the drug of choice and will reverse symptoms if overdose involves opiate. Commonly used narcotics such as heroin have relatively short half-lives, while methadone and propoxyphene have much longer half-lives; hence repeated administration of antagonist over 24 to 36 h may be required. Supportive treatment is important and consists mainly of assisting ventilation and oxygenation, supporting blood pressure, and maintaining circulation and airway.
Tricyclic antidepressants (Elavil, Endep, Aventyl, Vivactil, Tofranil, Norpramin, Pertofrane, Sinequan, and various others)	Cardiovascular effects are complex and often serious. Supraventricular tachycardias, premature ventricular contractions, ventricular tachycardia, and quinidine-like myocardial toxicity (e.g., bradycardia and heart block) are seen. Other serious symptoms include ileus, hypothermia, and convulsions.	Basic approach to treatment is supportive and symptomatic. Forced diuresis and dialysis are not effective in removing drug because of protein binding and large tissue distribution. ECG monitoring and checking vital signs are required for at least 48 to 72 h. Physostigmine may reverse central nervous system and cardiac toxicity but should only be used when coma, convulsions, or supraventricular tachycardias occur. Emesis or lavage followed by activated charcoal should be used as early as possible unless contraindicated. Convulsions intractable to physostigmine can be controlled

Table 33-7 Major Treatment Considerations in Poisoned or Overdosed Patients (*Continued*)

Agent	Comments	Treatment Considerations
		with diazepam IV. Quinidine and procainamide are contraindicated since they may worsen conduction defects. In severe overdose with tachyarrhythmia and heart block, cardiac pacing may be reasonable approach before physostigmine or other antiarrhythmics are used (e.g., lidocaine, phenytoin). Monitor arterial pH to keep greater than 7.45. Newer compounds (Asendin, Ludiomil) with antidepressant activity comparable to tricyclics in an overdose appear to produce more central stimulation activity, seizures, than cardiovascular and cardiac effects.
Phenothiazines (Thorazine, Mellaril, Stelazine, and Trilafon), thioxanthenes (Navane), butyrophenone (Haldol), and dibenzoxazepines (Loxitane)	Number of cases increasing among children and adults. Four common clinical syndromes: hypotension, arrhythmias, dystonic reactions, and atropism. Other effects include quinidine-like effects on ECG, dry mouth, hypothermia, ileus, and seizures. Although dilated pupils are commonly found, constricted pupils may be seen in more severely poisoned patients. Phenothiazines are radiopaque.	Dystonic reactions are seen occasionally; diphenhydramine 50 mg IV is given. Repeated (2 to 3) doses may be needed since phenothiazine is longer-acting than diphenhydramine. Hypotension often can be treated by expanding circulatory volume or placing patient in Trendelenburg position. Cardiac depressant effect can be reversed with phenytoin or, in more severe circumstances, with cardiac pacemaker.
Organophosphate insecticides (Parathion, Malathion, Diazinon, and Methyl Parathion)	Poisoning can occur from ingestion and absorption through the skin. Five important physical signs are characteristic: salivation, lacrimation, urination, defecation, and constriction of pupils. Response to large amounts of atropine confirms diagnosis.	2-Pralidoxime (2-PAM) should be used in organophosphate poisoning unresponsive to atropinization. Blood should be drawn for estimation of cholinesterase in red cells before 2-PAM is given. Thorough decontamination must be carried out.
Hydrocarbons and petroleum distillates	Vomiting and diarrhea often experienced. Central nervous system depression can occur. Aspiration pneumonitis is a serious complication. Chemical pneumonitis has occurred even after intravenous injection of hydrocarbon material (lighter fluid). Inhalation may cause euphoria, headache, and nausea. Chronic inhalation may result in hepatic and renal damage.	Emesis before central nervous system depression occurs, followed by cathartics, may provide some protection against absorption and major toxicities (hepatic, etc.). Avoid emesis of product with low viscosity. Lavage is reserved for patient with absent gag reflex, coma, or convulsion and *must* be preceded by intubation with cuffed endotracheal tube. Corticosteroid use in these circumstances is controversial. Treatment is supportive and symptomatic.

Table 33-7 Major Treatment Considerations in Poisoned or Overdosed Patients (*Continued*)

Agent	Comments	Treatment Considerations
Corrosives	Concentrated solutions of caustic material can cause burns of esophagus that characteristically progress from inflammatory phase to necrosis and constriction. *Sources:* liquid and crystalline corrosives, Clinitest tablets, certain household bleaches, dentifrices, and electric-dishwasher soaps.	Immediate treatment is dilution with copious amounts of water. Emesis and lavage should be avoided. Olive oil, vinegar, and juices should *not* be given. Patient should be evaluated by esophagoscopy and possible surgical follow-up.
Methanol	Ingestion (usually as substitute for ethanol) is highly toxic. May be a 6- to 30-h symptom-free period, followed by abdominal pain and muscle weakness. Hyperventilation and profound metabolic acidosis are seen. Toxic products may produce blindness. Other clinical effects include anorexia, acidosis, nausea, vomiting, dizziness, headache, muscle weakness, and malaise.	Blood methanol level should be determined. Methanol level greater than 50 mg per 100 ml is an indication for hemodialysis.
Ethylene glycol (antifreeze)	Ingestion is usually due to use as substitute for ethanol. Metabolism by alcohol dehydrogenase to oxalic acid produces renal damage with significant renal tubular necrosis and failure; ethanol can inhibit this reaction. Urine should be examined for oxylate crystals.	Renal status should be evaluated and hemodialysis begun in severe poisoning (marked acidosis, electrolyte abnormalities, and renal failure).
Household products	Cleaning agents, bleaches, solvents, and cosmetics constitute the largest group of toxins available in the home. Many products are relatively nontoxic, at least in amounts usually ingested.	All soaps and detergents can cause gastrointestinal irritation. Other toxic manifestations range from none (bar soaps) to severe mucous membrane damage, hypocalcemia (electric-dishwasher detergents), and shock. Treatment of severe intoxication should include immediate dilution and supportive care. Many liquid general-purpose cleaners and polishes contain petroleum distillates, and ingestion should be treated as hydrocarbon ingestion. Ammonia intoxication can be caused by exposure to its vapors, which can be decontaminated, or by ingestion, which should be treated as corrosive ingestion. Most bleaches are generally only moderately toxic and will not cause esophageal burns or strictures. Sodium perborate is highly toxic and management requires removal, support of vital functions, and control of seizures

Table 33-7 Major Treatment Considerations in Poisoned or Overdosed Patients (*Continued*)

Agent	Comments	Treatment Considerations
		if they occur. Common household solvents, such as acetone, have effects similar to those of ethanol when ingested except for more central nervous system depression. Treatment is supportive care, decontamination, and minimization of further absorption.
Mushrooms	The number of cases of mushroom poisoning is rising as a result of increasing popularity of wild mushroom consumption. Most nonlethal poisonous mushrooms produce symptoms (e.g., gastrointestinal disturbance, cholinergic activity, and hallucinations) soon after ingestion, and recovery occurs within 24 h, whereas those known to cause life-threatening reactions produce symptoms 6 to 24 h after ingestion. Symptoms of more toxic species occur characteristically in three stages: gastrointestinal effects during first 6 to 24 h; a 24- to 48-h period of symptom remission; finally, 3 to 4 days after ingestion, hepatocellular damage and renal impairment.	Treatment is primarily supportive. Induction of emesis is beneficial if done soon after ingestion. Numerous forms of therapy have been used, but none have been shown to be more effective than supportive care.

Source: M. Wiener and G. Pepper, *Clinical Pharmacology and Therapeutics in Nursing,* McGraw-Hill, New York, 1985, pp. 996–999. Used with permission.

ingestion because of the danger of central nervous system depression. If necessary, life-support measures and monitors are used. The nurse is also responsible for assisting with the many laboratory and other tests used, including (1) tests of electrolytes, blood sugar, blood type, and arterial blood gases; (2) a urinalysis; (3) x-rays; and (4) electrocardiograms. See the Nursing Care Plan at the end of this chapter.

The child who has ingested poison will be admitted to the hospital if the symptoms are severe, the poison is highly toxic, the child shows signs of toxicity such as decreased level of consciousness or abnormal vital signs, or if there are signs of tissue destruction such as oral ulcerations, salivation, or dysphagia.

If the ingestion appears to have been an intentional self-poisoning, the child will need reassurance that something will be done and that he or she is safe from such self-destructive impulses. At some point a detailed history will be needed. The family will also need help and counseling. The nurse should take the child seriously and find out the details of the child's intent, the substance ingested, the stress that the child is under, and the child's social setting and support system. Psychiatric consultation is usually necessary. Follow-up care is essential.

Teaching is an important part of caring for children who have been poisoned, especially since about half of them will have another ingestion accident. Parents should be reminded of the following safety measures.

1. Keep safety closures on medications and dangerous household products.
2. Keep all household products in their original containers.

Table 33-8 Signs and Symptoms as Aids in Differential Diagnosis of Poisoning

Signs and Symptoms	Substance
Abdominal colic	Corrosives, heavy metals, insect bites
Ataxia	Alcohol, barbiturates, anticonvulsants
Breath odor	Acetone, petroleum distillates
Coma and drowsiness	Narcotic opiates, barbiturates, tranquilizers
Convulsions and muscle twitching	Amphetamines, camphor, organic phosphate insecticides
Mouth dryness	Anticholinergics, atropine, or excessive salivation as in the case of organic phosphate insecticides
Nystagmus	PCP, barbiturates, anticonvulsants
Oliguria or anuria	Heavy metals, ethylene glycol
Paralysis	Botulism, organic phosphate insecticides, heavy metals
Pulse rate	Slow: digitalis; fast: atropine
Pupil size	Miosis: narcotic opiates; mydriasis: antihistamines and anticholinergics
Respiratory alterations	Rapid: salicylates; slow: narcotic opiates
Violent emesis, often with hematemesis	Aminophylline, iron, plants

Source: Joseph Greensher and Howard C. Mofenson, "Emergency Room Care of the Poisoned Child," *Issues in Comprehensive Pediatric Nursing* **4**(3):8 (June 1980).

3. Store all drugs and cleaners in locked cupboards or out of the reach of children.
4. Get rid of all old drugs by flushing them down the toilet.
5. Keep purses away from children.
6. Use anticipatory guidance based on the child's age and behavior.

Ingestion of poisonous substances

Corrosive substances Children who have ingested corrosive substances will probably experience one or more of the following: visible burns of the mouth; increased salivation; retching, vomiting, or both; pain; cardiovascular collapse; and airway stenosis. Many products contain both alkali and acid. Substances containing alkali are most frequently ingested; examples include lye, drain and oven cleaners, and Clinitest tablets. Substances containing acid include Lysol, hydrochloric acid, sulfuric acid, formaldehyde, and other acids.

Initial management is aimed at decreasing the chemical activity. Milk may be given for substances containing alkali. Acids are diluted by giving water and are neutralized by giving antacids. An esophagoscopy may be performed to identify the burned area. The ED nurse may administer prescribed drugs such as antibiotics to prevent infections and steroids to decrease inflammation and aid healing. Children who have ingested corrosive substances often require long periods of hospitalization and must undergo many dilatation procedures or reconstruction surgery to replace the esophagus. The physical, emotional, and financial stress placed on the child

Table 33-9 Poisons and Their Specific Antidotes

Poisons	Specific Antidote
Alcohol, methyl	Alcohol, ethyl
Amphetamines	Chlorpromazine
Anticholinergic poisonings	Physostigmine
Carbon monoxide	Oxygen
Coumarin anticoagulants	Vitamin K
Cyanide	Nitrites Thiosulfate
Ethylene glycol	Alcohol, ethyl
Heavy metals:	
Arsenic	Dimercaprol Penicillamine
Iron	Deferoxamine
Lead	Dimercaprol Calcium disodium edetate Penicillamine
Mercury	Dimercaprol Penicillamine
Narcotic opiate depressants:	Naloxone
Nitrates and nitrites	Methylene blue
Phenothiazines	Diphenhydramine (only idiosyncratic effect)
Phosphate ester insecticides	Atropine Pralidoxime

Source: Joseph Greensher and Howard C. Mofenson, "Emergency Room Care of the Poisoned Child," *Issues in Comprehensive Pediatric Nursing* **4**(3):12 (June 1980).

and the family is unimaginable and presents a tremendous nursing challenge.

Hydrocarbons Hydrocarbons include products such as gasoline, kerosene, lighter fluid, furniture polish, turpentine, and solvents for toxic materials such as pesticides and account for 3 percent of poison ingestions in children under 5 years of age. Hydrocarbons cause pulmonary symptoms due to aspiration, central nervous system depression, cardiomyopathy and arrhythmias, renal damage, hepatosplenomegaly, and occasional hypoglycemia. In up to 50 percent of cases there are pulmonary complications, including nonproductive cough, grunting respirations, tachypnea, dyspnea, and cyanosis. X-rays show basilar pneumonia, mottled densities in the midlung fields, and sometimes pleural effusions. Severe cases produce pulmonary edema and death. Central nervous system depression may or may not include irritability and convulsions; if it is severe, it may lead to coma and/or death.

The aim of treating a child who has ingested hydrocarbons is the same as that of treating a child who has ingested another poison. If a minimal amount of the substance has been ingested, vomiting should not be induced. Large quantities require removal of gastric contents. Oxygen may be required. Antibiotics are prescribed only when an infection is suspected.

Salicylates and acetaminophen Salicylates and acetaminophen are two of the most common substances that cause poisoning. Ingestion of 250 to 400 mg of salicylate per kilogram of body weight is fatal, while ingestion of 150 to 200 mg per kilogram of body weight is toxic. Salicylates are rapidly absorbed in the upper gastrointestinal tract. They produce hyperventilation through stimulation of the respiratory system, resulting in respiratory alkalosis. Salicylates also stimulate metabolism, causing a rise in body temperature. At the same time that they stimulate metabolism, they also disrupt the normal intracellular metabolism, resulting in ketone body production. Glucose metabolism is impaired.

Acetaminophen poisoning may be acute or chronic. Continuous improper dosages over time can lead to poisoning. The lethal dose in adults varies from 5 to 20 g. In children, 140 mg/kg or more is potentially toxic. Like salicylates, acetaminophen is rapidly absorbed in the upper gastrointestinal tract. It can cause necrosis of the liver, acute renal failure, and myocardial damage.

Management of both types of poisoning includes inducing emesis if the child is alert or performing a gastric lavage. Adequate hydration should be maintained. For salicylate poisoning, vitamin K may be given to correct hypothrombinemia. In cases of severe toxicity with acetaminophen, dialysis should be considered. N-acetylcysteine (Mucomyst) is an effective antidote for acetaminophen. It is given orally; 140 mg per kilogram of body weight is the loading dose; then 70 mg per kilogram of body weight is given every 4 h for 72 h.

Plants Plants are a frequent cause of accidental poisonings in children. The symptoms range from mild to severe and occur in only about 10 percent of victims. Table 33-10 lists the signs and symptoms of common plant poisonings.

Drowning

Drowning or near drowning is common in many parts of the country because of the presence not only of natural bodies of water but also of artificial lakes and swimming pools. Children of any age can be victims of drowning. Infants and toddlers can drown in toilets and fall in bathtubs and into pools and lakes. School-age children and teenagers may attempt to swim farther than they are able to. Some drownings are the result of games or dares.

The interval of anoxia and submersion should be determined. Any resuscitation efforts should be described. Other important aspects of the history include injuries, past medical and drug history, and tetanus immunization status.

When a near-drowning victim is brought to the ED, it is important to determine whether the accident occurred in fresh water or salt water. This information is vital because the physiological effects of salt water and fresh water are different and determine the type of treatment to be given.

A sample of the immersion fluid should be collected for chemical analysis and bacterial culture. Sometimes the water contains pulmonary toxins such as chlorine or hydrocarbons, which further complicate recovery.

Freshwater drowning In freshwater near drowning, the water aspirated into the lungs is

Table 33-10 Some Common Poisonous Plants

Common Name	Toxic Parts	Signs and Symptoms
Castor bean	All parts	Nausea, vomiting, burning in mouth and throat.
Precatory bean	Seeds	Nausea, vomiting, burning in mouth and throat.
Jequirity bean	Seeds	Nausea, vomiting, burning in mouth and throat.
Dieffenbachia	Stem and leaf	Burning of mouth, tongue, lips; may affect breathing. Sap in eye causes inflammation.
Philodendron	Stem and leaf	Burning of mouth, tongue, lips; may affect breathing. Sap in eye causes inflammation.
Oleander	All parts; sap, leaves, and seeds	Nausea, vomiting, blurred vision, headache, irregular pulse, arrhythmias.
Foxglove	All parts, especially leaves and seeds	Nausea, vomiting, blurred vision, headache, irregular pulse, arrhythmias.
Jimson weed	All parts	Intense thirst, urinary retention, dry mouth, rapid and weak pulse, hyperpyrexia, delirium, seizure.
Lantana	Berries (unripe)	Muscle weakness, lethargy, cyanosis, circulatory collapse.
Daffodil	Bulbs	Gastrointestinal upset, vomiting, diarrhea.
Narcissus	Bulbs	Gastrointestinal upset, vomiting, diarrhea.

Source: M. Wiener and G. Pepper, *Clinical Pharmacology and Therapeutics in Nursing,* McGraw-Hill, New York, 1985, p. 1000. Used with permission.

absorbed into the pulmonary capillaries by osmosis because it is hypotonic in relation to the 0.9% salinity of capillary blood. In significant amounts, the absorbed water causes intravascular overload, hemodilution of plasma, and hemolysis of red blood cells. The ruptured red blood cells release plasma-free hemoglobin, which can lead to acute renal tubular necrosis. Circulatory overload increases pulmonary hydrostatic pressure, and pulmonary edema results. In addition, water entering the lungs decreases surfactant, leading to alveolar collapse and atelectasis. Hypoxia is the end result.

Saltwater drowning When salt water enters the lungs, its hypertonicity draws fluid from the blood into the lungs, which then leads to increased intraalveolar fluid and fulminating pulmonary edema. Acidosis, hypoxemia, and hemoconcentration result.

Cold-water drowning Immersion in cold water should also be assessed with the drowning victim. Because children have a large body surface area relative to their weight, they lose heat rapidly, resulting in hypothermia. When treating a drowning victim who is also hypothermic (a temperature below 35.0° C), rewarming must be done, along with resuscitative measures.

Resuscitation of a cold-water drowning victim should be started immediately and continued until the victim has been thoroughly rewarmed. Successful resuscitations have occurred after 2 to 4 h of "clinical death," when the victim has been pulseless and apneic.

Both core and external rewarming should be done together to minimize the risk of ventricular fibrillation. Before rewarming, all wet clothing should be removed. Core warming can be accomplished with warmed intravenous fluids (a blood warmer is used); a warm peritoneal lavage with normal saline; a warm nasogastric or rectal lavage; warm, humidified oxygen; or cardiopulmonary bypass with heat exchange. External warming can be done using a thermal blanket or overhead radiant lamps or by immersing the child in a warm bath.

The most common clinical symptoms are related to asphyxia and pulmonary edema and include cyanosis, frothy sputum, tachypnea, tachycardia, and rales. Hemoglobinuria may result from liberation of plasma-free hemoglobin by ruptured (fresh water) or dehydrated (salt water) red blood cells.

Treatment and nursing management The treatment of serious submersion includes the establishment of an airway with a cuffed endotracheal tube, 100% oxygen, external cardiac massage, correction of acidosis, continuous monitoring, suctioning, treatment of arrhythmias, intravenous therapy, Foley catheterization, treatment of related injuries such as spinal cord compression, antibiotics, and evaluation of electrolytes and blood gases.

Frequently, near-drowning victims arrive at the hospital alert, oriented, and feeling "fine." Most children are very frightened and want to go home with their parents. Because of the secondary complications due to the aspiration of fairly large volumes of water, however, a thorough evaluation must be done. This evaluation includes blood gas analysis while the child is breathing room air, measurements of serum calcium and electrolytes, measurement of hemoglobin level, electrocardiogram, measurement of urine output, chest x-rays, and a thorough auscultation of the lungs. Some physicians admit all near-drowning victims to the hospital for overnight observation. However, if there are no apparent problems, some children are discharged to be closely watched by their parents and to be reevaluated the next day for any possible pulmonary complications.

Epistaxis

Etiology Epistaxis, or nosebleeds, almost always occurs in the anterior nares of children. The most common cause is digital exploration (nose-picking). Factors that increase the likelihood of bleeding include:

1. lack of humidity in the environment
2. allergy, rhinitis, and upper respiratory infections
3. forceful nose-blowing (or any other action that rapidly and significantly increases vascular pressure in the nose)
4. trauma
5. preexisting bleeding disorders, e.g., hemophilia

Clinical manifestations Unilateral bleeding from the nose most often confirms the diagnosis. Children may also have some bleeding down the back of the throat. A history of recent exacerbation of allergies or upper respiratory infections, especially if antihistamines have been used, is significant. Nosebleeds are more frequent in the winter, when heat in the home is not humidified. Copious bleeding down the posterior pharynx with hematemesis should alert the nurse to the possibility of a rare posterior epistaxis. Hemoglobin and hematocrit are usually normal unless frequent nosebleeds have occurred or an underlying blood dyscrasia exists.

Treatment and nursing management The triage nurse frequently receives a phone call prior to the child's arrival in the ED. The parents should be calmed first so that an accurate assessment can be made. Very little blood can create a nosebleed that looks massive, which is frightening to both the parents and the child. After quickly assessing for blood dyscrasias and a potential posterior bleed, the triage nurse should instruct the parent to apply firm pressure, "pinching" the anterior nose together continuously for 10 to 15 min with the child sitting up and leaning forward. Most parents apply pressure for too short a time. If bleeding persists or if the parent is very anxious, the child should be brought to the ED.

Initial treatment in the ED is the same while the nurse makes an assessment. A child who feels faint should be placed in a side-lying position. Cover the child with a plastic apron and keep an emesis basin handy for spitting out blood or in case of vomiting. An ample supply of tissues should be available.

Further treatment by the physician may be necessary. A cotton ball saturated with ¼ percent phenylephrine (Neo-Synephrine) can be inserted into the nostril, and external pressure is continued for 3 to 5 min. This causes vasoconstriction, which slows the bleeding. The nares can then be inspected to determine whether cautery is required. A local anesthetic consisting of 2 percent tetracaine (Pontocaine) or a mixture of cocaine and epinephrine is used before the blood vessel is cauterized with a silver nitrate stick. Cautery should never be done on children with a bleeding disorder. Rebleeding will occur and the cauterized area will slough off, producing worse bleeding. Instead, a petroleum gauze is used to pack the nose. This remains in place for several days, when it is removed by the physician.

Teaching Teaching is aimed at preventing further episodes. Humidification in the home keeps the mucous membranes moist. Children should be told that "nothing smaller than their elbows" should be placed in the nose. For the first 24 to 48 h the nose should be wiped, not blown. After that, only gentle blowing should be done. Quiet activities for the first 12 to 14 h should be planned to prevent increased vascular pressure in the nose. Susceptible children may need a daily application of a lubricant (petroleum jelly) to the nasal mucosa. The ED nurse should also review with the parents and the child the correct way to apply pressure to the nose if another nosebleed occurs.

SUDDEN INFANT DEATH SYNDROME

Incidence

Although accidents are the leading cause of death in children between the ages of 1 and 14 years, sudden infant death syndrome (SIDS) is the leading cause of death in infants 1 month to 1 year of age. SIDS is the sudden, unexpected death of an apparently healthy infant that remains unexplained after the performance of a complete case study and autopsy. The true incidence of SIDS is not clear because of confusion in reporting. The cause of death may be listed as pneumonia or as unknown, when the infant actually died of SIDS. Recent recognition of SIDS as a distinct entity has resulted in more accurate reporting. At present, the incidence of SIDS is estimated to be as high as 2 per 1000 to 3 per 1000 live births; the peak incidence is in children between the ages of 2 and 4 months. Parents who have had one baby die of SIDS have a 2 percent chance of having another baby die of SIDS, or a fivefold increase over the normal risk.

Etiology

While it is clearly accepted that SIDS is not caused by any lack of medical treatment or parental care, the exact etiology is still not known. Many years ago it was believed that the babies suffocated in their blankets. This was refuted because some babies died with their faces uncovered. Then evidence seemed to suggest a respiratory infection because a number of the infants displayed symptoms of a cold a day or two before they died and autopsy revealed occasional pulmonary infiltrates. But autopsies also demonstrated that the apparent respiratory infection was not severe enough to cause death. Other factors that are no longer considered to be causes of SIDs include an enlarged thymus, aspiration, allergy to cow's milk, and immunodeficiencies.

Some authorities believe that SIDS is related to an alteration in cardiorespiratory control. There is also speculation that the brain stem or carotid body does not respond appropriately to a buildup of carbon dioxide. Apnea has been observed in some infants who subsequently died of SIDS. Immaturity may be a factor in an infant who stops breathing and does not start again. When apnea occurs, the infant becomes hypoxic. Sixty percent of SIDS victims show signs of chronic lung underventilation and hypoxemia such as thickened musculature of the small pulmonary arteries.[9] Other common autopsy findings are intrathoracic petechiae and pulmonary edema. Nevertheless, at least one-third of the victims have no signs of hypoxia, and other infants with abnormal respiratory patterns do not die.

There is no such thing as a "typical SIDS infant," but researchers have found that certain characteristics are associated with SIDS. In about 40 percent of cases, there was a high-risk pregnancy and the baby was a high-risk infant. "These include infants who are premature, of low birth weight, and/or are products of multiple birth, or pregnancies associated with young maternal age, maternal drug use, short pregnancy interval, or lower socioeconomic status. However, 60% of infants appear healthy and thriving at birth and are the products of uneventful pregnancies," according to the Minnesota SIDS Center.[10] For purposes of research, this information is useful, but it still does not predict which infant will be a SIDS victim, and therefore prevention is almost impossible. Table 33-11 lists the characteristics of SIDS victims at death. Death occurs suddenly and without pain. The parents often discover the child dead in the morning or after a nap. Most infants die in the early morning hours.

Nursing management

Since approximately 50 percent of all SIDS victims and their families are seen in a hospital ED, the ED nurse has a significant role in their care. Most often, little can be done for the victim, since the child is already dead. If resuscitation was begun at home and was continued on the way to the ED, the physician will determine whether it should be continued. Usually it is terminated. Most states require an autopsy for any sudden

Table 33-11 Characteristics of SIDS Victims at Death

1. At the time of death, SIDS victims are usually in a good state of nutrition and hydration.
2. Generally, they appear to be well developed, although they may be small for their age.
3. They demonstrate no external signs of life-threatening injury.
4. There may be white or blood-tinged frothy fluids around the mouth or nostrils.
5. They generally exhibit the "natural" appearance of a dead baby.

Source: Minnesota SIDS Center Guidelines for Public Health Nursing, 1984, Minneapolis, Minn.

and unexpected death to determine the cause of death.

The ED nurse has several tasks to accomplish in a relatively short period of time. The first is to provide privacy for the parents. The nurse will need to obtain as much information as possible, while coordinating other personnel who are involved, such as the physician and law enforcement and ambulance personnel. Meanwhile, the parents will need to be informed about the death of their child and supported as they begin the grieving process. They should not be left alone.

The ED nurse should provide a separate, quiet environment for the parents where they will be able to begin to sort out what has happened. Many times the parents are not actually aware that the baby is dead. If resuscitation measures were begun in the home and were continued until the baby was admitted to the ED, the parents may be hoping to hear that the baby has been revived. The nurse should be present when the physician informs the parents that the infant is dead. The nurse listens to what they say and watches their reactions in order to ascertain that they really understand that the baby has died. If there is a language barrier, it is important to have an interpreter; this is not the time for sign language and guessing. After being informed of the death, it is essential that the parents be told that SIDS was the apparent cause and that nothing could have been done to prevent it. They should also be assured that their baby did not suffer and that the death was quick and painless. While the parents may not be able to fully integrate and comprehend what they are told, they need information to begin their mourning and to form a basis for handling the many emotions they will experience. It is recommended that the parents be given written information about SIDS to take home with them. The National Sudden Infant Death Syndrome Foundation has published a pamphlet entitled *Facts about SIDS*. It is available from the Foundation at 310 S. Michigan Ave., Chicago, Ill. 60604.

The nurse may act as a buffer when the parents are questioned by various professionals. The questions are occasionally lengthy but are necessary for records and reports. In their shock and grief the parents may have difficulty responding to the inquiries. The nurse can facilitate the process by keeping the questions simple and clear and by providing time for the parents to think before answering. It is essential that the atmosphere be one of understanding and empathy rather than of blame and accusation.

Determining whether SIDS was the cause of death requires an autopsy. Explain to the parents that an autopsy substantiates the cause of death as being unpreventable and not the parents' fault. Whenever possible, the parents should be encouraged to agree that an autopsy is necessary. However, if it is mandated by the state, the parents may not have a choice. The nurse and the physician should clearly explain to the parents the need for an autopsy and the benefits to them if one is performed.

Counseling

After the questioning, the parents must leave their baby and go home. It is essential to the grieving process that the parents begin with a separation from their *dead* baby. This is facilitated by having the parents see the baby after the body has been cleaned. It reinforces their awareness that the child is dead and gives them a chance to say good-bye in their own way. It also reassures them that the infant is whole and peaceful. If they desire, they should be given the opportunity to hold their baby. Some parents want to have other family members present. If this is possible, it should be encouraged. Privacy is of great importance, since this is a highly emotional time.

The nurse's knowledge of mourning and grief is of help to the family. The nurse is prepared for a variety of parental responses. An overwhelming feeling experienced by the parents is guilt. They wonder what they could have done to prevent the death. Unless this feeling is initially handled with information, as discussed earlier, it can leave the parents open to self-blame and distrust of themselves and others. Because the death is sudden and unexplained, the parents often are stunned, reacting with disbelief and denial. Again the nurse reinforces the facts of the death.

The intensity of the grief that accompanies SIDS has been described as almost unbearable. There is no warning or preparation, and the parents have no explanation to offer to other family members and friends. Often these people react with suspicion and blame at a time when their support is most needed.

The family of a baby who has died of SIDS has an overwhelming need for professional counseling and follow-up. The nursing care of the family does not end when they leave the ED. The nurse should make a referral to a social service agency, to a counseling facility, or to a community health nurse and arrange for a family follow-up or a home visit within 1 to 2 weeks. Often, other parents whose babies have died of SIDS are the most helpful resource to the family.

It is during the early period of grief that there may be a total disruption of family life. The parents may have difficulty carrying out their daily functions. They may report that they hear the baby cry or may go to check on the infant as if he or she were still there. They may fear that they are going crazy. Intervention at this time reassures the parents that what they are experiencing is normal. It may also mobilize other family members to provide specific types of support such as assisting with household duties. More information about SIDS can be given. In many states there are chapters of the National Sudden Infant Death Syndrome Foundation, or local support groups for parents who have lost a child. These organizations are composed of health professionals and of parents who have experienced a death from SIDS in their family. These groups are particularly helpful to parents.

The siblings are often overlooked in the trauma and pain of the death of the infant. They too will respond to the death. Their reactions will depend to a great extent on their stage of development. A toddler suffers most from a disruption of parenting. He or she is aware of the great changes in the family but does not understand the reason for them. The grief and sadness of the parents will disturb the toddler, as will the sudden lack of attention and routine. The toddler may react with aggressive, attention-getting behavior or with regressive behavior. A surrogate parent who provides affection and daily routine will often be of assistance to the toddler.

A preschooler realizes that the baby is gone but does not clearly understand where or why. He or she may ask many questions that the parents are unable to answer. Preschoolers often experience feelings of guilt, possibly because they wished at some time that the baby would go away so that they could have the parents exclusively. Now they may believe that the death was caused by this wish. Magical thinking and feelings of omnipotence are characteristic at this stage. Preschoolers may also fear that they will be the next victim of whatever happened to the baby. This is reinforced by the fact that one day the baby was there, apparently healthy, and the next day the baby was gone. A preschooler also needs reassurance, affection, and stability in daily life.

A school-age child, while beginning to have an understanding of death, is not fully aware of its finality and yet may be fascinated by the details of the preparations being made. The school-age child, who is greatly affected by the grief of the parents, needs reasonable explanations, as well as reassurance of love and signs of affection.

The professional who is making follow-up visits will assess the responses of all the family members and intervene appropriately. The immediate family may be too intimately involved to be aware of any disturbed relationships which might be developing. Thus it is essential that the ED nurse initiate the procedure for follow-up care.

SEXUAL ASSAULT

The first contact the nurse has with a child or adolescent who has been sexually assaulted often takes place in the ED. Because thousands of children are victims of this violent crime each year, the nurse must be cognizant of his or her role in providing initial care and follow-up treatment.

Incidence

Over 50 percent of rape victims are between 10 and 19 years of age. In most states the suspected rape of a minor child *must* be reported to the police. An adolescent over the age of consent can decide whether or not to report the crime. States also determine the age at which a minor can be treated for drug-related problems or gonorrhea or can be given contraceptives without parental consent. (Because laws and enforcement policies vary from state to state, the nurse must be familiar with those in the state where he or she is practicing.)

Criminal sexual conduct is legally defined as any sexual contact to which one party does not consent. Family sexual abuse, or *incest,* can be defined as the involvement of a minor child in sexual activity by his or her parent, a close relative, a guardian, or a caretaker. There are many more incestuous relationships involving children (some estimate 1 million per year) than are ever reported to the authorities.

It is estimated that only 1 in 5 to 10 cases of sexual abuse or rape is reported. Of those cases reported, 1 in 4 results in an arrest and 1 in 60 leads to a conviction. According to the task force of the National Commission on Causes and Prevention of Violence, 52 percent of rapists are strangers to their victims, and another 30 percent are slightly acquainted with them. However, when criminal sexual assault involves a younger adolescent or child, the rapist is known to the child or the family in more than 75 percent of cases.

Treatment and nursing management

Rape is a crime of aggression and violence, not sex. The victim, usually female but sometimes male, feels violated and humiliated by this highly stressful, often life-threatening experience. It is *not* the role of the health professional to determine whether rape or incest has occurred. It *is* the responsibility of the health professional to accept the victim's story in a nonjudgmental and supportive manner and to provide treatment and follow-up care. The nurse must realize that the quality of the initial treatment of the victim in the ED is crucial to the victim's long-term resolution of this crisis. The nursing goals for the sexual assault victim are summarized below:

1. Provide a safe, secure, and supportive environment.
2. Provide information about consent forms and rights, procedures to be done, reporting of the crime to the police, options that are available, community support services, and follow-up care.
3. Involve the victim in the decision making in regard to treatment and examinations.
4. Listen to the victim in an accepting, nonjudgmental manner.
5. Maintain an accurate legal record. Document the victim's description of the attack accurately in his or her own words, and record the observations made and the specimens collected.
6. Assist in evidence collection through a careful history, a physical examination, and collection of specimens.
7. Assist in the care of physical injuries.
8. Maintain the chain of custody of evidence collected. (All the people who participate in evidence collection—the nurse, the doctor, and laboratory personnel—must sign a slip stating that evidence placed in the collection kit came from the victim. The collection kit is kept refrigerated in a locked area and is monitored until it is turned over to the police upon written consent of the victim.)
9. Arrange for a change of clothes to be brought to the victim and for safe transportation home or to protective custody.

The child or adolescent who has been raped should be treated as a high-priority medical emergency. She should be quickly brought to a private examining room and not left alone. The very young child may need her mother present at all times. In cases of incest the child will also need to tell her story when the parents are not present. Older adolescents will also desire privacy when making statements and during the examination.

The victim may initially exhibit verbal or physical signs of anger, fear, and anxiety. She may rub her arms or other sore spots and may tend to hold her arms around her body for protection. She may be crying, shaking, and agitated. Some victims may appear calm and detached and even laugh. These are methods of denying their true feelings. They may also express statements of denial and self-blame. Because the victim has experienced the ultimate violation of self (other than murder), she feels fear, distrust, and loss of control.

During the whole ED examination and treatment process the nurse should use measures that enable an older victim to gain some control by involving her in decision making. Sometimes a very young child does not even realize what has happened, and then it is important not to make the situation any worse. Unless the victim is a minor, she has the right to refuse to be tested or treated, to report the incident to the police, and to prosecute the assailant. Consent must be given by an adolescent and the parents for examination and treatment, evidence collection, and reporting. If the victim is not sure about reporting the crime, the nurse will need to explain the value of collecting the evidence then so that it is not lost, in the event that she does decide to report the crime later.

Obtaining a history

The nurse must collect the regular identifying information in addition to a medical history, information about allergies, and data regarding menses. The length of the menstrual cycle, the last menstrual period, and the use of any birth control method should be noted. If intercourse occurred within 72 h preceding the assault, that should be recorded. It is wise to determine whether the girl has ever had a vaginal or rectal exam. Whether she showered, douched, or changed clothes should also be noted. If the victim is willing, other information needed regarding the attack includes date, time, place, witnesses, body orifices involved, occurrence of ejaculation, and injuries. If information about incest is needed, include when it started, other family members involved, and who knows about it.

When the victim is very young, every effort should be made not to upset the child any further. Dolls or illustrations can often help the child point out the affected areas or describe what happened.

Children under 10 frequently respond better to questions phrased in physical rather than sexual terms. The nurse should ask the parents what terms the family uses for body parts. When the child is interviewed, the nurse can assess the child's verbal ability as well as his or her psychological and physical reactions. Burgess, Holmshom, and McCausland suggest that early questions should be neutral in character.[11] Examples include the following: "Do you know why you were brought to the hospital?" "Were you able to tell your mother or father what happened?" "I would like you to tell me what happened so that I can help you." "Have you ever been to a hospital before?" "Do you know what will happen here?" "How do you feel about being here?"

Children should be allowed to use their own language. The nurse must be extremely careful not to make any judgments or put words into the child's mouth. Regardless of the age of the victim, questions should be neutral and not leading. "Show me where he touched you," is much better than "Did he touch your breasts?"

During the interview the child should be given the opportunity to talk about her feelings, since this will help her express them later on during the recovery phase.

The parents may also feel guilty and be more upset than the child. If family abuse is not involved, help the parents provide the strength and support that the child needs. Part of the nurse's role is to facilitate better communication between the child and the parents. The parents need to understand that it will be healing for the child to be able to talk about the assault later on.

When a family member is involved, the child must be protected from further injury. The child may feel betrayed by the parent who left the child unprotected as well as by the person who committed the act. The family may be divided between loyalty to the child and to the family member.

The physical examination

After the history is obtained and the vital signs are checked, the physician or nurse practitioner assesses the physical and gynecological trauma. The victim is also examined for the presence of sperm and indications of forcible rape. The skin is examined for bruises, scratches, lacerations, tooth imprints, pressure imprints, and tenderness. The findings of the examination and tests are termed *clinical evidence* of rape. They do not become legal evidence until they are turned over to the police.

The parents are often particularly concerned about their child's welfare and anxiously await the examination report. The examination can be very upsetting to the child, especially the gynecological examination. Sometimes doing a visual examination and swabbing the vagina will be sufficient for a very young child. A nasal speculum may also be used instead of the small vaginal speculum. Whatever is done must be done very gently and with a great deal of sensitivity.

Table 33-12 describes the equipment needed and the methods used to collect specimens from sexual assault victims.

The victim

The adolescent will need counseling about prevention of venereal disease and the possibility of pregnancy. Tests for syphilis and gonorrhea will

Table 33-12 Collection of Specimens: Examination of a Sexual Assault Victim*

Specimen	Equipment	Procedure	Comments
Clothing	*Paper* bags, labels	Have patient place each piece of clothing in separate paper bag. Handle as little as possible. Label.	Document in record who takes clothing. (Plastic bags may cause damp clothing to mold.)
Blood VDRL† Typing	Collection tubes, tourniquet, alcohol sponge, syringe, needle	Routine. Label.	Check for syphilis and repeat in 4 to 6 weeks. Check patient's blood type to differentiate it from assailant's.
Saliva test	Sterile gauze, forceps, sterile container, label	Place gauze in patient's mouth with forceps. Have patient wet gauze. Place on 4- by 4-in pad to dry. Place in sterile container. Label.	Do not touch gauze! Specimen will be examined for blood group antigens.
Oral washing	Sterile water, test tube, top, label	4 to 5 ml sterile water—rinse around mouth. Collect in test tube.	Examined for blood group antigens.
Fingernail scrapings	Sterile fingernail file, sterile gauze, envelope, label	Scrape under patient's fingernails. Place debris in gauze and then put in envelope. Label.	Specimen will be examined for blood, skin and clothing fibers belonging to assailant.
Hair			
Scalp	Forceps, envelopes, labels, comb	Pull 10 to 12 hairs from different parts of head. Place in envelope. Label.	The hair follicle is needed to make an accurate comparison of patient's hair with that of assailant.
Pubic		Pull 6 to 8 pubic hairs. Place in envelope. Label.	
		Comb pubic hair and place comb and hair in envelope.	Pubic combing is done to look for assailant's hair.
Pregnancy testing†	Urine container, label	Have patient collect urine specimen.	If patient is bleeding, obtain a midstream sample.
Vaginal smear	Sterile, dry swab; glass slide and holder; envelope	Swab vagina with dry swab. Make smear on slide. Dry slide and place in labeled envelope.	Do before introducing saline for sperm collection. May detect sperm. Useful for ABO typing.
Gonococcus (GC) culture†	Three to four Thayer-Martin plates, sterile swabs, labels	Collect specimens from: cervix, vagina, rectum, and throat if oral intercourse occurred. Label all specimens.	Repeat in 4 to 6 weeks.
Sperm			
Vaginal	Speculum, gloves, test tube, top, saline, aspirator, labels	Place saline in vagina and aspirate. Place aspirant in test tube. Label.	Sperm may be tested to determine blood type of assailant.
Dried semen and blood on skin	Saline, thread, test tube, top, label	Moisten spot with sterile saline and rub stain with thread. When dry, place in test tube. Label.	To be done on areas of body where dried semen or blood is noted. Be careful not to touch specimen.

*Prepared by Diane K. Olsen, R.N.

†The pregnancy test, GC culture, and VDRL are done in the hospital laboratory. They are repeated in 4 to 6 weeks. If results are positive, then they may be used as evidence in court.

Note: It is suggested that the nurse wear clean gloves when handling any specimens to avoid contaminating them. The nurse should explain to the patient that it is important for the nurse to avoid contamination because of the importance of identification of blood type, not because he or she fears touching the patient. *All specimens collected should be carefully documented in the medical record.*

need to be repeated 4 to 6 weeks after the attack. A written description of the symptoms of these venereal diseases may be given to the victim, and a return appointment may be made.

The possibility of becoming pregnant exists for the adolescent who is not using any birth control method. The physician may offer the victim several choices, such as menstrual extraction, insertion of an intrauterine device, diethylstilbestrol (the "morning after" pill), or abortion if pregnancy is determined to exist at a later date. Unfortunately, it may be very difficult for the victim to make a choice when she is experiencing the shock and confusion precipitated by the assault.

For a short time after the rape, most victims experience mixed feelings of shock, dismay, denial, anxiety, and anger. Nightmares and insomnia are common. These feelings are coupled with somatic complaints of loss of appetite, headache, dizziness, abdominal pain, and loss of libido. The reaction is one of grief and loss. This acute phase of disorganization may cause regressive behavior, but it also makes the victim more amenable to crisis intervention. The reorganization phase that follows lasts much longer, as the victim (and the family) comes to terms with the physical, emotional, and social disruption of her life. Depression is common in the reorganization phase.

The adolescent who has just begun to date may be concerned about the effect the rape will have on her relationship with young men. The parents must be cautioned against conveying the idea to her that she is somehow "altered" or "damaged" because of the rape. For the adolescent who is beginning to deal with her own sexuality, the rape may have a real effect on the way she feels about herself and others. Emotional counseling and support should be made available to the victim and her family through referral to a sexual assault counseling service and medical follow-up. During follow-up the victim will need to talk about the experience with those who cared for her during the immediate crisis.

Nursing Care Plan: Accidental Poisoning

Patient: Cindy Smith **Age:** 22 months **Date of Admission:** 7/7

ASSESSMENT HISTORY

Cindy, 22 months old, was rushed to the emergency department by her frightened, crying mother. Cindy apparently swallowed some diazepam about $\frac{1}{2}$ h previously while in the care of a baby-sitter. The baby-sitter thought the pill container was empty before Cindy began playing with it.

Mrs. Smith had left the pill container on the coffee table while preparing to leave to visit her own mother, who is terminally ill with cancer. Mrs. Smith estimated that she had used 15 to 20 tablets of the original thirty 5-mg tablets prescribed.

The mother appeared extremely upset, distraught, and frightened. She said, "I never should have gotten the Valium. Why did I leave it on the coffee table? Will Cindy be okay?" Later, she said, "I'll never leave her alone again."

Mrs. Smith held Cindy. The child was too sleepy and too weak to stand or walk by herself. Cindy responded to her name by opening her eyes.

PHYSICAL EXAMINATION

Temperature: 37.2°C. Apical pulse: 80. Respirations: 15 breaths per minute. Blood pressure: 80/56 mmHg. Weight: 11.8 kg (26 lb). *No treatment* was given at home for poisoning.

PHYSICIAN'S ORDERS

1. Vital signs q 15 min.
2. Neurological check q 30 min.
3. Orogastric tube.
4. Gastric lavage with 0.5 normal saline.
5. D5/0.2 NaCl IV at 40 ml/h.
6. Activated charcoal, 20 g per orogastric tube; 3 g of $NaSO_4$ 60 min later.
7. Endotracheal tube and oxygen available at bedside.
8. Routine laboratory tests.
9. Intake and output.
10. Transfer to pediatric ICU when stable.

Nursing Diagnosis	Outcome Criteria	Nursing Interventions	Evaluation and Modifications
1. Potential for central nervous system depression related to ingestion of diazepam	☐ Further central nervous system depression will be prevented, as evidenced by: **a.** Respiratory rate above 12 breaths per minute **b.** Blood pressure above 85/50 **c.** Response to verbal stimuli **d.** Absence of seizures	☐ Monitor vital signs with specific emphasis on respiratory status q 15 min. ☐ Notify physician if respiratory rate is less than 12 breaths per minute. ☐ Have endotracheal tube and oxygen available at bedside. ☐ Monitor neurological status (orientation, alertness, response, movement) q 30 min. ☐ Observe for seizure activity.	☐ Vital signs are stable. Pulse: 90; respirations: 18; blood pressure: 90/58. Respirations are easy; child continues to be drowsy but responds to name.

Nursing Diagnosis	Outcome Criteria	Nursing Interventions	Evaluation and Modifications
		☐ Assist with gastric lavage: **a.** Set up equipment. **b.** Observe level of consciousness, seizure activity, and gag reflex prior to insertion of orogastric tube; if unconscious or seizuring or if gag absent, child should be intubated prior to procedure. **c.** Position Cindy with head slightly down and to the side or flat. **d.** Restrain as needed during insertion of orogastric or nasogastric tube. **e.** Assist with insertion of orogastric or nasogastric tube. **f.** Check placement of tube. **g.** Collect specimen of initial gastric contents withdrawn. **h.** Record amount of fluid instilled and withdrawn. **i.** Record results of procedure, including color and consistency of fluid withdrawn. **j.** Prepare and administer dose of 30 g activated charcoal as ordered by physician after lavage. **k.** Prepare and administer $NaSO_4$ 60 min after charcoal is given. **l.** Maintain IV of D5/0.2 NaCl at 40 ml/h (to maintain blood pressure). **m.** Record strict intake and output. **n.** Recognize that symptoms of Valium overdose may persist for 24 to 48 h.	
2. Potential for anxiety and uncooperativeness related to intrusive procedures and separation from mother as primary support	☐ Cindy will cooperate during gastric lavage and will not be separated from her mother unnecessarily.	☐ Briefly explain procedures to Cindy in language comprehensible to her.	☐ Cindy needed minimal amount of restraint during gastric lavage because of sleepiness.

Nursing Diagnosis	Outcome Criteria	Nursing Interventions	Evaluation and Modifications
		☐ Inform Cindy of acceptable behavior during procedures, e.g., "It's okay to cry, but you must hold very still for a short time." ☐ Restrain child only as necessary. ☐ Allow mother to be present during procedures (if she can cope with situation) to provide support and comfort. Mother should *not* help restrain child during procedures. ☐ If mother is not able to cope with situation, comfort child through touch and language. ☐ Praise Cindy for appropriate behavior and cooperativeness during procedures.	☐ Mother was present during lavage, and she continually stroked Cindy's head, squeezed her hand, and talked to her, saying, "You will be all right. You have just got to be all right. Mommy loves you."
3. Parental guilt feelings and anxiety related to accidental poisoning and hospitalization	☐ Mother will exhibit increased coping through altered behaviors such as less crying, appropriate responses to questions, and increased ability to comfort Cindy.	☐ Explain purpose of procedures, how procedures are to be performed, and expected outcomes of procedures to mother. ☐ Allow mother to express anger directed at: **a.** Baby-sitter for allowing Cindy to play with pill container **b.** Herself for having diazepam available to child and leaving Cindy with baby-sitter **c.** Her mother for having terminal illness ☐ Allow mother to remain with Cindy to give support and comfort during procedures. ☐ Notify husband of incident and wife's need for support person. ☐ Prepare parents for transfer to pediatric ICU.	☐ Mother was very upset with herself for leaving Cindy with school-age baby-sitter and for leaving diazepam on coffee table by telephone. ☐ Father will be arriving shortly.
4. Lack of parental knowledge concerning prevention and emergency treatment of accidental poisoning	☐ Parents will be able to repeat information regarding prevention and treatment of poisoning.	☐ Discuss with parents the implications of growth and development as they pertain to poisoning.	☐ Mother remains too upset to understand this plan. Inform nurses in pediatric ICU of need to discuss prevention and treatment of poisoning.

Nursing Diagnosis	Outcome Criteria	Nursing Interventions	Evaluation and Modifications
		☐ Inform parents of services of local poison control center and telephone number. ☐ Recommend purchase of ipecac for home medicine chest. ☐ Explain use of ipecac. ☐ Discuss preventive measures: lock all cabinets containing medicine; place all medicine, household cleaning substances, and plants out of child's reach; do not store harmful (caustic) substances in food containers; and do not refer to medicine as "candy."	

*Prepared by Andrea Piens, R.N., M.S.

References

1. Nelson, K. G., "An Index for Severity of Acute Pediatric Illness," *American Journal of Public Health,* **70**(8): 804–807 (August 1980).
2. Murphy, Carol, *Quick Reference to Pediatric Nursing,* Lippincott, Philadelphia, 1984.
3. German, J. C., "Multiple System–Injured Children," *Topics in Emergency Medicine,* **6**(1):44–59 (April 1984).
4. Anderson, M. D., "Becky Needs Stitches," *Point of View,* **17**(1):20–21 (1980).
5. Greensher, Joseph, and Howard C. Mofenson, "Emergency Room Care of the Poisoned Child," *Issues in Comprehensive Pediatric Nursing,* **4**(3):1–21 (June 1980).
6. Ibid.
7. Hayden, G.F., and G. T. Sproul, "Baby Powder Use in Infant Skin Care: Parental Knowledge and Determinants of Powder Usage," *Clinical Pediatrics* **23**(3):163–165 (March 1984).
8. Sobel, Raymond, "Psychiatric Indications of Accidental Poisoning in Childhood," *Pediatric Clinics of North America,* **17**(3):653–685 (August 1970).
9. Naeye, R., "Sudden Infant Death," *Scientific American,* **242**(4):56 (April 1980).
10. *SIDS: Intervention Guidelines for Public Health Nurses,* Minnesota SIDS Center, Minneapolis, Minn., 1984, p. 5.
11. Burgess, Ann W., Lynda Holmshom, and Maureen McCausland, "Counseling the Child Rape Victim," *Issues in Comprehensive Pediatric Nursing* **1**(3):52–53 (November–December 1976).

PART IV

Alterations in Child Health: Psychosocial Emphasis

34

Marsha H. Cohen

The chronically ill child

Upon completion of this chapter, the student will be able to:

1 Differentiate between a chronic illness, a disability, and a handicap.
2 State the incidence of chronic illness in children.
3 List at least three causes of chronic conditions.
4 Identify at least two factors that influence the effects of a chronic illness on children.
5 Explain why a noncategorical approach to understanding the impact of chronic childhood illness is relevant to nursing.
6 Describe the reactions of the parents to a diagnosis of a chronic illness in their child as attempts to cope with its impact.
7 Identify at least four common problems of families with a chronically ill child.
8 Describe the interaction of a chronic illness and the development level of the child.
9 Identify at least four common problems of children who have a chronic illness.
10 List the nursing actions in the assessment and control of pain.
11 Describe the reactions of siblings to a chronically ill child.
12 Identify the important elements of discharge planning for a chronically ill child and his or her family.
13 Identify the need for in-home nursing care and respite care.
14 Describe the significance of Public Law 94-142 as it relates to nursing practice.

THE CONCEPT OF CHRONIC ILLNESS

Chronic illness has been defined as "a disorder with a protracted course which can be progressive and fatal, or associated with a relatively normal life span despite impaired physical or mental functioning."[1] Another frequently used definition is "a condition which interferes with daily functioning for greater than three months in a year, causes hospitalization for more than one month in a year, or (at the time of diagnosis) is likely to do so."[2] The terms *illness, disease, condition, impairment, defect,* and *disorder,* within the context of chronicity, are often used interchangeably, although each may have a slightly different meaning.[3] All these terms refer to the basic biological event that has occurred or is occurring.

Related concepts

The terms *disability* and *handicap* are used to convey a different meaning. A disability is an age-related, behavioral manifestation of an underlying condition; for example, a 10-month-old with cerebral palsy may be unable to sit unsupported, a 4-year-old with a cleft palate may have unintelligible speech, and an adolescent with cystic fibrosis may be unable to participate in competitive sports. All these children have a disability, but they are not handicapped. Handicap is a more complicated concept that involves the psychosocial consequences of a disability and interferes with the child's social roles, relationships, and goal-related activities. These aspects must be assessed before a child is considered to have a handicap. It is important for the nurse to recognize that children may achieve comparable developmental outcomes in a variety of different ways.

Incidence and prevalence

While the exact number of children who have a chronic illness is unknown, the incidence is high. If children with intellectual, sensory, learning, and behavioral impairments are included, the incidence may be as high as 30 to 40 percent of children in the United States. If children with these impairments are excluded, the incidence is estimated to be between 10 and 20 percent, with 1 to 2 percent of the total pediatric population having a severe chronic illness.[4,5,6] Although there has been little evidence of an increase in the *incidence* of chronic diseases, the increased survival rate of affected children, due to biomedical, surgical, and technological advances, has contributed to a dramatic increase in the *prevalence* of these diseases in the pediatric population. In fact, increasing numbers of survivors of previously fatal childhood illnesses are now young adults who are seeking health care from a system unfamiliar with their problems and needs.

Causes

Mattson classifies chronic conditions as follows:[7]

1. Diseases due to chromosomal abnormalities, such as Down syndrome
2. Genetic diseases, such as sickle cell anemia, cystic fibrosis, hemophilia, and diabetes mellitus
3. Disorders resulting from harmful intrauterine factors, such as drugs, infections, radiation, and hypoxia
4. Disorders resulting from birth trauma or perinatal infections, such as cerebral palsy and sepsis
5. Disorders due to postnatal infections, physical injuries, or neoplasms, such as meningitis, rheumatic fever, leukemia, and chronic renal disease

In addition, chronic disorders can result from prematurity (e.g., respiratory distress syndrome and bronchopulmonary dysplasia) and from medical therapy itself (e.g., retrolental fibroplasia). See Fig. 34-1.

Dimensions of chronic illness

Chronic childhood illness is a multidimensional phenomenon. The onset may occur at any time in the developmental history of the child and the family. With increasing frequency, chronic diseases are being diagnosed before birth. There is a great deal of current support for the belief that the specific medical diagnosis is not a very good predictor of the impact that the illness will have on the child and the family.[8,9] The dimensions that seem to be most related to the initial responses and ultimate outcomes in terms of adaptation are:

1. Whether the disease is life-threatening, stable in nature, or characterized by unpredictable crises

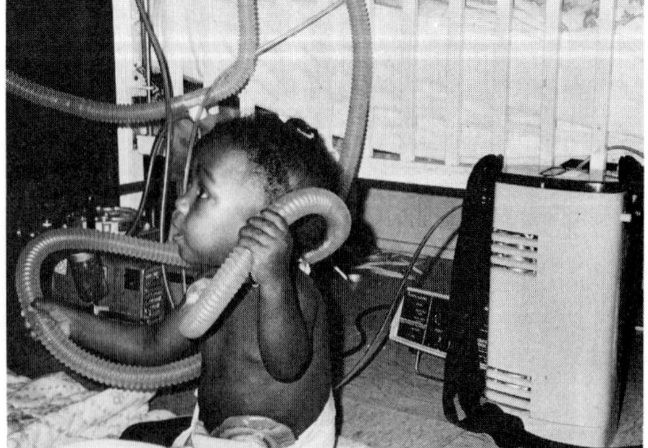

Figure 34-1 This child is confined to her room at home during most of the day due to oxygen dependence. Her mobility is impaired by decreased activity tolerance related to lung disease following a premature birth.

2. Whether the condition is visible and therefore obvious to others
3. What the child's care demands are and how much time and energy must be invested in meeting those demands
4. Whether mental deficiency is associated with the condition

Investigators have failed to demonstrate, with any reliability, that the severity of an illness is predictive of the response that the child or the family will have to it. The result of these findings has been a growing trend toward taking a noncategorical, or generic, approach to the study of chronic childhood illnesses, focusing on those dimensions which are common to all affected children and their families.

THE IMPACT OF CHRONIC ILLNESS

The parents

Reactions to the diagnosis The parents are generally unprepared to hear that their child has a chronic illness, even though they may have been aware, consciously or unconsciously, for some time that something was wrong. They often minimize the child's symptoms, interpreting them as not serious or as nuisances. Drawing on their past experience with similar problems, they may say, "I thought he was just trying to get out of going to school" or "It just seemed as if she had a bad cold." If the symptoms persist beyond what the parents think is a reasonable time or if the child does not respond to the usual remedies, the parent will generally seek medical care, often feeling a little foolish or apologetic for doing so. The nature and intensity of the initial response to the diagnosis of a chronic illness may be related to the parents' age, educational level, financial status, religion, and culture as well as to the child's sex and ordinal position in the family and the size and structure of the family unit. The amount and quality of social support available to the parents are another important factor influencing their reaction.

Shock and *disbelief* are common initial responses. Shock may distort the parents' perception of time and their ability to process information. As one mother described the experience, "It's like taking a blender and putting it in your brain and all of a sudden, nothing makes sense."[10] Conversely, the state of shock may create a feeling of detachment and lead to remarkable clarity and efficiency of thought and action.[11]

The use of *denial* as a defense mechanism may offer some momentary respite from the acute anxiety and fear that the diagnosis provokes. It permits the parents to limit the full impact of reality to levels that can be most effectively managed at the time, and, thus denial is adaptive. It does not necessarily mean that the parent who says, "This isn't really happening to me," or who will not talk to the nurse about the child's condition is disavowing the reality of the situation. This same parent may, moments later, experience intense grief or feelings of panic. The cycles of encounter or confrontation with the reality of the situation and retreat from it or denial of it occur frequently as the parents attempt to cope with the diagnosis.[12] The form of denial that is detrimental and requires active nursing intervention occurs when the parents refuse to accept or administer reasonable treatment because they are unable to acknowledge that there is anything wrong with their child, despite confirmatory evidence.

Guilt is perhaps the most universal reaction of parents as they search for a cause or a reason for the illness. Feelings of guilt and personal responsibility may be especially strong if the condition is genetic or due to accidental trauma, but all parents have these feelings to some degree, regardless of the cause. They may interpret the child's illness as a parenting failure, and it is not unusual for this feeling to be reinforced by others in the parents' network. A grandparent may admonish the mother for not having taken better care of herself during pregnancy; friends may relate stories of how they prevented similar illnesses in their children; and health professionals may ask routine questions during the initial assessment that the parents interpret as accusatory. It is imperative that nurses help parents express and cope with their feelings of guilt and that they suggest a referral for therapeutic counseling if these feelings seem unusually intense.

Anger is a normal response to the helplessness and loss of control that parents experience during the initial phases of coping. It may be directed toward the ill child, the spouse, the nursing or medical staff, or God. It may be internalized or repressed and be seen as depression, or a stress-induced illness, or it may be depersonalized and erupt in an exaggerated outburst over a seemingly inconsequential event, such as an unemptied wastebasket in the child's hospital room. The positive aspect of anger is that it can mobilize energy needed for coping. Unfortunately, expressed anger may cause a reactive withdrawal of persons who are crucial in the parents' support system.

Depression and *discouragement* are common, especially during periods of exacerbation or when treatment provides little visible evidence of improvement. Routines that must be followed every day may become monotonous, trying, and physically exhausting. Parents become discouraged when they see no end to the worry, disruption, expense,and continuing treatment for an illness that may never be cured. Olshansky noted that some parents who have a defective child experience *chronic sorrow* throughout their lives.[13] This reaction may be shown openly, but more often it is concealed or denied. It may be felt most acutely when the parents become aware that their child cannot do something that society expects other children of the same age to do, such as entering school or becoming independent of the parents.

Parents frequently cope with feelings of helplessness and lack of control over the illness by learning everything possible about the disease and its treatment. Some parents direct their energy toward raising money to find a cure through research. They may become so knowledgeable about the disease and its treatment that they are perceived as threatening by some of the medical and nursing staff. A secure and knowledgeable nurse will be able to discern when information seeking is a defense against emotional involvement and when it is a rational, intelligent behavior.

Living with a chronically ill child

Eventually, most parents accept the fact that their child has a chronic illness and develop a *dominant* pattern of interaction with the child that reflects their overall adjustment.

Overprotection occurs when the parents give excessive attention to the child in an attempt to compensate for the child's condition. Overprotective parents accept responsibility for the child's disease and devote themselves to caring for the child, often neglecting their other roles and responsibilities. They carefully regulate all aspects of the child's life and commonly are not aware of the child's real capabilities. They are oversolicitous and fearful of setting limits or disciplining the child, tending to overlook or neglect siblings.

Rejection does not occur as commonly as overprotection, but it has more serious consequences. A parent may deny the severity of the problem, withdraw from emotional involvement with the child, be excessively critical or punitive, and neglect necessary medical treatment.

Accepting parents have adjusted reasonably well to having a chronically ill child. They discipline consistently and encourage independence, self-care, school attendance, and play with peers. They enforce only those limits which are necessary, realistic, and age-appropriate. They are able to gain satisfaction from the child's accomplishments, and although they recognize the child's limitations, they do not dwell on them. They seek information about the disease and its physical and psychological effects in order to allay their own anxiety and anticipate the changing needs of the child.

The *noncategorical approach* to chronic illness recognizes that families with a chronically ill child not only have the same initial reactions but also have similar needs and concerns and confront common demands and problems throughout the course of the child's life. These factors result in predictable effects on family life.[14]

Marital distress has been reported with increasing frequency in families with a chronically ill child; however, the divorce rate has not increased.[15] It is plausible that different ways of responding to the diagnosis, conflicting opinions about treatment, and different rates and styles of adjustment might cause conflict between the parents. The nurse assesses not only how each parent is coping but also how each views the other's responses. One mother reported that her husband was a workaholic and that he was coping with their child's illness by spending more and more time at the office. She was left at home with the child, feeling alone and overwhelmed. She stated, "It's like we're both drowning and we can't save each other."[16]

Financial strain is common in all but the wealthiest families. Numerous surveys confirm that, regardless of the type and extent of coverage, parents may have out-of-pocket expenditures that are as high as 25 percent of the family income.[17] Expenses that are seldom covered include such things as transportation to and from medical centers or doctors' offices for appointments, special nutritional formulas, modifications that must be made to the home or car, and appliances or devices that are essential or are needed to improve the quality of the child's life. Loss of income due to time away from work, necessitated by the child's illness, is also a significant problem.

Sleep disturbances and physical exhaustion are relatively common experiences. One mother whose child had a tracheostomy and was a quadriplegic reported that she or her husband had to get up every 2 h during the night to turn and suction the child. They had been doing this for 4 years. Another mother who was a single parent reported being so exhausted from caring for her 5-year-old who had cystic fibrosis that she withheld the child's antibiotics for a few days, hoping that the child would become sick enough to be admitted to the hospital, thereby giving her a brief rest. Parental sleep deprivation and physical exhaustion have serious consequences for the well-being of the child as well as the parents.

The parents may experience *social isolation* in the form of curtailment of family activities such as outings and vacations, a breakdown in communication within the family, and isolation from neighbors, friends, and members of the extended family. Some families find themselves with a "courtesy stigma"; they sense that others are uneasy around them or reluctant to be with them because of their child's condition.[18] Some parents have increased somatic complaints and physical illnesses.

Ambiguity and *uncertainty* regarding the ultimate outcome or recurrent crises are major sources of stress for these parents. As one parent whose child had been in remission from leukemia for 4 years stated, "We're always aware of it. We still worry that she might have a relapse . . . especially if she gets a fever or looks tired."[19] The ways in which parents cope depend on how they appraise the situation and what resources are available to them. Ventors found that families were helped by the following coping strategies: (1) endowing the illness with meaning; (2) sharing the burdens of the illness with others, both inside and outside the family; and (3) anticipating the severity of the illness.[20]

The child

The duration of a chronic illness in children varies from a few months to many years. Some chronically ill children have had the condition all their lives. A child who was born with a chronic illness will construe the illness differently from the way a chronic illness is construed by a child who becomes ill at a later period, because the impairment has always been an integral part of the child's identity. The degree of disability varies from being able to participate in normal activities and having no visible stigma to being severely incapacitated, being visibly very different from other children, and needing frequent hospitalizations. The major factors that influence the consequences of a chronic illness are the child's age at the onset, the child's personality, and the family's attitudes. Other factors include the sex, intelligence level, and physical attractiveness of the child.

Influence of age

Infants A physical defect or serious illness that is present at birth may interfere with the normal parent-infant attachment process. (See Chaps. 8 and 9.) Sick infants often must be hospitalized for extended periods of time. Parents who are unable to see, hold, or care for their baby may have a decreased interest in nurturing.

The infant's socialization process begins in the immediate postpartum period, when pleasant feelings begin to be associated with persons who consistently respond to the baby's signals and satisfy his or her psychological and physical needs. If the infant's smile or other responses to the parents are delayed or modified by a physical defect or if the baby's cry is irritating and lacking in variation, interaction with the parents may be decreased and they may have difficulty interpreting the baby's cues. An irritable or unresponsive baby who is difficult to feed or cuddle makes the parents feel frustrated and inadequate. They may interpret the infant's behavior as negative feedback and withdraw from the child at the very time when the infant should be establishing trust in the responsiveness and predictability of the people in his or her environment.

Toddlers Toddlers are most vulnerable to separation from their parents. (See Chaps. 10 and 15.) Chronically ill toddlers who are repeatedly separated from their parents lack the ability to understand why this happens, they have no concept of time, and they lack confidence that the parents will return. They may receive messages that it is dangerous to venture outdoors or to initiate actions by themselves. Their protestations against such things as intrusive procedures, restraints, and swallowing medication are of no consequence, and they may soon learn that asserting themselves is ineffective. The increased restrictions that a chronic illness imposes on a toddler may impair the development of a sense of autonomy.

Preschoolers The feelings of initiative that began when the child was a toddler are stronger in the preschooler and directed more toward mastering certain tasks. The opportunity and the ability to play with peers are especially important in the preschool years. Other children help the child learn roles, cooperative and competitive behavior, independence, and appropriate ways to express aggression and other primitive emotions. The chronically ill child may have less opportunity to learn these social skills through peer interaction, and physical restrictions or decreased energy and agility may limit exploration of the environment, which is needed for normal cognitive development and mastery of motor skills. Sometimes the illness is such a dominating factor in the child's life that he or she does not have the experiences necessary to prepare for ordinary transitions, such as entering school. (See Chaps. 11 and 15.)

School-age children The task of school-age children is to master the skills required in a technological society by expanding beyond the family to the school, the peer group, and the outside world. It is during this period that the social consequences of a chronic illness become very evident. The inability to achieve in academics or sports and to be like others in the peer group may cause loss of self-esteem and feelings of inferiority or rejection.

One of the most striking characteristics of school-age children is their need to be like other children.[21] School-age children with a chronic illness tend to be apprehensive about their peers' reactions to their differentness. They may try to hide their impairment by withdrawing from social interaction. The chronically ill child may attend school sporadically or not at all. Repeated absences may cause the child to fail a grade, and repeating a grade further contributes to feelings of inferiority. For some chronically ill children, school is a place where they can achieve intellectually, develop their talents, and thus compensate for their impaired physical functioning. There is evidence from a number of studies that although the majority of children with a chronic illness are of normal intelligence, their academic performance is below that of their healthy peers.[22] These children are at risk for acquiring developmental handicaps related to social, emotional, and educational difficulties. These handicaps can evoke a more negative response from others than the illness itself.[23] (See Chaps. 12 and 15.)

Adolescents Adolescence is the most difficult developmental stage for many healthy teenagers because they are confronted with the need to establish their own unique identity, decide on a career, achieve independence, and cope with physical changes and with emerging sexual drives. These tasks may seem insurmountable to the chronically ill or disabled adolescent. Our society values physical beauty, mobility, athletic prowess, intelligence, and independence. Adolescence can become a nightmare for a teenager with a physical or intellectual impairment and limited family support.

Body image—the way people appear to themselves or believe they appear to others—has a special importance to adolescents. (See Chaps. 13 and 15.) Teenagers with chronic illnesses or disabilities commonly have a poor body image and low self-esteem, both because of their own responses to their health problems and because of the opinions of the peer group, which they accept as accurate. The teenage years are a time of rapid body changes, and chronically ill adolescents may experience them in an altered way. They may be small in stature, have delayed sexual development, have visible physical abnormalities that are due to the disease process or to therapy, and have limited mobility. If the impairment is of recent origin, the adolescent is confronted with a sudden loss of emerging identity and independence, and plans for the future may have to be changed; as a result, the adolescent may experience intense grief reactions.

A chronic illness interferes with the adolescent's need to achieve independence from the parents by creating feelings of helplessness and lack of control and threatening the sense of personal identity. A chronic illness also limits the adolescent's social experience and skills. The ability to compete for dates is jeopardized, since adolescents select dates who are most desirable according to the criteria of the peer group. This creates feelings of insecurity and inadequacy regarding sex roles in the ill adolescent.[24]

Adolescents can be helped to adjust to their

illness by their families, their peers, and the health care team. Peers, especially those who have experienced similar problems, can often provide help and insights during rap sessions and in support groups.[25] Organized groups of teenagers in the hospital facilitate the expression of feelings and adaptation.

Influence of personality

The influence of the individual child's personality is difficult to specify. Children cope with illness in various ways. Some are passive, some are stoical and courageous, and some are extremely fearful. (See Chap. 15.)

The number and type of life experiences that the child encounters and the emotional support provided by the parents in new situations are important in developing the child's coping capacity. As the child matures cognitively, past experiences and ways of coping can be recalled. (See the discussions of cognitive development in Chaps. 12 and 13.) Children who have developed coping skills that were successful in the past are likely to approach new situations with greater confidence.[26]

Influence of family attitudes

The family's feelings about, and attitudes toward, the child's competence and potential greatly determine the child's response to the illness. Solnit and Green describe a "vulnerable child syndrome" among children whose parents expect them to die because of a life-threatening illness.[27] A child who perceives and accepts the parents' assessment of his or her vulnerability may experience severe psychosocial and developmental disturbances.

The stress of chronic illness on the child

The multiple problems that confront most chronically ill children are similar across diagnostic groups, and the degree to which they are experienced by the child is a better predictor of adaptation than the specific type of illness. The types of problems most frequently encountered are:

Immobility and confinement
Stigma and social isolation
Pain
An altered body image
Sexual and reproductive concerns
Decreased stamina or energy
The threat of decreased life expectancy
Repeated hospitalizations and separation from family and friends
Increased academic, social, and emotional problems
Increased or prolonged dependency on the family

Immobility and confinement Mobility is very important in childhood. The ability to explore the environment is crucial in developing motor and social skills and in achieving a sense of mastery and control. Mobility is important because it permits expressing emotions, controlling anxiety, and learning to relate to people. It provides a way to obtain stimulation from friends and caregivers or to find solitude. It also serves a protective function, since it enables the child to escape from threats.

Immobility is the inability to move oneself physically from one place or position to another. Confinement differs from immobility in that a child who is confined is physically capable of movement but is restricted to a certain area. While immobility and confinement are not the same, they may have similar outcomes. They deprive the child of meaningful sensory stimulation and contact with peers, parents, and others. Confinement creates a barrier to exploration, thwarts attempts to master the environment, and isolates the child from other people. Confinement is imposed on chronically ill children in many ways. They are confined not only when they are hospitalized or must remain at home or in bed but also when the environment creates barriers to access. Immobility may result not only from the inability to crawl or walk but also from the unavailability of appropriate assistive devices. For example, externally imposed immobility that could be avoided occurs when a child whose leg has been amputated does not have a properly fitting prosthesis, and when an electric wheelchair is not substituted for a manually operated one when a child with muscular dystrophy develops increased weakness in the upper extremities. When freedom of movement is temporarily restricted or permanently impaired, the nurse must creatively design interventions that will reduce the negative consequences that may result.

Pain Pain, whether it is acute or chronic, severe or mild, has two major components: sensory and perceptual. The International Association for the Study of Pain has defined pain as "an unpleasant sensory and emotional experience associated with actual or potential tissue damage, or described in terms of such damage."[28] It has also been defined as "whatever the experiencing person says it is, existing whenever he says it does."[29,30] Children with a chronic illness frequently experience acute pain as a result of intrusive diagnostic procedures, treatments, or surgery. Widely accepted indicators of acute pain are listed in Table 34-1.[31] Acute pain is generally an immediate response to tissue injury or insult and serves a protective function by focusing attention on the site.[32] It is typically self-limiting and easily controlled pharmacologically with narcotic and nonnarcotic analgesics. However, undermedication is extremely common in the treatment of acute pain in children.

In the past, children were thought to have less pain than adults because their nervous systems are not mature. Recent evidence shows that this is not true. Haslam's study of children aged 5 to 18 years showed that the younger the child, the more susceptible he or she is to pain.[33] In a study that compared newborns undergoing circumcision, those who were not given a penile block displayed the physiological indicators of pain listed in Table 34-1.[34] Adults may also believe that children perceive less pain because they typically have difficulty describing their pain. A very young child may lack words; an older child may have come to accept pain as being normal. Children may be reluctant to talk about their pain because they are afraid of being given medicine and injections, because they want to avoid treatments, or because they do not want their peers to make them feel ashamed or be ridiculed by them.

A number of tools have been developed to help children describe the location and the intensity of their pain.[35] When asked to do so, children can point out the location of pain on drawings and indicate the intensity of pain by relating it to a color, or they can rate pain on a scale of 1 (mild discomfort) to 10 (severe or unbearable discomfort). In their drawings they may portray themselves as doing something to help cope with the pain or as frightened and helpless in the face of pain.[36] See Fig. 34-2. Cognitive level is im-

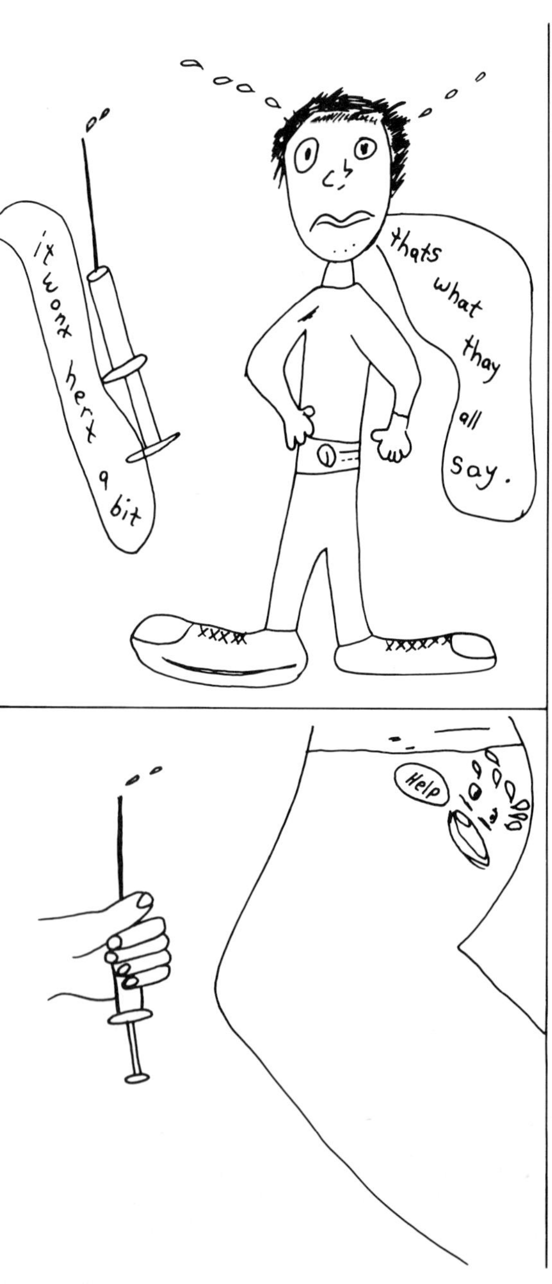

Figure 34-2 A drawing done by an 11-year-old asthmatic boy during his hospitalization.

Table 34-1 Indicators of Acute Pain

Physiological	Behavioral
Tachycardia	Irritability
Tachypnea	Restlessness
Diaphoresis	Guarding, rubbing, or pulling the affected part
Pallor	Anxiety
Decreased P_{O_2}	Unwillingness to eat
	Inability to sleep

portant when assessing the meaning that pain has for a child and the manner in which it is described. Children may believe that pain is a punishment for bad behavior. Some children have described pain as "abandonment," "being afraid," "when something hurts and no one comes," and "something you have no control over."

To help a very young child describe pain, the nurse might need to use other words, such as "sting" or "hurt," or to ask the child to point out the sore spot on his or her body or on a drawing. The nurse can ask a school-age child or adolescent to rate pain on a scale of 1 to 10. When this is possible, the nurse can learn how tolerant of pain the child is, as well as how the child expresses pain. This rating can be incorporated into a flowchart so that a record of the effectiveness of the various pain relief measures is available. In this way the child becomes part of the pain management process.

McCaffery lists several guidelines for pain relief. The nurse is advised to:[37]

1. Use a variety of pain relief measures.
2. Use the pain relief measures *before* the pain becomes severe.
3. Include what the child or the parent believes will be effective.
4. Consider whether the child will be active or passive in the application of pain relief measures.
5. Determine the potency of the pain relief measure on the basis of the child's behavior indicating the severity of the pain.
6. Encourage the child to try the pain relief measure at least one or two times more if it is ineffective the first time it is used.
7. Be open-minded about what may relieve pain.
8. Keep trying.
9. Do no harm.

Table 34-2 describes specific nonpharmacological nursing measures for the relief of pain.

Chronic pain differs from acute pain in that it no longer serves any useful purpose and it persists for an extended period of time (usually at least 6 months).[38] Many of the physiological and behavioral cues that nurses have customarily used to assess the intensity of pain are not present. Adaptation to pain occurs after varying lengths of time, and the physiological parameters return to normal or near normal. Chronic pain may manifest itself behaviorally as fatigue, decreased interest in the environment, delayed psychosocial development, decreased school performance, depression, or reluctance to cooperate with rules and the expectations of nurses. Social context, gender, ethnicity, psychological variables, and developmental factors may affect the expression of pain.

In addition to analgesics and the modalities listed in Table 34-2, chronic pain may be treated with antidepressants, nerve blocks, hypnosis, behavior modification, biofeedback, acupuncture, or transcutaneous nerve stimulation.[39,40] The management of chronic pain is often so complex that it is best dealt with by a multidisciplinary team operating from a pain clinic.[41]

Severe, unrelenting pain is common in children with terminal malignancies. Children with this type of pain have been found to respond well to a continuous subcutaneous infusion of morphine sulphate, which has permitted children to be cared for at home during the end stage of life.[42] (See Chap. 35.)

Social stigma and social isolation *Social stigma* is any known, deviant attribute of an individual that causes others to feel uneasy in a social interaction or causes them to avoid such interaction altogether. The uneasiness or the avoidance response may be due to irrational fears of contagion, feelings of personal vulnerability, or simply not knowing what to say or do. Children seem unaware of differences in other children when they are infants and toddlers. They are curious but accepting in the early preschool years and become increasingly critical and negative as they get older.[43] Chronically ill school-age children may be teased or ridiculed by their peers because they look different, cannot eat the same foods, are limited in mobility or stamina, have to take medication, or need assistance with toileting. They may be left out of activities and be rejected by their peer group. Teenagers may find that they are turned down for dates or not asked out on dates and that employers will not hire them for part-time or summer jobs.

A child whose impairment is not visible may take great pains to hide it, often to his or her own detriment. For example, one 12-year-old boy would not give himself insulin at school because he did not want his friends to find out that he was a diabetic, and a 14-year-old girl with cystic fibrosis was so embarrassed by the fact that her coughing attracted attention to herself and annoyed others that she tried hard to suppress it, with a resultant increase in pulmonary infections.

One young woman who had spent much of

Table 34-2 Nonpharmacological Pain Relief Measures Available to the Pediatric Nurse

Nurse's Relationship with the Child and Parents

1. Can be used to reduce anxiety with child and parents.
2. Provides the basis for collaboration in planning pain relief. Nurse can learn from child and from parents what has helped control child's pain in the past.

Teach about Pain

1. Have child touch and handle the actual equipment involved.
2. Have child meet physicians and nurses.
3. Have child play with dolls and other representations of the painful event.
4. Explain to child and parents when they will be separated and when they can be together during painful period.
5. Nurse should use hands to demonstrate location of pain and, by pressing and pulling the skin, quality of pain.

Teach Distraction Strategies

1. Child's involvement in the distraction needs to increase as the pain intensity increases, but with fatigue or higher intensity of pain, distraction needs to be less demanding. Younger child requires less complex distraction.
2. Distractions involving both rhythm and imagery tend to be most helpful; e.g., rhythmic, shallow breathing and making a sound with each exhalation can be coupled with image of steam locomotive ("choo-choo") taking child away from pain; train goes faster as pain increases. Nurse demonstrates method beforehand.

Use Cutaneous Stimulation

1. Simple rhythmic rubbing. Use of pressure; electric vibrator; massage with hand lotion, powder, or menthol cream; application of heat or cold.
2. Stimulation is most effective if rhythmic or constant and moderate in intensity.

Use Relaxation Techniques

1. Teaching child to relax may decrease painful stimuli, e.g., release tension on abdominal incision, or may act as distraction.
2. Ask child to take deep breath and "go limp as a rag doll" as he or she exhales slowly. Ask child then to yawn.
3. Older child may also need help into comfortable position (pillow under neck and knees), instruction in directing attention away from pain, and testing relaxation of limbs so that child will focus concentration on the task.

Use Desensitization and "Fading In"

1. Desensitization: Threatening stimuli (dressing trays, needles, etc., employed in painful procedure) are introduced gradually, beginning with least frightening items, and presented in pleasurable surroundings. When child shows fear, nurse retreats to nonthreatening stimuli and begins again, hoping to develop child's tolerance of fear-provoking stimuli. Requires several repetitions.
2. Fading in: If child continues to respond with anxiety, the object is placed far away and gradually brought closer while child is occupied with something pleasurable. If fear is again elicited, process is restarted with object farther away. Process needs to be repeated several times. Theoretically, child eventually will accept the object in his or her room and even be able to handle and discuss it.

Source: Adapted from Margo McCaffery, "Pain Relief for the Child: Problem Areas and Selected Nonpharmacological Methods." *Pediatric Nursing* **3**(4):11–12 (July–August 1977).

her childhood in hospitals for the correction of multiple congenital anomalies felt very accepted by the nursing staff but was critical of the nurses for not preparing her for the outside world, where she had to deal with people's negative reactions to her visible deformities. Like nurses, the parents may also accept the child as he or she is but find it hard to talk with the child about the impairment. In response, the child may sense that it is a taboo subject and be unable to question the parents. Children with a chronic impairment must learn how to make others comfortable enough to allow for the social exchange that is so necessary for their development and social survival. The nurse can help in this task by valuing the child as an individual who is like other children in *most* ways, but different in some other ways, and by not avoiding discussion of the differentness. Role playing and behavioral rehearsal are helpful in preparing children to deal with situations that they are likely to encounter. The nurse might say to a child who has lost his or her hair as a result of chemotherapy, "Pretend I'm one of your classmates at school and I come up to you and say, 'What happened to all your hair?' What will you say?" Younger children may be helped to develop these skills through the use of therapeutic play. Sensitivity and timing are most critical to any effective intervention. In addition to learning ways to explain their illness to others and to put others at ease, children should develop age-appropriate interests and participate in age-appropriate activities. The need for chronically ill children to dress attractively in clothes that are appropriate for their age and are like the clothes of peers cannot be overstressed; otherwise, they will not gain peer acceptance. Clothing designed for children with various handicaps is now available, including clothing which covers braces or which is designed to make dressing easier.

The siblings

The siblings of chronically ill children also have many common problems and concerns. They may feel embarrassed about having a brother or sister who is ill all the time or who does not look or act like other children. They may feel guilty because they believe that something they did or thought caused the illness, and often they are afraid that they will catch the disease.[44] Figure 34-3 was drawn by a child who had two siblings die of the same disease. Note the small figure that the child drew of himself and the enormity of the threat.

Another frequent problem is siblings' jealousy of the ill child and their envy of the time and energy that the parents devote to caring for the child. They resent the lenient and inconsistent discipline that the ill child is sometimes given and the fact that family interactions are centered on the ill child. They resent giving up their playtime to help care for their brother or sister and may feel that they have an unfair share of the chores and responsibilities. If they have been left with neighbors or friends during periods when the child was ill, they may feel angry and insecure. One extremely jealous older sister was heard to say, "I could care less what happens to her. No one pays any attention to me. Even the neighbors and people at church ask how she is. They never ask about me."

SUPPORTING THE CHILD AND THE FAMILY

No family is ever prepared for the multitude of problems caused by a chronically ill child. The family is in crisis; old solutions will not solve the present problems. The family members must reestablish their roles and seek new answers to their problems. The period of crisis is an optimal time for the nurse to intervene with the family as a family-advocate and coordinator of care.

The psychological effects of chronic illness can, at times, be more devastating than the physical condition. The overall objectives of nursing care are to maintain family unity; to promote optimal adjustment of *all* family members by helping them understand and accept the reality of the impairment, while ensuring that the child's primary needs for love and consistent discipline are met; and to integrate the child into the family in such a way that no family member feels victimized. To achieve this goal, the nursing process is used to continually assess, intervene, and evaluate the family's strengths and weaknesses, coping behaviors, and communication patterns; the quality of parent-child relationships; the child's de-

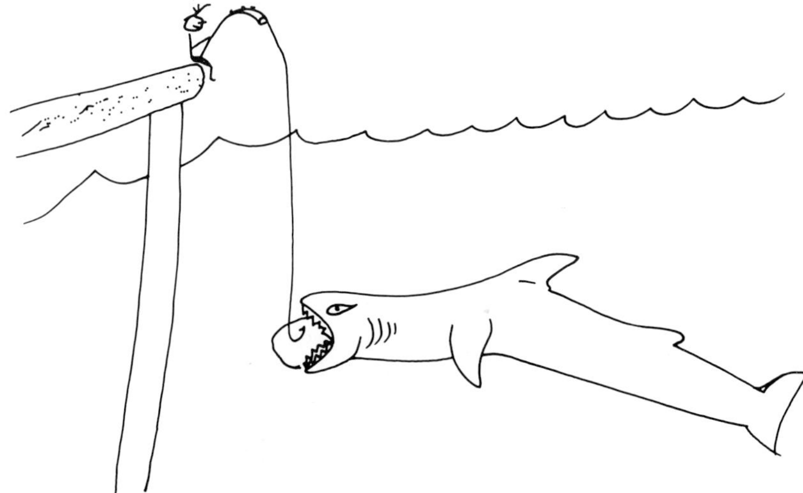

Figure 34-3 A drawing done by a child who had experienced the death of two siblings.

velopmental level, and place in the family; and the availability of resources (Fig. 34-4).

Making a comprehensive assessment of the impact of a chronic illness is difficult unless the nurse has some knowledge of the way the child and the family functioned prior to the illness. It is also difficult for the nurse to gain a long-term perspective on the child and the family during the brief hospitalizations for acute episodes of the illness. In order to gain insight into the ways in which the illness is experienced, explained, and managed, the nurse should seek out all sources of information. Assigning one primary nurse, if possible, adds stability to the family's care and builds trust between the nurse and the family. When one nurse coordinates and delivers care, arranges consultations, and is available to answer questions, clear communication and consistency can be more easily achieved.

The nurse needs to be honest, sensitive, compassionate, and understanding and to support the parents, rather than labeling or judging them harshly. Occasionally, a nurse is unable to deal with a particular child or a family's response to a child. When a cure is not possible, some nurses may feel unable to help the child and the family in any concrete way and find themselves focusing on tasks rather than dealing with the family's distress. Nurses may also find themselves repulsed by a child's physical appearance, frustrated by a child's behavior, or angered by a parent's reaction. When this happens, nurses must examine their underlying feelings and find someone who can offer insight and help. A trusting relationship develops when the family members feel that the nurse has a personal interest in them and the child, understands their distress, and is willing to talk with them about their problems.

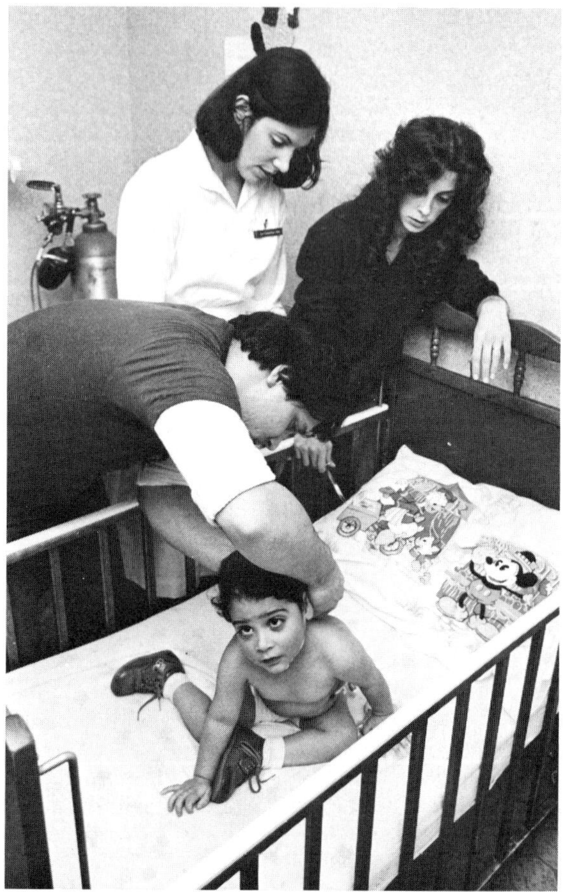

A

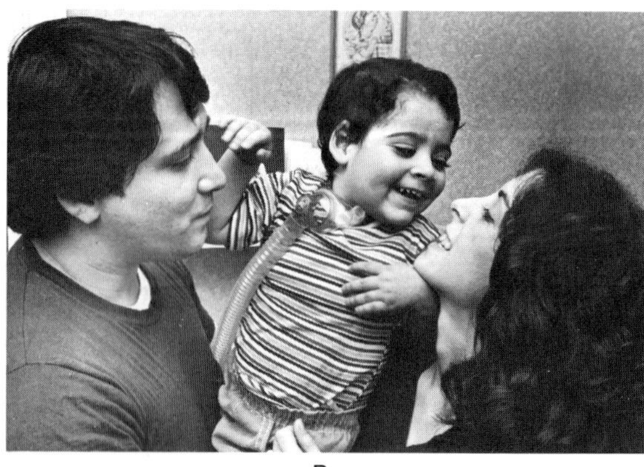

B

Figure 34-4 (*A*) A nurse teaches parents how to care for their chronically ill child. (*B*) The teaching can influence the successful integration of the child into the family.

Nursing management

The nurse uses knowledge of interviewing techniques, assessment skills, and a sensitive approach to the family to support the parents and the child, encouraging them to ask questions and supplying answers in simple, everyday language. The same questions may be asked repeatedly, and the parents and the child may need to hear the same information again and again before they can fully comprehend it. Using words that are legitimately interchangeable may be a source of confusion for the parents or the child and therefore a source of stress.

When the child or the parents are angry or frustrated, they should be encouraged to express their feelings and should be supported for revealing intense emotion. Anger is often directed at the nurse, who must realize that he or she may merely be the nearest, safest target and not the source of the anger.

Children often express their fears that the illness is a punishment for something they have done, and parents often feel guilty about genetic defects and the possibility that inadequate care caused the illness. It is important to let them express their feelings, to correct any misconceptions in their self-accusations, and to give understandable, factual information.

The nurse should positively reinforce the parents' ability to care for their child and the child's ability to care for himself or herself. The interventions described in Chap. 15 concerning teaching parents to care for their child should be used. Overprotective parents can be helped, after they have been allowed to express their feelings of anger and guilt, to recognize their child's capabilities. Assist them in developing realistic expectations and carefully noting the child's smallest achievements. Teach them to anticipate new developmental milestones and emphasize the child's potential, in spite of illness-imposed limitations. The support that parents can give during stressful procedures should not be underestimated, and they should be allowed to remain to support the child if they wish to.

Teaching should begin with the parents' and the child's area of greatest need, and the nurse should use simple, nontechnical language and base the teaching on the parents' educational level and knowledge. Assessing their knowledge prevents duplication and contradiction and allows for clarification if there has been any misunderstanding. The nurse provides the family members with information about treatment regimens, expected responses to treatments, ways to make treatments less stressful, the care and use of equipment, time management, and where to find available resources.

Nurses sometimes serve as parent-advocates and patient-advocates by teaching the child and the parents to be assertive, to exercise their right to review treatments, to speak up if they are angry or disturbed by the care that the child is receiving, and to seek clarification of unclear answers to their questions. This approach will help the parents and the child feel competent and see themselves as partners with the medical and nursing staff, rather than as powerless and victimized by the system.

The parents can also be helped to anticipate the siblings' response to the illness. Role playing verbal responses prepares the parents to answer the siblings' questions and to react to their feelings without evasion or anger. The nurse should encourage the parents to inform the siblings of the child's illness before they hear about it from others and to tell them if the child's condition changes. When explaining the illness the siblings' level of cognitive ability must be taken into account. Increasingly elaborate explanations will be needed as the siblings' ability to use more complex and abstract thought increases.

Support groups composed of the parents, friends, or relatives of children with similar conditions are tremendously helpful and tend to decrease the parents' and the child's feelings of isolation and powerlessness. Belonging to a group builds the parents' and the child's confidence in their ability to cope with the feelings of chronic grief and provides psychological support and information through discussion of common problems, experiences, and strategies that work. The members may role-play responses to insensitive comments or rejection by others. They also may invite professional speakers to share the latest results of research. The nurse should always be available as a resource to parent support groups.

Discharge planning

It is important for the nurse to recognize that bringing a chronically ill child home from the hospital is a vastly different experience for parents from bringing home a child whose illness has been successfully and completely treated during the hospital stay or a child who will need only a brief period of convalescence at home. The principles of discharge planning are discussed in Chap. 16.

All families with a chronically ill child should be referred to a community nurse at the time of discharge, and, if possible, the family and the referring nurse should meet with this nurse in the hospital prior to discharge. Decisions regarding what equipment, supplies, and services will be required when the child is at home should be made. If the child's care will require modifications in the home environment, the community nurse should plan to visit the home prior to discharge. A minor event, such as discovering that there are no three-pronged outlets for a piece of equipment, is enough to unnerve a family on the day they return home with the child. In the case of distant referrals, detailed information must be given over the telephone and in writing.

The most frightening period for families who bring a newly diagnosed chronically ill child home from the hospital is the first 24 h, particularly the first night. This is also true of the families of previously diagnosed children if their condition has significantly deteriorated since they were hospitalized or if new equipment or treatments are required at home. In these instances, it is essential that the nurse make a home visit within the first 24 to 48 h. The parents must be given 24-h access to a professional staff person who is knowledgeable about their child's problems. They should be encouraged to call if they have any concerns. Knowing that they have ready access to help reassures the parents and generally tends to allay their anxiety and decrease the number of calls they make.

Long-term planning for the chronically ill child must also take into account the aspects of child health that are routinely part of the nurse's domain when dealing with well children. Anticipatory developmental guidance, immunizations, vision and hearing screening, dental care, and nutritional assessment are all necessary components of the comprehensive care of the chronically ill child. These areas are frequently overlooked because of a preoccupation with the medical problem.

CURRENT ISSUES IN CHRONIC CHILDHOOD ILLNESS

Home care

The development or adaptation of equipment for home use and the rapid growth of home health agencies have made it possible to provide in-home care for children with a broad range of complex problems. These developments have been paralleled by an emerging societal trend toward deinstitutionalization and a growing awareness of the need to normalize the lives of chronically ill children. Continually rising hospital costs have added financial concerns to humanistic ones, resulting in a trend toward earlier discharge from the hospital and the transfer of care to the home, where a parent becomes the primary caregiver.

Children who require ventilatory assistance, continuous intravenous antibiotic therapy, peritoneal dialysis, parenteral nutrition, and a host of other complex treatments and support services are being successfully managed at home. For many of these children, home visits by a nurse may be scheduled daily, weekly, or less frequently. During these visits, the nurse assesses the child's and the family's ability to provide the necessary care. The nurse also provides counseling, teaching, support, and referral as needed. Other children may require from 4 to 24 h of in-home nursing care each day (Fig. 34-5).

Despite the feasibility and social desirability of maintaining chronically ill children at home, many families cannot take advantage of this alternative because they lack the resources to pay for in-home nursing care or supervision. The five major sources of third-party reimbursement for the health care of chronically ill children are private insurance companies, Medicaid, Crippled Children Service programs, disease-oriented voluntary organizations, and special state programs.[45] Frequently, home care is not covered, or coverage is restricted to a limited type or amount of service and does not adequately meet the family's needs. The best insurance covers only about 80 percent of expenses of a limited type.

Around-the-clock accessibility to nursing and medical care and consultation and sufficient respite care for the family are the most important components of a successful home care program. The home care role of the nurse is to teach skills, provide information, clarify issues, and help the

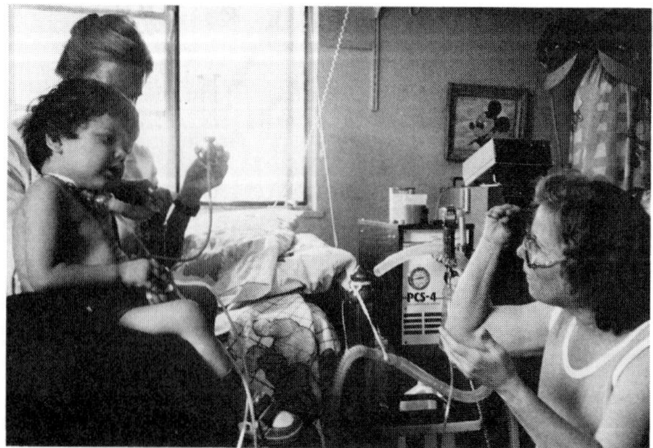

Figure 34-5 This family receives 16 hours of nursing care each day; 8 hours at night so family members can sleep. The grandmother is teaching the child sign language while the nurse administers oxygen therapy and gastrostomy feedings.

parents deal with their feelings so that they can accomplish the caretaking tasks more easily. The nurse must recognize that the parents are the primary caretakers and decision makers. The nurse assists the parents and the child by providing direct home nursing care to the child at the following times:

1. During the transitional phase after discharge, when the nurse helps stabilize the family environment and establish a routine.
2. When the parents cannot provide care because of employment or illness.
3. When a respite from caretaking activities is needed.
4. When a home death is planned and imminent. (See Chap. 35.)

Aided by data gathered during home observations, the nurse helps the family members communicate and prioritize caretaking responsibilities. If physical exhaustion and sleep deprivation are a problem, the nurse assists the family in finding respite care. Respite care, or relief from the responsibilities of caring for the chronically ill child, can be obtained through the help of a community nurse, a home health aide, or a homemaker; short-term care at a nursing home or a children's home is also possible. In addition, parent support groups can find couples who will act as foster parents, without charge, for short periods.

School

In November 1975, Congress passed the Education for All Handicapped Children Act (Public Law 94-142). It mandated that all school-age children in the United States were to have a free and appropriate public education available to them by September 1, 1978.[46] Furthermore, by September 1, 1980, such an education was to be made available to all handicapped children between the ages of 3 and 21 years.[47] This law means that any state that receives federal funds for the education of the handicapped cannot refuse to provide service to any handicapped child who is in need of special education, regardless of the severity of the child's condition or the parents' ability to pay. In addition to a free and appropriate education, handicapped children also have the right to nondiscriminatory testing, evaluation, and placement; procedural due process of law; and education in the least restrictive environment.[48] The concept of the right to an education in the least restrictive environment is based on the principle that special education systems or practices are inappropriate if they remove children from their expanded peer group without benefit of constitutional safeguards.[49] The least restrictive school placement is in the regular school, in the regular class, in the home school district. Education becomes more restrictive when it involves special classes, special education teachers, restricted programs, and tutoring at home or in the hospital; special residential school programs represent the most restrictive education.

Mainstreaming is a term frequently used to refer to the placement of handicapped children in a regular classroom in a regular school. Public Law 94-142 does not mandate mainstreaming for all handicapped children, nor does it abolish any special educational or residential setting.[50] Clearly, special settings are needed for some children. The intent of the legislation is to remove handicapped children from a regular classroom only when the severity of their impairment makes this necessary. In all other instances, additional school-related services should be provided to make it possible for the child to progress in school. See Table 34-3. The categories of children served under Public Law 94-142 are listed in Table 34-4.

Table 34-3 School-Related Services Available to the Chronically Ill Child

Support Therapies:
- Speech and language therapy
- Occupational therapy
- Physical therapy

Schedule modifications
Modified physical education
Transportation
Building accessibility
Toileting and lifting assistance
Counseling Services:
- School
- Career
- Personal

School Health Services:
- Administration of medications
- Implementation of medical procedures
- Emergency preparations
- Case coordination

Source: Adapted from D. K. Walker, "Care of Chronically Ill Children in Schools," *Pediatric Clinics of North America* **31:**229 (1984).

Table 34-4 Categories of Children Covered under the Education for All Handicapped Children Act (Public Law 94-142)

Mentally retarded
Speech-impaired
Visually handicapped
Learning-disabled
Multihandicapped
Otherwise impaired (heart disease, asthma, hemophilia, diabetes, and other conditions that adversely affect educational performance)
Hearing-impaired
Deaf
Deaf and blind
Emotionally handicapped
Orthopedically impaired

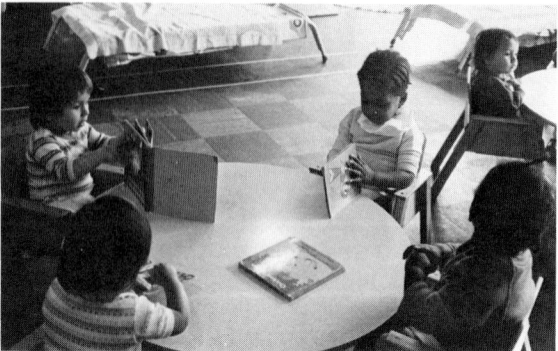

Figure 34-6 The blind preschooler fits in well with peers at the day-care center.

Integrating handicapped children into the regular classroom stimulates them to achieve more academically and socially and exposes them to a more realistic environment, in which there are normal role models for the patterning of behavior. This will help them cope better with the real world when they are adults. Exposure to handicapped children also helps normal children gain a better understanding of the wide range of individual differences.[51]

School can be a symbol of hope for the chronically ill child—a place where the child can think about and prepare for the future as other children do and where he or she can be free, for a time, of medical concerns.[52] Chronically ill children, like their peers, are concerned about their appearance and their grades and about being accepted by others and competing for rewards and praise.[53] These concerns take on heightened significance if their illness sets them apart and makes their psychosocial experiences different from those of their healthy peers.

Teachers frequently do not receive adequate education-related health information from parents and professionals. Information is withheld out of fear of discriminatory treatment, or the information that is given is not significant or helpful in the student-teacher relationship. Teachers do not need a detailed explanation of the physiological problem and the medical plan of care. Teachers do need to know:

1. Whether the child's activity must be restricted
2. Whether the child is taking any medication and how it is likely to affect behavior (e.g., whether it will cause drowsiness, hyperactivity, or inattentiveness
3. Whether the child's school day should be shortened or modified and whether rest periods are needed
4. Whether the child has dietary restrictions
5. Whether the child should have preferential seating in the classroom
6. Whether the child needs assistance with toileting
7. Whether the child needs physical, occupational, or speech therapy
8. Whether the child should receive special counseling or guidance
9. Whether the child needs any protective equipment or assistive devices
10. Whether school personnel need any special emergency training or knowledge of precautions
11. Whether the child's condition is improving, has stabilized, or is deteriorating
12. What the child's understanding of the problem is

A teacher who has insufficient information about the child's condition may be extremely fearful about having the child in the classroom and may be unnecessarily restrictive. The teacher may label a child who is experiencing side effects of drugs as disobedient or lazy or see a physically impaired child as also being intellectually impaired or "socially fragile" and therefore have lower expectations for that child.[54]

The nurse who works with chronically ill children must give teachers information that is child-specific and education-related, remain in contact with the school in order to answer questions, and provide updated information as circumstances change.

As a result of Public Law 94-142, more chronically ill children are being mainstreamed. These children require the constant presence of a nurse in the school. As this trend continues, the setting for nursing practice is moving out of the hospital and into the classroom. Nurses have new responsibilities to educate school personnel and provide the appropriate health-related services to chronically ill children. They also must promote the successful integration of chronically ill children into the school system by developing programs that will facilitate understanding and acceptance by healthy peers and by addressing the needs of students and teachers when one of these children dies. (See Chap. 35.)

As nurses work with chronically ill children in the future, their role as health care providers will continue to grow and change. The numbers of children who need care, the variety of disease processes, and the diversity of sites where care is provided—the clinic, the hospital, the long-term care facility, and the home—will all increase. Myers' six canons for chronic care are the foundation for good care in the present and in the future:[55]

Care Give genuine, personal, and professional care.
Communication Establish mutual trust.
Customize Remember that each child is unique.
Counsel Help the family members understand their choices.
Coordinate Facilitate and assist.
Continue Promote stability.

References

1. Mattson, Ake, "Long-Term Physical Illness in Childhood: A Challenge to Psychosocial Adaptation," *Pediatrics* **50**:801–811 (November 1972).
2. Hobbs, Nicholas, et al., "Chronically Ill Children in America," *Rehabilitation Literature* **45**:206–213 (July–August 1984).
3. Pless, I. B., and Philip Pinkerton, *Chronic Childhood Disorder: Promoting Patterns of Adjustment,* Year Book, Chicago, 1975, p. 21.
4. Gortmaker, Steven L., and William Sappenfield, "Chronic Childhood Disorders: Prevalence and Impact," *Pediatric Clinics of North America,* **31**:3–18 (February 1984).
5. Hobbs, et. al., op. cit., p. 208.
6. Pless, I. B., and K. J. Roghmann, "Chronic Illness and Its Consequences: Observations Based on Three Epidemiological Surveys," *Journal of Pediatrics,* **79**:351–359 (1971).
7. Mattson, op. cit., p. 802.
8. Stein, Ruth, and Dorthy Jessop, "A Noncategorical Approach to Chronic Childhood Illness," *Public Health Reports* **97**:354–362 (July–August 1982).
9. Stein, Ruth, and Dorthy Jessop, "General Issues in the Care of Children with Chronic Physical Conditions," *Pediatric Clinics of North America* **31**:189–198 (February 1984).
10. Martinson, Ida M., "Impact of Childhood Cancer Study," unpublished report, 1986.
11. Lazarus, Richard, and Susan Folkman, *Stress, Appraisal, and Coping,* Springer, New York, 1984.
12. Ibid., p. 145.
13. Olshansky, Simon, "Parent Responses to a Mentally Defective Child," *Mental Retardation* **4**:21–23 (August 1966).
14. Sabbeth, Barbara, "Understanding the Impact of Chronic Childhood Illness on Families," *Pediatric Clinics of North America* **31**:47–45 (February 1984).
15. Sabbeth, Barbara F., and John M. Leventhal, "Marital Adjustment to Chronic Childhood Illness: A Critique of the Literature," *Pediatrics* **73**:762–768 (June 1984).
16. Martinson, op. cit.
17. Perrin, J. M., et al., "The Organization of Services for Chronically Ill Children and Their Families," *Pediatric Clinics of North America* **31**:235–257 (February 1984).
18. Goffman, Irving, "Stigma," *Notes on the Management of Spoiled Identity,* Prentice-Hall, Englewood Cliffs, N.J., 1963, p. 30.
19. Martinson, op. cit.
20. Venters, M., "Familial Coping with Chronic and Severe Childhood Illness: The Case of Cystic Fibrosis," *Social Science and Medicine* **15**:289–297 (May 1981).
21. Weitzman, Michael, "School and Peer Relations," *Pediatric Clinics of North America* **31**:59–69 (February 1984).
22. Ibid.
23. Pless and Pinkerton, op. cit., pp. 59–86.
24. Yaros, Patricia S., and Jeanne Howe, "Responses to Illness and Disability," in Jeanne Howe (ed.), *Nursing Care of Adolescents,* McGraw-Hill, New York, 1980, p. 94.
25. Ibid., p. 103.
26. Vipperman, J., and P. Rager, "Childhood Coping: How Nurses Can Help," *Pediatric Nursing* **6**:11–18 (March–April 1980).
27. Solnit, M., and A. Green, "Reactions to the Threatened Loss of a Child: A Vulnerable Child Syndrome," In J. Schwartz and L. Schwartz (eds.), *Vulernable Infants: A Psychosocial Dilemma* McGraw-Hill, New York, 1977, pp. 183–189.

28. Schecter, Neil L., "Recurrent Pains in Children: An Overview and an Approach," *Pediatric Clinics of North America* **31**:949–969 (October 1984).
29. McCaffery, Margo, "Pain Relief for the Child: Problem Areas and Selected Nonpharmacological Methods," *Pediatric Nursing* **4**:11–16 (July–August 1977).
30. McCaffery, Margo, *Nursing Management of the Patient with Pain,* 2d ed., Lippincott, Philadelphia, 1979, pp. 35–49.
31. Hawley, D. D., "Postoperative Pain in Children: Misconceptions, Descriptions and Interventions," *Pediatric Nursing* **10**:20–23.
32. Schecter, op. cit., p. 95.
33. Haslam, D. R., "Age and the Perception of Pain," *Psychonomic Science* **15**:18 (1969).
34. Williamson, P. S., and M. L. Williamson, "Physiologic Stress Reduction by Local Anesthetic during Newborn Circumcision," *Pediatrics* **71**:36–40 (1983).
35. Abu-Saad, Huda, "The Assessment of Pain in Children," *Issues in Comprehensive Pediatric Nursing* **5**:327–335 (September–December 1981).
36. Unruh, Anita, et al., "Children's Drawings of Their Pain," *Pain* **17**:385–392 (1983).
37. McCaffrey, *Nursing management of the Patient with Pain,* pp. 35–42.
38. Lacouture, Peter G., et al., "Chronic Pain of Childhood: A Pharmacologic Approach," *Pediatric Clinics of North America* **31**:1133–1151 (October 1984).
39. Epstein, Mel H., and James Harris, Jr., "Children with Chronic Pain: Can They Be Helped?" *Pediatric Nursing* **4**:42–44 (January–February 1978).
40. Masek, Bruce J., et al., "Behavioral Approaches to the Management of Chronic Pain in Children," *Pediatric Clinics of North America* **31**:1113–1131 (October 1984).
41. Lacouture et al., op. cit., p. 1137.
42. Miser, Angela W., et al., "Continuous Subcutaneous Infusion of Morphine in Children with Cancer," *American Journal of Diseases of Children* **137**:383–385 (April 1983).
43. Strain, P. S., and M. M. Kerr, *Mainstreaming of Children in Schools: Research and Programmatic Issues,* Academic, New York, 1981.
44. Perrin, Ellen C., and Susan P. Gerrity, "There's a Demon in Your Belly: Children's Understanding of Illness," *Pediatrics* **67**:841–849 (June 1981).
45. Perrin, James M., and Henry T. Ireys, "The Organization of Services for Chronically Ill Children and Their Families," *Pediatric Clinics of North America* **31**:235–257 (February 1984).
46. Zettel, Jeffrey J., and Joseph Ballard, "The Education for All Handicapped Children Act of 1975 (P.L. 94-142): Its History, Origins, and Concepts," in J. Ballard et al. (eds.), *Special Education in America: Its Legal and Governmental Foundations,* Council for Exceptional Children, Reston, Va., 1982.
47. Zettel, Jeffrey J., "Implementing the Right to a Free Appropriate Public Education," in Ballard et al. op. cit., pp. 41–64.
48. Zettel and Ballard, op. cit., p. 16.
49. Walker, Deborah K., "Care of Chronically Ill Children in Schools," *Pediatric Clinics of North America* **31**:221–233 (February 1984).
50. Ibid., p. 222.
51. Ibid., p. 223.
52. Deasy-Spinetta, Patricia, "School as a Normalizing Factor in the Life of the Pediatric Cancer Patient," in D. R. Copeland et al. (eds.), *The Mind of the Child Who Is Said to Be Sick,* Charles C Thomas, Springfield, Ill., 1983, pp. 107–115.
53. Weitzman, op. cit., p. 64.
54. Walker, op. cit., pp. 226–227.
55. Myers, Gary J., "Myelomeningocele: The Medical Aspects," *Pediatric Clinics of North America* **31**(1) (February 1984).

35

Marlene S. Garvis
Ida M. Martinson

The terminally ill child

Upon completion of this chapter, the student will be able to:

1. List two characteristics of the child's concept of death at each developmental level.
2. Identify one coping response of a terminally ill child in each age group.
3. Identify two characteristics of a terminally ill child's awareness of dying.
4. Compare the responses of the parents to (*a*) the diagnosis, (*b*) remission, and (*c*) the terminal phase.
5. Explain the effects that a child's terminal illness may have on the parents' marital relationship.
6. Identify two responses of the siblings of a terminally ill child to the child's illness.
7. List three factors that may influence a child's adjustment to the loss of a sibling.
8. Identify two features of the grieving process.
9. Describe two feelings that may surface in the nurse who is caring for a terminally ill child.
10. List three resources that provide the nurse with support and skill in caring for a terminally ill child.
11. Give four examples of comfort care.
12. Give two reasons why the parents should be involved in planning and providing the care of a terminally ill child.
13. List four areas that are important to assess in the family of a terminally ill child.
14. List four symptoms of impending death.
15. Define the fear-pain-anxiety cycle and describe one appropriate nursing intervention.
16. Compare the roles of the parents, the nurse, and the physician in the home care of a dying child.

The word *terminal* is often confusing. It is sometimes synonymous with *fatal illness*, but there are differences. While a child who is terminal usually has a fatal illness, a child with a fatal illness is not always terminal. For the purposes of this chapter, the terminally ill child is defined as a child who has an illness from which he or she will soon die. There are many phases of a fatal illness, including diagnosis, remission, relapse, and even cure. The terminal phase brings the reality of death. Hopes for cure or long remissions can no longer be maintained. This phase can be quite short or may last for several weeks or even months.

Today, most childhood deaths result from accidents; however, cancer is the cause of the majority of deaths due to illness in children between the ages of 3 and 14 years.[1] The focus of this chapter is on the child with cancer, but the principles and concepts discussed apply to all children with terminal illnesses.

CHILDREN'S EXPERIENCES WITH DEATH

Scientific and medical advances have significantly reduced infant mortality as well as extended the average life span. Many diseases that were once devastating killers are now controlled or eradicated through the use of modern equipment and advanced technology. Also, palliative treatment is available to prolong survival while awaiting a new therapy or a cure. As a result, death now occurs less often early in life; it is increasingly seen as an experience of the aged.

Even in this age of scientific advances, death usually takes place in hospitals, where there are still likely to be restrictions on the presence of young children. Parents, in their efforts to protect their children, compound their children's limited opportunity to understand death. Thus most children never have the opportunity to see a person get sick, gradually grow worse, and die. When the death of a family member does occur, it is usually a new experience for the child. In the child's mind the person disappears into nowhere. Parents confuse their children by giving misleading answers to their questions, such as "Grandpa is permanently asleep," or answers which are difficult to grasp, such as "Grandma has gone to heaven."[2] In speaking of those who have died, people usually avoid the word *died,* saying instead that the person has "departed" or "passed away."

THE CHILD'S CONCEPT OF DEATH

Age, education, and experiences with death among family members, friends, and relatives influence the child's ideas about death. Cultural experiences and religious beliefs are also influential. For most children, death seems very far away, in the remote future. The child's reaction to his or her own dying is intimately related to the child's level of understanding and emotional maturity, how the disease process affects the child's self-concept, and the reactions of the people around the child. The child's awareness of the meaning of personal death changes.

Children under age 3

During the first 2 years of life, children have no understanding of death.[3] Young children live in the present and have little understanding of time. Dying has meaning to children under the age of 3 only as it affects the people around them. A very young dying child may feel sad and upset because the other family members are sad and upset, but the child is not really mourning because he or she does not realize the significance of death. Young children do not worry that their existence may come to an end. They do, however, react to the anguish and sadness of their parents and may become depressed.[4]

Preschoolers

During the preschool years, children come to understand the meaning of "myself" and "I," and while they appreciate that they are a "me," they sense that a person can become "not me." During the preschool period, children gradually develop the concept of nonexistence. It has been observed that "While the very young preschooler could readily crush an ant or destroy a flower, this same child a few years later may become very protective of living creatures."[5] Thus preschoolers understand the difference between "life" and "not life."

Preschoolers believe that their existence is unlimited by time. They understand that death is a departure. They believe that it is gradual and temporary, not a regular and final process. The child understands that one's condition can change periodically. Somewhat in the same way as one sleeps and wakes, so one "is made dead" and can return to ordinary life. The child believes that after death, breathing, eating, and living are still possible, although perhaps in a more restricted way than when the person was alive. For example, the child may believe that a dead person's eyes are closed to keep dirt out and that the dead do not move because the coffin restricts their mobility. The child often concludes that anyone who goes away is dead.[6,7,8]

Older preschoolers are prone to misinterpret superficial signals as being intrinsically involved with death. For example, they believe that if someone died in a hospital, one must stay away from hospitals. As children become increasingly aware that death is something that is both important and disruptive, they seek to isolate the phenomena which cause or mean death.

When a preschool child is threatened by a fatal illness, nightmares may increase. Games may become more violent, and the child may act out accidents, disasters, or even funeral rituals, complete with coffins. In play, figures die but come back to life. This type of play permits the child to reemphasize that his or her newly achieved independence will not come to an end. The dying preschooler may ask, "What will I look like when I die?" "Will I be able to breathe and have anyone to talk with?" "Will my death be painful?" "Have I been bad?" and "Maybe my parents do not want me—is that why I am dying?"[9]

The dying preschool child seeks comfort, reassurance, and support from the parents. They are the child's main protectors. The young child fears separation, pain, and bodily harm, but not death. Time has no meaning to the child except as it pertains to his or her needs. For example, the mother's absence during lunch may seem to last an eternity, while time seems to fly when the child is absorbed in a play activity.

For preschoolers, the emotional pain of separation from the parents may be far greater than actual physical pain. Often they think that the painful experiences and misery are a direct result of their misdeeds or bad thoughts. They need reassurances that good and bad private thoughts do not make things happen, that no one wants them to be sick and in pain, and that their parents do not want to be separated from them.

Evidence of a child's anxieties includes regressive behavior and increasing dependence on the parents, or the child may maintain independence and deal with private feelings by withdrawing into a daydream world of fantasy, wish fulfillment, and happy endings. While regression and withdrawal do occur, they are less than desirable. Reassurance and support from the staff and the parents can encourage the child to express his or her concerns and maintain independence.

Preschoolers should be approached on the basis of day-to-day reality. Questions should be answered when they are asked. When the end stage comes, dying children should be assured that they will not die alone but will be supported by their parents. Their anxieties and concerns need to be heard.

School-age children

Research has demonstrated that children between the ages of 5 and 9 years tend to personify death.[10] That is, they commonly think of death as a person, either living or dead and with either good or bad intentions, who causes people to die. At the same time, school-age children view death as removed from their lives. The child may say, "Only those die whom the deathman catches and carries off. Whoever can get away does not die."[11]

Piaget[12] observed that children up to 6 or 7 years of age equate life with general activity. That is, anything active is viewed as being "alive." At age 7 or 8, children begin to discriminate between things which are alive and things which are not. At first, they believe that all things which move, such as bicycles, are alive. Later, they attribute life only to things that move spontaneously, and they realize that bicycles are not alive. Finally, they learn that only humans, animals, and plants are alive.

Six-year-olds may worry about their own death and that of their parents, but unless they have had experiences with death, they usually relate death to old age. Seven-year-olds realize that they will die sometime. They are interested in the ceremonies which surround death—the coffin, the funeral, the burial, and the cemetery. Eight-year-olds explore the cause of death and what happens after death.[13]

Older school-age children, 10 to 12 years of age, understand that death is the cessation of bodily life. For example, they may explain that "It means the passing of the body"[14] or that death is something that no one can escape. "Everyone has to die once, but the soul lives on."[15] By age 10, most children have formulated a close approximation of the adult view of life and death. This gives them a framework within which the idea of death can be placed: death is one general principle among many other general principles. They see the world as a more comprehensible and predictable place.

Recent research indicates that three major components of the mature concept of death may actually be understood by children by the age of 7 years: (1) that death is irreversible, (2) that life-defining functions cannot be attributed to dead things, and (3) that everyone dies.[16,17] As they grow, grade-school children understand more and more that they may live and grow or may die and disappear. They begin to fantasize an alternative to death—heaven, paradise, or even hell. Even if this present existence is changed in some way, possibly by death, they believe that there will still continue to be a "me." Even hell is considered better than not existing at all. Heaven, of course, is by far the best solution.

Dying school-age children can understand the significance of a diagnosis and prognosis. Some children deduce their diagnosis on their own before they are even admitted or referred to a medical center. Children may feel that their illness is a punishment for something they said or did, since they still believe that every act involves a punishment or a reward. They have great difficulty with their feelings and tend to rely on authorities such as God, doctors, nurses, parents, or teachers for final protection. They know that they will die, but they also believe that they will still be secure and protected. School-age children mourn the loss of life, and worry about how their existence will end, and time begins to have meaning. Because they regard the prognosis more as a certainty than as a statement of possibility, they are usually eager to talk about and explore the meaning of death.

School-age children need their parents for support and security and for explanations of what is happening. It is important to help them maintain independence and control whenever possible. Separation from the family should be kept to a minimum because it makes them feel lonely, angry, and frustrated as well as depressed. When death is near and inevitable, their questions should be answered truthfully. School-age children have the emotional ability to face the prospect of death and to reach out to parents, family, and friends for comfort and understanding. Support by the persons they trust helps them through this final experience.

Adolescents

Adolescents think of death as both fearsome and fascinating. Studies indicate that they do not want to die without having had the opportunity to enjoy life's fulfillments. Some turn to religion as insurance against the risk of death. The majority repress and deny their anxiety.[18]

Adolescents live in an intense present. "Now" is so real to them that both the past and the future seem pallid by comparison. Everything that is important and valuable lies either in the immediate life situation or in the rather close future. Off in the distance stands death, the natural enemy to the developing self.

During adolescence, being accepted by others of one's own age is a high priority. Physical condition (strength, appearance, and ability to perform) has enormous influence on both peer acceptance and self-esteem. Terminally ill adolescents may express more concern over bodily changes, such as weight gain or hair loss, than over the course of the disease process itself.

The emotional growth and increasing independence of adolescence bring feelings of guilt. Terminally ill teenagers may believe that death is a punishment for their assertive or "grown-up" behavior. They may feel fearful and at the same time be unable to seek comfort from their parents, God, or society.

Friends may withdraw, emotionally if not altogether, when they are faced with the impending death of a peer. The resulting isolation emphasizes the adolescent's basic vulnerability and makes the adolescent extremely uncomfortable. Illness also forces the peer-oriented adolescent to become increasingly dependent on the parents. Adolescents treasure their independence and struggle to maintain it against the total passivity of death. In their effort to feel strong and powerful, they may well overtax their strength. While they long for understanding, their fear of losing their independence may produce behavior which forces other people away. Dying adolescents' responses to their fate include anger and bitterness.

Health team members should understand that emotional outbursts may well be a sign of adolescents' anger at dying. They may need physical outlets as well as visible evidence of love and support. While signs of attention from those they care for, such as visits, flowers, and letters, may be difficult to accept, they help adolescents understand that they are not really alone. These tokens make loneliness more bearable and, at times, bitterness less acute.

Providing ways to support adolescents' self-confidence, independence, and sense of control will help them accept the comfort and support of staff and parents as they face death. Terminally ill adolescents should be given information about the diagnosis, the prognosis, and the purpose and nature of treatments and procedures. Their questions will usually indicate how much information they can tolerate at any time. Adolescents should be encouraged to talk and ask questions about their illness. Like younger children, adolescents should be assured that dying is not a punishment, that they are loved and accepted, and that they will not die alone.

CHILDREN'S AWARENESS OF DYING

One of the tasks of the health team and of the parents of a terminally ill child is communicating with the child about his or her illness and about death. While developmental level is an important factor in approaching the child,[19] adults' understanding and their ability and willingness to communicate may actually determine how and when the child is approached. Parents and staff may wish to protect a child, stating "She really doesn't know how ill she is—why should I upset her?" This assessment is rarely accurate, however. Terminally ill children usually have some awareness that they are seriously ill, whether their parents or the health team has actually discussed this with them or not.

Early studies focused on anxiety as a sign of children's awareness of dying. In one study of leukemic children, children were observed to handle anxiety in one of three ways: younger children expressed the anxiety symbolically and physiologically; older boys tended to act out; and older girls tended to become depressed. Death anxiety was most often present in older children.[20]

In another study the primary source of anxiety in dying children was found to differ by age group. For children aged 10 years and older, fear of death and distress over the death of other children in the hospital were the most upsetting factors. In contrast, children aged 5 to 10 years found traumatic procedures, such as venipunctures, most distressing. Those up to 5 years found separation from their mothers the greatest cause of distress.[21] A third study of children with a fatal illness reported that anxiety varied with the prognosis.

A study of four groups of children aged 6 to 10 years found that the group with a poor prognosis showed more anxiety and more threat to body integrity than the comparison groups. Children with a poor prognosis included loneliness, separation, and death content in their stories, even when they had not talked about death with hospital staff and even if their parents believed that they did not know the prognosis. Death anxiety, while present, was not expressed overtly.[22]

Recent evidence suggests that the speed and completeness with which children develop an awareness of their terminal illness may be unrelated to age and intellectual ability. Bluebond-Langner reported that 3- to 9-year-old children with cancer acquire an awareness of their illness in similar stages (see Table 35-1). Progress from one stage to another depends on (1) acquisition of additional factual information and (2) personal disease-related experiences. Bluebond-Langner also observed changes in self-concept, as the children developed an awareness of their illness (see Table 35-1). Awareness occurred whether the children had been told about their disease and prognosis or not.[23,24]

Table 35-1 A Child's Growing Awareness of Dying

Stages of Awareness
1. The disease is a serious illness.
2. Names of drugs and side effects.
3. Purposes of the treatments and procedures.
4. The disease is a series of remissions and relapses.
5. The disease is a series of remissions and relapses which ultimately ends in death.
Changing Self-Concept
1. I am seriously ill.
2. I am seriously ill and will get better.
3. I am always ill and will get better.
4. I am always ill and will never get better.
5. I am dying.

Source: Myra Bluebond-Langner, *The Private Worlds of Dying Children*, Princeton, Princeton, N.J., 1978.

Adults should be honest and supportive in their approach to dying children. This helps establish a basis of trust and promotes dying children's ability to cope with future events. They are then able to ask as many or as few questions as they can emotionally handle. Evasive answers are not likely to shield them from the reality of their illness, since there are so many other cues that something serious is happening. In the end, informed children will be more comfortable and secure. While they may rely on their own resources, they also attempt to enlist the support of others, including parents, staff, and peers. Even when they know the prognosis, they do not always ask or always talk about dying. Rather, much of their time is spent in becoming aware, putting things together, and probing for more information. Children who are terminally ill may express themselves only in symbolic, not easily understood, ways. One has only to listen to dying children, however, to realize that they do know the truth about their illness.[25,26]

THE FAMILY AND THE DYING CHILD

Impact on the parents

Parents usually experience the need to care for and protect their children. Having a child who has a terminal illness threatens the fulfillment of this need and may even be perceived by the parents as an attack on their integrity and well-being.

The diagnosis The diagnosis is the event which may have the greatest impact on the family.[27] According to Gyulay, "Diagnosis marks the juncture of two radically different life styles: the one before diagnosis, which was normal, and the one after, in which the future is unknown and at the mercy of the child's illness."[28]

With the diagnosis, parents usually become depressed. Some parents blame themselves for the child's condition and critically review their attitudes and behavior toward the child. Most parents in our society have been reared to believe that conformity and good behavior will be rewarded; when their child is diagnosed as having a terminal illness, the parents may feel singled out and punished.

Health team members can help parents by being open and honest in their communication. An important factor in parents' ability to trust health care professionals is their perception of a willingness on the part of these individuals to be open and listen to them. Such interaction can help relieve anxiety and guilt, enable parents to participate in the care of their children, and give parents "confidence in their ability to master subsequent developments."[29] It is equally important that staff members support the decisions that parents make and maintain a hopeful outlook without giving unwarranted reassurances or promising too much.

While they may not always voice them, parents do have some general concerns that must be anticipated.[30]

1. What is the long-term significance of the fact that the diagnosis was not made earlier?
2. Will a previous illness or lack of a previous illness make any difference in the success of my child's treatment?
3. Will my child be able to go to school or continue normal activity?
4. What do I tell my other children, friends, and distant relatives?
5. What should I tell my child?
6. How long will my child be in the hospital?
7. Will my child be in much pain? How and when will my child die?
8. What are my child's chances for remission? When might remission begin? How long will it last?

The initial hospitalization involves induction therapy and repeated procedures for the child. The parents may be interviewed by a variety of professionals, such as a social worker, a psychologist, pediatric specialists, and many nurses. They may become frustrated by the intrusion of all these people in their lives. The parents may also experience such distressing symptoms as depression, nervousness, sleep difficulties, and loss of appetite.[31]

Continuity of nursing care helps the parents gain support and perspective at this time. Discharge from the hospital often comes before remission. While the parents are relieved to go home, they want to know who will help them, who will answer their questions, and who will relieve them when they are exhausted.

Remission Remission is a time when life becomes more normal again and the family begins to build a new life. During this period of "normalcy," the parents may deny the illness or vacillate between accepting the diagnosis and hoping that a mistake was made.[32] At this time, however, there is great concern about financial matters and the continued need for information about the child's condition.[33] There are also strong fears about the return of the disease. Parents often hope that by suppressing their thoughts of the disease, they can suppress the disease too.

Even when things outwardly begin to return to normal, the parents may become preoccupied with possible future developments. Any change in the medical or nursing procedure or routine causes alarm. The periodic trips to the hospital or clinic can accentuate fears and anxiety. Health team members can provide support by assuring the parents that their fears are normal and that other families experience the same concerns.[34]

Between clinic visits life is relatively normal; there is hope that the remission will continue. Parents report that the most difficult aspect of a child's illness is wondering how long the remission will last, whether there will be another treatment protocol, and when this will all be over.

Relapse Relapse brings back the reality of the diagnosis: "They were right." It sweeps away the dream of long-term remission and the hope for a cure. The anxieties and disruption of the diagnosis period reappear, including separation from the child's other parent, well siblings, and home. During relapse, the parents observe many emotional and physical changes in the child—anorexia, nausea, weight loss, bleeding, and fatigue.

Some parents may still hope for additional medication and treatment and a corresponding extension in life expectancy. This was well stated by one parent who said, "Where there's life, there's hope, so I'm looking forward."[35]

If the child again improves, family living can return to a semblance of normality. But living is likely to be on a day-to-day basis, and no long-term plans are made. Taking things a day at a time tends to minimize the parents' resentments and frustrations in adapting to the course of their child's illness.[36]

The terminal stage The terminal phase brings the parents face-to-face with the reality of impending death. While a few parents continue to deny or bargain, most give up hope for a cure, new therapy, and long remissions. Parents have many fears at this time, which usually include:

1. Fear of prolonging the inevitable and the pain
2. Fear of losing control or not being able to cope
3. Fear of being physically or emotionally isolated
4. Fear of having other people take over
5. Fear that death will occur while they are away or while they are alone with the child
6. Fear of not being able to love again

The parents, of course, also have many fears as they anticipate what the actual death will be like: Will the child bleed? Will the child just stop breathing? Will the pain be terrible? Will the child be alert? (Parents' wishes about this matter vary.) How much warning will they have?[37]

Knowing that death is near for a child with cancer may be a relief from the long period of stress created by the disease. However, it may instead precipitate further stress and abnormal grief reactions. Parents vary widely in this regard. Nevertheless, most seek to make the most of their child's final days of life. Even children who are close to death can have a "good day" with their families.

The actual death comes as a shock to the parents, no matter how long they have been prepared. Most parents want to be with their child at the time of death, although they may dread what it will be like and how they will react. Euphemisms, such as "critical" or "very bad," should be avoided. The parents should be told, "Your child is dying." If the parents wish, they should be allowed to hold their child.

When death comes, the parents, along with the other close family members, need some private time to say good-bye to the child. The parents should be encouraged to see their child before he or she is taken to the funeral home. Seeing the child dead is painful but helps the parents accept the fact that death has occurred; this acceptance is essential to the mourning process. After the child's death the parents must plan the burial ceremony. The religious and ceremonial aspects of death are, for many people, important means of confirming the reality of the loss and providing family members support in their mourning.

Family relationships during the illness

When the parents begin to appreciate the significance of their child's progressing illness, their relationship to the child can change in many ways. Initially, they may handle the child with greater care, have greater patience, and worry more about falls and bruises. As reality sets in, their expectations and hopes have to be altered. Whereas before the diagnosis the child was "the embodiment of a promise," after the illness is discovered that promise is "either gone or at least reduced in value."[38]

While it is important that the parents be aware of the child's actual physical limitations, it is equally important that they stimulate the child to achieve at a realistic level. As difficult as it may seem, the parents should maintain reasonable discipline practices. This provides the ill child with assurance that he or she is still normal in some respects. It also demonstrates to the well brothers and sisters that there are consequences for misbehavior even for the ill sibling.

A father faces tremendous stress when he is faced with the reality that his child has a terminal illness. Research on parents of children with leukemia has demonstrated that fathers find many ways of absenting themselves from painful involvement with their families. This is their way of coping, a way of avoiding the pain of ongoing involvement with the dying child. Such behavior can indicate a father's need for additional support.[39] A father's participation in the care of his dying child can be helpful to his wife as well as the child. A mother usually copes by becoming increasingly involved in the care of the child. She may give up employment and outside activities as well as isolate herself from friends and family in an effort to provide care and support to the ill child.

These coping behaviors place significant burdens on the husband-wife relationship. Financial concerns may limit social activities and necessitate increased time working to meet expenses. This combination of factors may reduce the amount of attention that the husband and wife can focus on their marital relationship. Consequently, both partners may feel an increasing sense of isolation and loss of support. An additional burden is placed on the marital relationship each time the child is hospitalized. While the mother may spend many hours at the child's bedside, the father may visit only infrequently. The mother may wish to protect him from the intensity of guilt, anger, and sadness she feels about their child's illness. At the same time, the husband may believe that it is necessary to protect his wife from his own quite similar feelings. In such a situation, each excludes and isolates the other.

One of the ways in which this gap in communication can be overcome is for the husband and wife to become aware of what is happening, to learn to focus on the common aspects of their situation, and to develop some practical ways to support each other in time of stress. Researchers have shown that family strength rather than weakness can be a result of coping with serious illness. Many parents have not only mastered the practicalities of their situation but also have appeared to grow together as people as a result of it.

Resources to assist the parents include discussion groups of parents of terminally ill children. Such groups provide information about the illness and also promote the sharing of feelings among parents. Group sessions can help the parents find ways for the family to cope with the child's illness. By hearing other parents discuss their experience with the death of a child, the parents can begin to feel that they can survive this devastating experience and that they will be able to go through the grief process reasonably well.

Four advantages of parent groups have been identified:[40]

1. Open communication among parents regarding their children's and their own personal problems relating to their special situation
2. Learning that they are not alone, as a result of informal sharing and mutual caring
3. Development of the ability to focus on individual situations
4. Provision of informational materials by the group which help parents face the course of their children's illness

Impact on other family members

While the parents suffer the greatest stress with the terminal illness of a child, other family members need special attention in such a situation: siblings and grandparents.

Siblings react to illness and death according to their age and ability to comprehend. Their relationship to the ill child and their own place and adjustment within the family both play a part. The honesty and appropriateness with which the parents communicate with them about the dying child and the nature of the problem are also important, that is, "how they are included, as a part of the family, in the family's adaptation to terminal illness."[41]

With the demands on the parents' energy, it is understandable that the needs of well siblings are given a lower priority. Brothers and sisters may grieve and fear that they will fall ill and die.[42] It is important that the parents be open and honest, provide age-appropriate and anxiety-reducing explanations, and listen to their children's questions.[43,44] Even when the parents try to protect siblings from sorrow by attempting to be cheerful and by giving evasive answers, they usually know that something is wrong. Young children, who believe in magic, may fear that they caused the death and must be reassured otherwise.

Communication about the disease between the parents and the well siblings is essential to minimize jealousy and promote cooperation. Siblings frequently feel isolated by the uniqueness of their experience. Siblings' visits to the ill child in the hospital will help eliminate fears and build up positive relationships. Siblings can also help care for an ill child at home. They will be able to learn about the ill child's needs, accept the illness, and participate in the family's concerns and activities.

When death is near, the siblings should be informed. The parents may decide to allow the siblings to be present when it occurs. If not, the parents should tell them that the child received the best care and did not suffer too much. The siblings should be encouraged to participate in the funeral and cemetery services.

The siblings' responses to the death can range from no apparent response to depression, nightmares, aggression, and physical complaints.[45] They may express a variety of feelings, including feelings of responsibility for the ill child's death, fear that they will die, resentment that the parents spent so much time with the ill child, and anger at the parents for allowing the child to die; they may also become preoccupied with fantasies about death.[46]

The parents should provide opportunities for the siblings to discuss the illness and death. Otherwise, their fears and anxieties will lie hidden below the surface and will continue to distress them. They may need to be reassured that the death was not their fault, that the illness was not contagious, that normally children grow up to be adults, and that the parents have many more years to live. As the parents are able to accept and express their grief and provide for the emotional needs of their surviving children, the children in turn will be able to accept their own feelings.

The terminal illness of a child has a significant impact on the grandparents. They grieve for the child, the parents, and also themselves. Initially, the grandparents may be angry with, and hostile toward, the parents ("Why didn't you take the child to the doctor sooner?"), or with themselves ("We should have realized the child was sick."). They may be less accepting of the diagnosis than the parents and thus complicate the parents' struggle to accept and cope with the reality of the illness. While the grandparents may wish to be included in the parents' grief and to help with the care of the child, some parents are reluctant to put the burden of their fears and feelings on the grandparents, who may be physically or emotionally frail.

Like other family members, the grandparents need to have effective means of gathering information and expressing their feelings in order to cope with their impending loss. They may find help in "grandparent groups," which provide information and support. When they can participate in the care of the dying child or the well siblings, the grandparents feel needed and have increased self-esteem.

Mourning after the death

Mourning for a dead child is an intense and lengthy experience for the family. Shock and numbness are usually the first responses, regardless of how well the family was prepared for the death. Family members may find it difficult to make judgments or function effectively. This phase of mourning is replaced by anger and guilt, restlessness and reality testing, depression, and awareness of the reality of the situation. Finally, after many months, family members may begin to experience a sense of relief and renewed energy. According to Davidson, the process of post-death mourning may last for at least 12 to 18 months.[47] For many families, mourning may continue longer.[48] Mourning may reoccur at times of special significance for the family: anniversary dates of the death, birthdays of the dead child, and religious holidays.

An important goal for the family is to rejoin the life of the community. Religious faith, support groups, and contact with the staff who cared for the dead child may be important in helping family members cope. The death of the child is an irrevocable fact, but life should continue to be enjoyed. As Harriet Schiff said, "As long as I live I will be sorry Robby is dead. That is a fact . . . I carry always. There are times . . . when I miss him still. But there are still good times. We share joys as a family that he did not live to share and I am sorry. But we still have joys. That is as it should be."[49]

THE IMPACT OF TERMINAL ILLNESS ON THE NURSE

Caring for a child who is dying can be a positive, rewarding component of the nurse's role. Nurses, like physicians, however, often tend to view terminal illness and death as failure because their usual goals of disease prevention and health promotion cannot be achieved.

In addition, working with dying children elicits many taxing emotional responses. Nurses, like family members and others who are close to the child, experience grief—denial, anger, guilt, and depression. Their frustration over the prognosis and their wish that the child would not die are confounded by the awareness that, at the same time, they wish death to come quickly so that all involved may be relieved of their suffering.

When the terminal state is the result of an accident, nurses may feel considerable anger at the parents or others who seem to be at fault for not having protected the child adequately. If the patient is an adolescent whose behavior has resulted in the accident, nurses may feel angry toward the patient. This blame setting can cause resentment, which in turn, can decrease the quality of nursing care.[50] Whether the terminal condition was caused by trauma or by an illness such as cancer, nurses may wish to alleviate their own suffering by withdrawing from the child and the family.

There are several approaches that nurses can take to deal with their own feelings and ensure effective care for both the child and the family. First, it is essential to recognize that denial, anger, guilt, frustration, and depression are normal for nurses, just as they are for family members and patients. Also, nurses can learn to accept their own reactions and to deal with them in ways that promote satisfaction and effectiveness in providing for the dying child and helping the family and friends.

A supportive work setting is of major importance in enabling nurses to cope with the stresses of caring for the terminally ill. Institutional mechanisms should be established to give nurses and other health team members a forum in which to share and confront their reactions to being involved in relationships that must be interrupted by a child's death. Staff members need to discuss the positive and negative aspects of the child and the child's care and must acknowledge and receive acceptance of their responses to the emotional and physical demands placed on them by caring for the child.

When such a support system is not available, there is a real danger that the nurse may attempt to cope by withdrawing from contact with the child and involvement with the parents. The problems tend to grow with each dying child, and a nurse can, in addition to being ineffective as a caregiver, become more angry, depressed, and cynical as a result of unresolved frustration and unresolved grief.[51]

Some ways in which a support system can be established in the practice setting have been suggested.[52]

1. During the report session, discuss the patients who are dying, the reactions of the staff, and the care plans. Discussing specifics will also help others implement effective means of care.
2. During staff meetings, identify those staff members who have, or will have, the greatest amount of involvement, thus alerting the other staff members to those who may be most in need of reinforcement.
3. During interactions with other staff members, give both verbal and nonverbal reinforcement whenever interpersonal or physical care has been done well.
4. Set aside some time for sharing knowledge, ideas, and plans and for evaluating goal achievement. In this way, the staff may come to feel a real sense of accomplishment.
5. Define and evaluate the purposes of care measures in order to measure each experience against the stated goal.
6. Take time to give a word of encouragement and to let someone cry with you or to discuss a patient. This will influence the quality of care as well as the well-being of the staff.
7. Encourage each staff member to find one other person with whom to share his or her experiences; this will be an enrichment and a support to both staff members and patients.

The nursing process itself provides the means by which nurses can avoid much of the frustration and distress that they might otherwise encounter in caring for dying children. When a child becomes terminal, the overall goal of nursing care is death with comfort and optimal functioning of the surviving family members. Comfort care is aimed at minimizing physical and psychological suffering and deterioration and at maximizing comfort. The nursing process breaks a complex situation into discrete, manageable subparts. For example, planning includes anticipation of needs in order to prevent unnecessary pain, skin breakdown, and complications. When such realistic goals are established, the success of nursing care is not linked to impossible objectives like cure and survival, and the evaluation phase of the nursing process allows the nurse to feel successful—even when the child dies—because provision for the best possible physical and emotional care has been made.

NURSING MANAGEMENT OF THE TERMINALLY ILL CHILD

Philosophy of terminal care

The decision to stop or continue cure-oriented treatment when children are at the end stage of a disease is often difficult to make. Frequently, the parents, the child, the doctor, and the nurse will have differing opinions. Many parents are reluctant to discuss stopping treatment with their physician. They wonder whether further treatment will help or whether making this request will jeopardize their relationship with the physician, and thus their child's care.

Once a good relationship with the parents has been established, the nurse can be alert for direct comments or subtle clues which indicate that the parents are considering discontinuing treatment.

The nurse also needs to listen for clues from children. This should be done with an especially attuned ear, since children often talk in symbolic language.[53] Most children do not like hospitalization and find their cancer treatment uncomfortable. Children know their diagnoses and understand the meaning of their illness, and they even know when they are dying.[54] If the nurse establishes a trusting relationship and listens carefully, the child will tell the nurse when further treatment and continued hospitalization are no longer desired. Allow children to discuss their thoughts, and share this information with both the parents and the physician.

The nurse can facilitate physician-family communication by sharing information with the physician about the family's preparedness for discussing the discontinuation of treatment. If the family appears reluctant to discuss their feelings with the physician, the nurse may need to provide support and encourage them to speak freely and honestly with the physician.

The nurse should feel free to discuss any feelings about discontinuing care with other health team members. It is important, however, to be aware of personal feelings and not to impose them on the parents. Instead, help the parents review all the alternatives so that they can decide what is the best choice for their child. If, after consultation with the medical staff, the parents decide to continue cancer treatment, the child's medical and nursing care should continue, with survival as the goal. The nurse should place a high priority on preventive nursing care and health maintenance and should utilize every opportunity to promote healing and prevent further physical deterioration.

If cure-oriented treatment is discontinued, the child's comfort is the primary goal. Once treatment is stopped, children can survive from several hours or days to a year or more, depending on the type of cancer. Comfort care should be provided when a child has only several days or weeks of life remaining. If it is predicted that the child will live longer, nursing care for the chronically ill child should be instituted.

Comfort care includes any measures that the family feels will make the child comfortable. Essentially, the child is provided with whatever he or she wishes during the final days. Many children, when they are ill and dying, refuse nutritious foods and fluids. Comfort care includes giving children whatever they want to eat, whenever they desire it, regardless of nutritional value.

Another important aspect of comfort care is effective pain control. It is important that the child be allowed to spend his or her last days free of pain. Whatever the source of the pain, the child should be adequately medicated so that the parents can hold the child. Months of valuable physical and emotional support can be lost if the child and the parents are not able to touch and hold each other. In many instances, methods of health maintenance such as antibiotics and blood replacements are discontinued unless the family desires these for the child's comfort.

Hospital care of the dying child

When treatment is discontinued, the family needs to decide where the child will spend his or her final days. There are many reasons why a family may choose to have their child die in the hospital. In some instances, the family may feel that the physical care is too difficult for them to provide or that the family social situation is not conducive to the child's dying at home. Parents of an infant may not feel that being "at home" is important to the child. Finally, the parents may not know that professional nursing care is available outside the hospital.

If the family chooses death in the hospital, health professionals should support this decision. The hospital nurses can greatly influence the quality of life of the child and the family during the final days of the child's life.

Assessment Once treatment has been discontinued, the nurse should complete a nursing assessment of the child's physical and emotional status, keeping the principle of comfort care in mind. The assessment should be completed as quickly as possible because hospitalized children who are not receiving medical therapy usually die within a short period of time. The nurse needs to plan for the child's complete comfort.

The physical assessment should include a review of all major systems, with an especially close look at sources of discomfort—pain from the disease, skin breakdown, contractures, constipation, and bleeding. Information from the parents regarding how they have solved problems and provided comfort at home can prove invaluable and should be elicited during the assessment phase. An emotional assessment of the child is of equal importance at this stressful time. It should include an appraisal of the child's knowledge of the illness and of his or her impending death. The child's current emotional status and ability to cope with this knowledge should also be assessed. The nurse should meet with and observe the child, in addition to discussing the child's emotional status with the parents.

The nurse usually has frequent contact with other family members—the parents, siblings, and grandparents—during the dying phase and provides them with emotional support and assistance. The nurse should assess the current emotional status and coping abilities of these other family members. A final important area for assessment is the family's desire for involvement in the dying process.

Table 35-2 outlines the assessment for care of a terminally ill child and his or her family. The nurse can use the information derived from this assessment to:

1. Identify and evaluate the present health status of the child and the other family members
2. Develop an appropriate nursing care plan for the dying child
3. Plan strategies to assist the other family members through this difficult time
4. Plan for the family's involvement in comfort care

Principles of planning care An individualized nursing care plan that addresses all pertinent physical and emotional health care needs is important for the dying child, just as it is for the chronically ill child or the child who will completely recover from a brief illness. The death of a child is a highly stressful event. Thorough, competent nursing care should be provided so that the child will be as comfortable as possible, both physically and mentally. This relieves the family of the worry or concern that their child is not receiving the best possible care.

When writing a nursing care plan, the nurse should first ascertain the life-support measures that the physician and the family have planned for the child. The nurse should ask what supportive measures are to be used, such as transfusions or oxygen, in order to develop a plan that includes sufficient time for teaching the child and the parents and preparing them emotionally.

The anticipated life expectancy should also be used as a guideline for writing the nursing care plan. For a child who may die in a few days, care should consist primarily of providing comfort. If the child wishes to remain in bed or curled up on a parent's lap eating popsicles and potato chips, the nurse should accept the child's choice. The nursing care plan for this child would not include the preventive and health-maintenance aspects included in the Nursing Care Plan at the end of this chapter, which involves a child whose death is expected 2 or more weeks in the future. Skin care and attention to muscle tone—including range-of-motion exercises, frequent turning, and getting out of bed several times a day—are included in this care plan to increase the child's comfort and prevent pain, contractures, and skin breakdown, which could occur over a period of time.

The care plan for each child needs to include information about the interventions that the parents have found to be successful prior to this time. For instance, a child might be able to prevent constipation by putting Metamucil on his or her cereal, taking milk of magnesia, or both, thereby avoiding suppositories and enemas.

Setting goals and planning care The family, including both the child and the parents, should participate in discussions to develop a plan of care, set goals, and outline plans to meet those goals. Families differ in the extent to which they wish to be involved in their children's care. There are three strong reasons why every child's parents (and perhaps other members of the family) should be included in planning and providing care: (1) separation of the parents from the child, which is stressful,[55,56,57,58] is diminished; (2) children experience less discomfort when their parents take part in planning and giving care; and (3) involvement in care helps the child and the parents regain some feeling of being in control.

From the time of diagnosis of a life-threatening disease and throughout the entire illness, the parents feel out of control of the destiny of their child. This feeling is very difficult to withstand; it often gives rise to other distressing reactions, such as frustration, despair, depression, and anger. The family may also have felt that much of their life-style was beyond their control during the illness, as they had to adjust many of their activities to provide care for the ill child. For example, a mother may have stopped working in order to care for the child, a father may have

Table 35-2 Assessment for Care of a Dying Child

I. Child's physical condition
  A. Prior to decision to discontinue treatment
  B. Present—length and duration of symptoms
    1. Pain
      a. Location, amount, and severity of pain
      b. Current pain medications, response to medications, and allergies
      c. Other comfort measures utilized (e.g., massage, distraction)
      d. Limitation of child's activity due to pain
      e. Limitation of parent–child contact due to pain
    2. Nutrition and hydration patterns
      a. Child's food and fluid routine—how often, how much
      b. Favorite foods and liquids or foods tolerated
      c. Food and fluid dislikes
      d. Recent changes
      e. Nausea and vomiting
      f. Family's mode of coping with feeding at the present time
      g. Current weight, weight change
      h. Swallowing ability
    3. Sleep patterns
      a. Recent changes
      b. Type of sleep: sound, restless, changes during hospitalization
      c. Support and comfort: blanket, bottle, toys, night-light, bedtime routine
    4. Elimination patterns
      a. Toilet-trained (when applicable)
      b. Urination:
        Frequency (how many diapers used, if applicable)
        Color and odor
        Foley or condom catheter
        Pain on urination
        Hematuria
        Recent changes, describe
      c. Defecation:
        Frequency
        Color and consistency
        Melena
        Pain on defecation
        Constipation—frequency, how managed
        Diarrhea—frequency, how managed
        Recent changes, describe
    5. Activity
      a. Walking, crawling, sitting
      b. Balance
      c. Amount of activity
      d. Limited by pain?
    6. Skin and mouth
      a. Turgor, color, temperature, bruises
      b. Area of breakdown or potential breakdown:
        Favorite position, place to sit, place to sleep
        Current preventive skin care
      c. Current skin care, if breakdown exists
      d. Tumor:
        Size, location
        Closed or draining
        Current care
        Painful?
      e. Mouth:
        Hydrated, dry
        Blisters
        Bleeding
    7. Respiratory status
      a. Color of skin
      b. Shortness of breath, rate and quality of respirations

Table 35-2 Assessment for Care of a Dying Child (*Continued*)

8. Neurological status
   a. Level of consciousness
   b. Speech, aphasia
   c. Seizures
   d. Paralysis
9. Special problems
   a. Vision
   b. Prosthesis

II. Emotional assessment
   A. Knowledge and understanding of child's current health status and prognosis by child, parents, siblings, extended family members
   B. Emotional status of child—from history and observation
      1. Previous
      2. Present
         a. Psychological behaviors, feelings exhibited, how often:

Angry	Anxious
Fearful	Crying
Depressed	Accepting
Calm	Flat or no affect

         b. Reaction to impending death—acceptance, denial, ambivalence
         c. Talks about illness and death with family, hospital staff
         d. Talks with family only
         e. Accepts emotional support from family, hospital staff, others
         f. Cooperates with hospital staff, parents
         g. Prefers one parent
         h. Discipline problems
   C. Emotional status of parents—from history and observation
      1. Previous
      2. Present
         a. Psychological feelings exhibited, how often:

Angry	Anxious
Fearful	Accepting
Depressed	Flat or no affect
Calm	Cries

         b. Reaction to impending death—acceptance, denial, ambivalence
         c. Talk about illness and death with child, family, hospital staff, others
         d. Accept emotional support from child, other family members, hospital staff, others
         e. Cooperate with hospital staff
   D. Emotional status of each sibling—from history and observation
      1. Previous
      2. Present
         a. Psychological feelings exhibited:

Angry	Accepting
Fearful	Flat or no affect
Depressed	Cries
Calm	Curiosity
Anxious	

         b. Reaction to impending death—acceptance, denial, ambivalence
         c. Talk about illness and death with child, parents, other siblings, hospital staff, others
         d. Relationship to dying sibling—close in age, play often, get along well
         e. Accepts emotional support from child, other family members, hospital staff, others
         f. Emotional problems relevant to disease and impending death of sibling

III. Family involvement in dying (includes child, parents, siblings, grandparents)
   A. How much involvement does family want?
   B. Does family want to provide physical care?
   C. Does family know how to provide physical care?
   D. Does family, including dying child, know signs and symptoms of impending death?
   E. Does family want to be present at time of death, stay during night?
   F. How often do siblings want to visit; do parents want siblings present at time of death?

been forced to change his job, or a mother may have had to go to work in order to cover the high cost of medical treatment. A recent study showed that during an illness one-fourth of the family's monthly income is spent on out-of-pocket, nonreimbursable expenses. These expenses include food, lodging, gasoline, clothing of different sizes, wigs, and many other items.[59]

These are only a few examples of the many changes and adjustments that a family may have to make during the illness. When the child is at the end stage of life, the nurse has the opportunity to help the parents and the child reestablish control. The nurse can begin to do this by including them in goal setting and the formulation of the nursing care plan.

Nursing care goals must be realistic. Explain that decreased healing occurs during the dying phase of a terminal illness so that the child and the parents will not become unduly distressed when, for example, a decubitus ulcer does not heal or a sore continues to drain. Stress the child's comfort as the most important goal. Goals should be simply written in terms of the child's condition or behavior "outcome"; for example, "The child will be able to move about in bed and be held by the parents without pain."

The nurse should select a quiet place where interruptions are at a minimum to discuss the care plan with the parents and also with the child if his or her age and emotional status permit. Share the plan that is developed, encourage questions, and request comments. Clarify specific nursing care measures that have been incorporated into the plan. This is very important because the child and the family may be unfamiliar with treatment measures and equipment that may be used to promote the child's comfort and well-being. Ask the parents when they will be available and what care they would like to provide. This should be noted on the child's care plan. Beds should be available for the parents so that they can stay with the child through the night if they desire. The nurse should make it clear that he or she is available to assist with the child's care whenever the parents wish.[60]

Implementing the nursing care plan *Teaching* It is important that the nurse evaluate the family's understanding of the child's care. The nurse may need to instruct the parents, the child, and the siblings in the correct way to provide care. Often, the nurse can offer suggestions that may improve the effectiveness of care provided by the family. It is important to realize that many parents feel inferior to hospital staff in their ability to perform medically oriented tasks. In addition, they may also be afraid of medical equipment and supplies. The nurse needs to anticipate these feelings and discuss them openly with the family. The nurse can support the family's desire to provide care by:

1. Providing teaching and having the parents give return demonstrations to demonstrate their competency
2. Praising the parents when they have learned a skill
3. Encouraging their involvement, pointing out that it is the parents who know the child's needs and desires better than anyone else

Information regarding the process of dying is essential for the parents and the child. Certainly, children about 10 years old and older need to know what to expect, and even children as young as 5 or 6 may ask questions about their death. Regardless of their age, all children should have their questions about death answered openly and honestly. The family should therefore receive information about the changes that occur as death approaches and about the child's changing needs. See Table 35-3.

It is helpful for the parents if the nurse asks the physician for an estimation of how long the child might live. Although no one can predict exactly when a child will die, an estimation helps the family regain some control and provides them with a time framework within which to make plans. If one or both parents want to remain in the hospital with the child, they need to arrange for the care of their other children, make arrangements regarding work, and organize their time so that they can get adequate rest and sleep during this stressful, exhausting time.

Physical care of the dying child Children who are dying of cancer often have numerous physical and mental symptoms caused by the disease process. Many of these symptoms (e.g., constipation, nausea and vomiting, temperature imbalance, and a sore mouth) can be managed using standard nursing care (see Chap. 32). The following are additional suggestions for nursing care of these routine problems as well as suggestions for specific problems related to cancer and dying. These measures may also be useful in providing care to children who are dying from other diseases.

Table 35-3 Signs and Symptoms of Approaching Death and Nursing Interventions

Signs and Symptoms	Nursing Interventions
External temperature decreases, beginning at distal extremities and progressing toward upper body; child will probably not feel cold; skin color may be pale, gray, bluish.	Offer to cover child with lightweight, loose-fitting bedding.
Internal temperature may increase.	Use lightweight blanket or sheet; have fresh circulating air in room.
Loss of sensation and movement, beginning in lower extremities and progressing toward upper body.	Use loose clothing and bedding; child may prefer no clothing; gentle change of positioning.
Decrease in muscle tone with resultant inability to swallow and cough, urinary and fecal incontinence, mouth breathing.	Atropine sulfate may be used to decrease oropharyngeal secretions; suctioning may be used; place absorbent padding under child if incontinent; give frequent mouth care.
Difficulty breathing, shortness of breath or "air hunger"; respirations may increase, then become shallow and irregular; Cheyne-Stokes respirations may occur.	Place child on side, head elevated and firmly supported; may administer oxygen.
Senses decrease; although vision and speech may cease, hearing may continue until death; although tactile sensation decreases, touch may become annoying.	Encourage family to continue communicating with child by speech until death; if child is comfortable, family and nurse should continue holding, caressing, touching child until death; if child is uncomfortable, it may be appropriate to stop bed baths and bed and clothing changes.
Child may indicate pain by restlessness and verbal utterances even when comatose; if in deep coma, probably will not feel pain.	Be alert for signs of pain and treat with pain medication.
Eyes may become sunken or bulging.	If child is comatose, place moist bandage over bulging eyes to prevent corneal drying and subsequent corneal ulceration.
Loss or faintness of pedal and radial pulses; apical pulse may become more rapid, then slower, irregular, and difficult to auscultate.	

Pain One of the areas of greatest concern for parents and children is pain. Pain is not new to dying children and their families. These children often experience pain associated with diagnostic or treatment procedures or the disease itself. The pain may become chronic. Many children with cancer also experience a sudden onset of severe pain in their final days of life. Past and current experiences and the anticipation of future pain can increase anxiety and fear in both the child and the family. Many terminal care facilities find that pain can be controlled effectively during the dying phase. These agencies give pain control top priority in providing comfort care.[61,62,63,64]

The most successful pain control is accomplished using a 24-h, around-the-clock schedule (see Table 35-4). This includes a hypnotic and a mood changer in addition to a narcotic. The around-the-clock schedule is used to prevent the fear-pain-anxiety cycle.[65,66] This cycle can occur if the child takes a pain medication that does not take effect for $\frac{1}{2}$ to $\frac{3}{4}$ h. After the medication takes effect, the child may worry about when the pain will begin again or about the period between the onset of pain and the time the next dose will provide relief. The fear and anxiety created by concern about the *next* pain often increase the *current* pain. When the child experiences this repetitive cycle, the usual dose of an analgesic is often inadequate for pain control. Unfortunately, this cycle occurs frequently, leading to more pain and increased dosages of medication.

It is essential that nurses get to know dying children well in order to evaluate and assess their complaints of pain. All health professionals and parents are aware that children can and do use pain to manipulate those around them and to get attention. Dying children often have real physical pain, which is aggravated by the knowledge that they are dying. Nurses must be very sensitive toward dying children who are in pain. They must be ready to administer around-the-clock total pain coverage, which will provide these chil-

Table 35-4 Around-the-Clock, 24-h Medication Schedules*

Medication	Dose	Route	Time
Dolophine (methadone hydrochloride)	0.7 mg/kg per day in 4 to 6 divided doses	PO	Every 6 to 8 h
Benadryl (diphenhydramine hydrochloride)	5 mg/kg per day in 4 divided doses	PO	Every 4 h
Vistaril (hydroxyzine pamoate)	2 to 5 mg/kg per hour in divided doses every 6 h and/or at bedtime	PO	HS: 7 pm

*Doses given in this table are minimum safe doses. The amount of pain medication given will vary greatly with the degree of pain, and drug tolerance and will need to be individually titrated to control pain and keep side effects of the drug at an acceptable level.

dren with physical and emotional comfort so that they can be active and alert and enjoy their final days with their loved ones.

Many different medications have been used successfully with children who are dying from cancer. Narcotics are usually necessary for moderate to severe pain in the final days. Tylenol (acetaminophen) with codeine, Demerol (meperidine hydrochloride), Dilaudid (hydromorphone), Dolophine (methadone hydrochloride), and morphine sulfate are examples of effective narcotics. All these drugs may be taken orally, the route preferred by children. Methadone hydrochloride has been used increasingly recently because it can be taken orally and is effective for 6 to 8 h. Specific dosage ranges of these drugs for achieving pain control in dying children have not yet been firmly established. Depending on the duration of the use of the drug and the child's physical and emotional reaction to pain, a much higher dosage than was given previously might be needed to achieve complete relief.

In order to assist the physician in planning pain management, the nurse needs to closely observe the child's response to medications. The parents can be very helpful in assessing pain relief because they know the child well. The nurse may need to alert the physician that the child's pain is not sufficiently controlled and that the child is still caught in the fear-pain-anxiety cycle. The child may need a large "loading" dose of a medication to break the cycle. Medications that are sometimes given in conjunction with around-the-clock pain medications to facilitate sleep include Vistaril (hydroxyzine pamoate), Benadryl (diphenhydramine hydrochloride), chloral hydrate, and phenobarbital. Tranquilizers such as doxepin hydrochloride and diazepam are also used.

The side effects of pain medications can be adequately controlled; they are a secondary consideration in the care of a dying child. Some parents and children express concern over the sedative effect of high doses of narcotics. In many instances, this sedation decreases after extended use of the drugs. The nurse should assist the family in discussing these concerns with the physician.

The following are additional measures that may be used when pain is mild or when emotional anxiety appears to cause more intense pain:

1. Changes in the room temperature and removal of some of the bedding or clothing; dying children often prefer little or no bedding or clothing.
2. Diversion with games, reading books, and visits from siblings or friends.
3. A change of environment, such as a wheelchair trip outdoors or to the hospital cafeteria.
4. A partial or total body massage; touching conveys closeness, caring, and love.
5. Muscle relaxation techniques, such as those used in yoga or for childbirth preparation.
6. Changes in equipment, such as a water bed, an alternating-pressure mattress, a gel flotation pad, or a foam mattress.

Some innovative methods of pain control that are being investigated and tested, such as hypnosis,[67,68] acupuncture, and electrical stimulation, may prove effective for dying children. Surgical procedures, such as a chordotomy, may also be used to control pain.

Bleeding Children with cancers that affect the bone marrow, such as leukemia and lymphoma, or children who have had chemotherapy are susceptible to bleeding. Although major hemorrhage is most often feared by parents and children, a more common problem is slight but persistent bleeding from the nose, mouth, or rectum.

Measures that can be utilized to stop the bleeding include:

1. Applying an ice pack over the bleeding area
2. Applying reasonable pressure by hand to the bleeding area
3. Using packing such as Gelfoam or gauze for epistaxis
4. Applying topical thrombin to the bleeding site
5. Applying salt pork to the nose and tea bags to bleeding gums

Measures to control bleeding may not be effective during the advanced stage of a disease. The nurse should share this information with the family.

Additional comfort measures for the child who is bleeding include:

1. Providing a good supply of tissues, towels, or disposable diapers to absorb the blood.
2. Quickly removing soiled tissues and linen from the child's environment.
3. Keeping the clothing and bedding clean in order to decrease the child's anxiety about the amount of blood lost.
4. Using a large basin rather than an emesis basin if the child is vomiting blood. This is more efficient and makes it easier to keep the child clean.

Transfusions of blood products may be used if the family so desires. See Chaps. 23 and 32 for further discussions of nursing management of the child who is receiving transfusions of blood products.

Respiratory Needs Respiratory pattern changes can occur as a result of tumor metastasis, infection, and fluid retention. Many families are afraid that their child will die while choking or fighting for breath. Respiratory difficulty can therefore create great anxiety in the parents and the child. The nurse needs to remain calm and reassuring and institute comfort measures that are designed to alleviate respiratory difficulty. Measures that improve respiration include:

1. Placing the child in an upright position
2. Increasing the moisture in the room air by using a humidifier
3. Suctioning
4. Using oxygen

Suctioning should be used judiciously because it often causes discomfort and anxiety that can further interfere with respiration. When oxygen is used, children and their families feel comforted because something is being done for the child. Children sometimes prefer nasal prongs to a face mask. Children who fear a face mask should be told that they can put it in their lap and hold it up to their face when they want to use it.

Seizures Children with leukemia or with brain tumors or tumors that metastasize to the brain, such as neuroblastomas, may develop seizures at any point during their illness. They often exhibit seizures when they are close to death; these seizures may be almost constant. Many parents and children express a desire for the child to be alert during the final days. Anticonvulsant medications may produce drowsiness, especially when they are used in conjunction with analgesics or tranquilizers. The nurse should alert the physician to the family's concern so that a medication regimen that produces the least amount of sedation can be provided. Sometimes families are willing to have the child experience numerous mild seizures in order to maintain the child's mental alertness.

Seizures are frightening to most people. If there is a possibility that the child will develop seizures, the nurse should tell the child and the parents what to expect and what to do in the event of a seizure. See Chap. 30 for a discussion of care of the child who has seizures.

Inadequate Nutrition and/or Hydration When children are in the dying phase of an illness, good nutrition is unlikely to prolong life. The child should therefore be allowed to eat what he or she wants, when he or she wants to eat it. The parents should be encouraged by the hospital staff to help in the preparation of the child's favorite foods.

During the last days of life, the dying child usually greatly decreases or stops eating and may drink only sips of fluid. Children often find the infusion of intravenous fluids painful and confining. Although it is traditional to use intravenous fluids for hydration of children who are dying in the hospital, the child or the parent may request that they be discontinued. It is important to honor this request. Conversely, the family may request intravenous fluids to increase the child's comfort.

Mouth Sores When children decrease their oral intake, their mouths may become dry and sore; cracks and blisters of the lips can also occur. A frequent problem for children with leukemia is superficial hematomas on the lips. These lesions are painful and may ooze blood.

The nurse should first try to treat these problems with standard measures such as petroleum jelly and normal saline or normal saline with bicarbonate mouth rinses. Additional measures to treat unrelieved pain include the use of topical agents such as viscous Xylocaine, Cetacaine, or a mixture of Kaopectate and Benadryl or milk of magnesia and Benadryl. Elixir of Benadryl (diphenhydramine hydrochloride) and mild narcotics may be used systemically.

Constipation Constipation is a common problem that may be caused by a combination of factors, such as inactivity, poor nutrition, and certain chemotherapeutic and analgesic medications. The nurse should be alert for the possible development of constipation and should institute treatment immediately. Diet changes and laxatives are often successful.

Enemas and digital removal of stool are usually avoided in children who are highly susceptible to bleeding and infection, but may be used if the child is experiencing pain caused by constipation or impaction. These procedures should be performed carefully and gently.

Skin Care Dying children are highly susceptible to skin breakdown because of their poor nutritional status, decreased physical activity, and neurological problems and because of the effects of chemotherapy on tissue repair. Preventive measures such as frequent turning, repositioning, skin massage, and the use of mechanical appliances such as an alternating-pressure mattress or heel protectors should be continued throughout the child's life. However, many children during the final days before death assume a specific posture of comfort and refuse to be moved. The dying child should be allowed to remain in this position if it provides comfort, and skin breakdown problems should be treated as they occur. It is important that the nurse teach the family that healing will probably be inadequate because of the advanced disease process and that comfort is the most important consideration.

Eye Care Tumors of the brain and cancers that metastasize to the brain can cause eye problems, such as crossed eyes, difficulty with vision, blindness, and protrusion of the eye from the socket. The latter may be caused by a tumor behind the eye, which presses the eye forward. Because of pressure on the lacrimal gland, the eye may not be adequately moistened. Artificial tears or normal saline should be applied to the eye as often as necessary. If the child cannot see or does not mind eye patches, the eye may be closed, and saline patches applied.

Activity Children should be encouraged to remain active for as long as possible. Activity will help maintain emotional health and prevent the physical complications of skin breakdown, constipation, and muscle weakness or tightening. The hospital should have a liberal pass policy that enables the child to leave the premises for brief periods. It is ideal if the hospital permits a nurse to accompany the child on brief visits home if the family feels that a nurse would be helpful to them. Dying children often want to go home "one more time," sometimes to say good-bye.

Emotional Care The emotional needs of dying children continue until the moment of death. Although children vary as greatly as adults in their acceptance of dying and their use of coping strategies, the nurse can anticipate some common basic emotional needs.

All dying children need to know that they are loved and cherished and will be missed after they die. A nurse who has a special, loving relationship with a child should feel free to express feelings of love for this child and sadness at the impending loss of the child. Dying children need to share in honest and open communication that creates a relationship of trust. Nurses can help families provide for these needs by establishing honest communication at the time of diagnosis and maintaining it throughout the dying period.

The question "Am I dying?" may be very difficult for the nurse or a parent to answer. Children deserve an honest answer and will know when the hospital staff or the family are being deceptive. Dying children need to know that they will be able to die in comfort, free of pain, and surrounded by the people and things they love. Liberal ward policies that allow families to room in, siblings and pets to visit, and toys to be brought from home will enhance the child's emotional comfort in the final days.

Dying children need to know that they will be supported by those they love through the moment of death. Children of all ages fear abandonment throughout their illness and especially at death. They may have already experienced changes in their relationships with their friends and relatives, who often become more distant in their relationships because they find it too difficult to be in frequent contact with the child and the family. Children who have already experienced these losses may fear that others will abandon them too. The hospital staff should assist the family to remain close to the child. Touching conveys closeness and warmth without words. The parents of a dying child should be permitted and encouraged to lie in the child's bed, holding and comforting the child. A parent can easily change positions if a treatment is necessary.

Other people in the hospital who are important to the child should also be encouraged to visit. Other patients on the ward who may themselves be dying can be especially helpful to the dying child and also to the parents. In addition, if these children are encouraged and allowed to visit other dying children, they will learn that they too will not be abandoned when they die.

Dying children are often placed in private rooms. However, private rooms are not always necessary. The child may want to be near friends, and the parents may benefit from the support of the other parents in the room. When the parents of a dying child request that the child remain in a "nonprivate" room, the nurse should speak with the parents of the other children and assess their feelings and those of their children. The nurse can then make a decision on the basis of the needs of everyone in the room.

Comfortable Environment Although the hospital can never be as comfortable as the child's home, many steps can be taken to make the environment as comfortable as possible. Throughout the illness, painful procedures and treatments should be performed in a treatment room away from the child's room. There should be a telephone in the child's room to help the child maintain contact with family and friends. The child should wear his or her own clothes and be encouraged to continue with normal activities as long as possible.

The child and the family will need to have adequate privacy to rest and relax, to share special feelings, and just to be alone as a family unit. The hospital environment is very noisy, highly stimulating, and demanding. It is emotionally exhausting for both the child and the family. Privacy helps limit stress from the environment at this very difficult time. Together, the nurse and the family can decide on time periods during which no treatments or procedures will be performed. If the child is in a private room, a sign can be placed on the door limiting entrance to only those persons who first check with the nurse. The nurse should also ask the parents whether they would prefer to be alone with their child at the time of death, or immediately thereafter, and communicate the parents' wishes to the ward staff.

Control The child and the parents suffer from the sense of loss of control. Active participation in care and decision making will help them gain some control over the situation. Throughout the illness and at the time of death, the nurse can find many opportunities for the child to make choices and participate in his or her own care.

Two important decisions that the child should participate in are the cessation of treatment and the choice of place of death. The dying child may also be permitted to choose the intravenous site, clothes to wear, foods to eat, whether to stay up all night, and when to get out of bed. If the child makes requests that seem unreasonable, the nurse should listen carefully, and if the nurse evaluates these requests as signs of the child's effort to regain control, they should be granted, if possible.

Information Information is very important during the dying process. The child can better cope with death when the fear of the unknown is decreased. The nurse should begin by eliciting the child's preconceived ideas about the act of dying and by correcting misconceptions. The nurse can then ask what questions the child has about dying.

Small children usually ask whether their parents will be with them when they die. The nurse might therefore want the parents present at these discussions so that they can reassure the child. Older children—those about 8 or 9 years of age and older—may want to know whether they will suffocate, have pain, or be conscious or unconscious at death. The nurse should answer these questions honestly, while also giving reassurance that everything will be done to keep them comfortable. Dying children should be told that someone will always be with them, and this promise must be kept.

Needs of Parents and Siblings Just as the child needs emotional support, so does the family. The nurse should get to know the family well in order to provide support according to their individual needs. The nurse's consistent interest and willingness to answer questions and to be involved in the family's sorrow can be very supportive. Often the best help the nurse can offer is a willingness to listen, regardless of when or how long. Sharing in the parents' anticipatory grieving and acknowledging that the nurse, too, loves and will miss the child are helpful.

Many parents are reluctant to leave their child's side or to sleep. They want to spend every remaining minute with their child and be present when the child dies. The emotional and physical strain that the parents experience is exhausting; the nurse should encourage them to rest. The nurse should offer to help find someone (perhaps a relative or a neighbor) to sit with the child while the parents sleep, assuring them that he or she will awaken them if any changes occur.

Many parents worry about their other children and feel that they are neglected at times during the illness. Siblings should be involved as much as possible in the family's and the dying child's activities.

Intervention after death occurs Many bereaved persons have remarked about their feelings during the period immediately after their loved one dies in the hospital. They often complain that they were not allowed enough time to be with their loved one after the death. Acceptance of death begins when the bereaved person sees the reality of the dead body. Parents who are allowed to remain with their dead child—to hold, touch, cry over, and say good-bye to the child—can begin to accept the reality of the death.

When children die at home, it is not unusual for the parents and siblings to sit with the dead child for 1 h or more. This experience should also be possible when the child dies in the hospital. The parents should be allowed to call in other family members who wish to see the child a last time. The nurse should be supportive of the family members' desires. They may want the nurse to sit with them, or they may ask to be left alone. The hospital should provide something to eat and drink before they leave.

The nurse who has established a good relationship with the family should attend the funeral, if at all possible. A follow-up visit to the home several weeks after the death or, minimally, a phone call to inquire about the family should be made. Some hospitals now have bereavement follow-up programs; the nurse calls or visits the family once a month for a year and on special days, such as the child's birthday and the anniversary of the death. The nurse can be helpful to the family during their grief by listening, answering questions, being willing to talk about the child (often others will not be able to), and making referrals if the family needs additional physical or emotional support.

Home care of the dying child

Care that facilitates the child's dying near loved ones in the familiar home surrounding is becoming increasingly available in the United States. Several hospice and home care programs for children are now in operation; these are based on the Martinson model, developed in the late 1970s and early 1980s.[69] Home care programs, in which visiting nurses and public health nurses work with physicians, make it possible for families to care for their children at home until the time of death.

Once the family and hospital staff have decided that treatment is to be discontinued, the family should have the option of choosing where the child will die. Many children request to return home. Frequently, the parents also want the child to be at home so that they can reunite the family. At this critical time, the other siblings also need their parents' presence. Brothers and sisters are usually fearful and upset about what is happening to their ill sibling. They need support and reassurance from their parents. The parents may also wish to re-create some normalcy in their lives. Home care enables the family members to reestablish considerable control over their lives, as the parents once again assume their role as primary caretakers of the child and managers of their household.[70] It may also facilitate the parents' adaptation following the child's death.[71,72]

Despite these important needs, the parents may be afraid to take their child home to die. They may fear that they are incapable of learning treatments and technical procedures, that they will give inadequate care, or that they will not be able to handle the actual death. They may fear the pressure of neighbors, relatives, and sometimes even health professionals, who may say that having a dying child at home is too much of a strain on the parents and may emotionally damage the siblings.

The hospital nurse can counsel the family that is considering home care for their dying child. Dying at home is a reasonable alternative to dying in the hospital. The nurse should address the fears the family is likely to have regarding home care, but the positive aspects should also be identified. The nurse needs also to explain the philosophy of quality home care and the services that are available so that the family can make a well-informed decision.

Philosophy of home care The home care team for the dying child usually consists of the parents, the home care nurse, and the physician. In order to enable the family members to regain control over their lives, a quality home care program must be structured so that the parents are the primary caregivers for the child. The professional must recognize the parents' need to be in control and must facilitate this in every possible manner.

The home care nurse functions primarily as a consultant to the family. The nurse assesses the child, discusses a care plan with the parents, teaches the family, provides emotional support, assesses medication effectiveness, and identifies equipment and supply needs. The nurse is a liaison between the family and the physician, other health care professionals, and health agencies. In addition, the nurse provides physical care, if the family desires, and medication, equipment, and supplies when necessary.

Quality home care ensures that the nurse is available to the family by telephone 24 h a day, 7 days a week, and that the nurse visits whenever and for whatever reason the family deems necessary. If the child is readmitted to the hospital, either temporarily or to die, the nurse continues to visit the family if they desire.

After discontinuation of active treatment, the home care physician generally functions as a consultant to the family. The physician is readily available to answer questions, make recommendations for care, or see the child if the parents or the nurse feel that the physician's opinion on the child's current status is needed. The physician also assures the family that readmission to the hospital is always an option.

Parents who take their child home to die often fluctuate from great confidence to ambivalence about their decision and their abilities. Home care programs organized as described above give parents a great deal of physical and emotional support. Whether the parents succeed in keeping the child home until death or decide to readmit the child, the time spent at home can be of great emotional benefit to the child and the whole family.

Assessment for home care *Hospital nurse assessment* Once the family has decided to take the child home, the hospital nurse should anticipate the physical and emotional care needs that the child will have at home in order to identify the teaching needs of he family. Once the decision is made to discontinue treatment, the family usually wants to leave the hospital immediately in order to spend as much time with the child at home as possible. The time for discharge teaching during hospitalization may be very limited; thus teaching should be started early. The parents' participation in the care of the child during the entire illness facilitates teaching them in preparation for going home.

The hospital nurse, either in conjunction with a home care coordinator or independently, should initiate a home care referral and, if possible, should have the home care nurse visit the child in the hospital. This enables the home care nurse to meet the family, observe teaching, and consult with the hospital staff. The family's needs can be discussed, and a home care plan can be developed that is consistent with the care given in the hospital.

Home care nurse assessment The home care nurse should telephone the parents on the day they take the child home and visit either that day or the next day. Because there are many differences between the home and the hospital setting, the nurse should complete a total family assessment. An assessment of the family's teaching needs should be made during the initial visit. The nurse then develops nursing diagnoses and establishes long- and short-term care goals for home care. See the Nursing Care Plan at the end of this chapter.

Planning home nursing care The process of developing a care plan differs when the parents are the primary caregivers and the nurse is the consultant. The home care nurse needs to inform the parents of the discharge recommendations sent by the hospital staff and of the nurse's recommendations for care based on the assessment. The parents, the child, and the nurse should discuss these recommendations and the care that the family desires for the child. A nursing care plan is then developed by the family and the nurse together.

There should be a clear understanding of who is to provide the care. If the family desires, the nurse can be included as a physical caregiver. Fathers are often excluded from care during hospitalization, and even at home, because they work outside the home. The nurse should encourage the father to assume specific care duties when he is not working. This will enable him to spend time with the child and provide support for the mother. If the family desires, the care plan can be written and left in the home. Parents also usually want to maintain flowcharts on which the child's status and the care given are recorded. The nurse's willingness to assist in any way and his or her around-the-clock availability should be made clear during this initial visit with the family as well as during subsequent visits. Knowing that the nurse is there to assist them whenever needed, regardless of the time or the apparent importance of the request, is very important and reassuring to the family members.

The concept of comfort care should be discussed at the initial visit. The nurse may need to explain the wide range of comfort care measures so that the family will know what is available at home. Comfort care at home can include medical measures such as intravenous fluids, oxygen, hypnosis, and hyperalimentation. Medications such as analgesics, psychotropics, anticonvulsants, steroids, antipruritics, antidiarrheals, and antipyretics may also be used.

The goals that the family and the nurse set depend on the child's life expectancy. If the child is expected to live for several months, disease-preventive and health-maintenance goals are appropriate. If the child's life expectancy is several days or a week, however, the child's comfort should be the only concern.

Implementing home care *Teaching* If the child's life expectancy is very short, the home care nurse should provide essential teaching about physical care during the initial visit.

The nurse should also begin, as soon as possible, to discuss what the dying process is like and to inquire about funeral arrangements. In many counties the county coroner must investigate deaths which occur outside a hospital or other institution where death is common. The home care nurse can help the family avoid the necessity of a police investigation in the home, which might involve the removal of the body to the county coroner's office for examination. With the family's permission, the nurse can call the medical examiner's or the coroner's office and say that the child is expected to die and that the home care physician will sign the death certificate. The nurse should also notify the funeral home of these arrangements. If the child's life expectancy is longer, e.g., several months, the nurse should discuss these topics when appropriate.

Home visits Once the home care tasks have been assumed by the various members of the family, the nurse can determine how often visits are needed. The frequency of visits depends on the condition of the child (Fig. 35-1). A child with a brain tumor who will live for 6 months might need only weekly visits after the initial assessment, planning, and teaching visits. If the child is in the final days of life, visits may be made every day, and more often if the family desires.

Physical care The provision of comfort care in the home is very similar to the provision of this care in the hospital. With the following few exceptions, the principles of hospital care of a dying child can be applied in the home.

Hospital equipment such as suction machines and alternating-pressure mattresses may be difficult to obtain. Equipment that can be borrowed for a brief time may be available in the community or surrounding communities.

Blood products are not commonly given in the home. The child may, however, go to an outpatient clinic or hospital emergency room in order to receive transfusions.

Emotional care of the child The child's greatest emotional need, to be surrounded by and cared for by the ones he or she loves, can be fulfilled when the child is cared for at home. The home care nurse is often not very involved with younger children, who usually prefer to be cared for by their parents. Older children and teenagers often strive to maintain their independence from their parents throughout the dying period at home. They are therefore usually more willing than young children to accept the nurse's involvement and assistance with their emotional needs.

The child who is dying at home has the same emotional concerns as the child who is dying in the hospital. The child may be fearful, depressed, or angry. (See the section "Emotional Care.")

The fear of abandonment does not disappear because the child is at home, although the possibility of abandonment is lessened when the family is together at home. The child still needs to be reassured that the family will always be close at hand. The nurse can offer to stay with

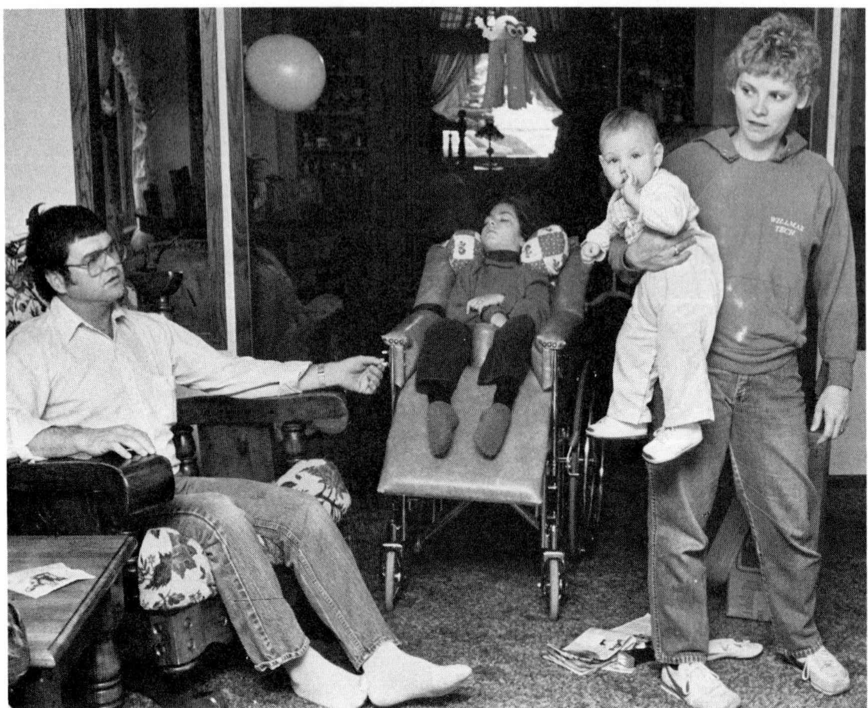

Figure 35-1 Leah, who is comatose as a result of a rare immunologic disease, is brought into the living room for social stimulation from her parents and sister. (*Photo used with permission of Minneapolis Star and Tribune.*)

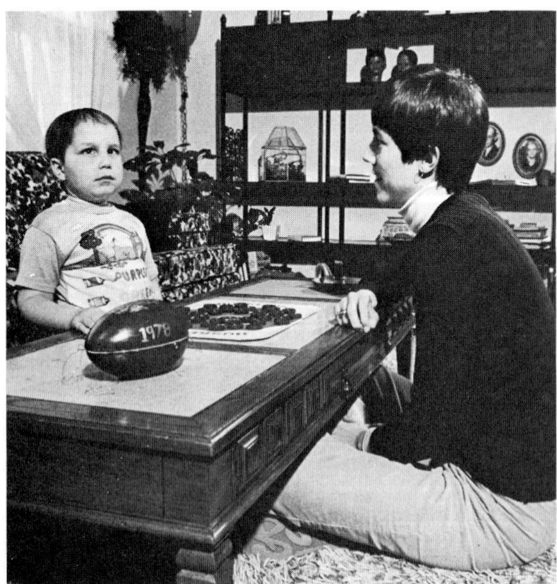

Figure 35-2 Jeremy, aged 8, at home with his home care nurse. (*From the film Time to Come Home, produced by Ida M. Martinson and Kenneth D. Greer.*)

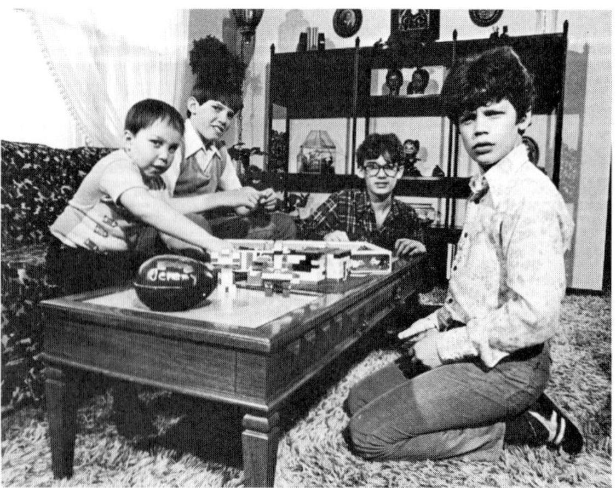

Figure 35-3 Jeremy, aged 8, and his brothers at home. (*From the film Time to Come Home, produced by Ida M. Martinson and Kenneth D. Greer.*)

the child while the parents rest or sleep or get away from the house for a while (Fig. 35-2).

Privacy is sometimes a problem if numerous friends and relatives wish to visit. The nurse can assist with this by suggesting that a sign be posted on the front door listing convenient visiting times.

Emotional needs of the parents and siblings The parents need the emotional support provided by the nurse's consistent interest and concern. Many parents also need reassurance throughout the home care period that they made the correct decision in taking their child home to die and that they are providing the best possible care. These parents are highly susceptible to feelings of guilt and remorse, and they need to be reassured repeatedly that they have made the correct decision for their family.

Home care can be exhausting. The nurse should help the family members plan for daily rest, sleep, and exercise.

As in the hospital, the siblings should be involved as much as possible, either providing direct care or helping by entertaining the dying child (Fig. 35-3). The siblings also need open and honest communication. They are astute and will be aware of the changes in the child and of the impending death. A trusting relationship with their family and the nurse is very important at this time.

Intervention after death occurs The family's need for emotional support continues through the many months that follow the child's death. The home care nurse should attend the funeral and participate in other burial activities and visit the family during the first week after the death. The nurse should telephone the family during the month and make a home visit 1 month after the child's death. If the family-nurse relationship is good, the nurse should continue visiting once a month for a year, or at least 6 and 12 months after the child's death.

Depression, guilt, anger, relief, low energy, and social isolation are but a few of the feelings and problems that the family members may experience in the months following the death of the child. The nurse can assist the family members by helping them cope with these feelings and problems or by referring them to a parent support group or a professional counselor.

Nursing Care Plan: Terminal Illness

Patient: Patty Gary **Age:** 8 years

ASSESSMENT HISTORY

Patty Gary is 8 years old. Her family consists of her mother, stepfather, and brothers, aged 4 and 6 years. Patty was first admitted to the hospital $1\frac{1}{2}$ years ago with symptoms of ataxia and petit mal seizures. A neuroblastoma with metastases to the brain and spine was diagnosed. During her first admission, a ventriculoperitoneal shunt was inserted to relieve intracranial pressure, and the maximum dose of radiation was given to the brain. Ten courses of chemotherapy were completed during the subsequent year.

Fourteen months after diagnosis, Patty demonstrated vomiting, irritability, and weakness in both lower extremities; she reported severe headaches. A repeat CT scan revealed recurring metastases. The physicians decided that cure-oriented therapy would no longer help Patty. This was discussed with Patty and her parents. The family decided that Patty should return home and that treatment should consist of supportive care to relieve her symptoms. At the time of discharge, Patty had no bowel or bladder control, weakness in both lower extremities, and a poor appetite, and she was very irritable.

A referral to the local community health nursing agency was made in anticipation of Patty's return home. The agency began visits immediately and provided 24-h coverage 7 days a week. Patty's family cared for her with the assistance of the community health nurses for 4 months. Although Patty became progressively worse, her family wanted to keep her at home as long as possible. Her illness advanced rapidly, resulting in total paralysis from the waist down and periods of unconsciousness lasting 1 or 2 days.

Patty's mother found it increasingly difficult to care for Patty at home and also care for other members of the family. The family's severe financial difficulties forced Mr. Gary to obtain a second job. Thus, he was not often able to assist his wife in caring for Patty or the other children. Signs of physical and emotional exhaustion were evident in Mrs. Gary. Last week, the community health nurse expressed her concerns about Mrs. Gary's ability to continue Patty's care at home. A long discussion followed. Mrs. Gary tearfully stated that she wanted Patty to spend her last days at home. The nurse offered to come daily and to arrange for a licensed practical nurse to come two nights a week to allow Mrs. Gary to get some needed rest.

Nursing Diagnosis	Outcome Criteria	Nursing Interventions	Evaluation and Modifications
1. Pain related to disease process	☐ Patty will indicate relief from pain and headache.	☐ Administer analgesic, as ordered. ☐ See nursing actions for impaired mobility, below.	☐ Obtains relief from analgesic administered q6h. ☐ Continue plan.
2. Impaired mobility related to lower extremity paralysis	☐ Skin will remain intact. ☐ Lower extremity muscles will remain firm and toned.	☐ Turn q1h when in bed. ☐ Use alternating-pressure mattress.	☐ Skin is smooth and intact. ☐ Muscles remain firm.

Nursing Diagnosis	Outcome Criteria	Nursing Interventions	Evaluation and Modifications
	☐ Joints of lower extremities will retain range of motion.	☐ When out of bed, use reclining wheelchair with flotation pad at least tid. ☐ Do range-of-motion exercises to all joints in both lower extremities, qid.	☐ Full flexion of lower extremities is possible with passive exercise. ☐ Continue plan.
3. Urinary incontinence related to paralysis	☐ Bladder will be sufficiently drained. ☐ Urine will be clear. ☐ Body temperature will be within normal limits.	☐ Use Foley catheter (No. 10) to straight drainage. ☐ Irrigate catheter with Renacidin, 50 to 100 ml, prn, if clogged. ☐ Change catheter once a week.	☐ Catheter is draining properly. ☐ No bladder distention is present. ☐ Urinary output averages within 200 ml of fluid intake. ☐ Urine is clear and pale straw color; nonodoriferous. ☐ Continue plan.
4. Bowel incontinence related to paralysis	☐ Patty will have a soft, formed bowel movement every 2 or 3 days.	☐ Give dioctyl sodium sulfosuccinate, 70 mg, PO, qd. ☐ Use a bisacodyl rectal suppository every third day if no bowel movement. ☐ Give pediatric (67.5 ml) sodium biphosphate–sodium phosphate enema and do digital removal, prn.	☐ No bowel movement for 3 days; suppositories ineffective. Enema yielded good amount of moderately hard stool. ☐ Continue plan.
5. Nutritional deficit related to poor appetite and disease process	☐ Daily caloric intake will be between 1800 and 2400 kcal.	☐ Offer small amounts of food frequently (Patty likes chocolate milk shakes, lemon soda, pickles, and spaghetti); do not force food. ☐ Administer nutrients via nasogastric feeding tube when Patty is unconscious.	☐ Eats only a few bites of food at a time. ☐ Average oral intake is 1000 kcal per day. ☐ Continue plan.
6. Fluid volume deficit related to poor appetite and disease process	☐ Daily fluid intake will be between 1500 and 1800 ml. ☐ Mucous membranes will be moist. ☐ Skin turgor will be good.	☐ Offer small sips of fluid frequently; offer popsicles. ☐ Administer supplemental IV fluids as ordered or prn. ☐ Administer mouth care with glycerin swabs and mouthwash at least qid. ☐ Apply petrolatum to lips, prn.	☐ Average oral fluid intake is 750 ml per day; requires supplemental IV fluids. ☐ Continue plan.
7. Periodic loss of consciousness related to disease process	☐ Clear respiratory passage will permit adequate ventilation; corneas will remain moist.	☐ Monitor vital signs. ☐ Check gag and swallow reflexes when awake q1h. ☐ Check corneal reflex q4h. ☐ Instill lubricating agent in both eyes, prn.	☐ Respiratory passages are clear on ausculation. ☐ Corneas remain moist. ☐ Continue plan.
	☐ Patty will not be injured.		

Nursing Diagnosis	Outcome Criteria	Nursing Interventions	Evaluation and Modifications
		☐ Keep both padded siderails up, unless responsible adult is at bedside. ☐ Provide supportive physical care as specified elsewhere in plan.	
8. Anticipatory grief of parents related to Patty's impending death	☐ Parents will verbalize their questions, concerns, and feelings with nurse. ☐ Parents will be able to provide care for Patty.	☐ Allow parents to provide as much of Patty's care as they are able to. ☐ Provide a private place and time for parents to discuss their feelings. ☐ Encourge parents to spend time with their sons. ☐ Encourage siblings to participate in Patty's care. ☐ Explain signs of death when parents are ready for this information.	☐ Parents able to express grief and feelings. ☐ Parents continue to provide Patty's care.
9. Financial stress related to medical expenses	☐ Family will receive any financial assistance for which they are eligible.	☐ Refer parents to hospital social worker.	☐ Parents met with social worker; applications for financial assistance were filed.
10. Sleep deprivation and exhaustion in Patty's mother related to caring for Patty for 24 h a day	☐ Patty's mother will receive help caring for Patty.	☐ Arrange for daily visits by registered nurse. ☐ Arrange for visits by licensed practical nurse twice a week.	☐ Mother is regaining her physical and emotional strength. ☐ Continue plan.

References

1. *Cancer Facts and Figures,* American Cancer Society, New York, 1984, p. 22.
2. Martinson, M., and G. D. Armstrong, "Death, Dying and Terminal Care: Dying at Home," in J. Kellerman (ed.), *Psychological Aspects of Childhood Cancer,* Charles C. Thomas, Springfield, Ill., 1980, p. 2.
3. Kastenbaum, R., "The Child's Understanding of Death: How Does It Develop?" in E. A. Grollman (ed.), *Explaining Death to Children,* Beacon Press, Boston, 1967, p. 94.
4. Easson, W. M., *The Dying Child,* Charles C. Thomas, Springfield, Ill., 1970, p. 24.
5. Ibid., p. 31.
6. Green-Epner, C. S., "The Dying Child," in R. E. Caughill (ed.), *The Dying Patient: A Supportive Approach,* Little, Brown, Boston, 1976, p. 131.
7. Pattison, E. M., *The Experience of Dying,* Prentice-Hall, Englewood Cliffs, N.J., 1977, pp. 20–22.
8. Nagy, M., "The Child's Theories concerning Death." *Journal of General Psychology* **73**:3 (1978).
9. Easson, op. cit., pp. 32–33.
10. Nagy, op. cit., p. 32.
11. Kastenbaum, op. cit., p. 103.
12. Piaget, J., *The Child's Conception of the World,* Routledge, London, 1929.
13. Gyulay, J., *The Dying Child,* McGraw-Hill, New York, 1978, p. 20.
14. Hostler, S. L., "The Development of the Child's Concept of Death," in Olle Jane Sahler (ed.), *The Child and Death,* Mosby, St. Louis, 1978, p. 20.
15. Kastenbaum, loc. cit.
16. Speece, M. W., and S. B. Brent, "Children's Understand-

ing of Death: A Review of Three Components of a Death Concept," *Child Development* **55**:1671–1686 (1984).
17. Raimbault, G., "Children Talk about Death," *Acta Paediatrica Scandindinavica* **70**:179–182 (1981).
18. Zeligs, R. (ed.), *Children's Experience with Death,* Charles C. Thomas, Springfield, Ill., 1974, p. 26.
19. Johnson-Soderberg, S., "The Development of a Child's Concept of Death," *Oncology Nursing Forum* **8**:23–26 (1981).
20. Morrissey, J. R., "Death Anxiety in Children with a Fatal Illness," in H. J. Parad (ed.), *Crisis Intervention,* Family Service Association of America, New York, 1965, pp. 324–338.
21. Natterson, J. M., and A. G. Knudson, "Observations concerning Fear of Death in Fatally Ill Children and Their Mothers," *Psychosomatic Medicine* **22**:456–465 (1960).
22. Waechter, E. H., "Children's Awareness of Fatal Illness," *American Journal of Nursing* **71**:1168–1172 (1971).
23. Blubond-Langner, M., *The Private Worlds of Dying Children,* Princeton University Press, Princeton, N.J., 1978, pp. 166–197.
24. Reilly, T. P., J. E. Hasazi, and L. A. Bond, "Children's Conceptions of Death and Personal Mortality," *Journal of Pediatric Psychology* **8**:21–31 (1983).
25. Reilly, T. P., J. E. Hasazi, and L. A. Bond, "I Know, Do You? A Study of Awareness, Communication and Coping in Terminally Ill Children," in B. Schoenbert et al. (eds.), *Anticipatory Grief,* Columbia, New York, 1974, p. 180.
26. Polcz, A., "Manifestations of Death Consciousness and the Fear of Death in Children Suffering from Malignant Disease," *Padeiatrica Academiae Scientiarum Hungaricae* **22**:89–97 (1981).
27. Woolsey, S. F., Doris S. Thornton, and Stanford B. Friedman, "Sudden Death," in Sahler, op. cit., p. 101.
28. Gyulay, op. cit., p. 83.
29. Friedman, S. B., "Epilogue to the Loss of a Child," in Sahler, op. cit., p. 279.
30. Martinson, I. M. (ed.), *Home Care for the Dying Child,* Appleton Century Crofts, New York, 1976, p. 201.
31. Burton, L. *The Family Life of Sick Children,* Routledge, London, 1975, p. 48.
32. Gyulay, op. cit., p. 91.
33. Smith, C. E., M. S. Garvis, and I. M. Martinson, "Content Analysis of Interviews Using a Nursing Model: A Look at Parents Adapting to the Impact of Childhood Cancer," *Cancer Nursing* **6**:269–275 (1983).
34. Ibid., p. 93.
35. Burton, op. cit., p. 225.
36. Ibid., p. 229.
37. Martinson, op. cit., p. 235.
38. Ibid., p. 139.
39. Binger, C. M., et al., "Childhood Leukemia: Emotional Impact on Patient and Family," *The New England Journal of Medicine* **280**:414–418 (1969).
40. Martinson, op. cit., p. 153.
41. Schoenbert, B. S., et al. (eds.), *Loss and Grief: Psychological Management in Medical Practice,* Columbia, New York, 1970, p. 96.
42. Burton, op. cit., p. 203.
43. Zelauskas, B., "Siblings: The Forgotten Grievers," *Issues in Comprehensive Pediatric Nursing* **5**:45–52 (1981).
44. Ibid., p. 48.
45. Munson, S. W., "Family Structure and the Family's General Adaptation to Loss: Helping Families Deal with the Death of a Child," in Sahler, op. cit., p. 40.
46. Ibid.
47. Davidson, G., "Mourning—Living with Dying," presentation at the University of Minneapolis, May 3, 1979.
48. Rando, T. A., "An Investigation of Grief and Adaptation in Parents Whose Children Have Died from Cancer," *Journal of Pediatric Psychology* **8**:3–20 (1983).
49. Schiff, H. S., *The Bereaved Parent,* Crown, New York, 1977, p. 146.
50. Schowalter, J. E., "The Reactions of Caregivers Dealing with Fatally Ill Children and Their Families," in Sahler, op. cit.
51. Reese, C. A., "Support Systems: A Necessity for Professionals in Health Care," in Martinson, op. cit., p. 89.
52. Ibid., pp. 92–93.
53. Kubler-Ross, E., "The Languages of Dying," *Journal of Clinical Psychology* 22–24 (Summer 1974).
54. Bluebond-Langner, op. cit.
55. Korsch, B. M., "Issues in Humanizing Care for Children," *American Journal of Public Health* **68**:831–832 (1978).
56. Jackson, P. B., "Child Care in the Hospital—A Parent/Staff Partnership," *The American Journal of Maternal-Child Nursing* **3**(2):104–107 (March–April 1978).
57. Ayer, A. H., "Is Partnership with Parents Really Possible?" *The American Journal of Maternal-Child Nursing* **3**(2):107–110 (March–April 1978).
58. Hardgrove, C. B., and Rosime Kermoian, "Parent-Inclusive Pediatric Units," *American Journal of Public Health* **68**:847–850 (1978).
59. Lansky, S., et al., "Childhood Cancer," *Cancer* **43**:403 (January 1979).
60. Arnold, J. H., and P. B. Gemma, *A Child Dies: A Portrait of Family Grief,* Rockville, Md., 1983.
61. Lamerton, R., "Drugs for the Dying," *St. Bartholomew's Hospital Journal,* (November 1974).
62. Lamerton, R., "Opiate Delusions," *World Medicine* 44–45 (January 1978).
63. Lack, S. A., "New Haven (1974)—Characteristics of a Hospice Program of Care," *Death Education* **2**:41–52 (Spring–Summer 1978).
64. Lamers, W. M., Jr., "Marin County (1976)—Development of Hospice of Marin," *Death Education* **2**:53–62 (Spring–Summer 1978).
65. Lamerton, "Opiate Delusions," p. 44.
66. Moldow, D. G., and Ida M. Martinson, *Home Care for Dying Children: A Manual for Parents,* Children's Hospice International, Alexandria, Va., 1979.
67. Olness, K., and G. G. Gardner, "Some Guidelines for the Uses of Hypnotherapy in Pediatrics," *Pediatrics* **62**(2):228–233 (August 1978).
68. La Baw, W., et al., "The Use of Self-Hypnosis by Children with Cancer," *The American Journal of Clinical Hypnosis* **17**(4):233–238 (April 1975).

69. Martinson, I. M., M. Nesbit, and J. Kersey, "Home Care for the Child with Cancer," in Adolph E. Christ et al. (eds.), *Childhood Cancer,* Plenum, New York, 1984, pp. 177–178.
70. Ibid, p. 177.
71. Lauer, M. E., Mulhern, J. M. Wallskog, and B. M. Camitta, "A Comparison Study of Parental Adaptation Following a Child's Death at Home or in the Hospital," *Pediatrics* **71**:107–112 (1983).
72. Binger, C. M., A. R. Ablin, J. H. Kushner, and G. A. Perin, "Terminal Care of Childhood Cancer: Home Care of the Dying," in John E. Schowalter et al. (eds.), *The Child and Death,* Columbia, New York, 1983, pp. 157–171.

36

Linda L. Jarvis

Developmental disabilities: focus on mental retardation

Upon completion of this chapter, the student will be able to:

1. Define mental retardation in terms of IQ scores and adaptive skills.
2. Define mental retardation in his or her own words.
3. State the term used for each degree of mental retardation.
4. Name four inherited abnormalities that are responsible for mental retardation.
5. Name four causes of acquired mental retardation in the prenatal, natal, and postnatal periods.
6. Describe the three stages of the parents' reaction to the diagnosis that their child is mentally retarded.
7. Describe the assistance that the nurse can give the siblings of a mentally retarded child to ease their feelings about the child.
8. Identify six roles for the nurse who is caring for children with developmental disabilities.
9. Discuss what the nurse can do to prevent handicapping conditions in the infant when dealing with expectant mothers.
10. Name the three major stages of casefinding.
11. List three characteristics of the counseling role.
12. Discuss the scope of a nurse's role as advocate for the mentally retarded.

Nurses who work in health care settings frequently care for mentally retarded children. In order to provide effective care, it is important for nurses to have a knowledge of mental retardation and to examine their own attitudes toward this condition. Primarily, nurses must remember that children who are mentally retarded are *children* first, with the same needs as all children (Fig. 36-1). The fact that they are mentally retarded certainly affects them and their future, but it is essential that their needs as children be met.

In the 1960s, President John F. Kennedy initiated the President's Committee on Mental Retardation. Since then, national interest, funds, and research have been directed toward the study, treatment, and understanding of mental retardation. To be mentally retarded in the United States often means relegation to second-class citizenship because educational, vocational, housing, and socialization options are severely restricted.

Nurses are involved in seeking ways to increase the intellectual and adaptive skill levels

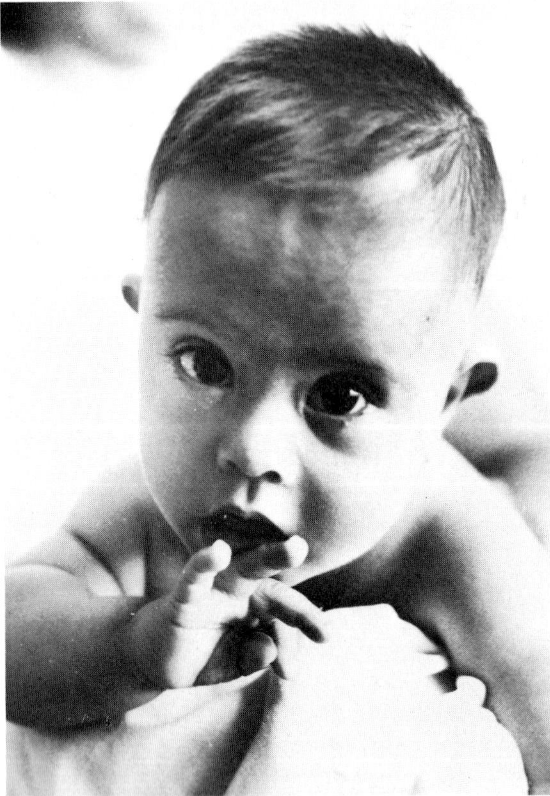

Figure 36-1 Mentally retarded children are first of all children, with the same needs of all children. (*Photo by Theresa Friedrich.*)

of mentally retarded children. Nurses assist families in developing effective ways of coping with the needs and demands of the mentally retarded family member. Educating health care peers and community members about the needs, abilities, and rights of the mentally retarded is another important role of the nurse. This chapter explores the impact of a mentally retarded child on the family unit, the nurse's role in providing care to mentally retarded children and their families, and the identification of helpful community resources.

DEFINITIONS OF MENTAL RETARDATION

The American Association on Mental Deficiency (AAMD) provides a definition of mental retardation in its *Manual on Terminology and Classification in Mental Retardation.*[1] This broad definition has been designed to reflect current thinking in education, medicine, and psychology (see Table 36-1).

Measurements of both intellectual and adaptive skills reflect a child's level of functioning at the time of a given evaluation. These scores may later change as a result of the child's maturation and learning. A diagnosis of mental retardation is valid *only* when the child demonstrates deficits in intellectual *and* adaptive functioning.

Intelligence

Intelligence measurement is an important component in the diagnosis of mental retardation. A score below 70 often is used to classify an individual as mentally retarded. Caution, however, is necessary because numerical designations are to be used as guidelines, not absolutes. Normative numerical scales may vary, depending on the intelligence test used. The accuracy of test results may be impaired if the child is uncooperative, is severely retarded, or is not given the right test. These tests must be administered and interpreted by individuals who are skilled in their use. A system for classifying mentally retarded children has been developed (See Table 36-2). It is important that caution be used before labeling a child as mentally retarded.

Adaptive behavior

Measurement of adaptive behavior is more difficult than measurement of intelligence because it is hard to identify what the child usually does

Table 36-1 Terms Related to Developmental Disabilities

Mental retardation Significantly subaverage general intellectual functioning existing concurrently with deficits in adaptive behavior and manifested during the developmental period

General intellectual functioning The results obtained by assessment with one or more of the individually administered general intelligence tests developed for that purpose

Significantly subaverage An IQ more than 2 standard deviations below the mean for the test

Adaptive behavior The effectiveness or degree with which an individual meets the standards of personal independence and social responsibility expected for the age and cultural group

Developmental period The period of time between birth and the eighteenth birthday

Source: Herbert J. Grossman (ed.). *Manual on Terminology and Classification in Mental Retardation.* American Association on Mental Deficiency, Washington, D.C., 1983, p. 1. Used with permission.

Table 36-2 Levels of Mental Retardation

Degree of Mental Retardation	IQ	Adaptive Skills
Mild ("educable")	50 or 55 to approximately 70	Usually masters basic academic skills; may live independently or semi-independently in the community.
Moderate ("trainable")	35 or 40 to 50 or 55	Can learn self-help, communication, social, and simple occupational skills and acquire limited academic or vocational skills.
Severe ("dependent retarded")	20 or 25 to 35 or 40	Requires continuing close supervision. May learn simple self-help skills and work skills with supervision.
Profound (needs "life support")	Below 20 or 25	Requires continuing close supervision. May learn simple self-help skills. Often has other handicapping conditions and requires total life support for maintenance.

Source: Adapted from Herbert J. Grossman, *Classification in Mental Retardation,* American Association on Mental Deficiency, Washington, D.C., 1983, p. 184. Used with permission.

on a day-to-day basis. Adaptive behavior includes the child's general affect and social and motor skills. Caution must also be used in interpreting the results of tests of adaptive behavior. A child's adaptive behavior may change rapidly as a result of maturation, learning, and environmental modification. Thus, the child should be reevaluated frequently.

Examples of tools that measure adaptive behavior include the AAMD Adaptive Behavior Scale, the Vineland Social Maturity Scale, the Camelot Behavioral Systems Checklist, and the Progress Assessment Chart. Any of these tests should be administered and interpreted only by qualified and licensed professionals.[2] In addition, testing must take into account such factors as culture, language, and hearing or visual impairment in order to be accurate and useful to the child, the parents, and professional health care providers.[3] It is not easy to reach a diagnosis of mental retardation. Although the AAMD advocates the utilization of both the intelligence and adaptive behavior criteria, others suggest using only one of these criteria.[4]

Public policy, developed over the last two decades, recognizes the needs and rights of the mentally retarded and mandates services that are to be provided to mentally retarded children and adults and their families. The most significant legislation has been Public Law 94-142, the Education for All Handicapped Children Act, which ensures school attendance for developmentally disabled children until the age of 21 (Table 34-4).[5] This act has enabled children to participate in an educational program designed for their learning needs and skills. For some children this means attending special classes in a particular subject during the school day. Other children might be mainstreamed in regular classrooms for certain subjects and then spend the rest of their day in special classes. Some children may need placement in special schools or programs outside the public school arena.

Developmental disabilities

Nurses should be aware of the definition of developmental disabilities in Public Law 95-602, signed into law by former President Jimmy Carter on November 6, 1978. It states:

> The term developmental disability means a severe, chronic disability which (a) is attributable to a mental or physical impairment or combination of mental and physical impairment (b) is manifested before the person attains age 22 years (c) is likely to continue indefinitely (d) results in substantial functional limitation in three or more of the following areas of major life activity—(1) self care (2) receptive and expressive language (3) hearing (4) mobility (5) self direction (6) capacity for independent living (7) economic self sufficiency and (e) reflects the person's need for a combination and sequence of special interdisciplinary or generic care, treatment or other services which are of a life long or extended duration and are individually planned and coordinated.[6]

This definition extends the focus of developmental disabilities further than previous definitions. It is not limited to a specific condition, such as cerebral palsy or mental retardation. The various components of the statement are critical to a clear understanding of the scope of the definition. Significantly, it means that physical, mental, or a combination of physical and mental impairments can occur prior to age 22 which interfere with the complete development of the individual. Although several developmental disabilities are present and identified at birth, deficits which are later identified or which result from illness, accidents, poisoning, or deprivation can also be included within the scope of developmental disabilities. This is important because it allows the child and the family to receive appropriate health and education services.

Because an age limit of 22 years is specified, children who become mentally retarded as a result of accident, trauma, or infectious disease during childhood and adolescence are included in the scope of services. This is particularly relevant, since the need for services for the mentally retarded probably will continue throughout their lifetimes. Although the ability of states to provide educational programs is curtailed at ages 21 to 22, other state services can be utilized. These include vocational rehabilitation, human services, and various kinds of institutional care ranging from community residences and halfway houses to the traditional institutional settings for more protective care and supervision.

This definition also recognizes that areas such as self-help, the ability to live independently, and self-mobility skills directly influence the learning and independence potential of the individual and therefore should be a focus of intervention. The final point of the definition is the need for individualized multidisciplinary services and programming. Professional input for treatment programs comes from nurses, social workers, physicians, physical and occupational therapists, educators, vocational counselors, nutritionists, and psychologists. Since mentally retarded children are identified at different chronological and developmental ages, their needs may vary considerably. Thus, the composition of the interdisciplinary team may also vary. Individualization ensures that the needs of the specific child and his or her family are identified and addressed. The team approach also allows these professionals to pool their knowledge and skills in order to identify and address the child's numerous needs in a comprehensive manner.

TERMINOLOGY AND LABELING

Terminology applied to the mentally retarded has changed over the years. This is due to increased knowledge about the complexity of various manifestations of mental retardation and sensitivity to the consequences of labeling for the child, the family, and the community. The term *developmental disability* or *disabilities* is now used for a large range of handicapping conditions affecting children, including mental retardation. It carries less social stigma than the terms *retardate, idiot, mentally deficient,* or others which have been used. Many parents find it far easier to say that their child is developmentally disabled than to say that he or she is mentally retarded.

The term *mentally retarded* has been used over the past decades to replace some of the older, less descriptive, and less accurate terms. It implies a degree of slowness in intelligence and adaptive skills, along with the hope that progress can be made in areas needing improvement. The term *mentally deficient* implies that something is missing and that replacement or improvement in areas in which there is a deficit is not likely to occur. This loss of hope can severely curtail the effort by the family members to provide for the special needs of the mentally retarded child. The term *developmentally disabled* rather than the label *mental retardation* allows families and professionals to focus on areas needing improvement.

Diagnostic labels are used by physicians primarily for identification and classification of the etiology and type of mental retardation. Once the diagnosis of mental retardation has been made, some labeling may occur if an intelligence quotient and adaptive rating are identified. Classification systems are applied to population groups and aid in identifying, classifying, and diagnosing individuals with mental retardation.[7] These systems aid in research activities and in program and service evaluation.[8] Labeling tends to be highly personal and informally conducted through interpersonal means.[9] Negative effects of labeling include stigmatizing children and their families; changed behavior toward, and expectations of mentally retarded children and adults; and incorrectly labeling children as a result of faulty testing procedures or incorrect use of testing tools.[10] Once a child has been labeled as mentally retarded, people often base their expectations and attitudes on the meaning of the label rather than on the child's behavioral and cognitive skills. Diagnostic labeling can be of help in designing educational activities for children and their families and in obtaining funds for these services.

Although labeling in itself is not negative, it can become detrimental to the progress of the child and his or her family if the labels are regarded as concrete and unchanging. As a result of appropriate interventions and child maturation, intellectual and life skills often show remarkable progress. The focus, therefore, should be on the *behavioral skills* which need to be developed rather than on the labels applied at a single, specific point in the child's life.

Labeling has long been a concern of parents and of educators who work with the mentally retarded. The general conclusion is that the label *mental retardation* has a negative impact which results in lowered expectations for the child. In 1974 an extensive review of the literature concerning this label was conducted. One conclusion was that research before 1970 did not support the negative effect of labeling.[11] The researchers found that individuals react to the label *mental retardation* on an individual basis and that the label is most important for the person functioning at the borderline level.[12] The impact of the label on children often depends on their ability to recognize the negative connotation of the label and their past history of success or failure in various endeavors. Mentally retarded children classified at the borderline level often know that they are labeled mentally retarded and are less capable in many areas than most of their peers. They are sensitive to the potential rejection by others both because of the label and because of their abilities. These children often have difficulty adjusting, particularly as they enter adolescence. They seek ways to look and behave like their nonretarded peers and actively resist placement in institutions or special classes.

Another study found that (1) labeling effects are less important when labels and other characteristics are combined for study, (2) the behavior exhibited by the children is often more biasing than the labels, and (3) children who interact with mentally retarded peers are more likely to respond to behavior than to labels.[13] The importance of the child's behavior was cited by one expert, who observed that behavioral characteristics and academic achievement often identify a child as mentally retarded before special class placement or labeling occurs.[14] For peers of the mentally retarded, academic performance is more important than the label.[15]

The effect of labeling is questionable. It appears that both academic performance and behavioral characteristics often identify the child prior to the use of labeling. One authority states that "clinical labels may provide a way for children to understand retarded children's poor performances or appearance."[16] If this is true, the clinical label will help protect retarded children from the abuse that children labeled *retard* may receive. The label *mentally retarded* appears more objective in terms of the individual child's problems than the term *retard*, which implies negative concerns.[17] The effects of labeling are likely to continue as an area of concern for parents, educators, health professionals, mentally retarded and non-mentally retarded children, and the community at large.

ETIOLOGY

Vulnerable periods

The causes of mental retardation vary, and the condition can occur at any time during the child's development. Handicapping conditions may appear singly or in multiples. The three periods during which mental retardation can occur are the prenatal period (conception to birth), the perinatal period (birth to 1 month of age), and the postnatal period (1 month to approximately 22 years of age). The causes of mental retardation are divided into two main categories—genetic conditions and acquired conditions. *Genetic conditions* are inherited from the parents through the gene pool. *Acquired conditions* are the result of toxic exposure, an accident, an infection, or deprivation. Table 36-3 lists common etiologies of mental retardation according to a developmental timetable.

Casefinding

Conditions of mental retardation may not be readily identifiable at birth. Because of this, regular visits to health care providers are essential for observing and recording individual neurological and developmental progress. This is particularly important during the first year. It takes time for the infant's neurological system to develop. Hasty decisions should therefore be avoided

Table 36-3 Causes of Mental Retardation

Prenatal			
Genetic	**Acquired**	**Natal (Acquired)**	**Postnatal (Acquired)**
1. Chromosomal abnormalities a. Autosomal abnormalities (1) Trisomy 21—Down syndrome (2) Trisomy 18—Edward syndrome (3) Trisomy 13—Patau syndrome (4) Cri-du-chat—Cat-cry syndrome b. Sex chromosome abnormalities (1) Klinefelter syndrome (2) Turner syndrome (3) XXX female (4) XYY male (5) Mosaic 2. Errors of metabolism a. Hurler syndrome b. Hunter syndrome c. Goitrous cretinism d. Phenylketonuria 3. Cranial abnormalities a. Anencephalus b. Microcephalus c. Hydrocephalus	1. Intrauterine environmental factors a. Viruses—rubella b. Chemical—LSD (?), alcohol (?), thalidomide c. Malnutrition d. Radiation e. Syphilis f. Anoxia g. Toxemia h. Blood type incompatibility	1. Birth a. Birth trauma b. Anoxia c. Prematurity d. Intracranial hemorrhage e. Kernicterus f. Infection g. Hydrocephalus	1. Exposure a. Radiation b. Toxic chemicals 2. Physical trauma or injury a. Head injury b. Asphyxia 3. Poisoning a. Lead b. Household cleaners c. Drugs and medications d. Insecticides e. Toxic chemicals 4. Infections a. Meningitis b. Encephalitis c. Viral or bacterial infections resulting in prolonged hyperpyrexia 5. Brain tumors a. Benign b. Malignant 6. Social and cultural factors a. Deprivation b. Abuse c. Malnutrition d. Emotional impairment

Sources: Herbert J. Grossman: *Classification in Mental Retardation,* American Association on Mental Deficiency, Washington, D.C., 1983, pp. 130–154; G. Scipien, M. U. Barnard, M. A. Chard, J. Howe, and P. J. Phillips (eds.), *Comprehensive Pediatric Nursing,* 3d ed., McGraw-Hill, New York, 1986, p. 641; Lucille F. Whaley, *Understanding Inherited Disorders,* Mosby, St. Louis, 1974, pp. 806–889; and Eugenia H. Waechter, Jane Phillips, and Bonnie Holaday, *Nursing Care of Children,* 10th ed., Lippincott, Philadelphia, 1985, pp. 1025–1095.

until substantial data have been collected to support the definite presence of a developmental deficit.

Prevention

Prevention of mental retardation is a primary focus of health professionals. The causes of many kinds of mental retardation are known. Therefore, it is possible to identify high-risk groups and encourage consistent prenatal care. Offering child development education programs in junior and senior high schools, in social service agencies, and for adults in the childbearing period should be encouraged. These efforts may be useful in preventing many acquired conditions.

Amniocentesis is a medical procedure involving puncture of the amniotic sac (via the abdominal wall) for the purpose of obtaining a sample of amniotic fluid. Laboratory tests performed on the fluid sample can aid in prenatal diagnosis of some chromosomal disorders accompanied by mental retardation.

If the results of an amniocentesis indicate that the fetus is defective, the parents may decide to terminate the pregnancy. The ethical and moral implications of abortion are substantial, and they permeate all areas of society. The decision to terminate a pregnancy should be made only after the parents have been given enough information to make an informed decision. Regardless of their decision, it is important that the nurse offer the parents support during this time of stress. Once a genetic disorder is identified or suspected, it is important that the parents obtain genetic counseling to help them make decisions regarding childbearing.[18] Genetic disorders and genetic counseling are discussed in Chap. 6.

The etiology of mental retardation is complex and may involve large numbers of factors. In many cases, the cause of mental retardation cannot be determined, but behavior and intellectual deficits indicate that it is present. Preventive efforts should be made where possible, and both lay and professional persons should be informed of actions that are effective. Current understanding of the etiology of mental retardation is incomplete, and more research and observation are necessary.

THE MENTALLY RETARDED CHILD IN THE FAMILY AND SOCIETY

Attitudes of society

Ever so slowly, society is becoming more tolerant of mentally retarded individuals and their families. Parents were once told to institutionalize their child upon confirmation of a diagnosis of mental retardation. Now, parents often keep their mentally retarded child at home in order to provide love, nurturing, and educational opportunities. Mentally retarded children often stay in their birth homes, play at the playground, attend school, get sick and see the doctor, and learn academic and self-help skills. They also laugh, cry, feel, and give, just as children without this disability do.

As families acknowledge the presence of mentally retarded children and care for them at home, the rest of society can develop an understanding of the special needs, issues, and contributions of these children. Indifference is slowly giving way to understanding of mental retardation and the provision of services. Although there is still a long way to go before the mentally retarded child or adult will be accepted into the mainstream of society, progress is being made in that direction. People are learning that mental retardation is not contagious, that it can occur in any family regardless of status, and that it has many causes which are not fully understood. Most important, mentally retarded children are first and foremost children, who have the same needs as their non-mentally retarded peers. Sensitivity opens the way for individualized, meaningful, and appropriate services for these children.

Parents' reaction

The reaction of families to the birth of a mentally retarded child is one of shock, disbelief, anger, and guilt. Whether it is the first or a subsequent child, parents generally approach the birth of a new child with dreams and fantasies of the "perfect" child.[19] Parents also give some thought to the possibility of having a disabled child. If the diagnosis of mental retardation is made at birth, the parents are immediately confronted with the loss of the fantasized perfect child. In many cases, however, a definitive diagnosis of mental retardation is not made until the the child is several months old and has demonstrated developmental delays. In some cases, the diagnosis is not made until the child is ready to enter school. Even when the parents suspect that their child is delayed in development, their active coping mechanisms are not utilized until the diagnosis is made. As they may do in the case of other chronic, disabling, or fatal conditions, the parents may "shop around" for other medical opinions before they are able to come to grips with the diagnosis of mental retardation.

Regardless of the time of the diagnosis, the parents need support, information, and access to helping persons in order to work through their feelings successfully before they can begin to provide care and services to their child.

The reaction of families to the diagnosis of mental retardation involves three stages of growth. Stage 1 is that of self-pity and subjective concern for themselves and the personal impact of the birth. Stage 2 is one of concern for the welfare and well-being of the child. Stage 3 is the time when the parents can examine and seek ways to serve other retarded children.[20]

This reaction to the diagnosis of mental retardation is often called *chronic sorrow*.[21,22,23] Some parents successfully reach stage 3, while others remain at stage 1 or 2 or move among all three stages. Parents also say that the diagnosis both confirms their worst fears and suspicions and provides relief. Once the diagnosis is made, the parents know that their observations are valid; something is wrong, but perhaps something can be done to help their child. Parents repeatedly express a sense of guilt about their child's condition.[24] They often say, "If only I had done this" or "If I hadn't done that," the mental retardation would not have occurred. The question "Why me?" also surfaces when parents are faced with the diagnosis. Once the diagnosis of mental retardation is made, the parents may be able to incorporate their mentally retarded child successfully into their home and family life. This mode of care is encouraged today. If this is not possible or feasible, a foster home or institutional placement may be necessary. Whatever their decision, the parents need support, encouragement, and guidance from professional health team members.

Siblings' reaction

Siblings of the mentally retarded child require special consideration because their lives, too, will be affected. They may be required to take on extra household or child care responsibilities. Siblings often need assistance in working through their own feelings about their brother or sister and may feel responsible for the condition. In addition, feelings of anger, fear, and resentment are common, and they should be discussed in an open, nonthreatening way. The mentally retarded child's condition must be explained to them in terms appropriate for their development level. Brothers and sisters also need reassurance that they will still be loved even if their mentally retarded sibling requires increased amounts of the parents' time. Involvement in the care and special programs required by the retarded child can help siblings feel that they are part of the family effort. It is also helpful if one or both parents can schedule their time so that all children in the family have the opportunity to have some "special" time with them without the presence of their mentally retarded sibling. This can provide all the family members with an opportunity to catch up on what each person is doing, to nurture and be nurtured, and to share some private time together. Keeping the family unit intact and functioning is an important nursing goal.

Family communication

The manner in which families communicate varies. Some find it easy to be open and honest and to share feelings, while others keep significant thoughts and feelings hidden, sharing only small parts of themselves. To aid families in communicating, the nurse should be aware of their past communication patterns. It is helpful to know how crises in the past have been resolved and which techniques were helpful. Honesty and openness should be encouraged. Because the parents often express a sense of pain and shock when they learn of their child's mental retardation, they may need several opportunities to clarify with the health care team the statements of the diagnosis and any specific information shared with them. It is not surprising to find that the parents did not hear any of the explanations or treatment plans when they first learned of the diagnosis. Therefore, it is essential that this critical information be repeated until the parents are able to demonstrate their understanding. Access to the health care team enables the parents to clarify information if it is made clear that questions are expected and encouraged.

Some families find it very helpful to join groups of parents who also have mentally retarded children so that they can share in discussing their feelings, concerns, fears, and objectives. Such support often helps the parents realize that others are coping with similar issues and that they are not alone. Groups for siblings of the mentally retarded exist in some areas. They provide an opportunity for siblings to share their feelings, fears, and concerns and to realize that other peers are dealing with similar issues.

It is vital that intrafamily and extrafamily communication be open and maintained if progress is to occur. Communication may be difficult at this time if the family members are not used to sharing their feelings and ideas. It is also important that health care providers be available for clarification of information about the child. They can also serve as a sounding board when necessary. The nurse often assists the family in establishing and maintaining communication channels for the family and the interdisciplinary team.

Institutional placement

From the time of the confirmed diagnosis, the potential for institutional placement exists. The decision to place the child depends on the attitude and abilities of the family, community resources, and the severity of the mental retardation. In situations in which the child has been cared for at home, institutional placement may be necessary if the parents are no longer able to provide sufficient care. A sibling may be able to take the mentally retarded family member into his or her own family, and for many this is a viable solution. However, problems may arise when the nuclear or extended family cannot provide the needed care.

In general, the first choice for child placement is in the home, as mentioned earlier. With various community services, including early infant stimulation, self-help training, and educational opportunities through special classes or school, family integrity can often be maintained. When relief from home care is needed because of fatigue or illness, residential respite care services are helpful. In such programs, the mentally retarded child can be cared for in an institution such as a school or in a foster home or residence. The time spent away from home varies with the needs of the family. It may range from a few days to 1 month. For many families, this kind of program provides sufficient relief from responsibilities to renew themselves and continue with the required care.

Foster home placement may be necessary on an extended or permanent basis. Residential programs, including schools for the mentally retarded, are another option. Children are often placed in such settings temporarily or permanently if the family is no longer able to provide care or if additional care and supervision are needed. Sometimes effective education and training can be obtained through placement in a school. The decision concerning institutional placement is not lightly made, and much ambivalence may be expressed by the parents regarding the wisdom of their decision. Some parents, after deciding on permanent placement, will reverse that decision, often on the basis of the perceived or actual level of care provided in the institution, a reevaluation of the family situation, and feelings of guilt. Regardless of the dynamics involved in the decision-making process, the parents should be encouraged to analyze the positive and negative aspects of the decision and to contact available professional health team members for support and discussions.

NURSING MANAGEMENT OF MENTALLY RETARDED CHILDREN

Nurses have played an increasingly significant role in developing an awareness of, and approaches to, dealing with the mentally retarded child and his or her family in a healthful, supportive, and individualized manner. This section explores in more detail some of the specifics of the nursing role with this client group. The exact role to be played depends in large measure on the nurse's educational and clinical preparation. Nurses who specialize in this field will need educational and clinical preparation beyond the baccalaureate level. Bean states that specialty preparation will be needed in such areas as pediatric neurology, orthopedics, cardiology, nutrition, assessment skills, anatomy and physiology, introductory genetics, child psychology, interpretation of growth and development parameters and data, techniques of child management and parenting, and counseling.[25] Nurses who do not have such specialized, in-depth knowledge but who are in contact from time to time with mentally retarded children and their families also do much to help.

Nurses often come in contact with this special population in three main hospital settings—the maternity-gynecological unit, the pediatric unit, and the outpatient department. Each of these settings provides the nurse with many opportunities for interviewing, counseling, teaching, and referring on questions of real or potential mental retardation. Although the nurse may not be able to provide the services directly, the need for such action can be identified, and an appropriate referral or referrals can be made. The depth of involvement will depend on the nurse's theoretical and clinical preparation, the availability of support services in the medical facility and community, and the extent of contact with the child.

Bean identifies six roles for the nurse: (1) casefinder, (2) teacher, (3) support source, (4) counselor, (5) coordinator of services, and (6) advocate.[26] In addition, Tudor specifies the importance of prevention and knowledge of community and state legislation when reviewing the scope of the nurse's role and responsibilities.[27] The following discussion will explore these specific activities.

Prevention and counseling

Prevention of handicapping conditions should be a primary goal of all nurses in all settings, particularly during the prenatal period. To this end, the encouragement of early, consistent, high-quality prenatal care is to be encouraged. Genetic counseling may be appropriate for couples who are hesitant about childbearing for such reasons as a previous birth of a child with mental retardation, a family history of mental retardation on one or both sides, or a high risk of carrying a disease which could cause mental retardation.[28] To the above list of concerns, Tudor also adds multiple spontaneous abortions.[29] The purposes of genetic counseling are to advise parents on the risks of pregnancy, identify special risk situations, and reduce the number of affected children.[30] A very detailed family history is obtained, including a pedigree chart. Analysis of findings and projected risk parameters are identified and shared with the involved couple.

Chapter 6 describes genetic counseling in more detail.

Genetic counseling may be spontaneously sought by the couple or recommended to them by a health care professional. As a result of the genetic counseling, couples may make a decision to parent biologically or not. One must be aware that the information provided during the genetic counseling session may not be understood. Therefore, follow-up contact with the couple should be initiated.[31]

When a couple have sought genetic counseling during a pregnancy, the information obtained as well as that derived from an amniocentesis may result in a decision to terminate the pregnancy. The issues involved in such a decision are too broad for inclusion in this chapter. However, it should be remembered that pregnancy termination is an option for many people faced with the birth of a defective child. The nurse may be sought out as a resource person as the couple struggle with this decision. The nurse's handling of such dilemmas is discussed in Chap. 4.

In addition to prenatal care and genetic counseling, adequate nutrition should be stressed. Cessation of smoking and alcohol consumption should be part of the pregnancy program to help ensure a strong, healthy baby of average birth weight. Alcohol consumption during pregnancy has been associated with fetal alcohol syndrome, which often leads to physical and intellectual deficits in infants.[32] The principal features of fetal alcohol syndrome include low birth weight, facial abnormalities, cleft lip and palate, nail dysplasia, ear and eye abnormalities, mild to moderate mental retardation, and central nervous system dysfunctions.[33] Teaching expectant mothers about the potential risks of alcohol consumption and cigarette smoking is a critical preventive activity for the nurse (Fig. 36-2). The ability of the nurse to give an appropriate rationale can increase the desired health behavior.

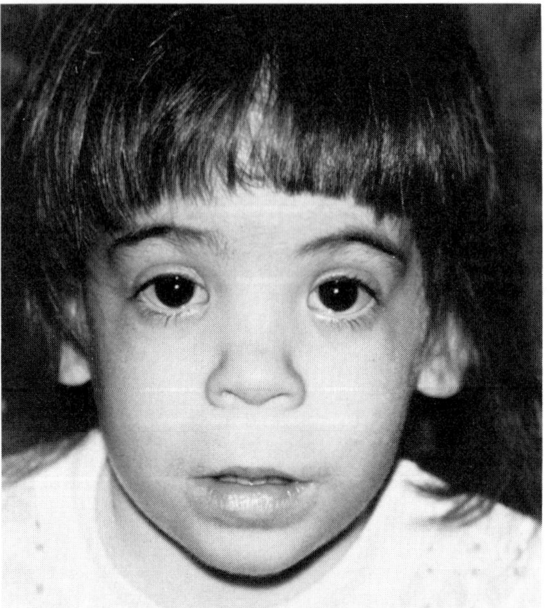

Figure 36-2 A child with typical facial features of fetal alcohol syndrome. These features include short palpebral fissures; a midface too long for the nasal length, giving the philtrum an elongated appearance; flat philtral furrows with a thinned upper vermilion border; and a flat midfacial structure. Additional features include epicanthal folds, a somewhat small jaw, prominent ears, and mild hirsutism. (*Source*: Sterling K. Clarren, M.D. From Clarren and Smith, "The Fetal Alcohol Syndrome." Reprinted by permission of *The New England Journal of Medicine*, 298:1063–1067, 1978. Used with permission.)

In the neonatal period especially and through infancy, attention should focus on adequate oxygenation and prevention of accidents and disease. Accepted childhood immunization should be started at 2 months of age and continued throughout the childhood years. High fever and infections should be carefully monitored and treated to prevent potential encephalitis or meningitis, which are sometimes the unfortunate result of some infections. Environmental safety at home, at school, and in the car should be stressed by the nurse.

Casefinding

Casefinding is a major focus for the nurse, regardless of the work setting. Again, the primary sites for such encounters are newborn nurseries, pediatric units, and pediatric outpatient units. Tudor states that referrals for developmentally disabled children are often not made until 18 months or later for two main reasons: (1) professionals often do not recognize or cannot define a developmental delay or abnormal physical or neurological finding, and (2) many are unaware of the existence or benefit of early intervention for infants and their parents.[34]

The first step to be taken in casefinding is the nursing assessment. A thorough history should be taken to determine attainment of developmental milestones, specific behavior patterns of the infant and child, and the child care and management techniques used by the parents. The date and duration of any high fever, illness, or trauma should be noted, as well as both routine and special medications given. All this information should be carefully recorded and available for future reference. This history should be updated after each contact with the child and the family. The style and format to be followed should be determined by the nursing team in each institutional setting, but the history needs to be clearly written and short enough to be usable.

Following the history, there should be a physical examination. Nurses who work in newborn nurseries are in a particularly critical setting in which they can observe infants for appropriate reflexes and neonatal behavior. Powell describes in some detail the use of the Neonatal Behavioral Assessment Scale, developed by T. Berry Brazelton. This scale measures six major categories of behavior: (1) habituation, (2) orientation, (3) motor maturity, (4) variation, (5) self-quieting activities, and (6) social behavior. (See Chaps. 8 and 14.) It allows the nurse to observe the infant's adaptation to the environment.[35] As the infant grows, other development assessment tools may be used. (See Table 14-8.)

Because of the immaturity of the infant's nervous system and the difficulty of drawing conclusions from one observation or encounter, the results of tests, observations of the nurse, and statements from the parents must be carefully recorded. Behaviors or lack of behaviors may be normal at 3 months of age, borderline at 6 months, and abnormal at 9 or 12 months. Any suspicions or abnormalities should be reported to the physician or other members of the multidisciplinary team for further investigation, observation, and evaluation.

In addition to the physical and developmental investigation which must be conducted, a thorough assessment of the family structure and functioning as well as parenting activities needs to be completed. Parent-child interaction should be observed directly by the nurse, including such points as eye contact, touch, methods of child management, efforts to teach the child, verbal communication, and attempts to play with the child.[36] The nurse should also determine the level of self-help skills present, which include self-feeding, dressing, and toilet training. The reactions of siblings and husband-wife interactions should be observed, with the recommendation of intervention where necessary.

Care planning and caregiving

When the mentally retarded child is admitted to the hospital for an illness, care needs to be planned on an individual basis, as it would be for any other child. The initial history that is taken should carefully define the skills the child demonstrates at home, communication practices used (including any special terms that the child uses for himself or herself), dressing, feeding, and toileting. An outline of the daily routine should be obtained. Because of the need for clarity and repetition with this client population, it is important that the teaching technique used at home be continued in the hospital when possible.

Conversations should be carried on with the child in a normal tone of voice, using appropriate terminology for his or her level of comprehension. Regression can occur with any child who is hospitalized and can be expected with the mentally retarded child. Behavioral expectations can be readjusted to compensate for this change. Procedures need to be explained, as would be done with any other child. Play activities appropriate for the child's functional age and health condition should be planned individually and with other children when possible.

Frequent checks of the child's condition should be made, with specific questions asked about how the child feels, what he or she wants, where it hurts, etc. Parents need to be informed of hospital rules and regulations, and special accommodations should be made where possible. The child should be placed in the mainstream of hospital activity, not in an isolated care area, unless this is warranted for medical or safety reasons.

Mentally retarded children require extra attention, patience, and time when they are hospitalized. Nurses, by careful planning, can make the hospital stay for mentally retarded children and their families a positive, supportive, and growing experience. The setting of nursing goals, the design and implementation of specific nursing interventions, and the reevaluation and revision of the nursing care plan are ongoing and should be available and shared with all involved persons.

Teaching

Teaching takes place in several areas. One is direct parent education, particularly during and after the specific diagnosis has been made. The parents should be provided with basic information about their child's condition, about the developmental prognosis if it is known, and about the various treatment approaches which might be used to treat and/or modify the disability. It is important that information given to parents be repeated; that simple, nonmedical terminology be used; that the parents be talked with and not to or down to; and that one or more resource persons be available at the health care site to clarify information and answer questions when they come up.

As the child grows, educational and training needs will change. It is important, particularly in the early years of childhood stimulation and training, that parental involvement be encouraged and reinforced. There should be no mystique about the site or equipment needed for adequate child stimulation. The parents should and can learn to work directly with infant stimulation programs, physical therapy programs, and self-help skills learning programs as the primary teachers in the home. Mothers can be taught the techniques to be utilized, observed for appropriateness of techniques, and then reinforced as they proceed to implement the techniques. They should be taught to watch for cues for training readiness in such areas as feeding, dressing, and toilet training. For example, they should observe for head and trunk support and the ability to grasp and release objects for feeding behavior; bladder continence for 2 h and sitting ability for toilet training; and attending to a task for about 5 min and a pincer grasp for dressing behavior.

When teaching the mentally retarded child, remember that the child will often have a short attention span, which may need to be increased before effective learning can occur. Teaching should be conducted in a familiar setting free from external stimuli. The child should be fed and well rested before the session. Terminology should be simple and concrete terms rather than abstract ones should be used when giving explanations. Tasks to be learned should be repeated frequently, and learning activities should be divided into component parts. Behavior modification techniques, such as fading, shaping, and positive reinforcement, are helpful and work successfully with these children. Behavior modification techniques can be used by the parents to teach their mentally retarded child many useful skills. Environmental modification can also help the child perform at a more independent level. Some modifications include feeding utensil adaptations such as padding the spoon or fork handle and using special suction cups or plates to keep them from sliding, cups with spill-proof tops, food of a size and consistency which will allow for self-feeding, and clothes which are not buttoned or zipped but rather pulled over the head, have elastic waistbands, and Velcro closures. Most of these and many other modifications are relatively simple to make and can significantly increase the independent functioning of the mentally retarded child.

Parents also need information about child management. Mentally retarded children need to have limits set for them, just as nonretarded children do. They need to know what is acceptable and what is nonacceptable behavior. Discipline should be encouraged. Where necessary, behavior modification techniques can be taught either to increase or to decrease specific behaviors. Mentally retarded children have enough special needs to cope with; they do not need to have disruptive or inattentive behavior further complicate their lives.

Providing emotional support

The nurse can furnish needed support at many points as the parents come to acknowledge and accept the mental retardation of their child. The parents need "to have their pain recognized, appreciated and validated," for they have experienced a loss, must grieve, and must reorganize their family unit to cope with the unanticipated needs of a mentally retarded child.[37] Providing a private area for expressing feelings is important in encouraging discussion of both the disappointments and the joys involved in caring for their mentally retarded child. The nurse should keep in mind that the parents may require frequent repetition of information before it is retained. The nurse often becomes the target of much of the parents' anger concerning their child. The ability to take this anger without backing away, retaliating, or becoming personally injured can often strengthen the bond between the nurse and the family. It is not particularly pleasant, at times, to be in such situations, but the nurse is often the professional at whom such anger can be safely vented. Quietly hearing the parents out and being available for future contacts will deliver the message that anger and disappointment are acceptable.

Counseling and referrals

As the parents deal with the many needs they face, referrals by the nurse to various agencies may be necessary. The nurse's availability by phone may provide the needed input or encouragement to deal with a major problem or a minor but irritating one. Nurses may be able to confirm the appropriateness of a decision and provide encouragement or simply to "be there" when needed. The day-to-day efforts and time involved in caring for a mentally retarded child can be exhausting, and knowing that there is a person available for discussion, encouragement, and reinforcement can be very helpful.

Counseling can take many forms and is dependent on the nurse's educational, clinical, and experiential preparation. Bean discusses three characteristics of the counseling role which must be present if such encounters are to be successful. The nurse must (1) present a professional apearance, (2) identify the parents' needs and help them meet these needs before discussing the child, and (3) listen to the parents discuss their concerns about their child.[38] Work with the parents to aid their mentally retarded child cannot adequately proceed if the parents see the nurse as a threat or an awesome figure. Such perceptions are detrimental to the helping process and must be identified and corrected. If the parents' energy is tied up in coping with their own needs, then the child's needs cannot be met. Again, by identifying these concerns and taking steps to meet them, the nurse can make efforts to meet the needs of the child. Once steps 1 and 2 have been taken, the nurse is in a position to explore with the parents their concerns about their child. These may run the gamut from confirming a disability to developing techniques to deal with a specific behavior issue. In all cases, the parents are ultimately responsible for the decisions they make.

Nurses educate and counsel prepubescent mentally retarded girls to prevent pregnancies. The parents also need education and counseling. When they realize that their daughter is maturing and is capable of childbearing, the parents must again acknowledge their daughter's abnormality. They must rework their original feelings of grief.[39] The parents should be counseled to educate their daughter and not wait for her to introduce questions about sex. Using simple language, repetition, and audiovisual aids, the girl should be taught the anatomic names of the parts of her body and should be told that sexual intercourse can result in a baby; she should also be instructed in socially acceptable behavior with members of the opposite sex. Mentally retarded adolescent girls are especially vulnerable to sexual exploitation because of their characteristic traits of dependency and respect for authority.[40]

The parents and their daughter should participate jointly in the choice of method of contraception. Appropriate options for a mentally retarded adolescent girl are (1) an intrauterine device (which has the drawback of requiring frequent checking for placement and menorrhagia), (2) intramuscular injections of medroxyprogesterone acetate every 3 months, and (3) sterilization (tubal ligation) or a hysterectomy (for a girl with an IQ under 40). The nurse and the parents can praise the girl for her choice of a method of contraception, which is necessary because of an increased risk of birth defects and the inability of mentally retarded adolescents to care for a child.[41]

The nurse can be most helpful in supporting those decisions. It is important to keep in mind that a family's values, ethics, and moral considerations may differ from those of the nurse. If the nurse cannot handle or therapeutically deal with the decisions made by a particular family, it would be most appropriate to refer the family to another nurse, who could be more supportive.

Coordinating services

Because the retarded child may have more than one problem and because of the multidisciplinary nature of the health care team, *coordination of services* is essential. The nurse is in an excellent position to provide this overseeing service. Appropriate referrals can be made through the health care team and to outside agencies for specific services. The nurse can explain and clarify the roles of various providers to the parents and may be able to correct any misunderstanding which may occur between the parents and agencies or team members. Such efforts can be invaluable in maintaining families in programs for the benefit of the child. If the parents develop concerns or difficulties with a specific agency, the nurse—because of his or her contact with, and knowledge of, the agency and its personnel and programs—may be able to resolve the problem, reevaluate the services, and/or make recommendations to the health care team concerning its appropriateness for services.

Advocacy

Advocacy for the mentally retarded child and his or her family is a much needed nursing role. This involves speaking out for and supporting the establishment of special services for the mentally retarded at the local, state, and federal levels. Education of the community, both lay and professional, concerning the special needs, skills, and qualities of the mentally retarded is a necessary function. Misunderstandings, fears, and prejudices still exist which need the dedicated efforts of many to correct and put to final rest. Nurses committed to the field of mental retardation are in a position to do this. Evaluation of agencies can aid in continuing those which provide beneficial services and closing those which are without value. Supporting educational programs for nurses at the generic and continuing education levels can improve the contribution that nursing makes to this field. As the pool of qualified nurses increases, the quality of the service should improve. Involvement in political lobbying efforts for the passage of pertinent legislation can have both a long- and a short-term impact on the mentally retarded and their families. Nurses can help by providing information, testimony, and assistance in the wording of legislation.

The final area of action, which often parallels that of advocacy, is *legislative action*. It is very important that the nurse be aware of state and federal legislation which will provide direct and indirect services to the mentally retarded. The nurse should be aware of state and federal senators and representatives and their position on legislation concerning the mentally retarded. Where there is negative support, educational efforts via letters, phone calls, and personal visits may be in order. Where there is support, reinforcement of the legislator's stance is appropriate. When new legislation needs to be written or old legislation must be modified, nurses can participate in such efforts. Sources of financial support for services, ranging from early childhood programs to vocational training, need to be identified and utilized. Support for nursing education at the generic, graduate, and continuing education levels needs to be encouraged and reinforced. Education of the public about the need for appropriate legislation is an ongoing process and must constantly be lobbied because of the large number of competing causes.

Summary

The nursing roles in mental retardation are many and varied. The depth of commitment made to the field will depend in large measure on the educational, clinical, and personal preparation of the nurse. In mental retardation nursing, as in other specialties, nurses must come to grips with personal feelings about the condition and its various manifestations and about the nursing role. Their effectiveness will be greatly compromised until they know and understand their feelings about working with the handicapped.

In mental retardation nursing, the nurse works with the parents, who are in the best position to implement treatment programs, identify needs, and set goals and objectives. The mental retardation will not disappear, but its impact on the child's life can be modified through consistent, diligent, goal-related actions. The nurse can help the family accept the handicapping condition, modify their life-style and expectations, and include their mentally retarded child in the family. It is time-consuming work filled with successes and failures, joys and disappointments, and the comforting knowledge that a service has been rendered to persons in real need.

COMMUNITY RESOURCES

The resources available to the family with a mentally retarded member depend on such factors as geographic location, state of residence, and medical and other resources. Services may be provided through such agencies as the state Crippled Children's Service, the United Cerebral Palsy Association, the Association for Children with Retarded Mental Development, the Association for Retarded Citizens, the Special Olympics, health departments, university-affiliated centers, public and private schools, residential houses, halfway houses, and respite care centers. Head Start provides early childhood training for many developmentally disabled children. Infant stimulation programs are often offered at the state level to parents with a mentally retarded child.

In addition to the above, services may be provided through the National Associations for Retarded Citizens, the Easter Seal Society for Crippled Children and Adults, and the National Foundation—March of Dimes. These organizations can be contacted at the local, state, or federal level, depending on access options. Special camps, day-care programs, and recreational and social activities are provided in many areas for the mentally retarded.

As the mentally retarded individual ages, vocational training and placement are needed. These services are often provided through state departments of vocational training. Work training preparation and work placement may be provided in sheltered workshops and various industrial settings. The exact type of work can vary but must consist of repetitive-type jobs and packaging activities.

Staying abreast of various community resources is time-consuming and requires persistence and frequent updating. Direct agency contact and visits, when possible, will aid in the evaluation of agencies. Developing a resource file which includes at a minimum each agency's name, the service provided, the telephone number, the name of the contact person, and any fee charged can be most useful and worthwhile.

In summary, community resources vary in quality and quantity from location to location. Before using any given agency as a resource, it is imperative to evaluate it in terms of the service rendered. No service is usually better than poor service. Nurses play an important role in identifying and evaluating community resources. Ideally, the social, educational, medical, residential, and recreational services that are available to the nonretarded should also be available to the developmentally disabled.

References

1. Grossman, Herbert J. (ed.) *Classification in Mental Retardation,* American Association of Mental Deficiency, Washington, D.C., 1983, p. 1.
2. Ibid., p. 54.
3. Ibid.
4. Taft, Lawrence T., "An Overview of the Etiology of Mental Retardation and Developmental Disabilities," in Michael K. McCormack (ed.), *Prevention of Mental Retardation and Other Developmental Disabilities,* Marcel Dekker, New York, 1980, pp. 4–5.
5. Mulliken, Ruth K., "Legal Constraints," in Ruth K. Mulliken and John J. Buckley (eds.), *Assessment of Multihandicapped and Developmentally Disabled Children,* Aspen, Rockville, Md., 1983, p. 17.
6. The Rehabilitation Comprehensive Services Act and Developmental Disabilities Amendments of 1978, Public Law 95-602.
7. Grossman, op. cit., p. 19.
8. Ibid., pp. 19–20.
9. Ibid, p. 20.
10. Mulliken, op. cit., p. 11.
11. MacMillan, Donald, and Reginald L. Jones, "The Mentally Retarded Label: A Theoretical Analysis and Review of Research," *American Journal of Mental Deficiency* **79**(3):253 (1974).
12. Ibid.
13. Freeman, Sheryl, and Bob Algozzine, "Social Acceptability as a Function of Labels and Assigned Attributes," *American Journal of Mental Deficiency* **84**(6):590 (June 1980).
14. Gottlieb, Jay, "Attitudes toward Retarded Children: Effects of Labeling and Academic Performance," *American Journal of Mental Deficiency* **79**(3):272 (1974).
15. Ibid.
16. Siperstein, Gary N., Milton Budoff, and John J. Bak, "Effects of Labels 'Mentally Retarded' and 'Retard' on the Social Acceptability of Mentally Retarded Children," *American Journal of Mental Deficiency* **84**(6):597 (June 1980).
17. Ibid.
18. Falek, Arthur, "Psychodynamics in Genetic Counseling of Families with Mental Retardation," in McCormack, op. cit., p. 502.
19. Paparella, Bonnie H. "Caring for the Severely Handicapped Newborn," *Nursing '82* **12**(12):61–62 (December 1982).
20. Boyd, Dan, *The Three Stages,* National Association for Retarded Children, New York, 1969.
21. Waisbren, Susan E., "Parents' Reaction after the Birth of a Developmentally Disabled Child," *American Journal of Mental Deficiency* **84**(4):345–351 (January 1980).
22. Solnit, Albert, and Mary H. Stark, "Mourning and the Birth of a Defective Child," reproduced by the U. S. Department of Health, Education, and Welfare, Social and Rehabilitation Service, Children's Bureau, with permission from *Psychoanalytic Study of the Child* **16**:523–537 (1961).
23. Olshansky, S., "Chronic Sorrow: A Response to Having a Mentally Defective Child," *Social Casework* **43**:191–194 (1962).
24. Falek, op. cit., p. 504.
25. Bean, Margaret R., "Nursing Roles in Developmental Disabilities," in Linda L. Jarvis (ed.), *Community Health Nursing: Keeping the Public Healthy,* Davis, Philadelphia, 1985, pp. 257–258.
26. Ibid., p. 258.

27. Tudor, Mary, "Nursing Intervention with Developmentally Disabled Children," *The American Journal of Maternal-Child Nursing* **3**(1):28–30 (January–February 1978).
28. Whaley, Lucille F., "Genetic Counseling," in Judith B. Curry and Katheryn K. Peppe (eds.), *Mental Retardation Nursing: Approaches to Care,* Mosby, St. Louis, 1978, p. 89.
29. Tudor, op. cit., p. 26.
30. Whaley, op. cit., p. 99.
31. Ibid., p. 105.
32. Chernoff, Gerald, "The Fetal Alcohol Syndrome: Clinical Studies and Strategies of Prevention," in McCormack, op. cit., pp. 321–322.
33. Ibid., p. 322.
34. Tudor, op. cit., pp. 27–28.
35. Powell, Marcene L., *Assessment and Management of Developmental Changes and Problems in Children,* Mosby, St. Louis, 1981, pp. 59–60.
36. Bean, op. cit., p. 260.
37. Tudor, op. cit., p. 25.
38. Bean, op. cit., p. 267.
39. Williams, Janet K., "Reproductive Decisions: Adolescents with Down Syndrome," *Pediatric Nursing* **9**(1):43–58 (January–February 1983).
40. Ibid. p. 43.
41. Ibid., p. 44.

37

Elizabeth C. Poster

Behavioral problems

Upon completion of this chapter, the student will be able to:

1. Compare children's and adults' responses to interviewing.
2. Compare the typical behavior of healthy children with that of disturbed children.
3. Describe the etiology and typical behavior associated with a reactive disorder.
4. Describe the behavioral and emotional responses of depressed children.
5. Identify the risk factors associated with childhood suicide.
6. Describe the nursing management of a depressed child.
7. Summarize the characteristic behavior, treatment, and nursing care of children diagnosed as having infantile autism, childhood-onset pervasive developmental disorder, and childhood psychosis.
8. Discuss the etiology and symptoms of elective mutism and stuttering and the nursing care of children with these disorders.
9. Describe the symptoms, treatment, and nursing care of children with enuresis and encopresis.
10. Compare and contrast the etiology of conduct disorders and attention deficit disorders (with and without hyperactivity) and the nursing management of children with these disorders.
11. Describe the nursing management of children with the eating disorders of anorexia nervosa, bulimia, and obesity.
12. Compare the etiology of separation anxiety (school refusal) and overanxious disorder, the behavior of children with these disorders, and the nursing management of these children.
13. Describe the symptoms and nursing care of children with stereotyped movement disorders (tics).
14. Describe the nursing care of chidren with sleep disorders.

Children with behavioral problems can appear in any pediatric nursing setting. The more severe disturbances are a mixture of neurological, perceptual, and behavioral problems. Symptoms are often observable from the beginning of a child's development. A definite organic (physiological) abnormality may underlie a severe disturbance. Other behavioral symptoms emerge as a result of stressful parent-child relationships. Poverty, a poor marriage, and job loss can precipitate dysfunctional (maladaptive) patterns of child rearing. For example, the parent may demand behavior that is beyond the child's developmental level. The pediatric nurse can assess these behavioral problems and recommend specialized treatment for the child and the family.

Pediatric nurses have a unique opportunity among health care professionals to prevent, at both the primary and secondary levels, behavioral problems in children and adolescents. Nurses who work with children and their families in schools, health maintenance organizations, outpatient departments, and hospitals are in an ideal position to assess behavior and the constantly changing environmental variables that affect children. Nurses can therefore identify children who are most vulnerable or who are at high risk for developing future mental and physical health problems. Research has identified the following groups of high-risk children: (1) those who have physical and intellectual handicaps, (2) those who are nutritionally and economically deprived, (3) those who are abused and neglected, (4) those who live in a disruptive family setting and have a disruptive life-style, and (5) those who have mentally ill or retarded parents.

It is generally agreed that mental health efforts should be directed toward primary (first-encounter) prevention among high-risk children. However, there are many unanswered questions about psychological and nursing interventions. Two major questions are (1) When should intervention be initiated? and (2) What specific nursing interventions are the most beneficial with specific behavioral problems? Until these questions are answered through nursing research, current nursing interventions will be employed. Current primary preventive nursing interventions include developmental counseling, anticipatory guidance, supervision of children's developmental progress, discussion of child-rearing practices and problems with parents, support of children and families who are in crisis and under stress, and consultation with teachers and school personnel.

Many nurses work in hospital and community settings where they intervene with children who are already exhibiting emotional distress and/or maladaptive behavior. Early intervention with these children and their families can significantly alter the children's subjective distress, socially inappropriate behavior, and developmental handicaps.

PSYCHOLOGICAL DEVELOPMENT

Psychological development is shaped by an individual's unique environment and by genetic endowment. Biological timetables determine the rate of certain behavioral capacities; maturation cannot be rushed. For example, an infant's capacity to remember images in the mind appears to begin near the end of the first year. Memory is an important tool in the child's psychological separation from parents and the process of individual development. (See Chaps. 10 and 11 for further discussion.) Environmental forces, particularly parental and other socialization experiences, shape a child's personality through the processes of internalization and identification.

A child *internalizes* (learns and later uses) the behavior of other people. For example, the ways a father expresses tenderness or handles angry feelings are internalized by a child as "emotional methods" to be used in relating to others. *Identification* is a complicated process of internalizing social, physical, and sexual roles enacted mainly by parents. (See Chap. 11 for a discussion of identification.) Absence of a role model (a parent) due to death or divorce can compromise the identification process. Behavioral symptoms may develop, depending on the child's vulnerability at the time the parent is lost. Age is one critical factor. The loss of a parent during a child's preschool years will have some impact on identification and the solidifying of self and role. The impact on a school-age child will vary with how effectively the remaining parent, the extended family, and other adults contribute the adult involvement needed for the child's development.

PSYCHOLOGICAL ASSESSMENT

Assessment of a child's developmental history and current functioning is essential when determining deviations from psychological health. There are three primary sources of information: (1) the developmental history (see Chap. 14 for guidelines); (2) interviews with the child, the family, and significant others such as teachers, extended family members, the police, and neighbors; and (3) diagnostic testing with psychometric and projective tests.

The child's reactions to interviewing differ from the adult's. The child is handicapped by:

1. Being less able to verbalize psychological distress. Younger children have more difficulty verbalizing internal conflicts.
2. Being less able to seek help independently.
3. Being cognitively immature and therefore lacking a fully developed ability to use abstract thought and to think symbolically.

These differences influence the interview process. If an interviewer questions a school-age child about school failure by asking, for example, "Why are you failing in your schoolwork?" the child will find the question symbolic and therefore too difficult to answer. The nurse instead asks concrete questions, such as, "What is your favorite subject?" or "What happens at school to make you unhappy?" or uses the techniques discussed in Chap. 15. There are numerous reasons for school failure. The length of the following list points up the thoroughness required of the nurse. Incomplete assessment may lead to an incorrect nursing diagnosis. Causes might include (1) conflicts within the child; (2) family problems to which the child is reacting; (3) a physical problem, such as poor eyesight, a hearing deficit, poor fine motor coordination, or interference with writing; (4) learning disabilities; and (5) a chronic illness.

After the patterns and possible causes of the child's behavior are assessed, encourage the parents to begin health screening. Always include a thorough physical examination and begin exploring with the family and the child possible internal psychological problems.

Usually, by the time a child's psychological problem attracts professional attention, a level of chaos has been reached that disturbs those in the child's immediate environment. Schools initiate the majority of psychological referrals. Disturbed children are often not identified before they start school for the following reasons:

1. Families tolerate unusual or peculiar habits in their children that are intolerable in a classroom.
2. School may provide the child's first contact with adults who are skilled in observing children.
3. Inability to pay attention or concentrate may not be noticed until the child goes to school, where these behaviors are required.
4. Children and adults express psychological pain differently (Table 37-1).

Table 37-1 Behaviors Expressing Psychological Pain

1. Runs away
2. Destroys family, school, or community property
3. Seeks the wrong kind of friend or group, enabling further acting out
4. Withdraws into a private fantasy world
5. Suicide
6. Homicide
7. Isolated incidents of bizarre behavior
8. Vague somatic symptoms: stomachaches, frequent upper respiratory illnesses, fatigue, or frequent visits to the school nurse

Some of the more frequent problems that emerge when a disturbed child enters school are listed in Table 37-2.

Helping the parents recognize their child's psychological difficulty requires a delicate balance between telling and facilitating. Parents rarely welcome outside authorities who investigate child abuse, neglect, or bizarre behavior. In addition, the parents may be unaware of or afraid to recognize their child's psychological difficulties. (See Chap. 34 for parental reactions to chronic illness.)

Reassuring and supporting the parents will increase the child's cooperation and trust. School-age children may be *fiercely loyal* to even the most chaotic families and disturbed parents. Once children feel that their parents trust the nurse, most of them are willing to begin relating to the new adult. The pediatric nurse who can identify problems and begin a trusting parent-family-nurse relationship is in an optimal position to refer the family and the child to more skilled psychological resources. The nurse can function as a *child-advocate* and as a *liaison* for a family until treatment begins.

Healthy behavior

Psychological health is a dynamic state of adaptation; the child responds to crises and to both unexpected and expected events. By the time a

Table 37-2 Problems Identified at School

Problems with Activity
Inability to concentrate
Inability to sit still in a chair or through an entire activity
Inability to follow directions
Impulsiveness: grabs others' materials, pushes, bites

Problems with Personal Habits
Tics, e.g., muscle twitches; head tilts or turning; strange shoulder, hand, or other body movements
Pulls hair out
Excessive nail-biting, thumb- or finger-sucking
Incomplete toilet training
  Daytime urine accidents (enuresis)
  Fecal soiling (encopresis)

Problems with Interpersonal Relationships
No friends: excessive shyness or behaviors causing others to avoid contact with the child
Attention-seeking behaviors: calling out and other disruptive actions
Provocative fighting
Seeks only adults as friends

child enters the school years, a number of developmental steps have been taken to some degree: separation from the parents, the autonomy struggle during toilet training, and the preschooler's attainment of initiative and sexual identity. Situational crises have occurred and been mastered, in a healthy way, as in the following example.

Example: Five-year-old Kathy was excited about beginning kindergarten and had attended an orientation session. She had talked about her new school all summer to everyone. On the first day, Kathy refused to get dressed and wanted to stay home and play. Her mother was bewildered but patient as she helped the child get ready to go. At school, Kathy cried and clung to her mother. The teacher helped both to separate by holding and comforting Kathy. Later that morning, Kathy complained of a "tummyache" and said that she "needed her mommy." The school nurse was consulted and talked with Kathy about how hard it was to begin school.

With support, Kathy's anxiety disappeared in a few days, and her original eagerness to attend school returned.

Disturbed behavior

Each culture identifies particular behaviors that it deems unhealthy. Problem behaviors generally have two characteristics: (1) they *interfere* with the child's development, and (2) they *continue* for a period of time. Any troublesome behavior that continues for 6 months should be investigated.

Example: Johnny, age 11, has always been a quiet, studious boy but has failed to make any close friends for several years. He has remained withdrawn and isolated from group projects at school, rarely participates in games, and has no regular neighborhood playmates.

This child is reaching adolescence without the interpersonal skills needed to negotiate the final separation from the parents. Peers and the accompanying activities provide this forum. His teacher, his parents, the school nurse, or the pediatrician needs to investigate the reasons behind Johnny's withdrawal, which will interfere with his development.

The disturbed behavior of most school-age children can be categorized into the five groups listed in Table 37-3. Each of these groups must be considered in terms of *frequency of occurrence, severity, duration,* and *impact on the child's growth and development*.

The pediatric nurse utilizes a working knowledge of major psychiatric problems of children

Table 37-3 Classification of Behavioral Symptoms

Problems with Bodily Functions
Anorexia or overeating, bizarre dietary practices
Sleep disturbances: insomnia, night terrors, excessive sleeping
Elimination difficulties: enuresis, encopresis
Changes in speech: mutism, stuttering, unclear speech

Problems with Motor and Perceptual Coordination
Very active, lethargic, or poorly coordinated
Tics

Problems with Cognitive Functions
Altered attention span
Language disorders
Difficulty with thinking and memory

Problems with Emotional Functions
Fears that interfere with daily life
Severe separation anxiety: cannot be separated from mother
Very anxious all the time: excessive worrying, anticipates the worst outcome in all new situations
Numerous physical complaints without clear physiological reasons: stomachaches, headaches, dizziness, colds, fatigue

Problems with Social Relationships
Unusual aggressiveness: rarely responds to limit setting; seems unable to control aggressive impulses
Antisocial behaviors: disregards other people and their property; shows little remorse or concern when reprimanded
Oppositional behaviors: always takes the opposite position even if this hurts the child
Isolates self from others
Depressed behaviors: aggressiveness or antisocial behavior; either high activity level different from usual pattern or more classic depressive symptoms of sadness, withdrawal, lethargy, anorexia, hopelessness, or discouragement; excessive clumsiness and poor motor coordination, which may be coupled with poor judgment; schoolwork becomes difficult: concentration is poor; thinking is slowed and indecisive; comments about wanting to die, disappear, go away forever, or symbolic stories, e.g., "the sun that went to sleep in the clouds and never came up"; multiple "accidental" injuries: falling out of windows or off roofs, pill ingestion, and self-inflicted injuries

Table 37-4 Psychiatric Problems of Children and Adolescents

1. Affective disorders
   a. Depression
   b. Suicide
2. Pervasive developmental disorders
   a. Infantile autism
   b. Childhood-onset pervasive developmental disorder
3. Childhood psychosis
   a. Schizophrenia
4. Disorders with physical manifestations
   a. Stuttering
   b. Elective mutism
   c. Enuresis
   d. Encopresis
   e. Sleepwalking disorder
   f. Sleep terror disorder
5. Stereotyped movement disorders
   a. Tic disorder
   b. Tourette disorder
6. Eating disorders
   a. Anorexia nervosa
   b. Bulimia
   c. Obesity
7. Conduct disorders
8. Attention deficit disorder (with or without hyperactivity)
9. Anxiety disorders
   a. Separation anxiety (school refusal)
   b. Overanxious disorder
   c. Shyness

Source: Diagnostic and Statistical Manual of Mental Disorders (DSM), 3d ed., American Psychiatric Association, New York, 1980.

in this age group, which are listed in Table 37-4 and discussed in this chapter. Table 37-4 is based on the newest classification system developed by the American Psychiatric Association (DSM III).[1] This broad developmental approach stresses observable signs and symptoms and avoids etiological considerations.

REACTIVE DISORDERS

Reactive disorders are behavioral reactions to *specific,* emotionally traumatic events. Reactions can be *adaptive,* such as short-term regression or withdrawal during an illness. The developmental milestones most recently mastered are temporarily lost as the child regresses; for example, bed-wetting and excessive fearfulness are common responses to traumatic events. Adults around a child often become alarmed at these reactions, but a healthy child usually uses these defense mechanisms temporarily.

Older children have a better command of language and, with support and encouragement from adults, can often verbally express their reactions to a traumatic event. But some children may be overwhelmed by the event or too frightened to put their feelings into words. They may be surrounded by adults who are struggling to cope with the same trauma. Referral for psychological intervention for both the child and the family is appropriate.

School-age children encounter a wide variety of social situations. They may have no opportunity to express their feelings about certain experiences. Secrecy is characteristic of school-age children. Frightening experiences may not be shared with parents.

Reactive responses may be precipitated by a traumatic separation from the parents or a direct threat to the child's integrity of self, such as an accident, school pressure, or ridicule from peers. For example, in gym class during baseball season, a student broke his leg. Later that week a teammate developed overwhelming malaise and mild fever and had to stay home. A physical examination revealed nothing specific and cultures were negative. The student dropped out of the school gym program for the rest of the year with the doctor's permission. This boy was unable to verbalize the overwhelming feelings he had about his classmate's accident. An astute school nurse connected the two events and arranged for the school psychologist to visit the family. Several family meetings and brief therapy with the student remedied the problem.

A psychologically traumatic event that is generally outside the range of children's experiences, such as a car accident, a kidnapping, or rape, can result in a reactive response termed a *posttraumatic stress disorder.*[2] The symptoms include a variety of physical, cognitive, social, and psychological behaviors (see Table 37-5).

The child who experiences this disorder reexperiences the traumatic event either immediately afterward, soon afterward, or at some time following the event. Symptoms range in intensity from mild to severe and include a number of the symptoms listed in Table 37-5. Associated symptoms of depression and anxiety are also common.

Nursing management

The nurse can use two guidelines in identifying behavioral problems: (1) Are these new problems interfering with development? and (2) Have the problem behaviors continued for 6 months?

Table 37-5 Symptoms of Posttraumatic Stress Syndrome

1. Existence of a stressor that would cause significant symptoms of distress in most individuals (e.g., rape)
2. Reexperiencing the trauma through recurrent and intrusive thoughts of the experience, dreams of the experience, and/or sudden acting or feeling as if the trauma were happening again
3. Numbing of responsiveness to, or reduced involvement with, the external environment, as evidenced by significant decrease of interest in previous activities, feeling detached from others, and/or constricted affect
4. At least two of the following symptoms not present before the traumatic experience:
   a. Hyperalertness or exaggerated startle reflex
   b. Sleep disturbance
   c. Guilt about surviving when others have not or about having exhibited the behavior required to survive the experience
   d. Memory impairment or trouble concentrating
   e. Avoidance of activities that arouse recollection of the event
   f. Intensification of symptoms after exposure to events that symbolize or resemble the traumatic event

If these two criteria are met, further assessment and intervention are needed. When assessing a child, the nurse should keep in mind the fact that a mild, unexpected incident may have a *profound* effect on the child. The child may misinterpret what happened or blame himself or herself for the event. The nurse can help a family trace through recent events that may have precipitated the child's current emotional distress. If the stress is not prolonged and emotional support is available, most children recover and develop new coping behaviors.

AFFECTIVE DISORDERS

Depression

Although an increased amount of research on depression in children has been done in recent years, much of the information is still based on research on, and theories of, depression in adults. One of the psychological explanations for childhood depression is the child's response to separation and loss.

The child must resolve the loss with the help of those close to him or her. The depression may deepen if the child's feelings are not relieved. A child needs opportunities to talk and to ask the same questions repeatedly. This may be painful to other family members who are also in mourning. Supportive counseling may help the family tolerate the child's continual questions.

The school-age child has the capacity to become deeply despondent. A child can have feelings of extreme hopelessness and helplessness and can even contemplate suicide. The younger suicidal school-age child may have an unclear understanding of the finality of death, but this does not influence the depth of the depression or the impulsive desire to end the hurt. While childhood depression is seen in this younger group, it occurs more commonly in prepubertal children, aged 9 to 12, and is still more common in adolescence.

Depressive symptoms may be masked by excessive aggressiveness and other antisocial behavior. Underneath this aggressiveness, which is a defense, the child feels sad, discouraged, and hopeless. (See Table 37-6 for symptoms of depression in children and adolescents.) Schoolwork becomes difficult: concentration is poor, thinking is slowed and indecisive, and excessive clumsiness may occur.[3]

Many childhood accidents and accidental deaths are masked suicide attempts. Adults have difficulty accepting the idea that a child's feelings of worthlessness could lead to suicide. When healthy children are very angry, they feel free to express their wishes to banish or hurt their parents. A suicidal child turns these feelings inside toward the self rather than toward others or the outside world.

Nurses can identify depression in hospitalized children using screening tools incorporated into their nursing assessment.[4] (See Chap. 15.) A mild depressive reaction can occur when the child is adjusting to the hospital. However, some children do not resolve these feelings and continue to be depressed after returning home. These children may show the following symptoms: anorexia, listlessness, loss of interest in the surroundings (toys, other children, and adults), altered speech or mutism, staring with blank despondency, failure to be comforted by physical tenderness, and overwhelming sadness expressed verbally or in drawings.

A severely depressed child may require hospitalization for safety while being treated. Antidepressants are used judiciously and require careful monitoring in a growing child. The environment must be kept safe. Medications and sharp objects must be removed from the room; bathroom doors should not lock and must be

Table 37-6 Symptoms of Depression in a Child or Adolescent

1. Dysphoric mood
   a. Makes statements about, or has appearance of, sadness, unhappiness, hopelessness, and/or helplessness
   b. Has mood swings; is moody
   c. Is irritable and easily annoyed
   d. Is hypersensitive; cries easily
   e. Is negative and difficult to please
2. Self-deprecatory ideation
   a. Has feeling of being worthless, useless, dumb, ugly, and/or stupid (negative self-concept)
   b. Has beliefs of persecution
   c. Has death wishes
   d. Wants to run away or leave home
   e. Has suicidal thoughts
   f. Makes suicide attempts
3. Aggressive behavior (agitation)
   a. Is difficult to get along with
   b. Is quarrelsome
   c. Disrespects authority
   d. Acts belligerent, hostile, and agitated
   e. Fights excessively; becomes suddenly angry
4. Sleep disturbances
   a. Has initial insomnia
   b. Sleeps restlessly
   c. Has terminal insomnia
   d. Has difficulty waking in the morning
5. Change in school performance
   a. Frequent complaints from teachers about daydreaming, poor concentration, poor memory
   b. Diminished work effort in school subjects
   c. Diminished interest in nonacademic school activities
6. Diminished socialization
   a. Shows decreased group participation
   b. Is less friendly and less outgoing
   c. Withdraws socially
   d. Loses social interests
7. Change in attitude toward school
   a. Does not enjoy school activities
   b. Does not want or refuses to go to school
8. Somatic complaints
   a. Has nonmigraine headaches
   b. Has abdominal pain
   c. Has muscle aches and pains
   d. Has other somatic concerns or complaints
9. Loss of usual energy
   a. Is no longer interested in pursuits other than school (e.g., hobbies)
   b. Has decreased energy; is mentally and/or physically fatigued
10. Has unusual change in appetite and/or weight

Source: Warren Wineberg et al., "Depression in Children Referred to an Educational Diagnostic Center: Diagnosis and Treatment," *Journal of Pediatrics*, **83:**1065–1072 (1973).

openable from the outside; and the child's room should be located near the nurses' station, away from elevators and exits.

Suicide in childhood and adolescence

The number of suicides has increased 11 percent in the last 20 years, and suicide is now the second leading cause of death among adolescents in the United States. The number of completed suicides among children is also increasing. Suicidal behavior in children as young as 5 or 6 years of age has been reported. Statistics show that while more females attempt suicide, males complete suicide more frequently because they use more lethal weapons, such as guns.

Children's attitudes toward, and beliefs about, death vary according to their level of cognitive development.[5] (See Chap. 35.) Children under 9 years of age believe that death is a reversible state. This belief may even continue into adolescence. During the latency period and earlier, children may, through the use of magical thinking, believe that suicide will reunite them with a pet or a loved one who has died. Children may attempt suicide to punish their parents or to retaliate against their parents' disciplinary actions. They are not aware that they will not be alive to observe the consequences of their action.

The major factors which increase the risk of attempted suicide in children and adolescents are:

1. Loss of a parent, a close family friend, or a pet or the end of a significant attachment as a result of death or separation. An event which leads to loss of self-esteem or perceived loss of peer support, particularly for an adolescent, may precipitate a suicidal crisis.
2. Family factors such as a family history of depression and suicide attempts, drug or alcohol abuse, marital relationships in which there is severe conflict with threats of separation, and hostile and defensive communication patterns with little expression of support or empathy.
3. A chronic illness (mental or physical) that alters body image and self-concept (including illnesses that, although not disfiguring, distinguish the child or adolescent from his or her peers, such as diabetes, epilepsy, and asthma).
4. Previous suicide attempts, particularly when successive attempts have involved increas-

ingly lethal means or increased painfulness. The child or adolescent may become desensitized to self-injury and eventually succeed in the suicide attempt.

5. A suicide plan. The risk of a suicide attempt increases as the suicide plan (e.g., the method, the time, and the place) becomes more specific.

No one factor has been found to explain the occurrence of suicide among children and adolescents, although a number of theories have emerged. Theories that propose a hereditary basis to suicidal behavior focus on the genetic predispositions within families to affective disorders such as depression. Depression, though not the sole reason for suicidal behavior, is highly correlated with suicidal behavior.

Social theorists suggest that a dysfunctional social network in which social supports are lacking may precipitate feelings of loneliness, isolation, and depression which lead to suicide. In addition, dysfunction within the family, including confusion of roles and feelings of powerlessness, may lead to the experience of hopelessness and helplessness. Actual or perceived rejection by family members or peers may also contribute to suicidal behavior.

Psychoanalytic theorists focus on the loss of self-esteem, the loss of a person or object, or the loss of especially meaningful experiences as the grounds for suicidal behavior. Because each individual attaches a special meaning to an experience, the loss can be of a symbolic nature. For example, a child who attempts suicide after being forbidden by a parent to ride a bicycle for a week is reacting to the loss of privileges and to the discipline rather than to the actual inability to ride the bicycle.

Nursing management Children and adolescents frequently attempt to alert others to their feelings prior to a suicide attempt. Warnings, regardless of their nature, should be taken seriously. A child who locks himself or herself in a closet and refuses to leave, stating, "I want to be left alone to die," is at risk for making a more serious suicidal attempt if the underlying problem is not dealt with by health professionals. A child who attempts suicide using a relatively less lethal weapon or method is at a greater risk for making a more serious attempt in the future, particularly if no psychological intervention is offered to the child. Children's warnings should *not* be interpreted as a barometer of the seriousness of their intention to harm themselves. The injuries listed at the bottom of Table 37-3 should alert the pediatric staff to the possibility of an attempted suicide.

Nursing assessment includes asking the child specific questions about the child's suicide plan, rescue fantasies, choice of method or weapon, and ideas about the consequences of the suicide attempt.[6] If the child is talking about how terrible life is, ask, "What would you do if things got worse?" It is also important for the nurse to ask what the child thinks will happen both during and after the attempt in order to explore the fantasies that the child has about suicide. For example, the child may fantasize about being saved by a parent in the midst of the attempt or might believe that he or she will become a very different person after demonstrating his or her unhappiness.

The acutely suicidal child in the hospital requires *constant* observation by the nurse to ensure the child's safety. This surveillance is called *suicide observation, suicide watch,* or *one-to-one observation*. The nurse must assess the environment each shift and remove all potential suicide weapons. The bathroom and closet doors must be unlockable, and visitors must be instructed not to bring in any potential weapons. The nurse should then talk with the child about alternative ways of meeting his or her needs. The nurse should precisely document on the chart the child's nonverbal and verbal behavioral responses. Whether the child is referred for psychological intervention on an inpatient or outpatient basis depends on the results of the psychological assessment, the lethality of the suicide plan, and the potential risk.

PERVASIVE DEVELOPMENTAL DEVIATIONS

Infantile autism

Pervasive developmental deviations are characterized by distortions in the development of the child's social skills, language, and cognitive functions. These distortions take the form of attention-seeking behavior, reality testing, and disturbances in perception and motor movements.[7] Developmental deviations are labeled *pervasive* because many psychological areas are affected at the same time. The child's behavior is extremely abnormal and would not be considered normal at any age. For example, the object twirling, high-pitched shrieks, hand flapping, and rhythmic rocking of autistic children would be very odd in a child of any age. *Infantile autism* is the major subgroup of pervasive developmental deviations. These severely disturbed children account for a small percentage of disturbed children. The incidence of autism is 2 in 10,000 to 4 in 10,000 children; it is more common in boys. Autistic children present a challenge to nurses when they are ill and hospitalized. A knowledge of their developmental struggle is essential in order to plan effective nursing care.

The cause of infantile autism remains unknown. Organic conditions associated with the disorder are phenylketonuria, congenital rubella, tuberous sclerosis, lead intoxication, congenital syphilis, and fragile X syndrome. Recent research has been geared toward finding and treating a relatively high blood serotonin concentration in children and adolescents with infantile autism.[8]

The diagnosis of infantile autism is made after thorough assessment. Mental retardation, schizophrenia, and language delays need to be ruled out during the differential diagnosis process. Neuropsychiatric interviews, psychological assessments, language samplings and assessments, and developmental inventories are used to differentiate infantile autism from other childhood disorders.

The following clinical manifestations, ranging from mild to severe, are exhibited by autistic children:[9,10]

1. *Disturbances of developmental rate* Arrests, delays, and regressions in motor, social, language, and cognitive development are common.
2. *Disturbances in the capacity to relate to people, events, and objects in the environment* Failure to develop appropriate reactions and relationships is a classic symptom of autism. The young child may show no evidence of attachment behavior: no stranger anxiety, no eye contact, no smiling, or even no molding to the caretaker's arms. The child makes odd, repetitive movements; ritualistic behavior is common, and the child cannot play cooperatively. If the child's routine or rituals are changed, he or she reacts with panic, crying, and rage.
3. *Disturbances of speech, language, and cognition* Speech may be delayed or absent. Immature articulation and syntax and odd inflections are common. The child uses symbols with difficulty and thinks concretely for a prolonged time. He or she frequently practices echolalia (repeating words spoken by another person). The use of inappropriate body gestures shows that the child does not understand the symbolic meaning of these body movements; this reflects a defect in cognition. For example, autistic children may tap an adult on the knee when they want to urinate, rather than attempting to pull down their pants.
4. *Disturbances of responses to stimuli* The child's behavior alternates between hyperactivity and hypoactivity within a wide time period of several hours to several months. One or more senses may be involved in the child's abnormal response to stimuli. For example, one child may not respond to verbal commands or loud noises but may become extremely upset and run away from an ordinary sound, such as a knock on the door. Another child might rub various materials together, apparently to feel different textures. Another child might disregard painful stimuli and not be sensitive to fine textural differences. The autistic child prefers varied smells and tastes. One child might smell and smear feces, while another might eat clay, both of which are offensive to most people.

The autistic infant is a "good baby," lying quietly in the crib, self-absorbed, crying little, and demanding minimal nurturing. The parent may unknowingly reinforce the infant's withdrawn behavior by leaving the baby alone. Failure to mold to the parent's body when held and failure to show anticipation of being picked up by the parent are common. The withdrawal from people influences other aspects of the child's development. Language and cognitive development lag. The autistic child repeatedly echoes words or phrases, avoids eye contact, and is negativistic. To maintain sameness of the environment, the child adopts certain rituals, such as touching walls. He or she withdraws from outside stimuli into an inner world (see Fig. 37-1). Self-stimulatory behavior increases: body rocking, head banging, object twirling, staring at lights, and moving to music.

Special nursery school stimulation and behavioral programming need to begin early. Educa-

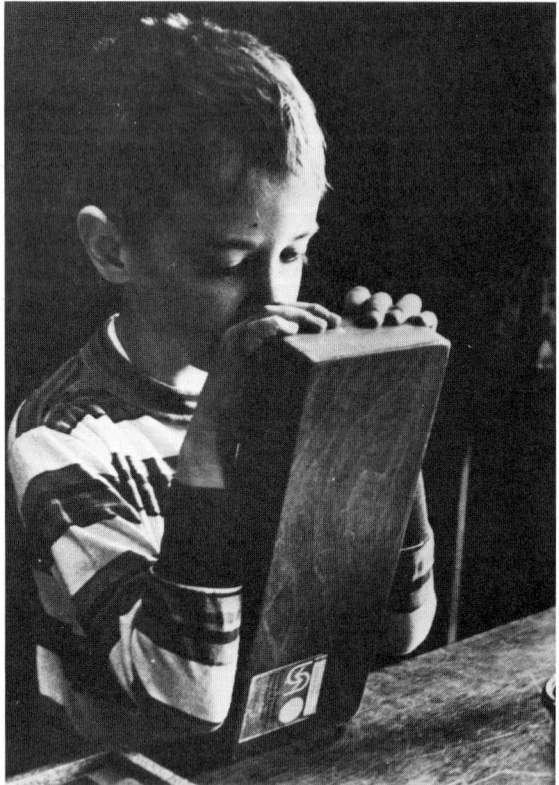

Figure 37-1 The autistic child is profoundly withdrawn from human relationships. (*Courtesy of Benhaven.*)

tional training is the primary form of treatment for school-age autistic children. It is difficult for the other family members to deal with sudden rage, fits of crying, strange fears, and other emotional outbursts. Autistic children lack the normal fears that promote safety, such as caution about cars and fire. Extra supervision must be provided. Family therapy may be needed to help the parents and siblings cope with the daily stress produced by having the child at home.

Nursing management Autistic children are usually quite healthy and require normal pediatric care. As such a child grows older, the question of placing the child in an institution may arise. The parents may try coping with the child at home and enrolling the child in special schools but may find that this does not work because the needs of the family outweigh those of the child. Locating appropriate placement for the child in the community may be very difficult. It may be necessary to put the child in an institution far from home and visit infrequently. A nurse may be able to help with such decisions by serving as a sounding board and by providing referral to a social service agency for placement or home services.[11,12]

Research has not supported the earlier belief that parents cause psychological disturbances in their children. During the 1950s and 1960s, parents were frequently blamed for their children's autistic behavior. These parents were characterized as highly intellectual, oriented toward abstractions rather than toward people, and emotionally aloof from their children. The infant was thought to enter a nonnurturing, nonsupportive, nonloving world. However, some poorly functioning families produce healthy children, and some healthy families have disturbed children. Therefore, many researchers now believe that environmental influences and both the parents' and the child's vulnerabilities interact to cause the child's disturbed behavior.

It is important for the nurse to assess the parents' beliefs about their role in their child's disorder. Reassuring them that they were not the cause of the child's autism will be supportive and help the parents accept their child's diagnosis. (See Chap. 34.)

Treatment A variety of treatments have been used with autistic children. *Milieu therapy* establishes an environment designed to promote growth. The child is encouraged to learn that the world is not destructive, to experience and manage destructive impulses and feelings, and gradually to form relationships with adults. *Behavior modification* techniques use the principles of reward and punishment to change the child's behavior. Behavior modification reduces tantrums and self-destructive behavior, teaches basic speech and social responses, increases the attention span, and teaches letter and word recognition.[13] Some success has been achieved with adolescents who are kept in regular classrooms and placed in carefully chosen work situations, with the aim of teaching them to live within the community.

Childhood-onset pervasive developmental disorder

This is an extremely rare disorder in which there is a severe impairment of emotional relationships. The child cannot make friends, clings to family members and caretakers, and lacks empathy with, and regard for, the feelings of others. Such tendencies are observable in infancy and the toddler years, but a diagnosis is usually confirmed between the ages of 3 and 12. The child is initially less disturbed and shows fewer of the autistic child's peculiar behaviors (see Table 37-7).

Several of the following behaviors must be present before a diagnosis of childhood-onset pervasive development disorder is made.[14]

1. *Acute, illogical anxiety* Unexplained panic attacks and hysterical reactions to everyday events (e.g., hearing a doorbell ring or seeing a series of blue cars).
2. *Distorted emotional responses* Inappropriate fears, unexplained rages, and extreme moodiness.
3. *Resistance to any change* The child requires special rituals and repetitive behavior to feel better: The same clothes are demanded each day, and furniture cannot be changed around, or routines varied; repetitive touching of a particular object (e.g., an ashtray or the corners of a desk) reduces the child's anxiety when relating to another person.
4. *Hyperactivity or hypoactivity, strange body postures* (unusual arching of the back or extending of the neck), and *special hand and finger movements*.
5. *Strange vocal quality* The voice has a sing-song or monotonous quality.
6. *Oversensitivity or undersensitivity to sensory and perceptual experiences* (touch, sound, and vision).
7. *Self-mutilation* The child bites himself or herself, bangs the head, or pulls the hair.

Widespread neurological abnormalities are present in many of the children afflicted with childhood-onset pervasive developmental deviations. These neurological problems show up as seizures, abnormal electroencephalograms (EEGs), visual problems, extreme sensitivity to noise and touch, abnormal reflexes, and medical histories of infections, tumors, poisoning, and severe head injuries. Some researchers believe that the child's behavioral symptoms result from an impairment in the reticular formation of the brain stem.

CHILDHOOD PSYCHOSES

Childhood psychoses are extremely rare; the incidence is 1 in 2600 children. Psychoses beginning in infancy occur even less often, with an incidence of 1 in 10,000 infants. Childhood schizophrenia is a form of childhood psychosis.

Childhood schizophrenia

Childhood schizophrenia is a label indicating a dramatic deviation from normal ego functioning. This classification is reserved for children exhib-

Table 37-7 Comparison of Autism and Childhood-Onset Pervasive Developmental Disorder

	Autism	Childhood-Onset Pervasive Developmental Disorder
Onset	Before 30 months	After 30 months; onset follows period of normal development
Language	Gross language deficits: echoing words and sounds, speaking in metaphors, being mute, reversing pronouns, using immature grammatical structure; demonstrates no abstract thinking	Language present but bizarre: sing-song, monotone, made-up words, rhyming (beyond the normal level of the preschool period)
Emotion	Lacks emotional responsiveness; does not mold to parents' bodies; is self-involved	Emotional responses present but abnormal; rage and panic attacks; molds and clings to parents' bodies
Anxiety	Acute anxiety *not* present	Acute, illogical anxiety present
Genetic family history	Parents have high intelligence, emotional stability, low divorce rate; low rate of family mental illness	More average background; higher rate of mental illness in family
Orientation	Is detached, self-absorbed	Is disoriented and confused
Motor coordination	Refined gross and fine motor coordination	Poor balance and coordination

iting a majority of classically schizophrenic behaviors. These children lack the normal guides necessary for self-regulation, for achieving an identity, and for differentiating inner (their own) from outer (others') experiences. The onset of a schizophrenic episode can be gradual, occurring from early childhood to adolescence. The relationship between childhood schizophrenia and adult schizophrenia continues to be a disputed topic.[15] Recent studies suggest that a genetic predisposition is involved in childhood schizophrenia.[16] The incidence of this form of mental illness is higher among identical twins than among ordinary siblings, for example, even when the children are reared in separate environments.

Childhood psychoses have been conceptualized on a continuum. At one end may be an organic or genetic cause; at the opposite end are harmful environmental influences. The children midway on the continuum have disturbed behavior caused by both organic and environmental influences; they disprove the single-causation theories. The multiple impact of these factors on a child may produce the more severe kinds of childhood psychoses.

Nursing management Early identification of these children is the most significant contribution that the nurse can make. A parent may complain to the nurse about a child's peculiar and troublesome habits. For example, the child's need for rituals can be exasperating; the hysterical screaming for no reason is embarrassing in public places; strange fears may limit a family's outside activities; and unusual movements and self-mutilation can be frightening, especially when the child is out of control. The nurse may detect the parent's need to avoid the painful awareness that the child is different and even bizàrre at times. The parent can be helped by critical, sensitive listening on the part of the nurse and can aid in identifying an area that can be managed through behavioral interventions.

Example: Three-year-old Ann arrived for a pre-nursery school physical. She was not toilet-trained, ran around touching all corners of the room, and would suddenly burst into screams without tears and cling to her mother's leg. The nurse noticed that Ann's hairline on her forehead was irregular. Ann's mother described a bedtime ritual: Ann banged her head on the crib and rocked herself to sleep.

Ann needed immediate referral for a developmental and psychiatric examination. Ann's mother was reluctant to follow through because she feared that her daughter would be labeled "crazy." She was also afraid of being blamed for Ann's peculiar behaviors. She had given up trying to toilet-train Ann because the child was so unmanageable in other areas.

The nurse offered suggestions for behavior modification based on Ann's developmental needs. Toilet training, it was explained, proceeds much as it would for a normal child. However, each step is broken down into smaller behaviors for the child to master. The nurse pointed out that mastering toilet training would help Ann gain control over a natural function. This control would be transferred to other behavioral areas that eventually would be mastered.

Ann's mother found these suggestions helpful and began voicing some of her feelings about Ann's development.

If the nurse can establish a trusting relationship, it can support the family while they begin the painful experience of learning their child's limitations and strengths.

Treatment approaches include a full range of therapies. The child will need special education. Depending on the child's level of functioning, this may be either a mainstream experience in a regular school or residential treatment. The trend today is toward intensive education, milieu therapy and the return of the child to the community, if possible. Individual psychotherapy focuses on the child's anxiety and inner experiences. The educational setting provides the forum for learning how to handle bizarre feelings and thoughts when the child is with others. Behavior modification is useful in controlling self-mutilating behaviors and eliminating the often strange body movements. Family therapy may be needed to help the whole family cope with the disturbed child and to identify any process within the family that may be fostering these peculiar behaviors.

The pediatric nurse plays an important role in the health maintenance of disturbed children. These special children and their families need extra support during routine health care procedures. Ordinary experiences are frightening to severely disturbed children. Blood tests, throat cultures, rectal examinations, and even being weighed become insurmountable problems. Patience and desensitizing through planning with a parent will go a long way toward providing routine health care.

DISORDERS WITH PHYSICAL MANIFESTATIONS

Stuttering

Stuttering is a complex behavioral disorder that results from an interaction of genetic and environmental factors. The fact that stuttering occurs in families has been known for centuries, and yet the reason is still not understood. Most research studies report a male/female ratio ranging from 2 to 1 to 5 to 1. Stuttering affects about 5 percent of children.

Most children begin to stutter before school age and spontaneously stop stuttering without treatment. Children who stutter mildly and only occasionally will not usually be at an emotional or vocational disadvantage. However, the incidence of persistent and more severe stuttering is 3 in 1000 children, and these children's life adjustments can be seriously affected by the disorder.

There are no conclusive theories that explain the cause of stuttering. A great deal of controversy also exists regarding the definition of stuttering. Young children normally have speech interruptions. It is difficult to assess early stuttering and differentiate it from the disfluencies of normally talking children.[17,18]

The earlier the stuttering is identified and treated, the better the child's prognosis for successful treatment and life adjustment will be. After the parents express concern to the nurse or other health professional about their child's stuttering, a differential evaluation by a speech and language therapist can determine whether (1) concern about the child's speech pattern is warranted and (2) what developmental and/or environmental factors need intervention to prevent the development or exacerbation of the stuttering, if a problem exists. This preventative approach considers and treats each child's individual problems and needs.[19]

Nursing management Parents and caretakers can be given two basic instructions to help a stuttering child. First, do not emphasize the expressive difficulty by calling attention to the stuttering, do not supply the word when the child is blocking, and do not tell the child to "start over and take it easy." Even offering praise is a type of negative labeling—"you aren't stuttering as much." Second, identify tension-producing situations in the child's life. Many families today are caught up in a hectic life-style that permits few relaxed moments. "Hurry up" may be frequently pressed upon a child, and the preschooler may find it impossible, under such pressure, to coordinate ideas and emerging speech patterns. Giving these children plenty of time, looking at them when they talk, and paying attention are important when they learn to talk.

Most young preschool children hesitate or repeat certain words or syllables, especially when excited or under stress. The parents may fail to realize that this hesitancy or repetition is normal, and they may unknowingly make matters worse by offering corrections or otherwise calling attention to the "problem." Tension between the parents and the child then builds. A parent's disappointment and confusion over "why my child can't speak" lead to mounting irritation with each verbal exchange. The child cannot understand the parent's feelings. Simple guidelines for parents can be invaluable and may be sufficient intervention when language is emerging and stuttering begins (see Table 37-8).

Elective mutism

Elective mutism is the term used to describe the behavior of children and adolescents who *choose* not to speak in specific environments or with specific people. The mute child typically speaks fluently with the immediate family but remains mute with teachers, peers, and others at school. Many therapists describe cases of elective mutism wherein the child is very communicative

Table 37-8 Guidelines for Parents of Preschoolers Who Are Beginning to Stutter

1. Ignore normal hesitation and repetitive sounds as speech emerges. Focus on intelligible sounds by reinforcing them through repetition and praise of clear words or sounds.
2. Focus on what the child is trying to communicate *without* questioning and guessing; interruptions discourage speech in any young child.
3. Slow your rate of speaking to the child's pace.
4. Simplify your language, speaking at the child's level.
5. Set aside time each day to do a few verbal exercises with your child. For example:
   a. Rhyming games, counting, naming all the blue objects in a room.
   b. When reading a story, ask the child to tell you about his or her favorite animal, person, or object in the story or ask the child to describe something happening on an eye-catching page.
   c. Play together for a short time and then ask the child to tell you what is happening.

nonverbally, using gestures and pantomime. These children clearly understand what is being said to them. This disorder usually occurs before the age of 5 years or when the child enters school. However, elective mutism has been reported among older children and adolescents.

Elective mutes characteristically demonstrate the following behaviors: hypersensitivity, shyness, and familial speech (usually articulation) disturbances. Besides mutism, they may also show excessive shyness or sensitivity over being teased, may cling to the mother, may refuse to go to school, and may wet the bed, soil themselves, and engage in temper tantrums and other controlling or oppositional behavior, especially at home.

The causes of mutism continue to be debated by mental health professionals. Behavioral therapists believe that mutism is a learned behavior pattern, while psychoanalysts claim that psychological and social processes are the cause. Stressful trauma before 3 years of age, physical trauma involving the mouth, and early hospitalization are among the predisposing factors associated with elective mutism. Other factors include pathological family interactions such as excessive marital strife (the use of silence by the parents to express their hostility and their disapproval of each other's behavior), passive-aggressive behavior to express hostility, and symbiotic parent-child relationships. A mother who speaks a foreign language and remains isolated at home may have a child who simply refuses to speak the new language.[20]

The different etiological theories have resulted in various programs of treatment for elective mutism. The majority of recently reported treatments for elective mutism are behavioral.[21] Positive reinforcement and stimulus fading, aversive conditioning, prompting and modeling, shaping, and using tokens to reward behavior are all examples of behavioral techniques reported as successful treatment approaches. Psychodynamic intervention strategies, in contrast, are highly individualized and focus on the intrapsychic and social causes of the child's mutism.

Nursing management The nurse's role is to prevent and identify elective mutism. Adequate preparation and support of a family with a young hospitalized child can prevent this symptom choice. The nurse can identify vulnerable families, for example, an immigrant family isolated from the larger community. Most young children are constantly talking and making sounds. By being alert to the excessively quiet child or to the parents' comment that their child does not talk much or talks less than before, the nurse will help the child receive early treatment. An experienced clinician should differentially diagnose this disorder to rule out mental retardation, language disorders, childhood depression, anxiety disorders, and adjustment problems. The nurse can assess the child's mutism by asking, "Does the child use any syllables or gestures?" "Are there special people to whom the child directs some words or sounds?" Psychotherapy, often with the family as a unit, is warranted when the diagnosis of elective mutism is established.

Enuresis

Enuresis is the *persistent, involuntary* voiding of urine either day or night after the age of 4 years at least once a month. Both nocturnal and daytime enuresis tend toward self-correction or spontaneous remission. *Primary enuresis* is enuresis, either during the day or at night, in a child who was never fully toilet-trained. *Secondary enuresis* is incontinence that occurs at least once a month after urinary continence (toilet training) has been established for at least 1 year. The chance of developing secondary enuresis decreases with age. The birth of a sibling, divorce of the parents, or hospitalization may precipitate secondary enuresis as a stress response in the younger child.[22]

Primary enuresis is due to delayed development of the neurological system. Boys are affected more often than girls, and there is a familial tendency. Every enuretic child should be evaluated for organic causes such as urinary tract infections *before* psychological treatment is begun.

Enuresis affects families in a variety of ways. Parents who wish or demand that their child stop the inconvenient wetting are losing a maturational battle. Their child's neurological system needs further development. Some normal preschool children become absorbed in play, forget to heed the cues from their bladder, and void before reaching the toilet. Many children with psychiatric disorders of childhood have persistent enuresis. However, not all children with enuresis have emotional problems. If a thorough physical examination, including an emotional assessment, has linked no emotional difficulties to the enuresis, the parents need the nurse's support to understand that their child will gradually outgrow the problem.

Some parents unwisely continue using diapers to avoid inconvenience and extra laundry; this carries a clear message of "my child the baby." Most children who have been toilet-trained feel belittled or confused if diapered. The child's feeling of having been belittled is accentuated if there is a younger, diapered child in the home. A particularly frustrating situation may exist when there is an older enuretic son and a younger daughter who is day- and night-trained. Careful consideration of the child's feelings is important for the development of self-esteem. Any accusations by the parents, venting of anger while changing the sheets, or stating that the enuresis is voluntary or deliberate will only confuse and create unnecessary feelings of guilt in the child.

After medical and possible surgical interventions have been ruled out, the parents may request medication to control the bed-wetting. Tofranil (imipramine), an antidepressant, is the primary medication used to control enuresis. Tofranil controls the child's involuntary voiding by affecting the muscles surrounding the bladder. This medication has serious side effects and should be used with caution.

Research has shown that behavior modification techniques using an alarm device are more successful than medication. Mechanical bells and alarm devices used at night are successful in treating nocturnal enuresis.[23] The sleeping child is awakened by a bell when voiding. These devices *must* be used according to the manufacturer's instructions; the nurse should review the instructions with the parents. However, behavior modification techniques such as the devices cannot hasten the child's neurological maturation.

Nursing management The stresses of hospitalization and separation from the family frequently cause enuresis in the ill child. Helping the parents anticipate the problem may be useful. Nurses should instruct the parents in the following methods of decreasing the child's voiding during sleep: (1) decrease the child's fluid intake before he or she goes to bed, (2) have the child void just prior to going to bed, and (3) get the child up to void before the parents go to bed. The nurse should also try to decrease the child's stress associated with hospitalization as much as possible.[24,25] (Chapter 15 discusses methods of reducing the stress of hospitalization.)

Encopresis

Encopresis is the voluntary or involuntary passage of feces of near-normal consistency in an inappropriate place. Most children are fully bowel- and bladder-trained by age 5. Children usually master first bowel and then bladder control. (See Chap. 10 for a discussion of toilet training.) The former is easier to achieve because it is a more predictable physiological function. There are two types of encopresis: primary and secondary. In *primary encopresis,* training is not completed by 5 years of age, and soiling continues at least once per month. Primary encopresis is associated with poor and inconsistent toilet training. However, most children achieve bowel control by 3 years of age with minimum help and maximum patience on the part of the family.

Secondary encopresis occurs when a child who has achieved bowel control begins withholding feces. This is usually associated with family problems, tensions, or life stresses. In most cases it is transient unless the family members focus on it rather than alleviating the family problem or tension.

Encopresis is more common in boys. Unlike enuresis, encopresis does not run in families, but bathroom habits may be unusual in many family members. The parents may excessively emphasize cleanliness related to bowel habits, or they may go to the other extreme and not have demanded regular toileting of the child during the training period.

Soiling refers to the most common symptom of encopresis, defecating into underwear. Loose stools may seep around a bolus of impacted stool formed by withholding defecation. Some children are embarrassed to use public bathrooms and school toilets and attempt to "hold" their bowel movements until they get home. Some children also refuse to wipe themselves and therefore soil their underwear. While this may seem less serious, it is still considered a form of encopresis, and a closer look by the parents and the nurse is warranted.

Many encopretic children defecate in unusual places, such as shoes or closet corners, to hide their bowel movements. Others develop severe constipation and overflow diarrhea. If soiling or inappropriate withholding of stool occurs beyond the age of 3 years, a careful assessment of the child and the family system should begin (see Table 37-9). Prolonged withholding can produce distention of the large bowel and result in other medical complications.[26]

Table 37-9 Guide for Assessing an Encopretic Child

1. When did bowel training begin, and by whom was it given?
2. Methods used: How long was each used, and why did several methods need to be used?
3. Child's response to questions 1 and 2: Was there self-initiated interest in bowel training?
4. Presence of urinary incontinence.
5. Presence of other behavioral disturbances or parents' concerns:
   a. Temper tantrums.
   b. Dietary patterns.
   c. Child is too active by parents' standards.
6. Bowel habits and attitudes of other family members.
   a. Demands of excessive cleanliness.
   b. Unusual toilet habits of parents: regular use of laxatives, enemas, or other measures.

Nursing management The focus of nursing intervention is on alleviating both the physical symptoms and the psychosocial stressors associated with the disorder.[27] Pediatric nurses also help cleanse an impaction using enemas and medication. This is obviously a very sensitive situation for the child because both the symptom (encopresis) and the treatment (enemas) involve the same body part. Supportive talking and handling of the equipment, through doll play, are very useful for letting a child "play out" feelings of bodily intrusion. A surprising amount of enema fluid may be absorbed by the child's bowel; careful monitoring of the quantity of fluid instilled and returned and careful monitoring of vital signs must be done and documented on the chart. Other useful play media are clay and paints (see Chap. 15). However, care must be exercised with these materials; encopretic children often have a strong aversion, despite their encopresis, to "messing" consciously. Offering a child a choice of several play activities is a more sensitive approach until the child's strengths and vulnerabilities are assessed.

Behavior modification techniques are used successfully by nurses to alter bowel habits. Instruct the parents to have the child sit on the toilet for perhaps 10 min 1 to 2 h after meals, on arising, or both to establish a regular stooling pattern. Give the child hugs, praises, and rewards after each successful stool and when the pants are clean. For example, a nurse helped one family establish a reward system. The preschooler received hugs, kisses, and a sticker after each normal stool and at the end of the day if the pants were clean. If the pants had been clean for a week, the child received a package of sugarless gum. Star charts also work well; the child is given a star for each day that the pants are clean. As the child achieves more success, 2 or 3 "clean" weeks can be rewarded with a coveted toy.

School nurses can support the encopretic child by providing a private place where the child can wash and change his or her underpants without being ridiculed by other children. One encopretic boy who smelled like stool was called "Frankenstein" by his classmates and was ostracized from the peer group. Having a safe place to change his clothes would have decreased the ridicule. A child who is embarrassed to use public bathrooms may also be helped if he or she is allowed to use the nurse's bathroom.

Sleep disorders

Sleep disorders are a recurring complaint of parents.[28] The child awakens at night, has nightmares, and is reluctant to go back to sleep. Sleepwalking and sleep terror disorder are less common than sleep problems. Sleep problems are caused by environmental factors (such as stress, fatigue, watching violent television shows before bedtime, or engaging in stimulating play before going to bed), central nervous system immaturity, and psychological factors (such as fear of separation from the parents).[29] The nursing management of children with sleep disorders is discussed in Chap. 10.

Sleepwalking Approximately 15 percent of children between 6 and 12 years of age have isolated experiences of *sleepwalking* (somnambulism). Boys sleepwalk more frequently than girls. Sleepwalking usually disappears by adolescence. Episodes occur during the first 1 to 3 h of sleep and last from a few moments to 30 min.

The child typically sits up, gets out of bed, dresses, eats, or goes to the bathroom during a sleepwalking episode. The child can be injured by walking through a window or falling down stairs, even though the eyes are open while sleepwalking. Apparently, the sleepwalker cannot judge potential hazards. The child may return to bed or fall asleep in a different location. The child has no memory of sleepwalking upon awakening.

Fatigue, stress, and sleep medications have been related to sleepwalking. The cause remains uncertain, even though physiological, environmental, and genetic factors have been considered.

Sleep terror disorder *Sleep terror disorder* (pavor nocturnus) affects 1 to 4 percent of children between 4 and 12 years of age. It occurs more frequently in males and usually disappears by adolescence. The other family members are commonly affected and the cause remains unknown.

Episodes of sleep terror disorder differ from nightmares in the following ways:

1. Each episode may last up to 20 min and is not followed by waking.
2. The child commonly clings to objects, screams, runs, and jumps, and the eyes are open.
3. The child is unresponsive to comfort and reassurance.
4. The child exhibits signs and symptoms of severe anxiety: profuse perspiration, rapid breathing and pulse, dilated pupils, agitated movements, and a fearful facial expression.

Nursing management Sleep disorders frequently occur in children during hospitalization and during periods of illness and stress. Separation from the family, fatigue, pain, side effects of medication, and waking in the strange hospital environment are factors contributing to sleep disturbances in the hospital.

The child's sleep habits and nighttime routines are an important part of the nurse's admission assessment and should be written on the nursing care plan. The parents (or the child, if he or she is old enough) can describe bedtime comfort measures such as a favorite toy or blanket or a night-light. Specific fears associated with the hospitalization must be assessed and alleviated. For example, a child who feels unsafe in the hospital without the parents' protective presence will have difficulty sleeping. Allowing a parent to sleep in the room will help considerably.

The child should be reassured that the nurse will make frequent checks during the night. Tell the child that he or she can change the dream content; for example, "During a nightmare, dream that you are very powerful and can frighten away any monsters with a magic sword!" Increasing the child's feelings of control during sleep decreases frightening dreams. Neuromuscular relaxation techniques are another effective nursing intervention to induce sleep in children.[30] The nurse can purchase relaxation tapes or develop them. The parents can also be taught by the nurse to provide bedtime relaxation sessions for their child.[31] (See Chap. 15 for additional suggestions for inducing sleep.)

CONDUCT DISORDERS

Conduct disorders are characterized by repetitive and persistent patterns of antisocial behavior that infringes on the rights of others. These behaviors are not mere pranks or occasional mischievous acts. Children with conduct disorders fail to establish the normal bonds of friendship with peers and often use others exploitively. Their language is abusive. Persistent lying, truancy, vandalism, and early sexual activity are common. Frustration tolerance is low. For example, temper outbursts may occur when these children are simply asked to wait their turn. Aggression may be direct and violent or manipulative to meet the child's own self-centered needs.[32] Some children are relatively healthy but engage in acts that fall under the classification of conduct disorders. These children are often members of a group or gang and are influenced toward deviant behavior.

Etiology

The psychosocial concept of conduct disorder and the legal concept of delinquency make it difficult to identify the incidence and causes of conduct disorders. The label *delinquent* depends on the community's definition of morality and whether the deviant behavior falls within the scope of law enforcement. Each community has its own criteria and tolerance for acceptable behaviors.

Research points to the behavioral similarities between children with attention deficit disorder (with hyperactivity) and children with conduct disorders. The hyperactivity, short attention span, impulsiveness, low frustration tolerance, irritability, inability to delay gratification, and unusual aggressiveness are problems in both groups. Learning disabilities commonly occur in children with attention deficit disorder and with conduct disorders; dyslexia, a reading disability, is prominent.[33] (See Chap. 30.)

In attempting to explain the cause of conduct disorders, some investigators emphasize that the family is the most important socializing influence. The families of these children have a high incidence of severe marital problems, such as divorce, separation, and ongoing parental conflict. Adult supervision and control over the child's behavior are the key factors missing in these families.

While studies have linked delinquency to low socioeconomic status, the important factor actually appears to be deprivation: economic, social, and cultural. Socially deviant behavior is learned from peers and adults. If these relationships are the only ones that the child has, deviant behaviors are learned, and because they are not counterbalanced by more socially acceptable behaviors, they are incorporated into the child's general behavior. A child can be psychologically healthy and seemingly well adjusted and still act in a socially deviant way.

The emphasis on environmental influences in the development of conduct disorders is significant. However, the question of why some children in a disturbed family and a deprived social setting develop conduct disorders while others become well socialized remains unanswered.

Psychodynamic explanations of conduct disorders view the central problem as defects in conscience development. Traumatic experiences and faulty identification contribute to a weakened character structure in the child's developing personality. The child develops the need to discharge impulses directly because his or her personality cannot delay or discharge them in an appropriate, more indirect way. Some children may act out their parents' impulsiveness as well as their own.

While the causes of conduct disorders are not precisely known, it is clear that every child with a conduct disorder has difficulty with *self-control.* Punishments have not deterred the child; anxiety to avoid punishment was not sufficient to cause self-control. Constitutional differences are believed to contribute to some children's vulnerability to develop a conduct disorder if the environmental influences are sufficiently stressful.

Nursing management

Children with conduct disorders can wreak havoc on pediatric units with their aggressive destruction and disregard for other children's feelings and rights. Careful attention must be paid to safety, especially regarding drug paraphernalia, pranks, and leaving the hospital unit impulsively.

Developing a relationship with these children is difficult but not impossible. Endless testing of limits, rules, and the nurse's patience can be met by firm, authoritative discipline without inflicting punitive measures on the child or displaying angry feelings. More specifically, the pediatric nurse can:

1. Facilitate the child's experience with his or her body by helping the child through painful and uncomfortable hospitalization experiences, listening to the child's complaints, and offering concrete ways of handling the discomfort.
2. Teach the child about the body. This is a safe way to begin building trust between the nurse and the child (see Chap. 15).

The nurse must be aware that all people have their own biases about deviant behavior. Morality and values are subjective. A child's conduct may make a nurse uncomfortable because it is in conflict with the nurse's and the community's value systems. The nurse can provide socialization experiences for children with conduct disorders without showing harsh prejudice and expecting them to fail.

ATTENTION DEFICIT DISORDER (WITH AND WITHOUT HYPERACTIVITY)

Attention deficit disorder (ADD) is a clinical syndrome in children characterized by inattention, restlessness, and impulsivity. It was previously referred to as *hyperactivity* and *minimal brain dysfunction.* ADD commonly occurs in 8- to 10-year-old males; the male/female ratio is 10 to 1.

Children with ADD can have some of the following problems: hyperactivity, learning disorders, speech and language disorders, conduct problems, lack of insight into the consequences of their behavior, minor physical malformations, and abnormal EEGs. Children with ADD have increased gross motor activity that is haphazard, lacks goal direction, is poorly organized, and is *never-ending.* They have low self-esteem, have temper tantrums, and can be very stubborn.[34] These children run and climb continuously, are always moving and fidgeting, and tax the parents' patience and resources. Children with ADD, with or without hyperactivity, have the same behaviors. Fewer learning disabilities exist in chil-

Table 37-10 Characteristics of Children with Attention Deficit Disorder*

Hyperactivity	Inattention	Impulsivity
Excess running or climbing	Often fail to finish things started	Often act before thinking of consequences
Difficulty sitting still	Do not seem to listen	Excessive shifting from one activity to another
Fidgeting	Are easily distracted	Difficulty organizing work
Restlessness during sleep	Have difficulty concentrating on schoolwork, play, or any activity requiring sustained attention	Need a lot of supervision
"Always on the go"		Find it hard to take turns in games

*Children defined as hyperactive usually demonstrate two or three of the behaviors described in each column.

Source: Adapted from B. Shaywitz et al., "New Diagnostic Terminology for Minimal Brain Dysfunction," *Journal of Pediatrics* **95:**(1)735 (November 1979).

dren who have ADD without hyperactivity. (See Table 37-10.)

Classroom problems result from the child's short attention span, impulsive behavior, and noncompliance with adult authority and discipline. Fooling around, interrupting others, not paying attention to others, not completing tasks, fighting, and bullying are frequent problems in school. Low academic achievement usually results, even though the child has the intellectual ability to succeed in school.

Detection

Early diagnosis permits careful management and counseling. A thorough evaluation of the child's physical and neurological status, behavioral patterns, social interactions, and learning skills is necessary for a diagnosis. An accurate EEG is advisable to help rule out any neurological disease.

Etiology

ADD is believed to have a genetic predisposition because it is more common in some families.[35] Alcoholism and antisocial personality disorders are more prevalent among families with children who have ADD. Perinatal risk factors are not related to ADD. Although food additives have been purported to cause ADD, research has not supported this claim.[36]

Treatment

ADD with hyperactivity is the only childhood behavioral disorder that requires a trial use of Ritalin, a central nervous system stimulant. Ritalin is the most commonly used drug for the treatment of ADD with hyperactivity; it decreases the child's hyperactivity by an unknown physiological action.[37] A multimodality treatment approach consisting of behavior modification, social training, and educational strategies is used to manage the various symptoms and problems of the child with ADD (see Table 37-11).

Nursing management

Hyperactive hospitalized children frequently challenge the nurse's communication and discipline skills. Parents and nurses need to collaborate to maintain consistent discipline. These children must be closely monitored to prevent injuries, to ensure their safety, and to promote the safety of other children on the unit.

Table 37-11 Central Nervous System Stimulants Used in the Treatment of Attention Deficit Disorder

Drug	Average Daily Dose*	Side Effects
Methylphenidate (Ritalin)	15 to 60 mg	Insomnia Anorexia
Pemoline (Cylert)	56.25 to 75 mg	Insomnia Anorexia Skin rash Depression
Dextroamphetamine sulfate (Dexedrine)	10 to 40 mg	Insomnia Anorexia Reduction of growth Headache Moodiness

*Therapy is begun with the lowest dose possible. The therapeutic effect takes 2 to 3 weeks. A child on long-term drug therapy will usually benefit from a drug-free trial periodically to assess the necessity of continuing the medication.

A primary nurse and a consistent, predictable environment will increase the child's sense of control and decrease frustration. Short-term tasks and activities using large muscles are helpful.

Nutritional status should be observed closely. Height and weight graphs are kept. Children eat better if breakfast is served before the drug's action begins and if they are given several small, high-calorie meals during the day.

The parents should be helped to understand that the mild alterations in brain function will cause behavioral, motor, and learning problems. Suggestions for the parents include:

1. Reduce distraction and stimuli in the child's environment.
2. Set reasonable limits and rules, and be firm in their enforcement.
3. Provide stable and predictable routines.
4. Learn and use behavioral modification techniques. Reward desirable behavior and promote the child's self-esteem.
5. Provide short lists of tasks to help the child remember what is expected.
6. Try to remain calm, noncritical, and nonirritable.
7. Remember that the child will be absent-minded and accept it, while being alert to problems that it might cause in care of belongings, toys, etc.
8. Do not ask the child to make many decisions about unimportant items; instead, involve the child in major ones.

The parents need support in their role as limit setters and help in developing parenting skills to manage their child. They need to understand the treatment program and the side effects of drug therapy. For example, the parents need to know that Ritalin will not stunt their child's growth. They also need to understand that a child on Ritalin will be more active during the evening and during sleep as a result of a rebound response to the morning dose of Ritalin. The nurse is the ideal professional for educating families and coordinating services between health and educational professionals.

ANXIETY DISORDERS

Anxiety disorders are characterized by excessive anxiety. The anxiety may be focused on specific concerns or may be a generalized response to most situations.

Separation anxiety

The child with *separation anxiety* experiences severe distress when separated from the family and home. Abnormal separation anxiety occurs from the school-age period through adolescence and adulthood, *beyond* the periods when concern about separating from the parents is appropriate, under 3 years. School-age children with separation anxiety are preoccupied with horrible fantasies of harm that may occur to the parents, usually the mother, or to themselves if separated. Preschool children have more vague concerns.

School refusal (previously called *school phobia*) becomes severe at around 10 to 11 years of age but begins earlier for many children when forced separation occurs through mandatory schooling. These children are usually "model children" in the home and conscientious students, but they are fear-ridden about leaving home.[38]

Pediatric nurses and school nurses see these severely anxious children because somatic symptoms frequently develop. Extensive work-ups are often done for gastrointestinal problems, headaches, and influenza-like symptoms that plague the child and worry the parents. If school is missed too often, academic performance is compromised, and lowered self-esteem further troubles the child.

Care must be taken in talking with the families of severely anxious children. Interviewing must be conducted carefully because most of the mothers are highly ambivalent about separating from their anxious children. Coordination with the school-age child's teacher and school nurse may help the child feel safe, despite eruptions of somatic symptoms. The nurse must be careful not to focus on the symptoms or accuse the child of malingering. *Anxiety is the root of the problem.*[39]

A pediatric-psychiatric liaison service is ideal for coordinating the physical findings and the therapeutic approach for the child and the family. The pediatric nurse and the school nurse may be included in helping the child and the parents tolerate the symptoms while trust is developed and anxiety is reduced. Helping a parent to feel separate and secure through psychiatric treatment may be the first step before a child can stop fearing that the parent will be harmed if the parent is out of sight. The older school-age child has more specific fears and will need individual treatment. By the time a child reaches the age of 10 to 11 years, internalized and fixed fears are more difficult to help with support alone.

Example: Nine-year-old Rosie was referred by her school for excessive absenteeism. Rosie was from a close Hispanic family and had three older brothers. Rosie's mother worked in her daughter's school and could monitor Rosie and the teachers. Rosie knew her mother was nearby. They traveled to and from school together because the mother felt that the city was dangerous. Their residing in an unsafe neighborhood only reinforced their mutual fear of separation.

Rosie was placed in a different class and finally in a Catholic school because both she and her mother did not like the public school teachers. Physical symptoms began to emerge in the second grade. Rosie became dizzy, had persistent headaches and stomach upsets, and "fainted in bed." Rosie had always missed many school days, but her absenteeism rapidly escalated to months.

Rosie's symptoms were treated by a pediatrician, but the etiology was uncertain. Finally, an EEG revealed a nonspecific abnormal wave pattern. This finding had no relationship to her physical symptoms, but her mother seized on the abnormality and again "doctor-shopped" until she found a physician who prescribed a low dosage of phenobarbital. At this point, a coordinated effort was made to help this family focus on the central issue of separation anxiety. Rosie was assigned to an individual psychotherapist. Her mother was seen individually after attempts to involve the whole family for at least one interview failed.

These interviews revealed that Rosie's mother had also stopped school at the second to third grade level for the same reason: a desire to be close to her mother.

Rosie was referred to a pediatric neurologist for examination and another EEG. While the results were explained endlessly to Rosie's mother, she was unwilling to give up her image of Rosie as "the sick child." A pediatric examination was arranged. All pediatric care was consolidated in hopes of discouraging Rosie's mother from seeking other advice.

Rosie was enrolled in home instruction even though this reinforced her desire to stay home. However, the problem was long-standing and symptoms had been present for 2 years. Rosie needed to continue learning basic skills and to complete the school year. Many therapy appointments were missed, a pattern similar to the school absenteeism. This was tolerated as long as more appointments were kept than were broken.

A final treatment plan emerged after building trust with this approach for 6 months. Rosie was enrolled in the day treatment school program, a combination of school and psychotherapy. A school bus picked her up, alleviating her mother's anxiety about safety. Somatic symptoms occur occasionally, especially in the winter, but the plan remains in effect. Rosie shows gradual but definite progress.

Overanxious disorder

Overanxious disorder is a generalized worrying and concern that is not focused on specific situations, such as school or problems with relating to peers. Children with this disorder worry about almost everything related to current and future events. Excessive anticipation, questions about the future, and overconcern about examinations and possible dangers plague them. Tasks are avoided through endless questions and stalling.

Characteristic somatic complaints—"lump in the throat," gastrointestinal problems, headaches, shortness of breath, feeling cold, and dizziness—appear when deadlines or dreaded events approach. Nail biting, hair twirling, and other nervous habits are displayed by these highly verbal and often precocious children. Academic and social difficulties arise when school performance drops or the child misses trips, events, and games because of fearfulness. The physical symptoms and treatment for them can confirm the "sick" role. When the anxiety disorder is recognized as the cause of the somatic complaints, a nurse can reassure the child that the physical problems will subside as self-confidence grows. Encouraging the child to explore new experiences, planning small steps toward new experiences, and talking about fears and failures can build a trusting nurse-child relationship.

Shyness

Shyness is often accepted by parents as a behavior peculiar to their child, unless the shyness begins to interfere with schoolwork or infringes on the parents' independence. For example, a teacher may observe a child's reluctance to participate in most activities, or a parent may notice that the child always clings when a baby-sitter arrives. Usually these children are warm and friendly within the family, but they are almost mute, may pale or blush excessively, stammer unintelligibly, and show excessive embarrassment outside the family setting. Participating in play, school, and other events is minimal, and clinging to parents is the child's usual response.

With support and encouragement, a child may gradually break out into the world. If the shyness increases and isolates the child further as adolescence approaches, the new pressures of adolescent development may be unusually stressful. The parents may share this concern with the nurse during a routine health checkup. The nurse can assess this area of the preadolescent's development by questioning his or her social adjustment. The nurse can observe how a school-age child contributes and answers questions during the examination.

EATING DISORDERS

An *eating disorder* exists when food is used to deal with anxiety, unhappiness, or a life problem. The major eating disorders are anorexia nervosa, bulimia, and obsesity. Common factors associated with all of them are low self-esteem, depression, and dysfunctional food habits.

For all eating disorders the nursing assessment of the problem includes measurement of height and weight and a developmental assessment. A basic nutritional assessment (see Chap. 14) includes a 24-h and a 3-day dietary recall, factors and feelings associated with eating, skinfold measurements, and exercise pattern. A careful history emphasizes family eating disorders, menstrual history, life problems, and coping mechanisms; it should be followed by a general physical examination and appropriate laboratory tests (a urinalysis and tests of serum triglycerides, cholesterol, and electrolytes).

Anorexia nervosa

The major characteristic of *anorexia nervosa* is a relentless drive to become thin and a corresponding dread of gaining weight and becoming "fat." Although many teenagers go on diets and are dissatisfied with their bodies, teenagers with this disorder carry the typical fad diet and exercise program to extremes of obsessive dieting and preoccupation with food. The DSM criteria for this disorder include:[40]

1. An intense fear of becoming obese, which does not diminish as the weight loss progresses
2. A disturbance of body image, e.g., claiming to "feel fat" even when emaciated
3. A weight loss of at least 25 percent of original body weight or, in the case of children under 18 years of age, a weight loss plus an original weight gain that could be expected on the basis of growth charts equaling 25 percent
4. A refusal to maintain body weight over a minimal normal weight for the child's age and height
5. The absence of a physical illness that would account for the weight loss

Anorexia nervosa is most common in females between the ages of 12 and 18 years, but it has been reported in males as well.[41] Because of the severe weight loss, hospitalization is often required to prevent death from starvation. The physical signs and symptoms associated with starvation are listed in Table 37-12.

Although the etiology of anorexia nervosa is unknown, a number of theories have been proposed, including biological factors (such as hypothalamic dysfunction), psychodynamic factors, family system dysfunction, behavioral factors, and social factors. The onset of adolescence may cause feelings that the teenager attempts to control. Control seems to be a primary issue in anorexia nervosa. A desire to control body changes and the feelings associated with puberty, as well as a desire to control parental relationships, may be an underlying factor. Sometimes a phobic fear of food that becomes associated with fear of maturation and body change exists. Another factor may be the family's use of food as a means of control.

A major social factor is the pressure on teen-

Table 37-12 Physical Signs and Symptoms Associated with Anorexia Nervosa

Marked weight loss (20 to 40%)
Muscle weakness
Fat and muscle tissue loss
Cardiac irregularities
Poor circulation to extremities
Inefficient temperature regulation (hypothermia)
Decreased metabolic rate, blood pressure, and heart rate
Amenorrhea
Sleep disturbances
Lanugo
Ankle edema

age girls to be thin and attractive. The current emphasis on appearance and thinness are thought to influence the adolescent's initial dieting and subsequent development of anorexia nervosa. Initially, the peer group and the family positively reinforce the weight loss, causing continuation of the diet.

The anorexic child is often unusually compliant and is described by the parents as having been a "perfect child" during early development. The anorexic teenage girl perceives her weight and her body as the only things she can control. Not eating is a way of asserting independence. Symbolically, the lack of physical development which results from the starvation is proposed to be an expression of the need to remain a child rather than become a sexual adult. Currently, all the above theories are considered when planning treatment for the anorexic child and his or her family.[42]

Nursing management The immediate goal of hospitalization of the anorexic child is weight gain and the prevention of death from starvation. Tube feedings, intravenous therapy, and total parenteral nutrition may be utilized as lifesaving techniques. Meals and snacks are regularly scheduled and vitamin and mineral supplements are given in order to achieve weight gain. Supervision of the child by the nurse during and after meals is important because the anorexic child typically hides food or induces vomiting to avoid weight gain. The child also must be watched closely to prevent excessive exercise.[43,44,45] (See the Nursing Care Plan at the end of this chapter.)

The anorexic child is weighed daily at the same time, and intake and output are carefully recorded. Activity may be restricted to promote weight gain. As the child gains weight, he or she is given more control over diet and activities, both in and out of the hospital. Behavior modification techniques are used with clearly established guidelines, rewards, and expected behaviors. Medications may be used to decrease preoccupation with food or to reduce depression.

These children can be difficult to work with because of their anxiety and their distorted and desperate behavior around food. Consistent, firm nursing care, combined with clear limits and rewards for eating, is helpful to the anorexic child and the nurse.

Individual psychotherapy, which continues after hospitalization, and family therapy are important in the treatment of anorexia nervosa. The nurse should refer the child to an eating disorder clinic if the diagnosis of an eating disorder is being considered.

Bulimia

Bulimia is generally seen in the older adolescent. It is characterized by episodic binges during which large quantities of food are consumed (10,000 to 20,000 cal) followed by self-induced vomiting. Bulimia usually remains hidden, and the adolescent does not seek medical help. It can persist for many years, unnoticed by the adolescent's family and friends, because he or she seems to be in good health and maintains a normal weight. Characteristically, the adolescent with bulimia (1) goes on recurrent binges, during which large amounts of food are consumed rapidly; (2) eats high-calorie, easily ingested foods during binges; (3) eats alone rather than in the presence of others; (4) terminates binges because of abdominal pain or social interruption or by sleeping or vomiting; (5) experiences frequent weight fluctuations of more than 10 lb in a relatively short period of time; (6) is aware that the eating pattern is abnormal and fears not being able to control the behavior; and (7) is in a depressed mood and thinks self-deprecating thoughts following the binges.[46]

It is estimated that 19 percent of all female college students and 5 percent of all male college students have this disorder. Approximately 50 percent of all children with anorexia nervosa will develop bulimia.[47] The binge-eating pattern can begin early in childhood and progress to a binge-eating–purging pattern during adolescence or early adulthood. After a lengthy period of time the disorder will usually manifest itself in various physical symptoms that require medical attention (see Table 37-13).

Researchers have proposed a variety of causes of bulimia. Biological causes include hypothalamus dysfunction and "set-point" disturbance. Familial factors, social pressure to be thin, and psychological factors may also play a role. Low self-esteem and depression also contribute to the onset and maintenance of bulimic behavior. Commonly, the bulimic patient expresses such feelings as "I can never do anything right." Wanting to be perfect but being unable to achieve perfection contributes to the low self-esteem and the self-destructive behavior.

Treatment measures similar to those used with

Table 37-13 Physical Signs and Symptoms Associated with Bulimia

Electrolyte imbalance and dehydration
Muscle weakness and lethargy
Syncope
Cardiovascular failure
Renal failure
Gastric distention
Tooth erosion
Enlargement of salivary glands
Menstrual irregularities
Abrasions and callus formation on knuckles of hand used to induce vomiting
Changes in bowel and bladder habits (indicating cathartic and diuretic use)

the anorexic child are helpful. Support groups have proved valuable in the long-term management of these patients.

Obesity

Obesity is the most common nutritional problem of children, affecting between 12 and 30 percent of the pediatric population. Because criteria for obesity vary, it is difficult to establish the exact number of obese children. Being overweight during childhood increases the individual's chances of being overweight in adulthood. Obesity in both children and adults is associated with many health problems and has various psychological and social consequences.

Variables that affect the development of obesity include lack of self-confidence, decreased activity levels, rapid consumption of food without proper chewing, genetic predisposition, and the use of food as a primary source of pleasure and reward.

Progressive obesity begins prior to the age of 6 months. The parents are usually obese and are the role models for eating behavior. *Developmental obesity* is also related to the family but is due more to problems of control of eating associated with hyperemotional stress. Developmental tasks may be affected in these children. Parents' use of cookies, ice cream, and candy as rewards for good behavior may create an association between food and feeling loved and valued. In some children there is a direct relationship between unhappiness and overeating.

The causes of obesity are complex and probably multiple. A prominent biological causative theory is the "set-point" theory, according to which

Table 37-14 Clinical Manifestations of Stereotyped Movement Disorder

Transient Tic Disorder

1. Onset is sudden and spontaneous.
2. Onset is before age 12; most common in boys; peaks at 6 to 7 years.
3. Bilateral or unilateral eye blinks or facial movements are common.
4. Voluntary suppression is possible for minutes to hours (rebound of movements may result).
5. Vocalizations such as throat clearing may also occur.
6. Stress increases frequency and duration of tic.
7. Tic usually disappears without intervention.

Chronic Motor Tic Disorder

1. Is less common than transient tic disorder.
2. Usually begins before age 15 or after age 40.
3. Involves three or fewer muscle groups at one time.
4. Intensity is usually constant over weeks or months.
5. Vocalizations are not common.
6. Voluntary suppression of movements is possible for minutes to hours.
7. Duration is greater than 1 year; often is lifelong.

Tourette Disorder

1. Onset is usually before age 13.
2. Male/female ratio is 3 to 1.
3. Usually is lifelong.
4. Phases of the disorder are consistent:
   a. *Stage 1: motor tics* Muscular jerking of the eyes, face, neck, and shoulders.
   b. *Stage 2: verbal cries* Motor tics accompanied by involuntary verbalizations such as throat clearing, barking noises, coughs, and sniffing.
   c. *Stage 3: coprolalia (obscenities) and echolalia (echoing others' words)* Coprolalia accompanies motor tics in approximately 50% of patients.
5. EEG findings are abnormal in approximately 50% of patients.
6. Learning disabilities are common.
7. Intelligence is average or better.
8. Psychosis is unusual.
9. Compulsive impulses to touch things or to perform movements such as squatting or twirling may occur.
10. Suicide may be attempted because of disruption in social or occupational functioning.

Atypical Stereotyped Movement Disorder

1. Head-banging, rocking, and repetitive hand movements or finger movements are common.
2. Movements are voluntary rather than spasmodic.
3. Usually the person derives pleasure from the activity.
4. Usually is seen in children.
5. Is seen in individuals with mental retardation, pervasive developmental disorders, and inadequate social stimulation.

the body has a specific, "ideal" set point (weight), even if this weight is greater than would be considered normal. It is especially difficult to alter this set point because the body continually adjusts its metabolic rate to maintain it.

The adipose cellularity (fat cell) theory is also widely supported. This theory is based on the concept that the size of fat cells changes but that the actual number of cells does not. Although research based on this theory is continuing, there are limited data to support it conclusively at this time.

In addition to biological factors, social and psychological factors are believed to have a significant influence on the development and maintenance of obesity.[48] For many people, food is a symbol of love and nurturance, and eating is a major source of pleasure in life. Poor food habits also contribute to excessive weight.

Nursing management The goal of managing an obese child is to normalize his or her eating and exercise patterns. A plan to balance food intake, activity, and rest is essential. Changing food habits, rather than going on fad diets, is important for the long-term maintenance of weight loss.

Assessing the psychosocial components of obesity is the first step in attaining the goal of weight loss. It is important to determine whether the child is experiencing depression or low self-esteem and whether there have been traumatic precipitating events or family problems.[49, 50] Overeating can become a compulsive behavior pattern that the child uses to cope with the difficulties of growing up. Asking the child about the ways in which he or she copes with stress can elicit information for planning interventions.

Education regarding caloric intake, appropriate foods, and the relationship of exercise to weight control is basic to the management of obesity. Group therapy is extremely helpful in achieving long-term results, especially for adolescents. Ego support and approval from the group increase self-esteem, providing reinforcement for changes in diet and life-style.

STEREOTYPED MOVEMENT DISORDERS

Stereotyped movement disorders, or *tics*, are involuntary movements of skeletal muscles that may be accompanied by involuntary speaking or grunting. Four types of tics have been described:[51] (1) transient tic disorder, (2) chronic tic disorder, (3) Tourette syndrome, and (4) atypical stereotyped movement disorder. See Table 37-14.

The cause of these disorders is unknown. Some researchers believe that tics result from emotional tension, while others believe that they are learned behaviors. Others believe that tics have an organic basis and result from dysfunction of the central nervous system. A specific biochemical dysfunction has not been found.

Nursing management

Early intervention is the key to preventing and reducing the psychological and social consequences of stereotyped movement disorders.[52] The nurse can educate the child and the family about tics. Often the parents believe that the child is "crazy," is mentally retarded, or is simply seeking attention. Because overly punitive, threatening, and restrictive child-rearing practices increase the tic activity, the parents will benefit from learning a variety of behavioral approaches such as behavior modification techniques. Relaxation techniques, biofeedback, and psychotherapy have also been beneficial for some children. Haldol is the drug of choice for children with Tourette syndrome. Monitoring the drug's side effects and teaching the child and the other family members about it contribute to the management of the disorder.

Anticipatory guidance can help the child and his or her family deal with their feelings of shame and embarrassment. The nurse should find ways to help the family increase the child's self-esteem and avoid social isolation. When psychiatric symptoms or family disruption occurs, psychiatric consultation and treatment should be sought.

Nursing Care Plan: Anorexia Nervosa*

Patient: Denise Kline **Age:** 15 years **Date of Admission:** 10/14

ASSESSMENT

Denise was admitted to the adolescent unit with a diagnosis of dehydration secondary to anorexia nervosa. She also has a 1-month history of laxative abuse and self-induced vomiting to expedite weight reduction.

During the initial chart review and interview with Denise and her parents, the primary nurse obtained the following information. Denise is the oldest of three children. She has a 12-year-old brother and a 7-year-old sister. Both are healthy. The father is a 45-year-old aerospace engineer; he travels extensively. The mother is a 39-year-old homemaker. Before Denise's birth, the mother taught high school English. She currently is active in her community. Both parents stated that until recently the family was close, with few problems or conflicts. The present conflict revolves around Denise and her dieting. The family is very concerned about Denise's recent dramatic weight loss and her isolation from friends.

Denise was then interviewed alone by the nurse. Denise takes ballet lessons for recreation, is an accomplished ballerina, and wishes to pursue this as a career. Her grades have always been A's. She has one girlfriend from school with whom she occasionally talks on the telephone. Denise has no boyfriend at present because she is not allowed to date. Her parents constantly insist that she eat and nag her about losing weight.

During the past month she began taking laxatives and inducing vomiting in order to lose more weight. She has not had a menstrual period for the past 4 months. Denise stated, "I object to being in the hospital. I only feel a little tired and am not really sick. I look fine. My parents are making a fuss over nothing. I am eating enough."

Denise's nurse observed that she appeared calm, perhaps even detached, during the interview. She was clean and stylishly dressed. Denise appears emaciated. Her skin is pale and dry with poor turgor. There is lanugo hair on her arms and back. Her hair is long, blond, lusterless, and dry. Her eyes appear sunken with dark circles around them. Her lips are dry, cracked, and sticky. There is an odor suggestive of vomitus on her breath. She is 5 ft 4 in tall and weighs 80 lb (her weight 3 months ago was 105 lb).

PHYSICAL EXAMINATION

Temperature: 96°F. Pulse: 50 and regular. Respirations: 18 and regular. Blood pressure: 75/50.

*Prepared by Kitty Miller, R.N., M.S.N., and Susan Rabinovitz, R.N., B.A. The authors wish to thank Joan Shapiro, Ph.D., Richard Mackenzie, M.D., and Lawrence Neinstein, M.D., for their assistance with this Nursing Care Plan.

Nursing Diagnosis	Outcome Criteria	Nursing Interventions	Evaluation and Modifications
1. Alteration in nutrition; inadequate body requirements related to anorexia nervosa	☐ Denise will have an adequate nutritional intake and weight stabilization and gain, as evidenced by compliance with the health care plan.	☐ Participate in multidisciplinary case conferences to establish treatment goals and a medical and therapeutic plan and to formulate patient contract. Participate in a weekly review to evaluate effectiveness and modify the plan as needed.	☐ Denise is meeting her contracted goals for weight stabilization and gain.

Nursing Diagnosis	Outcome Criteria	Nursing Interventions
	☐ Honesty and trust will be promoted in Denise's relationship with all members of the health care team.	☐ Organize and chair a weekly team conference to review and project new goals of each discipline and member. ☐ Fulfill the nursing component of the comprehensive treatment plan: **a.** Monitor weight daily (every morning or three times per week before breakfast). **b.** Maintain calorie count if ordered. **c.** Record nutritional intake. **d.** Note food preferences on the Kardex. **e.** Provide one-on-one nursing supervision for 2 h after meals. ☐ Offer Denise information on nutritional requirements and diet planning to achieve the desired weight gain goal. (A nutritionist may do this, and the nurse will then reinforce the plan.) ☐ Assure that the appropriate level of contract (i.e., matching appropriate behaviors with specific privileges) is carried out by the health team members. (For example, at level 4, when Denise drinks three 8-oz glasses of fluid and eats 80% of her meal, she may make one phone call lasting 20 min, or when she attains a weight of 84 lb, she may make one phone call lasting 20 min.) ☐ Promote Denise's compliance with the health care team's care plan by establishing an effective nurse-patient therapeutic relationship. ☐ Meet daily with Denise at a scheduled time to discuss her progress and encourage expression of her feelings; e.g., "How do you feel about . . .?" Validate her feelings; e.g., "This must be very difficult for you." Verbalize the nonverbal; e.g., "You're so quiet this morning. Are you angry with me?" ☐ Provide verbal and nonverbal support to Denise even if her established weight gain goals are not met. ☐ Avoid conflict and power struggles with Denise by: **a.** Offering her choices within the confines of the care plan. **b.** Avoiding a parental judgmental and authoritarian role. **c.** Encouraging a sense of self-control and of having options (e.g., some

Nursing Diagnosis	Outcome Criteria	Nursing Interventions	Evaluation and Modifications
		patients with anorexia nervosa *choose* not to gain weight for almost 2 weeks and thus prolong their hospitalization and isolation from friends and school). ☐ Actively collaborate and communicate with all members of the health care team and unit nursing staff in order to prevent Denise from splitting or manipulating team members and sabotaging treatment goals.	
2. Fluid volume deficit related to abnormal fluid loss	☐ Further abnormal fluid loss will be prevented. ☐ Fluid replacement (intake) will be adequate, as evidenced by a return to normal hydration status.	☐ Monitor: **a.** Vital signs for change, particularly decreased blood pressure and increased pulse and pulse pressure **b.** Laboratory values (i.e., urine specific gravity, electrolytes, and PCV) ☐ Assess for signs of dehydration: **a.** Dry, cracked lips **b.** Dry mucous membranes and tongue **c.** Poor skin turgor **d.** Sunken eyeballs **e.** Decreased urine output **f.** Decreased tearing **g.** Urine specific gravity above 1.025 ☐ Strict intake and output. ☐ Administer IV fluid therapy as ordered and provide PO fluid replacement as per health team's care plan. ☐ Monitor behavior for 2 h after meals on a one-on-one basis (to prevent self-induced vomiting). ☐ Encourage and reinforce positive behaviors (such as increased oral intake). ☐ Allow for independent decision making within the confines of the therapeutic plan (e.g., choosing cranberry juice instead of orange juice). ☐ Encourage discussion of feelings related to the therapeutic regimen.	☐ Normal fluid balance has returned; signs of dehydration are absent.

Nursing Diagnosis	Outcome Criteria	Nursing Interventions	Evaluation and Modifications
3. Alteration in body image related to inaccurate perception of self as overweight	☐ Denise will have a more appropriate body image, as evidenced by: **a.** Ability to talk about what weight loss lets her do and not do **b.** Ability to talk about the impact of weight loss on appearance, clothes, etc. ☐ Denise will have decreased negative behaviors that encourage further weight loss: **a.** Restrictive eating **b.** Laxative use **c.** Excessive physical activity **d.** Self-induced vomiting ☐ Denise will develop a positive sense of self.	☐ Encourage and reinforce positive self-statements; ignore negative ones. ☐ Reinforce the medical, nutritional, and psychosocial plan to enable Denise to engage in appropriate behaviors. ☐ Have Denise engage in a series of tasks that are designed to improve her body image and self-esteem. Allow her to choose a task, such as keeping a daily journal focused on how she experiences each day. ☐ Set aside 15 min daily with Denise for interaction focusing on her feelings, followed by writing down five things she likes about herself, what others like about her, and her future-oriented goals; fantasizing her life in 1 year and 5 years; and making a collage from magazine ads which are concerned with body image.	☐ Denise talks about her weight loss—its meaning and impact on her life. ☐ Denise makes one positive statement about herself daily. ☐ Denise complies with the health team's therapeutic plan. ☐ Denise is keeping the contract for task completion.
4. Social isolation related to obsession with weight loss	☐ Denise will achieve social reintegration with her peers, as evidenced by establishing appropriate peer relationships and engaging in appropriate social activities.	☐ Select appropriate roommates for Denise while she is on the unit (i.e., ones that are outgoing and friendly). Avoid roommates who also have eating disorders. ☐ Encourage participation in unit activities and/or playroom activities. Allow Denise to choose activities according to the contract. ☐ Encourage a renewed interest in hobbies and previously enjoyed activities. ☐ Encourage socialization with peers on the unit. ☐ According to Denise's contract and level, encourage phone calls and visits from peers and discuss with the parents car pools to bring friends to the hospital. (These are privileges earned according to the therapeutic plan. Denise should choose whom to see and when, etc., in order to give her control.)	☐ Denise has renewed social interaction with peers and is participating in appropriate activities.

References

1. *Diagnostic and Statistical Manual of Mental Disorders*, 3d ed., American Psychiatric Association, New York, 1980, pp. 35–99.
2. Ibid., pp. 236–239.
3. Wineberg, Warren, et al., "Depression in Children Referred to an Educational Diagnostic Center: Diagnosis and Treatment," *Journal of Pediatrics* **83**:1065–1072 (1973).
4. Brady, Margaret A., "Childhood Depression: Development of a Screening Tool," *Pediatric Nursing* **9**(3):222–225 (May–June 1984).
5. Betz, Cecily Lynn, and Elizabeth C. Poster, "Children's Concepts of Death: Implications for Pediatric Practice," *Nursing Clinics of North America* **19**:(2)341–349 (1984).
6. Valente, Sharon, "Suicide in School Aged Children," *Pediatric Nursing* **4**(1):25–29 (January–February 1983).
7. *Diagnostic and Statistical Manual of Mental Disorders*, p. 89.
8. Ritvo, Edward, et al., "Effects of Fenfluramine on 14 Outpatients with the Syndrome of Autism," *Journal of the American Academy of Child Psychiatry* **22**(11):549–558 (November 1983).
9. Ritvo, Edward, and B. J. Freeman, "National Society for Autistic Children Definition of the Syndrome of Autism," *Journal of Pediatric Psychology* **2**:146–158 (1977).
10. Rutter, Michael, and Eric Schopler (eds.), *Autism—A Reappraisal of Concepts and Treatment*, Plenum, New York, 1978, pp. 1–26.
11. Dudziak, Diane, "Parenting the Autistic Child," *Journal of Psychosocial Nursing and Mental Health Services* **20**:11–16 (1982).
12. Bernheimer, Lucinda, and Pamela Winton, "Stress over Time: Parents with Young Handicapped Children," *Journal of Developmental and Behavioral Pediatrics* **4**:177–181 (September 1983).
13. Hebert, Martin, *Behavioral Treatment of Problem Children*, Academic, New York, 1981.
14. *Diagnostic and Statistical Manual of Mental Disorders*, p. 91.
15. Howells, John, and Waguih Guirguis, "Childhood Schizophrenia 20 Years Later," *Archives of General Psychiatry* **41**:123–129 (February 1984).
16. Gottesman, Irving I., and James Shields, *Schizophrenia: The Epigenetic Puzzle*, Cambridge, New York, 1982, pp. 37–98.
17. Costello, J. (ed.), *Speech Disorders in Children: Recent Advances*, College-Hill Press, San Diego, Calif., 1984.
18. Goldberg, Robin, "Identifying Speech and Language Delays in Children," *Pediatric Nursing* **10**(4):252–259 (July–August 1984).
19. Perkins, William (ed.), *Current Therapy of Communication Disorders: Stuttering Disorders*, Thime-Stratton, New York, 1984.
20. Jaso, Hector, "Disorders Usually First Evident in Infancy, Childhood, or Adolescence," in *Diagnostic and Statistical Manual of Mental Disorders*, pp. 18–19.
21. Sanok, Richard, and Frank Ascione, "Behavioral Interventions for Childhood Elective Mutism: An Evaluative Review," *Child Behavior Therapy* **1**:49–68 (Spring 1979).
22. Cohen, Michael, "Enuresis," in Robert Hoekelman et al. (eds.), *Principles of Pediatrics: Health Care of the Young*, McGraw-Hill, New York 1978, pp. 475–481.
23. Doleys, D. M., "Behavioral Treatments for Nocturnal Enuresis in Children: A Review of the Recent Literature," *Psychological Bulletin* **84**:30–54 (1977).
24. Poster, Elizabeth C., "Stress Immunization: Techniques to Help Children Cope with Hospitalization," *Maternal Child Nursing Journal* **12**(3):119–134 (Summer 1983).
25. Poster, Elizabeth C., and Cecily Lynn Betz, "Allaying the Anxiety of Hospitalized Children Using Stress Immunization Techniques," *Issues in Comprehensive Pediatric Nursing* **6**:227–233 (Summer 1983).
26. Levine, Melvin, "Encopresis: Its Potentiation, Evaluation, and Alleviation," *Pediatric Clinics of North America* **29**:315–330 (April 1982).
27. Crowley, Angela, "A Comprehensive Strategy for Managing Encopresis," *The American Journal of Maternal-Child Nursing* **9**(6):395–400 (November–December 1984).
28. Deni, Laura, "The Nightmare of Sleep Problems," *Journal of Nursing Care* **13**(5):8–10 (May 1980).
29. Segal, Julius, "A Child's Secret Nightlife," *Health* **14**:28–32 (May 1982).
30. Schumann, Mary Jean, "Neuromuscular Relaxation—A Method of Inducing Sleep in Young Children," *Pediatric Nursing* **7**(5):9–13 (September–October 1981).
31. Poster, op. cit., pp. 126–127.
32. Jaso, op. cit., pp. 10–11.
33. Bakker, D. J. (ed.), *Treatment of Hyperactive and Learning Disordered Children*, University Park Press, Baltimore, 1980.
34. Cantwell, Dennis, "Recognition, Evaluation and Management of Hyperactive Children," *Pediatric Nursing* **5**(5):11–22 (September–October 1979).
35. McMahon, Robert, "Genetic Etiology in Hyperactive Child Syndrome: A Critical Review," *American Journal of Orthopsychiatry* **50**:145–150 (January 1980).
36. Harley, J. Preston, et al., "Hyperkinesis and Food Additives: Testing the Feingold Hypothesis," *Pediatrics* **61**:818–828 (1978).
37. Cantwell, Dennis, "A Clinician's Guide to the Use of Stimulant Medication for Psychiatric Disorders of Children," *Developmental Pediatrics* **1**:133–140 (September 1980).
38. Varley, Christopher, and Gail Borigard, "A Clinical Nurse Specialists's Role in the Comprehensive Management of Attention Deficit Disorder," *Children's Health Care* **13**:139–142 (1985).
39. Hersov, L., and I. Berg (eds.), *Modern Perspectives in School Refusal*. Wiley, New York, 1980.
40. *Diagnostic and Statistical Manual of Mental Disorders*, p. 68.

41. Glaser-Kiecolt, J., and K. Dixon, "Post Adolescent Onset Male Anorexia Nervosa." *Journal of Psychosocial Nursing and Mental Health Services* **22**(1):11–20 (January 1984).
42. Johnson, Martha, "Anorexia Nervosa: Framework for Early Identification and Intervention," *Issues in Mental Health Nursing* **4**(2):87–100 (April–June 1982).
43. Grossniklaus, D. M., "Nursing Interventions in Anorexia Nervosa," *Perspectives in Psychiatric Care* **18**(1):11–16 (January–February 1980).
44. Gardner, D. M., and P. E. Garfinkel (eds.), *Handbook of Psychotherapy for Anorexia Nervosa and Bulimia*, Guilford Press, New York, 1985.
45. Sanger, Elaine, and Therese Cassino, "Eating Disorders: Avoiding the Power Struggle," *American Journal of Nursing* **84**(1):31–34 (January 1984).
46. Potts, Nicki Lee, "Eating Disorders: The Secret Pattern of Binge-Purge," *American Journal of Nursing* **84**(1):33–35 (January 1984).
47. Garfinkel, P. E., and D. M. Gardner (eds.), *Anorexia Nervosa: A Multidimensional Perspective*, Bruner/Mazel, New York, 1982.
48. Baum, Cynthia G., and Rex Forehand, "Social Factors Associated with Adolescent Obesity," *Journal of Pediatric Psychology* **9**(9):293–302 (September 1984).
49. Hoover, Michele L., "The Self Image of Overweight Adolescent Females: A Review of the Literature," *Maternal Child Nursing Journal* **13**(3):125–137 (Summer 1984).
50. White, J. H., "An Overview of Obesity: Its Significance to Nursing," *Nursing Clinics of North America* **17**:191–198 (June 1982).
51. *Diagnostic and Statistical Manual of Mental Disorders*, pp. 73–77.
52. Golden, G. S., and O. J. Hood, "Tics and Tremors," *Pediatric Clinics of North America* **24**:95–103 (February 1982).

38

Mona Clare Lotz Finnila

Child abuse and neglect

Upon completion of this chapter, the student will be able to:

1. Define child abuse, neglect, sexual abuse, emotional abuse, and institutional abuse.
2. Describe six hospital or community resources designed to assist abused children and their families.
3. Describe his or her emotional reaction to acutely injured or severely neglected infants and their parents.
4. State how this reaction may affect communication with abused or neglected children and their families.
5. Identify 10 common environmental problems which contribute to the abuse of children.
6. Detail 10 predictive signs prior to labor or after delivery of potential abuse of the infant by the parents.
7. Construct a support plan for a young family to prevent child abuse from occurring, utilizing a variety of community resources.
8. List 10 assessment findings about a child and his or her family that indicate that abuse has occurred.
9. State five examples of patient goals and nursing actions for giving adequate care to the abused child.
10. List five common diagnostic procedures and their rationale for use with the nonaccidentally injured child.
11. Identify five common physical signs or symptoms of failure to thrive due to environmental neglect.
12. List six assessment behaviors that indicate sexual abuse of a child.
13. Describe the nursing management of a sexually abused child and his or her family.
14. Outline the nursing management of emotionally abusive (verbally assaultive) parents.

Child abuse comprises a group of clinical health problems in children of all ages caused by incompetent or hostile adult caretakers, hazardous environments, or inadequate health services. Child abuse represents part of a larger problem—violence within families, the community, and society. The children who are most vulnerable to child abuse are children from infancy to 3 years (50 percent of cases reported) and children aged 13 to 15 years (33 percent of cases reported).[1] The health problem may be acute (e.g., a duodenal rupture from a blow to the stomach) or chronic (e.g., verbal assault over many years, resulting in a poor self-concept). The clinical picture may be minor, such as welt marks on a child's back, or severe, such as a fractured skull, which can cause death. The emotional, physical, social, and psychological health of the child may be impaired temporarily, as in the case of a burn that will heal, or permanently, as when there is severe mental retardation due to a head injury. Abuse occurs in children of all ages, from the fetal stage to late adolescence, and in *all socioeconomic classes*. Children of all races, religions, ethnic groups, and nationalities are abused. Adult and child abuse may also occur concurrently in families. Adults, including parents and elderly relatives, can be victims of violence and neglect.

The major categories of child abuse include fetal abuse, nonaccidental injury, neglect, sexual abuse, emotional abuse, and institutional abuse.

Child abuse is a tremendous problem in the world today. It is estimated that 2 million children in the United States are abused (e.g., kicked, bitten, burned, or punched) each year. In addition, many children experience moderate to severe failure to thrive as a result of environmental deprivation. One-fourth of the women and one-tenth of the men in the United States have reported that they were sexually abused as children. Sibling abuse, which is a violent attack by one child on a sibling, occurs in four out of five families with children between the ages of 3 and 17 years. Approximately 50 percent of these attacks are severe, and a gun or a knife is used in 0.3 percent of the cases.[2] When the number of children who have experienced toxic ingestions, burns, near drownings, fetal abuse, and emotional abuse is added to the statistics, it becomes obvious that many children have suffered some degree of abuse. All children are mildly abused during their childhood from various environmental influences, such as lead intoxication and smog exposure. Like the United States, many other nations are beginning to study child abuse problems.

As people have begun to look at how children are raised and to study the end results of various child care practices, parenting practices and children's environments are being modified to produce healthier, happier children. Although child abuse has been recognized as a problem for about 100 years, most of the progress has occurred during the last 20 years. Great strides have been made in helping families in which children suffered from nonaccidental injury and neglect. Work is under way in sexual abuse, while work in emotional, institutional, and environmental abuse has barely begun.

Nurses have a role in identifying and treating abused children. In addition, nurses help prevent child abuse through careful assessment and treatment of parents, including preventive health education. As nurses continue to work in cooperation with persons in other disciplines for the long-term health benefits of families, major contributions will be made to the health of children.

HISTORICAL PERSPECTIVES

In ancient Greece and Rome, unwanted infants were left exposed in an open place. Mythology includes tales of heroes who began life in this manner. Infanticide (baby killing) may have been used as a form of birth control. Before 1900, Eskimos encouraged the killing of female babies who were born before the birth of a male infant. This was a tribal economic policy thought necessary for survival in their harsh environment. In certain African tribes, twin children were viewed as unlucky omens and were killed. In many cultures, physically handicapped children were destroyed at birth. Children who were biracial were also in danger. In some countries even today, some infants are deliberately maimed so that they will become beggars and help support the family.

In the nineteenth century, during the industrial revolution, children were put to work in the fields and factories. Four- and five-year-olds worked in dungeon-like factories or mines 14 h a day, 6 days a week. Farm children worked just as hard. The average life span for people at that time was 17 years. Malnutrition and epidemics of tuberculosis, cholera, typhoid, and typhus were rampant, especially among the poor and very young.[3] In 1916 a major law, the Child Labor Act, was passed, prohibiting children younger than 9 years of age from engaging in certain hazardous forms of labor. Not until 1938 were the present child labor policies enacted.[4] Children of migrant farm workers are still not adequately protected against excessive work, exposure to noxious chemicals, and poor housing and education. Some of the historical landmarks which signaled relief for children are listed in Table 38-1.

FETAL AND POSTPARTAL ABUSE

Fetal abuse is exposure of the child before birth to influences in the maternal environment. These agents compromise the child's potential for a healthy life or even cause death, either before or after birth. Inadequate maternal education, inadequate health care resources, and exposure to noxious drugs or infection are three major causes. The mother can prevent fetal abuse by not smoking cigarettes, ingesting alcohol, or using street drugs (see Chap. 39). Maternal cigarette smok-

Table 38-1 Historical Landmarks

1869	New York Foundling Hospital was established to care for unwanted babies (1060 infants were received the first year, 61% in critical condition).
1875	American Humane Society child protective services were established.
1900 to 1920	Abused children were removed from their homes, and their parents imprisoned.
1920 to the present	Social workers began assisting families in the home setting. Foster care was used extensively.
1960 to 1970	Kempe coined the term *battered child syndrome* and established some multidisciplinary approaches to treatment. Laws requiring that child abuse be reported were established in all states. Experimental programs were funded by the federal government.
1974	The Child Abuse and Prevention Act was passed by Congress; $85 million was earmarked for treatment of abused youngsters and their parents.
1979	Multiple local parent and child treatment centers were operating throughout the country.

Sources: C. H. Kempe, "Approaches to Preventive Child Abuse: The Health Visitor Concept," *American Journal of Diseases of Children* **130:**941 (1976); and Vincent DeFrancis, "Progress and Problems in Protecting the Abused Child," *Speaking Out for Child Protection,* American Humane Association, Englewood, Colo., 1973, pp. 19–72.

ing may result in a low-birth-weight infant or a premature birth. The mother's chronic, moderate drinking of alcohol can cause fetal alcohol syndrome; affected infants are malnourished and small for gestational age and have mild to moderate mental retardation. Drug abuse during pregnancy can result in an addicted infant with neurological disturbances, including irritability, tremors, and difficulty in feeding and sleeping.[5] The causes and consequences of fetal abuse are discussed in more detail in Chaps. 6 and 17.

Nursing management

The health care team's management of the abusive mother and the abused fetus or infant varies greatly according to the health problem. For example, when the nurse, in collaboration with the physician, suspects substance abuse in the mother or its effects in the infant, the nurse should obtain urine specimens from both for a drug toxicity scan. If the tests are positive for illicit substances, *immediate* referral must be made to the child protective services and the hospital's child abuse team.

Long-term management is necessary to minimize the emotional sequelae and learning problems that occur in abused preschoolers and school-age children. For example, an addicted mother is likely to be inadequately prepared emotionally for childbirth and childrearing. Drug-abusing parents were frequently abused as children. It is not unusual for such parents to exhibit poor bonding behavior and even hostility toward the newborn. The nurse can help the parents safeguard their unborn child by providing good health care, education, and supervision. Parents who abuse drugs will need referral for specialized services such as those provided by Alcoholics Anonymous, stop-smoking clinics, dietitians, and Parents Anonymous.

Within the community, nurses can support and establish programs to decrease noxious substances in the environment, to improve the nutritional status of adolescents and women of childbearing age, to provide adequate health care programs for women, and to educate the public about healthy life-styles and parenting.

PREVENTION OF CHILD ABUSE

Adults in high-risk categories for child abuse can often be identified before, after, or during the birth of their child. The nurse, functioning as a parent health educator, can observe the parents' verbal and nonverbal behavior toward the baby even before it is born. An informal interview with the parents should follow. The nurse assesses their emotional and physical preparation for childbirth and their responses to the child. Maintaining a nonjudgmental attitude toward the parents increases their cooperation and promotes the infant's safety. A partial list of warning signs for the nurse to observe is given in Table 38-2.

When the nurse observes one or more of these warning signs, the behavior should be noted on the patient's record. Plans for further action can also be detailed. An example follows:

Example: 3 P.M.: Mary fed John 1 oz and then returned him to his crib within 5 min of receiving him from the nursery and went to the visitors' room. She was found smoking and laughing loudly with a friend. When asked, "Why did you stop feeding John?" she replied, "He stinks and I needed a smoke." John was returned to the nursery, still clean and dry. He was alert and hungry (drank $1\frac{1}{2}$ oz more).

Nursing Diagnosis: Alteration in parenting related to lack of knowledge manifested by inappropriate parenting behaviors.

Plan

1. Spend time with Mary tomorrow during a feeding period and some time with her alone.
2. Gather data: How does Mary handle John, how does she feed him, and what are her current attitudes toward John and her plans for him? What personal problems is she having? How has she prepared her home for John?
3. Gather data from other health care personnel who have given care to Mary.
4. Develop an intervention plan alone or with other nurses for Mary and John based on the above data.
5. Develop an evaluation and follow-up plan for Mary and John.

Failure of the nurse to recognize or deal with parents' problems and poor parent-infant bonding can result in abuse or even the death of the child. In health care facilities today, it is common for many health care personnel to ignore parents' problems for reasons such as the following:

She's only here for 2 days. I can't change anything.
There are too many patients with too many problems.
Her problems are unsolvable.
It's the doctor's responsibility.

But nurses who do take the responsibility for communicating with patients effectively and helping them establish an adequate support system to deal with their problems can facilitate a better quality of life. Consider the contrast between these two examples:

Example: A single teenager, alone with a dog, moved to a large city in the late stages of pregnancy. She secured a small, unfurnished apart-

Table 38-2 Predictive Signs of Potential Child Abuse

In the Prenatal Period

1. Mother is living alone or with small children without supportive family and friends.
2. Father is uninterested in the outcome of the pregnancy.
3. Mother is living with a man unrelated to the infant.
4. Mother is overly concerned about the sex of the child.
5. Mother is hostile toward the biological father.
6. Pregnancy was unplanned, and comments suggest that the child is unwanted.
7. Pregnancy was planned, but mother wants the baby in order to have "someone to love me."
8. Parents considered an abortion.
9. Parents were children of abusing, neglectful parents.
10. There is no telephone in the home.
11. Parents seem poorly educated, have learning and emotional problems, seem immature for their age, are underemployed, have marital conflicts, are depressed, and have inadequate housing.
12. Parents do not prepare a "nest" for the child—crib, clothing.
13. Mother denies pregnancy, e.g., is late in seeking medical care, refuses to wear maternity clothes, and fails to gain weight.
14. Mother is under 16 years of age.
15. Mother repeatedly misses doctor's appointments.

In the Labor and Delivery Suite

1. Mother speaks angrily about the baby's "causing" her to be in pain.
2. Parents do not touch, hold, or examine their baby, or they make disparaging remarks about the sex or appearance of the child and exhibit lack of joy about the birth.
3. Mother is alone or father is remote or dutiful without affection.
4. Difficult or complicated labor.

In the Postpartum Period

1. Mother spends minimal time caring for the infant and rarely touches or cuddles the infant.
2. Mother does not enjoy or play with her baby.
3. Mother avoids eye contact with her child.
4. Mother feeds her child with minimal body contact.
5. Mother is bothered by her child's crying and messiness.
6. Child has congenital anomalies and requires a special-care nursery.
7. Husband shows jealous behavior.
8. Mother names the child after her former boyfriend.

Sources: Jane D. Gray et al., "Prediction and Prevention of Child Abuse and Neglect," in M. L. Lauderdale et al. (eds.), *Child Abuse and Neglect: Issues on Innovation and Implementation,* vol. 1, Department of Health, Education, and Welfare, Washington, D.C., Publication No. (OHDS) 78-30147, 1977, pp. 246–254; and Raymond H. Starr, *Child Abuse Prediction,* Ballinger, Cambridge, Mass., 1982, pp. 135–152.

ment. She applied for welfare, but payments were delayed. She had no money to prepare the home for the baby. She did not know anyone in her apartment building. She delivered a son after normal labor and was hospitalized for 2 days.

On her discharge day, she returned home with the baby. The dog had not eaten for 3 days. She put the child on the floor and left to get some dog food. On her return, she found that the dog had killed the baby.

Example: Pregnant 17-year-old Jennifer came to a prenatal clinic 1000 miles from her family's home. The physical examination indicated that she was in her sixth month of pregnancy. The clinic nurse who interviewed her discovered that the girl had many problems, including infrequent illegal drug use, insufficient funds, a poor education, poor nutrition, no close friends, and a great deal of hostility; also, she had made no preparations for the baby. On the positive side, the girl revealed that she was dissatisfied with her previous life-style and wanted a better life for herself and the baby. She was willing to accept counseling from the nurse and other health care personnel. The clinic nurse worked closely with her for the next 3 months, introducing resources to Jennifer. The clinic nurse prepared the obstetrical unit to support Jennifer. A pediatric clinic continued to follow up Jennifer and her son, Jimmy, for the next 5 years. Largely as a result of concerned health care personnel, Jennifer was able to utilize multiple resources to resolve her life problems. At 23 years of age, Jennifer had a stable marriage, two healthy, normal children, and a junior college education.

When the nurse develops an intervention program and cooperates with other health care personnel in the hospital and the community, better family functioning and increased safety for children are the results.

NONACCIDENTAL INJURY

Nonaccidental injury (NAI) is physical injury to the child as a result of hostile actions of an adult caretaker, such as when a parent dips a 1-year-old boy in hot water to punish him for soiling his diapers. NAI may also be due to failure to protect a child when injury will result from inaction, such as when a toddler falls from an open and unscreened second-story window or when an infant drowns in the bathtub because a parent has left the baby to answer the phone.

Characteristics of nonaccidental injuries

Whenever a child is injured, NAI must be considered as a possible cause. There are some factors that a nurse can assess when developing a nursing diagnosis. One is whether the injury makes sense in terms of the child's age. For example, an infant under 1 year of age rarely fractures a femur by falling out of a crib or high chair. It takes 150 lb of direct or twisting pressure to break an infant's femur. X-rays may reveal that the femur was fractured by a severe twisting movement which requires adult muscle strength. X-ray findings of old healed fractures along with a fresh injury suggest repeated abuse.

Another factor is whether the parent's explanation is compatible with the injury. Inconsistency or inappropriateness should alert the nurse to the possibility of abuse. The following case history is an example.

Example: An 11-month-old girl is admitted with a fractured skull (a cracked eggshell appearance on x-ray). The parents report that she fell off a couch while napping. A fractured skull is unlikely to result from a short fall. The x-ray finding of a cracked eggshell appearance usually means that the child was violently slammed against a wall. The injury does not match the parents' explanation.

When assessing an injury, collect and scrutinize all relevant data. Consider the child with bruises. Small bruises on a toddler's forehead, chin, and knees are normal consequences of learning to walk. Bruises on multiple surfaces (the cheeks, back, trunk, and extremities) suggest that a toddler has been slapped (Fig. 38-1). If the bruises are in different stages of healing, multiple beatings may have occurred. Mongolian spots on the young child's lower back can resemble bruises but are normal findings. Do the bruises suggest the use of a weapon, such as a belt or electric cord? Using a weapon to hit a child is a reportable problem. Slapping sometimes leaves characteristic petechial marks (Fig. 38-2).[6]

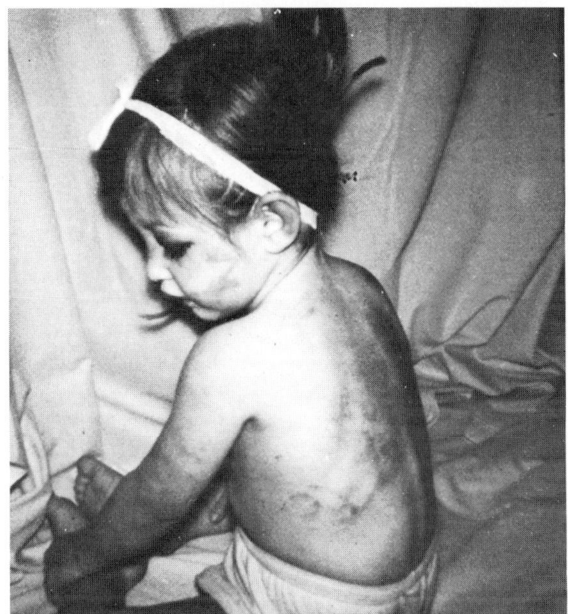

Figure 38-1 A nurse thoroughly assesses the undressed child for signs of injury. Note the welt mark on the child's body. (*Courtesy of Vincent J. Fontana, M.D., The New York Foundling Hospital.*)

Reporting suspected abuse

It is not necessary for the nurse or other health care workers to know whether abuse has definitely occurred, who did it, or how the injury was inflicted. A nurse who only *suspects* that child abuse has occurred is *required* by law to report the suspicion to the local police or protective child care service agency. The child has been injured under suspicious circumstances and needs protection until an investigation has taken place.

A nurse (as well as certain other professionals, including teachers and physicians) who fails to report suspected child abuse may be charged with a misdemeanor. Nurses have immunity from being sued when reporting suspected child abuse. In most emergency rooms, the physician will take the responsibility for contacting the police or protective child care service worker. Every hospital and community health care agency needs a written policy concerning how the abused child will be admitted, assessed, treated, and returned to the general community and concerning who is responsible for reporting the abuse to authorities. In many hospitals, this responsibility is assigned to the medical or psychiatric social worker. In some states, a doctor can be charged with a felony for failing to report an obvious case of child abuse if the child is readmitted for another injury.

Some hospitals are developing suspected child abuse and neglect (SCAN) teams, which participate in identifying, reporting, assessing, treating, and following up abused children and their families. Team members have the very difficult task of informing the parents that child abuse is suspected and that the hospital staff, by law, must report the child's problem to the police. They also tell the parents that they wish to help the family through the process of assessment and treatment. The team members know that some of the parents' responses will be anger, denial, and depression. Sometimes a team member will support the family during the juvenile court or criminal court proceedings.

Absolute honesty with the parents regarding

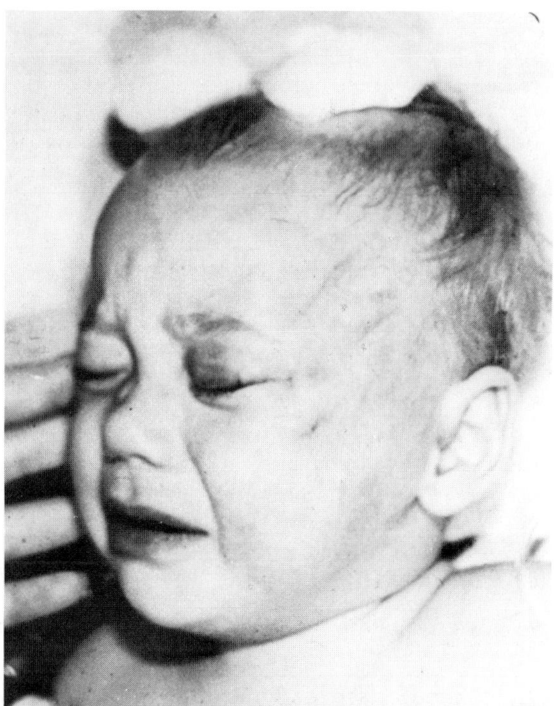

Figure 38-2 Hand slaps to the face of this 6-month-old child resulted in visible linear marks from the fingers and a subdural hematoma. (Cotton balls are routinely placed on the scalp after subdural taps are done.) [*Courtesy of Robert W. ten Bensel, M.D.*]

the court process and treatment recommendations is required. Empathic and nonjudgmental team members are a great comfort to the family members. The courts respect the written reports of the team members and most often follow their recommendations about treatment plans for the child and the family. The child's primary nurse is also part of the team and provides data on the child and the family, as well as the nurse's observations, nursing diagnoses, nursing actions, and recommendations for discharge planning. All members of the team are responsible for accurately recording pertinent data in the child's record.

Some child abuse teams utilize community resources for treatment and review the family's progress only at specified periods. Other teams, in addition to making community referrals, participate in a therapy program for families during and after hospitalization. This participation may include supervising lay therapists (who work with families mainly at home) and conducting individual and group therapy sessions for children, siblings, and parents. Nurses often see great progress and experience a sense of satisfaction as families make tremendous gains in the quality of their child care. The threat of reinjury to a child is greatly reduced when a family participates actively in a treatment program designed by a multidisciplinary team.

Children within the health care system

Table 38-3 outlines the movement of an abused or neglected child through the health care system. The rehabilitation unit mentioned in the table is a special type of hospital unit. Children (and sometimes their parents) are housed in an informal, homelike setting. Children are dressed in their regular clothes and eat family style. Many health professionals, including nurses, psychologists, physicians, and physical and occupational therapists, work cooperatively for the benefit of the families.

Nurses' participation in the court process

The nurse's role in the investigation of abuse or neglect is rarely complicated, and court appearances are infrequently required. Usually the court wants accurate written data documenting the child's health problems, including injuries and illnesses. The nurse should not include value judgments in the chart, since these may invalidate it.[7] A sample of how data should be recorded on the chart follows:

Table 38-3 The Path of Abused and Neglected Children in the Health Care System

Entry
Report by relative, neighbor, or friend
Is brought in by school nurse
Child's self-report
Parent's report
"Accident story" in emergency room
Is brought in by police or protective service worker
Private physician's report
Where Decisions Are Made
Emergency room
Acute inpatient unit
Rehabilitation unit
Outpatient unit (usually a nonreportable mild abuse and neglect problem)
Exit
Home without court supervision
Home with court supervision (3 months to 18 years)
Shelter care facility until investigation is completed
Group home for mentally retarded or mentally ill children
Foster care, adoption, or other short-term or long-term relinquishment of child by parent
Death

Example: A large, dark-purple bruise (approximately 6 cm in diameter and irregularly shaped) is on the upper right quadrant of Tommy's abdomen. Tommy's father said, "Tommy fell out of a tree, hitting a large rock on the ground." Tommy reported, when his father was out of the examining room, "My dad hit me."

Court processes vary in different cities. Usually the atmosphere in juvenile court is more casual than that in civil or criminal court. A treatment plan is evolved, sometimes with the aid of the hospital child abuse team, that permits adequate supervision of the child and rehabilitation of the family.

The child may be placed in a foster home or referred to an adoption agency. Foster placement can cause emotional disturbances in the child. Sometimes the child is placed with relatives or at home, under supervision. The child may stay under court supervision for months or until adulthood. Reevaluation is required approximately every 6 months to determine how the child is progressing. If the parents do not show evidence of healthier coping mechanisms and child-rearing patterns, the child may be released for adoption.

Causative factors in nonaccidental injury

Any parents, regardless of socioeconomic status, religion, race, or culture, can become child abusers. People in the lower socioeconomic groups, who use impersonal health care facilities, are reported most often. Private physicians have been hesitant to report families in the past. This is gradually changing, as physicians have become more familiar with the usual court process and aware of the development of treatment centers.

Many researchers in different locations are attempting to delineate the multiple causes of child abuse.[8] There are some common findings. Parents are the abusers in 85 percent of cases. The mother is more often the perpetrator with children aged 1 to 3 years, and the father with children aged 13 to 15 years. Mothers' "boyfriends," stepfathers, and baby-sitters are also frequent abusers.

Often, parental psychosocial pathology is present, with a history of abuse or neglect going back three or four generations. The parent has learned violent methods of child discipline, such as beating with a belt or hitting with a board. Rigid, restrictive religious beliefs and strict, authoritarian discipline are related to child abuse. Abusive parents have low self-esteem and unmet dependency needs and are unable to handle stress. They may feel hostile, angry, and overwhelmed. The incidence of child abuse increases with family stress—more children than the parents can cope with, unemployment, isolation, inadequate financial resources, overcrowding, and marital discord. Many abusive parents feel socially isolated or receive little, if any, support from their spouses or other family members.

Parents may also have inadequate knowledge of normal growth and development. They have inappropriate expectations of their child. Instead of taking care of the child, they expect the child to function as a little adult, meeting the parents' needs. In other situations, parents are physically or psychologically absent because of alcoholism or mental illness. In most instances, education and psychotherapy will assist these families to function better.

Often, the abused child is considered different from other children. This perception may be based on a physical problem (e.g., prematurity, a crippling disorder, retardation, or a heart defect). A negative emotional tie may result if the child has been named after a disliked person or is a symbol of a former spouse. The abused child can also be highly valued or "wanted."

When episodes of abuse are carefully studied, a precipitating stressor is often found. Although this stressor may seem minor to the nurse, it may be perceived as severe by the parent. For example, lack of sleep or the crying of an irritable infant may trigger an episode of abuse. One author has noted three common situations that cause abusive parents to erupt with anger. In the first situation, the parent considers the infant's crying to be excessive. The parent is unable to stop the crying, becomes angry and impatient, and reacts violently toward the baby. It is very important that the nurse discuss infants' crying with parents who have been identified as at risk for becoming abusive (Table 38-2). Normal crying patterns should be described (see Chap. 9), and the parents need to be taught to interpret why the baby is crying (because of pain, hunger, boredom, fear, etc.) and what to do about it. The parent needs to have a backup plan for times when the baby's crying becomes intolerable; for example, perhaps a neighbor can care for the infant while the mother takes a walk. Babies who cry excessively need evaluation to rule out organic disease as a cause of the irritability.

The second situation that can lead to abusive episodes results when toilet training is started too early or when the parents have a poor understanding of what can and cannot be expected of the child. For example, if a $2\frac{1}{2}$-year-old child defecates in his or her pants or behind the couch, the parent may perceive the act as hostile or as deliberately defiant and react violently. As another example, a parent may try to toilet-train a 1-year-old child and react with anger to the inevitable failure. Obviously, as a teacher, the nurse can identify the parents' expectations for, and attitudes toward, toilet training and help them modify unrealistic expectations.

In the third situation, a hyperactive school-age child may provoke child abuse. Excessive talking and moving and reduced sleep needs produce stress for the parents. Child abuse may be prevented by referring hyperactive children, or active children who are perceived by the parents as hyperactive, to a counselor.

Nursing management When a child with a suspected NAI is admitted to the hospital, the immediate priorities are to assess, describe parent-child behavior in writing, and treat injuries; to provide physical and psychological comfort; and to protect the child from further injury or removal from the hospital by the parents. Long-range goals deal with changing the family's functioning to prevent further abuse.

Usually by the time the child reaches the inpatient unit from the emergency room, the police have been notified and custody of the child has been assigned to the hospital, pending a court hearing. The parents must be told about the custody and must be informed that they are not to take the child from the hospital.

Gentleness is important during the physical examination and any other handling of the child. Explanations and reassurance must be provided at the child's level of understanding. In addition to the usual apprehension that all children experience when they come to the hospital, children who have been abused may have a generalized mistrust of adults. These children usually scan the environment (exhibiting "on-guard" behavior) and are fearful not only of health care personnel but also of their parents. In spite of their apprehension, they passively submit to caregiving activities and protest or cry very little, because they have learned that complaining and resisting lead to punishment.

From the outset of nursing care, a major objective is to enable the child to establish a sense of security and trust. Consistent kindness and sustained interaction with the same staff members encourage the child's confidence in people and diminish anxiety. It is also critically important to remember that these children, like others (especially young children), have strong affectional and dependency ties to their parents; they are distressed by separation from the parents and need sustained contact with them and reassurance that the parents have not abandoned them.

The initial interview with the parents should deal with the child's present stage of development in order to provide the nurse with data on which to construct the care plan. (See Appendix D for a personal history form.) Parents need to be oriented to the hospital unit and its routines. They are told at this initial interview that the nurse will work closely with them and with the other members of the child abuse team to help the family change ineffective patterns and to increase the well-being of the parents and the child. The parents are generally upset at admission, and lengthy or sensitive aspects of the interview are deferred until a later visit. It is important to convey the idea that the nurse wants to work with—not against—the parents and that many families in similar situations have found ways to work out their problems. Visits to the hospital are encouraged (appointments with the nurse should be scheduled if the parents do not routinely come in) so that intervention care can take place.

Nursing intervention with the parents involves identifying and recording both the negative aspects and the positive resources of the abusive family.

Example: A 7-year-old girl is admitted to an inpatient unit because of welts and bruises on her back, upper thighs, and left cheek. A school nurse brought her to the emergency room. In gathering data for assessment, the nurse learned the following:

1. The stepfather, who admitted hitting the child, recently became unemployed.
2. The mother is a passive person and is unable to stop the stepfather; she is 7 months pregnant.
3. The child displays hyperactive behavior and sleeps only 4 h a night.
4. The child was a premature twin and, because of hospitalization for prematurity, was not touched by her mother for 3 months after her birth.
5. The child is considered possessed (of devils) by her mother.
6. The child was jumping from a dresser onto a bed where her sister was sleeping at 3 A.M. when the incident occurred.
7. The stepfather is remorseful about the incident.
8. The parents are asking, "How can we help our child?"
9. The parents are willing to come in for appointments.

With these data, the nurse was able to collaborate with the hospital child abuse team in an effective intervention approach. Guidelines for the nursing care of children with NAIs are presented in Table 38-7.

Communication patterns When a nurse sees a severely abused child, an emotional response occurs. This reaction is based on the nurse's personal family history, childrearing beliefs, and

Table 38-4 Common Diagnostic Tests Performed on Children Who Have Suffered a Suspected Nonaccidental Injury

Blood and Urine Tests	Radiological Examinations	Consultations
Bleeding tests to rule out underlying diseases which cause bleeding: Platelet count Prothrombin time Ivy bleeding time Partial thromboplastin time Complete blood count Urinalysis Serum amylase for traumatic pancreatitis	Skeletal survey (particularly in children under 3 years of age) of all bones to identify fractures Serial x-rays to date healing, identify fracture not initially seen (chip fracture) X-rays of bones to rule out pathology which allows for abnormal fracturing Contrast studies of gastrointestinal tract (useful for children with forced ingestion of caustics or duodenal or jejunal injury from blunt trauma) CAT scans of brain and trunk when trauma is suspected, e.g., to identify subdural hematoma Radioactive scan for liver, spleen, or kidney trauma	Psychologist: Psychometric testing Parent interview Interviews with child and siblings Psychiatrist: Parent interview Child interviews Neurologist: May order EEG Physical and occupational therapist to do developmental examination Pediatrician specializing in child abuse Photographer to document evidence of abuse

protective or rescue fantasies. The nurse's reaction affects the communication patterns with the child and other members of the family. In order to be an objective and effective nurse, it is vital to recognize this reaction, determine whether it is blocking communication, and find a resource to help. The members of the nursing staff often will gather for a conference to share their thoughts and learn from one another. An effective intervention program depends on a trusting relationship and bonding of the family to the hospital staff, and nonjudgmental behavior clearly will enhance this. Greet the parents when they visit their child. Praise them for correct actions. Gather data on their knowledge of growth and development, discipline problems, the emotional climate in the home, financial resources, and support systems within the family.

Diagnostic tests Several diagnostic tests are commonly administered to NAIs who have bruises, fractures, or suspected neurological damage. Table 38-4 is a brief guide to these tests.

NEGLECT

Neglect, which is another form of child abuse, occurs when an adult caretaker either deliberately or unintentionally fails to provide the supports necessary for the development of a child's physical, intellectual, and emotional capacities.[9] These supports are the basic necessities of life: food, housing, clothing, protection and supervision, love, and medical and dental care. Neglect is more widespread than abuse, and its consequences are equally serious. The different types of neglect which will be discussed in this section are environmental (nonorganic failure to thrive), physical, and emotional.

Parents' characteristics

Neglectful parents have many of the psychological characteristics of abusing parents, listed in Table 38-2. They are perpetuating the cycle of abuse that they learned as abused or neglected children. They often feel rejected by their parents and lack good parenting role models. They experience role reversal and expect the child to meet their needs. They have low self-esteem and often expect their child to reject them; for this reason, they also have few friends. Many parents are burdened by multiple stresses which deplete the energy reserves needed to raise children. They often have inadequate housing, money, food, and medical care and may have limited coping abilities. It is therefore understandable that these parents are frequently harried, anxious, and depressed and have many psychosomatic illnesses.

Environmental neglect

Failure to thrive Environmental neglect may cause a syndrome called *nonorganic failure to thrive*. In this disorder, the child's height and weight are below the 3d percentile, and the child experiences delays in emotional, social, motor, language, and intellectual development.[10] The child's head circumference is also smaller than normal for the child's age. The growth retardation is thought to result from emotional deprivation, which causes the hypothalamus and pituitary gland to secrete decreasing amounts of growth hormone.[11] The emotional deprivation is believed to result from a disturbed mother-child relationship.[12] Emotional deprivation is discussed in the section "Emotional Neglect." The parents relate less to their child, cuddling and holding the child less.[13] The lack of stimulation and nurturing causes other clinical manifestations, which are listed in Table 38-5. Most of the examples of clinical manifestations listed in Table 38-5 are reportable problems. Even parents who fail to protect young children in motor vehicles can be ticketed in some states. Many children show several manifestations (Table 38-6). When in doubt, the nurse should contact the SCAN team or child protective service workers.

The many organic (physical) causes of failure to thrive must be carefully ruled out before a child can be considered to suffer from nonorganic failure to thrive. Those disorders that cause organic failure to thrive, such as malabsorption and cardiac anomalies, are discussed elsewhere in this book.

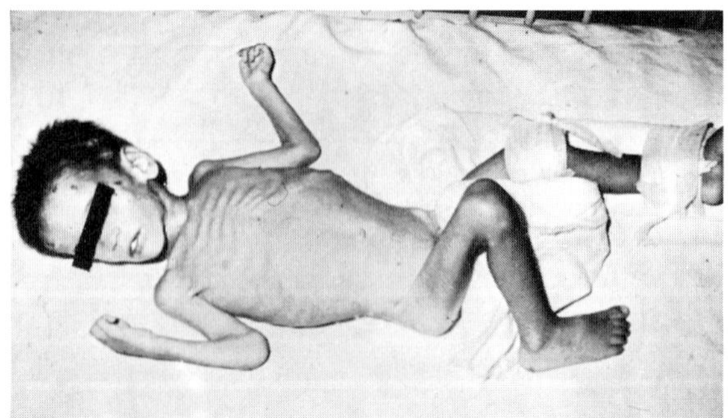

Figure 38-3 This 18-month-old infant was hospitalized for failure to thrive. No organic basis was found for the failure to gain weight. The findings of the physical examination included a dislocated knee. (*Courtesy of Robert W. ten Bensel, M.D.*)

Some physicians advocate hospitalization of infants who fail to thrive or to grow (the term preferred by some) so that their nutritional intake can be increased by $2\frac{1}{2}$ times the normal amount. Once growth begins, there is time enough to pursue the cause of the failure to thrive or grow.

Nursing management The child who suffers from nonorganic failure to thrive is usually treated on an outpatient basis. The three highest-priority areas for assessment are the child's dietary pattern and eating behaviors, developmental delays, and apathetic emotional behavior. The nurse and the dietitian assess the child's diet history and eating habits and the family's food purchases and conduct a calorie count.[14]

Table 38-5 Clinical Manifestations of Neglect

1. Delayed development for age
2. Poor growth pattern
3. Poor or absent dental care
4. Chronic malnutrition, including eating excessive junk food and inadequate essential growth foods; cooks own meals
5. Repressed personality
6. Evidence of poor supervision, e.g., repeated falls downstairs, repeated ingestions, child locked out of the house
7. Poor immunization pattern
8. Lack of medical attention for illnesses
9. Not protected in motor vehicles
10. Inadequate stimulation for speech development
11. Skin problems, e.g., poor cleansing, seborrhea, impetigo, and diaper rash
12. Is left home alone (under 13 years)
13. Unsanitary, unsafe, or filthy home environment
14. Feeding difficulties: rumination, pica, ravenous appetite
15. Refusal to suck, arching, spitting, or sleeping to avoid nipple
16. Chronic vomiting and/or diarrhea

Table 38-6 Characteristic Problems of Neglected Children

Short-Term Problems	Long-Term Problems
Malnutrition	Poor "catch-up growth" (motor, language, social, intellectual)
Pneumonia	Abnormally sad, apathetic
Repeated nonaccidental injuries	Behavior problems (exaggerated fears, cajoles others for attention and affection)
Disruption in brain development (decreased intellect)	Social problems (antisocial behavior, drug and alcohol abuse, delinquency)
Short stature; is underweight	Poor bonding with parents

The nurse also assesses the parents' feeding techniques during several visits. The nurse should also assess the child's developmental delays and the parents' knowledge of growth and development, appropriate stimulation, and parenting techniques. The nurse may use the Neonatal Perception Inventory, the Degree of Bother Inventory, or the Carey Infant Temperament Questionnaire to objectively assess the parent-child interaction.[15] Finally, the nurse should assess the child's apathetic behavior, which may be caused by lack of stimulation and maternal deprivation. Physicians should avoid elaborate, strenuous diagnostic evaluations during this assessment phase.

The most important nursing intervention for these parents is to provide nurturance. The nurse meets their unmet dependency needs and acts as a role model for additional parenting methods. The assessment phase should be ongoing while the nurse builds a trusting relationship during home visits. The nurse and the dietitian collaborate to provide the parents with a specific feeding guide and instructions for providing a high-calorie diet. They conduct calorie counts, obtain a dietary history, and teach the parents about correct nutrition, feeding techniques, and food purchasing. The nurse teaches appropriate stimulation, toy selection, and parenting skills on the basis of continued developmental evaluations. The nurse praises and rewards the parents for appropriate behaviors in order to increase their self-esteem. The nurse also assesses support systems and stresses within the family during long-term follow-up. Table 38-7 defines common problems and suggests nursing interventions. These families need continued support from the health care team because many children continue to be below the 50th percentile in weight and to have delayed development.

With continued support, these parents can bond to the SCAN team members, which is necessary before they can bond to their child. Frequently, the parents will rapidly form social relationships if a support system is created within the family.[16] Many parents respond quickly to the nurse's expressed acceptance of, and concern for, them and their child.

Example: A 3-month-old boy was admitted to a medical facility because of poor weight gain, difficulty in feeding, seborrhea, severe diaper rash, and general irritability. The child was given a minimum of diagnostic tests (a complete blood count, urinalysis, history, and physical examination). The 16-year-old mother, who lived alone, stated that the pregnancy, labor, and delivery had been normal (birth weight was 3.15 kg and length was 52.5 cm). Weight was now 3.37 kg, and length was 53.7 cm. The child was given well-child care (regular feeding or formula, baths, and regular sleeping and cuddling periods). The mother visited her child infrequently and for short periods. She seemed to resent the baby's obvious return to health. The child gained 0.45 kg and grew 1.25 cm within a week. His skin problems and irritability disappeared.

He was transferred to a rehabilitation unit, and the nursing staff worked intensively with both the mother and the child, using a variety of techniques, such as putting a radio in the child's room so that the mother would be more comfortable with her favorite music stations while feeding her baby and praising the mother when she exhibited positive mothering techniques. The nurse compared the child's handsomeness to the mother's beautiful features, giving the mother a sense of having produced a beautiful baby from her own beauty. Within 2 weeks the baby was discharged home to his mother. A support system was developed that included a lay home visitor and a special high school where the mother was enrolled while her baby was cared for in a school nursery. One year later, both mother and child were thriving.

Physical neglect

Physically neglected children have not been provided with the basic physical necessities of life, such as clothing, food, shelter, and medical care. They frequently have the clinical manifestations listed in Table 38-5. For example, the child who is given inadequate, irregular meals may receive insufficient nutrients and have an insufficient caloric intake to maintain metabolism, promote growth, and support motor activity. The child may lack the energy to explore the environment, and the malnutrition may result in limited energy to walk or stand. The parents' characteristics were discussed earlier in this chapter.

Emotional neglect

Emotional neglect occurs when the caregiver is unable to provide adequate emotional stimulation, nurturing, and guidance for the infant or child. Emotional deprivation occurs when the caregiver has not firmly bonded to the infant. Much of the infant's behavior is geared toward bringing the parent's face into direct view. The

Table 38-7 General Guidelines for Nursing Care of Children Who Have Suffered Neglect or Nonaccidental Injury

Patient Problem and Goal	Nursing Actions
Growth delay Child will gain weight during hospitalization	Develop a baseline assessment and assessment of admission height and weight. Interview parents regarding feeding patterns and types and amount of food taken at home. Feed child a balanced diet appropriate for his or her age. Feed on demand unless child does not communicate hunger; then feed on schedule. Weigh child daily. Document food intake and response to feeding. Hold infant for all feedings. Provide eye contact and verbal communication during feeding. Observe and record parent's feeding behavior with child. Gently teach parent successful feeding behavior. Reward successful feeding behavior when demonstrated by parent.
Developmental delay Child will show age-appropriate developmental milestones	Interview parents regarding developmental history (especially milestones). Assess and document current activity pattern, muscle strength, and usual play interests and activities. Provide verbal, tactile, and motor stimulation appropriate for child's age. Vary toys, stimulation, and location regularly.
Physical trauma Child will have maximum healing, recovery, and protection from bodily injury	Observe and document unusual physical findings. Record parent's explanation of child's injuries. Monitor all visitors in a discreet manner. Observe and record parent-child communication. Maintain a friendly, accepting attitude when dealing with parents. Maintain a calm, gentle approach when giving care to child. Identify and document family problems. Teach normal well child care, effective and safe discipline, and realistic expectations of behavior for child's age. Guide parents in safety and accident prevention.
Emotional deprivation and trauma Child will develop trust in, and attachment to, significant people	Assess and document parent-child interaction, child's affect, child's attachment behavior, and sibling interaction. Assign consistent nursing personnel. Secure social history, especially any problems promoting parental mistreatment, e.g., loss of job or a drinking problem. Provide substitute parenting and emotional stimulation. Cuddle, hold, touch, and make eye contact for planned periods each day. Respond immediately to crying. Teach parent by example to comfort and play with child.
Inadequate social situation Parents will have resources to utilize during crises	Introduce family to resources to use as lifelines in stress and crisis situations. Help parents to utilize psychotherapy and self-help groups for more effective family function. Help parents identify physical environmental problems, e.g., housing or finances. Help parents solve environmental problems.
Parenting inabilities and inadequacy	Assess and document parents' capabilities and inabilities by observing their behavior. Accept parents as worthy human beings capable of change. Develop parents' trust: assign a staff person on each shift to act as a liaison. Identify parents' characteristics that prevent nurturing. Reinforce parents' self-image. Teach parents behaviors that strengthen their weak areas.

Table 38-7 General Guidelines for Nursing Care of Children Who Have Suffered Neglect or Nonaccidental Injury (*Continued*)

Patient Problem and Goal	Nursing Actions
Home care and long-term follow-up Parents will provide a safe, stimulating, and pleasant home environment for the child	Introduce parents to long-term treatment program while child is still in hospital. Participate in discharge planning for child. Inform parents that child abuse is a long-term problem and needs long-term treatment. Provide opportunities for parents and child regularly to discuss details of the treatment program. Utilize the juvenile court social workers to promote compliance with the treatment plan. Encourage parents to utilize foster care and adoption services if they decide not to participate in a treatment program and do not wish to keep their child. Give them support if they make this decision.

Sources: Mary Andrews and Audrey H. Beatty, "Standards of Care for Children with Failure to Thrive Syndrome," unpublished paper, Children's Hospital, Los Angeles, 1977; and Audry Edberg and Judy Cohen, "Standards of Care for Children with Battered Child Syndrome," unpublished paper, Children's Hospital, Los Angeles, 1981.

infant repeatedly seeks to bond to the parent, so great is the child's hunger for physical and emotional closeness. When mother-seeking efforts fail, the infant withdraws from social contact. The emotionally neglected infant becomes a highly anxious, withdrawn, and anorexic child; refuses to play (a sign of high anxiety); and is developmentally delayed. The child will lag behind his or her peers in psychological, intellectual, language, and motor development.

Psychologists and pediatricians became interested in studying maternal and emotional deprivation in the 1930s. Researchers observed that institutionalized and hospitalized children who were physically cared for by various caretakers literally emotionally starved to death. The infants became apathetic, listless, pale, anorexic, and immobile. When they were approached by nurses, they did not move or have a brighter facial expression, which is typical when infants anticipate being held or played with. Many infants thus lost interest in the environment and in eating and died. The living infants were delayed developmentally and had difficulty trusting adults.

Nursing management The nurse's primary goal is to strengthen the parent-child bond. The nurse slowly establishes a trusting relationship with the mother while assessing the family's communication patterns, support systems, knowledge of growth and development, appropriate discipline and parenting techniques, and community activities. The nurse may encourage the mother to join support groups within the community such as nursery schools in which parents participate, neighborhood play groups, or Head Start nursery schools. The nurse should act as a role model for alternative methods of communicating with and disciplining children. Too many children are expected to be "seen and not heard" and are allowed to raise themselves. The nurse talks with parents and children in an interested manner.

SEXUAL ABUSE

Sexual abuse is defined as the use of a child for sexual gratification by an adult or by another child who is at least 5 years older than the abused child. In 1982 approximately 170,000 children were abused sexually, and other studies report the figure to be higher, at 360,000 each year.[17] Only 10 percent of child molestations are believed to be reported. Children from all socioeconomic classes are abused, 75 percent of the time by a close family member (e.g., the father or a brother) or a close family friend.

Sexual abuse of children takes various forms, including having lewd conversation, genital viewing, fondling of the genitals and breasts, masturbating, oral copulation (which may progress to vaginal intercourse), and anal penetration. Fingers or instruments may be inserted into body orifices, and children may be tortured and even murdered. (See Table 38-8 for clinical manifestations of sexual abuse.) The longer the abuse continues, the more profound the psychological consequences will be. The child may conceal the psychological trauma for years until it emerges at a psychosexual crisis point at a later time. Abused children blame themselves and feel guilty, depressed, humiliated, and self-depreciating. Children suffer the same symptoms as adults do after rape. (See Chap. 33.)

The sexual abuser was often sexually abused as a child and is part of a dysfunctional family unit. A sexually abused girl becomes a mother with a sexually abused daughter; a sexually abused boy becomes an adult child abuser. In many homes the parents no longer communicate well or have sexual intercourse. The daughter may take on many of the mother's roles, including meeting the sexual needs of the father. The mother consciously or unconsciously condones this to keep the family intact. The daughter does not discuss it in order to protect the father. In a second type of family there are multiple problems such as drug or alcohol abuse, physical abuse, and imprisonment of family members. The father, who is often dominant or violent, perceives all women as sexual objects to be exploited. In a third type of family the father may have a weak identity and inadequate coping mechanisms. He may cope with stress through substance abuse. The behaviors in this type of family are less typical. The family members need intensive, long-term psychotherapy, both on an individual and a family basis.[18]

Table 38-8 Clinical Manifestations of Sexual Abuse

Physical Manifestations	Behavioral Manifestations
Genital area: Abrasions, lacerations, ecchymosis, bleeding, itching	Behavior indicates psychological conflict in the home, but child refuses to discuss it or withdraws from help.
Vagina: Discharge, bleeding, lacerations	Inappropriate modesty; child refuses to remove underwear or clothing at school.
Anus: Discharge, bleeding, scarring (from stretching)	Child refuses to bathe or shower.
Breasts: Bruises, lacerations	Child expresses anxiety: nail-biting, facial tics, excessive clinging and crying when separated, sleep disturbances, change in eating habits.
Sexually transmitted diseases (genitals, anus, mouth, eyes)	Inappropriate knowledge of sexual acts; child behaves seductively toward adults and undresses or fondles adults.
Dysuria, enuresis, encopresis	Poor peer relationships.
Pregnancy (especially if victim refuses to name father)	Change in school performance or attendance.
Semen evident in genital area, on underwear, or on skin	Acting-out behavior, delinquency.
	Truancy; child runs away from home.
	Alcohol or drug abuse.
	Child withdraws from close contact with people.
	Increased, exaggerated fears.
	Multiple, vague psychosomatic complaints (e.g., abdominal pain).

Nursing management

Nurses may encounter a sexually abused child in an emergency room or a clinic. The nurse should call the hospital's child abuse team and proceed as with an abused child workup. The child is examined as in the case of a rape. (See Chap. 33, Table 33-12.) The parents should be interviewed separately from the child, since the child may believe that he or she is the focus of their anger.[19] When interviewing the parents, use open-ended questions and do not attempt to elicit a confession. Show support and be realistic by saying, for example, "You should be angry. The most important thing now is to protect your child from any future abuse." Encourage the parents to express their greatest concerns.

When interviewing the child, show an interest in the child and ask about neutral areas first, such as friends, pets, and school. Ask the child to validate (or deny) your observations by saying, for example, "You have been awfully quiet these past few months, and you have had a lot of stomachaches. What's bothering you?" Do not promise to keep a secret, and if the child confesses, assure the child that he or she is doing the right thing by telling you and that you will provide absolute protection. If the child is too young to describe the abuse, use dolls with realistic genitalia. Ask the child to play with the dolls or to touch them "where he touched you," for example. Finally, document the child's exact words, movements of the dolls, and precise nonverbal behavior; this will become part of a court record.[20,21]

Only increased public awareness and stricter laws will decrease the sexual abuse of children. Nurses are involved in public education programs held in schools, preschools, and churches. Parents must be taught how to protect children. Instruct parents (1) to enforce strict boundaries and curfews for children—they should be home by dark; (2) not to allow children to roam the neighborhood—they should be required to inform the parents where they are and with whom they are playing; (3) not to allow children to bring guests into the home when they are alone; (4) not to use male baby-sitters; and (5) not to allow children to go for extended excursions with an opposite-sex adult. Children should be taught (1) that they must decide who hugs, kisses, and touches them; (2) that touching should feel all right and that if it does not, they should tell someone they trust; (3) that secrets are not the same as surprises—that they should never keep a secret if it makes them feel scared or unhappy; (4) that they should never go with a stranger and that if a stranger grabs them, they should scream as loud as they can and run away fast toward someone they know; (5) that they should never allow a stranger to undress them or show them "what big people do to play"; and (6) that if they feel uncomfortable in someone's presence, they should leave and tell a trusted adult about it.[22]

EMOTIONAL ABUSE

Emotional abuse is intellectual and psychological damage, inflicted either deliberately or as a result of neglect, which is evidenced by observable damage to the child's ability to perform.[23] Common clinical manifestations of emotional abuse are listed in Table 38-9. Emotional abuse is included in most state child abuse laws, but laws concerning emotional abuse have been utilized very little to protect children. Over the next decade, as the process of emotional abuse is studied further, more children will be protected. Emotional abuse accompanies physical abuse and neglect.

Clinical manifestations

When discussing the child's signs and symptoms and the behavior of the parents, the terms *emotional disturbance* and *emotional abuse* become inseparable. Not all childhood emotional disturbances are linked to abuse, of course; a child's chronic grief reaction to a parent's death, for example, clearly does not involve emotional abuse. Moreover, mentally retarded parents and others may not understand that they are damaging their child with their childrearing methods.

Health care personnel who can communicate with families in a friendly, nonjudgmental manner, expressing interest in both the parents and the child, will succeed in improving the emotional health of the child. Some families refuse to be treated. The family that is emotionally bat-

Table 38-9 Parental Behaviors That Lead to Emotional Abuse of Children

	Child's Behavior	
Parent's Behavior	**If Parent Gives Too Little**	**If Parent Gives Too Much**
Love	Poor growth Poor self-esteem Depression Withdrawal	Overconfidence Overprotection Passivity
Intellectual stimulation	Academic failure Development delay	Hyperactivity Stress in relation to school
Stability	Lack of trust	Inflexibility
Limits (moral and social)	Tantrums Antisocial behavior	Fearfulness Lack of creativity

Source: Ira S. Lourie and Lorrain Stephana, "On Defining Emotional Abuse: Results of a NIMH/NCCAN Workshop," *Child Abuse and Neglect* **1**:201–208 (April 1977).

tering a child and refuses help or ignores pleas from concerned friends, relatives, and health and educational personnel will require legal intervention.

Nursing management with verbally assaultive parents

Verbal abuse is one common form of emotional abuse. A large number of children are exposed to ridicule, shaming, threatened violence, and threatened withdrawal of love. The following statements are examples of assaultive language:

"My God, you're clumsy."
"I'm going to kill you!"
"What are you, deaf or something?"
"You're going to get hit till you're black and blue."
"I'm going to beat the shit out of you!"
"When you grow up, you're not going to amount to a hill of beans."
"Come here, stupid."
"Mommy won't love you anymore if you're bad."
"I don't want you, I don't love you, get lost!"

Sometimes only one child is selected for abuse in a family, and the siblings join the parents in attacking that child. The end result of many years of this can be an adult with a very poor self-concept, little motivation for educational achievement or gainful employment, and some emotional disturbance.

Example: Bob's mother, Barbara, was a lonely 25-year-old woman with a poor educational background (in relation to her family) when she met Joe at a roadside coffee stand. She conceived a child by him and subsequently married him, despite her family's concern about his suitability as a husband. Bob was a difficult child to feed and comfort from birth. Barbara's parents were ashamed of the inappropriate timing of the birth and offered limited support. The marriage broke up after 2 years, and Barbara quickly married again. She bore three children by her second husband. Verbal assault had begun when Bob was 1 year old and starting to walk. The siblings quickly learned to continue the parents' verbally abusive pattern when communicating with Bob, but they themselves were rarely verbally abused. Bob did poorly in school but was "pushed along" until he graduated from high school. At 21 years of age, he is living at home with his parents, is unemployed, has few friends, and aspires to become a writer of murder mysteries. He physically abuses his mother if she opposes him. She admits that she is afraid of him. Both Bob's parents and Bob refuse to go for counseling.

When the nurse identifies a parent who is verbally abusive to a child, intervention is needed. The following are some suggestions for dealing with the parent after a trusting relationship has been established:

1. Encourage the parents to join Parents Anonymous, a parent self-help group which very effectively helps parents who are verbally abusive. To do this, of course, parents must realize the consequences of this type of behavior and wish to change it.
2. Give time and attention to the parents, using interviewing techniques and allowing them freedom to express their concerns, worries, and doubts.
3. Provide a lay volunteer, preferably a parent of about the same age, who will spend time with the parents and show them alternative responses to children, a different life-style, and an improved self-concept.
4. Teach or encourage the parents to attend parent education classes where child care theories and practices are taught.
5. Encourage enrollment in a nursery school in which the parents observe and practice under the guidance of a skilled teacher.
6. Talk with a child protective service worker about the family, filing a formal report if requested.

Verbal abuse is usually considered a mild form of child abuse and is not ordinarily prosecuted by the juvenile court. The long-range effects of this behavior can be crippling to a child and should be prevented or stopped if possible. The parent who verbally abuses a child is usually a needy person who will respond to an empathetic, caring nurse.

INSTITUTIONAL ABUSE

Institutional abuse is abuse or neglect of a child who is permanently or temporarily under the care of some group other than his or her family. Such care settings include hospitals, schools, shelters, detention centers, camps, and communes. The following are examples of institutional abuse.

1. A 5-year-old boy in a group home for emotionally disturbed boys has his arm fractured by an attendant.
2. A 10-year-old girl taken to a shelter facility suffers a detached retina during a fight with another child.
3. A 7-year-old moderately retarded boy lies in a crib all day and night without stimulation and with minimal care.
4. A child in a religious commune is taken to a pit near a jungle and is threatened with fake snakes and told gruesome stories for being "bad."
5. A 9-year-old girl is belt-whipped in a public school for using foul language.
6. A child is placed in restraints to prevent night wandering in an institution for mentally retarded children.

Abuse and neglect should be reported to the supervisor. Suggestions of ways to improve care should be included in the written and oral reports and discussed in nursing clinical education classes. Reporting abuse creates a difficult situation for a nurse, since harassment and loss of a job may result. The American Nurses' Association can offer assistance to the nurse.

References

1. Thomas, J. N., C. M. Rogers, D. Lloyd, and R. Sihlangu, *Child Sexual Abuse: Implications for Public Health Practice,* U.S. Department of Health and Human Services, Division of Maternal and Child Health, Washington, D.C., July, 1985, p. 3.
2. Warner, Carmen, G., and G. Richard Braen, *Management of the Physically and Emotionally Abused,* Appleton Century Crofts, New York, 1982, pp. 3–311.
3. Burchell, S. C. (ed.), *Age of Progress,* Time-Life, New York, 1966, pp. 72–82.
4. *Encyclopedia Americana,* international ed., vol. 6, Americana Corporation, New York, 1964, pp. 461–464.
5. Hoekelman, Robert A., et al. (eds.), *Principles of Pediatrics: Health Care of the Young,* McGraw-Hill, New York, 1978, p. 356.
6. O'Doherty, Neil, *The Battered Child,* Saunders, Philadelphia, 1982, pp. 1–52.
7. Helberg, June L., "Documentation in Child Abuse," *American Journal of Nursing* **83**(11):236–239 (November 1983).
8. Starr, Raymone H. (ed.), *Child Abuse Prediction,* Ballinger, Cambridge, Mass., 1982, pp. 1–217.
9. Polansky, C., C. Hally, and N. F. Polansky, *Profile of Neglect: A Survey of the State of Knowledge of Child Neglect,* U.S. Department of Health, Education, and Welfare, Community Services Administration, Washington, D.C., 1975, p. 5.
10. Yoos, Lorrie, "Taking Another Look at Failure to Thrive," *The American Journal of Maternal-Child Nursing* **9**(1):32–36 (January–February 1984).
11. Ibid., p. 32.
12. Ibid.
13. Ibid., pp. 32–33.
14. Ibid., p. 34.
15. Ibid.
16. Finnila, Mona C., Robert Jacobs, and William Bucher, "Failure to Thrive Protocol," unpublished paper, Children's Hospital, Department of Psychiatry, Los Angeles, 1974, p. 3.
17. American Humane Society, Children's Division, statistics gathered by National Study of Official Child Abuse and Neglect Reporting, in Marjorie T. Ryan, "Identifying the Sexually Abused Child," *Pediatric Nursing* **10**:419–433 (November–December 1984).
18. Waechter, Eugenia H., et al., "Child Abuse," in *Nursing Care of Children,* Lippincott, Philadelphia, 1985, p. 633.
19. Ryan, op. cit., p. 420.
20. Ibid., p. 421.
21. Miller, Elissa L., "Interviewing the Sexually Abused Child," *The American Journal of Maternal-Child Nursing* **10**(2):103–105 (March–April 1985).
22. Robertson, Katherine C., and Jean A. Wilson-Walker, "A Program for Preventing Sexual Abuse of Children," *The American Journal of Maternal-Child Nursing* **10**(2): 100–102 (March–April 1985).
23. Barnett, Henry L., and Arnold H. Einhorn, *Pediatrics,* 15th ed., Appleton Century Crofts, New York, 1972, pp. 575–577.

39

Connie L. Tooley

Substance abuse

Upon completion of this chapter, the student will be able to:

1. Identify four responsibilities of a health care professional in the prevention of substance abuse.
2. List four patterns of drug use and give an example of each.
3. Name three categories of drugs that are commonly abused and give one health implication of each.
4. List four factors which contribute to substance use by adolescents.
5. Identify three factors which affect the blood alcohol level.
6. Define and give an example of primary, secondary, and tertiary prevention of substance abuse.

Watching television for even a short time gives one a view of the drug-oriented society in which American children are being raised. "Extra strength," "long-acting," "faster-acting," "no unpleasant taste," and "doctor-recommended," for example, are used to describe an unprecedented number of substances that are designed to keep people from hurting, feeling upset, not sleeping, or not breathing freely. In addition, concerned parents give their children orange-flavored aspirin, cherry-flavored cough syrup, and vitamins in a vast array of shapes, colors, and flavors. With the message, "This will make you feel better," or "This is good for you," parents give their children their earliest education in drug use. This, combined with the parents' substance use, from aspirin to alcohol, initiates the child into a culture that accepts and encourages mood altering by "taking something." It is predictable that some young people will experience problems with substance use. Nurses have a responsibility to (1) understand the potential for abuse of chemical substances, (2) provide responsible role modeling in the use and dispensation of such substances, (3) recognize potential and developing substance abuse problems in children in all age groups, and (4) provide intervention for problems that have developed. Nurses also need to work with other professionals to address this major health problem.

DEFINITIONS

Substance abuse is defined as a pattern of use of psychoactive (mood-altering) substances that involves hazards to health.[1] As defined in Chap. 1, health includes physical, emotional, and psychological well-being. The term *substance abuse* is used here to refer to both alcohol abuse and the abuse of other drugs. Alcohol is frequently not thought of as a drug, and yet it is the most widely used mood-altering substance in American society and is consumed by both adults and adolescents (see Fig. 39-1).

In regard to involvement with substances, it is useful to categorize people as (1) abstainers, (2) experimental and occasional users, (3) social or recreational users, (4) abusers, or (5) substance-dependent users.

Abstainers

Abstainers are those who avoid the use of mood-altering substances. Some may consume caffeine-containing beverages and may perhaps use tobacco products. They may take mood-altering drugs that are prescribed for a specific illness or problem. Any substance use problem would probably be the result of an untoward reaction to a drug.

Experimenters and occasional users

The infrequent use of alcohol or other drugs, usually in a social or recreational setting, characterizes *experimenters* and *occasional users*. *Experimentation*, or the first use of a particular

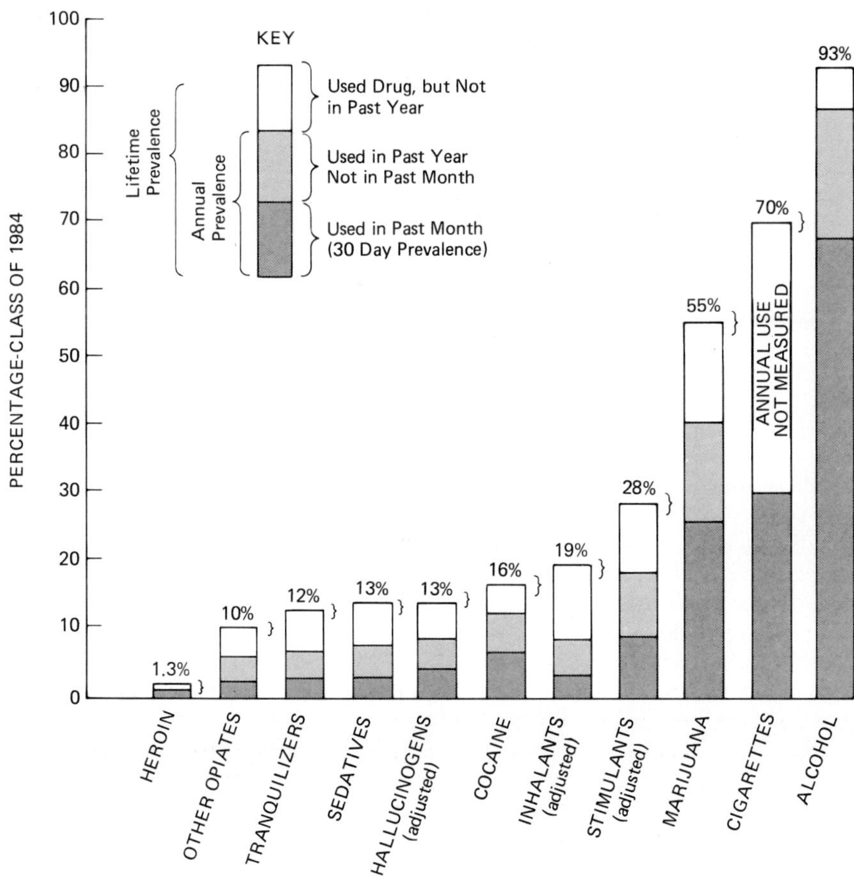

Figure 39-1 The prevalence and recency of use of 11 types of drugs among high school seniors in 1984. The bracket near the top of a bar indicates the lower and upper limits of the 95 percent confidence level.

substance, often occurs by the sixth or seventh grade. In a 1983 study, 56 percent of eighth graders reported using alcohol in the sixth and seventh grades. This was an earlier age at initial use than was reported by tenth and twelfth graders.[2] A downward trend in the age at first marijuana use appears to be holding now at the sixth-grade level.[3]

The range of experimentation that nurses have encountered includes third graders who sniff felt-tip markers and deodorant spray; sixth graders who sell a mixture of flour and salt, claiming that it is cocaine; children who bring alcoholic beverages from home to school, parties, or summer camp; children who sell prescription and over-the-counter medications that they find in the family medicine cabinet; and children who roll oregano in cigarette papers and sell it as "pot." Experimentation with drugs, which can lead to acute intoxication or a medical emergency, appears to be a norm. Almost 60 percent of adolescents experiment with an illicit drug before finishing high school.[4]

Social or recreational users

Social or *recreational users* have integrated regular drug use into their life-style. There is great variety in terms of the frequency of use and the quantity and kinds of substances used. The person has individual standards and appropriate control over usage that reflect the surrounding culture. The recreational user may experience an occasional problem requiring medical services. In 1982, 27 percent of young people between the ages of 12 and 17 used drugs or alcohol at least once a month.[5]

Abusers

Abusers allow the use of drugs to interfere with their health. The American Psychiatric Association identifies substance use disorders as substance abuse and substance dependence.[6] Three criteria must be met in order for the diagnosis of substance abuse to be made: (1) the pattern of use must be pathological—the person is unable to cut down or reduce use and has made repeated efforts to control or reduce use; (2) there is impairment of social or occupational functioning as a result of use; and (3) disturbances occur that last for at least a month. Abusers are sometimes referred to as *problem users* because their substance use causes problems with their health, their family life, their interpersonal relationships, school, work, the law, or their finances. A *polydrug abuser* uses more than one psychoactive substance.

Substance abuse has been identified as a major contributor to the increased death rate among those aged 15 to 24.[7]

> With increasing frequency, intoxicated youths are being diverted from the juvenile justice system to health care facilities. This is consistent with the decriminalization of public drunkenness and the general "medicalization" of alcohol problems. On the other hand, because adolescent abusers of alcohol and other drugs rarely evidence the physiological effects of long-term abuse, they are frequently not recognized unless they are seriously intoxicated or exhibit gross antisocial behavior.[8]

Observing patterns of behavior, such as those listed in Table 39-1, helps the nurse who works with the family and the school to identify those young people who are progressing in their substance use to abusive levels.[9]

Chemical dependence

In the past, *chemical dependence* (or *substance dependence*) referred to *addictive* or *compulsive* use of drugs. The World Health Organization's definition of addiction is:

> . . . a state of periodic or chronic intoxication produced by the repeated consumption of a drug (natural or synthetic), which produces the following characteristics: (1) an over-powering desire or compulsion to continue taking the drug and to obtain it by any means; (2) a tendency to increase the dosage, showing body tolerance; (3) a psychic and, generally, a physical dependence on the effects of the drug; and (4) the creation of an individual and social problem.

Psychological dependence is defined as "a strong tendency to continue the use of a drug because of the pleasure it provides and/or the feeling that the drug is needed to alleviate discomfort."[10]

Physical dependence exists when stopping or reducing drug use results in acute withdrawal symptoms and the "user exhibits an overwhelming desire to use the drug again as the maintenance of normal body function requires its use."[11] The American Psychiatric Association's criteria for substance dependence include the three cri-

Table 39-1 Indications of a Potential Substance Abuse Problem

Physical Indications

Change in physical hygiene Becomes more sloppy, wears same clothes frequently.

Weight change Has drastic weight loss or gain.

Coming home drunk or high Smells of marijuana or alcohol, seems unusually giddy, has slurred speech.

Loss of initiative Has decreased energy, sleeps more than usual.

Emotional and Behavioral Indications

Emotional highs and lows Is easily upset, emotional state changes rapidly, seems less happy than usual.

Becoming more secretive Does not share any personal problems or only a few.

Isolation Spends a lot of time in his or her room.

Short-temperedness Becomes angry often, has "short fuse"

Defensiveness Is defensive when confronted about behavior or other concerns.

Abusive behavior Is verbally or physically abusive to another family member.

Social and Family Indications

Switching friends Has a different set of friends, has more friends that the parents object to, does not make any new friends.

Defiance of rules and regulations Pushes limits at home, does not do chores around the house.

Withdrawing from family functions Is not interested in camping, trips, church, or meals.

Many excuses for staying out late Does not come home on time, does not come home at all, makes constant excuses.

Money or alcohol missing Takes money or alcohol belonging to parents or siblings.

Selling possessions Sells clothing, records, or gifts; seems to have money but no job.

Manipulative and bargaining behavior Plays parents against each other.

Owning drug paraphernalia Has papers, pipes, clips, drugs, bottles.

Academic and Legal Indications

Drop in grades A *slow* decrease in grades over a period of 6 months to 1 year or a *sudden* decrease.

Not informing parents of school activities Fails to tell parents about open houses, times to meet teachers, suspensions, warnings.

Calls from school Reports of skipping classes, sleeping in class, poor work performance, not doing homework.

Legal problems Driving while intoxicated, curfew violations, being at parties that are broken up by the police.

Source: Minnesota School District 281 Chemical Awareness Advisory Committee, "Never Too Early Never Too Late," Hazelden, Center City, Minn., 1983. Used with permission.

teria for abuse as well as the presence of (1) *tolerance*, which is a markedly diminished effect with regular use of the same amount, or (2) *withdrawal*, which is the development of physiological responses to the cessation of, or a reduction in, use.[12] Substance dependence is categorized by the substance used, e.g., alcohol dependence and barbiturate dependence. Difficulty in defining substance dependence among adolescents has created concern about overreporting and overidentification or underidentification of young people whose use is becoming progressively harmful. Care must be taken to differentiate dependent adolescents from adolescents who are experiencing primary emotional or psychological problems.

PREVALENCE AND PATTERNS OF USE

Nationwide surveys of drug use by high school seniors have been conducted since the mid-1970s by the Institute for Social Research at the University of Michigan. These studies clearly show trends and current use patterns. They are useful in formulating social policies and plans for prevention. Findings from a 1984 nationwide survey of high school seniors are presented in Table 39-2.

In the *1984 National Strategy for Prevention of Drug Abuse and Drug Trafficking*, the following was reported:[13]

1. In 1982, 27 percent of young people between the ages of 12 and 17 used drugs or alcohol at least once a month.
2. Sixty percent of young Americans try an illicit drug before they finish high school.
3. By 1982, the use of cocaine by young people under the age of 18 had leveled off, after

Table 39-2 Findings from a 1984 Nationwide Survey of High School Seniors

	Used Once or More in Lifetime	Used in Past Month
Alcohol	92.6%	67.2%
Marijuana and hashish	54.9%	25.2%
Cocaine	16.1%	5.8%
Tranquilizers	12.4%	2.1%
Stimulants	27.9%	8.3%
Cigarettes	69.7%	29.3%

Source: The Monitoring the Future Study, Institute for Social Research, University of Michigan, Ann Arbor.

showing sharp increases between 1976 and 1979. Approximately 2 million cocaine users are between the ages of 18 and 25.
4. Alcohol-related accidents are the leading cause of death among 16- to 24-year-olds.

Factors contributing to substance use

Adolescents use mood-altering substances for many of the same reasons that adults do. They use alcohol and other drugs to enhance their enjoyment at social gatherings, to help them relax, to alleviate anxiety, and to produce pleasurable states of euphoria. Mood-altering substances have been and are being used in almost all cultures, past and present. Some factors that contribute to the use of drugs by children and adolescents are:

1. *Curiosity* The illegal and forbidden nature of drugs heightens curiosity and attracts the novice user. Curiosity is a leading factor in experimentation.
2. *Peer group influence* Peer group influence is an important factor in drug use among adolescents. Areas in which adolescents' choices are influenced by peers are (in order of importance) clothing and appearance; use of leisure time; personal style, language, and "presentation of self"; and use of alcohol and drugs. According to Hedin, "The best single predictor of an adolescent's use of alcohol and drugs is to look at the use pattern of his/her best friend."[14] The peer group approves, protects, reinforces, and sometimes even defines the members' drug-seeking and drug-using behavior. Substance use may admit a teenager to, and establish the teenager within, a peer group.
3. *Developmental limitations of adolescence* Adolescents generally lack the maturity necessary to use alcohol and other drugs successfully and appropriately. The adolescent's egocentricity compounds the possible problems. The capacity to form mature judgments is not fully developed, nor are values and goals clearly formulated. In addition, risk-taking behavior is expected and reinforced. Adolescents also need immediate gratification. They may also believe that they are immune from any negative effects.
4. *Escape* Many adolescents use mood-altering substances to escape boredom and psychological or physical pain resulting from family, school, or socioeconomic problems. Children from families with a history of alcoholism, incest, physical abuse, or rigid, moralistic expectations are more likely to abuse alcohol or other drugs.
5. *Imitation of adult behavior* Adolescents copy parents' use of alcohol and drugs to cope with stress and problems. An adolescent child of an alcoholic parent has less opportunity to observe mature methods of coping with life's stresses.

Although the progression of substance use in adolescents is unclear, experts agree on several common elements:[15]

1. There are distinct stages of drug use, and the use of drugs at one stage increases the probability of use at a subsequent stage.
2. The more extensive the involvement with a drug at an earlier stage of development, the greater the likelihood of experimentation with drugs at the next stage or at subsequent stages of development.
3. Two factors that contribute to the progression through advancing stages of drug use are continuing association with friends and acquaintances who are drug users and involvement in selling and distributing drugs.

THE ACTION OF DRUGS

Psychopharmacology deals with the effects of psychoactive (mood-altering) drugs. These drugs are classified according to their specific pharmacological properties and according to society's attitude toward them.[16] Four basic facts are true of all drugs:

1. *No drug is all good or all bad* Tranquilizers, narcotics, barbiturates, and amphetamines are beneficial when used under medical supervision but can be very dangerous when self-administered for nonmedicinal purposes. Volatile substances, such as aerosol deodorants and hair sprays, and solvents, such as glue and gasoline, while useful products, are potentially harmful when inhaled.
2. *Every drug has multiple effects* All drugs act on different parts of the central nervous system to produce a wide range of effects. Depressants produce some excitatory effects, and stimulants ultimately produce depression.

Hallucinogens cause complex emotional responses in addition to perceptual alterations.

3. *The effects of a drug depend on the dose* Varying the dose changes both the magnitude and the character of its effects. The potential for abuse of a drug increases in proportion to the dose. Certain dose levels constitute abuse, while others do not.
4. *The effects of a drug depend on the individual user and the circumstances under which it is taken* The effects of any psychoactive drug are influenced by the user's environment, history, and physical makeup. Body size, time of administration, psychological state, physiological state,and rate of absorption all affect a drug's action.

Table 39-3 Guide for Estimating How Much Alcohol Must Be Consumed in Order to Reach a Level of Impairment or Intoxication According to Body Weight*

	Body Weight							
Drinks	100	125	150	175	200	225	250	
1	0.03	0.03	0.02	0.02	0.01	0.01	0.01	
2	0.06	0.05	0.04	0.04	0.03	0.03	0.03	Sober
3	0.10	0.08	0.06	0.06	0.05	0.04	0.04	
4	0.13	0.10	0.09	0.07	0.06	0.06	0.05	
5	0.16	0.13	0.11	0.09	0.08	0.07	0.06	
6	0.19	0.16	0.13	0.11	0.10	0.09	0.08	Impaired
7	0.22	0.18	0.15	0.13	0.11	0.10	0.09	
8	0.26	0.21	0.17	0.15	0.13	0.11	0.10	
9	0.29	0.24	0.19	0.17	0.14	0.13	0.12	
10	0.33	0.26	0.22	0.18	0.16	0.14	0.13	Illegal
11	0.36	0.29	0.24	0.20	0.18	0.16	0.14	
12	0.39	0.31	0.26	0.22	0.19	0.17	0.16	

*To estimate your blood alcohol concentration, match the number of drinks consumed to your body weight. Subtract 0.015 for each hour since drinking began. One drink equals 1 oz of 86-proof liquor, a 12-oz beer, or a glass of wine. Check your weight and find the number of drinks it takes you to become impaired or intoxicated. Fill in the spaces below so that you will be reminded to quit while you are still ahead.

I weigh ______ lb.

I can drink ___ 12-oz beers **or** ___ oz of 86-proof liquor **or** ___ glasses of wine before I become impaired.

I can drink ___ 12-oz beers **or** ___ oz of 86-proof liquor **or** ___ glasses of wine before I go over 0.10 blood alcohol concentration.

Remember that black coffee or fresh air will not sober you up; only time does that.

Note: This is only a guide and is not accurate enough to be legal evidence. Individuals vary in their personal alcohol tolerance. The figures are averages.

Source: Minnesota Department of Public Safety, St. Paul.

CLASSIFICATION OF PSYCHOACTIVE DRUGS

The many varieties of psychoactive drugs can be classified according to their method of procurement or availability and according to their pharmacological properties.

Procurement classification

1. *Social drugs* These drugs are readily available in homes and social settings, e.g., nicotine, alcohol, and caffeine.
2. *Illegal drugs* These substances are restricted by legislation (controlled substances) or other legal constraints on the basis of the potential for abuse. Street drugs usually belong to this category. Uncertainty about the actual content of these drugs is a cause of concern and makes treatment of an overdose or adverse reactions more difficult. Alcohol is both a legal and an illegal drug, depending on the age of the consumer and the blood alcohol level, or concentration. Table 39-3 presents a method for estimating the amount of alcohol that must be consumed before the blood alcohol level exceeds 0.1 percent.
3. *Over-the-counter drugs* These substances are readily available for self-medication of minor illnesses. They include analgesics, appetite control products, cold products, sleep-inducing preparations, and sedatives. Misuse and abuse of these drugs, often consisting of overuse or use in combination with alcohol and other drugs, as well as adverse effects of the drugs are common.
4. *Natural drugs* These are substances that occur in nature and have psychoactive properties. They include certain mushrooms, seeds such as those of morning-glory plants, and spices such as nutmeg.

Pharmacological classification

Drugs can also be classified according to their pharmacological properties. Table 39-4 summarizes the properties and actions of commonly abused drugs.

Cannabis Marijuana ("grass," "pot," or "weed") is the common name for the hemp plant, *Cannabis sativa*. The main mind-altering ingredient in marijuana, THC, comes from the flowering

Table 39-4 Commonly Abused Drugs

Category	Drugs	Sample, Trade, or Other Names	Medical Uses	Dependence: Physical	Dependence: Psychological	Effects in Hours	Possible Effects	Effects of Overdose	Withdrawal Symptoms
Cannabis	Marijuana	Pot, grass, reefer, sinsemilla	Under investigation				Euphoria, relaxed inhibitions, increase in heart and pulse rate, reddening of the eyes, increased appetite, disoriented behavior	Anxiety, paranoia, loss of concentration, slower movements, time distortion	Insomnia, hyperactivity, decreased appetite occasionally reported
	Tetrahydrocannabinol	THC							
	Hashish	Hash	None						
	Hash oil	Hash oil		Unknown	Moderate	2 to 4			
Depressants	Alcohol	Liquor, beer, wine	None	High	High	1 to 12	Slurred speech, disorientation, drunken behavior	Shallow respiration, cold and clammy skin, dilated pupils, weak and rapid pulse, coma, possible death	Anxiety, insomnia, tremors, delirium, convulsions, possible death
	Barbiturates	Secobarbital, Amobarbital, Butisol, Tuinal	Anesthetic, anticonvulsant, sedative, hypnotic	High to moderate	High to moderate	1 to 16			
	Methaqualone	Quaalude, Sopor, Parest	Sedative, hypnotic	High	High	4 to 8			
	Tranquilizers	Valium, Librium, Equanil, Miltown	Anti-anxiety, anti-convulsant, sedative	Moderate to low	Moderate				
Stimulants	Cocaine	Coke, flake, snow	Local anesthetic				Increased alertness, excitation, euphoria, increase in pulse rate and blood pressure, insomnia, loss of appetite	Agitation, increase in body temperature, hallucinations, convulsions, possible death, tremors	Apathy, long periods of sleep, irritability, depression
	Amphetamines	Biphetamine, Dexedrine	Hyperactivity, narcolepsy	Possible	High	$\frac{1}{2}$ to 2			
	Nicotine	Tobacco, cigars, cigarettes	None	High	High	2 to 4			
	Caffeine	Coffee, tea, cola drinks, No-Doz	None	Low	Low			Agitation, increase in pulse rate and blood pressure, loss of appetite, insomnia	

Hallucinogens	LSD	Acid	None	None	Degree unknown	8 to 12	Illusions and hallucinations, poor perception of time and distance	Drug effects becoming longer and more intense, psychosis	None
	Mescaline and peyote	Button, Cactus							
	Phencyclidine	PCP, angel dust	Veterinary anesthetic	Unknown	High	Variable			
	Psilocybin, psilocin	Mushrooms	None	None	Degree unknown	6			
Inhalants	Nitrous oxide	Whippets, laughing gas	Anesthetic				Excitement, euphoria, giddiness, loss of inhibitions, aggressiveness, delusions, depression, drowsiness, headache, nausea	Loss of memory, confusion, unsteady gait, erratic heartbeat and pulse, possible death	Insomnia, decreased appetite, depression, irritability, headache
	Butyl nitrite	Locker room, rush	None						
	Amyl nitrite	Poppers, snappers	Heart stimulant						
	Chlorohydrocarbons	Aerosol paint, cleaning fluid	None	Possible	Moderate	Up to ½ hr			
	Hydrocarbons	Aerosol propellants, gasoline, glue, paint thinner	None						
Narcotics	Opium	Paregoric	Antidiarrheal, pain relief	High	High		Euphoria, drowsiness, respiratory depression, constricted pupils, nausea	Slow and shallow breathing, clammy skin, convulsions, coma, possible death	Watery eyes, runny nose, yawning, loss of appetite, irritability, tremors, panic, chills and sweating, cramps, nausea
	Morphine	Morphine, Pectoral Syrup							
	Codeine	Codeine, Empirin Compound with codeine, Robitussin A-C	Pain relief, cough medicine	Moderate	Moderate	3 to 6			
	Heroin	Horse, smack	Under investigation						
	Methadone	Dolophine, Methadose	Heroin substitute, pain relief	High	High	12 to 24			

Source: For Parents Only: What You Need to Know about Marijuana, U.S. Department of Health and Human Services, National Institute of Drug Abuse, Publication No. ADM 80-909, Washington, D.C., 1980.

tops of the plant. A marijuana cigarette (joint) is made from the dried particles of the whole plant, except for the main stem and the roots. The user is affected by the amount of THC in the cigarette.

Hashish, or "hash," is made by extracting the resin from the leaves and flowers and pressing it into cakes or slabs. Hash may contain 5 to 10 times as much THC as marijuana. "Hash oil" may contain up to 50 percent THC. Pure THC is unavailable, and substances sold as THC often are found to be something else. The marijuana available today is as much as 10 times as potent as the marijuana used in the early 1970s.

Many professionals are concerned that marijuana alters a person's motivation. Teachers feel that adolescents who use it regularly exhibit loss of motivation and difficulty coping with school responsibilities.

A review of the research reveals the following health concerns related to marijuana use:

1. Researchers believe that regular marijuana use may interfere with the normal process of growing up. Adolescents stay at the developmental level that they were at when heavy use began.
2. Marijuana can be particularly harmful to the lungs because users typically inhale the unfiltered smoke deeply and hold it in their lungs as long as possible.
3. Marijuana use can increase the heart rate as much as 50 percent, depending on the amount of THC in the cigarette. Marijuana use is particularly dangerous for people with high blood pressure or heart problems.
4. Presently, there is no substantial evidence to suggest that marijuana causes damage to an unborn baby or to the genes provided by the parent. However, marijuana does pass through the placenta and may cause prematurity and low birth weight.
5. Studies of users have shown that marijuana alters hormonal levels, causing irregular menstrual cycles as well as temporary loss of fertility in both men and women.
6. To date, there is no evidence to show that marijuana is related to permanent brain damage.
7. Marijuana smoke has been found to contain cancer-causing agents. One report strongly suggests that tobacco and marijuana smoke together are more carcinogenic than the smoke of either drug alone.
8. Marijuana use can impair driving ability by affecting judgment, caution, concentration, and perception.
9. Regular marijuana users are more likely to experiment with other drugs, such as amphetamines.

Depressants These drugs depress the central nervous system by inhibiting the sending and receiving of messages by the nerve cells. Alcohol, tranquilizers, barbiturates, and sedative-hypnotics are depressants. They are prescribed for relief of acute anxiety, irritability, tension, and insomnia.

Alcohol Alcohol is the major social lubricant of our culture. The use of beer, wine, or liquor to enhance social occasions has been accepted and promoted for thousands of years. Alcohol is the only drug sanctioned by our society for social use. Its use varies widely from appropriate moderate usage to addiction, or *alcoholism*.

Alcohol is absorbed through the stomach and small intestine and then travels throughout the body. The rate of absorption is influenced by the amount of alcohol ingested, the speed of ingestion, the presence or absence of food in the stomach, and body weight. The effect of alcohol on the body is determined primarily by its concentration in the blood, not just by the amount ingested. The blood alcohol level, or BAL, is the number of grams of alcohol in each 100 ml of blood and is expressed as a percentage: 100 mg of alcohol in 100 ml of blood is reported as 0.1 percent and is the legal level of intoxication in most states. Behavioral impairment is noted when the BAL is 0.05 percent. A BAL of 0.2 to 0.25 percent results in extreme intoxication, and a BAL of 0.3 percent and over produces stupor or coma and, potentially, death (see Table 39-5).

Other depressants Sedative-hypnotics are drugs that depress the body's functions. They include drugs that "calm the nerves" and produce sleep, such as barbiturates, benzodiazepines, and the major tranquilizers.

Barbiturates, commonly referred to as "barbs" and "downers," are used in the treatment of anxiety, tension, sleeplessness, and illnesses in which seizures and convulsions occur. These drugs are sold in the form of white powder contained in capsules and tablets, in liquid form that is injected or swallowed, and in the form of suppositories.

Table 39-5 Blood Alcohol Levels Correlated with Behavioral Changes

Blood Alcohol Level	Drinks Consumed	Behavioral Effects
0.04%	1 to 2	Lowered alertness, release of inhibitions, relaxation, increased heart rate
0.06%	3 to 4	Impaired judgment, loss of coordination, apathy
0.10%	5 to 6	Impaired motor function, exaggerated emotions, clumsiness, impaired vision, impaired ability to drive a car
0.16%	6 to 8	Staggering, slurred speech, blurred vision, serious loss of judgment, and coordination
0.20%	8 to 10	Sensory depression, mood swings, difficulty maintaining balance, double vision
0.30%	10 to 15	Uninhibited behavior; stupor and confusion; rowdy, unrestrained, or combative behavior; reality disorientation
0.40 to 0.50%	15 to 25	Loss of feeling, unconsciousness, shock
Above 0.50%	More than 25	Coma, death

Source: Adapted from Brent Q. Hafen, *Alcoholism: The Crutch That Cripples*, West, St. Paul, Minn., 1977. p. 41.

Benzodiazepines, which are minor tranquilizers, include Valium, Librium, and Miltown. They are manufactured as capsules and tablets in various sizes, shapes, and colors.

Of these drugs, the barbiturates have the highest rate of abuse and misuse. They are the most dangerous drugs and are a major factor in suicides, suicide attempts, and accidental drug poisonings. Suddenly discontinuing their use may lead to restlessness, anxiety, and possibly death. Withdrawal is usually accomplished by gradually decreasing the dosage levels, under a doctor's supervision. One of the most commonly abused nonbarbiturate drugs is methaqualone, or Quaalude. It was originally marketed as an alternative to barbiturates because it seemed to have fewer harmful side effects and less potential for abuse than barbiturates. Benzodiazepines, especially Valium, are commonly abused; the rate of abuse and misuse is increasing.

Stimulants Stimulants are drugs that affect the central nervous system by increasing alertness and activity. Caffeine, cocaine, and amphetamines are examples. Stimulants are used to treat only a few medical conditions: chronic sleepiness, childhood hyperactivity, and obesity. Cocaine is sometimes used as a local anesthetic.

Amphetamines On the street, amphetamines are called "speed," "white crosses," "uppers," "dexies," "bennies," and "crystal." In their pure form, amphetamines consist of yellowish crystals which can be swallowed in the form of tablets or capsules, sniffed, or injected.

When amphetamines are injected, a "rush" is immediately felt throughout the body. This sensation can lead a person to take the drug repeatedly. However, self-prepared solutions can become contaminated, and injecting them may lead to potentially fatal disease.

"Look-alike" stimulants are manufactured as capsules or pills and are made to closely resemble prescription amphetamines. Look-alikes are sold on the street as "speed" and "uppers" and cost more than one would pay for the same thing in a drugstore.

Cocaine Cocaine, a drug extracted from the leaves of the coca plant, is available in the form of a fine, white, crystal-like powder or sometimes as chunks of white material, called "rocks" or "crack." In most cases, cocaine is inhaled, although some users inject or smoke it. Physiologically cocaine increases adrenalin, heart rate, and blood pressure. Cocaine intoxication can also cause sudden death.

"Freebase" is a form of cocaine which enables the drug to be smoked; this is the fastest way to get cocaine to the brain. Freebasing increases the risk that the user will become fearful or anxious or will develop serious psychological symptoms. When smoked, cocaine produces an immediate "rush," or sense of well-being and confidence. Higher doses may produce confusion, slurred speech, and anxiety. Freebase smokers appear to be less able or willing than other cocaine users to control their use, which suggests that smoking cocaine can produce a strong form of psychological dependency.

Cocaine is *highly addictive psychologically*. People use the drug repeatedly because of the euphoria it produces and because of its short action and the lack of a subsequent depression. Mild withdrawal symptoms may still be experienced.

With frequent cocaine use, the feelings of euphoria and well-being are gradually replaced by feelings of restlessness, irritability, sleeplessness, and sometimes paranoia. Some regular users experience hallucinations of touch, sight, taste, or smell. A mental condition called *cocaine psychosis* may result, but it is reversible if cocaine use is discontinued. The physical effects of both short-term and heavy cocaine use include a chronic stuffy and runny nose and nostril and nasal membrane irritation. Injecting cocaine with nonsterile equipment can cause hepatitis, AIDS, or other infections.

Caffeine Caffeine may be the world's most popular drug. It is a white, bitter, crystal-like substance and is found in coffee, tea, cocoa, and cola drinks as well as in aspirin, nonprescription cough and cold remedies, soft drinks, diet pills, and some street drugs.

Hallucinogens Hallucinogens, or psychedelics, are drugs which affect a person's perceptions, feelings, thinking, self-awareness, and emotions. They include such drugs as LSD, mescaline, psilocybin, and MDA. LSD is the most popular and the best studied of the psychedelics.

LSD LSD is a partly synthetic drug made from lysergic acid. It is odorless, colorless, and tasteless. LSD is sold on the street in tablet, capsule, and occasionally liquid form. Often it is added to gelatin sheets or blotting paper. It is usually taken orally but can be sniffed or injected.

Mescaline Mescaline comes from the peyote cactus, and although it is not as strong as LSD, its effects are similar. Most of what is sold on the street as mescaline is really LSD or PCP (phencyclidine). Rarely injected, mescaline can be smoked or swallowed in the form of capsules or tablets.

Psilocybin Psilocybin is a white, crystal-like material derived from certain mushrooms. It is distributed in tablet or capsule form and is taken orally or by injection. The mushrooms, fresh or dried, may be eaten. Like mescaline, psilocybin is often misrepresented on the street and may actually be LSD or PCP.

DMT DMT is another psychedelic drug that acts like LSD. Its effects begin almost immediately and last for 30 to 60 min. Because its effect is of short duration, DMT has acquired the nickname "businessman's trip."

Researchers do not yet know whether the use of psychedelics, particularly LSD, causes damage to chromosomes, birth defects, or long-lasting changes in personality, beliefs, or values. Some users who experience abnormal thought processes and disorganized personalities have a history of mental or emotional problems.

Inhalants Inhalants are a diverse group of breathable chemicals. They include solvents, aerosols, some anesthetics, and other chemicals. Solvents include plastic cement, model airplane glue, nail polish remover, lighter fluid, and gasoline. Cookware-coating agents, deodorants, hair sprays, insecticides, medications, and paints sold in aerosol form are inhalants.

Inhalants are depressants and produce effects similar to those of alcohol. Inhaled vapors from solvents and aerosols rapidly enter the bloodstream from the lungs and then go to the brain and liver. The initial excitement and euphoria, or "high," tends to be short-lived (from a few minutes to several hours) and mild. Deep breathing of these vapors or continuous use over a short period of time can cause loss of touch with the surroundings, loss of self-control, unconsciousness, seizures, and slow or delayed reflexes. Other effects include nosebleeds, bloodshot eyes, unpleasant breath, and sores in the nose and mouth.

Inhaling a spray can either interfere directly with breathing or produce an irregular heartbeat leading to heart failure and death. The risk of death increases when users sniff concentrated spray fumes from a paper bag. Most deaths have been connected with the propellant gases used in aerosol sprays.

Narcotics The term *narcotic* refers to opium and opium derivatives or synthetic substitutes used to relieve pain and induce sleep. Opium is available in the form of dark-brown chunks or powder that is smoked or eaten. Heroin is a powder that can be dissolved in water and injected. Most street preparations of heroin are diluted, or "cut," with other substances such as sugar or quinine. Other opiates come in a variety of forms.

The physical dangers depend on the specific drug used, its source, and the way it is used. Most physical dangers are caused by overuse of the drug, the use of unsterile needles, contamination of the drug itself, or use of the drug in combination with other substances. Over a period of time, users of opium and opium derivatives may develop an infection of the heart lining and valves, skin abscesses, and congested lungs. Infections from unsterile solutions, syringes, and needles cause illnesses such as liver disease, tetanus, AIDS, and serum hepatitis.

The use of barbiturates in combination with other depressant drugs, such as alcohol, multiplies their effects and greatly increases the risk of respiratory depression and death. The use of barbiturates and alcohol together, either deliberately or accidentally, is the most common cause of overdose that results in death.

ETIOLOGY AND INCIDENCE OF CHEMICAL DEPENDENCE

Chemical dependence is a primary, progressive, chronic, and ultimately fatal disease process.[17] The theories of causation of chemical dependence are divergent. Research continues, but it is clear that no one cause is known at this time. Psychological theories centered on tension reduction, reinforcement, transactional factors, and personality characteristics have been studied. Sociocultural investigations have explored cultural groups and subgroups; sex roles; societal practices, including advertising; alienation from society; and society's attitude toward use of chemicals. Biological factors researched include body function and genetic factors. Identification of a morphine-like substance in the brain of some alcoholics has encouraged the search for a biochemical cause of alcoholism.

Studies of families have provided strong evidence that there is a genetic factor in alcoholism. These findings may permit the identification of "prealcoholics," who can be monitored as the disease process develops.[18] Psychological and social factors also contribute to the development of the disease.

An estimated 10 million adults and 3 million adolescents between the ages of 14 and 17 years are problem drinkers.[19] In the general population, it is estimated that 3 to 5 percent of males and 0.1 to 1.0 percent of females are alcoholics during the course of their lifetime. The rate of alcoholism among relatives of alcoholics is as much as 6 times higher than that among people in the general population. The male relatives of alcoholics are most prone to developing a dependence on alcohol. The rate of dependence among the siblings of alcoholics is also higher than the rate among people in the general population.[20]

ASSESSMENT AND MANAGEMENT OF SUBSTANCE ABUSE

The assessment process

The use and abuse of psychoactive substances by adolescents need to be of concern to all nurses. In the emergency room, nurses see trauma, overdose, inappropriate or withdrawn behavior, and potentially life-threatening situations related to substance abuse. Nurses in pediatric, medical, and surgical units see adolescents with a substance use problem who were originally admitted for medical or surgical treatment. In public health departments, school systems, mental health centers, and industrial environments, nurses see adolescents and their families who are struggling with issues related to adolescent substance use.

In each nursing area, the assessment process provides a method for evaluating the needs of the adolescent and his or her family. Figure 39-2 provides a framework for determining the extent of use, abuse, or possible dependence on drugs.

Assessment tools A survey of facilities in which adolescents are treated for alcohol and other drug problems identified a variety of assessment tools. Most have been adapted from those used for adults or were developed in-house to meet specific needs. Findings of the survey led to the development of the Chemical Dependency Adolescent Assessment Project, which was begun in 1982 to develop standardized instruments for use with adolescents.* The assessment package includes a separate screening tool.[21]

Two screening tools specifically developed for adolescents and used over a period of time are the Adolescent Alcohol Involvement Scale (AAIS), published in 1979, and the Youth Diagnostic Screening Test (YDST), published in 1978. The AAIS, which is a 14-item paper-and-pencil test, has been widely used to gather information about

*Additional information can be obtained from Chemical Dependency Adolescent Assessment Project, 919 Lafond Ave., St. Paul, Minn. 55104.

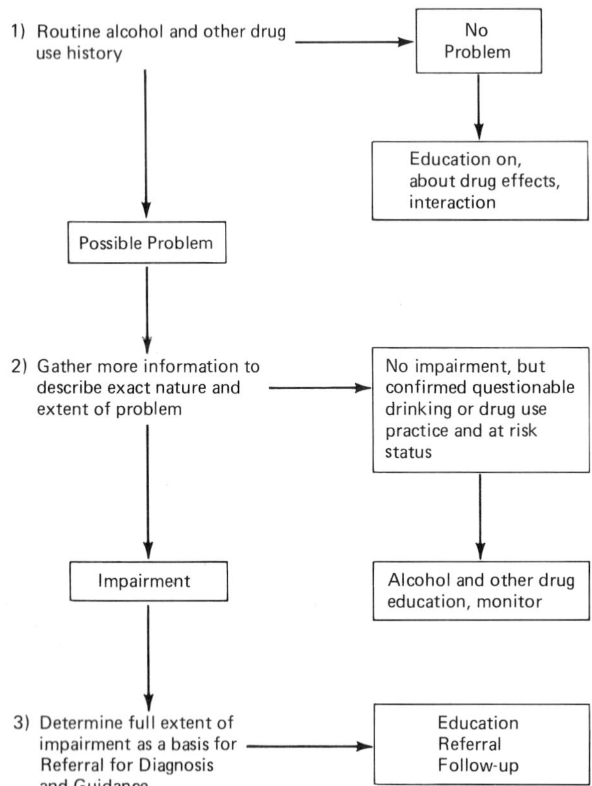

Figure 39-2 A framework for determining the extent of use, abuse, or possible dependence on drugs. (*Adapted from the Community Health Nurse and Alcohol Related Problems, The National Center for Alcohol Education, National Institute on Alcohol Abuse and Alcoholism, Rockville, Md., 1978.*)

quantity and frequency of alcohol use, the context in which use occurs, and the effects and consequences of use. Research has validated the accuracy of the AAIS, although concern has been expressed regarding the age norms used and its reliability with heavy users.[22,23]

The YDST is a 36-item paper-and-pencil test that uses information about pathological styles of drinking, problematic alcohol consumption, and consequences of consumption to identify problem drinkers. The score on this test indicating a diagnosis of alcoholism has not been empirically demonstrated as valid.

The nature of adolescents' use of chemicals continues to change. There are still unanswered questions regarding the similarities and differences between adults' and adolescents' chemical abuse and dependence. Nurses need to monitor research reports as more valid screening and diagnostic tools are developed.

Personal assessment Nurses must examine closely their own attitudes toward psychoactive substances, adolescents who use or abuse the substances, and substance dependence in order to provide care to adolescents effectively. Attitudes can be examined in terms of their cognitive, affective, and behavioral components. What nurses believe, feel, and do combine to influence their utilization of the assessment, planning, intervention, and evaluation process. The nurse's attitude is quickly perceived by adolescents, and if it is not open and nonjudgmental, it may inhibit the communication and relationship formation needed for therapeutic intervention.

Nurses must also examine their own substance use patterns. One often judges the deviance of another person's substance use by comparing it with one's own use. This can distort judgment by exaggerating or minimizing the nurse's perception of the adolescent's behavior. Only after accurately evaluating their own substance use and finding it nondestructive to themselves and others can nurses respond to adolescents' challenging statements in an objective, nondefensive, and constructive manner.

Self-exploration and change are often difficult. As nurses examine their own attitudes and chemical use patterns, they need to review their own experiences and relationships with substance use as children in a family, as adolescents in one or more peer groups, as adults with friends or a spouse, and as professional nurses. Unresolved issues need to be identified and addressed. Positive attitudes can be attained through education and discussion with other concerned and informed individuals.

The physical examination and interview*

A physical examination, laboratory tests, and an interview with the adolescent and his or her family provide information pertinent to identifying the drug and providing care to the substance-abusing or substance-dependent adolescent. The physical examination addresses the signs and symptoms of drug use, the level of intoxication, the potential for withdrawal, management of an overdose, and the complications or side effects of drug use. Table 39-6 lists the aspects of the general physical examination that are relevant to young people who use drugs.

Frequently, the observed physical or behavioral symptoms of drug use are not specific enough to identify the drug or drugs being taken. Laboratory testing of serum, urine, or gastric contents helps identify the drugs that are present in the body. Unlike conventional blood counts and urinalyses, which do not detect or identify drugs, drug screenings and drug surveys can identify substances and provide data about the type of drug and the amount present. The presence of some drugs can be detected by laboratory tests long after the adolescent's behavior and mental status have returned to normal.

*This section, "Nursing Management," and the Nursing Care Plans at the end of this chapter were prepared by Shari Brumm, R.N., B.S.N., clinical educator, Rochester Methodist Hospital, Rochester, Minn.

Interviews with the adolescent and the family provide data that the nurse requires for a psychosocial assessment. The adolescent's drug use history is one component of the process (Table 39-6). The interviews are conducted after the physical assessment has been completed and the young person's physiological condition has stabilized. Data collection may begin when the nurse first has contact with the adolescent. Completion of the assessment, however, requires that the young person be alert and involved. This is essential because the adolescent will accept further drug education, assessment, or treatment only if an accurate self-assessment demonstrates the need for, and benefits of, change. (Table 14-4 describes additional components of a health history.)

Nursing management Nurses who work in inpatient assessment or treatment units need to have a thorough understanding of child and adolescent development, family dynamics, and chemical dependence. Nurses who work in chemical dependence units may be expected to seek certification through state chemical dependence associations or to gain further education. Sometimes additional training and supervision are provided by physicians and psychologists. Nurses are expected to become skillful at facilitating group therapy, family conferences, multiple family group sessions, and educational presentations (see Fig. 39-3). Nurses lead group activities for the siblings of adolescents who are undergoing treatment; they also provide information and support for the members of the adolescent's extended family during planned activities.

Adolescents in an inpatient setting need a structured daily program. A typical day in a hospital treatment unit begins early with 15 min of group exercise. Popular music and staff participation in the exercises enhance everyone's sense of unity and reinforce the concept that "each day is a new beginning." At breakfast a topic is presented for reflection. Often headlines and introductions to stories from the morning newspaper are "broadcast" by the residents. This is one of the many daily activities that support the adolescents' connectedness to the community. Learning new and current information also helps them develop conversational skills and broaden their interests. As the day progresses, nurses coordinate recreational, educational, assessment, social, spiritual, and physical activities. These

Table 39-6 A Nursing Assessment Guide for Adolescent Substance Abuse*

Physical Assessment

1. General
   a. Vital signs: compare with normal values.
   b. Height and weight: look for evidence of malnutrition.
   c. Muscular development: note emaciation.
   d. Teeth and gums: look for evidence of cavities, infection, or trauma.
2. Skin
   a. Appearance: assess color, hydration, and personal cleanliness.
   b. Assess for trauma: injection sites, needle tracks or scar tissue over veins in antecubital spaces, beneath tongue, in groin or penis, between fingers and toes, and along arms, hands, feet, and legs. Examine for cigarette burns, bruises, and old lacerations.
   c. Assess for acne, lice, and scabies.
3. Eyes
   a. Note presence of redness, irritation, or jaundice.
   b. Assess pupil size and response: miotic with opiates; normal with alcohol, barbiturates, and marijuana; mydriatic with amphetamines.
   c. Note lateral, vertical, or horizontal nystagmus.
4. Central nervous system
   a. Assess reflexes and coordination: note depression or hyperexcitability.
   b. Assess for seizure potential related to withdrawal or intoxication.
5. Cardiorespiratory system
   a. Note evidence of secondary complications resulting from drug use: arrhythmias, pulmonary infections, and excessive nasal discharge.
6. Genitalia and pelvic examination†
   a. Assess for signs of trauma.
   b. Assess for pain, lesions, or discharge associated with sexually transmitted diseases.

Psychosocial Assessment

1. Drug history
   a. Determine the nature and quantity of drugs used and the frequency of use: systematically explore use of prescription and nonprescription medications, alcohol, marijuana, and all other frequently abused psychoactive substances, including inhalants.
   b. Determine the date and time of last use: assess potential for withdrawal symptoms.
   c. Explore favorable and unfavorable experiences that the young person has had while using drugs.
   d. Determine whether attempts have been made to stop or control use, tolerance has increased, or blackouts (temporary periods of amnesia while using alcohol) have occurred.
   e. Determine whether prior counseling or hospitalization for drug-related problems has occurred.
   f. Systematically explore the young person's functioning within various life areas: identify problems and determine what changes have occurred in relation to the family, friends, the school setting, leisure or play activity, job experiences, and the legal system. Assess for correlation between problems in life areas and drug use.
   g. Determine the adolescent's perception of drug use and why it is or is not viewed as problematic.
2. Mental and emotional status
   a. Reality orientation: assess for the presence of hallucinations, confusion, or preoccupation.
   b. Mental activity and level of consciousness: assess for alertness, responsiveness, and comprehension. Note slowed or agitated thought processes and characteristics of speech.
   c. Emotional state: assess mood, using both objective and subjective data. Note depression, euphoria, or hostility. Assess potential for suicide by asking, "Have you ever thought of killing yourself?" "Are you thinking of killing yourself now?" and "What is your plan?"
   d. Stress factors: determine what is of major concern to the adolescent (e.g., family relationships, school performance, or acceptance by peers).
   e. Coping strategies: determine the typical response to stress; assess for use of chemicals to obtain relief.
   f. Defense mechanisms: assess for frequent or repetitive use of denial, minimization, rationalization (excuses), or projection of blame onto others.

Family Status and History

1. Membership
   a. Assess communication and relationship patterns.
   b. Assess leadership role and style.
   c. Assess support function.
   d. Assess values.
   e. Assess chemical use patterns and attitudes.
   f. Assess attitudes toward change.
2. Changes
   a. Identify changes in membership or relationships.
   b. Identify changes in the physical and emotional health of the family members.
   c. Identify changes in the adolescent's relationship to his or her family.

*Prepared by Shari Brumm, B.S.N.

†During the physical examination, the nurse can observe for drugs hidden in the clothing, hair, axillae, vagina, or anus.

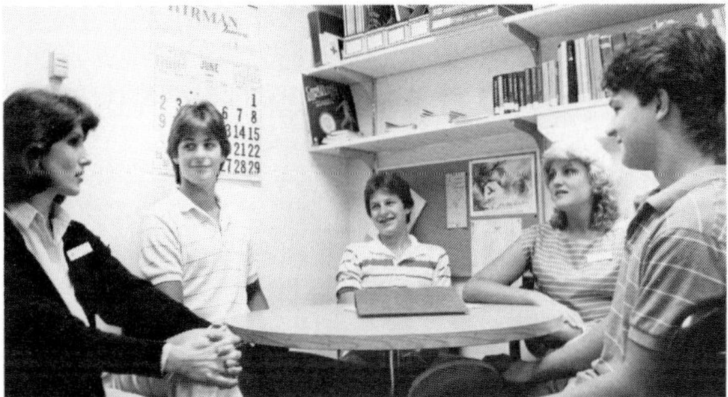

Figure 39-3 Small groups are ideal for building trust and learning about drugs. These group members are identifying problem-solving methods as alternatives to drug use. (*Photo courtesy of Rochester Methodist Hospital, Rochester, Minn.*)

activities help the adolescent in the recovery process (see Figs. 39-4 and 39-5 and the Nursing Care Plans at the end of this chapter).

CONTINUUM OF SERVICES

> Chemical use (particularly alcohol) has become so commonplace and so well-entrenched in American social life that it seems naive to expect any force (family, church, school, law enforcement, courts, youth organizations) to be able to intervene effectively. Only strategies which are based on cooperation and shared responsibility among many community forces are likely to have a significant impact.[24]

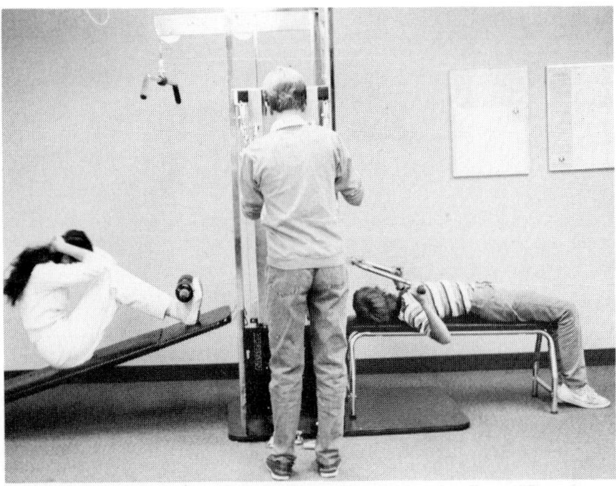

Figure 39-4 A sense of well-being and fitness can be achieved through a daily exercise program. These adolescents are working on their individual fitness goals. (*Photo courtesy of Rochester Methodist Hospital, Rochester, Minn.*)

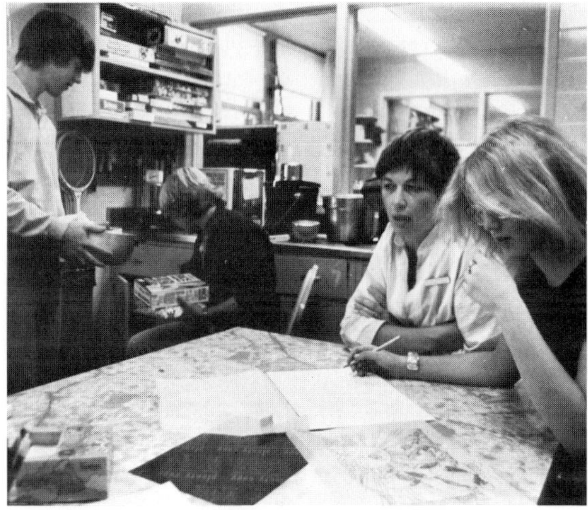

Figure 39-5 Building the adolescent's self-esteem is the foundation for successful treatment. These teenagers are learning basic living skills in the occupational therapy department. (*Photo courtesy of Rochester Methodist Hospital, Rochester, Minn.*)

Responding to substance abuse necessitates action at many levels. By viewing the need for services as a continuum (see Fig. 39-6), the health care professional can identify opportunities to intervene with individuals, families, communities, and human service systems. Although often identified as linear, in reality the continuum of services needed is *circular.*

Prevention

Primary prevention of substance use problems involves efforts to define and promote a particular family's, individual's, or "community's" idea of chemical health. While the causes of substance abuse are not clear, some at-risk populations have been identified. Education and exploration of social policy can play an important role for all families. Developing decision-making skills and promoting informed decisions concerning all types of chemical use are basic steps. Increasing coping skills and self-esteem help children respond to our chemically oriented society.

Comprehensive chemical health curricula for use in elementary schools, junior high schools, and high schools have been developed and researched. "It is unlikely that school-based drug education courses will have a major impact unless the information provided in these courses is constantly reinforced by parents, other role models, and community and religious organizations."[25] Some success is being achieved by peer-led programs. A curriculum for use with children of confirmation age and their families has been developed by some interdenominational groups.

The decrease in cigarette smoking is indicative of the potential for change when education and social policy are joined. Current efforts to raise the legal drinking age, curb drunken driving, introduce low-alcohol or alcohol-free beverages, and control cigarette and other drug advertising are all potentially positive influences on decreasing substance abuse.

Parent and neighborhood groups are organizing to bring about more involvement at the grass-roots level. "Neighborhood action groups" form to "generate a neighborhoodwide uniform code of action for children and to implement such a code once it is agreed upon."[26]

Identification and intervention

While individual responses to chemical substances may vary widely, a pattern of increasingly dysfunctional behavior becomes apparent in most young people after a period of continued substance use and abuse (see Table 39-1). Because the behavioral changes occur when the child is also experiencing the physical and emotional changes associated with puberty and adolescence, they are often dismissed or overlooked, rather than viewed as signs of potential substance abuse. Few health care professionals think to caution 13- or 14-year-olds that no alcohol should be consumed while they are taking certain prescriptions or cold preparations. In order for intervention to be effective, potential use problems must be identified in all health-related services as well as in human service agencies. Young people who are involved in accidents, overdose situations, or episodes of intoxication should be assessed to determine the extent of their involvement with substances and should be referred to appropriate community services for the level of intervention they need (Fig. 39-6).

Parents, juvenile justice workers, youth agency staff members, church workers, school personnel, and health care professionals need to be educated to recognize young drug abusers. These professionals can mobilize communities to develop the appropriate services.

When a drug use problem is identified, a concerted effort is needed to direct the child and his

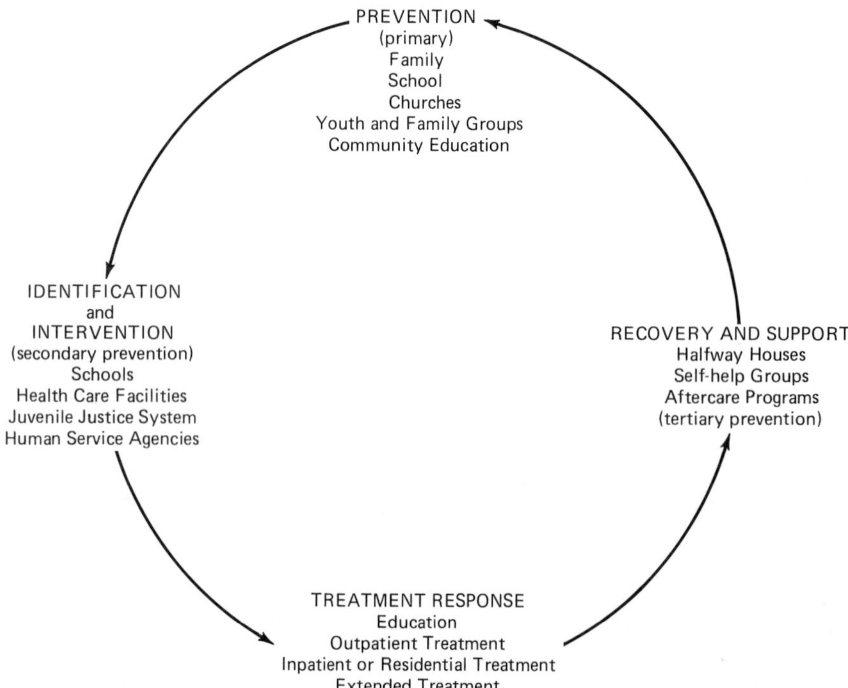

Figure 39-6 The continuum of services for adolescents and their families.

or her family to the most appropriate community service. Secondary prevention takes place as efforts are made to alter the cause of harmful usage.

Children of chemically dependent parents *Secondary* prevention also occurs when children of alcoholic parents and other drug-dependent parents are recognized and supported. An estimated 15 million school-age children in the United States live with alcoholic parents.[27]

In responding to the dysfunction of the substance-dependent parent, a child often assumes patterns of behavior or "roles" that help the child survive. These survival roles provide a framework for interpersonal relationships and bring some sense of stability to the child's existence. Often, if caregivers are aware of the problem, they may perceive the child as coping very well with the parent's chemical abuse.

Black[28] has identified the roles that children adopt and the difficulties that these roles cause in interpersonal and intrapersonal relationships in adulthood. The role of "responsible one" is often assumed by an only child or the oldest child in a family. These children accept a large part of the responsibility for parenting the parents and the siblings and for maintaining family life in general. Well organized and used to setting their own goals, they learn to rely completely on themselves. They are often rewarded and reinforced for their leadership roles. As adults, they have difficulty trusting others and attempt to maintain control over most situations.

"Adjusters" tend to be very flexible in their response to life. They find it easier simply to adjust to whatever happens. They are the most detached from their families, and their response appears to be, "I can't do anything about it anyway." In social settings, adjusters do not assume leadership roles. In school, they remain on the outer edges of involvement with others. As adults, they continue to see themselves as powerless over their own lives and therefore have difficulty taking responsibility for their lives.

Children who assume the role of "placater" are perceived as sensitive and emotionally involved with family events. They like to make others feel better and attempt to "fix" family problems in order to make life easier for everyone. As adults, they continue to please others and are well liked for their listening ability and their empathetic nature. While meeting others' needs, they have difficulty accepting their own needs without guilt.

"Acting-out" children are the ones who most often come to the attention of the family, the school, or a human services agency. They use negative behavior to attract attention to themselves, thereby providing distractions from the parents' chemical abuse problems. These children are frequently seen in correctional facilities, treatment programs for mental health or chemical abuse problems, or other social service institutions. They may drop out of school, become pregnant in midadolescence, or drink or use drugs at an early age. As adults, they continue to experience conflict, and their low self-esteem causes them to seek out peers with similar problems. Their tendency to use and abuse chemicals early in life frequently leads to a premature death.

Awareness of these roles and combinations of roles can help the nurse understand the effects of chemical abuse on the entire family. Children in this high-risk group can benefit from all efforts to address the dysfunctional life-style and prevent them from being affected by mental health and chemical abuse issues.

Dr. Robert ten Bensel, of the University of Minnesota, has identified the relationship between chemical abuse and violence against children. He states that "50–70 percent of all cases involving incest, rape, child abuse, and homicide are alcohol related."[29] In addition to the situations mentioned above, the damage done to children "comes not from what their parents actually do, but from how the children interpret events in the home."[30] Nurses can join other professionals to reach out to these children and help them reinterpret their experiences without waiting for the parents to be helped. Group work has proved especially helpful in supporting these children. In such groups, children are identified as being from "families in change," not from chemically dependent families. Working with other children who are experiencing changes such as a move, a death, a divorce, or the birth of a new sibling, they learn to develop problem-solving skills, build self-esteem, communicate feelings, and reduce stress. Table 39-7 presents suggested means of support when working with an individual child, a family, or a group.

Treatment response

Young substance abusers are usually treated in outpatient clinics, day-care centers, halfway houses, nonhospital residential settings, or hospital settings.[31] Intensive educational programs involving the adolescent and his or her family

Table 39-7 Support for Children of Alcoholics

1. *Let them know that they are not alone* Assure them that others share their experiences and understand their feelings.
2. *Validate their experiences* Help them sort out their confusion and explain that although they may feel "crazy," they are not. They are reacting to a parent who downplays or ignores the severity of his or her own problems, denies that certain events ever took place, and behaves inconsistently.
3. *Help them gain some perspective on how the parent's alcoholism has affected them* It has often been said that children of alcoholics fall into predictable, unhealthy patterns of behavior as a reaction to this problem. Some become overly responsible in order to compensate for the irresponsibility of a parent; others act out constantly to get attention from an otherwise inattentive parent; and so forth. Groups for children of alcoholics can help them identify and consider ways of changing their patterns of behavior.
4. *Absolve them of blame* Convince them of the fact that their mother's or father's drinking is not their fault and that they cannot control it.
5. *Help them separate the parent from the drunken behavior* Make it clear that the parent's drinking is not a sign that the parent does not love them. Ask them to remember, if they can, what it was like at home before the parent started drinking heavily.
6. *Offer them hope* Let them know that alcoholism is a disease from which the parent can recover.
7. *Urge them to take care of themselves* Encourage them to do positive things for themselves and stop any behavior that enables the parent to continue drinking. Sometimes making a contract with these children helps them achieve their goals.
8. *Provide them with a safe outlet for dealing with their anger* Help them deal with their anger at both the alcoholic parent and the nonalcoholic parent (who has not protected them or made things better).
9. *Explain the risks related to chemical dependency* Make them aware that they are at high risk of becoming chemically dependent or of marrying a chemically dependent person. If they are about to leave home, they may believe that their troubles will soon be over. They need to know that they are likely to encounter certain problems that children raised in families in which alcoholism is not an issue do not have to deal with. This has to be handled very judiciously. Be careful not to use the label "children of alcoholics" as though that particular aspect of their lives totally defines their present identity and future actions. Nonetheless, it is clear that, for a variety of reasons, the children of alcoholics are at high risk of becoming chemically dependent, and at the proper time and in the proper way, they should be made aware of that fact.
10. *Build their self-esteem* Help raise the self-esteem of these children in whatever way possible. Simply having an adult listen closely to them can boost the self-esteem of many of these children.

Source. James F. Crowley, *Alliance for Change*, Community Intervention, Minneapolis, Minn., 1984, pp. 152–153.

may be recommended. Outpatient treatment programs may be provided by youth or family agencies or health care facilities. These programs often have the advantages of costing less and causing less disruption of the family system. A residential program is often used for heavy drug users who need a long-term, structured, controlled environment. Inpatient assessment units are needed when the adolescent cannot be successfully evaluated in an outpatient setting or is at serious medical risk.

Recovery and support

The treatment program serves as a beginning step in changing the pattern and effect of chemical abuse. Children and their families need a supportive network as they become healthier, more functional units. Aftercare services are often provided by treatment programs and other youth and/or family service agencies. Self-help groups such as Families Anonymous, Al-Anon, Alcoholics Anonymous, and Narcotics Anonymous are very helpful and are available in most communities.

While the goal of most recovery programs is abstinence from mood-altering substances, others base their criteria for recovery on improved functioning and the reduction of consequences related to substance use. In either case, *tertiary* prevention consists of directing services, providing education, and giving support in order to decrease the likelihood of a return to chemical use problems and to promote chemical health.

The nurse plays an important role in providing education, influencing social policy, advocating needed services, assessing adolescents and their families, and referring adolescents for diagnostic workup or treatment. In addition, nurses can act as role models for chemically healthy behavior and responsible use of chemical substances.

Nursing Care Plan: Substance Abuse

Patient: Joan Reily | Age: 16 years | Date of Admission: 4/18

IDENTIFYING DATA AND ASSESSMENT

Joan was admitted to the emergency department at 8 P.M. She was escorted to the desk by three girlfriends who provided her name, age, address, and parents' telephone number and stated that she was having a "bad trip." They refused to provide further information and left quickly.

GENERAL APPEARANCE

Joan is well nourished and well hydrated and is attentive to grooming and self-care needs. She screamed loudly, "It's crazy. I'm losing it. I can't stop it." She paced by the desk, wringing her hands and pulling at her clothing. She sat for several minutes when asked to. Calls were placed to the physician and Joan's family.

PHYSICAL EXAMINATION

Respiratory rate: 30 breaths per minute. Pulse: 110 and regular. Temperature: 38.0°C. Blood pressure: 140/90. Blood and urine tests (drug abuse screen) will be done after the initial attempt to calm the patient.

Nursing Diagnosis	Outcome Criteria	Nursing Interventions	Evaluation and Modifications
1. Panic related to drug-induced sensory and perceptual alterations	☐ Joan will regain non-fear-provoking sensory and perceptual function within 6 h, as evidenced by: **a.** Absence of screams, pacing, hand wringing, and clothes pulling **b.** Verbalizing feeling comfortable and unafraid	☐ Provide a quiet, secure, nonstressful environment: **a.** Adjust the lighting for the comfort of the patient. **b.** Remove harmful objects (those which might injure the patient or others if grabbed or thrown). **c.** Determine the safety of exits and doors (windows should be secure, and bathroom and room doors should unlock from the outside).	☐ 9 P.M.: When seated in a small, well-lit but not bright room, Joan appeared less frightened and consented to rest on the bed. Pushed the over-the-bed table into the wall. Exhibits potential for destructive or assaultive behavior at times. The door remains open, and additional staff members are nearby. Pacing and screams have ended. ☐ Data from the initial interview with Joan's family and evidence of drug-induced panic suggest a possible substance abuse and dependence disorder. Nurse will collaborate with the health care team to determine an appropriate referral for Joan and her family for outpatient chemical use assessment.

Nursing Diagnosis	Outcome Criteria	Nursing Interventions	Evaluation and Modifications
		☐ Reassure Joan using a calm manner, an informative approach, an empathetic attitude, and an evenly modulated voice. ☐ Assign one nurse to remain with Joan at all times. ☐ Assure Joan that this experience is drug-related and temporary. ☐ Orient Joan to reality: persons, place, time, and events (if the perceptual experience becomes pleasant and Joan is calm, allow this to continue without offering support for hallucinations).	☐ Joan is oriented to persons, time, and place and is calm when reassured of the temporary nature of the experience. A rapid approach to the bedside or physical touching increases agitation.
		☐ When necessary, give short, clear directions with an attitude of expecting cooperation.	☐ Joan responds positively to directives when they are given by the assigned nurse and when she is allowed several minutes for increased comprehension and encouragement.

Nursing Care Plan: Possible Substance Dependence, and Possible Withdrawal

Patient: John Williams **Age:** 17 years **Date of Admission:** 9/12

IDENTIFYING DATA AND ASSESSMENT

John arrived in the emergency department following an automobile accident last night. An injury to the left foot, slurred speech, and an alcohol smell to the breath were evident. He was admitted to the surgical unit following repair of foot and ankle lacerations. His physical condition is stable. His blood alcohol level on admission was 0.09; a drug screen (blood and urine) showed that he was positive for THC (marijuana) and a common barbiturate. John appears well nourished and well hydrated. His arms and legs evidence numerous old bruises and minor lacerations. He is talkative and friendly and frequently asks in a joking manner for "better pain meds." He is receiving 50 mg of Demerol intramuscularly every 4 h or prn. His parents are both employed and will visit only in the evening. The nurses' notes indicate a need for assessment of substance use pattern and order close monitoring for withdrawal symptoms.

PHYSICAL EXAMINATION

Temperature: 38.4°C. Pulse: 68. Respirations: 18 breaths per minute. Blood pressure: 118/74.

Nursing Diagnosis	Outcome Criteria	Nursing Interventions	Evaluation and Modifications
1. Possible withdrawal symptoms related to sudden cessation of alcohol and/or barbiturate intake	☐ John will maintain his present level of physical comfort for the next 24 h, as evidenced by: **a.** Absence of excessive anxiety (restlessness and agitation) **b.** Absence of tremors **c.** Ability to sleep 6 h consecutively **d.** Maintenance of present appetite and elimination pattern **e.** Absence of seizures	☐ Assess, document, and report the following indicators of withdrawal: **a.** An increase in blood pressure, pulse, respiration, or temperature **b.** Signs of restlessness or agitation (hurried speech, rapid movement, and insomnia) **c.** Shakiness or tremors (of the upper extremities, hands or tongue). **d.** Nausea, vomiting, or diarrhea ☐ Request and administer a physican-prescribed withdrawal medication following a gradual reduction schedule if: **a.** Results of the drug history indicate a high po-	☐ There was no evidence of agitation, tremors, inability to sleep, or alteration in appetite or elimination patterns. Vital signs are unchanged. John's drug history indicates that alcohol and barbiturates are used infrequently. The drug of choice, marijuana, is used on a daily basis. Continue to monitor for signs of withdrawal during the next 24 h. The reliability of John's use report has not been determined. Anxiety may increase as the amount of Demerol and the frequency of administration are decreased.

Nursing Diagnosis	Outcome Criteria	Nursing Interventions	Evaluation and Modifications
		tential for withdrawal syndrome. **b.** Signs and symptoms of withdrawal appear	
2. Possible ineffective individual coping related to drug abuse and dependence	☐ When interviewed today, John and his family will verbally identify John's drug use pattern (types and quantities of drugs used and frequency of use). ☐ John and his family will verbally identify consequences of drug use that John has experienced in various areas of his life. ☐ John and his family will verbally identify resources available for assessment and/or treatment of adolescent substance abuse.	☐ Involve John in frequent one-to-one conversations. Designate one nurse to establish a trusting relationship. ☐ Complete the drug history and psychosocial assessment during an uninterrupted time and in a quiet, private environment. ☐ Communicate with John's parents about their son's drug use. Seek information related to alterations in family function, legal involvement, school experiences, the peer group, and attitude and behavioral changes. ☐ Collaborate with the health care team to identify appropriate referral options to recommend to John and his family. ☐ Plan a meeting with John and his family. Ask John to share with his parents what he has been experiencing. (Do not violate John's right to confidentiality.) Ask the parents to share with John what they have observed. Present specific recommendations for further education about substance use and provide additional assessment or treatment as determined by the health care team.	☐ John and his family give conflicting reports of John's drug use and its consequences. Both John and his family have identified problems in school, at home, and within the legal system. They have been provided with written information describing community drug use assessment services. John and his family have expressed a desire to have an assessment done during this hospitalization. Nurse will contact the agency selected by the family and arrange a meeting. Depending on the findings, the health care team will help make a referral to a treatment provider.

References

1. Bennett, Gerald, Christine Vourakis, and Donna S. Woolf (eds.), *Substance Abuse: Pharmacologic, Developmental, and Clinical Perspectives,* Wiley, New York, 1983, p. xiii.
2. *Report on 1983 Minnesota Survey on Drug Use and Drug-Related Attitudes,* Search Institute, Minneapolis, Minn., 1983, p. 12.
3. Bennett, Vourakis, and Woolf, op. cit., p. 165.
4. *1984 National Strategy for Prevention of Drug Abuse and Drug Trafficking.* Drug Abuse Policy Office, GPO, Washington, D.C., 1984, p. 18.
5. Ibid.
6. *Quick Reference to the Diagnostic Criteria from Diagnostic and Statistical Manual of Mental Disorders,* 3d ed., American Psychiatric Association, Washington, D.C., 1980, pp. 91–101.
7. *1984 National Strategy for Prevention of Drug Abuse and Drug Trafficking.*
8. Stephenson, John N., D. Paul Moberg, Beverly J. Daniels, and Joan F. Robertson, "Treating the Intoxicated Adolescent: A Need for Comprehensive Services," *Journal of the American Medical Association* **252**(14): 1884–1888 (October 1984).
9. Milgram, Gail Gleason, *What, When, and How to Talk to Children about Alcohol and Other Drugs: A Guide for Parents,* Hazelden, Center City, Minn., 1983, p. 60.
10. Ibid., p. 65.
11. Ibid.
12. *Quick Reference to the Diagnostic Criteria from Diagnostic and Statistical Manual of Mental Disorders.*
13. *1984 National Strategy for Prevention of Drug Abuse and Drug Trafficking.*
14. Minnesota Institute of Public Health, "As Young People Grow: A Look at Adolescent Development," *Impact,* Minnesota Prevention Resource Center, Anoka, Minn. (Fall 1984).
15. *1984 National Strategy for Prevention of Drug Abuse and Drug Trafficking,* p. 104.
16. Oakley, Ray, *Drugs, Society, and Human Behavior,* Mosby, St. Louis, 1978, pp. 59–61.
17. Johnson, Vernon E., *I'll Quit Tomorrow,* Harper & Row, New York, 1980, pp. 15–24.
18. Schuckit, Marc A., *Drug and Alcohol Abuse: A Clinical Guide to Diagnosis and Treatment,* 2d ed., Plenum, New York, 1984.
19. *1984 National Strategy for Prevention of Drug Abuse and Drug Trafficking,* p. 17.
20. Pickens, Roy W., *Children of Alcoholics,* Hazelden, Center City, Minn., 1984.
21. Moberg, Paul D., "Identifying Adolescents with Alcohol Problems: A Field Test of the Adolescent Alcohol Involvement Scale," *Journal of Studies on Alcohol* **44**(4):701–721 (1983).
22. Riley, Kate, and Alan J. Klockars, "A Critical Reexamination of the Adolescent Alcohol Involvement Scale," *Journal of Studies on Alcohol* **45**(2):184–187 (1984).
23. Filstead, William J., and John E. Mayer, "Validity of the Adolescent Alcohol Involvement Scale: A Reply to Riley and Klockars," *Journal of Studies on Alcohol* **45**(2):188–189 (1984).
24. *Report on 1983 Minnesota Survey on Drug Use and Drug-Related Attitudes,* p. 104.
25. Ibid., p. 90.
26. Kim, Sehwan, and Stephen H. Newman, "Synthetic-Dynamic Theory of Drug Abuse: A Revisit with Empirical Data," *The International Journal of the Addictions* **17**(5):921 (1982).
27. Deutsch, Charles, *Children of Alcoholics: Understanding and Helping,* Health Communications, Hollywood, Fla., 1983, p. 1.
28. Black, Claudia, *It Will Never Happen to Me,* M. A. C. Printing and Publication Division, Denver, 1981, pp. 14–27.
29. Minnesota Institute of Public Health, "Dr. Robert ten Bensel: A Man among Children," *Impact,* Minnesota Prevention Resource Center, Anoka, Minn.: (Summer 1984).
30. Deutsch, op. cit., p. 3.
31. Freidman, A. S., "Referral and Diagnosis of Adolescent Substance Abusers," in *Treatment Services for Adolescent Substance Abusers,* National Institute on Drug Abuse, 1985.

PART V

Appendices

Appendix A: Metric conversion tables

Table A-1 Celsius and Fahrenheit Equivalents: Body Temperature Range

C°	F°	C°	F°	C°	F°	C°	F°	C°	F°
34.0	93.20	35.5	95.90	37.0	98.60	38.5	101.30	40.0	104.00
34.1	93.38	35.6	96.08	37.1	98.78	38.6	101.48	40.1	104.18
34.2	93.56	35.7	96.26	37.2	98.96	38.7	101.66	40.2	104.36
34.3	93.74	35.8	96.44	37.3	99.14	38.8	101.84	40.3	104.54
34.4	93.92	35.9	96.62	37.4	99.32	38.9	102.02	40.4	104.72
34.5	94.10	36.0	96.80	37.5	99.50	39.0	102.20	40.5	104.90
34.6	94.28	36.1	96.98	37.6	99.68	39.1	102.38	40.6	105.08
34.7	94.46	36.2	97.16	37.7	99.86	39.2	102.56	40.7	105.26
34.8	94.64	36.3	97.34	37.8	100.04	39.3	102.74	40.8	105.44
34.9	94.82	36.4	97.52	37.9	100.22	39.4	102.92	40.9	105.62
35.0	95.0	36.5	97.70	38.0	100.40	39.5	103.10	41.0	105.80
35.1	95.18	36.6	97.88	38.1	100.58	39.6	103.28		
35.2	95.36	36.7	98.06	38.2	100.76	39.7	103.46		
35.3	95.54	36.8	98.24	38.3	100.94	39.8	103.64		
35.4	95.72	36.9	98.42	38.4	101.12	39.9	103.82		

Table A-2 Fahrenheit and Celsius Equivalents: Body Temperature Range

F°	C°	F°	C°	F°	C°	F°	C°	F°	C°
94.0	34.44	97.0	36.11	100.0	37.78	103.0	39.44	106.0	41.11
94.2	34.56	97.2	36.22	100.2	37.89	103.2	39.56	106.2	41.22
94.4	34.67	97.4	36.33	100.4	38.00	103.4	39.67	106.4	41.33
94.6	34.78	97.6	36.44	100.6	38.11	103.6	39.78	106.6	41.44
94.8	34.89	97.8	36.56	100.8	38.22	103.8	39.89	106.8	41.56
95.0	35.00	98.0	36.67	101.0	38.33	104.0	40.00	107.0	41.67
95.2	35.11	98.2	36.78	101.2	38.44	104.2	40.11	107.2	41.78
95.4	35.22	98.4	36.89	101.4	38.56	104.4	40.22	107.4	41.89
95.6	35.33	98.6	37.00	101.6	38.67	104.6	40.33	107.6	42.00
95.8	35.44	98.8	37.11	101.8	38.78	104.8	40.44	107.8	42.11
96.0	35.56	99.0	37.22	102.0	38.89	105.0	40.56	108.0	42.22
96.2	35.67	99.2	37.33	102.2	39.00	105.2	40.67		
96.4	35.78	99.4	37.44	102.4	39.11	105.4	40.78		
96.6	35.89	99.6	37.56	102.6	39.22	105.6	40.89		
96.8	36.00	99.8	37.67	102.8	39.33	105.8	41.00		

Table A-3 Length Conversions

Meters	Centimeters	Yards	Feet	Inches
1	100	1.094	3.281	39.37
0.01	1	0.01094	.0328	0.3937
0.9144	91.44	1	3	36
0.0348	30.48	1/3	1	12
0.0254	2.54	1/36	1/12	1

Table A-4 Weight Conversions (Metric and Avoirdupois)

Grams	Kilograms	Ounces	Pounds
1	0.001	0.0353	0.0022
1000	1	35.3	2.2
28.35	0.02835	1	1/16
454.5	0.4545	16	1

Table A-5 Pound-to-Kilogram Conversion Table*

Pounds	0	1	2	3	4	5	6	7	8	9
0	0.00	0.45	0.90	1.36	1.81	2.26	2.72	3.17	3.62	4.08
10	4.53	4.98	5.44	5.89	6.35	6.80	7.25	7.71	8.16	8.61
20	9.07	9.52	9.97	10.43	10.88	11.34	11.79	12.24	12.70	13.15
30	13.60	14.06	14.51	14.96	15.42	15.87	16.32	16.78	17.23	17.69
40	18.14	18.59	19.05	19.50	19.95	20.41	20.86	21.31	21.77	22.22
50	22.68	23.13	23.58	24.04	24.49	24.94	25.40	25.85	26.30	26.76
60	27.21	27.66	28.12	28.57	29.03	29.48	29.93	30.39	30.84	31.29
70	31.75	32.20	32.65	33.11	33.56	34.02	34.47	34.92	35.38	35.83
80	36.28	36.74	37.19	37.64	38.10	38.55	39.00	39.46	39.91	40.37
90	40.82	41.27	41.73	42.18	42.63	43.09	43.54	43.99	44.45	44.90
100	45.36	45.81	46.26	46.72	47.17	47.62	48.08	48.53	48.98	49.44
110	49.89	50.34	50.80	51.25	51.71	52.16	52.61	53.07	53.52	53.97
120	54.43	54.88	55.33	55.79	56.24	56.70	57.15	57.60	58.06	58.51
130	58.96	59.42	59.87	60.32	60.78	61.23	61.68	62.14	62.59	63.05
140	63.50	63.95	64.41	64.86	65.31	65.77	66.22	66.67	67.13	67.58
150	68.04	68.49	68.94	69.40	69.85	70.30	70.76	71.21	71.66	72.12
160	72.57	73.02	73.48	73.93	74.39	74.84	75.29	75.75	76.20	76.65
170	77.11	77.56	78.01	78.47	78.92	79.38	79.83	80.28	80.74	81.19
180	81.64	82.10	82.55	83.00	83.46	83.91	84.36	84.82	85.27	85.73
190	86.18	86.68	87.09	87.54	87.99	88.45	88.90	89.35	89.81	90.26
200	90.72	91.17	91.62	92.08	92.53	92.98	93.44	93.89	94.34	94.80

*The numbers in the first column are 10-lb increments; the numbers across the top row are 1-lb increments. The kilogram equivalent of weight in pounds is found at the intersection of the appropriate row and column. For example, to convert 54 lb, read down the first column to 50 and then across that row to 4; 54 lb = 24.49 kg.

Table A-6 Gram Equivalents for Pounds and Ounces: Conversion Table for Weight of Newborns*

	Ounces																
Pounds	0	1	2	3	4	5	6	7	8	9	10	11	12	13	14	15	Pounds
0	—	28	57	85	113	142	170	198	227	255	283	312	430	369	397	425	**0**
1	454	482	510	539	567	595	624	652	680	709	737	765	794	822	850	879	**1**
2	907	936	964	992	1021	1049	1077	1106	1134	1162	1191	1219	1247	1276	1304	1332	**2**
3	1361	1389	1417	1446	1474	1503	1531	1559	1588	1616	1644	1673	1701	1729	1758	1786	**3**
4	1814	1843	1871	1899	1928	1956	1984	2013	2041	2070	2098	2126	2155	2183	2211	2240	**4**
5	2268	2296	2325	2353	2381	2410	2438	2466	2495	2523	2551	2580	2608	2637	2665	2693	**5**
6	2722	2750	2778	2807	2835	2863	2892	2920	2948	2977	3005	3033	3062	3090	3118	3147	**6**
7	3175	3203	3232	3260	3289	3317	3345	3374	3402	3430	3459	3487	3515	3544	3572	3600	**7**
8	3629	3657	3685	3714	3742	3770	3799	3827	3856	3884	3912	3941	3969	3997	4026	4054	**8**
9	4082	4111	4139	4167	4196	4224	4252	4281	4309	4337	4366	4394	4423	4451	4479	4508	**9**
10	4536	4564	4593	4621	4649	4678	4706	4734	4763	4791	4819	4848	4876	4904	4933	4961	**10**
11	4990	5018	5046	5075	5103	5131	5160	5188	5216	5245	5273	5301	5330	5358	5386	5415	**11**
12	5443	5471	5500	5528	5557	5585	5613	5642	5670	5698	5727	5755	5783	5812	5840	5868	**12**
13	5897	5925	5953	5982	6010	6038	6067	6095	6123	6152	6180	6290	6237	6265	6294	6322	**13**
14	6350	6379	6407	6435	6464	6492	6520	6549	6577	6605	6634	6662	6690	6719	6747	6776	**14**

*1 lb = 453.59 g. 1 oz = 28.35 g. Grams can be converted to pounds and tenths of a pound by multiplying the number of grams by 0.0022.

Appendix B: Growth charts

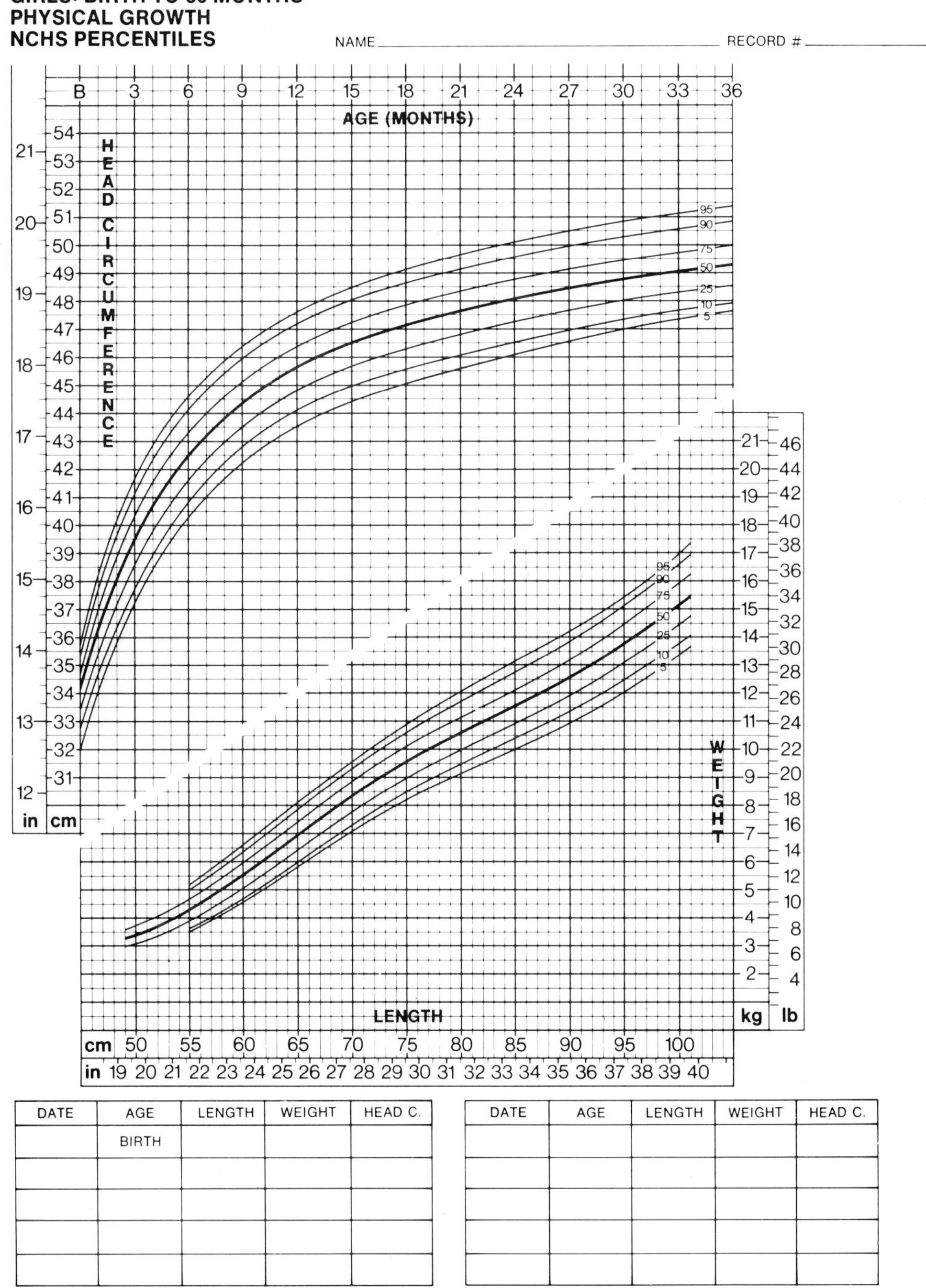

DATE	AGE	LENGTH	WEIGHT	HEAD C.
	BIRTH			

DATE	AGE	LENGTH	WEIGHT	HEAD C.

Figure B-1 Female infant growth chart: head circumference–age and length-weight relationships from birth to 36 months. See also Fig. 14-5. (*Adapted from the NCHS Growth Charts, 1976.*)

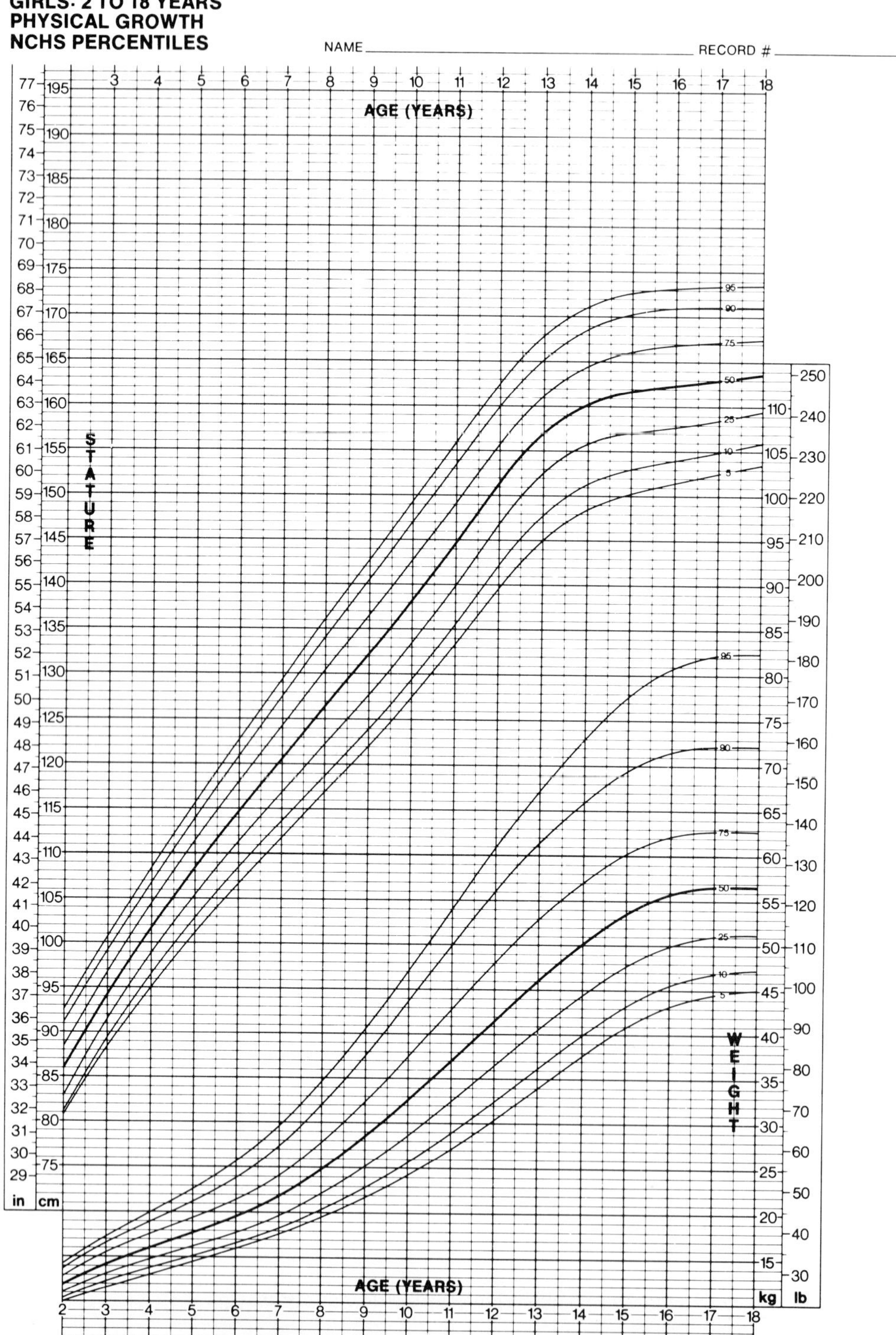

Figure B-2 Female growth chart: age-weight-stature relationships from 2 to 18 years. (*Adapted from the NCHS Growth Charts, 1976.*)

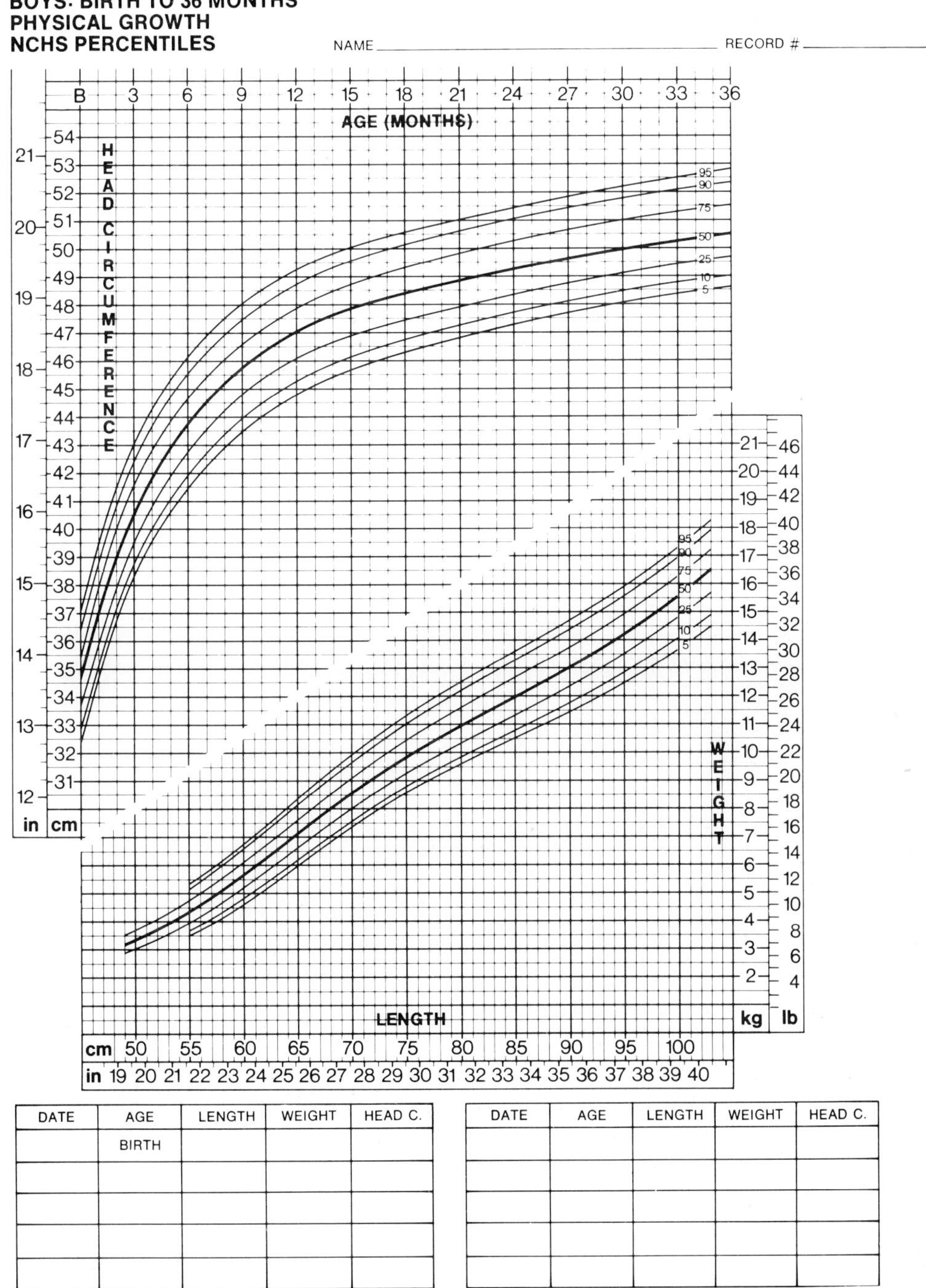

DATE	AGE	LENGTH	WEIGHT	HEAD C.
	BIRTH			

DATE	AGE	LENGTH	WEIGHT	HEAD C.

Figure B-3 Male infant growth chart: head circumference–age and length-weight relationships from birth to 36 months. (*Adapted from the NCHS Growth Charts, 1976.*)

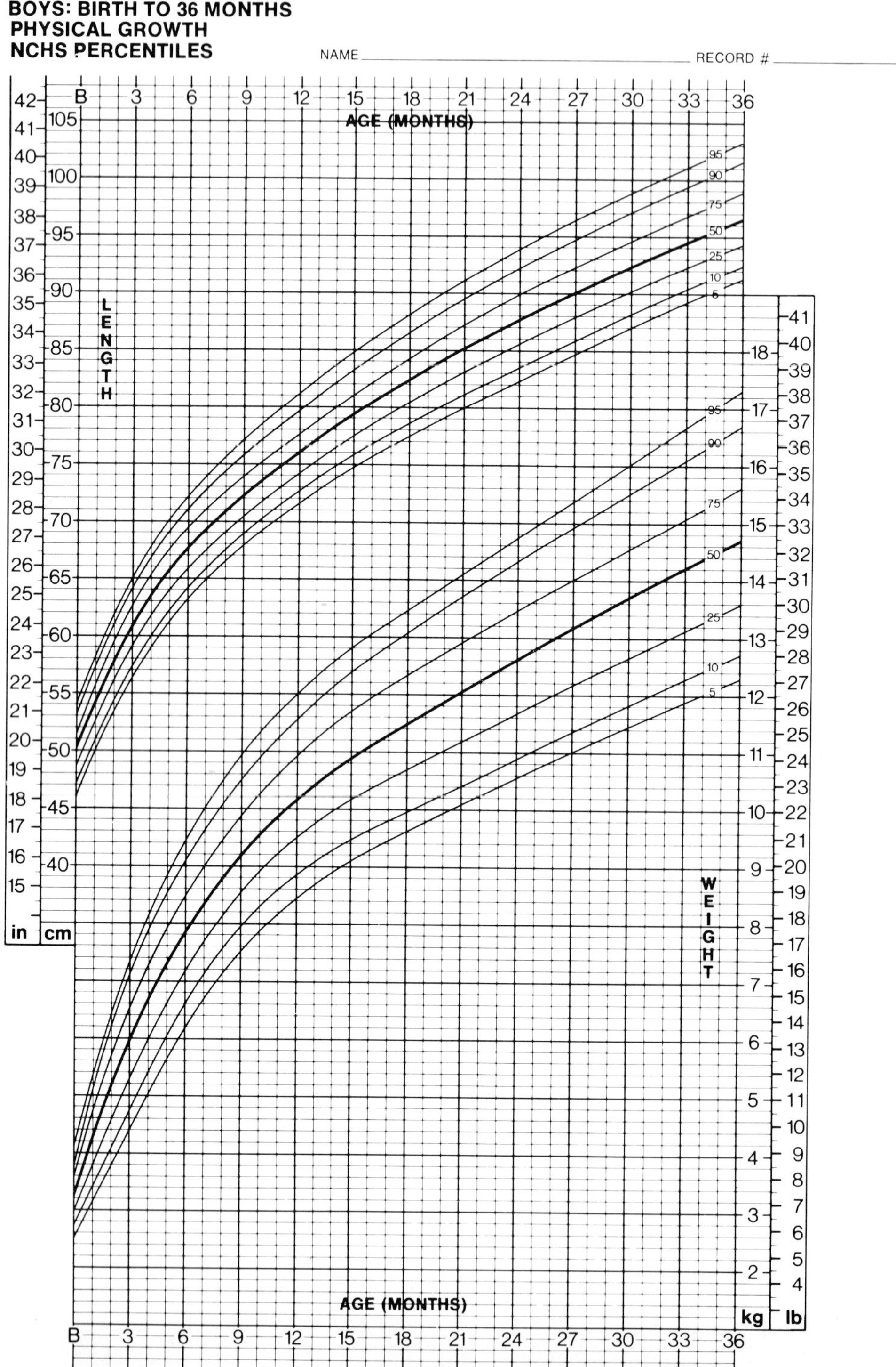

Figure B-4 Male infant growth chart: length-age and weight-age relationships from birth to 36 months. (*Adapted from the NCHS Growth Charts, 1976.*)

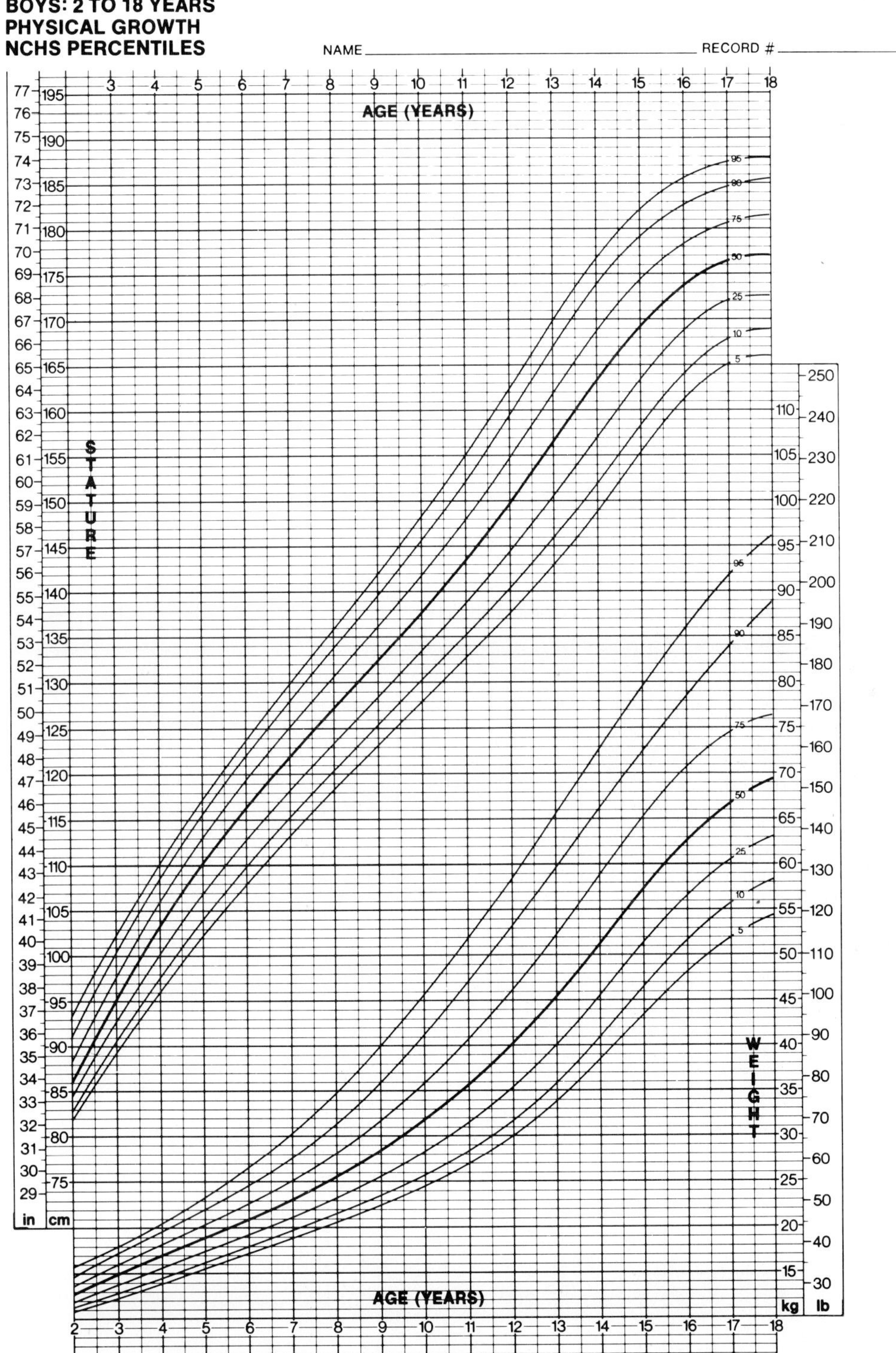

Figure B-5 Male growth chart: age-weight-stature relationships from 2 to 18 years. (*Adapted from the NCHS Growth Charts, 1976.*)

Appendix C: Nutrition

Table C-1 Nutrition History Form

Name

Date

Age

Informant

Current weight ________ Height or length ________ Skinfold measurement ________

Birth weight ________ Length ________

Was the child breast-fed ________ or bottle-fed ________

Bottle-fed: Formula used
Frequency of feedings
Amount taken
Age of child when formula was discontinued

Breast-fed: Frequency of feedings
Length of time for feedings
Were supplemental bottles given? Give specifics.
Age of weaning and to what child was weaned

Was the infant given a vitamin and/or mineral supplement? Specify.

When did the child stop taking middle-of-the-night feeding?

At what age were solids introduced?
Problems encountered
Length of time for a meal

At what age did the child start eating table foods?
Problems encountered

At what age did the child feed himself or herself?

At what age did the child begin to drink from a cup?

List previous medical or nutritional problems.

Are there any current medical and/or nutritional problems? (Obtain all necessary data.)

Current Nutritional Data

Do you use any vitamin or mineral supplements regularly? Specify.

Do you now or have you (child) ever followed a special diet? Explain.

What did you eat yesterday?

Time	Food	Amount

Table C-1 Nutrition History Form (*Continued*)

Do you eat at similar times every day?

What was different about your meals yesterday compared with your meals today or the day before?

Do you snack in the morning ______, afternoon ______, before supper ______, after supper ______, before bed ______?

What kinds of snack foods do you eat?

Do you ever skip meals? Which ones and why?

Do you eat lunch at school? If yes: Do you carry your lunch to school ______ or buy it at school ______?

Do you help prepare meals at home? Which ones?

Name some of your favorite foods.

Name some of the foods you do not like.

Have you ever eaten nonfoods (clay, dirt, or starch)?

Family Nutritional Data

In which room do you eat at home?

Do you eat meals with your family?

Is anyone in the family following a special diet? Specify.

Who purchases the food for the family?

Who prepares the food for the family?

Table C-2 Recommended Daily Dietary Allowances (1980 Revision)[a]

		Weight		Height			Fat-Soluble Vitamins		
	Age	(Kg)	(Lb)	(Cm)	(In)	Protein (G)	Vitamin A (μg RE)[b]	Vitamin D (μg)[c]	Vitamin E (mg α-TE)[d]
Infants	Birth to 6 months	6	13	60	24	kg × 2.2	420	10	3
	6 months to 1 year	9	20	71	28	kg × 2.0	400	10	4
Children	1 to 3 years	13	29	90	35	23	400	10	5
	4 to 6 years	20	44	112	44	30	500	10	6
	7 to 10 years	28	62	132	52	45	700	10	7
Males	11 to 14 years	45	99	157	62	45	1000	10	8
	15 to 18 years	66	145	176	69	56	1000	10	10
Females	11 to 14 years	46	101	157	62	46	800	10	8
	15 to 18 years	55	120	163	64	46	800	10	8
Pregnant women						+30	+200	+5	+2
Lactating women						+20	+400	+5	+3

Table C-2 Recommended Daily Dietary Allowances (1980 Revision)[a] (*Continued*)

	Age	Weight (Kg)	Weight (Lb)	Height (Cm)	Height (In)	Water-Soluble Vitamins: Vitamin C (Mg)	Thiamin (Mg)	Riboflavin (Mg)	Niacin (Mg NE)[e]	Vitamin B_6 (Mg)	Folacin[f] (μg)	Vitamin B_{12} (μg)
Infants	Birth to 6 months	6	13	60	24	35	0.3	0.4	6	0.3	30	0.5[g]
	6 months to 1 year	9	20	71	28	35	0.5	0.6	8	0.6	45	1.5
Children	1 to 3 years	13	29	90	35	45	0.7	0.8	9	0.9	100	2.0
	4 to 6 years	20	44	112	44	45	0.9	1.0	11	1.3	200	2.5
	7 to 10 years	28	62	132	52	45	1.2	1.4	16	1.6	300	3.0
Males	11 to 14 years	45	99	157	62	50	1.4	1.6	18	1.8	400	3.0
	15 to 18 years	66	145	176	69	60	1.4	1.7	18	2.0	400	3.0
Females	11 to 14 years	46	101	157	62	50	1.1	1.3	15	1.8	400	3.0
	15 to 18 years	55	120	163	64	60	1.1	1.3	14	2.0	400	3.0
Pregnant women						+20	+0.4	+0.3	+2	+0.6	+400	+1.0
Lactating women						+40	+0.5	+0.5	+5	+0.5	+100	+1.0

	Age	Weight (Kg)	Weight (Lb)	Height (Cm)	Height (In)	Minerals: Calcium (Mg)	Phosphorus (Mg)	Magnesium (Mg)	Iron (Mg)	Zinc (Mg)	Iodine (μg)
Infants	Birth to 6 months	6	13	60	24	360	240	50	10	3	40
	6 months to 1 year	9	20	71	28	540	360	70	15	5	50
Children	1 to 3 years	13	29	90	35	800	800	150	15	10	70
	4 to 6 years	20	44	112	44	800	800	200	10	10	90
	7 to 10 years	28	62	132	52	800	800	250	10	10	120
Males	11 to 14 years	45	99	157	62	1200	1200	350	18	15	150
	15 to 18 years	66	145	176	69	1200	1200	400	18	15	150
Females	11 to 14 years	46	101	157	62	1200	1200	300	18	15	150
	15 to 18 years	55	120	163	64	1200	1200	300	18	15	150
Pregnant women						+400	+400	+150	[h]	+5	+25
Lactating women						+400	+400	+150	[h]	+10	+50

[a]The allowances are intended to provide for individual variations among most normal persons as they live in the United States under usual environmental stresses. Diets should be based on a variety of common foods in order to provide other nutrients for which human requirements have been less well defined.

[b]Retinol equivalents. 1 retinol equivalent = 1 μg retinol or 6 μg β carotene.

[c]As cholecalciferol. 10 μg cholecalciferol = 400 IU of vitamin D.

[d]α-tocopherol equivalents. 1 mg *d*-α tocopherol = 1 α-TE

[e]1 NE (niacin equivalent) is equal to 1 mg of niacin or 60 mg of dietary tryptophan.

[f]The folacin allowances refer to dietary sources as determined by *Lactobacillus casei* assay after treatment with enzymes (conjugates) to make polyglutamyl forms of the vitamin available to the test organism.

[g]The recommended dietary allowances for vitamin B_{12} in infants are based on average concentration of the vitamin in human milk. The allowances after weaning are based on energy intake (as recommended by the American Academy of Pediatrics) and consideration of other factors, such as intestinal absorption.

[h]The increased requirements during pregnancy cannot be met by the iron content of habitual American diets or by the existing iron stores of many women; therefore, the use of 30 to 60 mg of supplemental iron is recommended. Iron needs during lactation are not substantially different from those of nonpregnant women, but continued supplementation of the mother for 2 to 3 months after parturition is advisable in order to replenish stores depleted by pregnancy.

Source: Food and Nutrition Board, National Academy of Sciences—National Research Council, Washington, D.C.

Table C-3 Estimated Safe and Adequate Daily Dietary Intakes of Selected Vitamins and Minerals*

	Age	Trace Elements†					
		Copper (Mg)	Manganese (Mg)	Fluoride (Mg)	Chromium (Mg)	Selenium (Mg)	Molybdenum (Mg)
Infants	Birth to 6 months	0.5–0.7	0.5–0.7	0.1–0.5	0.01–0.04	0.01–0.04	0.03–0.06
	6 months to 1 year	0.7–1.0	0.7–1.0	0.2–1.0	0.02–0.06	0.02–0.06	0.04–0.08
Children and adolescents	1 to 3 years	1.0–1.5	1.0–1.5	0.5–1.5	0.02–0.08	0.02–0.08	0.05–0.1
	4 to 6 years	1.5–2.0	1.5–2.0	1.0–2.5	0.03–0.12	0.03–0.12	0.06–0.15
	7 to 10 years	2.0–2.5	2.0–3.0	1.5–2.5	0.05–0.2	0.05–0.2	0.10–0.3
	Over 11 years	2.5–3.0	2.5–5.0	1.5–2.5	0.05–0.2	0.05–0.2	0.15–0.5

	Age	Electrolytes		
		Sodium (Mg)	Potassium (Mg)	Chloride (Mg)
Infants	Birth to 6 months	115–350	350–925	275–700
	6 months to 1 year	250–750	425–1275	400–1200
Children and adolescents	1 to 3 years	325–975	550–1650	500–1500
	4 to 6 years	450–1350	775–2325	700–2100
	7 to 10 years	600–1800	1000–3000	925–2775
	Over 11 years	900–2700	1525–4575	1400–4200

	Age	Vitamins		
		Vitamin K (μg)	Biotin (μg)	Pantothenic Acid (Mg)
Infants	Birth to 6 months	12	35	2
	6 months to 1 year	10–20	50	3
Children and adolescents	1 to 3 years	15–30	65	3
	4 to 6 years	20–40	85	3–4
	7 to 10 years	30–60	120	4–5
	Over 11 years	50–100	100–200	4–7

*Because there is less information on which to base allowances, these figures are not given in the main table of RDA and are provided here in the form of ranges of recommended intakes.

†Since the toxic levels for many trace elements may be only several times usual intakes, the upper levels for the trace elements given in this table should not be habitually exceeded.

Source: Food and Nutrition Board, National Academy of Sciences—National Research Council, Washington, D.C.

Table C-4 Mean Heights and Weights and Recommended Energy Intake*

Age and Sex Group	Weight Kg	Weight Lb	Height Cm	Height In	Energy Needs MI	Energy Needs Kcal	Energy Range in Kcal
Infants:							
Birth to .5 years	6	13	60	24	kg. × 0.48	kg. × 115	95–145
6 months to 1 year	9	20	71	28	kg. × 0.44	kg. × 105	80–135
Children:							
1 to 3 years	13	29	90	35	5.5	1,300	900–1,800
4 to 6 years	20	44	112	44	7.1	1,700	1,300–2,300
7 to 10 years	28	62	132	52	10.1	2,400	1,650–3,300
Males:							
11 to 14 years	45	99	157	62	11.3	2,700	2,000–3,700
15 to 18 years	66	145	176	69	11.8	2,800	2,100–3,900
Females:							
11 to 14 years	46	101	157	62	9.2	2,200	1,500–3,000
15 to 18 years	55	120	163	64	8.8	2,100	1,200–3,000
Pregnant women						+300	
Lactating women						+500	

*The data in this table have been assembled from the observed median heights and weights of children. Energy allowances for children through age 18 are based on median energy intakes of children in these ages followed in longitudinal growth studies. Ranges are the 10th and 90th percentiles of energy intake, to indicate range of energy consumption among children of these ages.

Source: From *Recommended Dietary Allowances*, rev. ed., Food and Nutrition Board, National Academy of Sciences—National Research Council, 1980, Washington, D.C.

Table C-5 The Basic Four Food Groups throughout the Growing Years

Food Group	Servings Per Day	Average-Size Servings for Age: Toddlers	Preschoolers	School-age Children	Adolescent
Milk or Equivalent ½ cup milk equals: 2 tbsp of powdered milk 1 oz of cheese ¼ cup of evaporated milk ½ cup of cottage cheese 1 serving of custard (4 servings from 1 pt. of milk) ½ cup of milk pudding ½ cup of yogurt	4	½–¾ cup	¾ cup	¾–1 cup	1 cup
Meat, Fish, Poultry, or Equivalent 1 oz of meat equals: 1 egg, 1 frankfurter 1 oz of cheese,* 1 cold cut 2 tbsp of peanut butter, cut meat ¼ cup of tuna fish or cottage cheese* ½ cup of dried peas or beans	2 or more	3 tbsp	4 tbsp	3–4 oz (6–8 tbsp)	4 oz or more

Table C-5 The Basic Four Food Groups throughout the Growing Years (*Continued*)

		Average-Size Servings for Age			
Food Group	Servings Per Day	Toddlers	Preschoolers	School-age Children	Adolescents
Vegetables and Fruits	4 or more				
Citrus fruit or equivalent 1 citrus fruit serving equals: ½ cup of orange or grapefruit juice ½ grapefruit or cantaloupe ¾ cup of strawberries *1 medium orange ½ citrus fruit serving equals: ½ cup of tomato juice or tomatoes, broccoli, chard, collards, greens, spinach, raw cabbage, brussels sprouts, 1 medium tomato, 1 wedge of honeydew	1 or more	4 oz	4 oz	4–6 oz	4–6 oz
Yellow or Green Vegetable or Equivalent 1 serving equals: ½ cup of broccoli, greens, spinach, carrots, squash, pumpkin 5 apricot halves ½ medium cantaloupe	1 or more	4 tbsp	4 tbsp	⅓ cup	½ cup
Other Fruits and Vegetables Other vegetables including potatoes Other fruit including apples, bananas, pears, peaches	2 or more	2–3 tbsp ½ medium apple	4 tbsp ½–1 medium apple	⅓–½ cup 1 medium apple	¾ cup 1 medium apple
Breads and Cereals or Whole Grain or Enriched Equivalent 1 slice of bread equals: ¾ cup of dry cereal ½ cup of cooked cereal, rice, spaghetti, or macaroni 1 roll, muffin, or biscuit	4 or more	½ slice ½ cup 2 tbsp	1 slice ¾ cup ¼–½ cup	1–2 slices 1 oz ½–1 cup	2 slices 1 oz 1 cup or more

*If cottage or cheddar cheese is used as a milk equivalent, it should not also be counted as a meat equivalent.

Sources: Infant Feeding Guide, Washington State Department of Social and Health Services, Health Services Division, Local Health Services, Nutrition Unit, 1972; and G. Scipien, M. U. Barnard, M. A. Chard, J. Howe, and P. J. Phillips (eds.), *Comprehensive Pediatric Nursing,* 3rd ed., McGraw-Hill, New York, 1986. Used with permission.

Appendix D: Personal information forms

Table D-1 Sample Personal Information Form: Birth to 6 Years

Help Us Know Your Child

Name ____________ Nickname ____________ Age ____________

Has your child been away from home before? ____________

Why? ____________ For how long? ____________

Who cares for your child at home? ____________

Has your child been told the reason for this hospitalization? ____________

By whom? ____________

Do you plan to stay with your child? ____________

If not, when can you visit? ____________

Is your child afraid of anything in particular? ____________

What comforts your child best (bottle, toy, your arms, and so forth)? ____________

____

Eating

Is or was your child breast-fed? ____________

Is your child on a bottle? ____________ When? ____________

Does your child have any food allergies? ____________

____

Has feeding ever been a problem? ____________

What food or foods does your child especially like or dislike? ____________

____

Toilet Training

Does your child stay dry during the day? ____________ At night? ____________

Is your child toilet trained for bowel movements? ____________

Does your child use a potty chair? ____________ A toilet? ____________

What word or words does your child use when he or she needs to go to the bathroom? ____________

____

Sleeping

Does your child sleep alone? ____________ If not, with whom does your child share a bed or a room? ____________

Would a doll or stuffed animal comfort your child at bedtime? ____________

What? ____________

Table D-1 Sample Personal Information Form: Birth to 6 Years (*Continued*)

Play

Does your child have a favorite toy? ________ Did you bring it along? ________ Is there a pet in your home? ________

What is it? ________________ What are your child's favorite games, special interests, or hobbies? ________________

Speech

Can your child speak well enough to make wants and needs understood with words? ________________

What language is spoken in your home?

School

Does your child attend nursery school? ________________

A Head Start Program? ________________ A day-care center? ________________

Is there anything else you would like us to know? ________________

Source: Committee on Hospital Care, *Hospital Care of Children and Youth*, American Academy of Pediatrics, Evanston, Ill., 1978, pp. 90–93. Used with permission.

Table D-2 Sample Personal Information Form: 6 to 12 Years

Help Us Know Your Child

Name ________________ Nickname ________________ Age ________________

Birthday ________________

How does your child take care of his or her own needs?

Dressing ________________ Eating ________________ Schoolwork ________________

Toileting ________________ Is your child on a special diet? ________________

What? ________________

Does your child know the reason for hospitalization? ________________

Did your child tour the hospital before admission? ________________

What interests your child most (toys, games, people, and so forth)? ________________

Does your child prefer groups? ________________ Is your child a loner? ________________

Name of your child's school ________________

Grade ________________Is your child in any special program? ________________

Has your family moved recently? ________________ Was the move within the same city? ________________

Does your child have any particular fears? ________________

Is there anything special you would like us to watch for? ________________

____

We and your child want you to visit as much as possible. How can we help you with this? ________________

Source: Committee on Hospital Care, *Hospital Care of Children and Youth*, American Academy of Pediatrics, Evanston, Ill, 1978, p. 90–93. Used with permission.

Table D-3 Sample Personal Information Form: Teenagers

Help Us Know You: Tell Us about Yourself

Name ______________________ Nickname ______________ Age ______________

Birthday (we would like to celebrate it with you if you are here). ______________

Who lives in your household? ______________

Names and ages of your brothers and sisters ______________

Have you ever been in the hospital before? ______________

When? ______________ Why? ______________

Are you on a special diet at home? ______________ What is it? ______________

____

Do you eat breakfast? ______________

What are your special interests and hobbies? ______________

____

How can we provide for them here? ______________

How can we help you keep in touch with your friends or school? ______________

Is there anything else that might make your hospital stay easier? ______________

Source: Committee on Hospital Care, *Hospital Care of Children and Youth,* American Academy of Pediatrics, Evanston, Ill., 1978, pp. 90–93. Used with permission.

Appendix E: Poison treatment

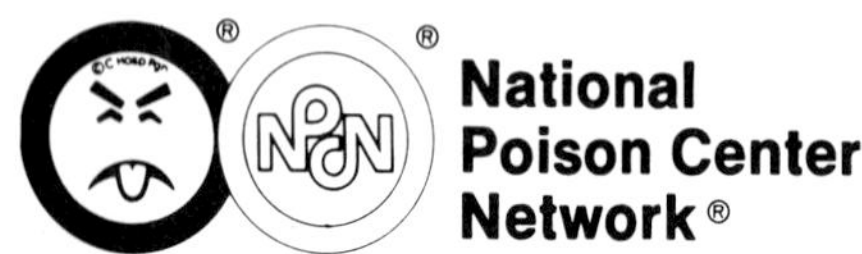

Poison Treatment Chart

Suggested general treatment for poisoning management*

1. There should be no problem in small amounts.
NO TREATMENT NECESSARY.
Fluids may be given.†

2. Call the poison center. Induce vomiting. Give syrup of ipecac in the following dosages:

   UNDER ONE YEAR OF AGE:
   Not recommended for use.

   ONE YEAR AND OVER:
   Give 1 tbsp followed by at least two or three glasses of fluid.

   DO NOT INDUCE VOMITING IF THE PATIENT IS SEMICOMATOSE, COMATOSE, OR CONVULSING.

   Call the poison center for additional information.

3. Dilute or neutralize with water or milk.
DO NOT INDUCE VOMITING. Gastric lavage is indicated. Call the poison center for specific instructions.

4. Treat symptomatically unless botulism is suspected. Call the poison center for specific information regarding botulism.

5. Dilute or neutralize with water or milk.
DO NOT INDUCE VOMITING. Gastric lavage should be avoided. This substance may cause burns of the mucous membranes. Consult an ENT specialist following emergency treatment. Call the poison center for specific information.

6. Immediately wash skin thoroughly with running water. Call the poison center for further treatment.

7. Immediately wash eyes with a gentle stream of running water. Continue for 15 min. Call the poison center for further treatment.

8. A specific antagonist may be indicated. Call the poison center.

9. Remove the patient to fresh air. Support respirations. Call the poison center for further treatment.

10. Call the poison center for specific instructions.

11. Give symptomatic and supportive treatment.
DO NOT INDUCE VOMITING for ingestions. IV Naloxone Hydrochloride (Narcan) to be given as indicated for respiratory depression.

    Dosage:
    Adult—0.4 mg IV
    May be repeated at 2- to 3-min intervals.
    Child—0.01 mg/kg IV.
    May be repeated at 5- to 10-min intervals.

---

*Always call the poison control center if there is *any* question about appropriate treatment.

†The numbers preceding these instructions correspond to the numbers following the poisonous substances listed on p. 1361.

- **Acetaminophen** ... 2, 8
- Acetone ... 2
- Acids
  - Ingestion ... 5
  - Eye contamination ... 7
  - Topical ... 6
  - Inhalation if mixed with bleach ... 9
- Aerosols
  - Eye contamination ... 7
  - Inhalation ... 9
- Aftershave lotions ... See Cologne
- Airplane glue ... 10
- Alcohol
  - Ingestion ... 2
  - Eye contamination ... 7
- Ammonia
  - Ingestion ... 5
  - Eye contamination ... 7
  - Inhalation ... 9
- Amphetamines ... 2
- Analgesics ... 10
- Aniline dyes
  - Ingestion ... 2, 8
  - Inhalation ... 8, 9
  - Topical ... 6, 8
- Antacids ... 1
- Antibiotics
  - Less than 2 to 3 times total daily dose ... 1
  - More than 3 times total daily dose ... 2
- Antidepressants
  - Tricyclic ... 2, 8
  - Others ... 2
- Antifreeze (ethylene glycol)
  - Ingestion ... 2
  - Eye contamination ... 7
- Antihistamines ... 2, 8
- Antiseptics ... 2
- Ant traps
  - Kepone type ... 1
  - Others ... 2
- Aquarium products ... 1
- Arsenic ... 2, 8
- Aspirin ... 2
- **Baby oil** ... 1
- Ballpoint ink ... 1
- Barbiturates
  - Short-acting ... 10
  - Long-acting ... 2
- Bathroom bowl cleaners
  - Ingestion ... 5
  - Eye contamination ... 7
  - Inhalation if mixed with bleach ... 9
  - Topical ... 6
- Batteries
  - Dry cell (flashlight) ... 1
  - Mercury (hearing aid) ... 2
  - Wet cell (automobile) ... 5
- Benzene
  - Ingestion ... 10
  - Inhalation ... 9
  - Topical ... 6
- Birth control pills ... 1
- Bleaches
  - Liquid ingestion ... 1
  - Solid ingestion ... 5
  - Eye contamination ... 7
  - Inhalation when mixed with acids or alkalies ... 9
- Boric acid ... 2
- Bromides ... 2
- Bubble bath ... 1
- **Caffeine** ... 1
- Camphor ... 2
- Candles ... 1
- Caps
  - Less than one roll ... 1
  - More than one roll ... 2
- Carbon monoxide ... 9
- Carbon tetrachloride
  - Ingestion ... 2
  - Inhalation ... 9
  - Topical ... 6
- Chalk ... 1
- Chlorine bleach ... See Bleaches
- Cigarettes
  - Less than one ... 1
  - One or more ... 2
- Clay ... 1
- Cleaning fluids ... 10
- Cleanser (household) ... 1
- Clinitest tablets ... 5
- Cold remedies ... 10
- Cologne
  - Less than 15 cc ... 1
  - More than 15 cc ... 2
- Contraceptive pills ... 1
- Corn and wart removers ... 5
- Cosmetics ... See specific type
- Cough medicines ... 10
- Crayons
  - Children's ... 1
  - Other ... 2
- Cyanide ... 8
- **Dandruff shampoo** ... 2
- Dehumidifying packets ... 1
- Denture adhesives ... 1
- Denture cleansers ... 5
- Deodorants
  - All types ... 1
- Deodorizer cakes ... 2
- Deodorizers, room ... 10
- Desiccants ... 1
- Detergents
  - Liquid and powder (general) 1
  - Electric-dishwasher and phosphate free ... 5
- Diaper rash ointment ... 1
- Dishwasher detergents ... See Detergents
- Disinfectants ... 3
- Drain cleaners ... See Lye
- Dyes
  - Aniline ... See Aniline dyes
  - Others ... 2
- **Electric dishwasher detergents** ... See Detergents
- Epoxy glue
  - Catalyst ... 5
  - Resin or when mixed ... 10
- Epsom salts ... 2
- Ethyl alcohol ... See Alcohol
- Ethylene glycol ... See Antifreeze
- Eye makeup ... 1
- **Fabric softeners** ... 2
- Fertilizers ... 10
- Fishbowl Additives ... 1
- Fluoride ... 10
- Food poisoning ... 4
- Foreign body ... 10
- Furniture polish ... 10
- **Gas (natural)** ... 9
- Gasoline ... 10
- Glue ... 10
- Gun products ... 10
- **Hair dyes**
  - Ingestion ... 3
  - Eye contamination ... 7
  - Topical ... 6
- Hallucinogens ... 10
- Hand cream ... 1
- Hand lotions ... 1
- Herbicides ... 10
- Heroin ... 8, 11
- Hormones ... 1
- Hydrochloric acid ... See Acids
- Hydrogen peroxide ... 1
- **Inks**
  - Ballpoint pen ... 1
  - Indelible ... 2
  - Laundry marking ... 2
  - Printer's ... 2
- Insecticides
  - Ingestion ... 8
  - Topical ... 6, 8
- Iodine ... 5, 8
- Iron ... 10
- Isopropyl alcohol ... See Alcohol
- **Kerosene** ... 10
- **Laundry marking ink** ... 2
- Laxatives ... 2
- Lighter fluid ... 10
- Liniments ... 2
- Lipstick ... 1
- Lye
  - Ingestion ... 5
  - Eye contamination ... 7
  - Inhalation when mixed with bleach ... 9
  - Topical ... 6
- **Magic markers** ... 1
- Makeup ... 1
- Markers
  - Indelible ... 2
  - Water soluble ... 1
- Matches
  - Fewer than 12 wood or 20 paper ... 1
  - More than the above ... 2
- Mercurochrome
  - Less than 15 cc ... 1
  - More than 15 cc ... 2
- Mercury
  - Metallic (thermometer) ... 1
  - Salts ... 2
- Metal cleaners ... 10
- Methadone ... 8, 11
- Merthiolate
  - Less than 15 cc ... 1
  - More than 15 cc ... 2
- Methyl alcohol ... 2, 8
- Methyl salicylate ... 2
- Mineral oil ... 1
- Model cement ... 10
- Modeling clay ... 1
- Morphine ... 8, 11
- Mothballs ... 2
- Mushrooms ... 2, 8
- **Nail polish** ... 1
- Nail polish remover
  - Less than 15 cc ... 1
  - More than 15 cc ... 2
- Narcotics ... 8, 11
- Natural gas ... 9
- Nicotine ... See Cigarettes
- **Oil of wintergreen** ... 2
- Opium ... 8, 11
- Oven cleaners ... See Lye
- **Paint**
  - Acrylic ... 10

Paint, *continued*

  - Latex ... 10
  - Lead base ... 10
  - Oil base ... 10
- Paint chips ... 10
- Paint thinner ... 10
- Pencils ... 1
- Perfume ... See Cologne
- Permanent wave solution
  - Ingestion ... 5
  - Eye contamination ... 7
- Pesticides
  - Ingestion ... 8
  - Topical ... 6, 8
- Petroleum distillates ... 10
- Phenol
  - Ingestion ... 3
  - Eye contamination ... 7
  - Topical ... 6
- Phosphate free detergents ... 5
- Pine oil ... 10
- Plants ... 10
- Plant food ... 1
- Polishes ... 10
- Printer's ink ... 2
- Putty ... 1
- **Quaternary ammonium compounds** ... 3
- **Record cleaners** ... 10
- Rodenticides ... 10
- Rubbing alcohol ... See Alcohol
- **Saccharin** ... 1
- Sachet ... 1
- Sedatives ... 10
- Shampoo
  - Ingestion ... 1
  - (See also Dandruff shampoo)
- Shaving cream ... 1
- Shaving lotion ... See Cologne
- Shoe dyes ... 2
- Shoe polish ... 2
- Sleep aids ... 10
- Soaps ... 1
- Soldering flux ... 5
- Starch, washing ... 1
- Steroids ... 10
- Strychnine ... 10
- Sulfuric acid ... See Acids
- Suntan preparations ... 10
- Swimming pool chemicals ... 5
- **Talc**
  - Ingestion ... 1
  - Inhalation ... 10
- Teething rings ... 1
- Thermometers (all types) ... 1
- Toilet bowl cleaners ... See Bathroom bowl cleaners
- Toilet water ... See Cologne
- Toothpaste ... 1
- Toys, fluid filled ... 1
- Tranquilizers ... 2, 10
- Tricyclic antidepressants ... 2, 8
- Turpentine ... 10
- Typewriter cleaners ... 10
- **Varnish** ... 10
- Vitamins
  - Water-soluble ... 1
  - Fat-soluble ... 2
  - With iron ... 10
- **Wart removers** ... 5
- Weed killers ... 10
- Window cleaners ... 10
- Windshield washer fluid ... 2, 8
- Wood preservatives ... 5

Source: National Poison Center Network.

INDEX

Blood chemistries

Factor	Normal Range		
	Newborn		Child
Acid phosphatase	7.4–19.4 IU/ml		6.4–15.2 IU/ml
Alkaline phosphatase	20–266 IU/l		70–160 IU/l
Alpha fetoprotein		10 mg/dl	
Bicarbonate	20–26 mEq/l		
Bilirubin	2–6 mg/dl (24 h) 6–7 " (48 h) 4–12 " (3–5 days)		1 mg/dl
BUN		5–25 mg/dl	
Calcium (total)	7–12 mg/dl		8–11 mg/dl 4.4–5.4 mg/dl (ionized)
Chloride		94–106 mEq/l	
Cholesterol	50-120 mg/dl		135–270 mg/dl
Creatinine (serum)	0.2–0.5 mg/dl		0.3–0.8 mg/dl
Fibrinogen		200–400 mg/dl	
Glucose	40 mg/dl		60–110 mg/dl
Iron	110–270 μg/dl		53–119 μg/dl
Magnesium	1.52–2.33 mEq/l		1.4–1.9 mEq/l
Phenylalanine		3mg/dl	
Phospholipids	0.48–1.6 gms/l		1.66–2.47 gms/l
Phosphorus	4–10.5 mg/dl		3.6–6.8 mg/dl
Potassium	3.5–7 mEq/l		3.5–5.5 mEq/l
Proteins	6.4 gm/dl		7.4 gm/dl
Sodium		135–145 mEq/l	
Triglycerides		29–154 mg/dl	
Urea nitrogen		6–23 mg/dl	
Zinc	74–146 μg/dl		65–125 μg/dl

Normal arterial blood gas values*

Factor	Range
pH	7.35–7.45
P_{CO_2}	34–45 mmHg
P_{O_2}	80–100 mmHg
HCO_3^-	25–35 mmHg
Base excess (BE)	±2 mEq
O_2 saturation	95–100%

Average range of normal blood values

Measure	Birth-1 mo Newborn	1 mo-2 yr Infant	2 yr-12 yr Child	Adolescent/Adult Male	Adolescent/Adult Female
Hemoglobin (g/100 ml blood)	14–24	10–15	11–16	14–16	13–15.5
Hematocrit (ml packed cells/ 100 ml blood)	43–63	30–42	34–37	42–52	37–47
Red blood cells (RBCs) millions per cubic millimeter	4.8–7.1	4.5–5.1	3.8–5.5	4.8–5.5	4.4–5
Reticulocytes (% of total RBCs)	4–6 decreasing to 0.5–1.6 by 2 weeks	0.5–1.6	0.5–1.6	0.5–1.6	0.5–1.6
Erythrocyte indices					
MCH (mean corpuscular Hb), μμg	32–34	27–31	27–31	29–32	29–32
MCV (mean corpuscular volume) μm³ per RBC	96–108	82–96	82–96	82–96	82–96
MCHC (mean corpuscular Hb concentration), percent	32–33	32–36	32–36	32–36	32–36
White blood cells (WBC) (number per cubic millimeter)	9000–30,000	5000–17,000	5000–10,000	5000-11,000	
Differential count					
Neutrophils (%)	40–80	30–50	55–60	38–70	38–70
Basophils (%)	0–0.5	0–0.5	0–3	0–3	0–3
Eosinophils (%)	5	2–3	2	1–5	1–5
Lymphocytes (%)	30–35	40–50	40–45	15–45	15–45
Monocytes (%)	5–10	5–10	1–8	1–8	1–8
Platelets (thrombocytes) (number per cubic millimeter)	140,000–300,000	200,000–473,000	150,000–450,000	200,000–400,000	